Experience Partnering with Families Through the Eyes of a Nurse

The relationship you create with your clients and their families is the most essential and rewarding part of your nursing career. You will enjoy your job and be more effective in it when you develop these bonds. *Through the Eyes of a Nurse* shows you how one nurse establishes a connection with a couple throughout the pregnancy and after the birth of their baby. We believe that seeing this partnership develop—in your textbook and on the videos on your Prentice Hall Nursing MediaLink DVD-ROM—will help you understand how this wonderful process works.

Resources for Student Success

COMPANION WEBSITE
http://www.prenhall.com/davidson

- Audio Glossary
- NCLEX-RN®-style questions with rationales
- Case Studies
- Care Plans
- MediaLink Applications
- MediaLink Web Links
- Nursing Tools
- Thinking Critically
- Student Success
- *and more . . .*

PRENTICE HALL NURSING MEDIALINK DVD-ROM

- NCLEX-RN®-style questions with rationales
- Through the Eyes of a Nurse videos
- Critical Thinking in Action videos and graphic animations with questions
- Newborn Reflex videos
- Nursing Tools
- *and more . . .*

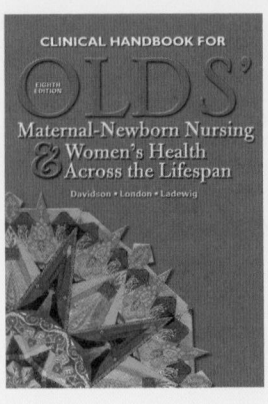

CLINICAL HANDBOOK FOR OLDS' MATERNAL-NEWBORN NURSING & WOMEN'S HEALTH ACROSS THE LIFESPAN
ISBN: 0-13-232441-5

This pocket guide serves as a portable, quick reference to maternal-newborn nursing care. Covering from pregnancy through the postpartum and newborn stages, this handbook allows you to take the information you learn in class into any clinical setting.

STUDENT WORKBOOK FOR OLDS' MATERNAL-NEWBORN NURSING & WOMEN'S HEALTH ACROSS THE LIFESPAN
ISBN: 0-13-240149-5

This popular study tool incorporates strategies for you to focus your study and increase comprehension of concepts of nursing care. It contains a variety of activities, MediaLinks referencing the DVD-ROM and Companion Website, and more.

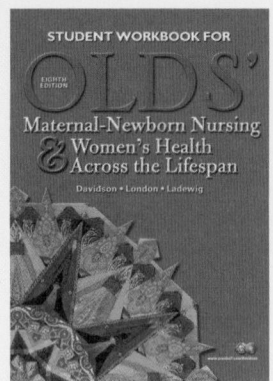

NATIONAL LEAGUE FOR NURSING (NLN) TESTS

Prentice Hall and the National League for Nursing are pleased to offer you unique practice tests that correlate directly to your Prentice Hall Nursing textbooks. Each test is a comprehensive examination intended for students who have completed their course work and provides feedback regarding comprehension of the course content. The access code gives you access to two unique practice tests—use them to prepare for your course final exams or for NCLEX-RN®. Go to http://www.mypearsonstore.com and search for the National League for Nursing to find practice tests in any of your core nursing courses or to accompany the Prentice Hall Reviews & Rationales Series.

Student Assessment . . . Real Nursing Skills . . . Customized Study Plans . . . The path to student success and nursing excellence in maternal-newborn nursing!

MyNursingLab is a user-friendly site that gives students the opportunity to test themselves on key concepts and skills in maternal-newborn nursing. By using *MyNursingLab,* students can track their own progress through the course and use their customized, media-rich, study plan activities to help them achieve success in the classroom, in clinical, and ultimately on the NCLEX-RN®. *MyNursingLab* can also help you, the instructor, to monitor class progress as students move through the curriculum.

To take a tour and see the power of **mynursinglab**, go to http://www.prenhall.com/nursing.

Resources for Faculty Success

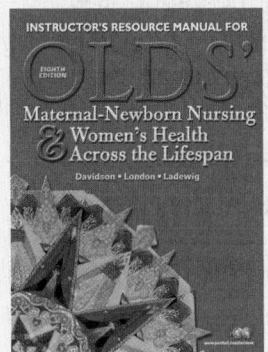

INSTRUCTOR'S RESOURCE MANUAL

This manual contains a wealth of material to help instructors plan and manage the maternity nursing course. For each learning objective, there are correlating lecture notes, numbered PowerPoint slides, and suggestions for classroom and clinical activities. Also in the manual is an entire test bank of chapter-specific NCLEX-RN®-style questions, complete with rationales and classification ratings.

INSTRUCTOR'S RESOURCE DVD-ROM

This media-rich DVD-ROM provides all of the tools faculty need for ease in classroom preparation and evaluation.

Test Generator—Equipped with TestGen 7.3, the Instructor's Resource DVD-ROM provides a test bank with peer-reviewed NCLEX-RN®-style questions including the new alternate item formats written at the analysis or application cognitive level. Instructors can search for test items by level and chapter or topic and can preview answers, rationales, NCLEX-RN® Test Plan, and cognitive level for all questions. TestGen 7.3 can output either print or electronic tests.

Integrated Text and Image PowerPoint Presentations—The Instructor's Resource DVD-ROM provides chapter-specific, integrated PowerPoint presentations with approximately 1,000 customizable text slides and an image library with art from the book.

Animation and Video Library—With a rich store of animations and videos, the Instructor's Resource DVD-ROM enables faculty to view and select resources to show in the classroom. Included are the Through the Eyes of a Nurse videos and other videos from the Prentice Hall Nursing MediaLink DVD-ROM. New to this edition are Newborn Reflex Videos.

Classroom Response System—Prentice Hall is pleased to offer PowerPoint content on the Instructor's Resource DVD-ROM to support instructors who use Classroom Response Systems to engage students and provide instant feedback in the classroom. Ask your Prentice Hall sales representative for more information.

▶ *See your Prentice Hall sales representative to request Instructor's Resource CD-ROMs.*

Online Course Management Systems

Prentice Hall OneKey is an open-access, integrated online course cartridge for schools using Blackboard and WebCT platforms and provides you with the following:

For Students	**For Instructors**	**For a Preview, go to:**
NCLEX-RN® Review questions	Test Item Files	
Case Studies	PowerPoint Presentations	http://cms.prenhall.com/webct/ index.html
Care Plan Activities	Media Gallery Resources	
MediaLinks	Discussion Board	
E-mail Communication	Class Announcements	**Bb** http//cms.prenhall.com/ blackboard/index.html

Brief Table of Contents

OLDS'

EIGHTH EDITION

Maternal-Newborn Nursing
& Women's Health
Across the Lifespan

Davidson • London • Ladewig

Michele R. Davidson, PhD, CNM, CFN, RN
Associate Professor of Nursing and Women's Studies
GEORGE MASON UNIVERSITY
Fairfax, Virginia
STAFF MIDWIFE WOMEN'S HEALTHCARE ASSOCIATES
Lansdowne, Virginia

Marcia L. London, RNC, MSN, APRN, CNS, NNP
Senior Clinical Instructor and Director of Neonatal Nurse Practitioner Program
BETH-EL COLLEGE OF NURSING AND HEALTH SCIENCES
UNIVERSITY OF COLORADO
Colorado Springs, Colorado
Staff Clinical Nurse
URGENT CARE AND AFTER HOURS CLINIC
Colorado Springs, Colorado

Patricia A. Wieland Ladewig, PhD, RN
Professor and Academic Dean
RUECKERT-HARTMAN SCHOOL FOR HEALTH PROFESSIONS
REGIS UNIVERSITY
Denver, Colorado

PEARSON

Prentice Hall

Upper Saddle River, New Jersey 07458

Library of Congress Cataloging-in-Publication Data

Davidson, Michele R.
  Olds' maternal-newborn nursing & women's health across the
lifespan / Michele R. Davidson, Marcia L. London, Patricia Wieland
Ladewig.—8th ed.
    p.; cm.
  Rev. ed. of: Maternal-newborn nursing & women's health care /
Sally B. Olds . . . [et al.]. 7th ed. c2004.
  Includes bibliographical references and index.
  ISBN-13: 978-0-13-220873-4
  ISBN-10: 0-13-220873-3
  1. Maternity nursing. I. London, Marcia L. II. Ladewig, Patricia
W. III. Olds, Sally B., 1940- IV. Maternal-newborn nursing &
women's health care. V. Title. VI. Title: Maternal-newborn nursing &
women's health across the lifespan. VII. Title: Olds' maternal-
newborn nursing and women's health across the lifespan.
  [DNLM: 1. Maternal-Child Nursing—methods. 2. Neonatal
Nursing—methods. 3. Nursing
Assessment—methods. 4. Pregnancy Complications—nursing. 5.
Women's Health. WY 157.3
D253o 2008]
  RG951.04327 2008
  618.2′0231—dc22   2006100508

Publisher: Julie Levin Alexander
Assistant to Publisher: Regina Bruno
Editor-in-Chief: Maura Connor
Executive Acquisitions Editor: Pamela Lappies
Associate Editor: Michael Giacobbe
Development Editor: Alan Sorkowitz
Managing Editor, Development: Marilyn Meserve
Editorial Art Manager: Patrick Watson
Media Product Manager: John J. Jordan
Director of Marketing: Karen Allman
Senior Marketing Manager: Francisco del Castillo
Marketing Specialist: Michael Sirinides
Managing Editor, Production: Patrick Walsh
Production Editor: Heather Willison, Carlisle Publishing Services

Production Liaison: Anne Garcia
Media Project Manager: Stephen Hartner
Manufacturing Manager: Ilene Sanford
Manufacturing Buyer: Ilene Sanford
Senior Design Coordinator: Maria Guglielmo
Printer/Binder: RR Donnelley, Willard
Composition: Carlisle Publishing Services
Interior Design: Rae Grant
Cover Design: Cheryl Asherman
Cover Illustration: *Kaleidoscopic VIII: The Sun, the Moon . . . and the Stars.* A quilt designed and made by Paula Nadelstern, copyright 1991
Cover Printer: Phoenix Color

Pearson Education LTD.
Pearson Education Australia PTY, Limited
Pearson Education Singapore, Pte. Ltd
Pearson Education North Asia Ltd
Pearson Education Canada, Ltd.

Pearson Educación de Mexico, S.A. de C.V.
Pearson Education—Japan
Pearson Education Malaysia Pte. Ltd
Pearson Education, Upper Saddle River, New Jersey

10 9 8 7 6 5 4 3 2 1
ISBN-13: 978-0-13-220873-4
ISBN: 0-13-220873-3

Dedication

Sally B. Olds is the quintessential nurse and teacher—

She sees possibilities where others see problems, abilities where others
see limitations.

She cares passionately about childbearing families and has a clear vision
of what excellent nursing means.

She stresses the importance of clinical skill and acumen but never loses sight
of the human side of caregiving.

She is committed to students, to helping them to learn and grow,
to develop their own sense of the difference a nurse can make.

She is the best of the best of nursing. . .

And so, with the deepest affection and respect we dedicate this book to Sally,
our dear friend and colleague. Thank you for the inspiration you provided,
the warmth you brought, and the expertise you shared.

We hope you enjoy many days of sunshine, blessings, and joy.

And, as always, to our beloved families

To Nathan Davidson, Hayden, Chloe, Caroline, and Grant
To David London, Craig, and Matthew
To Tim Ladewig, Ryan, Amanda, and Reed,
and Erik, Kedri, and Emma

About the Authors

MICHELE DAVIDSON

Michele Davidson received an ADN degree from Marymount University in 1990 and upon graduation began working in postpartum and the newborn nursery in Washington, DC. Because of her interest in educating expectant and new families, she began an education and consulting service providing childbirth education classes, lactation consulting services, and newborn care courses. During this time she also worked as a reproductive endocrinology/infertility nurse while she obtained a BSN from George Mason University. Dr. Davidson then attended Case Western Reserve University where she earned her MSN and a nurse-midwifery certificate. She worked as a nurse-midwife at Columbia Hospital for Women in Washington, DC, while completing her PhD in nursing administration and healthcare policy from George Mason University (GMU). Dr. Davidson began teaching at GMU in 1999. Dr. Davidson maintains a part-time clinical practice at Women's Healthcare Associates of Loudoun because of her strong belief that active clinical practice is essential to provide students with current clinical and critical-thinking skills. Dr. Davidson has developed an immersion clinical experience for GMU students on a remote island in the Chesapeake Bay, where she teaches community health nursing to students who reside in the community. In 2003, she founded the Smith Island Foundation, a nonprofit organization in which she serves as executive director. In her free time, Michele enjoys spending time with her mother, gardening, reading, and spending time at their home on Smith Island with her nurse practitioner husband, Nathan, and their four young children, Hayden, Chloe, Caroline, and Grant. Dr. Davidson recently received certification as a Certified Forensic Nurse. Her research interests include maternal-newborn and forensic nursing issues.

MARCIA L. LONDON

Marcia L. London has been able to combine her two greatest passions by being both a nurse caring for children and families and a teacher for almost 35 years. She received her BSN and school nurse certificate from Plattsburgh State University in Plattsburgh, New York. After graduation, she began her nursing career as a pediatric nurse at St. Luke's Hospital in New York City, then moved to Pittsburgh, where she began her teaching career. Mrs. London accepted a faculty position at Pittsburgh's Children's Hospital Affiliate Program and received her MSN in pediatrics as a clinical nurse specialist from the University of Pittsburgh. Mrs. London began teaching at Beth-El School of Nursing and Health Science in 1974 after opening the first intensive care nursery at Memorial Hospital of Colorado Springs. She has served in many administrative and faculty positions at Beth-El, including coordinator for nursing care of children for 32 years. Mrs. London maintains her clinical skills working in an urgent care and after-hours clinic and doing undergraduate pediatric clinical supervision. She obtained her postmaster's neonatal nurse practitioner certificate in 1983 and subsequently developed the neonatal nurse practitioner (NNP) program and the master's NNP program at Beth-El. She is active nationally in neonatal nursing and was involved in the development of the Neonatal Nurse Practitioner Educational Program Guidelines. She has contributed five chapters to various neonatal nursing texts. Mrs. London is active in nurse practitioner education in general. She was involved in the revision of the Core Competency for Nurse Practitioners and Curriculum Guidelines for Nurse Practitioner Education, as a member of the Education Committee of the National Organization of Nurse Practitioner Faculties, and participated as part of the Core Competency Validation Expert Panel. Mrs. London has also pursued her interest in college student learning by taking doctoral classes in higher education administration and adult learning at the University of Denver in

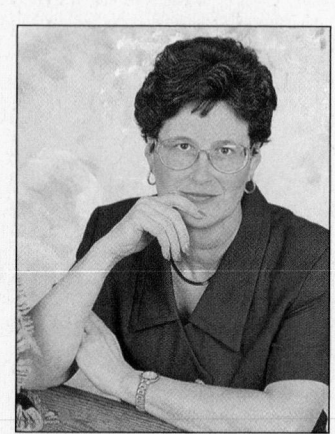

Colorado. She feels fortunate to be involved in the education of her future colleagues. Her teaching philosophy is that, with support, students can achieve more than they may initially believe they are capable of achieving. She believes in life-long learning and applying it to her nursing care of clients as part of her faculty practice. Mrs. London and her husband have two sons and one dog (Reilly, daughter by proxy). Her two sons, Craig and Matthew, are involved in computer informatics, as well as media arts and animation, and are more than willing to give Mom helpful hints.

PATRICIA A. WIELAND LADEWIG

Patricia A. Wieland Ladewig received her BS from the College of Saint Teresa in Winona, Minnesota. After graduation, she worked as a pediatric nurse before joining the U.S. Air Force. After completing her tour of duty, Dr. Ladewig relocated in Florida, where she accepted a faculty position at Florida State University. There she embraced teaching as her calling. Over the years, she taught at several schools of nursing while earning her MSN in maternal-newborn nursing from Catholic University of America in Washington, DC, and her PhD in higher education administration from the University of Denver in Colorado. In addition, she became a women's health nurse practitioner and maintained a part-time clinical practice. In 1988 Dr. Ladewig became the first director of the nursing program at Regis College in Denver and, in 1991, when the college became Regis University, she became dean of the Rueckert-Hartman School for Health Professions. Under her guidance, the Department of Nursing has added a graduate program and the school has added three departments: the Department of Physical Therapy, the Department of Health Services Administration and Management, and the Department of Health Care Ethics. Dr. Ladewig feels that teaching others to be excellent, caring nurses gives her the best of all worlds because it keeps her in touch with the profession she loves and enables her to help shape the future of the nursing profession. When not at work or writing textbooks, Pat and her husband, Tim, enjoy skiing, baseball games, and traveling. However, their greatest pleasure comes from their family: son Ryan, his wife, Amanda, and grandson Reed; and son, Erik, his wife Kedri, and granddaughter Emma.

Contributors

We are grateful to the contributors to the eighth edition of *Olds' Maternal-Newborn Nursing & Women's Health Across the Lifespan.*

Nancy Benner RNC, BSN
Presbyterian/St. Luke's Medical Center
Denver, Colorado
Chapter 30: The Normal Newborn: Needs and Care

Laura Bonazzoli MFA
Medical Writer
Chapter 3: Complementary and Alternative Therapies

Barbara Cheuvront MS, RN
Regis University Denver, Colorado
Chapter 2: Care of the Family in a Culturally Diverse Society
Chapter 14: Physical and Psychologic Changes of Pregnancy
Chapter 15: Antepartal Nursing Assessment

Marian C. Condon RN, DeD
York College of Pennsylvania
Chapter 8: Women's Care: Social Issues

Alyssa Consigli RD
University of Vermont
Chapter 18: Maternal Nutrition

Kim Eby PhD
George Mason University
Chapter 9: Violence Against Women

Cathy Emeis CNM, PhD(c)
Beth-El College of Nursing and Health Sciences
University of Colorado at Colorado Springs
Chapter 34: Postpartal Family Adaptation and Nursing Assessment

Victoria Flanagan RN, MS
Dartmouth-Hitchcock Medical Center
Chapter 19: Pregnancy at Risk: Pregestational Problems

Dee Ann Lucky Gallegos MS, RN
Regis University
Denver, Colorado
Chapter 6: Women's Health: Commonly Occurring Infections

Brigitte Hall MSN, IBCLC
LifeSpan Home Health and
Director of Maternal/Infant and Pediatric Services
Lackland AFB
Chapter 31: Newborn Nutrition

Carol Ann Harrigan RNC, MSN, NNP
Banner Desert Medical Center
Mesa, Arizona
Chapter 32: The Newborn at Risk: Conditions Present at Birth

Jennifer Hensley, CNM, MSN, WHCNP, EdD, LCCE
University of Colorado Health Sciences Center
Chapter 5: Women's Health: Family Planning

Stephanie Holaday, RN, DrPH
George Mason University
Fairfax, Virginia
Chapter 22: Processes and Stages of Labor and Birth

Nancy Houck RNC, BSN, NNP
Banner Desert Medical Center
Mesa, Arizona
Chapter 32: The Newborn at Risk: Conditions Present at Birth

Janet Houser PhD, RN
Regis University
Denver, Colorado
Research boxes
Evidence-Based Practice boxes

Vanessa Howell BSN
Memorial Health Care Systems
Colorado Springs, Colorado
Chapter 29: Nursing Assessment of the Newborn

Joanne Jonell MSN, RN
Regis University
Denver, Colorado
Chapter 17: Adolescent Pregnancy

Cheryl Pope Kish RNC, MSN, EdD, WHNP
Georgia College & State University
Chapter 38: The Postpartal Family at Risk

Deborah Cooper McGee RNC, MSN, PNNP, RDMS
Obstetrix Medical Group of Colorado
Chapter 20: Pregnancy at Risk: Gestational Onset

Julie Nadeau RN, MS
University of the Incarnate Word
San Antonio, Texas
Chapter 35: The Postpartal Family: Needs and Care
Chapter 36: Home Care of the Postpartal Family

Laura Riedel RN, MS
Perinatal Clinical Nurse Specialist/Consultant
Professional Health Consulting
Burke, Virginia
Chapter 23: Intrapartal Nursing Assessment

Susan Saindon RNC, MSN
Chapter 4: Women's Health Across the Lifespan

Candice Schoeneberger RNC, PhD
Regis University
Denver, Colorado
Chapter 16: The Expectant Family: Needs and Care

Kelly E. Shields RNC, BS, NCBF
Healing Through Hope
Lakewood Ranch, Florida
Chapter 37: Grief and Loss in the Childbearing Family

Lisa Smith-Pedersen APRN, MSN, CNNP
Denver Children's Hospital
Chapter 33: The Newborn at Risk: Birth-Related Stressors

Kelly A. Timbers MSN, CRNP
University of Pennsylvania Medical
Chapter 12: Special Reproductive Concerns: Infertility and Genetics

Karen Zimmerman RN, MSN, PNNP
Rocky Mountain Women's Care
Denver, Colorado
Chapter 7: Women's Health Problems

Instructor's Resource Manual with Test Bank

Anne Krouse BSN, MBA, MSN, PhD
Widener University

Pamela Hamre RN, MS, CNM
The College of St. Catherine

Prentice Hall Nursing MediaLink DVD-ROM

Sharon Lytle AAS, BSN, MSN
Carl Sandburg College

Brenda Ludwig EdD, RNCS
Bob Jones University

Kathryn Magorian BS, MSN
Mount Marty College

Companion Website

Mary Ann McLaughlin MSN, RN
University of Pennsylvania

Elizabeth Loeper RNC, MSN
Eastern University

Thank You!

We are grateful to all the nurses, both clinicians and educators, who reviewed the manuscript of this textbook. Their insights, suggestions, and eye for detail helped us prepare a more relevant and useful textbook, one that will prepare caring and competent nurses in the field of maternal-newborn and women's health nursing.

Patricia Annear
Butler County Community College

Joanne Barnes
Director, Laurel Regional Hospital
Laurel, Maryland

Kathleen Beebe
Dominican University of California

Laura Bernaix
Southern Illinois University - Edwardsville

Kate Brennan
Radford University

Mary Ann Burnam
Otterbein College

Beverly Bye
Towson University

Darlene Cantu
San Antonio College

Katrina Carter
McNeese State University

Nancy Darland
Louisiana Tech University

Adele Dean
Northern Kentucky University

Patricia Duclos-Miller
Capital Community College

Susan Escoto-Lloyd
California State University - Los Angeles

Patricia Frank
Radford University

Karolyn Givens
Radford University

Bobbe Gray
Wright State University

Sandra M. Grinnell
Northern Kentucky University

Donna Hallas
Pace University - Pleasantville

Margaret Hamilton
Florida International University

Jeffery Hanes
Hinds Community College

Janice Harris
Columbia State University

Lovena Haumann
The College of New Jersey

Debra Hrelic
Mount St. Mary's College

Linda Johnson
Sinclair Community College

Teresa Johnson
University of Wisconsin - Milwaukee

Holly Kailani
Hawaii Pacific University

Joan Keller-Maresh
Viterbo University

Brenda Lenz
Saint Cloud State University

Judith Lewis
Virginia Commonwealth University

Mary Lynd
Wright State University

Carol Mailloux
University of Massachusetts - Dartmouth

Susan Mayer
Glendale Community College

Mary McKelvey
Otterbein College

Shahnaz Moezzi
University of Utah

Christine Nelson
SUNY - Buffalo

Ann Nguyen
Oklahoma State University

Michelle Offutt
St. Petersburg College

Kathy O'Leary Oller
FCCJ North

Lynne Peterson
Montana Technical College – Butte

Melissa Powell
Eastern Kentucky University

Connie Powe-Watts
Michigan State University

Kristen Priddy
University of Texas - Arlington

Anne Rameika
Community College of Rhode Island - Warwick

Linda Reid
University of Louisiana - Monroe

Nicole Robert
McNeese State University

Mary Terhaar
Johns Hopkins University

Susan Theobald
Jefferson Community College

Rosalena Thorpe
Community College of Allegheny County - Allegheny

Donna Tilley
Texas Tech University

Kimberly Veney
Prince Georges Community College

Janice Vincent
University of Alabama - Birmingham

Iris Warren
University of Alabama - Huntsville

Cindy Welch
University of Southern Mississippi

Barbara West
Broward Community College - North

Preface

Most often, pregnancy and childbirth are times of great joy, a celebration of life, and a promise of the future. But they may also be times of deepest sorrow as families deal with illness, complications, and loss. Nurses play a central role in all aspects of the childbearing experience, from the earliest days of pregnancy, through the moments of birth, and during the early days of parenthood. Often the quality of the nursing care that a family receives profoundly influences their perceptions of the entire experience—for better or for worse. However, the changes occurring in the healthcare delivery system are altering the way we practice nursing and have staggering implications for nurses everywhere, even nurses caring for childbearing women and their families.

Now, more than ever, nurses must be flexible, creative, and open to change. They must be able to think critically and problem solve effectively. They must be able to meet the teaching needs of their clients so that their clients can, in turn, better meet their own healthcare needs. They must be open to an increasingly multicultural population. They must understand and use the technology available in their chosen area of practice. Most crucially, they must never lose sight of the importance of excellent nursing care in improving the quality of people's lives.

The underlying philosophy of *Olds' Maternal-Newborn Nursing & Women's Health Across the Lifespan* remains unchanged. We believe that pregnancy and birth are normal life processes and that family members are coparticipants in care. We believe that women's health care is an important aspect of nursing. We remain committed to providing a text that is accurate and readable; a text that helps students develop the skills and abilities they need now and in the future in an ever-changing healthcare environment.

NURSING EXCELLENCE IN MATERNAL-NEWBORN AND WOMEN'S HEALTH

Truly effective nurses have both a solid understanding of underlying nursing theory and excellent clinical skills. Perhaps equally important, they have a deep appreciation of the essential need to partner with childbearing women and their families to ensure optimum outcomes for all. But how do we help students develop this level of expertise? We believe that nursing excellence as it relates to women's health and to childbearing families starts here, in the pages of this text. This book provides essential theoretical content within a holistic, family-centered context. Our goal is to lay a foundation that you can build on with each clinical experience you have.

Women's Health Care

In this edition there is an increased emphasis on women's health care across the lifespan. The women's healthcare chapters have been expanded significantly to include new content on women's health maintenance, societal trends such as body piercing and tattooing, increased depth about menopause and healthy aging, and discussion of pressing social issues. Within Chapter 7, Women's Health Problems, we have added all new content on polycystic ovary syndrome as well as updated content on infections. In addition, the updated information in Chapter 11, Conception and Fetal Development, is especially relevant for nurses today as is Chapter 17, Adolescent Pregnancy. Moreover, because of the text's focus on community-based care, gynecologic cancers are addressed briefly in the text.

Commitment to Diversity

As nurses and as educators, we recognize the importance of honoring diversity and of providing culturally competent care. Thus, we continually strive to make our text ever more inclusive. Chapter 2, Care of the Family in a Culturally Diverse Society, provides the theoretical basis for the consideration of cultural factors that influence a family's expectations of their healthcare providers and their experience with the healthcare system. We elaborate upon this information throughout the text in a boxed feature entitled Developing Cultural Competence. In addition, we have worked hard to ensure that our photos, illustrations, charts, and case scenarios are inclusive in their appearance and in the information they provide. As our society becomes more global in nature, nurses need to cultivate their awareness of these issues because they ultimately do affect how we deliver health care in this country.

Partnering with Families Through Teaching

Developing a partnership with women and their families is a pivotal aspect of maternal-newborn nursing, and one key element of that partnership is client and family teaching. It is a crucial responsibility of the maternal-newborn nurse to find opportunities to educate clients and their families, and we continue to emphasize and highlight this in the eighth edition. Again, the focus is on the teaching that nurses do at all stages of pregnancy and the childbearing process including the important postpartal teaching that is done before and immediately after families are discharged.

Because we believe that nursing excellence must include partnering with women and their families for all outcomes, we have added a new chapter to this edition, Chapter 37, Grief and Loss in the Childbearing Family. It is designed to assist nurses to support families as they deal with the painful losses that sometimes turn moments of great joy into times of deep sorrow. We know that it often takes time for nurses to find authentic ways to support grieving families. Our aim in adding this chapter is to help you understand the dynamics of loss and to offer concrete guidance about effective nursing approaches.

Community-Based Nursing Care

By its very nature, maternal-newborn nursing is community-based nursing. Only a brief portion of the entire pregnancy and birth is spent in a birthing center or hospital. Moreover, because of changes in practice, even women with high-risk pregnancies are receiving more care in their homes and in the community and spending less time in hospital settings. Similarly, most aspects of women's health care are addressed in ambulatory settings.

The provision of nursing care in community-based settings is a driving force in health care today and, consequently, is a dominant theme throughout this edition. We have addressed this topic in several ways. Community-Based Nursing Care is a heading used throughout the text to assist you in identifying specific aspects of this content. Because we consider Home Care to be one form of community-based care, it is often a separate heading under Community-Based Nursing Care. Even more important, Chapter 36, Home Care of the Postpartal Family, provides a thorough explanation of home care as an important aspect of care for childbearing families.

ORGANIZATION: A NURSING CARE MANAGEMENT FRAMEWORK

Whereas some books cover the role of the medical community in childbirth as a separate topic, our book gives an overview of all aspects of the childbearing process with a specific emphasis on nursing care throughout pregnancy, labor, and birth, and the postpartal period. The plans and pathways help you become familiar with these two approaches to managing care so that they are better equipped for variations in clinical settings.

NURSING CARE MANAGEMENT

The *Nursing Care Management* head delineates the important care management role of the nurse within the organizing framework of the nursing process to help you understand what nursing actions are needed. Numerous special features reinforce the nursing care management role.

 NURSING CARE PLAN

Nursing Care Plans address nursing care for clients who have complications, such as a woman with preeclampsia. We designed this feature to help you approach care from the nursing process perspective. These care plans use a nursing diagnosis approach in planning and providing care when pregnancy-related and newborn complications arise.

 CLINICAL PATHWAY

Clinical Pathways describe nursing actions as women are integrated into care of other health professionals. They help you organize care for healthy women and evaluate its effectiveness.

 ASSESSMENT GUIDE

Assessment Guides help you organize your questions and steps during a physical assessment, and provide normal findings, alterations, and possible causes, as well as guidelines for nursing interventions.

THROUGH THE EYES OF A NURSE

To help you prepare for clinical experiences, your textbook provides an unfolding story of an expecting couple and their nurse. **Through the Eyes of a Nurse** vignettes show the interaction between the nurse and the couple surrounding a typical topic of concern for expecting women and their partners. Viewing the partnership that develops will prepare you for success in clinical encounters and in practice.

First, read the **Family Experience** section. The question presents a common concern of women and their partners.

Next, read how the nurse answers in the **Nurse's Response,** taking the opportunity to educate the client.

Finally, the **Nurse's Actions and Rationale** explains why the nurse responded as she did and points out the evidence for the response.

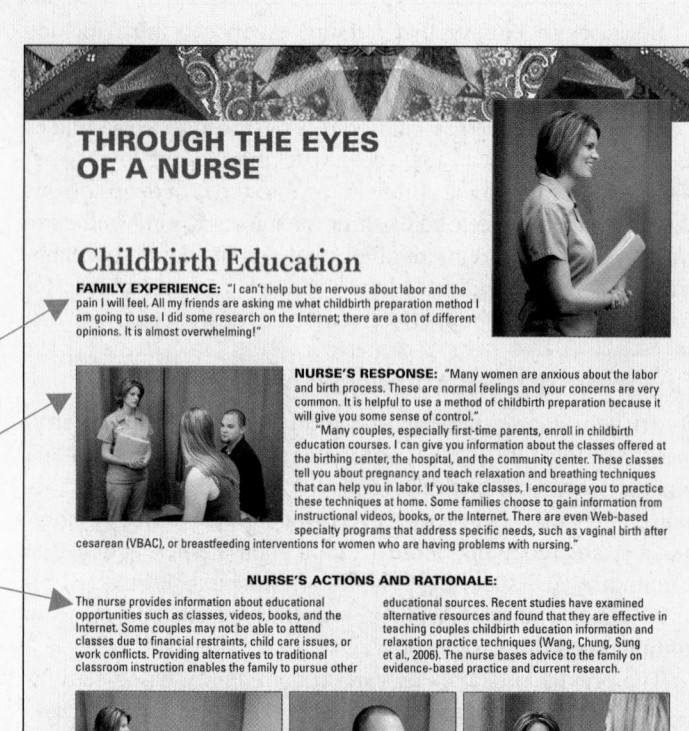

THROUGH THE EYES OF A NURSE

Childbirth Education

FAMILY EXPERIENCE: "I can't help but be nervous about labor and the pain I will feel. All my friends are asking me what childbirth preparation method I am going to use. I did some research on the Internet; there are a ton of different opinions. It is almost overwhelming!"

NURSE'S RESPONSE: "Many women are anxious about the labor and birth process. These are normal feelings and your concerns are very common. It is helpful to use a method of childbirth preparation because it will give you some sense of control."

"Many couples, especially first-time parents, enroll in childbirth education courses. I can give you information about the classes offered at the birthing center, the hospital, and the community center. These classes tell you about pregnancy and teach relaxation and breathing techniques that can help you in labor. If you take classes, I encourage you to practice these techniques at home. Some families choose to gain information from instructional videos, books, or the Internet. There are even Web-based specialty programs that address specific needs, such as vaginal birth after cesarean (VBAC), or breastfeeding interventions for women who are having problems with nursing."

NURSE'S ACTIONS AND RATIONALE:

The nurse provides information about educational opportunities such as classes, videos, books, and the Internet. Some couples may not be able to attend classes due to financial restraints, child care issues, or work conflicts. Providing alternatives to traditional classroom instruction enables the family to pursue other educational sources. Recent studies have examined alternative resources and found that they are effective in teaching couples childbirth education information and relaxation practice techniques (Wang, Chung, Sung et al., 2006). The nurse bases advice to the family on evidence-based practice and current research.

Reference:
Wang, H. H., Chung, U. L., Sung, M. S., & Wu, S. M. (2006). Development of a Web-based childbirth education program for vaginal birth after C-section (VBAC) mothers. *Journal of Nursing Research, 14*(1), 1–8.

With your book is a DVD-ROM that features the interaction between Kaitlyn and Kyle and their nurse during four examinations at various stages throughout their childbirth experience. Author Michele Davidson introduces each segment to help you notice the important communication and client education that takes place. View the partnership that develops and use it to help you prepare for clinical by answering the questions about what you have seen.

The DVD-ROM includes videos of four examinations to model nurse-client interaction:

- **Through the Eyes of a Nurse:** The First Trimester
- **Through the Eyes of a Nurse:** The Second Trimester
- **Through the Eyes of a Nurse:** The Third Trimester
- **Through the Eyes of a Nurse:** The Postpartal Visit: *Welcoming the New Arrival*

CRITICAL THINKING IN ACTION

PREMENSTRUAL SYNDROME

View the Critical Thinking in Action video for Chapter 4.

Linda Knoll, 35 years old, presents to you at the GYN clinic for her annual physical and pelvic exam. You obtain the following menstrual history: LMP 8 days ago. Periods occur every 29 days and last 5 days. She tells you that she uses superabsorbent tampons during the first 2 days of her period and then changes to regular absorbency tampons for the duration, and that she currently has an IUD in place for contraception. She tells you that her husband has been complaining for the last few months that she seems irritable, tense, and moody near "that time of the month." Linda admits that she doesn't feel well before her period and describes having low pelvic discomfort, breast tenderness, "bloating," and some constipation. She seems to cry easily 2 to 3 days before her period. She has noticed this pattern over the last 4 or 5 months. You recognize these symptoms as related to premenstrual syndrome (PMS). Linda asks you if these changes are due to female hormones.

1. How would you answer Linda's question concerning female hormones?

2. After reviewing Linda's diet with her, what would you recommend to help?

3. Linda has an IUD in place. What other type of contraceptive might help reduce the symptoms of PMS?

4. What other activities can you suggest to help Linda reduce PMS symptoms?

5. What should you tell Linda about using tampons during heavy menstrual flow?

◀ Critical Thinking in Action

The abilities needed to think critically and problem solve effectively are learned skills that you can cultivate and develop. New Critical Thinking in Action exercises at the end of each chapter present brief client scenarios with questions that help you apply concepts. To further enhance the true-to-life nature of the case study, the Prentice Hall Nursing MediaLink DVD-ROM continues the exercise with a video enactment of the situation, followed by questions. Not only can you review chapter content in an easy, quick-view format, but you can also apply the concepts used in preparation for clinical work, ensuring success in partnering with your clients.

Client Teaching

The teaching that nurses do at all stages of pregnancy and childbearing and throughout the life of a woman is one of the most important aspects of their work. The Client Teaching boxes in the textbook help you plan and organize your client teaching.

Teaching Cards and Chart

The tear-out Client/Family Teaching Cards are also handy tools for you to use while studying or for quick reference in the clinical setting. Furthermore, a foldout, full-color Maternal-Fetal Growth and Development Chart depicts maternal/fetal development month by month and provides specific teaching guidelines for each stage of pregnancy. You can use this chart as another tool for study or as a quick clinical reference.

CLIENT TEACHING   Using a Method of Contraception

CLIENT GOALS At the completion of the teaching, the woman will be able to

1. Confirm for herself that the chosen method of contraception is appropriate for her.

2. List the advantages, disadvantages, and risks of the chosen method.

3. Describe (or demonstrate) the correct procedure for using the chosen method.

4. Cite warning signs that should be reported to the caregiver.

TEACHING PLAN

CONTENT	TEACHING METHOD
Discuss the factors that a woman should consider in choosing a method of contraception (see Table 5–1). Stress that the different methods may be appropriate at different times in the woman's life. Review the woman's reasons for selecting a particular method and confirm any contraindications to specific methods.	Contraception is a personal decision, so the discussion should take place in a private area free of interruptions. Create a supportive, warm, and comfortable atmosphere by attitude and communication style—both verbal and nonverbal. Provide accurate information in an open, nonjudgmental way.
Discuss the advantages, disadvantages, and risks of the chosen method.	Focus on open discussion. It may help to have written information about the method chosen. If a signed permit is required (as with sterilization or IUD insertion), the physician should also discuss the advantages, disadvantages, and risks.
Describe the correct procedure for using a method. Go through step by step. Periodically stop and have the woman review the information. If a technique is to be learned (as with inserting a diaphragm or charting basal body temperature), demonstrate and then have the woman do a return demonstration as appropriate. (*Note:* If certain aspects are beyond the nurse's level of expertise, the nurse can review the content and confirm that the woman has the opportunity to do a return demonstration. For example, an office nurse who does not do cervical cap fittings may cover information on its use, have the woman try inserting the cap herself, and then have the placement checked by the nurse practioner or physician.)	Learning is best accomplished when material is broken down into smaller steps. Have a model or chart available to enable the woman to visualize what is being described. Have a sample of the chosen method available: a package of oral contraceptives, an open IUD, or a symptothermal chart.
Provide information on what the woman should do if unusual circumstances arise (she forgets a pill or misses a morning temperature).	Provide a written handout identifying the warning signs of her chosen method and listing the actions a woman should take. The handout should also cover actions the woman should take if an unusual situation develops. For example, what should she do if she vomits or has diarrhea while taking oral contraceptives?
Stress warning signs that require immediate action on the part of the woman and explain why these signs indicate a risk. Carefully delineate the actions the woman should take.	Arrange to talk with the woman again soon, either on the phone or at a return visit, to determine if she has any questions about the method and to ensure that no problems have arisen.

EVALUATION

Evaluate the woman's learning by asking her to describe the method she has chosen, its contraindictions and warning signs, and the procedure for using it correctly. In some cases, a return demonstration is useful.

First Page of Chapter

Vignette—Each chapter begins with a personal vignette that helps set the tone for the chapter.

Objectives—Learning objectives introduce you to the topics covered in each chapter.

Key Terms—Key terms introduce each chapter, with page numbers showing where each term first appears in the chapter, in bold type.

MediaLink and EXPLORE MediaLink—The MediaLink box at the start of each chapter reminds you of the chapter-related content on the Prentice Hall Nursing MediaLink DVD-ROM that accompanies your textbook. Special MediaLink icons appear in the margins throughout the chapter to refer you to related videos, animations, or other learning material that appears on the DVD-ROM or Companion Website at http://www.prenhall.com/davidson. At the end of each chapter, EXPLORE MediaLink sections encourage you to use these tools to apply what you have learned in case studies, to practice NCLEX-RN®-style questions, and to use additional resources.

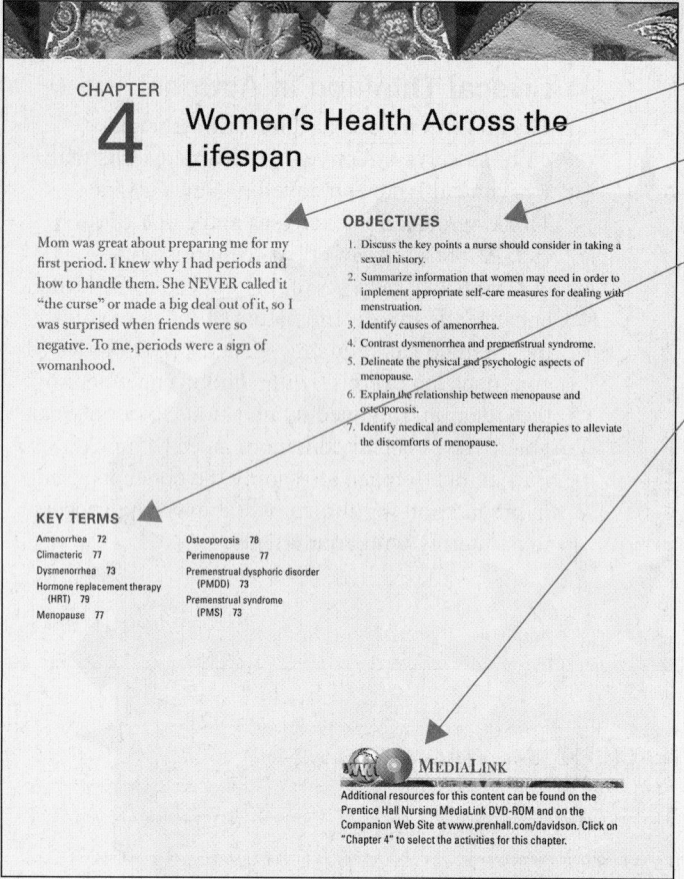

CHAPTER 4

Women's Health Across the Lifespan

Mom was great about preparing me for my first period. I knew why I had periods and how to handle them. She NEVER called it "the curse" or made a big deal out of it, so I was surprised when friends were so negative. To me, periods were a sign of womanhood.

OBJECTIVES

1. Discuss the key points a nurse should consider in taking a sexual history.
2. Summarize information that women may need in order to implement appropriate self-care measures for dealing with menstruation.
3. Identify causes of amenorrhea.
4. Contrast dysmenorrhea and premenstrual syndrome.
5. Delineate the physical and psychologic aspects of menopause.
6. Explain the relationship between menopause and osteoporosis.
7. Identify medical and complementary therapies to alleviate the discomforts of menopause.

KEY TERMS

Amenorrhea 72
Climacteric 77
Dysmenorrhea 73
Hormone replacement therapy (HRT) 79
Menopause 77
Osteoporosis 78
Perimenopause 77
Premenstrual dysphoric disorder (PMDD) 73
Premenstrual syndrome (PMS) 73

MEDIALINK

Additional resources for this content can be found on the Prentice Hall Nursing MediaLink DVD-ROM and on the Companion Web Site at www.prenhall.com/davidson. Click on "Chapter 4" to select the activities for this chapter.

Evidence-Based Practice and Research in Practice

To help you understand the use of reliable information to plan and provide effective nursing care, Evidence-Based Practice boxes relate research evidence to women's health and maternal-newborn nursing. We also include Research in Practice boxes that provide strong examples of relevant clinically focused research.

RESEARCH IN PRACTICE

EFFECTS OF MUSIC THERAPY ON WOMEN'S PHYSIOLOGIC MEASURES, ANXIETY, AND SATISFACTION DURING CESAREAN DELIVERY

What is this study about? Cesarean birth is major surgery and may cause considerable stress, resulting in an unsatisfying birth experience. Music therapy, or the systematic application of music to aid in healthcare treatment, may be effective in reducing anxiety and improving satisfaction with the birth experience. Researchers have demonstrated the effectiveness of music therapy in a variety of settings for a range of physiologic conditions. Specifically, music has been shown to ease anxiety, distract attention, and increase the threshold of pain during operative procedures. The purpose of this

author-developed questionnaire. Physiologic indices included pulse hemoglobin oxygen saturation, finger temperature, respiratory and pulse rates, and blood pressure. Women in the experimental group were also asked to evaluate the level of satisfaction with the music therapy. Measures were collected before anesthesia, upon the end of maternal contact with the newborn, and after completion of the skin sutures.

What were the results of the study? There were no differences on any of the measures between the groups before the birth. No differences were found at any point between the experimental and control groups on any of the physiologic measures. Women in the music listening group had lower anxiety than the women in the [group] in the intraoperative period and after completion of [the sutu]res. The participants in the music group also reported [measure]s related to satisfaction with the cesarean birth experience. [The] majority of women who experienced music therapy [rated their] sense of satisfaction with the therapy as high.

[Addi]tional questions might I have? Can the re[searcher s]eparate the effects of continuous presence of the nurse [from the eff]ects of the music therapy? Are there any potential neg[ative conseq]uences from music therapy during cesarean birth?

[Can I] use this study? Music therapy is consistent with the [holist]ic support for the mother during birth. This type of ther[apy is] cost and noninvasive and may help mothers have a more [positive expe]rience during cesarean birth. Nurses should consider [using mu]sic therapy to mothers to reduce anxiety and improve [satisfaction] with the birth experience.

[Source: ...], S., & Chen, C. (2005). Effects of music therapy on women's [physiologic meas]ures, anxiety, and satisfaction during cesarean delivery. *Research in [Nursing & Hea]lth, 28,* 453–461.

EVIDENCE-BASED PRACTICE

HORMONE THERAPY AND CARDIOVASCULAR DISEASE

Clinical Question

What are the effects of hormone therapy on cardiovascular morbidity and mortality in postmenopausal women?

The Evidence

At one time, it was believed that hormone therapy produced a cardioprotective effect for postmenopausal women. These findings were based primarily on observational studies. Recently, data from several randomized controlled trials produced evidence suggesting that hormone therapy is not associated with any beneficial effect for cardiovascular disease and may actually increase risk. These reviewers aimed to provide a more precise estimate of the cardiovascular effects of hormone therapy using meta-analysis and systematic review. Four reviewers appraised seven large-scale, multisite randomized clinical trials comparing hormone therapy of duration greater than 1 year to placebo. The seven trials together comprised a sample size of more than 32,000 women. Outcomes of interest were mortality from any cardiovascular cause; nonfatal acute myocardial infarction (AMI); coronary heart disease (CHD); and all strokes. The studies were independently appraised by at least two of the reviewers and effect-size statistics were calculated using meta-analysis.

What Is Effective?

The use of hormone therapy had no significant effect—protective or harmful—on mortality from all causes, nonfatal AMI or CHD. The risk of stroke was significantly higher for the hormone groups, including both fatal and nonfatal strokes that were either ischemic or hemorrhagic. The women who were receiving hormone therapy had a 29% increased risk of stroke, and this risk was higher for younger women (under the age of 65) than for older women.

What Is Unclear?

There were insufficient data to determine which type of stroke—ischemic or hemorrhagic—was higher in the hormone group. The suggested physiologic mechanism underlying stroke was ischemic, but these reviewers were unable to determine if there was a difference. There is conjecture as to why the observational studies produced paradoxical results from the randomized trials. It is hypothesized that women who participated in the observational studies (e.g., the Nurses' Health Study) were demographically more likely to have healthier lifestyles than the general population. The effects of these demographic modifiers require more study to determine if the risk of stroke can be modified with health-related behaviors.

Best Practice

It is difficult to directly compare the benefits of hormone therapy in preventing menopausal symptoms, reducing the rate of osteoporosis, and improving quality of life to a 29% increase in the risk of stroke. The balance of risk and benefit of hormone therapy must be weighed individually for each woman. When women are given hormone therapy for more than a short time period (1 year) the risk of stroke does increase, but there is no protective or harmful effect as reflected in nonfatal AMI, CHD, or cardiovascular mortality. Women should be given accurate information about the risks and benefits of this therapy so that they can make a personal decision based on reliable research.

Critical Thinking

What assessments would indicate to the nurse that a woman would be at higher risk of stroke and should avoid hormone therapy altogether? How can these findings be incorporated into the health teaching plans of women who are postmenopausal?

REFERENCE Magliano, D., Rogers, S., Abramson, M., & Tonkin, A. (2006). Hormone therapy and cardiovascular disease: A systematic review and meta-analysis. *British Journal of Obstetrics and Gynecology, 113,* 5–14.

◄ Complementary and Alternative Therapies

Complementary and alternative therapies have become a credible component of holistic care. To help you become familiar with this content, we have included these boxes to inform you about therapies your clients might be using or therapies you might safely suggest. In all cases, research is cited for safe practice of these therapies.

Developing Cultural Competence ▶

The Developing Cultural Competence boxes foster your awareness of cultural factors that influence a family's expectations of and responses to their healthcare provider and their experiences with the healthcare system.

◄ Drug Guide

Drug Guide boxes for selected medications commonly used in maternal-newborn nursing guide you in correctly administering the medications and evaluating your actions.

PROCEDURE 7-1 Assisting with a Pelvic Examination

NURSING ACTION	RATIONALE
Preparation	
• Ensure that the room is sufficiently warm by checking room temperature and adjusting thermostat if necessary. If overhead heat lamps are available, turn them on.	
• Explain the procedure to the woman. If she has never had a pelvic examination, show her the equipment to be used as part of the explanation.	*Explaining the procedure helps reduce anxiety and increase cooperation.*
• Ask the woman to empty her bladder and to remove clothing below the waist.	*An empty bladder promotes comfort during the internal examination.*
• Have padding on the stirrups. If stirrups are not padded, the woman may prefer to leave her shoes on during the procedure.	*Stirrups are padded to ease the pressure of the feet against the metal and to decrease the discomfort associated with cold stirrups. If they are not padded, wearing shoes accomplishes the same purpose.*
• Give the woman a disposable drape or sheet to use during the exam. Ask her to sit at the end of the examining table with the drape opened across her lap.	
• Position the woman in the lithotomy position with her thighs flexed and abducted. Place her feet in the stirrups. Her buttocks should extend slightly beyond the edge of the examining table.	*This position provides the exposure necessary to conduct the examination effectively.*
• Drape the woman with the sheet, leaving a flap so that the perineum can be exposed.	*The drape helps preserve the woman's sense of dignity and privacy.*

NURSING ACTION	RATIONALE
Equipment and Supplies	
• Vaginal specula of various sizes, warmed with water or on heating pad prior to insertion	
• Sterile gloves	
• Water-soluble lubricant	
• Materials for Pap smear or *ThinPrep* Pap test and cultures	
• Good light source	
Note: Lubricant may alter the results of tests and cultures and is not used during the speculum examination. Its use is reserved for the bimanual examination.	
Procedure: Sterile Gloves	
1. The examiner dons gloves for the procedure. Explain each part of the procedure as the certified nurse-midwife, nurse practitioner, or physician performs it. Let the woman know that the examiner begins with an inspection of the external genitalia. The speculum is then inserted to allow visualization of the cervix and vaginal walls and to obtain specimens for testing. After the speculum is withdrawn the examiner performs a bimanual examination of the internal organs using the fingers of one hand inserted in the woman's vagina while the other hand presses over the woman's uterus and ovaries. The final step of the procedure is generally a rectal examination.	
2. Ask the woman to breathe slowly and regularly and to use any method she finds effective in helping her to remain relaxed.	*Relaxation helps decrease muscle tension. Bearing down helps open the*

◀ Procedures

Procedure boxes offer step-by-step techniques that show you the tasks expected of a nurse in clinical situations, preparing you for your clinical experiences. Included in each box are the preparation steps with rationales, equipment and supplies needed, and steps for the procedure itself, with rationales for the nurse's actions.

RESOURCES FOR STUDENT SUCCESS

Prentice Hall Nursing MediaLink DVD-ROM—Packaged with this book is a DVD-ROM with NCLEX-RN®-style questions with rationales, an audio glossary, animations, Through the Eyes of a Nurse videos, Newborn Reflex videos, Critical Thinking in Action videos, and other material to prepare you for success in the classroom, in clinicals, and on the NCLEX-RN® exam.

Companion Website (http://www.prenhall.com/davidson)—This site offers study tools to enrich your learning. Included are additional NCLEX-RN®-style questions with rationales, case studies, care plans, critical thinking exercises, activities, Web links, and other tools to help you succeed.

Clinical Handbook for Old's Maternal-Newborn Nursing & Women's Health Across the Lifespan (ISBN: 0-13-232441-5)—This pocket guide serves as a portable, quick-reference to maternal-newborn nursing care. Covering from pregnancy through the postpartum and newborn stages, this handbook allows you to take the information you learn in class into any clinical setting.

Student Workbook (ISBN: 0-13-240149-5)—This popular study tool incorporates strategies for you to focus your study and increase comprehension of concepts of nursing care.

RESOURCES FOR FACULTY SUCCESS

Instructor's Resource Manual—This manual contains a wealth of material to help instructors plan and manage the maternity nursing course. Lecture concepts and PowerPoint slides are grouped under learning objectives for each chapter, along with suggestions for classroom and clinical activities. Included is a test bank of chapter-specific NCLEX-RN®-style questions, complete with rationales and classification ratings for each question.

Instructor's Resource DVD-ROM—This media-rich DVD-ROM provides the tools faculty need for ease in classroom preparation and evaluation. Included are the Test Generator with peer-reviewed NCLEX-RN®-style questions, integrated PowerPoint presentations, an image library, and animations and videos from the Prentice Hall Nursing MediaLink DVD-ROM.

 Online Course Management Systems—Prentice Hall OneKey is available for schools using Blackboard and WebCT platforms. It provides the student and faculty resources in an open-access, integrated course cartridge.

Acknowledgments

Our goal with every revision is to incorporate the latest research and information from the literature of nursing and related fields to make our text as relevant and useful as possible. This would not be possible without the support and encouragement of our colleagues in nursing. The comments and suggestions we have received from nurse educators and practitioners around the country have helped us keep this text accurate and up to date. Whenever a nurse takes the time to write or to speak to one of us at a professional gathering, we recognize again the intense commitment of nurses to excellence in practice. And so we thank our colleagues.

We are grateful, too, to our students, past, present, and future. They stimulate us with their interest; they reinvigorate us with their enthusiasm; they challenge us with their questions to make each edition of this text clear and understandable. We learn so much from them.

In publishing, as in health care, quality assurance is an essential part of the process. That is the dimension our reviewers have added. Some reviewers assist us by validating the accuracy of the content, some by their attention to detail, and some by challenging us to examine our ways of thinking and to develop a new awareness about a given topic. Thus, we extend our sincere thanks to all those who reviewed the manuscript for this book. Their names and affiliations are listed on the preceding pages.

We are also grateful to the contributors to the eighth edition of *Olds' Maternal-Newborn Nursing & Women's Health Across the Lifespan*. Their knowledge of clinical practice and current literature in their areas of expertise helps make the chapters relevant and accurate. They, too, are listed on the preceding pages.

The success of a project of this scope requires the skills and dedication of many people. We would personally like to thank the following people:

A new editor joined us for this edition. Pamela Lappies is a delight—supportive, enthusiastic, experienced, and astute. She brings a wealth of publishing experience to challenge us, a fresh eye to refocus us, and a warmth and responsiveness that has already enabled us to bond as a team. We are so pleased to work with you, Pam.

Our editor-in-chief, Maura Connor, deserves our sincere thanks. In her leadership role she ensures that we have the support and resources we need to produce an exceptional text, one designed to support students and foster the profession of nursing. Maura's energy and enthusiasm are contagious.

Julie Alexander, our publisher, has played an important role in the development of our text. Her leadership of Prentice Hall Health has resulted in the growth of a company committed to excellence, to technology, and to student support. She is a visionary in publishing.

We are grateful to Alan Sorkowitz, our developmental editor. Alan played an important role in coordinating our chapter revisions and updates. His mean eye for detail helped us produce a tight, accurate manuscript. Many thanks, Alan.

Thanks, too, to Marilyn Meserve, executive managing editor, who oversaw the overall development of the book. She stayed unfailingly calm as we dealt with many new changes,

Our thanks to Maria Guglielmo and Cheryl Asherman for the stunning interior and cover design; to Anne Garcia for the production support; to Patrick Watson, who skillfully managed our photographs and illustrations; and to Heather Willison of Carlisle Publishing Services. Without support in these crucial areas, our work would not be as visually appealing and accurate as it is.

We are especially grateful to Kim Mohler, RN, and to Kaitlyn and Kyle Kersey—and their beautiful baby, Braeden—for their participation in the Through the Eyes of a Nurse features and videos. This edition benefits immensely because they were willing to share with nursing students this special time of their lives.

During these times of uncertainty in the healthcare environment, we are sustained by our passion for nursing and our vision of what childbirth means. Time and again, we have seen the difference a skilled nurse can make in the lives of people in need. We, like you, are committed to helping all nurses recognize and take pride in that fact. Thank you for your letters, your comments, and your suggestions. We are renewed by your support.

Michele R. Davidson
Marcia L. London
Patricia W. Ladewig

Special Features

Developing Cultural Competence

 ## Clinical Pathways

Assessment Guides

 ## Complementary and Alternative Therapies

Drug Guide

Procedures

Research in Practice

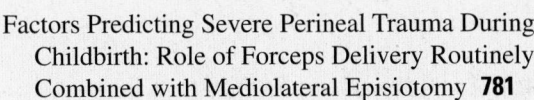

Contents

UNIT 4

PREGNANCY

UNIT 7

POSTPARTUM

UNIT

1

Contemporary Maternal-Newborn Nursing

Current Issues in Maternal-Newborn Nursing

Our daughter just told us that she is 3 months pregnant with our first grandchild. As a labor and delivery nurse for 25 years, I've helped with hundreds of births, but it still seems magical to me, especially now. I'm excited for her and a little worried because I know all the risks as well as the joys. She is so happy; when I am with her I just want to laugh out loud. I already know I love being a grandmother, even though I really am too young!

OBJECTIVES

1. Relate the concept of the expert nurse to nurses caring for childbearing families.

2. Discuss the impact of the self-care movement on contemporary childbirth.

3. Compare the nursing roles available to the maternal-newborn nurse.

4. Identify specific factors that contribute to a family's value system.

5. Delineate significant legal and ethical issues that influence the practice of nursing for childbearing families.

6. Evaluate the potential impact of some of the special situations in contemporary maternity care.

7. Contrast descriptive and inferential statistics.

8. Relate the availability of statistical data to the formulation of further research questions.

9. Delineate the benefits of evidence-based nursing practice to the client, the institution, and the profession of nursing.

KEY TERMS

Assisted reproductive technology (ART)   15
Birth rate   17
Certified nurse-midwife (CNM)   8
Certified registered nurse (RNC)   8
Client   5
Clinical nurse specialist (CNS)   8
Evidence-based practice   20
Infant mortality rate   18
Informed consent   11
Intrauterine fetal surgery   14
Maternal mortality rate   19
Nurse practitioner (NP)   8
Professional nurse   8
Therapeutic insemination (TI)   14

MEDIALINK

Additional resources for this content can be found on the Prentice Hall Nursing MediaLink DVD-ROM and on the Companion Website at http://www.prenhall.com/davidson. Click on "Chapter 1" to select the activities for this chapter.

The practice of most nurses is filled with special moments, shared experiences, times in which they know they have practiced the essence of nursing and, in doing so, have touched a life. What is the essence of nursing? Simply stated, nurses care for people, care about people, and use their expertise to help people help themselves.

I like working with students. I enjoy the enthusiasm they bring, the questions they ask, the ways they cause me to examine my practice. I love being a nurse. I am passionate about the importance of what I do, and I feel the need to seize every chance to influence those who will be practicing beside me someday. Last week was a perfect example. I had a nursing student working with me in one of our birthing rooms. It was her first day caring for a laboring woman, and she was scared and excited at the same time. We were taking care of a healthy woman who had two boys at home and really wanted a girl.

As labor progressed, the student and I worked closely together monitoring contractions, teaching the woman and her husband, doing what we could to ease her discomfort. Sometimes the student would ask how I knew when to do something, a vaginal exam, for example, and I'd have to think beyond "I just do" to give her some clues. At the birth the student stayed close to the mother, coaching and helping with breathing. The student was excited but felt she had an important role to play, and she handled it beautifully. At the moment of birth the student and the dad were leaning forward watching as the baby just slipped into the world. There wasn't a sound until the student said in a voice filled with awe, "Oh, it's a girl!" Then we all laughed and hugged each other. What a day—using my expertise to help others and helping a future nurse recognize the importance of what we do!

All nurses who provide care and support to childbearing women and their families can make a difference. But how does this happen? How do nurses develop expertise and become skilled, caring practitioners?

In her classic work, Benner (1984) suggested that as nurses develop their skills in making clinical judgments and intervening appropriately, they progress through five levels of competence. Beginning as a novice, the nurse progresses to advanced beginner and then to competent, proficient, and finally, expert nurse.

In the preceding situation, the student was clearly a novice. Lacking experience, the novice relies on rules to guide actions. As nurses gain experience, they begin to draw on that experience to view situations more holistically, becoming increasingly aware of subtle cues that indicate physiologic and psychologic changes. Expert nurses, like the nurse in the preceding situation, have a clear vision of what is possible in a given situation. This holistic perspective is based on a wealth of knowledge bred of experience and enables nurses to act "intuitively" to provide effective care. In reality nurses' intuition reflects their internalization of information. When faced with a clinical situation, nurses draw almost subconsciously on their stored knowledge and judgment.

This intuitive perception is integral to the "art of nursing," especially in areas such as maternal-newborn nursing, where change occurs quickly and families look to the nurse for help

and guidance. Labor nurses become attuned to a woman's progress or lack of progress; nursery nurses detect subtle changes in their infant charges; antepartal and postpartal nurses become adept at assessing and teaching. Similarly, nurses who are cross-trained as labor, delivery, recovery, and postpartum (LDRP) nurses become skilled at caring for childbearing families during all phases of childbirth. Thus skilled nursing practice depends on a solid base of knowledge and clinical expertise delivered in a caring, holistic manner.

Control develops as nurses learn to handle their own emotions and to master clinical situations by making and acting on client care decisions. Control issues are often difficult for advanced beginners, who can demonstrate only marginally acceptable performance (Benner, 1984) and they may look to expert nurses for guidance. As nurses provide good nursing care and develop a knowledge base, they gain competence. From this competence flows credibility as others begin to trust and believe in them. Nurses in turn become self-reliant and gain confidence in their judgment. Finally a sense of comfort develops and nurses feel able to predict probable outcomes.

My first pregnancy ended in spontaneous abortion at 8 weeks, so this time I decided not to tell anyone I was pregnant until I was 3 months along. We had just told both families the news the preceding day when it happened again. I began bleeding heavily, and we rushed to the ER. Here I was, a maternal-newborn nursing instructor, and I couldn't seem to handle a pregnancy. I was in the bathroom when I passed the fetus into the Johnny cap. My poor baby—so small, maybe 3 or 4 inches long. I began to sob uncontrollably as I rang for the nurse. I told her what happened, and she helped me to bed. My husband sat with his arm around me as I cried while the nurse took our baby out. A few minutes later, she came back and said, "I saw on your record that you are Catholic. Would you like me to baptize your baby?" I said, "Oh, yes, please," and she left. I've never forgotten how that made me feel. She saw me as a total person. I'm still teaching, and now I have two children. Whenever I teach high-risk pregnancy, I tell that story to the students. I want them to know what a difference a nurse can make.

We believe that many nurses who work with childbearing families are experts: They are sensitive, intuitive, knowledgeable, critical thinkers. They are technically skilled, empowered professionals who can collaborate effectively with others and advocate for those individuals and families who need their support. Such nurses do make a difference in the quality of care that childbearing families receive.

CONTEMPORARY CHILDBIRTH

The scope of practice of maternal and newborn nurses has changed dramatically in the past 25 years. Today's maternal-newborn nurses have far broader responsibilities and focus more on the specific goals of the individual childbearing woman and her family (Figure 1–1 ◆).

Not only has maternal-newborn nursing changed, so has the whole experience of childbirth. No longer do laboring women leave their partners and family at the labor room door while they

Figure 1–1 ◆ Individualized education for childbearing couples is one of the prime responsibilities of the maternal-newborn nurse.

work to give birth without the family's loving presence; no longer are newborns routinely whisked away for a prescribed period, to reappear magically for feedings every 4 hours and then return to the safe atmosphere of a central nursery; no longer are young siblings treated like walking sources of infection that threaten every infant. Today fathers are active participants in the birth experience. Families and friends are also often included. Siblings are encouraged to visit and meet their newest family member and may even attend the birth. Today the concept of "family-centered childbirth" is accepted and encouraged.

In addition, new definitions of family are evolving as discussed in Chapter 2. ∞ For example, the family of the single mother may include her mother, sister, another relative, a close friend, or the father of the child. Many cultures also recognize the importance of extended families, where several family members often provide care and support.

The family can generally make choices about many aspects of the childbirth experience, including the place of birth (hospital, free-standing birthing center, or home birth); the primary caregiver (physician, certified nurse-midwife, or certified midwife); and birth-related experiences (methods of childbirth preparation, use of analgesia and anesthesia, and position for labor and birth, for example).

As recently as the early 1990s, women who gave birth vaginally remained in the hospital for approximately 3 days. This provided ample time for nurses to assess the family's knowledge and skill and complete essential teaching. By the mid-1990s, in an effort to control costs, hospitals were routinely discharging new mothers within 12 to 24 hours or less following birth. For women with supportive families, thorough prenatal preparation, and adequate resources for necessary follow-up

care, this practice did not necessarily pose a problem. However, because early discharge severely limits the time available for client teaching, women with little knowledge, experience, or support were at greater risk of being inadequately prepared to care for themselves and their newborn infants.

Fortunately, the negative impact of this practice gained recognition nationwide. As a result, Congress passed the Newborns' and Mothers' Health Protection Act of 1996, which took effect in January 1998. This act provides for a postpartum stay of up to 48 hours following vaginal birth and up to 96 hours following cesarean birth at the discretion of the mother and her healthcare provider. However, it does not contain a provision for home care follow-up if a new mother chooses to leave the birthing facility earlier than the length of stay mandated by the act. Some states have developed home care provisions that strengthen the federal legislation.

It seems likely that home follow-up nursing care will continue to gain acceptance because it is a cost-effective approach with favorable long-term family outcomes. In addition, families can access a variety of community resources, from local programs focusing on specific topics such as parenting or postpartal exercise to the widely recognized support provided by national organizations such as La Leche League.

For families with access to the Internet, a wealth of information and advice is available. For example, the Department of Health and Human Services' Office on Women's Health offers a wide variety of educational resources designed to help promote women's health and well-being. Web links to a variety of other organizations and consumer publications also exist.

Interest in complementary and alternative medicine (CAM) practices is growing nationwide and is having an impact on the care of childbearing families. In response to this trend, the National Institutes of Health now has an Office of Alternative Medicine. Nurses caring for childbearing families need to recognize that a significant percentage of Americans are using some form of unconventional or alternative practice although they may not share this information with their healthcare provider. Thus it is important for nurses to communicate a willingness to work with the client to recognize and respect these alternative approaches. To assist nurses caring for these childbearing families we have included a chapter—Chapter 3 ∞—on complementary and alternative therapies.

Many women elect to have their pregnancy and birth managed by a certified nurse-midwife (CNM), a registered nurse who is also prepared as a midwife. Accreditation of the CNM is offered through the American College of Nurse-Midwives (ACNM). The preparation and role of the CNM is described on page 8.

Some women choose to receive care from a direct-entry certified midwife or even a lay midwife (an unlicensed or uncertified midwife who is trained through an informal route such as apprenticeship or self-study rather than a formal educational program [Midwives Alliance of North America{MANA}, 2006]). Midwives who complete a direct-entry midwifery education program that meets the standards established by ACNM may take a certification exam to become a *certified midwife (CM)*. ACNM has mandated that, by 2010, a master's or doctoral degree will be required for entry into clinical practice as either a CNM or CM (ACNM, 2005).

The North American Registry of Midwives (NARM) is also a certification agency. Midwives certified through NARM may become midwives through a formal educational program at a college, university, or midwifery school, or through apprenticeship or self-study. They are eligible to use the credential *certified professional midwife (CPM)*.

Some women choose to give birth at home although healthcare professionals do not generally recommend this approach. The concern of the healthcare professional is that, in the event of an unanticipated complication that threatens the well-being of the mother or her infant, delay in obtaining emergency assistance might result. Some CNMs do attend home births; however, the majority of home births are attended by CMs, CPMs, or lay midwives.

THE SELF-CARE MOVEMENT

The self-care movement began to emerge in the late 1960s as consumers sought to understand technology and take an interest in their own health and basic self-care skills. More and more people have begun to exercise, control their diet, monitor their psychologic and physiologic status, and in some cases even do their own diagnostic tests. They thus assume many primary care functions. Furthermore, today's healthcare consumers are requiring greater information and accountability from their healthcare providers. These consumers recognize that knowledge, indeed, is power.

Practicing self-care—assuming responsibility for one's own health—often requires assertiveness and taking an active role in seeking necessary information. Nurses can foster self-care by providing information readily and by acknowledging people's right to ask questions and become actively involved in their own care.

Maternal-newborn care offers a special opportunity to promote active participation in health care because it is essentially health focused; in most cases, clients are well when they enter the system. The consumer movement that has already influenced childbirth encourages people to speak up for preferences in dealing with healthcare providers.

Self-care has gained an even broader appeal in recent years because research suggests that it can significantly reduce healthcare costs. We believe that self-care will be a vital part of health care for years to come. Obviously, self-care is not always realistic or appropriate, especially in acute emergencies, but in many situations it is appropriate. With this in mind, throughout this book we have attempted to suggest ways in which nurses might offer health education that would enable the childbearing family to meet their own healthcare needs. We see this as one of nursing's most important functions and one that nurses are especially well qualified to perform.

Because of our support of self-care, we have used the term *client* rather than *patient* when referring to the childbearing woman. The term **client** implies an active, rather than a passive, role. The client seeks assistance from professionals who have special skills and knowledge that the client does not. The healthcare professional offers information and suggestions for a plan of action regarding the client's particular situation. The client can choose not to accept the professional's advice. Furthermore, the healthcare professional cannot proceed with the plan of action without the client's consent. In this relationship, clients assume responsibility for their decisions.

The nursing profession has been at the forefront in recognizing that people who are able to do so should take an active role in their own health care, and the term *client* best fits this concept. Nurses must understand that it is their professional expertise and skill that the client is seeking. Any attempt to make decisions for the client is inappropriate.

THE HEALTHCARE ENVIRONMENT

Healthcare issues are at the top of policy and legislative agendas. Cost, access, and quality of health care have become the "bywords" of the times. In 1960, healthcare costs in the United States accounted for approximately 5% of the gross domestic product (GDP). In 2004 the healthcare share of the GDP was 16%, a staggering percentage. Currently the United States spends a greater portion of the GDP on health than any other major industrialized nation worldwide. In actual dollars in 2004 the United States spent $1.9 trillion on health care (Smith, Cowan, Heffler, & Catlin, 2006).

Despite this increase in spending, however, not all pregnant women and children in the United States have access to health care. In 2005, 16% of people under age 65 (41 million) were without health insurance (Figure 1–2 ◆). People with incomes below or near the poverty level were significantly more likely to be uninsured, as were people of Hispanic origin (Cohen & Martinez, 2006). For people living in poverty, Medicaid is the most prevalent form of insurance. Together Medicaid, the State Children's Health Insurance Program (SCHIP) (a federally funded program to provide states with funds for low-income, uninsured children), and Medicare account for one third of healthcare spending as shown in Figure 1–3 ◆ (Centers for Medicare and Medicaid Services [CMS], 2006).

For women who become pregnant, early prenatal care is one of the most important approaches available to reduce adverse

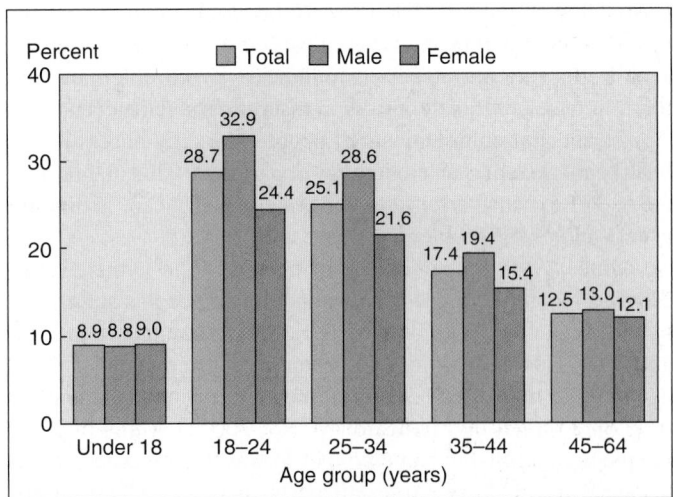

Figure 1–2 ◆ No health insurance coverage among persons under 65 years of age by selected characteristics, United States, 2005. SOURCE: CDC. National Center for Health Statistics. *Health Insurance Coverage: Estimates from the National Health Interview Survey, 2005.*

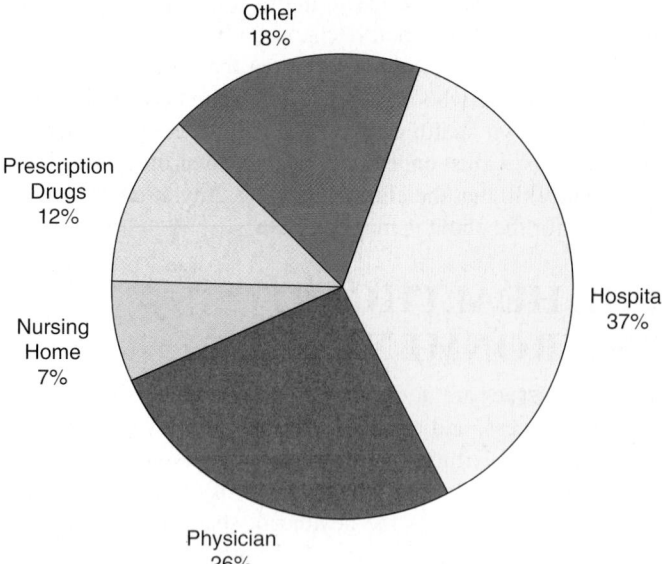

NOTE: The "Other" category includes visits to nonphysician medical providers, medical supplies, and other health services.

Figure 1–3 ◆ The nation's health dollar for calendar year 2004.
SOURCE: Centers for Medicare and Medicaid Services, Office of the Actuary, National Health Statistics Group.

pregnancy outcomes. In 2003, 84.1% of pregnant women in the United States began prenatal care in the first trimester. However, these percentages vary significantly among groups, with black, Hispanic, and Native American women less likely to receive early and adequate prenatal care than white and Asian women (National Center for Health Statistics [NCHS], 2005a).

The United States spends more per capita than any other country in the world on health care; nevertheless, compared with other industrialized nations, the United States has higher infant mortality rates, similar life expectancy, and less access to care. Many people who have insurance fear changing or losing jobs because they may lose healthcare benefits and access to insurance. They may be denied insurance in the future because of preexisting conditions. The increase in serious, debilitating illnesses, such as AIDS and tuberculosis, and in chronic illnesses, such as diabetes and hypertension, makes this problem of "job lock" and lack of transferability of insurance benefits even more significant. For some uninsured people, the only access to the healthcare system is an emergency department. This inappropriate use of expensive services for basic primary care is both an access and a cost problem.

Since 1998 the percentage of people in the United States covered by employment-based health insurance has stayed between 69% and 73%, although the percentage decreased in 2002 and 2003. However, little actual change occurred in the percentage of those uninsured because of the increase in the percentage of people served by Medicaid (NCHS, 2005a). Many of these people are enrolled in some type of managed care organization because, in an effort to curtail costs, many employers have moved from fee-for-service coverage to some form of managed care. Thus managed care is now the dominant form of healthcare delivery in the United States. The move toward managed care has sparked concerns about the quality of health care. Because a fee-for-service model allows the consumer to register dissatisfaction by choosing to seek care elsewhere, quality is a high priority among fee-for-service providers. A managed care model, in contrast, limits consumer choice and, in turn, potentially affects quality. Establishing managed care's effects on quality poses a problem because in the US system, quality indicators such as outcomes of care usually have not been well determined. An outcome-based system is essential if there is to be comprehensive healthcare reform.

Changing the current system requires a new way of thinking and providing services. Primary healthcare services should be the base on which all other secondary and tertiary services are built. Today in the United States the opposite is still the case. The system emphasizes high-technology care rather than prevention. However, morbidity and mortality from disease are reduced significantly when people use preventive health services. There are some areas of improvement. For example, between 1990 and 2003, the percentage of pregnant women who received prenatal care increased from 76% to 84%. Similarly, between 1987 and 2003, the percentage of women age 40 and over who had had a mammogram in the preceding 2 years more than doubled, increasing from 29% to 69.5% (NCHS, 2005a).

The new *Health Insurance Portability and Accountability Act (HIPAA)* of 1996, which was fully implemented in 2002, has also had an impact on health care. HIPAA has two areas of focus: it protects the health insurance coverage of employees and their family if they lose a job or change jobs. It also addresses the privacy and security of health information and requires that national standards be established for the electronic transmission of healthcare data. The *privacy rule* is the federal regulation developed to meet HIPAA requirements. It defines the policies and procedures to be followed to safeguard an individual's protected health information. It also guarantees people access to their medical records and provides recourse for them if their medical privacy is violated. HIPAA regulations have caused healthcare facilities to take a wide variety of actions to ensure client/patient privacy. It has also empowered individuals by giving them access to information about their health care. Academic programs that prepare nurses, physicians, and other healthcare professionals have had to develop tools and resources to ensure that their students understand privacy requirements and comply with them.

Providing all segments of the population with access to primary health care should be the chief criterion for meaningful reform of the US healthcare system. This includes a focus on health promotion, prevention, and individual responsibility for one's own health. In this model, secondary healthcare services would use a smaller proportion of the healthcare dollar.

The current emphasis on healthcare reform has yielded an unexpected benefit: Many healthcare providers and consumers have become more aware of the vitally important role nurses play in providing excellent care to clients and families. The emerging shift in the US healthcare system presents a significant opportunity for the nursing profession. However, this opportunity for responding to and creating change in nursing and healthcare delivery requires a new way of thinking. Nurses must clearly articulate their role in the changing environment. They must define and differentiate practice roles and the educational preparation required for those new roles, especially in community-based nursing practice and advanced practice roles such as nurse practitioners (NPs) and CNMs. Nurses must delineate roles of caregiver and care manager. Nurses must also assume greater roles in promoting health and preventing disease. In reality, in many settings nurses assume the primary responsibility for preventive healthcare services and screening programs.

Healthcare reform is influencing women's health and maternal-newborn nursing. Several factors, including demographic changes, the nationally recognized need to improve access to care, public demand for more effective healthcare options, new research findings, and women's preferences for health care, are contributing to changes in the field. Changes are predicted in clinical procedures, provider roles, care settings, and financing of care. As access to health care and the need to control costs increase, so will the need for, and utilization of, nurses in advanced practice roles.

CULTURALLY COMPETENT CARE

The US population has a varied mix of cultural groups, with ever-increasing diversity. More than one third of all children less than 20 years of age are from families of minority populations. Culture develops from socially learned beliefs, lifestyles, values, and integrated patterns of behavior that are characteristic of the family, cultural group, and community. The cultural background and values of childbearing families are often quite different from those of the nurse.

Specific elements that contribute to a family's value system include the following:

- Religion and social beliefs
- Presence and influence of the extended family, as well as socialization within the ethnic group
- Communication patterns
- Beliefs and understanding about the concepts of health and illness
- Permissible physical contact with strangers
- Education

Specific differences in beliefs between families and healthcare providers are common in the following areas:

- Help-seeking behaviors
- Pregnancy and childbirth practices
- Causes of diseases or illnesses
- Death and dying
- Caretaking and caregiving
- Childrearing practices

These elements in differing degrees influence the cultural beliefs and values of an ethnic group, making the group unique. Misunderstandings may occur when the healthcare professional

DEVELOPING CULTURAL COMPETENCE

VALUES CONFLICTS

Conflicts can occur with a childbearing woman and her family when traditional rituals and practices of the family's elders do not conform with current healthcare practices. Nurses need to be sensitive to the potential implications for the woman's health and that of her newborn, especially after they are discharged home. When cultural values are not part of the nursing care plan, a woman and her family may be forced to decide whether the family's beliefs should take priority over the healthcare professional's guidance.

and the family come from different cultural groups. In addition, past experiences with care may have made the family angry or suspicious of providers. Nurses need to be able to recognize, respect, and respond to ethnic diversity in a way that leads to a mutually desirable outcome. The nurse needs to identify culturally relevant facts about the client to provide culturally appropriate and competent care.

When the family's cultural values are incorporated into the care plan, the family is more likely to accept and comply with the needed care, especially in the home care setting. It is important for nurses to avoid imposing personal cultural values on the women and families in their care. By learning about the values of the different ethnic groups in the community—their religious beliefs that have an impact on healthcare practices, their beliefs about common illnesses, and their specific healing practices—nurses can develop an individualized nursing care plan for each childbearing woman and her family.

Because of the importance of culturally competent care, this topic is discussed in more depth in Chapter 2 ∞ and throughout the book as well.

PROFESSIONAL OPTIONS IN MATERNAL-NEWBORN NURSING PRACTICE

As a man, I don't always find it easy to be a labor and delivery nurse. I have three children of my own and attended all their births. It meant a lot to me to be there, and I like helping others to have good childbirth experiences, too. I don't fit some people's image of a nurse; so they refer to me as a "male nurse" as opposed to a real nurse, and they ask why I didn't go into medicine instead. Why can't they understand that I'm a nurse because it's what I really want to be—and I'm darned good at it, too. More men are choosing nursing now, and I think that will help. I hope to see the day when we don't have "female doctors" and "male nurses," but doctors and nurses, period!

Maternal-newborn nurses are found in the maternity departments of acute care facilities, in physicians' offices, in clinics, in college health services, in school-based programs dealing with sex education or adolescent pregnancies, in community health services, and in any other setting where a client has a need for maternity care. The depth of nursing involvement in various settings is determined by the qualifications and the role or function of the nurse employed. Many different titles have evolved to describe the professional requirements of the nurse in various maternity care roles. These titles include the following:

- A **professional nurse** is a graduate of an accredited basic program in nursing who has successfully completed the nursing examination (NCLEX-RN) and is currently licensed as a registered nurse (RN). Professional nurses are typically educated as generalists.

- A **certified registered nurse (RNC)** has shown expertise in a particular field of nursing such as labor and delivery by taking a national certification examination.

- A **nurse practitioner (NP)** is a professional nurse who has received specialized education in either a master's degree program or a continuing education program and thus can function in an expanded role. Nurse practitioners often provide ambulatory care services to the expectant family (women's health nurse practitioner, family nurse practitioner); some NPs also function in acute care settings (neonatal nurse practitioner, perinatal nurse practitioner). NPs focus on physical and psychosocial assessment, including health history, physical examination, and certain diagnostic tests and procedures. The nurse practitioner makes clinical judgments and begins appropriate treatments, seeking physician consultation when necessary. The emerging emphasis on community-based care has greatly increased opportunities for NPs.

- A **clinical nurse specialist (CNS)** is a professional nurse with a master's degree who has additional specialized knowledge and competence in a specific clinical area. CNSs assume a leadership role within their specialty and work to improve client care both directly and indirectly.

- A **certified nurse-midwife (CNM)** is educated in the two disciplines of nursing and midwifery and is certified by the American College of Nurse-Midwives (ACNM). The certified nurse-midwife is prepared to manage independently the care of women at low risk for complications during pregnancy and birth and the care of normal newborns (Figure 1–4 ◆). In 2001 the American College of Obstetricians and Gynecologists (ACOG) and the ACNM issued a joint statement describing the independent, collaborative, and interdependent responsibilities of both groups, namely obstetricians/gynecologists and certified nurse-midwives/certified midwives. This agreement affirms that the "quality of care is enhanced by the interdependent practice of the obstetrician/gynecologist and the certified nurse-midwife/certified midwife working in a relationship of mutual respect, trust and professional responsibility." This agreement does not require the physical presence of an OB/GYN physician but does include the use of mutually agreed-upon written medical guidelines/protocols (ACOG, 2001).

Figure 1–4 ◆ A certified nurse-midwife confers with her client.
SOURCE: Photographer, Jenny Thomas.

The term *advanced practice nurse* is used to describe nurses who, by education and practice, function in an expanded nursing role. The term, often used in a legal sense in state nurse practice acts, most frequently applies to NPs, CNSs, CRNAs (certified registered nurse anesthetists), and CNMs. As NPs assume a more prominent role in providing care, the distinctions between the roles of the nurse practitioner and the clinical nurse specialist are beginning to blur and these roles may ultimately merge.

Collaborative Practice

Managed care has led to a rethinking of care delivery. One approach that is becoming increasingly popular is collaborative practice. Collaborative practice is a comprehensive model of health care that uses a multidisciplinary team of health professionals to provide cost-effective, high-quality care. In maternal-newborn settings, the team generally includes CNMs and NPs in practice with physicians (often obstetricians or family practice physicians) and may include other health professionals, such as lactation consultants, social workers, or CNSs (Figure 1–5 ◆).

Successful teams have certain characteristics (Simpson & Knox, 2001):

- They have established consensus about their mission and vision, their goals, and their objectives and strategies.

- They recognize, respect, and value the unique contributions of each team member.

- They share a sense of mutual accountability—the team, not an individual, is responsible for success or failure.

- They are part of an organization that has strong, well-delineated performance standards and expectations.

- They have established effective communication.

In a successful team, each individual has autonomy but functions within a clearly defined scope of practice. In such a collaborative approach, no single profession "owns the client." Rather, the team seeks to empower clients and families and include them as partners in their care and in decision making.

Figure 1–5 ◆ A collaborative relationship between nurse and physician contributes to excellent client care.
SOURCE: Photographer, Elena Dorfman.

Community-Based Nursing Care

Many advocates of a new direction for health care support the increasing emphasis on primary care. Primary care includes a focus on health promotion, illness prevention, and individual responsibility for one's own health. These services are best provided in community-based settings. Third-party payers and managed care organizations are beginning to recognize the importance of primary care in containing costs and maintaining health. Community-based health services providing primary care and some secondary care will be available in schools, workplaces, homes, churches, clinics, transitional care programs, and other ambulatory settings.

The growth and diversity of managed care plans offer both opportunities and challenges for women's health care. The potential exists for managed care organizations to work with consumers to provide a model for coordinated and comprehensive well-woman care that includes improved screening and preventive services. One challenge managed care organizations will face is how to relate to essential community providers of care—organizations such as family planning clinics or women's health centers—that offer a unique service or serve groups of women with special needs (adolescents, disabled women, ethnic or racial minorities). Community-based care remains an essential element of health care for uninsured and underinsured individuals as well as for those individuals who benefit from programs such as Medicare or state-sponsored health-related programs. Some of these programs, such as those offered through public health departments, are broad based; others, such as parenting classes for adolescents, are geared to the needs of a specific population.

Community-based care is also part of a trend initiated by consumers, who are asking for a "seamless" system of family-centered, comprehensive, coordinated health care, health education, and social services. This seamless system requires coordination as clients move from primary care services to acute care facilities and then back into the community. The shortened length of hospital stays further mandates the need for coordination of services. Nurses can assume this care management role and perform an important service for individuals and families.

Maternal-newborn nurses are especially sensitive to these changes in healthcare delivery because the vast majority of health care provided to childbearing families takes place outside hospitals in clinics, offices, and community-based organizations. In addition, maternal-newborn nurses offer specialized services such as childbirth preparation classes or postpartal exercise classes. In essence, we are already experts at providing community-based nursing care. However, it is important that we remain knowledgeable about current practices and trends and open to new approaches to meet the needs of women and children.

HOME CARE

The provision of health care in the home is emerging as an especially important dimension of community-based nursing care. The shortened length of hospital stays has resulted in the discharge of individuals who still require support, assistance, and teaching. Home care can help fill this gap. Conversely, home care also enables individuals to remain at home with conditions that formerly would have required hospitalization.

Nurses are the major providers of home care services. Home care nurses perform direct nursing care and also supervise unlicensed assistive personnel who provide less skilled levels of service. In a home setting, nurses can use their skills in assessment, therapeutics, communication, teaching, problem solving, and organization to meet the needs of childbearing families. They also play a major role in coordinating services from other providers, such as physical therapists or lactation consultants.

Postpartum and newborn home visits are becoming a recognized way of ensuring that childbearing families make a satisfactory transition from the hospital or birthing center to the home. We see this trend as positive and hope that this method of meeting the needs of childbearing families becomes standard practice. Chapter 36 ∞ discusses home care in more detail and provides guidance about making a home visit. In addition, throughout the text we have provided information on how home care can meet the needs of women with health problems such as diabetes or preterm labor, which put them at risk during pregnancy. We believe that home care offers nurses the opportunity to function in an autonomous role and make a significant difference for individuals and families.

LEGAL AND ETHICAL CONSIDERATIONS

Professional nursing practice requires full understanding of practice standards, institutional or agency policies, and local, state, and federal laws. Professional practice also requires an understanding of the ethical implications of those standards, policies, and laws that impact care, care providers, and care recipients. Every professional nurse is responsible for obtaining and maintaining current information regarding ethics and laws related to nursing practice and health care.

Scope of Practice

State nurse practice acts protect the public by broadly defining the legal *scope of practice* within which every nurse must

MEDIALINK Application: Scope of Practice

function and by excluding untrained or unlicensed individuals from practicing nursing. Although some state practice acts continue to limit nursing practice to the traditional responsibilities of providing client care related to health maintenance and disease prevention, most state practice acts cover expanded practice roles that include collaboration with other professionals in planning and providing care, diagnostic and prescriptive privilege, and the delegation of client care tasks to other specified licensed and unlicensed personnel. Specified care activities for certified nurse-midwives and women's health, perinatal, or neonatal nurse practitioners may include diagnosis and prenatal management of uncomplicated pregnancies (CNMs may also manage births) and prescribing and dispensing medications using protocols in specified circumstances. A nurse must function within the scope of practice or risk being accused of practicing medicine without a license.

Correctly interpreting and understanding state practice acts enables the nurse to provide safe care within the limits of nursing practice. State boards of nursing may provide official interpretation of practice acts when the limits are not clear. On occasion hospital policy may conflict with a state's nurse practice act. It is important to recognize that hospital or agency policy may restrict the scope of practice specified in a state practice act, but such policy cannot legally expand the scope of practice beyond the limits stated in the practice act.

Nurse practice acts are subject to change. One component of professional nursing practice is the responsibility of each nurse to remain up-to-date regarding scope of practice and even to participate actively in promoting appropriate changes.

Nursing Negligence

Negligence is defined as omitting or committing an act that a reasonably prudent person would not omit or commit under the same or similar circumstances. Negligence consists of four elements:

1. There was a duty to provide care.
2. The duty was breached.
3. Injury occurred.
4. The breach of duty caused the injury (proximate cause).

Duty may be breached by omission—failing to give a medication, failing to assess properly, failing to notify a physician of a change in a laboring woman's condition, and so on. Duty may also be breached by commission—giving the wrong medication, placing an infant in the wrong crib, and so on. The injury that results may be physical or mental (pain and suffering). In determining whether nursing negligence occurred, the care that was given is compared with the standard of care. If the standard was not met, negligence occurred.

Standards of Nursing Care

Standards of care establish minimum criteria for competent, proficient delivery of nursing care. Such standards are designed to protect the public and are used to judge the quality of care provided. Legal interpretation of actions within standards of care is based on what a reasonably prudent nurse with similar education and experience would do in similar circumstances.

SOURCES OF CARE STANDARDS

Written standards of care are provided by a number of different sources. The American Nurses Association (ANA) has published standards of professional practice since 1950. In 1973, the ANA Congress for Nursing Practice began to write generic standards for all nurses in all settings. In addition, the ANA Divisions of Practice have published standards that include nursing practice for maternal-child health. The Council of Perinatal Nurses has published standards for perinatal nursing. Other specialty organizations, such as the Association of Women's Health, Obstetric, and Neonatal Nurses (AWHONN), the Association of Operating Room Nurses (AORN), and the National Association of Neonatal Nurses (NANN), have developed standards of specialty practice. Agency policies, procedures, and protocols also provide appropriate guidelines for care standards. The Joint Commission on Accreditation of Healthcare Organizations (JCAHO), a private, nongovernmental agency that audits the operation of hospitals and healthcare facilities, has also contributed to the development of nursing standards.

Agency policies, procedures, and protocols also provide appropriate guidelines for care standards. For example, *clinical practice guidelines* and clinical pathways are comprehensive interdisciplinary care plans for a specific condition that describe the sequence and timing of interventions that should result in expected client outcomes. Clinical practice guidelines or clinical pathways are adopted within a healthcare setting to reduce variation in care management, to limit costs of care, and to evaluate the effectiveness of care.

Some standards carry the force of law; others, although not legally based, still carry important legal significance. Any nurse who fails to meet appropriate standards of care invites allegations of negligence or malpractice. (*Malpractice* is negligent action of a professional person.) However, any nurse who practices within the guidelines established by agency, local, or national standards is assured that clients are provided with competent nursing care, which, in turn, diminishes the potential for litigation.

ETHICAL COMPONENTS OF CARE STANDARDS

Standards of care are based on a legal model rather than on ethics. However, they incorporate important ethical components that extend the narrow legal interpretation of the term *standard*. Although there is a great deal of interplay between the two disciplines, each has a different perspective.

Law is based primarily on a rights model that establishes rules of conduct to define relationships among individuals. Law may also define relationships to impersonal entities like formal organizations, agencies, or hospitals.

Ethics, in contrast, is based on a responsibility or duty model that considers a wider range of factors than the rights model of law. Ethics incorporates factors such as risks, benefits, other relationships, concerns, and the needs and abilities of persons affected by and affecting decisions.

Law and ethics are interrelated; they share a similar decision process and standards. Both disciplines incorporate fact-finding, conflict negotiation, prioritization of related issues and values, and the application of resolutions of particular cases in decision making. Professional nurses must consider the ethical implications of legal decisions and the legal implications of ethical decisions.

Understanding the distinctions among medical or healthcare decisions, legal decisions, and ethical decisions is important. Consider the case in which parents from a culture unfamiliar to the nurse refuse surgery for their newborn based on a deeply held spiritual belief that intentional cutting of a body will result in spiritual death. Such a decision to forgo surgery may be viewed as negligent in the eyes of the law, unwise and inappropriate from a medical perspective, yet fully justifiable ethically. Similarly, legally sanctioned maintenance of life support for a severely damaged newborn with little hope for meaningful existence may remain a medically viable alternative, but to many it is not ethically justifiable. Recognizing the type of decision to be made often helps measure the worth and outcome of a decision more appropriately.

Clients' Rights

Law and ethics impact all of nursing practice, and several topics have specific implications for maternal-child nursing practice. Clients' rights encompass such topics as informed consent, privacy, and confidentiality.

CLIENT/PATIENT SAFETY

The Joint Commission on the Accreditation of Healthcare Organizations (JCAHO) (2006) has identified patient safety as an important responsibility of healthcare providers and established the following patient safety goals as requirements for accreditation in 2007.

1. Improve the accuracy of patient identification.
2. Improve the effectiveness of communication among caregivers.
3. Improve the safety of using medications.
4. Reduce the risk of healthcare-associated infections.
5. Accurately and completely reconcile medications across the continuum of care.
6. Reduce the risk of patient harm resulting from falls.
7. Reduce the risk of influenza and pneumococcal disease in institutionalized older adults.
8. Reduce the risk of surgical fires.
9. Implementation of applicable National Patient Safety Goals and associated requirements by components and practitioner sites.
10. Encourage patients' active involvement in their own care as a patient safety strategy.
11. Prevent healthcare-associated pressure ulcers (decubitus ulcers).
12. The organization identifies safety risks inherent in its patient population.

INFORMED CONSENT

Informed consent is a legal concept designed to allow clients to make intelligent decisions regarding their own health care. In-

formed consent means that a client, or a legally designated decision maker, has granted permission for a specific treatment or procedure based on full information about that specific treatment or procedure as it relates to that client under the specific circumstances of the permission. Although this policy is usually enforced for such major procedures as surgery or regional anesthesia, it pertains to any nursing, medical, or surgical intervention. To touch a person without consent (except in an emergency) constitutes battery.

Several elements must be addressed to ensure that the client has given informed consent. The information must be clearly and concisely presented in a manner understandable to the client and must include risks and benefits, the probability of success, and significant treatment alternatives. The client also needs to be told the consequences of receiving no treatment or procedure. Finally, the client must be told of the right to refuse a specific treatment or procedure. Each client should be told that refusing the specified treatment or procedure does not result in the withdrawal of all support or care.

The individual who is ultimately responsible for the treatment or procedure should provide the information necessary to obtain informed consent. In most instances, this is a physician. In such cases, the nurse's role may be to witness the client's signature giving consent. A nurse who knows the client and the procedure may certainly help the physician obtain the client's consent by clarifying the information the physician provides. It is also part of the nurse's role to determine that the client understands the information before making a decision. Anxiety, fear, pain, and medications that alter consciousness may influence an individual's ability to give informed consent. An oral consent is legal but written consent is easier to defend in a court of law.

Society grants parents the authority and responsibility to give consent for their minor children. Parents are presumed to possess what a child lacks in maturity, experience, and capacity for judgment in life's difficult decisions. Although the age of majority is 18 years in most states, variations in certain states require that nurses be aware of the law in the state where they practice. Children under 18 or 21 years of age, depending on state law, can legally give informed consent in the following circumstances:

* When they are minor parents of the infant or child client
* When they are *emancipated minors* (self-supporting adolescents under 18 years of age, not subject to parental control)
* When they are adolescents between 16 and 18 years of age seeking birth control, mental health counseling, or substance abuse treatment (Dickey & Deatrick, 2000)

Mature minors (14- and 15-year-old adolescents who are able to understand treatment risks) can give consent for treatment or refuse treatment in some states.

Special problems can occur in maternity nursing when a minor gives birth. It is possible, depending upon state law, that a minor may be able to consent to treatment for her infant but not for herself. In some states, however, a pregnant teenager is considered an emancipated minor and may therefore give consent for herself as well.

Additionally, some states require a married woman to obtain the consent of her spouse when a procedure involves sterilization or threatens the life of a fetus. Although child-bearing women sign a general consent form on admission to an agency, separate informed consent is often required for surgery, cesarean birth, the administration of anesthesia, tubal ligation, or participation in research.

Refusal of a treatment, medication, or procedure after appropriate information also requires that a client sign a form to release the physician and agency from liability. Jehovah's Witnesses' refusal of blood transfusion or Rh immune globulin is an example of such refusal.

Nurses are responsible for educating clients about any nursing care provided. Before each nursing intervention, the maternal-child nurse lets the individual and/or family know what to expect, thus ensuring cooperation and obtaining consent. Afterward, the nurse documents the teaching and the learning outcomes in the person's record. The importance of clear, concise, and complete nursing records cannot be overemphasized. These records are evidence that the nurse obtained consent, performed prescribed treatments, reported important observations to the appropriate staff, and adhered to acceptable standards of care.

RIGHT TO PRIVACY

The *right to privacy* is the right of a person to keep his or her person and property free from public scrutiny. Maternity nurses need to remember that this includes avoiding unnecessary exposure of the childbearing woman's body. In the context of health care, the right to privacy dictates that only those responsible for a client's care should examine the client or discuss the client's case.

Most states have recognized the right to privacy through statutory or common law, and some states have written that right into their constitution. The ANA, the National League for Nursing (NLN), and JCAHO have adopted professional standards protecting clients' privacy. Healthcare agencies should also have written policies dealing with client privacy. HIPAA, discussed previously, also has a provision to guarantee the security and privacy of health information.

Laws, standards, and policies about privacy specify that information about clients' treatment, condition, and prognosis can be shared only by the health professionals responsible for their care. Authorization for the release of any client information should be obtained from competent clients or their surrogate decision maker. Although it may be legal to reveal vital statistics such as name, age, occupation, and prognosis, such information is often withheld because of ethical considerations. The client should be consulted regarding what information may be released and to whom. When a client is a celebrity or is considered newsworthy, inquiries may be best handled by the public relations department of the agency.

CONFIDENTIALITY

Given the highly personal and intimate information requested of clients, the need for maintaining confidentiality is extremely crucial for the development of trust in the relationship between client and provider. Privileged communications exist between client and physician, client and attorney, husband and wife, and clergy and those who seek their counsel. In some states, laws of privilege also protect nurses. Nurses should become well informed about privileged communication laws in their state.

A client may waive the right to confidentiality of medical records by action or words. For example, if a childbearing woman sues a physician, hospital, or other care provider, she waives the right to confidentiality of the medical record because the record becomes a source of evidence. Clients commonly consent to disclose information to insurance companies or to their employers. Computerization of medical records has created a greater concern for the integrity of records and the potential invasion of privacy.

In some instances, the public good takes precedence over an individual's right to privacy. For example, state laws require that care providers report gunshot wounds, child abuse, elder abuse, and some communicable diseases.

The Federal Patient Self-Determination Act requires all healthcare institutions that are reimbursed by Medicare or Medicaid to provide all hospitalized individuals with written information about their rights, which include expressing a preference for treatment options and making *advance directives* (writing a living will or authorizing a durable power of attorney for healthcare decisions on the individual's behalf). This often comes as a surprise to young women and couples of childbearing age who may have no experience of hospitals. However, with an advance directive in place, a childbearing woman can be certain that, even if she becomes incompetent, she can retain her autonomy about healthcare decisions. Nurses often discuss these issues with clients and their families and can help them explore their beliefs and values about treatment options and dying.

CLINICAL TIP

Breaching confidentiality is a potential problem for pregnant adolescents, who are just learning whom they can trust in the healthcare system. Make sure you openly discuss the limits of confidentiality for such things as mandatory reporting requirements with the client and family. Inadvertent disclosure of personal information may lead to psychologic, social, or physical harm for some clients.

Ethical Decision Making

Healthcare and bioethical literature are filled with examples of ethical decision-making models and frameworks. Decision-making models help nurses and other care providers confront seemingly unresolvable conflicts among the rights, duties, theories, principles, values, and individuals impacted by the ethical dilemmas of practice. There are six critical components of ethical decision making; they are very similar to the components of the nursing process.

1. Establish a means of determining who is involved in the dilemma, who is involved in the decision, and who will be affected by the outcome of the decision. This data-gathering step allows the nurse to identify and define the issue and determine who owns the problem, the information, the decision, and the consequences of it.

2. Establish a mechanism for obtaining all the information relevant to the conflict, including data related to diagnosis, prognosis, treatment options, available health

care, and psychosocial, spiritual, financial, and other appropriate resources.

3. Formulate a plan to outline all potential options and the consequences of each option. Be sure that opposing viewpoints are presented and considered. Set individual values aside during this phase to encourage divergent views.

4. In the conflict resolution process that follows, review driving and restraining forces, assess risks and benefits, and assess the likelihood of a successful outcome with each option. At this stage, be sure that the moral values of everyone involved are addressed. In addition, review peripheral issues—such as the possible impact on other individuals or systems related to the decision, changes in client condition, pertinent laws, or new information—within the context of general and individual moral principles.

5. Select and act on a plan to resolve the conflict. Before acting on the resolution, determine who is ultimately responsible for the decision, who is most impacted by the outcome, and whether consensus is required.

6. Evaluate the resolution, its consequences, and the decision process itself. This step is critically important to avoid making similar decisions in isolation.

Ethical decisions in maternal-child nursing are often complicated by moral obligations to more than one client. Straightforward solutions to the ethical dilemmas nurses encounter in caring for childbearing families are often, quite simply, not available. By using a formal decision-making structure, nurses may, however, increase the likelihood of addressing multiple needs in complex care situations in an ethically appropriate and legal manner.

SPECIAL ETHICAL SITUATIONS IN MATERNITY CARE

Maternity care is fraught with unique circumstances in which an ethical dilemma may arise. These include situations of maternal-fetal conflict, issues related to termination of pregnancy, embryonic and fetal research, reproductive assistance, and cord blood banking. Additionally, the use of data from the Human Genome Project may give rise to ethical challenges.

Maternal-Fetal Conflict

Until fairly recently, the fetus was viewed legally as a nonperson. Mother and fetus were viewed as one complex client—the pregnant woman—of which the fetus was an essential part. However, advances in technology have permitted the physician to treat the fetus and monitor fetal development. The fetus is increasingly viewed as a client separate from the mother, although treatment of the fetus necessarily involves the mother. This type of approach, by nature adversarial, tends to emphasize the divergent interests of the mother and her fetus rather than focus on their shared interests. This focus on the fetus intensified in 2002 when President George W. Bush announced that "unborn children" would qualify for government healthcare benefits. The move was designed to promote prenatal care, but it represented the first time that any US federal policy had defined childhood as starting at conception.

Most women are strongly motivated to protect the health and well-being of their fetus. In some instances, however, women have refused interventions on behalf of the fetus, and forced interventions have occurred. These include forced cesarean birth, coercion of mothers who practice high-risk behaviors such as substance abuse to enter treatment, and, perhaps most controversial, mandating experimental in utero therapy or surgery in an attempt to correct a specific birth defect. These interventions infringe on the autonomy of the mother. They may also be detrimental to the baby if, as a result, maternal bonding is hindered, the mother is afraid to seek prenatal care, or the mother is herself harmed by the actions taken (Hornstra, 1999). These forced interventions raise two thorny questions: (1) What practices should be monitored? and (2) Who will determine when the behaviors pose such a risk to the fetus that the courts should intervene?

Attempts have also been made to criminalize the behavior of women who fail to follow a physician's advice or who engage in behaviors that are considered harmful to the fetus. For example, in 2003 a woman in Great Falls, New York, was prosecuted for child endangerment when her son tested positive for alcohol at birth. Her conviction was successfully appealed. In 1999, in South Carolina a 22-year-old homeless woman, who used cocaine regularly during her pregnancy and subsequently gave birth to a stillborn infant, became the first woman in the United States to be convicted of homicide because of her behavior during her pregnancy. She was sentenced to 12 years in prison. The South Carolina Supreme Court upheld the conviction and the US Supreme Court declined to hear the case (ACOG, 2005a).

The American College of Obstetricians and Gynecologists (ACOG) (2004) and the American Academy of Pediatrics (AAP) Committee on Bioethics (1999) both affirm the fundamental right of pregnant women to make informed, uncoerced decisions about medical interventions. Moreover, in 2005 ACOG's Committee on Ethics took a direct stand against coercive and punitive approaches to the maternal-fetal relationship, citing the following "overwhelming rationale for avoiding such approaches.

1. Coercive and punitive legal approaches to pregnant women who refuse medical advice fail to recognize that all competent adults are entitled to informed consent and bodily integrity. . . .

2. Court-ordered interventions in cases of informed refusal, as well as punishment of pregnant women for their behavior that may put a fetus at risk, neglect the fact that medical knowledge and predictions of outcomes in obstetrics have limitations. . . .

3. Coercive and punitive policies treat medical problems such as addiction and psychiatric illness as if they were moral failings. . . .

4. Coercive and punitive policies are potentially counterproductive in that they are likely to discourage prenatal care and successful treatment, adversely affect

infant mortality rates, and undermine the physician-patient relationship. . . .

5. Coercive and punitive policies directed toward pregnant women unjustly single out the most vulnerable women. . . .

6. Coercive and punitive policies create the potential for criminalization of many types of otherwise legal maternal behavior" (ACOG, 2005a, pp. 6–9).

ACOG and AAP recognize that cases of maternal-fetal conflict involve two clients, both of whom deserve respect and treatment. Such cases are best resolved by using internal hospital mechanisms including counseling, the intervention of specialists, and consultation with an institutional ethics committee. Court intervention should be considered a last resort, appropriate only in extraordinary circumstances.

Abortion

Since the 1973 Supreme Court decision in *Roe v. Wade*, abortion has been legal in the United States. It can be performed until the period of viability, after which abortion is permissible only when the life or health of the mother is threatened. Before viability, the mother's rights are paramount; after viability, the rights of the fetus take precedence.

Personal beliefs, cultural norms, life experiences, and religious convictions shape people's attitudes about abortion. Ethicists have thoughtfully and thoroughly argued positions supporting both sides of the question. Nevertheless, few issues spark the intensity of response seen when the issue of abortion is raised.

At present, decisions about abortion are made by a woman and her physician. Nurses (and other caregivers) have the right to refuse to assist with the procedure if abortion is contrary to their moral and ethical beliefs. However, if a nurse works in an institution where abortions may be performed, the nurse may be dismissed for refusing. To avoid being placed in a situation contrary to their values and beliefs, nurses should determine the philosophy and practices of an institution before going to work there. A nurse who refuses to participate in an abortion because of moral or ethical beliefs does have a responsibility to ensure that someone with similar qualifications is able to provide appropriate care for the client. Clients may never be abandoned, regardless of the nurse's beliefs.

Fetal Research

Research with fetal tissue has been responsible for remarkable advances in the care and treatment of fetuses with health problems and advances in the treatment of progressive, debilitating adult diseases such as Parkinson disease, Alzheimer disease, and DiGeorge syndrome. Therapeutic research with living fetuses has been instrumental in the treatment of Rh-sensitized infants, the evaluation of lung maturity using the lecithin/sphingomyelin ratio, and the treatment of pulmonary immaturity in the newborn. Because it is aimed at treating a fetal condition, therapeutic fetal research raises fewer ethical questions than does nontherapeutic fetal research. To be approved, nontherapeutic research requires that the risk to the fetus be minimal, that the knowledge to be gained be important, and that the information be unobtainable by any other means. Control over

research standards and attention to state and federal regulations remain foci of debate regarding fetal research.

Intrauterine fetal surgery, which began in 1981 and developed through therapeutic research, is a therapy for anatomic lesions that can be corrected surgically and are incompatible with life if not treated. Intrauterine fetal surgery involves opening the uterus during the second trimester (before viability), treating the fetal lesion, and replacing the fetus in the uterus. The risks to the fetus are substantial, and the mother is committed to cesarean births for this and subsequent pregnancies because the upper, active segment of the uterus is incised during the surgery. The parents must be informed of the experimental nature of the treatment, the risks of the surgery, the commitment to cesarean birth, and alternatives to the treatment.

As with other aspects of maternity care, the pregnant woman's autonomy must be respected. The procedure does involve health risks to the woman, and she retains the right to refuse any surgical procedure. In 2001, ACOG issued a news release calling fetal surgery "experimental." Speaking specifically about fetal surgery for open neural tube defects, ACOG reported that long-term neurologic outcomes have not yet been demonstrated and the surgery exposes the mother to the risks of anesthesia, hemorrhage, preterm labor, and uterine rupture and also poses additional risk to the fetus (ACOG, 2001).

Healthcare professionals are generally encouraged to provide a clear summary of the risks and benefits of a given approach and to follow the principle of nondirectiveness, in which only the client's values are discussed during the decision-making process. However, it is likely that some "slippage" in approach occurs, which can result in a blurring of the boundaries between choice and coercion. This may be complicated by the reality that many women are influenced by their views about what it means to be a "good" mother, to behave responsibly. As a result some women may feel that they must opt for a risky procedure to avoid a sense of blame for failing to do their "duty" (Williams, 2006). The dilemmas associated with the consideration of fetal surgery are challenging and complex. Healthcare providers must be careful that their zeal for new technology does not lead them to focus unilaterally on the fetus at the expense of the mother.

Reproductive Assistance

The number and sophistication of reproductive assistance techniques continue to grow. Infertile couples now have available a wide range of reproductive options, from therapeutic insemination to in vitro fertilization and beyond. The ethical dimensions of such techniques are discussed here. The techniques themselves are identified and described in detail in Chapter 12. ∞

Therapeutic insemination (TI) is accomplished by depositing into a woman sperm obtained from her husband, partner, or other donor. Some women who are single are choosing TI as a childbearing option. No states prohibit therapeutic insemination using a husband's sperm because there is no question of the child's legitimacy. Legal problems may occur with TI using donor sperm, however. Because the child is the biologic child of the mother, legal concerns center on the donor. A donor must sign a form waiving all parental rights. The donor must also furnish accurate health information, particularly regarding genetic traits or diseases. Donor sperm must be tested for HIV. Husbands often are requested to sign a form to agree to the insemination and to assume parental responsibility for the child. Some men legally adopt the child so there is no question of parental rights and responsibilities. Several states have enacted legislation regarding paternity of the child conceived by insemination with donor sperm.

A variety of procedures such as testicular sperm aspiration (TESA) have been developed to address severe male factor infertility. Although these procedures have been quite promising, they do raise questions about the increased risk of genetic defects related to bypassing of certain aspects of the process of natural selection. In the United States there are no established barriers to the use of these procedures.

Assisted reproductive technology (ART) is the term used to describe any fertility treatment in which both the egg and sperm are handled. Treatments in which only the sperm are handled (e.g., therapeutic insemination) or in which a woman takes medication to stimulate egg production without subsequent egg retrieval are not included in the definition of ART. In vitro fertilization and embryo transfer (IVF-ET), a therapy offered to selected infertile couples, is perhaps the best known ART technique. Some effort has been made legislatively to address consumer concerns about ART. In the United States, the Federal Fertility Clinic Success Rate and Certification Act (FCSRCA) of 1992 addresses issues related to laboratory quality and the standardized reporting of pregnancy success rates associated with ART programs. The act requires all clinics performing ART in the United States to report their success rates annually to the Centers for Disease Control and Prevention (CDC). However, it does not contain provisions to deal with the unethical practices that may occur, nor does it address false reporting of success rates. To help ensure data accuracy, a validation process, which includes site visits to a portion of reporting clinics, is completed.

The success rates of the ART procedures vary significantly. Specifically, in 2002, the highest success rate—50% live births—occurred when donor eggs and freshly fertilized embryos were used. However, the largest percentage of ART procedures occurred among women who used their own eggs. Freshly fertilized embryos from the woman's own eggs resulted in a live birth 34.8% of the time, although this varied by maternal age, ranging from 43% for women under 35 years to 7% for women over age 42. The lowest success rate occurred among women using their own eggs and thawed embryos—24.8% resulted in a live birth (Wright, Schieve, Reynolds, & Jeng, 2005). Of the births that resulted from ART in 2002, about 53% included more than one fetus (45.7% twins, 7.6% triplets or greater) (Wright et al., 2005). Multiple pregnancy occurs because the use of ovulation-inducing medications typically triggers the release of multiple eggs, which, when fertilized, produce multiple embryos that are then implanted. Multiple pregnancy increases the risk of miscarriage, preterm birth, and neonatal morbidity and mortality. It also increases the mother's risk of cesarean birth and of complications such as hypertensive diseases of pregnancy, gestational diabetes, and hemorrhage. To help prevent a high-level multiple pregnancy, the American Society for Reproductive Medicine has issued guidelines to limit the number of embryos transferred. ACOG (2005b) supports the effort to lower the risk of multiple pregnancy with ART. The ethical dilemma of what to do with the unused embryos remains a consideration.

When a multiple pregnancy does occur, the physician may suggest that the woman abort some of the embryos—nonselective embryo reduction—to give the remaining embryos a better chance for survival. This procedure does raise ethical concerns about the sacrifice of some so that the remainder can survive (ACOG, 2002).

Surrogate childbearing is another approach to addressing the issue of infertility. Surrogate childbearing occurs when a woman agrees to become pregnant for another woman or for a couple who are usually childless. Depending on the infertile woman's or couple's needs, the surrogate may be therapeutically inseminated with the male partner's sperm or a donor's sperm, or she may even receive a gamete transfer. If fertilization occurs, the woman carries the fetus to term and then releases the infant to the couple after birth.

These methods of resolving infertility raise many ethical questions, including the problem of religious objections to artificial conception, the question of who will assume financial and moral responsibility for a child born with a congenital defect, the issue of candidate selection, and the threat of genetic engineering. Other ethical questions include the following:

- What should be done with surplus fertilized oocytes?

- To whom do frozen embryos belong—parents together or separately? The hospital or infertility clinic?

- Who is liable if a woman or her offspring contracts HIV disease from donated sperm?

- Should children be told the method of their conception?

Our son was born after artificial insemination. Nick, my husband, was sterile because of radiation therapy, so his cousin was the donor for us. I thought that might be awkward but the whole family was so excited that there was a way to help us after Nick's battle with cancer that it has been OK. Every time we look at Vincent Joseph (he is named for his grandfathers) and see him smile, we know that we would do it again in an instant.

Embryonic Stem Cell Research

Human stem cells can be found in embryonic tissue and in the primordial germ cells of a fetus. Research has demonstrated that in tissue cultures these cells can be made to differentiate into other types of cells such as blood, nerve, or heart cells, which might then be used to treat problems such as diabetes, Parkinson and Alzheimer diseases, spinal cord injury, or metabolic disorders. The availability of specialized tissue or even organs grown from stem cells might also decrease society's dependence on donated organs for organ transplants.

In 2001, President George W. Bush decided to permit federal funding of embryonic stem cell research, but only on the 64 existing cell lines identified by the National Institutes of Health (NIH). The president also announced the creation of a

President's Council on Bioethics, which is to oversee all federally funded embryonic stem cell research and study the range of ethical issues found in the biomedical and behavioral sciences. Later that year the National Academy of Sciences released a report on the subject. In the report the academy stated that public funding should be provided for further stem cell research and that, ultimately, new embryonic stem cell lines will have to be developed (American Association for the Advancement of Science, 2002).

Positions about embryonic stem cell research vary dramatically, from the view that any use of human embryos for research is wrong to the view that any form of embryonic stem cell research is acceptable, with a variety of other positions that fall somewhere in between these extremes. Other questions also arise: What sources of embryonic tissue are acceptable for research? Is it ever ethical to clone embryos solely for stem cell research? Is there justification for using embryos remaining after fertility treatments?

The question of how an embryo should be viewed—with status in some way as a person or in some sense as property (and, if property, whose?)—is a key question in the debate. Ethicists recognize that it is not necessary to advocate full moral status or personhood for an embryo to have significant moral qualms about the instrumental use of a human embryo in the "interests" of society. The issue of consent, which links directly to an embryo's status, also merits consideration. The Bush policy, like many proposed approaches, requires parental consent (Cameron, 2006). In truth, the ethical questions and dilemmas associated with embryonic stem cell research are staggeringly complex and require careful analysis and thoughtful dialogue.

Cord Blood Banking

Cord blood, which is taken from a newborn's umbilical cord by the physician or nurse-midwife assisting with the birth, may play a role in combating leukemia, certain other cancers, metabolic disorders, and other immune and blood system disorders such as sickle cell anemia, thalassemia, and severe aplastic anemia. However, umbilical cord blood cannot be used to treat leukemia or inborn errors of metabolism in the same child who donated it at birth (Moise, 2006). Cord blood, like bone marrow, contains regenerative stem cells, which are able to replace diseased cells in the affected individual. The value of bone marrow transplants has long been recognized, and a national registry of potential bone marrow donors has been established. The process of collecting bone marrow is expensive and uncomfortable, however, and the National Marrow Donor Registry often has difficulty finding a matching bone marrow donor.

Cord blood has some advantages over bone marrow:

- Collecting cord blood is less invasive and involves no risk to mother or infant.
- Large-scale cord blood banking would increase the availability of stem cells for minority groups, who are seriously underrepresented in bone marrow registries.
- Cord blood is less likely than bone marrow to trigger a potentially fatal rejection response.

- Cord blood works with a less-than-perfect match.
- Cord blood is available for use more rapidly than bone marrow.

Cord blood banks that process and store cord blood have now been established in the United States. Cord blood banks may be public or private. Public banks receive cord blood units given on a volunteer basis and are designed to support unrelated-donor transplant programs. Private banks are for-profit entities designed primarily for families who plan to use the cord blood for the infant who provided the blood (autologous donation) or for another family member who might need transplantation therapy in the future because of a genetic blood condition, cancer, bone marrow failure, or inborn error of metabolism, for example. In 2005 the Institute of Medicine (IOM) completed a study for the Health Resources and Services Administration (HRSA) focused on identifying the best way to organize public cord blood banking and distribution to individuals in need. The IOM study recommended that HRSA establish contracts with eligible public banks to procure approximately 150,000 new units of cord blood from ethnically diverse unrelated donors over the next 5 years and list them on a computerized Web-based system to allow searching of all unrelated cord blood units (Kurtzberg, Lyerly, & Sugarman, 2005). Legislation authorizing funding passed in 2005.

Ethical issues associated with cord blood banking include the following (Smith & Thomson, 2000):

- Who owns the blood? The donor? The parents? Private blood banks? Society?
- How will informed consent be obtained and by whom?
- How will confidentiality be ensured? Family members need to understand that, if they choose to donate, the mother will be asked to provide a blood sample and a detailed history about her health and infectious disease status.
- How will obligations to notify the family and donor be addressed if testing of the blood reveals infectious diseases or genetic disorders? Should there be any ongoing assessment of donors so that if health problems develop, recipients can be notified?
- How can the harvested blood be distributed fairly, so that it is available to individuals from all races, ethnic groups, and income levels?

Implications for Nursing Practice

The complex ethical issues facing maternal-newborn nurses have many social, cultural, legal, and professional ramifications. Nurses, like all healthcare professionals, need to learn to anticipate ethical dilemmas, clarify their own positions and values related to the issues, understand the legal implications of the issues, and develop appropriate strategies for ethical decision making. To accomplish these tasks, they may read about bioethical issues, participate in discussion groups, or attend courses and workshops on ethical topics pertinent to their areas of practice. Most nurses develop solid skills in logical thinking and critical analysis. These skills, coupled with theoretical knowledge about ethical decision making, can serve nurses well in dealing with the many ethical dilemmas found in health care.

STATISTICAL DATA AND MATERNAL-INFANT CARE

Increasingly nurses are recognizing the value and usefulness of statistics. Health-related statistics provide an objective basis for projecting client needs, planning use of resources, and determining the effectiveness of treatment.

There are two major types of statistics: *descriptive* and *inferential. Descriptive statistics* describe or summarize a set of data. They report the facts—what is—in a concise and easily retrievable way. How the data are compiled and presented is determined by the question being asked. An example of a descriptive statistic is the birth rate in the United States. Although no conclusion may be drawn from these statistics about why some phenomenon has occurred, they can identify certain trends and high-risk "target groups" and generate possible research questions.

Inferential statistics allow the investigator to draw conclusions or inferences about what is happening between two or more variables in a population and to suggest or refute causal relationships between them. For example, descriptive statistics reveal that the infant mortality rate in the United States has declined over the past decade. Exactly why that trend has

occurred cannot be answered by simply looking at these data, however. More data and inferential statistics using smaller samples of the population of pregnant women are needed to determine whether this finding is because of earlier prenatal care, improved maternal nutrition, use of electronic fetal monitoring during labor, and/or any number of factors potentially associated with maternal-fetal survival.

Descriptive statistics are the starting point for the formation of research questions. Inferential statistics answer specific questions and generate theories to explain relationships between variables. Theory applied in nursing practice can help change the specific variables that may cause or contribute to certain health problems.

This section discusses descriptive statistics that are particularly important to maternal-newborn health care. Inferences that may be drawn from these descriptive statistics are addressed as possible research questions that may help identify relevant variables.

Birth Rate

Birth rate refers to the number of live births per 1000 people. In 2004, the US birth rate was 14 per 1000, a slight decrease from the 2003 rate of 14.1. Table 1–1 provides valuable information

Table 1–1   LIVE BIRTHS AND BIRTH RATES BY AGE, RACE, AND ORIGIN OF MOTHER: UNITED STATES, 2003 AND 2004

Age and Race and Hispanic Origin of Mother	2004 Number	2004 Rate	2003 Number	2003 Rate
All races and origins[1]				
Total[2]	4,112,052	66.3	4,089,950	66.1
10–14 years	6781	0.7	6661	0.6
15–19 years	415,262	41.1	414,580	41.6
15–17 years	133,980	22.1	134,384	22.4
18–19 years	281,282	70	280,196	70.7
20–24 years	1,034,454	101.7	1,032,305	102.6
25–29 years	1,104,485	115.5	1,086,366	115.6
30–34 years	965,663	95.3	975,546	95.1
35–39 years	475,606	45.4	467,642	43.8
40–44 years	103,679	8.9	101,005	8.7
45–54 years[3]	6122	0.5	5845	0.5
Non-Hispanic white[2]	2,296,683	58.4	2,321,904	58.5
Non-Hispanic black[2]	578,772	67	576,033	67.1
American Indian or Alaska Native total[4,5]	43,927	58.9	43,052	58.4
Asian or Pacific Islander total[2,5]	229,123	67.1	221,203	66.3
Hispanic	946,349	97.8	912,329	96.9

[1]Includes origin not stated.

[2]The total number includes births to women of all ages, 10–54 years. The rate shown for all ages is the fertility rate, which is defined as the total number of births, regardless of age of mother, per 1000 women aged 15–44 years.

[3]The number of births shown is the total for women aged 45–54 years. The birth rate is computed by relating the number of births to women aged 45–54 years to women aged 45–49 years, because most of the births in this group are to women aged 45–49.

[4]Includes births to Aleuts and Eskimos.

[5]Data for persons of Hispanic origin are included in the data for each race group according to the mother's reported race, see "Technical Notes."

[6]Includes all persons of Hispanic origin of any race; see "Technical Notes."

NOTES: Race and Hispanic origin are reported separately on birth certificates. Persons of Hispanic origin may be of any race. Race categories are consistent with the 1977 Office of Management and Budget (OMB) standards. Fifteen states reported multiple-race data for 2004. The multiple-race data for these states were bridged to the single race categories of the 1977 OMB standards for comparability with other states; see "Technical Notes" and references 1 and 2.

SOURCE: Hamilton, B. E., Ventura, S. J., Martin, J. A., & Sutton, P. D. (2005, October 28). Preliminary births for 2004. Health E-Stats. Hyattsville, MD: National Center for Health Statistics.

Table 1–2   LIVE BIRTH RATES AND INFANT MORTALITY RATES FOR SELECTED COUNTRIES

Country	Birth Rate	Infant Mortality Rate
Afghanistan	46.6	160.2
Argentina	16.7	14.7
Australia	12.1	4.6
Cambodia	26.9	68.8
Canada	10.8	4.7
China	13.3	23.1
Egypt	22.9	31.3
Germany	8.3	4.1
Ghana	30.5	55
India	22	54.6
Iraq	32	48.6
Japan	9.4	3.2
Mexico	20.7	20.3
Russia	10	15.1
United Kingdom	10.7	5.1
United States	14	6.9

SOURCE: Data from *The World Fact Book 2006.* Washington, D.C.: The Central Intelligence Agency.

Table 1–3   INFANT DEATHS AND INFANT, NEONATAL, AND POSTNEONATAL MORTALITY RATES: UNITED STATES 1982–2002. (2005)

		Infant Mortality Rate				
			Neonatal (under 28 days)			Postneonatal (28 days – 11 months)
Year	Infant Deaths	Total	Total	Under 7 Days	7–27 Days	
2002[1]	28,042	7	4.7	3.7	0.9	2.3
2001	27,568	6.8	4.5	3.6	0.9	2.3
2000	28,035	6.9	4.6	3.7	1	2.3
1999	27,937	7.1	4.7	3.8	1	2.3
1998	28,371	7.2	4.8	3.8	1	2.4
1997	28,045	7.2	4.8	3.8	0.9	2.5
1996	28,487	7.3	4.8	3.8	0.9	2.5
1995	29,583	7.6	4.9	4	0.9	2.7
1994	31,710	8	5.1	4.2	0.9	2.9
1993	33,466	8.4	5.3	4.3	0.9	3.1
1992	34,628	8.5	5.4	4.4	1	3.1
1991	36,766	8.9	5.6	4.6	1	3.4
1990	38,351	9.2	5.8	4.8	1	3.4
1989	39,655	9.8	6.2	5.1	1.1	3.6
1988	38,910	10	6.3	5.2	1.1	3.6
1987	38,408	10.1	6.5	5.4	1.1	3.6
1986	38,891	10.4	6.7	5.6	1.1	3.6
1985	40,030	10.6	7	5.8	1.2	3.7
1984	39,580	10.8	7	5.9	1.1	3.8
1983	40,627	11.2	7.3	6.1	1.2	3.9
1982	42,401	11.5	7.7	6.4	1.3	3.8

[1]Partially edited data processed through January 2004.

SOURCE: Health E-Stats. Supplemental Analysis of Recent Trends in Infant Mortality. www.cdc.gov/nchs.

about births in the United States in 2003 and 2004. In 2004 there were 4.1 million births. The number of births to white (non-Hispanic) women decreased, whereas the number of births to black women remained essentially unchanged. Births to Hispanic, Native American, and Asian/Pacific Islander women increased. Teenage birth rates decreased for all race and ethnic groups, whereas birth rates for women ages 30 to 44 increased (Hamilton, Ventura, Martin, & Sutton, 2006).

Childbearing by unmarried women continued to increase in 2004, reaching record highs—almost 1.5 million births—an increase of 4%. In fact, 35.7% of all births were to unmarried women. Moreover, these increases occurred in all ages, races, and Hispanic-origin subgroups (Hamilton, Ventura, Martin, & Sutton, 2005). The cesarean birth rate reached record levels, increasing by 6% to 29% of all births in 2004. Concurrently the rate of vaginal birth after cesarean (VBAC) dropped 13% from 10.6% in 2003 to 9.2% in 2004 (National Center for Health Statistics [NCHS], 2005b).

Birth rates also vary dramatically from country to country. Table 1–2 identifies the birth rates for selected countries.

- Is there an association between birth rates and changing societal values?

- Do the differences in birth rates between various age groups reflect education? Changed attitudes toward motherhood?

- Do the differences in birth rates among various countries reflect cultural differences? Do they represent availability of contraceptive information? Are there other factors at work?

Infant Mortality

The **infant mortality rate** is the number of deaths of infants under 1 year of age per 1000 live births in a given population. In 2003 the US infant mortality rate was 6.85, a decrease over 2002. The year 2002 was marked by the first increase in infant mortality in more than 40 years (Table 1–3). However, the infant mortality rate varied widely by race of the mother, from 5.17 for infants of white mothers to 14.01 for infants of black mothers (Hoyert, Heron, Murphy, & Kung, 2006). *Neonatal mortality* is the number of deaths of infants less than 28 days of age per 1000 live births. *Perinatal mortality* includes both neonatal deaths and fetal deaths per 1000 live births. (*Fetal death* is death in utero at 20 weeks' or more gestation.) Figure 1–6 ◆ shows the leading causes of deaths of infants in the United States from 1940 to 2003.

The US infant mortality rate has continued to be of concern because the United States has fallen to 22nd place among industrialized nations in infant mortality rankings. Healthcare professionals, policy makers, and the public have continued to stress the need in the United States for better prenatal care, coordination of health services, and the provision of comprehensive maternal-child services.

Table 1–2 identifies infant mortality rates for selected countries. As the data indicate, the range is dramatic among the coun-

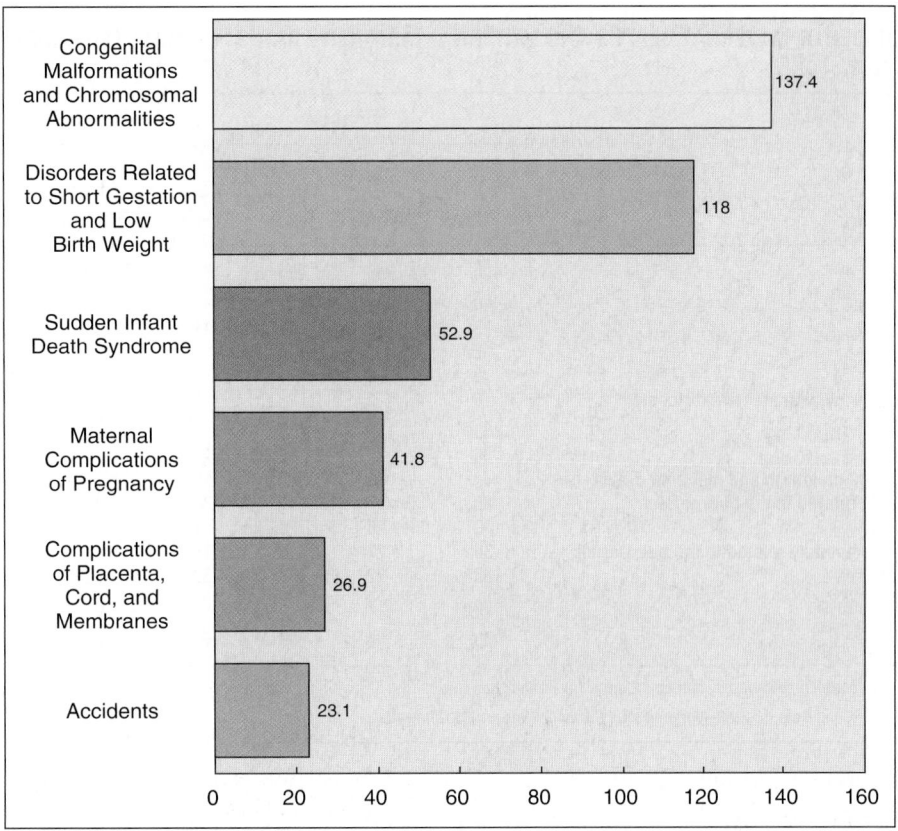

Figure 1–6 ◆ Leading causes of death for infants in the United States, 2003.
SOURCE: Adapted from Hoyert, Heron, Murphy, & Hsiang-Ching. (2006). Deaths: Final data for 2003. *National Vital Statistics Report, 54*(13), 1–27.

tries listed. Unfortunately, information about birth rates and mortality rates is limited for some countries because of a lack of organized reporting mechanisms.

The information prompts questions about access to health care during pregnancy and following birth, standards of living, nutrition, sociocultural factors, and more. Additional factors affecting the infant mortality rate may be identified by considering the following research questions:

- Does infant mortality correlate with a specific maternal age?
- What are the leading causes of infant mortality in each country?
- Is there a difference in mortality rates among racial groups? If so, is it associated with the availability of prenatal care? With educational level of the mother or father?

Maternal Mortality

The **maternal mortality rate** is the number of deaths from any cause related to or aggravated by pregnancy or its management during the pregnancy cycle (including the 42-day postpartal period) per 100,000 live births. It does not include accidental or unrelated causes. Between 2002 and 2003 maternal deaths increased by 138 deaths, resulting in a maternal mortality rate of 12 per 100,000 live births. This increase in part reflects the fact that a growing number of states are using a separate item on the death certificate to help identify pregnancy-related deaths (Hoyert et al.,

2006). Table 1–4 identifies the number of maternal deaths and maternal mortality rates for 2003. In general, maternal mortality rates are significantly lower than they were 25 years ago. Factors influencing the decrease in maternal mortality include the increased use of hospitals and specialized healthcare personnel by antepartal, intrapartal, and postpartal maternity clients; the establishment of care centers for high-risk mothers and infants; the prevention and control of infection with antibiotics and improved techniques; the availability of blood and blood products for transfusions; and the lowered rates of anesthesia-related deaths.

Additional factors to consider may be identified by asking the following research questions:

- Is there a correlation between maternal mortality and age?
- Is there a correlation with availability of health care? Economic status?

Implications for Nursing Practice

Nurses can use statistics in a number of ways. For example, statistical data may be used to:

- Determine populations at risk
- Assess the relationship between specific factors
- Help establish databases for specific client populations
- Determine the levels of care needed by particular client populations

Table 1–4   NUMBER OF MATERNAL DEATHS AND MATERNAL MORTALITY RATES FOR SELECTED CAUSES BY RACE: UNITED STATES, 2003

	Number				Rate			
			All Other				All Other	
	All Races	White	Total	Black	All Races	White	Total	Black
Maternal causes	495	280	215	183	12.1	8.7	24.9	30.5
Pregnancy with abortive outcome	40	18	22	18	1	*	2.5	*
Ectopic pregnancy	23	12	11	11	0.6	*	*	*
Spontaneous abortion	6	2	4	1	*	*	*	*
Medical abortion	3	2	1	1	*	*	*	*
Other and unspecified pregnancy with abortive outcome	8	2	6	5	*	*	*	*
Other direct obstetric causes	338	180	158	135	8.3	5.6	18.3	22.5
Eclampsia and pre-eclampsia	68	33	35	29	1.7	1.0	4.1	4.8
Hemorrhage of pregnancy and childbirth and placenta previa	47	28	19	16	1.1	0.9	*	*
Complications predominately related to the puerperium	88	47	41	34	2.2	1.5	4.7	5.7
Obstetric embolism	49	26	23	18	1.2	0.8	2.7	*
Other complications predominately related to the puerperium	39	21	18	16	1	0.7	*	*
All other direct obstetric causes	135	72	63	56	3.3	2.2	7.3	9.3
Obstetric death of unspecified cause	22	17	5	4	0.5	*	*	*
Indirect obstetric causes	95	65	30	26	2.3	2	3.5	4.3

*Figure does not meet standards of reliability followed by National Center for Health Statistics.

SOURCE: Hoyert et al. (2006). Deaths: Final Data for 2003. *National Vital Statistics Report, 54*(13), 1–40.

- Evaluate the success of specific nursing interventions
- Determine priorities in caseloads
- Estimate staffing and equipment needs of hospital units and clinics

Statistical information is available through many sources, including professional literature; state and city health departments; vital statistics sections of private, county, state, and federal agencies; special programs or agencies (family-planning and similar agencies); and demographic profiles of specific geographic areas. Most of these sources are accessible via the Internet. Nurses who use this information will be better prepared to promote the health needs of maternal-newborn clients and their families.

EVIDENCE-BASED PRACTICE IN MATERNAL-CHILD NURSING

Evidence-based practice—that is, nursing care in which all interventions are supported by current, valid research evidence—is emerging as a force in health care. It provides a useful approach to problem solving/decision making and to self-directed, client-centered, lifelong learning. Evidence-based practice builds on the actions necessary to transform research findings into clinical practice by also considering other forms of evidence that can be useful in making clinical practice decisions. These other forms of evidence may include, for example, statistical data, quality improvement measurements, risk management measures, and information from support services such as infection control.

As clinicians, nurses need to meet three basic competencies related to evidence-based practice:

1. To recognize which clinical practices are supported by sound evidence, which practices have conflicting findings as to their effect on client outcomes, and which practices have no evidence to support their use
2. To use data in their clinical work to evaluate outcomes of care
3. To appraise and integrate scientific bases into practice

Unfortunately, some agencies and clinical units where nurses practice still operate in the old style, which often generates conflict for nurses who recognize the need for more responsible clinical practice. In truth, market pressures are forcing nurses and other healthcare providers to evaluate routines to improve efficiencies and provide better outcomes for clients.

Nurses need to know what data are being tracked where they work and how care practices and outcomes are improved as a result of quality improvement initiatives. However, there is more to evidence-based practice than simply knowing what is being tracked and how the results are being used. Competent, effective nurses learn to question the very basis of their clinical work.

Throughout this text we have provided *snapshots* of evidence-based practice related to childbearing women, children, and families such as the one on page 80. We believe that these snapshots will help you understand the concept more clearly. We also expect that these examples may challenge you to question the usefulness of some of the routine care you observe in clinical practice. That is the impact of evidence-based practice—it moves clinicians beyond practices of habit and opinion to practices based on reliable, valid, current science.

Nursing Research

Research is vital to expanding the science of nursing, fostering evidence-based practice, and improving client care. Research also plays an important role in advancing the profession of nursing. For example, nursing research can help determine the psychosocial and physical risks and benefits of both nursing and medical interventions.

The gap between research and practice is being narrowed by the publication of research findings in popular nursing journals, the establishment of departments of nursing research in hospitals, and collaborative research efforts by nurse researchers and clinical practitioners. Interdisciplinary research between nurses and other healthcare professionals is also becoming more common. This ever-increasing recognition of the value of nursing research is important because well-done research supports the goals of evidence-based practice. Most chapters of this text, therefore, include Research in Practice boxes such as the one shown on p. 37.

Clinical Pathways and Nursing Care Plans

One result of nursing research into the nursing process has been the creation of clinical pathways. *Clinical pathways* specify essential nursing activities and provide basic guidelines about expected outcomes at specified time intervals. These guidelines are research based and enable the nurse to determine whether a client's responses meet expected norms at any given time. In the text, we have provided sample clinical pathways for a woman experiencing a normal vaginal birth and a cesarean birth. We have also provided sample clinical pathways for the normal newborn and for a woman in the postpartal period.

Nursing care plans, which use the nursing process as an organizing framework, are also invaluable in planning and organizing care. Care plans are especially valuable for nursing students and novice nurses. To help organize care, this text also provides several examples of nursing care plans such as those found in Chapter 19. ∞

Evidence-Based Practice: An Example

In using evidence-based practice, nurses draw on a variety of tools such as statistical data, nursing research and other research, standards of care, statistics, and critical analysis skills.

These tools can exist separately, but in practice they overlap and build upon each other. An example of just one possible situation is presented in the following case study.

Two birthing unit nurses express concerns to each other about the seemingly high number of adolescents who have been giving birth in their unit. At the next staff meeting, they voice their concerns and raise questions about whether the number of teenage mothers seen in their unit is higher than normal. After the discussion, the nurses decide they need to formulate a plan to gather more information. Each nurse volunteers to pursue a particular aspect of the plan of action. Their plan includes contacting the local public health department for local and national statistics on this age group; looking at the availability of health care for adolescents in their community; investigating the particular health problems of pregnant teenagers and risks to their infants; checking the availability of prenatal education groups for adolescents; finding out whether their community has school health programs and what the program content is; looking at national statistics identifying when adolescents seek prenatal care; talking with local certified nurse-midwives, physicians, and prenatal clinic personnel to see if the national statistics apply to their community; collecting information about current legislative issues affecting adolescent health care; seeking further information about the needs of adolescents during pregnancy and birth by doing a library search; and looking for continuing education programs dealing with the pregnant adolescent client.

At subsequent staff meetings, nurses share information and investigate other areas as the need is identified. How they evaluate the data and apply them will depend on the requirements of their maternal-newborn unit and the unique needs of their community. Possible outcomes may include developing a research study, volunteering in local adolescent clinics, developing and teaching prenatal classes for adolescents, volunteering to teach in community school health programs, organizing a continuing education program on the adolescent mother for community hospitals, and forming a network within their professional nursing organization to stay informed about legislative issues pertaining to adolescents.

As the example illustrates, the application of tools of evidence-based practice assists the nurse in analyzing data and planning a course of action.

CHAPTER REVIEW

FOCUS YOUR STUDY

- Many nurses working with childbearing families are expert practitioners who are able to serve as role models for nurses who have not yet attained the same level of competence.

- Contemporary childbirth is family centered, offers choices about birth, and recognizes the needs of siblings and other family members.

- The self-care movement, which emerged in the late 1960s, emphasizes personal health goals, a holistic approach, and preventive care.

- The US healthcare system is facing a variety of challenges including the high cost of health care and the need for cost containment while retaining quality; the large numbers of uninsured and underinsured people; high infant mortality rates as compared with other industrialized nations; and a high incidence of poverty, especially among children and women-headed households.

- The nurse who provides culturally competent care recognizes the importance of the childbearing family's value system, acknowledges that differences occur among people, and seeks to respect and respond to ethnic diversity in a way that leads to mutually desirable outcomes.

- A nurse must practice within the scope of practice or be open to the accusation of practicing medicine without a license. The standard of care against which individual nursing practice is compared is that of a reasonably prudent nurse.

- Nursing standards provide information and guidelines for nurses in their own practice, in developing policies and protocols in healthcare settings, and in directing the development of quality nursing care.

- Informed consent—based on knowledge of a procedure and its benefits, risks, and alternatives—must be secured before providing treatment.

- State constitutions, statutes, and common law protect the right to privacy.

- Maternal-fetal conflict may arise when the fetus is viewed as a person of equal rights to those of the mother's and external agents attempt to force the mother to accept a therapy she wishes to refuse, or similarly attempt to restrict a mother's actions to support the well-being of the fetus.

- Abortion can be performed until the age of viability. Caregivers have the right to refuse to perform an abortion or assist with the procedure.

- A variety of procedures are available to help infertile couples achieve a pregnancy. However, some of these procedures provoke serious ethical dilemmas.

- Embryonic stem cell research using human stem cells obtained from a human embryo is marked by controversy. On the one hand, it raises the possibility of treatment for a variety of major diseases such as diabetes, Parkinson disease, and Alzheimer disease. On the other hand, ethicists question the ethical implications of using embryonic tissue—especially tissue obtained specifically for stem cell research.

- Cord blood banking provides the opportunity to make stem cells available to treat a variety of cancers and blood system disorders. Its growing popularity has revealed several ethical issues, such as: Who owns the blood? How will informed consent be obtained and by whom? How will confidentiality be ensured? How can the harvested blood be distributed fairly, so that it is available to individuals from all races, ethnic groups, and income levels? And so forth.

- Descriptive statistics describe or summarize a set of data. Inferential statistics allow the investigator to draw conclusions about what is happening between two or more variables in a population.

- Evidence-based practice—that is, nursing care in which all interventions are supported by current, valid research evidence—is emerging as a positive force in health care.

- Nursing research plays a vital role in adding to the nursing knowledge base, expanding clinical practice, and expanding nursing theory.

EXPLORE MEDIALINK

http://www.prenhall.com/davidson

NCLEX review questions, case studies, and other interactive resources for this chapter can be found on the Web Site at http://www.prenhall.com/davidson. Click on "Chapter 1" to select the activities for this chapter.

For tutorials including animations and videos, more NCLEX review questions, and an audio glossary, access the accompanying Prentice Hall Nursing MediaLink DVD-ROM in this book.

PRENTICE HALL NURSING MEDIALINK DVD-ROM
Audio Glossary
NCLEX Review

COMPANION WEBSITE
Additional NCLEX Review
Case Study: *Cord Blood Banking*
Care Plan Activity: *Request for Second Trimester Abortion*
Applications: *Scope of Practice; Standards of Care*
Critical Thinking

CRITICAL THINKING IN ACTION

CULTURALLY COMPETENT CARE

View the Critical Thinking in Action video in Chapter 1 of the DVD-ROM. Then answer the questions that follow.

You are working as a prenatal nurse in a local clinic. Before entering a client's room, you review the chart for pertinent information such as cultural background, significant family members, weeks of gestation, test results, birth plan, and education for health promotion. You greet each client and family member by name and ask how they are coping with the pregnancy. Depending on the trimester of the pregnancy, you review the discomforts or concerns of the mother/family and what they may expect.

You examine the mother, including fundal height, fetal heart rate and fetal position if appropriate, maternal blood pressure, weight gain, and urine analysis. With each client, you discuss the community resources available such as prenatal classes, lactation consultants, and prenatal exercise/yoga classes. Based upon the information you obtain, you might refer the mother to social services or the WIC program as appropriate. At the end of the clinic session, you review the clients with the collaborating physician.

1. How would you define the terms *family* and *family-centered care?*

2. Describe how the nursing process provides the framework for the delivery of direct nursing care.

3. How would you describe the concept of community-based care?

4. How would you describe culturally competent care?

REFERENCES

American Academy of Pediatrics, Committee on Bioethics. (1999). Fetal therapy—Ethical considerations (RE9817). *Pediatrics, 103*(5), 1061–1063.

American Association for the Advancement of Science. (2002). *Stem cell research* (Policy Brief). Washington, DC: Author.

American College of Nurse-Midwives. (2005). *Mandatory degree requirements for midwives.* Retrieved March 13, 2006, from http://www.midwife.org

American College of Obstetricians and Gynecologists. (2001). *Joint statement of practice relationships between obstetrician-gynecologists and certified nurse-midwives/certified midwives* (ACOG Statement of Policy). Washington, DC: Author.

American College of Obstetricians and Gynecologists. (2001, February 28). *ACOG calls fetal surgery experimental.* ACOG press release retrieved April 27, 2002, from http://www.acog.com/from_home/publications/press_releases/nr02-28-01-1.html

American College of Obstetricians and Gynecologists. (2002). *Nonselective embryo reduction: Ethical guidance for the obstetrician-gynecologist* (Committee Opinion). Washington, DC: Author.

American College of Obstetricians and Gynecologists. (2004). *Ethics in obstetrics and gynecology* (2nd ed.). Washington, DC: Author.

American College of Obstetricians and Gynecologists. (2005a). *Maternal decision making, ethics, and the law* (Committee Opinion No. 321). Washington, DC: Author.

American College of Obstetricians and Gynecologists. (2005b). *Perinatal risks associated with assisted reproductive technology* (Committee Opinion No. 324). Washington, DC: Author.

Benner, P. (1984). *From novice to expert.* Menlo Park, CA: Addison-Wesley.

Cameron, N. M. de S. (2006). Research ethics, science policy, and four contexts for the stem cell debate. *Journal of Investigative Medicine, 54*(1), 38–42.

Centers for Medicare and Medicaid Services (CMS). (2006). *National health care expenditure data: Historical.* Retrieved July 27, 2006, from http://www.cms.hhs.gov

Cohen, R. A., & Martinez, M. E. (2006). *Health insurance coverage: Estimates from the National Health Interview Survey, 2005.* Retrieved July 25, 2006, from http://www.cdc.gov/nchs

Dickey, S. B., & Deatrick, J. (2000). Autonomy and decision making for health promotion in adolescence. *Pediatric Nursing, 26*(5), 461–467.

Hamilton, B. E., Ventura, S. J., Martin, J. A., & Sutton, P. D. (2005, October 28). *Preliminary births for 2004.* Health E-Stats. Hyattsville, MD: National Center for Health Statistics. Retrieved March 8, 2006, from http://www.cdc.gov/nchs/products/pubs/pubd/hestats/prelim_births/prelim_births04.htm

Hamilton, B. E., Ventura, S. J., Martin, J. A., & Sutton, P. D. (2006, July 6). *Final births for 2004.* Health E-Stats. Hyattsville, MD: National Center for Health Statistics. Retrieved July 25, 2006, from http://www.cdc.gov/nchs/products/pubs/pubd/hestats/finalbirths04/finalbirths04.htm

Hornstra, D. (1999). A realistic approach to maternal-fetal conflict. *Neonatal Intensive Care, 12*(2), 24–31.

Hoyert, D. L., Heron, M., Murphy, S. L., & Kung, H. C. (2006, January 19). Deaths: Final data for 2003. *National Vital Statistics Reports, 54*(13), 1–40.

Joint Commission on the Accreditation of Healthcare Organizations (JCAHO). (2006). *2007 patient care safety goals.* Retrieved July 25, 2006, from http://www.jointcommission.org

Kurtzberg, J., Lyerly, A. D., & Sugarman, J. (2005). Untying the Gordian knot: Policies, practices, and ethical issues related to banking of umbilical cord blood. *The Journal of Clinical Investigation, 115*(10), 2592–2597.

Midwives Alliance of North America (MANA). (2006). *Definitions.* Retrieved March 13, 2006, from http://www.mana.org/definitions.html

Moise, K. J. (2006). What to tell patients about banking cord blood stem cells. *Contemporary OB/GYN, 51*(Suppl. 4), 42–52.

National Center for Health Statistics (NCHS). (2005a). *Health, United States, 2005.* Retrieved March 14, 2006, from http://www.cdc.gov/nchs

National Center for Health Statistics (NCHS). (2005b). *2004 preliminary birth data: Maternal and infant health.* Health E-Stats. Retrieved July 26, 2006, from http://www.cdc.gov/nchs/products/pubs/pubd/hestats/highlights/2004prebirth.htm

Simpson, K. R., & Knox, G. E. (2001). Perinatal teamwork: Turning rhetoric into reality. *AWHONN Lifelines, 5*(5), 56–59.

Smith, C., Cowan, C., Heffler, S., & Catlin, A. (2006). National health spending in 2004: Recent slowdown led by prescription drug spending. *Health Affairs, 25*(1), 186–196.

Smith, F. O., & Thomson, B. G. (2000). Umbilical cord blood collection, banking, and transplantation: Current status and issues relevant to perinatal caregivers. *Birth, 27*(2), 127–135.

Williams, C. (2006). Dilemmas in fetal medicine: Premature application of technology or responding to women's choice? *Sociology of Health & Illness, 28*(1), 1–20.

Wright, V. C., Schieve, L. A., Reynolds, M. A., & Jeng, G. (2005, June 3). Assisted reproductive technology surveillance—United States, 2002. *Mortality and Morbidity Weekly Reports, 54* (SS-2), 1-23.

Care of the Family in a Culturally Diverse Society

I can't imagine going through pregnancy, birth, or those initial few weeks after my daughter was born without my family. My brother called regularly throughout my pregnancy to check on me. Dad gave me pep talks on eating right and taking care of myself. My husband and my mom were both with me during my labor and my unexpected cesarean birth. After Rosario was born, my husband accompanied our new daughter to the nursery and mom stayed with me, talking and holding my hand. What a difference a family can make.

OBJECTIVES

1. Explore factors that influence the values, decision making, and roles within the family unit.
2. Summarize employment, marital, and economic trends affecting the contemporary family.
3. Distinguish among different types of families.
4. Identify major developmental tasks to be completed by the childbearing family.
5. Delineate the advantages of using a family assessment tool.
6. Discuss the impact of culture in caring for the childbearing family.
7. Identify prevalent cultural norms related to childbearing and childrearing.
8. Summarize the importance of cultural competency in providing nursing care.
9. Discuss the use of a cultural assessment tool as a means of providing culturally sensitive nursing care.
10. Identify the key considerations in providing spiritually sensitive nursing care.

KEY TERMS

MEDIALINK

Additional resources for this content can be found on the Prentice Hall Nursing MediaLink DVD-ROM and on the Companion Website at http://www.prenhall.com/davidson. Click on "Chapter 2" to select the activities for this chapter.

$\mathbf{A}$lthough a woman may arrive for her healthcare appointment physically alone, in another sense, she is always accompanied by her family. Her parents, partner, spouse, or in-laws may accompany her in the form of internalized messages about her body, contraception, sex, or childbearing, or in the form of their expectations for her behavior. In addition, her family's culture and religious beliefs will influence her healthcare practices, decisions, and needs. Thus, a nurse may provide expert teaching about condom use to an adolescent, but the teaching may not be put into practice because the client's partner objects. Or a nurse may encourage a pregnant client to increase her consumption of cow's milk, but a religious proscription against consuming animal products may prohibit this behavior. The goal of effective, holistic nursing care requires nurses to recognize that their clients' values, behaviors, decisions, and needs do not exist in a vacuum; instead, nurses must actively seek to learn about and care for the entire childbearing family.

In this chapter, we provide a perspective on the childbearing family in a culturally diverse society. We begin by discussing family values, power, and roles, as well as key social changes affecting the contemporary family. We then identify a variety of different family types the nurse is likely to encounter, and explore the developmental tasks of these varied families. Because families cannot be considered in isolation from their culture, we introduce several concepts essential to culturally competent nursing care. We close the chapter with a brief look at the influence of a family's religious beliefs on health outcomes, and identify key considerations in providing spiritually sensitive nursing care.

DEFINING FAMILY

A number of definitions of families can be found in the literature. For example, a nurse researcher defines **family** as "two or more persons who are joined together by bonds of sharing and emotional closeness and who identify themselves as being part of a family" (Friedman, Bowden, & Jones, 2003, p. 10). The US Census Bureau defines *family* in more traditional terms as individuals joined together by marriage, blood, adoption, or residence in the same household (US Census Bureau, 2006).

Family Values

Families have values that guide their behavior and interactions within society and their own family units. In a classic study of families in crisis, **family values** are defined as a "system of ideas, attitudes, and beliefs about the worth of an entity or concept that consciously or unconsciously bind together the members of the family in a common culture" (Parad & Caplan, 1965, p. 55). These values are greatly influenced by external factors including cultural background, social norms, education, environmental influences, socioeconomic status, and beliefs held by peers, coworkers, political and community leaders, and other individuals outside of the family unit. Because of the influence of these external factors, a family's values may change significantly over the years.

Family Power and Decision Making

Within each family, there is an individual or group who possesses **family power**; that is, the potential or actual ability to change the behavior of other family members (Olson & Cromwell, 1975, p. 143). This individual or group may affect how a client responds to a healthcare provider, a diagnosis, treatments, or health teaching. Research has shown that many families make health-related decisions only with the aid of other family members. For example, in the Korean culture, in which elders are highly respected and play a key role in family matters, family power may rest with the grandfather. If the son wanted to make a health-related change in the family's diet, for example, he would first seek the advice and approval of his grandfather. Similarly, many Chinese identify themselves in relation to other members of the family and believe that personal independence is not as important. Thus, a Chinese client may avoid taking action regarding a health matter unless a family leader gives permission (Galanti, 2004).

In many traditional families, the father figure is the decision maker. In traditional Cuban culture, for example, the father may be aggressive and dominant and is critical to all family decisions (Galanti, 2004). In contrast, the mother typically remains at home, passive and dependent. However, Cubans in the United States have become much more egalitarian because women are usually the first ones able to find jobs and contribute to their families. Thus, among Cubans who have assimilated, one may find equal decision-making power.

Filipino families also consider the father to be the major decision maker in most cases. However, the mother has an equal say with the father about issues of health, welfare, and money (St. Hill, Lipson, & Meleis, 2003).

In many immigrant families, the child is first to learn the new language and may be used as an interpreter in healthcare settings. In families in which the father is considered the power holder, this situation can cause problems if the family perceives that the healthcare provider is relating only to the child. They may feel that their child is being placed in a superior position, which may be unacceptable to them. Children appear to acculturate more rapidly than adults, which can lead to stress within the family unit (Lau, McCabe, Yeh, Garland, Wood, & Hough, 2005).

Family Roles

Family roles are "homogeneous sets of behaviors that are normatively defined and expected of an occupant of a given social position. Roles are based on role expectations or prescriptions defining what individuals in a particular situation should do in order to meet their own or another's expectations of them" (Nye & Gecas, 1976, p. 7).

Roles vary depending on age, position within the family, conflict within the family, stressors, cultural backgrounds, health status of family members, and demographic trends. However, within each family, roles commonly encountered include breadwinner, homemaker, nurturer, social planner, and peacemaker. Although roles are sometimes perceived to be gender specific, they are more accurately assigned to the family member who performs that specific function. In the majority of US households in the 1950s, a male was the sole breadwinner and a female performed all homemaker functions. In contemporary society, these roles are often shared. For example, both parents may be employed and may participate equally in the care of the children. Segregated roles are more evident in certain cultures where roles are defined more sharply based on gender.

Any one individual within a family may have two or more roles. In nuclear families, roles are typically paired and consist of father-husband, wife-mother, son-brother, and so forth. In extended families the number of paired roles increases, whereas in single-parent families the numbers are less.

Increasingly important in the contemporary US family is the role of the grandparent. High adolescent pregnancy rates have created a sizable population of young grandparents (as young as the 30s), and increased life expectancy rates have created a sizable population of great-grandparents. Grandparents vary in how they express their role. Role functions may include: (1) witness who is simply present for the grandchildren, (2) protector who provides care and ensures safety when needed, (3) peacemaker who helps resolve conflicts between parents and children, and (4) active participant who maintains involvement in family life in the past, present, and future.

Grandparents can offer a great deal to children and provide substantial support and advice to parents (Figure 2–1 ◆). Often grandparents are able to spend more quality time with grandchildren than they did with their own children. Many grandparents are retired and use this opportunity to build lasting bonds with grandchildren. Although extended families are often geographically separated, many grandparents have identified alternative means to stay connected with grandchildren when frequent visits are not possible. These alternatives include phone calls, emails, and letters, as well as sharing journals, photos, and videotapes.

Computers, emails, and cell phones were not the kinds of communication I grew up using, however, I decided to learn so that I could communicate with my grandchildren who don't live close by. My grandchildren send me jokes and digital photos and it has helped me to feel like I am more a part of their lives. They think I am 'cool'

because I have learned to use their technology. We exchange cards electronically now for many special occasions and we communicate much more often than we did before I knew how to use my computer. It sure doesn't replace being together face-to-face but it does help me feel like I know them better!

Changes Affecting the Contemporary Family

The contemporary family has changed dramatically from the family unit of the 1950s, which typically consisted of a working father and a stay-at-home mother who cared for the children and ran the family home (Figure 2–2 ◆). Today, the mother may be working outside the home and the father may be the stay-at-home parent. According to the US Census Bureau (2004), 26% of the stay-at-home parents were mothers and 0.7% were fathers. Affecting the contemporary family are employment trends, changes in marriage rates, and economic trends.

EMPLOYMENT TRENDS

Employment trends have changed with the shift from a male-dominated workforce to a mixed male-female workforce. In 2003, 32.4% of women earned more than their spouses (US Census Bureau, 2003). Today, the majority of households consist of dual-earner families in which both the mother and father have employment outside of the home. Dual-earner families may have different needs than traditional families. For example, when a child becomes ill in a dual-earner family, the parents must decide who will take off work to care for the child. In traditional families, the mother would care for the child and work stresses from illness-related absences would not be a concern.

CHANGES IN MARRIAGE RATES

Since World War II, there has been a consistent decline in marriage rates. In 2003, 68% of all US households were occupied

Figure 2–1 ◆ Grandparents can offer nurturing and guidance to their grandchildren, not to mention lots of fun.
SOURCE: Paul Barton/CORBIS.

Figure 2–2 ◆ The traditional family of the mid-20th century consisted of a father who worked outside of the home, a mother who performed all homemaking and childrearing functions, and one or more children.
SOURCE: Getty Images, Inc.–Hulton Archive Photos.

by a two-parent family unit compared with 87% in 1970. It is interesting to note that households with children make up only one third of all US households. The proportion of single mothers rearing children grew to 26% in 2003, up from 12% in 1970. Single-parent father families have grown from 1% in 1970 to 6% in 2003. These changes reflect changing society norms including a delay in the age at first marriage, which increases the rate of nonmartial births, and a high percentage of marriages that result in divorce (Fields, 2003).

Along with the high proportion of single-parent families, there is also a higher proportion of never-married individuals in the United States than ever before, and those who do marry tend to do so at a later age than in the past. A combination of factors has led to delayed childbearing (see Chapter 8 ∞). There is also a growing trend for women to remain childless. In 1980, 10% of women ages 40 to 44 were childless compared with 18% in 2002 (US Census Bureau, 2003). American women spend fewer childbearing years in marriage, which increases the likelihood of nonmarital childbearing.

Other trends in the United States include increasing acceptance of single women giving birth. In 1950, 3% of births were to unmarried women. Today, 29.1% of all births are to unmarried women (Fields, 2003). Although this trend is increasing in the United States, in some cultures, an unmarried woman giving birth is viewed negatively. We discuss cultural views on birth outside of marriage later in this chapter.

ECONOMIC TRENDS

Changes in income levels have directly affected families. The household income of most American families increased by 25% between 1973 and 2001 (Mishel, Bernstein, & Boushey, 2003). Families who experienced the most economic growth had two wage earners and higher educational preparation. Median incomes are 64% higher for white workers than for black workers (Mishel et al., 2003). Although family median income levels fell in 2001 after the September 11, 2001, terrorist attacks, income levels have contiuned to rise since that time and unemployment statistics have remained relatively stable.

TYPES OF FAMILIES

Various types of families—both traditional and nontraditional—exist in contemporary society.

Nuclear Family

The *nuclear family* consists of a husband provider, a wife who stays home, and children (see Figure 2–2). Although the nuclear family was once the norm in the United States, it is no longer the most common type of family.

Dual-Career/Dual-Earner Family

The *dual-career/dual-earner family* is now considered the norm in modern society. Today, two thirds of all two-parent families have both parents working. Although many women work outside the home because of financial necessity, other women work either full or part time out of personal choice. Dual-career/dual-earner families have specific challenges. Because both

Figure 2–3 ◆ Today, 5% of married couples voluntarily choose to remain childless.
SOURCE: Michael Keller/CORBIS.

parents are working, child care, household chores, and spending time with other family members are priorities that need to be addressed.

Childless Family

A growing trend exists for couples to remain childless (Figure 2–3 ◆). Although as many as 10% of couples experience infertility problems, 5% of married couples are voluntarily without children. This trend is continuing to grow with the increased opportunities available to women in the workplace, delayed marriage, availability of contraceptives to prevent unwanted pregnancy, and wider acceptance of women's choosing not to become mothers.

Extended Family

Extended families consist of a couple who shares household responsibilities, chores, and expenses with parents, siblings, or other relatives. Multigenerational family living arrangements are more common in non-US cultures and in working-class families. Children are reared by parents and other relatives. Extended families are also common when an elderly or ill relative requires care by the younger family members.

Extended Kin Network Family

An *extended kin network family* is a specific form of an extended family in which two nuclear families of primary or unmarried kin live in close proximity to each other. The family shares a social support network, chores, goods, and services. This type of family model is common in the Latino community (Figure 2–4 ◆).

Single-Parent Family

Single-parent families are headed by only one parent (Figure 2–5 ◆). Although rare in the past, by the year 2003 there were 12 million such families in the United States, almost one third of all families. Since 1970 there has been a 14% increase in single-mother families and a 5% increase in single-father families (Fields, 2003).

Figure 2–4 ◆ In an extended kin network family, two nuclear families live in close proximity to each other and share responsibilities and resources.
SOURCE: Getty Images, Inc.

Figure 2–5 ◆ Single-parent families account for nearly one third of all US families.
SOURCE: Joyce Choo/CORBIS.

In the traditional single-parent family the head of the household is widowed, divorced, abandoned, or separated. In the nontraditional single-parent family the head of the household, most often the mother, was never married. Single-parent families often face difficulties because the sole parent may lack social and emotional support, need assistance with childrearing issues, and face financial strain. Mothers who have never married tend to have more financial difficulties, less educational achievement, and are younger in age than those who are divorced (Fields, 2003).

Stepparent Family

With divorce rates exceeding 50% and rates of remarriage at 75%, *stepfamilies* have become increasingly common (Stepfamily Association of America, 2005). Stepfamilies include a biologic parent with children, and a new spouse who may or may not have children. These families are also known as *remarried families, reconstituted families,* or *blended families.* It is estimated that 75% of all divorced individuals eventually remarry. Sixty-five percent of these remarriages involve children from a prior marriage (Stepfamily Association of America, 2005).

Stepfamily models have both strengths and weaknesses. Although marriage is often a new opportunity for success in a marital relationship for the parents, the relationship between stepparents and stepchildren can be strained. Stresses can include discipline issues, adjustment problems, role ambiguity, strain with the other biologic parent, and communication issues. Although stepfamilies may have fewer financial issues and may actually offer the child a new support person and role model, open communication is imperative to ensure a smooth transition.

Binuclear Family

A *binuclear family* is a postdivorced family in which the biologic children are members of two nuclear households, both that of the father and that of the mother. The children alternate between the two homes, typically spending a week with the father and a week with the mother. This is also called *coparenting,* and involves joint custody. Legally, *joint custody* refers to situations in which both parents have equal responsibility and legal rights, regardless of where the children live. Although this type of family represents a small number as yet, there has been an increase in this type of household as fathers assume a more active role in parenting. The increased recognition of the importance of having both a maternal and paternal presence has encouraged more parents to actively raise their children together, regardless of their relationship with each other. The benefits of a binuclear family include the ability to have both the mother and father involved in the child's upbringing, a model for effective communication (in a successful family model), and additional support and role models from extended family members.

Nonmarital Heterosexual Cohabitating Family

A *nonmarital heterosexual cohabitating family* is a heterosexual couple who may or may not have children and live together outside of marriage. This may include never-married individuals, as well as divorced or widowed persons. Unmarried cohabitating couples made up 4.6% of all US households in 2003. There are 4.2 million families classified as cohabitating, but it is estimated that this number is underreported (Fields, 2003).

CLINICAL TIP

It is important to establish which parent has legal custody, current visitation policies, and other legal variables (restraining orders, supervised visitation, etc.) when communicating information to parents about their children. Certain legal issues may prohibit the nurse from sharing some information with the noncustodial parent.

Figure 2–6 ◆ Some gay and lesbian couples choose to adopt children in need of loving homes.
SOURCE: Dana White/PhotoEdit.

Although some individuals may choose this model for personal reasons, others may do so for financial reasons or to seek companionship. For example, a widow may fear losing her pension if she remarries, or an individual who owns significant assets may fear losing these assets to a spouse, especially if residing in a community-property state.

Gay and Lesbian Families

Gay and *lesbian families* include those in which two or more people who share a same-sex orientation live together (with or without children), as well as families consisting of a gay or lesbian single parent rearing a child (Figure 2–6 ◆). The number of gay and lesbian families is underreported. Between 1990 and 2000, the number of gay or lesbian families rose by 319% (Smith & Gates, 2001). Of the 598,209 same-sex families, 301,148 are

male couples and 297,061 are female couples. These couples reside in 99.3% of all counties in the United States (Gates & Ost, 2004). It is estimated that 6 to 10 million children are being raised by at least one gay or lesbian parent (Gates & Ost, 2004).

Small studies have evaluated children raised by gay and lesbian couples and have found that they show no significant differences from children raised in other types of families. These children get along with their parents and peers the same as children raised in heterosexual households. Children raised in gay or lesbian families may face unique issues in interacting with peers and in revealing their parents' sexual orientation. In cases where the biologic parents divorced or separated because of one parent's newfound sexual orientation, children may be particularly vulnerable during the adjustment phase (Tasker, 2005).

CONTEMPORARY FAMILY DEVELOPMENT FRAMEWORKS

Family development refers to the dynamics or changes that families experience over time. It includes relationships, communication patterns, roles, and changes in interactions. Although each family is unique, the members must go through a set of fairly predictable changes. The amount of time in each stage and the duration between stages vary within each family unit.

Multiple family models and frameworks have been proposed over the years to facilitate an understanding of the complexities of family development. These developmental frameworks observe a family's progression over time by identifying specific stages in family life. Contemporary models, primarily based on the developmental framework by Duvall (1977), have embraced the trends and changes of contemporary society and family life. Duvall developed an eight-stage family life cycle that describes the developmental process that each family encounters. This model is based on a nuclear family (Table 2–1). The oldest child serves as a marker for the family's

Table 2–1	THE EIGHT-STAGE FAMILY LIFE CYCLE	
Stage I	Beginning families	Marriage between partners, identification as partners, establishing goals for future interaction, and building relationships with kin.
Stage II	Childbearing families	Birth of first child, new role as parents, integrating new family member into existing family.
Stage III	Families with preschool children	Establishing family network, socialization of children, reinforcing independence in children when separating from parents.
Stage IV	Families with school-age children	Facilitating peer relationships while maintaining family dynamics, adjusting to outside influences.
Stage V	Families with teenagers	Increase in children's independence and autonomy; parents' concerns shift to aging parents, careers, and marital relationship.
Stage VI	Families launching young adults	Readjustment of marital relationship; parents and children establish separate identities outside the family unit.
Stage VII	Middle-aged parents	Renewed marital relationship, new outside interests, fewer family responsibilities, new roles as grandparents and as in-laws, increased concern for aging parents, death, and disability of older generation.
Stage VIII	Retirement and old age	End of career, shift to retirement, maintain functioning during the aging process, maintain marital relationship, adjust to potential loss of spouse, friends, and siblings, prepare for eventual death.

SOURCE: FRIEDMAN, MARILYN M., FAMILY NURSING: RESEARCH, THEORY, AND PRACTICE, 4th ed., © 1998. Reproduced with permission of Pearson Education, Inc., Upper Saddle River, New Jersey. From Evelyn Duvall *Marriage and Family Development*, 5e. Published by Allyn and Bacon, Boston, MA. Copyright © 1977 by Pearson Education. Reprinted by permission of the publisher.

developmental stage except in the last two stages when the children are no longer present. Couples with more than one child may be in overlapping stages with developmental advances occurring simultaneously.

Model of the Childbearing Family

Multiple tasks exist for the childbearing family. The couple must first arrange the home to meet the needs of the newborn. This entails preparing for the infant by providing a safe environment, a safe clean place to sleep, and appropriate clothing and supplies.

At the time of birth of the first child, the childbearing family will engage in behaviors aimed at identifying responsibility and accountability for the newborn. Couples are rapidly faced with the realization that infants require 24-hour care. Although fathers are taking a more active role in childrearing, the mother is frequently the primary care provider, especially if she is breastfeeding. Although a breast pump can be used and milk can be given by bottle, the breastfeeding mother still assumes the majority of the feeding responsibilities. The father may assume other household tasks or other baby care activities, such as changing, bathing, and putting the infant down to sleep. Many facilities are now offering special classes just for fathers that help them learn to care for their infants. During the early stages, new roles will be identified as couples strive to establish a daily routine that includes the new family member.

Another task of the childbearing family is reestablishing a satisfying sexual relationship. Nurses can play an active role in teaching couples about normal changes during this period of family life. For example, in the postpartum period, sexual activity typically declines or ceases. The parents are transitioning to new roles, especially the mother. Fatigue is common. Women may also feel discomfort because of the birth and may fear pain with resumption of sexual intercourse. Reduced desire and vaginal dryness due to low estrogen levels are especially common in breastfeeding women. Counseling can provide the couple with reassurance that these changes are a common part of this developmental stage.

Couples need to communicate effectively and share thoughts and feelings as they adjust to their new roles. Fathers may feel isolated or "left out" as the mother embraces her new role. New mothers may feel overwhelmed with the responsibility of caring for an infant when alone. Even dual-career families typically have a transition period in which the mother is at home caring for the newborn and the father is working. For some women who previously worked full-time, being at home may cause feelings of isolation.

I thought I would love being at home with my beautiful new son. It wasn't that I didn't love him and want to be with him, I just felt like I was losing part of myself. I wasn't me anymore, and I missed talking with other adults and working. I felt tremendously guilty when I returned to work at 3 months; however, it made my time with him so much more special and I regained my self-confidence and felt like a real person again.

As the new family adapts to their changing roles and responsibilities, the role of other family members also emerges. Some extended families take an active role, whereas others may be more passive. Family members frequently provide guidance, advice, and assistance with child care. Both sets of grandparents may have strong beliefs about childrearing and may attempt to promote their own beliefs and rituals. Couples must effectively communicate with each other and other family members to avoid conflict. Although both families may want their traditions followed in terms of childrearing, the couple may wish to develop new traditions and rituals within their own family unit.

Along with changes in family relationships, the childbearing family may also experience changes in personal relationships and outside activities. After the birth of an infant, couples are typically more involved with their home life, may stay home more often, and may engage in different activities. Many women, especially women who formerly worked outside of the home, may feel like they have less in common with previous coworkers or friends who do not have children. This may lead to new friendships with other families who have more in common with the new family unit.

Allie and I met in high school, and from then on, we were inseparable. Even after I got married, we stayed close, going out to lunch or shopping together every couple of weeks, and talking on the phone every few days. When she found out I was pregnant, she threw a surprise shower for me, but as my due date approached, we started to drift apart. Since my daughter's birth, we've gotten together just once. Allie says she feels excluded and that all I ever talk about is the baby. I guess she's right—my daughter is the center of my world now, so it's hard to talk about anything else. I haven't seen Allie for several months now. It makes me sad when I think about it.

Childbearing families face multiple changes and challenges as they embark into new parenthood. The nurse can assist the childbearing family by providing teaching about family-planning issues, infant care and appropriate development, and safety concerns. The nurse can also offer guidance to the couple as they transition into parenthood by identifying interventions that can assist in meeting the emotional and physical needs of caring for a newborn. The nurse can provide support by actively listening as the couple expresses their feelings related to current role transition and changes in personal and family relationships. Resources can be provided to the new parents that will enable them to establish new relationships within their community.

Model Incorporating the Unattached Young Adult

Other models have been created to encompass the changes in contemporary families. For instance, Carter and McGoldrick (2005) modified the Duvall (1977) model to include the unattached young adult. This stage begins when the young adult leaves the family home and becomes financially independent, and lasts throughout young adulthood as long as the individual remains unmarried. Developmental tasks in this stage include differentiating self from the family unit, developing intimate peer relationships, and establishing a career and financial independence.

Because the median age at first marriage continues to rise, it is important to include the unattached young adult in family models. In 1970 the median age at first marriage was 23.2 years for men and 20.8 years for women. By 2003 the median age had increased to 27.1 and 25.3 years, respectively (Fields, 2003). Because of this increased age at first marriage, it is less common for adolescents to go directly from their parental home to a marital relationship. However, there is also a trend for young adults to reside with their parents well into their 20s. This is especially true for young men. In 2003, 55% (7.6 million) of men and 46% of women aged 18 to 24 lived at home with a parent or parents (Fields, 2003). It was fairly uncommon for young adults in the 18- to 24-year-old age group to live alone (5%).

Model Incorporating Divorce and Remarriage

Carter and McGoldrick (2005) devised another developmental model to describe issues encountered in undergoing divorce and in postdivorce (Table 2–2). Both emotional and developmental issues are encountered as families dissolve during the divorce process. Family members not only mourn the loss of a two-parent family, they also must adjust to a single-parent family model. Child visitation, financial issues, guilt, and attachment difficulties all play a major role in the changing family dynamics. Remarriage, which is becoming increasingly common, is another transitional stage in which family members must adjust to new roles and expectations (Table 2–3).

Model of the Lesbian or Gay Family

Lesbian or gay families face unique challenges in completing their developmental tasks. For example, they are frequently faced with discrimination and disapproval from mainstream society. For this reason, many gay or lesbian families opt to keep their sexual orientation a secret. In most states, they do not have the option of legal marriage and therefore do not have many of the benefits of marriage that heterosexual couples have such as insurance benefits, rights to property, custody issues, and family leave benefits associated with family illness or childbirth (Giger & Davidhizar, 2004). Chapter 8 ∞ provides an overview of obstacles faced by lesbians.

Slater (1995) developed a model specific to the stages of family life for lesbian and gay families (Table 2–4). The model identifies five stages in the development of the gay or lesbian family and addresses different issues and tasks in each stage.

Table 2–2   STAGES IN DIVORCE AND POSTDIVORCE

Stage	Issues
Divorce	
I. Decision to divorce	Accepting responsibility/part of responsibility for failed marriage.
II. Planning the breakup	Collaboratively working to resolve marital issues: financial, child care/custody. Communicating dissolution of marriage to relatives and friends.
III. Separation	Adapting to loss of previously established family unit, reorganizing relationships with spouse and children, restructuring finances, adapting to living apart, addressing issues related to attachment to spouse, maintaining bonds with extended family and spouse's extended family.
IV. Divorce	Grieving related to loss of prior family unit, accepting that the marriage is over, retrieving positive aspects of marriage (hopes, memories, dreams, expectations), overcoming negative feelings (anger, guilt, hurt, disappointment), maintaining relationships with extended family members.
Postdivorce	
I. Single parent (custodial)	Dealing with issues related to visitation and custody, rebuilding social relationships. Ensuring financial stability.
II. Single parent (noncustodial)	Continuing parenting role, identifying new means to relate to children, facilitating relationship between ex-spouse and children, providing support with childrearing decisions, providing financial support to ex-spouse for children, establishing new social relationships.

SOURCE: From Carter, Betty and McGoldrick, Monica (Eds). *The Changing Family Life Cycle: A Framework for Family Therapy*, 2ed. Published by Allyn and Bacon, Boston, MA. Copyright © 1989 by Pearson Education. Reprinted by permission of the publisher.

Table 2–3   STAGES IN REMARRIAGE

Stage	Issues
I. Establishing a new relationship	Resolve feelings from divorce, determine new marriage is desired, evaluate emotional readiness for new family, commit to new family.
II. Planning new marriage and family	Deal with personal fears and fears of new spouse and children, establish openness and open communication, determine financial obligations and coparenting roles with former spouses, plan for adjustment to new roles for parents and children, set new boundaries, resolve loyalty conflicts, maintain relationships with extended family members of ex-spouses, foster relationships between extended family and new spouse.
III. Remarriage and reconstitution of family	Include new spouse into family unit, dissolve previous attachment to former spouse and image of the "ideal family," restructure family system to include stepparent role, incorporate both families into a system to support children, foster all family relationships with extended family (including ex-spouses), share special memories to enhance family bonding and integration.

SOURCE: FRIEDMAN, MARILYN M., FAMILY NURSING: RESEARCH, THEORY, AND PRACTICE, 4th ed., © 1998. Reproduced with permission of Pearson Education, Inc., Upper Saddle River, New Jersey. From Carter, Betty & Monica McGoldrick (Eds.) *The Changing Family Life Cycle: A Framework for Family Therapy*, 2e. Published by Allyn and Bacon, Boston, MA. Copyright © 1989 by Pearson Education. Reprinted by permission of the publisher.

Table 2–4	LESBIAN AND GAY FAMILY STAGES
Stage	**Issues**
I. Formation of couple	Establish themselves as a couple versus individuals, combine two lives together, develop trust, reveal details about self, respond empathetically to partner to encourage further risk taking in relationship, tell others about their relationship.
II. Ongoing couplehood	Move from a physical passionate relationship to a stable relationship that includes passion and dailiness, manage differences between partners and handle conflict, increase sense of security and belonging as a couple.
III. Middle years	Progress into a long-term relationship with commitment, continue sense of security, make efforts to keep relationship fresh and new, rework rewards and disappointments.
IV. Generativity	Create a legacy beyond their own self-identity that will endure.

SOURCE: FRIEDMAN, MARILYN M., FAMILY NURSING: RESEARCH, THEORY, AND PRACTICE, 4th ed., © 1998. Reproduced with permission of Pearson Education, Inc., Upper Saddle River, New Jersey. Reprinted with the permission of The Free Press, a Division of Simon & Schuster Adult Publishing Group, from *THE LESBIAN FAMILY LIFE CYCLE* by Suzanne Slater. Copyright © 1995 by Suzanne Slater. All rights reserved.

FAMILY ASSESSMENT

The nurse's understanding of the family structure helps provide insight into the family's support systems and needs. A **family assessment** is a collection of data regarding the family's current level of functioning, support systems, sociocultural information, environmental information, type of family, family structure, and needs.

To obtain an accurate and concise family assessment, the nurse needs to establish a trusting relationship with the woman and her family. Data are best collected in a comfortable, private environment, free from interruptions. The nurse can use therapeutic communication skills, such as active listening, reflection, and silence, to encourage the woman and family to verbalize information. Basic information should include:

- Name, age, sex, and family relationship of all family members residing in the household

- Cultural associations, including cultural norms and customs related to childbearing, childrearing, and infant feeding (discussed shortly)

- Religious affiliations, including specific religious beliefs and practices related to childbearing

- Support network, including extended family, friends, and religious and community associations

- Family type, structure, roles, and values

- Communication patterns, including verbal and written language barriers

Health History

The health of individual family members can have a great impact on the health, well-being, and functioning of the family as a whole. The nurse should gather data about acute and chronic illnesses, genetic conditions, history of family violence, and mental health. A personal history beginning with pregnancies, pregnancy losses, infant health concerns, or deaths is also obtained. The nurse completes a comprehensive review of current health practices and health promotion behaviors to assess the family's ability to prevent accidents and chronic health conditions and performs a brief nutritional assessment. Families with nutritional excesses or deficits are provided with nutritional education to reduce the risk of nutrition-related illnesses.

The health history should also assess current exercise and activity patterns, sleep patterns, occupational exposures, use of prescription and nonprescription drugs, herbal remedies, alcohol consumption, smoking, and use of illegal drugs.

Environmental Considerations

A family's home environment can be assessed through home visits. Although not always possible, multiple home visits will yield more information than a single visit. A home visit enables the nurse to observe the family directly in their own environment and personal space. It also provides a more realistic view of family relationships, roles, parenting styles, and family needs. Often, the first visit serves as an introduction for the nurse to lay the foundation for a therapeutic relationship.

Observations should include the availability of personal space for all family members, including a place to sleep. The home should have basic necessities for daily living such as safe drinking water, a working waste-disposal system, electricity, and heat. The nurse can ensure that adequate cooking facilities, including a stove and refrigerator, are available for safe meal preparation. The availability of a phone is important so family members have access to healthcare providers and emergency services as needed.

The childbearing family should have resources available for the new baby, including a safe place to sleep, appropriate clothing, blankets, hygienic equipment, and age-appropriate resources for other children.

The home should also be inspected for potential hazards. Childproofing the home is a topic generally covered during the home visit. A safe place to bathe the infant should be identified. Parents should be taught never to leave the infant unattended during bathing and never to leave the infant in a location where a fall can occur. Environmental hazards such as open stairs, uncovered electrical outlets, fragile items that could harm the infant or other children if the items were broken, and unattended electrical appliances need to be discussed. Many new childbearing families may not recognize the potential environmental dangers and will benefit from a brief review.

During the home visit, the nurse can also assess the neighborhood in which the family lives. Observations should include availability of resources (drug store, grocery store, closest medical facility, child care resources, and schools), characteristics of the neighborhood (safety issues, proximity of public transportation), and community resources (new mothers' groups, breastfeeding support groups, and availability of infant development/first aid classes).

Upon completion of the home visit(s), the nurse can make recommendations and identify community resources and sources of support for the new family. Families can also be counseled on the availability of social services, such as the Special Supplemental Food Program for Women, Infants, and Children (WIC), and financial support programs. Parents without health insurance coverage should be encouraged to apply for Medicaid coverage for their infant. Community health programs, such as local health department immunization clinics, should also be discussed.

Family Assessment Tool

Multiple tools are available to assist the nurse in collecting data regarding the family. The Friedman Family Assessment tool is a comprehensive assessment of family functioning and other essential family data (Figure 2–7 ◆). It can be used during the home visit to obtain pertinent information and provide a framework for the nurse when planning and implementing interventions for the family.

CULTURAL INFLUENCES AFFECTING THE FAMILY

When caring for families, it is critical to consider the influence of culture, which may affect how a family reacts and responds to health-related issues. Cultural beliefs that may seem strange to a person born and raised in Ohio might have significant meaning for an immigrant from West Africa. Developing knowledge about cultural beliefs and traditions can increase the nurse's appreciation of diversity, prevent violation of cultural norms, and most important, improve the family's healthcare experience.

Within the United States there is tremendous cultural diversity. The 2000 census reported that 12.5% of Americans are Hispanic or Latino, 12.3% are of African descent, 3.6% are of Asian descent, and 0.9% are American Indian or Alaska Native. Thus it is important for nurses to have an understanding of how culture can influence family care.

Cultural Concepts

Culture can be defined as the beliefs, values, attitudes, and practices that are accepted by a population, a community, or an individual. Culture is learned and not ingrained in our genetic material, yet it can be passed on from generation to generation by means of *enculturation*. When a group is isolated, whether geographically or economically, culture is often reinforced.

Ethnicity is a social identity that is associated with shared behaviors and patterns. These include family structure, religious affiliation, language, dress, eating habits, and health behaviors.

Many Americans define ethnicity by physical characteristics such as skin color. However, many individuals consider themselves "biracial" or identify themselves with a specific ethnic group not because of skin color but because of a shared ideology or attitude. Many Americans are blends of ethnic backgrounds and it is often difficult to assign a specific ethnic identity to someone. Although some beliefs and cultural practices are common among certain ethnic groups, one must be careful to avoid stereotyping individuals. It is important not to assume that because individuals identify themselves as a specific ethnicity, they must practice a certain custom.

Within the United States, cultures have in the past been forced to blend. When people from one culture are transported to another place with new cultural norms, many adapt to these new behaviors. This process by which people adapt to a new cultural norm is called **acculturation**. Moreover, when a group completely changes their cultural identity to become part of the majority culture, **assimilation** occurs.

Acculturation

Many immigrants acculturate, and sometimes the acculturation process has an effect on the family's health. Acculturation is frequently associated with improved health status and health behaviors; however, this does not suggest that the American lifestyle is somehow more healthful. Instead, it seems that many factors contribute to the improved health status of acculturated immigrants. Primary among these are socioeconomic factors. Many immigrants are financially better off in the United States than they were in their country of origin, particularly those who have immigrated from developing nations.

Despite economic resources, acculturation plays a major role in immigrants' use of preventive care services. It appears that the length of time in the United States is a predictor for utilization of health services. One study showed that newly arrived refugees were at risk for not having breast and cervical cancer screening when compared with women who lived in the United States, despite comparable economic resources (Barnes & Harrison, 2004). In a study that examined the use of lay educators or *promotoras,* among Hispanic immigrants, Hispanic women who had been educated by a *promotora* from their own culture were 35% more likely to obtain a mammogram or a Pap smear (Hansen, Feigl, Modiano, Lopez, Escobedo, Moinpour, Pauler, & Meyskens, 2005). Another study that examined women from Southeast Asia found that the less acculturated women were, the less likely they were to obtain cervical cancer screenings (Gupta, Kumar, & Stewart, 2002).

Sometimes health declines with acculturation. One study examined Mexican American immigrants and found that they had superior birth outcomes when compared with American-born women. The positive outcomes were associated with familial support, religious beliefs, avoidance of smoking and alcohol use, and a healthy diet. As acculturation increased, the superior health outcomes decreased (Page, 2004). Obesity is another problem that is growing rapidly within the United States, particularly among immigrant populations.

Meeting of Physical, Emotional, and Spiritual Needs of Members

- Ability to provide food and shelter
  Space management as regards living, sleeping, recreation, privacy
  Crowding if over 1.5 persons per room
  Territoriality or control of each member over lifespace
  Access to laundry, grocery, recreation facilities
  Sanitation including disposal methods, source of water supply, control of rodents and insects
  Storage and refrigeration
  Available food supply
  Food preparation, including preserving and cooking methods (stove, hotplate, oven)
  Use of food stamps and donated foods as well as eligibility for food stamps
  Education of each member as to food composition, balanced menus, special preparations or diets if required for a specific member
- Access to health care
  Regularity of health care
  Continuity of caregivers
  Closeness of facility and means of access such as car, bus, cab
  Access to helpful neighbors
  Access to phone
- Family health
  Longevity
  Major or chronic illnesses
  Familial or hereditary illnesses such as rheumatic fever, gout, allergy, tuberculosis, renal disease, diabetes mellitus, cancer, emotional illness, epilepsy, migraine, other nervous disorders, hypertension, blood diseases, obesity, frequent accidents, drug intake, pica
  Emotional or stress-related illnesses
  Pollutants that members are chronically exposed to such as air, water, soil, noise, or chemicals that are unsafe
- Neighborhood pride and loyalty
- Job access, energy output, shift changes
- Sensitivity, warmth, understanding between family members
  Demonstration of emotion
  Enjoyment of sexual relations
  Male: Impotence, premature or retarded ejaculation, hypersexuality
  Female: Frigidity (inability to achieve orgasm), enjoyment of sexual relations, feelings of disgust, shame, self-devaluation; fear of injury, painful coitus
  Menstrual history, including onset, duration, flow, missed periods and life situation at the time, pain, euphoria, depression, other difficulties
- Sharing of religious beliefs, values, doubts
  Formal membership in church and organizations
  Ethical framework and honesty
  Adaptability, response to reality
  Satisfaction with life
  Self-esteem

Childrearing Practices and Discipline

- Mutual responsibility
  Joint parenting
  Mutual respect for decision making
  Means of discipline and consistency
- Respect for individuality
- Fostering of self-discipline
- Attitudes toward education, reading, scholarly pursuit
- Attitudes toward imaginative play
- Attitudes toward involvement in sports
- Promotion of gender stereotypes

Communication

- Expression of a wide range of emotion and feeling
- Expression of ideas, concepts, beliefs, values, interests
- Openness
- Verbal expression and sensitive listening
- Consensual decision making

Support, Security, Encouragement

- Balance in activity
- Humor
- Dependency and dominance patterns
- Life support groups of each member
- Social relationship of couple: go out together or separately; change since marriage mutually satisfying; effect of sociability patterns on children

Growth-Producing Relationships and Experiences Within and Without the Family

- Creative play activities
- Planned growth experiences
- Focus of life and activity of each member
- Friendships

Responsible Community Relationships

- Organizations, including involvement, membership, active participation
- Knowledge of and friendship with neighbors

Growing with and Through Children

- Hope and plans for children
- Emulation of own parents and its influence on relationship with children
- Relationship patterns: authoritarian, patriarchal, matriarchal
- Necessity to relive (make up for) own childhood through children

Unity, Loyalty, and Cooperation

Positive interacting of members toward each other

Self-Help and Acceptance of Outside Help in Family Crisis

Figure 2–7 ◆ The Family Assessment tool.
SOURCE: Murray, R. B., & Zentner, J. P. (2001). *Health promotion strategies through the lifespan* (7th ed.). Upper Saddle River, NJ: Prentice Hall, p. 200, Figure 4–2 Family Assessment Tool.

Some studies have also shown that there is very little difference in health status related to the level of acculturation within an ethnic group if strong traditional ties remain within a culture. One study examined the unhealthy behaviors and risk factors for cardiovascular disease among recent immigrants from Sweden and found no difference in those who were acculturated and those who were not. The researchers concluded that the lifestyle factors from their native country dominated norms in their new culture; therefore their risk factors remained unchanged (Gadd, Sundquist, Johansson, & Wandell, 2005).

Impact of Culture on Family Structure

Traditional family structure within the United States usually consists of a nuclear family with an extended family living separately. However, many immigrants to the United States live together with and rely on a network of grandparents and even aunts, uncles, and cousins. For example, Cuban families are often multigenerational and consider grandmothers to be part of the nuclear family. Further, godparents (or *compadrazgos*) are often considered part of the family even if they are not related by blood (Giger & Davidhizar, 2004).

Many Islamic families from West Africa practice polygamy. Although they do not often freely admit this when in the United States, sometimes women live in households with their co-wives. Sometimes the co-wives work well together and get along, and in some cases they do not. Often children view each co-wife as their own mother.

> **CLINICAL TIP**
>
> When caring for a family in which grandparents play a key role in family decision making, the nurse should include the grandparents in the decision-making and teaching sessions because their views are highly respected within the family unit.

Cultural Influences on Childbearing and Childrearing

A family's culture may influence its beliefs about and practices surrounding many aspects of childbearing and childrearing, including beliefs about the importance of children, beliefs and attitudes about pregnancy, health practices, and infant feeding behaviors.

BELIEFS REGARDING THE IMPORTANCE OF CHILDREN

Children are generally valued all over the world, not only for the joy they bring, but also because they ensure continuation of the family and cultural values. This valuing of children may manifest in different ways, however. Families in the United States and many Western countries commonly only have one or two children, often out of a desire to provide the children with the best home and education they can afford, and to spend as much free time with them as possible. Many fear that additional children would too greatly dilute their financial and emotional resources. In contrast, in many cultures throughout the world, it is common to have as many children as possible. In Mali, West Africa, for example, the average woman has about seven children in her lifetime.

An understanding of the meaning of children in a culture may explain reactions of joy or shame to pregnancy. Pregnancy is a joyful event in a culture that values children. In some cultures, a woman who gives birth achieves higher status, especially if the newborn is male (Safadi, 2005). The latter is especially true in traditional Chinese culture and some Middle Eastern cultures (Do, 2005). Similarly, in the western United States, people of the Mormon faith view motherhood as the most important aspect of a woman's life, comparable with the male role of priesthood. In Mexican American society and among many other Hispanic groups, having children is evidence of the male's virility and is a sign of manliness, or *machismo,* a desired trait.

In cultures that value children only when they are born to a legally married couple, however, pregnancy is a shameful event if it occurs outside of marriage. In some Middle Eastern countries, for example, a woman who conceives outside of marriage would be permanently banned from her family. Pregnancy outside of marriage may even be dangerous. In many Muslim countries, an unmarried pregnant woman may seek a clandestine abortion because the consequences of carrying an illegitimate child can be social ostracism or even death—in some cases, even when the pregnancy has resulted from rape. It is not unheard of for women to be killed if the family discovers she engaged in sexual intercourse outside of marriage and became pregnant.

There are also many culturally influenced beliefs related to contraception. Many Muslims from the Middle East may use birth control but do not believe in sterilization because it is a permanent method (Hammoud, White, & Fetters, 2005). Other Muslims may not practice contraception because children are highly valued and it is believed that the traditional role of the woman is to bear children.

In a culture in which children are highly valued, a woman's self-esteem may be related to her childbearing ability. In such cultures, women may even be made to feel that it is their fault if they are unable to bear children. Such women may go to great lengths to preserve their fertility. In Zambia, for example, it is believed that to preserve a woman's fertility, the placenta must be buried so that witches cannot unearth it and harm the mother or the baby (Maimbolwa, Yamba, Diwan, & Ransjö-Arvidson, 2003).

BELIEFS AND ATTITUDES ABOUT PREGNANCY

Beliefs and attitudes about pregnancy may also be culturally influenced and may influence a woman's health behaviors. Thus certain health behaviors can be expected if a culture views pregnancy as a sickness, whereas other behaviors can be expected if pregnancy is viewed as a natural occurrence. Prenatal care may not be a priority for women who view pregnancy as a natural occurrence. For example, in India, pregnancy is considered a normal physiologic event. The husband is rarely involved in attending prenatal visits and has little knowledge of pregnancy and childbirth. The woman gives birth with female family members in attendance, with the husband coming to see his wife only after she has given birth (Fisher, Bowman, & Thomas, 2003).

Attitudes about pregnancy do vary somewhat among cultures. Americans of African descent, for example, usually consider pregnancy as a state of wellness. Mexican Americans generally view pregnancy as a natural and desirable condition, and most Native American groups consider pregnancy a normal process. Although pregnancy is perceived as a natural occurrence in many cultures, it may also be viewed as a time of increased vulnerability. Individuals with European/Western ideas might expect the woman to be away from work before and right after childbirth. In Orthodox Judaism, it is a man's responsibility to procreate, but it is a woman's right, not her obligation, to do so. This is because, according to Orthodox Jewish law, the health of the mother, both physically and mentally, is of primary concern, and she should never be obliged to do something that threatens her life (Semenic, Callister, & Feldman, 2004).

Individuals of many cultures take certain protective precautions based on their beliefs. For example, many women of Malawi, Africa, avoid preparing clothes for the infant during the prenatal period because they believe that this action will lead to the birth of a stillborn infant. Similarly, many Southeast Asian women fear that they will have a complicated labor and birth if they sit in a doorway or on a step. Thus they tend to avoid areas near doors in waiting rooms and examining rooms. For many Vietnamese women, lifting the arms above the head is believed to increase the risk of preterm birth. Vietnamese women are also discouraged from sitting or lying down for lengthy periods because doing so might allow the baby to become too large.

In the Mexican American culture, the concept of *mal aire,* or bad air, is sometimes related to evil spirits. It is thought that air, especially night air, may enter the body and cause illness. Preventive measures, such as keeping the windows closed or covering the head, are used. Some Latinos may place a raisin on the cord stump of a newborn to prevent drafts from entering the baby's body.

For many Southeast Asians, the wind (or *vata*) is a potentially negative force that can disturb the body's internal harmony when a person is in a vulnerable state, such as during and after childbirth or during surgery. The natural forces thought to be more desirable during pregnancy include the earth, for groundedness, and water, for fluidity. Thus, in addition to avoiding wind and drafts, the pregnant woman is encouraged to eat creamy, oily, and other heavy foods, retire early and sleep until dawn, avoid stimulants and stress, and drink plenty of water.

Taboos refer to behaviors or things that are avoided. Many cultures, including those found in the United States, have taboos centered around the unborn baby that are meant to ensure that the baby will survive. Many of these beliefs stem from the fear of injuring an unborn child or the worry that a baby might die. In developing countries, mortality rates among infants and young children are extremely high; thus, certain traditions have centered around preventing early death. For example, it is common among Muslims to avoid naming babies until after birth and to ensure that the first words a baby hears are from God. In the western part of Mali, babies' faces are covered in mud and they are called ugly names to ward off evil spirits. Taboos also emanate from the fear that a pregnant woman has evil powers. For this reason, pregnant women are sometimes prohibited from taking part in certain activities with other people.

Many cultures ascribe to the *equilibrium model of health,* which is based on the concept of balance between light and dark, heat and cold. As described in Chapter 3 ∞, Far Eastern philosophical belief systems focus on the notion of yin and yang. Yin represents the female, passive principle—darkness, cold, and wetness. Yang is the masculine, active principle—light, heat, and dryness. When the two are combined, they are all that can be.

The hot-cold classification is also seen in cultures in Latin America, the Near East, and Southeast Asia. The dimensions and meanings of this classification vary, however, and require further investigation. Spanish priests brought the concept of "hot" and "cold" to Mexico, where it was combined with ancient Aztec beliefs. Consequently, some Mexican Americans may consider illness to be an excess of either hot or cold (Galanti, 2004). To restore health, imbalances are often corrected by the proper use of foods, medications, or herbs. These substances are also classified as hot or cold. For example, an illness attributed to an excess of coldness will be treated only with hot foods or medications. The classification of foods is not always consistent, but it does conform to a general structure of traditional knowledge. Certain foods, spices, herbs, and medications are perceived to cool or heat the body. These perceptions do not necessarily correspond to the actual temperature; some hot dishes are said to have a cooling quality.

Southeast Asians believe it is important to keep the woman "warm" after the birth because blood, which is considered "hot," has been lost, and the woman is at risk of becoming "cold." Therefore, they avoid cold drinks and foods following birth (Holroyd, Twinn, & Yim, 2004). In addition, many women in India consider pregnancy a hot period and eat cool foods to counterbalance the hot state (Holroyd et al., 2004). The concepts of hot and cold are not as important in Native American or African American beliefs. There are some similarities, however, in all of these groups because of the emphasis on a balance in nature.

CLINICAL TIP

When caring for a woman of Asian descent, ask her if she would prefer hot water or ice water at her bedside. This can help ensure that proper oral hydration is maintained and cultural beliefs are supported.

HEALTH PRACTICES DURING PREGNANCY

Health practices during pregnancy are influenced by numerous factors, such as the prevalence of traditional home remedies and folk beliefs, the importance of indigenous healers, and the influence of professional healthcare workers. In an urban setting the age of the family members, length of time in the city, marital status, and strength of the family may affect these patterns. Socioeconomic status is also important because modern medical services are more accessible to those who can afford them.

An awareness of alternative health sources is crucial for health professionals because these practices affect health outcomes. For example, many members of the Mexican American community utilize the *partera,* a lay midwife, as a healer who gives advice and treats illnesses during pregnancy as well as being in attendance during labor and birth.

Indigenous healers are also important in some cultures. In the Mexican American culture the healer is called a *curandero* or *curandera.* In some Native American tribes the medicine man may fulfill the healing role. Herbalists are often found in Asian cultures; and faith healers, root doctors, and spiritualists are sometimes consulted in the African American culture.

CULTURAL NORMS REGARDING INFANT FEEDING PRACTICES

Culture can greatly affect new mothers' as well as experienced mothers' choices in feeding decisions. For example, in the His-

RESEARCH IN PRACTICE

HISPANIC WOMEN'S PERCEPTIONS OF CLIENT-CENTEREDNESS DURING PRENATAL CARE: A MIXED-METHOD STUDY

What is this study about? There is evidence that the quality of prenatal care (e.g., client education, psychosocial support, and behavioral coaching) may affect the outcomes of pregnancy. Client-centered prenatal care means that the provider is responsive to the cultural needs, values, and preferences of the client. The Hispanic population is rapidly growing in the United States, with a higher live birth rate than other racial/ethnic groups. Prior studies have shown that Hispanic mothers do not use healthcare services at the same rate as non-Hispanic groups. These researchers speculate that this may be due in part to perceptions that prenatal care is not responsive to Hispanic cultural and language needs. This study assessed whether Hispanic mothers perceive their prenatal care as patient centered; compared these perceptions with non-Hispanics'; and sought explanations for these perceptions.

How was this study done? A total of 427 mothers in 10 Florida hospitals were interviewed within 48 hours of giving birth. Of these, 359 initiated prenatal care in the first trimester and 68 initiated prenatal care in the third trimester. Of these mothers, 29% were Hispanic, and the rest were classified as white/non-Hispanic, black/non-Hispanic, or Haitian. Five interviewers completed 2 days of training on the interview protocol before conducting the semistructured interviews. The interviews addressed three aspects of client-centered prenatal care: whether nurses and doctors treated them with respect, whether office staff treated them with respect, and the occurrence of communication or language problems with the nurse or physician. Answers were recorded as yes or no, with any response indicating a negative perception followed by exploratory interviewing. The yes/no answers were analyzed using chi square statistics and odds ratios were calculated. Responses to the exploratory interviews were analyzed using constant comparison and qualitative open coding.

What were the results of the study? The majority of Hispanic mothers felt that they were treated with respect by doctors and nurses (86%) and by office staff (80%) and reported no communication or language problems (73%). However, Hispanic mothers responded negatively to all three questions at a higher rate than did non-Hispanic mothers. Hispanic mothers were less likely to perceive that nurses, doctors, and office staff treated them with respect and were more likely to report communication or language problems. The mothers explained that perceiving a lack of respect was related to feeling that the visit was rushed and impersonal, and that their questions were not adequately addressed. The mothers reported that these perceptions affected their ability to understand information given during the visit and reduced their desire to return for subsequent visits.

What additional questions might I have? Do these findings relate to other Hispanic groups that may have a different cultural makeup than Hispanics in Florida? Hispanic mothers in this sample were less educated, younger, and less likely to have insurance; could this affect the outcomes? Does self-report after birth based on recall accurately represent what happened during the prenatal period?

How can I use this study? Cultural and linguistically competent care may benefit Hispanic mothers in the prenatal period. The nurse who is responsive to cultural norms will provide care that is perceived as more patient centered. Responsiveness to the cultural needs of Hispanic mothers may include valuing close interpersonal relationships; a warm, personalized style of interaction; a relaxed sense of time; and a comfortable, informal environment for the prenatal visit. Hispanic mothers may benefit from group prenatal care sessions in which they can discuss their norms and attitudes, ask questions freely, and experience prolonged interaction with providers without feeling rushed.

SOURCE: Tanson, S., Parillo, K., & Keefer, M. (2005) Hispanic women's perceptions of patient-centeredness during prenatal care: A mixed-method study. *Birth*, 32(4), 312–317.

panic culture, women often believe that newborns need to be supplemented with infant formula before the milk comes in. Although colostrum provides vital antibodies for the infant, many Hispanic women refuse to nurse until their milk supply is established. It is important for the nurse to understand cultural norms and make recommendations that complement these norms, rather than conflict with them. In the preceding example, the nurse may advise the woman to first nurse her newborn at the breast and then offer the infant formula.

The majority of research on formula-feeding behavior has been conducted among Hispanic mothers and African American mothers. One common practice in these cultural groups is the addition of foods to the formula bottle, usually after 2 to 3 months, but for some, as early as 2 weeks into a baby's life. The kinds of food added vary from nonnutritive, high-calorie substances like sugar to adult foods like rice, beans, cereal, potatoes, yams, and eggs. Once the food is added, the nipple is often enlarged so that the baby can consume the food, creating a potential choking hazard.

Such supplementation may be done for a variety of reasons. Hispanic mothers report that it is important to add these foods to the formula to help the baby grow to be large. In Latin American culture, many people believe that "the bigger the baby, the better," so parents supplement the breast or formula hoping for a big and healthy baby. Unfortunately, the parents are usually unaware of the fact that the addition of these foods can hurt the growth and health of the infant. Indeed, if a mother does not feed her child in the culturally accepted way, she may appear to be unfit or irresponsible in the community.

A second reason why foods are added to formulas lies in the belief that the addition of traditional foods at a very young age will prepare children to accept and enjoy their traditional foods when they are older. Food is an extremely important component of many Hispanic cultures; it ties people together and is usually the centerpiece of religious events and holidays. This relates to the third reason why foods are added to formula. During the holidays, it is considered important that everyone eat the same thing and participate equally; thus, infants are often included by being given the same foods the adults are eating.

African American mothers have also reported adding foods like cereal, potatoes, evaporated milk, or even extra scoops of powdered formula to thicken the formula. As with Hispanic families, the addition of these foods is thought to be necessary to help the child grow to be big and healthy, but more immediately, it is thought that this thickened formula will better satisfy a baby, so that he or she will sleep better through the night and allow the mother to do so as well. Thin formulas are associated with making a baby cry at night.

Overfeeding is a common cultural behavior as well. Hispanic mothers are reported to often overfeed their infants. Some mothers have reported to feed a child until he or she spits up. That is the indication that a child is eating in a healthful manner. Puerto Rican mothers believe overfeeding to be a protective care behavior that keeps a child healthy, well fed, and safe from illness or harm.

Many immigrants choose formula-feeding over breastfeeding. Although this choice may be partly due to their busy lives, it also can be due to cultural beliefs, particularly among immigrants from developing countries, where the ability to formula-feed is a status symbol because it is so expensive. In Mali, for example, a can of formula can cost the equivalent of $2, although the average individual only earns $200 per year. In the United States, formulas are more affordable and available to the poor; however, when additional cultural practices come into play, such as overfeeding and adding extra formula, the subsidized formulas can run out quickly, and mothers may choose to substitute cow's milk, use canned evaporated or condensed milk, dilute the formula, or purchase unsafe formulas on the "black market." Obviously, these choices have dangerous health implications for the infant.

A nurse may educate a mother in her native language about appropriate infant feeding practices, but the influences from her family and their cultural beliefs may have a greater impact than the health teaching on her feeding behavior. Understanding parents' beliefs and traditions can help nurses to educate families more effectively about healthful feeding behaviors.

Cultural Diversity in Family Nursing Care

Cultural attitudes, behaviors, and beliefs that are related to health can greatly affect how a client will respond to and comply with health advice (Table 2–5). Thus it is critical that nurses develop a holistic understanding of their clients' needs. Healthcare providers are often unaware of the cultural characteristics they themselves demonstrate. Without cultural awareness, caregivers tend to project their own cultural responses onto foreign-born clients; clients from different socioeconomic, religious, or educational groups; or clients from different regions of the country.

This leads caregivers to assume that clients are demonstrating a specific behavior for the same reason that they themselves would. Moreover, healthcare providers frequently fail to recognize that medicine has its own culture, which has been dominated historically by traditional, middle-class values and beliefs.

Ethnocentrism is the conviction that the values and beliefs of one's own cultural group are the best ones or the only acceptable ones. It is characterized by an inability or unwillingness to understand the beliefs or worldview of another group or culture. To a certain extent, most people are guilty of ethnocentrism, at least some of the time. Thus the nurse who values stoicism during labor may be uncomfortable with the more vocal response of a Latin American woman. Another nurse may be disconcerted by the Southeast Asian woman who believes that pain is something to be endured rather than alleviated and is very intent on maintaining self-control in labor (Andrews, Boyle, & Carr, 2003).

Healthcare providers sometimes believe that if members of other cultures do not share Western values, they should adopt them. This is especially difficult for a nurse caring for childbearing families if the nurse is a firm believer in the equality of the sexes and feminism. The nurse may find it difficult to remain silent if a woman from a Middle Eastern culture defers to her husband in decision making. It is important to remember that pressure to defy cultural values and beliefs can be stressful and anxiety provoking for these women.

To address issues of cultural diversity in the provision of health care, emphasis is being placed on developing **cultural competence**—that is, the skills and knowledge necessary to appreciate, understand, and work with individuals from different cultures. It requires self-awareness, awareness and understanding of cultural differences, and the ability to adapt clinical skills and practices as necessary (Tate, 2003).

The nurse can begin developing cultural competence by becoming knowledgeable about the cultural practices of local groups. For example, is it considered courteous to avoid eye contact? Should last names be used in conversation as a sign of respect? Is a female healthcare provider necessary? Do communication and language barriers exist? If so, how can they be addressed?

Giger and Davidhizar (2004) have suggested that care providers conduct a "cultural assessment" to glean information about health practices based on the client's beliefs, values, and customs. This kind of assessment might include questions such as:

1. Who in the family must be consulted before decisions are made about a person's care?

2. Does the client see primarily in the present or does he or she have a futuristic time orientation?

3. What type of health provider is most appropriate for the client?

4. Does the client have beliefs or traditions that may impact the care plan?

Several cultural assessment tools are in use to assist the nurse in obtaining cultural information. Giger and Davidhizar

Table 2–5 CULTURAL RESOURCES

Networks: Health-Related Organizations

National Black Child Development Institute
1023 Fifteenth Street, NW
Suite 600
Washington, DC 20005
(202) 387-1281

National Center for the Advancement of Blacks in the Health Professions
(NCABHP)
P.O. Box 21121
Detroit, MI 48221
(313) 345-4480

American Indian Health Care Association
1550 Larimer Street
Suite 225
Denver, CO 80202
(303) 607-1048

National Indian Health Board
1385 South Colorado Blvd.
Suite A-708
Denver, CO 80222
(303) 759-3075

Asian American Health Forum
116 New Montgomery Street
Suite 531
San Francisco, CA 94105
(415) 541-0866

Asian Pacific Center on Aging
1511 Third Avenue
Seattle, WA 98101
(206) 624-1221

Association of Asian Pacific Community Health Organizations
(AAPCHO)
1212 Broadway, Suite 730
Oakland, CA 94612
(510) 272-9536

Hispanic Health Council
9648 Cedar Street
Hartford, CT 06106
(203) 527-0856

National Coalition of Hispanic Health and Human Services Organizations (COSSMHO)
1501 Sixteenth Street, NW
Washington, DC 20036
(202) 387-5100

American Public Health Association
African American, Asian, Hispanic, and Native American Caucus
1015 Fifteenth Street, NW
Washington, DC 20005
(202) 789-5600

National Council for International Health
1701 K Street, NW
Suite 600
Washington, DC 20006
(202) 833-5903

National Multicultural Institute
3000 Connecticut Avenue, NW
Suite 438
Washington, DC 20008
(202) 483-0700

Cross-Cultural Health Care Program
1200 Twelfth Avenue S
Seattle, WA 98144
(206) 621-4161
http://www.xculture.org/

The Center for Cross-Cultural Health
1313 SE Fifth Street, Suite 100B
Minneapolis, MN 55414
(612) 379-3573
http://www.crosshealth.com/

Web Sites

Ethnomed
This site provides health information for a variety of ethnic groups.
http://ethnomed.org/

Culture Clues

Culture Clues are tip sheets for clinicians designed to increase awareness about concepts and preferences of patients from the diverse cultures served by the University of Washington Medical Center. Currently there are five cultures represented, with additional ones in progress.
http://depts.washington.edu/pfes/cultureclues.html

Transcultural and Multicultural Health Links
This site provides general resources for a variety of ethnic and special population groups.
http://www.iun.edu/~libemb/trannurs/trannurs.htm

(2004) developed a transcultural assessment tool that identifies the cultural background, communication patterns, issues related to personal space, social organization, time, roles within the environment, biologic variations, and a nursing assessment (Figure 2–8 ◆).

Culturally Influenced Responses

It is imperative when caring for families that nurses provide culturally sensitive care that supports cultural differences. The nurse who respects cultural diversity is an asset to the childbearing family as they adjust to their new role. Establishing a trusting relationship enables the nurse to assist the family in meeting educational needs. The nurse who considers the woman's personal values, beliefs, and customs will be a far more effective caregiver than the nurse who does not.

BIOLOGICAL DIFFERENCES

Genetic and physical differences occur among cultural groups and can lead to disparities in needs and care. African Americans are more likely to experience hypertension, strokes, obesity, di-

abetes, and sickle cell anemia. Thalassemia, another type of anemia, occurs primarily in individuals of Mediterranean descent. African Americans and Native Americans tend to have higher rates of tuberculosis than the general population. On the other hand, African Americans have higher bone mass than Caucasians and lower rates of osteoporosis. Caucasians have higher rates of heart disease. Caucasians from certain geographic regions have higher rates of cystic fibrosis, celiac disease, and Crohn's disease. Hispanics have higher rates of diabetes and lactose intolerance. Asians and Native Americans often do not metabolize alcohol readily and are more prone to either injury after alcohol ingestion or to alcohol abuse. Otitis media, or infection of the middle ear, is common in Native American and Alaskan Native children. Diabetes, liver disease, and injuries are common in Native American groups (Spector, 2004). Metabolism of certain drugs is also linked to genetics in certain groups.

Nurses must understand other genetic characteristics in order to provide culturally competent nursing assessments and interventions. Differences in skin color may make cyanosis, pallor,

---

A Transcultural Assessment Model

CULTURALLY UNIQUE INDIVIDUAL

1. Place of birth
2. Cultural definition
   What is . . .
3. Race
   What is . . .
4. Length of time in country

COMMUNICATION

1. Voice quality
   A. Strong, resonant
   B. Soft
   C. Average
   D. Shrill
2. Pronunciation and enunciation
   A. Clear
   B. Slurred
   C. Dialect
3. Use of silence
   A. Infrequent
   B. Often
   C. Length
      (1) Brief
      (2) Moderate
      (3) Long
      (4) Not observed
4. Use of nonverbal
   A. Hand movement
   B. Eye movement
   C. Moves entire body
   D. Kinesics (gestures, expressions, or stances)
5. Touch
   A. Startles or withdraws when touched
   B. Accepts touch without difficulty
   C. Touches others without difficulty

6. Ask these and similar questions:
   A. How do you get your point across to others?
   B. Do you like communicating with friends, family, and acquaintances?
   C. When asked a question, do you usually respond (in words or body movements, or both)?
   D. If you have something important to discuss with your family, how would you approach them?

SPACE

1. Degree of comfort
   A. Moves when space invaded
   B. Does not move when invaded
2. Distance in conversations
   A. 0 to 18 inches
   B. 18 inches to 3 feet
   C. 3 feet or more
3. Definition of space
   A. Describe degree of comfort with closeness when talking with or standing near others
   B. How do objects (e.g., furniture) in the environment affect your sense of space?
4. Ask these and similar questions:
   A. When you talk with family members, how close do you stand?
   B. When you communicate with coworkers and other acquaintances, how close do you stand?
   C. If a stranger touches you, how do you react or feel?
   D. If a loved one touches you, how do you react or feel?
   E. Are you comfortable with the distance between us now?

SOCIAL ORGANIZATION

1. Normal state of health
   A. Poor
   B. Fair
   C. Good
   D. Excellent

Figure 2–8 ◆ Cultural assessment tool.

2. Ask these and similar questions:
   A. How do you define social activities?
   B. What are some activities that you enjoy?
   C. What are your hobbies, or what do you do when you have free time?
   D. Do you believe in a Supreme Being?
   E. How do you worship that Supreme Being?
   F. What is your function (what do you do) in your family unit/system?
   G. What is your role in your family unit/system (father, mother, child, advisor)?
   H. When you were a child, what or who influenced you most?
   I. What is/was your relationship with your siblings and parents?
   J. What does work mean to you?
   K. Describe your past, present, and future jobs.
   L. What are your political views?
   M. How have your political views influenced your attitude toward health and illness?

TIME

1. Orientation to time
   A. Past-oriented
   B. Present-oriented
   C. Future-oriented
2. View of time
   A. Social time
   B. Clock-oriented
3. Physiochemical reaction to time
   A. Sleeps at least 8 hours a night
   B. Goes to sleep and wakes on a consistent schedule
   C. Understands the importance of taking medication and other treatments on schedule
4. Ask these and similar questions:
   A. What kind of timepiece do you wear daily?
   B. If you have an appointment at 2 PM, what time is acceptable to arrive?
   C. If a nurse tells you that you will receive a medication in "about a half hour," realistically, how much time will you allow before calling the nurses' station?

ENVIRONMENTAL CONTROL

1. Locus-of-control
   A. Internal locus-of-control (believes that the power to affect change lies within)
   B. External locus-of-control (believes that fate, luck, and chance have a great deal to do with how things turn out)
2. Value orientation
   A. Believes in supernatural forces
   B. Relies on magic, witchcraft, and prayer to affect change
   C. Does not believe in supernatural forces
   D. Does not rely on magic, witchcraft, or prayer to affect change
3. Ask these and similar questions:
   A. How often do you have visitors at your home?
   B. Is it acceptable to you for visitors to drop in unexpectedly?
   C. Name some ways your parents or other persons treated your illnesses when you were a child.
   D. Have you or someone else in your immediate surroundings ever used a home remedy that made you sick?
   E. What home remedies have you used that worked? Will you use them in the future?

F. What is your definition of "good health"?
G. What is your definition of illness or "poor health"?

BIOLOGIC VARIATIONS

1. Conduct a complete physical assessment noting:
   A. Body structure
   B. Skin color
   C. Unusual skin discolorations
   D. Hair color and distribution
   E. Other visible physical characteristics (e.g., keloids, chloasma)
2. Ask these and similar questions:
   A. What diseases or illnesses are common in your family?
   B. Describe your family's typical behavior when a family member is ill.
   C. How do you respond when you are angry?
   D. Who (or what) usually helps you to cope during a difficult time?
   E. What foods do you and your family like to eat?
   F. Have you ever had any unusual cravings for:
      (1) White or red clay dirt?
      (2) Laundry starch?
   G. When you were a child what types of foods did you eat?
   H. What foods are family favorites or are considered traditional?

NURSING ASSESSMENT

1. Note whether the client has become culturally assimilated or observes own cultural practices.
2. Incorporate data into plan of nursing care:
   A. Encourage the client to discuss cultural differences; people from diverse cultures who hold different worldviews can enlighten nurses.
   B. Make efforts to accept and understand methods of communication.
   C. Respect the individual's personal need for space.
   D. Respect the rights of clients to honor and worship the Supreme Being of their choice.
   E. Identify a clerical or spiritual person to contact.
   F. Determine whether spiritual practices have implications for health, life, and well-being (e.g., Jehovah's Witnesses may refuse blood and blood derivatives; an Orthodox Jew may eat only Kosher food high in sodium and may not drink milk when meat is served).
   G. Identify hobbies, especially when devising interventions for short or extended convalescence or for rehabilitation.
   H. Honor time and value orientations and differences in these areas. Allay anxiety and apprehension if adherence to time is necessary.
   I. Provide privacy according to personal need and health status of the client (Note: the perception and reaction to pain may be culturally related).
   J. Note cultural health practices
      (1) Identify and encourage efficacious practices.
      (2) Identify and discourage dysfunctional practices.
      (3) Identify and determine whether neutral practices will have a long-term ill effect.
   K. Note food preferences
      (1) Make as many adjustments in diet as health status and long-term benefits will allow and that dietary department can provide.
      (2) Note dietary practices that may have serious implications for the client.

Figure 2–8 ◆ Cultural assessment tool. *continued*

SOURCE: Reprinted from *Transcultural Nursing: Assessment and Intervention,* by J. N. Giger and R. E. Davidhizar, Copyright © 1991, with permission from Elsevier.

and jaundice difficult to recognize and describe. Mongolian spots are darkened skin spots on the lower back and buttocks of some babies with dark skin. Variations in texture of hair require different approaches to hygiene among various racial groups.

COMMUNICATION PATTERNS

Communication is a method by which members of culture groups share information and preserve their beliefs, values, norms, and practices. To ensure effective nursing care, it is essential for nurses to be able to communicate with the family. This becomes an issue when the family and nurse do not speak the same language. In such cases, translators should be provided. The Joint Commission of Accreditation of Hospital Organizations (JCAHO) requires that hospitals provide a mechanism for clients to communicate in their own language. This reduces medical errors and increases effective communication (Illinois Hospital Association, 2006). The use of children and other family members to act in the role of translator is not recommended because of confidentiality issues (Spector, 2004). Written instructions, signs, and brochures should be offered in the individuals' native language.

Language can also affect health literacy skills. A large number of instructions are given in writing. Examples include prescriptions and directions on medication bottles, signs hanging in health facilities, consent forms for procedures and surgery, insurance forms, directions for techniques or procedures, future appointment dates, and health promotion materials. Nurses need to verify that the client and family can read and whether alternate methods are needed. Nurses can verbally give the information and provide paper and pencil so that the family can write it down in their own language. Translation services should be available in all healthcare settings.

Variations in communication among cultures are reflected in their word meaning, voice inflection and quality, and verbal styles. Culture not only influences the manner in which feelings are expressed, but also which verbal and nonverbal expressions of communication are considered appropriate. An individual's willingness to discuss certain topics or to express or conceal certain thoughts and feelings are also influenced by the cultural norms. For example, Native Americans and people of Asian descent may feel it is appropriate to remain quiet when experiencing pain, whereas people of Italian, Jewish, and Latino descent may feel that it is best to express pain more vocally.

Use of names varies among cultural groups. Assuming that each person wishes to be called by a first name can be disrespectful. Address family members respectfully, usually using terms such as Mr., Mrs., and Ms. If the person has a title such as doctor, judge, or senator, it should be used. Ask what the person prefers to be called and record this in the health record for future reference. In some cultures such as Korean, Cambodian, and Filipino, the first name used is actually the family name. Asking for the "family name" rather than the "last name" may clarify this practice.

Nonverbal Communication

Nonverbal communication patterns may hinder or help communication. For example, gestures and body language may be misunderstood or misinterpreted. Similarly, eye contact has different meanings among cultures. European Americans, for example, value eye contact with communication and interpret this as a sign of sincerity and interest. In other cultures, such as Asian and Native American, sustained eye contact may be considered rude or disrespectful.

Silence may also be considered a sign of respect in some cultures. Among those groups, offering an immediate response to a question may be viewed as being disrespectful because an instant reply could indicate that no thought was given to the matter. Nurses should watch for patterns in various cultures and alter their own approach to be more congruent. For example, many nurses commonly nod and say "yes" or "oh, I see" when a healthcare client is speaking. This may seem disruptive to some cultures. Noting that the listener is silent and does not use such patterns of agreement helps the nurse alter his or her own response to match more closely the acceptable method of communication for the family. Nurses need to learn that silence and quiet listening can be perceived as positive approaches.

Touch

The appropriateness of touch varies with each culture. For example, an Asian may consider touching an unfamiliar person of the opposite gender to be inappropriate, whereas touch between men and women may be viewed as appropriate by another culture. Adults commonly feel that it is acceptable to touch children of all ages but this may not be accurate. Nurses should look for responses from family to touch and progress accordingly.

Space

Depending on an individual's specific culture, the use of space has different meanings. "Space," as defined in this context, refers to the relationship between the individual and other persons and objects in the environment. Cultures may have specific spatial preferences, such as personal distance and social distance. Some cultures tend to prefer close contact with less space because they use touch as a form of communication. Nurses should be alert for how close a childbearing woman or a child comes to them and other individuals and try to maintain this space in their interactions. Nursing procedures often cause the space barrier to be broken. Nurses need to touch clients to take vital signs, administer injections, change dressings, and the like. This does not mean that close touch is appropriate at all times. Telling all clients before touching them for procedures will help them understand what is happening.

TIME ORIENTATION

Time orientation can vary significantly among cultures. Cultural groups may place emphasis on the events of the past, those events that occur in the present, or those events that will occur in the future. Time is also influenced by development so that young children sometimes do not understand the use of clocks, the importance ascribed to being "on time," or other time orientations.

Cultures that are oriented predominantly to the past may want to begin healthcare encounters with lengthy descriptions of past healthcare treatments, family history of diseases, or individual past experiences with health. There may be little interest in learning methods of adapting to or maintaining a new plan of care.

For cultures that are oriented predominantly to the present, little consideration may be given to either the past or the future. For example, adolescents commonly focus on the present and may not engage in preventive health practices for long-term health. Short-term goals often provide more incentive to adolescents.

Cultures that are oriented predominantly to the future, such as European Americans, may not focus on what is important at the present time. For example, the family focusing on the future may focus on the dreams they had for a child's education or sports performance and have trouble setting present goals for treatment of a disease such as juvenile rheumatoid arthritis. One commonly hears that it was a big adjustment to learn to "take one day at a time." Not living up to the family's expectation for their future success may be difficult for a child who has developed an illness that has a chronic course.

Time also refers to punctuality about schedules and appointments. In the United States and Canada, the predominant culture respects promptness and considers time valuable and not to be wasted. Other cultures may not reflect this same concern for time. This may be manifested by a family's inability to follow timed medication schedules or treatments, or to show up as scheduled for an appointment. In these cases, it is not intended as a sign of disrespect.

IMPACT OF RELIGION AND SPIRITUALITY

The goal of truly holistic care of the childbearing family requires that the nurse understand the influence that religion and spirituality may have on their childbearing experience.

Diverse Meanings of Religion and Spirituality

The terms *religion* and *spirituality* mean very different things to different people. Although many people think of **religion** as an institutionalized system that shares a common set of beliefs and practices, others define it more simply as a belief in a transcendent power. The latter definition approaches most people's understanding of **spirituality** as a concern with the spirit or soul.

Philosophers and mystics have debated the meaning of religion for millennia, but within the last 200 years, technologic advances and the ascendance of rationalism and postmodernism have led many influential thinkers to condemn religion as mere wishful thinking. For example, in 1844, philosopher Karl Marx famously decried religion as "the opium of the people" (Marx, 1971), and in 1932, in his *New Introductory Lectures on Psychoanalysis,* psychologist Sigmund Freud stated: "Religion is an illusion . . . an attempt to get control over the sensory world, in which we are placed, by means of the wish-world . . ." (Freud, 1965). More recently, however, religious teachers as diverse as the Buddhist monk Thich Nhat Hanh, Benedictine monk Brother David Steindl-Rast, and the mystic J. Krishnamurti

have offered new visions of a religious life grounded in day-to-day experience. For Hanh (1995), "Religious life is life." According to Krishnamurti (1989), "To be religious is to be sensitive to reality."

Range of Religious Beliefs

These diverse meanings and approaches to religion and spirituality are reflected in the diversity of religious beliefs encountered in contemporary childbearing families. Some may belong to large institutionalized religious organizations; others may feel deeply religious yet have no formal affiliation or practice. Many clients are *agnostic,* or doubtful about the existence of a transcendent being, or truly *atheist,* meaning that they believe there is no higher power. Internationally and in the United States, Christianity is the largest organized religious group, with over 2.1 billion members worldwide accounting for approximately 33% of the world's population. Another 21% of people worldwide are Islamic, and 14% are Hindu. Whatever their religious affiliation, Americans are overwhelmingly religious: fully 95% state that they believe in a higher power (Hunter, 2005).

A childbearing family's religious beliefs, affiliation, and practices can influence deeply their experience and attitudes toward health care, childbearing, and childrearing. Members of certain religious groups such as Christian Scientists may attempt to avoid all medical interventions, whereas others such as Jehovah's Witnesses may refuse specific interventions, such as blood transfusions. Roman Catholics may refuse contraception. Many religions promote childbearing as a sacred right and responsibility, and some prescribe childrearing practices as well. In most cases, the woman and her family gain comfort from acknowledgment of and respect for their religious beliefs and practices in the healthcare setting. However, the agnostic or atheist family may be offended if care providers assume that references to God or a higher power will be comforting.

Provision of Spiritually Sensitive Nursing Care

For all these reasons, nurses are increasingly committed to providing spiritually sensitive nursing care to childbearing families. On admission to the clinic or labor setting, a religious or spiritual history is now included when assessing the childbearing family. Many clients specify a religious affiliation on admission to an acute care facility, but more specific information is also needed. The assessment can include questions about current spiritual beliefs and practices that will affect the mother and baby during the hospital stay, or preferences for religious rituals during labor and birth.

Whenever possible, the nurse and other healthcare providers should attempt to accommodate religious rituals and practices requested by the childbearing family. Most such requests, such as for certain music, foods, or keeping a statue or picture by the bed, can be accommodated without causing danger; however, some, such as lighting candles, could present a risk in an acute care setting. In these circumstances, the family should be given a clear explanation of why the particular action cannot safely be carried out. In addition, nurses can provide clients with resources to meet their religious needs, such as consultation with on-staff chaplains. In settings where chaplains are not readily available, the nurse should be familiar with community resources in the area and offer referral as needed. In circumstances of spiritual distress, such as with severe fetal deformity or loss of a newborn, the family may prefer to meet with their personal religious adviser, and the nurse can arrange for that visit.

Considering the diversity of religious beliefs, it is not unusual for nurses to encounter childbearing families whose beliefs conflict with their own. This is not problematic as long as the nurse avoids attempts to influence the client's decision making. For example, a nurse who does not believe in baptism should avoid revealing this belief to a Catholic client seeking baptism for her stillborn infant. Nurses should also examine their religious beliefs related to genetic screening procedures, use of assisted reproductive technology to achieve pregnancy, use of technology to support life in a severely compromised newborn, abortion, and even less dramatic issues such as methods of contraception, circumcision, and infant feeding. In many institutions, nurses can ask to be reassigned to a different client if their religious beliefs are in conflict; however, if other personnel are not available, it is the nurse's responsibility to provide sensitive, appropriate, and nonjudgmental care to that client.

CHAPTER REVIEW

FOCUS YOUR STUDY

- Family values, power, and roles are important to consider when attempting to provide holistic health care to contemporary families.

- Multiple trends have influenced changes in the traditional family, including employment trends, changes in marital status patterns, and economic trends.

- Nuclear families consist of a mother, father, and children.

- Dual-career/dual-earner families make up the majority of contemporary families in the United States.

- Childless families are a growing trend in American culture.

- Extended family members can play an active role in family life, decision making, and family roles.

- Single-parent families account for almost a third of all US families, and stepparent and binuclear families are increasingly common.

- The developmental framework looks at a family over time as it progresses through predictable stages within the life cycle.

- A family assessment provides an in-depth tool to collect pertinent family life information that can assist the nurse in planning care.

- Culture plays a significant part in a family's development, roles, and observance of traditions, customs, and taboos.

- Cultural norms influence a family's beliefs about the importance of children, pregnancy, health practices, and infant feeding.

- A cultural assessment can assist the nurse in identifying cultural norms and providing culturally appropriate nursing care.

- A religious history is included when assessing contemporary families. Whenever possible, the nurse accommodates the family's religious-based preferences for care.

EXPLORE MediaLink

http://www.prenhall.com/davidson

NCLEX review questions, case studies, and other interactive resources for this chapter can be found on the Web Site at http://www.prenhall.com/davidson. Click on "Chapter 2" to select the activities for this chapter.

For tutorials including animations and videos, more NCLEX review questions, and an audio glossary, access the accompanying Prentice Hall Nursing MediaLink DVD-ROM in this book.

PRENTICE HALL NURSING MEDIALINK DVD-ROM
Audio Glossary
NCLEX Review

COMPANION WEBSITE
Additional NCLEX Review
Case Study: Family Assessment
Care Plan Activity: *Effects of Hispanic Culture on Infant Feeding Practices*
Applications: *Ethnocentrism and Health Care— Providing Culturally Sensitive Care; Examine Your Cultural Influences*
Critical Thinking

CRITICAL THINKING IN ACTION

CULTURAL BELIEFS AND HEALTH PRACTICES

View the Critical Thinking in Action video in Chapter 2 of the DVD-ROM. Then answer the questions that follow.

While working in an inner-city clinic for adolescents, you meet a new client, a 14-year-old Latina girl named Juanita. She is accompanied by her parents. None of them speak English. Through a translator, Juanita tells you that she recently moved here with her parents. They have brought her here today because she has a sore throat. The *curandero* they took her to see pre-scribed the herbal remedy echinacea, but her throat is still sore. The rapid test you perform for strep throat is positive, and the nurse practitioner prescribes an antibiotic.

1. According to the national standards for culturally and linguistically appropriate services in health care set by the government, what are examples of important standards of care that you, as the nurse, can provide in the care of this adolescent?

2. How can you, as the nurse, take steps to achieve cultural competence?

3. How would you, as the nurse, be able to address some of the disparities that can exist when this client comes to the clinic?

4. What are some examples of common food preferences in the Latino American culture?

REFERENCES

Andrews, M. M., Boyle, J. S., & Carr, T. J. (2003). *Transcultural concepts in nursing care* (4th ed.). Philadelphia: Lippincott Williams & Wilkins.

Barnes, D. M., & Harrison, C. L. (2004). Refugee women's reproductive health in early resettlement. *Journal of Obstetric, Gynecologic, & Neonatal Nursing, 33*(6), 723–728.

Carter, E. A., & McGoldrick, M. (Eds.). (2005). *The expanded family life cycle: Individual, family, and social perspectives* (3rd ed.). New York: Allyn & Bacon.

Do, H. (2005). *Chinese culture.* Ethnomed. Retrieved November 29, 2005, from http://ethnomed.org/ethnomed/cultures/chinese/chinese_cp.html

Duvall, E. M. (1977). *Marriage and family development* (5th ed.). New York: Harper Row.

Fields, J. (2003). *America's families and living arrangements: 2003s. Current population reports.* (No. P20–553). Washington, DC: US Census Bureau.

Fisher, J. A., Bowman, M., & Thomas, T. (2003). Issues for South Asian Indian patients surrounding sexuality, fertility, and childbirth in the US healthcare system. *Journal of the American Board of Family Medicine, 16,* 151–155.

Freud, S. (1965). *New introductory lectures on psychoanalysis* (lecture 35). New York: W. W. Norton. (Original work published 1932.)

Friedman, M. M., Bowden, V. R., & Jones, E. (2003). *Family nursing: Research, theory and practice* (5th ed.). Upper Saddle River, NJ, Prentice Hall Health.

Gadd, M., Sundquist, J., Johansson, S. E., & Wandell, P. (2005). Do immigrants have an increased prevalence of unhealthy behaviours and risk factors for coronary heart disease? *European Journal of Cardiovascular Prevention & Rehabilitation, 12*(6), 535–541.

Galanti, G. A. (2004). *Caring for patients from different cultures* (3rd ed.). Philadelphia: University of Pennsylvania Press.

Gates, G. J., & Ost, J. (2004). *The gay and lesbian atlas.* Washington, DC: Urban Institute Press.

Giger, J. N., & Davidhizar, R. E. (2004). *Transcultural nursing: Assessment and interventions* (4th ed.). St. Louis, MO: Mosby.

Gupta, A., Kumar, A., & Stewart, D. E. (2002). Cervical cancer screening among South Asian women in Canada: The role of education and acculturation. *Health Care for Women International, 23*(3), 123–134.

Hammoud, M. M., White, C. B., & Fetters, M. D. (2005). Opening cultural doors: Providing culturally sensitive healthcare to Arab American and American Muslim patients. *American Journal of Obstetrics & Gynecology, 193*(4), 1307–1311.

Hanh, T. N. (1995). *Living Buddha, living Christ.* New York: Riverhead Books.

Hansen, L. K., Feigl, P., Modiano, M. R., Lopez, J. A., Escobedo S. S., Moinpour, C. M., et al. (2005). An educational program to increase cervical and breast cancer screening in Hispanic women: A Southwest oncology group study. *Cancer Nursing, 28*(1), 47–53.

Holroyd, E., Twinn, S., & Yim, I. W. (2004). Exploring Chinese women's cultural beliefs and behaviours regarding the practice of "doing the month." *Women's Health, 40*(3), 109–123.

Hunter, P. (2005). *Largest religious groups in the U.S.A.* Retrieved January 17, 2006, from http://www.Adherants.com

Illinois Hospital Association. (2006). *Quality improvement and performance reporting updates.* Chicago: Author.

Krishnamurti, J. (1989). *Think on these things.* New York: Harper Perennial.

Lau, A. S., McCabe, K. M., Yeh, M., Garland, A. F., Wood, P. A., & Hough, R. L. (2005). The acculturation gap-distress hypothesis among high-risk Mexican American families. *Journal of Family Psychology, 19*(3), 367–375.

Maimbolwa, M. C., Yamba, B., Diwan, V., & Ransjö-Arvidson, A. (2003). Cultural childbirth practices and beliefs in Zambia. *Journal of Advanced Nursing, 43*(3), 263–274.

Marx, K. (1971). *Critique of the Hegelian Philosophy of Right.* Cambridge, England: Cambridge University Press. (Original work published 1844.)

Mishel, L., Bernstein, J., & Boushey, H. (2003). *The state of working America: 2002/2003.* Ithaca, NY: Cornell University Press.

Murray, R. B., & Zentner, J. P. (2001). *Health promotion strategies through the lifespan* (7th ed.). Upper Saddle River, NJ: Prentice-Hall.

Nye, F. I., & Gecas, V. (1976). The role concept: Review and delineation. In F. I. Nye (Ed.), *Structure and analysis of the family.* Beverly Hills, CA: Sage.

Olson, D. H., & Cromwell, R. E. (1975). Methodological issues in family power. In R. E. Cromwell & D. H. Olson (Eds.), *Power in families.* New York: Sage.

Page, R. (2004). Positive pregnancy outcomes in Mexican immigrants: What can we learn? *Journal of Obstetric, Gynecologic, & Neonatal Nursing, 33*(6), 783–790.

Parad, H. J., & Caplan, G. (1965). A framework for studying families in crisis. In H. J. Parad (Ed.), *Crisis intervention: Selected readings.* New York: Family Services of America.

Safadi, R. (2005). Jordanian women: Perceptions and practices of first-time pregnancy. *International Journal of Nursing Practice, 11*(6), 269–276.

Semenic, S. E., Callister, L. C., & Feldman, P. (2004). Giving birth: The voices of Orthodox Jewish women living in Canada. *Journal of Obstetric, Gynecologic, & Neonatal Nursing, 33*(1), 80–87.

Slater, S. (1995). *The lesbian family life cycle.* New York: The Free Press.

Smith D. M., & Gates, G. J. (2001). *Gay and lesbian families in the United States: Same-sex, unmarried partner households.* A preliminary analysis of 2000 United States Census data. A Human Rights Campaign Report. Washington, DC: Human Rights Campaign.

Spector, R. E. (2004). *Cultural diversity in health and illness* (6th ed.). Upper Saddle River, NJ: Prentice Hall Health.

Stepfamily Association of America. (2005). *Stepfamily factsheet.* Lincoln, NE: Author. Retrieved November 29, 2005, from http://www.saafamilies.org

St. Hill, P., Lipson, J. G., & Meleis, A. I. (2003). *Caring for women cross-culturally.* Philadelphia: F. A. Davis.

Tasker, F. (2005). Lesbian mothers, gay fathers, and their children: A review. *Journal of Developmental and Behavioral Pediatrics, 26*(3), 224–240.

Tate, D. M. (2003). Cultural awareness: Bridging the gap between caregivers and Hispanic patients. *Journal of Continuing Education in Nursing, 34*(5), 213–217.

US Census Bureau. (2003). *Fertility of American women: June 2002.* Retrieved November 6, 2004, from http://www.census.gov/prod/2003pubs/p20-548.pdf

US Census Bureau. (2004). *America's family and living arrangements: 2003.* Retrieved November 6, 2004, from http://www.census.gov/population/www/socdemo/hh-fam/cps2002.html

US Census Bureau. (2006). American Fact Finder: Glossary. Retrieved on September 2, 2006, from http://factfinder.census.gov/home/en/epss/glossary-2.html

CHAPTER
3

Complementary and Alternative Therapies

As part of a continuing education course on body-based therapies for nurses, I was giving a back massage to one of my classmates. At one point, I felt a buzz of energy shoot up my hands and arms. At that exact moment, the other student said, "Wow!" Our instructor just laughed and said, "Oh, you're just exchanging friendly energy." That experience changed forever my views as a nurse and educator. I like the fact that nursing is based in science, but I remain open to the mysteries of the human body, mind, and spirit.

KEY TERMS

Acupressure   60
Acupuncture   60
Alternative therapy   48
Aromatherapy   60
Ayurveda   54
Biofeedback   55
Chiropractic   56
Complementary therapy   48
Guided imagery   55
Hatha yoga   58
Homeopathy   53

Hypnosis   55
Integrative medicine   50
Massage therapy   56
Naturopathy   53
Reflexology   57
Reiki   61
Therapeutic Touch   61
Traditional Chinese medicine (TCM)   53
Visualization   55

OBJECTIVES

1. Distinguish between *complementary* and *alternative therapies.*
2. Identify several factors that have contributed to the rise in popularity of complementary and alternative therapies in the United States and Canada.
3. Describe the role of the National Center for Complementary and Alternative Medicine.
4. Explain the role of complementary and alternative therapies in promoting wellness, disease prevention, and holistic healing.
5. Delineate the risks of using complementary and alternative therapies.
6. Compare the basic principles and components of naturopathy, homeopathy, traditional Chinese medicine, and ayurvedic medicine.
7. Describe the use of mind-body therapies in promoting the well-being of childbearing families.
8. Contrast the different manipulative and body-based therapies.
9. Explain the advantages and disadvantages to childbearing women of therapies involving ingestion of substances such as foods, dietary supplements, herbs, and homeopathic remedies.
10. Distinguish between acupressure and acupuncture.
11. Distinguish between Reiki and Therapeutic Touch.
12. Discuss complementary therapies appropriate for the nurse to use with childbearing families.

 MEDIALINK

Additional resources for this content can be found on the Prentice Hall Nursing MediaLink DVD-ROM and on the Companion Website at http://www.prenhall.com/davidson. Click on "Chapter 3" to select the activities for this chapter.

Until the latter part of the 20th century in the United States, it was rare for European American childbearing families to consult anyone except their obstetrician for advice about their pregnancy, birth, and postpartum. Though such clients are still encountered today, perinatal nurses are more likely to care for childbearing families who integrate other types of practitioners and therapies with traditional Western medicine. Families choosing complementary and alternative therapies may include those whose health practices are rooted in their cultural heritage, as well as European Americans who have explored one or more of the vast number of non-Western healing approaches available today. The nurse may even encounter families who consider alternative approaches superior to the diagnostics and treatments that conventional Western medicine offers, and who enter a clinic or hospital environment only reluctantly.

Because the use of complementary and alternative therapies has become so widespread, all nurses need to have at least a fundamental understanding of their benefits and risks and guidelines for their safe use. The chapter begins with an overview of the evolution of complementary and alternative therapies. A brief description of the most common therapies currently used by childbearing families is also provided.

EVOLUTION OF COMPLEMENTARY AND ALTERNATIVE THERAPIES

A **complementary therapy** may be defined as any procedure or product that is used together with conventional medical treatment (National Center for Complementary and Alternative Medicine [NCCAM], 2005). For example, a childbearing woman might request aromatherapy to help her cope with the discomfort she anticipates following a scheduled cesarean birth. Although complementary therapies were entirely absent from clinics and hospitals until the last few decades, they are now often used in conjunction with surgery, pharmaceuticals, and other conventional treatments for a variety of injuries and illnesses. They are also being more and more frequently integrated with conventional perinatal care.

In contrast, an **alternative therapy** is used in place of conventional medicine (NCCAM, 2005). For example, a woman with a postterm pregnancy may refuse medication to induce labor, and instead ingest an herb she believes will stimulate contractions. Because alternative therapies are used in place of medically prescribed treatments, clients may be reluctant to discuss them with a conventional physician or registered nurse.

The very terms *complementary* and *alternative* suggest the contemporary view that herbs, homeopathy, chiropractic, and other such healing techniques are peripheral to conventional Western medicine, which is the "primary" treatment. How did we come to hold this view? And what has contributed to the resurgence in complementary and alternative therapies in the last few decades?

Historical Perspective

Five hundred years ago, a Native American woman drinking hot water steeped with chamomile to settle her stomach would never have described her beverage as a complementary or alternative therapy. She was merely following a custom handed down to her by her ancestors and practiced widely in her tribe. If her symptoms continued, she would likely have consulted a medicine woman or medicine man, who might have performed a healing ritual using other herbs, stones, chanting, and/or communion with the "animal spirits" or ancestors who had passed on. Such forms of self- and community-based treatment, though varying somewhat from one culture to another, are thought to have been the norm around the world for thousands of years.

Many therapies that are today considered complementary or alternative grew out of indigenous cultures' use of the herbs, spices, flowers, fruits, and other plants and natural materials available in the region, and reflected their health concerns. For example, it has been proposed that one rationale for the highly spiced cuisine of India is that the spices used, in addition to being widely available, have an antimicrobial effect. This would have been important for a hot region of the world where food could not be preserved without fear of spoilage. In contrast, people in colder regions of the world, such as northern Europe, developed techniques such as salting, drying, and freezing foods during long winters to preserve them from microbial decay.

Many other complementary and alternative therapies developed from cultures' spiritual beliefs. Thousands of years ago, most cultures held the belief that illnesses and injuries—as well as therapies to heal them—were spiritually based. For example, peoples from ancient China, India, and the Americas shared the belief that all animals, plants, and even minerals contain a spiritual "essence," a vibrational life force that could be employed in healing. European peoples once believed that disease was caused by supernatural forces either to punish human beings or to teach them spiritual lessons. Others, such as the people of ancient India, believed that illness demonstrated a lack of alignment of the mind and body with God. For Patanjali, who wrote the *Yoga Sutras* in the third century BCE, a healthy body was a precondition for spiritual wholeness. In some cultures, spiritual healers performed rituals to exorcise the evil spirit from the diseased body.

Around 400 BCE, Hippocrates became the first practitioner in the West known to challenge the idea that illnesses and injuries have spiritual causes and remedies. His school of medicine investigated impurities in the individual's food, water, and environment as causes of disease, and attempted to base healing practices in the known laws of nature. Students began to investigate systematically the healing properties of local plants and other substances, and to develop standards of practice.

Over the next millennium, indigenous peoples worldwide continued to hand down the knowledge of healing plants and practices. Shamans, alchemists, and midwives were highly respected members of their communities and were relied upon for their cures. However, between the 13th and 17th centuries in Europe, Church-led inquisitions sought out and killed indigenous healers, typically burning them as "witches." At the same time, the new philosophy of rationalism became popular, and community leaders began to demand empirical evidence for healing practices. During the 17th century, the scientific method gained ascendancy, single-celled organisms were discovered, and the first experiments challenging the idea of spontaneous generation of life were conducted.

From the 18th to the 19th centuries, several scientific achievements further advanced the supremacy of empirically based medical techniques. High-powered microscopes were developed that could allow detection of microorganisms such as bacteria. In 1796, the English physician Edward Jenner developed the first effective vaccine, which used material from cowpox lesions to stimulate immunity to smallpox. In the mid-1800s, the French scientist Louis Pasteur conducted experiments that led to the formulation of the *germ theory of disease,* that is, the theory that microbes can cause human disease. In the 1860s, the English surgeon Joseph Lister introduced aseptic techniques using phenol and dramatically reduced the mortality rate following surgery. His techniques were widely adopted by other surgeons and led to increased acceptance of surgery as a viable treatment. By 1875, the German scientist Robert Koch had established postulates to prove whether a certain organism was pathogenic and what disease it caused. Thus, people learned that infectious disease, which was the leading cause of death at that time, was not due to spiritual flaws.

At the same time, European colonization of countries in Asia, Africa, Australia, and the Americas brought European medical practices as well. Indigenous healers and their therapies, such as the ayurvedic system of India and the nature-based therapies of Africa, were prohibited by the colonial powers and replaced with Western procedures and pharmaceuticals. In the United States, the American Medical Association (AMA) grew in prominence, replacing female midwives with male obstetricians, and homeopathic physicians (estimated to comprise about 50% of US physicians in the mid-19th century) with medical doctors who had graduated from AMA-approved schools of medicine.

In the early 20th century, several factors combined to ensure a virtual monopoly of conventional medicine in the United States. First, antimicrobial drugs and vaccines were developed that dramatically reduced morbidity and mortality due to infectious disease. Second, pharmaceutical companies began dominating medicine by heavily subsidizing US medical schools, giving rewards and subsidies to physicians who used their drugs, and lobbying US legislators for statutes and regulations favorable to their industry. Third, two world wars led to advances in both pharmaceuticals and surgical techniques that helped convince legislators of the superiority of the AMA's approach to health care.

Resurgence of Complementary and Alternative Therapies

Complementary and alternative therapies never entirely died out in the United States. Even in the 1950s, some people were able to eke out a living as chiropractors or herbalists. The social upheavals and "back to the land" movements of the 1960s and 1970s led to a renewed study of the therapies of indigenous cultures and an increased interest in herbs, massage, sound, and crystals as healing therapies. Still, even at the close of the millennium, such therapies were not mainstream.

The dramatic increase in complementary and alternative therapies in the past decade has probably resulted from a combination of several factors:

- Increased consumer awareness of the limitations of conventional Western medicine
- Increased international travel
- Increased media attention
- Advent of the Internet

America's love affair with conventional Western medicine began to cool in the latter part of the 20th century as costs increased, health care began to be seen as more technologic and less "human," and access to healthcare professionals' time became strictly limited. Childbearing families in particular began to seek more "natural" birth experiences, without anesthesia, in homelike settings attended by female certified nurse-midwives. Americans began to recognize that many health problems, such as back pain, headaches, cancer, diabetes, heart disease, autoimmune diseases, and others, could not be cured simply by swallowing a pill or "going under the knife." Such disorders came to be seen as complex, involving lifestyle factors, cultural factors, emotional elements, and—many people believed—spiritual aspects that were ignored by conventional approaches. Increasingly, people with such diseases turned to the complementary and alternative healing community.

As Americans began to engage more widely in international work, study, and travel, their exposure to other healing systems and practices increased. Indeed, several American physicians, disillusioned by the limitations of conventional Western medicine, traveled to Asia and other regions to study alternative therapies.

At the same time, the US media was beginning to pay attention to the complementary and alternative movement. The publication of Bill Moyers's *Healing and the Mind* in 1993, with its accompanying public television series, brought credibility to complementary and alternative therapies because all of Moyers's interviewees were respected scientists or physicians. For the same reason, the dramatic success of books on complementary therapies by Dr. Deepak Chopra, Dr. Andrew Weill, Dr. Joan Borysenko, and many others helped move complementary and alternative therapies into the forefront of public attention. Respected mainstream newspapers and national magazines began regularly to report on research and developments in complementary and alternative therapies, and television commercials began advertising nutritional supplements, homeopathic remedies, and other alternative products and services.

But perhaps the most explosive element in the resurgence of complementary and alternative therapies in the 1990s was the development of the Internet. With a computer and modem, current information on complementary and alternative products and services was now just a few mouse clicks away. For example, a paper presented at a conference in Germany on the health benefits of reflexology might become available to Internet users worldwide the next day. The Internet increased not only information, but also communication among people with similar health concerns. A pregnant woman who had just begun to experience first trimester nausea could join a chat group debating the advantages and disadvantages of ginger tea. Infertile couples could share a technique claiming to increase fertility that they had learned on a trip to Asia, or describe a fertility ritual they had learned from their Mexican grandmother. Suddenly, it became easy for people to integrate complementary and alternative therapies into their own unique approach to their healthcare concerns.

Growing Integration with Conventional Western Medicine

In this new century, it seems clear that the future of American health care will see an ever increasing integration between conventional medicine and complementary therapies. Some obvious examples of this new integration in perinatal settings include the acceptance of certain herbal teas for antepartal discomforts; the use of massage, Reiki, or therapeutic touch during the first stage of labor; the use of music and aromatherapy during labor and childbirth; and the increased emphasis on skin-to-skin, mother-to-baby bonding in the immediate postpartum period.

Further evidence of this increased integration was the establishment in 1992 of the Office of Alternative Medicine (OAM) at the National Institutes of Health. The OAM was mandated by Congress to promote research into complementary and alternative therapies and dissemination of information to consumers. In 1998 the OAM was incorporated into a new National Center for Complementary and Alternative Medicine (NCCAM) with an expanded mission and increased funding. NCCAM is dedicated to exploring complementary and alternative healing practices in the context of rigorous science, training CAM researchers, and disseminating authoritative information to the public and professionals (NCCAM, 2005). Recently, NCCAM recognized a new domain of integrative medicine. **Integrative medicine** is an approach that combines mainstream medical therapies with complementary therapies for which there is some high-quality scientific evidence of safety and effectiveness (NCCAM, 2005). Many studies of complementary and alternative therapies are currently under way at the NCCAM, which can be accessed via the Internet.

BENEFITS AND RISKS OF COMPLEMENTARY AND ALTERNATIVE THERAPIES

Complementary and alternative therapies undisputedly have many benefits for the childbearing family and other healthcare consumers. However, many of these remedies have associated risks that must be considered thoughtfully before a decision is made to use them.

Benefits

Many complementary and alternative therapies emphasize prevention and wellness, and place a higher value on holistic healing than on physical cure. In addition, many are noninvasive and have few side effects, and many are more affordable and available than conventional therapies.

EMPHASIS ON PREVENTION AND WELLNESS

The therapies of conventional Western medicine—pharmaceuticals and surgery—are typically prescribed after a disease has already manifested in symptoms. These therapies are of course entirely appropriate—and may be lifesaving—in certain circumstances; for example, albuterol for an acute asthma attack or appendectomy for appendicitis. However, they may be limited in effectiveness for subacute conditions.

In contrast, most complementary and alternative therapeutic systems emphasize maintenance of wellness and prevention of illness. For example, a woman consulting a medical doctor for fatigue might be tested for iron deficiency anemia. If the lab test came back negative, the woman might be advised simply to try to get more sleep, and the physician might prescribe a sedative to help achieve a full night's rest. In contrast, a woman consulting a practitioner of naturopathy, homeopathy, traditional Chinese medicine, or ayurveda (these systems are described shortly) would likely be asked dozens of questions about every aspect of her life, including her childhood, relationships, work habits, diet, lifestyle, stressors, and even how she feels about sunny days versus rainy days. These questions would attempt to unearth the underlying cause of even the most subtle complaints, and to prescribe remedies in several domains (acupuncture, homeopathic treatments, herbs, nutritional modifications, lifestyle modifications, massage, color therapy, and so forth) early enough in the process of breakdown to restore wellness before significant disease manifests.

EMPHASIS ON HEALING VERSUS CURE

The complementary therapeutic systems attempt to assess, diagnose, and treat the whole person. For example, the homeopathic physician and author Dr. Andrew Lockie and his associate Dr. Nicola Geddes (2000) have identified a breadth of concerns of the holistic healer that might seem astonishing—and even irrelevant—to someone familiar with only conventional approaches (Table 3–1).

This holistic approach extends to the goal of therapy as well; that is, the goal of many complementary therapies is not curing an illness but rather healing the client's psyche, spirit, body, and even community. The physician and author Dr. Rachel Naomi Remen describes healing as "a process we're all involved in all the time." She states that healing includes education, the leading forth of wholeness in people. "Sometimes people heal physically, and they don't heal emotionally, or mentally, or spiritually. And sometimes people heal emotionally, and they don't heal physically. . . . People can heal and live, and people can heal and die" (Moyers, 1993, p. 344).

Table 3–1	CONCERNS OF THE HOLISTIC HEALER

The holistic healer may be concerned with the following aspects of the client's life:

- Exercise, breathing, and posture
- Self-care, including dental care
- Nutrition, hydration, use of dietary supplements, and method of food preparation
- Digestion and elimination
- Sleep/wake cycles
- Stress and emotional responses
- Purity of air, food, water, and environment
- Use of alcohol, tobacco, caffeine, and other substances
- Employment and unemployment
- Hobbies, sports, and other recreational activities
- Home life and relationships
- Spirituality
- Type and age of bed and bedding
- Types of clothing, cosmetics, and personal care products used
- Pets
- Exposure to and use of sound and music
- Reactions to weather and seasons
- Electromagnetic phenomena and exposure to radiation
- Exposure to sunlight and artificial light
- Travel
- Personality and temperament
- Fears (e.g., of heights, of death, etc.)

SOURCE: Compiled from data in Lockie, P., & Geddes, N. (2000). *Complete guide to homeopathy: The principles and practice of treatment.* New York: DK Publishing.

NONINVASIVE APPROACHES

In part because of this emphasis on healing versus cure, many of the therapeutic techniques offered by complementary systems are noninvasive and potentially enriching on many levels. For example, imagery is often used to help people with cancer enhance their immune function, but also to help increase their optimism and gain new access to feelings of love and nurturance that may have been buried by fear of their diagnosis. Meditation, hypnosis, and biofeedback are other mind-based therapies that are entirely noninvasive and can affect the client on several levels. Massage and the other body-based therapies noninvasively promote healing of both the physical body and the client's psyche. Music, light, colors, magnets, gems, and fragrances are also noninvasive and likely achieve their effects by subtly influencing the neurochemistry, circulation, memories, and/or emotions of the client. Indeed, only a very few of the complementary therapies are invasive: these include acupuncture, certain techniques used in ayurveda, foods and dietary supplements, herbs, homeopathic remedies, and flower essences, the latter two of which are highly diluted substances.

COST AND ACCESS

Complementary and alternative therapies may be less expensive and more readily available than conventional remedies. For example, most homeopathic remedies cost less than $10 for a vial of 100 pellets or tablets. Flower essences, essential oils, herbs, and dietary supplements also tend to be far less expensive than most conventional pharmaceuticals. In fact, some complementary and alternative therapies—including meditation, prayer, visualization, self-massage, dietary modifications, regular physical exercise, music therapy, and color therapy—are free.

Visits to complementary healers are usually somewhat less expensive than visits to medical doctors; however, most insurance carriers do not cover complementary therapies unless the primary care physician has prescribed them. On the other hand, in some cases it is far easier to access complementary healers than conventional physicians—and at little or no expense to the consumer. Many neighborhood pharmacies and even grocery stores now have on staff herbalists, nutritionists, and others trained in a wide range of complementary therapies. No appointment is necessary to consult with them and no fee is charged. The same is true for complementary healers who have Web sites: by searching the Internet, it is possible for a childbearing family to glean tips on everything from relieving first-trimester nausea, to managing pain during childbirth without drugs, to preventing plugged ducts during breastfeeding.

Risks

These benefits of complementary and alternative therapies notwithstanding, it is critical that all consumers—and especially childbearing families—be aware of their not-insignificant risks. These include lack of standardization, lack of regulation and research substantiating safety and effectiveness, inadequate training and certification of some healers, and financial and health risks of unproven methods.

LACK OF STANDARDIZATION

Pharmaceuticals prescribed by a Western physician or nurse practitioner have been approved by the Food and Drug Administration (FDA). All preparations of an FDA-approved pharmaceutical, whether a brand-name drug or a generic version, have to contain identical quantities of certain precisely regulated, purified substances. In contrast, herbs, dietary supplements, and other non-FDA-approved ingested remedies may vary dramatically from one manufacturer to another. For example, preparations of herbs may use the flowers, leaves, or stems, all of which vary in potency, and preparations may contain various concentrations of the actual herb versus carrier materials. Additionally, some manufacturers use such harsh chemicals to process herbs that their healthful properties are reduced or lost. Some herbs lose their potency over time with different types of storage, whereas others vary in strength according to the soil in which they were grown or the season in which they were harvested. This lack of standardization means that one preparation may be highly potent, whereas another is ineffective.

LACK OF REGULATION AND RESEARCH

Complementary and alternative remedies are largely unregulated, and their claims may not be backed by valid, reliable research. NCCAM cautions: "While some scientific evidence exists regarding some CAM therapies, for most there are key questions that are yet to be answered through well-designed scientific studies—questions such as whether these therapies are safe and whether they work for the diseases or medical conditions for which they are used" (NCCAM, 2005).

Approval by the FDA guarantees that a drug has been subjected to—and passed—a rigorous process requiring, in most cases, development under strictly controlled conditions, precise molecular delineation of all components, and double-blind research studies substantiating the safety and effectiveness of the drug for the purpose under investigation. For this reason, when a childbearing client is told that a certain drug will safely induce labor, or when a breastfeeding mother is told that a drug will relieve her breast tenderness without harming her infant, she can accept these statements with confidence.

In contrast, the claims to effectiveness and safety of some complementary therapies may be largely unsubstantiated, resting on flawed or inadequate research, testimonials, tradition, or merely the healer's say-so. Thus, the consumer choosing these therapies often has little valid and reliable evidence that they will work effectively and safely.

The current inadequacy of research into complementary and alternative therapies is often due to lack of funding. When drug manufacturers commit millions of dollars to research and development of new pharmaceuticals, they do so knowing that, if they succeed in developing a safe and effective drug, their financial gain will more than cover their investment. In contrast, no one profits financially from consumers who use meditation, prayer, visualization, dietary modifications, exercise, water therapy, music, or sunlight. Even the profits from essential oils, flower remedies, herbs, and the body-based therapies are minimal compared with the costs of research studies to substantiate their use. Fortunately, as noted earlier, NCCAM is now funding research into several of these therapies.

Research into complementary and alternative therapies is also hindered by the very nature of these therapies. It is comparatively easy to provide a control group with either the drug being studied or a placebo and then to measure reduction in symptoms, but how does one design a reliable, valid study of therapies that attempt to maintain wellness or prevent illness, that value healing rather than cure, that claim to work on subtle, vibrational levels, or that admit to the necessity of a therapeutic relationship with the healer? Currently there is so little understanding of the cultural, psychologic, emotional, and spiritual aspects of healing that investigators trained in quantitative research methodologies may be unprepared even to design studies of complementary and alternative therapies. On the other hand, it is interesting to note that several qualitative nursing research studies over the past decade have studied complementary and alternative therapies with some success.

INADEQUATE TRAINING AND CERTIFICATION

Many complementary therapies do have rigorous training and testing requirements that applicants must fulfill before they receive certification as practitioners. For example, naturopathic, homeopathic, and chiropractic physicians usually complete a typical undergraduate premedical program before enrolling in a 4-year graduate school in their specialty. Acupuncturists, certified massage therapists, Reiki practitioners, sound healers, and

many other complementary therapists must complete a course of study at an approved school, achieve a certain number of hours of practice, and pass an exam before they are certified.

In contrast, many titles are unregulated. For example, many states do not require that people calling themselves "counselors," "nutritionists," "healers," "intuitives," or "consultants" have any particular education or license. Thus, consumers who purchase the services of such therapists must beware.

FINANCIAL AND HEALTH RISKS OF UNPROVEN METHODS

As noted earlier, complementary and alternative remedies and techniques may cost considerably less than conventional pharmaceuticals and procedures. However, consumers may make a considerable investment in unproven methods and products that may not, in the end, improve their well-being, prevent illness, or promote healing.

Although few complementary and alternative therapies actually harm consumers directly, consumers' health may indeed suffer if their belief in the therapy or healer causes them to delay or forgo conventional medical treatments. Tragically, each year in the United States, cases of fetal demise occur among childbearing families who choose to use unlicensed birth attendants in home settings.

TYPES OF COMPLEMENTARY AND ALTERNATIVE THERAPIES

The following review of complementary and alternative therapies is meant as an introduction. The list is not exhaustive, and the descriptions are exceedingly brief. For more information, consult the Web sites listed in Table 3–2.

The categories under which particular therapies are discussed here are somewhat arbitrary. For example, homeopathy is categorized as a complementary therapeutic system, but it could also be considered an energy therapy. Therapeutic touch and Reiki are both energy based and body based. Massage is a sense therapy in that it approaches the client through touch, yet it is classified with the body-based therapies. In truth, the holistic nature of these therapies means that they affect the client in many different ways.

Complementary Therapeutic Systems

The complementary therapeutic systems described here are complex and multidimensional, incorporating several different techniques into a holistic approach to wellness, prevention, and healing.

HOMEOPATHY

Homeopathy is best understood in contrast to conventional Western medicine, which is also called *allopathic medicine.* The term *allopathy* is derived from the Greek words *allos,* meaning "different," and *pathos,* meaning "suffering." Thus, allopathic medicine, which has been dominant in the United States for over 100 years,

Table 3–2	SOURCES OF INFORMATION ON COMPLEMENTARY AND ALTERNATIVE THERAPIES	
CAM Modality	**Organization**	**Web Site**
Acupressure	Acupressure Institute	www.acupressure.com
Acupuncture	National Acupuncture Oriental Medical Alliance	www.acuall.org
Acupuncture and Oriental medicine	National Certification Commission for Acupuncture and Oriental Medicine	www.nccaom.org
Alexander technique	North American Society of Teachers of the Alexander Technique	www.alexandertech.org
Aromatherapy	National Association for Holistic Aromatherapy	www.naha.org
Biofeedback	Association for Applied Psychophysiology and Biofeedback	www.aaph.org
Chiropractic	American Chiropractic Association	www.amerchiro.org
Craniosacral therapy	Craniosacral therapy (Upledger)	www.Upledger.com
Feldenkrais	Feldenkrais Guild of North America	www.feldenkrais.com
Herbs	American Botanical Council	www.herbalgram.org
Homeopathy	National Center for Homeopathy	www.homeopathic.org
Massage therapy	National Certification Board for Therapeutic Massage and Bodywork	www.ncbtmb.com
Massage therapy	American Massage Therapy Association	www.amtamassage.org
Meditation	Meditation Institute of Noetic Sciences	www.noetic.org
Reflexology	Reflexology Association of America	www.reflexology-usa.org
Sound	Sound Healers Association	www.healingsound.com
Therapeutic touch	Therapeutic Touch Nurse Healers Professional Association	www.therapeutic-touch.org

NOTE: The authors do not officially endorse any of these Web sites.

uses remedies that produce effects differing from—or in opposition to—those of the disease being treated. For example, allopathic healthcare practitioners may prescribe an anti-inflammatory to reduce swelling or a sedative to relieve insomnia.

In contrast, the term **homeopathy** is derived from the Greek word *homos,* meaning "the same." Thus, it is often described as a healing system that uses like to cure like; that is, homeopathic remedies are minute dilutions of substances that, if ingested in larger amounts, would produce effects *similar* to the symptoms of the disorder being treated. For example, *Cantharis vesicatoria* is a species of beetle (commonly called Spanish fly) whose poison causes, among other things, burning urinary tract pain and a continuous urge to urinate. Homeopathic *Cantharis* is a minute dilution of this toxin and is thus a remedy of choice for women suffering from cystitis.

Founded by the German physician Samuel Hahnemann in the late 18th century, homeopathy traces its roots to Hippocrates, who was the first physician known to have observed the principle of like curing like. Homeopathic remedies are believed to achieve their effects by stimulating the client's immune system to mount a response against the diluted substance. Thus, it is the individual's own body, rather than the ingested remedy, that opposes the symptoms. Indeed, homeopathic physicians advise that an initial worsening of symptoms indicates that the correct remedy has been given.

It is important to note that, although homeopaths do rely on certain standard remedies such as *Cantharis* for cystitis, they believe that physical symptoms manifest disturbances on far deeper levels. Thus, they work to peel away ever-more subtle layers of disturbance, beginning with the obvious physical symptoms and moving deeper to those that may have originated in the client's childhood. Thereby, homeopaths work to effect holistic healing.

NATUROPATHY

Naturopathy is commonly referred to as *natural medicine.* It is more precisely defined as a healing system that combines safe and effective traditional means of preventing and treating human disease with the most current advances in modern medicine (American Association of Naturopathic Physicians, 2005). Many naturopathic physicians are eclectic, employing a variety of therapies in their practice. These might include clinical nutrition, botanical medicine, homeopathy, natural childbirth, traditional Chinese medicine, hydrotherapy, naturopathic manipulative therapy, pharmacology, minor surgery, and counseling for lifestyle modification (American Association of Naturopathic Physicians, 2005). For example, a naturopath might counsel a woman with vaginitis to eliminate from her diet all refined foods, to reduce her intake of sugars and fats, to consume lactobacillus-culture yogurt, to take B-complex vitamins and other supplements, to cleanse with a calendula preparation, and to avoid sexual intercourse.

TRADITIONAL CHINESE MEDICINE

Traditional Chinese medicine (TCM) developed more than 3000 years ago in the Chinese culture and then gradually spread with modifications to other Asian countries including Japan, Vietnam, Tibet, and Korea. Its goal is to promote health and well-being, so the underlying focus of TCM is prevention although diagnosis and treatment of disease also play an important role.

TCM seeks to ensure the balance of energy, which is called *chi* or *qi* (pronounced "chee"). Chi is the invisible flow of energy in the body that maintains health and energy and enables the body to carry out its physiologic functions. Chi flows along certain pathways or meridians, which are discussed on p. 60 under acupuncture and acupressure.

Figure 3–1 ◆ Traditional Chinese symbol of the opposing forces of *yin* and *yang* in perfect balance, representing integration and wholeness.

Another important concept in TCM (mentioned briefly in Chapter 2 ∞) is that of *yin* and *yang,* opposing internal and external forces that, together, represent the whole (Figure 3–1 ◆). Yin is the female force—passive, cool, wet, and close to the earth. Yang is the masculine force—aggressive, hot, dry, and celestial. Yin and yang cannot exist independently because they are complementary and both are essential. Certain foods, behaviors, and environmental factors are believed to increase yin, whereas others increase yang. Well-being occurs when these two opposing forces are in balance, and illness can result if this balance is disturbed over a period of time.

TCM includes the following therapeutic techniques:

* Acupuncture (described shortly)
* Herbal therapy
* Nutrition
* Acupressure (Chinese massage) (described shortly)
* *Moxibustion,* which involves the application of heat from a small piece of burning herb called *moxa* (*Artemisia vulgaris,* commonly called "mugwort")
* *Qigong* (pronounced "chee-goong"), which is a self-discipline that involves the use of breathing, meditation, self-massage, and movement. Typically practiced daily, the movements are nontiring and are designed to stimulate the flow of chi (Figure 3–2 ◆).
* T'ai chi (pronounced "ty chee"), which is a form of martial art. It originally focused on physical fitness and self-defense but is currently used more as a health discipline. T'ai chi resembles a cross between slow-motion dancing and shadow boxing and is helpful in improving balance in older adults.

I am so glad that complementary therapies are becoming more accepted. I don't plan to stop going to see my doctor, but now that I am pregnant I like doing things on my own to improve my health. I used acupressure wrist bands early on and felt they really helped my nausea. I'm taking prenatal yoga classes now and I feel terrific! I think I will definitely continue doing yoga after the baby is born.

AYURVEDA

The classical system of Hindu medicine is known as **ayurveda.** The term *ayurveda* is derived from the Sanskrit words *ayus,* meaning "life, health, and vitality," and *veda,* meaning "science" or "knowledge." Thus, ayurveda is the knowledge of how to live a vital, healthful life. Ayurvedic physicians believe that

Figure 3–2 ◆ Pregnant woman practices the movements of *Qigong.*

the five elements of ether, wind, fire, water, and earth take form in the body as three tendencies, called *doshas:* vata, pitta, and kapha. Each person's constitution is believed to reflect some combination of these three doshas. For example, vata reflects the elements of ether and wind; thus, a person in whom vata is dominant may be flighty, ungrounded, and anxious, with dry skin, eyes, and respiratory membranes. The primary element in kapha is water, and so it is not surprising that pregnancy is considered a kapha condition.

An important part of the ayurvedic physician's job is to balance the doshas to achieve harmony and holism. The physician does this by suppressing the dosha that is dominating the client and stimulating the dosha that is sluggish. For example, a fatigued woman in whom kapha is too dominant may be prescribed hot foods, spices, warm colors, energizing music, pungent aromas, and other therapies to stimulate her internal fire (pitta) and burn away some of her internal water (kapha). This is a simplistic example of a highly complex system, but the important thing to bear in mind about ayurveda is that, like homeopathy, naturopathy, and TCM, it approaches the client holistically, through the diet, the senses, breathing, posture, sleep patterns, and even through examination and alteration of the client's work life, home routine, relationships, and spirituality.

Mind-Body Therapies

This section discusses therapies engaging the mind in activities such as imagination, reflection, communication, and relaxation.

BIOFEEDBACK

Biofeedback is a method used to help individuals learn to control their physiologic responses based on the concept that the mind controls the body. An individual is hooked up to a system of highly sensitive instruments that relay information about the body back to that person. The effectiveness of biofeedback has been proven in countless studies and it is now considered a conventional therapy more than a complementary one. For example, biofeedback may focus on temperature or thermal feedback, especially in treating certain vascular diseases or in promoting relaxation. It may focus on galvanic skin response, which measures sweat gland activity in the fingers or palms, in helping people learn to deal with stress or excessive perspiration. It may use electromyography (EMG) to provide feedback about muscle tension to help in the treatment of muscle spasm, tension headache, and pain reduction. It may use electroencephalography (EEG) to gain information about brain wave activity to help with insomnia, pain management, and substance abuse.

Currently biofeedback has more than 150 applications for disease prevention and the restoration of health, including stress-related disorders such as insomnia, anxiety, headaches, hypertension, and asthma; gastrointestinal disorders such as ulcers and irritable bowel syndrome; temporomandibular joint syndrome; and hyperactivity in children (*Nurse's Handbook,* 2002).

HYPNOSIS

Hypnosis, whether guided by a trained hypnotherapist or induced through self-hypnosis, is a state of great mental and physical relaxation during which a person is very open to suggestions. Because hypnosis cannot make people do something against their will, hypnosis will not work unless an individual is really interested in changing. Studies have shown that some people are able to anesthetize themselves using hypnosis, and studies have shown that self-hypnosis during invasive medical procedures significantly reduces individuals' pain, anxiety, drug use, and number of complications (ClinicalTrials.gov, 2005). Pregnant women who receive hypnosis before childbirth have reported shorter, less painful labors and births (*Nurse's Handbook,* 2002).

MEDITATION AND PRAYER

Many people think of meditation as sitting quietly with the legs crossed and eyes closed, repeating a *mantra* or counting one's breaths to still the mind and bring peace. In contrast, the great spiritual teacher J. Krishnamurti (1895–1986) defined *meditation* far more simply, as something one can do every day at any moment. For Krishnamurti (2000), "Meditation is to perceive the truth each second. . . . When the mind has seen the fallacy of [accumulated knowledge] completely, then it is in a constant state of 'not knowing.' Such a mind can then receive that which is not measurable and which only comes into being from moment to moment." When clients allow their family values, education, social conditioning, knowledge, desires, expectations, and all other "accumulations" to fade away, and listen receptively in a state of not knowing, they experience an emptiness that is itself transformative and healing (Figure 3–3 ◆).

Figure 3–3 ◆ Meditation does not have to be practiced in a particular pose, but can be incorporated into each day. People who meditate regularly find it helpful to assume a comfortable position in a quiet area free of distractions. Eyes may be open or closed. This woman, 8 months pregnant, has chosen a comfortable position with her arms and legs supported. She is gazing into the distance, unfocused. Her goal is to open her mind and move into a receptive state.

Whereas meditation is often likened to listening, *prayer* is an act of silently or vocally addressing a deity such as Allah, Jesus, Shiva, or the Great Spirit, or for clients outside of a particular religious tradition, simply "talking to the Universe." Prayer specifically for health reasons is the most commonly used complementary therapy (Barnes, Powell-Griner, McFann, & Nahin, 2004). The effect of prayer on healing has been studied and documented and more research is under way.

Nurses need to be cognizant of the spiritual needs of the people for whom they care because religion is so often a part of people's lives. Thus nurses, and all healthcare workers, need to be respectful of an individual's belief system and choices about issues of doctrine. Healthcare professionals also must avoid pushing religion onto people or attempting to convert clients to a particular faith.

VISUALIZATION AND GUIDED IMAGERY

Visualization, a complementary therapy, has been used since ancient times. In visualization a person goes into a relaxed state and focuses on or "visualizes" soothing or positive scenes such as a beach or a mountain glade. Visualization helps reduce stress and encourage relaxation. For example, a therapist may work with a woman before childbirth to help her create positive images of labor.

Guided imagery is a state of intense, focused concentration used to create compelling mental images. It is sometimes considered a form of hypnosis. Guided imagery is useful in imagining a desired effect such as weight loss or in mentally rehearsing a new procedure or activity. Skill in using guided imagery improves with practice so people who wish to use it should set aside 5 to 20 minutes of quiet time once or twice daily and practice creating images that are personal and meaningful.

Manipulative and Body-Based Therapies

Therapies requiring practitioner manipulation of the body are discussed here, along with hydrotherapy, hatha yoga, and regular physical exercise.

CHIROPRACTIC THERAPY

Chiropractic, the third largest independent health profession in the United States (behind medicine and dentistry), is based on concepts of manipulation. It was developed by Daniel David Palmer, a self-taught American healer, in the late 19th century. Palmer believed that many diseases and illnesses were the result of abnormal nerve transmissions (subluxation) caused by misalignment of the spine. He postulated that spinal manipulation could correct these vertebral misalignments. In 1898 he founded the Palmer Chiropractic Institute in Iowa and began training others in his approach. For many years, chiropractic was viewed with scorn by traditional medical doctors, who refused to refer clients to chiropractors. In the early 1990s, however, a Supreme Court ruling against the American Medical Association (AMA) required medical doctors to cooperate with the chiropractic profession (Bratman, 1998).

Currently chiropractors are licensed in all 50 states and are regulated by state boards. Chiropractors continue to focus on the close relationship between structure and function but also stress the importance of proper nutrition and regular exercise to good health. Chiropractic is widely available, and popular demand has earned it a higher level of insurance coverage than most other alternative therapies.

A number of studies have shown chiropractic to be effective in treating problems such as lower back pain. Some women find chiropractic effective in managing the backache and physical stress resulting from spinal realignment secondary to increased body weight and changing body contours during pregnancy (Cole, 1998).

Clients who are considering chiropractic therapy should consider the following recommendations (Mayo Clinic, 2001):

- They should ask their primary caregiver for referral to the appropriate professional, which may be a chiropractor, physical therapist, or osteopathic physician.
- If they seek chiropractic care without referral, they should choose someone who has completed a training program at a school accredited by the Council on Chiropractic Education.
- They should see only chiropractors who are willing to give them a written treatment plan, who send a written report to the primary physician or care provider, and who allow the care provider to observe the chiropractic treatment, if desired.
- They should avoid chiropractors who order frequent x-rays and who ask them to extend treatment indefinitely.

- They should avoid chiropractors who consider spinal manipulation a cure for "anything that ails you." No research supports this notion.

CRANIOSACRAL THERAPY

Craniosacral therapy, developed by Dr. John Upledger in the 1970s, is a variation of cranial osteopathy, which is the belief that the bones of the skull do not fuse completely during childhood and that rhythmic impulses can be detected. The craniosacral therapist uses light touch—generally no more than the weight of a nickel—to test for restrictions in the craniosacral system. This is done by holding a client's head and other designated parts of the body and focusing on monitoring the subtle rhythm of the cerebrospinal fluid as it flows through the system. According to the Upledger Institute (1998), the therapist's light, hands-on approach assists the hydraulic forces inherent in the craniosacral system to improve the body's internal environment and strengthen its ability to heal itself.

ALEXANDER TECHNIQUE

The focus of the *Alexander technique* is on proper alignment of the head, neck, and trunk. This movement education technique was developed by F. M. Alexander, an Australian actor, in the late 1900s. After completing an assessment, an Alexander instructor uses touch, instructions (verbal cuing), and activities to guide clients into the correct use of their bodies. The Alexander technique is used by many schools of music and acting worldwide, but it is becoming more commonly used by people in other professions to improve their posture, alignment, and ease of movement.

The Alexander technique, though not in itself a therapy, has been proven to help problems related to poor posture, other musculoskeletal complaints, and even certain respiratory and digestive problems. Secondarily, it is useful in reducing both physical and mental stress. Consequently it is often recommended for stress-related disorders.

FELDENKRAIS

The *Feldenkrais method,* another movement-oriented therapy, was developed by the Russian-born physicist, educator, and judo expert, Moshe Feldenkrais. It is based on the belief that health is improved by establishing new connections between the brain and body through movement reeducation. The Feldenkrais practitioner uses verbal instruction and hands-on assistance to help clients become aware of their movements and to develop alternate ways of moving that improve posture, flexibility, and range of motion, as well as physical performance and well-being. The movements also help relieve certain forms of discomfort such as backache, muscle tension, shoulder pain, and jaw pain. Feldenkrais did not view his approach as a medical therapy but rather a training method (*Nurse's Handbook,* 2002).

MASSAGE THERAPY

Massage has been used for centuries as a form of therapy. **Massage therapy** involves the manipulation of the soft tissues of the body to reduce stress and tension, increase circulation,

Figure 3–4 ◆ Pregnant woman receiving massage. Massage is often useful in helping a pregnant woman cope with the discomforts of pregnancy.
SOURCE: Steve Mason/Getty Images, Inc.

Figure 3–5 ◆ Infant massage.

REFLEXOLOGY

Reflexology is a form of massage that involves the application of pressure to designated points or reflexes on the client's feet, hands, or ears using the thumb and fingers. Eunice Ingham, a physical therapist, mapped the specific reflex zones and is credited with spreading the practice of reflexology.

Reflexology most often involves manipulation of the feet. Practitioners believe that distinct areas of the feet correspond to particular organs or body systems. The stimulation of the appropriate region is intended to eliminate energy blockages thought to produce pain or disease. Organs on the right side of the body are represented on the right foot and organs on the left side are represented on the left foot (Figure 3–6 ◆). Although they are used less frequently, the hands and ears have also been mapped.

diminish pain, and promote a sense of well-being. Different techniques have been developed, including for example, Swedish massage, shiatsu massage, Rolfing, trigger point massage, Thai massage, and sports massage. Most forms of massage use approaches such as pressing, kneading, gliding, circular motion, tapping, and vibrational strokes.

Certification and/or licensure for massage therapists varies from state to state although most states require at least 500 hours of training. Massage therapists who have passed the written examination given by the National Certification Board for Therapeutic Massage and Bodywork (NCBTMB) are nationally certified. Continuing education is then required for recertification.

Certain massage therapists specialize in massage for women during pregnancy (Figure 3–4 ◆). Massage is often helpful as women adapt to the discomforts of their changing bodies. In addition, certified nurse-midwives often use perineal massage before labor to stretch the muscles of the perineum around the vaginal opening and thereby prevent tearing of the tissues during childbirth. During labor, massage of the back and buttocks by the nurse, labor coach, or doula can help the woman relax and may help decrease her discomfort.

Infant massage has become increasingly popular in the United States (Figure 3–5 ◆). The calm, soothing strokes of baby massage can help soothe an infant and minimize crying. In addition, research has demonstrated that massage can improve immune function, relieve pain, reduce anxiety, and promote relaxation and sleep (Sinclair, 2005).

I got into infant massage when Ryan was born. I loved that time we spent together and I am convinced it was part of the reason he was such a good baby.

Figure 3–6 ◆ Foot reflexology points.
SOURCE: Fontaine, K. L. Complementary and Alternative Therapies for Nursing Practice, 2nd ed., 2005. p. 225. Reprinted by permission of Pearson Education, Upper Saddle River, NJ.

HYDROTHERAPY

Hydrotherapy is the term used to describe therapy that makes use of hot or cold moisture in any form. Hydrotherapy is used to relax muscles, promote rest, decrease pain, reduce swelling, promote healing, cleanse wounds and burns, reduce fever, lessen cramps, and improve well-being. The major types of hydrotherapy include the following:

- *Compresses* (ice packs, hot water packs, towels or dressings soaked in hot or cold water and wrung out). Compresses are applied locally and are often alternated between hot and cold compresses. They are especially effective in improving circulation to a given area, thereby reducing swelling and promoting healing. They are also helpful in reducing pain or achiness in a given area.

- *Baths* (local, such as a foot bath or sitz bath, or full immersion bath). Baths serve many of the same functions as compresses but also are effective in cleansing. Full immersion baths are often used in treating extensive burns and in rehabilitation.

- *Sweat baths* (steam bath or sauna). Sweat baths are used to open pores and induce sweating because sweating is a type of detoxification that is helpful in promoting the elimination of toxins, drugs, and salts from the body. Because high heat has been associated with neural tube defects, pregnant women should not do steam baths or saunas, especially in the first trimester (Fontaine, 2005).

HATHA YOGA

When they hear the word *yoga,* most people think of people in leotards moving through a series of postures, such as the cat stretch or the salute to the sun. In reality, the term *yoga* comes from the Sanskrit word for "union," and implies a path toward union with God. **Hatha yoga** is the physical branch of yoga, and in the United States, it is commonly practiced for wellness, illness prevention, and healing. In hatha yoga, the client moves through a series of gentle stretches and postures (called *asanas*), coordinated with deep, rhythmic breathing techniques that promote oxygenation of all body tissues.

Certain yoga positions are especially beneficial during pregnancy and can be practiced safely by most women. These techniques coordinate breathing with movement while increasing strength and suppleness, providing valuable preparation for childbirth. In many communities, yoga teachers offer classes specifically designed for pregnant women (Figure 3–7 ♦).

REGULAR PHYSICAL EXERCISE

As more and more people are recognizing, regular physical exercise plays an important role in maintaining health and fitness. Exercise is important in maintaining muscle tone and strength, controlling weight, promoting cardiovascular health, improving digestion and elimination, reducing stress, promoting sleep, preventing a variety of chronic health problems, and providing an overall sense of fitness and well-being. In addition, exercise programs are an important component of ongoing therapy for a variety of health conditions such as arthritis, diabetes, and osteoporosis. Exercise is

Figure 3–7 ♦ Pregnant woman doing a hatha yoga stretch.
SOURCE: Ryan McVay/Getty Images, Inc.

also crucial as part of recovery from heart attacks, fractures, orthopedic surgery, and stroke.

For further discussion of exercise during pregnancy, please refer to Chapter 16. ∞

Nutritional and Herbal Therapies

The nutritional and herbal therapies include the use of particular foods as remedies; the use of vitamins, minerals, and other supplements; and the use of herbs.

DIETARY THERAPIES

It has long been recognized that certain foods have properties that are necessary for health, for healing, and for well-being. For example, caregivers have long known that people who are weak and easily fatigued often benefit from a diet rich in iron. Sailors learned to avoid the tissue damage caused by scurvy by consuming foods rich in vitamin C such as citrus fruits. However, the value of a nutritious diet in maintaining health is becoming more widely recognized and concerns are growing about the quality of some of the food products available today.

As part of their quest for optimum health, people make choices about their diets: whether to choose vegetarianism, a high-protein, low-carbohydrate diet, or a more balanced combination based on the USDA's MyPyramid (see Chapter 18 ∞);

whether to consume alcohol in moderation or no alcohol at all; whether to include processed foods in the diet or not; whether to incorporate regular fasting or not, and so forth. The literature offers a wealth of information about nutrition and diet therapy. Some of this information is grounded in data and research; other relies more on tradition and hearsay.

Diet therapy is also an important part of treatment for many health conditions such as coronary artery disease, gout, kidney stones, gallbladder disease, Crohn's disease, anemia, diverticulitis, and so forth. The importance of good nutrition for pregnant women and for infants and children cannot be overemphasized. Please refer to Chapter 18 ∞ for a discussion of nutrition for women during pregnancy and the postpartum period and to Chapter 31 ∞ for a discussion of newborn nutrition.

USE OF SUPPLEMENTS

A *dietary supplement* is any product (excluding tobacco) intended to supplement the diet. It may be available for ingestion in the form of a powder, capsule, geltab, liquid, extract, and so forth, and it contains one or more of the following ingredients: a mineral, vitamin, herb, amino acid, other botanical supplements, or extracts and ingredients of animal and plant origin. Dietary supplements are not presented as conventional food products and they are not intended to be the sole item of a meal or of the diet (National Institutes of Health, 2001).

Dietary supplements, sometimes called natural food supplements, are used to achieve a specific purpose. Perhaps the most widely used form of supplement is a multivitamin tablet or capsule. Table 3–3 provides information on selected dietary supplements. Women who are pregnant should discuss the use of supplements with their caregiver or with a registered dietitian.

HERBAL THERAPIES

Herbal therapy or herbal medicine has been used since ancient times to treat illnesses and ailments. In fact, the oldest surviving prescription for garlic use was found on a clay tablet that dates from 3000 BCE (Fontaine, 2005). Like vitamins and minerals, herbs are a form of dietary supplement, but they are often used to treat the symptoms of specific ailments rather than simply to enhance overall health (Mayo Clinic, 2002). Certain herbs have become better known because of specific claims about their use. For example, many people have used St. John's wort over the counter to help treat mild to moderate depression. However, a recent study indicates that St. John's wort is no more effective than a placebo in dealing with major depression of moderate severity (Davidson, Kishore, Fairbank, et al., 2002). Further study about its effectiveness for mild depression is needed. Other well-known herbal remedies include, for example, ginger, rosemary, ginseng, ginkgo, chamomile, oil of evening primrose, echinacea, garlic, lemon balm, and black cohosh.

Currently about 1500 botanical substances are sold in the United States as dietary supplements or as part of traditional ethnic medications. However, herbal formulations are not subject to Food and Drug Administration (FDA) premarket testing for safety and effectiveness (National Toxicology Program, 2002). Thus, these products can be sold over the counter with only little control. The FDA does have the authority to pull a product off the market if it is proven to be dangerous. Consequently most of what is known about herbs comes from Europe, where they have been studied for some time. Herbal products from Germany, France, England, and Australia are reasonably safe because in these countries herbs are regulated as if they were drugs (Graedon & Graedon, 2001).

The use of herbs during pregnancy and breastfeeding is an especially important consideration for nurses working with childbearing families. Pregnant and lactating women interested in using herbs are best advised to consult with their healthcare provider before taking any herbs, even as teas. Lists identifying common herbs that women are advised to avoid or use with caution during pregnancy and lactation are available.

Table 3–3	NATURAL FOOD SUPPLEMENTS
Supplement	**Benefit**
Alfalfa	Rich in minerals and vitamins
Aloe vera	Used for digestive complaints; can also be used as a skin moisturizer
Bee by-products* (bee pollen, honey, Royal bee jelly)	Contains minerals, proteins, and vitamins
Brewer's yeast	Amino acids, B vitamins, and minerals
Coenzyme A	Helps to produce the energy the body needs
Coenzyme Q10	Helps with fat and energy metabolism
Colostrum (cow's)	Helps boost the immune system
Fish oil	Protects the heart and blood vessels
Garlic	Acts as an immune system stimulant; also a natural antibiotic
Green papaya	Enzymes, minerals, and vitamins
Kelp (type of seaweed)	Rich in vitamins (especially B vitamins) and minerals
Wheat germ	Source of vitamin E and most B vitamins, minerals

*Bee pollen should not be used by children, or by pregnant or lactating women (Gastelu, 2000).

SOURCE: Adapted from Balch and Balch, 2000; Graedon and Graedon, 2001; Gastelu, 2000; Hobbs and Keville, 1998.

DEVELOPING CULTURAL COMPETENCE

HERBAL THERAPIES

The World Health Organization estimates that 80% of the Earth's population depends on plants to treat common ailments. Herbalism is an essential part of ayurvedic (Indian), traditional Asian, Native American, and naturopathic medicines. Many homeopathic remedies are also developed from herbs.

Sense Therapies

Most practitioners who use the sense therapies are trained in several. For example, to boost immunity, one healer might prescribe a varied menu of aromas, colors, and sounds.

AROMATHERAPY

Aromatherapy is the use of certain essential oils, derived from plants, whose odor or aroma is believed to have a therapeutic effect. Essential oils are typically diluted in a carrier oil such as sweet almond oil, olive oil, or vegetable oil before they are applied to the skin. Essential oils can also be inhaled (a few drops in warm water) or added to bath water. Essential oils are used for many purposes such as the following (Fontaine, 2005):

- Aid in restful sleep
- Help reduce stress
- Mood regulation—some oils are sedating, others are stimulating
- Reduce weight
- Enhance the immune system
- Refresh a room

Opinion varies about the use of essential oils during pregnancy because certain oils may pose a risk to the woman or her fetus. A pregnant woman who is considering aromatherapy should first discuss it with a healthcare provider who is knowledgeable about aromatherapy or a skilled aromatherapist (Fontaine, 2005).

COLOR AND LIGHT THERAPIES

Chromotherapy or *color therapy* is designed to use colors to help restore the body to harmony. Color therapists believe that, because all matter is a form of energy, the application of energy to the body in the form of light can have therapeutic results. Because light can be split into colors, it is possible to deliver this energy at very precise levels and in easily controlled doses. After assessment, the color therapist exposes the client to a particular color of light to promote healing.

Although sunlight has been used for healing purposes since ancient times, Western scientists have only recently begun to explore how exposure to light affects human functioning (*Nurse's Handbook*, 2002). *Light therapy* has become accepted treatment for jaundice in newborns (see Chapter 33 ∞). Light

therapy is also used in treating individuals with seasonal affective disorder.

MUSIC AND SOUND THERAPIES

Sound therapy is based on the premise that when the body is exposed to the correct sound frequency (including some very low and very high frequencies that humans cannot normally hear) the body restores itself. Thus sounds from Tibetan and crystal bowls, vibrating tuning forks, *mantras* (such as "Om"), and handheld machines that transmit sound waves through the skin are used to promote healing. It is suggested that certain sounds have a healing influence on the body because they influence the geometric patterns and organization of cells and living systems (Gerber, 2001). A simple application of sound therapy is to encourage a woman in childbirth to moan on as low a pitch as possible during contractions. This opens the jaw, throat, and chest, and many women report that it promotes feelings of relaxation and power. In contrast, high-pitched squealing or screaming tightens the body and may promote feelings of fear.

Music therapy can be considered a form of sound therapy. Music has been used during pregnancy and labor and birth to help soothe women and decrease their anxiety by stimulating endorphin release. Similarly, research involving low-birth-weight premature and newborn infants revealed that those infants who were played hour-long tapes of lullabies and children's songs lost 50% less weight and spent an average of 5 fewer days in the hospital (Gaynor, 1999). See Research in Practice.

Energy Therapies

The energy therapies work at the most subtle level of the body to enhance immunity, reduce allergy, improve circulation, and improve neural integration. Although acupressure and acupuncture are familiar to most healthcare professionals, many of the energy therapies are very new, and some are not widely available.

ACUPRESSURE AND ACUPUNCTURE

Both acupressure and acupuncture were originally part of traditional Chinese medicine. These practices are based on the traditional Eastern belief that the body's life energy, chi, which was discussed previously, flows along certain pathways known as meridians. The meridians—14 in number—connect all parts of the body. The places where the meridians pass close to the skin's surface are called pressure points. Stimulating specific pressure points can promote wellness, relieve pain, and even cure certain illnesses.

Acupressure (sometimes called Chinese massage) uses pressure from the fingers and thumbs to stimulate pressure points. Acupressure is easy to learn and is often used for self-treatment of tension-related ailments such as headaches, muscle aches, and tension due to stress. Pregnant women often use acupressure wristbands to help relieve the nausea of early pregnancy.

Acupuncture, considered the stronger technique, uses very fine (hairlike) stainless steel needles to stimulate specific points depending on the client's medical assessment and condition. A treatment typically involves the placement of 6 to 12 needles. Acupuncture has become more widely available in most countries since the 1970s when China became more open

RESEARCH IN PRACTICE

EFFECTS OF MUSIC THERAPY ON WOMEN'S PHYSIOLOGIC MEASURES, ANXIETY, AND SATISFACTION DURING CESAREAN DELIVERY

What is this study about? Cesarean birth is major surgery and may cause considerable stress, resulting in an unsatisfying birth experience. Music therapy, or the systematic application of music to aid in healthcare treatment, may be effective in reducing anxiety and improving satisfaction with the birth experience. Researchers have demonstrated the effectiveness of music therapy in a variety of settings for a range of physiologic conditions. Specifically, music has been shown to ease anxiety, distract attention, and increase the threshold of pain during operative procedures. The purpose of this study was to assess the effectiveness of music therapy in improving physiological and psychological indices of stress and the level of birth satisfaction in mothers undergoing cesarean birth.

How was this study done? A total of 64 women were recruited from two hospitals in Taiwan. All of the births were at term and were planned cesareans for nonemergent indications. Women were randomly assigned to a treatment group that received music therapy and a control group that did not. Both groups received standard obstetric care. The women in the experimental group were asked to choose one of the following types of music: Western classical; new age; or Chinese religious music. The researcher accompanied the participants to the surgical suite and provided earphones and a compact disc player. The experimental participants listened to music for at least 30 minutes from the start of anesthesia to the end of surgery. The volume was low enough to allow for communication with the researcher and the healthcare team. In both groups, anxiety was measured with a visual analogue scale, and satisfaction with the birth experience was measured with an author-developed questionnaire. Physiologic indices included pulse hemoglobin oxygen saturation, finger temperature, respiratory and pulse rates, and blood pressure. Women in the experimental group were also asked to evaluate the level of satisfaction with the music therapy. Measures were collected before anesthesia, upon the end of maternal contact with the newborn, and after completion of the skin sutures.

What were the results of the study? There were no differences on any of the measures between the groups before the birth. No differences were found at any point between the experimental and control groups on any of the physiologic measures. Women in the music listening group had lower anxiety than the women in the control group in the intraoperative period and after completion of the skin sutures. The participants in the music group also reported higher scores related to satisfaction with the cesarean birth experience. The majority of women who experienced music therapy rated their sense of satisfaction with the therapy as high.

What additional questions might I have? Can the researchers separate the effects of continuous presence of the nurse from the effects of the music therapy? Are there any potential negative consequences from music therapy during cesarean birth?

How can I use this study? Music therapy is consistent with the idea of holistic support for the mother during birth. This type of therapy is low cost and noninvasive and may help mothers have a more positive experience during cesarean birth. Nurses should consider offering music therapy to mothers to reduce anxiety and improve satisfaction with the birth experience.

SOURCE: Chang, S., & Chen, C. (2005). Effects of music therapy on women's physiologic measures, anxiety, and satisfaction during cesarean delivery. *Research in Nursing and Health, 28,* 453–461.

to the West. Nurses can recommend that women considering the use of acupuncture check with local, state, and national health organizations for qualified acupuncturists.

MAGNETIC THERAPY

Like the Earth itself, all the body's cells act as magnetic fields radiating energy outward and ultimately becoming part of other magnetic fields. Within the body electrical energy is apparent in electrocardiogram (ECG) and electroencephalogram (EEG) tracings, for example, which provide data about the magnetic fields of the heart and brain. As with other magnetic fields, the energy level is highest at its core and dissipates with distance. For humans this energy field is called "aura" and surrounds the body from head to foot. *Magnetic therapy* is believed to work by increasing blood flow and circulation to infected areas. This increased blood flow, in turn, helps relieve swelling and inflammation. Magnetic therapy is used for diagnosis and treatment of movement disorders (electromyography). It is also used for pain relief (transcutaneous electrical nerve stimulation [TENS]) and to treat insomnia and hypertension (low-energy emission therapy). Magnets should not be used during pregnancy, especially over the abdominal area (Balch & Balch, 2000).

REIKI

Reiki, a Tibetan-Japanese technique, is a form of hand-mediated therapy designed to promote healing, reduce stress, and encourage relaxation. Reiki practitioners place their hands on or above specific problem areas and transfer energy from themselves to their clients to restore the balance of the client's energy fields (Fontaine, 2005).

THERAPEUTIC TOUCH

Therapeutic Touch is a complementary therapy designed to interface with conventional medical care. It was developed in the early 1970s by Dr. Delores Krieger, a nursing professor at New York University, and Dora Kunz, a clairvoyant healer. Therapeutic Touch is grounded in the belief that people are a system of energy with a self-healing potential. The Therapeutic Touch practitioner, often a nurse, can modulate his or her energy

Table 3–4   FACTS ABOUT THERAPEUTIC TOUCH (TT)

Therapeutic Touch is taught in more than 100 colleges and universities worldwide and has been taught to more than 40,000 healthcare providers.

The North American Nursing Diagnosis Association (NANDA) recognizes "energy field disturbance" as a nursing diagnosis, and professional organizations such as the American Nurses Association and the National League for Nursing have supported TT as a nursing intervention.

TT is used as a complementary therapy for virtually all medical and nursing diagnoses as well as for surgical procedures.

TT is best known for its ability to relieve pain and anxiety.

SOURCE: *Nurse's handbook of alternative and complementary therapies.* Springhouse, PA: Springhouse Corporation. (1999.)

field with that of the client's, directing it in a specific way to promote well-being and healing. Proponents of Therapeutic Touch believe that a strong desire to help the recipient is essential as is a conscious use of self to act as a link between the universal life energy and the other person (Fontaine, 2005).

Krieger asserted that healing is an innate human potential and believed that people could be trained to do healing. Her research has demonstrated that the Therapeutic Touch interaction could increase hemoglobin levels in people in the same way that chlorophyll content could be increased in healer-treated plants. This finding was one of the first that allowed quantitative biochemical measurements in humans to detect the effects of healing energy (Gerber, 2001).

Therapeutic Touch has been used for a wide variety of medical and nursing diagnoses but is best known for its use to relieve pain and anxiety. Therapeutic Touch is not difficult to learn nor does it require a lengthy training process. In fact, family members have been taught to use Therapeutic Touch to help their loved ones. There are more specific requirements, including standards and scope of practice and a credentialing process for healthcare workers. Table 3–4 provides a brief description of the elements of the procedure for Therapeutic Touch.

Like many other conventional and complementary therapies, Therapeutic Touch should be applied cautiously to pregnant women and newborns by trained providers (Figure 3–8 ◆).

NURSING CARE OF THE CHILDBEARING FAMILY USING COMPLEMENTARY THERAPIES

Some form of complementary and alternative medicine (CAM) is currently being used by 36% of adults in the United States. When prayer for health reasons and megavitamin therapy are added to the definition, that number increases to 62%. Women use CAM more often than men do, as do people with higher educational levels and people who have been hospitalized within the past year. By race, when megavitamin therapy and prayer are included in the definition, blacks are the greatest users of CAM. When those elements are excluded, Asians are the greatest users followed by whites (NCCAM, 2004). (See Figure 3–9 ◆.)

Figure 3–8 ◆ During pregnancy, Therapeutic Touch is often helpful in easing pain and reducing anxiety.
SOURCE: Nurse Healers—Professional Associates International, The official organization for Therapeutic Touch. www.therapeutic_touch.org.

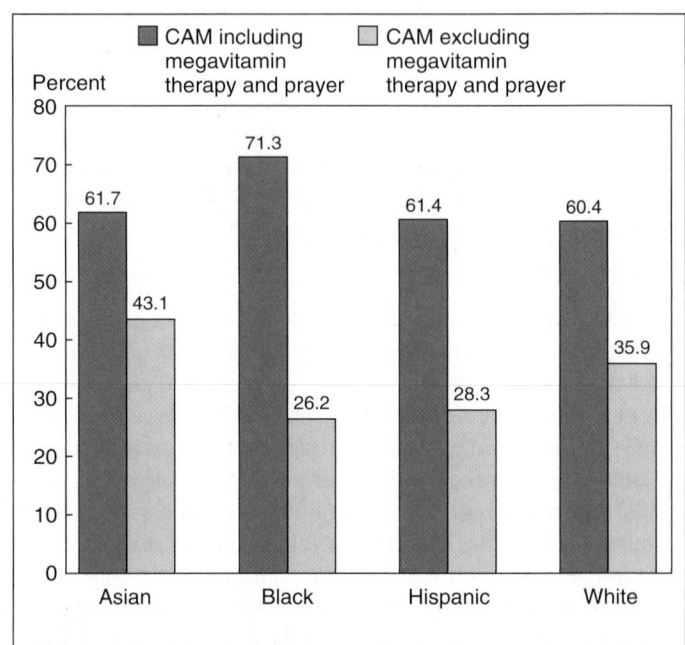

Figure 3–9 ◆ Complementary and alternative medicine (CAM) use by race/ethnicity.
SOURCE: NCCAM. (2004). The Use of Complementary and Alternative Medicine in the United States.

As knowledge of complementary and alternative therapies grows, the number and type of people using one or more of them will probably increase as well. Thus, it is likely that the majority of childbearing families are using some form of CAM even though they do not share that information.

Assessing a Client's Use of Complementary Therapies

The reality that women may use CAM and not reveal it raises some concern. Certain CAM modalities such as biofeedback, acupuncture, aromatherapy, massage, and prayer are not likely to cause adverse effects during pregnancy. However, the possibility exists that there might be interactions between herbal therapies and other medications prescribed by the caregiver. Similarly, complications might develop from the use of vitamin supplements immediately before or after surgery (Olson, 2001).

Nurses who create a climate of respect and openness tend to be more effective in gathering information about a woman's use of complementary or alternative therapies. The following recommendations may be useful to nurses in taking a history (Cady, 2002):

- Ask questions that are direct and nonjudgmental in seeking information about the client's use of CAM.

- Ask questions about specific therapies, including the use of herbal therapy and homeopathy. Because many people consider herbs to be natural substances and because they are often sold as dietary supplements, clients may not think to mention them.

- Avoid making negative or disparaging comments about CAM. Such comments send the message that CAM is not desirable and may discourage people from disclosing their use of CAM therapies.

All nurses practicing today need to have at least an awareness of complementary and alternative therapies. The NCCAM Web site is an excellent resource for healthcare providers and for childbearing women and their families.

Incorporating Complementary Therapies into Maternal-Newborn Nursing Care

Because the practice of nursing is holistic in nature, many nurses are open to and supportive of the use of complementary and alternative therapies. However, nurses in the United States need to know whether the nurse practice act in their state specifically addresses CAM therapies because some states do, whereas others do not. For example, in Louisiana RNs may initiate and use complementary therapies for clients who seek the therapies as part of the nursing plan of care to meet goals such as relief of pain, comfort, reduction of stress, relaxation, improved coping mechanisms, and increased sense of well-being, if the individual has given informed consent. Written policies are required in all practice settings that permit the RN to per-

form such modalities (Cady, 2002). Nurses also need to be knowledgeable about any legal requirements that govern their use of CAM.

In working with childbearing families, or indeed with any clients, nurses who use CAM therapies should choose those methods that are within the scope of nursing practice in their state and not limited by the licensure of other providers (such as massage therapists). Nurses are also best advised to use CAM therapies that are considered somewhat mainstream and that are supported by evidence about their safety and effectiveness (Gaydos, 2001). For example, nurses working with a pregnant woman might safely suggest acupressure wristbands for the treatment of nausea. Other therapies nurses often employ include progressive relaxation, exercise and movement, Therapeutic Touch, visualization and guided imagery, prayer, meditation, music therapy, massage, hydrotherapy, storytelling, aromatherapy, and journaling.

Nurses who use complementary modalities should document their use within the context of nursing practice. This is most effective when the modality is identified as an intervention to address a specific nursing diagnosis or identified client need (Frisch, 2001). Thus, music therapy might be used for a laboring woman to address the identified nursing diagnosis of pain. Other modalities that might be used include progressive relaxation, massage, aromatherapy, and visualization.

Many certified nurse-midwives incorporate complementary and alternative therapies into their clinical practice with childbearing families. Research suggests that CNMs who prescribe CAM do so for the following reasons: nausea and vomiting, labor stimulation, perineal discomfort, lactation disorders, postpartum depression, preterm labor, postpartum hemorrhage, and labor analgesia. The methods most frequently used included herbal therapy, massage therapy, chiropractic, acupressure, and mind-body interventions. To a lesser degree they also recommend aromatherapy, homeopathy, spiritual healing, acupuncture, and bioelectric or magnetic applications (Allaire, Moos, & Wells, 2000). Research on CAM sparks great interest in the public, and momentum is increasing to design and carry out well-developed research on alternative modalities. Nurses have a role in conducting and supporting research of this type. Because of the variety of CAM therapies in use, research is needed in a host of areas.

The results of research sometimes support the use of a given modality; at other times they raise questions about the use of modalities that have enjoyed great popularity. For example, many people consume large doses of vitamin C to prevent the common cold. However, several large-scale, controlled studies have yielded no conclusive data that large doses of vitamin C prevent colds (National Institute of Allergy and Infectious Diseases, 2004). On the other hand, several research studies have demonstrated the effectiveness of moxibustion (described earlier) in treating breech presentation. Although less well known in the West than acupuncture and other forms of TCM, moxibustion has been used in China for centuries to treat pregnant women with a breech presentation. The goal is to get the fetus to turn so that birth occurs in a vertex (headfirst) position. In an analysis of research on CAM therapies in obstetrics, Anderson and Johnson (2005) confirmed that at least three randomized, controlled studies demonstrated that groups receiving moxibustion therapy had a significantly higher percentage of fetuses convert to a vertex presentation than the control groups.

The results of research on CAM can be found in professional journals and at the NCCAM Web site. As the evidence supporting the use of certain interventions grows, nurses and other healthcare providers are incorporating the results as part of their evidence-based practice.

CHAPTER REVIEW

FOCUS YOUR STUDY

- A complementary therapy is an adjunct to conventional medical treatment, whereas an alternative therapy is used in place of prescribed medical therapy.

- The National Center for Complementary and Alternative Medicine (NCCAM) promotes research into complementary and alternative therapies and disseminates the information to consumers and professionals.

- Integrative medicine combines mainstream medical therapies with complementary therapies for which there is some high-quality scientific evidence of safety and effectiveness.

- CAM therapies have several benefits. Many of them emphasize prevention and wellness, place a higher value on holistic healing than on physical cure, are noninvasive, and have few side effects. In addition, many are more affordable and available than conventional therapies.

- Risks include lack of standardization, lack of regulation and research substantiating safety and effectiveness, inadequate training and certification of some healers, and financial and health risks of unproven methods.

- The term *homeopathy* is derived from the Greek word *homos,* meaning "the same." It is a healing system that uses like to cure like; that is, homeopathic remedies are minute dilutions of substances that, if ingested in larger amounts, would produce effects *similar* to the symptoms of the disorder being treated.

- Traditional Chinese medicine (TCM) seeks to ensure the balance of energy, called *chi* or *qi*. Techniques of TCM include acupuncture, moxibustion, herbal therapy, nutrition, acupressure, Qigong, and t'ai chi.

- Ayurveda is the classical system of Hindu medicine. It promotes balance of the three primary forces thought to influence human health and well-being.

- Biofeedback is a method used to help individuals learn to control their physiologic responses based on the concept that the mind controls the body.

- Hypnosis, whether guided by a trained hypnotherapist or induced through self-hypnosis, is a state of great mental and physical relaxation during which a person is very open to suggestions.

- Guided imagery is a state of intense, focused concentration used to create compelling mental images.

- Chiropractic, a profession practiced by licensed chiropractors, is based on concepts of manipulation, especially spinal manipulation.

- Massage therapy involves the manipulation of the soft tissues of the body to reduce stress and tension, increase circulation, diminish pain, and promote a sense of well-being. Reflexology is a specific form of massage that involves the application of pressure to designated points or reflexes on the client's feet, hands, or ears using the thumb and fingers.

- Hydrotherapy is any therapy that makes use of hot or cold moisture in any form to relax muscles, promote rest, decrease pain, reduce swelling, promote healing, cleanse wounds and burns, reduce fever, lessen cramps, and improve well-being.

- Hatha yoga, the physical branch of yoga, is commonly practiced to improve health and well-being, to prevent illness, and to promote healing.

- A *dietary supplement* is any product (excluding tobacco) intended to supplement the diet. It contains one or more of the following ingredients: a mineral, vitamin, herb, amino acid, other botanical supplements, or extracts and ingredients of animal and plant origin.

- Herbs, a form of dietary supplement, are used to treat the symptoms of specific ailments or to enhance overall health. Pregnant and lactating women should inform their primary care provider about any herbs they plan to take.

- Acupressure (sometimes called Chinese massage) uses pressure from the fingers and thumbs to stimulate pressure points. Acupuncture, considered the stronger technique, uses very fine (hairlike) stainless steel needles to stimulate specific points depending on the client's medical assessment and condition.

- Therapeutic Touch is based on the belief that people are a system of energy with a self-healing potential. The Therapeutic Touch practitioner, often a nurse, can unite his or her energy field with that of the client's, directing it in a specific way to promote well-being and healing.

- Many nurses are open to and supportive of complementary and alternative therapies. Nurses who incorporate such therapies into the practice must be certain that they are practicing within the framework of their nurse practice act and with the informed consent of their clients.

EXPLORE MediaLink

http://www.prenhall.com/davidson

NCLEX review questions, case studies, and other interactive resources for this chapter can be found on the Web Site at http://www.prenhall.com/davidson. Click on "Chapter 3" to select the activities for this chapter.

For tutorials including animations and videos, more NCLEX review questions, and an audio glossary, access the accompanying Prentice Hall Nursing MediaLink DVD-ROM in this book.

PRENTICE HALL NURSING MEDIALINK DVD-ROM
Audio Glossary
NCLEX Review
Video: *Massage for Pregnancy*

COMPANION WEBSITE
Additional NCLEX Review
Case Study: *Complementary Therapies*
Care Plan Activity: *Use of CAM in High-Risk Adolescent Pregnancy*
Applications: *Complementary Therapies; Internet Information on Complementary Therapies*
Critical Thinking

CRITICAL THINKING IN ACTION

COMPLEMENTARY AND ALTERNATIVE THERAPIES

View the Critical Thinking in Action video in Chapter 3 of the DVD-ROM. Then answer the questions that follow.

Rommy Startorius, a 34-year-old woman who has never been pregnant, is being seen for her annual gynecologic examination. As part of the health history you ask her whether she is using any forms of treatment for her health that are new since she was seen last year. Initially she reports that she has been getting massage therapy for low back pain and then, as the conversation progresses, she reports that she has been having acupuncture as well. She asks you how "regular" doctors feel about acupuncture and other forms of alternative therapy.

1. How would you describe the role of CAM in health care today?

2. What information could you provide about the use of acupuncture?

3. Ms. Startorius asks you how she can learn about CAM therapies that have some research support for their effectiveness. How would you reply?

REFERENCES

Allaire, A. D., Moos, M. K., & Wells, S. R. (2000). Complementary and alternative medicine in pregnancy: A survey of North Carolina certified nurse-midwives. *Obstetrics and Gynecology, 95*(1), 19–23.

American Association of Naturopathic Physicians. (2005). *What is naturopathic medicine?* Retrieved December 7, 2005, from http://www.naturopathic.org/naturopathic_medicine/whatis.aspx

Anderson, F. W. J., & Johnson, C. T. (2005). Complementary and alternative medicine in obstetrics. *International Journal of Gynecology and Obstetrics, 9*, 116–124.

Balch, P. A., & Balch, J. F. (2000). *Prescription for nutritional healing* (3rd ed). New York: Penguin Putnam.

Barnes, P., Powell-Griner, E., McFann, K., & Nahin, R. (2004, May 27). *CDC Advance Data Report #343. Complementary and alternative medicine use among adults: United States, 2002.* Retrieved December 7, 2005, from http://nccam.nih.gov/news/camsurvey.htm

Bratman, S. (1998). *The alternative medicines ratings guide.* Rocklin, CA: Prima Health.

Cady, R. (2002). Are there legal issues of concern for nurses when patients use complimentary [sic] and alternative medicine? *The American Journal of Maternal/Child Nursing, 27*(2), 119.

ClinicalTrials.gov. (2005). *Self-hypnotic relaxation therapy during invasive procedures.* (Last updated July 25, 2005.) Retrieved December 7, 2005, from http://clinicaltrials.gov/show/NCT00087841

Cole, R. L. (1998). *The gentle greeting.* Naperville, IL: Sourcebooks.

Davidson, J. R. T., Kishore, M. G., Fairbank, J. A., Krishnan, K. R. R., Califf, R. M., & Binanay, C., et al. (2002). Effect of *Hypericum perforatum* (St. John's wort) in major depressive disorder: A

randomized, controlled trial. *Journal of the American Medical Association, 287,* 1807–1814.

Fontaine, K. L. (2005). *Complementary and alternative therapies for nursing practice* (2nd ed.). Upper Saddle River, NJ: Prentice Hall Health.

Frisch, N. C. (2001). Nursing as a context for alternative/complementary modalities. *Online Journal of Issues in Nursing, 6*(2). Retrieved June 19, 2001, from http://www.nursingworld.org.ojin/topic15/tpc15_2.htm

Gastelu, D. (2000). *The complete nutritional supplement buyer's guide.* New York: Three Rivers Press.

Gaydos, H. L. (2001). *Complementary and alternative therapies in nursing education: Trends and issues.* Retrieved June 19, 2001, from http://www.nursingworld.org.ojin/topic15/tpc15_5.htm

Gaynor, M. L. (1999). *Sounds of healing.* New York: Broadway Books.

Gerber, R. (2001). *Vibrational medicine* (3rd ed). Rochester, VT: Bear & Company.

Graedon, J., & Graedon, T. (2001). *The people's pharmacy guide to home and herbal remedies.* New York: St. Martin's Griffin.

Hobbs, C. L., & Keville, K. (1998). *Women's herbs, women's health.* Loveland, CO: Interweave Press.

Krishnamurti, J. (2000). *To be human.* (D. Skitt, Ed.). Boston: Shambhala.

Lockie, A., & Geddes, N. (2000). *Complete guide to homeopathy: The principles and practice of treatment homeopathy.* New York: DK Publishing.

Mayo Clinic. (2001). *Chiropractic treatment.* Retrieved September 2, 2002, from http://www.mayoclinic.com

Mayo Clinic. (2002). *Using herbal supplements wisely.* Retrieved September 2, 2002, from http://www.mayoclinic.com

Moyers, B. D. (1993). *Healing and the mind.* New York: Doubleday.

National Center for Complementary and Alternative Medicine. (2004, May 27). More than one-third of adults use complementary and alternative medicine [press release]. Retrieved May 26, 2006, from http://nccam.nih.gov/news/2004/052704.htm

National Center for Complementary and Alternative Medicine. (Last modified July 12, 2005.) *What is complementary and alternative medicine (CAM)?* Retrieved December 7, 2005, from http://nccam.nih.gov/health/whatiscam/

National Institute of Allergy and Infectious Diseases. (2004, December). *The common cold.* Retrieved July 14, 2005, from http://www.niaid.nih.gov/factsheets/cold.htm

National Institutes of Health (NIH), Office of Dietary Supplements. (2001). *What are dietary supplements?* Retrieved September 2, 2002, from http://ods.od.nih.gov/whatare/whatare.html

National Toxicology Program. (2002). Herbal medicines. *NTP Factsheets—Year 2002.* Retrieved September 2, 2002, from http://ntp-server.niehs.noh.gov/htdocs/liason/factsheets/HerbMedFacts.html

Nurse's handbook of alternative and complementary therapies (2nd ed.). (2002). Springhouse, PA: Springhouse Corporation.

Olson, G. L. (2001). When your pregnant patient uses alternative medicine. *Contemporary OB/GYN, 46*(9), 45–58.

Sinclair, M. (2005). *Pediatric massage therapy* (2nd ed., p. 2). Baltimore: Lippincott Williams & Wilkins.

Upledger Institute. (1998). *Discover craniosacral therapy* [Pamphlet]. Palm Beach Gardens, FL: Author.

UNIT 2

Women's Health

Women's Health Across the Lifespan

Mom was great about preparing me for my first period. I knew why I had periods and how to handle them. She NEVER called it "the curse" or made a big deal out of it, so I was surprised when friends were so negative. To me, periods were a sign of womanhood.

OBJECTIVES

1. Discuss the key points a nurse should consider in taking a sexual history.

2. Summarize information that women may need in order to implement appropriate self-care measures for dealing with menstruation.

3. Identify causes of amenorrhea.

4. Contrast dysmenorrhea and premenstrual syndrome.

5. Delineate the physical and psychologic aspects of menopause.

6. Explain the relationship between menopause and osteoporosis.

7. Identify medical and complementary therapies to alleviate the discomforts of menopause.

KEY TERMS

Amenorrhea   72

Climacteric   77

Dysmenorrhea   73

Hormone replacement therapy (HRT)   79

Menopause   77

Osteoporosis   78

Perimenopause   77

Premenstrual dysphoric disorder (PMDD)   73

Premenstrual syndrome (PMS)   73

MEDIALINK

Additional resources for this content can be found on the Prentice Hall Nursing MediaLink DVD-ROM and on the Companion Website at http://www.prenhall.com/davidson. Click on "Chapter 4" to select the activities for this chapter.

A woman's healthcare needs change throughout her lifetime. As a young girl she requires health teaching about menstruation, sexuality, and personal responsibility. As a teen she needs information about reproductive choices and safe sexual activity. During this time she should also be introduced to the importance of healthcare practices such as breast self-examination and regular Pap smears. The mature woman may need to be reminded of these self-care issues and prepared for physical changes that accompany childbirth and aging. By educating women about their bodies, their healthcare choices, and their rights and responsibilities, nurses can help women be knowledgeable consumers who assume responsibility for the health care they receive.

This chapter, the first of six devoted to women's health, focuses primarily on wellness care. Chapter 5 ∞ then considers issues related to family planning. Chapter 6 ∞ focuses on infections women may encounter, and Chapter 7 ∞ addresses some of the common gynecologic issues and conditions a woman may face. Chapter 8 ∞ explores some of the major social issues women face, and Chapter 9 ∞ focuses on violence against women.

COMMUNITY-BASED NURSING CARE

Women's health refers to a holistic view of women and their health-related needs within the context of their everyday lives. It is based on the awareness that a woman's physical, mental, and social status are interdependent and determine her state of health or illness. The woman's perception of her situation, her assessment of her needs, her values, and her beliefs are valid, important factors to be incorporated into any healthcare intervention.

CLINICAL TIP

Remember that a woman's views frequently influence the health care of her entire family because women typically coordinate the family's healthcare needs.

Nurses can provide health teaching and information about self-care practices in schools, during routine examinations in a clinic or office, at senior centers, at meetings of volunteer organizations, through classes offered by the local health department or community college, or in the home. Nurses can also help women with various forms of disability to address their unique healthcare needs and optimize their state of wellness. This community-based focus is the key to providing effective nursing care to women of all ages.

In reality, the vast majority of women's health care is provided outside of acute care settings. Nurses oriented to community-based care are especially effective in recognizing the autonomy of each individual and in dealing with clients holistically. This approach is important in addressing not only physical problems but also major health issues such as violence against women, which may go undetected unless care providers

DEVELOPING CULTURAL COMPETENCE

DEVELOPING EFFECTIVE COMMUNICATION

In the course of your work as a nurse, you are bound to encounter people different from yourself. Even with the best of intentions, you may say or do something your client or the client's family finds offensive or inappropriate. Often it is due to a misunderstanding, misinterpretation, or miscommunication of information. Body language and facial expressions from the client or family will give you a clue that this has occurred. Asking the client if she has any questions or concerns related to information you are trying to convey may open up communication and allow the woman or her family to express concerns or misunderstandings. You could ask about their cultural traditions, which shows respect for their personal belief system. This allows for a trusting relationship to develop, which in turn will encourage and facilitate improved communication and therapeutic relationships.

ask women specifically about violence and are alert for signs of it. See Developing Cultural Competence.

The Nurse's Role in Addressing Issues of Women's Wellness and Sexuality

Women expect the nurses who care for them to be knowledgeable not only about gynecologic health, but about a wide variety of health topics. Thus it is important that nurses expand their knowledge about the issues healthy women and their families may face. These include, for example, a general knowledge of normal growth and development; recommended screening procedures for both women and men, and the ages at which these procedures are indicated; signs and symptoms of substance abuse, including alcoholism; health issues that well men face; signs of emotional stress and depression; community resources; and a variety of other topics. By keeping abreast of issues well families may face, the nurse becomes a more complete resource and acts to promote overall health.

On occasion, most women experience concern and even anxiety about some aspect of menstruation, contraception, or sexual activity. Societal standards and pressures can cause girls and adolescents to evaluate and compare with others their experiences with menstruation, sexual attractiveness, and beliefs and values about engaging in sexual activity. Young adults may be more concerned about the reproductive and health implications of sexual intercourse. The desire to achieve or avoid pregnancy and the fear of sexually transmitted infections may cause many women to modify their sexual practices and activities. Although older women share many of these same concerns, they may also experience anxiety about the onset of menopausal changes and wonder how these changes will affect their sexuality. Furthermore, throughout the lifespan women may have concerns, problems, and questions about sex roles, sexual orientation, be-haviors, inhibitions, morality, and related areas such as family planning. Recently divorced women who have been in a long-term marriage may need education about sexual activity and sexually transmitted infections if they are reentering the dating world. Women frequently voice these concerns to the nurse in a clinic or ambulatory setting. Thus the nurse may need to assume the role of counselor on sexual and reproductive matters.

Nurses who assume this role must be secure about their own sexuality. They must also develop an awareness of their own feelings, values, and attitudes about sexuality so that they can be more sensitive and objective when they encounter the values and beliefs of others. Nurses also need to know about the structures and functions of female and male reproductive sys-tems. In addition, they should have accurate, up-to-date infor-mation about topics related to menstruation, sexuality, sexual practices, cultural differences, menopause, and common gyne-cologic problems.

Staying up-to-date on issues of sexuality and women's health requires constant vigilance: regular journal review, atten-dance at reputable conferences, library and Internet searches, and diligent perusal of women's health literature are essential activities. Continuing education for the practicing nurse and ap-propriate courses in undergraduate and graduate nursing educa-tion programs can also help nurses achieve and maintain the requisite knowledge. These activities enhance the nurses' knowledge about these topics and improve their effectiveness in teaching and providing care for their clients.

Taking a Sexual History

Nurses today are often responsible for taking a woman's initial history, including her gynecologic and sexual history. To be ef-fective in this role, the nurse must have good communication skills and should conduct the interview in a quiet, private place free of distractions. The sexual history is one part of a lengthier health history and covers personal and intimate topics.

CLINICAL TIP

When taking a history, start your interview with less intimate areas, such as medical and surgical history, and then proceed to the sexual history toward the end of the history-taking session. This approach helps the woman develop a comfort level with you before disclosing personal information.

Opening the sexual history discussion with a brief explana-tion of the purpose of such questions is often helpful. For exam-ple, the nurse might say, "As your nurse I'm interested in all aspects of your well-being. Often women have concerns or questions about sexual issues, especially as their life situations change. I will be asking you some questions about your sexual history as part of your general health history." This explanation will help women understand the nature of this part of the history and allow for more open, honest answers.

It may be helpful to use direct eye contact as much as pos-sible unless the nurse knows it is culturally unacceptable to the woman. The nurse should do little, if any, writing during this

part of the interview. Open-ended questions are often useful in eliciting information. For example, "What, if anything, would you change about your sex life?" will elicit more information than "Are you happy with your sex life now?" The nurse should also clarify terminology to ensure accurate information is be-ing conveyed. Proceeding from easier topics to those that are more difficult will help a natural flow of information. Through-out the interview, the nurse should be alert to the client's body language and nonverbal cues. It is essential that the nurse lis-ten, react in a nonjudgmental manner, and use teachable mo-ments to educate women about their bodies. It is also important that the nurse not assume the client is heterosexual. Nurses should be respectful of all clients when discussing their sexu-ality; some clients are open to this discussion whereas others will be very reserved until a sense of trust in the caregiver is established.

After completing the sexual history, the nurse assesses the information obtained. If there is a concern that requires further medical tests and assessments, the nurse refers the woman to a nurse practitioner, certified nurse-midwife, physician, or counselor as necessary. In many instances the nurse alone will be able to develop a nursing diagnosis and then plan and im-plement an appropriate intervention. For example, if the nurse determines that a woman who is interested in conceiving a child does not have a clear understanding of when she ovu-lates, the nurse may formulate the nursing diagnosis *Deficient Knowledge* related to lack of information about the timing of ovulation. The nurse can then implement a plan of care to eval-uate the woman's knowledge, and then provide the necessary education.

The nurse must be realistic in making assessments and planning interventions. It requires insight and skill to recognize when a woman's problem requires interventions that are beyond a nurse's preparation and ability. In such cases, the nurse must make appropriate referrals.

MENSTRUATION

Girls today begin to learn about puberty and menstruation at a surprisingly young age. Unfortunately, the source of their "edu-cation" is sometimes their peers and sometimes the media; thus the information is frequently incomplete, inaccurate, and sensa-tionalized. Nurses who work with girls and adolescents recog-nize this and are working hard to provide accurate health teaching and to correct misinformation about *menarche* (the on-set of menses) and the menstrual cycle.

Cultural, religious, and personal attitudes about menstrua-tion are part of the menstrual experience and often reflect nega-tive attitudes toward women. In the past, many misconceptions surrounded menstruation. Women were often isolated or re-stricted to the company of other women during their monthly flow because they were considered "unclean." Currently in the Western world there are few customs associated with menstru-ation, although some women remain uncomfortable about dis-cussing it. Sexual intercourse during menstruation is a common practice and is not generally contraindicated. For most couples, the decision is one of personal preference. (The physiology of menstruation is discussed in Chapter 10 ∞).

Counseling the Premenstrual Girl about Menarche

The average age of menarche is about 12.5 years for girls in the United States, but it may occur between the ages of 8 and 16. For about 2 years before menarche, a girl experiences a series of physical changes as her body develops. Maturity level and self-concept often influence a young girl's comfort in discussing these changes. However, the most critical factor in successful adaptation to menarche is the preteen's or adolescent's level of correct information and preparedness. The nurse is an excellent source of information about puberty and menarche. Information should be clear and straightforward and offered as it relates to each girl's individual situation and maturation level. The following basic information is helpful for young clients:

- *Cycle length.* Cycle length is determined from the first day of one menses to the first day of the next menses. Initially, cycle length may be irregular. It is not unusual for cycles to be unpredictable for the first year. Once established, the cycle is about 29 days, but the normal length may vary from 21 to 35 days. Cycle length often varies by a day or two from one cycle to the next, although greater normal variations may also occur.
- *Amount of flow.* The average flow is approximately 25 to 60 mL per period. Usually women characterize the amount of flow in terms of the number of pads or tampons used. Flow often is heavier at first and lighter toward the end of the period. Blood loss over 80 mL is generally considered abnormal but estimating that can be challenging because women may over- or underestimate the amount of their flow (Varney, Kriebs, & Gregor, 2004).
- *Length of menses.* Menses usually lasts from 2 to 8 days, although the length may vary.

The nurse should make it clear that variations in age at menarche, length of cycle, and duration of menses are normal, because girls are likely to be concerned if their experience varies from that of their peers. It also is helpful to acknowledge the negative aspects of menstruation (messiness and embarrassment) while stressing its positive role as a symbol of maturity and womanhood.

Educational Topics

The nurse's primary role is to provide accurate information and assist in clarifying misconceptions so that girls will develop positive self-images and progress smoothly through this phase of maturation.

PADS AND TAMPONS

Since early times women have made pads from cloth or rags, which required washing but were reusable. Some women made them from gauze or cotton balls. Commercial tampons were introduced in the 1930s.

Today adhesive-stripped minipads and maxipads and flushable tampons are readily available. However, the deodorants and increased absorbency that manufacturers have added to both sanitary napkins and tampons may prove harmful. The chemicals used to deodorize and increased absorbency can create irritation of the vulva and inner aspects of the vagina. This irritation may cause an external rash or internal sores from trauma to the tender mucosal lining of the vagina.

When taking a menstrual history, the nurse should attempt to determine the amount of bleeding each month. The woman can be asked what type of pad or tampon she uses, how frequently she changes, and how much blood has been absorbed. Women should be advised to change pads frequently, every 3 to 6 hours when awake, regardless of the amount of blood that is absorbed. If a woman reports that she supersaturates a maxipad every 1 to 2 hours for 2 to 3 days, she may be experiencing a gynecologic problem. Heavy menstrual flow is a leading cause of anemia in women.

The use of superabsorbent tampons has been linked to the development of toxic shock syndrome (TSS). Women may prevent problems by using tampons with the minimum absorbency needed to control menstrual flow, changing them every 3 to 6 hours, and avoiding using them for vaginal discharge or abnormal bleeding. Women should be instructed on proper hygiene techniques for insertion and removal of tampons to decrease the risk of bacterial toxins being spread from hands to the vagina. Specifically, a woman should wash her hands before inserting or removing a tampon. After the tampon is unwrapped she should avoid touching the portion of the tampon to be inserted into the vagina. Most toilet systems become clogged if tampons are flushed. Thus, when a tampon is removed, it should first be wrapped in toilet tissue or placed in a disposable bag and then discarded in a trash receptacle or designated container. Finally the woman should again wash her hands.

In the absence of a heavy menstrual flow, tampons absorb moisture, leaving the vaginal walls dry and subject to injury; therefore, their use should be discouraged when the flow is too light to warrant a tampon. The absorbency of regular tampons varies. If the tampon is hard to pull out or shreds when removed, or if the vagina becomes too dry, the tampon is probably too absorbent. If a woman is worried about accidental spotting, she can check the diagrams on the packages of regular tampons. Those that expand in width are better able to prevent leakage without being too absorbent.

A woman may want to use tampons only during the day and switch to pads at night to avoid vaginal irritation. If a woman experiences vaginal irritation, itching, or soreness or notices an unusual odor while using tampons, she should stop using them and be evaluated for infection.

The choice of sanitary protection must meet the individual's needs and feel comfortable, whether it be pads or tampons. Cultural factors may play a role in this decision for a woman. See the accompanying Developing Cultural Competence box. Young women should be taught to track their periods and to carry feminine hygiene products when their menses is due so that they are prepared for its onset.

VAGINAL SPRAYS AND DOUCHING

Vaginal sprays are unnecessary and can cause itching, burning, rashes, and other problems. Healthcare providers do not generally recommend that women use them. If a woman chooses to

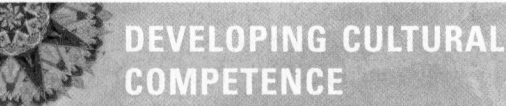

DEVELOPING CULTURAL COMPETENCE

CULTURAL PROHIBITIONS ABOUT TAMPON USE

Among Arab people, a girl's virginity is highly valued. As a result, unmarried Arab women do not use tampons during menstruation for fear of breaking the hymen. They use only sanitary pads or napkins (Al-Oballi Kridli, 2002).

The avoidance of tampons by unmarried women may also be advocated by other religious groups or sects. Thus it is wise to ask the young woman (or her mother if the girl is uncertain) about the issue.

use a spray, she needs to know that these sprays are for external use only, should be used infrequently, and should never be applied to irritated or itching skin.

Douching as a hygiene practice is unnecessary, because the vagina has numerous glands that provide a natural cleansing. Caregivers generally advise against it. The vagina has naturally occurring bacteria that aid in maintaining a pH balance to keep fungal and bacterial growth at bay. Douching upsets this vaginal ecology, which can make the vagina more susceptible to infection. Douching with one of the perfumed or flavored douches can cause an allergic reaction. Propelling water up the vagina may force bacteria and germs from the vagina into the uterus. It is essential that women avoid douching during menstruation, because the cervix is dilated to permit the downward flow of menstrual fluids from the uterine lining. Douching is also contraindicated during pregnancy.

CLEANSING THE PERINEUM

The secretions that continually bathe the vagina are completely odor free while they are in the vagina; only when they combine with perspiration and become exposed to the air does odor develop. Keeping one's skin clean and free of bacteria with plain soap and water is the most effective method of controlling odor. Bathing is as important (if not more so) during menses as at any other time. A long leisurely soak in a warm tub may also help to relieve cramps.

A woman can ensure herself of adequate ventilation by wearing cotton panties and clothes loose enough to allow air to circulate. After using the toilet, a woman should always wipe herself from front to back and, if necessary, follow up with a moistened paper towel or toilet paper.

The most important thing to remember is that if an unusual odor persists despite these efforts, a visit to one's healthcare provider is indicated. Certain conditions, such as vaginitis, produce a foul-smelling discharge.

Associated Menstrual Conditions

A variety of menstrual irregularities have been identified. Several of them are discussed in Chapter 7 ∞ in the section on dysfunctional uterine bleeding. Others are addressed in the following sections.

The following terms are used to describe variations in uterine bleeding:

- *Hypomenorrhea*—short duration of menstrual flow or, in other words, uterine bleeding at normal intervals but in decreased amounts
- *Hypermenorrhea*—an abnormally long or heavy menstrual flow at normal menstrual intervals (sometimes used interchangeably with menorrhagia)
- *Oligomenorrhea*—bleeding, often irregular, occurring at intervals greater than 40 days
- *Polymenorrhea*—bleeding, either regular or irregular, occurring at intervals of less than 22 days
- *Menorrhagia*—bleeding that is excessive in amount and duration, which occurs at regular intervals (see hypermenorrhea)
- *Metrorrhagia*—bleeding, usually of a normal amount, occurring at irregular intervals
- *Menometrorrhagia*—bleeding that is excessive in amount and duration, which occurs at either regular or irregular intervals
- *Intermenstrual bleeding*—bleeding occurring between regular menstrual cycles

AMENORRHEA

Amenorrhea, the absence of menses, is classified as primary or secondary. Primary amenorrhea is said to occur if menstruation has not been established by 16 years of age. Secondary amenorrhea is said to occur when an established menses (of longer than 3 months) ceases. Typically, the causes of amenorrhea are categorized into one of four groups:

1. *Hypothalamic dysfunction.* Several types of hypothalamic disorders can occur. Some are very rare disorders and may be related to a failure of the central structures of the hypothalamus to develop properly. Other disorders may be caused by a tumor. More common forms of hypothalamic dysfunction are triggered by systemic stress related to marked weight loss (anorexia, bulimia, fad dieting), excessive exercise (associated with long-distance runners, dancers, and other athletes with a low body fat ratio), and severe or prolonged stress.

2. *Pituitary dysfunction.* Pituitary disease and pituitary tumors, such as a pituitary adenoma, can cause changes in the many hormones, including prolactin, that the pituitary manufactures. A variety of medications, including several used to treat anxiety and other psychiatric disorders, can induce a mild increase in prolactin levels, resulting in amenorrhea. Amenorrhea may also be related to low prolactin levels resulting from pituitary failure. Sheehan's syndrome, head trauma, and cancer are also serious causes of hypopituitarism.

3. *Chronic anovulation or ovarian failure.* Some forms of ovarian failure are caused by genetic disorders often related to the sex chromosomes and are not treatable. Turner syndrome (see Chapter 12 ∞) is one of the most

common genetic disorders. Causes of chronic anovulation include polycystic ovarian syndrome or thyroid or adrenal disorders. Ovarian failure is related to exposure to radiation, chemotherapy, viral infection, and surgical removal of the ovary.

4. *Anatomic abnormalities.* This category includes a variety of structural disorders such as congenital absence of the uterus, ovaries, or vagina; congenital obstruction; or imperforate hymen.

Diagnosis begins with a thorough history and careful physical examination. For women who have had periods, this evaluation begins with a pregnancy test. For a woman who has never menstruated, the pelvic examination is a crucial assessment tool in determining that she has a normal vagina, uterus, and ovaries. Regardless of type of amenorrhea, based on initial findings, further, more specific tests are usually done. To evaluate pituitary function, a serum prolactin level is often obtained as a screening test. If serum prolactin levels are elevated, magnetic resonance imaging (MRI) will be ordered to rule out a pituitary tumor. Other pituitary hormones can be evaluated if necessary. Similarly, elevated serum follicle-stimulating hormone (FSH) levels indicate ovarian failure. A thyroid-stimulating hormone (TSH) level is assessed to rule out thyroid disease, and a 2-hour postprandial, 75-gram-load glucose tolerance test is done to rule out polycystic ovarian syndrome.

Treatment is dictated by the causative factors. Some conditions, such as imperforate hymen, are easily corrected. Other causes are not treatable. The nurse can explain that once the underlying condition has been corrected—for example, when the client gains sufficient body weight—menses will resume. Female athletes and women who participate in strenuous exercise routines may be advised to increase their caloric intake or reduce their exercise levels for a month or two to see whether a normal cycle resumes. If it does not, medical referral is indicated.

DYSMENORRHEA

Dysmenorrhea, or painful menstruation, occurs at, or a day before, the onset of menstruation and disappears by the end of menses. Dysmenorrhea is classified as primary or secondary.

Primary dysmenorrhea is defined as cramps without underlying disease. Prostaglandins F_2 and $F_{2\alpha}$, which are produced by the uterus in higher concentrations during menses, are the primary cause. They increase uterine contractility and decrease uterine artery blood flow, causing ischemia. The end result is the painful sensation of cramps. Dysmenorrhea typically disappears after a first pregnancy and does not occur if cycles are anovulatory.

Treatment of primary dysmenorrhea includes oral contraceptives (which inhibit ovulation); nonsteroidal anti-inflammatory drugs (NSAIDs) (such as ibuprofen, aspirin, and naproxen), which act as prostaglandin inhibitors; and self-care measures such as regular exercise, rest, application of heat, and good nutrition. Biofeedback has also been used with some success.

Secondary dysmenorrhea is associated with pathology of the reproductive tract and usually appears after menstruation has been established. Conditions that most frequently cause secondary dysmenorrhea include endometriosis, residual pelvic inflammatory disease (PID), cervical stenosis, uterine fibroids, ovarian cysts, benign or malignant tumors of the pelvis or abdomen, or the presence of an intrauterine device (IUD). Because primary and secondary dysmenorrhea may coexist, accurate differential diagnosis is essential for appropriate treatment.

Dysmenorrhea sometimes occurs in women who are also experiencing menometrorrhagia. In such cases, a careful examination is necessary to determine what is causing both symptoms. Testing may include transvaginal ultrasound, hysterosalpingography, and hysteroscopy. If the examination shows an endometrial polyp, treatment is removal of the polyp with a dilation and curettage (D&C) of the uterus.

For women with severe dysmenorrhea, use of continuous oral contraceptive therapy, which does not allow ovulation or menstruation to occur, may be of benefit. Hysterectomy may be the treatment of choice if there are anatomic disorders and childbearing is not desired. Presacral neurectomy may control severe dysmenorrhea caused by endometriosis.

Self-Care Measures for Dysmenorrhea

Some nutritionists suggest that vitamins B and E help relieve the discomforts associated with menstruation. Vitamin B_6 may help relieve the premenstrual bloating and irritability some women experience. Vitamin E, a mild prostaglandin inhibitor, may help decrease menstrual discomfort. Avoiding salt can decrease discomfort from fluid retention.

Heat is soothing and promotes increased blood flow. Any source of warmth, from sipping herbal tea to soaking in a hot tub or using a heating pad, may be helpful during painful periods. Massage can also soothe aching back muscles and promote relaxation and blood flow.

Daily exercise can ease existing menstrual discomfort and help prevent cramps and other menstrual complaints. Aerobic exercise—jogging, cycling, aerobic dancing, swimming, and fast-paced walking—is especially helpful (Figure 4–1 ◆). Persistent discomfort should be medically evaluated.

PREMENSTRUAL SYNDROME

Premenstrual syndrome (PMS) refers to a symptom complex associated with the luteal phase of the menstrual cycle (2 weeks before onset of menses). An estimated 70% to 90% of women of reproductive age report physical or emotional changes premenstrually. A diagnosis of PMS is made when women report at least one affective (emotional) or somatic (physical) symptom that occurs after ovulation and before the onset of menses in three consecutive menstrual cycles. This incorporates approximately 20% to 40% of all women. **Premenstrual dysphoric disorder (PMDD)** affects an even smaller percentage of women, 3% to 8%. Women with PMDD must experience five or more symptoms in the given time frame, which are relieved with menstruation and have occurred during most cycles during the previous year. PMDD markedly interferes with work, school, and relationships and must not merely be worsened symptoms of another disorder such as major depressive disorder, panic disorder, or personality disorder (Shulman, 2005).

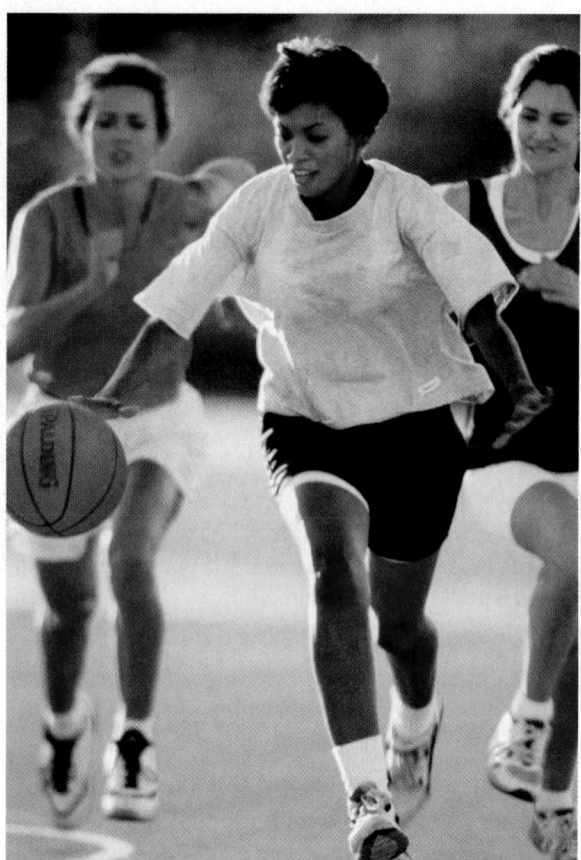

Figure 4–1 ◆ Regular exercise is an important part of therapy for dysmenorrhea.
SOURCE: Tim Pannell-CORBIS.

Premenstrual symptoms include, but are not limited to, the following:

- *Psychologic:* irritability, lethargy, depression, low morale, anxiety, sleep disorders, crying spells, hostility, decreased concentration
- *Neurologic:* classic migraine, vertigo, syncope
- *Respiratory:* rhinitis, hoarseness
- *Gastrointestinal:* nausea, vomiting, constipation, abdominal bloating, increased appetite or food cravings
- *Urinary:* retention and oliguria
- *Dermatologic:* acne
- *Mammary:* swelling and tenderness
- *Musculoskeletal:* joint or muscle pain

The exact cause of PMS is unknown, although a variety of theories have been put forth to explain it. These include, for example, hormone imbalance, nutritional deficiency, prostaglandin excess, and endorphin deficiency. Researchers currently speculate that PMS is related to decreased serotonin levels, and selective serotonin reuptake inhibitors (SSRIs) are the most common treatment supported by the literature (Shulman, 2005).

Diagnosis is generally made after having the woman keep a menstrual calendar for 3 months on which she carefully records daily symptoms, rating them on a scale of 0 to 4, with 0 used for no symptoms and 4 used for severe, debilitating symptoms. The information provided by the diary should be very helpful. In some cases, the diary may reveal that a woman has psychologic symptoms that are present throughout her cycle but intensify premenstrually. This is not a diagnosis of PMDD but an exacerbation of an underlying disease that should be referred for psychiatric evaluation. Except in very severe cases, treatment focuses, at least initially, on lifestyle changes and natural approaches. These are discussed in the following section. In addition to vitamin supplements, pharmacologic treatments for PMS include diuretics, calcium supplementation, and prostaglandin inhibitors. All have been effective in some women and not in others. There is little evidence to support the use of oral contraceptives for the successful treatment of PMS (Shulman, 2005). Previously progesterone had been used to treat PMS but it is no longer recommended. Research suggests that it is no more effective than a placebo and it may actually increase symptoms in some women (Dell, Moskowitz, & Sondheimer, 2001).

NURSING CARE MANAGEMENT

The nurse can help the woman identify specific symptoms and develop healthy behavior. After assessment, the nurse may advise the woman to restrict her intake of foods containing methylxanthines, such as chocolate, cola, and coffee. It is advisable for the woman to restrict her intake of alcohol, nicotine, red meat, animal fats, and foods containing salt and sugar. Concurrently, she should increase her intake of complex carbohydrates (such as whole grains, brown rice, oatmeal), protein, fruits, vegetables, and vegetable oils and increase the frequency of meals. A multiple vitamin and mineral supplement may also be helpful.

Supplementation with B complex vitamins, especially B_6, may decrease anxiety and depression. Vitamin E supplements may help reduce breast tenderness. Supplementation with 1200 mg calcium carbonate is often effective in reducing physical and psychologic symptoms of PMS. Magnesium supplements of 200 mg daily may help reduce fluid retention and breast tenderness. Herbal remedies such as black cohosh, ginger, red raspberry leaf, and evening primrose oil may reduce the effects of PMS. Underlying health conditions may contraindicate the use of herbal or vitamin supplements, however, and must be considered when recommending them (Mayo Clinic Staff, 2004).

A program of aerobic exercises such as fast walking, jogging, or aerobic dancing is generally beneficial. In fact, women who exercise regularly tend to have fewer, less severe symptoms.

An empathic relationship with a healthcare professional to whom the woman feels free to voice concerns is highly beneficial. The nurse can also encourage the woman to keep a journal to help identify life events associated with PMS. Stress reduction education, self-care groups, and self-help literature can also help women gain control over their bodies.

HEALTH MAINTENANCE FOR WELL WOMEN

Healthcare providers are becoming increasingly aware of the value of health maintenance and disease prevention, as are many consumers of healthcare services. Women can make lifestyle choices that promote health and well-being. These choices involve a variety of factors including:

- Eating a nutritious, balanced diet
- Maintaining normal weight for height (no fad dieting)
- Performing regular aerobic exercise and weight training several times a week
- Getting adequate sleep
- Avoiding smoking and/or stopping smoking
- Consuming alcohol in moderation
- Managing stress effectively
- Developing enjoyable hobbies and leisure activities
- Developing an inner life in some form through religion, spirituality, personal reflection, yoga, and so forth
- Fostering bonds of support and affection with family and friends
- Obtaining regular health screenings and assessments
- Ensuring that immunizations are up-to-date

Health screening recommendations vary by age. Table 4–1 from the National Women's Health Information Center (2006) identifies general screening and immunization guidelines for low-risk women based on their age. Nurses can share this information with well women so that they can be aware of indicated screening procedures.

Body Piercing, Tattoos, and Branding

Body piercing and tattooings, often called *body art*, are rapidly becoming commonplace in today's culture among people of all ages (Figure 4–2 ◆). Branding is a more controversial and riskier expression of body art.

Tattooing is the application of minute amounts of pigments into the skin with indelible inks. It has a rich history, beginning as early as 200 BC in Egypt. Over the years in various cultures, it represented social standing, family affiliation, or achievements (Knutson, 2002).

Body piercing sites include earlobes and ear cartilage, lips, nose, tongue, eyebrow, nipples, umbilicus, and the external genitalia for the purpose of displaying some form of adornment or jewelry. Estimates suggest that, in the United States, as many as 50% of undergraduates have had some form of body piercing (Donohoe, 2006).

Branding is the application of intense heat to tissue, resulting in a scar two to three times the width of the instrument used. The procedure is very painful, causing third-degree burns. Historically, it has been used to label prisoners, slaves, or social outcasts (Knutson, 2002).

Each of these forms of body art carries with it an element of health risk. For tattooing and body piercing, risks include infections such as HIV and hepatitis B and C because of the use of inadequately sterilized equipment, as well as allergic reactions, local swelling and burns, granulomas, and keloid formation (more common in people of African descent). Tattooing has also been associated with a variety of risk-taking behaviors in adolescents (Donohoe, 2006). Oral piercing has been associated with tooth and gum damage. Among pregnant or breastfeeding women, nipple piercing has been associated with mastitis, damaged milk ducts, difficulty with breastfeeding, and galactorrhea (Camann, 2006).

Educating clients about the risks associated with these practices should include information about infection, permanent

A

B

Figure 4–2 ◆ Tattoos vary greatly in size, complexity, and meaning to the individual. A. This tattoo, on the ankle of a young woman, is purely decorative. B. This tattoo, on the shin of a young man, is the Chinese symbol for honor. He chose it to express a personal commitment to live a life of integrity.

Table 4–1	RECOMMENDED SCREENINGS AND IMMUNIZATIONS FOR WOMEN AT AVERAGE RISK FOR MOST DISEASES			
Screening Tests	**Ages 18–39**	**Ages 40–49**	**Ages 50–64**	**Ages 65 and Older**
General Health: Full checkup, Including weight and height	Discuss with your doctor or nurse.	Discuss with your doctor or nurse.	Discuss with your doctor or nurse.	Discuss with your doctor or nurse.
Thyroid test (TSH)	Start at age 35, then every 5 years	Every 5 years	Every 5 years	Every 5 years
Heart Health: Blood pressure test	At least every 2 years	At least every 2 years	At least every 2 years	At least every 2 years
Cholesterol test	Start at age 20, discuss with your doctor or nurse.	Discuss with your doctor or nurse.	Discuss with your doctor or nurse.	Discuss with your doctor or nurse.
Bone Health: Bone mineral density test		Discuss with your doctor or nurse.	Discuss with your doctor or nurse.	Get a bone mineral density test at least once. Talk to your doctor or nurse about repeat testing.
Diabetes: Blood sugar test	Discuss with your doctor or nurse.	Start at age 45, then every 3 years	Every 3 years	Every 3 years
Breast Health: Mammogram (x-ray of breast)		Every 1-2 years. Discuss with your doctor or nurse.	Every 1-2 years. Discuss with your doctor or nurse.	Every 1-2 years. Discuss with your doctor or nurse.
Reproductive Health: Pap test & pelvic exam	Every 1-3 years if you have been sexually active or are older than 21	Every 1-3 years	Every 1-3 years	Discuss with your doctor or nurse.
Chlamydia test	If sexually active, yearly until age 25. Ages 26-39, if you are at high risk for chlamydia or other STDs, you may need this test.	If you are at high risk for chlamydia or other sexually transmitted diseases (STDs) you may need this test.	If you are at high risk for chlamydia or other sexually transmitted diseases (STDs) you may need this test.	If you are at high risk for chlamydia or other sexually transmitted diseases (STDs) you may need this test.
Sexually Transmitted Disease (STD) tests	Both partners should get tested for STDs, including HIV, before initiating sexual intercourse.	Both partners should get tested for STDs, including HIV, before initiating sexual intercourse.	Both partners should get tested for STDs, including HIV, before initiating sexual intercourse.	Both partners should get tested for STDs, including HIV, before initiating sexual intercourse.
Colorectal Health: Fecal occult blood test			Yearly flexible sigmolidoscopy (with fecal occult blood test is preferred)	Every 5 years (If not having a colonoscopy) Every 5 years (If not having a colonoscopy)
Double Contrast Barium Enema (DCBE)			Every 5-10 years (if not having a colonoscopy or sigmolidoscopy)	Every 5-10 years (if not having a colonoscopy or sigmolidoscopy)
Colonoscopy			Every 10 years	Every 10 years
Rectal exam	Discuss with your doctor or nurse.	Discuss with your doctor or nurse.	Every 5-10 years with each screening (sigmolidoscopy, colonoscopy, or DCBE)	Every 5-10 years with each screening (sigmolidoscopy, colonoscopy, or DCBE)
Eye and Ear Health: Eye exam	Get your eyes checked if you have problems or visual changes.	Every 2-4 years	Every 2-4 years	Every 1-4 years
Hearing test	Starting at age 18, then every 10 years	Every 10 years	Discuss with your doctor or nurse.	Discuss with your doctor or nurse.
Skin Health: Mole exam	Monthly mole self-exam; by a doctor every 3 years, starting at age 20.	Monthly mole self-exam; by a doctor every year.	Monthly mole self-exam; by a doctor every year.	Monthly mole self-exam; by a doctor every year.
Oral Health: Dental exam	One to two times every year	One to two times every year	One to two times every year	One to two times every year
Mental Health Screening	Discuss with your doctor or nurse.	Discuss with your doctor or nurse.	Discuss with your doctor or nurse.	Discuss with your doctor or nurse.
Immunizations: Influenza vaccine	Discuss with your doctor or nurse.	Discuss with your doctor or nurse.	Yearly	Yearly
Pneumococcal vaccine				One time only
Tetanus-Diphtheria Booster vaccine	Every 10 years	Every 10 years	Every 10 years	Every 10 years

SOURCE: The National Women's Health Information Center. (2006). Office of Women's Health, U.S. Department of Health and Human Services, Washington, DC.

scarring, keloid formation, and care afterward. It is important for the nurse to avoid passing judgment or making generalizations about clients who have these types of body alterations.

MENOPAUSE

Menopause, defined as the absence of menstruation for 1 full year, is a time of transition for a woman, marking the end of her reproductive abilities. Although it usually occurs between 45 and 52 years of age, the current median age of menopause in the United States is 51.3 years. Not all of the physiologic mechanisms initiating menopause are precisely understood; however, it is known that the onset occurs when estrogen levels drop because of cessation of ovarian function. In addition, most researchers agree that the age of onset is influenced by such factors as the woman's overall health, weight, nutrition, lifestyle, culture, and genetic factors.

Climacteric, or *change of life* (often used synonymously with *menopause*), refers to the host of psychologic and physical alterations that occur around the time of menopause. These aspects are discussed separately.

Perimenopause

Perimenopause refers to the period of time before menopause during which the woman moves from normal ovulatory cycles to cessation of menses. Perimenopause typically lasts from 2 to 8 years. It is characterized by decreasing ovarian function, unstable endocrine physiology, and highly variable, unpredictable hormone profiles.

In the United States, the number of women entering their perimenopausal years (40 to 49) has never been higher. This is due to the aging of the post-World War II baby boomers. Currently nearly 22 million women are in their perimenopausal years.

Symptoms of perimenopause range from nonexistent to quite bothersome. PMS, hot flashes, irregular periods, insomnia, and mood changes may be problematic. Other concerns include anovulatory dysfunctional uterine bleeding, vasomotor instability, loss of bone density, and gynecologic cancers.

Contraception remains a major concern for many perimenopausal women. In reality, although a growing number of women are choosing to delay childbearing, just over half (51%) of pregnancies for women ages 40 and higher are unplanned (*The Contraception Report* [TCR], 2001). As women age fertility decreases and the risk of spontaneous abortion increases significantly so that it is over 50% in women by age 45 (Wild, 2005). In women who delay pregnancy until after age 40, risks for pregnancy complications are approximately twofold to sixfold higher. These complications include hypertensive disorders, diabetes, placenta previa, and placental abruption. These complications in turn increase the rate of preterm birth, intrauterine growth restriction, and serious neonatal complications. Women of this age have a two times greater risk of pregnancy-related death than their younger counterparts (Joseph, Allen, Dodds et al., 2005).

In the United States, female sterilization is, in general, the most commonly used method of contraception among US couples over age 30 (Hatcher, Trussell, Stewart et al., 2004). However, combined hormonal contraceptives (the pill, patches, and vaginal rings) are gaining popularity for contraception during this time in a woman's reproductive life. Combined hormonal contraceptives prevent pregnancy and provide noncontraceptive benefits. Healthy nonsmokers benefit from effective contraception; regulation of menses; treatment of anovulatory bleeding; relief of symptoms of estrogen deficiency and variability such as hot flashes, sleep disturbances, menorrhagia, and vaginal dryness; and a decreased risk of endometrial and ovarian cancer. They may also experience less acne and hirsutism (abnormal hair growth, often on the face and neck) and decreased osteopenia. Thus they are considered by many to be an optimal approach to this transition, even when contraception is not a concern. Other contraceptive options for perimenopausal women include sterilization, contraceptive IUDs, progestin-only methods of contraception, and barrier methods of contraception such as male and female condoms, diaphragm, cervical cap, and spermicides (Hatcher et al., 2004). (See Chapter 5 ∞ for a discussion of these methods).

Women describing problems that suggest perimenopause should be referred to their care provider. If oral contraceptives are not an option, other alternatives are available. Exercise, calcium and vitamin D, and other medications may be effective.

Psychologic Aspects

A woman's psychologic adaptation to menopause and the climacteric is multifactorial. It is often further complicated because women of this age may be dealing with other life circumstances such as adjustment to an "empty nest" or caring for aging parents. Numerous personal factors influence a woman's ability to transition and cope with these changes, such as self-concept, physical health, marital stability, relationship with others, and cultural values. Some women express disappointment in approaching this time of their life, whereas others may see it as a positive transition that offers freedom from menses or concern about contraception. Women who are dealing with aging, ill parents may have increased stressors that affect their emotional health and ability to deal with their symptoms. Often night sweats and insomnia affect a woman's capability to cope because of increased fatigue.

As a nurse, understanding the basic physiology of menopause offers an opportunity to provide education, supportive resources, and encouragement to women at this time of their life. Suggesting exercises and teaching on proper nutrition are critical for overall health and may help these women improve the emotional aspects associated with menopause. It is important to help women understand the changes that come with menopause and deal with their feelings during this period. Moreover, caregivers need to be alert for signs that distinguish between the mood swings that are related to hormonal changes and true clinical depression.

In reality the average woman in the United States will live one third of her life after menopause. The changing perceptions of menopause and beyond are enabling menopausal women to cope more effectively and to view menopause as a time of personal growth.

MEDIALINK   Application: Menopause

My personal response to menopause has surprised me a little. Suddenly 52 doesn't really seem old. I look at pictures of my mother in her early fifties and she seems so much older. I imagine each generation looks back and thinks the same thing. I do wish I had known at 22 what I know now, but I still see myself as learning and growing. Now I am being more selective about my goals for the future—maybe I'll try writing a novel, or I'll take a gourmet cooking class. One thing I am committed to—I intend to do my very best to live each day as it comes and enjoy it to the hilt!

Physical Aspects

CHANGES IN THE REPRODUCTIVE SYSTEM

The physical characteristics of menopause are linked to the shift from a cyclic to a noncyclic hormonal pattern. Beginning 2 to 8 years before menopause, women experience episodes of anovulation, reduced fertility, decreased or increased flow, irregular frequency of menses, and then ultimately, amenorrhea. Generally ovulation ceases 1 to 2 years before menopause, but individual variations exist. FSH levels rise, and ovarian follicles cease to produce estrogen. As estrogen levels decline, physiologic changes occur within the reproductive organs. The uterine lining, or endometrium, thins and the uterine muscle layer, or myometrium, atrophies. The fallopian tubes and ovaries atrophy. The vaginal mucosa loses its elasticity and becomes thinner and smoother. The loss of cervical gland function leads to dryness of the mucous membranes of the vagina, which can lead to burning and itching. The vaginal pH level increases as the number of Döderlein's bacilli decreases. This change in the vaginal ecology can lead to a condition known as atrophic vaginitis and increases the woman's risk of vaginal infections.

Pubic hair thins, turns gray or white, and may ultimately disappear. The labia shrink and lose their heightened pigmentation. Pelvic fascia and muscles atrophy, resulting in decreased pelvic support. Kegel exercises and regular sexual activity help prevent this change. The breasts become pendulous and decrease in size and firmness.

Postmenopausal women can remain orgasmic, although they may require the use of water-soluble lubricants during intercourse because of vaginal dryness and decreased elasticity. Some women report that sexual interest and activity increase as the need for contraception disappears and personal growth and awareness increase. Other women report a decrease in libido following menopause, which may be related to lower estrogen and testosterone levels.

Sexual function is complex and is influenced by physiologic and interpersonal factors. A caring, communicative relationship is crucial to sexual desire. Other factors that may influence sexual function include body image, general health, and stressors at work or with family. Her partner's health or inability to perform may also influence a woman's sexual desire (Shifren, 2005). Completing a good sexual history will help the nurse to assess the client's sexual health and allow the woman to ask questions and express concerns or frustrations.

VASOMOTOR CHANGES

As many as 80% to 90% of women who are perimenopausal or menopausal experience a vasomotor disturbance commonly known as a *hot flash,* which makes it the most commonly reported menopausal symptom (Varney et al., 2004). Hot flashes are typically described as a feeling of heat rising from the chest and spreading to the neck and face. Hot flashes at night are often accompanied by sleep disturbances triggered by profuse sweating (*night sweats*) in which a woman awakens with drenched night clothes and bedding. These episodes may occur as often as 20 to 30 times a day and generally last 3 to 5 minutes or less. Some women also experience dizzy spells, palpitations, and weakness. Many women find their own most effective ways to deal with the hot flashes. Some report that dressing in layers, using a fan, avoiding alcoholic beverages, or drinking a cool liquid helps relieve distress. Still others seek relief through hormone replacement therapy or complementary therapies such as herbs.

CHANGES IN THE MUSCULOSKELETAL SYSTEM AND SKIN

Osteoporosis, a decrease in bone strength related to diminished bone density and bone quality, is a major health concern for women. It is estimated that 20% of Caucasian and Asian women have osteoporosis and 52% have the beginning of bone loss or osteopenia (Minkin, 2005). This change is associated with lowered estrogen levels; however, the greatest influencing factor is family history of osteoporosis. Osteoporosis puts an individual at increased risk for fractures of the hip, forearm, and vertebrae. Risk factors associated with osteoporosis are identified in Table 4–2.

As skin ages, collagen and elastin, which are what maintain firmness of the skin, weaken. The skin appears looser and thinner, and wrinkles. Past sun exposure and tobacco use influence the amount of skin changes that occur. As women age, skin becomes drier and may need increased moisturizing. Nurses, as a part of general counseling, can remind women to wear sunscreen with an SPF of at least 15 to protect their skin from further damage. Recommending annual dermatologic screening for serious skin changes is also important.

During menopause there is a change in body fat distribution. Shifts occur from the lower to the upper body, as well as internal organs such as the heart, lungs, liver, kidneys, and intestine (Hamilton & Lovejoy, 2003). This shift in fat distribu-

Table 4–2   RISK FACTORS FOR OSTEOPOROSIS
• Middle-aged and elderly women
• European American or Asian ethnic origin
• Small-boned and thin body type
• Low body weight (less than 127 lb)
• Family history of osteoporosis
• Lack of regular weight-bearing exercise
• Nulliparity
• Early onset of menopause
• Consistently low intake of calcium
• Cigarette smoking
• Moderate to heavy alcohol intake
• Use of certain medications such as anticonvulsants, corticosteroids, or lithium

tion increases a woman's risk for chronic illness, such as diabetes, heart disease, or hypertension. Body Mass Index is a measurement tool for determining obesity. Nurses should be especially concerned for central obesity, which is a more accurate index to predict the development of chronic illness. This is done by calculating a waist-to-hip ratio, or dividing the woman's waist measurement by the hip measurement. Women should maintain a waist-to-hip ratio of less than 0.85 to decrease their risk for chronic disease (Freeman, 2005).

CHANGES IN THE CARDIOVASCULAR SYSTEM

An important long-range physical change of menopause is a shift in lipid and lipoprotein levels. Estrogen has a protective mechanism that fosters elevated levels of high-density lipoprotein (HDL) and lower low-density lipoprotein (LDL). As estrogen levels fall during menopause, this protective mechanism ceases, which potentially places a woman at increased risk for coronary heart disease, hypertension, and strokes.

Although viewed as a higher risk in men, cardiovascular disease (CVD) is the number one killer of women in the United States. Coronary heart disease (CHD), the major cause of heart attacks in women, kills more women than the next seven causes of death in women combined. Approximately 300,000 women in the U.S. die each year from CHD, or one death every minute. This is six times higher than those deaths caused by breast cancer. Women are more apt than men to die in the first year after a heart attack by a 3-to-1 ratio (Caboral, 2004). Risk factors for CHD are identified in Table 4–3.

Metabolic syndrome is a major predisposing factor for CHD and is defined through a collection of risk factors. Clinical characteristics are waist measurement greater than 35 inches, triglycerides greater than 150 mg/dL, HDL less than 50, blood pressures over 130/85, and fasting glucose levels greater than 110 mg/dL (Ansell, 2003).

CHANGES IN COGNITIVE FUNCTION

Memory and cognitive function change with advancing age. There is suggestion that the brain benefits from circulating estrogen and that declining estrogen levels might contribute to loss of this function as well as to the development of dementia (Henderson, 2005). This change is also influenced by lifestyle, genetics, and socioeconomic status. In the United States, Alzheimer's disease (AD) is the most commonly occurring form of dementia, estimated to affect 4.5 million Americans. The number of new cases of AD is projected to more than dou-

Table 4–3   RISK FACTORS FOR CHD IN WOMEN
• Family history of heart disease
• Advancing age—over 55 or postmenopausal
• Overweight and obesity
• Cigarette smoking and/or tobacco use
• Sedentary lifestyle
• Hypertension
• Diabetes
• Elevated cholesterol
• Race (highest incidence in African American women)

ble between the years 2010 and 2050. Beyond age 65, the number of persons with AD doubles every 5 years. Estimates suggest that half of people over 85 have AD. The causes of AD are not certain; however, besides advanced age, family history is a major factor. Other potential risk factors being explored currently are increased cholesterol, hypertension, and diabetes (Reynolds & Mintzer, 2005).

Numerous treatments for AD have been explored, including ginkgo biloba, estrogen therapy, cholesterol-reducing medications, nonsteroidal anti-inflammatory drugs, and antioxidants. None of these treatments have proven effective, however, and some, such as ginkgo biloba and estrogen, may prove harmful. At present there are no therapies available that consistently reduce symptoms or slow the progress of the disease. Cholinesterase inhibitors are the only medications approved by the Food and Drug Administration (FDA) to treat cognitive dysfunction (Reynolds & Mintzer, 2005).

Premature Menopause

Spontaneous premature menopause (also called premature ovarian insufficiency) is a devastating event and is not well understood, although family history is a major influencing factor. It occurs in about 1% of women under age 40 (Thacker, 2005) and is demonstrated by the development of amenorrhea, a sharp decline in estrogen levels, and a rise in follicle-stimulating hormone (FSH). After the initial diagnosis, an estimated 5% to 10% of cases will spontaneously reverse. For those women whose diagnosis is permanent, and who are anticipating pregnancy, it is emotionally traumatizing and requires extra sensitivity from caregivers (Nelson, 2004). Premature menopause is treated with estrogen and progesterone therapy until the usual age of menopause (Thacker, 2005). Other forms of premature menopause occur with anorexia, chemotherapy or radiation treatments, and oophorectomy (surgical removal of the ovaries).

Medical Therapy
HORMONE REPLACEMENT THERAPY (HRT)

Hormone replacement therapy (HRT) refers to the administration of specific hormones to alleviate symptoms associated with the changes of menopause. Estrogen (ET) and combined estrogen-progestogen therapy (EPT) are the individual types currently in use. ET is given to women who have undergone hysterectomy (surgical removal of the uterus), whereas EPT is used for women with an intact uterus for the relief of vasomotor symptoms (hot flashes) and urogenital and vaginal symptoms, as well as osteoporosis prevention. Estrogen alone, in a woman with a uterus (unopposed estrogen), increases the risk of endometrial (the lining of the uterus) cancer by eightfold and therefore is never given without progesterone in these women.

In 2002 the advisability of HRT, specifically EPT, was called into question because of the results of the Women's Health Initiative (WHI) study, which suggested that the risks of HRT outweigh its benefits, especially for long-term use, because of the slightly increased risk of breast cancer, thromboembolic disease, and stroke (Writing Group for the Women's Health Initiative Investigators, 2002).

Previously HRT was thought to provide protection against cardiovascular disease, the number one cause of death for women over age 50. However, a second study, the Heart and Estrogen/Progestin Replacement Follow-up Study (HERS II), indicated that HRT does not decrease the risk of heart attack. Moreover, women taking HRT experienced adverse effects including gallbladder disease and blood clots in the legs and lungs (Grady, Herrington, Bittner et al., 2002). Thus all major professional groups in the United States agree that HT/ET should not be started or continued solely to prevent heart disease (Thacker, 2005).

Furthermore, the beneficial effect of long-term estrogen use in reducing the incidence of Alzheimer's disease (AD) was called into question by the Women's Health Initiative Memory Study (WHIMS), which found a 105% increase in AD with estrogen use (Shumaker, Legault, Rapp et al., 2003). However, the WHIMS study participants were all 65 years or older when they began therapy. Thus, it is possible that those women already had brain changes related to AD (Gambrell, 2004). Other research about AD risk indicates that the age when estrogen is initiated is crucial. When estrogen is begun at menopause and used for more than 10 years, there is a reduction of up to 83% in lifetime risk (Gambrell, 2004; Zandi, Carlson, Plassman et al., 2002).

Consequently, the picture about HRT is somewhat clouded. Currently HRT is recognized as the most effective short-term (1 to 4 years) therapy for women who experience severe menopausal symptoms. However, women considering HRT should clearly understand the associated risks so that they can make an informed decision about using it. HRT is not indicated for the prevention of coronary heart disease, and women at risk of osteoporosis should explore alternative treatments (see later discussion).

HRT can be prescribed in a number of ways, including orally; transdermally (patch); topically as a gel, lotion, or vaginal creams; and through a vaginal ring. It is given in a continuous manner, daily administration of both estrogen and progestogen, or as a cyclic or sequential therapy, with estrogen

EVIDENCE-BASED PRACTICE

HORMONE THERAPY AND CARDIOVASCULAR DISEASE

Clinical Question

What are the effects of hormone therapy on cardiovascular morbidity and mortality in postmenopausal women?

The Evidence

At one time, it was believed that hormone therapy produced a cardioprotective effect for postmenopausal women. These findings were based primarily on observational studies. Recently, data from several randomized controlled trials produced evidence suggesting that hormone therapy is not associated with any beneficial effect for cardiovascular disease and may actually increase risk. These reviewers aimed to provide a more precise estimate of the cardiovascular effects of hormone therapy using meta-analysis and systematic review. Four reviewers appraised seven large-scale, multisite randomized clinical trials comparing hormone therapy of duration greater than 1 year to placebo. The seven trials together comprised a sample size of more than 32,000 women. Outcomes of interest were mortality from any cardiovascular cause; nonfatal acute myocardial infarction (AMI); coronary heart disease (CHD); and all strokes. The studies were independently appraised by at least two of the reviewers and effect-size statistics were calculated using meta-analysis.

What Is Effective?

The use of hormone therapy had no significant effect—protective or harmful—on mortality from all causes, nonfatal AMI or CHD. The risk of stroke was significantly higher for the hormone groups, including both fatal and nonfatal strokes that were either ischemic or hemorrhagic. The women who were receiving hormone therapy had a 29% increased risk of stroke, and this risk was higher for younger women (under the age of 65) than for older women.

What Is Unclear?

There were insufficient data to determine which type of stroke—ischemic or hemorrhagic—was higher in the hormone group. The suggested physiologic mechanism underlying stroke was ischemic, but these reviewers were unable to determine if there was a difference. There is conjecture as to why the observational studies produced paradoxical results from the randomized trials. It is hypothesized that women who participated in the observational studies (e.g., the Nurses' Health Study) were demographically more likely to have healthier lifestyles than the general population. The effects of these demographic modifiers require more study to determine if the risk of stroke can be modified with health-related behaviors.

Best Practice

It is difficult to directly compare the benefits of hormone therapy in preventing menopausal symptoms, reducing the rate of osteoporosis, and improving quality of life to a 29% increase in the risk of stroke. The balance of risk and benefit of hormone therapy must be weighed individually for each woman. When women are given hormone therapy for more than a short time period (1 year) the risk of stroke does increase, but there is no protective or harmful effect as reflected in nonfatal AMI, CHD, or cardiovascular mortality. Women should be given accurate information about the risks and benefits of this therapy so that they can make a personal decision based on reliable research.

Critical Thinking

What assessments would indicate to the nurse that a woman would be at higher risk of stroke and should avoid hormone therapy altogether? How can these findings be incorporated into the health teaching plans of women who are postmenopausal?

REFERENCE: Magliano, D., Rogers, S., Abramson, M., & Tonkin, A. (2006). Hormone therapy and cardiovascular disease: A systematic review and meta-analysis. *British Journal of Obstetrics and Gynecology, 113*, 5–14.

use daily and a progestogen added on a set sequence (North American Menopause Society, 2003). Combination estrogen-progestogen preparations are also available.

Research, though still preliminary, does seem to indicate that postmenopausal women experiencing decreased libido experience improved sexual desire, responsiveness, and frequency when testosterone is added to their HRT. Options for providing testosterone in doses low enough for women are still limited. Estratest, a combined estrogen-androgen pill, is used by some women. Custom-compounded testosterone preparations are available by prescription and work is under way on low-dose testosterone patches (Shifren, 2006).

A great deal of attention has been given to "bioidentical" hormones lately because of current views, which are not supported by medical literature, that these "more natural" hormones are safer and more effective. A bioidentical hormone refers to a hormone that is structurally identical to those found in the body, more specifically, those produced by the ovaries (Wysocki, 2005).

In light of the findings from the WHI and HERS II studies, the North American Menopause Society (NAMS) convened an advisory panel to develop recommendations about the clinical management of postmenopausal hormone therapy. Among their recommendations they suggested the following (NAMS, 2003):

- The treatment of menopausal symptoms such as hot flashes and urogenital symptoms is the primary indication for HRT and estrogen therapy (ET).

- Progestogen is prescribed only to protect the endometrium from unopposed estrogen. Thus women with a uterus who are taking estrogen should also have a prescription for adequate progestogen coverage (HRT). Women without a uterus who are taking estrogen (ET) should *not* have a progestogen prescribed.

- No estrogen therapy regimen (ET or EPT) should be used to prevent coronary heart disease. Alternative prevention regimens should be used instead (weight control, regular exercise, no smoking, healthy diet, etc.).

- HRT and ET have been used for the prevention of osteoporosis. However, because of the associated risks, alternative approaches to preventing and treating osteoporosis should be considered.

- HRT and ET use should be limited to the shortest duration feasible in light of treatment goals, benefits, and risks for an individual woman.

- Lower-than-standard doses of HRT and ET should be considered for symptom relief.

- Alternate routes of administration of HRT may provide advantages, but at present the long-term risk benefit ratio has not been shown.

- Therapy decisions should be made individually based on each woman's symptoms and identified risks.

Women should be informed of the known risks.

At present, HRT is still recognized as the most effective therapy for women who experience severe menopausal symp-toms. For women taking short-term (1 to 4 years) HRT therapy to relieve symptoms, the benefits are likely to outweigh the risks (National Association of Nurse Practitioners in Women's Health, 2002).

Before starting HRT the woman should undergo a thorough history; physical examination including Pap smear; measurement of cholesterol, lipids, and liver enzyme levels; and baseline mammogram. An initial endometrial biopsy is no longer routinely recommended for all women beginning HRT; however, biopsy is indicated for women with an increased risk of endometrial cancer and if excessive, unexpected, or prolonged vaginal bleeding occurs. Caregivers who prescribe HRT should teach their clients to report immediately any signs of complications such as headaches, visual changes, signs of thrombophlebitis, or signs of myocardial infarction that are common in women (see later discussion).

PREVENTION AND TREATMENT OF OSTEOPOROSIS

Osteoporosis is rapidly becoming a significant health risk for older adults (see Table 4–2). According to the American College of Obstetricians and Gynecologists (2004) 13% to 18% of US women over 50 years of age have osteoporosis and another 37% to 50% have osteopenia, or low bone mass. These numbers are especially worrisome because osteoporosis is a largely preventable disease and a source of significant risk for fracture and subsequent health decline.

Bone mineral density (BMD) testing is useful in identifying individuals who are at risk for osteoporosis. A variety of guidelines are available for BMD testing. The American College of Obstetricians and Gynecologists (ACOG) (2004) recommends BMD testing for the following:

- All postmenopausal women aged 65 or older

- All postmenopausal women with fractures

- Postmenopausal women under age 65 with one or more risk factors

BMD testing may also be indicated for premenopausal or postmenopausal women with certain medical conditions such as eating disorders, thyroid disorders, leukemia, rheumatoid arthritis, and multiple sclerosis, and for those women on certain medications such as corticosteroids or anticonvulsants.

This quick, painless test assesses whether a woman has normal bone mass or has decreased bone density (osteoporosis) or increased bone porosity or softening (osteomalacia). Optimum screening is done using a central dual-energy x-ray absorptiometry (DEXA) scan to measure bone density at the hip and lumbar spine. Figure 4–3 ◆ shows a sample bone density testing result.

The woman's height should be measured at each visit, because a loss of height is often an early sign that vertebrae are being compressed because of reduced bone mass. A variety of conditions, including malabsorption syndrome, cancer, cirrhosis of the liver, chronic use of cortisone, and rheumatoid arthritis, can cause secondary arthritis, which resembles osteoporosis. If these secondary causes are ruled out, treatment for osteoporosis is instituted.

Name:	**Doe, Jane**	Sex:	Female	Height:	66.5 in.
Patient ID:	Case A004	Ethnicity:	White	Weight:	165.0 lb
Age:	66	Date of Birth:	09/02/1933	Menopause Age:	53

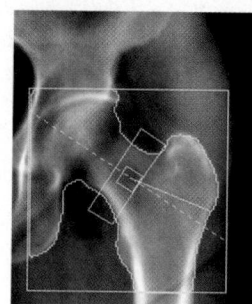

Scan Date: May 01, 2000
Scan ID: A0501000M

Scan Type: f Left Hip

Scan Date: May 01, 2000
Scan ID: A0501000K

Scan Type: f Lumbar Spine

Scan Date: May 01, 2000
Scan ID: A0501000Q
Scan Type: f SE R/L Lateral Image

Scan Date: May 01, 2000
Scan ID: A0501000O
Scan Type: f SE AP Image

Results:

	BMD (g/cm²)	T-Score	PR (%)	Z-Score	AM (%)
Left Hip (Neck)	0.773	-0.7	91	0.9	115
Left Hip (Total)	0.870	-0.6	92	0.7	111
Spine (Total)	1.027	-0.2	98	1.7	122

Total BMD CV 1.0%

Summary:

	Classification
Left Hip BMD (Neck)	Normal
Left Hip BMD (Total)	Normal
Spine BMD (Total)	Normal
Vertebral Evaluation:	Severe Wedge Deformity at L2

A spine fracture indicates 5X risk for subsequent spine fracture and 2X risk for subsequent hip fracture.

World Health Organization criteria for BMD interpretation classify patients as Normal (T-score above -1), Osteopenic (T-score between -1 and -2.5), or Osteoporotic (T-score at or below -2.5).

HOLOGIC®
OSTEOPOROSIS ASSESSMENT

Figure 4–3 ◆ For osteoporosis assessment, published studies demonstrate that up to 30% of clients needing treatment are missed using BMD results of the spine and hip alone. The standard of care for assessing osteoporotic fracture risk is combining BMD results with imaging of the thoracic-lumbar spine. The osteoporotic assessment examination presented here shows a 66-year-old postmenopausal woman who has not received hormone replacement therapy because of a personal history of breast cancer. Although her bone mineral density (BMD) results are within normal limits, she does have an identifiable vertebral fracture at L2. This fracture places her at increased risk for future vertebral fractures and therefore in need of treatment for osteoporosis.

SOURCE: Scan provided courtesy of Hologic, Inc., Osteoporosis Assessment Division, Bedford, MA. Mary Ann Barrick, Product Specialist, Hologic, Inc., mbarrick@hologic.com.

Prevention of osteoporosis is a primary goal of care. Thus, women are advised to maintain an adequate calcium intake. Because a woman's calcium requirement increases at menopause, NAMS (2006) recommends that peri- and postmenopausal women have a daily calcium intake of 1200 mg/day. Most women require supplements to achieve this level. Calcium supplementation is most efficient when single doses do not exceed 500 mg and when taken with a meal. Research suggests that vitamin D deficiency is a major factor in women with osteoporosis. Worldwide, over half of postmenopausal women with osteoporosis have a vitamin D deficiency regardless of age, season (summer or winter), or latitude (Loewy, 2005). Thus vitamin D supplements are also indicated.

Women are also advised to participate regularly in weight-bearing exercise, to consume only modest quantities of alcohol and caffeine, and to stop smoking. This is especially important because alcohol and smoking have a negative effect on the rate of bone resorption.

The effectiveness of estrogen in preventing osteoporosis is well documented. Women with no contraindications to estrogen who are showing evidence of bone loss are good candidates for HT. For women who are unable or unwilling to take estrogen, other medications available to treat or help prevent osteoporosis include the following:

1. *Bisphosphonates* reduce bone resorption and bone loss by inhibiting osteoclast activity (ACOG, 2004). The two most common, alendronate (Fosamax) and risedronate (Actonel), are both taken upon arising in the morning on an empty stomach with a large glass of water. The woman should sit upright or stand for about 30 minutes after taking the medication and before eating. New bisphosphonates may offer women alternatives that eliminate the undesirable gastrointestinal side effects. For example, in 2002, an intravenous bisphosphonate, zoledronic acid (Zometa), was approved by the FDA for use in the treatment of metastatic bone cancer. However, some clinicians are using it to treat osteoporosis. The drug, administered IV once a year, seems to achieve the same results in treating osteoporosis as other bisphosphonates taken daily or weekly without the troublesome side effects (Reid, Brown, Burckhardt et al., 2002).

2. *Selective estrogen receptor modulators (SERMs)* have estrogen-like properties. The SERM approved for osteoporosis treatment, raloxifene (Evista), acts like estrogen by protecting against osteoporosis but does not stimulate uterine or breast tissue. Raloxifene does not relieve other menopausal symptoms and may increase hot flashes, so it is indicated in asymptomatic women who want preventive therapy for osteoporosis.

3. *Salmon calcitonin* is a calcium regulator that may inhibit bone loss and is approved for use to treat osteoporosis in women who are 5 years postmenopause. Administered as a nasal spray, its value is less clear than that of the other medications listed.

4. *Parathyroid hormone,* a daily subcutaneous injection, activates bone formation, which results in substantial increases in bone density.

5. *Ultra-low-dose estrogen patches* (Menostar) have proven to treat osteoporosis and can be used without a progestogen. These small doses are found to demonstrate effective prevention of fracture without the increased side effects or risks of endometrial stimulation found in larger dose estrogen patches (Ettinger, 2004).

The National Osteoporosis Foundation (NOF) provides a wealth of information about osteoporosis diagnosis and management.

PREVENTION OF CORONARY HEART DISEASE

Prevention is the key to dealing with CHD. Prevention begins with lifestyle choices and with lifestyle modifications as necessary. This includes maintaining ideal body weight, exercising regularly, eating a nutritious diet, avoiding smoking, managing stress effectively, obtaining regular healthcare screenings as indicated, and developing a strong social support system.

It is critical that women be familiar with the signs of myocardial infarction (heart attack) that are commonly seen in women. These include pain in the neck, back, or epigastric region; loss of appetite; shortness of breath; nausea or vomiting; and weakness in the shoulder, arms, and chest. Research indicates that women are more likely than men to delay seeking treatment. They are also more likely to die from the attack (Arslanian-Engoren, 2002). Thus it is important for nurses to stress the need to seek immediate treatment if symptoms develop.

Complementary and Alternative Therapies

As women evaluate their feelings about the use of HT in light of the recent findings in clinical trials, they may wish to explore alternative therapies for control of their symptoms. A variety of therapeutic modalities have been proposed as alternative or complementary treatment or prevention measures for the discomforts and ailments of the perimenopausal and postmenopausal years. These include nutrition supplements, such as a diet rich in calcium and vitamins E, D, and B complex.

According to the National Center for Complementary and Alternative Medicine (NCCAM) (2006), there is little high-quality research currently available about the effectiveness and long-term safety of CAM therapies for treating or relieving menopausal symptoms. Thus more research is needed. It is important that women who are considering using CAM discuss them with their healthcare provider to help ensure that their treatment plan is comprehensive.

Phytoestrogens are plant products that have estrogen-like properties and may help relieve some menopausal symptoms, although it is not clear whether the relief comes from estrogens or other substances in the plants (NCCAM, 2006). Examples of foods rich in phytoestrogens include carrots, yams, and soy products. Women who have or who are at increased risk for diseases affected by hormones (uterine, breast, or ovarian cancer; uterine fibroids, and endometriosis), women who are taking medications that increase their estrogen levels (birth control pills, HRT), and women who are on cancer medications such as

Figure 4–4 ◆ Regular exercise is important, especially for post-menopausal women.
SOURCE: Ariel Skelley-CORBIS.

tamoxifen should be especially careful about taking phytoestrogens (NCCAM, 2006).

Herbal supplements include black cohosh, dong quai, red clover, soy isoflavones, ginseng, and kava. About 10% of women have tried herbal remedies, which have been used in traditional Chinese medicine for years (Osmers, Friede, Liske et al., 2005). These therapies are not regulated by or approved for use by the Food and Drug Administration (FDA), and their safety is unknown. See "Complementary and Alternative Therapies: Use of Botanicals for Menopausal Symptoms" for a summary of NCCAM findings on these substances.

Conversely, menopausal women should avoid foods that may trigger symptoms, including caffeine, alcohol, and spicy foods.

Weight-bearing exercise, including such activities as walking, jogging, tennis, and running, is a means of increasing bone mass and potentiating the effect of estrogen on bone mass. Exercise also improves cholesterol profiles and contributes to overall health (Figure 4–4 ◆). Pelvic floor, or Kegel, exercises can help maintain vaginal muscle tone and increase blood circulation to the perineal area. Vaginal lubricants and adequate foreplay can be helpful in maintaining a satisfactory sexual experience.

Relaxation techniques including yoga, meditation, deep breathing, visualization, massage, or acupuncture may provide a sense of well-being. Overall, healthy lifestyle, proper nutrition, and adequate exercise will maximize health and decrease health risks and symptoms.

NURSING CARE MANAGEMENT

Some menopausal women may need counseling to adjust successfully to this developmental phase of life. Others have no difficulty with this life transition. Reaction to menopause is determined to a large extent by the kind of life the woman has lived, by the security she has in her feminine identity, by her feelings of self-worth and self-esteem, and by her relationships with others.

Nurses and other healthcare professionals may be able to help the menopausal woman achieve high-level functioning at this time in her life. Of paramount importance is the nurse's ability to understand and provide support for the woman's views and feelings. Whether the woman expresses relief and delight or tearfulness and fear, the nurse needs to use an empathetic approach in counseling, health teaching, or providing physical care.

Women may discuss areas of deep concern, including a history of sexual abuse, current distress, or life problems. Nurses should have appropriate referrals to domestic violence hotlines and to professional therapists who work with women. Women may also be dealing simultaneously with chronically ill parents, divorce or the death of a spouse, troubled or handicapped children, children leaving home, job stressors, and/or generalized fear and anxiety. Nurses can be of assistance with referrals to support groups and counselors who are specific to each woman's need. Although this is a challenge, it is the responsibility of the nurse caring for women to be prepared to meet their needs.

Nurses should explore the question of the woman's comfort during sexual intercourse. In counseling, the nurse may say, "After menopause many women notice that their vagina seems drier, and sex of any kind can be uncomfortable. Have you noticed any changes?" This gives the woman information and may open discussion. The nurse can then go on to explain that the woman can address dryness and shrinking of the vagina by us-

ing a water-soluble lubricant to help provide relief. Use of estrogen, orally or in vaginal creams, may also be indicated. Increased frequency of sexual activity will maintain some elasticity in the vagina. When assessing the menopausal woman, the nurse needs to address the question of sexual activity openly but tactfully, because the woman may have been socialized to be reticent in discussing sex. Heterosexual women who do not wish to become pregnant should be counseled to use a method of contraception for 1 year after their last menstrual period. They should also be advised to report any bleeding after 1 year of amenorrhea because this may indicate a problem and requires evaluation.

The crucial need of women in the perimenopausal period of life is for adequate information about the changes taking place in their bodies and their lives and support in adjusting to the changes that occur. Supplying that information and providing support as needed present both a challenge and an opportunity for nurses.

Additional information about the most current approaches to the management of menopause and the postmenopausal period can be found at the Web site of the North American Menopause Society.

CLINICAL TIP

Women respond differently to the experience of menopause, so it is important to avoid generalizations. However, in working with menopausal women—and indeed, any women—touch, listening, and caring, as nursing measures, may enhance your self-actualization and that of your client.

CHAPTER REVIEW

FOCUS YOUR STUDY

- Nurses should provide girls and women with clear information about menstrual issues, such as the use of pads and tampons (including warnings regarding deodorant and absorbency); vaginal spray and douching practices; and self-care comfort measures during menstruation, such as maintaining good nutrition, exercising, and applying heat and massage.

- Dysmenorrhea usually begins at, or a day before, the onset of menses and disappears by the end. Hormone therapy (e.g., combined oral contraceptives), nonsteroidal anti-inflammatory drugs, or prostaglandin inhibitors can alleviate dysmenorrhea. Self-care measures include improving nutrition, exercising, applying heat, and getting extra rest.

- Premenstrual syndrome occurs most often in women over 30. The most pronounced symptoms occur 2 to 3 days before onset of menstruation and subside as menstruation

starts, with or without treatment. Medical management usually includes prostaglandin inhibitors and calcium supplementation. Self-care measures include improving nutrition (taking vitamin B complex and E supplements and avoiding methylxanthines, which are found, for example, in chocolate and caffeine), undertaking a program of aerobic exercise, and participating in self-care support groups. In some cases, pharmacologic agents such as selective serotonin reuptake inhibitors may be indicated.

- During her adult years, a healthy woman should make healthful lifestyle choices such as avoiding smoking and exercising regularly. She should also participate in regular health screenings, following a recommended schedule.

- Menopause is a physiologic, maturational change in a woman's life. Physiologic changes include the cessation of menses and a decrease in circulating hormones. Hormonal changes sometimes bring unsettling emotional responses. The more common physiologic symptoms are "hot flashes," palpitations, dizziness, and increased perspiration at night. The woman's anatomy also undergoes changes, such as atrophy of the vagina, reduction in size and pigmentation of the labia, and myometrial atrophy. Osteoporosis becomes an increasing concern.

- Osteoporosis is becoming a significant health problem in the United States. Prevention is the preferred approach to addressing the issue. This includes adequate calcium intake, regular weight-bearing exercise, and HT. For women who have already developed osteoporosis, medications are available as a treatment option.

- Coronary heart disease is the number one killer of women in the United States. Prevention is the goal of therapy.

- Current management of menopause centers around hormone replacement therapy, complementary therapies, and client healthcare education. Decisions regarding the use of HRT should be made individually based on each woman's symptoms and risks, and women should be advised of the known risks.

EXPLORE MEDIALINK

http://www.prenhall.com/davidson

NCLEX review questions, case studies, and other interactive resources for this chapter can be found on the Web Site at http://www.prenhall.com/davidson. Click on "Chapter 4" to select the activities for this chapter.

For tutorials including animations and videos, more NCLEX review questions, and an audio glossary, access the accompanying Prentice Hall Nursing MediaLink DVD-ROM in this book.

PRENTICE HALL NURSING MEDIALINK DVD-ROM

Audio Glossary

NCLEX Review

COMPANION WEBSITE

Additional NCLEX Review

Case Study: *Premenstrual Girl*

Care Plan Activity: *Bone Injuries in a Postmenopausal Woman*

Applications: *Teaching Adolescents How to Keep a Period Calendar; Menopause*

Critical Thinking

CRITICAL THINKING IN ACTION

PREMENSTRUAL SYNDROME

View the Critical Thinking in Action video in Chapter 4 of the DVD-ROM. Then answer the questions that follow.

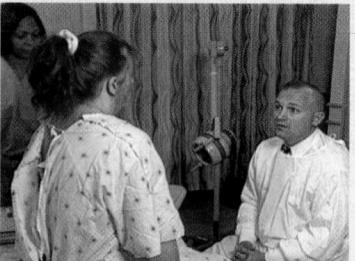

Linda Knoll, 35 years old, presents to you at the GYN clinic for her annual physical and pelvic exam. You obtain the following menstrual history: LMP 8 days ago. Periods occur every 29 days and last 5 days. She tells you that she uses superabsorbent tampons during the first 2 days of her period and then changes to regular absorbency tampons for the duration, and that she currently has an IUD in place for contraception. She tells you that her husband has been complaining for the last few months that she seems irritable, tense, and moody near "that time of the month." Linda admits that she doesn't feel well before her period and describes having low pelvic discomfort, breast tenderness, "bloating," and some constipation. She seems to cry easily 2 to 3 days before her period. She has noticed this pattern over the last 4 or 5 months. You recognize these symptoms as related to premenstrual syndrome (PMS). Linda asks you if these changes are due to female hormones.

1. How would you answer Linda's question concerning female hormones?

2. After reviewing Linda's diet with her, what would you recommend to help?

3. Linda has an IUD in place. What other type of contraceptive might help reduce the symptoms of PMS?

4. What other activities can you suggest to help Linda reduce PMS symptoms?

5. What should you tell Linda about using tampons during heavy menstrual flow?

REFERENCES

Al-Oballi Kridli, S. (2002). Health beliefs and practices among Arab women. *American Journal of Maternal/Child Nursing, 27*(3), 178–182.

American College of Obstetricians and Gynecologists (ACOG). (2004). *Osteoporosis Practice Bulletin,* Number 50. Washington, DC: Author.

Ansell, B. (2003). The metabolic syndrome in postmenopausal women. *Contemporary OB/GYN, 48*(5), 71–83.

Arslanian-Engoren, C. (2002). Recognizing heart disease: Helping women seek treatment faster. *AWHONN Lifelines, 5*(2), 114–122.

Caboral, M. (2004). Women: The target of the new American Heart Association, Guidelines on cardiovascular prevention. *Topics in Advanced Practice Nursing, eJournal, 4*(3). Retrieved October 27, 2005, from http://www.medscape.com/viewarticle/487462-print

Camann, W. (2006). Obstetric and anesthetic implications of "body art" (piercing and tattooing). *Medscape OB/GYN & Women's Health, 11,* 1–3. Retrieved April 17, 2006, from http://www.medscape.com/viewarticle/527920_print

Contraception for women in perimenopause. (2001). *The Contraception Report, 12*(1), 4–12.

Dell, D. L., Moskowitz, D., & Sondheimer, S. J. (2001). PMS and PMDD: Identification and treatment. *Contemporary OB/GYN, 46*(4), 15–30.

Donohoe, M. (2006). Beauty and body modification. *Medscape OB/GYN & Women's Health, 11,* 1–6. Retrieved April 26, 2006, from http://www.medscape.com/viewarticle/529442_print

Ettinger, B. (2004) Unopposed ultra-low-dose estradiol: A new approach to osteoporosis prevention. *OBG Management* (Suppl.), 17–19.

Freeman, S. (2005). The metabolic syndrome: Diagnosis and management. *Women's Health Care, 4*(5), 11–18.

Gambrell, R. D., Jr. (2004). The women's health initiative reports in perspective: Facts or fallacies? *Climacteric: The Journal of the International Menopause Society, 7*(3), 225–228.

Grady, D., Herrington, D., Bittner, V., Blumenthal, R., Davidson, M., Hlathy, M., et al. (2002). Cardiovascular disease outcomes during 6–8 years of hormone therapy. Heart and Estrogen/Progestin Replacement Study Follow-up (HERS II). *Journal of the American Medical Association, 288,* 49–57.

Hamilton, M., & Lovejoy, J. (2003). *Helping middle-aged patients lose weight.* Retrieved October 27, 2005, from http://www.contemporaryobgyn.net

Hatcher, R. A., Trussell, J., Stewart, F., Nelson, A., Cates, W., Guest, F., et al. (2004). *Contraceptive technology* (18th ed.). New York: Ardent Media.

Henderson, V. (2005). Memory complaints. *The Female Patient, 30*(8), 39–40.

Joseph, K. S., Allen, A. C., Dodds, L., Turner, L., Scott, H., & Liston, R. (2005). The perinatal effects of delayed childbearing. *Obstetrics and Gynecology, 105*(6), 1410–1418.

Knutson, M. C. (2002, November 27). *Tattooing, piercing and branding: A review for clinicians.* Medscape conference coverage, based on selected section at the Women's Health Care in the New Millennium: Fifth Annual Meeting of the Association of Nurse Practitioners in Women's Health. Retrieved October 20, 2005, from http://www.medscape.com

Loewy, M. A. (2005). Vitamin D deficiency common among postmenopausal osteoporotic women. *Reuters Health Information.* Retrieved November 8, 2005, from http://www.medscape.com/viewarticles/515690_print

Mayo Clinic Staff. (2004). *Premenstrual syndrome.* Retrieved October 14, 2005, from http://www.mayoclinic.com

Minkin, M. J. (2005, February). New strategies for prevention of osteoporosis. *Innovative Options of Patient Care, a New Way of Thinking* (CE Monograph). Washington, DC: National Association of Nurse Practitioners in Women's Health.

National Association of Nurse Practitioners in Women's Health. (2002). Hormone replacement therapy: From the National Association of Nurse Practitioners in Women's Health. *Topics in Advanced Practice Nursing eJournal, 2*(3). Retrieved July 31, 2002, from http://www.medscape.com/viewarticle/439106_print

National Center for Complementary and Alternative Medicine (NCCAM). (2006). *Do CAM therapies help menopausal symptoms?* Retrieved March 8, 2006, from http://nccam.nih.gov/health/menopauseandcam/

National Women's Health Information Center. (2006). *Recommended screenings and immunizations for women at average risk for most diseases.* Washington, DC: Office of Women's Health, U.S. Department of Health and Human Services.

Nelson, L. (2004, November 1). Grand rounds: What's the best approach to spontaneous premature ovarian failure? *Contemporary OB/GYN.* Retrieved October 28, 2005, from http://www.obgyn.adv/100.com

North American Menopause Society (NAMS). (2006). The role of calcium in peri- and postmenopausal women: 2006 position statement of the North American Menopause Society. *Menopause, 13* (6), 862–877.

North American Menopause Society (NAMS). (2003). *Amended report from the NAMS Advisory Panel on postmenopausal hormone therapy.* Retrieved October 13, 2002, from http://www.menopause.org

Osmers, R., Friede, M., Liske, E., Schnitker, J., Freudenstein, J., & Henneicke-von Zepelin, H.

(2005). Efficacy and safety of isopropanolic black cohosh extract for climacteric symptoms. *Obstetrics and Gynecology, 105*(5, Part 1), 1074–1083.

Reid, I. R., Brown, J. P., Burckhardt, P., Horowitz, Z., Richardson, P., Trecksel, U., et al. (2002, February 28). Intravenous zolehydronic acid in postmenopausal women with low bone mineral density. *New England Journal of Medicine, 346,* 653–661.

Reynolds, J., & Mintzer, J. (2005). *Alzheimer's disease update: New targets, new options.* Retrieved October 28, 2005, from http://www.medscape.com/viewart/500169-print

Shifren, J. L. (2005). Hypoactive sexual desire disorder in postmenopausal women: Treatment options. *OBG Management* (Suppl.), 15–21.

Shifren, J. L. (2006). Testosterone therapy in postmenopausal women. *The Female Patient, 21*(4), 29–31.

Shulman, L. P. (2005, February). Unique progestational impact on PMS/PMDD. *Innovative Options of Patient Care, a New Way of Thinking* (CE Monograph).

Shumaker, S. A., Legault, C., Rapp, S. R., Thal, L., Wallace, R. B., Ockene, J. K., et al. (2003). Estrogen plus progestin and the incidence of dementia and mild cognitive impairment in postmenopausal women: The Women's Health Initiative Memory Study: A randomized, controlled trial. *Journal of the American Medical Association, 289*(20), 2651–2662.

Thacker, H. L. (2005). Menopausal hormone therapy: The symptomatic patient. *The Female Patient, 30*(3), 16–21.

Varney, H., Kriebs, J. M., & Gregor, C. L. (2004). *Varney's midwifery* (4th ed.). Sudbury, MA: Jones and Bartlett Publishers.

Wild, R. A. (2005). Fertility changes during perimenopause. *The Female Patient, 30*(12), 22–23.

Writing Group for the Women's Health Initiative Investigators. (2002). Risks and benefits of estrogen plus progestin in healthy postmenopausal women: Principal results from the Women's Health Initiative randomized controlled trial. *Journal of the American Medical Association, 288,* 321–333.

Wysocki, S. (2005). Bioidentical hormones for menopause hormone therapy: An overview. *Women's Health Care, 4*(2), 9–17.

Zandi, P. P., Carlson, M. C., Plassman, B. L., Welsh-Bohmer, K. A., Mayer, L. S., Steffens, D. C., et al., (2002). Hormone replacement therapy and incidence of Alzheimer disease in older women: The Cache County Study. *Journal of the American Medical Association, 288*(17), 2123–2129.

Women's Health: Family Planning

I was 15 when I fell in love with Joe, a handsome, 17-year-old senior on our high school basketball team. My friends were so envious. We didn't plan on becoming sexually involved. It just happened. I knew I should use some method of birth control, but I didn't know where to go. I couldn't talk to my mother. She wouldn't understand. Joe tried condoms, but he didn't like the way they felt. Several months went by and nothing happened. Then one month my period was late. I was SCARED. It really hit me that a pregnancy would be so hard to handle. I was only a sophomore. My best friend took me to see her nurse practitioner. My pregnancy test was negative. The nurse practitioner encouraged me to talk. She taught me about my body and how to protect myself. She helped me build my self-esteem. I realize now that I'm not ready to be in a sexual relationship yet.

OBJECTIVES

1. Describe the reasons why women and couples choose to use contraception.

2. Discuss types of fertility awareness-based methods such as natural family planning.

3. List the spermicides currently available in the United States.

4. Compare the barrier methods of contraception with regard to correct use and advantages and disadvantages.

5. Summarize the key points women who use combined oral contraceptives should know, including the correct procedure for taking pills, common side effects, warning signs, and noncontraceptive benefits.

6. Compare other hormonal methods of birth control, including Depo-Provera, NuvaRing, Ortho Evra, and the minipill.

7. Identify the appropriate time frame for initiating postcoital emergency contraception (EC).

8. Delineate the advantages and disadvantages of an IUD as a method of contraception.

9. Contrast the forms of sterilization—tubal ligation, Essure, and vasectomy—with regard to risk, effectiveness, advantages, and disadvantages.

10. Compare medical and surgical approaches to pregnancy termination.

KEY TERMS

MEDIALINK

Additional resources for this content can be found on the Prentice Hall Nursing MediaLink DVD-ROM and on the Companion Website at http://www.prenhall.com/davidson. Click on "Chapter 5" to select the activities for this chapter.

Family planning refers to actions an individual or a couple takes to avoid a pregnancy, to space future pregnancies for a specific reason, or to gain control over the number of children conceived. Thus at a given time a woman may choose one method of contraception and at a later time may elect to use a different approach. For example, birth control pills are an excellent method of contraception for women who are healthy and have no contraindications. A married woman in a stable sexual relationship may choose to use an intrauterine device (IUD), whereas a woman who has no desire for further children may elect permanent sterilization for herself or her male partner may choose such for himself. Although women have several contraceptive options available, currently, contraceptive approaches for men are limited to condoms and vasectomy. This chapter focuses on methods of contraception that are currently available including the advantages and disadvantages of each.

OVERVIEW OF FAMILY PLANNING

Demographics

Approximately 62 million women in the United States are of childbearing age (15 to 44 years). Of these women, 62% practice contraception whereas 31% do not because they are not sexually active, are infertile, are pregnant or trying to become pregnant, are postpartum, or have never had intercourse. Only 7% of these women at risk of becoming pregnant are not using contraception (Alan Guttmacher Institute [AGI], 2006a.)

Nevertheless, in the United States nearly half of all pregnancies are unintended, and of these, 4 in 10 are terminated by abortion. Among women who have abortions, 52% are younger than 25. Latino women are 2.5 times more likely to have an abortion than white women, while black women are 4 times more likely to do so. Two thirds of all abortions are for women who have never been married (AGI, 2006b).

Family planning is an important component of women's health. Worldwide, women who are able to plan the number of pregnancies they have and the interval between pregnancies benefit in several ways (Donovan & Wulf, 2002).

• They enjoy improved health.

• They have lower rates of induced, sometimes unsafe, abortions.

• They have fewer unwanted pregnancies and births.

• They have the opportunity to get more education and to find jobs, which enhances their economic and social status and improves the well-being of their families.

Maternal morbidity and mortality remain a major health challenge in developing countries. Three hundred million of these women will suffer pregnancy-related problems, and 529,000 will die annually. Fewer than 1% of these deaths occur in developed countries (WHO, 2005).

In the developing world, 137 million women have an unmet need for contraception, and an additional 64 million have an unmet need for a modern contraceptive method. This is especially apparent in sub-Saharan Africa where maternal mortality rates are very high (Sonfield, 2006).

Most of the causes of maternal mortality are treatable or preventable with adequate health care including contraceptive services. Thus, it is essential that maternal healthcare services improve if maternal mortality and morbidity are to be reduced. Up to 100,000 maternal deaths per year could be avoided if contraception was available and used by women who did not desire children (WHO, 2005).

In the United States, 34 million women are in need of contraceptive services and supplies (AGI, 2005). These women obtain health coverage that may or may not cover contraceptive services in one of three ways: their employers, the private market, or government-subsidized programs (Sonfield, Gold, Frost, & Darroch, 2004). More than 17 million women need subsidized family-planning services. The largest funding source for this subsidy comes from the joint federal-state Medicaid program. Research suggests that this is money well spent. For every $1 spent on family-planning services, an average of $3 is saved in pregnancy-related care and care of newborns. Moreover, without these publicly supported services an additional 1.3 million pregnancies would occur, leading to approximately 632,300 abortions (AGI, 2005).

Choosing a Method of Contraception

The decision to use a method of contraception may be made individually by a woman (or, in the case of condoms or vasectomy, by a man) or jointly by a couple. Attitudes about contraceptive methods vary considerably. The two leading contraceptive methods in the United States are the pill for women younger than 30 years of age and sterilization for women over the age of 35 (AGI, 2006a). Use of the condom and other barrier methods has increased because of the prevalence of sexually transmitted infections (Maher, Harvey, Bird et al., 2004).

Decisions about contraception should be made voluntarily, with full knowledge of advantages, disadvantages, effectiveness, side effects, contraindications, and long-term effects. Many outside factors influence this choice, including cultural practices, religious beliefs, personality, cost, effectiveness, availability, misinformation, practicality of method, and self-esteem. Different methods of contraception may be appropriate at different times in a couple's life (Table 5–1). In choosing a specific method, consistency of use outweighs the absolute reliability of the given method.

FERTILITY AWARENESS-BASED METHODS

Fertility awareness-based methods (FAB) are based on an understanding of the changes that occur throughout a woman's menstrual cycle and require recording of certain events to identify fertile days. FAB takes into account the lifespan of sperm (2–7 days) and the ovum (1–3 days) in the female reproductive tract. Maximum fertility for the woman occurs approximately 5 days before ovulation and decreases rapidly the day after (Speroff & Darney, 2005). Therefore, the couple must abstain from

Table 5–1 FACTORS TO CONSIDER IN CHOOSING A METHOD OF CONTRACEPTION	
Effectiveness of method in preventing pregnancy	Personal preferences, biases
Safety of the method:	Lifestyle:
Are there inherent risks?	How frequently does client have intercourse?
Does it offer protection against STIs or other conditions?	Does she have multiple partners?
Client's age and future childbearing plans	Does she have ready access to medical care in the event of complications?
Any contraindications in client's health history	Is cost a factor?
Religious or moral factors influencing choice	Partner's support and willingness to cooperate
	Personal motivation to use method

intercourse, or use a barrier method, during the fertile days (Hatcher et al., 2004).

If the couple using an FAB method also uses a barrier method during fertile days, it is known as fertility awareness-combined methods. If the couple abstains completely from intercourse during fertile days, it is known as natural family planning (NFP) (Hatcher et al., 2004).

NFP is free, safe, and acceptable to many whose religious beliefs prohibit other methods; it provides an increased awareness of the body; it involves no artificial substances or devices; it encourages a couple to communicate about sexual activity and family planning; and it is useful in helping a couple plan a pregnancy.

All FAB methods require extensive initial counseling to be used effectively; they may interfere with sexual spontaneity; they require the couple to maintain records for several cycles before beginning use; they may be difficult or impossible for certain groups of women to use, including those with irregular cycles and women who are breastfeeding or perimenopausal; and they may not be as reliable in preventing pregnancy as other methods.

In conjunction with FAB or NFP, women may choose to identify their fertile days by use of an ovulation prediction kit available over the counter (e.g., OvuKit). They may also choose

to use a temperature computer (e.g., Bioself) or a hormone computer (e.g., Persona) (Hatcher et al., 2004).

Basal Body Temperature Method

The *basal body temperature (BBT)* method is an objective, FAB method for a woman to record and determine her fertile days. BBT is incorporated into the symptothermal method. The BBT method is used to detect ovulation by temperature changes during the menstrual cycle. It requires that the woman take her temperature every morning upon awakening (before any activity) and record the readings on a temperature graph. After 3 to 4 months of recording her temperatures, if she has regular cycles, she should be able to predict when ovulation will occur by a retrospective review of her temperature charts. This method is based on the fact that the temperature almost always rises and remains elevated for several days after ovulation because of the production of progesterone, which is thermogenic (heat producing). Figure 5–1 ◆ shows a sample BBT chart.

To avoid conception, the woman and her partner abstain from intercourse or use a barrier method on the day of the temperature rise and for 3 days following. Because the temperature rise does not occur until after ovulation, if the woman had intercourse just before the rise she may be at risk of pregnancy.

Ovulation Method

The *ovulation method,* sometimes called the *cervical mucus method* or the *Billings method,* is an FAB method that involves the assessment of cervical mucus changes that occur during the menstrual cycle. The amount and character of cervical mucus change because of the influence of estrogen and progesterone. During the follicular phase of the cycle (from the end of menses until just before ovulation) cervical mucus is thin and scanty and may even be entirely absent. This progesterone-dominant mucus is not friendly to sperm and is known as "hostile" mucus. At the time of ovulation, the mucus (estrogen-dominant mucus) is clearer, more stretchable (a quality called *spinnbarkheit*), and more permeable to sperm. It has an "egg-white" appearance and is known as "fertile mucus"; it is friendly to sperm, because it assists passage through the cervix and uterus up into the fallopian

Figure 5–1 ◆ Sample basal body temperature chart.
SOURCE: Data from Crooks/Baur: *Our Sexuality,* 5th ed, 1993, Wadsworth.

tubes. It also shows a characteristic fern pattern when placed on a glass slide and allowed to dry.

During the luteal phase, cervical mucus is again thick and sticky (progesterone-dominant mucus) and forms a network that traps sperm, making their passage difficult.

Before using the cervical mucus method, the woman abstains from intercourse for one entire menstrual cycle, during which time she assesses her cervical mucus daily for amount, feeling of slipperiness or wetness, color, clearness, and spinnbarkheit. Abstinence is essential during this time, not only so that the woman avoids pregnancy, but also because the presence of ejaculate in the vagina in the hours following intercourse could interfere with the woman's assessment of her cervical mucus.

When using this method, the woman assumes that the peak day of wetness and clear, stretchable mucus is the day of ovulation. However, she abstains from intercourse from the time she *first* notices that the mucus is becoming clear, more elastic, and slippery until 4 days *after* the peak wet mucus (ovulation) day. Because this method evaluates the effects of hormonal changes, women with irregular cycles can use it. Women who feel uncomfortable testing their mucus should be encouraged to use another method.

Calendar Rhythm Method

The *calendar rhythm method (CRM)* is an FAB method based on the assumptions that ovulation tends to occur 14 days (plus or minus 2 days) before the start of the next menstrual period, that sperm are viable for up to 7 days, and that the ovum is viable for up to 3 days. To use this method, the woman must record her menstrual cycle for 6 months to identify the shortest and longest cycles. The first day of menstruation is the first day of the cycle. The fertile phase is calculated from 18 days before the end of the shortest recorded cycle through 11 days from the end of the longest recorded cycle. For example, if a woman's cycle lasts from 24 to 28 days, the fertile phase would be calculated as day 6 through day 17. Once this information is obtained, the woman can identify the fertile and infertile phases of her cycle. For effective use of this method, she must abstain from intercourse during the fertile phase or use a barrier method. CRM is the *least reliable* of the FAB methods and has largely been replaced by approaches based on objective data.

Symptothermal Method

The *symptothermal method* is an FAB approach that consists of various assessments made and recorded by the couple. These include information about cycle length; frequency and timing of coitus; cervical mucus changes; secondary signs of ovulation such as increased libido, abdominal bloating, mittelschmerz (midcycle abdominal pain); and change in BBT. In retrospect, through the various assessments, the couple learns to recognize signs that indicate ovulation. This combined approach tends to improve the effectiveness of FAB as a method of birth control and is best taught by an expert in the method. For couples interested in the FAB natural family planning method (NFP), training courses are available through the Couple to Couple League.

Other Options

The *standard days method* is good for women with regular cycles between 26 and 32 days. Intercourse is avoided, or a barrier method used, between cycle days 8 through 19 (Hatcher et al., 2004).

The *lactational amenorrhea method* is based on a woman's breastfeeding exclusively for the first 6 months after childbirth. High levels of prolactin in the woman's body during breastfeeding should prevent ovulation. The woman should breastfeed on demand and the newborn should empty both breasts of milk to prevent ovulation. If a formula supplement is used often, a barrier method should be used concurrently. When the woman stops breastfeeding, resumes her menses, or her newborn becomes 6 months old, she should select another method of contraception. This method is most reliable in the United States when used with a barrier method. In developing countries, it is a useful method of "pregnancy spacing" (Hatcher et al., 2004).

SITUATIONAL CONTRACEPTIVES

Certain practices such as coitus interruptus (withdrawal) and douching are considered situational contraceptives because they are activities an individual uses in a given situation to avoid pregnancy without benefit of clinical guidance or medical care. Abstinence, a lifestyle choice, is also considered a situational contraceptive.

Abstinence

Abstinence can be considered a method of contraception and, partly because of changing values and the increased risk of infection with intercourse, it is gaining increased acceptance among people of all ages, but especially among adolescents and young adults. In the past several years, the popular media has featured several stories about film stars, sports heroes, and other personalities who are choosing abstinence, and support groups and Web sites for abstinent teens and adults have become popular. As a result of these and other factors, more and more young people are embracing abstinence and making a commitment to delay sexual intercourse until marriage. Some have even signed pledges to that effect or have purchased and wear a "purity ring."

Abstinence may be culturally dictated before marriage. Abstinence is also the norm in some cultures for women during the postpartum period.

Coitus Interruptus

Coitus interruptus, or withdrawal, is one of the oldest and least reliable methods of contraception. This method requires that the male withdraw from the female's vagina when he feels that ejaculation is impending. He then ejaculates away from the external genitalia of the woman. Failure tends to occur for two reasons:

- This method demands great self-control on the part of the man, who must withdraw just as he feels the urge for deeper penetration with impending orgasm.

- Some preejaculatory fluid, which can contain sperm, may escape from the penis during the excitement phase before ejaculation. Because the quantity of sperm in this preejaculatory fluid is increased after a recent ejaculation, this is especially significant for couples who engage in repeated episodes of orgasm within a short period of time.

Couples who use this method should be aware of postcoital emergency contraceptive options should the man fail to withdraw in time.

Douching

Douching after intercourse is an ineffective method of contraception and is *not* recommended. Moreover, it may actually facilitate conception by pushing sperm farther up the birth canal.

SPERMICIDE

The **spermicide** approved for use in the United States, nonoxynol-9 (N-9), is available as a cream, jelly, foam, vaginal film, and suppository. A spermicide is inserted into the vagina before intercourse. It destroys sperm by disrupting the cell membrane. A spermicide that effervesces in a moist environment offers more rapid protection, and coitus may take place immediately after it is inserted. A suppository may require up to 30 minutes to dissolve and will not offer protection until it has done so. The nurse instructs the woman to insert any of these spermicide preparations high in the vagina and maintain a supine position.

N-9 is minimally effective when used alone, but its effectiveness increases in conjunction with a barrier method of contraception such as the diaphragm, cervical cap, contraceptive sponge, and male and female condoms. The major advantages of spermicides are wide availability, lack of systemic side effects, and low local toxicity.

In the past, N-9 was thought to offer a modest level of protection against several sexually transmitted infections. However, recent research suggests that N-9 does not offer protection against the organisms that cause gonorrhea and chlamydia, or against human immunodeficiency virus (HIV), the organism that causes HIV/AIDS (Centers for Disease Control and Prevention [CDC], 2002). Moreover, N-9 may actually increase a woman's risk of HIV infection because it has a negative effect on the integrity of vaginal cells, making them more susceptible to invasion by organisms such as HIV.

Other forms of spermicidal agents are available for use outside the United States. *Protectaid,* a contraceptive sponge made in Canada, contains F-5 gel (N-9, benzalkonium chloride and sodium cholate). It is available over the Internet.

BARRIER METHODS OF CONTRACEPTION

Barrier methods of contraception prevent the transport of sperm to the ovum, immobilize sperm, or are lethal against them. Barrier methods are often used in conjunction with a spermicide, which some authorities consider a form of chemical barrier.

Barrier methods are clearly related to an individual's sexual behavior. Each act of intercourse demands that one or both partners consciously decide whether to use a barrier contraceptive and then take action. Thus these methods require motivation on the part of the user and cooperation from the partner. They may be used less consistently than non-coitus-related methods of contraception, for example, use of the diaphragm only during a woman's fertile days vs. taking a pill every day. They are very safe methods and do offer a level of protection against some bacterial sexually transmitted infections.

Barrier methods of contraception are a good choice for women who:

- Have a contraindication to using a specific method such as combined oral contraceptives (COCs), the intrauterine device (IUD), subdermal implants (Norplant, currently off the market in the United States), and the like

- Are opposed to taking systemic medications or chemicals such as COCs, monthly injections (Lunelle; currently off the market in the United States), and so forth

- Are in early postpartum or are lactating

- Need a backup method of contraception for a period of time such as when beginning COCs, after an IUD has been inserted, or when a male partner has just had a vasectomy

- Have intercourse rarely or sporadically

- Are perimenopausal but smoke and thus are not good candidates for COCs

Before inserting any female barrier contraceptive, a woman should wash her hands with soap and water to prevent the introduction of organisms. Women who use vaginal barrier methods should avoid using oil-based products such as mineral oil or baby oil and vaginal medications such as Monistat cream (for yeast infection) and estrogen creams because they can have a negative effect on latex.

Many barrier methods are made of latex, so women who are allergic should avoid products made of this material and tell their healthcare provider. Nonlatex barrier methods made of silicone, polyurethane, and lambskin are available.

Barrier methods such as the diaphragm, cervical cap, and Lea's Shield can be worn for 24 to 48 hours, should be cleaned with soap and water after use, and should not be shared with other women. After the last act of intercourse, these devices should remain in place for a minimum of 6 or 8 hours to prevent pregnancy.

In general, female barrier methods are more effective when used with a male condom. However, a male condom should not be used with a female condom. Women who use barrier methods should be alert for signs of toxic shock syndrome (TSS) such as high fever, sore throat, vomiting and/or diarrhea, faintness, weakness, muscle aches, and a rash (see Chapter 7 ∞).

Male Condom

The male **condom** offers a viable means of contraception when used consistently and properly (Figure 5–2 ◆). Acceptance has been increasing because a growing number of men are assum-

Figure 5–2 ◆ *A,* An unrolled condom with reservoir tip. *B,* Correct use.

ing responsibility for regulation of fertility. The condom is applied to the erect penis, rolled from the tip to the end of the shaft, before vulvar or vaginal contact. Most condoms have a reservoir tip to allow for collection of ejaculate. When using a condom without a reservoir end, a small space must be left at the end to collect the ejaculate, so that the condom does not break at the time of ejaculation. If the condom or vagina is dry, water-soluble lubricants, such as K-Y jelly or Astroglide, should be used to prevent irritation and possible condom breakage. Care must be taken in removing the condom after intercourse. For optimal effectiveness, the man should withdraw his penis from the vagina while it is still erect and hold the condom rim to prevent spillage. If after ejaculation the penis becomes flaccid while still in the vagina, the man should hold onto the edge of the condom while withdrawing to avoid spilling the semen and to prevent the condom from slipping off.

The effectiveness of male condoms is largely determined by their use. The condom is small, lightweight, disposable, and inexpensive. It has no side effects (if not allergic to latex), requires no medical examination or supervision, and offers visual evidence of effectiveness. Most condoms are made of latex. Thus, their use is contraindicated if the male or his partner has a latex allergy. Polyurethane and silicone rubber condoms are also manufactured and recommended for individuals allergic to latex. Condoms are available with ribbed or smooth sides, tapered or straight-sided, lubricated or unlubricated, with or without spermicide. They come in a variety of colors, sizes, and flavors. "Natural skins" (lambs' intestines) are available; they are used primarily by individuals with latex allergies. All condoms except natural skin condoms offer protection against sexually transmitted infections (STIs). Moreover, a systematic research review indicates that consistent use of condoms results in an 80% reduction of the incidence of HIV (Weller & Davis, 2006). Concurrent use of a vaginal spermicide does in-

crease the overall effectiveness of all condoms in the prevention of pregnancy.

The male condom is becoming increasingly popular because of the protection it offers from STIs. For women, regardless of age, an STI increases the risk of pelvic inflammatory disease (PID) and resultant infertility. Many women are beginning to insist that their sexual partners use condoms, and many women carry condoms with them.

Misplacement, risk of breakage, perineal or vaginal irritation, and dulled sensation are possible disadvantages of male condoms. Condoms should not be stored in hot conditions because heat accelerates their deterioration, making them more susceptible to breaking. Thus, men should avoid placing them in their car glove box or in their wallets in a rear pants pocket.

Female Condom

The *Reality female condom* (Figure 5–3 ◆) is a thin polyurethane sheath with a flexible ring at each end. The inner ring, at the closed end of the condom, serves as the means of insertion and fits over the cervix like a diaphragm. The second ring remains outside the vagina and covers a portion of the woman's perineum. It also covers the base of the man's penis during intercourse. A woman needs to be careful not to twist the sheath when she inserts the condom because twisting makes male penetration impossible.

Available over the counter and designed for one-time use, the condom may be inserted up to 8 hours before intercourse. The inner sheath is prelubricated but does not contain spermicide and is not designed to be used with a male condom. Because it also covers a portion of the vulva it probably provides better protection against some of the pathogens that cause STIs than other methods. High cost, noisiness during intercourse, and the cumbersome feel of the device make acceptability a problem for some couples.

Figure 5–3 ◆ *A,* The female condom. To insert the condom: *B,* Remove condom and applicator from wrapper by pulling up on the ring. *C,* Insert condom slowly by gently pushing the applicator toward the small of the back. *D,* When properly inserted, the outer ring should rest on the folds of skin around the vaginal opening, and the inner ring (closed end) should fit loosely against the cervix.

SOURCE: From *Our Sexuality,* 5th edition by Crooks/Baur. © 1993. Reprinted with permission of Wadsworth, a division of Thomson Learning: www.thomsonrights.com. Fax 800 730-2215.

Diaphragm

The **diaphragm** is a barrier method that consists of a steel band that forms a ring and is covered with rubber so that when the diaphragm is inserted, the ring lodges high in the vagina with the rubber covering the cervix. It is used with spermicidal cream or jelly and offers a good level of protection from conception. The diaphragm was the first effective method of contraception available to women and was the mainstay of contraception for women until the development of the IUD and oral contraceptives (Sobrero, 2002). Currently it is used by only about 0.3% of US women (AGI, 2006a).

Three types of diaphragms are available—the flat spring, the coil spring, and the arcing spring. Each type has its own advantages, and the type of coil makes the different diaphragms better suited to some women than to others. A woman must be fitted with a diaphragm and given instructions by trained per-

sonnel. The diaphragm should be rechecked for correct size after each childbirth and whenever a woman has gained or lost 10 to 15 pounds or more. Most diaphragms are made of latex; for allergic women, Milex® produces the WIDE-SEAL Silicone Diaphragm.

The diaphragm must be inserted before intercourse, with approximately one teaspoonful (or 1.5 inches from the tube) of spermicidal jelly placed around its rim and in the cup (Figure 5–4 ◆). This chemical barrier supplements the mechanical barrier of the diaphragm. The diaphragm is inserted through the vagina and covers the cervix. The last step in insertion is to push the edge of the diaphragm under the pubic symphysis, which may result in a "popping" sensation. When fitted properly and correctly in place, the diaphragm should not cause discomfort to the woman or her partner. Correct placement of the diaphragm can be checked by touching the cervix with a fingertip through the cup. The cervix feels like a small rounded structure and has

Figure 5–4 ◆ Inserting the diaphragm. *A,* Apply jelly to the rim and center of the diaphragm. *B,* Insert the diaphragm. *C,* Push the rim of the diaphragm under the pubic symphysis. *D,* Check placement of the diaphragm. The cervix should be felt through the diaphragm.

a consistency similar to that of the tip of the nose. The center of the diaphragm should be located over the cervix.

If more than 6 hours elapse between insertion of the diaphragm and intercourse, additional spermicidal jelly should be inserted into the vagina, although no evidence supports this (Hatcher et al., 2004). It is necessary to leave the diaphragm in place for at least 6 hours after coitus. If intercourse is desired again within the 6 hours, another type of contraception must be used or additional spermicidal jelly placed in the vagina with an applicator, taking care not to disturb the placement of the diaphragm. The diaphragm should not remain in the vagina for more than 24 hours; other barrier methods can be left in place for up to 48 hours.

Periodically the diaphragm should be held up to the light or filled with water and inspected for tears or holes. If properly maintained, it can last for several years, so it is a cost-effective method of contraception. The diaphragm should be washed and dried well after each use and then stored in a clean dry container. Talcum powder should not be used with a diaphragm because it contributes to the deterioration of the rubber.

Some couples feel that the use of a diaphragm interferes with the spontaneity of intercourse. The nurse can suggest that the partner insert the diaphragm as part of foreplay or the woman may choose to insert it herself before intercourse. Diaphragm use potentially reduces the incidence of cervical gonorrhea and chlamydia. Its use does protect against human papilloma virus (HPV) infection, which can cause cervical neoplasia (Hatcher et al., 2004).

Women who object to touching their genitals to insert the diaphragm, check its placement, and remove it may find this method unsatisfactory. Women who are very obese or who have short fingers may find the diaphragm difficult to insert. It is not recommended for women with a history of urinary tract infection (UTI), because pressure from the diaphragm on the urethra may interfere with complete bladder emptying and lead to recurrent UTIs. They should be given information about other methods of contraception. As mentioned previously, women with a history of toxic shock syndrome should not use diaphragms or any of the barrier methods because they are left in place for prolonged periods. For the same reason, the diaphragm should not be used during a menstrual period or if a woman has abnormal vaginal discharge.

Cervical Cap

The Prentif Cavity Rim **cervical cap** (Figure 5–5 ◆) is a latex cup-shaped device, used with spermicidal cream or jelly, that

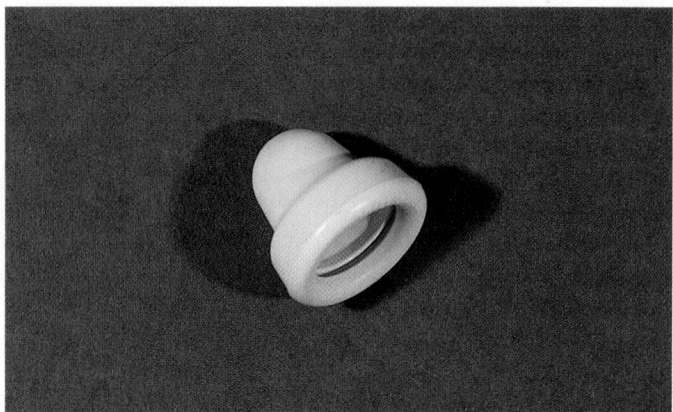

Figure 5–5 ◆ A cervical cap.

fits snugly over the cervix and is held in place by suction and by positive abdominal pressure. The method of insertion is similar to that for the diaphragm. The cap may be left in place for up to 48 hours, and repeated acts of intercourse do not require additional spermicide. The cervical cap should be inserted without rushing, ahead of possible intercourse. Advantages, disadvantages, and contraindications are similar to those associated with the diaphragm. It tends to be more difficult for some women to insert and remove, because it is smaller than the diaphragm. Some women complain about unpleasant odor and discoloration of the cap, especially as the cap ages.

The *FemCap* looks like a small sailor's cap and is made of soft silicone. The "dome" of the cap fits over the cervix, while the soft "brim" flares out slightly and conforms to the shape of the vagina. A strap placed over the dome permits easier removal. It is available in three sizes and was approved for use in the United States in 2003.

A systematic research review indicates that the Prentif cervical cap is comparable to the diaphragm in preventing pregnancy; however, the FemCap is not as effective as a diaphragm. Both forms of cap are medically safe to use (Gallo, Grimes, & Schulz, 2006).

Lea's Shield, a reusable, silicone, one-size-fits-all vaginal barrier method that completely covers the cervix, has been available over the counter in several European countries for over a decade. It contains a centrally located valve that permits the passage of cervical secretions and air. It is held in place by the vaginal walls. In the United States, the woman must see her practitioner to obtain one. A spermicide should be used with it and it should not be worn for more than 48 hours.

Vaginal Sponge

The *vaginal sponge,* available without a prescription, is a pillow-shaped, soft, absorbent synthetic sponge containing a spermicide. It is made with a concave or cupped area on one side, which is designed to fit over the cervix. It also has a loop to permit easy removal. The sponge acts as a contraceptive by releasing the spermicide N-9 gradually over a 24-hour period. The *Today* contraceptive sponge, whose production was halted in 1994 because of manufacturing problems, has been reintroduced on the US market and is once again available for purchase over the Internet.

Figure 5–6 ◆ The contraceptive sponge is moistened well with water and inserted into the vagina with the concave portion positioned over the cervix.

The sponge is moistened thoroughly with water before use to activate the spermicide and is then inserted into the vagina so that the cupped side fits snugly against the cervical os (Figure 5–6 ◆). This decreases the chances of the sponge being dislodged during intercourse. The sponge may be worn for up to 24 hours. It should be left in place for at least 6 hours after intercourse and then removed and discarded.

Advantages of the sponge include the following: professional fitting is not required; it may be used for multiple acts of coitus for up to 24 hours; one size fits all; and it acts as both a barrier and a spermicide. Problems associated with the sponge include difficulty removing it and irritation or allergic reactions. Some women also report a problem because the sponge absorbs vaginal secretions, contributing to vaginal dryness. For women without children the failure rate is comparable to that of the diaphragm and cervical cap. It is higher for women who have borne children, possibly because of changes in the shape of the cervix.

Intrauterine Devices

Both of the **intrauterine devices** available in the United States are designed to be inserted into the uterus by a qualified healthcare provider and left in place for an extended period, providing continuous contraceptive protection. The Copper IUD (ParaGard T380A) provides effective contraception for 10 years, whereas the Mirena levonorgestrel intrauterine system (LNG-IUS) provides 5 years of protection. The exact mechanism of either IUD is not clearly understood. Traditionally, it was believed to act by preventing the implantation of a fertilized ovum. Thus, it was considered an abortifacient or abortion-causing method. This belief is not accurate; both IUDs are truly contraceptive. The Copper IUD is known to have local inflammatory effects on the endometrium and to impair sperm from functioning properly. The Mirena IUD causes the lining of the uterus (endometrium) to become atrophic. It also produces thick cervical mucus that is "hostile" or unfriendly to sperm. Both IUDs produce a spermicidal intrauterine environment (Speroff & Darney, 2005).

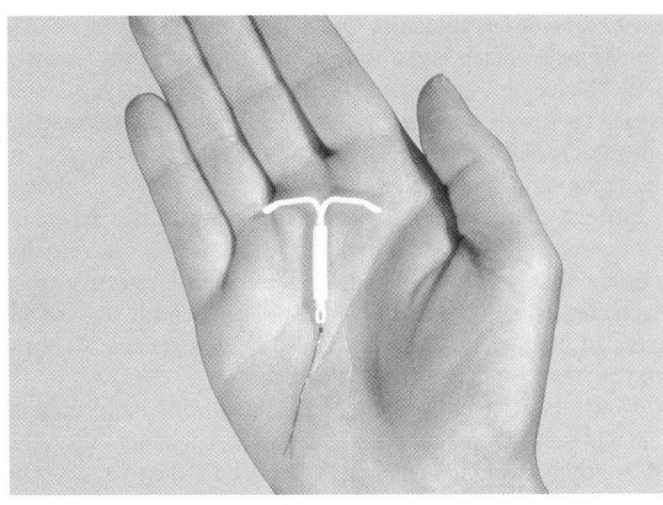

Figure 5–7 ◆ The Mirena Intrauterine System, which releases levonorgestrel gradually, may be left in place for up to 5 years.
SOURCE: Berlex Laboratories, Wayne, NJ.

Both IUDs available today, contrary to common myth, do not increase the risk of ectopic pregnancy or cause pelvic inflammatory disease (PID). In reality, infections in IUD users are probably related more to the woman's lifestyle than to the presence of the IUD. Advantages of both include high rate of effectiveness, continuous contraceptive protection, non-coitus-related activity, and relative inexpensiveness over time. Possible adverse reactions to both IUDs include discomfort to the wearer, increased bleeding during menses, increased risk of pelvic infection for about 3 weeks following insertion, perforation of the uterus during insertion, intermenstrual bleeding, dysmenorrhea, and expulsion of the device.

The Copper IUD (ParaGard T380A) is a small T-shaped device that has copper covering parts of its stem and arms. This IUD is not an option for women allergic to copper but is an excellent choice for women who have medical conditions that preclude use of other contraceptives, hormonal or barrier. The Mirena (LNG-IUS) (Figure 5–7 ◆) is a small, T-shaped frame with a reservoir that releases levonorgestrel on a daily basis. After 3 months of Mirena use, bleeding and length of menstrual cycles are reduced. In fact 14% to 20% of women have amenorrhea, which they often welcome once they are advised that the absence of menses is safe and not an indication of pregnancy. The LNG-IUS is an excellent choice for women who are allergic to copper or who have heavy menses and desire amenorrhea.

IUDs are recommended for women who have at least one child, have no history of PID, and are in a stable, mutually monogamous relationship, because they have the lowest risk of contracting an STI. Women who have not had children but have a medical condition that precludes use of hormonal contraception can be a candidate for insertion of the IUD if the cavity of their uterus is deep enough. After the birth of a child, the inside of the uterus is usually deep enough to be able to fit an IUD. Neither is recommended for women with multiple sexual contacts, because they are at risk for sexually transmitted infections (STIs). However, because the Mirena causes thick cervical mucus, it may have a protective effect against STIs (Hatcher et al., 2004).

The IUD is inserted into the uterus with its string or tail protruding through the cervix into the vagina. It may be inserted at any time during the woman's cycle, providing she is not pregnant, or during the 4- to 6-week postpartum check. The Copper IUD may be inserted up to 5 days after unprotected intercourse as a method of emergency contraception. After insertion, the clinician instructs the woman to check for the presence of the string once a week for the first month and then after each menses. She does this by inserting her index finger or middle finger into her vagina to feel the string. She is told that she may have some cramping or bleeding intermittently for 2 to 6 weeks and that her first few menses may be irregular. Follow-up examination is suggested 4 to 8 weeks after insertion.

Women with IUDs should contact their healthcare providers if they are exposed to an STI or if they develop the following warning signs: late period, abnormal spotting or bleeding, dyspareunia (pain with intercourse), abdominal pain, abnormal discharge, signs of infection (fever, chills, malaise), or missing string. If a woman becomes pregnant with an IUD in place, the device should be removed as soon as possible to prevent infection.

HORMONAL CONTRACEPTIVES

Hormonal contraceptives are available in a variety of forms. They may be progestin-only hormones, most often using a synthetic form of progesterone, or a combination of estrogen and a progestin.

Combination Estrogen-Progestin Approaches

The use of a combination of the hormones estrogen and a progestin is a highly successful, very safe birth control method. Hormonal contraceptives work by inhibiting the release of an ovum, by creating an atrophic endometrium, and by maintaining a thick cervical mucus that slows sperm transport and inhibits the process that allows sperm to penetrate the ovum. There are several forms available, including combined oral contraceptives (COCs), transdermal patches, vaginal rings, and injections (such as Lunelle, which is currently off the market in the United States).

COMBINED ORAL CONTRACEPTIVES

Combined oral contraceptives (COCs)—commonly called birth control pills or "the pill"—are a combination of a synthetic estrogen and a progestin. COCs are one of the most popular contraceptive options available to women in the United States because they are safe, highly effective, and rapidly reversible. COCs are taken daily for 21 days, following one of these methods:

1. *Day 1 start.* The woman begins taking the pill on the first day of her menstrual cycle. This method prevents ovulation in the first cycle, so no backup method of contraception is needed.

2. *Sunday start.* The woman begins taking the pill on the Sunday after the first day of the menstrual cycle and

MediaLink ● Oral Contraceptive Animation

ending on a Saturday. In most cases a hormonally mediated menses (known as a "withdraw" bleed) will occur 1 to 4 days after the last pill is taken. The Sunday start is common because it tends to prevent periods on weekends. However, a backup method of contraception is necessary during the first 7 days of use.

3. *Quick start.* The woman begins taking the pill in the practitioner's office if she is reasonably certain she is not pregnant. A backup method is necessary for 7 days.

With any of the methods, 7 days after taking her last pill, the woman restarts the next cycle of pills. Thus the woman always begins the pill on the same day. Some companies offer a 28-day pack with seven "blank" pills so that the woman never stops taking a pill. The pill should be taken at approximately the same time each day—usually on arising or before retiring in the evening.

Seasonale® is the one COC that is marketed for extended use. Women who choose this COC take 84 active pills followed by 7 "blank" pills. Women taking Seasonale® have 4 withdrawal bleeds per year rather than 12. Extended use reduces the side effects of COCs such as bloating, headache, breast tenderness, cramping, and swelling (Hatcher et al., 2004).

Irregular pill taking is one of the major causes of breakthrough bleeding, a side effect that leads many women to discontinue COCs. Also, although they are highly effective when taken correctly, improper use of the pill can contribute to an unintended pregnancy. COCs may also be less reliable in obese women. (See Evidence-Based Practice.)

Birth control pills have been available for more than 45 years. In the United States, the estrogen component of the pill is either ethinyl estradiol (EE) or mestranol. Of the two, EE is by far the more commonly used estrogen. Initially, COCs con-

---

EVIDENCE-BASED PRACTICE

OBESITY AND CONTRACEPTIVE FAILURE

Clinical Question

What is the effect of body mass index (BMI) and weight on the risk of pregnancy while using oral contraceptives?

The Evidence

Three large studies described the association between BMI and weight and the incidence of unintended pregnancy among oral contraceptive users. All three studies were from large, multisite research projects. One study used data from the 1995 National Survey of Family Growth to examine the relationship between BMI and oral contraceptive failure, as measured by unintended pregnancy while using hormonal contraceptives among 1916 women. A second study evaluated the association between body weight and unintended pregnancy in 18,445 women enrolled in the multistate Pregnancy Risk Assessment Monitoring System. A case/control study was conducted using information from the monitoring system about pregnancy intention, consistency of contraceptive use, and body weight. A third study relied on data from 248 health maintenance organization enrollees who became pregnant while using oral contraceptives, and compared their pregnancy rate with that of 533 age-matched enrollees who were nonpregnant oral contraceptive users during the same period. All studies calculated odds ratios to examine the relationship, yielding statistics that allow the researcher to estimate the comparative probability of pregnancy as it relates to BMI and weight.

What Is Effective?

Women with a BMI greater than 30 had a significantly greater risk of having an oral contraceptive failure, resulting in an unintended pregnancy. In one study, this difference was smaller when the sample results were adjusted for age, marital status, education, parity, and dual method use. In the other studies, adjustment for demographic factors made no difference in the results. Obese women were between 50% and 70% more likely to have an unintended preg-

nancy while consistently using oral contraceptives. One study was able to quantify that the risk was 60% higher when BMI was greater than 27.3 and 70% higher when BMI was greater than 32.2. The risk of unintended pregnancy when using oral contraceptives was nearly doubled for women weighing more than 86.2 kg (approximately 190 pounds). No association was found between body weight and unintended pregnancy among noncontraceptive users, so it is suggested that the effect of obesity on unintended pregnancy is limited to contraceptive failure.

What Is Unclear?

All of these studies used measures of association or correlation, so it is possible that an extraneous variable or confounding effect is present. None of these studies can draw a conclusion about whether the higher BMI actually causes contraceptive failure or whether higher BMI and contraceptive failure are both attributed to some other characteristic or physiologic process.

Best Practice

The evidence would suggest that women who must avoid pregnancy and who have a BMI greater than 30 should be advised to use methods in addition to hormonal contraceptives alone. Women with a high BMI should be advised to lose weight if they will rely solely on oral contraceptives to avoid an unintended pregnancy.

Critical Thinking

What additional kinds of contraceptive methods can women use who have a higher BMI but want to avoid unintended pregnancy?

REFERENCES: Brunner, L., & Hogue, C. (2005). The role of body weight in oral contraceptive failure: Results from the 1995 National Survey of Family Growth. *Annals of Epidemiology, 15,* 492–499.
Holt, V., Scholes, D., Wicklund, K., Cushing-Haugen, K., & Daling, J. (2005). Body mass index, weight, and oral contraceptive failure risk. *Obstetrics and Gynecology, 105* (1), 46–52.
Huber, L., & Hogue, C. (2005). The association between body weight, unintended pregnancy resulting in a live birth, and contraception at the time of conception. *Maternal and Child Health Journal, 9* (4), 413–420.

tained high levels of estrogen and were linked with an increased risk for myocardial infarction (MI), thromboembolic disorders (blood clots), and stroke. Lowering the estrogen dose in the formulation decreased these risks. Based on this understanding, over the years the estrogen component of COCs has been decreased from 150 mcg/day to the lowest dose currently available—20 mcg/day (Speroff & Darney, 2005).

Currently nine different formulations of progestins are available. These progestins vary with respect to their biologic activity including their inhibition of ovulation. Synthetic progestins can have androgenic, antiandrogenic, estrogenic, and antiestrogenic effects. These effects are responsible for the varying progestin-related side effects.

COCs are among the most studied medications available. The current generation of low-dose pills is very safe and would be even safer if smokers over age 35 did not take them. In an effort to reduce complications such as myocardial infarction, stroke, blood clots, and hypertension, regimens have been developed that use very low doses of estrogen (20 or 25 mcg) and progestins that are less androgenic in effect. These very-low-dose pills may result in weaker cycle control, which leads to more irregular or "breakthrough" bleeding. These low-dose pills do provide the same noncontraceptive benefits as the pills that contain 30 to 35 mcg of EE, and it is recommended that smokers of all ages who wish to take the pill be prescribed 20 mcg COCs to reduce serious complications.

Side effects are generally identifiable as estrogen related or progestin related. Thus it is possible to modify some side effects by choosing a different oral contraceptive preparation. The side effects associated with COCs are identified in Table 5–2.

Absolute contraindications to the use of oral contraceptives include pregnancy, previous history of thrombophlebitis or thromboembolic disease, acute or chronic liver disease of cholestatic type with abnormal function, presence of estrogen-dependent carcinomas, undiagnosed uterine bleeding, heavy smoking, gallbladder disease, hypertension, diabetes, migraine with visual disturbances, hypercoagulable disorders, and hyperlipidemia. Women with the following relative contraindications may initiate COC use; however, they require close and frequent monitoring. These include women with migraine headaches without visual disturbances, epilepsy, depression, oligomenorrhea, and amenorrhea. Women who choose this method of contraception should be fully advised of the potential side effects and complications.

Oral contraceptives have several important noncontraceptive benefits. Many women who use COCs experience relief of uncomfortable menstrual symptoms and premenstrual syndrome. Cramps diminish, flow decreases, and the cycle becomes more regular. Mittelschmerz is eliminated, and the incidence of functional ovarian cysts decreases. More important, there is a reduction in the incidence of ectopic pregnancy, PID, ovarian cancer, endometrial cancer, colorectal cancer, iron deficiency anemia, and benign breast disease. Currently, oral contraceptives are considered a wonderful solution to the physiologic problems some women experience during the perimenopause and can be used by nonsmoking women until they transition to hormone replacement therapy at menopause, if necessary to control vasomotor symptoms, such as hot flashes (Hatcher et al., 2004). Because of an increased risk of MI (heart attack), women over age 35 who smoke should not take oral contraceptives.

The woman using oral contraceptives should contact her healthcare provider if she becomes depressed, develops a breast lump, becomes jaundiced, or experiences any of the following warning signs: severe abdominal pain, severe chest pain or shortness of breath, severe headaches, dizziness, changes in vision (vision loss or blurring), speech problems, or severe leg pain.

Another oral contraceptive is the progesterone-only pill, also called the *minipill*. It is used primarily by nursing mothers, because it does not interfere with breast milk production. It is also used by women who have a contraindication to the estrogen component of the combination preparation, such as history of thrombophlebitis or hypertension, but are strongly motivated to use this form of contraception. The major problems with progesterone-only pills are amenorrhea or irregular bleeding patterns. They are slightly less effective than a COC. They must be taken consistently at the same time every day (Hatcher et al., 2004).

TRANSDERMAL HORMONAL CONTRACEPTION

Combined hormonal contraception can now be provided transdermally using a weekly *contraceptive skin patch* called Ortho Evra. Roughly the size of a silver dollar, but square, this patch is applied weekly for 3 weeks on one of four sites: the woman's abdomen, buttocks, upper outer arm, or trunk (excluding the breasts). During the fourth week, no patch is applied and menses typically occurs. The patch is highly effective in women who weigh less than 198 pounds (Hatcher et al., 2004). Patch users apply their first patch on the first day of their menses, or on the the Sunday following; if the latter is chosen a backup method for 7 days is necessary.

Table 5–2 SIDE EFFECTS ASSOCIATED WITH ORAL CONTRACEPTIVES

Estrogen Effects	Progestin Effects
Alterations in lipid metabolism	Acne, oily skin
Breast tenderness, engorgement or increased breast size	Breast tenderness; increased breast size
Cerebrovascular accident	Decreased libido
Changes in carbohydrate metabolism	Decreased high-density lipoprotein (HDL) cholesterol levels
Chloasma	
Fluid retention; cyclic weight gain	Depression
Headache	Fatigue
Hepatic adenomas	Hirsutism
Hypertension	Increased appetite; weight gain
Leukorrhea, cervical erosion, ectopia	Increased low-density lipoprotein (LDL) cholesterol levels
Nausea	
Nervousness, irritability	Oligomenorrhea, amenorrhea
Telangiectasia	Pruritus
Thromboembolic complications—thrombophlebitis, pulmonary embolism	Sebaceous cysts

The patch is as safe and effective as COCs and has a better rate of user compliance. Generally, women who are candidates for COCs are candidates for the patch unless they are obese (weight greater than 198 pounds) or have skin disorders that may result in reactions at the site of application. Recently the manufacturer, Ortho-McNeil, has worked with the federal Food and Drug Administration (FDA) to reword the product labeling. Because skin absorption of transdermal estrogen is 60% greater than oral absorption of a 35 mcg COC, it is unknown if this increases a woman's risk of serious side effects or complications (US FDA, 2005b). Women using the patch still have a 25% lower blood level of estrogen than those using COCs. Research as to whether the patch increases serious side effects is ongoing. In the meantime, this method remains a safe birth control option.

VAGINAL CONTRACEPTIVE RING

NuvaRing vaginal contraceptive ring (manufactured by Organon), another form of low-dose, sustained-release combined hormonal contraceptive, is a flexible, soft vaginal ring that is inserted monthly (Figure 5–8 ◆). The ring is left in place for 21 days and then removed for 7 days (Hatcher et al., 2004). (One size ring fits virtually all women.) Women with marked vaginal prolapse should be cautioned to check for expulsion of the ring during early use. Women who use the NuvaRing should begin its use in the same way as described for the patch. Replacement rings should be kept in the refrigerator to maintain integrity.

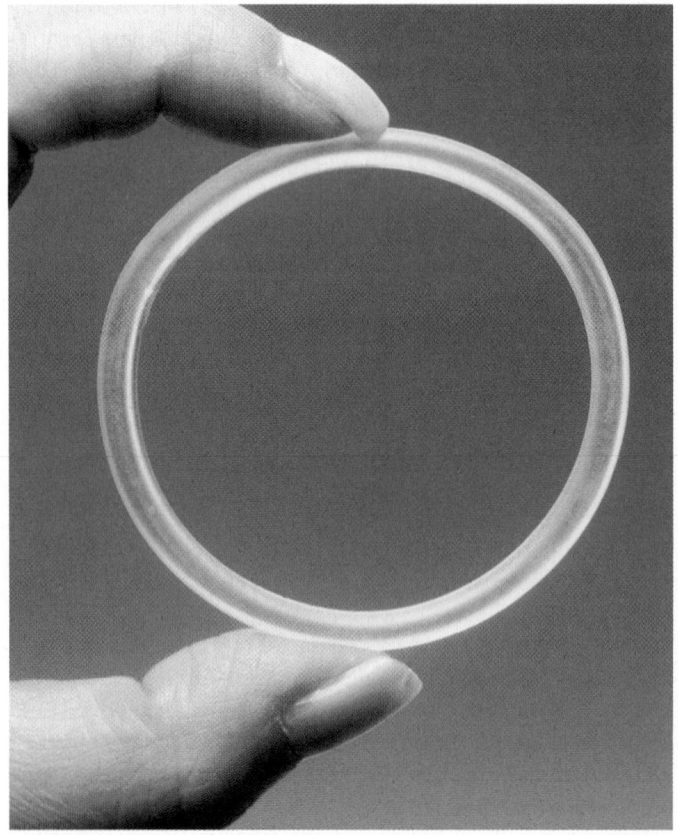

Figure 5–8 ◆ The NuvaRing vaginal contraceptive ring.

INJECTABLE COMBINATION CONTRACEPTIVE

Lunelle, a combination of medroxyprogesterone acetate and estradiol cypionate (MPA/E₂C), now off the market in the United States because of manufacturing problems, was administered every 28 to 30 days (not to exceed 33 days) as an intramuscular (IM) injection. Women who used Lunelle had regular menstrual bleeding patterns and rapid return to fertility when the medication was stopped. Its contraindications and side effects are the same as those of oral contraceptives.

Long-Acting Progestin Contraceptives

With the exception of the progestin-only pill, or minipill, discussed previously, depot-medroxyprogesterone acetate (DMPA), or Depo-Provera, is the only progestin-only contraceptive on the market in the United States today.

Depot-medroxyprogesterone acetate (DMPA) (**Depo-Provera** 150 mg), a long-acting progestin, provides highly effective birth control for 3 months (every 10 to 14 weeks) when administered as a single IM injection of 150 mg, preferably in the deltoid muscle. DMPA, which acts primarily by suppressing ovulation, is safe, convenient, private, and relatively inexpensive. It also separates birth control from the act of coitus. It can be given to nursing mothers, because it contains no estrogen. DMPA provides levels of progesterone high enough to block the luteinizing hormone (LH) surge, thereby suppressing ovulation. It also thickens the cervical mucus to block sperm penetration. Side effects include menstrual irregularities, headache, weight gain, breast tenderness, hair loss, and depression. Return of fertility may be delayed for an average of 9 months (Hatcher et al., 2004). Depo-Provera is not recommended for use longer than 2 years without specific informed consent by the woman. It has been associated with calcium loss from the bones that may not resolve after discontinuing use. Women who remain on DMPA longer than 2 years must be educated about this serious side effect and must exercise and take 1200 mg of calcium daily.

Depo-Provera 104 mg SQ is an alternative to Depo-Provera 150 mg. Originally approved by the FDA for the treatment of endometriosis, it subsequently was approved as a contraceptive. Because there is 30% less drug available compared with the 150 mg preparation, it may result in less bone density loss for long-term users. It is administered every 10 to 13 weeks, only it is given subcutaneously.

The original **subdermal implants,** called *Norplant,* consist of six silastic capsules the size of a matchstick containing levonorgestrel, a progestin, which are implanted in the woman's upper underarm. They are effective for up to 5 years. Norplant is *now off the market in the United States.* Norplant II, which consists of two rods, was never introduced in the United States. This two-rod preparation is available as *Jadelle* in other countries and is effective for up to 5 years. Women who weigh more than 154 pounds are not good candidates for implants (Hatcher et al., 2004).

Subdermal implants prevent ovulation in most women. They also stimulate the production of thick cervical mucus, which inhibits sperm penetration. These implants provide effective continuous contraception that is removed from the act of coitus. Possible side effects include spotting, irregular bleeding or amenorrhea, an increased incidence of ovarian cysts, weight gain, headaches, fluid retention, acne, hair loss, mood changes, and depression.

Implanon is a single-capsule implant also inserted under the skin of the arm. It is impregnated with etonogestrel, another of the progestins. It is good as a contraceptive for 3 years, and its mechanism of action is similar to Norplant and Jadelle. Its release in the United States has been postponed but remains anticipated.

Implants are mentioned in this chapter because some women may not have had their Norplant rods removed or the nurse may care for women from foreign countries who use Jadelle. A minor surgical procedure is required to insert and remove the implants.

POSTCOITAL EMERGENCY CONTRACEPTION

Postcoital emergency contraception (EC) is indicated when a woman is worried about pregnancy because of unprotected intercourse, sexual assault, or possible contraceptive failure (e.g., broken condom, slipped diaphragm, missed oral contraceptives, or too long a time between DMPA injections). Research indicates that oral hormonal EC taken within 72 hours can reduce the risk of pregnancy after a single act of unprotected intercourse by 75% to 89%. Placement of the Copper IUD within 5 days after unprotected intercourse may reduce pregnancy risk by as much as 99% (Hatcher et al., 2004).

Two hormonal regimens for EC include a combined hormonal approach (levonorgestrel and ethinyl estradiol) and Plan B, a progestin-only approach (levonorgestrel). Though sometimes called the "morning-after pill," the phrase is misleading because the woman actually takes her first dose as soon after intercourse as possible and a second dose 12 hours later. The combined hormonal approach uses high-dose oral contraceptives. The high dose of estrogen may lead to nausea and vomiting. A prophylactic antiemetic may be useful.

Plan B (progestin-only) is more effective than the combined hormonal EC; it also has a much lower incidence of associated nausea and vomiting. Thus, if it is available it should be used instead of the combined regimen effective (American College of Obstetricians and Gynecologists [ACOG], 2005a). Although the package insert for Plan B instructs women to take the two doses 12 hours apart, research indicates that taking both pills at the same time or taking the pills 24 hours apart is equally as effective as the 12-hour regimen and does not increase the risk of side effects (ACOG, 2005a).

The combined regimen remains an option because many women knowledgeable about EC can use their unused COCs, if necessary, after consulting with their healthcare provider. COCs are prescriptions that must be obtained from a healthcare provider.

In 2006 Plan B was approved by the FDA for over-the-counter sale to women 18 years and older. A prescription for Plan B is still required for use by teenagers under age 18.

Both regimens must be initiated within 72 hours after unprotected intercourse, although most research indicates they could be effective up to 5 days after coitus. Emergency contraceptive pills are safe for almost all women. The only contraindication is a diagnosed pregnancy because the pills are ineffective (Hatcher et al., 2004).

Currently there is considerable debate about the best ways to improve access to EC. It is essential that healthcare providers counsel women about the availability of EC during routine screenings and appointments. This approach ensures that women are familiar with the method before an emergency occurs. It is also helpful to have printed literature on EC available in the waiting area. Information about postcoital emergency contraception is available through the Emergency Contraception Hotline (1-888-NOT-2-LATE), and on the World Wide Web. (See Research in Practice).

OPERATIVE STERILIZATION

Operative **sterilization** is an inclusive term that refers to surgical procedures that permanently prevent pregnancy. In the man, sterilization is achieved through a procedure called *vasectomy*. In the woman, sterilization is done by *tubal ligation.*

Before sterilization is performed on either partner, the clinician provides a thorough explanation of the procedure to both. Each needs to understand that sterilization is not a decision to be taken lightly or entered into at times of psychologic stress, such as separation or divorce. Even though both male and female procedures are theoretically reversible, the permanency of the procedure should be stressed and understood.

Vasectomy

Male sterilization is achieved through a relatively minor procedure called a **vasectomy.** This involves surgically severing the vas deferens in both sides of the scrotum. It takes about 4 to 6 weeks and 6 to 36 ejaculations to clear the remaining sperm from the vas deferens. During that period, the couple is advised to use another method of birth control and to bring in two or three semen samples for a sperm count. When the sperm count is negative the couple can safely have unprotected sex. The man is rechecked at 6 and 12 months to ensure that fertility has not been restored by recanalization. Side effects of a vasectomy include pain, infection, hematoma, sperm granulomas, and spontaneous reanastomosis (reconnecting).

Vasectomies can sometimes be reversed by using microsurgery techniques. Restored fertility, as measured by subsequent pregnancy, ranges from 38% to 82% (Hatcher et al., 2004).

Tubal Ligation

Voluntary female sterilization is accomplished by **tubal ligation.** Three procedures are common in the United States:

- Laparotomy following a cesarean birth or other abdominal surgery
- Minilaparotomy in the postpartum period soon after a vaginal birth
- Laparoscopy done postabortion or during an "interval period," when the woman is not pregnant or postpartum

RESEARCH IN PRACTICE

DIRECT ACCESS TO EMERGENCY CONTRACEPTION THROUGH PHARMACIES AND EFFECT ON UNINTENDED PREGNANCY AND STIS: A RANDOMIZED CONTROLLED TRIAL

What is this study about? Estimates suggest that half of unintended pregnancies could be averted if emergency contraception was easily accessible and used. Emergency contraception is a method of preventing pregnancy after intercourse. It may be used in situations when a condom fails or in cases as extreme as rape. Opinions vary widely as to whether it is appropriate for teens and young women. Proponents see the use of emergency contraception as a method to reduce the adolescent pregnancy rate. Critics are concerned that access to emergency contraception will result in high-risk sexual behavior, increased rates of sexually transmitted infections, and decreased use of other types of contraception. This study undertook the analysis of the relationships among three different methods of accessing emergency contraception and the rates of risky sexual behaviors and sexually transmitted infections.

How was this study done? More than 2100 young women aged 15 to 24 from four California family-planning clinics were randomized into one of three treatment groups. All of the women were at the clinics seeking family-planning services or were already users of hormonal contraception. One treatment group was given pharmacy access, meaning they could receive emergency contraception at nearby pharmacies; one group had advance provision of three packs of emergency contraception, meaning they were given the emergency contraception before they needed it; and one group was able to get emergency contraception from a clinic. The outcomes of interest were self-report of high-risk sexual practices, screening for sexually transmitted infections, and self-reported use of contraception. Statistical analysis was used to determine if there were differences among the three groups on the three outcome variables.

What were the results of the study? Overall, fewer than half of study participants who had unprotected intercourse used emergency contraception at any point during the study period. Eight percent of participants became pregnant and 12% acquired a sexually transmitted infection, but there were no differences in these rates among the three groups. Women in the pharmacy access group were no more likely to use emergency contraception than the women with clinic access. The women in the advance access group—those who had emergency contraception "on hand" in case they needed it—were almost twice as likely to use the emergency contraception as those in either of the other two groups. There were no significant differences in the rates of high-risk sexual practices or sexually transmitted infections among any of the groups.

What additional questions might I have? Are these findings similar for women of all ages? Is the self-report method accurate and reliable for this information? Are there emotional or psychologic needs involved in emergency contraception that aren't met when the medications are obtained without counseling or advice?

How can I use this study? Teens and young women who are given convenient access to emergency contraception will use the treatment without an associated increase in their high-risk sexual behaviors. Use of emergency contraception is not associated with sexually transmitted infection or decreased use of contraception. The nurse can recommend this contraception method to teens and young women without concern that he or she is contributing to risky sexual behaviors.

SOURCE: Haine, T., Harper, C., Rocca, C., Fischer, R., Padian, N., Klausner, J., et al. (2005). Direct access to emergency contraception through pharmacies and effect on unintended pregnancy and STI's: A randomized controlled trial. *Journal of the American Medical Association, 293*(1), 54–59.

Tubal ligation may be done at any time. However, the postpartal period is an ideal time to perform a tubal ligation because the uterus is enlarged and the tubes are easy to locate. During these procedures the tubes are ligated, clipped, electrocoagulated, banded, or plugged. This interrupts the patency of the fallopian tube, thus preventing the ovum and the sperm from meeting.

Complications of female sterilization procedures include coagulation burns on the bowel, bowel perforation, pain, infection, hemorrhage, and adverse anesthesia effects. Reversal of a tubal ligation depends on the type of procedure performed. A pregnancy can be achieved up to 75% of the time after mechanical occlusion as compared with electrocoagulation, because more tissue is destroyed in the latter procedure (Berek, 2002).

Nonoperative Sterilization

The *Essure* method of permanent sterilization by Conceptus requires no surgical incision. Under hysteroscopy, a stainless steel microinsert is placed into the proximal section of each fallopian tube. Within 3 months, these microinserts create a benign tissue response that occludes the fallopian tubes. Three months after placement, tubal occlusion is confirmed by hysterosalpingogram. One of the materials used in the production of the implants is a nickel-titanium alloy; therefore, *women allergic to nickel should consult their healthcare provider before placement.* It is the only sterilization method approved in the United States that will yield no surgical scar (Magos & Chapman, 2004).

MALE CONTRACEPTION

The vasectomy and the condom, discussed previously, are currently the only forms of male contraception available in the United States. Developing reversible methods of contraception for men is a challenge because healthy men produce sperm continuously, whereas women produce eggs cyclically. It is easier to devise a reversible method that interrupts a cyclic process than it is to find ways to interrupt continuous fertility.

Hormonal contraception for men has yet to be developed, although studies are under way using weekly injections of testosterone, a synthetic hormone that significantly inhibits sperm production in most men. These injections have significant side effects of feminization of the male, which make them largely unacceptable. A combination injection of testosterone and DMPA, the progestin found in Depo-Provera, is also under way. If it is successful, injections may only be needed monthly. Investigational approaches include gonadotropin-releasing hormone analogues and sex steroids (Hatcher et al., 2004; Speroff & Darney, 2005).

I think I'm like a lot of women. During my life I've used a variety of contraceptive methods. I took the pill back when doses were higher; I used foam alone and had a baby, then used spermicidal cream and condoms more successfully. I never wanted a tubal, and my husband refuses to consider a vasectomy, so the IUD was a perfect alternative for us. I am 47 and I like something I don't have to think about every time we want to make love. Maybe someday there will be more contraceptives for men—it seems only fair—but I'm glad that at least I've had some choices.

NURSING CARE MANAGEMENT

In most cases, the nurse who provides information and guidance about contraceptive methods works with the woman, because most contraceptive methods are female oriented. Because a man can purchase condoms without seeing a healthcare provider, only in the case of vasectomy does a man require counseling and interaction with a nurse. However, men should be encouraged to participate in contraceptive services. The nurse can play an important role in helping a woman or couple choose a method of contraception that is acceptable to both partners.

In addition to completing a history and assessing for any contraindications to specific methods, the nurse can spend time with a woman learning about her lifestyle, personal attitudes about particular contraceptive methods, religious and cultural beliefs, personal biases, and plans for future childbearing to help the woman select a particular contraceptive method. (See Developing Cultural Competence.)

Once the woman chooses a method, the nurse can help her learn to use it effectively. "Client Teaching: Using a Method of Contraception" provides guidelines for helping women use a method of contraception effectively.

The nurse also reviews any possible side effects and warning signs related to the method chosen and counsels the woman about what action to take if she suspects she is pregnant. In many cases, the nurse is involved in telephone counseling of women who call with questions and concerns about contraception. Thus it is vital that the nurse be knowledgeable about this topic and have resources available to find answers to less common questions.

DEVELOPING CULTURAL COMPETENCE

BIRTH CONTROL PRACTICES

Attitudes about birth control may be influenced by cultural factors. Although it is impossible to attribute one attitude to an entire group of people, the following general information may be helpful as a starting point in working with women from a particular ethnic group (Cefalo & Dominguez, 2002):

- Among women from China the IUD is the most popular form of birth control although sterilization is common.

- Oral contraceptives are the most common form of birth control among African Americans.

- Birth control is an issue that causes mixed emotions for some African Americans. Those who wish to avoid pregnancy or space children see contraception as a blessing; however, some view contraception as a form of genocide.

- Although many African Americans are opposed to abortion because of religious or cultural beliefs, the high rates of teen pregnancy have decreased opposition to abortion somewhat.

- Among many Hispanic women, abstinence and rhythm are the only acceptable forms of contraception and abortion is seen as morally wrong. Prolonged breastfeeding may be used to protect against pregnancy.

- Among many American Indians and Native Alaskans, large families are valued and, traditionally, birth control is not used.

CLINICAL TIP

Have informational handouts available for the various methods of contraception. Describe correct use, side effects, warning signs, and important tips for effective use. Women can then refer to the sheets at home. Be sure to include the office or clinic phone number.

CLINICAL INTERRUPTION OF PREGNANCY

Abortion, the termination of a pregnancy, was legalized in the United States in 1973. However, the associated controversy over moral and legal issues continues. This controversy is as readily apparent in the medical and nursing professions as in other groups.

Many women are strongly opposed to abortion for religious, ethical, or personal reasons. Other women feel that abortion provides a legally available alternative to a pregnancy. A number of physical and psychosocial factors influence a woman's decision to seek an abortion. The presence of a disease or health state that jeopardizes the mother's life and serious, life-threatening fetal problems are frequently suggested as indications for abortion. In other instances, the timing or circumstance of the pregnancy creates an inordinate stress on the woman, prompting her to choose an abortion. Some of these

MediaLink Case Study: Family Planning

MediaLink Application: Contraceptive Services for Minors

CLIENT TEACHING Using a Method of Contraception

CLIENT GOALS   At the completion of the teaching, the woman will be able to

1. Confirm for herself that the chosen method of contraception is appropriate for her.

2. List the advantages, disadvantages, and risks of the chosen method.

3. Describe (or demonstrate) the correct procedure for using the chosen method.

4. Cite warning signs that should be reported to the caregiver.

TEACHING PLAN

CONTENT

Discuss the factors that a woman should consider in choosing a method of contraception (see Table 5–1). Stress that the different methods may be appropriate at different times in the woman's life. Review the woman's reasons for selecting a particular method and confirm any contraindications to specific methods.

Discuss the advantages, disadvantages, and risks of the chosen method.

Describe the correct procedure for using a method. Go through step by step. Periodically stop and have the woman review the information. If a technique is to be learned (as with inserting a diaphragm or charting basal body temperature), demonstrate and then have the woman do a return demonstration as appropriate. (*Note:* If certain aspects are beyond the nurse's level of expertise, the nurse can review the content and confirm that the woman has the opportunity to do a return demonstration. For example, an office nurse who does not do cervical cap fittings may cover information on its use, have the woman try inserting the cap herself, and then have the placement checked by the nurse practioner or physician.)

Provide information on what the woman should do if unusual circumstances arise (she forgets a pill or misses a morning temperature).

Stress warning signs that require immediate action on the part of the woman and explain why these signs indicate a risk. Carefully delineate the actions the woman should take.

TEACHING METHOD

Contraception is a personal decision, so the discussion should take place in a private area free of interruptions.

Create a supportive, warm, and comfortable atmosphere by attitude and communication style—both verbal and nonverbal.

Provide accurate information in an open, nonjudgmental way.

Focus on open discussion. It may help to have written information about the method chosen. If a signed permit is required (as with sterilization or IUD insertion), the physician should also discuss the advantages, disadvantages, and risks.

Learning is best accomplished when material is broken down into smaller steps.

Have a model or chart available to enable the woman to visualize what is being described. Have a sample of the chosen method available: a package of oral contraceptives, an open IUD, or a symptothermal chart.

Provide a written handout identifying the warning signs of her chosen method and listing the actions a woman should take. The handout should also cover actions the woman should take if an unusual situation develops. For example, what should she do if she vomits or has diarrhea while taking oral contraceptives?

Arrange to talk with the woman again soon, either on the phone or at a return visit, to determine if she has any questions about the method and to ensure that no problems have arisen.

EVALUATION

Evaluate the woman's learning by asking her to describe the method she has chosen, its contraindictions and warning signs, and the procedure for using it correctly. In some cases, a return demonstration is useful.

situations may involve contraceptive failure, sexual assault, or incest. Usually the decision is best made by the woman or couple involved. A woman whose life is threatened by the pregnancy may choose to continue the pregnancy, whereas one with no obvious threat may choose abortion.

Globally, the legal status of abortion varies greatly. It ranges from complete prohibition to abortion at a pregnant woman's request. Among the 6 billion people who inhabit the Earth, national attitudes and laws about abortion can be classified into three broad categories (Henshaw, 2002):

- About one fourth of the world's people live in countries where abortion is absolutely forbidden or where it is only allowed to save the life of a pregnant woman. These include most Muslim countries of Asia, the majority of African countries, about two thirds of the Latin American countries, and one European country—Ireland.

- About one tenth live in a country where abortion is allowed to protect a woman's physical health or her mental health, and where social factors such as unmarried status, substandard housing, and inadequate income can be considered. Major countries in this group include Japan, Great Britain, and India.

- About two fifths of world countries permit abortion on request, generally without specifying a reason, although this is sometimes limited to the first trimester. Abortions for medical reasons are often allowed beyond the limits specified for an elective abortion. Countries in this category are a varied group and include the People's Republic of China, Austria, Denmark, Cuba, France, Italy, Sweden, Denmark, the United States, and most of the formerly socialist republics of Central and Eastern Europe.

Worldwide, abortion rates decline when women have access to modern methods of contraception, whether a country has legalized abortion or not.

Medical Interruption of Pregnancy

Medical abortion is now available in the United States and provides an effective alternative to surgical abortion for many women with unintended pregnancies. FDA approved in 2000, *mifepristone* (Mifeprex), originally called RU 486, was originally given FDA labeling to medically induce abortion during the first 7 weeks of pregnancy or 49 days following the first day of the last menstrual period. Complete abortion success rates are higher when the medication is taken earlier in pregnancy— approximately 96% to 98% in pregnancies up to 42 days and 91% to 95% in pregnancies from 43 to 49 days' gestation (ACOG, 2005b). Some clinicians support the use of a slightly modified dosage regimen through 63 days' gestation (Creinin, Blumenthal, & Shulman, 2006; Hatcher et al., 2004).

Mifepristone blocks the action of progesterone, thereby altering the endometrium. After the length of the woman's gestation is confirmed, she takes a dose of oral mifepristone in her caregiver's office. One to 3 days (depending upon gestation) later she returns to her caregiver and takes an oral or vaginal dose of the prostaglandin misoprostol, which induces contrac-

tions that expel the embryo/fetus. About 14 days after taking the misoprostol, the woman is seen a third time to confirm that the abortion was successful.

Since 2001, seven deaths that may possibly have been related to the oral mifepristone-vaginal misoprostol regimen have been reported to the distributing company and to the FDA. Four of these deaths were related to an infection caused by a rare organism, *Clostridium sordelli* (Creinin et al., 2006). The FDA has issued an advisory warning for its use. Therefore, *any* woman who has decided on a medical abortion and has taken the oral mifepristone-vaginal misoprostol regimen within the last 24 hours who develops stomach pain, weakness, nausea, vomiting or diarrhea, with or without fever, should contact her healthcare provider *immediately* (US FDA, 2005a). Currently, mifepristone is still considered safe and use of routine prophylactic antibiotics is not recommended.

Although methotrexate is not labeled for medical abortion, 20 years of experience with it has led to its use in the first 7 weeks of pregnancy. Methotrexate stops cell division, and when used with misoprostol, it can be up to 96% effective in terminating a pregnancy (Hatcher et al., 2004). However, ACOG (2005b) states that mifepristone-misoprostol regimens are preferable to those using methotrexate-misoprostol or misoprostol alone for medical abortion.

Surgical Interruption of Pregnancy

Surgical abortion in the first trimester (less than 13 weeks' gestation) is technically easier and safer than abortion in the second trimester. The technique most widely used is vacuum curettage (Speroff & Darney, 2005). The cervix is anesthetized with local anesthesia using a paracervical block. It then must be dilated either mechanically with metal dilators or laminaria or medicinally with misoprostol or mifepristone. A cannula is placed through the cervix and suction is applied to recover all the products of conception. The major risks include perforation of the uterus, laceration of the cervix, systemic reaction to the anesthetic agent, hemorrhage, retained products of conception, and infection.

Second trimester abortion (greater than 13 weeks' gestation) may be done medically or surgically. Medical termination includes the use of a mifepristone-misoprostol regimen and the intra-amniotic injection of hypertonic saline or urea to euthanize the fetus. The woman will need to labor and pass the fetus in the hospital. Surgical termination is done using dilation and evacuation (D&E). This procedure combines vacuum aspiration with the use of forceps. Risks are similar to a first trimester termination but greater (Hatcher et al., 2004).

NURSING CARE MANAGEMENT

The woman deciding to terminate a pregnancy may choose to do so based on an unwanted/unintended pregnancy, sexual assault, lack of finances, her health, or the health of the fetus. The nurse should assess the woman's need for support and/or counseling. If the decision was difficult for the woman, the nurse should assist her in finding postprocedure support.

Client selection is an important factor in medical abortion. Pregnancy needs to be verified early, by 5 weeks' gestation if possible. The woman needs to understand clearly that medical abortion takes time and follow-up is important. Moreover, women need accurate information about the cramping, bleeding, and pain that occur so that they are prepared to deal with both the discomfort and the sight of the blood and possible uterine contents.

In general, important aspects of nursing care for a woman who chooses to have an abortion include providing information about the methods of abortion and associated risks; counseling regarding available alternatives to abortion and their implications; encouraging the woman to verbalize her feelings; providing support before, during, and after the procedure; monitoring vital signs, intake, and output; providing for physical comfort and privacy throughout the procedure; and teaching the client self-care, the importance of the postabortion checkup, and contraception review.

CHAPTER REVIEW

FOCUS YOUR STUDY

- The fertility awareness-based method (FAB), natural family planning (NFP), is a "natural," noninvasive method of contraception often used by people whose religious beliefs prevent them from using other methods.

- Other FAB methods can be used in conjunction with a barrier method during the woman's fertile days.

- Situational contraceptives such as coitus interruptus (withdrawal) and douching are activities an individual uses in a given situation to avoid pregnancy without benefit of clinical guidance or medical care. Abstinence is also considered a situational contraceptive.

- Barrier contraceptives such as the contraceptive sponge, diaphragm, cervical cap, FemCap, Lea's Shield, and condom act by blocking the transport of sperm. These methods are often used in conjunction with a spermicide.

- N-9, the spermicide available in the United States, is far less effective in preventing pregnancy when it is not used with a barrier method.

- The Copper IUD is a mechanical contraceptive. Although its exact method of action is not clearly understood, research suggests it acts by immobilizing sperm or by impeding the progress of sperm from the cervix to the fallopian tubes. In addition, the IUD does have a local inflammatory effect.

- The Mirena levonorgestrel-releasing IUS (LNG-IUS) is both a hormonal and mechanical contraceptive. Its action is similar to that of the Copper IUD; it also secretes a progestin, etonogestrel, that helps the endometrium to become atrophic, the cervical secretions to become "hostile" to sperm, and the menstrual flow to be decreased.

- Combined oral contraceptives (the "pill") are combinations of estrogen and a progestin. When taken correctly, they are one of the most effective reversible methods of fertility control.

- Suspended hormonal options, once available on the US market, include the injection containing estrogen and progestin, Lunelle, and the progestin-only implants (Norplant).

- The one progestin-only subdermal implant, Implanon, is being awaited in the United States.

- Other combined hormonal options (estrogen and progestin) such as the patch (Ortho Evra) and the vaginal ring (NuvaRing) have broadened the range of contraceptive options available.

- The "patch" is under investigation for its potential role in increased complications associated with greater systemic absorption of estrogen.

- The long-acting progestin-only injection, Depo-Provera, is now recommended only for short-term use (less than 2 years) because of loss of bone mineral density (BMD) (calcium bone loss). There is a subcutaneous form, Depo 104 mg, that may cause less BMD loss.

- Permanent sterilization is accomplished by tubal ligation for women and vasectomy for men. Although theoretically reversible, clients are advised that the method should be considered irreversible. Essure offers a nonoperative approach to permanent blockage of the fallopian tubes.

- The termination of pregnancy through abortion may now be achieved by either medical or surgical means.

EXPLORE MediaLink

http//www.prenhall.com/davidson

NCLEX review questions, case studies, and other interactive resources for this chapter can be found on the Web Site at http://www.prenhall.com/davidson. Click on "Chapter 5" to select the activities for this chapter.

For tutorials including animations and videos, more NCLEX review questions, and an audio glossary, access the accompanying Prentice Hall Nursing MediaLink DVD-ROM in this book.

PRENTICE HALL NURSING MEDIALINK DVD-ROM

Audio Glossary

NCLEX Review

Oral Contraceptive Animation

Videos: *Vasectomy; Through the Eyes of a Nurse—Welcoming the New Arrival at the First Postpartal Visit*

COMPANION WEBSITE

Additional NCLEX Review

Case Study: *Family Planning*

Care Plan Activity: *Fertility Awareness*

Applications: *Abstinence Support Resources; Contraceptive Services for Minors*

Critical Thinking

CRITICAL THINKING IN ACTION

REDUCING ANXIETY DURING A FIRST PELVIC EXAM

View the Critical Thinking in Action video in Chapter 5 of the DVD-ROM. Then answer the questions that follow.

You are working at a local clinic when Joy Lang, age 20, presents for her first pelvic exam. You obtain the following GYN history: menarche age 12, menstrual cycle 28–30 days lasting 4–5 days, heavy one day, then lighter. She tells you that she needs to use super-absorbent tampons on the first day of her period and then she switches to a regular absorbency tampon for the remaining days. She confirms that she changes the tampon every 6 to 8

hours, never leaving it in overnight. She denies premenstrual syndrome, dysmenorrhea, or medical problems and says that she is not taking any medication on a regular schedule. She tells you that she recently got married, but would like to wait before getting pregnant. She'd like to discuss birth control methods. Joy tells you that doctors make her nervous and she admits to being anxious about her first pelvic exam.

1. What steps would you take to reduce Joy's anxiety relating to the pelvic exam?

2. What position is best to relax Joy's abdominal muscles for the pelvic exam?

3. What precaution should be taken when obtaining a Pap smear?

4. Explain the purpose of the Pap smear.

5. What factors do you include in a discussion of the type of birth control that Joy could practice?

REFERENCES

Alan Guttmacher Institute (AGI). (2005). Contraceptive services. *Facts in Brief.* Retrieved May 30, 2006, from http://www.guttmacher.org

Alan Guttmacher Institute (AGI). (2006a). Contraceptive use. *Facts in Brief.* Retrieved May 30, 2006, from http://www.guttmacher.org

Alan Guttmacher Institute. (2006b). Facts on induced abortion in the United States. *Facts in Brief.* Retrieved May 30, 2006, from http://www.guttmacher.org

American College of Obstetricians and Gynecologists (ACOG). (2005a). *Emergency contraception* (ACOG Practice Bulletin No. 69). Washington, DC: Author.

American College of Obstetricians and Gynecologists (ACOG). (2005b). *Medical management of abortion* (ACOG Practice Bulletin No. 67). Washington, DC: Author.

Berek, J. (2002). *Novak's gynecology* (13th ed.). Philadelphia: Lippincott Williams & Wilkins.

Cefalo, R. C., & Dominguez, L. (2002). *Culture, women, and healthcare: A multicultural approach to patients* (A continuing education monograph).

New York: Medical Education Collaborative and Creative 4 Media Inc.

Centers for Disease Control and Prevention (CDC). (2002, May 10). Nonoxynol-9 spermicide contraceptive use—United States, 1999. *Mortality and Morbidity Weekly Reports, 51*(18), 389–392.

Creinin, M., Blumenthal, P., & Shulman, L. (2006). Mifepristone-misoprostol medical abortion mortality. *Medscape General Medicine, 8*(2), 26. Retrieved May 6, 2006, from http://www.medscape.com/viewarticle/529318_print

Donovan, P., & Wulf, D. (2002). Women and societies benefit when childbearing is planned. *Issues in Brief.* Retrieved May 30, 2006, from http://www.guttmacher.org

Gallo, M. F., Grimes, D. A., & Schulz, K. F. (2006). Cervical cap versus diaphragm for contraception (Accession No. 2009134249). *Cochrane Library, 2006*(1).

Hatcher, R. A., Trussell, J., Stewart, F., Nelson, A., Cates, W., Guest, F., et al. (2004). *Contraceptive technology* (18th ed.). New York: Ardent Media.

Henshaw, S. K. (2002). Induced abortion: Epidemiologic aspects. In J. J. Sciarra (Ed.), *Gynecology and obstetrics* (Vol. 6, chap. 115, pp. 1–11). Philadelphia: Lippincott Williams & Wilkins.

Magos, S., & Chapman, L. (2004). Hysteroscopic tubal sterilization. *Obstetrics & Gynecology of North America, 31,* 705–719.

Maher, J., Harvey, S., Bird, S., Stevens, V., & Bechman, L. (2004). Acceptability of the vaginal diaphragm among current users. *Perspectives on Sexual and Reproductive Health, 36*(2), 64–71.

Sobrero, A. J. (2002). Use and effectiveness of barrier and spermicidal contraceptive methods. In J. J. Sciarri (Ed.), *Gynecology and obstetrics 2002* (Vol. 6, chap. 17). Philadelphia: Lippincott Williams & Wilkins.

Sonfield, A. (2006). Working to eliminate the world's unmet need for contraception. *Guttmacher Policy Review, 9*(1), 10–13.

Sonfield, A., Gold, R., Frost, J., & Darroch, J. (2004). US insurance coverage of contraceptives and the impact of contraceptive coverage mandates, 2002. *Perspectives on Sexual and Reproductive Health, 36*(2), 72–79.

Speroff, L., & Darney, P. (2005). *A clinical guide for contraception* (4th ed.). Philadelphia: Lippincott Williams & Wilkins.

US Food and Drug Administation (FDA). (2005a). *Mifeprex information.* Retrieved November 20, 2005, from http://www.fda.gov.cder/drug/infopage/mifepristone/default/htm

US Food and Drug Administration (FDA). (2005b). *Ortho Evra: New labeling information.* Retrieved November 19, 2005, from http://www.fda.gov/bbs/topics/news/2005/NEW01262.html

Weller, S., & Davis, K. (2006). Condom effectiveness in reducing heterosexual HIV transmission (Accession No. 2009134003). *Cochrane Library, 2006*(1).

World Health Organization. (2005). *Facts and figures from the world health report, 2005.* Retrieved November 28, 2005, from http://www.who.org

CHAPTER

6 Women's Health: Commonly Occurring Infections

I guess I was what you would call a wild kid. I took way too many chances, even sexually, and eventually I got herpes. Now I am 32, with two children, and married to a great man who loves me. He has never had herpes but we are very careful because I don't want him infected because of me. How much simpler life would be if I didn't carry that virus. Too bad that we can't change the past.

OBJECTIVES

1. Compare vulvovaginal candidiasis and bacterial vaginosis.
2. Summarize modes of transmission, treatments, and descriptions of the most commonly occurring sexually transmitted infections (STIs).
3. Summarize the health teaching that a nurse needs to provide to a woman with an STI.
4. Relate the implications of pelvic inflammatory disease (PID) for future fertility to its pathologic origin, signs and symptoms, and treatment.
5. Contrast cystitis and pyelonephritis.
6. Compare the different types of viral hepatitis.

KEY TERMS

MEDIALINK

Additional resources for this content can be found on the Prentice Hall Nursing MediaLink DVD-ROM and on the Companion Website at http://www.prenhall.com/davidson. Click on "Chapter 6" to select the activities for this chapter.

Many women seek health care because of infections of one sort or another including those that are sexually transmitted. The nurse caring for a woman with an infection can be most helpful by providing accurate, sensitive, and supportive health care and health information. Additionally, the nurse is uniquely able to provide nonjudgmental health promotion, education, and counseling to influence the woman's future health behaviors positively. To meet the woman's needs, the nurse needs to have up-to-date information about a variety of infections, including how they are spread, diagnosed, and treated, and their long-term implications.

This chapter focuses on several types of infections, with an emphasis on sexually transmitted infections. It is designed to provide current information to help nurses provide more effective health care for women and their families.

CARE OF THE WOMAN WITH A LOWER GENITAL TRACT INFECTION (VAGINITIS)

Vaginitis is the most common reason women seek gynecologic care. Symptoms of vaginitis, or vulvovaginitis, may include increased vaginal discharge, vulvar irritation and pruritus, external dysuria, or a foul odor. Women with vaginitis may have either infectious abnormal organisms or an abundance or overgrowth of vaginal microorganisms such as *Gardnerella vaginalis, Mycoplasma hominis, Ureasplasma urealyticum, Mobiluncus, Bacteroides,* and *Peptostreptococcus* species (Owen & Clenney, 2004; Riggs & Klebanoff, 2004).

Bacterial Vaginosis

Bacterial vaginosis (BV) is the most prevalent form of vaginal infection in the United States and worldwide. BV is more prevalent in sexually active women; however, the debate continues as to whether BV is a sexually transmitted infection, because it has also been detected in virginal women. Newer studies link BV as a sexually transmitted infection between heterosexual couples. In the past, studies of male sexual partner treatment did not reveal a decrease in the BV reoccurrence rate of their female partners. However, colonization of the male genital tract with BV-associated microorganisms with consequent nongonococcal urethritis is significantly correlated with recurrent BV of the female partner (Schwebke & Desmond, 2005). Other studies have revealed a high prevalence of BV in adolescent girls and higher rates in women with human immunodeficiency virus (HIV) infection (Plitt et al., 2005).

Previously referred to as nonspecific vaginitis, or *Gardnerella* vaginitis, BV is an alteration of normal vaginal bacterial flora resulting in the loss of hydrogen-producing lactobacilli and an overgrowth of predominantly anaerobic bacteria. This process is poorly understood and the causes leading to overgrowth are not clear. Frequent sexual intercourse without condom use (sperm and seminal fluid has pH greater than 7), trauma from douching, and an upset in normal vaginal flora are

all predisposing or contributing factors. Research also suggests that increased psychosocial stress is associated with an increased incidence and greater prevalence of BV (Nansel et al., 2006). The *Gardnerella vaginalis* and *Mycoplasma hominis* organisms have been found in the vast majority of cases, along with an increased concentration of anaerobic bacteria.

The infected woman often notices an excessive amount of thin, watery, white or gray vaginal discharge, with a foul odor sometimes described as "fishy." The characteristic "clue cells" are seen on a wet-mount preparation, and leukocytes are conspicuously absent (Figure 6–1 ◆). The addition of a 10% potassium hydroxide (KOH) solution to the vaginal secretions, called the "whiff" test, releases a strong, fishy, aminelike odor. The vaginal pH is usually greater than 4.5 (normal vaginal pH should be between 3.8 and 4.2). Women with BV have an increased risk of pelvic inflammatory disease (PID), abnormal cervical cytology, postoperative cuff infections after hysterectomy, and postabortion PID. The pregnant woman with BV is at risk for premature rupture of the membranes (PROM), preterm labor, chorioamnionitis, and postcesarean endometritis (Centers for Disease Control and Prevention [CDC], 2006b).

The nonpregnant woman who is symptomatic is generally treated with metronidazole (Flagyl) 500 mg orally twice a day for 7 days (see Drug Guide: Metronidazole [Flagyl]) or one full applicator of metronidazole gel, 0.75% intravaginally, once daily for 5 days. Both these routes are equally effective. Alternatively the woman can be treated with 2% clindamycin (Cleocin) vaginal cream, one full applicator at bedtime for 7 days. This treatment is slightly less effective (CDC, 2006b). Follow-up visits are not necessary unless symptoms recur.

For many years, metronidazole was regarded as a potential teratogen, especially in the first trimester, and its use was generally avoided, especially in early pregnancy. However, the CDC (2006b) now reports that multiple studies have not demonstrated a consistent relationship between metronidazole use during preg-

Figure 6–1 ◆ The characteristic "clue cells" seen in bacterial vaginosis.
SOURCE: Courtesy Centers for Disease Control and Prevention.

DRUG GUIDE   Metronidazole (Flagyl)

Overview of Action

Metronidazole is an antiprotozoal and antibacterial agent. It possesses direct trichomonacidal and amebicidal activity against *T vaginalis and E histolytica*. Metronidazole is active in vitro against most obligate anaerobes but does not appear to possess any clinically relevant activity against facultative anaerobes or obligate aerobes. It is used in the treatment of various infections caused by organisms that are sensitive to this drug. It is used predominantly to treat the following infections in women: *T vaginalis*, bacterial vaginosis, endometritis, endomyometritis, tubo-ovarian abscess, and postsurgical vaginal cuff infection.

Route, Dosage, Frequency

Trichomoniasis—non-pregnant woman: 1 day treatment 2 g orally in a single dose, 7-day treatment: 500 mg orally twice a day for 7 consecutive days (CDC, 2006b).

Amebiasis—Adults: 750 mg orally three times a day for 5–10 days; children: 35–50 mg/kg/24 hours orally divided into three doses for 10 days.

Bacterial vaginosis—non-pregnant woman: 500 mg orally twice a day for 7 consecutive days or one full applicator of metronidazole gel 0.75% intravaginally, once daily for 5 days (CDC, 2006b).

Contraindications

Blood dyscrasias

Breastfeeding women (drug secreted in breast milk)

Impaired kidney or liver function

Active CNS disease

Side Effects

Convulsive seizures	Weakness
Peripheral neuropathy	Insomnia

Nausea/Vomiting	Cystitis
Headache	Dysuria
Anorexia	Reversible neutropenia and
Diarrhea	thrombocytopenia
Epigastric distress	Flattening of the T wave on ECG
Abdominal cramping	Polyuria
Constipation	Incontinence
Metallic taste in	Pelvic pressure
mouth	Proliferation of *Candida* in the vagina
Dizziness	and mouth
Vertigo	Joint pains
Uncoordination	Decreased libido
Ataxia	Dryness in the mouth, vulva, and vagina
Confusion	Dyspareunia
Irritability	Depression

Nursing Considerations

- Inform woman about potential side effects.
- Stress the importance of contraceptive compliance during course of treatment.
- Obtain baseline renal and liver function tests as ordered.
- Teach woman about the signs, symptoms, and treatment of vulvovaginal candidiasis.
- Counsel the woman to avoid alcoholic beverages while taking the medication.
- If the woman is taking oral contraceptives, a backup nonhormonal contraceptive method is recommended during treatment.
- Take thorough history to rule out the woman's exposure to this medication within the last 6 weeks.
- Teach woman to monitor the signs and symptoms of her infection.
- Encourage cooperation with the entire course of treatment.

nancy and teratogenic effects on the newborn. Thus, currently the recommended treatment during pregnancy is metronidazole 500 mg orally twice a day or metronidazole 250 mg orally three times a day or clindamycin 300 mg orally twice daily. All these regimens should be taken for 7 days (CDC, 2006b). Some providers recommend screening of all pregnant women for BV because it has been associated with preterm labor and birth; others recommend screening only those pregnant women at increased risk for preterm birth. In either case, if a pregnant woman is found to be positive for BV she should be treated.

Vulvovaginal Candidiasis

Vulvovaginal candidiasis (VVC), also known as a candidiasis, or fungal and yeast infection, is a very common vaginal infection. It is estimated that in their lifetime, 75% of women will have at least one episode of VVC, whereas 40% to 45% of women will have two or more episodes (CDC, 2006b). *Candida albicans* is responsible for the vast majority of vaginal yeast infections. Non-*albicans* species of *Candida*, such as *C glabrata*, *C tropicalis*, and *C krusei*, can also cause vulvovaginal symptoms and they are becoming more prevalent. There is evidence that some of these strains are developing resistance to therapies such as fluconazole. Predisposing factors to yeast infections include glycosuria, use of oral contraceptives, use of antibiotics, pregnancy, diabetes mellitus, and the use of immunosuppressant drugs.

The woman with VVC often complains of thick, white vaginal discharge, severe itching, dysuria, and dyspareunia. A male sexual partner may experience a rash or excoriation of the skin of the penis, and possibly pruritus. The male may be symptomatic and the female asymptomatic.

On physical examination, the woman's labia may be swollen and excoriated if pruritus has been severe. A speculum examination usually reveals thick, white, tenacious, curdy patches adhering to the vaginal mucosa. The diagnosis is made by observing mycelia or pseudohyphae upon direct microscopy in a 10% KOH preparation (Figure 6–2 ◆). A Gram stain or culture positive for the fungus is a more accurate way of diagnosing

Figure 6–2 ◆ Hyphae and spores of *Candida albicans.*
SOURCE: Courtesy Centers for Disease Control and Prevention.

the causative organism. The pH of the vagina remains 4.5 or less (the normal pH of the vagina is about 3.8 to 4.2).

Local vaginal treatment with intravaginal butoconazole, clotrimazole, miconazole, nystatin, terconazole, or tioconazole cream, tablets, or suppositories is recommended. Single-dose and short-course approaches (3 days) are effective for 80% to 90% of women with uncomplicated VVC. Oral fluconazole, 150 mg in a single dose, is also effective for mild VVC (CDC, 2006b). Women with severe symptoms who are treated with oral fluconazole may need a repeat dose in 4 days (Mead, 2001). If the vulva is also infected, the cream is applied topically. Women with recurrent infections may be advised to use long-term clotrimazole or fluconazole therapy. The use of vaginal application of boric acid capsules and lactobacilli products remains unproven and controversial (Owen & Clenney, 2004). Some of these medications are available over the counter. They are indicated for women with a history of yeast infections who are able to correctly recognize true VVC symptoms.

Treatment of the male partner is generally not indicated although it may be recommended for partners of women who have recurrent infection. For men who have candidal balanitis (inflammation of the glans penis) treatment with a topical antifungal medication is indicated (CDC, 2006b).

Recurrent VVC, defined as four or more episodes of symptomatic VVC in 1 year, affects less than 5% of women (CDC, 2006b). If a woman experiences frequent recurrences of monilial vaginitis, she should be tested for an elevated blood glucose level to determine whether a diabetic or prediabetic condition is present. Women at high risk for sexually transmitted infections should also be tested for HIV infection. In the absence of other risk factors, recurrent VVC treatment should include confirmation of the organism by culture, then an intensive regimen of topical agents for 7 to 14 days or oral doses of fluconazole every third day for 3 doses (days 1, 4, and 7), followed by maintenance antifungal therapy using oral fluconazole weekly for 6 months or clotrimazole suppository once weekly for 6 months (CDC, 2006b).

Pregnant women with VVC should be treated only with topical azole preparations applied for 7 days (CDC, 2006b). Infection at the time of birth may cause thrush (a *candidal* infection of the mouth) in the newborn.

NURSING CARE MANAGEMENT
Nursing Assessment and Diagnosis

The nurse caring for the woman should suspect VVC if the woman complains of intense vulvar itching and a thick nonodorous, white discharge. Because HIV-positive women and pregnant women with diabetes mellitus are especially susceptible to this infection, the nurse should be alert for symptoms in these women. In some areas nurses are trained to do speculum examinations and wet-mount preparations and can confirm the diagnosis themselves. In most cases, however, the nurse who suspects a vaginal infection reports it to the woman's healthcare provider.

Nursing diagnoses that might apply to the woman with VVC include the following:

- *Risk for Impaired Skin Integrity* related to scratching secondary to discomfort of the infection
- *Health-Seeking Behaviors:* Information about yeast infection related to an expressed desire to know about ways of preventing the development of VVC

Nursing Plan and Implementation

If the woman is experiencing discomfort because of pruritus, the nurse can recommend gentle bathing of the vulva with a weak sodium bicarbonate solution. If a topical treatment is being used, the woman will need to bathe the area before applying the medication.

The nurse also discusses with the woman the factors that contribute to the development of VVC and suggests ways to prevent recurrences, such as wearing cotton underwear, cotton-crotch pantyhose, and avoiding douching and vaginal powders or sprays that may irritate the vulva. Women taking antibiotics should be advised about the possibility of developing VVC and encouraged to seek treatment early if symptoms develop.

Evaluation

Expected outcomes of nursing care include the following:

- The woman's symptoms are relieved, and the infection is cured.
- The woman is able to identify self-care measures to prevent further episodes of VVC.

CARE OF THE WOMAN WITH A SEXUALLY TRANSMITTED INFECTION

The occurrence of **sexually transmitted infection (STI),** or sexually transmitted disease (STD), has increased over the past few decades. In fact, vaginitis and STIs are the most common reasons for outpatient, community-based treatment of women. More than one STI can occur at the same time. All symptomatic women should be tested for other infections. Table 6–1 provides a summary of VVC and BV as well as the common STIs.

Table 6–1   SUMMARY OF SEXUALLY TRANSMITTED INFECTIONS*

Disease	Organism	Diagnosis	Treatment Nonpregnant	Pregnant
Vulvovaginal candidiasis (VVC)	*Candida albicans*	Wet-mount hyphae	Topically applied azole drugs	Topically applied azole drugs
Bacterial vaginosis (BV)	*Gardnerella vaginalis* and *Mycoplasma hominis*	Wet-mount clue cells	Metronidazole	Metronidazole or clindamycin
Trichomoniasis	*Trichomonas vaginalis*	Wet-mount trichomonads	Metronidazole	Metronidazole
Syphilis	*Treponema pallidum*	Dark-field examination VDRL, RPR, or MHA-TP	Benzathine Penicillin G	Benzathine Penicillin G
Herpes genitalis	Herpes simplex virus	Herpes culture or titer	Acyclovir	Acyclovir
Chlamydia	*Chlamydia trachomatis*	Chlamydia culture	Doxycycline or azithromycin*	Azithromycin or amoxicillin
Gonorrhea	*Neisseria gonorrhoeae*	Gonorrhea culture	Cefixine, ciprofloxacin, ofloxacin, or levofloxacin plus doxycycline or azithromycin	Ceftriaxone or cefixime with Azithromycin or amoxicillin
Acquired immunodeficiency syndrome	Human immunodeficiency virus	ELISA test and Western blot	Varies	Varies
Condylomata acuminata	Human papilloma virus	Virapap, biopsy, Pap smear, colposcopy	Cryotherapy, TCA, BCA, Podophyllum, podofilox, excision	Cryotherapy Trichloroacetic acid
Pediculosis pubis	*Phthirus*	Microscopic identification of lice or nits	Permethrin 1% creme rinse or lindane 1% shampoo	Permethrin 1% creme rinse
Scabies	*Sarcoptes scabiei*	Confirmation of symptoms or scraping of furrows	Lindane 1% lotion or permethrin 5% cream	Crotamiton 10% lotion or permethrin 5% cream

*Note: VVC and BV are included for comparison even though they are not spread primarily by sexual contact.

Prevention of Sexually Transmitted Infections

Effective prevention and control of STIs is based on the following concepts (CDC, 2006b):

1. Education and counseling for people at risk on ways to practice safer sexual behavior.
2. Identification of infected, asymptomatic individuals and of people with symptoms of STI who are not likely to seek diagnostic and treatment services.
3. Effective diagnosis and treatment of people with an STI.
4. Evaluation, treatment, counseling, and education for individuals who are the sex partners of people with an STI.
5. Preexposure vaccination of individuals at risk for vaccine-preventable STIs.
6. Expedited partner therapy (EPT), whereby partners are treated, is recommended by the CDC (2005). Infected individuals deliver medications or prescriptions to their partners to manage and decrease the reinfection rates of STIs. The legal status of EPT has not been determined in all states.

Individuals are at lowest risk for an STI if they abstain from sexual intercourse (whether vaginal, anal, or oral sex) and if they are in a long-term, monogamous relationship with a partner who is free of infection. Ideally, before entering a new sexual relationship, both partners should be tested for STIs, including HIV infection. If a person decides to have sex without knowing the partner's infection status, a new condom should be used before each act of intercourse (CDC, 2006b).

Nurses can play an important role in educating and counseling individuals who have an STI, who are at risk for one, or who are the partners of an infected individual. Information should be tailored to individual needs and specific risk factors. It can include details about actions a person can take to avoid exposure to an STI or to avoid transmitting one. Nurses need to be nonjudgmental and respectful and draw on their counseling skills in sharing information.

Trichomoniasis

Trichomoniasis is a commonly occurring STI caused by *Trichomonas vaginalis,* a microscopic motile protozoan that thrives in an alkaline environment. Among females in general the reported prevalence ranges from 5% to 13%; the prevalence among female sex workers is 50% to 60% (Schachter, 2005). The single-celled parasite, called a trichomonad, is an anaerobe that has the ability to generate hydrogen, which combines with oxygen to create an anaerobic environment. Most infections are acquired through sexual intimacy. Fomite transmission by shared bath facilities, wet towels, or wet swimsuits may also be possible.

Often women with trichomoniasis are asymptomatic or have only mild symptoms. More pronounced symptoms of trichomoniasis may include a yellow-green, frothy, odorous discharge and vulvar itching. The woman may also complain of dysuria and dyspareunia. Occasionally, subepithelial hemorrhages on the cervix (strawberry-like red spots) can be seen with the naked eye; smaller areas of hemorrhage are generally visible with a colposcope. Microscopic visualization of mobile trichomonads and increased leukocytes, a vaginal pH of 4.5 or

RESEARCH IN PRACTICE

A RANDOMIZED TRIAL OF CLINICIAN-DELIVERED INTERVENTIONS PROMOTING BARRIER CONTRACEPTION

What is this study about? Women are more likely to acquire sexually transmitted infections (STIs) than men, and the consequences are more dire in terms of disease and infertility. Thus efforts to develop risk-reduction interventions for young women are increasing. The primary focus of intervention is promoting the use of condoms. Few studies have evaluated intervention effectiveness using STI outcomes; fewer still use clinicians to deliver the intervention. This study sought to determine if a highly structured intervention provided by a clinician was superior to the provision of basic information in promoting condom use and preventing STIs.

How was this study done? Clinicians were trained to deliver a scripted counseling intervention and were certified through a process of observation, video-taped role playing, and systematic feedback. The actual intervention consisted of a 19-minute videotape, a 30-minute counseling session, free condoms, and additional take-home items to reinforce condom use. The "basic intervention" consisted of a 3- to 5-minute discussion about the effectiveness of condoms, free supplies of condoms, and brochures about correct use. Women were recruited from an STI clinic and 427 were randomized to either the experimental or basic intervention group. Af-

ter the interventions were applied, subjects kept a diary about the number and type of sexual partners, frequency and type of sexual activity, and condom use. At each clinic visit, a physical examination was conducted and subjects were tested for STIs.

What were the results of the study? Condom use rates were 69% for the experimental intervention group and 49% for the basic intervention group. However, STI rates did not differ significantly between the groups. Regardless of the intervention, perfect condom use was associated with a dramatic decrease in STI rates. The enhanced intervention increased perfect use of condoms, but only modestly.

What additional questions might I have? Are the diaries a good way of recording this sensitive information? Is there a concern for honesty in reporting these data? Why did the increased use of condoms not result in an associated decrease in STIs?

How can I use this study? In-depth counseling by a clinician can increase the usage rates of condoms, even if STI rates are unaffected. The clinician should focus on encouraging women to use condoms every time they have sexual activity, because perfect condom use was associated with dramatically reduced STI rates.

Lynn, A., Maurizio, M., Meinzen-Derr, J., Kelaghan, J., Harland, A., Fleenor, M., Hook, E., & Brill, I. (2005). A randomized trial of clinician-delivered interventions promoting barrier contraception for sexually transmitted disease prevention. *Journal of the American Sexually Transmitted Disease Association, 32*(11), 672–679.

Figure 6–3 ◆ Microscopic appearance of *Trichomonas vaginalis.*
SOURCE: Centers for Disease Control and Prevention (CDC).

higher, and a positive whiff test are diagnostic of *T. vaginalis* (Figure 6–3 ◆). Pregnant women with trichomoniasis may be at increased risk for premature rupture of membranes, preterm birth, and low birth weight. Pregnant women who are symptomatic should be treated with a single 2-g dose of metronidazole orally to relieve their symptoms (CDC, 2006b).

Recommended treatment for trichomoniasis is metronidazole (Flagyl) administered in a single 2-g dose, tinidazole in a single 2-gm dose; alternatively, metronidazole 500 mg twice daily for 7 days for both male and female sexual partners (CDC,

2006b). Partners should avoid intercourse until both are cured (therapy is completed and both are symptom free). The woman and her partner should be cautioned to avoid alcohol while taking metronidazole; the combination has an effect similar to that of alcohol and disulfiram (Antabuse)—abdominal pain, nausea, flushing, or tremors.

Chlamydial Infection

Chlamydial infection, caused by *Chlamydia trachomatis*, is the most common bacterial STI in the United States. It is found most frequently in sexually active adolescents and young adults. Transmission commonly occurs through vaginal sex. The organism is an intracellular bacterium with several different immunotypes. Immunotypes of chlamydia are responsible for lymphogranuloma venereum and trachoma, which is the world's leading cause of preventable blindness.

Chlamydia is a major cause of nongonococcal urethritis (NGU) in men. In women it can cause infections similar to those that occur with gonorrhea. However, asymptomatic infection is common in both men and women. In women, chlamydia can infect the fallopian tubes, cervix, urethra, and Bartholin's glands. Severe sequelae can result from untreated chlamydial infection, including PID, infertility, and ectopic pregnancy. In men, chlamydial infection may result in epididymitis and infertility. In the United States, newborn exposure to chlamydia in the birth canal of the mother is the most common cause of ophthalmia neonatorum (CDC, 2006b). This chlamydial conjunctivitis responds to erythromycin ophthalmic ointment but not to silver nitrate eye prophylaxis. The newborn may also develop chlamydial pneumonia.

Symptoms of chlamydia include a thin or mucopurulent discharge, cervical ectopia, friable cervix (bleeds easily), burning and frequency of urination, and lower abdominal pain. However, up to 70% of women are asymptomatic (Walsh & Irwin, 2002). Of the laboratory tests currently available to diagnose chlamydia, nucleic acid amplification testing (NAAT) is the most sensitive. Other tests used for diagnosis include culture, direct immunofluorescince, EIA, and nucleic acid hybridization tests (CDC, 2006b). Diagnosis is frequently made after treatment of a male partner for NGU or in a symptomatic woman with a negative gonorrhea culture.

The recommended treatment is a single dose of azithromycin 1 g orally or doxycycline 100 mg by mouth twice a day for 7 days. Doxycycline costs less than azithromycin and has been used for a longer period. However, azithromycin administered at the clinic or office visit is an excellent choice for people who do not comply well with treatment or who are erratic about completing a course of medication. Sexual partners should also be treated and the couple should abstain from intercourse for 7 days after taking the single-dose treatment or for the entire 7 days of the doxycycline therapy (CDC, 2006b). Doxycycline is contraindicated during pregnancy, but preliminary data on azithromycin, a category B drug, suggest that it is safe and effective, and many caregivers prescribe it. Currently the CDC (2006) recommends that pregnant women be treated with azithromycin or amoxicillin. For pregnant women, repeat testing is recommended 3 weeks after completion of the prescribed medication as a test of cure. Because so many males and females who have chlamydia are asymptomatic, the CDC and medical specialty organizations such as the American College of Obstetricians and Gynecologists (ACOG) recommend screening as the primary method of decreasing the incidence of chlamydia. Specifically, annual screening is recommended for the following groups (CDC, 2006b; Walsh & Irwin, 2002):

- All sexually active adolescent females and women ages 20 to 25 even if they are asymptomatic.

- Women over age 25 who are at risk for chlamydia (history of STIs, multiple sexual partners, new sexual partner, inconsistent use of barrier contraceptives).

- ACOG also recommends screening for high-risk pregnant women at their first prenatal visit, during the third trimester of pregnancy, or both. Some practitioners routinely screen all pregnant women.

Screening using a nucleic amplification test can be done on endocervical, urethral, or urine specimens. The urine tests are an attractive alternative for women who are not comfortable with pelvic exams or in clinics where access to gynecologic examination facilities is limited or lacking (Walsh & Irwin, 2002).

Gonorrhea

Gonorrhea, an infection caused by the bacterium *Neisseria gonorrhoeae,* is the second most commonly reported STI in the United States with an estimated 600,000 people infected each year (Little, 2006). Most men seek treatment for gonorrhea early because of symptoms but many women with the infection are asymptomatic until complications such as PID occur. Transmission can occur through vaginal, anal, or oral sex.

If a pregnant woman becomes infected after the third month of gestation, the mucous plug in the cervix will prevent the infection from ascending, and it will remain localized in the urethra, cervix, and Bartholin's glands until the membranes rupture. Then it can spread upward. A newborn exposed to a gonococcal-infected birth canal is at risk of developing ophthalmia neonatorum. Eye prophylaxis for all newborns is provided to prevent this complication.

About 80% of women with gonorrhea are asymptomatic (Little, 2006). Thus it is accepted practice to screen for this infection by doing a cervical culture during the initial prenatal examination. For women at high risk, the culture may be repeated during the last month of pregnancy. Cultures of the urethra, throat, and rectum may also be required for diagnosis, depending on the body orifices used for intercourse.

The most common symptoms of gonorrheal infection, when they occur, include a purulent, greenish-yellow vaginal discharge, dysuria, and urinary frequency. Some women also develop inflammation and swelling of the vulva. The cervix may appear swollen and eroded and may secrete a foul-smelling discharge in which gonococci are present. Bilateral lower abdominal or pelvic pain may also occur.

Treatment for nonpregnant women consists of antibiotic therapy with cefixime, ciprofloxacin, ofloxacin, or levofloxacin orally (or ceftriaxone administered intramuscularly) plus doxycycline or azithromycin administered orally if chlamydia has not been ruled out. This combined approach provides dual treatment for gonorrhea and chlamydia because the two infections frequently occur together (CDC, 2006b). Additional treatment may be required if the cultures remain positive 7 to 14 days after completion of treatment. All sexual partners must also be treated, or the woman may become reinfected. Pregnant women should be treated with a recommended cephalosporin, usually ceftriaxone intramuscularly or cefixime orally. This is combined with azithromycin or amoxicillin to address the risk of co-infection with chlamydia (CDC, 2006b).

Women should be informed of the need for reculture to verify cure and the need for abstinence or condom use until cure is confirmed. Both sexual partners should be treated if either has a positive test for gonorrhea. Women should also be informed of signs that the infection is worsening (sharp abdominal pain, fever, or chills) and encouraged to seek further care if any of these develop.

Herpes Genitalis

The herpes simplex virus (HSV) causes herpes infections, which are recurrent, lifelong infections. Two serotypes of HSV cause human infections: HSV-1 and HSV-2. HSV-2 causes most cases of recurrent genital herpes and is spread through vaginal, anal, or oral sex. It can also be spread through skin-to-skin contact with an infected site such as a finger (herpetic whitlow). The clinical symptoms and treatment of both types are the same. At least 50 million people in the United States have been diagnosed with genital HSV-2 infection—**herpes genitalis.** Even so, most people infected with genital herpes have not been diagnosed because they have mild or unrecognized infections but shed the virus intermittently (CDC, 2006b).

The primary episode (first outbreak) of herpes genitalis is characterized by the development of single or multiple blister-like vesicles, which usually occur in the genital area and sometimes affect the vaginal walls, cervix, urethra, and anus. The vesicles may appear within a few hours to 20 days after exposure and rupture spontaneously to form very painful, open, ulcerated lesions. Inflammation and pain secondary to the presence of herpes lesions can cause difficult urination and urinary retention. Enlargement of the inguinal lymph nodes may be present. Flulike symptoms and genital pruritus or tingling also may be noticed. Primary episodes usually last the longest and are the most severe. Lesions heal spontaneously in 2 to 4 weeks.

After the lesions heal, the virus enters a dormant phase, residing in the nerve ganglia of the affected area. Some individuals never have a recurrence, whereas others have regular recurrences. Recurrences are usually less severe than the initial episode and seem to be triggered by emotional stress, menstruation, ovulation, pregnancy, frequent or vigorous intercourse, poor health status or a generally run-down physical condition, tight clothing, or overheating. Diagnosis is made on the basis of the clinical appearance of the lesions, culture of the lesions, polymerase chain reaction (PCR) identification, and glycoprotein G-based type-specific assays (Herpe Select™, Biokit HSV-2, & Sure Vue HSV-2) (CDC, 2006b).

No known cure for herpes exists; however, medications are available to provide relief from pain and prevent complications from secondary infection. The recommended treatment of the first clinical episode of genital herpes is oral acyclovir, valacyclovir, or famciclovir. These same medications, in somewhat different dosages, are also recommended for recurrent herpes infection and for daily suppressive therapy for people who have frequent recurrences. Therapy should be started during the prodromal period (time before the onset of lesions) for the greatest benefit. Recent research suggests that a 1-day, high-dose (2 g) treatment with famciclovir initiated within 6 hours of an outbreak is as effective as longer therapy in accelerating healing in people with a healthy immune system. This approach, which is self-initiated, is convenient and enables individuals to control their own infection (Whitley, 2005).

The safety of acyclovir, valacyclovir, and famciclovir in pregnancy has not been established. However, because there is more documented information on acyclovir during pregnancy, it may be administered orally to pregnant women with first episode genital herpes or severe recurrent herpes. Its use in the third trimester may reduce the frequency of cesarean births by decreasing the incidence of recurrences at term (CDC, 2006b). Self-care suggestions include cleansing with povidone-iodine (Betadine) solution to prevent secondary infection and with Burow's solution to relieve discomfort. Use of vitamin C or lysine is frequently suggested to prevent recurrence, although studies have not documented the effectiveness of these supplements. Sometimes 2% lidocaine (Xylocaine) is used to decrease intense pain at the site of the lesions. Keeping the genital area clean and dry, wearing loose clothing, taking sitz baths, and wearing cotton underwear or none at all will promote healing. Primary or recurrent lesions will heal without treatment.

If herpes is present in the genital tract of a woman during childbirth, it can have a devastating, even fatal, effect on the newborn. See Chapter 20 ∞ for more detail.

Syphilis

Syphilis is a chronic infection caused by the spirochete *Treponema pallidum*. Syphilis is commonly acquired through vaginal, oral, or anal sex. Less commonly, it can result from nonsexual exposure to exudates from an infected individual. Congenital transmission through transplacental inoculation may also occur. The incubation period varies from 10 to 90 days, and even though no symptoms or lesions are noted during this time, the woman's blood contains spirochetes and is infectious.

Syphilis is divided into early and late stages. During the early stage (primary), a chancre (painless ulcer) appears at the site where the *T pallidum* organism entered the body. Symptoms include slight fever, loss of weight, and malaise. The chancre persists for about 4 weeks and then disappears. In 6 weeks to 6 months, secondary symptoms appear. Skin eruptions called condylomata lata, which resemble wartlike plaques and are highly infectious, may appear on the vulva. Other secondary symptoms are acute arthritis, enlargement of the liver and spleen, nontender enlarged lymph nodes, iritis, and a chronic sore throat with hoarseness. Transplacentally transmitted syphilis is as high as 95% in the primary and secondary stages, but decreases to 10% in the late latent phase. Congenital syphilis may cause intrauterine growth restriction, preterm birth, and stillbirth.

As a result of the disease's impact on the fetus in utero, serologic testing of every pregnant woman is recommended; some state laws require it. Testing is done at the initial prenatal screening and repeated in the third trimester. Blood studies may be negative if blood is drawn too early in the pregnancy.

During the early primary stage, the diagnosis is made by dark-field microscopic examination of the chancre for spirochetes. Blood tests such as VDRL (Venereal Disease Research Laboratories), RPR (Rapid Plasma Reagin), or the more specific FTA-ABS (fluorescent treponemal antibody absorption test) are commonly done.

For pregnant and nonpregnant women with syphilis of less than a year's duration (early latent syphilis), the CDC (2006b) recommends 2.4 million units of benzathine penicillin G intramuscularly in a single dose. If syphilis is of long duration (more than 1 year) or of unknown duration, 2.4 million units of benzathine penicillin G is given intramuscularly once a week for 3 weeks. If a woman is allergic to penicillin, and nonpregnant, doxycycline or tetracycline can be given. Clients who are allergic to penicillin whose cooperation with treatment and follow-up is questionable should be desensitized to penicillin and then treated with it. Similarly, the pregnant woman with syphilis who is allergic to penicillin should be desensitized and then treated (CDC, 2006b). Maternal serologic testing may remain positive for 8 months, and the newborn may have a positive test for 3 months.

Human Papilloma Virus/Condylomata Acuminata

Condylomata acuminata, also called genital or venereal warts, is a common STI caused by the human papilloma virus (HPV). Transmission can occur through vaginal, oral, or anal sex.

Annually 1 million new cases of condylomata acuminata are diagnosed. Of these, two thirds are in women. Estimates suggest a prevalence rate of 15% in the US population (Scheinfeld & Lehman, 2006). Because of the increased evidence of a link between HPV and cervical and anorectal cancers, the condition is receiving increasing attention. Over 120 HPV subtypes have been identified; of these, about 30 types can infect the genital tract. Most HPV infections are unrecognized, asymptomatic, or subclinical. HPV types 6 and 11 most commonly cause visible genital warts but they are rarely associated with anogenital cancers. Eleven specific types of HPV are considered intermediate risk, whereas HPV types 16 and 18 are strongly associated with high-grade cervical dysplasia and anogenital cancer (Scheinfeld & Lehman, 2006). Clients with visible genital warts can be infected concurrently with different HPV types.

Often a woman seeks medical care after noticing single or multiple soft, grayish pink, cauliflower-like lesions in her genital area (Figure 6–4 ◆). These warts are often asymptomatic; however, depending on their location and size, they may cause itching (pruritus), be friable (bleed easily), or be painful. The moist, warm environment of the genital area is conducive to the growth of the warts, which may be present on the vulva, perineum, vagina, cervix, urethra, and anus. The incubation period following exposure is 3 weeks to 3 years, with the average being about 3 months.

Because condylomata sometimes resemble other lesions and may become cancerous, all atypical, pigmented, and persistent warts should be biopsied and treatment instituted promptly. Diagnosis is usually made by visual appearance. However, vaginal and cervical warts are more common than warts of the external genitalia. Most of these are flat lesions visible only by colposcopy. Subclinical diagnosis can be made if characteristic changes are present on a Pap smear.

The CDC (2006b) does not specify a treatment of choice for genital warts but recommends that treatment be determined based on client preference, available resources, and experience of the healthcare provider. No single treatment is best for all warts or for all clients. Client-applied therapies include podofilox solution or gel or imiquimod cream. For these methods to be effective, the client must be able to reach and identify the warts being treated. Provider-administered therapies include cryotherapy with liquid nitrogen or cryoprobe; topical podophyllin; trichloroacetic acid (TCA); bichloroacetic acid (BCA); and surgical removal by tangential scissors excision, shave excision, curettage, or electrosurgery. Alternative therapies include intralesional interferon or laser surgery (CDC, 2006b). Imiquimod, podophyllin, and podofilox are not used during pregnancy because they are thought to be teratogenic and in large doses have been associated with fetal death.

Women with HPV infections should have frequent Pap smears to monitor cervical cellular changes. Sex partners are probably infected and do not require treatment unless large exophytic lesions are present. Moreover, no research to date indicates that reinfection plays a role in recurrence (CDC, 2006b). The use of condoms may reduce the risk of transmitting the virus to an uninfected partner. In 2006 the U.S. Food and Drug Administration approved the first vaccine designed to protect against four HPV types, which, when considered together, are responsible for 90% of genital warts and 70% of cervical cancers. The vaccine—Gardasil®—given in three doses, is recommended for 11- and 12-year-old girls (typically before they are sexually active) although it can be given to girls as young as 9. At present it is also recommended for females 13 to 26 who have not been vaccinated (CDC, 2006a).

I've finally come to terms with the fact that I carry HPV. I know I will always run the risk of recurrence, but it's just a virus. It doesn't define me as a person.

Pediculosis Pubis (Pubic or Crab Lice)

Pediculosis pubis is caused by *Phthirus,* a grayish, parasitic "crab" louse that lays eggs that attach to the hair shaft. Transmission is primarily by sexual contact, although shared towels and bed linens are also possible sources.

Symptoms include itching, usually in the pubic area. It is treated by applying 1% permethrin creme rinse to the affected area and washing it off after 10 minutes. Some caregivers recommend combing the pubic hair with a fine-toothed comb before rinsing off the permethrin. Lindane shampoo applied for 4 minutes and then washed off well can also be used. However, lindane is not recommended for pregnant or lactating women. Over-the-counter medications can also be used. Retreatment may be necessary. Both partners must be treated and tested for

Figure 6–4 ◆ Condylomata acuminata on the vulva.
SOURCE: Copyright Kenneth Greer/Visuals Unlimited.

MediaLink   Case Study: Pediculosis Pubis

COMPLEMENTARY AND ALTERNATIVE THERAPIES

HEPATITIS C TREATMENT ALTERNATIVES

Hepatitis C virus (HCV) infection has become the most common bloodborne infection in the United States with about 35,000 new cases diagnosed annually. People at high risk for the infection include IV drug users, people who received a blood transfusion or organ transplant before 1992, healthcare workers who receive a needle stick, and people with multiple sexual partners. Newly infected individuals have acute hepatitis C. For a small percentage (15% to 40%), the infection lasts a short time then goes away permanently. The majority, however, develop chronic hepatitis C although they may not know it because the majority of people who are infected show no symptoms for up to 20 to 30 years. Most people with HCV develop chronic liver disease such as cirrhosis, liver cancer, and liver failure.

Some people with chronic HCV choose to try regular injections with interferon combined with an antiviral drug called ribavirin, which is effective in eliminating the virus in about 55% of infected individuals. However, interferon has many severe side effects, including anemia; sudden hearing loss; headaches; liver, heart, kidney, or eye problems; and psychologic disorders including depression.

To date, no complementary therapies have been proven safe or effective to cure HCV or even ease the symptoms. The following substances have received the most attention:

- Milk thistle (*Silybum marianum*), a plant of the aster family, may protect the liver from injury by toxins such as viruses, radiation, alcohol, and poisonous mushrooms and limit the damage these toxins can cause. Milk thistle may also improve the way in which the liver functions in people with cirrhosis. Systematic reviews of the literature have found that it is generally safe, but conclusions about its effectiveness cannot be drawn as yet. It is available as a dietary supplement in capsule form.
- Licorice root (*Glycyrrhiza glabra*), taken as a tea, shows antiviral properties and may help manage some of the effects of HCV on the liver. Randomized studies suggest that it may help prevent liver cancer in people with chronic HCV and may also reduce some of the long-term complications of HCV in those who do not respond to interferon. If taken for a prolonged period, however, licorice root has been associated with high blood pressure, sodium and fluid retention, low potassium levels, and so forth.
- Other herbals that have been used for HCV include ginseng and schisandra. Both may have beneficial effects on the liver but have not been studied in humans with HCV.

SOURCE: National Center for Complementary and Alternative Medicine. (2004). *Research Report: Hepatitis C and Complementary and Alternative Medicine: 2003 Update.* Retrieved June 4, 2006, from http://nccam.nih.gov.

---

other STIs. Bed linens, towels, and clothing should be machine washed and dried in a hot dryer, dry-cleaned, or removed from body contact for at least 72 hours.

Scabies

Sarcoptes scabiei is a parasitic itch mite. The female mite burrows under the skin to deposit her eggs. Transmission by intimate sexual contact is common in adults but scabies in children is not generally sexually acquired (CDC, 2006b).

Symptoms include itching that worsens at night or when the individual is warm. Noticeable erythematous, papular lesions or furrows may be present. The recommended treatment for scabies is permethrin cream 5% applied to all body areas from the neck down and washed off after 8 to 14 hours. Alternate therapy includes lindane 1% lotion or cream (Kwell) applied in a thin layer to all areas of the body from the neck down and then washed off after 8 hours. Lindane is not recommended

for pregnant or lactating women, for people with extensive dermatitis, or for children under age 2 years. Although lindane is less expensive than permethrin, it has more associated risk, and, in some parts of the world, including portions of the United States, lindane resistance has been reported (CDC, 2006b). Permethrin 5% is used in pregnant women. Clothing and bed linens should be washed and dried in a hot dryer or dry-cleaned.

Viral Hepatitis

Hepatitis is an inflammatory process of the liver caused by infection by one of the five distinct viruses: A, B, C, D, and E. Currently, immunizations are only available for hepatitis A and B. Table 6–2 compares the five forms of viral hepatitis.

Hepatitis A is characterized by symptoms of jaundice, anorexia, nausea, vomiting, malaise, and fever. It is self-limiting and is not a chronic condition. A vaccine is available to prevent hepatitis A.

Table 6–2   TYPES OF VIRAL HEPATITIS

Form	Primary Route of Transmission	Incubation Period	Chronic Infection	Immunization Available?
Hepatitis A	Fecal-oral, contaminated food/water	15–50 days	No	Yes
Hepatitis B	Blood/body fluids	45–160 days	Yes	Yes
Hepatitis C	Blood/blood products	14–180 days	Yes	No
Hepatitis D	Blood/body fluids	45–160 days	Yes	No
Hepatitis E	Fecal-oral	15–60 days	No	No

Hepatitis B, C, and D have symptoms similar to those of hepatitis A and can also include arthralgias, arthritis, and skin eruptions or rash. Unlike hepatitis A infection, those of B, C, and D infections are chronic. See Complementary and Alternative Therapies: Hepatitis C Treatment Alternatives.

Hepatitis E occurs primarily in South Central Asia and the Middle East, and its symptoms are like those of hepatitis A. It is also a self-limiting disease and not a chronic condition.

Acquired Immunodeficiency Syndrome (AIDS)

Acquired immunodeficiency syndrome (AIDS) is a fatal disorder caused by HIV, which may be transmitted sexually. A medical-surgical text will more fully describe this condition. However, because the diagnosis of HIV/AIDS or the presence of the HIV antibody has implications for a fetus if the woman is pregnant, HIV/AIDS is discussed in greater detail in Chapter 19. ∞

NURSING CARE MANAGEMENT
Nursing Assessment and Diagnosis

The nurse working with women must become adept at taking a thorough history and identifying women at risk for STIs. Risk factors include multiple sexual partners; a partner's involvement with other partners; high-risk sexual behaviors, such as intercourse without barrier contraception or anal intercourse; partners with high-risk behaviors; and young age at onset of sexual activity. The nurse should be alert for signs and symptoms of STI and be familiar with diagnostic procedures if it is suspected.

Although each STI has certain distinctive characteristics, the following complaints suggest the possibility of infection and warrant further investigation:

- Presence of a "sore" or lesion on the vulva
- Increased vaginal discharge or malodorous vaginal discharge
- Burning with urination
- Dyspareunia
- Bleeding after intercourse
- Pelvic pain

In many instances the woman is asymptomatic but may report symptoms in her partner, especially painful urination or urethral discharge. It is often helpful to ask the woman whether her partner is experiencing any symptoms.

Nursing diagnoses that may apply to a woman with an STI include the following:

- *Interrupted Family Processes* related to the effects of a diagnosis of sexually transmitted infection on the couple's relationship
- *Health-Seeking Behaviors:* Information on preventing STIs related to an expressed desire to avoid infection

Nursing Plan and Implementation

In a supportive, nonjudgmental way, the nurse provides the woman who has an STI with information about the infection, methods of transmission, implications for pregnancy or future fertility, and importance of thorough treatment. If treatment of her partner is indicated, the woman must understand that it is necessary to prevent a cycle of reinfection. She should also understand the need to abstain from sexual activity, if necessary, during treatment.

Some STIs, such as trichomoniasis or chlamydia, may cause a woman concern but, once diagnosed, are rather simply treated. Other STIs may also be fairly simple to treat medically but may carry a stigma and be emotionally devastating for the woman. Thus the nurse should stress prevention with all women and encourage them to require partners, especially new partners, to use a condom.

The sensitive nurse can be especially helpful in encouraging the woman to explore her feelings about the diagnosis. She may experience anger or feel "betrayed" by a partner; she may feel guilt or see her diagnosis as a form of "punishment"; or she may feel concern about the long-term implications for future childbearing or ongoing intimate relationships. She may experience a myriad of emotions that she never expected. Opportunities to discuss her feelings in a nonjudgmental environment can be especially helpful. The nurse can offer suggestions about support groups, if indicated, and assist the woman in planning for her future with regard to sexual activity.

More subtly, the nurse's attitude of acceptance and matter-of-factness conveys to the woman that she is still an acceptable person who happens to have an infection. Table 6–3 provides a summary of basic information the nurse should share with women who have an STI. STIs that can have an impact on pregnancy or the fetus/newborn are discussed in Chapter 20. ∞

Evaluation

Expected outcomes of nursing care include the following:

- The infection is identified and cured, if possible. If not, supportive therapy is provided.
- The woman and her partner can describe the infection, its method of transmission, its implications, and the therapy.
- The woman copes successfully with the impact of the diagnosis on her self-concept.

CARE OF THE WOMAN WITH AN UPPER GENITAL TRACT INFECTION (PELVIC INFLAMMATORY DISEASE)

Pelvic inflammatory disease (PID) occurs in approximately 1% of women between ages 15 and 39, although sexually active young women between 15 and 24 have the highest infection rate. In the United States, an estimated 1 million cases of PID are diagnosed annually, and more than 100,000 women become

Table 6–3   PREVENTING STIs AND THEIR CONSEQUENCES

The risk of contracting an STI increases with the number of sexual partners. Because of the extended time between infection with HIV and evidence of infection, intercourse with an individual exposes a female or male to all the other sexual partners of that individual for the past 5 or more years. Because of this risk, it is important to take the following actions:

- Plan ahead and develop strategies to refuse sex (especially important for adolescents who may be less confident about saying "no" to casual sexual encounters), because abstinence is the best method of preventing STIs.
- Limit the number of sexual contacts and practice mutual monogamy.
- The condom is the best contraceptive method currently available (other than abstinence) for protection from STIs. Use one for every act of vaginal and anal intercourse. Other contraceptives such as the diaphragm, cervical cap, and spermicides also offer some protection against STIs.
- Plan strategies for negotiating condom use with a partner.
- Reduce high-risk behaviors. Use of recreational drugs and alcohol can increase sexual risk taking.
- Refrain from oral sex if your partner has active sores in mouth, vagina, or anus or on penis.
- Seek care as soon as you notice symptoms and make sure your partner gets treatment if indicated. Absence of symptoms or disappearance of symptoms does not mean that treatment is unnecessary if you suspect an STI. Take all prescribed medications completely.
- The presence of a genital infection may lead to an abnormal Pap smear. Women with certain infections should have more frequent Pap tests according to a schedule recommended by their caregiver. Ask your healthcare provider if you need more frequent Paps.

infertile as a result of it (CDC, 2004). The disease is more common in women who have had multiple sexual partners, a history of PID, early onset of sexual activity, or recent insertion of an intrauterine device (IUD) and in women who douche regularly (Mayo Clinic, 2005). It usually produces a tubal infection (salpingitis) that may or may not be accompanied by a pelvic abscess. However, perhaps the greatest problem of PID is postinfection tubal damage, which is closely associated with infertility.

PID is defined as a clinical syndrome of inflammatory disorders of the upper female genital tract that includes any combination of endometritis, salpingitis, tubo-ovarian abscess, pelvic abscess, and pelvic peritonitis (CDC, 2006b). The organisms most frequently identified with PID include *C trachomatis* and *N gonorrhoeae* with a co-infection rate (both organisms are present) of 60%. Bacterial vaginosis may facilitate the ascending spread of pathogens. Often PID is the result of polymicrobial infection, involving other aerobic and anaerobic organisms that are often part of the normal vaginal flora (Scott & Hasik, 2001).

Symptoms of PID include bilateral sharp, cramping pain in the lower quadrants, fever greater than 101F, chills, mucopurulent cervical or vaginal discharge, irregular bleeding, cervical motion tenderness during intercourse, malaise, nausea, and vomiting. However, it is also possible to be asymptomatic and have normal laboratory values.

Diagnosis consists of a clinical examination to define symptoms. Laboratory tests include vaginal, cervical, and possibly rectal cultures for *N. gonorrhoeae* and *C. trachomatis* as well as blood tests including a complete blood count (CBC) with differential, and RPR or VDRL to test for syphilis. A woman with PID often has an elevated C-reactive protein and

elevated sedimentation rate. Microscopic examination of the vaginal secretions may reveal white blood cells. Physical examination usually reveals direct abdominal tenderness with palpation, and on bimanual examination, adnexal tenderness, and cervical and uterine tenderness with movement (Chandelier sign). A palpable mass is evaluated with ultrasonography. In confounding cases, laparoscopy may be used to confirm the diagnosis and to enable the examiner to obtain cultures from the fimbriated ends of the fallopian tubes.

Currently, there is no evidence comparing parenteral versus oral treatment, and outpatient treatment is an option. The decision to hospitalize a woman is based on clinical judgment. The woman should be hospitalized if the diagnosis is uncertain, ectopic pregnancy or appendicitis is suspected, the woman is severely ill (nausea, vomiting, high fever, dehydration), there has been little response to oral therapy after 48 to 72 hours, the client is an adolescent, or the woman is unable to return for follow-up care. Treatment includes intravenous (IV) fluids, pain medication, and administration of IV antibiotics. Intravenous cefotetan or cefoxitin, plus doxycycline, is one treatment regimen. Another is clindamycin plus gentamicin (CDC, 2006b). Ambulatory or outpatient treatment includes levofloxacin or ofloxacin orally with or without oral metronidazole both for 14 days. This combination is highly effective in treating both gonorrhea and chlamydia, as well as BV. An alternative regimen would include intramuscular injection of ceftriaxone or cefoxitin, plus doxycycline orally, plus metronidazole (CDC, 2006b). Other supportive measures that may be helpful include increased oral fluids (up to 2 liters per day), continued bed rest or pelvic rest, acetaminophen for fever, and naproxen sodium for relief of pain. Follow-up visits are important within 48 to 72 hours, sooner if symptoms worsen. The sexual partner should also be treated. If the woman has an IUD, it is generally removed 24 to 48 hours after antibiotic therapy is started.

NURSING CARE MANAGEMENT
Nursing Assessment and Diagnosis

The nurse is alert to factors in a woman's history that put her at risk for PID. Even though fewer types of IUDs are available, many women still have them, and the nurse should question the woman about possible symptoms, such as aching pain in the lower abdomen, foul-smelling discharge, malaise, and the like. The woman who is acutely ill has obvious symptoms, but a low-grade infection is more difficult to detect.

Nursing diagnoses that may apply to a woman with PID include the following:

- *Acute Pain* related to peritoneal irritation
- *Deficient Knowledge* related to a lack of information about the possible effects of PID on fertility

Nursing Plan and Implementation

The nurse plays a vital role in helping to prevent or detect PID. Accordingly, the nurse spends time discussing risk factors related to this infection. The woman who uses an IUD for contraception and has multiple sexual partners needs to understand clearly the risk she faces.

The nurse should strongly recommend that the IUD be removed and another method of contraception used. The nurse discusses signs and symptoms of PID with women at high risk and stresses the importance of early detection.

The woman who develops PID needs to understand the importance of completing her antibiotic treatment and of returning for follow-up evaluation. She should also understand that one outcome of the infection may be decreased fertility.

Evaluation

Expected outcomes of nursing care include the following:

- The woman describes her condition, her therapy, and the possible long-term implications of PID on her fertility.
- The woman completes her course of therapy and the PID is cured.

CARE OF THE WOMAN WITH A URINARY TRACT INFECTION

Urinary tract infection (UTI) is defined as significant bacteriuria in the presence of symptoms. Approximately 50% to 70% of women will experience a UTI in their lifetime and 20% to 30% will have a recurrent UTI (Dwyer & O'Reilly, 2002). A UTI may be life threatening or a mere inconvenience. Bacteria usually enter the sterile environment of the urinary tract by way of the urethra. The organisms are capable of migrating against the downward flow of urine. The shortness of the female urethra facilitates the passage of bacteria into the bladder. Other conditions that are associated with bacterial entry are relative incompetence of the urinary sphincter, frequent enuresis (bed-wetting) before adolescence, pregnancy, and urinary catheterization. Wiping from back to front after urination may transfer bacteria from the anorectal area to the urethra.

Voluntarily suppressing the desire to urinate is also a predisposing factor. Retention overdistends the bladder and can lead to an infection. There also seems to be a relationship between recurring UTI and sexual intercourse. General poor health or lowered resistance to infection can increase a woman's susceptibility to UTI. Factors that may inhibit bacterial growth include a low pH (5.5 or less) resulting in more acidic urine, high urea concentration, and the presence of organic acids from food such as fruits and proteins.

Asymptomatic bacteriuria (ASB) refers to bacteria in the urine actively multiplying without accompanying clinical symptoms. It occurs in about 2% to 9% of UTIs (Dwyer & O'Reilly, 2002). This becomes especially significant if the woman is pregnant because it is found in up to 11% of pregnancies, and as many as 40% of pregnant women with untreated ASB will develop pyelonephritis (Varney, Kriebs, & Gegor, 2004). ASB is almost always caused by one organism. If more than one type of bacteria are cultured, the possibility of urine-culture contamination must be considered. The most common cause of ASB is *Escherichia coli*. Other commonly found causative organisms include *Klebsiella* and *Proteus*, and less commonly, *Pseudomonas* and *Staphylococcus* species.

A woman who has had a UTI is susceptible to recurrent infection. Although the role of ASB in pregnancy complication remains controversial, the majority of evidence supports the view that bacteriuria does not, as an isolated factor, lead to low birth weight or prematurity. However, ASB is associated with low birth weight, preterm birth, hypertension, preeclampsia, maternal anemia, and symptomatic UTI (Thorsen & Poole, 2002). UTIs are more frequently encountered in pregnant women in part because of dramatic physiologic changes. Muscle tone and activity of the ureters decrease, resulting in reduced passage of urine through the urinary system. The bladder experiences decreased tone, increased capacity, and incomplete emptying. Urinary pH is elevated along with glycogen levels. All of these changes contribute to the increased risk for urinary tract disorders. The US Preventive Services Task Force (2004) strongly recommends that all pregnant women be screened for ASB by urine culture at 12 to 16 weeks' gestation. Women at increased risk for bacteriuria, such as women with a history of UTIs, sickle cell trait, diabetes, renal calculi, chronic renal disease, or significant hypertension, should be screened every 6 to 12 weeks via clean-catch urine sample for ASB. Treatment in pregnant women includes amoxicillin, nitrofurantoin, cephalexin, trimethoprim-sulfamethoxazole, and sulfisoxazole.

Lower Urinary Tract Infection (Cystitis and Urethritis)

Because UTIs ascend, it is important to recognize and diagnose a lower UTI early to avoid the sequelae associated with upper UTI. One common lower UTI is cystitis, or infection of the urinary bladder. Several factors place a woman at increased risk for cystitis, including sexual intercourse, the use of a diaphragm and a spermicide, delayed postcoital micturition, pregnancy, and a history of a recent UTI.

E. coli is present in 80% of women with UTIs. *Staphylococcus saprophyticus, Klebsiella, Proteus, Enterobacter,* and *Pseudomonas* are also causative pathogens. Infections without bacteriuria may indicate urethritis and are usually caused by *C. trachomatis, N. gonorrhoeae,* and herpes simplex.

When cystitis develops, the classic initial symptoms are often acute and include dysuria, specifically at the end of urination, as well as urgency and frequency. Suprapubic or low back pain may also occur. Cystitis is usually accompanied by a low-grade fever (38.3C, or 101F, or lower), and hematuria is occasionally seen. Urine specimens often contain an abnormal number of leukocytes and bacteria and may contain protein. Urethritis symptoms usually have a gradual onset and are associated with a cervicitis or vulvovaginal herpetic lesion.

The diagnosis can be made with a urine culture. Bacteriuria dipstick screening tests are quick office screening tests; however, they have high false-positive and false-negative rates. Before treatment the diagnosis should be confirmed by clinical evaluation and urine culture and sensitivity results. The treatment depends on the causative pathogen. Oral trimethoprim-sulfamethoxazole, fluoroquinolones, and fomycin tromethamine are frequently used in single-dose, 3-day, and 7-day regimens.

Upper Urinary Tract Infection (Pyelonephritis)

Pyelonephritis (inflammatory disease of the kidneys) is less common but more serious than cystitis and is often preceded by lower UTI. It is more common during the latter part of pregnancy or early postpartum and poses a serious threat to maternal and fetal well-being. Women with pyelonephritis during pregnancy are at significantly increased risk of preterm labor, preterm birth, development of adult respiratory distress syndrome and septicemia, and in some instances intrauterine growth restriction (Samuels & Colombo, 2002). Acute pyelonephritis has a sudden onset with chills, high temperature of 39.6C to 40.6C (103F to 105F), and costovertebral angle tenderness or flank pain, which may be unilateral or bilateral. The right side is almost always involved if the woman is pregnant because the large bulk of intestines to the left pushes the uterus to the right, putting pressure on the right ureter and kidney. Nausea, vomiting, and general malaise may ensue. With accompanying cystitis, the woman may experience frequency, urgency, and burning with urination.

Edema of the renal parenchyma or ureteritis with blockage and swelling of the ureter may lead to temporary suppression of urinary output. This is accompanied by severe colicky (spastic, intense) pain, vomiting, dehydration, and ileus of the large bowel. The woman with acute pyelonephritis will generally have increased diastolic blood pressure, positive fluorescent antibody titer (FA-test), low creatinine clearance, significant bacteremia in urine culture, pyuria, and presence of white blood cell casts.

Often the woman is hospitalized and started on IV antibiotics. Therapy also includes IV hydration, urinary analgesics such as Pyridium, pain management, and medication to manage fever. In the case of obstructive pyelonephritis, a blood culture is necessary. The woman is kept on bed rest. If signs of urinary obstruction occur or continue, the ureter may be catheterized to establish adequate drainage.

Initial IV treatment options include ampicillin plus gentamicin, ceftriaxone, trimethoprim-sulfamethoxazole, aztreonam, and cefazolin. With appropriate drug therapy, the woman's temperature should return to normal. The pain subsides, and the urine shows no bacteria within 2 to 3 days. Follow-up urinary cultures are needed to determine that the infection has been eliminated completely.

NURSING CARE MANAGEMENT
Nursing Assessment and Diagnosis

During the woman's visit, the nurse obtains a medical history, including a sexual history, to determine whether she is at risk for UTI. Additionally, the nurse notes any complaints from the woman of painful urination or other urinary difficulties, and systemic complaints such as fever, chills, nausea, vomiting, or back pain. If the nurse is concerned, a clean-catch urine sample is obtained to evaluate for the presence of bacteriuria.

Nursing diagnoses that may apply to the woman with a UTI include the following:

- *Acute Pain* related to dysuria, systemic discomforts, or back pain secondary to lower or upper urinary tract infection
- *Health-Seeking Behaviors:* Information about preventing UTIs related to an expressed desire to avoid recurrence
- *Fear* related to the possible long-term effects of the disease

Nursing Plan and Implementation

Most bacteria enter through the urethra after having spread from the anal area. Therefore, the nurse should make sure the woman is aware of good hygiene practices and provide information on other ways to avoid UTI (Figure 6–5 ◆ and Table 6–4.) Additionally, the nurse provides the woman with information to help

Figure 6–5 ◆ The nurse counsels the woman about measures for preventing urinary tract infection.

Table 6–4   MEASURES FOR PREVENTING CYSTITIS
If you use a diaphragm for contraception, try changing methods or using another size diaphragm.
Avoid bladder irritants, such as alcohol, caffeine products, and carbonated beverages.
Increase fluid intake, especially water, to a minimum of six to eight glasses per day.
Make regular urination a habit, avoid long waits.
Practice good genital hygiene, including wiping from front to back after urination and bowel movements.
Be aware that vigorous or frequent sexual activity may contribute to urinary tract infection.
Urinate before and after intercourse to empty the bladder and cleanse the urethra.
Complete medication regimens even if symptoms decrease.
Do not use medication left over from previous infections.
Drink cranberry juice to acidify the urine. This has been found to relieve symptoms in some cases.

her recognize the signs and symptoms of a UTI to facilitate early identification and treatment of future infections. The nurse should also reinforce instructions and answer any additional questions the woman may have regarding the prescribed antibiotic, the type and amount of liquid to ingest, and the reasons for these treatments. UTIs usually respond quickly to treatment, but follow-up clinical evaluation and urine cultures are important.

Evaluation

Expected outcomes of nursing care include the following:

- The woman implements self-care measures to help prevent recurrent UTI as part of her personal routine.
- The woman completes her prescribed course of antibiotic therapy.

- The woman can identify signs of recurrent UTI, or signs and symptoms of worsening urinary symptoms that would require follow-up care.
- The woman's infection is cured.

CLINICAL TIP

To avoid contamination of a clean-catch urine in a woman with a suspected UTI, you might try having her place a cotton ball or gauze square just inside her vagina. After she obtains the urine specimen and closes the container, she then removes the cotton or gauze and discards it in the trash receptacle.

CHAPTER REVIEW

FOCUS YOUR STUDY

- Vulvovaginal candidiasis (moniliasis), a vaginal infection most often caused by *Candida albicans,* is most common in women who use oral contraceptives, are taking antibiotics, are currently pregnant, or have diabetes mellitus. It is generally treated with intravaginal miconazole or clotrimazole suppositories or fluconazole orally.

- Bacterial vaginosis (*Gardnerella vaginalis* vaginitis), a common vaginal infection, is diagnosed by its characteristic fishy odor and by the presence of "clue" cells on a vaginal smear. It is treated with metronidazole.

- Chlamydial infection is difficult to detect in a woman but may result in PID and infertility. It is treated with antibiotic therapy.

- Gonorrhea, a common sexually transmitted infection, may be asymptomatic in women initially but may cause PID if not diagnosed early. The treatment of choice is ceftriaxone and doxycycline or azithromycin.

- Herpes genitalis, caused by the herpes simplex virus, is a recurrent infection with no known cure. Acyclovir (Zovirax) may reduce the symptoms.

- Syphilis, caused by *Treponema pallidum,* is a sexually transmitted infection that is treatable if diagnosed. The

characteristic lesion is the chancre. Syphilis can also be transmitted in utero to the fetus of an infected woman. The treatment of choice is penicillin.

- Condylomata acuminata (venereal warts) are transmitted by the human papilloma virus (HPV). Treatment is indicated, because research has identified seven strains of HPV linked with high-grade abnormal cervical changes. The treatment chosen depends on the size and location of the warts.

- Pelvic inflammatory disease may be life threatening and may lead to infertility. The organisms that cause PID most frequently include *C trachomatis* and *N gonorrhoeae.*

- Women with an abnormal finding on a pelvic examination will need careful explanation of the finding and techniques of diagnosis and emotional support during the diagnostic period.

- The classic symptoms of a lower UTI are dysuria, urgency, frequency, and sometimes hematuria. Oral sulfonamides are the treatment of choice except in middle to late pregnancy.

- An upper UTI is a serious infection that can permanently damage the kidneys if untreated. Generally the woman is acutely ill and may require supportive therapy as well as antibiotics.

EXPLORE MediaLink

http//www.prenhall.com/davidson

NCLEX review questions, case studies, and other interactive resources for this chapter can be found on the Web Site at http://www.prenhall.com/davidson. Click on "Chapter 6" to select the activities for this chapter.

For tutorials including animations and videos, more NCLEX review questions and an audio glossary, access the accompanying Prentice Hall Nursing MediaLink DVD-ROM in this book.

PRENTICE HALL NURSING MEDIALINK DVD-ROM
Audio Glossary
NCLEX Review

COMPANION WEBSITE
Additional NCLEX Review
Case Study: *Pediculosis Pubis*
Care Plan Activity: *Gynecologic Infection*
Applications: *Sexually Transmitted Infections; Preventing Urinary Tract Infections*
Critical Thinking

CRITICAL THINKING IN ACTION

GONORRHEA IN WOMEN

View the Critical Thinking in Action video in Chapter 6 of the DVD-ROM. Then answer the questions that follow.

Cherelle Latkowski, age 18, was just diagnosed with gonorrhea by the nurse practitioner at the clinic where you work. Although she had been asymptomatic, she had come in for evaluation after her boyfriend was diagnosed with gonorrhea and

started on antibiotics. Cherelle is treated with ceftriaxone administered intramuscularly plus doxycycline by mouth.

1. Cherelle asks you why she received two medications. How would you reply?
2. Cherelle asks you whether she is now immune to gonorrhea. Is she?
3. Cherelle asks whether she can now have sex with her boyfriend. Can she do so?

REFERENCES

Centers for Disease Control and Prevention (CDC). (2004). *Fact sheet: Pelvic inflammatory disease*. Retrieved February 20, 2006, from http://www.cdc.gov/std/PID/STDFact-PID.htm

Centers for Disease Control and Prevention (CDC). (2005). *Expedited partner therapy (EPT)*. [Letter to Health Care Providers, May 11, 2005]. Atlanta: Author.

Centers for Disease Control and Prevention (CDC). (2006a). HPV vaccine questions and answers. Retrieved October 1, 2006 from http://www.cdc.gov.

Centers for Disease Control and Prevention (CDC). (2006b). Sexually transmitted diseases treatment guidelines 2006. *Morbidity and Mortality Weekly Report, 55*(RR-11), 1–94.

Dwyer, P., & O'Reilly, J. (2002). Recurrent urinary tract infection in the female. *Current Opinion in Obstetrics and Gynecology, 14*(5), 537–543.

Little, J. W. (2006). Gonorrhea: Update. *Oral Surgery, Oral Medicine, Oral Pathology, Oral Radiology, and Endodontology, 101*(2), 137–143.

Mayo Clinic. (2005). *Pelvic inflammatory disease*. Retrieved February 20, 2006, from http://www.mayoclinic.com/health/pelvic-inflammatory-disease/DS00402/DSECTION-4

Mead, P. B. (Moderator). (2001). Symposium: What's new in vaginitis diagnosis and treatment? *Contemporary OB/GYN, 46*(11), 14–42.

Nansel, T. R., Riggs, M. A., Yu, K. F., Andrews, W. W., Schwebke, J. R., & Klebanoff, M. A. (2006). The association of psychosocial stress and bacterial vaginosis in a longitudinal cohort. *American Journal of Obstetrics & Gynecology, 194*(2), 381–386.

Owen, M., & Clenney, T. (2004). Management of vaginitis. *American Academy of Family Physicians, 70*(11), 2125–2132.

Plitt, S., Garfein, R., Gaysos, C., Strathdee, S., Sherman, S., & Taha, T. (2005). Prevalence and correlates of *Chlamydia trachomatis, Neisseria gonorrhoeae, Trichomonas vaginalis* infections, and bacterial vaginosis among a cohort of young injection drug users in Baltimore, Maryland. *Journal of the American Sexually Transmitted Disease Association, 32*(7), 446–453.

Riggs, M., & Klebanoff, M. (2004). Treatment of vaginal infections to prevent preterm birth: A meta-analysis. *Clinical Obstetrics and Gynecology, 47*(4), 796–807.

Samuels, P., & Colombo, D. F. (2002). Renal disease. In S. G. Gabbe, J. R. Niebyl, & J. L. Simpson (Eds.), *Obstetrics: Normal and problem pregnancies* (4th ed., pp. 1065–1080). New York: Churchill-Livingstone.

Schachter, J. (2005). *Sexually transmitted infections.* Paper presented at the 45th Interscience Conference on Antimicrobial Agents and Chemotherapy, Washington, DC, December 16–19. Retrieved February 9, 2006, from http://www.medscape.com/viewprogram5017_pnt

Scheinfeld, N., & Lehman, D. S. (2006). An evidence-based review of medical and surgical treatments of genital warts. *Dermatology Online Journal, 12*(3), 1–19. Retrieved May 1, 2006, from http://dermatology.cdlib.org/123/reviews/warts/scheinfeld.html

Schwebke, J., & Desmond, R. (2005). Risk factors for bacterial vaginosis in women at high risk for sexually transmitted diseases. *Journal of the American Sexually Transmitted Disease Association, 32*(11), 654–658.

Scott, L. D., & Hasik, K. J. (2001). The similarities and differences of endometritis and pelvic inflammatory disease. *Journal of Obstetric, Gynecologic, & Neonatal Nursing, 30*(3), 332–341.

Thorsen, M., & Poole, J. (2002). Renal disease in pregnancy. *Journal of Perinatal and Neonatal Nursing, 15*(4), 13–26.

US Preventive Services Task Force. (2004). *Recommendation statement: Screening for asymptomatic bacteriuria.* Retrieved February 20, 2006, from http://www.ahrq.gov/clinic/3rduspstf/asymbac/asymbacrs.htm

Varney, H., Kriebs, J. M., & Gegor, C. L. (2004). *Varney's midwifery.* Sudbury, MA: Jones and Bartlett.

Walsh, C. M., & Irwin, K. L. (2002). Combating the silent chlamydia epidemic. *Contemporary OB/GYN, 47*(4), 90–98.

Whitley, R. (2005, December). *Advances in diagnosis and treatment of herpesviruses.* Paper presented at the 45th Interscience Conference on Antimicrobial Agents and Chemotherapy, Washington, DC, December 16–19. Retrieved February 9, 2006, from http://www.medscape.com/viewprogram5017_pnt

CHAPTER 7

Women's Health Problems

A friend was turning 41 years old a few months ago and knew that it was time for her annual gynecology exam. She had been putting off having her first mammogram because she had heard stories about how much it hurt. Finally, knowing that her nurse practitioner would ask her if she had gotten a mammogram, she scheduled the test the week before her annual gynecology exam. The mammogram detected a suspicious mass and she had a biopsy that confirmed intraductal carcinoma. She never had a palpable lump, she was not considered high risk for breast cancer, and she was an active, health-conscious woman. It never occurred to her that she could get breast cancer.

OBJECTIVES

1. Contrast the common benign and malignant breast disorders.

2. Briefly describe the emotional reactions a woman may experience in regard to a diagnosis of breast cancer.

3. Discuss the signs and symptoms, medical therapy, and implications for fertility of endometriosis.

4. Discuss the signs and symptoms, diagnosis criteria, treatment options, and health implications of polycystic ovarian syndrome.

5. Discuss abnormal uterine bleeding and abdominal masses.

6. Identify the implications of an abnormal finding during a pelvic examination.

7. Summarize behaviors that help to minimize recurrence of some of the common lesions of the vulva.

8. Discuss the importance of an annual Pap smear and appropriate follow-up for an abnormal finding.

9. Briefly discuss the role that human papilloma virus plays in abnormal Pap smears.

10. Delineate the psychosocial responses a woman may experience when facing any of the common gynecologic procedures.

KEY TERMS

Breast self-examination (BSE) 127

Colposcopy 141

Cystocele 149

Dysfunctional uterine bleeding (DUB) 144

Dyspareunia 146

Endometriosis 145

Fibrocystic breast change 130

Galactorrhea 131

Hysterectomy 150

Mammogram 127

Pap smear 139

Polycystic ovarian syndrome (PCOS) 147

Toxic shock syndrome (TSS) 142

 MEDIALINK

Additional resources for this content can be found on the Prentice Hall Nursing MediaLink DVD-ROM and on the Companion Website at http://www.prenhall.com/davidson. Click on "Chapter 7" to select the activities for this chapter.

From early childhood, through adolescence, the active reproductive years, into menopause and the years beyond, a woman will likely face a variety of gynecologic or urinary problems. Some may be minor, whereas others have the potential to be quite serious, provoking a wide array of physical and psychologic responses. This chapter provides information about selected gynecologic problems that a woman may encounter during her lifetime, with an emphasis on problems commonly addressed in community-based settings. Some of the issues are addressed in detail, and other topics are discussed more briefly. The chapter concludes with a brief description of common gynecologic surgical procedures. For a detailed discussion of gynecologic cancers, for more detailed information on any of the subjects covered in this chapter, or for more in-depth discussion of gynecologic procedures, please consult a specialized text.

CARE OF THE WOMAN WITH A DISORDER OF THE BREAST

Throughout her lifetime a woman may experience a variety of breast disorders. Some, like mastitis, which is discussed in Chapter 38 ∞, are acute disorders, whereas others, such as fibrocystic breast changes, are chronic. This section begins with breast screening techniques and then deals with some of the common breast disorders a woman may experience.

Screening Techniques for the Breasts

Despite their limitations, breast examination and mammography remain the most effective screening techniques available for disorders of the breast.

BREAST EXAMINATION

Like the uterus, the breast undergoes regular cyclic changes in response to hormonal stimulation. Each month, in rhythm with the cycle of ovulation, the breasts become engorged with fluid in anticipation of pregnancy and the woman may experience sensations of tenderness, lumpiness, or pain. If conception does not occur, the accumulated fluid drains away via the lymphatic network. *Mastodynia* or *mastalgia* (premenstrual swelling and tenderness of the breasts) is common and usually lasts for 3 to 4 days before the onset of menses. Some women may also experience mastalgia at the time of ovulation, about 14 days into her cycle; for other women the symptoms may persist throughout the month.

After menopause, connective breast tissue atrophies and is replaced by adipose tissue. The breasts lose elasticity and may droop and become pendulous. The recurring breast engorgement associated with ovulation ceases. If hormone replacement therapy (HRT) is used to counteract other symptoms of menopause, breast engorgement may resume.

Monthly **breast self-examination (BSE)** has been advocated for years as a good method for detecting breast masses early, and, in truth, a large percentage of women discover their breast cancer accidentally or during a BSE. Women at high risk for breast cancer are specifically encouraged to be attentive to the importance of early detection through routine BSE. BSE

may also be of real value for younger women (under age 40) who do not yet get regular mammograms. Nevertheless, several research studies have questioned the value of BSE. BSE does not appear to decrease mortality and has associated risks and costs. These include the reality that false-positives require clinical follow-up, resulting in unnecessary mammograms and diagnostic biopsies, cause psychologic distress, and increase the actual financial cost of BSE screening. Consequently recommendations about the use of BSE conflict (Howard & Scott-Findlay, 2006). The American Cancer Society (ACS) (2006) and the Canadian Cancer Society (2005) both recommend that women begin performing monthly BSE at age 20. The US Preventive Services Task Force has not made a recommendation about BSE because of insufficient evidence, and the Canadian Task Force on Preventive Health recommended that the teaching of BSE be eliminated from regular health examinations (Howard & Scott-Findlay, 2006).

Despite the conflicting recommendations, in the course of a routine physical examination, or during an initial visit to the caregiver, women are generally taught BSE technique. The effectiveness of BSE is determined by the woman's ability to perform the procedure correctly, by her knowledge of her own breast tissue, and by the density of her breast tissue. (See Client Teaching: Breast Self-Examination.)

Advocates of BSE advise that it be performed on a regular monthly basis about 1 week after the onset of each menstrual period, when the breasts are typically not tender or swollen. BSE is most effective when it uses a dual approach incorporating both inspection and palpation. After menopause, BSE should be performed on the same day each month (chosen by the woman for ease of remembrance). During pregnancy and lactation, BSE is not performed routinely; however, new, abnormal findings should be reported to the woman's clinician.

Clinical breast examination (CBE) by a trained healthcare provider, such as a physician, nurse practitioner, or nurse-midwife, is an essential element of a routine gynecologic examination. Experience in differentiating among benign, suspicious, and worrisome breast changes enables the caregiver to reassure the woman if the findings are normal or move forward with additional diagnostic procedures or referral if the findings are suspicious or worrisome. The ACS (2006) recommends CBE every 3 years for women age 20 to 39 with no abnormal findings or history of breast-related problems and CBE annually for women age 40 and older. In clinical practice, however, many caregivers advocate annual CBE for all women over age 20.

MAMMOGRAPHY

A **mammogram** is a soft-tissue x-ray image of the breast taken without the injection of a contrast medium. It can detect lesions in the breast before they can be felt and has gained wide acceptance as an effective screening tool for breast cancer. Research indicates that mammography detects about 90% of breast cancers in women who are symptom free, although it is slightly more accurate in postmenopausal women, as compared with premenopausal women (ACS, 2006). Currently the ACS (2006) guidelines recommend that all women age 40 and over have an annual mammogram and, as discussed previously, an annual

CLIENT TEACHING Breast Self-Examination

CLIENT GOALS   At the completion of the teaching, the woman will be able to:

1. Discuss her risk of breast cancer
2. Describe the use of BSE in breast cancer detection
3. Demonstrate the correct procedure for BSE
4. List warning signs of breast cancer to be reported to the caregiver
5. Incorporate monthly BSE into her personal routine

TEACHING PLAN

CONTENT

Discuss the risk factors associated with breast cancer.

Stress the unique risk factors associated with the woman's personal history and lifestyle.

Discuss the use of BSE in breast cancer detection.

TEACHING METHOD

Breast cancer should be discussed in a private area free of interruptions. The room needs to have a mirror; bed, couch, or examining table; pillows; a patient gown; and private area for the woman to disrobe.

Create a supportive, warm, and comfortable atmosphere by attitude and communication style—both verbal and nonverbal. A discussion of breast cancer may bring forth many emotions in the woman, including grief for previous breast cancer-related losses.

Focus on open discussion. A brochure with statistics and illustrations may be useful. Stress the positive outcomes of early detection to counterbalance fears.

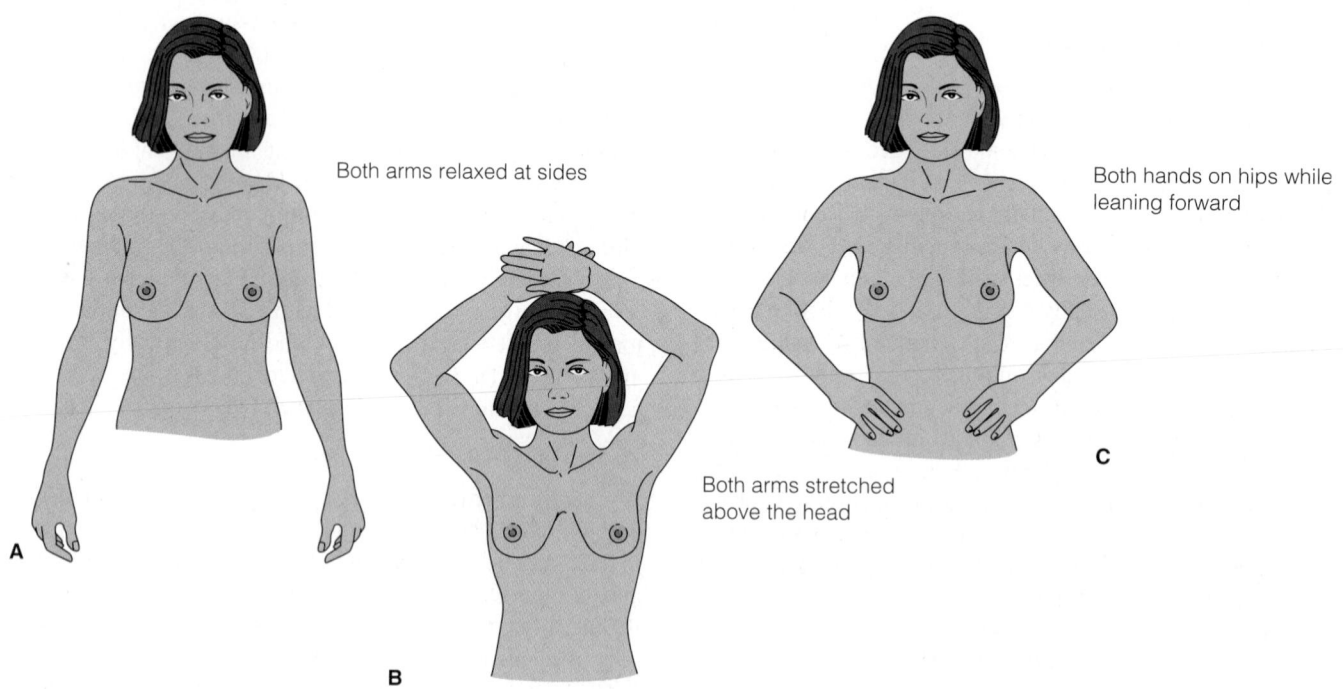

Both arms relaxed at sides

Both arms stretched above the head

Both hands on hips while leaning forward

A

B

C

Figure 7–1 ◆ Positions for inspection of the breasts. *A,* Both arms relaxed at sides. *B,* Both arms stretched above the head. *C,* Both hands on hips while leaning forward.

CLIENT TEACHING   Breast Self-Examination   continued

Describe and demonstrate the correct procedure for BSE.

A. Instruct the woman to inspect her breasts by standing or sitting in front of a mirror. She needs to inspect her breasts in three positions: with both arms relaxed down at her sides, both arms stretched straight over her head, and both hands placed on her hips while leaning forward (Figure 7–1 ◆).

B. Advise the woman to look at her breasts individually and in comparison with one another. Note and record the following characteristics for each position:

SIZE AND SYMMETRY OF THE BREASTS

1. Breasts may vary, but the variations should remain constant during rest or movement—note abnormal contours.
2. Some size difference between the breasts is normal.

SHAPE AND DIRECTION OF THE BREASTS

1. The shape of the breasts can be rounded or pendulous with some variation between breasts.
2. The breasts should be pointing slightly laterally.

COLOR, THICKENING, EDEMA, AND VENOUS PATTERNS

1. Check for redness or inflammation.
2. A blue hue with a marked venous pattern that is focal or unilateral may indicate an area of increased blood supply due to tumor. Symmetric venous patterns are normal.
3. Skin edema observed as thickened skin with enlarged pores ("orange peel") may indicate blocked lymphatic drainage due to tumor.

SURFACE OF THE BREASTS

1. Skin dimpling, puckering, or retraction (pulling) when the woman presses her hands together or against her hips suggests malignancy.
2. Striae (stretch marks) red at onset and whitish with age are normal.

NIPPLE SIZE AND SHAPE, DIRECTION, RASHES, ULCERATIONS, AND DISCHARGE

1. Long-standing nipple inversion is normal, but an inverted nipple previously capable of erection is suspicious. Note any deviation, flattening, or broadening of the nipples.
2. Check for rashes, ulcerations, or discharge.

C. Instruct the woman to palpate (feel) her breasts as follows:

1. Lie down. Put one hand behind your head. With the other hand, fingers flattened, gently feel your breast. Press lightly (Figure 7–2 ◆, A). Now examine the breast.
2. Figure 7–2, B shows you how to check each breast. Begin as you see in B and follow the arrows, feeling gently for a lump or thickening. Remember to feel all parts of each breast.
3. Now repeat the same procedure sitting up, with the hand still behind your head (Figure 7–2, C).
4. Squeeze the nipple between your thumb and forefinger. Look for any discharge—clear or bloody (Figure 7–2, D).

D. Take the woman's hand and help her to identify her "normal lumps" (e.g., mammary ridge, ribs, and nodularity in the upper outer quadrants).

E. After she examines her breasts and identifies her normal lumps, instruct her to palpate her breasts once more to identify any areas that she may have questions about. If questions arise, the nurse should palpate the area and attempt to identify whether it is normal.

Learning is best accomplished when material is broken down into smaller steps and presented with multiple approaches. Prior to asking the woman to perform BSE, use a model or a chart to demonstrate the procedure. Then have the woman perform BSE. Be very supportive and give a lot of positive feedback because some women may be embarrassed. Demonstrate a nonjudgmental, accepting attitude.

With one hand behind your head, flatten your fingers and press lightly on your breast, feeling gently for a lump or thickening.

A

Check each breast in a circular manner, feeling all parts of the breast.

B

Figure 7–2 ◆ Procedure for breast self-examination.

Demonstrate "normal lumps" on the woman herself while guiding her hand and identifying the area. This will increase confidence that she will recognize an abnormal finding. Checking her immediately afterward will positively reinforce her and diminish the fear associated with BSE.

F. If a breast model is available, instruct the woman to palpate it and identify the lumps.

G. Provide information on the warning signs of breast cancer and what she should do if she identifies any of these signs during BSE.

(Continued on next page)

CLIENT TEACHING   Breast Self-Examination   continued

TIMING

Instruct the woman to perform BSE on a monthly basis. Be specific based on whether she is premenopausal, pregnant, postmenopausal, or postmenopausal receiving hormone replacement therapy.

DOCUMENTATION

Documentation of client teaching should include the teaching information discussed, the client's verbalization of understanding, and specific interventions or warning signs that were given, along with the client's understanding of follow-up if needed in the future.

EVALUATION

Evaluate the woman's learning through discussion and return demonstration. Learning has occurred if the woman performs BSE correctly and can identify timing, normal and abnormal findings, and follow-up activities.

Provide a written handout on the warning signs of breast cancer. The handout should also cover actions that the woman should take if a warning sign is discovered. Stress the positive effects of early detection.

Provide the woman with a reminder symbol for monthly BSE. The American Cancer Society provides such items to hang in the shower, place on a refrigerator, and so forth. Praise her commitment to do monthly BSE. Give the woman a follow-up telephone number (e.g., American Cancer Society) to use if she needs additional information or has questions.

Repeat the same procedure sitting up with your hand still behind your head.

C

Squeeze your nipple between your thumb and forefinger; look for any clear or bloody discharge.

D

Figure 7–2 ◆ Procedure for breast self-examination.
SOURCE: Data from American Cancer Society. (1973). *Breast self-examination and the nurse* (No. 3408 PB).

CBE. The National Cancer Institute (NCI) (2006) recommends mammograms every 1 to 2 years for women age 40 and older. The NCI also recommends that "women who are at higher than average risk of breast cancer should talk with their health care providers about whether to have mammograms before age 40 and how often to have them." If a woman has a history of breast cancer in a close relative (i.e., mother, sister) and the cancer was diagnosed before the relative was age 40, many clinicians advocate that the client begin mammograms 10 years before the age of her close relative's diagnosis.

Negative consequences of mammography do exist. Thirty percent of women age 40 to 49 are likely to have a false-positive result requiring biopsy. Moreover, mammograms miss more than 25% of invasive breast cancers in women in this age group (Love, 2000). Furthermore, in some women, especially women who are quite elderly, the cancer tissue type may be so slow-growing that it would not cause morbidity or mortality within the woman's lifetime.

Breast sensitivity seems to vary from woman to woman and may be a factor in a woman's reluctance to have a mammogram.

To help prevent any discomfort, the nurse can suggest that this x-ray study be scheduled when their breasts are least sensitive, which is about 2 weeks after the onset of menses. In some cases, the woman can obtain relief by reducing caffeine intake from 5 to 7 days before the test. In most cases, a mammogram causes feelings of compression but not pain (Figure 7–3 ◆). All women should be instructed to refrain from applying lotions, powders, deodorant, or other cosmetic substances to the torso on the day of the exam because the substances may appear as questionable areas on the mammogram and may interfere with accurate interpretation. The risk of radiation exposure with mammograms is low but it does become more significant depending on the age of the woman at her initial mammogram and the number of mammograms she has (Love, 2000).

BENIGN BREAST CONDITIONS

Fibrocystic breast change, the most common of the benign breast conditions, is most prevalent in women 20 to 50 years of age and results from fluctuating hormone levels. It is rare in postmenopausal women who are not taking HRT. Fortunately,

Figure 7–3 ◆ Recommended position for mammogram.
SOURCE: Philip Bailey/CORBIS.

fibrocystic breast changes are not a risk factor for breast cancer in most women. In some women, however, the fibrocystic change is proliferative, resulting in a *hyperplasia* or buildup of the cells of the breast ducts. When atypia is associated with this hyperplasia, there is a fivefold increase in the risk of breast cancer (Gemignani, 2003).

Fibrocystic changes may produce an asymptomatic mass but more often are accompanied by pain or tenderness and sometimes nipple discharge. Fluctuations in size and rapid appearance or disappearance of breast masses are common. Bilateral, cyclic breast pain is the most common symptom, and the nodularities may be unilateral or bilateral, often in the upper outer quadrants of the breasts.

The woman often reports pain, tenderness, and swelling that is cyclic, worsening in the late luteal phase of the menstrual cycle (just before menses), and improving about 1 to 2 days into the menstrual cycle. Physical examination may reveal only mild signs of irregularity, or the breasts may feel dense, with areas of irregularity and nodularity. Women often refer to this as "lumpiness." Some women may also experience spontaneous nipple discharge, which should be evaluated separately.

If the woman has a large, fluid-filled cyst, she may experience a localized painful area as the capsule containing the accumulated fluid distends coincident with her cycle. However, if small cysts form, the woman may experience not a solitary tender lump but a diffuse tenderness. Several characteristics help differentiate a cyst from a cancerous lesion. Cysts tend to be mobile and tender and do not cause skin retraction (pulling) in the surrounding tissue, whereas cancerous lesions tend to be fixed and painless and may cause skin retraction.

Mammography, sonography, magnetic resonance imaging (MRI), palpation, and fine-needle aspiration may be used to confirm fibrocystic breast changes. Often, fine-needle aspiration provides treatment as well as relief from the tenderness or pain. Palpable cysts are often treated conservatively with medical management; however, all discrete masses should have a tissue sample sent for biopsy. Women with mild symptoms may benefit from restricting sodium intake and taking a mild diuretic during the week before the onset of menses. This counteracts fluid retention, relieves pressure in the breast, and helps decrease the

pain. In other cases, a mild analgesic is necessary. Some studies report that the use of vitamins A and E may be helpful (Gemignani, 2003). Oral contraceptives help alleviate symptoms for the majority of women, but, unfortunately, symptoms tend to recur when the oral contraceptives are discontinued.

In severe cases, the hormone inhibitor danazol is often helpful although it can cause several undesirable side effects including masculinization. A 3- to 6-month course of danazol may significantly reduce symptoms and the beneficial results may last for several months. Women who do not respond to other treatment approaches may be given a trial of bromocriptine, a prolactin inhibitor. The antiestrogen medication tamoxifen may be used although this is an "off-label" use because tamoxifen has not been approved by the Food and Drug Administration (FDA) for this purpose. Tamoxifen relieves symptoms in about 70% of women and has fewer side effects, but it can cause proliferation of endometrial tissue, increasing the risk of endometrial cancer, so women taking it should be monitored closely (Eskin & Sepilian, 2001). Women of childbearing age should be advised that tamoxifen has been associated with birth defects.

Some researchers suggest that methylxanthines (found in caffeine products, such as coffee, tea, colas, chocolate, and some medications) and the use of tobacco may contribute to the development of fibrocystic breast changes and that limiting use of these substances will help decrease fibrocystic changes. Other research fails to demonstrate a clear association between methylxanthines and fibrocystic breast changes.

Fibroadenoma is the second most common benign breast lesion over all and the most common breast lesion in women under age 25. Fibroadenoma is most commonly seen in women in their teens and into their early 30s and is rarely associated with breast cancer (Gemignani, 2003). A fibroadenoma is an asymptomatic, mobile, well-defined, painless, palpable mass with a rubbery texture.

If there are any disquieting features to the appearance of a lump, ultrasound, MRI, fine-needle biopsy, or excision of the mass may be indicated. Caution is exercised when deciding on biopsy because excision of the mass in a young girl may interfere with normal breast development. Watchful observation, including monthly BSE and annual CBE, is the most appropriate treatment. Surgery is often deferred but is indicated if the mass continues to enlarge, if there are suspicious findings on imaging or cytology, or if the client wants it removed (Gemignani, 2003). Surgical removal of the fibroadenoma, when advisable, concludes its treatment.

The term for nipple discharge not associated with lactation (production of milk for breastfeeding) is **galactorrhea.** It is a common breast problem and has been reported in 10% to 15% of women with benign breast disease and in 2.5% to 3% of women with breast cancer (Gemignani, 2003). Galactorrhea may be physiologic (as in the case with fibrocystic changes), drug induced, idiopathic, or pathologic. Physiologic discharge, usually associated with benign conditions, is characterized by clear, milky, straw-colored, or greenish fluid obtained by manual compression. Pathologic discharge, sometimes associated with malignancy, is spontaneous, unilateral, and often bloody or serosanguineous. Most providers recommend cytologic evaluation of all nipple discharge, regardless of its character; however, the absence of malignant cells does not exclude cancer, and a positive result does not distinguish in situ cancer from invasive cancer (Gemignani, 2003; Morrow, 2000).

Intraductal papillomas are tumors growing in the terminal portion of a duct or, sometimes, throughout the duct system within a section of the breast. Symptoms may include a unilateral mass or a spontaneous, and often bloody, nipple discharge.

The majority of papillomas present as solitary nodules. These small ball-like lesions may be detected on mammography but often are nonpalpable. The presence of a papilloma is often frightening to the woman, because her primary symptom is a discharge from the nipple that may be serosanguineous or brownish green because of old blood. The location of the papilloma within the duct system and its pattern of growth determine whether nipple discharge will be present. They are typically benign but they are generally excised to rule out the possibility of cancer (Gemignani, 2003).

Duct ectasia (comedomastitis), an inflammation of the ducts behind the nipple, commonly occurs during or near the onset of menopause and is not associated with malignancy. The condition typically occurs in women who have borne and nursed children. It is characterized by a thick, sticky nipple discharge of various colors and by burning pain, pruritus, and inflammation. Nipple retraction may also be noted, especially in postmenopausal women. Treatment is conservative, with drug therapy aimed at symptomatic relief. The major central ducts of the breast occasionally have to be excised.

Table 7–1 provides a comparison of the most frequently seen benign breast disorders.

Malignant Breast Disease

The lifetime risk of breast cancer in the United States is 1 out of 8. The risk increases with age. Excluding skin cancer, breast cancer accounts for one third of female cancers and is the most frequently diagnosed cancer in women (ACS, 2006). Only lung cancer causes more cancer deaths in women (ACS, 2006).

PREDISPOSING FACTORS

Factors that predispose a woman to breast cancer include the following:

- Age. Incidence increases steadily with age. In fact, over 95% of new cases of breast cancer are diagnosed in women age 40 and over (ACS, 2006).
- Female gender.
- History of previous breast cancer.
- Family history of mother, sister, or daughter with breast cancer. The risk increases if two or more relatives develop breast cancer or if the relative developed breast cancer premenopausally or in both breasts.
- Long-term (more than 5 years) postmenopausal combined estrogen and progestin HRT (ACS, 2006)
- Being overweight or obese after menopause.
- Alcohol consumption. This risk increases with the amount of alcohol consumed (ACS, 2006).
- No history of pregnancy or first pregnancy after age 30.
- Never breastfeeding a child.

Table 7–1   SUMMARY OF BENIGN BREAST DISORDERS

Condition	Age	Pain	Cancer Risk	Nipple Discharge	Location	Consistency and Mobility	Diagnosis and Treatment
Fibrocystic breast changes	30–50	Yes	Yes with proliferative disease and atypical hyperplasia	Varies: none at all or may be clear, milky, straw colored, or green	Upper outer quadrant	Multiple lumps occurring bilaterally, influenced by menstrual cycle, nodular	Needle aspiration, Pap smear of nipple discharge, observation, biopsy if unresolved mass exists or mammographic changes, sonography
Fibroadenoma	15–25, median age 20	No	No	No, but milky discharge in pregnancy	Nipple or upper outer quadrant along the lateral side	Solid, well defined, sharply delineated, rounded rubbery mobile	Mammography, observation, surgical excision
Intraductal papilloma	Menopausal 50–60	Yes on palpation	Yes with multiple papillomas	Yes: serous bloody, or brownish green	No specific location	Nonpalpable or small, ball-like, poorly delineated	Pap smear of nipple discharge, mammography, ductogram; surgical excision
Duct ectasia	45–55	Yes: burning and itching around the nipple	No	Yes in perimenopausal women: thick, sticky, green, greenish brown or bloodstained	Mass behind or around the nipple	Poorly circumscribed, inflammation, nipple retraction, axillary lymphadenopathy	Pap smear of breast discharge, mammography, drug therapy for symptoms, surgical excision, observation.

DEVELOPING CULTURAL COMPETENCE

BREAST CANCER SURVIVAL RATES

After age 40, white women are more likely to be diagnosed with breast cancer than black women, but black women with breast cancer have lower 5-year survival rates (72% versus 87%). About half of this difference is related to the fact that breast cancer in African American women tends to be diagnosed later and the tumors diagnosed tend to be more aggressive forms that are less responsive to treatment (ACS, 2006).

- Longer reproductive phase (early menarche [before age 12] and late menopause [after age 55]).
- History of high-dose radiation to the chest before age 30 (ACS, 2006).
- Physical inactivity.
- Ashkenazi Jewish descent.

PREVENTION

Women should be encouraged to take action to reduce modifiable risks for breast cancer. These include, for example, avoiding obesity, exercising regularly, reducing dietary fat, and limiting alcoholic intake. Women at high risk of breast cancer may choose to begin chemoprevention using the drug tamoxifen. Women at very high genetic risk may consider bilateral prophylactic mastectomy. It has been shown to reduce the risk of breast cancer by 90% (Beattie, 2005).

Diagnosis

A malignant neoplasm may originate either in a duct or in the epithelium of the breast lobes. About 50% of breast cancers originate in the upper outer quadrant and spread or metastasize to the axillary lymph nodes. Common sites of distant metastasis are the lymph nodes, lungs, liver, brain, and bone.

As previously discussed, a cancerous lump may be discovered by the woman herself, by the clinician who palpates or observes an abnormality, or by mammogram. A painless mass or lump is the most important physical symptom of breast cancer, although up to 10% of women have breast pain but no palpable mass (ACS, 2006). Early detection greatly improves the treatment options available and increases women's long-term survival rates.

Worrisome findings that point to a higher risk of breast cancer include dimpling of the breast tissue, recent or acute nipple inversion, change in breast size or shape, increase of size in breast mass, skin erosion or ulceration, or presence of axillary lump. Routine mammography screening detects masses 2 to 3 years before clinical appearance. Other diagnostic modalities include fine-needle biopsy, ultrasonography, thermography, and MRI. Biopsy is essential for a diagnosis. Once the diagnosis is made and lymph node involvement is evaluated, clinical staging of the disease is determined and a treatment plan that coincides with the stage is initiated.

Clinical Therapy

Once breast cancer is diagnosed, the woman and her physician make treatment decisions together. The decision is based on a consideration of the following factors:

- Stage of cancer
- Optimal treatment for that stage
- Woman's age
- Personal preferences
- Risks and benefits of each treatment protocol

Most women diagnosed with breast cancer have some form of surgery. The primary goal of the surgery is to remove the cancer from the breast and the lymph nodes, if they are involved. Surgical treatment may consist of *simple or total mastectomy,* which involves removal of the entire breast. A *modified radical mastectomy* involves the removal of the breast and the axillary lymph nodes but does not include removal of any of the pectoral muscles of the chest wall. Women who undergo mastectomy are generally given the option of having breast reconstruction surgery. This surgery may be done at the time of the mastectomy or delayed until the prescribed chemotherapy and/or radiation is completed. *Lumpectomy,* or the removal of the cancerous tissue plus a rim of normal tissue, is a breast-sparing approach that is often used for women with stages I or II breast cancer. It is almost always followed by several weeks of radiation therapy to destroy any remaining cancerous cells.

Adjunctive therapy for breast cancer includes chemotherapy, radiation, and hormone therapy. Chemotherapy typically involves a combination of drugs known to combat breast cancer. As indicated previously, radiation is often used to destroy remaining cells following surgery but it may also be used to reduce the size of a cancerous tumor before surgery. Hormone therapy is based on the knowledge that the hormone estrogen, which is produced by the ovaries, stimulates certain types of breast cancer. Women who have a form of breast cancer that tests positive for estrogen receptors can be given the antiestrogen drug tamoxifen. Tamoxifen therapy has produced a 26% annual reduction in breast cancer recurrence and a 14% annual reduction in deaths (ACS, 2006).

Research is also under way evaluating the effectiveness of tamoxifen as a preventive measure to reduce the incidence of breast cancer in women at high risk for the disease. In addition, a second-generation antiestrogen drug called raloxifene is under study. Raloxifene, a selective estrogen receptor modulator (SERM), is used to prevent osteoporosis. However, it was shown to be even more effective than tamoxifen in decreasing the risk of breast cancer in postmenopausal women who were taking it for osteoporosis. Other research focuses on the use of monoclonal antibodies such as Herceptin, which works against a protein (HER2/neu) found in some breast tumors. Clinical trials are under way using Herceptin in combination with standard chemotherapy in newly diagnosed women whose cancer cells show high levels of this protein. It is also being used for women who have a recurrence of breast cancer or when the cancer progresses during chemotherapy (ACS, 2006).

Some women prefer a combined approach to treatment that draws on both allopathic and complementary medicine. These women elect to use complementary therapies, such as herbal remedies, therapeutic touch, acupuncture, aromatherapy, and massage, in combination with medical treatments.

When a woman is confronted with a breast cancer diagnosis, she must decide which therapy is worth what personal risk for her. Although prompt treatment is indicated, a second opinion is encouraged. Care of the woman with breast cancer involves a multidisciplinary approach, including a primary care provider, radiotherapist, surgeon, medical oncologist, and nursing specialists.

Psychologic Adjustment

The emotional feelings a woman experiences can range from fear of the loss of a body part, to fear of the ill effects of treatments, to fear of death. The nurse should encourage the woman to discuss her feelings and concerns, informing her of all procedures, their pros and cons, and alternative options.

The course of adjustment confronting the woman with cancer has been described in four phases: shock, reaction, recovery, and reorientation. In the *shock* phase, women make statements such as "Everything is unreal" or "I can't understand why this is happening to me." Shock generally extends from the discovery of the lump through the process of diagnosis.

Reaction occurs in conjunction with the initiation of treatment. As treatment begins, the woman is compelled to face what has occurred and begins to take in what has happened. Coping mechanisms become evident during this phase. Reaction coincides with the length of treatment. For many women, radiation treatment or chemotherapy prolongs this period to months. Treatment reinforces the diagnosis of cancer and the immediate consequences of the disease. Denial of breast loss, if a mastectomy is done, and denial of the reality of the illness are common responses by the woman during the periods of diagnosis and treatment. Denial protects the woman, making therapy tolerable.

Recovery begins during convalescence following the completion of medical treatment. Anxiety about her illness diminishes and the woman looks to the future once more. She turns outward and gradually resumes her former activities. Conversely, depression and social isolation occur if the woman is unable to negotiate the recovery phase successfully.

A woman's family and friends significantly influence her recovery. Women often perceive their partners as their primary source of support. Both members of a couple must adjust to the woman's condition and its implications as well as to the effect of therapy on their sexual intimacy. Difficulties with psychosocial adjustment to breast cancer tend to be similar for women and their partners except in the area of role adjustments, where women have more difficulties. Many hospitals and community agencies sponsor support groups for women with breast cancer. Online support groups are also available and are of particular value to women in rural areas and in areas that lack adequate community support. In addition, the ACS sponsors support groups for cancer survivors and their families. They also have a highly successful program, "Reach to Recovery," for women following surgery.

Reorientation follows recovery and is unending. It is accomplished when the woman can acknowledge that breast cancer is part of her life; yet living, for her, has returned to or perhaps exceeded its former fullness and meaning.

For additional information on breast cancer, refer to a medical-surgical text.

The physician also felt the lump and thickening and now I'm waiting to have my mammogram. My thoughts and feelings since I first felt the lump have been like a roller coaster. I'm 46 and I'm wondering if this is it. Am I dying? Now? I am afraid as I have not been afraid since one of our children was very ill.

NURSING CARE MANAGEMENT

Nursing care of the woman with breast cancer is multidimensional. It involves meeting the educational, psychosexual, and physical needs of the woman and, to a certain extent, those of her family. In meeting these needs, the nurse functions as a caregiver, counselor, educator, liaison, and advocate. Nurses need to support women in their efforts to provide self-care. This increases their self-esteem and sense of control. Nursing care changes as the woman progresses from the period of diagnosis to the recovery period.

Nursing Assessment and Diagnosis

During the period of diagnosis of any breast disease, the woman may be extremely anxious. The nurse can use therapeutic communication to assess the significance the woman places on her breasts; her current emotional status, coping mechanisms used during periods of stress, and knowledge and beliefs about cancer; and other variables that may influence her coping and adjustment.

Assessment is an ongoing process. Sufficient data must be obtained to provide the nurse and other members of the healthcare team with increasing insight into the woman's physical, mental, emotional, and social situation.

Nursing diagnoses that may apply to a woman with a disorder of the breast include the following:

- *Health-Seeking Behavior:* Information about diagnostic procedures for suspected breast cancer related to an expressed wish for information

- *Anxiety* related to threat to body image or her life

Nursing Plan and Implementation

During the prediagnosis period, the nurse should provide emotional support, clarify misconceptions, encourage the woman to express her anxiety, and urge her to ask many questions. Once a diagnosis has been made, the nurse should ensure that the woman clearly understands her condition, its association to breast malignancy, and treatment options. The nurse can also locate appropriate resources in the community and encourage the woman to make use of them as she deals with this difficult time. The woman and her partner or support person should discuss the treatment alternatives with her healthcare provider. Nursing advocacy involves supporting the woman's right to make the best treatment decision for her. With the assistance of the nurse, the woman can explore her fears, clarify her values, and identify the treatment options that would be personally acceptable. The nurse can provide psychologic support for the woman with a troublesome diagnosis, supply her with client education materials, and refer her to professional support groups.

For women who must undergo surgery, nursing care focuses on necessary perioperative interventions. Refer to a medical-surgical nursing textbook for detailed information on these aspects of nursing care.

Evaluation

Expected outcomes of nursing care include the following:

- The woman is able to discuss her fears, concerns, and questions during the period of diagnosis.
- The diagnosis is made quickly and accurately, and treatment initiated, if indicated.

CARE OF THE WOMAN DURING A PELVIC EXAMINATION

Women have a pelvic examination performed for a variety of reasons ranging from health maintenance to disease diagnosis. Many women perceive the pelvic exam as an uncomfortable and embarrassing procedure. These negative feelings may cause women to delay having yearly gynecologic examinations, and this avoidance may pose a threat to life and health.

A woman's first pelvic examination is especially important because a positive experience can help allay anxiety and make subsequent pelvic exams less threatening. Because the initial pelvic examination is typically done when a young woman is a teenager, nurses should be sensitive to a teen's attitudes and concerns. Teens are often shy about revealing their bodies and may feel very embarrassed by the procedure. Nurses can also help by being alert for atypical responses that might indicate a history of sexual abuse.

To make the pelvic exam less threatening, and hopefully improve the woman's health-seeking behavior, it is important to create a trusting atmosphere and incorporate practices that help the woman maintain a sense of control. Additionally, it is important for the nurse to assist in facilitating a nonjudgmental and safe environment in which the woman can be honest in response to the medical providers' inquiries. Some healthcare providers are offering to perform what is called an educational pelvic exam. During this type of exam the woman becomes an active participant and has an opportunity to learn about her body, voice her concerns, and share decisions about her care.

The educational exam includes offering the woman a mirror to watch the procedure, pointing out anatomic parts to her, and positioning and draping her to allow eye-to-eye contact with the practitioner. The woman is encouraged to participate by asking questions and giving feedback. The nurse can assist the woman by encouraging her to relax with specific advice such as "Keep your bottom flat against the table" and "Wiggle your toes if you find yourself beginning to tense your muscles."

Nurse practitioners, certified nurse-midwives, and physicians all perform pelvic examinations. Nurses assist the practitioner and the woman during the examination. Procedure 7–1 provides information on assisting with a pelvic examination.

PROCEDURE 7–1   Assisting with a Pelvic Examination

NURSING ACTION	RATIONALE
Preparation	
• Ensure that the room is sufficiently warm by checking room temperature and adjusting thermostat if necessary. If overhead heat lamps are available, turn them on.	
• Explain the procedure to the woman. If she has never had a pelvic examination, show her the equipment to be used as part of the explanation.	*Explaining the procedure helps reduce anxiety and increase cooperation.*
• Ask the woman to empty her bladder and to remove clothing below the waist.	*An empty bladder promotes comfort during the internal examination.*
• Have padding on the stirrups. If stirrups are not padded, the woman may prefer to leave her shoes on during the procedure.	*Stirrups are padded to ease the pressure of the feet against the metal and to decrease the discomfort associated with cold stirrups. If they are not padded, wearing shoes accomplishes the same purpose.*
• Give the woman a disposable drape or sheet to use during the exam. Ask her to sit at the end of the examining table with the drape opened across her lap.	
• Position the woman in the lithotomy position with her thighs flexed and abducted. Place her feet in the stirrups. Her buttocks should extend slightly beyond the edge of the examining table.	*This position provides the exposure necessary to conduct the examination effectively.*
• Drape the woman with the sheet, leaving a flap so that the perineum can be exposed.	*The drape helps preserve the woman's sense of dignity and privacy.*

(Continued on next page)

PROCEDURE 7–1 Assisting with a Pelvic Examination continued

NURSING ACTION	RATIONALE

Equipment and Supplies

- Vaginal specula of various sizes, warmed with water or on heating pad prior to insertion
- Sterile gloves
- Water-soluble lubricant
- Materials for Pap smear or *ThinPrep* Pap test and cultures
- Good light source

Note: Lubricant may alter the results of tests and cultures and is not used during the speculum examination. Its use is reserved for the bimanual examination.

Procedure: Sterile Gloves

1. The examiner dons gloves for the procedure. Explain each part of the procedure as the certified nurse-midwife, nurse practitioner, or physician performs it. Let the woman know that the examiner begins with an inspection of the external genitalia. The speculum is then inserted to allow visualization of the cervix and vaginal walls and to obtain specimens for testing. After the speculum is withdrawn the examiner performs a bimanual examination of the internal organs using the fingers of one hand inserted in the woman's vagina while the other hand presses over the woman's uterus and ovaries. The final step of the procedure is generally a rectal examination.

2. Ask the woman to breathe slowly and regularly and to use any method she finds effective in helping her to remain relaxed.

3. Let her know when the examiner is ready to insert the speculum and ask her to bear down.

4. After the speculum is withdrawn, lubricate the examiner's fingers prior to the bimanual examination.

5. After the examiner has completed the examination and moved away from the woman, move to the end of the examination table and face the woman. Cover her with the drape. Apply gentle pressure to her knees and encourage her to move toward the head of the table. Assist her to remove her feet from the stirrups, then offer your hand to her and assist her to sit up.

6. Provide her with tissues to wipe the lubricant from her perineum.

7. Provide the woman with privacy while she dresses. Be sure that she is not dizzy and that she is standing or sitting safely before leaving the room.

Relaxation helps decrease muscle tension. Bearing down helps open the vaginal orifice and relaxes the perineal muscles.

Lubrication decreases friction and eases insertion of the examiner's fingers.

Assistance is important because the lithotomy position is an awkward one and many women, but especially those women who are pregnant, obese, or older, may find it difficult to get out of the stirrups.

Vaginal secretions and lubricant may be discharged from the vagina when the woman sits upright.

Lying supine may cause postural hypotension.

> **CLINICAL TIP**
>
> With the examiner's consent (obtained beforehand), offer the woman a hand mirror so that she can watch all or part of the examination. This practice removes the "mystery" from the procedure and enables the woman to become familiar with the appearance of her body.

The pelvic examination consists of three segments: inspection of the vulva; inspection of the vagina and the cervix via a speculum examination; and palpation of the cervix, uterus, and ovaries via a bimanual examination. Often a Papanicolaou smear is obtained during the speculum examination. The Pap smear is discussed in the section on abnormal Pap smear results, which begins on page 139.

Vulvar Self-Examination

During the pelvic examination many caregivers also provide education about self-examination of the vulva. This procedure, like BSE (discussed previously), permits early detection of abnormalities, thereby maximizing the possibility of early diagnosis and treatment.

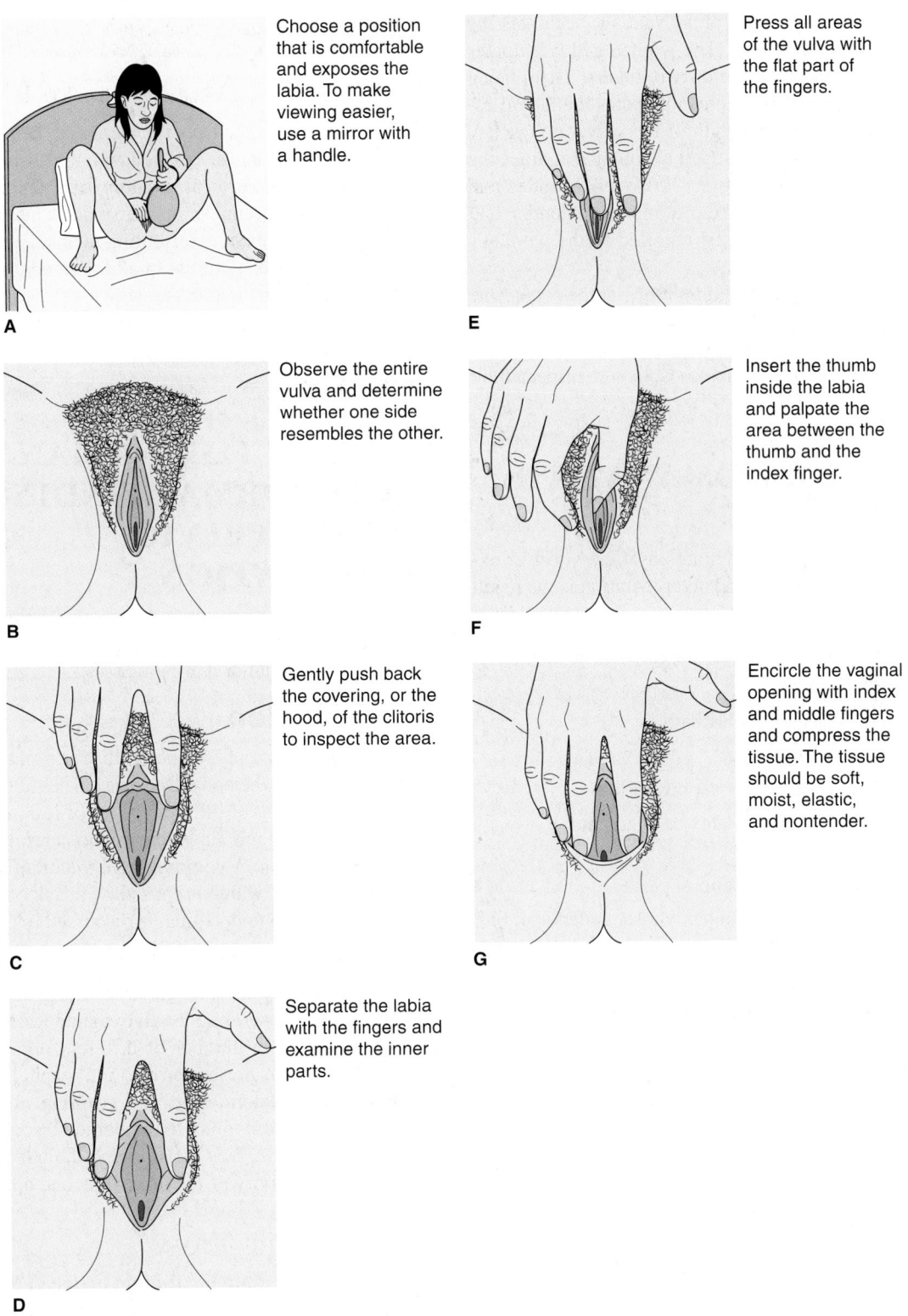

Choose a position that is comfortable and exposes the labia. To make viewing easier, use a mirror with a handle.

A

Observe the entire vulva and determine whether one side resembles the other.

B

Gently push back the covering, or the hood, of the clitoris to inspect the area.

C

Separate the labia with the fingers and examine the inner parts.

D

Press all areas of the vulva with the flat part of the fingers.

E

Insert the thumb inside the labia and palpate the area between the thumb and the index finger.

F

Encircle the vaginal opening with index and middle fingers and compress the tissue. The tissue should be soft, moist, elastic, and nontender.

G

Figure 7–4 ◆ Steps to follow to perform vulvar self-examination.

Self-examination of the vulva is simple to perform. The woman is advised to assume a sitting position on a bed or a chair. In good light she holds a mirror in one hand and uses the other hand to expose the tissues of her perineum while she carefully inspects and palpates the area. Pregnant or obese women may find it easier to inspect this area in a standing position with one foot elevated on a low stool. Figure 7–4 ◆ shows the correct procedure for vulvar self–examination.

Initially, the woman inspects the entire perineum for symmetry, discharge, and lesions. She then gently pushes back the hood of the clitoris to inspect this area. Next she separates the labia to examine the inner tissues. The woman gently palpates the vulva using the flat part of one or two fingers. Then, using her thumb and index finger, the woman palpates the lateral aspects of the genitalia along the length of the vulva, noting any tenderness, masses, or lesions. Lastly, the woman examines the vaginal opening, compressing the tissues between the index and middle fingers. The tissues should be soft, moist, nontender, and elastic. Any abnormalities should be reported to the woman's healthcare provider.

This exam should be performed monthly, at the same time as the BSE, in all sexually active asymptomatic women or women over the age of 18. Women with a history of vulvar lesions or women with adverse symptoms should inspect their vulva more frequently.

CARE OF THE WOMAN WITH VULVITIS

The term *vulvitis* refers to an inflammation of the vulva or external female genitalia. Sometimes vulvar irritation is the result of nonpathologic factors such as:

- Frequent douching or use of over-the-counter douches
- Feminine deodorant spray
- Detergents, harsh soaps, or bubble bath
- Colored or perfumed toilet paper
- Contraceptive creams, foams, or suppositories
- Condoms, possibly related to a latex or nonoxynol-9 (spermicide) sensitivity
- Dye, such as found in new clothing
- Synthetic clothing, such as nylon pantyhose, underwear, or synthetic slacks that may trap moisture
- Tight clothing, such as jeans
- Some repetitive motion exercise, such as running or biking
- Frequent shaving of the perineum
- Frequent intercourse or intercourse without adequate lubrication
- Deodorant menstrual pads or tampons, or frequent use of menstrual pads or tampons
- Estrogen deprivation due to menopause, surgical menopause, or medication-induced menopause (such as chemotherapy)

Other times, external genital irritation may be the result of inflammation or infection of the vagina or cervix. The irritation results when increased vaginal or cervical secretions flow distally and create inflammation of the vulvar tissues. This condition is called *vulvovaginitis.*

Often it is difficult to differentiate, by symptoms alone, vulvitis from vaginitis. The nurse needs to understand that vulvitis can occur as a distinct entity from vaginitis, and the previously mentioned practices may be significant contributing factors to both.

NURSING CARE MANAGEMENT

The nurse gathers data from the woman to help differentiate behaviors that may cause isolated vulvitis from those that may cause vaginal and cervical inflammation. Once the assessment of vulvitis has been made, the nurse plays a crucial role in providing education about contributing factors that may have led to the development of vulvitis. In addition, educating the woman about behaviors to avoid, strategies or therapies to improve symptoms, and signs of a worsening condition that require further evaluation are all part of the nurse's responsibilities.

CARE OF THE WOMAN WITH AN ABNORMAL FINDING DURING PELVIC EXAMINATION

An abnormal finding resulting from pelvic examination may involve tissues of the vulva, vagina, or cervix; abnormal uterine bleeding; or ovarian or uterine masses.

Vulvar Lesion

The skin of the vulva is subject to diseases and changes, just as skin elsewhere on the body. Because cancer of the vulva may be present in a variety of different types of lesions it is important that the external genitalia be examined carefully at the time of pelvic examination. A common benign condition of the vulva, atrophic vaginitis, which is caused by a lack of estrogen stimulation to the vulva and vagina, is discussed in Chapter 4.∞

BARTHOLIN'S GLAND CYST

Infection of the Bartholin's gland resulting in inflammation of the gland itself is a common vulvovaginal lesion. The infection can be caused by a number of different organisms, the most common of which are gonorrhea and staphylococcus. Symptoms include unilateral pain and swelling of the Bartholin's gland, ranging from mild to moderate discomfort to severe pain. Treatment involves incision and drainage of the abscess, culture and sensitivity of the discharge, and appropriate antibiotic therapy.

VITILIGO OF THE VULVA

Vitiligo is a fairly common finding on the vulva. It is a depigmentation of the skin resulting in white patchy areas because of the absence of melanin. Vitiligo may appear anytime after puberty and anywhere on the body, but it is never associated with a systemic disorder. However, it can cause significant disfiguring cosmetic changes, particularly in dark-skinned individuals.

LICHEN SCLEROSUS

Lichen sclerosus is a benign disorder of the vulva that can occur at any age, but is more common in girls less than 10 years old and in postmenopausal women. The initial symptoms are bluish white papules that coalesce and become white plaques. The skin becomes thin, and small fissures or ulcerations may develop. Children and adults often experience pruritus, and sexually active women may have pain during intercourse related to shrinkage of the labial tissues. Diagnosis is made by clinical exam and confirmed by biopsy. Treatment includes high-dose topical steroid cream twice daily for 2 to 3 weeks, and then decreased to once or twice weekly thereafter. In postmenopausal women there has been some benefit to topical progesterone or testosterone use, but women may experience undesired side effects like hair growth, acne, or clitoral enlargement.

VULVAR VESTIBULITIS

Women with *vestibulitis* experience local irritation and inflammation of the vulvar vestibule, severe pain with vaginal penetration (tampons or intercourse), burning and itching, and sometimes urinary frequency or dysuria. The cause is unknown. No definitive treatment exists so therapies are directed at comfort measures to relieve symptoms. Therapies include vaginal and introital lubricants, topical anesthetics (2% lidocaine gel or 5% Xylocaine ointment), local interferon injections, oral antifungal medications, oral tricyclic antidepressants, biofeedback techniques, and in severe cases, surgical intervention (Wilkinson, 2003).

MALIGNANT TUMORS OF THE VULVA

Cancer of the vulva can occur at any age but is more common in postmenopausal women, usually older than 70 years of age. The woman may present with pruritus, a lump, or a flat lesion, or may be relatively asymptomatic. Some risk factors include chronic vulvar inflammation, immunosuppression from chronic steroid use, smoking, diabetes, history of sexually transmitted infections (STIs) such as human papilloma virus (HPV) or human immunodeficiency virus (HIV), and history of lower genital tract cancer.

Clinical appearance can vary greatly. Some lesions are scaly with a red background, some are flat and almost totally white or red, and others are irregularly pigmented and may be flat or raised. For these reasons, it is necessary to biopsy many vulvar lesions to confirm or rule out malignancy. Treatment usually involves surgery to remove the lesions and often the tissue surrounding the lesion, but the extent varies greatly depending on findings and degree of the lesion (Gould, Walker, & Mannel, 2003).

Cervicitis

Acute inflammation of the cervix is usually the result of infection from *Neisseria gonorrhoeae* or *Chlamydia trachomatis*. It may be caused by other organisms such as *Candida, Gardnerella vaginalis, Trichomonas,* herpes, staphylococci, or enterococci. Other causes may include use of intravaginal feminine hygiene products, frequent tampon use, frequent intercourse, or presence of a foreign body (such as an intrauterine device [IUD], contraceptive sponge, diaphragm, or tampon).

Symptoms often include a yellowish white vaginal discharge or copious purulent discharge that is sometimes malodorous, depending on the etiology. Dyspareunia is a common complaint, with postcoital bleeding, and occasional irregular vaginal bleeding. Sometimes there is a sense of pelvic heaviness and urinary symptoms such as urgency, frequency, and burning. Diagnosis and evaluation consists of a clinical pelvic examination, wet-mount smear, cultures, and a Pap smear. Treatment depends on the identified problem. It may include antibiotics to treat positive cultures (see Chapter 6 ∞), cryotherapy to treat some lesions of the cervix, removal of foreign bodies, and in some instances treatment of nonspecific inflammation with local medication (metronidazole gel or clindamycin cream).

Abnormal Pap Smear Results

Women tend to expect a normal Pap smear report but various abnormal findings are common. Notification of an abnormal result may cause significant anxiety in the woman. Therefore, results should be provided in a caring manner, with an accurate explanation of the findings, reassurance that early detection of a problem allows early intervention, and information about expected further evaluation, treatment, and follow-up. The woman should be encouraged to ask questions and to voice her concerns.

PAP SMEAR

The purpose of the Papanicolaou smear (**Pap smear**) is to screen for the presence of cellular abnormalities by obtaining a sample containing cells from the cervix and the endocervical canal. Precancerous and cancerous conditions, as well as atypical findings and inflammatory changes, can be identified by microscopic examination. Estimates suggest that, annually in the United States, about 50 million women have a Pap smear done. Of these women, approximately 7% (3.5 million) are diagnosed with an abnormal finding that requires follow-up (Wright, Cox, Massad et al., 2002).

Traditionally the test has been performed by preparing a Pap smear slide. However, the smear was often difficult to read because of obscuring factors such as blood, mucus, overlapping cells, and so forth. More recently, another test—the liquid-based medium Pap smear—was approved by the FDA. In this test, no slide is prepared; instead, the cervical cells are transferred directly to a vial of preservative fluid, thereby preserving the entire specimen. The specimen is sent to a laboratory where a special processor prepares a slide.

Liquid-based Pap smear preparations have become the method of choice for cervical cancer screening. These types of preparations allow for removal of debris from the sample, such as blood and mucus, thereby increasing the accuracy of the test. Additionally, these preparations allow for HPV screening and for some STI screening. The Pap smear is a screening tool. A definitive diagnosis of cervical cancer is made by studying tissue samples obtained by biopsies.

CLINICAL TIP

Pap Smear Preparation

Whenever you teach about pelvic examination and Pap smear, be certain that the woman understands that she should avoid having anything in her vagina for 24 hours before the examination—no intercourse, no tampons, no female hygiene products, and no douching—because this might interfere with the accuracy of the test. Specimens should not be obtained during menstruation or when visible cervicitis exists.

Currently, both the ACS and the American College of Obstetricians and Gynecologists (ACOG) recommend that all women begin having Pap smears when they reach the age of 18 or when they become sexually active, whichever comes first. ACOG recommends annual Pap smears thereafter. Alternatively, the ACS states that, following three consecutive negative Pap smears, the Pap smear may sometimes be done less frequently at the discretion of the caregiver. Less frequent Pap smears might be suggested, for example, for a woman with no history of STI or gynecologic cancer who is in a stable, monogamous relationship with a partner who is also monogamous and infection free. Some caregivers are reluctant to extend the time between Pap smears, however, because they worry that women may delay the test beyond the recommended time frames.

THE BETHESDA SYSTEM

The *Bethesda System* (Table 7–2) is a standardized method of reporting cytologic Pap smear findings. The most widely used

---

 Table 7–2   THE BETHESDA SYSTEM FOR CLASSIFYING PAP SMEARS

Specimen Type:

Indicate conventional smear (Pap smear) vs. liquid based vs. other

Specimen Adequacy

Satisfactory for evaluation *(describe presence or absence of endocervical/transformation zone component and any other quality indicators; e.g., partially obscuring blood inflammation, etc.)*

Unsatisfactory for evaluation. . . *(specify reason)*

   Specimen rejected/not processed *(specify reason)*

   Specimen processed and examined, but unsatisfactory for evaluation of epithelial abnormality because of (specify reason)

General Categorization (optional)

Negative for intraepithelial lesion or malignancy.

Epithelial cell abnormality. See interpretation/result *(specify 'squamous' or 'glandular' as appropriate).*

Other: See interpretation result *(e.g., endometrial cells in a woman greater than or equal to 40 years of age).*

Automated Review

If case examined by automated device, specify device and result.

Ancillary Testing

Provide a brief description of the test methods and report the result so that it is easily understood by the clinician.

Interpretation/Result

Negative for intraepithelial lesion or malignancy (when there is no cellular evidence of neoplasia, state this in the General Categorization above and/or in the Interpretation/Result section of the report, whether or not there are organisms or other nonneoplastic findings)

   ORGANISMS:

      Trichomonas vaginalis

      Fungal organisms morphologically consistent with *Candida* spp.

      Shift in flora suggestive of bacterial vaginosis.

      Bacteria morphologically consistent with *Actinomyces* spp.

      Cellular changes associated with herpes simplex virus.

   OTHER NONNEOPLASTIC FINDINGS (*Optional to report list not inclusive*).

Reactive cellular changes associated with

   —inflammation (includes typical repair)

   —radiation

   —intrauterine contraceptive device (IUD)

Glandular cells status posthysterectomy

Atrophy

Other

Endometrial cells (in a woman greater than or equal to 40 years of age) (Specify if negative for squamous intraepithelial lesion)

Epithelial Cell Abnormalities
   SQUAMOUS CELL

   Atypical squamous cells

      —of undetermined significance (ASC-US)

      —cannot exclude HSIL (ASC-H)

   Low-grade squamous intraepithelial lesion (LSIL)

      —encompassing HPV/mild dysplasia/CIN-1

   High-grade squamous intraepithelial lesion (HSIL)

      —encompassing: moderate and severe dysplasia CIS/CIN-2 and CIN-3

      —with features suspicious for invasion (*if invasion is suspected*)

      Squamous cell carcinoma

GLANDULAR CELL

   Atypical

      —endocervical cells (*NOS or specify in comments*)

      —endometrial cells (*NOS or specify in comments*)

      —glandular cells (*NOS or specify in comments*)

   Atypical

      —endocervical cells, favor neoplastic

      —glandular cells, favor neoplastic

   Endocervical adenocarcinoma in situ

   Adenocarcinoma

      —endocervical

      —endometrial

      —extrauterine

      —not otherwise specified (NOS)

Other Malignant Neoplasms (specify)

Educational Notes and Suggestions (optional)

Suggestions should be concise and consistent with clinical follow-up guidelines published by professional organizations (references to relevant publications may be included).

SOURCE: Courtesy of National Cancer Institute.

method system in the United States for reporting Pap smear results, it provides a uniform format and classification of terminology based on current understanding of cervical disease.

Cervical Abnormalities

Cervical cancer is the sixth most common cancer in women in the United States, after lung, breast, colorectum, endometrium, and ovary (Bristow, 2003). However, 50 years ago cervical cancer was the leading type of cancer in women. Since the use of Pap smear screening, in the United States and other countries that have a system of Pap smear screening, the incidence of and mortality due to cervical cancer have decreased dramatically. Nevertheless, worldwide cervical cancer remains the most common cancer among women.

Cervical cancer is considered a preventable disease because it is slow-growing, has a lengthy preinvasive state, has inexpensive and available screening programs, and has effective treatment approaches for preinvasive lesions. Unfortunately, several subgroups of women in the United States have never been screened or are not screened at regular intervals. One half of women with newly diagnosed cervical cancer have never had a Pap smear, and 10% have not had a Pap smear in the last 5 years (Bristow, 2003).

Factors that place a woman at high risk for cervical cancer include:

- Coitus at an early age (first intercourse before 16 years of age increases the risk of cervical cancer twofold)
- History of multiple sexual partners
- Sex partner with a history of numerous sexual partners
- Exposure to STIs
- History of HPV infection
- History of immunosuppressive therapy (chemotherapy) or immunocompromised state (HIV)
- Long-term oral contraceptive use (greater than 5 years)
- Smoking
- Antenatal exposure to diethylstilbestrol (DES)
- History of dysplasia

A growing body of evidence has developed linking HPV infection with cervical dysplasia and carcinoma. As discussed in Chapter 6 ∞, over 120 different types of HPV have been identified; 30 types are known to infect the genital tract. To date, 11 specific types of HPV strains are considered intermediate risk for high-grade cervical dysplasia and cervical cancer while two strains (HPV types 16 and 18) are strongly associated with those disorders (Scheinfeld & Lehman, 2006). Recently a vaccine has been approved by the FDA that has been shown to be effective in preventing HPV-16 and HPV-18–related moderate and high-grade cervical intraepithelial neoplasia.

Several years ago I was treated for HPV—I got the infection from my husband—and seemed to be doing well. But now I've had some abnormal Pap smears and my doctor is talking about doing a LEEP procedure. I was a virgin when I got married but my husband wasn't. I've done a lot of reading and I know how common HPV is, so I guess I can't be too hard on the guy. Still I have to admit that I feel a little nudge of resentment—I'm the one with problems. He is symptom free.

The 2001 Bethesda System (Solomon et al., 2002) identifies three categories for premalignant squamous cell lesions: atypical squamous cells (ASC), low-grade squamous intraepithelial lesion (LSIL), and high-grade squamous intraepithelial lesion (HSIL), as well as squamous cell carcinoma (see Table 7–2). The focus of the Pap smear is on the detection of high-grade cervical disease, especially *cervical intraepithelial neoplasia* (CIN). CIN refers to a lesion that may progress to invasive carcinoma (cancer). It is synonymous with the term *dysplasia*. To further support this objective, the ASC category is subdivided into two qualifiers that recognize the importance of detecting HSIL:

- Atypical squamous cells of undetermined significance (ASC-US)
- Atypical squamous cells—cannot exclude HSIL (ASC-H)

The ASC-US category acknowledges equivocal results. This is considered essential because a large number of women with CIN are identified during a work-up for an equivocal finding (Solomon et al., 2002).

Evaluation of Abnormal Cytology

Evaluation of an abnormal Pap smear finding varies. If the results of a Pap smear indicate the presence of an infection other than HPV, the woman should be reassessed with a repeat Pap after receiving appropriate treatment for the infection (CDC, 2002).

The following points summarize the primary guidelines developed by the 2001 Consensus Conference (Wright et al., 2002) for managing ASC-US, ASC-H, LSIL, and HSIL:

- Women with ASC-US can be treated in one of three ways: (a) immediate referral for colposcopy; (b) repeat the Pap at 4- to 6-month intervals until two negative results are obtained with referral for colposcopy if the repeat Pap shows ASC or higher; or (c) testing for HPV infection with referral for colposcopy if the testing reveals a high-risk strain of HPV. If the HPV testing is negative, the woman should have a repeat Pap in 12 months.
- Women with ASC-H are at greater risk for CIN than women with ASC-US and should be referred directly for colposcopy.
- Women with either LSIL or HSIL are also referred directly to colposcopy. (Previously LSIL was managed with repeat Paps but this approach is no longer recommended because of the risk of CIN, the likelihood that the repeat Pap would continue to be abnormal, and the risk that women would not return for follow-up multiple times.)

Based on the results of the colposcopy, of endocervical curettage of the tissue, and of biopsy if performed, further treatment may be indicated or follow-up with repeat Pap smears may be recommended. These tests are discussed next.

Colposcopy, the direct, detailed visualization and examination of the cervix, is done in most gynecologic offices. A speculum is placed in the vagina and the cervix is isolated. A 3%

acetic acid solution applied on the cervix causes the abnormal epithelial cells to take on a characteristic white appearance. The colposcope, with its bright light and various color filters, provides a 6 to 40 times magnification of the cervical tissues. Lesions or other abnormalities are identified and documented, and directed biopsies can be obtained at this time, if indicated. Sometimes, the biopsy itself can be therapeutic as well as diagnostic if the entire lesion can be removed.

Endocervical curettage (ECC) may also be done at this time to evaluate for extension into the cervical canal. This involves a scraping of the endocervix from the internal os to the external os to obtain endocervical cells for cytology. Histologic evaluation of tissue biopsies and ECC samples is necessary for a definitive diagnosis.

The woman may experience moderate to severe cramplike pains during and after the biopsy and/or ECC. To help alleviate this discomfort, nurses can advise women to premedicate with 600 mg ibuprofen about 30 minutes before the procedure. A small amount of bleeding, initially bright red and then becoming darker, is normal for up to 2 weeks. Bleeding as heavy as a menstrual period is not normal and should be reported to the woman's care provider.

Surgical Treatment for Abnormal Cytology

Premalignant (precancerous) and malignant (cancerous) lesions are often treated with surgical procedures, varying from simple biopsy of the cervix to radical surgery of the pelvic organs, depending on the diagnosis and extent of the disease. A diagnosis of cancer can only be made after a pathologic evaluation of tissue obtained via biopsy. The goals of management are to exclude the presence of invasive cancer, to determine the extent and distribution of noninvasive cancer, and to provide appropriate treatment.

The treatment of cervical cancer depends on the stage of the disease, which is determined by the extent of its spread to other tissues or structures. Surgical treatment of cervical cancer may include a total abdominal hysterectomy (TAH), bilateral salpingo-oophorectomy (BSO), and bilateral lymphadenectomy. It may also include radiation therapy and chemotherapy.

LOOP ELECTROSURGICAL EXCISION PROCEDURE

Loop electrosurgical excision procedure (LEEP) can be used to treat cervical, vaginal, and vulvar intraepithelial neoplasia. When an abnormal Pap smear and a colposcopic evaluation indicate a premalignant lesion, a small electrically hot wire loop can be used to excise the entire lesion, squamocolumnar junction, and transformation zone. The cutting effect is created by a steam envelope that develops between the wire loop and the water-laden tissue. This procedure can be performed on an outpatient basis, often in the gynecologic office, under local anesthesia. Complications following LEEP are usually minimal, and it is virtually painless and bloodless. The woman can expect some slight bleeding, and possibly a malodorous dark brown discharge for 1 to 2 weeks after the procedure. The woman needs to know that moderate to heavy bleeding would be abnormal and should be reported to her care provider.

CRYOSURGERY

Cryosurgery is used to treat women with a small ectocervical lesion who have a negative ECC and no endocervical gland involvement. A double freezing method is advocated, using nitrous oxide or carbon dioxide to freeze the tissue below $-20°C$ $(-4°F)$, resulting in tissue destruction and necrosis. Although cryosurgery is less widely used since the development of LEEP, it is less expensive, produces similar results, and can easily be done in a gynecologic office or clinic without anesthesia. The woman may experience some mild cramping and should be told to expect a thin, watery, persistent, and sometimes heavy vaginal discharge for up to several weeks as the frozen tissue is sloughed. She should avoid tampon use and sexual intercourse while the discharge is present to minimize further damage to the cervix.

LASER THERAPY

The carbon dioxide (CO_2) laser is used to treat cervical, vaginal, and vulvar intraepithelial lesions. The laser is used when all boundaries of the lesion are visible on colposcopy and when the ECC is negative. The invisible, highly concentrated beam is absorbed by water in the tissues, elevating the temperature in the tissues to above 100C (212F). The targeted tissue "boils" and the exploded cells are vaporized, leaving the normal tissue intact. Laser treatment can be done in outpatient or office settings without anesthesia. The woman may experience mild cramping and a slight discharge for 5 to 7 days; however, bleeding is minimal. She should avoid tampon use, intercourse, and douching for 2 weeks; complete healing may take up to 12 weeks. In many clinical settings, laser therapy has become less common with the advent and effective use of LEEP.

CONIZATION

A cold knife *conization* of the cervix (also known as a "cone") is most commonly performed when the entire lesion cannot be visualized by colposcopic examination or when there is a positive ECC sampling. In this procedure, a cone-shaped section of cervical tissue is excised. The width and depth of the tissue removed varies depending on the extent of the lesion. A large amount of normal tissue is removed, as well as the abnormal tissue, and this procedure can often be diagnostic as well as therapeutic if the entire lesion is excised. Conization is usually done under general anesthesia with the woman in a lithotomy position (Sheets, 2003). Immediate postoperative risks include infection and hemorrhage; long-term risks include spontaneous abortion, incompetent cervix, or preterm labor with future pregnancies. A prolonged or profuse menstrual period may occur in two or three cycles following the procedure. Conization is used less frequently today because of the availability of LEEP.

CARE OF THE WOMAN WITH TOXIC SHOCK SYNDROME

Although **toxic shock syndrome (TSS)** has been reported in children, postmenopausal women, and men, it is primarily a disease of women in their reproductive years, especially women at or near menses or during the postpartum period. In most cases, the causative organism is a strain of *Staphylococcus aureus*. The use of superabsorbent tampons has been widely related to an increased incidence of TSS. However, occluding the cervical os with a contraceptive device such as a diaphragm or cervical cap, especially if it is left in place for more than 48 hours, may also increase the risk of TSS.

Early diagnosis and treatment are important in preventing a fatal outcome. The most common signs of TSS include fever (often greater than 38.9C, or 102F); rash on the trunk initially followed by desquamation of the skin, especially the palms and soles, which usually occurs 1 to 2 weeks after the onset of symptoms; hypotension; and dizziness. Systemic symptoms often include vomiting, watery diarrhea, severe myalgia, and inflamed mucous membranes (oropharyngeal, conjunctival, or vaginal). Disorders of the central nervous system, including alterations in consciousness, disorientation, and coma, may also occur. Evidence of renal, hepatic, and hematologic involvement can be seen in abnormal laboratory findings, which reveal elevated blood urea nitrogen (BUN), creatinine, aspartate aminotransferase (AST), alanine aminotransferase (ALT), and total bilirubin, while platelets are often less than 100,000/mm^3.

Women with TSS are generally hospitalized and given supportive therapy, including intravenous (IV) fluids to maintain blood pressure. Severe cases may require renal dialysis, administration of vasopressors, and intubation. Penicillinase-resistant antibiotics, although of limited value during the acute phase, do help reduce the risk of recurrence from 30% to 50% (Eschenbach, 2003).

Two years ago a friend died of toxic shock syndrome. It happened so quickly. Within days she was on life support until the family had it turned off. Until that happened I was oblivious to the risk factors, especially leaving tampons in too long, one of my big offenses. I have changed that for myself and I am making it a point to tell other women about toxic shock and ways to prevent it. Such a senseless death!

NURSING CARE MANAGEMENT

Nurses play a major role in helping to educate women about ways to prevent the development of TSS. Women should understand the importance of avoiding prolonged use of tampons. They should change tampons every 3 to 6 hours, avoid using superabsorbent tampons, and never use more than one tampon at a time. Some women may choose to use other products, such as sanitary pads or minipads. The woman who chooses to continue using tampons may reduce her risk by alternating them with pads and avoiding overnight use of tampons.

Women who are postpartum should avoid the use of tampons for 6 to 8 weeks after childbirth. Women with a history of TSS should be advised of the risk of recurrence and should never use tampons. Women who use diaphragms or cervical caps should not leave them in place for prolonged periods and should not use them during the postpartum period or when they

are menstruating. Nurses can also help make women aware of the signs and symptoms of TSS so that they can seek treatment promptly if symptoms occur.

Abnormal Uterine Bleeding

During the many years of a woman's reproductive period, she is likely to experience some form of abnormal uterine bleeding. It may occur as spotting between periods, missing several cycles followed by a heavy bleed, or menses that occur every 2 to 3 months. Heavy, unpredictable menstrual periods can cause a woman to experience fatigue, anemia, and embarrassment. Abnormal bleeding may be a symptom that accompanies infertility.

Abnormal uterine bleeding (AUB) is a common gynecologic problem. Estimates suggest that it may account for 20% of visits to women's healthcare providers and 25% of gynecologic surgeries (Bradley, 2005). AUB, with or without ovulation, that is caused by organic problems is generally classified as either a systemic or reproductive disorder. Systemic diseases that cause AUB include thyroid dysfunction, coagulation disorders, and cirrhosis. AUB may also result from trauma including accidental injury, sexual abuse, or intercourse-related trauma. Diagnosticians often use the mnemonic PHIMIC (pregnancy, hormones, iatrogenic, mechanical, infection, and cancer) to help focus evaluation (London, 2003):

- *Pregnancy* including normal pregnancy, ectopic pregnancy, miscarriage, hydatidiform mole (see Chapter 20 ∞).
- *Hormonal disorders* can be classified as thyroid disorders, prolactin disorders, chronic anovulation (the most common cause), and coagulation disorders. Coagulation disorders, although relatively rare, most commonly occur in girls within the first year of their menstrual cycle and might include von Willebrand disease (the most common bleeding disorder in women [Bradley, 2005]), leukemia, aplastic anemia, and idiopathic thrombocytopenia purpura.
- *Iatrogenic causes* ("caregiver caused"; usually related to the effects of medications or treatment). Medications associated with AUB include heparin, coumadin, prednisone, tamoxifen, and Depo-Provera.
- *Mechanical causes* may include leiomyomata (fibroids), endometrial polyps, adenomyosis.
- *Infection* resulting in endocervicitis (often related to chlamydia or gonorrhea infection), herpes, or endometritis.
- *Cancer* including endometrial and cervical cancer.

Evaluation of AUB begins with a thorough history and physical examination including a careful pelvic exam and Pap smear. The diagnosis is made by excluding organic causes, specifically pregnancy, uterine or ovarian pathology, medications, or systemic disease. Based on the information gained, specific laboratory tests such as pregnancy test, liver and renal function tests, thyroid tests, coagulation studies, or prolactin levels may be indicated. Based on the woman's age and findings, other tests that may be indicated include transvaginal ultrasound, saline infusion sonography (SIS), hysteroscopy, MRI, and endometrial biopsy. Endometrial biopsy to rule out endometrial cancer is indicated for all women over age 35 (Bradley, 2005).

The goals of treatment are to control bleeding, prevent or treat anemia, prevent endometrial hyperplasia or cancer, and restore quality of life. Pharmacologic treatment for AUB varies depending on the woman's desire for pregnancy and whether she is premenopausal, perimenopausal, or postmenopausal. Combined oral contraceptives (COCs) are the most common treatment for women who are not actively trying to conceive. COCs help regulate cycles while also providing contraception. Other options include short-term, high-dose estrogen therapy, cyclic progesterone to regulate cycles in women with contraindications to estrogen therapy, Depo-Provera, danazol, gonadotropin-releasing hormone (GnRH) therapy, and the levonorgestrel intrauterine system (LNG-IUS) (see Chapter 5 ∞). If conservative measures are not effective, the woman and her provider may consider surgical interventions, such as myomectomy, uterine artery embolization, endometrial ablation, or hysterectomy (Bradley, 2005).

Dysfunctional uterine bleeding (DUB) is characterized by anovulatory cycles with AUB that does not have a demonstrable organic cause. Oligomenorrhea, polymenorrhea, menorrhagia, metrorrhagia, menometrorrhagia, and intermenstrual bleeding are all forms of DUB (see Chapter 4 ∞). DUB can occur at any age but is most common at either end of the reproductive age span. Adolescents account for 20% of DUB cases due to hypothalamic immaturity after menarche. Perimenopausal women account for 50% of cases due to waning ovarian function. The remaining cases occur among women of reproductive age, generally as a result of polycystic ovary syndrome, hyperprolactinemia, or hypothalamic dysfunction. It is typically treated medically. Surgical intervention is generally limited to cases in which medical therapy is contradicted or has failed.

Ovarian (Adnexal) Masses

An *adnexal mass* most commonly refers to an ovarian abnormality but it can also refer to masses found in the fallopian tubes, broad ligament, or bowel, or even a lateral mass of the uterus. Between 70% and 80% of ovarian masses are benign. More than 50% are functional cysts (cysts that develop from ovarian follicles, from the corpus luteum, or from the theca luteum) occurring most commonly in women 20 to 40 years of age. Functional cysts are rare in women who take oral contraceptives.

Ovarian cysts usually represent physiologic variations in the menstrual cycle. Nearly all perimenopausal women have ovarian cysts, and about 15% of postmenopausal women have them. Dermoid cysts (cystic teratomas) comprise 10% of all benign ovarian masses. Cartilage, bone, teeth, skin, or hair can be observed in these cysts. Endometriomas, or "chocolate cysts," are another common type of ovarian mass.

No relationship exists between benign ovarian masses and ovarian cancer. Unfortunately, at present, no adequate techniques exist for ovarian cancer screening. Some risk factors for ovarian cancer include increased age (mean age is 59), history of treatment with fertility drugs, and early menarche or late menopause. Asbestos and talc exposure may be causative agents. The risk of ovarian cancer is slightly increased in women with family members diagnosed with the disease, but fewer than 10% of women with ovarian cancer have a positive family history (Le, 2003).

Family transmission and increased lifetime risk of ovarian cancer is most commonly related to hereditary breast-ovarian cancer, which is associated with a mutation in specific genes (BRCA1 and BRCA2 genes). It is now possible to identify many of these mutations. If a mutation of BRCA1 is found, for example, estimates suggest that a woman's lifetime risk of ovarian cancer is between 28% and 44%. In addition, in women with these mutations, ovarian cancer tends to develop at an earlier age. Thus increased screening is recommended for women with these mutations. This includes the measurement of CA-125 and transvaginal ultrasounds beginning in the mid-20s (Le, 2003).

In reality, ovarian cancer is the most fatal of all cancers in women because it is difficult to diagnose and often has spread throughout the pelvis before it is detected. Symptoms are often vague and nonspecific and may include abdominal swelling and heaviness or bloating, pelvic pressure, mild constipation, and increased abdominal girth.

A woman with an ovarian mass may be asymptomatic; the mass may be noted on a routine pelvic examination. She may experience a sensation of fullness or cramping in the lower abdomen (often unilateral), dyspareunia, irregular bleeding, or delayed menstruation.

Diagnosis is made on the basis of a palpable mass, with or without tenderness, and other related symptoms. Radiography or ultrasonography may be used to assist or confirm the diagnosis.

The woman is frequently kept under observation for a month or two because most cysts will resolve on their own and are harmless. Oral contraceptives may be prescribed for 1 to 2 months to suppress ovarian function. If this regimen is effective, a repeat pelvic examination should yield normal findings. If the mass is still present after 60 days of observation and oral contraceptive therapy, a diagnostic laparoscopy or laparotomy may be considered. Tubal or ovarian lesions, ectopic pregnancy, cancer, infection, or appendicitis also must be ruled out before a diagnosis can be confirmed.

Surgery is not always necessary but will be considered if the mass is larger than 6 to 7 cm in circumference; if the woman is over 40 years of age with an adnexal mass, a persistent mass, or continuous pain; or if the woman is taking oral contraceptives. Surgical exploration is also indicated when a palpable mass is found in an infant, a young girl, or a postmenopausal woman. Women may need clear explanations about why the initial therapy is observation. A discussion of the origin and resolution of ovarian cysts may clarify this treatment plan. If a surgical treatment removes or impairs the function of one ovary, the woman needs to be assured that the remaining ovary can be expected to take over ovarian functioning and that pregnancy is still possible.

Women who are taking oral contraceptives should be informed of their preventive effect against ovarian masses.

Uterine Masses

Endometrial polyps are pedunculated (growing on a stalk) overgrowths of the endometrium. They may develop as soft tumors, composed of hyperplastic endometrium, and they can occur as single or multiple growths. Polyps are common, occurring in women between the ages of 12 and 81, and often they are identified incidentally during pelvic ultrasound, curettage, or hysterectomy. Polyps are benign, but they can coexist with carcinoma of the endometrium in about 10% of postmenopausal women. Treatment is curettage, or hysteroscopy and removal, in the postmenopausal woman or if bleeding persists after diagnosis.

Fibroid tumors, or *leiomyomas,* are among the most common benign disease entities in women and are the most common reason for gynecologic surgery. Between 20% and 50% of women develop leiomyomas by 40 years of age. The potential for cancer is minimal. Leiomyomas are more common in women of African heritage.

Fibroid tumors develop when smooth muscle cells are present in whorls and arise from uterine muscles and connective tissue. The size varies from 1 to 2 cm to the size of a 12- to 14-week fetus. Frequently the woman is asymptomatic. Lower abdominal pain, fullness or pressure, menorrhagia, metrorrhagia, or increased dysmenorrhea may occur, particularly with large leiomyomas. As a result, anemia may develop. Ultrasonography revealing masses or nodules can assist and confirm the diagnosis. Leiomyoma is also considered a possible diagnosis when masses or nodules involving the uterus are palpated on a pelvic examination.

The majority of these masses require no treatment and will shrink after menopause. Close observation for symptoms or an increase in size of the uterus or the masses may be the only management most women will require. Routine pelvic examinations every 3 to 6 months are recommended unless new symptoms appear.

If a woman notices symptoms, or pelvic examination reveals that the mass is increasing in size, surgery is generally recommended. Myomectomy is indicated if future childbearing is a consideration. Otherwise, a hysterectomy is generally performed. The surgical approach is individualized and may be vaginal, abdominal, or laproscopically assisted. There are no medications or therapies to prevent fibroids. The use of GnRH agonists can decrease the volume of the leiomyoma by 35% to 50%, but most fibroids quickly return to pretreatment size when the GnRH agonist is discontinued. The main goal of medical suppression with GnRH agonists is to stop excessive vaginal bleeding before surgery (Haney, 2003). If a myomectomy is performed, a woman can preserve her fertility. However, if there is a uterine incision, subsequent children would be born by cesarean.

Endometrial cancer, the most common female genital tract cancer, has a high rate of cure if detected early. Although the overall incidence is lower in black women than in white women, black women have a poorer survival rate; it is not clear whether this is related to lack of access to care, delayed treatment, or a higher likelihood that the cancer has more serious characteris-

tics (American College of Obstetricians and Gynecologists [ACOG], 2005). Risk factors include white race; obesity; nulliparity; history of infertility or menstrual irregularities; history of diabetes, hypertension, thyroid disease, or gallbladder disease; long-term use of unopposed estrogen; early menarche or late menopause; and use of tamoxifen (ACOG, 2005).

The majority of endometrial cancer occurs in postmenopausal women. The hallmark sign is vaginal bleeding in postmenopausal women not treated with HRT. Diagnosis is made occasionally by Pap smear, by endometrial biopsy, by transvaginal ultrasound, or by posthysterectomy pathologic examination of the uterus. Exploratory laparotomy is performed to establish the stage of the cancer. Uterine tissues are biopsied, lymph nodes are sampled, and peritoneal washings are collected for cytology.

Once staging of the cancer is completed, a plan of treatment is proposed. Treatment for all stages of endometrial cancer involves TAH and BSO. This may be adequate treatment for stage I disease without lymph node involvement. Women with stage II may undergo TAH and BSO and extensive dissection of the lymph nodes. Stage III or IV cancer is extrauterine. Therapy includes all of the previously listed surgical treatment plus therapeutic pelvic radiation; postoperatively hormone therapy with progestins or systemic chemotherapy may also be used (ACOG, 2005).

NURSING CARE MANAGEMENT

Only nurses with special training perform pelvic examinations and Pap smears. In most cases, nursing assessment is directed toward evaluating the woman's understanding of the findings and their implications and her psychosocial response.

The woman needs accurate information on the etiology of the disorder, its symptoms, and treatment options. She should be encouraged to report symptoms and keep appointments for follow-up examination and evaluation. The woman needs realistic reassurance if her condition is benign; she may require counseling and effective emotional support if a malignancy is likely. If the management plan includes surgery, she may need the nurse's support in obtaining a second opinion and making her decision. The nurse can also provide information on available community resources including support groups.

CARE OF THE WOMAN WITH ENDOMETRIOSIS

Endometriosis is a condition characterized by the presence of endometrial tissue outside the uterine cavity. The exact prevalence of endometriosis is unknown but it is found in 12% to 32% of reproductive-age women who undergo laparoscopy to determine the cause of pelvic pain (Schenken, 2003). Endometriosis has been found almost everywhere in the body, including the vagina, lungs, cervix, central nervous system, and gastrointestinal tract. The most common location, however, is the pelvis. This tissue responds to the hormonal changes of the menstrual cycle and bleeds in a cyclic fashion. The bleeding results in inflammation, scarring of the peritoneum, and formation of adhesions.

Endometriosis may occur at any age after puberty, although it is most commonly diagnosed in women between ages 20 and 45 and is rare in postmenopausal women. The exact cause of endometriosis is unknown. Proposed causative factors include retrograde menstrual flow of the endometrium, physiologic disruption following gynecologic surgery or cesarean birth, hereditary tendency, and a possible immunologic defect (Schenken, 2003). Endometriosis is thought to be an autoimmune condition. It is associated with an increased risk of breast cancer, ovarian cancer, melanoma, and non-Hodgkin's lymphoma, as well as hypothyroidism, fibromyalgia, chronic fatigue syndrome, autoimmune diseases, allergies, and asthma (Sinaii, Cleary, Ballweg et al., 2002).

Although endometriosis can be asymptomatic, the most common symptom of endometriosis is pelvic pain, which is often dull or cramping although it can be debilitating. Usually the pain is related to menstruation and is thought to be dysmenorrhea by the affected woman. **Dyspareunia** (painful intercourse) and abnormal uterine bleeding are other common signs. The condition is often diagnosed when the woman seeks evaluation for infertility. Bimanual examination may reveal a fixed, tender, retroverted uterus and palpable nodules in the cul-de-sac. Diagnosis is confirmed by laparoscopy.

Treatment may be medical or surgical, or a combination of the two. In women with minimal disease and symptoms, treatment includes observation, analgesics, and nonsteroidal anti-inflammatory drugs (NSAIDs). Medical therapy aims at interrupting cyclic ovarian hormone production.

The woman who desires pregnancy and has been unsuccessful in her attempts to conceive is often treated for a designated period of time with a medication that suppresses estrogen synthesis. This causes an atrophy of endometrial implants. Medications commonly used to treat endometriosis include oral contraceptives, progestins, antiprogestins, and GnRH analogs.

- COCs create a "pseudopregnancy" state that leads to decreased menstrual bleeding and possible amenorrhea. Treatment with COCs is cost effective and can relieve dysmenorrhea and pelvic pain.

- Progestins such as medroxyprogesterone acetate (MPA) exert an antiendometriotic effect and ultimate atrophy. The medication is administered intramuscularly every 3 months, and the effectiveness of the treatment is evaluated every 3 to 6 months. Side effects may include nausea, weight gain, fluid retention, and breakthrough bleeding.

- The antiprogestin danazol is sometimes used to treat endometriosis. It suppresses GnRH and has high androgen and low estrogen effects that do not support the growth of the endometrium. It suppresses ovulation and causes amenorrhea. In effect, danazol and the other GnRH analogs (discussed next) induce a "pseudomenopausal" state. Danazol does have some significant side effects, including hirsutism, vaginal bleeding, acne, oily skin, weight gain,

reduced libido, voice changes and hoarseness, clitoral enlargement, and decreased breast size.

- GnRH analogs such as nafarelin acetate (given as a metered nasal spray twice daily) and leuprolide acetate (Lupron, given once a month as an intramuscular injection), are gaining popularity because many women tolerate them better than danazol and their results in treating endometriosis are comparable. GnRH analogs suppress the menstrual cycle through estrogen antagonism. This may result in the hypoestrogen side effects of hot flashes, vaginal dryness, headache, breast reduction, and loss of bone density.

Surgical treatment may be conservative (laparoscopy) or definitive (hysterectomy). It is conservative when the uterus and as much of the ovaries as possible are preserved. During the laparoscopic examination, the physician may surgically resect any visible implants of endometrial tissue, taking care to avoid damaging any organs. Laser vaporization can be used for all but the deepest implants. This allows for more exact removal of tissue, less damage of adjacent tissue, and decreased bleeding. If the woman is experiencing severe dyspareunia or dysmenorrhea, the surgeon may perform a presacral neurectomy. In advanced cases in which childbearing is not an issue, treatment may be a hysterectomy with bilateral salpingo-oophorectomy (removal of the uterus, fallopian tubes, and ovaries).

NURSING CARE MANAGEMENT
Nursing Assessment and Diagnosis

The nurse should be aware of the common symptoms of endometriosis and elicit an accurate history if a woman mentions these symptoms. If a woman is being treated for endometriosis, the nurse should assess the woman's understanding of the condition, its implications, and the treatment alternatives.

Nursing diagnoses that may apply to a woman with endometriosis include the following:

- *Acute Pain* related to peritoneal irritation secondary to endometriosis
- *Compromised Family Coping* related to depression secondary to infertility

Nursing Plan and Implementation

The nurse can be available to explain the condition, its symptoms, treatment alternatives, and prognosis. The nurse can help the woman evaluate treatment options and make appropriate choices. If the woman begins taking medication, the nurse can review the dosage, schedule, possible side effects, and any warning signs. Women are often advised to avoid delaying pregnancy because of the risk of infertility. The woman may wish to discuss the implications of this decision on her life choices, relationship with her partner, and personal preferences. The nurse can be a nonjudgmental listener and help the woman consider her options. In addition, the nurse can refer the woman to the Endometriosis Association. This group, founded in 1980, offers women support and education.

EVIDENCE-BASED PRACTICE

PAIN MANAGEMENT FOR WOMEN WITH ENDOMETRIOSIS

Clinical Question

What are the most effective pain management strategies for women with pelvic pain associated with endometriosis?

The Evidence

A substantial number of systematic reviews related to managing the pain of endometriosis have been done and at least two descriptive studies of the qualitative experience of pelvic pain. Four reviews explored the effects of various medications, including progestagens, danazol (an androgenic), nonsteroidal anti-inflammatory drugs (NSAIDs), and oral contraceptives. There were four randomized controlled trials of danazol and one trial each of the other medications. One review described the results of trials of laparoscopic surgery. Two qualitative studies explored the meaning of living with endometriosis pain.

What Is Effective?

Laparoscopic surgery is effective in the long-term relief of moderate to severe pelvic pain from endometriosis. Danazol and progestagen were both more effective than placebo. The experience of endometrial pain was consistent among the qualitative studies. The dominant feature of the qualitative studies was the experience of severe and chronic pain impacting all aspects of life. Analysis of this overarching theme resulted in the identification of subthemes including symptoms of pain, controlling pain, dyspareunia, and impact on social relationships. These experiences, coupled with the limited effectiveness of treatments, affected relationships with partners and family, work, and sexual relationships.

What Is Unclear?

Only one study each was available for the analysis of oral contraceptives and NSAIDs, but neither demonstrated effectiveness over placebo. The studies had samples that were quite small, so these findings cannot be considered conclusive evidence that these less expensive alternatives are not helpful. More research is needed on these treatment options.

Best Practice

Medical or surgical management of moderate and severe pain associated with endometriosis is the most effective in the long term. Specifically androgenic and progestagenic drugs are most effective in relieving pain. These drugs had side effects that were, in some cases, poorly tolerated by the women. Androgenic changes and mood affect were the most commonly reported undesirable side effects. Laparoscopic surgical removal of tissue is also effective and has few long-term adverse effects. Nurses can help women who are affected by endometriosis pain understand their options and make informed treatments about pain management.

Critical Thinking

How can the nurse design counseling plans that help women make informed decisions about pain management associated with endometriosis?

REFERENCES: Allen, C., Hopewell, S., & Prentice, A. (2006). Non-steroidal anti-inflammatory drugs for pain in women with endometriosis. *The Cochrane Database of Systematic Reviews(1)*.

Denny, E. (2004). Women's experience of endometriosis. *Journal of Advanced Nursing, 46*(6), 641–648.

Huntington, A., & Gilmour, J. (2005). A life shaped by pain: Women and endometriosis. *Journal of Clinical Nursing, 14*(9), 1124–1132.

Jacobson, T., Barlow, D., Garry, R., & Koninckx, P. (2006). Laparoscopic surgery for pelvic pain associated with endometriosis. *The Cochrane Database of Systematic Reviews(1)*.

Prentice, A., Deary, A., & Bland, E. (2006). Progestagens and anti-progestagens for pain associated with endometriosis. *The Cochrane Database of Systematic Reviews(1)*.

Evaluation

Expected outcomes of nursing care include the following:

- The woman is able to discuss her condition, its implications for fertility, and her treatment options.
- After considering the alternatives, the woman chooses appropriate treatment options.

CARE OF THE WOMAN WITH POLYCYSTIC OVARIAN SYNDROME

Many women struggle with the short-term and long-term effects of a condition known as **polycystic ovarian syndrome,** or **PCOS.** This complex syndrome, with no clear etiology, is the most common endocrine disorder affecting women of reproductive age, with a suggested incidence of 3.5% to 11.2% of women (Tsilchorozidou, Overton, & Conway, 2004). The true incidence of PCOS may well be underestimated because of the broad range of signs, symptoms, and lifetime effects that may never be labeled PCOS.

As early as 1921, Achard and Thiers cited the link between insulin and elevated androgens in the medical literature in their description of a "bearded woman with diabetes." In 1935, Stein and Leventhal described a triad of symptoms in some women— obesity, hirsutism, and amenorrhea—and additionally, pathologic ovarian findings. As ultrasound techniques became more refined in the 1970s and 1980s, the ability to see polycystic ovaries more clearly further complicated the diagnostic process. Over time, it became evident that not all women with PCOS had polycystic ovaries, and it became recognized that many "normal" women did have polycystic ovaries noted by ultrasound. For these reasons, the term "polycystic ovarian syndrome" is a bit misleading because PCOS is a complex disorder with many confounding variables and multisystem effects.

Signs and Symptoms of PCOS

The most common clinical signs and symptoms of PCOS include menstrual dysfunction, androgen excess, obesity, hyperinsulinemia, and infertility.

Menstrual dysfunction. Irregular menses, including total absence of periods (amenorrhea), intermittent or infrequent periods (oligomenorrhea), and very frequent heavy periods (menorrhagia), are the hallmark of PCOS (Jackson, 2004/2005). In women of reproductive age, 85% to 90% of oligomenorrhea and 30% to 40% of amenorrhea are attributed to PCOS. Anovulation is usually a chronic problem with PCOS, but it often presents as a long history of menstrual irregularities. However, some women with PCOS can have regular periods and still be chronically anovulatory.

Hyperandrogenism. Women with PCOS consistently have elevated serum androgen levels, specifically testosterone and androsterone. These elevated androgen levels often lead to clinical manifestations such as acne, alopecia (male-patterned hair loss), hirsutism, deepening voice, increased muscle mass, and menstrual irregularities. Estimates suggest that 70% to 80% of women with PCOS have hirsutism (Hill, 2003). Generally, PCOS-related hirsutism is found on the upper lip, chin, and cheeks; between the breasts and around the areola of the breast; and on the inner thighs, lower back, and intergluteal area. Additionally, the higher levels of circulating androgens stimulate sebaceous gland cell activity, increasing the incidence of PCOS-related acne.

Obesity. About 50% of women with PCOS are clinically obese (Hill, 2003). In PCOS women who struggle with obesity, it is generally of the android type, with an increased hip-to-waist ratio.

PCOS-related obesity is consistent with increased androgen levels, glucose intolerance, insulin resistance, and abnormal lipoprotein profiles. Unfortunately, women with PCOS obesity have difficulty losing weight, which is probably related to hyperinsulinemia and carbohydrate cravings.

Hyperinsulinemia. Women with PCOS are insulin resistant. This insulin resistance, characterized by the failure of insulin to enter the cells appropriately, leads to an increased level of circulating insulin. These high insulin levels coupled with obesity often seen with PCOS place these women at increased risk for impaired glucose tolerance and type 2 diabetes mellitus (Legro & Azziz, 2003).

Infertility. Nearly 75% of women who have been diagnosed with PCOS struggle with some degree of infertility related to anovulation, and obese women with PCOS have even higher rates of infertility (Hill, 2003). (See Chapter 12 ∞, Special Reproductive Concerns: Infertility and Genetics).

Diagnosis of PCOS

Endocrinologists and obstetrician/gynecologists have found it difficult to agree on diagnostic criteria for PCOS, and the diagnosis has become one of exclusion. If a woman presents with complaints of hirsutism, menstrual irregularities, acne, difficulty conceiving, and unexplained weight gain, several other disorders must be ruled out. Important disorders to consider include hyperthyroidism or hypothyroidism, congenital adrenal hyperplasia, Cushing's syndrome, hyperprolactinemia, and androgen-producing tumors. The diagnostic process is fourfold: history, physical examination, laboratory studies, and imaging (Table 7–3).

Table 7–3   DIAGNOSTIC PROCESS FOR PCOS

History:

- Medical history—onset, timing, duration of symptoms (acne, hirsutism, menstrual problems)
- Surgical history
- Menstrual history—frequency, duration, regularity of periods; perception of pain and amount of bleeding
- Medications history (some medications may cause hirsutism, acne, menstrual irregularities)
- Family history—close attention to diabetes, menstrual problems, hirsutism, infertility

Physical Examination:

- Blood pressure, weight, height, and calculation of body mass index (BMI)
- Waist-to-hip ratio—if greater than 0.72, abnormal, suggestive of android obesity
- Evaluate for signs of hyperandrogenism: acne, coarse hair in unlikely places for women (lip, chin, chest, back, abdomen, breasts), male-pattern hair loss, deep voice, and so on.
- Evaluate for signs of hyperinsulinemia: acanthosis nigricans (velvety dark skin changes of neck, axilla, medial thighs), skin tags of neck

NOTE: Findings of moon face and abdominal striae are not typical in PCOS but suggestive of Cushing's syndrome.

- Pelvic examination—evaluate size, shape, and location of uterus; evaluate ovaries

LABORATORY STUDIES: (remember, PCOS is diagnosis of exclusion, so tests should rule out other disorders)

- Pregnancy test—urine and quantitative serum β-human chorionic gonadotropin (β-hCG)
- Thyroid testing—initially thyroid-stimulating hormone (TSH)
- Prolactin level
- Two-hour glucose tolerance test (2-hr GTT)—to evaluate for type 2 diabetes
- Fasting insulin level
- Total testosterone level—to assess for androgen-producing ovarian tumor
- Dehydroepiandrosterone sulfate (DHEAS)—to assess for androgen-producing adrenal tumor
- Cholesterol and triglyceride levels—to assess risk for developing cardiovascular disease

Imaging:

- Many providers will include endovaginal ultrasound to evaluate the uterus and ovaries

NOTE: The finding of polycystic ovaries is not beneficial in diagnosing PCOS because 20% to 25% of normally ovulating women will have this finding, and 10% of women with PCOS will not have polycystic ovaries (Hill, 2003).

Clinical Therapy

Once the diagnosis of PCOS is made several options are available to the clinician for management. First, the goals for treatment should be established. These include decreasing the effects of hyperandrogenism (hirsutism, acne, etc.), restoring reproductive functioning for women desiring pregnancy, protecting the endometrium (increased risk for uterine cancer), and reducing long-term risks, specifically type 2 diabetes and cardiovascular disease.

If pregnancy is not an immediate goal, menstrual irregularities can be treated with a COC or cyclic progesterone. COCs help to regulate menstrual cycles; provide a balance between estrogen and progesterone, thereby protecting the endometrium and decreasing the risk of uterine cancer; and may improve acne by inhibiting ovarian androgen production (Jackson, 2004/2005). If pregnancy is an immediate goal then another option is the use of medications that improve insulin sensitivity and utilization.

Although no medications have been approved for the treatment of PCOS, the most common drug used to decrease circulating insulin is metformin (Glucophage®). Metformin inhibits glucose production in the liver and improves glucose uptake by fat and muscle cells. In the presence of better insulin levels and glucose metabolism, metformin thereby improves ovarian function, improves the degree of hyperandrogenism, restores normal ovulation in women with PCOS, and is associated with an improved ability to lose weight (Marshall, 2001). In addition, lifestyle changes should also be a major component in the treatment of PCOS. Modifications should include weight loss, regular exercise, balanced diet, and cessation of smoking.

Long-Term Implications

PCOS may increase a woman's risk for developing overt type 2 diabetes, dyslipidemia, hypertension, cardiovascular disease, endometrial cancer, breast cancer, and ovarian cancer. Additionally, and very importantly, the woman with PCOS may struggle with significant emotional responses to this chronic disorder. She will likely face, throughout her lifetime, issues related to body image, infertility, problematic menses, and depression.

NURSING CARE MANAGEMENT

The nurse plays a vital role in the identification, evaluation, management, and follow-up when caring for a woman with PCOS. Sometimes it is the nurse who puts the bigger picture together, especially in a community health setting where knowledge of PCOS may be lacking. Women with PCOS may present with complaints such as weight gain, excess hairiness, difficult periods, inability to get pregnant, depression, or expressing feelings like, "What is wrong with me? Why am I not normal like other women?"

Research suggests that the signs of PCOS, especially hirsutism, negatively impact women's feelings of femininity and lead them to invest considerable time and effort in hair removal treatments. Women with PCOS also feel a strong desire to "be normal," with regular menstrual cycles and a more feminine appearance, and struggle with a sense of guilt over their difficulty losing weight (Snyder, 2006). Nurses can help women recognize these feelings and find ways to develop a more positive body image. The nurse also has an important role in providing accurate information, education, and counseling for a woman diagnosed with PCOS. Finally, because the woman with PCOS is at great risk for developing long-term complications, the nurse can play a key role in follow-up and continuity of care throughout the life of a woman facing this challenging disorder.

CARE OF THE WOMAN WITH PELVIC RELAXATION

The muscles of the pelvic floor form a supportive layer that prevents the abdominal and pelvic organs from prolapsing or sagging downward into the genital tract. If these muscles are weakened or damaged, a variety of conditions may develop, including cystocele, rectocele, and uterine prolapse. Factors that may contribute to diminished pelvic floor muscle tone include damage to these structures related to childbirth, deterioration with age, metabolic diseases that affect muscle functioning, prolonged lifting, or even chronic coughing due to chronic pulmonary disease (DeLancey & Strohbehn, 2003).

Cystocele

A **cystocele** is the downward displacement of the bladder, which appears as a bulge in the anterior vaginal wall. Arbitrary classifications of mild to severe are frequently given. Genetic predisposition, childbearing, obesity, and increased age are factors that may contribute to cystocele.

Women with a cystocele commonly show symptoms of stress incontinence including loss of urine with coughing, sneezing, laughing, or sudden exertion. Vaginal fullness, a bulging out of the vaginal wall, or a dragging sensation may also be noticeable.

If pelvic relaxation is mild, Kegel exercises are helpful in restoring tone (see Chapter 16 ∞). The exercises involve contracting and relaxing the pubococcygeal muscle. Women have found these exercises helpful before and after childbirth in maintaining vaginal muscle tone. Estrogen may improve the condition of vaginal mucous membranes—especially in menopausal women. Vaginal pessaries or rings may be used if surgery is undesirable or impossible, or until surgery can be scheduled. Surgery may be considered for cystoceles considered moderate to severe.

The nurse can instruct the woman in the use of Kegel exercises. Providing information on causes and contributing factors and discussing possible alternative therapies greatly assists the woman.

Rectocele

A rectocele may develop if the posterior vaginal wall is weakened. The anterior wall of the rectum sags forward, ballooning

MEDIALINK   Application: Cystocele

into the vagina, pushing the weakened posterior wall of the vagina in front of it. When the woman strains to have a bowel movement, a pocket of rectum develops that traps stool, and constipation results. The harder a woman with rectocele strains, the larger the pocket becomes. To defecate, women with a rectocele may find it necessary to press the tissue between the vagina and rectum, which elevates the rectocele.

Diagnosis is based on history and physical examination. Decisions about treatment are based on the size of the prolapse, the presence and severity of symptoms, and the woman's individual situation including her overall health status. Surgery is often indicated.

Uterine Prolapse

Because the vagina and the uterus are attached to one another, prolapse of the uterine cervix is associated with prolapse of the upper vagina. The extent of the prolapse is determined by the location of the cervix in the vagina. In severe cases the cervix may prolapse below the vaginal introitus. The woman may report a "dragging" sensation in her groin and a backache over the sacrum, which is caused by pulling on the uterosacral ligaments. Typically these sensations are relieved when the woman lies down. Furthermore, with pronounced prolapse, exposure of the moist vaginal walls may cause a sensation of perineal wetness that the woman might mistake for incontinence. As with cystocele, conservative treatment includes the use of topical or systemic estrogen and vaginal pessaries. Surgery for uterine prolapse often involves hysterectomy and repair of the prolapsed vaginal walls.

CARE OF THE WOMAN REQUIRING GYNECOLOGIC SURGERY

Gynecologic surgeries—particularly hysterectomies—are some of the most common surgical procedures being done in the United States. Many new techniques have been developed for treating a variety of gynecologic and reproductive disorders, and controversy remains as to the high number of procedures being done annually. For these reasons, it is important for the woman considering medical or surgical management of a given gynecologic problem to be well informed.

There are many components to an informed decision to undergo reproductive tract surgery. Questions that should be addressed include, for example: What are the indications for having the surgery? What are the risks? What is the success rate? Are there other alternative therapies to try before proceeding to surgery? An explanation of the surgical procedure and the reasons it is recommended over other possible therapies should be given to the woman. Effects on childbearing ability and potential impact on sexual performance should be addressed, as well as effects on the general functioning of the body. A discussion of the risks and benefits should be presented, and the risks should include the common risks, the nonserious risks, the rare or unusual complications, and the risk of death.

The question of whether to seek a second opinion about the recommended treatment is somewhat controversial. In the case of elective surgery, different physicians may have very different opinions. A woman should be encouraged to consult other physicians when there is controversy about a treatment (as in the treatment of early cervical cancer) or when the surgeon is unknown to the woman. A specialist in gynecology is the preferred source for a second opinion. Some third-party payment plans require second opinions. The woman can analyze the information and discuss her concerns with the nurse or physician before signing a written consent acknowledging that the information has been given and authorizing the surgery.

Other concerns that may influence the decision to have reproductive surgery may be categorized as general concerns about surgery and specific concerns related to gynecologic surgery. General concerns may include:

- Fear of general anesthesia because of loss of control or fear of "not waking up"; fear of regional anesthesia because of possible postoperative problems and concern about being awake during surgery
- Fear of death or disability
- Concerns about limitation of normal functioning and dependency during recovery
- Financial coverage for hospitalization, and potential financial loss if it is necessary to take extensive time off from work
- Concerns about welfare of family members while undergoing surgery (such as child care, loss of wages, help with household work)

Specific concerns related to gynecologic surgery are related to the significance of the reproductive organs for the woman. Surgery to alter or remove reproductive organs may be perceived as a threat to self-concept.

Body image is affected whenever a body part is lost. The degree of mourning for that loss is related to the significance attached to it. Even though there is no outwardly apparent change with a hysterectomy and most other gynecologic procedures, the loss may be felt very strongly. Many women fear postoperative changes such as masculinization, weight gain, loss of sexuality, and permanent loss of the ability to have a child. Reproductive surgery may also be seen as a threat to femininity in any social or cultural group that emphasizes childbearing and motherhood.

Hysterectomy

Hysterectomy is the removal of the uterus. In the United States, approximately 650,000 hysterectomies are performed each year, making it the most common nonpregnancy-related surgical procedure that women in the United States undergo (Kim & Lee, 2001). Removal of the uterus through an abdominal incision is called a *total abdominal hysterectomy (TAH)* and removal of both fallopian tubes and ovaries is called a *bilateral salpingo-oophorectomy (BSO);* when both procedures are done at the same time it is termed a TAH-BSO. When the uterus is removed through the vagina it is termed a *total vaginal hysterectomy (TVH).*

RESEARCH IN PRACTICE

FROM HYSTERECTOMY TO HISTORICITY

What is this study about? Hysterectomy is the second most common major surgery, performed on one in three women by the age of 60. This surgical rate has remained essentially unchanged for the past 20 years. Hysterectomy is performed for a variety of reasons and affects women without respect to race, age, or socioeconomic status. Yet women's lived experience after hysterectomy has not been well documented and contradictory findings are reported in the literature. Many of the studies that do exist have a discernible negative stereotype of the experience. This study sought to describe the recovery experiences of women who underwent a hysterectomy for a noncancer-related condition.

How was this study done? This was a qualitative study using a phenomenological method. Data were analyzed from interviews with women at four intervals during 1 year post-hysterectomy. Participants were recruited from two hospitals in the south central United States. Sixty-five women were recruited into the study and provided data for the first three data collection periods. Seven women were lost to follow-up at the 1-year point, resulting in a total sample size of 58 women who completed all interviews. At each data point, women completed a semistructured interview that included questions about how the hysterectomy had affected their life; how they felt since the surgery; if they would change anything about the surgery; and what advice they would give other women considering a hysterectomy. Women were interviewed over the telephone, and the interviews were transcribed verbatim. Data were analyzed using a systematic process of descriptive content analysis.

What were the results of the study? Women identified four common elements of the recovery experience: physical symptoms, emotional well-being, activity levels, and decision making. Early in the healing process, physical symptoms and labile emotions char-

acterized the experience. As physical restrictions decreased and emotional lability diminished, the informants described feeling better than before the surgery. This happened commonly at 8 weeks' postsurgery. Most of the women were glad they had had the surgery, and the majority of emotional responses were positive. Concerns about having made the right decision to have the surgery diminished. By 6 months, physical healing occurred and activity levels were greater than before the surgery. Many of the women reported an improved quality of life. By 1 year postsurgery, most of the women had resolved the experience of recovery and the surgery was no longer of primary interest.

Consistent with this process, the authors identified four phases of recovery: measuring health; comparing the past with the present; renewal; and growth through healing. The authors' overarching theme of "from hysterectomy to historicity" refers to a process whereby an event of personal historical significance no longer influences daily life but becomes part of one's life experience.

What additional questions might I have? Were these women typical of all women who have hysterectomies? How did the authors control their bias in trying to find positive outcomes of hysterectomy?

How can I use this study? Healthcare providers must better understand the recovery process after hysterectomy if they are to provide adequate support for these women. This study can provide a framework for understanding the experiences of women who have a hysterectomy, and how these experiences change over time. Preoperative and early postoperative teaching plans can include a description of the recovery phases so women are aware of what to expect.

SOURCE: Linenberger, H., & Cohen, S. (2004). From hysterectomy to historicity. *Health Care for Women International, 25,* 349–357.

A common technique to perform this surgery is a laparoscopic-assisted vaginal hysterectomy (LAVH). In this technique, the surgeon inserts the laparoscope through an incision near the umbilicus and uses it to assist with visualization and dissection to facilitate vaginal removal of the uterus. The benefit is that the surgeon can achieve results similar to those of a TAH without a large abdominal incision. Theoretically the recovery time should be shorter as compared with a TAH. Some controversy exists because there is often added expense from increased time in the operating room and the risks associated with prolonged anesthesia exposure.

Hysterectomy is the usual treatment for several conditions, although there is no medical consensus about absolute indications. Abdominal hysterectomy is generally recommended for cancer of the cervix, endometrium, or ovary; large fibroids; severe endometriosis; chronic pelvic inflammatory disease (PID); and adenomyosis. TAH is preferred when malignancy is suspected or confirmed because the procedure allows exploration of the abdomen and pelvis to determine the degree and extent of involvement. This approach is also helpful when large uterine

masses are present, requiring a larger incision. Disadvantages include more scarring, more postoperative pain, slower recovery, and more problems with bowel function.

Vaginal hysterectomy is generally done for pelvic relaxation, abnormal uterine bleeding, or small fibroids. An anterior and posterior repair of the vaginal walls may also be performed during TVH. Sometimes this repair is done when weakened pelvic supports have displaced one or more of the pelvic organs (such as the urethra, bladder, or rectum), sometimes causing urinary incontinence, constipation, or defecation problems. Advantages include earlier ambulation, less postoperative pain, less anesthesia and operative time, less blood loss, no visible scar, and a shorter hospital stay. This approach is preferred for the elderly, obese, or debilitated woman who is a poor risk for abdominal surgery. The major disadvantage is increased risk of trauma to the bladder.

Removal of the ovaries at the time of hysterectomy remains controversial. In premenopausal women, without evidence of ovarian pathology, the ovaries are generally left to avoid forced surgical menopause. Because of the risk of ovarian cancer, some physicians recommend removal of ovaries in all women over 40 years old who undergo hysterectomy. Still others recommend removal of the ovaries in any woman with a family history of ovarian cancer. In any case, removal of the ovaries is not considered routine, and when a BSO is performed in a premenopausal woman, supplemental estrogen replacement therapy is recommended.

Dilation and Curettage

In the United States, dilation and curettage (D&C) is the most frequently performed minor gynecologic procedure. Indications for a D&C may be diagnostic or therapeutic. Diagnostic indications include evaluation for uterine malignancy, infertility evaluation, and investigation of DUB. Therapeutic indications include elective abortion, treatment of heavy bleeding, incomplete abortion, dysmenorrhea, and removal of polyps. Sometimes D&C is done after hysteroscopy, which is a procedure that allows visualization of the endometrial cavity and minor surgical procedures. Another procedure that can be done at the time of hysteroscopy is an endometrial ablation, which cauterizes endometrial tissue, preventing regeneration and further bleeding. This procedure is not recommended for women who desire pregnancy, and so a simple D&C may be more appropriate. All of these procedures can be done under general anesthesia, intravenous sedation, and/or regional anesthesia, and most are done as an outpatient procedure.

Uterine Ablation

Several newer techniques and instruments have been developed to treat DUB. One form of therapy gaining wider acceptance is *uterine ablation,* which is a procedure using a variety of specialized instruments to destroy the innermost layer of the endometrium. The instruments often involve some type of heat source, such as cautery or a balloon filled with hot water. In most cases, this procedure is done in a day-surgery setting, and it will often immediately follow a hysteroscopy/D&C, if these procedures confirm the diagnosis of simple endometrial hyperplasia. The success rate varies, depending on the device used and the experience of the operator of the device, but some manufacturers quote as high as a 75% success rate with uterine ablation.

Salpingectomy

The unilateral or bilateral removal of the fallopian tube is called a salpingectomy. Indications include diseases of the tubes, sepsis, malignancy, and ectopic pregnancy of the fallopian tube. Salpingectomy for an ectopic pregnancy is generally an emergency procedure. The developing placental tissue erodes the fallopian tube and can cause rupture and hemorrhage once the tube is completely eroded. This procedure can be done via laparoscopy or via an open abdominal approach.

Oophorectomy

Oophorectomy is the unilateral or bilateral removal of the ovary. Indications include severe PID, malignancy, ectopic pregnancy, and symptomatic ovarian cysts. When both ovaries are removed in a premenopausal woman, abrupt surgical menopause occurs. In this case the woman will experience the same symptoms she might in natural menopause: decreased libido, decreased vaginal lubrication, hot flashes and/or night sweats, and decreased sensation in the lower vaginal tract. These symptoms can be treated with estrogen replacement.

Vulvectomy

A *simple vulvectomy* is the removal of the labia majora, labia minora, and clitoris. *Radical vulvectomy* is the removal of the entire vulva, including the skin and the fat of the femoral triangle, and the pelvic lymph nodes. Skin grafts may be necessary. A simple vulvectomy is performed for leukoplakia and intractable pruritus, whereas a radical procedure is done for malignant disease.

This disfiguring procedure is associated with marked psychosexual disturbances. Most women report decreased sexual arousal levels and low self-image. Sexual activity can be resumed within 3 months; however, significant adjustments will be necessary owing to the loss of sensory perception for foreplay. Stimulation of breasts, thighs, buttocks, or anterior abdominal wall can be suggested.

Pelvic Exenteration

A pelvic exenteration is performed for recurrence of cervical cancer. Only about 5% of women with recurrence are candidates for this procedure, which is not performed if there is any evidence of tumor outside of the pelvis, if the cancer has metastasized to the lymph nodes, or if all of the tumor cannot be removed.

Exenteration can be of the anterior or posterior pelvis, or of the total pelvis. Anterior exenteration is the removal of the uterus, ovaries, fallopian tubes, vagina, bladder, urethra, and pelvic lymph nodes. Urine is diverted through an ileal conduit. Posterior exenteration is the removal of the uterus, fallopian tubes, ovaries, descending colon, rectum, and anal canal. A colostomy is created. A total exenteration is a combination of the anterior and posterior procedures. A vagina can be reconstructed from split-thickness skin grafts or a segment of small bowel.

Complications associated with exenteration include intestinal and urinary obstruction, thrombophlebitis, pulmonary embolism, pyelonephritis, hypovolemia, peritonitis, pneumonia, and wound infection.

NURSING CARE MANAGEMENT
Nursing Assessment and Diagnosis

Nursing assessment for all of these surgical procedures includes identifying the woman's physiologic, psychosocial, and sexual needs as she approaches her surgery. Additionally, it is important to understand her learning needs about the procedure and its effects. Some factors to consider are the age of the woman, her cultural background and educational level, the attitude of her partner and family, her preoperative status (physically and emotionally), and whether or not this involves a cancer diagnosis.

The significance of her reproductive health to her self-image will be reflected in her attitudes about menstruation, childbearing, body image, and sexuality. Many of these procedures have the potential to involve loss, so grieving, anger, sadness, and loss of control are just a few of the feelings the woman may experience.

Nursing diagnoses that may apply to a woman facing gynecologic surgery include the following:

- *Deficient Knowledge* related to lack of information about preoperative routines, postoperative activities, and expected postoperative changes
- *Fear* related to the unknown outcome and long-term implications of the surgery

Nursing Plan and Implementation

Preoperative teaching may be brief in the instance of a simple D&C, or quite extensive in the instances of hysterectomy or pelvic exenteration. In any case, preoperative teaching should include information about the procedure, expected preparation, type of anesthesia to be used, possible risks and complications, postoperative care routines, and expected recovery time. See Figure 7–5 ◆.

Routine postoperative care includes monitoring of physiologic responses, emotional responses, and nursing interventions to facilitate physical and emotional well-being specific to the procedure performed. The woman should be aware of potential postoperative complications and when to follow up with her surgeon. Additionally, it is important to discuss those psychosocial issues identified preoperatively, such as support at home, potential for sadness or depression related to the loss she has experienced, and expected sexual and self-image fears. In some instances, it may be necessary to refer the woman to a professional therapist who can help her adjust to these dramatic changes.

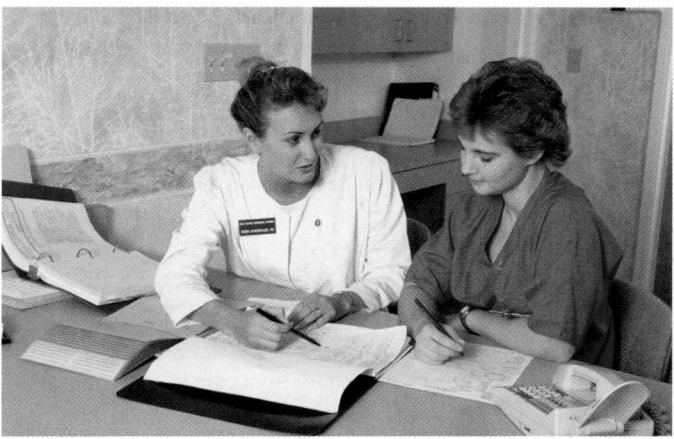

Figure 7–5 ◆ The nurse provides information for the woman during preoperative teaching.

Evaluation

Expected outcomes of nursing care include:

- The woman can discuss the reasons for her surgery, the alternatives, and the aspects of self-care after surgery.
- The woman has an uneventful recovery without complications.
- The woman feels she is able to ask questions and obtain support.
- The woman participates in decision making about her care.
- The woman is aware of available resources if she has physical or emotional concerns in the postoperative period.

CHAPTER REVIEW

FOCUS YOUR STUDY

- With fibrocystic breast changes, the cysts tend to be round, mobile, and well delineated. The woman generally experiences increased discomfort premenstrually.
- Because of the increased risk of breast cancer, women with fibrocystic changes should understand the importance of monthly breast self-examination (BSE).
- Galactorrhea (nipple discharge not associated with lactation) should be evaluated with cytologic testing.
- Breast cancer affects one in eight women in the United States. Biopsy is essential for a diagnosis, and prompt treatment is critical.

- Endometriosis is a condition in which endometrial tissue occurs outside the endometrial cavity. This tissue bleeds in a cyclic fashion in response to the menstrual cycle. The bleeding leads to inflammation, scarring, and adhesions. The prime symptoms include dysmenorrhea, dyspareunia, and infertility.
- Treatment of endometriosis may be medical, surgical, or a combination. For the woman not desiring pregnancy at present, oral contraceptives are used. Women desiring pregnancy are treated with danazol or the GnRH analogs.
- Toxic shock syndrome, a rare but potentially fatal disease, is usually caused by a toxin of *Staphylococcus aureus* and is

most common in women of childbearing age. There is an increased incidence in women who use superabsorbent tampons or barrier methods of contraception, such as the diaphragm and cervical cap, especially if the woman leaves them in place for extended periods of time.

- Vulvitis is an inflammation of the vulva often caused by external irritants such as tight clothing, feminine hygiene products, and some harsh soaps.

- Vulvar lesions range from slight irritation to vulvar cancer. A common vulvar lesion found in postmenopausal women is atrophic vaginitis. All vulvar lesions should be closely evaluated because cancer of the vulva can have various presentations.

- Pap smear screening is recommended for all women who are sexually active or who have reached the age of 18 years. Several factors put a woman at high risk for an abnormal Pap: intercourse at a young age, multiple partners, history of

immunotherapy, long-term COC use, smoking, and previous history of dysplasia. HPV is highly associated with abnormal Pap smears.

- Abnormal uterine bleeding can occur with or without organic pathology. Treatment is geared toward controlling bleeding, preventing anemia, and detecting pathology.

- There are three common forms of pelvic relaxation: A cystocele is a downward displacement of the bladder into the vagina. Often it is accompanied by stress incontinence. Kegel exercises may help restore tone in mild cases. A rectocele is displacement of the rectum into the vagina. Prolapse of the uterus is displacement of the uterine cervix into the vagina.

- Gynecologic surgeries are some of the most common surgical procedures performed in the United States. It is important for the nurse to understand the purpose of the procedure, to know the alternatives to surgery, and to assess the woman's emotional response.

EXPLORE MediaLink

http//www.prenhall.com/davidson

NCLEX review questions, case studies, and other interactive resources for this chapter can be found on the Web Site at http://www.prenhall.com/davidson. Click on "Chapter 7" to select the activities for this chapter.

For tutorials including animations and videos, more NCLEX review questions, and an audio glossary, access the accompanying Prentice Hall Nursing MediaLink DVD-ROM in this book.

PRENTICE HALL NURSING MEDIALINK DVD-ROM
Audio Glossary
NCLEX Review
Video: *Breast Self-Examination*

COMPANION WEBSITE
Additional NCLEX Review
Case Study: *Toxic Shock Syndrome*
Care Plan Activity: *Irregular Bleeding in Perimenopausal Woman*
Applications: *Preparing an Adolescent for Her First Pelvic Examination; Cystocele*
Critical Thinking

CRITICAL THINKING IN ACTION

FIBROCYSTIC BREAST CHANGES

View the Critical Thinking in Action video in Chapter 7 of the DVD-ROM. Then answer the questions that follow.

Mercedes de Martini is a 32-year-old gravida 2, para 2 who has a well-documented history of fibrocystic breast changes. Mercedes's breast symptoms typically increase premenstrually, when her breasts become markedly nodular and dense. She is

being seen today because she has a palpable "lump" in her left breast that she describes as painful and easily movable. Mercedes reports that her menses is due in 5 days. Based on history and physical examination, the physician suspects that Mercedes has developed a cyst and decides to complete a fine-needle aspiration.

1. Identify findings on examination that might help distinguish a cyst from breast cancer.

2. Why is a fine-needle aspiration done?

3. What steps can Mercedes take to help decrease the discomfort associated with her fibrocystic breast changes?

REFERENCES

American Cancer Society (ACS). (2006). *Breast cancer facts and figures 2005–2006*. Atlanta: Author.

American College of Obstetricians and Gynecologists (ACOG). (2005). *Management of endometrial cancer* [ACOG Practice Bulletin No. 65]. Washington, DC: Author.

Beattie, M. S. (2005). Breast cancer risk reduction. *The Female Patient, 30*(10), 16–18.

Bradley, L. D. (2005). Abnormal uterine bleeding. *The Nurse Practitioner, 30*(10), 38–50.

Bristow, R. E. (2003). Cervical cancer. In J. R. Scott, R. S. Gibbs, B. Y. Karlan, & A. F. Haney (Eds.), *Danforth's obstetrics and gynecology* (9th ed., pp. 923–939). Philadelphia: Lippincott Williams & Wilkins.

Canadian Cancer Society. (2005). *Canadian cancer statistics 2005*. Retrieved November 26, 2005, from http://www.cancer.ca

Centers for Disease Control and Prevention (CDC). (2002). Sexually transmitted diseases treatment guidelines 2002. *Morbidity and Mortality Weekly Report, 51*(RR-6), 1–84.

DeLancey, J. O. L., & Strohbehn, K. (2003). Pelvic organ prolapse. In J. R. Scott, R. S. Gibbs, B. Y. Karlan, & A. F. Haney (Eds.), *Danforth's obstetrics and gynecology* (9th ed., pp. 791–817). Philadelphia: Lippincott Williams & Wilkins.

Eschenbach, D. A. (2003). Pelvic infections and sexually transmitted diseases. In J. R. Scott, R. S. Gibbs, B. Y. Karlan, & A. F. Haney (Eds.), *Danforth's obstetrics and gynecology* (9th ed., pp. 581–603). Philadelphia: Lippincott Williams & Wilkins.

Eskin, B. A., & Sepilian, V. (2001). Common benign conditions of the breast. *The Female Patient, 26*(10), 44–49.

Gemignani, M. L. (2003). Disorders of the breast. In J. R. Scott, R. S. Gibbs, B. Y. Karlan, & A. F. Haney (Eds.), *Danforth's obstetrics and gynecology* (9th ed., pp. 889–910). Philadelphia: Lippincott Williams & Wilkins.

Gould, N. S., Walker, J. L., & Mannel, R. S. (2003). Vulvar and vaginal cancer. In J. R. Scott, R. S. Gibbs, B. Y. Karlan, & A. F. Haney (Eds.), *Danforth's obstetrics and gynecology* (9th ed., pp. 911–922). Philadelphia: Lippincott Williams & Wilkins.

Haney, A. F. (2003). Leiomyomata. In J. R. Scott, R. S. Gibbs, B. Y. Karlan, & A. F. Haney (Eds.), *Danforth's obstetrics and gynecology* (9th ed., pp. 869–887). Philadelphia: Lippincott Williams & Wilkins.

Hill, K. (2003). Update: The pathogenesis and treatment of PCOS. *The Nurse Practitioner, 28,* 8–23.

Howard, F., & Scott-Findlay, S. (2006). Breast self-examination: When research contradicts accepted practice. *AWHONN Lifelines, 10*(1), 66–70.

Jackson, M. L. (2004/2005). Ovarian syndrome: What nurses need to know about this misunderstood disorder. *AWHONN Lifelines, 8*(6), 512–518.

Kim, K. H., & Lee, K. A. (2001). Symptom experience in women after hysterectomy. *Journal of Obstetric, Gynecologic, & Neonatal Nursing, 30*(5), 472–480.

Le, L. V. (2003). Management of the adnexal mass. In J. R. Scott, R. S. Gibbs, B. Y. Karlan, & A. F. Haney (Eds.), *Danforth's obstetrics and gynecology* (9th ed., pp. 1007–1018). Philadelphia: Lippincott Williams & Wilkins.

Legro, R. S., & Azziz, R. (2003). Androgen excess disorders. In J. R. Scott, R. S. Gibbs, B. Y. Karlan, & A. F. Haney (Eds.), *Danforth's obstetrics and gynecology* (9th ed., pp. 663–683). Philadelphia: Lippincott Williams & Wilkins.

London, S. N. (2003). Abnormal uterine bleeding. In J. R. Scott, R. S. Gibbs, B. Y. Karlan, & A. F. Haney (Eds.), *Danforth's obstetrics and gynecology* (9th ed., pp. 643–651). Philadelphia: Lippincott Williams & Wilkins.

Love, S. M. (2000). *Dr. Susan Love's breast book* (3rd ed.). Boulder, CO: Perseus.

Marshall, K. (2001). Polycystic ovary syndrome: Clinical considerations. *Alternative Medicine Review, 6,* 272–292.

Morrow, M. (2000). The evaluation of common breast problems. *American Family Physician, 61*(8), 2371–2378.

National Cancer Institute (NCI). (2006). *Screening mammograms: Questions and answers*. Fact sheet retrieved July 6, 2006, from http://www.cancer.gov/cancertopics/factsheet/Detection/screening-mammograms

Scheinfeld, N., & Lehman, D. S. (2006). An evidence-based review of medical and surgical treatments of genital warts. *Dermatology Online Journal, 12*(3), 1–19. Retrieved May 1, 2006, from http://dermatology.cdlib.org/123/reviews/warts/scheinfeld.html

Schenken, R. S. (2003). Endometriosis. In J. R. Scott, R. S. Gibbs, B. Y. Karlan, & A. F. Haney (Eds.), *Danforth's obstetrics and gynecology* (9th ed., pp. 713–720). Philadelphia: Lippincott Williams & Wilkins.

Sheets, E. E. (2003). Management of the abnormal Pap smear. In J. R. Scott, R. S. Gibbs, B. Y. Karlan, & A. F. Haney (Eds.), *Danforth's obstetrics and gynecology* (9th ed., pp. 941–950). Philadelphia: Lippincott Williams & Wilkins.

Sinaii, N., Cleary, S. D., Ballweg, M. L., Nieman, L. K., & Stratton, P. (2002). High rates of autoimmune and endocrine disorders, fibromyalgia, chronic fatigue syndrome and atopic diseases among women with endometriosis: A survey analysis. *Human Reproduction, 17*(10), 2715–2724.

Snyder, B. S. (2006). The lived experience of women diagnosed with polycystic ovary syndrome. *Journal of Obstetric, Gynecologic, & Neonatal Nursing, 35*(3), 385–392.

Solomon, D., Davey, D., Kurman, R., Moriarity, A., O'Connor, D., Prey, M., et al. (2002). Consensus statement: The 2001 Bethesda System—Terminology for reporting results of cervical cytology. *Journal of the American Medical Association, 287*(16), 2114–2119.

Tsilchorozidou, T., Overton, C., & Conway, G. S. (2004). The pathophysiology of polycystic ovary syndrome. *Clinical Endocrinology, 60*(1), 1–17.

Wilkinson, E. J. (2003). Benign vulvovaginal disorders. In J. R. Scott, R. S. Gibbs, B. Y. Karlan, & A. F. Haney (Eds.), *Danforth's obstetrics and gynecology* (9th ed., pp. 605–623). Philadelphia: Lippincott Williams & Wilkins.

Wright, T. C., Cox, J. T., Massad, L. S., Twiggs, M. D., & Wilkinson, E. J. (2002). Consensus statement: 2001 consensus guidelines for the management of women with cervical cytological abnormalities. *Journal of the American Medical Association, 287*(16), 2120–2129.

CHAPTER
8
Women's Care: Social Issues

There has never been a more exciting time for women. Although we face many challenges—work, wage, and role issues; safety in pregnancy and childbearing; and conflict over women's rights—we have never been more active and involved in issues that affect us. Moreover, the men who care about us, and recognize the importance of fairness for all, are beginning to join us in speaking out. Together, men and women of integrity and vision are making a difference in women's lives.

KEY TERMS

Civil unions   171
Comparable worth   161
Disability   169
Domestic partnership   171
Elder abuse   168
Environmental toxin   164

Female genital mutilation (FGM)   173
Feminization of later life   167
Feminization of poverty   157
Polypharmacy   169

OBJECTIVES

1. Define the phrase *feminization of poverty*.
2. Identify factors that contribute to the wage gap between women and men.
3. Discuss poverty's effect on women's health care.
4. Discuss the impact of the Family and Medical Leave Act (FMLA) of 1993 on maternity and paternity leave.
5. Identify environmental hazards that may be present in the workplace or home of a woman of childbearing age.
6. Identify factors that contribute to older women's economic vulnerability.
7. Identify four different categories of elder abuse.
8. Discuss the implications of aging on women's health and health care.
9. Explain the implications of homophobia for lesbian and bisexual women's health care.
10. List the five main types of disability.
11. Discuss ways in which a woman's disability may affect her health care.
12. Identify types of discrimination commonly faced by lesbian and bisexual women.
13. Discuss the cultural implications of female genital mutilation.

 MEDIALINK

Additional resources for this content can be found on the Prentice Hall Nursing MediaLink DVD-ROM and on the Companion Website at http://www.prenhall.com/davidson. Click on "Chapter 8" to select the activities for this chapter.

In the 21st century, many women in developed nations are creating and experiencing new opportunities for personal and professional growth. Despite these unparalleled opportunities, other women still struggle daily to overcome poverty, age discrimination, abuse, the economic and interpersonal effects of disability, and unequal treatment because of sexual orientation. Even the most successful and satisfied working women face wage discrimination, lack of safe and nurturing day care for their children, and failure of their governments to support paid maternity and paternity leave.

Every day in their clinical practice, nurses working with women are confronted with these issues and their impact on women's health and well-being. To help nurses better understand their clients' concerns and problems, this chapter addresses some of the serious social issues facing women today.

SOCIAL ISSUES AFFECTING WOMEN LIVING IN POVERTY

For impoverished women, life is a day-by-day struggle fraught with anxiety and hardship.

> *I never thought this would happen to me. Two months after I became pregnant with our second child, it was over. My husband left us. Suddenly, I am the sole support of myself and my children. Since he left I haven't been able to get a job, so I don't have medical insurance or any benefits to help with this pregnancy. Applying for Medicaid has to be one of the most humiliating experiences I have ever had. I'm an intelligent woman with a college degree, and yet I couldn't figure out the forms. I felt so dumb. The lines and the impersonal treatment that you hear about are real. I felt like a number, shuttled from one place to the next. I know they don't do it on purpose; they've heard so many awful stories. Still, it hurt. It will take 6 weeks to qualify for assistance, and by then I will be more than halfway through my pregnancy. What's more, only two doctors here accept Medicaid, and they are clear across town—that means three bus transfers with a 2-year-old in tow. I'm thankful that I can get some help, but it is so hard. I never dreamed I'd be in this position. I just never dreamed.*

The Feminization of Poverty

The fact that many more women than men live below the poverty level is reflected in the phrase **feminization of poverty,** which was coined by Diana Pearce in 1993. Increasing numbers of US women and their children are attempting to live on $19,350 or less, which is the current income that defines the poverty level for a family of four. In 2003, the number of women living in poverty totaled 13.8 million, or 12.4% of all women 18 years of age or older (Department of Health and Human Services [DHHS], 2005a).

Women raising children alone are especially likely to be impoverished. In 2003, only 5.2% of families headed by a married couple lived in poverty, but among households headed by single mothers the percentage was 24.4% (DHHS, 2005a). With a divorce rate of approximately 38%, an out-of-wedlock birth rate of

about 34%, and the median age at first marriage rising for men and women, the reality is that many children will spend at least a portion of their lives in a single-parent family (DHHS, 2005a).

The number of children in the United States living in poverty is disturbing. Seventeen percent live below the poverty level. No other age group, not even the elderly, has a higher poverty rate. The two demographic factors most strongly associated with children's poverty are female-headed family and race. Parental gender is important because men earn more money overall than women; men who are single heads of households have an average income of $41,959, whereas the average income of women raising their families alone is $29,307 (DeNavas-Walt, Proctor, & Mills, 2004). More than 50% of impoverished children live in female-headed homes (DHHS, 2005b). Parental race is related to poverty in children because ethnic minority parents tend to have less education and lower incomes, on average, than Caucasian parents. Twenty-eight percent of black children and 25% of Hispanic children live in poverty, but only 12% of Caucasian children do. For children parented by single, ethnic-minority mothers, the situation is even grimmer: 43% of black and 43% of Hispanic children are impoverished, whereas 28% of Caucasian children are (US Census Bureau, 2005). Currently, two thirds of all poor people in the United States are women and children; in other words, women and children account for most of the people living in poverty (Figure 8–1 ◆).

The feminization of poverty is also evident in the rising trend for women to declare bankruptcy. In 2005, new bankruptcy laws were passed that reduce consumer protection and give lenders more leverage to push for repayment. These new laws have hurt women who are divorced, separated, or widowed, particularly single mothers. Single mothers often work in low-wage jobs and have been shown to be 50% more likely to file for *bankruptcy* than married parents and three times more likely than childless couples (Gardner, 2005).

The feminization of poverty extends beyond the United States. Although there are many scales used to measure global

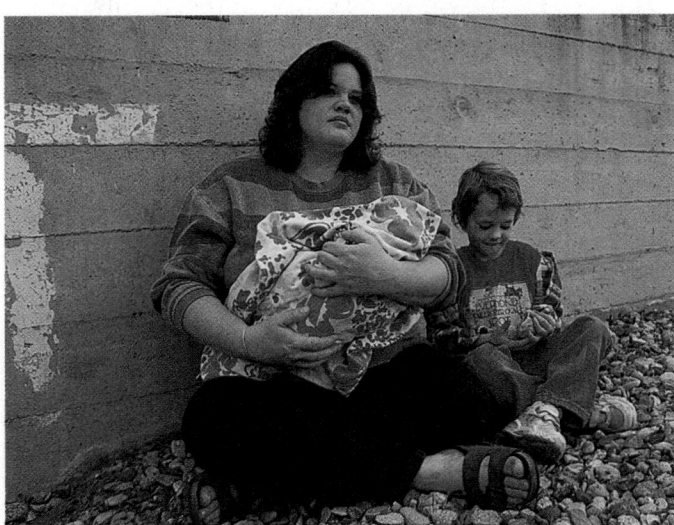

Figure 8–1 ◆ Two thirds of Americans living in poverty are women and children.
SOURCE: Photographer, Elena Dorfman.

poverty, the Purchasing Power Parity (PPP) scale uses calculations based on money available for purchasing. It is estimated that 1.1 billion people in the world live on less than $1 per day, and an additional 2.7 billion live on less than $2 per day (PovertyNet, 2005). Globally, women must cope with some unique challenges. They typically work more hours than men but are paid less for the same work; they are often expected to bear and raise many children, sometimes in addition to performing a job outside the home; they are frequently abused and beaten in their own homes; and often they have few legal rights.

Both globally and in the United States, poverty has been directly linked to literacy and educational attainment. The literacy rate for females is lower than that for males, and education—when available—is more frequently provided for men even though economic returns on investment in women's education are found to exceed those for men. Also, women who use their skills to increase their income invest more in their children's health and education (PovertyNet, 2005).

Economic Effects of Divorce

The increase in the number of female-headed families is closely associated with divorce. Almost one out of every two marriages ends in divorce. As a result of divorce, a woman's standard of living generally decreases significantly, whereas a man's increases. This dramatic change in the standard of living is usually associated with the lower earning capacity of women, the fact that women receive custody of the children in 80% of cases, and that women often accept lower support payments in exchange for a guarantee of custody (Kelly, Redenback, & Rinanman, 2005). Although only about one half of divorced women receive the full amount of promised child support payments, tightened enforcement policies at the national level have increased the percentage of men who meet their obligations, either partially or in full, through improved rates of paternity establishment, support order initiation, and support collection. The United States Department of Justice actively investigates and prosecutes individuals who cross state lines to avoid paying child support, and the federal government now intercepts delinquent parents' income tax refunds. To make it easier to track delinquent parents across state lines, employers are required to report all newly hired employees to state agencies, which then transmit the information to the national directory. Moreover, states are required to establish central registries of child support orders and centralized collection and disbursement units. States are permitted to implement tough collection techniques, including garnishing wages, seizing assets, revoking driver's and professional licenses, and, in some cases, requiring mandatory community service of individuals who are delinquent in making child support payments (DHHS, 2005c). Information about the enforcement program may be found on the DHHS Office of Child Support Enforcement's Internet home page.

Factors Contributing to Poverty in Working Women

Women have steadily increased their participation in the labor force. The number of working women has risen from 5.1 million in 1900, to 18.4 million in 1950, to nearly 65 million in 2003 (Department for Professional Employees, AFL-CIO, 2005).

Along with their participation in the labor market, women have steadily increased their earnings; however, a significant wage discrepancy still exists. In 2002, women employed full-time earned only 76.5% of men's median weekly wages, and for women of color, the gap was wider: African American women earned 67%, and Latina women 55%, of men's weekly earnings. Although Asian Pacific American women do better, they still earn only 83.5% as much as men (Department for Professional Employees, AFL-CIO, 2005). The disparity between men's and women's wages may be attributed to several factors:

- About one third of women work in a cluster of "pink collar" occupations, which tend to be poorly paid when compared with male-dominated positions requiring comparable levels of responsibility, skill, and education (Haignere, Inc., 2005).

- Women are paid less than men for comparable work in virtually all occupations: In 2003, professional and technical women earned almost 27% less than their male counterparts, whereas women in office and administrative support occupations earned over 12% less. Even women in female-dominated fields (teaching, office work, clerical work) are outearned by male peers (Department for Professional Employees, AFL-CIO, 2005).

- Because women are paid less when they work, they receive smaller pensions and social security benefits when they retire. Less than half of all employed women in the United States participate in a pension plan, and half of all older women with private pensions receive less than $5600 a year. Older men, in contrast, receive an average of $10,340 a year. Part-time workers, most of whom are women, often have no benefits such as sick leave and health insurance (Department for Professional Employees, AFL-CIO, 2005).

For working divorced or single women with children, the issue of child care is especially difficult. Child care is expensive and places a tremendous burden on the single parent's household budget. Moreover, with no partner to bear the burden, divorced or single mothers without social support must miss work when their children become ill, causing employers to view them as unreliable or uncommitted. Currently, more enlightened employers are beginning to recognize and accommodate the needs of mothers in the workforce. Like other areas of reform, however, this trend tends to benefit women in better paying, more secure positions far more than it benefits women who are poor and in low-paying positions.

Public Assistance

The US welfare system was originally designed to provide assistance to those in need—in many cases, single female heads of households and their children. Unfortunately, the system often failed to provide adequate assistance to raise families above poverty levels and, in many cases, actually provided disincentives for women to work.

In 1996, growing national concern over the failure of the system led to welfare reform via the passage of the Personal Responsibility and Work Opportunity Reconciliation Act. As part of the act, a block grant known as the Temporary Assistance for Needy Families (TANF) was created. The TANF grant replaced the Aid to Families with Dependent Children (AFDC) program, which had provided cash welfare to poor families with children since 1935 (DHHS, 2005d).

TANF is implemented through block grants to the states. States use these funds to operate their own programs in whatever fashion they choose, provided they are congruent with the four TANF purposes set out in federal law:

- Provide assistance to needy families so that children may be cared for in their own homes or in the homes of relatives.
- End the dependence of needy parents on government benefits by promoting job preparation, work, and marriage.
- Prevent and reduce the incidence of out-of-wedlock pregnancies and establish annual numerical goals for preventing and reducing the incidence of these pregnancies.
- Encourage the formation and maintenance of two-parent families.

Under TANF, states are granted unprecedented flexibility in designing welfare programs to meet the needs of their recipients, but they must demonstrate measurable results in moving families toward self-sufficiency and work. With few exceptions, recipients are required to find employment after they have received assistance for 2 years. Work requirements may be met through participation in subsidized or unsubsidized employment, community service, on-the-job training, or 12 months of vocational education. Recipients can also meet the requirement by providing child care services to others who are involved in community service. After 5 cumulative years of assistance, families become ineligible for cash aid, although states can exempt up to 20% of their cases from the time limit provision. States can also choose to use state funds or social security block grant dollars to provide additional noncash assistance and vouchers for families who have reached the time limit. TANF provides $14 billion (an increase of $4 billion) in child care funding to enable mothers to provide for adequate child care as they move into jobs. Women on welfare are guaranteed continued health-care coverage for their families, including at least 1 year of transitional Medicaid as they leave the welfare rolls for work.

- The law also mandates that unmarried teenage parents live at home (or in an adult-supervised setting) and stay in school in order to receive assistance (DHHS, 2005e). As discussed previously, the act also contains several provisions designed to crack down on noncustodial parents who fail to pay child support.

Several trends have emerged as a result of the welfare reform efforts. A comparison of welfare recipients' pre-TANF status in 1996 to their post-TANF status in 2003 reveals the following: more single women on welfare are living with partners, a decrease in the poverty rate, a decrease in the poverty gap (the amount of income necessary to lift poor families out of poverty), and an increase in the number of families that include at least one working parent (DHHS, 2005e). Although results appear favorable, it is too early to judge more long-term effects of welfare reform; many parents who have entered the workforce have not yet escaped poverty.

Homelessness

For many people the thought of a homeless person conjures up a vision of an older man curled in a doorway or making a home under a bridge. However, this vision is less accurate today than in the past; today's homeless people have very different characteristics. It is estimated that by 2010, 1.7 billion people in the United States will have been homeless at one time in their lives. Homeless families represent the fastest growing group of homeless, having increased to 40%. Many of these families are composed of single mothers and their children. In addition, single childless women make up 14% of the homeless population (National Alliance to End Homelessness, 2005).

FACTORS CONTRIBUTING TO HOMELESSNESS

Because of the nature of homelessness, it is very difficult to come up with a number that reliably reflects the number of people who experience homelessness. The most recent national count, conducted in 1996, suggested that between 2.3 and 3.5 million people experienced homelessness over the course of that year. Data collected by various local jurisdictions since that time indicate that the number has risen and is continuing to rise each year. Approximately 90% of homeless families are headed by a single mother. A major factor contributing to the incidence of homelessness is a lack of housing that low-income people can afford. During the past 20 years, housing costs have increased far more than wages or other income sources, especially for women. In many communities, low-income housing has waiting lists of several hundred families (National Alliance to End Homelessness, 2005). Another factor contributing to homelessness is domestic violence. Research suggests that many homeless women and their children are fleeing from an abusive situation. Domestic violence and lack of affordable housing are interrelated factors contributing to women's homelessness. Women often return to abusive living situations following unsuccessful attempts to find adequate affordable housing. Many women who have been victims of domestic violence lack rental and employment histories or have poor credit; all are barriers to finding adequate housing and can lead to homelessness (Marcos & Lima, 2003).

Other factors that contribute to homelessness (in order of frequency) include low-paying jobs, substance abuse, untreated mental illnesses, domestic violence, unemployment, poverty, prison release, and changes and cuts in public assistance programs. Race, education, and the number of children a woman has borne also influence the likelihood that she will experience homelessness. In one study of more than 4000 women, 20% of all the African American women had a documented homeless episode during the 7-year period of the study, compared with much lower rates for Caucasian (1.2%), Asian (0.9%), and Hispanic (4.8%) women. Years of education varied inversely with episodes of homelessness, and women who had given birth to more children experienced homelessness more often than women who had fewer children. The incidence of homelessness is also related to the extent of a woman's social support system. Because middle-class women typically have relatives and friends with more space and resources, they are able to avoid becoming homeless to a greater extent than poorer women (Webb, Robbins, Culhane et al., 2003). A rising concern exists that the nation's weak economy and the job losses associated with the terrorist attacks of September 11, 2001, are also having a negative impact on the incidence of homelessness.

HEALTH RISKS OF HOMELESS WOMEN AND CHILDREN

Homeless women and children experience greater health risks and problems than do people in the general population. Malnutrition predisposes homeless people to a variety of respiratory and nutritional disorders. Moreover, a disproportionately high number of homeless women and children have not received preventive healthcare services, such as screening tests and immunizations.

Homeless women who are pregnant are a special challenge for healthcare providers. Inadequate prenatal care, limited access to general health care, poor nutrition, and inadequate housing lead to poor birth outcomes, including an increased incidence of low-birth-weight newborns and a higher rate of infant mortality. In addition, as a group they are at risk for many illnesses that could negatively affect their pregnancies, including substance abuse, sexually transmitted infections, and hepatitis A, B, and C (Lewis, Andersen, & Gelberg, 2003).

Effects of Poverty on Women's Health Care

The effects of poverty on women's health care are extensive. Since 1981, many funding cuts have reduced or eliminated programs that used to help families in poverty access health care. Funding has not been restored, even though adequate nutrition and prenatal care have been proven to yield significant healthcare benefits.

Medicaid is the major US program providing health care to low-income people in four categories: children, adults in families, the elderly, and blind and disabled people. Traditionally Medicaid has played an important role in financing maternity care, covering the costs of about 40% of births in the United States. Because welfare reform measures eliminate the automatic connection between TANF and Medicaid and mandate that women apply for Medicaid separately, the number of women that Medicaid serves may be shown to have decreased over the years since the inception of TANF. Although such an outcome would certainly be undesirable, the overall effect of welfare reform on women's health is not yet clear. Some research suggests that because women on Medicaid are served in managed care programs that typically stress preventive care, poor women's health will improve. Nason, Alexander, Pass et al. (2003) found that both black and Caucasian women enrolled in an Alabama Medicaid-managed maternity care program were more likely to take advantage of WIC (Women, Infants and Children nutrition program) than women not enrolled in the managed care program, and that black women in the managed care program had a reduced risk of giving birth to babies who were small for their gestational age. Investigators in

another study found that women enrolled in Ohio Medicaid HMO (Health Maintenance Organization) for prenatal care had more prenatal visits and a lower smoking incidence, but no better birth outcomes, than poor women not served by the HMO (Kenney, Sommers, & Dubay, 2005).

Lack of health insurance is also a major problem for the poor. In 2004, 45.8 million people were without health insurance coverage of any kind. The numbers of uninsured citizens increased by 3.8 million between 2003 and 2004, even though the numbers of people covered by government programs such as Medicaid and The State Children's Health Insurance Program have increased over that same time period. Lack of employment is responsible for these trends: The percentage of people covered by private health insurance decreased from 64% in 2003 to 59.8% in 2004 (DeNavas-Walt, Proctor, & Mills, 2005). Decreases in health insurance coverage have led to declines in preventive health care that are costing dollars and even lives. Women who do not receive prenatal care are three times more likely to have low-birth-weight babies, and the incidence of low-birth-weight babies is increasing. Women who receive adequate prenatal care are less likely to develop severe complications, such as preterm labor. Moreover, lack of prenatal care is a risk factor for infant morbidity and mortality.

The issue of women and poverty is critical, and the implications for childbearing care are very real. A pregnant woman who is suffering economically may also suffer physically and psychologically. In the end, it is often the children who suffer the most, bearing the physical and psychologic scars of their mothers' struggles. As healthcare professionals, nurses should be concerned about the issue of women and poverty. The limited resources available to impoverished women often frustrates nurses' efforts to provide quality care. Nurses need to explore their own beliefs about poverty and public assistance programs and inform others about the barriers poor women face.

Assessing women's financial status is a nursing responsibility, because some women may not have the economic resources to buy infant supplies or other medical supplies that may be needed in the home setting. The nurse asks questions in a sensitive manner and refers women with insufficient resources to social workers or appropriate agencies. A nurse who is knowledgeable about community resources and who can provide the woman with follow-up contacts and phone numbers provides an immeasurable service to impoverished clients.

Nurses can also assist impoverished women by working with community groups and organizations and becoming actively involved in the political process. Many nurses use their work experience to present their views to legislators, support various childbearing programs, and alert legislators to legislation that would benefit mothers and families. Finally, nurse researchers can explore medical and social issues related to the impact of poverty on families.

SOCIAL ISSUES AFFECTING WOMEN IN THE WORKPLACE

In 2004, women made up 40% of the total US workforce. Seventy-four percent worked full-time, whereas 26% worked part-time (US Department of Labor, Women's Bureau, 2005). As a result of political and social changes that began in the early 1970s, women's career options have expanded dramatically. Although many women still choose careers traditionally entered into by women (office work, nursing, etc.), or choose to stay home full-time to raise children, others are entering occupations that until recently were reserved for men. More women than ever have joined the ranks of lawyers and judges, authors and artists, managers and corporate heads, scientists, engineers, legislators, construction workers, plumbers, and electricians, and thus are sharing in the benefits that come with these positions.

Progress has its costs, however. For example, the woman with both a career and a family may experience tremendous day-to-day stress in attempting to fulfill both her professional and mothering roles. The woman who would like nothing more than to be a stay-at-home mother may be forced by financial pressures to work outside the home and entrust the care of her children to others. Women who do stay at home to raise their children sacrifice earnings, retirement savings, and social security benefits, and have decreased opportunities for social contact and intellectual stimulation. In contrast, the woman who has devoted her prime childbearing years to establishing a career rather than a family may feel a deep sense of loss as she ages.

Several social issues affect women in the workplace. Key among these are wage discrepancy, maternity/paternity leave issues, child care, and environmental hazards.

Wage Discrepancy

In 2004, the male-to-female earnings ratio was 76.5%. This means that in that year, women, on average, earned about 76.5 cents for every dollar earned by men. To keep this percentage in perspective, however, it is well to realize that 40 years ago, the wage discrepancy between men and women was much greater. Over the past four decades, women have entered the labor market in great numbers and have also substantially increased their level of educational attainment. For example, in 1970, only 8% of workers classified as professionals (physicians, executives, lawyers, etc.) were women, but by 2001, the percentage had soared to 28%. At the same time, the wage gap between professional workers and blue-collar workers (laborers, service workers, etc.) rose considerably. Consequently, the overall wage discrepancy between men and women declined as women's educational attainment grew and their workforce participation increased. Nevertheless, a wage gap remains, and, ironically, it is widest between well-educated women and men. As of 2003, blue-collar women had closed 31% of the gap, whereas professional women had closed only 15% and white-collar women only 5%. Moreover, highly educated men are 50% more likely than educated women to join the ranks of professional workers (Eckstein & Nagypál, 2004). The decreasing, but tenacious, discrepancy between men's and women's wages is thought to be related to a number of factors: deliberate wage discrimination against women, undervaluing of women's work, and women's socialization.

In the past deliberate and blatant wage discrimination against women was ubiquitous and generally accepted. Women's wages were purposely set lower than men's because it was assumed that men needed substantial funds to support families whereas women did not. In the 1960s and 1970s, women's groups and unions pushed for legislation that would end wage discrimination by mandating that compensation for various types of work be based on **comparable worth,** which means equal pay for work that is of comparable value and requires comparable skills, responsibility, education, and experience. Comparable worth legislation was opposed by business leaders, who argued that wage disparities were rooted not in discrimination against women, but in differences in educational level and seniority, and that basing wages on comparable worth would decrease US manufacturers' ability to compete with foreign manufacturers and reallocate limited salary resources away from lower-class, minority men to middle-class, Caucasian women. Such arguments prevailed, and comparable worth legislation proposed during the Carter administration was never implemented. Comparable worth has not been raised as a serious issue in recent years, even though research has demonstrated that neither worker nor job characteristics fully account for the wage differences between men and women and that the gender of individuals performing a given job is the best single predictor of the salary associated with that job; surveys of wage trends show that when the proportion of women in a given occupational field increases, the average weekly salary level decreases (Gibelman, 2003).

Labor classified as "women's work" has been historically undervalued, and that pattern continues and contributes to the wage gap. In 2004, the mean hourly wage for occupations classified under construction and extraction (e.g., brick masons, construction laborers, paving equipment operators), in which male workers predominate, was $18.04. In contrast, the mean hourly wage for the largely female workers in healthcare support occupations (e.g., home health aides, medical assistants, and nursing aides) was $11.17 (Bureau of Labor Statistics, 2005). Whether wage discrimination favoring males exists in the nursing profession is not clear. Although it is known that overall, male nurses outearn female nurses, Jones and Gates (2004) attribute that phenomenon to the fact that male nurses are overrepresented in high-paying nursing specialties such as anesthesia. The small numbers of men in the profession make it difficult to determine whether men working in the less well-compensated areas of nursing practice are also better compensated, overall, than women.

Women can combat wage discrimination in several ways. First, they can refuse to contribute to the secrecy about wages that allows some employers to get away with paying women less than men for doing the same job. Women can also actively push for wage equity by making community leaders and legislators aware of wage discrepancies and by urging legislators to support legislation that enhances equal employment and wages for women.

Women's socialization has long been thought to contribute to the wage gap. Although most boys are encouraged to develop a competitive spirit, first in sports and then in other areas of their lives, girls may lack this early introduction to healthy competition, because the willingness and ability to compete has not been seen as an important or desirable trait for a girl to have. Also, some girls learn from their parents, the media, their peers, and others that physical attractiveness, rather than intelligence and hard work, is the key to popularity and success. And, until relatively recently, another significant factor was women's tendency to settle for lower levels of education than men and then choose to work in poorly compensated "women's fields." Since 1982, however, more American women than men have earned bachelor's degrees, and parents, educators, and other concerned citizens have lobbied successfully for programs that encourage girls to explore a wide range of academic pursuits and career options, especially in fields not traditionally seen as welcoming to women. For example, the Department of Labor has developed a mentoring program that encourages schoolgirls to seek nontraditional, higher paying careers. Currently, several factors make it likely that the current wage gap between men and women will be narrowed in years to come:

- As noted earlier, more women are entering professions previously dominated by men. For example, women have outnumbered men in law and medical schools since the early 1990s (*The Economist*, 2005).

- More working women are holding jobs for extended, rather than short, periods and are thus gaining in experience, productivity, and eligibility for promotion.

- More and more women own their own businesses. In 2004, nearly half (48%) of all privately held firms were owned or co-owned by women (Center for Women's Business Research, 2005).

- Women are contributing more money than in the past to political campaigns, thus increasing their influence on public policy. The number of women who donated $10,000 or more to federal candidates was 78% higher in 2004 than in 2000 (*USA Today*, 2005).

> **CLINICAL TIP**
>
> Speaking out about issues that affect women, children, and families is an integral part of maternal-child nursing. It is difficult for many nurses to do this, so you should practice with friends and family frequently. Be prepared with accurate information, and try various techniques for presenting the information. A friendly, supportive audience helps you get started.

Maternal and Paternal Leave Issues

Combining full-time employment with motherhood has always been challenging. In the past, women who took official or unofficial maternity leave to bear a child often lost benefits, missed out on promotions, or lost their jobs completely. Paternity leave for fathers was unheard of, and remains rare, even in developed countries.

Parenthood and employment became a bit more compatible in 1993 when President Clinton signed the Family and Medical Leave Act (FMLA) into law. FMLA permits employees to take up to 12 weeks of unpaid leave from work following the birth or adoption of a child or the placement of a foster child. Employees may also take leave if faced with serious illness, or the illness of a spouse, child, or parent. Health insurance benefits must be continued during the leave, and employees are entitled to return to their former position or one considered comparable. Because the FMLA applies only to companies with 50 or more employees, however, the vast majority of companies are not subject to the law. Moreover, coverage is not mandated for employees who work fewer than 25 hours per week, or who have been employed less than 1 year. Thus, about 25 million employees are not covered by FMLA and must rely on whatever policies their employers have established. Even though FMLA applies to men, US fathers often fail to take advantage of it. Studies have shown that American men often forgo paternity leave because they fear that taking it will hinder their careers, and that men who do take it feel stigmatized. Companies often send out subtle messages to men that paternity leave exists only on paper; men who do take paternity leave are often seen as pioneers even though the law has been in effect since 1993.

Despite the advances made in this country by the FMLA, parental leave benefits in the United States are meager in comparison with benefits provided in other countries. In other parts of the world, paid parental leave is the rule, rather than the exception, and the funding source is often public rather than the private employer. In Sweden, for example, the Swedish Parental Insurance Benefit provides Swedish women with up to 14 weeks of maternity leave, which may begin 7 weeks before the birth, and fathers with up to 2 weeks of paternity leave after the birth. The parents' salaries are reimbursed on a prorated basis, and many workers receive 100% of their salaries for the first 4 months (Lund, 2004). Paid maternity leave, and often paternity leave as well, are standard in most European countries and Canada. The United States remains one of the few countries that have no legislation requiring a national *paid* maternity leave program.

Discrimination Against Pregnant Women

Discrimination against pregnant women by employers who cling to false stereotypes about them (that they cannot do their jobs; that they take more sick leave than other employees; that they fail to return to work after having given birth) remains an issue in some areas. Each year, the Equal Employment Opportunity Commission receives complaints from pregnant women who were turned down for jobs, denied transfers to positions for which they were qualified, or fired unjustly (US Equal Employment Opportunity Commission, 2006). Thus, it is important that pregnant women be aware of their legal rights. The Pregnancy Discrimination Act of 1978 guarantees the following:

- A pregnant woman cannot be denied a job if she is able to perform major job functions.

- The same procedure for using sick leave pay or disability benefits must be used for the pregnant woman as for other employees.

- Employee medical coverage must include pregnancy benefits.

- The mother can use all her maternity benefits without penalty.

When a woman is planning a pregnancy, she should acquire information about pregnancy benefits in her work setting. The state in which she lives also has guidelines or regulations about pregnancy.

I was thrilled when I found out I was pregnant! Although I had a high-stress job and worked long hours, I rejoiced in the thought of being a mother. As my pregnancy became apparent, my boss started "worrying about me." He feared I could not keep up with my demanding schedule and that the "emotional strain" would be hard on the baby. By the time I reached 28 weeks, I learned that a coworker would be taking over some of my responsibilities and 2 weeks later I was laid off. My boss felt that my current workload would be too difficult for a "very pregnant woman or a new mother." I immediately started fighting for my right to keep my position. I was the perfect employee previously with flawless evaluations. Sure there may be legal protection in place, but right now I have no income, am paying high insurance premiums to maintain my health insurance, and am rapidly depleting my savings. I am angry and cry all of the time. I have been diagnosed with depression and am now taking antidepressants. I never missed a minute of work, my performance remained flawless . . . their only complaint, I was pregnant! This should be the happiest time of my life but instead I'm in counseling and taking Prozac; it's so unfair!

Child Care

In 1947, only 12% of mothers with small children were employed. By 2003, that percentage had jumped to 72% (US Census Bureau, 2003). Although some fathers are actively involved in meshing work and family responsibilities, child care remains predominantly a woman's issue, both because of the traditional belief that child care is "women's work," and because of the high percentage of single-parent households headed by a woman (Figure 8–2 ◆). In 1970, only 11% of families with children were headed by single women, but in 1998, 26% were. Finding high-quality, affordable child care is a critical issue for many American women (National Network of Child Care Resources [NACCRRA], 2005).

In contemplating starting a family, I never dreamed that child care would top my list of primary stressors. The decision to work is hard enough, but then you are faced with the inability to find safe, nurturing child care. The turnover is constant, the settings never ideal. I used to think the trick was to pay more. I was wrong there. It doesn't seem to matter how much you pay or how much you investigate, it is an unending struggle. It leaves you wishing away your children's preschool years, just so you can get past the point in their lives when you are constantly dealing with child care!

Child care costs in the United States range from $4000 to $13,000 per child per year, with an average of $6750 per year per child. Families with multiple children can quickly consume a large amount of their income on child care costs. These costs hit low-income families especially hard; families with an income of $18,000 per year or less spend an average of 22.8% of their earnings on child care, whereas families with an income of $54,000 or more spend only 3.9% (NACCRRA, 2005).

Numerous studies have demonstrated the benefits of early, high-quality child care that features frequent, positive staff-child interactions and a strong educational component (Figure 8–3 ◆). Children who receive such care tend to do better in school and are more likely to graduate, and have lower rates of juvenile crime and adolescent pregnancy when they are older. In

Figure 8–2 ◆ Some women rely on the father to provide full-time child care at home while they pursue their career. Stay-at-home fathers provide only 1.5% of care to children under the age of 5 in the United States.
SOURCE: Corbis RF.

Figure 8–3 ◆ Childhood education centers provide preschoolers with advanced skills for early education and provide care while parents work outside of the home.
SOURCE: Tom and Dee Ann McCarthy/CORBIS.

contrast, low-quality child care is associated with strained maternal-child relationships, higher incidence of insecurity, more problem behaviors, and lower scores on cognitive, language, and school readiness scales (American Academy of Pediatrics, 2005).

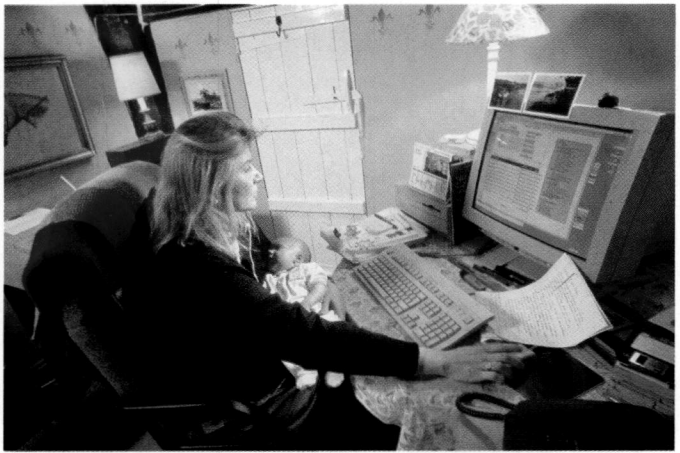

Figure 8–4 ◆ Some mothers are able to combine professional careers with motherhood by telecommuting from a home office.
SOURCE: Getty Images, Inc.

Mothers who have a college education and work outside of the home are more likely to enroll their children in these types of programs. Currently some employers provide support for employees' child care needs through such mechanisms as referral programs, on-site or near-site centers, or financial assistance programs. Other creative approaches to handling child care are also gaining in popularity: flex-time scheduling, part-time work, job sharing, and telecommuting (working at home via email, phone, and fax) (Figure 8–4 ◆). Some parents choose to work alternating shifts to eliminate the need for day care or other forms of nonparental care. Although this option has its advantages, it can be stressful for the family because the parent who is at home may not get enough sleep.

Grandparents can be an invaluable source of child care assistance to working families. In the United States about 7% of grandparents, usually grandmothers, provide extensive care (more than 30 hours per week, or more than 90 nights per year) to their grandchildren. Approximately 10% of grandparents, many of whom are African American grandmothers, act as full-time, surrogate parents. Grandmothers who take on such daunting responsibility are at risk for neglecting their own health and are at greater risk for depression than grandmothers who do not act as primary care providers for their grandchildren (Mawthorpe, 2003).

Until quite recently, grandparents and other relatives who assume responsibility for one or more of the approximately 2,000,000 children whose parents are unable to care for them have not been eligible for the financial aid routinely provided to nonrelated foster parents. As of 2004, however, 35 states and the District of Columbia had instituted *Subsidized Guardianship,* a mechanism by which custodial relatives may receive funds through a variety of local, state, and federal programs (Children's Defense Fund, 2004).

Advocacy for Working Women

Nurses can act as advocates for working women by serving as role models, providing positive reinforcement and support, and working actively to establish woman-friendly workplace policies. All women, including nurses, who must balance work and family responsibilities should inquire about maternity and paternity leave, child care benefits, the possibility of working flexible hours, and whether on-site, discounted day care is provided before accepting employment. Women should also inquire about the flexibility of break periods to express their milk for nursing infants. Many employers now have special areas specifically designed for women who need to express milk throughout the workday. Nurses, and women in general, must support other women who are fighting for their rights in the workplace and must demand that legislators pass family and woman-friendly employment laws. Solidarity and the willingness to actively oppose unfair or discriminatory practices are twin keys to equal rights and treatment for working women.

Environmental Hazards in the Workplace and at Home

Women in developed countries such as the United States are increasingly exposed to **environmental toxins,** chemical compounds found in air, food, and water, whose bioaccumulation can lead to adverse health effects. These substances can affect their reproductive and general health and the health of their children. Those of greatest concern include gases that may contaminate indoor air, toxic chemicals to which women may be exposed at work and at home, and various poisonous or otherwise harmful substances that contaminate produce, fish, and meats. Women who are nurses are also exposed to potentially harmful chemical and biological agents associated with the healthcare industry.

Air pollution is an environmental hazard caused by the release of toxins into the air. Both indoor and outdoor air pollution can cause minor problems such as eye, nose, and throat irritation and headaches, as well as serious problems such as lung and heart disease. Indoor air pollution, however, poses the more serious threat to women's health, because most Americans spend 90% of their time indoors. Most indoor air pollution is caused by gases (fumes) released from lit cigarettes, burning candles (especially those scented with synthetic chemicals), wood-burning stoves, kerosene lamps, oil-burning furnaces, cleaning products, paint, varnish, and carpets made from synthetic materials. Pressed-wood products, such as fiberboard, used in flooring, shelving, and paneling, may release a colorless, odorless gas known as *formaldehyde gas,* which is known to cause cancer in animals and may eventually be shown to cause it in humans. *Radon,* a naturally occurring radioactive gas, may seep into homes from certain types of bedrock beneath the foundation and is the second leading cause of lung cancer (smoking is the first), which kills more women than any other type of cancer, including breast cancer. Special kits for detecting radon gas are available, as are devices for removing it from homes. Other common sources of indoor air pollution are cat dander, molds and mildew, dust mites, and cockroaches. Asthma, an increasingly common and serious problem in children, is worsened by most forms of indoor air pollution (National Women's Health Information Center, 2005a).

RESEARCH IN PRACTICE

DURATION OF BREAST MILK EXPRESSION AMONG WORKING MOTHERS ENROLLED IN AN EMPLOYER-SPONSORED LACTATION PROGRAM

What is this study about? There is little doubt that breastfeeding provides numerous, positive health benefits for both mother and baby. The American Academy of Pediatrics recommends exclusive breastfeeding for the first 6 months of life, with breast milk and the gradual addition of solids from 6 months to 1 year. The *Healthy People 2010* objective for breastfeeding is that 50% of babies receive breast milk until 6 months of age. The breastfeeding rate in 2001 was 32.5%, so it is clear that this objective may be challenging to meet. A common barrier to breastfeeding is maternal employment. Lack of knowledge about how to maintain breastfeeding after returning to work, a workplace that is not supportive of breastfeeding, and problems pumping breast milk are frequent reasons that working women wean their babies early. The purpose of this descriptive study was to measure the rate of initiation and duration of breast milk expression in women who were employed in an organization with an employer-sponsored lactation program.

How was this study done? This retrospective study involved a chart review of 462 women who participated in an employer-sponsored lactation support program in one of five corporations. The lactation program specifically included a class on the benefits of breastfeeding, the services of a certified lactation consultant, and a private room in the workplace for expressing breast milk. The employees used regularly scheduled breaks and mealtimes to pump breast milk. Equipment was provided that allowed the employee to pump both breasts simultaneously, and the mothers were provided with a pump for 2 weeks before maternity leave ended so they would be comfortable with the procedure. Accessories were provided to each mother, including an insulated tote bag for transporting milk, bottles to collect and transport milk, flanges that fit over the breast, and pump tubing. All but one of the companies provided the accessories at no cost to the employee. Data were collected from consultant charts, including demographic data, length of postnatal maternity leave, percent of mothers who were breastfeeding at hospital discharge, percent of mothers who successfully expressed their milk at work, and the number of months the women expressed milk at work.

What were the results of the study? Breastfeeding was initiated by 97.5% of the women in the sample, with 57.8% breastfeeding for at least 6 months. Of the mothers who returned to work, 79% attempted to express milk at work and 98% of them were successful. Mothers expressed milk at work for an average of 6.3 months. Breastfeeding was discontinued at an average infant age of 9.1 months, and 24.4% of the mothers expressed milk until the baby was 12 months old. Salaried women were more likely to express milk at work than hourly workers.

What additional questions might I have? Although the benefits for the mothers were clear, what were the benefits for the organization? This information is important to justify the expenses associated with the program and to encourage corporations to adopt similar programs.

How can I use this study? The workplace can create one of the greatest barriers to breastfeeding. This research demonstrates that women who receive the right support can successfully continue breastfeeding after returning to work. Nurses involved in employee health are in a particularly strong position to recommend corporate policies that support breastfeeding for working mothers. All nurses can provide support, education, and direction for mothers who want to continue breastfeeding after they return to work. Providing comprehensive lactation information and supportive programs are needed if this country is to reach the *Healthy People 2010* goals.

Ortiz, J., McGilligan, K., & Kelly, P. (2004). Duration of breast milk expression among working mothers enrolled in an employer-sponsored lactation program. *Pediatric Nursing, 30*(2), 111–119.

Women may be exposed to potentially harmful chemicals and other toxic substances at work and at home. Of the approximately 80,000 chemicals used today in industry and found in various consumer products, only about 1500 have been tested to find out whether they are likely to cause cancer or have toxic effects on the immune and/or reproductive systems or on children's pre- and postnatal growth and development. Even when testing is done, chemicals are tested individually, not in combination. The interactive and cumulative effects of the thousands of chemicals to which adults and children may be exposed are unknown (Pesticide Action Network North America, 2005).

Some types of employment expose women to chemical toxins that may harm them or their unborn children. Women who work around paints, varnishes, sealants, dry cleaning chemicals, synthetic perfumes, hair or clothing dyes, and organic solvents (such as benzene and acetone) are at increased risk.

Women may be exposed to toxic chemicals in their homes as well. Some plastics, such as polyvinyl chloride (PVC), release harmful chemicals (e.g., dioxin and phthalates) when heated. *Dioxin* is a highly toxic compound that occurs as impurities in petroleum-containing pesticides and has been linked to cancer, birth defects, and neurological disorders. *Phthalates*, salt compounds with known toxic qualities, have been linked to a number of adverse effects on health; they are known carcinogens and sufficient levels of exposure can cause male fetuses to be born with undescended testicles and other abnormalities of the sex organs. Recently, they have been shown to damage the DNA in adult men's sperm (Duty et al., 2003). The softer a plastic container or bottle is, the more likely it is to release toxic chemicals when heated. It is safer to store foods in nonplastic materials, such as glass, and to reheat foods in nonplastic containers. Plastic wrap should not be used to cover foods about to be reheated or cooked in a microwave oven (Wolf, 2003).

Beauty products may also contain harmful chemicals. Studies funded by the nonprofit organization Environmental Working Group have revealed that many brands of nail polish, fragrances, deodorants, lotions, hair spray, and other hair care products contain phthalates. The Food and Drug Administration (FDA) maintains that phthalate levels in cosmetic products are too low to be of concern and does not regulate them, nor does it mandate safety testing of personal care products before they are marketed. Some companies voluntarily submit some or all of their products to the Cosmetic Ingredient Review (CIR) panel for testing. CIR is an industry-established and policed body that has no direct ties to the FDA. According to a study done by the Environmental Working Group, 89% of the nearly 11,000 ingredients used in personal care products have never been tested by the CIR or the FDA (Environmental Working Group, 2004).

Many *pesticides,* chemicals used to kill unwanted pests, are commonly used on public and private lawns and gardens and are potentially dangerous to women and their children. Currently, there are over 1200 such chemicals registered for use in the United States. These chemicals, in various combinations, make up the hundreds of products used by the public to control insects. Of the 30 most frequently used pesticide chemicals, 26 have been found to cause liver or kidney damage; 21 have been linked to various reproductive problems in men or women, or both; 19 have been found to be carcinogenic; 15 are known to be toxic to the nervous system; 13 have been linked with birth defects; and 11 disrupt the hormone systems of human beings (National Coalition for Pesticide-Free Lawns, 2005). Few of us escape exposure to these dangerous chemicals. We may breathe them in if we are downwind when insecticide sprays are being applied to crops or golf courses or along highways, or we may inadvertently consume them when we eat nonorganic fruits and vegetables. We may track them from our lawns into our homes, where they degrade more slowly in the absence of rain and sunlight, and where children who play on the floor will come into contact with them. In 2005, scientists at the Pesticide Action Network North America (PAANA) analyzed data collected by the Centers for Disease Control and Prevention (CDC) and found that more than 90% of the individuals tested had a mix of pesticides in their bodies. One pesticide chemical subtype, the *organochlorines* (a combination of dioxin, malathion, chlorpyrifos, and lindane) degrade very slowly and remain in the environment for many decades. Thus, even if these dangerous pesticides were banned today, exposures would not cease entirely. The fact that organochlorines persist in the environment has implications for women of childbearing age, because organochlorines can be passed from mothers to babies in the womb and through breast milk. It is imperative that women not increase their own and their children's exposure to pesticides by applying them to their own lawns and gardens. Infants' and children's rapid rates of growth from conception through adolescence make them particularly susceptible to the effects of toxic chemicals. Pound for pound, children eat more food, drink more water, and breathe more air than do adults, which increases their potential exposure to harmful chemicals in the environment (American Association of Women's Health, Obstetric, and Neonatal Nurses [AWHONN], 2005). Moreover, children's organ systems are not fully developed and are therefore more susceptible to damage from exposures to toxins. The National

Coalition for Pesticide-Free Lawns provides information about effective alternatives to the use of dangerous pesticides and herbicides. The plethora of dangerous pesticides sold and used in this country is a problem women should take very seriously. A study done in 2002 (Perera, Rauh, Tsai, Kinney, Camann, Barr, Bernert, Garfinkel, Tu, Diaz, Dietrich, & Whyatt, 2002) linked elevated blood levels of an organophosphate pesticide in pregnant New York City women with smaller birth weight and head circumference in their babies.

Produce, fish, and meats can also be contaminated with substances that are not good for women and their children. Nonorganic fruits and vegetables carry *pesticide residue* (trace amounts of pesticides left on produce after washing) on their surfaces. Some fruits and vegetables typically carry more residue than others. Bananas, canned peaches, grape juice, and broccoli tend to have low levels. Organic produce has been shown to have much lower levels of pesticide residue than nonorganic produce. Data from the United States Department of Agriculture (USDA) indicate that almost 75% of nonorganic produce tested contained residue, whereas only 23% of organic produce tested did. Because winds can blow pesticides from nonorganic farms to organic farms, it is important to wash all produce before ingesting it (National Coalition for Pesticide-Free Lawns, 2005). Although the FDA maintains that pesticide levels in the US food supply are safe, critics charge that the FDA is excessively influenced by the food industry and other industries as well.

Nearly all fish and shellfish contain some amount of *mercury,* a silvery white metallic element that can cause birth defects when consumed in large quantities. Most fish do not contain enough mercury to be of concern. Because larger amounts of mercury can harm the nervous systems of fetuses and small children, however, pregnant women and toddlers should not eat the flesh of large, predator fish that can have a large buildup of mercury in their fat, for example, shark, tilefish (white or golden snapper), swordfish, and king mackerel. Because tuna are also large, predator fish, pregnant women should not eat more than 6 ounces of white, albacore tuna per week or more than 12 ounces per week of "light" tuna. Salmon is typically low in mercury, but it may be contaminated with industrial chemicals known as *polychlorinated biphenols (PCBs).* PCBs are different types of compounds that are used to replace hydrogen atoms in biphenol with chlorine. These industrial chemicals were banned 30 years ago, but they still linger in the environment. PCBs are known carcinogens, at least in animals. Farmed salmon contains much higher PCB levels than wild salmon, but wild salmon is available only at certain times of the year and is expensive. The farmed fish industry is being pressured by environmental and consumer groups to lower the PCB levels in its products. Meanwhile, there are still quite a few varieties of tasty, uncontaminated fish, for example, cod, mahi-mahi, ocean perch, whitefish, pollock, halibut, haddock, flounder, sole, tilapia, and striped bass (Salmon, 2004).

Meat animals, such as cattle, hogs, and chicken, are dosed with antibiotics to prevent diseases from spreading because of the generally overcrowded conditions in which these animals are kept. The antibiotics given to farm animals are the same ones used to control disease in human beings—sulfa drugs, penicillin, and others. Because the flesh of commercially raised meat animals contains antibiotic residues, humans who eat meat may develop antibiotic-resistant bacterial strains in their bodies. The emergence of difficult-to-treat urinary infections in women has been attributed to the pervasive and indiscriminate use of antibiotics by the meat industry (Union of Concerned Scientists, 2005). Organic meats are free of antibiotic residues.

Questions regarding the safety of exposure to video display terminals (VDTs) have arisen in recent years, and various studies have produced contradictory results. However, at present there is no documented evidence of increased risk of spontaneous abortion or overall fetal loss in women whose work exposed them regularly to VDTs. Until more is known about the possibility of other biologic effects of chronic exposure to the low-frequency electromagnetic fields found with VDTs, women should avoid chronic exposure. Because the strength of the field decreases significantly with distance, women can decrease their exposure by sitting at least 50 cm (20 inches) from the screen and at least 1 m (3.25 feet) from the sides or back of adjacent machines (electromagnetic field strength is typically higher from the back and sides). Exposure is also decreased by turning off VDTs, printers, and other electrical devices when they are not in use.

The exposure to various biological and chemical toxins inherent in providing care for sick people constitutes an occupational hazard for nurses. Exposure to toxoplasmosis, rubella, cytomegalovirus, herpes simplex, and hepatitis B may adversely affect pregnancy and fetal outcome. The risk of exposure to HIV infection via needle sticks and contact with blood and other body fluids also exists. Latex allergy is rapidly becoming a significant problem among healthcare workers, with 8% to 12% demonstrating hypersensitivity symptoms ranging from mild contact dermatitis to severe systemic reactions and anaphylactic shock (American Nurses Association, 2005).

Two governmental agencies have primary responsibility for addressing workplace safety. The Occupational Safety and Health Administration (OSHA), part of the Department of Labor, is responsible for creating and enforcing workplace health and safety regulations. The National Institute for Occupational Safety and Health (NIOSH), which is part of the Department of Health and Human Services, is primarily a research agency. However, it also disseminates information on preventing workplace injury and illness, provides training to occupational safety and health professionals, and investigates potentially hazardous working situations when requested by employers or employees.

Environmental hazards are an area of particular interest and importance to maternal-newborn nurses, both personally and professionally. Nurses need to be aware of the risks that they face in their own environment and the risks that childbearing women (and all women) face in theirs. Nurses can encourage administrators to investigate potential hazards in their clinical environment, and they can encourage clients to take similar action to protect themselves from environmental hazards in their workplaces. The Internet can provide information and resources on specific hazards and preventive strategies to decrease risk of exposure. Nurses can also lobby community leaders and legis-

lators to support positions that protect childbearing women from environmental toxins. Nurse researchers can investigate workforce and environmental hazards, recording, analyzing, and publishing findings.

SOCIAL ISSUES AFFECTING OLDER WOMEN

In the United States and other developed nations, women tend to outlive men. Thus, women are overrepresented in the ranks of older people. This phenomenon is referred to as the **feminization of later life.** There are 20.8 million women aged 65 or older living in the United States. Among people aged 80 or older, 65% are female (Maternal and Child Health Bureau, 2005).

Economic Vulnerability of Older Women

The feminization of later life means that older women are more likely than their male counterparts to be widowed, to live alone, to be disabled, and to be poor. However, of all the elderly in the United States, women of color have the highest poverty rates. Factors that contribute to the increased economic vulnerability of women include the following (Davis & Huber, 2004):

- Women must stretch their financial resources further than men because of their longer life expectancy.
- Older women tend to have less educational preparation than older men.
- Historically women have been economically dependent on men and may have intermittent or nonexistent employment histories.
- Women typically earn less than men and often work in jobs without pension benefits or have only limited benefits.
- Intermittent employment is more common in women, which decreases their social security and retirement benefits.
- Women generally have more family caregiving responsibilities than men.
- Historically, public pension systems have been designed with an expectation that men would be the primary economic providers. Older women who worked outside their homes may have only meager pensions.

Even middle-class women face the risk of "cycling into poverty" should they become widows. A drastic decline in financial circumstances is particularly likely if a woman's husband had a long, costly illness or if his pension is decreased or discontinued following his death. To help keep elderly women from spending their final years in poverty, it is necessary for governments to develop solutions to the economic concerns caused by a fixed income, to deal with problems of pension inequity, and to address the potentially disastrous effects of staggering healthcare costs for the uninsured or underinsured. Because women are living longer than men and the average age has continued to climb, the need for additional income sources is imperative (Table 8–1).

Table 8–1	YEARS OF LIFE EXPECTANCY AT BIRTH FOR SELECTED COUNTRIES, 2004 (ROUNDED TO NEAREST YEAR)	
Country	**Male Life Expectancy**	**Female Life Expectancy**
Afghanistan	42	43
Argentina	72	80
Australia	77	83
Canada	77	84
China	70	73
Egypt	63	67
Ethiopia	40	41
France	76	83
India	62	64
Japan	78	85
Mexico	72	78
Russia	60	73
Tanzania	43	44
United Kingdom	76	81
United States	75	80

SOURCE: U.S. Census Bureau. (2005). International Programs Center, International Data Base.

Table 8–2	DEFINITIONS OF ELDER ABUSE

Physical abuse: Any physical pain or injury that is intentionally inflicted upon an elderly person by a caregiver or individual who has custody of, or stands in a position of trust with, that elder. Sexual assault, physical attacks, unreasonable physical restraint, and prolonged deprivation of food and water all constitute physical abuse.

Financial abuse: Any theft or misuse of an elderly person's money or property by a caregiver or person in a position of trust.

Neglect: Failure on the part of a caregiver, or any person having custody of an elder, to provide reasonable care, which is the degree of care that a reasonable person would provide. Reasonable care includes, but is not limited to, assistance with personal hygiene; protection from health and safety hazards; and provision of shelter, food, clothing, health needs, and medical care except in instances when the elder refuses treatment.

Self-neglect: Failure to provide adequate self-care because of inability or inattention.

Psychologic abuse: The intentional infliction of mental suffering on an elder by a caregiver or person in a position of trust. Psychologic abuse includes, but is not limited to, verbal assaults, threats, humiliation, intimidation, or isolation of the elder.

Abandonment: The desertion of an elder by any person responsible for the care and custody of that elder, under circumstances in which a reasonable person would continue to provide care.

SOURCE: Adapted from *Definitions of Elder Abuse,* 2005, with permission from the National Center on Elder Abuse.

Elder Abuse

Elder abuse includes any deliberate action, or lack of action, that causes harm to an elderly person. It is difficult to determine how many elderly women in the United States are victims of abuse, because perpetrators are usually careful to conceal their behavior, but elderly women are believed to be more at risk than elderly men. Currently in the United States, it is estimated that 3% to 5% of the total elderly population, or approximately 500,000 individuals, are abused annually. Experts anticipate that the problem will continue to grow as the population ages and as illness and financial burdens strain family relationships (National Center on Elder Abuse [NCEA], 2005).

Five different categories of elder abuse have been recognized: psychologic abuse, physical abuse (including sexual abuse), neglect (by self or caregiver), financial abuse, and abandonment (Table 8–2). Multiple forms of abuse may occur simultaneously and tend to intensify with time unless intervention occurs.

The prototypical victim of elder abuse is a white woman over 80 years old who lives in her own home or the home of a family member. The abuser is most often a spouse, followed by family members and then primary caregivers. Elder abuse by staff in nursing homes and long-term care facilities is also well documented. On average, elderly black Americans are more at risk for abandonment than older white Americans. Abandonment statistics are much lower for Asians and Hispanics. Factors that increase the risk of elder abuse include shared living arrangements, family history of violence, lack of financial resources, dependence, isolation, poor health, and cognitive impairment. Substance abuse and stressful events in the life of the abuser may also contribute to the risk (NCEA, 2005).

A full discussion of this growing problem, its identification, and treatment is beyond the scope of this textbook. It is imperative, however, that nurses who care for the elderly be alert for signs of abuse and take steps to address the problem when it is identified.

Implications of Aging for Women's Health and Health Care

Older women often face health problems that become more common as people age: hypertension, coronary artery disease, arthritis, diabetes, osteoporosis, dementia, and depression. Heart disease, cancer, and stroke are the leading causes of death for all women age 65 or older. Among white women, lung disease is the fourth leading cause of death, but for minority women it is diabetes. By age 65, half of all women have developed two or more chronic diseases. Minority and low-income women are more likely than white, higher income women, to have serious health problems; African American women are twice as likely as white women to have coronary heart disease (Maternal and Child Health Bureau, 2005).

Unfortunately, older women, particularly those who are poor, face multiple barriers in obtaining adequate healthcare services. For some, lack of transportation to healthcare facilities is an issue. Many older women are no longer able to drive because of failing eyesight or diminished reflexes. Although public transportation may be available in larger cities, many rural areas have no bus, train, or cab service, and even if public transportation is available, poorer women may not be able to afford the costs involved.

Lack of private health insurance coverage or excessive medical costs not covered by Medicare are major problems for many older women. Too often, women on limited incomes must choose between paying rent and purchasing food and paying for needed medicines or other forms of health care. Thus, nurses must remain aware of the possibility that a client's noncompliance may be economically driven.

Another problem common in older women with multiple health problems is a phenomenon known as **polypharmacy,** which means "multiple medicines." A woman who sees two or more specialists for the treatment of multiple medical conditions may well be taking a half-dozen or more powerful drugs, each with its own array of side effects and with the potential for dangerous interactions with one or more of the others, and perhaps several over-the-counter drugs as well. Sometimes polypharmacy is justified by the woman's medical needs, but often it is inadvertent; nurse practitioners and physicians are sometimes unaware that a given woman is taking medications prescribed by a different provider. Elderly people may not remember what medications they are taking or may not think to keep caregivers apprised of them. Also, many people assume that herbs, and various other products classified as *nutritional supplements,* are safe because they are sold without a prescription. Although such products are generally much less potent than prescription drugs, many can and do interact with drugs elderly people commonly take. For example, the herbal supplement St. John's wort, often taken to relieve mild depression, can increase or decrease the effects of oral contraceptives, blood thinners, and some prescription antidepressants (Mathuna, 2003). Sometimes, symptoms in an elderly person are related to drug effects or interactions rather than to disease or illness. Nurses must advise elderly clients to keep a list of the medications they take and provide each of their providers with a copy, and to fill all their prescriptions at the same pharmacy. Pharmacists are increasingly alert to the potential risks posed by multiple drug prescriptions and will warn patients and providers of likely negative effects and interactions (Figure 8–5 ◆).

Some drugs have known potential for causing cognitive impairment in elderly persons who have diminished kidney and liver function. Drugs that alter the central nervous system (anti-cholinergics, antihistamines, antidepressants, anxiolytics, antipsychotics, and antiepileptics) may cause such symptoms as forgetfulness, confusion, disorientation, and inability to concentrate (March, 2005). Nurses can play a key role in identifying older women's concerns as well as the onset of new symptoms. In collaboration with other providers, they can improve an older woman's chances of receiving optimal health care.

SOCIAL ISSUES AFFECTING WOMEN WITH DISABILITIES

Approximately 19.1 million US women and girls have some type of mental or physical disability, and, of these, 15.4% are unable to perform basic self-care activities. Women are more likely than men to be disabled because of longer life expectancy rates, and disabilities are most prevalent in women over the age of 85. The majority of women with disabilities (56%) are in this age group, whereas another 44% are over the age of 65 (National Center on Birth Defects and Developmental Disabilities [NCBDDD], 2005).

Definitions of Disability

A **disability** is a chronic physical or mental health problem or impairment that restricts an individual's ability to perform one or more major activities. Whether a given activity is considered major depends on the circumstances and responsibilities of the woman in question. For example, if a middle-aged woman cannot care for her home and children because of a disability, that disability would be considered major. If an elderly woman's disability makes independent self-care impossible, that disability would be considered major. Disabilities may also be categorized as "work" and "severe." *Work disabilities* restrict individuals from employment; a nurse who sustains a back injury that becomes chronic and prevents her from returning to her position as a staff nurse has a work disability. *Severe disabilities* prohibit individuals from performing basic activities of daily living without assistance.

Types of Disabilities

Disabilities are categorized as developmental, learning, neurological, psychiatric, and sensory. *Developmental disabilities* such as autism, cerebral palsy, epilepsy, and spina bifida are ongoing and manifest before the age of 22. They create severe limitations in three or more of the following areas: self-care, receptive and expressive language, learning, mobility, self-direction, ability to live alone, and financial independence. More than 4 million individuals are affected with some type of developmental disability, and mental retardation is the most common (Center on Birth Defects and Developmental Disabilities, 2005) (Figure 8–6 ◆).

Learning disabilities, such as dyslexia and attention-deficit hyperactivity disorder, can inhibit educational attainment and employment. *Common neurological disabilities* include spina bifida, multiple sclerosis, and Alzheimer's disease. Spina bifida, or congenital malformation of the spinal cord, can cause partial paralysis. Multiple sclerosis, which affects a disproportionately

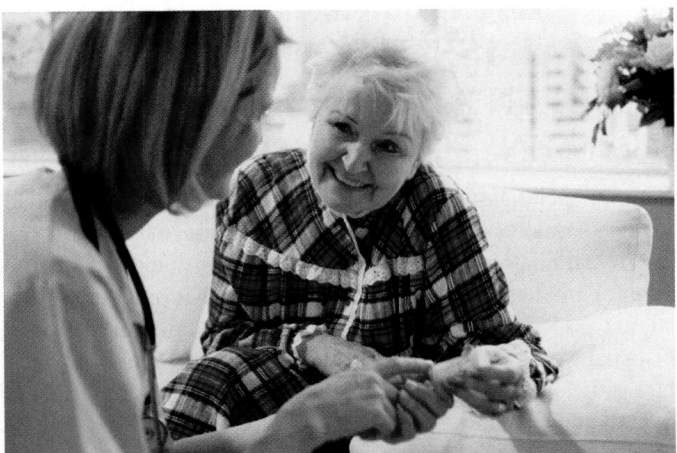

Figure 8–5 ◆ Older women are more likely to have multiple medical conditions that require medication. Careful instructions should be given to prevent medication interactions.
SOURCE: Dann Tardif/CORBIS.

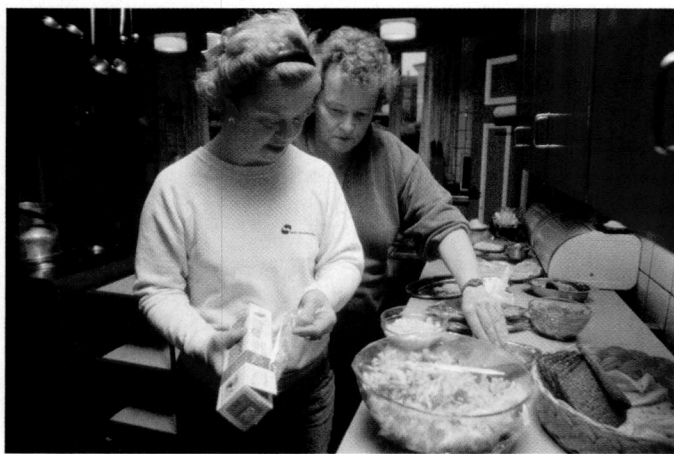

Figure 8–6 ◆ Mental retardation is the most common developmental disability.
SOURCE: Stephanie Maze/CORBIS.

high number of women in comparison with men, can cause severe mental and physical disability through degeneration of nerve fibers in the brain and spinal cord. Alzheimer's disease causes ongoing, incurable dementia that culminates in death. *Psychiatric disabilities* can cause significant impairment and significantly alter an individual's quality of life. Women's rates of depression, anxiety, panic disorders, and phobic disorders are 50% higher than men's. *Sensory disabilities* such as hearing loss and visual impairments can dramatically impair a woman's ability to interact socially and to live independently (National Women's Health Information Center, 2002).

Economic Vulnerability of Women with Disabilities

Only about 31% of women with a disability are employed, in contrast with 62% of disabled men. Many disabled women can only manage part-time employment, which severely restricts their income potential. An additional problem is that disabled people face formidable barriers to employment: Some cannot drive or easily access public transportation. Many buildings are still without ramps and wide door openings that facilitate wheelchair access, and employers are sometimes reluctant to hire disabled persons. The Americans with Disabilities Act (ADA) of 1990 was intended to reduce such barriers by mandating modest improvements in building accessibility and forbidding unjustified hiring discrimination against disabled persons (Department of Justice, 2005). Although the ADA has brought about some improvements, many barriers to employment still exist, including transportation barriers, architectural obstacles, and discrimination in general.

Even when disabled women are able to work and find work, they typically do not earn as much as women who are not disabled. Census data indicate that the median wages for disabled and nondisabled women in 2000 was $25,201 and $28,164, respectively. Men with disability earned $32,345. When disabled women cannot work, or cannot find a job, they often lose the ability to care for themselves and their families financially. Although many people assume that social security benefits keep disabled individuals out of poverty, this is simply not the case. More than a fourth of all women with disabilities live in poverty, and, in all age groups, more disabled women live in poverty than disabled men (NCBDDD, 2005).

Violence Against People with Disabilities

Both men and women with developmental disabilities are 4 to 10 times more likely to be victims of crime than people without disabilities. Women who have developmental disabilities are 50% more likely to be sexually assaulted in their lifetime than women of normal intelligence. Disabled women may have difficulties escaping from or fighting off an attacker, may be unable to communicate well enough to report crimes, and/or may be unable to positively identify an attacker because of sensory or cognitive limitations (National Women's Health Information Center, 2002).

Effects of Disability on Women's Health Care

Women with disabilities need routine gynecologic care and preventive health education, as do all women, but healthcare services for disabled women are often suboptimal. Many women with disabilities report that various barriers prevent them from obtaining routine healthcare services. On one survey that explored disabled women's perceptions of barriers that prevented them from receiving optimal health care, 37% of respondents reported having difficulty getting onto examination tables and 29% said their physician was not empathetic regarding issues related to their disability (National Women's Health Information Center, 2002).

An additional problem is that many healthcare providers assume incorrectly that women with severe disabilities are not sexually active. Because of these false assumptions, many disabled women are not offered screening for sexually transmitted infections (STIs), education regarding STI prevention, contraceptive counseling, or preconception counseling.

SOCIAL ISSUES AFFECTING LESBIAN AND BISEXUAL WOMEN

Various social issues can detract from lesbian and bisexual women's quality of life. These include employment and housing discrimination, discrimination involving domestic life and parenting issues, and general social discrimination based on the stigma associated with homosexuality. In addition, lesbian and bisexual women face perceived and actual discrimination on the part of healthcare providers that negatively affects both access to and quality of health care.

Employment Discrimination

Employment discrimination is the most frequent complaint the American Civil Liberties Union (ACLU) receives from gay and lesbian individuals. An act that would have prohibited termina-

Table 8–3	U.S. STATES WITH LEGISLATION PROTECTING HOMOSEXUAL WORKERS AGAINST DISCRIMINATION BY PUBLIC AND PRIVATE EMPLOYERS

California	Nevada
Connecticut	New Hampshire
District of Columbia	New Jersey
Hawaii	New York
Maryland	Rhode Island
Massachusetts	Vermont
Minnesota	Wisconsin

tion of employment on the basis of sexual orientation, the 1997 Employment Non-Discrimination Act, was defeated by one vote. An updated version of the bill was introduced in 2002 but has yet to be passed. At present, it is still legal in 34 states to fire a lesbian woman (or gay man) on the basis of sexual orientation alone (Human Rights Campaign, 2005). Table 8–3 lists those states that do provide legal protection for homosexual employees.

Discrimination exists not only in the private sector, but also in the military. The battle over homosexuals in the military has raged on since President Clinton enacted the "don't ask, don't tell" policy in 1994. Although this legislation removed sexual orientation as a contraindication to military service, it has been far from successful in protecting gay and lesbian service members from expulsion; homosexual conduct is still grounds for terminating their service. Homosexual conduct includes not only homosexual acts, but also statements that demonstrate a propensity or intent to engage in homosexual acts. In short, lesbian women can serve in the military, but if their sexual orientation becomes known, they can be asked to resign. In 2004, the number of military discharges based on sexual orientation was lower (770) than at any time since 1996, comprising a small fraction of total unplanned discharges (US Military, 2005).

Lesbians face additional discrimination in the area of spousal benefits. Although individuals who are legally married can receive health insurance coverage, life insurance benefits, retirement pensions, and disability coverage for their partners, lesbian partners who are not legally married (the vast majority) cannot. Currently, only one state—Massachusetts—recognizes marriage between same-sex individuals. Three states however, Vermont, New Jersey, and Connecticut, permit **civil unions:** legally recognized partnerships that involve rights and responsibilities comparable with those enjoyed by married couples. Couples who enter into civil unions are generally subject to the same laws and processes regarding inheritance, property rights, child custody, and medical decision making as married couples. Same-sex couples who wish to enter into a civil union must obtain a special license and have a solemnization ceremony. Civil union dissolution proceedings are handled in much the same manner as divorces (Lambda Legal Defense Fund, 2005).

Domestic partnership recognition is another mechanism by which public and private employers can provide insurance coverage and pension rights benefits to the partners of gay and lesbian employees. Twenty-five state governments (and the Dis-

trict of Columbia) provide such benefits to employees, as do increasing numbers of city and county governments and private employers (Lambda Legal Defense Fund, 2005).

Housing Discrimination

Lesbians also face housing discrimination. Although *Fair Housing laws* protect members of various groups (minorities, pregnant women, and families with children) from being denied housing, they do not generally apply to homosexuals. Except in the few states and municipalities in which antidiscrimination-in-housing laws cover sexual orientation, landlords can refuse to rent, and homeowners can refuse to sell, to gay and lesbian people. The mechanisms by which housing discrimination on the basis of sexual orientation work are often subtle; leases may forbid "immoral" (code for homosexual) activities and/or restrict occupancy to those "related by blood or marriage." Some homeowner association boards reserve the right to refuse prospective purchasers on the basis of "inappropriate lifestyle." Another housing-related problem gay and lesbian couples face is that, unlike married couples, they may not be able to use their combined income to determine their eligibility for a mortgage and may have to settle for cheaper housing than they can actually afford. Ironically, gay and lesbian couples who are not well off often wind up at the bottom of eligibility lists for public housing because they are not considered to constitute a "family" ("Understanding Discrimination Against Gays and Lesbians," 2004).

Parenting Issues

Many lesbian women wish to become adoptive parents. Both single women and couples often desire the presence of children in their lives, and women who are coparenting their partner's child may want to formally adopt that child. Gay and lesbian people who wish to adopt, however, often face formidable barriers. Some child placement agencies have policies restricting adoption to married couples and in a few states, legislation specifically bars homosexuals from adopting. Even in the absence of such policies or statutes, however, prejudice on the part of judges, social workers, and others who make decisions about child placement often makes it almost impossible for gay and lesbian people to adopt children or even become foster parents. Foreign adoptions may be no easier, because some agencies that facilitate them refuse gay and lesbian applicants. A small number of states, however, have laws prohibiting child custody or adoption discrimination against homosexuals, and some states make what is known as *second parent adoption* available to lesbian women who are coparenting the biological children of their partners. This option allows coparents to adopt children legally, thus ensuring stability for them, should the biological parent become incapacitated or die (American Civil Liberties Union [ACLU], 2005).

Although there are societal concerns about children that are being raised by same-sex parents, there is no objective evidence supporting such concern. The American Academy of Pediatrics (AAP) reviewed decades of research data on children raised by heterosexual parents and children raised by lesbian or gay

Figure 8–7 ◆ Lesbian families face discrimination that more traditional families do not commonly encounter.
SOURCE: Vanessa Vick/Photo Researchers, Inc.

parents, and in 2002 it issued a policy statement stating that no differences were observed (AAP, 2002) (Figure 8–7 ◆).

Although sexual orientation per se has no effect on the quality of parenting, discriminatory tax laws can adversely affect lesbian couples' ability to provide for their children. If one of the partners is employed and the other remains at home to care for the children, the working partner may not be able to claim either her partner or their children as dependents because the partners are not legally married ("Understanding Discrimination Against Gays and Lesbians," 2004).

Social Barriers

Lesbian and gay individuals and couples often face discrimination—and even danger. They may be treated rudely in stores, motels, restaurants, and other public facilities and ostracized by business networks, churches, neighbors, and even families. There are reports of newspapers having refused to accept advertisements from gay people or gay organizations, and Disneyland (not Disney World) has a policy banning same-sex couple dancing. When homosexual people are made to feel uncomfortable in establishments that cater to the general public, they are forced to congregate in *gay bars,* where they may become inviting targets for violently homophobic individuals. In 2003, 1430 hate crimes based solely on sexual orientation (16.4% of total hate crimes) were reported to the Federal Bureau of Investigation (Hate Crime Network, 2005). Although those numbers may seem relatively small, it must be kept in mind that hate crime reporting by law enforcement officials is voluntary, and hate crimes motivated by homophobia are considered to be significantly underreported. Many lesbian women are reluctant to be open about their lifestyle because of social discrimination and the possibility of violence.

Although the goal of equality for all women is still unmet and the burden of discrimination is even greater for lesbian than heterosexual women, there is reason for optimism. Acceptance of gay men and lesbian women is on the rise, with sympathetic

portrayals (*Will and Grace; Ellen*) in the media. Ongoing research by the American Enterprise Institute indicates that 80% of Americans now believe homosexual people should be allowed to serve in the military (Ricci & Biederman, 2004).

Effects of Discrimination on Lesbian and Bisexual Women's Health Care

In its *Healthy People 2010* action plan, the US Department of Health and Human Services acknowledged sexual orientation as a risk factor for inferior health care, citing reasons such as lack of insurance, fear of discrimination on the part of providers, and provider ignorance of gay and lesbian people's healthcare needs. The first two factors limit access to health care, and the third has a negative effect on healthcare quality (Thayer, 2004).

Lesbian and bisexual women are less likely than heterosexual women to have health insurance because, unlike heterosexual women, they are usually not eligible for insurance benefits based on a partner's employment. Lack of coverage can cause women to forgo health screening procedures such as Pap smears and mammography, and delay treatment until illnesses have become serious. The fear that providers may harbor antigay sentiments, or be uncomfortable around gay people, is, unfortunately, well-founded. In a study published in 2005 (Hinchliff, Gott, & Galena), investigators reported that over half of primary care physicians surveyed said they would find it embarrassing to discuss issues related to sexual health with gay or lesbian women. Healthcare providers may also assume that all clients are heterosexual, thus creating an uncomfortable atmosphere for homosexual clients. The assumption of heterosexuality, revealed in questions such as, *What kind of birth control do you use?* and intake forms that list only *single, married, widowed, or divorced* as lifestyle options, alienate lesbian women and may cause them to conceal their sexual orientation. A study done in 2002 by Witeck-Combs Communications and Harris Interactive found that only 55% of lesbian women surveyed had disclosed their orientation to their healthcare provider. Lesbian women's reluctance to disclose their sexual orientation can lower the quality of health care they receive. For example, women who do not admit that they live with a partner will not be screened for domestic violence, which is a routine screening for women in heterosexual relationships (Thayer, 2004).

An additional problem that lesbian women face is that providers tend to not be knowledgeable about lesbian women's healthcare needs. Providers may not realize, for example, that lesbians are thought (but not yet proven) to be at increased risk for breast cancer because they are more likely than heterosexual women to have never given birth, to be overweight, to be stressed, and to smoke and drink alcohol. Many providers also believe that lesbian women are not at risk for sexually transmitted diseases (STDs) and cervical cancer, both of which are untrue. Lesbian sexual contact can transmit a number of STDs and the virus that causes cervical cancer, because it involves exposure to vaginal secretions (National Women's Health Information Center, 2005b).

FEMALE GENITAL MUTILATION (FGM)

Female genital mutilation (FGM), also known as *female genital cutting, female circumcision,* and *genital circumcision,* refers to the practice of removing all or parts of a girl's or woman's genitalia for cultural reasons. It is a phenomenon with which nurses who provide health care to women, especially immigrant women from certain parts of the world, must be familiar. The damage done to a woman's anatomy in the more severe versions of the practice can cause a variety of health problems, including bleeding, infection, infertility, painful intercourse, and difficulties related to childbearing.

Origin and Demographics of FGM

FGM is a very old practice; evidence of it is present in the female mummies of Egyptian royalty. It survives in at least 28 countries in Northern Africa, parts of the Middle East (Oman, Yemen, United Arab Emirates), and Asia (Indonesia, Malaysia, Sri Lanka, India). In some countries, a high percentage of women undergo the procedure, and in others only a minority does. FGM is not associated with any particular religion and is found among Christians, Muslims, Animists, and one Jewish sect. FGM is practiced in male-dominated societies in which patriarchal authority and control of women's bodies and fertility are taken for granted. In such societies, girls receive little education and are valued primarily as sources of labor and for their future role as producers of children. Fathers in many such societies sell their daughters into marriage, the payment being known as the *brideprice.*

The original reason for FGM is thought to have been the prevention of sexual intercourse before or outside of marriage, thus ensuring men that the children their wives bear are theirs. In societies in which genital mutilation has become the norm, the procedure has become heavily enculturated and is supported by both men and women. It is women, in fact, who actively promote and carry out FGM. Myths about the clitoris (that it will grow very long if not amputated; that if it touches a baby during childbirth, the baby will die) are widely believed, and uncircumcised women are seen as impure, unclean, and ugly. They are generally cut off from marriage, motherhood, and full female identity and may be ostracized. Because FGM is so closely associated with female identity, even the educated women in a given society may support it. The age at which FGM procedures are performed varies from culture to culture, with the most common range being from 5 to 12 years. A few societies carry out the procedure on infants or on teenagers just before marriage (Ben-Ari, 2003).

Nature of the Procedure(s)

In the most extreme form of FGM, known as *infibulation,* the clitoris, the labia minora, and most of the labia majora are removed and the raw surfaces of the remaining stumps of the labia majora are sewn together over the vaginal opening, leaving only a small hole for the passage of urine and menstrual blood. The opening is widened (deinfibulated) somewhat at the time of marriage, either rapidly, with a knife, or gradually, to permit sexual intercourse. Further deinfibulation is done to permit childbirth, and women are sewn up again afterward. Of all circumcised women in Djibouti, the Sudan, and Somalia, 80% to 90% are infibulated. The least extreme form of FGM is *partial clitoridectomy,* in which the tip of the clitoris is removed. The most common procedure (80% to 85% of all procedures) involves complete removal of the clitoris, with partial or complete removal of the labia minora.

FGM procedures are generally carried out in villages, by a female birth attendant or elder, as part of an elaborate ritual. Very primitive instruments may be used and no anesthesia is provided. The procedure lasts approximately 20 to 30 minutes, depending on its nature and the skill of the person carrying it out. Girls are restrained by female relatives, usually including their mothers. Young girls do not usually realize what is about to happen to them; older girls may undergo the procedure willingly to conform to societal expectations. In urban areas, affluent parents may have the procedure done in a hospital (Ben-Ari, 2003).

Health Implications

Data on the number of deaths from shock and infection that occur following FGM are hard to come by, because mortality is often attributed to some other cause. Hemorrhage is the most common immediate complication of all procedures, followed by infection and urinary retention related to swelling. Infibulation causes the most severe long-term complications, most of which are related to the urinary tract and childbirth. Chronic urinary infections caused by inadequate emptying of the bladder are common; although a woman with intact genitalia can usually empty her bladder in 5 to 10 seconds, it may take an infibulated woman as long as 5 minutes to do so. Some women develop chronic reproductive tract infections related to retained vaginal fluid and blood. Such infections can lead to infertility, which is thought to affect 25% to 30% of infibulated women. Urinary incontinence in the form of dribbling is another common problem, as is genital pain. Many infibulated women experience pain during sexual intercourse (dyspareunia), some because they have developed a neuroma in their scar tissue. Infibulation-related complications associated with childbirth include obstructed labor, nonreassuring fetal status, postpartum hemorrhage, and postpartum sepsis. The psychologic trauma caused by FGM may persist throughout a woman's life. It is related not only to personal suffering, but also to knowing that daughters and granddaughters will undergo the procedure too (Little, 2003).

Efforts to Eradicate FGM

FGM has been denounced as a form of child abuse by the World Health Organization and by many other international and national organizations. Healthcare-related organizations, including the American Medical Association and the American Nurses Association, have denounced it as well. FGM has been outlawed in 14 African countries and some Arab countries in which it has traditionally been practiced. It is illegal in many North American and European countries that have sizable immigrant populations. The United States and Great Britain have laws forbidding parents from taking girls to another country for the purpose of having an FGM procedure performed. Grassroots organizations in many countries combat FGM by providing education about its dangers to parents and village elders. Nevertheless, FGM persists, even in countries in which it is illegal. Entrenched cultural values and practices are exceedingly difficult to change and can only be changed from within a given society. In time, FGM will no doubt go the way of foot-binding in China, but until it does, nurses must respond appropriately and professionally to women who have been subjected to it (Little, 2003).

Responding Appropriately to Circumcised Women

It is estimated that 130,000 women worldwide have had an FGM procedure. Given the increasingly multicultural nature of American society, it is likely that nurses who provide physical care to female clients will encounter women and/or girls whose genitalia have been surgically altered. Nurses must be prepared for this eventuality and refrain from behavior that may insult or alienate the client. Exhibiting shock, revulsion, or pity at the sight of altered genitalia, for example, is inappropriate. Nurses must also understand that women brought up in cultures in which FGM is a fact of life may not consider themselves to have been mutilated or victimized. In fact, such a woman may be offended if her nurse uses the term *mutilation* or expresses disapproval of genital alteration. If a woman shares her indecision regarding some aspect of FGM, for example, whether to be sewn up again after delivery, the nurse should listen nonjudgmentally.

CHAPTER REVIEW

FOCUS YOUR STUDY

- The number of women living in poverty is increasing. Childbearing women seem to be at particular risk because of current trends in the divorce rate, the frequency with which the mother gains custody of children, and factors in the work environment that make it difficult for women to earn an adequate wage.

- The number of homeless families is increasing.

- Women's wages have always been lower than men's because of demand, education, skills, discrimination, and underlying philosophies that deem women's work less valuable. Many people are working to change the wage system by pushing for comparable worth legislation.

- Employee benefits that affect women include maternity leave, paternity leave, and child care. The Family and Medical Leave Act mandates parental leave for childbirth or adoption but applies only to companies with 50 or more employees. Insurance coverage for childbirth varies by company.

- Elder abuse includes physical abuse, financial abuse, neglect, self-neglect, psychologic abuse, and abandonment.

- Older women may face multiple barriers when obtaining health care, including transportation difficulties; lack of health coverage; lack of research regarding chronic conditions affecting women; and symptom-specific, rather than holistic, care.

- There are multiple types of disabilities. All have the potential for limiting a woman's quality of life, her ability to care for herself, and the quality of her health care.

- Lesbian and bisexual women face various forms of discrimination, some of which can negatively affect their health and health care.

- Nurses must provide culturally sensitive care to women who have undergone procedures involving genital mutilation.

EXPLORE MediaLink

http://www.prenhall.com/davidson

NCLEX review questions, case studies, and other interactive resources for this chapter can be found on the Web Site at http://www.prenhall.com/davidson. Click on " Chapter 8 " to select the activities for this chapter.

For tutorials including animations and videos, more NCLEX review questions, and an audio glossary, access the accompanying Prentice Hall Nursing MediaLink DVD-ROM in this book.

PRENTICE HALL NURSING MEDIALINK DVD-ROM

Audio Glossary
NCLEX Review

COMPANION WEBSITE

Additional NCLEX Review
Case Study: *Social Issues Affecting Women*
Care Plan Activity: *Pregnancy in a Disabled Client*
Applications: *How to Find Good Day Care; Elder Abuse*
Critical Thinking

CRITICAL THINKING IN ACTION

DOMESTIC VIOLENCE IN THE ELDERLY

View the Critical Thinking in Action video in Chapter 8 of the DVD-ROM. Then answer the questions that follow.

Grace Abbey, an 83-year-old woman, presents for irregular bleeding to the gynecologist. Mrs. Abbey, a widow, has been living with her son, a 54-year-old unemployed retail manager, for the last 2 years when her husband died. Her son accompanies her to the visit and is reluctant to leave his mother's side. You ask the son to wait in the waiting room and begin your assessment of Mrs. Abbey. When you roll up her sleeve to take her blood pressure, you note bruises on her wrist and forearm. When you question her about the eti-ology of the bruises, she looks down at the floor and avoids making eye contact. She then states she cannot remember how the bruises occurred. After obtaining her vital signs, you escort her into the exam room and note additional bruises on her back as you assist her with her gown. When you question her about those bruises, she breaks down sobbing, saying, "Don't say anything. Don't tell my son you saw them."

1. Discuss how you would assess Mrs. Abbey for other forms of elder abuse.

2. Mrs. Abbey describes physical violence that started occurring after her son lost his job and his wife left him. She admits, "I have been more trouble with my health problems lately." What factors can increase the risk of elder abuse?

3. Mrs. Abbey begins crying and says, "I know this has never happened to anyone else. I don't understand why this is happening." What is your reply?

REFERENCES

American Academy of Pediatrics (AAP). (2002). Technical report: Coparent or second-parent adoption by same-sex parents. *AAP Policy Statement, 109*(2), 341–344.

American Academy of Pediatrics. (2005). Quality of early education and child care from birth to kindergarten. *Pediatrics, 15*(1). Retrieved September 16, 2005, from the Academic Search Premier database.

American Association of Women's Health, Obstetric, and Neonatal Nurses (AWHONN). (2005). *Protecting the health of women and children from environmental toxins.* (Policy Statement Approved 2001). Retrieved September 17, 2005, from http://www.awhonn.org

American Civil Liberties Union (ACLU). (2005). *Adoption and foster care.* Retrieved September 9, 2006, from http://www.aclu.org/GetEqual/par/adopt.htm

American Nurses Association. (2005). *Latex allergy an occupational health hazard for nurses.* Retrieved September 23, 2005, from http://www.nursingworld.org/dlwa/osh/latex.htm

Ben-Ari, N. H. (2003). Villagers join campaigns against FGM. *Horizons, 16*(4). Retrieved October 18, 2005, from the Academic Search Premier database.

Center for Women's Business Research. (2005). *Top facts about women-owned businesses.* Retrieved September 3, 2005, from http://www.womensbusinessresearch.org/topfacts.html

Children's Defense Fund. (2004). *States' subsidized guardian laws at a glance.* Retrieved September 16, 2005, from http://www.childrensdefense.org/childwelfare/kinshipcare/guardianship_laws.pdf

Davis, R., & Huber, K. (2004). Class, ethnicity, age, physical status, and sexual orientation: Implications for health and healthcare. In M. Condon (Ed.), *Women's health: An integrated approach to wellness and illness* (pp. 21–38). Upper Saddle River, NJ: Prentice Hall Health.

DeNavas-Walt, C., Proctor, B. D., & Mills, R. (2004). *Income, poverty and health insurance coverage in the United States: 2003.* Retrieved August 29, 2005, from http://www.census.gov/prod/2004pubs/p60-226.pdf

DeNavas-Walt, C., Proctor, B. D., & Mills, R. (2005). *Income, poverty and health insurance coverage in the United States: 2004.* Retrieved September 3, 2005, from http://www.census.gov/prod/2005pubs/p60-229.pdf

Department for Professional Employees, AFL-CIO. (2005). *Professional women: Vital statistics* (Fact Sheet 2004-1). Retrieved August 29, 2005, from http://www.dpeaflcio.org/policy/factsheets/fs_2004_Professional_Women.htm

Department of Health and Human Services (DHHS). (2005a). The 2005 HHS poverty guidelines. *Federal Register, 70,* 33. Retrieved August 27, 2005, from http://aspe.hhs,gov/poverty/05poverty.html

Department of Health and Human Services (DHHS). (2005b). *Women's health, 2005.* Retrieved August 27, 2005, from http://mch10.hrsa.gov/_05/pages/0308wp.htm

Department of Health and Human Services (DHHS), Office of Child Support Enforcement. (2005c). *Child support enforcement, FY 2004 preliminary report.* Retrieved August 29, 2005, from http://www.acf.dhhs.gov/programs/cse/pubs/2005/reports/preliminary_report/

Department of Health and Human Services (DHHS), Office of Family Assistance. (2005d). *TANF final rule regulations.* Retrieved August, 29, 2005, from http://www.acf.dhhs.gov/programs/ofa/

Department of Health and Human Services (DHHS), Office of Family Assistance. (2005e). *TANF 6th annual report to Congress, November 2004.* Retrieved August 29, 2005, from http://www.acf.hhs.gov/programs/ofa/annualreport6/ar6index.htm

Department of Justice. (2005). *ADA regulations and technical assistance materials.* Retrieved October 1, 2005, from http://www.usdoj.gov/crt/ada/publicat.htm#Ancho-14210

Duty, S. M., Singh, N. P., Silva, M. J., Barr, D. B., Brock, J. W., Ryan, L., et al. (2003). The relationship between environmental exposures to phthalates and DNA damage in human sperm using the neutral comet assay. *Environmental Health Perspectives, 111*(9), 1164–1210.

Eckstein, Z., & Nagypál, É. (2004). The evolution of U.S. earnings inequality: 1961–2002. *Quarterly Review (Federal Reserve Bank of Minneapolis, 28*(2). Retrieved September 3, 2005, from the EBSCOhost database.

Environmental Working Group (EWG). (2004). Skin deep: A safety assessment of ingredients in personal care products. Retrieved September 18, 2005, from http://www.ewg.org/reports/skin-deep

Gardner, M. (2005). Bankruptcy reform hits women hard. *Christian Science Monitor, 97*(90). Retrieved August 29, 2005, from the Ebsco Host Research databases.

Gibelman, M. (2003). So how far have we come? Pestilent and persistent gender gap in pay. *Social Work, 48*(1), 34–39.

Haignere, Inc. (2005). What is pay equity/comparable worth? Retrieved August 29, 2006, from http://www.payequityresearch.com/worth.htm

Hate Crime Network. (2005). *Hate crime information and statistics.* Retrieved October 8, 2005, from http://www.infoplease.com/ipa/A0004885.html

Hinchliff, S., Gott, M., & Galena, E. (2005). I do say I might find it embarrassing: General practitioners' perspectives on discussing sexual health issues with gay and lesbian patients. *Health & Social Care in the Community, 13*(4), 345–353.

Human Rights Campaign. (2005). *Employment non-discrimination act.* Retrieved October 1, 2005, from http://www.hrc.org/Template.cfm?Section5Employment_Non-Discrimination_Act&Template5/TaggedPage/TaggedPageDisplay.cfm&TPLID523&ContentID513319

Jones, C. B., & Gates, M. (2004). Gender-based wage differentials in a predominantly female profession: Observations from nursing. *Economics of Education Review, 23*(6), 615–617, 631.

Kelly, R. F., Redenback, L., & Rinanman, R. C. (2005). Family law custody research: Determinants of sole and joint custody arrangements in a national sample of divorces. *American Journal of Family Law, 19*(1), 25–29.

Kenney, G., Sommers, A., & Dubay, L. (2005). Moving to mandatory Medicaid managed care in Ohio: Impacts for pregnant women and infants. *Medical Care, 43*(7), 683–690.

Lambda Legal Defense Fund. (2005). *Partial summary of domestic partner benefit legislation.* Retrieved October 8, 2005, from http://www.lambdalegal.org/cgi-bin/iowa/news/resources.html?record=21

Lewis, J. H., Andersen, R. M., & Gelberg, L. (2003). Populations at risk: Health care for homeless women's unmet needs and barriers to care. *Journal of General Internal Medicine, 18*(11), 921–928.

Little, C. M. (2003). Female genital circumcision: Medical and cultural considerations. *Journal of Cultural Diversity, 10*(1). Retrieved October 22, 2005, from the Academic Search Premier database.

Lund, K. (2004). *International best practices for maternity and parental benefits.* Retrieved September 11, 2006, from http://www.wnpei.org/international.pdf

March, A. (2005). A cognitive conundrum. *American Journal of Nursing, 105*(10), 33–35.

Marcos, P. A., & Lima, N. R. (2003). Homelessness in the United States and its effect on children. *Guidance & Counseling,18*(3). Retrieved August 27, 2005, from the Academic Search Premier database.

Maternal and Child Health Bureau. (2005). *Women's health USA 2005.* Retrieved September 23, 2005, from http://mchb.hrsa.gov/whusa_05/pages/0434ow.htm

Mathuna, D. (2003, April). Herb-drug interactions. *Alternative Medicine Alert, 6*(4), 37–48.

Mawthorpe, J. (2003). Mothers' helpers? *Nursing Older People, 15*(9). Retrieved September 16, 2005, from the Academic Search Premier database.

Nason, C. S., Alexander, G. R., Pass, M., & Bolland, J. M. (2003). Women's Health. *Journal of Health & Human Services Administration, 26*(2), 239–267.

National Alliance to End Homelessness. (2005). *Family homelessness.* Retrieved August 31, 2005, from http://www.endhomelessness.org/back/FamiliesFacts.pdf

National Center on Birth Defects and Developmental Disabilities (NCBDDD). (2005). *Women with disabilities.* Retrieved September 30, 2005, from http://www.cdc.gov/ncbddd/women/links/ctrresearch.htm

National Center on Elder Abuse (NCEA). (2005). *Frequently asked questions.* Retrieved September 23, 2005, from http://www.elderabusecenter.org/default.cfm

National Coalition for Pesticide-Free Lawns. (2005). *Pesticide alert.* Retrieved September 17, 2005, from http://www.beyondpesticides.org

National Network of Child Care Resources (NACCRRA). (2005). *Child care in America.* Retrieved September 8, 2006, from http://nrc.uchsc.edu/RESOURCES/list.htm

National Women's Health Information Center. (2002). *Illness and disabilities.* Retrieved June 16, 2006, from http://www.4women.gov/WWD

National Women's Health Information Center. (2005a). *The environment and women's health.* Retrieved September 17, 2005, from http://www.4women.gov/faq/environment.htm

National Women's Health Information Center. (2005b). *Lesbian health.* Retrieved September 8, 2006, from http://www.4woman.gov/faq/lesbian.htm#1

Perera, F., Rauh, V., Tsai, W. Y., Kinney, P., Camann, D., Barr, D., et al. (2002). Effects of transplacental exposure to environmental pollutants on birth outcomes in a multi-ethnic population. *Environmental Health, 112*(12), 1293–1297.

Pesticide Action Network North America (PANNA). (2005). *Research update data analysis.* Retrieved September 17, 2005, from http://www.panna.org

PovertyNet. (2005). *Poverty overview.* Retrieved August 29, 2005, from http://web.worldbank.org/ WBSITE/EXTERNAL/TOPICS/EXTPOVERTY/ 0,,contentMDK:20153855~menuPK:373757~ pagePK:148956~piPK:216618~theSitePK: 336992,00.html

Ricci, J., & Biederman, P. W. (2004, March 30). Acceptance of gays on rise, polls show. *The Los Angeles Times.* Retrieved October 8, 2005, from http://www.sodomylaws.org/usa/usnews094.htm

Salmon, M. (2004). Down on the farm. *University of California, Berkeley Wellness Letter, 20*(7), 8–9.

Sex changes. (2005). *The Economist, 375*(8429). Retrieved September 3, 2005, from the EBSCOhost database.

Thayer, L. (2004, May–June). For better lesbian health, fewer barriers to care. *The Women's Health Activist,* 6–7.

Understanding discrimination against gays and lesbians. (2004). Retrieved October 1, 2005, from http://faculty.ncwc.edu/toconnor/soc/355lect07.htm

Union of Concerned Scientists. (2005). *Urinary tract infections in women may be difficult to treat because of overuse of antibiotics in food animals* [Press release]. Retrieved September 23, 2005, from http://www.ucsusa.org/news/press_release/ urinary-tract-infections-in-women-may-be-difficult-to-treat-because-of-overuse-of-antibiotics-in-food-animals.html

USA Today. (2005, May 19). Female business owners gain more political clout. Retrieved September 3, 2005, from the Academic Search Premier database.

US Census Bureau. (2003). *Percentage of childless women 40 to 44 years old increases since 1976* [Census Bureau Reports]. Retrieved January 21, 2006, from http://www.census.gov/ Press-Release/www/releases/archives/fertility/ 001491.html.

US Census Bureau. (2005). *Poverty. Historical poverty tables. Table 4. Poverty status of families, by type of family, presence of related children, race, and hispanic origin: 1959 to 2003.* Retrieved August 29, 2005, from http://www.census.gov/ hhes/www/poverty/histpov/hstpov4.html

US Department of Labor, Bureau of Labor Statistics. (2005). *National occupational employment and wage estimates for May, 2004.* Retrieved September 9, 2006, from http://www.bls.gov/oes/current/oes_00Al.htm

US Department of Labor, Women's Bureau. (2005). *Statistics and data.* Retrieved September 11, 2005, from http://www.dol.gov/wb/stats/ main.htm

US Equal Employment Opportunity Commission. (2006). *Pregnancy discrimination charges.* Retrieved May 2, 2006, from http://www.eeoc.gov/stats/pregnanc.html

US Military. (2005). *Homosexual discharge rates drop.* Retrieved October 8, 2005, from http://usmilitary.about.com/od/gaylesbians/a/ gaydischarge.htm

Webb, D. A., Robbins, J. M., Culhane, J., Metraux, S., & Culhane, D. (2003). Prevalence of episodic homelessness among adult childbearing women in Philadelphia, Pa. *American Journal of Public Health, 93*(11). Retrieved August 27, 2005, from the Academic Search Premier database.

Wolf, P. (2003 July–August). Plastics: Everything you need to know to improve your health and the environment. *Beginnings,* 9–11.

CHAPTER 9

Violence Against Women

To my friends I'm living the American dream. My husband is a successful broker and our life looks ideal. Even if I told them about the occasional slap, the shove, the forced sex they would probably think it was worth it. Sometimes I think about leaving, but it would mean admitting I failed. I know it doesn't make sense—he does the hitting, but I feel ashamed. I'm not a battered wife; I can't be. My husband just has a quick temper.

KEY TERMS

Acquaintance rape   191
Cycle of violence   182
Date rape   191
Domestic violence   179
Drug-facilitated sexual
    assault   191
Post-traumatic stress
    disorder   192
Rape   189
Rape trauma syndrome   191
Sexual assault   189

OBJECTIVES

1. List the social, psychologic, political, and cultural factors that contribute to the occurrence of domestic violence and sexual assault.

2. Describe ways in which psychologic, physical, and sexual abuse are used by batterers to maintain power and control in abusive relationships.

3. Identify factors that contribute to domestic violence.

4. Dispel the common myths about domestic violence and sexual assault.

5. Identify the phases of the cycle of violence.

6. Summarize the characteristics of batterers and perpetrators of sexual assault.

7. Delineate the role of the nurse in caring for women who have experienced battering.

8. Articulate proper procedures for the screening, assessment, and documentation of abuse.

9. Specify physical and psychologic signs that may indicate a woman is in an abusive relationship.

10. Discuss strategies for providing more culturally aware, competent care to survivors of domestic violence or sexual assault survivors.

11. Describe the needs that women with abusive partners and their children may have beyond the healthcare setting.

12. Compare the types of sexual assault.

13. Identify the phases of the rape trauma syndrome.

14. Identify drugs commonly used in drug-facilitated sexual assault.

15. Explain the reasons why nurses who care for survivors of sexual assault and domestic violence should explore their personal values and beliefs.

16. Discuss the nurse's role as client advocate and counselor with domestic violence and sexual assault survivors.

17. Summarize the procedures for collecting and preserving physical evidence of sexual assault.

18. Discuss the legal responsibilities of the community to prevent and address violence against women.

MEDIALINK

Additional resources for this content can be found on the Prentice Hall Nursing MediaLink DVD-ROM and on the Companion Website at http://www.prenhall.com/davidson. Click on "Chapter 9" to select the activities for this chapter.

Violence against women has become endemic in society today. Experts suggest that as many as one in three women will be abused at some time in their lives. Violence affects women of all ages, races, ethnic backgrounds, and religions, from all socioeconomic levels, all educational levels, and all walks of life. Two of the most common forms of societal violence are domestic violence (also called *intimate partner violence* or *IPV*) and sexual assault, the topics of this chapter. Perhaps surprisingly, these two types of violence are primarily perpetrated by intimate partners or persons known to the victim. Further, evidence indicates that a significant proportion of all female homicide victims are killed by their intimate partners. For example, national statistics indicate that for the years 1998 through 2002, approximately one third of female murder victims were killed by intimate partners or ex-partners (Fox & Zawitz, 2004).

Violence against women is a major health concern. Intimate partner violence results in nearly 2 million injuries and 1300 deaths nationwide every year (Centers for Disease Control & Prevention [CDC], 2003). In addition to injuries sustained during violent episodes, physical, sexual, and psychologic violence are linked to a number of adverse physical and mental health outcomes. The estimated health-related costs of violence against women exceed $5.8 billion *annually* in the United States (CDC, 2003).

Healthcare providers play a critical role in identifying and reducing violence, even in homicide prevention efforts. One study found that 44% of women murdered by their intimate partner had visited an emergency department within 2 years of the homicide. Of these women, 93% had at least one injury visit (Crandall, Nathens, Kernic et al., 2004).

Since the early 1980s healthcare providers and organizations have recognized the importance of their role and worked to address this issue. Over the past three decades there have been a number of notable changes in healthcare policy and practices aimed at responding to violence against women. In 1990 the Joint Commission on Accreditation of Healthcare Organizations (JCAHO) mandated the development of protocols for the identification and treatment of women who have been abused by their intimate partners. *Healthy People 2010* (2005), a national health promotion and disease prevention project, cites intervention and prevention for violent behavior as a national priority. In 1991 the American Nurses Association (ANA) authored a position statement which was revised in 2000, advocating education for all nurses in identifying and preventing violence against women (Table 9–1). Significantly, nursing has played and continues to play a key role in developing and evaluating innovative healthcare practices aimed at identifying and reducing violence against women.

HISTORICAL FACTORS CONTRIBUTING TO VIOLENCE AGAINST WOMEN

Violence against women is not new. Throughout history, for thousands of years in patriarchal societies, women have been victims of violence. Within the institution of marriage, wives

Table 9–1   ACTIONS SUPPORTED BY THE ANA TO COMBAT VIOLENCE AGAINST WOMEN

- Routine education of all nurses and healthcare providers in the skills necessary to prevent violence against women.
- Routine assessment and documentation for physical abuse of all women in any healthcare institution or community setting.
- Targeted assessment of women at increased risk of abuse, including pregnant women and women presenting in emergency rooms.
- Education of all women as to the cycle of violence, the potential for homicide, and community resources for primary, secondary, and tertiary prevention and care.
- Inclusion of the topic of violence against women in every undergraduate nursing curriculum.
- Education of school-age children and adolescents in public schools about relationships without violence and community resources for help.
- Research on violence against women, including the development and evaluation of nursing models for preventive assessment, intervention, and treatment for abused women, their children, and perpetrators of violence.

SOURCE: Reprinted with permission from American Nurses Association, *ANA Position Statement on Physical Violence Against Women,* © 1991, American Nurses Association, Silver Spring, MD.

MediaLink Video: Spousal Abuse

were considered the property of husbands, subject to their wishes and demands. A husband had the right—even the duty—to "keep her in line," to have sex on demand, even to kill her. Outsiders were expected to "keep out of it"; battering and sexual assault were family matters. The legal status of women has improved over the years in many cultures. However, many people still hold to the traditional views of male dominance in marriage or any intimate relationship, which can contribute to the occurrence of domestic violence and sexual assault.

Traditionally, rape outside of marriage was not viewed as an act of a man against a woman, but as an act of aggression against another man—the woman's husband, father, or brother, whoever was considered her "owner." On conclusion of a battle, rape of the wives and daughters of the losers symbolized the triumph of the conquerors and the humiliation of the vanquished. Unfortunately, women's bodies are still being used today to establish dominance, assert authority, and punish the enemy during armed conflicts.

DOMESTIC VIOLENCE

Domestic violence is defined as a pattern of coercive behaviors and methods used to gain and maintain power and control by one individual over another in an adult intimate relationship. This chapter focuses on domestic violence experienced by women in heterosexual relationships, although gay and lesbian individuals do experience domestic violence in their relationships as well. Among heterosexual couples, estimates indicate that in at least 95% of all domestic violence cases the perpetrators are men. Domestic violence occurs in relationships in which the partners are dating, living together, married, separated, or divorced.

Domestic violence is staggeringly common in the United States although the incidence has decreased significantly in the last decade. Currently it accounts for 20% of violent crimes against women. In the United States, one in four women will experience domestic violence (National Coalition Against Domestic Violence, 2005), whereas worldwide as many as one in three women will be the victim of violence or sexual coercion at some point in her life (United Nations Population Fund, 2005).

Forms of abuse vary, but are typically described as falling into the following categories, which the batterer uses to maintain control over his partner's behavior and the relationship: psychologic abuse, physical abuse, sexual abuse, and threats of physical or sexual violence. In addition, stalking, a course of conduct directed at a specific person that would cause a reasonable person to feel fear, is another way that women with abusive partners are threatened.

Psychologic abuse includes a range of behaviors such as:

- *Emotional abuse:* putting her down, making her feel bad about herself, calling her names, negatively comparing her to other women, making unreasonable demands, using things that matter to her against her

- *Isolation:* controlling who she sees and where she goes, using jealousy to justify restricting her actions, interfering with her job, forbidding her to see family and friends, limiting her outside involvement

- *Obfuscation:* denying responsibility for his actions, blaming her, minimizing her concerns, distorting the truth, lying to her

- *Using others:* using the children against her, using visitation to harass her, threatening to take the children away from her, using religion to control her

- *Male privilege:* treating her like a servant, defining rigid men's and women's roles, making all of the decisions or rules in the household

- *Economic abuse:* preventing her from getting or keeping a job, making her ask for money, controlling her money, destroying her property, making all the financial decisions

- *Coercion threats:* making and/or carrying out threats to harm her or her family and friends, threatening to commit suicide, pressuring her to drop charges, threatening negative consequences if she does not cooperate with his wishes, pressuring her with gifts/promises/apologies

- *Intimidation:* making her afraid through looks and gestures, smashing things, harming pets, displaying weapons, yelling, stalking her, driving recklessly

Often, in addition to psychologic abuse, the batterer will use physical and sexual abuse to maintain power and control within the relationship. Physical abuse can include acts such as pushing, shoving, slapping, hitting the woman with a fist or object, kicking, choking, threatening with a gun or knife, or using a gun or knife against her. Sexual abuse occurs any time the batterer forces or tries to force sex (including vaginal, oral, or anal intercourse). It also includes the forced use of objects, or forcing a woman to have sex with someone else against her will. Figure 9–1 ◆, the power and control wheel, illustrates how batterers use these tactics in relationships.

Typically these forms of abuse begin slowly and subtly after some form of commitment, such as engagement, onset of a

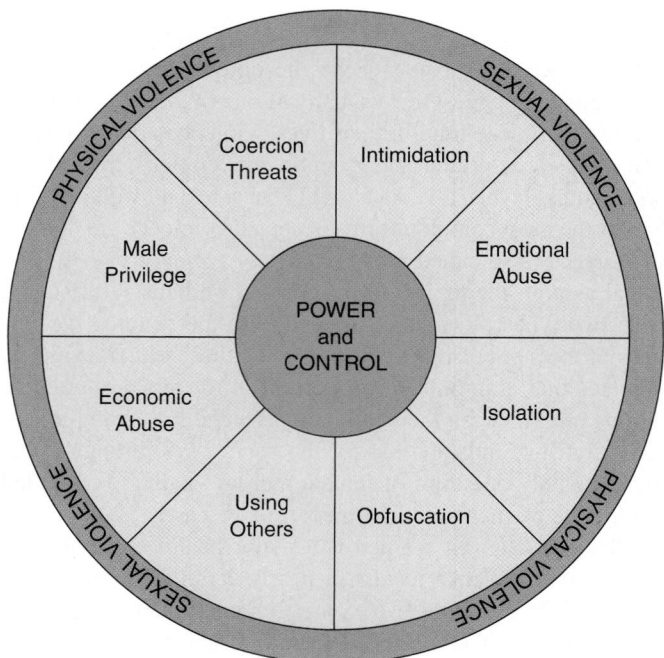

Figure 9–1 ◆ The power and control wheel.
SOURCE: Adapted from the Domestic Abuse Intervention Project, Duluth, Minnesota.

sexual relationship, marriage, pregnancy, first childbirth, or first statement of commitment. Sometimes the woman will not recognize that she is in an abusive relationship.

The consequences of the abuse can be profound. In addition to the physical consequences, which are outlined later in this chapter, a woman may experience adverse psychologic consequences, such as symptoms of post-traumatic stress disorder, depression, antisocial behavior, anxiety, suicidal behavior, low self-esteem, and fear of intimacy. Women sometimes face social consequences as well, including restricted access to services, isolation from social networks, and strained relationships with health providers and employers (Heise & Garcia-Moreno, 2002; Plichta, 2004). Clearly it is important to understand the factors that contribute to domestic violence and the role of the nurse in caring for women who have experienced battering.

Contributing Factors

Domestic violence is a result of the complex and dynamic interaction of social, cultural, political, and psychologic factors. Although none of these factors alone is sufficient to explain why domestic violence occurs, there is substantial research to suggest that the following factors are significantly related to experiences of domestic violence.

- *Childhood experiences.* Children who witness or experience abuse and battering are more likely to become batterers (men) or to be abused (women) in their own relationships. Exposure to domestic violence, however, is not a prerequisite for future abuse. Perhaps more importantly, not all children who witness violence in the home as children find themselves in abusive relationships as adults.

- *Male dominance in the family.* Worldwide, male economic and decision-making authority in the family is one of the strongest predictors of societies that demonstrate high violence against women, including domestic violence. This notion is also supported by research that demonstrates that men raised in patriarchal families (those that encourage traditional gender roles) are more likely to engage in domestic violence.

- *Marital conflict.* Relationships that are characterized by high levels of conflict, including verbal disagreements, are more likely to include the use of violence than are those relationships with lower levels of marital conflict.

- *Unemployment/low socioeconomic status.* Domestic violence occurs in all socioeconomic classes; however, it is more common in families with low incomes and unemployed men. The reasons for this have not yet been determined. It may not be a lack of income, but some other variable related to living in poverty—stress, frustration, feelings of inadequacy in filling the male role of provider, overcrowding, or a lack of community institutions and norms that would create quality community social interactions—that explains this relationship.

- *Traditional definitions of masculinity/hypermasculinity.* Cultures that link definitions of manhood to dominance, toughness, or male honor are more likely to demonstrate violence against women. This may result because socialization into traditional male norms includes telling young boys to be tough, not to shy away from violence, and to hide their feelings, particularly those that are associated with traditional notions of femininity.

Often healthcare providers view domestic violence as primarily a problem of younger women and believe that the violence decreases with age. Research indicates, however, that domestic violence does exist in older couples and that it will become an ever-increasing health problem as the population of baby boomers ages (Straka, 2006).

Common Myths about Battering and Women with Abusive Partners

Both professionals and the public believe numerous myths about battering and about women with abusive partners. These myths often reinforce misunderstanding of battering, furthering a woman's sense of victimization. Nurses need to recognize and counteract these myths. Some commonly accepted myths are discussed here.

- *Battering occurs in a small percentage of the population.* The statistics on reported cases under-represent the true incidence. As many as 1 in 3 women may be the victim of assault by her partner in her lifetime; however, it is estimated that only 1 in 10 women will report battering assaults.

- *Women who are abused provoke men to beat them; women push men beyond the breaking point and incite physical violence.* It is important to recognize that people are individually responsible for their own behavior. Batterers become violent because of their own internal inadequacies, not because of what their partners did or did not do.

- *Alcohol and drug abuse cause battering.* Studies do show a relationship between battering incidents and alcohol or drug use by batterers, and many batterers have a history of alcoholism or drug addiction. However, claims that substance abuse *causes* domestic violence are false and only serve to shift the responsibility away from the batterer. Some researchers suggest that batterers use alcohol as an excuse to carry out a violent act and shift the blame from themselves to the alcohol. Others suggest that alcohol or drugs reduce the batterer's inhibitions, increasing the likelihood of violent acts. Battered women sometimes think the abuse will stop if their partners stop drinking or using drugs. Unfortunately, this usually does not happen.

- *Battered women can easily leave the situation.* Leaving is easier said than done. Society encourages women to take greater responsibility for their marriages and children. In addition, battered women may still love their partners or husbands and believe the promises of change, rely on them for financial support, and feel their children need a father. Women with physically abusive partners nearly always experience psychologic abuse as well and have been told repeatedly by their batterers that the family's problems are their fault. They often are isolated by their abuser from family, friends, and agencies that could assist them. Women may also experience a lack of support from family members, friends, and their religious community. Some family members or friends may send the message that they warned the woman about the batterer and now it is her problem. Others may think that the batterer is a wonderful person, either not believing the woman's accounts or blaming her for the violence she experiences. Many women with children have no place to go, and shelters sometimes have long waiting lists. Moreover, battered women are at greatest risk for injury or domestic homicide when they leave the abuser. A woman may fear for her safety, her children's safety, and the safety of those who help her.

- *Domestic violence is a low-income or minority issue.* Domestic violence occurs among all sectors of society. It happens to women of all socioeconomic statuses, races, ethnicities, and religious faiths. It is true that lower income women are more likely to seek assistance from public agencies, such as hospitals and emergency rooms, because they have fewer private resources than women with greater incomes do. Therefore, they are more likely to be counted in various reporting statistics.

- *Battered women will be safer when they are pregnant.* Battering may occur for the first time during pregnancy or may escalate in intensity if the woman is already being abused. The injury is frequently aimed at the breasts, abdomen, or vagina. Many researchers and advocates believe that batterers are threatened by a pregnancy because the fetus interferes with the abuser's ability to maintain power and control within the relationship. Pregnancy is often a time during which a woman receives extra attention from family, friends, and healthcare providers. The intensified violence that some women experience merits serious attention. Alarmingly, pregnant and recently pregnant women are more likely to be victims of homicide than to die of any other cause (Horon & Cheng, 2001).

Miles hit me for the first time when I was 5 months pregnant. I was stunned. My father never laid a hand on my mother or any of us. Women who stayed in abusive situations had always appalled me but suddenly I found myself making excuses for him and rationalizing that he hadn't meant it, that he would never do it again. Three months later he shoved me so hard I fell against an end table. I was pretty bruised but I didn't go into labor. Somehow I found the courage to call my dad. He came and got me that night. My baby is 3 months old now and Miles keeps calling, telling me how sorry he is and that he loves me. Oh how I want to believe him when he says he is changed but I just can't take the chance.

Cycle of Violence

Walker (1984), in an effort to better explain the experience of battered women, developed the theory of the **cycle of violence,** which postulates that battering takes place in a cyclic fashion through three phases.

1. In the *tension-building phase,* the batterer demonstrates power and control. This phase is characterized by anger, arguing, blaming the woman for external problems, and possibly minor battering incidents. As the stress builds and communications break down, the woman often senses growing danger. She may also blame herself for the battering and believe she can prevent the escalation of the batterer's anger by her own actions, hoping that the relationship will somehow change for the better. The length of this phase varies considerably across individual cases, ranging from weeks to years.

2. The *acute battering incident* is typically triggered by some external event or internal state of the batterer. It is an episode of acute violence distinguished by lack of predictability and major destructiveness. The batterer blames the woman for the abuse, and the woman may accommodate him in order to survive, believe that escape is futile, or escape and return when the crisis is over. This is generally the briefest of the three phases, lasting from a few hours to a few days.

3. The *tranquil phase* is also sometimes called the *honeymoon period.* This phase may be characterized by extremely loving, kind, and contrite behaviors by the batterer as he tries to make up with the woman, or it may simply be manifested by an absence of tension and violence. The couple or family is often relieved that the crisis is past, and the woman may accept the batterer's promises and gifts because she is worn down and wants to believe that the violence will not happen again. Without intervention this phase will end at some point, and the cycle of violence will repeat. Over time, the cycle of violence often increases in severity and frequency.

Characteristics of Batterers

Batterers come from all racial, ethnic, and religious groups and all professions, occupations, and socioeconomic strata. They may have only a sixth-grade education or hold a doctorate. What they have in common are feelings of insecurity, inferiority, powerlessness, and helplessness that conflict with their assumptions of male supremacy. Because they tend to be emotionally immature and aggressive, they have a tendency to express their overwhelming feelings of inadequacy through violence.

Many batterers feel undeserving of their partners, yet they blame and punish the very person they value. Extreme jealousy and possessiveness are the hallmarks of abusers. They characteristically express their ambivalence by alternating episodes of unmerciful beatings with periods of remorse and loving attention. Extremes in behavior and overreacting are typical patterns.

Batterers may be very calculating and select a partner they feel may be vulnerable. Over a period of time they slowly and purposefully isolate the woman, creating a situation of increased dependence.

Women often describe their abusive husbands or partners as lacking respect toward women in general, having come from homes where they have witnessed abuse of their mothers or were themselves abused as children, and having a hidden rage that erupts occasionally. Batterers accept conventional "macho" values, yet when they are not angry or aggressive, they may appear childlike, dependent, seductive, manipulative, and in need of nurturing. They may be well respected in the community. This is important because it is one of the reasons why women are sometimes not believed or taken seriously when they seek support and assistance from friends, family members, and other resources. This dual personality of batterers reflects the conflict between their belief that they must live up to their macho image and their feelings of inadequacy and insecurity in the role of husband or provider. Combined with low tolerance for frustration and poor impulse control, their pervasive sense of powerlessness leads them to strike out at life's inequities by abusing women.

NURSING CARE MANAGEMENT

Increased publicity, public sensitivity, and heightened awareness of domestic violence are encouraging women with abusive partners to seek resources and community assistance. In the past decade, many communities have developed domestic violence programs, shelters, and resources for women with abusive partners. However, the needs of women who have been abused and their children are still insufficiently met.

Women in abusive relationships enter the healthcare system in many different settings. Nurses may see them in the physician's office with minor trauma or in the emergency department (ED) with multiple severe injuries. They are frequently seen in obstetric services because battering often begins or escalates during pregnancy. Nurses in psychiatric-mental health services frequently counsel women who have been battered, and community health nurses may find women reporting

EVIDENCE-BASED PRACTICE

SCREENING FOR DOMESTIC VIOLENCE

Clinical Question

Who should be screened for domestic violence? How should the screening be conducted and documented?

The Evidence

A systematic review and a practice guideline were developed to guide screening for domestic violence. An expert panel at Brigham and Women's Hospital in Boston, Massachusetts, evaluated the literature and developed a practice guideline for selecting subjects for screening, the actual content of the screening, and the documentation processes. The Canadian Task Force on Preventive Health Care sponsored two reviewers in developing systematic reviews for prevention and treatment of violence against women. The final pool of studies included 97 papers, 22 of which met criteria for critical appraisal; the remaining studies were considered for descriptive review regarding individual preferences and values.

What Is Effective?

Universal screening is the best way to identify abuse. All women should be asked about the incidence of domestic violence as part of routine care, whether or not signs, symptoms, or behaviors suggest the presence of abuse. Pregnant women should be screened at the initial visit and in the third trimester. Even if a woman does not disclose abuse, the simple act of asking is an intervention. The woman should be screened when alone, because she may be at risk for retaliation by an abusive partner if she is witnessed disclosing abuse to a healthcare provider. The screening should be documented in the medical record. If the person answers "no," the nurse can let her know support is available if she should ever need it, and note that " . . . abuse is not an issue at present time." Documenting that the woman denied abuse can create legal doubt later about her credibility. A suggested way of screening women is with the state-ment, "I'm so concerned about family violence that I ask every client about this, just as I ask about other health issues. . . . "

What Is Unclear?

Interpersonal issues, lack of access to information and resources, and some institutional barriers may prevent a woman from admitting she is in an abusive situation. Women may actively hide an abusive situation out of shame or fear. There are some clear clinical symptoms that suggest that a woman may be experiencing abuse, but signs may be subtle. Screening tools are available but their reliability in correctly identifying those women who may be in abusive situations is not well documented. It is also unclear if there are useful screening tools that can be used when screening men as perpetrators of domestic violence.

Best Practice

Screen all women who come in contact with the healthcare system. A woman is more likely to admit a domestic violence situation if she perceives that the provider is actively listening and concerned for her welfare, and if she feels assured that the disclosure will not be reported back to the abuser. The clinical evaluation should include a thorough history, an assessment of psychologic symptoms and behavioral indicators of abuse, and examination for physical findings that are characteristic of injuries caused by domestic violence. Use of a domestic violence assessment tool may be helpful in identifying suspected abuse situations.

Critical Thinking

How can the nurse incorporate an assessment of domestic violence into the standard client assessment in women's health?

REFERENCES: Brigham and Women's Hospital. (2004). Domestic violence: A guide to screening and intervention. Boston: Author.

Wathen, C., & Macmillan, H. (2004). Prevention of violence against women: Recommendation statement from the Canadian Task Force on Preventive Health Care. *Canadian Medical Association Journal, 169*(6), 582–584.

abuse during home visits. Unfortunately, emergency departments, hospitals, and social service agencies do not routinely screen for, recognize, and report battering cases to the legal authorities for action and follow-up, although some states are initiating this policy.

Nurses in many different healthcare settings often come in contact with women who have experienced abuse but fail to recognize them, especially if they have no visible injuries. Nurses who wish to help battered women need advanced knowledge of the dynamics of battering; assessment skills for recognizing and documenting abuse; and appropriate intervention skills in counseling, safety planning, and referral.

Working with women who have been abused is sometimes frustrating, and many healthcare providers feel puzzled when women return to their abusive situations. Nurses must realize that they cannot rescue women with abusive partners; women must decide on their own how to handle the situation, which is often incredibly complex and dangerous. Research has shown that women's risk for homicide and additional violence are greatest during separation or attempts at separation. The effective nurse provides women who have been abused with information that empowers them in decision making and provides critical assistance in safety planning for women and their children.

Nursing Assessment and Diagnosis

Because domestic violence is so prevalent and yet frequently remains unidentified by healthcare providers, experts and caregivers now advocate *universal screening of all female clients at every healthcare encounter.* See Evidence-Based Practice: Screening for Domestic Violence. Unfortunately, impediments to universal screening exist that range from a lack of institutional or organizational support to the attitudes of individual nurses.

A majority of the reasons cited by nurses indicate a lack of education about domestic violence in general and a lack of confidence in their own skills specific to domestic violence intervention. This fact underscores the importance of and need for comprehensive domestic violence education and training for healthcare providers, a policy recommendation that was affirmed by the 2000 National Violence Against Women (NVAW) Survey and the ANA Position Statement on Physical Violence Against Women (see Table 9–1). In addition to factual information about domestic violence and its impact on women's physical, psychologic, and sexual health, comprehensive education and training should include opportunities to practice skill development (e.g., in screening, assessment, empathic listening, diagnosis, planning, and communication across diverse age and ethnic/cultural groups) as well as opportunities to explore one's personal responses, attitudes, and values related to abuse.

Nurses may also be hesitant to ask because they presume the woman may be offended by the questions. However, women are rarely offended by questions about abuse, particularly if prefaced by a statement such as, "Because violence is so common in many people's lives, I've begun routinely asking all the women I care for about it." Showing knowledge about and familiarity with the issue of domestic violence not only increases a nurse's effectiveness in identifying women who have experienced abuse, but also fulfills an important health education function for women who have not experienced abuse.

Four basic screening questions, identified in Figure 9–2 ◆, are useful in identifying women who are experiencing abuse. If a woman responds affirmatively to the questions, she is asked to mark the area(s) of injury on the body map. Screening for women experiencing domestic violence must be done privately, with only the nurse and client present, in a safe and quiet place (Figure 9–3 ◆). The nurse needs to reassure the woman that her responses will be kept confidential. The nurse should also strive for a calm and reassuring tone. Although tone, body language, and other nonverbal signs are important in establishing trusting relationships with all women, nurses should be especially aware of these issues in interventions with women from cultural and linguistic minority groups. Women from cultural and linguistic minority groups are often sensitized to these cues because they have used them as a survival strategy against discrimination and prejudice.

A number of signs that may not be related to a woman's presenting injuries can indicate the possibility that a woman is in a violent relationship. Although no single one of these signs necessarily indicates abuse, the occurrence of several of these signs certainly merits an at-risk diagnosis. Nurses must exercise their professional judgment and communicate their conclusions to their clients. Signs that may indicate a woman is in an abusive relationship include the following:

- *Neurologic signs.* Headaches, including headache following trauma or concussion, tension headache, and migraines; dizziness; paresthesias; unexplained stroke from strangulation; hearing loss; detached retina
- *Gynecologic signs.* Dyspareunia (painful intercourse), sexually transmitted infections (STIs), frequent vaginal infections, sexual dysfunction, menstrual disorders, pelvic pain
- *Obstetric signs.* Late onset of prenatal care, premature labor, low-birth-weight infant, excessive concern over fetal well-being, recurrent therapeutic abortion, recurrent spontaneous abortion
- *Gastrointestinal signs.* Dyspepsia, irritable bowel syndrome, globus (sensation of a lump in the throat)
- *Musculoskeletal signs.* Arthralgias (painful joints), chronic pain, osteoarthritis, fibromyalgia
- *Psychiatric signs.* Anxiety, panic, post-traumatic stress disorder, mood disorders, depression, suicide attempts, somatization, eating disorders, substance abuse, child abuse and neglect
- *Constitutional signs.* Fatigue, weight loss, weight gain, multiple somatic complaints, contusions, abrasions, sleep and appetite disturbances, decreased concentration, frequent use of pain medication or tranquilizers
- *Trauma.* Any injury to the female organs, extensive accident history, old fractures, sexual trauma
- *Other signs.* History of missed appointments or frequently changed appointments; low self-esteem, as seen in the woman's dress, her appearance, and the way she relates to healthcare providers

When a woman seeks care for an injury, the nurse should be alert to the following cues of abuse:

- Hesitation in providing detailed information about the injury and how it occurred
- Inappropriate affect for the situation
- Defensive injuries
- Delayed reporting of symptoms or of seeking care for injuries
- Pattern of injury consistent with abuse, including multiple injury sites involving bruises, abrasions, or contusions to the head (eyes and back of neck), throat, chest, breast, abdomen, or genitals (Nonbattered women's injuries are usually located at one or two sites and on the extremities, such as sprains and strains. Women in abusive relationships may have scars and evidence of old injuries that have healed.)
- Inappropriate explanation for the injuries, such as being "accident prone"
- Vague complaints without accompanying pathology
- Lack of eye contact
- Signs of increased anxiety in the presence of the possible batterer, who frequently does most of the talking or hovers around the woman

As with the universal screening, if the nurse observes these potential cues, then the nurse should arrange for a private place in which the woman can feel safe. If a man is with the woman, the nurse should tell him to remain in the waiting room while the woman is examined. It is good practice to ask the same of family members or friends because it can be difficult for women in abusive relationships to talk candidly about their situation with others present. The nurse can encourage the woman to talk about her injuries and home situation by asking, "How did this happen to you?" or by saying, "We often see injuries like yours when a woman has been beaten. Has this happened to you?" Directly confronting the injuries and possible abuse may provide

Abuse Assessment Screen

Universal Screening is recommended for all women during ED visits, Hospital admission, Prenatal visits, Routine PE and GYN screening, and Well Child visits of children to their pediatricians.

Note: Some agencies have nurses and/or physicians verbally ask questions, others include them in a written health questionnaire given to all patients, and others do both.

INTRODUCTION AND QUESTIONS:

Because violence is so common in many people's lives, I've begun to ask all my patients about it routinely:

1. **WITHIN THE LAST YEAR**, have you been hit, slapped, kicked, or   YES   NO
otherwise physically hurt by someone?

    If YES, by whom?_____

    Total number of times _____

2. **SINCE YOU VE BEEN PREGNANT**, have you been hit, slapped,   YES   NO
kicked, or otherwise physically hurt by someone?

    If YES, by whom?_____

    Total number of times _____

**MARK THE AREA OF INJURY ON THE BODY MAP
SCORE EACH INCIDENT ACCORDING TO THE FOLLOWING SCALE**

SCORE

1 = Threats of abuse including use of a weapon

2 = Slapping, pushing; no injuries and/or lasting pain

3 = Punching, kicking, bruises, cuts, and/or continuing pain

4 = Beating up, severe contusions, burns, broken bones

5 = Head injury, internal injury, permanent injury

6 = Use of weapon; wound from weapon

If any of the descriptions for the higher number apply, use the higher number.

3. **WITHIN THE LAST YEAR**, has anyone forced you to have   YES   NO
sexual activities?

    If YES, by whom?_____

    Total number of times _____

4. Are you afraid of anyone at home or an ex-partner?   YES   NO

Developed by the Nursing Research Consortium on Violence and Abuse.
Readers are encouraged to reproduce and use this assessment tool.

Figure 9–2 ◆ Abuse assessment screen.
SOURCE: Developed by the Nursing Research Consortium on Violence and Abuse. Reprinted from the Web site of the Nursing Network on Violence Against Women International (http://www.nnvawi.org).

an opening for the woman who is trying to cope in private. A woman may continue to deny her battering. The nurse should encourage her to talk but should avoid badgering her. When culturally appropriate, it is important to maintain eye contact and avoid excessive note taking. The nurse should assure the woman that her privacy will be respected. It is essential that the nurse remains nonjudgmental; creates a warm, caring climate conducive to sharing; and demonstrates a willingness to talk about violence. A woman will often interpret the nurse's willingness to discuss violence as permission for her to discuss it as well.

Figure 9–3 ◆ Screening for domestic violence should be done privately.

No one had ever asked me about my "injuries" until I was in the ER one night and the nurse asked me right out if I had been beaten. It gave me real hope to think that people might see what was happening to me.

Assessment is a complex process. It is important for the nurse to gather information about the woman's history of abuse. Getting a sense of the pattern of abuse is key to determining the degree of danger she might face. The nurse can help the woman assess whether or not the cycle of violence is becoming more frequent or severe. Determining whether or not there are weapons in the home, and whether or not her batterer has used or threatened to use weapons might also be warranted. In cases of severe abuse, it is important for the nurse to address the connection between homicide and domestic violence. Finally, the nurse should ask about the presence of sexual abuse within the relationship, another factor that indicates severe abuse.

Equally important, however, the assessment of the woman who may be experiencing abuse should include information about her strengths and her support system. Strengths may include education, employment history, activities in the home, community involvement, and her ability to cope with past problems. The woman's support system may include her family, friends, neighbors, and community agencies or organizations. It is helpful to consider assessing a woman's strengths in a cultural context. If the nurse is aware of strong values that a particular cultural group holds, then he or she should look for opportunities to recognize and affirm those strengths as valuable.

CLINICAL TIP

Actually recording a woman's strengths in her medical record and showing her that they are an official part of the record lets her know that the nurse believes that her strengths are as significant as any problems that were noted.

During the assessment phase, the nurse begins building a relationship with the woman based on trust, understanding, and ad-

vocacy. A woman may feel ashamed and embarrassed about her injuries and her situation. It is important to tell her the purpose of the assessment and to communicate what level of confidentiality she can expect. Clearly, nurses need to be informed about the confidentiality policies of the organization where they work and aware of any mandatory reporting policies that exist. Trust begins as the nurse conveys an attitude of unconditional acceptance, empathy, and positive regard for the woman's worth and dignity. Nurses should show that they recognize the woman's feelings and that they accept her right to feel as she does.

In cases in which the woman states she has been beaten, kicked, punched, or attacked but does not identify the assailant, the nurse should record the extent of injuries (e.g., size, shape, color, where they are located on her body), note the woman's exact words, and describe the incident with a diagnosis of probable battering. Full documentation of specific information is critical, because the nurse might be called to testify in court or the medical records might be subpoenaed as evidence in legal proceedings such as custody disputes, stay-away/restraining orders, or other civil or criminal proceedings. Moreover, documenting the abuse works to ensure a woman's continuity of care. Those cases in which the woman states she was beaten by a husband or partner may be diagnosed as battering with all evidence recorded, including the woman's statements. In both cases, taking photographs of the injuries can be of great value. However, to further protect the woman's confidentiality and safety, it is critical that the nurse or other medical personnel do not refer to domestic violence or abuse on any discharge papers.

When abuse or battering is suspected or determined, the nurse should formulate nursing diagnoses based on the assessment findings. Nursing diagnoses related to nonphysical components of abuse or battering may include the following:

- *Self-Esteem Disturbance* related to feelings of worthlessness and powerlessness
- *Health-Seeking Behavior:* Information about community resources to assist battered women related to an expressed desire to learn about alternatives

Nursing Plan and Implementation

A woman who is experiencing abuse needs to reestablish a feeling of control over her world. She needs to regain a sense of predictability by knowing what to expect from her disclosure. The nurse should provide sufficient information about what to expect in terms the woman can understand. Simple explanations about how long she will stay, whom she will see, and what will be done are important. Giving the woman control can be accomplished by asking her permission before any activities or procedures and by providing her with choices whenever possible.

Supportive counseling and reassurance are professional skills nurses use throughout each phase of the nursing process with a battered woman. The nurse should do the following:

- Acknowledge and support the woman for talking about her situation. Reporting abuse is a risk.
- Let the woman work through her story, problems, and situation at her own pace.

DEVELOPING CULTURAL COMPETENCE

CULTURAL FACTORS INFLUENCING SURVIVORS OF VIOLENCE

Providing nursing care to women who are from a different cultural community, who speak a different language, or who are immigrants can be challenging. This is especially true when providing care to women who are in abusive relationships. When assisting survivors from different cultural or linguistic backgrounds, consider the following:

- It is often difficult for women in certain cultural communities to seek help outside their families for a variety of reasons, ranging from cultural notions about the role of women, to fear of being ostracized within or isolated from her community, to a loss of social respect that includes her entire family (Orloff & Little, 1999).

- Language can be a powerful barrier to effective communication. Thus it is important to have bilingual nurses and personnel available and to translate assessment tools, such as those found in Figure 9–2.

- Have information available about language-specific and culturally appropriate community resources including legal services that specialize in family and immigration law, individual and family counseling services, and shelters with bilingual and bicultural staff.

- Immigrant women may have inaccurate perceptions of law enforcement and the legal system, either because of negative experiences with law enforcement in their country of origin or because of misinformation about the US legal system from their abusers (Shetty & Kaguyutan, 2002).

- Abusers may threaten women with deportation if they seek help for the abuse. Women may be fearful of jeopardizing their financial or immigration status and that of their children, their family, or their abuser. For a more complete list of tactics used to control immigrant women experiencing domestic violence, see Table 9–2.

- Women in some cultures may have deeply held religious beliefs that conflict with standard legal remedies. It is vital to find creative remedies that do not ask a woman to choose between religious and spiritual convictions and much needed legal remedies (Orloff & Little, 1999).

- Avoid cultural stereotyping—there are many subcultures and traditions within any cultural community. Create a safe space for the woman to share her needs, fears, and any cultural barriers that she must overcome (Orloff & Little, 1999).

- Educate yourself. Become aware of your own biases and stereotypes and make a commitment to learn about the practices of others from various minority communities.

- Let the woman know that she is believed and that her feelings are reasonable and normal.
- Anticipate her ambivalence in the love-hate relationship with the batterer. She knows he may be loving and contrite after the incident if she has been through the cycle of violence before.
- Respect the woman's capacity to change and grow when she is ready.
- Assist her in identifying specific problems, and support realistic ideas for reducing or eliminating those problems.
- Help clarify the woman's beliefs and myths, and provide information to change her false beliefs.
- Stress that no one should be abused and that the abuse is not her fault.

The appropriate intervention is not to tell an abused woman what to do, but to help her recognize her options and resources and make her own decisions. Even advising or encouraging a woman to leave an abusive situation is not always in the woman's best interest; leaving the home is a major decision with long-lasting consequences. The woman may be economically unable to leave the situation, especially if she has young children. If the woman leaves and then later returns home, both husband and wife may become more frustrated, in-

creasing the possibility of further beatings and even homicide. The most acceptable course of action is one that the woman freely chooses.

TEACHING FOR SELF-CARE

If the woman returns to an abusive situation, the nurse should encourage her to develop an exit, or safety, plan for herself and her children, if she has any. As part of the plan, she should pack a change of clothes for herself and the children, including toilet articles and an extra set of car and house keys. She should store these away from the house with a friend or neighbor and ask a neighbor to call the police if violence begins. If possible, she should have money, identification papers (driver's license, social security cards), checkbook, bank account information, other financial records (such as mortgage papers, rent and utility receipts, automobile title, insurance policies and numbers), and information about the children to help her enroll them in school. She should also plan where she will go, regardless of the day or time. It is also helpful to identify friends and family who know about the situation and will help her. Ask that she establish a code word for danger with those family and friends. The nurse should ensure that the woman has a planned escape route and emergency telephone numbers she can call, including personal numbers, the local police, a phone hotline, and a women's shelter if one is available in the community.

MediaLink   Video: Going Back?

Table 9–2   TACTICS USED TO CONTROL IMMIGRANT WOMEN IN ABUSIVE RELATIONSHIPS

Isolation	Keeping her isolated from family, friends, community and religious leaders, or people who speak her native language; not allowing her to learn English.
Threats	Threatening to report the victim to the US Immigration and Naturalization Service (INS) or threatening to withdraw a petition to legalize immigration status. The abuser often threatens to seek sole custody of the children if the woman reports the abuse or attempts to leave.
Intimidation	Hiding or destroying important papers such as passports and green cards, documentation for the children, destroying her only property from the country of origin such as mementos or photographs.
Citizenship or residency privilege	Failing to file papers to legalize immigration status, lying to the woman that her immigration is legal, and/or withdrawing such papers altogether.
Economic abuse	Not letting her obtain job training, work, or schooling; threatening to report the victim for working "under the table"; taking money she wants to send abroad to family; forcing the woman to work illegally.
Emotional abuse	Lying about immigration status, threatening to harm the children or other family members, calling her racist or abusive names.
Spiritual abuse	Misusing religious teachings and/or personal beliefs and values.

SOURCE: From *Immigrant Victims of Domestic Violence*, National Coalition Against Domestic Violence (NCADV). Reprinted with permission.

National Coalition Against Domestic Violence

MEDIALINK

COMMUNITY-BASED NURSING CARE

Besides offering emotional support, medical treatment, and counseling, the nurse should inform any woman who may be in an abusive situation of the services available in the hospital, through agencies, and in the community. The nurse can also provide the woman with the phone number of any local resources, as well as the number for the National Domestic Violence Hotline. (See the Companion Web Site for a range of Internet and phone resources for the nurse to explore and potentially share with the woman who has experienced domestic violence.)

Specifically, a woman who has been abused may need:

- Medical treatment for injuries
- Temporary shelter to provide a safe environment for herself and her children
- Legal assistance for protection or prosecution of the batterer
- Financial assistance to provide shelter, food, and clothing
- Job training or employment counseling
- Counseling to raise her self-esteem and help her understand the dynamics of domestic violence, or an ongoing support group for herself and her children

A network of community agencies can meet the numerous, varied needs of women, children, and batterers. It is important that employees in these agencies understand the complex dynamics of domestic violence as well as how their services and those of other agencies can assist women and

their children. An overview of resources available to women with abusive partners and their children is presented in the following sections.

Emergency Department Services

Many women who are experiencing abuse are first seen and diagnosed in the EDs of their neighborhood hospitals. ED nurses and personnel need to be alert to symptoms of battering, recognize these cues, and encourage women to seek assistance from community agencies. The most innovative and effective domestic violence programs in hospitals and urgent care facilities work collaboratively with domestic violence service agencies, develop a comprehensive community referral network, and work with multidisciplinary intervention teams. Some states require that suspected cases of abuse and battering be reported to the legal authorities or social service agencies.

Shelter

Because domestic violence has been recognized as a major social problem, many community agencies have sought federal and state funds to provide shelters. These shelters differ in the services they provide, depending on the governing body, financial resources and funding agencies, organizational structure, staff qualifications, and range of available community services. Typical shelters provide women in abusive relationships and their children with a room, beds, food, clothing, and other basic necessities. If professional staff is available, the shelter may offer crisis counseling, individual and group counseling, and information about community agencies such as legal aid, welfare, job training, financial and employment agencies, and women's counseling or support groups.

For safety reasons, the location of most shelters is undisclosed, but they can be contacted through a community crisis line. Admission requirements vary from shelter to shelter, so it is wise for nurses to become familiar with local shelters and the resources available if the shelter is full and the woman and her children are in need of a safe place to stay.

Legal Services and Options

During incidents of domestic violence, the woman or her neighbors may summon the police. Domestic violence typically occurs on the weekend or in late evening, when most social service agencies are closed; therefore, the police department is often one of the first major agencies involved, in addition to those that provide medical services.

Legal options for women with abusive partners vary according to state laws and services. In some states a woman may seek a restraining order from the family court or a domestic relations court to protect herself from the batterer. This restraining order specifies that the man must stay a specified distance away from the woman and may not physically abuse any family members, but it does not give him a criminal record. Unfortunately, many abusive men violate the restraining order and continue to stalk, harass, intimidate, and abuse their female partner. If the woman decides to prosecute, and if her case meets the legal requirements for an indictment, the case is usually heard in criminal court, which handles crimes of assault, harassment, and battery. Criminal court hearings may result in a fine, probation, or a jail sentence if the batterer is convicted, giving the man a criminal record. The prosecution process is often lengthy and may last more than a year. Some state judicial systems are introducing other options, such as mandatory counseling in a Batterer Intervention Program (BIP) in lieu of prosecution. Unfortunately, this counseling does not show great promise for permanent change. Divorce is another legal recourse a woman may choose, but divorce often takes several months to a year.

Many women who are abused are unaware of their legal options. They fear further beatings if they prosecute the batterer. Limited financial resources may also keep them from seeking legal assistance. Some women report lack of sensitivity or awareness about domestic violence on the part of some members of the legal and criminal justice systems, further limiting their ability or willingness to seek help. Currently, some communities provide legal advocacy services to help women understand the judicial process, their options within that system, and the possible consequences for the woman, her children, and the batterer.

Financial Services

Once women who have been in a battering relationship leave their homes or seek legal assistance, they usually receive no financial support from the batterer. Without funds, women and their children are at the mercy of community social service agencies, and it usually takes weeks for papers to be processed before any money is forthcoming. Agencies that may provide financial assistance include their county welfare department, federal programs (e.g., Temporary Assistance for Needy Families), the United Way, women's support groups, religious organizations, and, possibly, the Salvation Army. There may be other local groups who assist abused women in other ways, such as by providing food or clothing.

Employment Training or Placement

Some women who experience abuse are full-time mothers who may lack advanced education, training, and job experience. Minimal or out-of-date skills and inadequate transportation often make it difficult for these women to obtain employment with an adequate salary. Women who have children must consider where to place them during working hours as well as the added cost of child care. Often, the woman's choice is restricted to accepting welfare or taking a low-paying job. Either choice usually means lowering the standard of living to mere subsistence.

Some women do seek job training if the opportunities are available, but training provides no guarantee of future job placement. A woman may still have to arrange for financial support and child care while obtaining advanced employment skills or an education.

Counseling

Women who have experienced domestic violence may be offered a variety of counseling services, such as crisis intervention, short-term individual therapy, group therapy, or peer support groups, over an extended period. Specially trained nurses, social workers, psychologists, mental health specialists, or clergy may provide counseling and therapy.

Evaluation

Expected outcomes of nursing care include the following:

- The woman receives compassionate, respectful, and individualized medical attention.
- The woman recovers from the physical effects of physical and sexual abuse.
- The woman has the information she needs to make a decision about her future based on thoughtful consideration of alternatives.
- The woman is able to identify culturally appropriate community resources available to her and develops strategies for keeping herself, her children, and her family as safe as possible.
- If the woman chooses to apply for a restraining order or to prosecute her assailant, all necessary documentation is recorded in her medical records, leading to a more successful prosecution.

SEXUAL ASSAULT

Sexual assault is a broad term that refers to a variety of types of unwanted sexual touching or penetration without consent, from unwanted sexual contact or touching of an intimate part of another person to forced anal, oral, or genital penetration. Rape is, therefore, one type of sexual assault. Although the specific definition of rape varies from state to state, the National Crime Victimization Survey defines it as follows: "**Rape** is forced sexual intercourse and includes both psychologic coercion as well as physical force. Forced sexual intercourse means vaginal, anal, or oral penetration by the offender(s)." The rapist may be a stranger, acquaintance, spouse or other relative, or an employer. Rape is an act of violence expressed sexually—most commonly, a man's aggression and rage acted out against a woman.

Sexual assault remains one of the most underreported violent crimes in the United States. In 2004 approximately 35.8% of sexual assaults were reported to the police (Catalano, 2005). Research indicates that one in six American women over age 12 has been the victim of an attempted or completed sexual assault or rape (Rape, Abuse, and Incest National Network [RAINN], 2006). However, the incidence of sexual assault is down by 64% since 1993. In 2004 there were 204,370 sexual assaults and rapes compared with 485,000 in 1993 (Catalano, 2005). Experts attribute this dramatic decline to two trends (RAINN, 2003):

1. *Tough-on-crime policies with longer sentences and three-strike laws.* All types of criminals commit rapes and rapists often commit other forms of crime.
2. *Generational changes.* Over three fourths of rape victims are under 30 years of age and have grown up knowing that "no means no." These young women are more cautious about potentially risky situations and more willing to express their wishes forcefully.

MEDIALINK

Video: Parental Sexual Abuse

RAINN (2006) estimates that every two and a half minutes, somewhere in the United States, someone is sexually assaulted. Reporting varies by the type of rape or sexual assault. Rapes and sexual assaults committed by strangers are more likely to be reported to the police than rapes and sexual assaults committed by "nonstrangers," including intimate partners, other relatives, and friends or acquaintances (Hart & Rennison, 2003).

Although both men and women can be sexually assaulted, the 2004 National Crime Victimization Survey reported that 9 out of every 10 rape victims were female (Catalano, 2005). Sexual violence often occurs early in life. Over half (54%) of all female rapes occur before age 18; of these, 22% occur before age 12 (National Center for Injury Prevention and Control [NCIPC], 2006). No woman of any age, cultural or ethnic background, or socioeconomic status is immune, but statistics indicate that young, unmarried women, women who are unemployed or have low family income, and students have the highest incidence of sexual assault or attempted assault.

Common Myths about Rape

As with domestic violence, many myths about rape exist. These myths can have a negative impact on women who are assaulted and can hinder their ability to receive optimum health care following their attack. Some of the most commonly cited myths include the following:

- *Only certain types of women are raped.* No woman is safe from a rape attempt. Women of all ages, races, ethnicities, classes, religious backgrounds, occupations, ability levels, sexual and gender identities, or appearances are raped; rape is a very "democratic" form of violence.

- *Men rape women because that is men's nature and biological role.* Rape is not universal to all societies and not all men rape women. This suggests that rape is an act that can be encouraged or discouraged. Research has found positive correlations between rates of sexual assault and societies and individuals who glorify violence, objectify women, and encourage toughness and aggression in boys and men (Greensite, no date [n.d.]).

- *Women who party hard, drink, and do drugs are setting themselves up to be sexually assaulted.* No one asks for or deliberately "sets herself up" to be sexually violated. The misunderstanding that rape is about sex perpetuates this myth. Rape is sexual violence and a crime of power. Blaming the victim for the crime is not only inappropriate, it serves to excuse the behavior of the perpetrator. Because alcohol and drugs may affect judgment, feelings, and perceptions, as well as lower inhibitions, a woman may be in a more vulnerable position when she drinks. However, it is not a crime to wear particular clothes, show naivete, use poor judgment, or even engage in reckless behavior. The victim's behavior before the crime is irrelevant.

- *If a woman just relaxes, it will all be over with soon. She might even find it isn't so bad after all.* Rape is an act of violence in which the perpetrator uses sex as a weapon to control, intimidate, and violate the victim. Survivors of sexual violence feel very clearly that rape and consensual sex are worlds apart. Rape involves persistent pressure, taking advantage of a person's inability to say "no," calculated drugging with alcohol or other substances, and/or threats, sometimes against the woman's life, her livelihood, her academic career, even her family members and friends. Many survivors recall being in fear for their lives, even if a weapon was not present.

- *Most rapes are interracial.* The overwhelming majority of rapes and other sexual assaults, between 80% and 90%, involve people of the same racial background. Unfortunately, media reports tend to play up the race of accused criminals, further encouraging racist misconceptions in our society. When men rape women of other races and ethnicities, it is more often a white assailant raping a woman of color than a man of color raping a white woman (Greensite, n.d.).

- *A rapist is easy to spot in a crowd.* There is no way to distinguish men who commit sexual assault from men who do not on the basis of race, ethnicity, socioeconomic status, educational level, or religious background. They can be large or small, able-bodied or disabled, married or single.

- *Women lie about rape as an act of revenge or guilt.* False rape charges are infrequent. According to the Federal Bureau of Investigation (FBI), false charges are reported at the same rate for rape as for other felonies; that is, about 2% of all rape charges. Furthermore, it is important to remember that simply because there is not enough evidence to prosecute **does not** mean the woman was lying.

- *Fighting back incites a rapist to violence.* Most assailants pick out potential victims they believe may be good targets without a fight. They may even test women nonverbally or verbally before determining whether or not to assault. Both verbal and physical resistance may actually lessen the severity of injury in some instances. Recent studies of rape avoidance behavior have shown that women who recognize that they have options for responding to their assailant are less likely to be paralyzed by fear and more likely to resist. However, no one should tell another person what to do in a dangerous situation. Only the woman knows her abilities and can assess the assailant's behavior. Evaluating her options realistically may help the survivor understand that submission is also a viable form of self-protection.

Characteristics of Perpetrators

Like their victims, rapists come from all ethnic, racial, and religious backgrounds; socioeconomic statuses; educational levels; and professions. Clinicians and researchers who work with rapists, both convicted and not convicted, report that many rapists are married and engage in regular sexual relationships, both inside and outside of marriage. A substantial number of perpetrators are quite young. One study by the Bureau of Justice Statistics found that 23% of all sexual offenders are under the age of 18 (Snyder, 2000). Unfortunately, so few perpetrators are arrested and convicted that clear characterizations of assailants have not been developed.

Attitudes toward women do seem to influence who is likely to be a rapist and who is not, especially when it comes to believing that men have a right to sexual access of women (Greensite, n.d.). Perpetrators tend to be impulsive and have antisocial tendencies. They may prefer impersonal sex and feel hostility toward women. Additional individual risk factors for perpetration include alcohol and drug use, hypermasculinity, an emotionally unsupportive family environment, childhood history of physical and sexual abuse, having witnessed family violence as a child, and a belief in societal norms that support male entitlement and female inferiority and sexual submissiveness as well as strict gender roles with male dominance (NCIPC, 2006).

Types of Rape

Rape has been categorized in different ways, which are not mutually exclusive. Specifically, rape may be categorized according to the rapist's possible motives or purposes for the assault, according to the relationship between the victim and perpetrator, or according to the number of assailants.

- In *power rape,* the purpose of the assault is control or mastery. The assailant uses sexual intercourse to place a woman in a powerless position so that he can feel dominant, potent, and strong. He often believes his victim enjoys the assault, and he exerts only the amount of force necessary to subdue his victim. Often power rape is a planned stranger attack, but most acquaintance rapes are also power rapes.

- In *anger rape,* the sexual assault is used to express feelings of rage and to retaliate for what the attacker perceives as wrongs against him. These perceived wrongs most often have nothing to do with the rape victim. Considerable brutality and degradation can characterize this type of rape. Attacks on older women often are a form of anger rape.

- In *sadistic rape,* the assailant has an antisocial personality and delights in torture and mutilation. In this type of rape, the victim and assailant are generally strangers, and the assault is planned. Most rape homicides are sadistic rapes.

- In *stranger rape,* the assailant and victim are strangers, and the rape is sudden and unexpected. The rapist is more likely to use a weapon and threaten violence or murder.

- In *acquaintance rape,* the assailant is someone with whom the victim has had previous nonviolent interaction. The attacker uses deception and trust to gain access to the victim and then betrays that trust. Marital rape and **date rape** are included in this category. In date rape, the male has usually planned to have sex and will do what he feels is necessary if denied. **Acquaintance rape** is significantly more frequent than stranger rape. Approximately 67% of female rape victims know their assailant as an acquaintance, friend, relative, or intimate (Catalano, 2005).

- In *gang rape,* the rape is used as a reinforcing mechanism for membership in a particular group of men; therefore, assailants are more commonly younger men responding to peer pressure. Participation in the rape provides a means for individuals to prove their sexual ability to others and underscore their status in the group. Generally the group leader will initiate the rape and then incite the others to follow. Often gang rape can escalate to severe violence as the young men seek to outdo each other.

I always knew that rape was a terrifying experience physically but I never really thought about the horror that comes from being helpless and in someone else's control.

Role of Drugs in Sexual Assault

In some cases, a perpetrator uses alcohol or other drugs to sedate his intended victim— **drug-facilitated sexual assault.** Flunitrazepam (Rohypnol), a potent sedative-hypnotic that is legal in 80 countries worldwide but illegal in the United States, received considerable attention as the "date rape drug of choice" in the late 1990s. Typically Rohypnol, which dissolves easily and is odorless, is slipped into the drink of an unsuspecting woman. More recently, gamma hydroxybutyrate (GHB), ketamine, MDMA (Ecstasy), clonazepam, and scopolamine have been identified as date rape drugs that are used to incapacitate a woman. Because these drugs frequently produce amnesia, the woman may be unable to remember details of her assault, thereby making prosecution more difficult. She may be left uncertain about the perpetrator's identity, the events of the assault, the presence of birth control, and possible injury or risk for contracting STIs. See Table 9–3 for indicators of possible drug-facilitated sexual assault.

Rape Trauma Syndrome

Rape is viewed as a situational crisis, that is, an unanticipated traumatic event that the victim generally is unprepared to handle because it is unforeseen. Following rape, the survivor may experience a cluster of symptoms originally described by Burgess and Holmstrom (1979) as the **rape trauma syndrome.** Burgess and Holmstrom described this syndrome as having two phases: the acute phase and the adjustment, or reorganization, phase. Other authors added a third phase: an intermediate, outward adjustment phase. Recently a fourth phase—integration and recovery—has been suggested (Holmes, 1998). Although the phases of response

Table 9–3   INDICATORS OF POSSIBLE DRUG-FACILITATED SEXUAL ASSAULT
• Becoming intoxicated very rapidly, especially after accepting a drink from someone else or drinking a drink she left unattended
• Having just one or two drinks, and then suddenly feeling "very drunk"; feeling more intoxicated than usual after drinking an amount of alcohol she is used to consuming
• Feeling drowsy, dizzy, agitated, weak, confused, or nauseous; experiencing an increased heart rate or blood pressure, slurred speech, or a lack of motor coordination
• Waking up suspecting she may have been raped because of vaginal soreness, finding herself in an unfamiliar place, or other indicators
• Being told that she suddenly appeared drunk, drowsy, dizzy, or confused, with impaired motor skills, judgment, and amnesia or partial amnesia

MEDIALINK   Application: Rohypnol

are discussed individually in the following sections, they often overlap, as do individual responses and their duration.

ACUTE PHASE (DISORGANIZATION)

The acute phase of rape trauma syndrome begins during the rape and may last for a few days or up to 3 weeks. The woman may experience fear, shock, disbelief, and, sometimes, denial. The woman may feel humiliated, guilty, and unclean; her wish to cleanse herself by bathing or douching may be overpowering, even if she knows that by doing so she is destroying evidence. She may feel angry or anxious, powerless or helpless.

The rape survivor may suppress her emotions or may reveal them by crying, sobbing, or acting tense and restless. Survivors who control or mask their emotions may appear calm, composed, or subdued. Many rape survivors also experience alterations in sleep patterns, such as insomnia, nightmares, or crying out at night.

OUTWARD ADJUSTMENT PHASE (DENIAL)

Once the acute stage has passed, the survivor may appear adjusted. She returns to work or school and resumes her usual roles. But although she appears composed, she is actually coping by denial and suppression. The survivor needs the outward adjustment phase to cope with the experience of rape; it is a means of regaining control of her life. During this time, she may move to a different residence or may institute security measures, such as installing extra locks or requesting an unlisted telephone number. She may buy a weapon or take a course in self-defense. These activities do not resolve her emotional trauma; they simply push it further into her subconscious. In addition she may get less support from others who perceive her as being "over it."

REORGANIZATION

Denial and suppression cannot sustain the survivor for long. As these coping mechanisms deteriorate, she becomes depressed and anxious and feels a strong urge to talk about the rape. At this point, the woman enters the reorganization phase of the rape trauma syndrome. She must alter her self-concept and resolve her feelings about the rape.

During this phase, the rape survivor may develop phobias. Fears of being indoors or outdoors or of being attacked from behind—depending on how the attack took place—are common. Because of these fears, the woman may alter her lifestyle. If she is afraid of crowds, of being out after dark, or of returning to an empty house, she may become a virtual recluse.

Rape survivors frequently report menstrual or other gynecologic disorders, as well as sexual dysfunction. Some women become totally averse to sexual activity. Those who do try to engage in sex often report a decrease in vaginal lubrication, an inability to be aroused, unusual sensations in the genital area, and an inability to achieve orgasm.

There are a number of long-term physical and psychologic health consequences of sexual assault. Long-term physical consequences include chronic pelvic pain, premenstrual syndrome, gastrointestinal disorders, gynecologic and pregnancy complications, migraines and other frequent headaches, back pain, and facial pain. Chronic psychologic consequences include depression, attempted or completed suicide, alienation, post-traumatic stress disorder, and/or unhealthy diet-related behaviors (e.g., fasting, vomiting, abusing diet pills, overeating) (NCIPC, 2006). Sleep disorders persist. Survivors report repeated nightmares in which they either relive the rape or thwart the rapist's attempt. In either case the dream contains disturbing violence. The woman repeatedly replays the role of victim until she comes to terms with the experience.

INTEGRATION AND RECOVERY

This final phase brings resolution for the woman. She is able to recognize that the blame for her assault lies with her assailant. She begins to trust others again and begins to feel safe in her life and day-to-day activities. She may be filled with a sense of righteous anger and become an advocate for other women (Holmes, 1998).

SILENT REACTION

Women who do not report the rape go through the phases of the rape trauma syndrome without using available support systems. Their reasons for keeping silent vary. A woman may be embarrassed, she may accept society's "temptress view" and blame herself, or she may fear retaliation. Her experience may be discovered much later, perhaps when she seeks professional help in resolving a different crisis.

Some women seek medical help for their physical injuries without disclosing that a rape was the cause. The nurse who suspects that a woman has been raped should seek validation through sympathetic questioning.

Rape as a Cause of Post-Traumatic Stress Disorder

Rape survivors may exhibit high levels of **post-traumatic stress disorder** (PTSD), the same disorder that developed in many of the veterans of the Vietnam War. To be diagnosed as having PTSD, a person must:

- Have been exposed to a traumatic event that triggered feelings of intense fear, horror, or helplessness
- Reexperience the event in recurrent, intrusive thoughts, images, perceptions, and flashbacks
- Persistently avoid stimuli associated with the trauma and demonstrate a generalized "numbing" of responsiveness
- Demonstrate persistent signs of increased arousal, such as exaggerated startle response, difficulty falling asleep, hypervigilance or outbursts of anger, emotional detachment, and sleep disturbances that were not present before the trauma occurred

PTSD is marked by varying degrees of intensity. One mitigating factor is individual resiliency. Not surprisingly, the intensity of the PTSD is often greatest for women who had psychiatric disorders before their sexual assault.

PTSD is difficult to treat. Because the symptoms keep an individual from addressing the problem, she cannot integrate the event into her life, and healing is blocked. Recovery depends on empowering the woman to seek to regain control of her life within the context of healing relationships and professional counseling.

Physical Care of the Sexual Assault Survivor

Following a sexual assault, a primary purpose of care is to meet the needs of the survivor. This is accomplished by evaluating and treating injuries; conducting prompt examinations; providing support, crisis intervention, and advocacy; providing prophylaxis against STIs; assessing for pregnancy risk and discussing treatment options; and providing follow-up care for medical and emotional needs ("National Protocol for Sexual Assault Medical Forensic Examinations: Adults/Adolescents," 2004). As many as 42% of women who are sexually assaulted sustain injuries, although often the injuries are minor; more severe physical consequences may also occur (NCIPC, 2006; Tjaden & Thoennes, 2006).

Because sexual assault is a crime as well as a traumatic emergency, however, the other purpose of health care is to collect and preserve legal evidence for use in prosecuting the assailant. It is important to note that even though evidence is collected, it does not necessarily mean that the survivor has to prosecute; the survivor always has the right to reconsider her decisions. In collecting legal evidence, healthcare providers must respect the rights of the survivor. Sexual assault survivors have the right to immediate, compassionate, and comprehensive medical-legal examination and treatment by a trained professional who has the experience to anticipate their needs during this time of crisis.

Unfortunately, in many communities the treatment of a woman immediately following a sexual assault has been almost as traumatic as the assault itself. Often referred to as "the second rape" or as "secondary victimization," it is reflected in victim blaming, insensitive, and prying care. To address this concern, many emergency departments use multidisciplinary teams to provide effective care to sexual assault survivors and their families. Sexual assault nurse examiner (SANE) programs and sexual assault response teams (SART) are two examples of successful multidisciplinary community programs that coordinate teams of medical, legal, and social service professionals with effective advocacy on behalf of sexual assault survivors. Other communities provide rape victim advocates, who help survivors in hospital EDs and in dealing with the police. Research suggests that rape survivors who have the assistance of an advocate in the ED report less emotional distress from the experience, have fewer negative interactions with hospital staff, and receive more medical services such as prophylaxis against STIs and emergency contraception (Campbell, 2006).

DETAILED HISTORY

Obtaining a detailed history is an essential first step in acquiring necessary medical and forensic data, but it can also be a therapeutic tool if done in a sensitive, caring way. Because a

sexual assault survivor may appear relaxed and normal when first seen, caregivers may underestimate her needs, but it is essential that she receive immediate attention. Immediately after the woman has received any necessary emergency care, the nurse takes an explicit history of the event in the woman's own words to aid in evidence collection and examination of injuries. Many agencies use a standardized forensic chart containing a history flow sheet to record information obtained. The caregiver should use a nonjudgmental approach and must avoid leading or coaching the woman.

COLLECTION OF EVIDENCE

The collection of evidence may, in itself, be traumatic for the woman. It is valuable to have someone available to provide support and act as an advocate. This person may be a family member or close friend, but often it is a nurse. An interpreter should also be provided as necessary.

The woman should receive a thorough explanation of the procedures to be carried out and should sign an informed consent form. An important legal concept when dealing with rape survivors is the need to preserve the *chain of evidence,* meaning that all physical evidence and specimens must remain in the hands of a professional until they are turned over to a police officer. The evidence that the nurse or forensic examiner collects has four primary uses (Ledray, 1999): (1) to confirm recent sexual contact; (2) to show that force or coercion was used; (3) to identify the assailant; and (4) to corroborate the survivor's story. Most agencies have special sexual assault kits that contain all necessary supplies for collecting and labeling evidence.

A careful examination of the entire body is necessary. Vaginal and rectal examinations are performed, along with a complete physical examination for trauma. Any lacerations of the vaginal wall are repaired and noted. A colposcope with photographic capability can be used to document injuries to the genitalia.

Clothing

Each piece of clothing and foreign material dislodged from clothing is marked, placed in an individual paper bag, sealed, and labeled.

Swabs of Stains and Secretions

Swabs of body stains and secretions are analyzed for semen or sperm. The absence of sperm, however, does not signify that no sexual assault has occurred. Many assailants do not ejaculate because of sexual dysfunction, or they may use a condom. Because victims are often forced to commit fellatio, oral swabs are also examined for semen. Gonorrhea and chlamydia cultures also are taken from vaginal, rectal, and oral cavities.

Hair and Scrapings

Clippings or scrapings of the woman's fingernails are examined for blood or tissue from the assailant. Approximately 20 to 25 hairs are pulled from her head and pubic area to analyze the root structure and identify foreign hairs. Her pubic hair is also combed to check for loose hairs that may have been transferred from the rapist.

RESEARCH IN PRACTICE

HUMAN IMMUNODEFICIENCY VIRUS POSTEXPOSURE PROPHYLAXIS IN CHILD AND ADOLESCENT VICTIMS OF SEXUAL ASSAULT

What is this study about? The sexual assault of children and adolescents carries with it the risk of transmission of sexually transmitted infections, including human immunodeficiency virus (HIV). The Centers for Disease Control and Prevention published guidelines for prophylaxis for occupational and nonoccupational exposure to HIV, but the guidelines do not clearly identify indications for HIV prophylaxis in individual cases of sexual assault. Limited studies have been done on the use of HIV prophylactic drugs, but there is only indirect evidence supporting its value for victims of sexual assault. This was a descriptive study of the experience of providing HIV prophylaxis for sexual assault victims at a Midwest child abuse center.

How was this study done? Two reviewers performed a retrospective chart review of 2685 children and adolescents presenting at a pediatric emergency department and child abuse clinic. Information was gathered from the charts about the indications for HIV prophylaxis, the type of sexual assault, the type of prophylaxis dispensed, compliance with the prophylaxis and with follow-up visits, and the incidence of positive tests for HIV.

What were the results of the study? Thirty-four individuals received HIV prophylaxis (1%). Ages ranged from 12 weeks to 18 years, with a mean age of 12 years. The most common indications for HIV prophylaxis were stranger assault, reported known drug abuse by the perpetrator, or assault by multiple perpetrators. Prophylaxis most often followed genital-to-genital contact, although oral-genital and genital-anal contact also prompted preventive measures. Only eight individuals were known to have finished their medication completely. The reason cited most frequently for noncompliance was the incidence of side effects, the most common of which were nausea and vomiting, abdominal pain, and headache. The majority were discharged to the custody of their biologic parents, but six were placed into foster care. Children who were placed into foster care were more likely to finish the medication regimen and keep all follow-up appointments. None of the children tested positive for HIV during the follow-up period.

What additional questions might I have? What was the rate of positive tests for HIV among the majority of children who were lost to follow-up? What was the rate of positive tests for HIV among the children who were not treated with HIV prophylaxis?

How can I use this study? Evaluation of the child or adolescent who has experienced sexual abuse is a complicated, emotional process. The decision to initiate HIV prophylaxis adds complexity to the situation. During the evaluation of a sexual assault victim, it is rarely known if the perpetrator is infected with HIV. A high level of fear of HIV compounds the anguish of the child or teen and the family. Information that is known about the perpetrator is important to gather, because it often drives the decision to apply HIV prophylaxis. These children and adolescents are frequently lost to follow-up, and compliance with both medication use and follow-up healthcare visits is poor. The nurse should ensure that the family understands the importance of completing the prophylactic regimen and of getting adequate treatment for the child or adolescent.

Schremmer, R., Swanson, D., & Kraley, L. (2005). Human immunodeficiency virus postexposure prophylaxis in child and adolescent victims of sexual assault. *Pediatric Emergency Care, 21*(8), 502–506.

Blood Samples

Blood is drawn to test for syphilis and to determine the woman's blood type. Additional blood may be drawn for a pregnancy test if the woman indicates that she wants to take emergency contraception (see discussion in Chapter 5) to prevent pregnancy. She has to have a negative pregnancy test to receive the medication.

Urine Samples

Urine should be collected in cases in which a drug-facilitated sexual assault is suspected and the drug was ingested within 96 hours of the evidentiary exam. It is important to document in the record the time the survivor believes that the drug was ingested and the number of urinations between the ingestion and the exam. A forensic laboratory with the capability of conducting toxicology tests should be identified because not all crime labs have the specialized equipment needed to test for rape drugs. Moreover, because of the increased sensitivity of deoxyribonucleic acid (DNA) tests, many jurisdictions are extending the standard cutoff time for evidence collection in their jurisdictions ("National Protocol for Sexual Assault Medical Forensic Examinations: Adults/Adolescents," 2004).

Photographs

Photographs should be taken of injured areas if possible. Before taking any photos, the healthcare provider should ask the woman to sign an informed consent form.

PREVENTION OF SEXUALLY TRANSMITTED INFECTIONS

Among women who have been sexually assaulted, trichomoniasis, bacterial vaginosis, gonorrhea, and chlamydia are the most frequently diagnosed infections. Thus, during the initial examination, cultures for *Neisseria gonorrhoeae* and *Chlamydia trachomatis* should be obtained from any body sites of penetration or attempted penetration. However, because these infections are fairly prevalent among sexually active women, the diagnosis of one or more of these infections following an assault does not necessarily indicate that it was acquired during the assault. If any STI is diagnosed, it is treated (Centers for Disease Control and Prevention [CDC], 2002). Most clinicians recommend routine preventive therapy after a sexual assault with follow-up referral to a clinic specializing in the treatment of STIs to evaluate the effectiveness of the therapy. The CDC (2002) recommends a prophylaxis regimen that includes a single dose of ceftriaxone intramuscularly plus a single oral dose of metronidazole and a single oral dose of azithromycin. If the survivor chooses not to receive prophylactic antibiotic treatment, the nurse should instruct her to be seen by her caregiver in 2 weeks for assessment for any STIs. In addition, because hepatitis B is a risk, the woman who has never been immunized should be given hepatitis B immune globulin; she should also begin the hepatitis B three-dose immunization series immediately (CDC, 2002).

If the assailant's human immunodeficiency virus (HIV) status is not known, consideration should be given to offer postexposure prophylaxis with HIV antiviral medications. If postexposure HIV prophylaxis is considered, consultation with an HIV specialist is advised (CDC, 2002).

PREVENTION OF PREGNANCY

The woman is questioned about her menstrual cycle and contraceptive practices. If she is at risk for pregnancy and a pregnancy test is negative, she should receive information about her treatment options. Women of different ages, social, cultural, and religious/spiritual backgrounds will have diverse feelings about acceptable treatment options. The nurse needs to be sensitive and nonjudgmental when discussing various reproductive health services. If the woman wishes, emergency postcoital contraception is provided. (See Chapter 5 for further discussion.)

NURSING CARE MANAGEMENT

Because sexual assault survivors frequently enter the healthcare system by way of the ED, nurses are often the first to counsel them. Because the caregiver's values, attitudes, and beliefs will necessarily affect the competence and focus of the care, nurses who work with survivors must understand their own attitudes and beliefs about sexual assault and sexual assault survivors and resolve any conflicts that may exist.

In addition to examining their own attitudes and beliefs, nurses must be mindful of the potential for increased complexity of treatment with sexual assault survivors who are members of different ethnic or cultural backgrounds. For example, a woman's membership in a particular ethnic or cultural group could affect her willingness to disclose all the details of an assault, her willingness to follow up with community resources or to seek counseling, and her willingness to prosecute. Being aware of potential cultural differences is important when discussing future courses of action available.

Nursing Assessment and Diagnosis

Policies for admitting and examining sexual assault survivors vary among institutions. A woman who has been assaulted is under great stress and needs the sensitive care of professionals who are aware of her special needs. The first priority is creating a safe, secure milieu. Professionals should gather admission information in a quiet, private room and reassure the woman that she is not alone, will not be abandoned, and is safe from a second attack.

A full mental status examination should be performed, both for the purpose of planning care and as possible courtroom evidence. Scrupulous documentation is essential because the survivor's medical record is often used in the courtroom to verify her testimony if the rapist is prosecuted.

Examples of nursing diagnoses that may apply to the sexual assault survivor include the following:

- ***Fear*** related to invasion of personal space secondary to assault
- ***Powerlessness*** related to inability to regain sense of control secondary to assault

Nursing Plan and Implementation

Table 9–4 outlines the general nursing actions that are appropriate during each of the phases of recovery. It is imperative that control be returned to the woman as quickly as possible. When feasible, the woman should decide on the sequence of forensic events, such as pulling her own hair (head and pubic), having blood drawn after clothes are collected rather than before, and so forth. In this way the nurse helps her deal with her crisis in small, manageable increments. The nurse should encourage the woman to express her feelings and reassure her that anger and fear are normal, appropriate responses. The nurse can also address expressed or unexpressed guilt by assuring the woman that the sexual assault was not her fault.

By explaining the forensic examination and the general sequence of events in the ED, the nurse can alleviate the client's anxiety related to fear of the unknown. The woman should know what is going to happen and why and how she can assist in each phase of the examination. Throughout the experience, the nurse acts as the survivor's advocate, providing support without usurping decision making. The nurse need not agree with all the survivor's decisions but should respect and defend her right to make them. A survivor also has the right to have a victim advocate, family member, or friend with her throughout the examination process.

The family members or friends on whom the survivor calls also need nursing care. Like those of the survivor, the reactions of the family will depend on the values to which they ascribe.

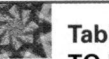

Table 9–4 NURSING ACTIONS APPROPRIATE TO PHASES OF RECOVERY FOLLOWING RAPE

Acute phase	Create a safe milieu.
	Explain the sequence of events in the healthcare facility.
	Allow the woman to grieve and express her feelings.
	Provide care for significant others.
Outward adjustment phase	Provide advocacy and support at the level requested by the woman.
	Provide assistance to significant others.
Reorganizational phase	Establish a trusting relationship.
	Assist the woman to understand her role in the assault.
	Clarify and enhance the woman's feelings.
	Assist the woman in planning for her future.
Integration and recovery	Acknowledge survivor's success in overcoming trauma; support advocacy efforts.

MEDIALINK

Case Study: Teenage Rape Victim

Some family members or partners may blame the survivor for the sexual assault and feel angry with her for not having been more careful. They may also incorrectly view the assault as a sexual act rather than as an act of violence. They may feel personally wronged or attacked and see the survivor as being devalued or unclean. Their reactions may compound the survivor's crisis. By spending some time with family members before their first interaction with the survivor, the nurse can reduce their anxiety and help them examine and reconcile their feelings, sparing the woman further trauma. In some cases, the nurse may want to refer them to a sexual assault advocate who can help them address their needs.

> **CLINICAL TIP**
>
> Strive to listen nonjudgmentally. Impartial listening can often make the difference in a victim's readiness to disclose the full details of the assault and assist her in the recovery process.

COMMUNITY-BASED NURSING CARE

As the woman enters the reorganization phase, she usually feels a strong urge to discuss and resolve her feelings about herself and her assailant. During this phase, the survivor may benefit from talking with a specially trained sexual assault advocate or counselor. If she is not certain that she wants counseling, or denies any need for counseling, it is appropriate to respect her current wishes and to provide her with referral information for possible future use.

Counseling, provided by qualified nurses or other counselors, is a valuable tool in helping the sexual assault survivor come to terms with her attack and its impact on her life. In counseling, the woman is encouraged to explore and identify her feelings and determine appropriate actions to resolve her problems and concerns. It is important for the counselor to assist the woman to realize that the sexual assault was not her fault. The fault lies with the perpetrator. With the counselor, the woman explores her thoughts and feelings about self-care and celebrates her victories. It is important to emphasize that the loss of control that occurred during the assault was temporary and that she does have control over other aspects of her life.

Preventive Education

Local high schools, colleges, or rape awareness groups may offer courses in preventive strategies. Some classes focus on increasing women's awareness of situations in which they are at risk, whereas others are concerned with changing societal and men's attitudes about sexual assault and sexual assault survivors. Because sexual assault is a considerable risk for any woman, courses in what to do during and after an attack and how family members and friends can support a survivor are also helpful. Table 9–5 provides general guidelines for helping victims of sexual assault. Nurses who have completed additional education and are thoroughly prepared are well qualified to initiate or participate in preventive instruction.

Sexual Assault Counseling and Information

Most sexual assault centers operate 24 hours a day, 7 days a week. Their services are invaluable. Properly trained counselors

Table 9–5   GENERAL GUIDELINES FOR HELPING VICTIMS OF SEXUAL ASSAULT

- Believe the victim—one of the greatest fears of sexual assault survivors is that they will not be believed.
- Listen and be patient—let the person talk and tell the story at her/his own pace.
- Reinforce the fact that the sexual assault was not the victim's fault.
- For recent assaults, encourage the victim to report the assault and preserve evidence.
- Encourage the person to seek medical attention.
- Suggest seeking counseling and other support services.
- Help the victim to organize her/his thoughts, but let the survivor make her/his own decision on how to proceed.
- Take care of yourself—assisting a friend or family member can be stressful. Set aside time for yourself so that you don't feel overwhelmed by the survivor's problems.
- Acknowledge your limits and realistically identify your abilities to assist the survivor.

SOURCE: From *General Guidelines for Helping Victims of Sexual Assault.* George Mason University Sexual Assault Services. Reprinted with permission.

can help the survivor regain control early in the crisis. Many sexual assault centers offer free counseling to survivors or can refer them to qualified counselors. Information on STIs and pregnancy alternatives may also be obtained from these centers. In addition, there are many Web resources that provide information for survivors and their family members and friends, as well as for professionals seeking information about how to better assist survivors of sexual assault. See the Companion Web Site for a list of hotline information and Internet-based resources about sexual assault.

Evaluation

Expected outcomes of quality nursing care include the following:

- The survivor receives prompt, compassionate, respectful, and individualized medical attention.
- The woman recovers from the physical effects of the sexual assault.
- The woman is able to verbalize her recognition that sexual assault is a crime of violence expressed sexually.
- The woman is able to identify culturally appropriate community resources available to her as she works to adjust psychologically to the assault.
- The woman makes a decision about whether to prosecute her assailant.
- If a survivor decides to prosecute her assailant, all necessary forensic evidence will have been collected, leading to a more successful investigation and prosecution.

Prosecution of the Assailant

Legally, sexual assault, like any criminal action, is considered a crime against the state rather than against the victim. Therefore, prosecution of the assailant is a community responsibility in which the district attorney will act on the victim's behalf. The victim, however, must initiate the process by reporting the crime and pressing charges against her assailant. Once authorities have apprehended the alleged attacker, the judicial system is set into motion.

Procedures vary from state to state. A judge or magistrate generally conducts a hearing to determine whether there is sufficient evidence to hold the defendant over for a grand jury. If so, the grand jury will determine whether the evidence is sufficient to indict the defendant. If not, he is acquitted. If indicted, a defendant must stand trial unless he waives this right. Either a judge or a jury will find the defendant guilty or not guilty, and he will be retained or set free accordingly.

Many sexual assault survivors who have gone through the judicial process refer to it as a second rape—and sometimes a more damaging one. The survivor will be repeatedly asked to identify the assailant and describe the assault in intimate detail. Throughout the pretrial period, the defense attorney may use delaying tactics, further frustrating the survivor and her support system. Publicity may intensify her feelings of humiliation, and if the assailant is released on bail, she may fear retaliation.

During the trial itself, cross-examination by the defense attorney can be a severely degrading experience in which the "victim as temptress" myth may be continually evoked. The defense attorney may try to discredit her testimony, causing her to feel victimized a second time. Fortunately, rape shield laws have become quite common, and nearly every state has passed legislation that prohibits the publicizing of a victim's sexual history. Moreover, despite the difficulties of prosecution, many victims feel a sense of justice in taking their case to court.

The nurse acting as a counselor needs to be aware of the judicial sequence to anticipate rising tension and frustration in the survivor and her support system. They will need consistent, effective support at this crucial time.

Responding to Violence Against Women: Vicarious Trauma

Vicarious trauma, or secondary trauma effect, can occur as a result of working with people who are trauma victims. It refers to a gradual internal transformation that can negatively affect commitment to one's work, reduce any sense of accomplishment, and lead to a questioning of personal belief systems. Nurses who treat and assist domestic violence and sexual assault survivors should be aware of this phenomenon so that they are able to periodically assess the effect of their work on their lives. When the lives of nurses—and indeed of all healthcare professionals—are balanced and there is equal time for self, family, friends, work, play, and rest, then they are better able to provide compassionate and sensitive health care.

CHAPTER REVIEW

FOCUS YOUR STUDY

- Domestic violence is very common. One in three to one in four women will experience violence at the hands of an intimate partner during their lifetime.

- Batterers use psychologic, physical, and sexual abuse to maintain power and control in abusive relationships.

- Battering occurs in a cyclic pattern called the cycle of violence, which increases in frequency and severity over time.

- Women in abusive relationships who belong to cultural and linguistic minority communities and immigrant women face additional barriers when attempting to access services. The nurse must work to provide culturally aware and competent care.

- Nurses are in an excellent position to intervene and assist women with abusive partners by recognizing their cues,

diagnosing their problems appropriately, and understanding the complex dynamics of the battering family. The nurse provides information about available culturally appropriate community resources, medical attention, and emotional support.

- Estimates suggest that over 60% of sexual assaults are not reported to the police. Rapes and sexual assaults committed by strangers are more likely to be reported to the police than rapes or sexual assaults committed by "nonstrangers," including intimate partners, other relatives, and friends or acquaintances.

- Rape is an act of violence acted out sexually. Most sexual assaults are expressions of anger or power.

- Following sexual assault, the survivor will usually experience an assortment of symptoms known as the rape trauma syndrome. Recent research also links the effects of rape to the post-traumatic stress disorder. Nursing actions to assist rape survivors are encompassed in the roles of advocate, educator, and counselor.

- Nurses inform the woman of the sequence of events involved in providing her care and developing the chain of evidence, and support the survivor's decisions.

- Widespread education is needed to abolish societal myths surrounding domestic violence and sexual assault.

EXPLORE MediaLink

http://www.prenhall.com/davidson

NCLEX review questions, case studies, and other interactive resources for this chapter can be found on the Web Site at http://www.prenhall.com/davidson. Click on "Chapter 9" to select the activities for this chapter.

For tutorials including animations and videos, more NCLEX review questions, and an audio glossary, access the accompanying Prentice Hall Nursing MediaLink DVD-ROM in this book.

 PRENTICE HALL NURSING MEDIALINK DVD-ROM
Audio Glossary
NCLEX Review
Videos: *Spousal Abuse; Parental Sexual Abuse; Going Back?*

 COMPANION WEBSITE
Additional NCLEX Review
Case Study: *Teenage Rape Victim*
Care Plan Activity: *Suspicious Injury and Bruises*
Applications: *Domestic Violence; Rohypnol*
Critical Thinking

CRITICAL THINKING IN ACTION

COUNSELING THE SURVIVOR OF DOMESTIC VIOLENCE

View the Critical Thinking in Action video in Chapter 9 of the DVD-ROM. Then answer the questions that follow.

Marishka Devonowski, a 28-year-old G2P2, has a 9-year-old daughter and a 3-month-old daughter at home. Mrs. Devonowski has been seen at the emergency department several times for a variety of problems including a broken arm, sprained ankle, and multiple contusions from reportedly "walking into a door" when she got up during the night but did not turn on a light. She describes herself as clumsy and accident-prone. At each visit her husband, a computer analyist, who appears thoughtful and protective of his wife, accompanies her.

Today she is being seen for a severe laceration of her cheek and a mild concussion. You observe that she also has a black eye and bruising of her upper arm and chest. At each previous visit the nurse had managed to spend time alone with Mrs. Devonowski and had asked specifically about domestic violence. However, Marishka denied it vehemently each time. Today, when you are alone with her you ask about abuse. This time she admits that her husband caused her injuries. She states, "His job is so stressful and sometimes he just loses his temper. But he seems to get more angry no matter what I do. I hate it but I can't leave him. I don't know how I would manage alone."

1. In talking with Marishka, what information would you focus on initially?

2. What specific information should you share about preparing an exit or safety plan?

REFERENCES

American Nurses Association (ANA). (1991, Revised March 24, 2000). *Position statement on physical violence against women.* Retrieved November 10, 2005, from http://nursingworld.org/readroom/position/social/scviol.htm

Burgess, A. W., & Holmstrom, L. L. (1979). *Rape: Crisis and recovery.* Englewood Cliffs, NJ: Prentice Hall.

Campbell, R. (2006). Rape survivors' experiences with the legal and medical systems: Do rape victim advocates make a difference? *Violence Against Women, 12*(1), 30–45.

Catalano, S. M. (2005). *Criminal victimization, 2004.* Bureau of Justice Statistics National Crime Victimization Survey. Retrieved July 1, 2006, from http://www.ojp.usdoj.gov/bjs

Centers for Disease Control and Prevention (CDC). (2002, May 10). Sexually transmitted diseases treatment guidelines 2002. *Morbidity and Mortality Weekly Report, 51*(RR-6).

Centers for Disease Control and Prevention (CDC). (2003). *Costs of intimate partner violence against women in the United States.* Retrieved November 10, 2005, from http://www.cdc.gov/ncipc/pub-res/ipv_cost/ipv.htm

Crandall, M., Nathens, A. B., Kernic, M. A., Holt, V. L., & Rivara, F. P. (2004). Predicting future injury among women in abusive relationships. *Journal of Trauma-Injury Infection and Critical Care, 56*(4), 906–912.

Fox, J. A., & Zawitz, M. W. (2004). *Homicide trends in the United States.* Washington, DC: US Department of Justice. Retrieved November 10, 2005, from http://www.ojp.usdoj.gov/bjs/homicide/homtrnd.htm

George Mason University Sexual Assault Services. (2005). *General guidelines for helping victims of sexual assault.* Retrieved July 1, 2006, from http://www.gmu.edu/facstaff/sexual/Helping_GenGuid.htm

Greensite, G. (n.d.). *Rape myths.* California Coalition Against Sexual Assault [CALCASA]. Retrieved July 1, 2006, from http://www.calcasa.org/34.0.html

Hart, T. C., & Rennison, C. M. (2003, March). *Reporting crime to the police, 1992–2000.* Bureau of Justice Statistics Special Report, US Department of Justice (NCJ-195710). Retrieved November 14, 2005, from http://www.ojp.usdoj.gov/bjs/pub/pdf/rcp00.pdf

Healthy People 2010. (2005). Leading health indicators: Priorities for action. Retrieved November 14, 2005, from http://www.healthypeople.gov

Heise, L. L., & Garcia-Moreno, C. (2002). Violence by intimate partners. In E. Krug, L. L. Dahlberg, J. A. Mercy, et al. (Eds.), *World report on violence and health* (pp. 87–121). Geneva, Switzerland: World Health Organization.

Holmes, M. M. (1998). The clinical management of rape in adolescents. *Contemporary OB/GYN, 43*(5), 62–78.

Horon, I. L., & Cheng, D. (2001). Enhanced surveillance for pregnancy-associated mortality—Maryland, 1993–1998. *Journal of the American Medical Association, 285*(11), 1455–1459.

Ledray, L. E. (1999). *Sexual Assault Nurse Examiner (SANE) development and operations guide.* Washington, DC: US Department of Justice, Office for Victims of Crime and Minneapolis, MN: Sexual Assault Resource Service.

National Center for Injury Prevention and Control (NCIPC). (2006). *Sexual violence: Fact sheet.* Centers for Disease Control and Prevention. Retrieved July 1, 2006, from http://www.cdc.gov/ncipc/factsheets/svfacts.htm

National Coalition Against Domestic Violence. (2005). *Domestic violence facts.* NCADV Public Policy Office. Retrieved July 1, 2006, from http://www.ncadv.org

National Coalition Against Domestic Violence. *Immigrant victims of domestic violence.* NCADV Public Policy Office. Retrieved November 10, 2005, from http://www.ncadv.org

Orloff, L. E., & Little, R. (1999). *Immigrant women: A "how to" manual for battered women's advocates and service providers.* Ayuda, Inc. Retrieved November 10, 2005, from http://www.vawnet.org/DomesticViolence/ServicesAndProgramDev/ServiceProvAndProg/BIW99-c1.php

Plichta, S. B. (2004). Intimate partner violence and physical health consequences: Policy and practice implications. *Journal of Interpersonal Violence, 19*(11), 1296–1323.

Rape, Abuse, and Incest National Network (RAINN). (2003). RAINN News: New report shows dramatic increase in willingness to report rape to the police. Retrieved December 6, 2003, from www.rainn.org/news/ncvs 2002.html.

Rape, Abuse, and Incest National Network (RAINN). (2006). *Statistics.* Retrieved July 1, 2006, from http://www.rainn.org/statistics

Shetty, S., & Kaguyutan, J. (2002, February). Immigrant victims of domestic violence: Cultural challenges and available legal protections. *Applied Research Forum, VAWNet.* Retrieved November 10, 2005, from http://www.vawnet.org/DomesticViolence/Research/VAWnetDocs/AR_immigrant.pdf

Snyder, H. (2000). *Sexual assault of young children as reported to law enforcement: Victim, incident, and offender characteristics.* Washington, DC: Bureau of Justice Statistics, US Department of Justice (NCJ-182990).

Straka, S. M. (2006). Responding to the needs of older women experiencing domestic violence. *Violence Against Women, 12*(3), 251–267.

Tjaden, P., & Thoennes, N. (2006). *Extent, nature, and consequences of rape victimization: Findings from the National Violence Against Women Survey.* [Special Report]. Retrieved July 1, 2006, from http://www.ojp.usdoj.gov/nij

United Nations Population Fund. (2005). *State of the world population 2005.* Retrieved July 1, 2006, from http://www.unfpa.org

US Department of Justice. (2004). *National protocol for sexual assault medical forensic examinations: Adults/adolescents.* US Department of Justice, Office on Violence Against Women (NCJ-206554). Washington, DC: Author.

Walker, L. (1984). *The battered woman syndrome.* New York: Springer.

UNIT
3

Human
Reproduction

CHAPTER 10

The Reproductive System

I always thought it was so boring to study anatomy and physiology. Who cares how many bones there are in the pelvis or the muscles involved. But now I'm with mothers having babies, and now it all makes sense.

~ A Nursing Student ~

KEY TERMS

OBJECTIVES

1. Describe the differentiation of the male and female reproductive organs during embryonic development.

2. Summarize the major changes in the reproductive system that occur during puberty.

3. Identify key aspects of the female and male reproductive systems that are important to reproduction and conception.

4. Discuss the significance of specific female reproductive structures during pregnancy and childbirth.

5. Identify the actions of the hormones that affect reproductive functioning.

6. Identify the two phases of the ovarian cycle and the changes that occur in each phase.

7. Describe the phases of the menstrual cycle, their dominant hormones, and the changes that occur in each phase.

MEDIALINK

Additional resources for this content can be found on the Prentice Hall Nursing MediaLink DVD-ROM and on the Companion Website at http://www.prenhall.com/davidson. Click on "Chapter 10" to select the activities for this chapter.

Understanding childbearing requires more than understanding sexual intercourse or the process by which the female and male sex cells unite. The nurse must also become familiar with the structures and functions that make childbearing possible and the phenomena that initiate it. This chapter considers the anatomic, physiologic, and sexual aspects of the female and male reproductive systems. It also provides information regarding basic embryonic development of the reproductive structures.

The female and male reproductive organs are *homologous;* that is, they are fundamentally similar in function and structure. The primary functions of both the female and male reproductive systems are to produce sex cells and transport them to locations where their union can occur. The sex cells, called *gametes,* are produced by specialized organs called *gonads.* A series of ducts and glands within both the male and female reproductive systems contributes to the production and transport of the gametes.

EMBRYONIC DEVELOPMENT OF REPRODUCTIVE STRUCTURES AND PROCESSES

Although the genetic sex of an embryo is determined at fertilization, the male and female reproductive systems are undifferentiated for about the first 8 weeks of gestation. This undifferentiated period is followed by a period of rapid, dramatic changes as the reproductive organs differentiate into recognizable structures.

Ovaries and Testes

During the 5th week of gestation, a primitive gonad arises from the intermediate mesoderm tissue known as gonadal ridges (Figure 10–1 ◆, top). The gonad develops a medulla (inner part of the organ) and cortex (outer part of the organ), which appear in the underlying mesenchyme (embryonic tissue from which connective and muscle tissue arises; see Table 11–2). In genetic males during the 7th and 8th weeks, the medulla develops into a testis, and the cortex regresses. In genetic females by about the 10th week, the cortex develops into an ovary, and the medulla regresses.

Every egg available for maturation in a woman's reproductive life is present at her birth. During fetal life the ovary produces oogonia, cells that become primitive eggs called **oocytes,** by the process of **oogenesis** (see Chapter 11 ∞). No oocytes are formed after fetal development. About 150,000 oocytes are contained in the ovaries at birth. Each oocyte is contained in a small ovarian cavity called a *primitive follicle.*

Every month during a female's reproductive years, one of the oocytes undergoes a process of cellular division and maturation that transforms it into a fertilizable egg, or **ovum.** At ovulation, the ovum is released from its follicle. The remaining follicles and oocytes degenerate over time.

Each testis produces the male gametes, called **spermatozoa** or *sperm,* by a process called **spermatogenesis.** This process is described in Chapter 11. ∞ Spermatogenesis of mature sperm does not occur until the onset of puberty. Figure 10–1 illustrates the embryologic development of the gonads and other internal reproductive organs.

Other Internal Structures

During the undifferentiated period—the first 7 weeks—two pairs of genital ducts develop: the mesonephric and paramesonephric ducts (Cunningham, Leveno, Bloom et al, 2005).

In genetic females the fallopian tubes are formed from the unfused portions of the paramesonephric ducts, and the fused portions give rise to the epithelium and uterine glands. The endometrial stroma and the myometrium (thick layer of smooth muscle in the wall of the uterus) develop from the adjacent mesenchyme.

The vagina is derived from more than one embryologic structure. The vaginal epithelium develops from the endoderm of the urogenital sinus, and the musculature develops from the uterovaginal primordium.

The urethral and paraurethral glands develop from outgrowths of the urethra into the surrounding mesenchyme. Bartholin's glands arise from similar structures.

In genetic males the fetal testes secrete two hormones. The first hormone, testosterone, stimulates the mesonephric ducts to develop into the male genital tract. The other hormone, Müllerian regression factor, suppresses the development of the paramesonephric ducts, which would otherwise develop into the female genital tract.

From the mesonephric ducts comes development of the efferent ductule, vas deferens, epididymis, seminal vesicle, and ejaculatory duct. Both the prostate and the bulbourethral glands develop from endodermal outgrowths of the urethra.

External Structures

Genetic males and females possess the same external genitals until the end of the 9th week. By the 12th week, differentiation of the external genitals is complete.

If fetal testosterone is not present, the undifferentiated external genitals are feminized. The phallus becomes the clitoris, and the urogenital folds remain open, forming the labia minora. The labioscrotal folds form the labia majora.

If fetal testosterone is present, the undifferentiated external genitals become masculine. The phallus elongates, forming the penis. The fusion of the urogenital folds on the ventral surface of the penis forms the penile urethra, with the urethral meatus moving forward toward the glans penis.

PUBERTY

The term **puberty** refers to the developmental period between childhood and attainment of adult sexual characteristics and functioning. Generally, boys mature physically about 2 years later than girls. Puberty lasts from 1.5 to 5 years and involves profound physical, psychologic, and emotional changes. These changes include an altered body image, changing roles, and changing societal expectations and responses as the child matures into an adult.

Figure 10–1 ◆ Embryonic differentiation of male and female internal reproductive organs.

Major Physical Changes

In both girls and boys, puberty is preceded by an accelerated growth rate called adolescent spurt. Widespread body system changes occur, including maturation of the reproductive organs.

Girls experience a broadening of the hips, then budding of the breasts, the appearance of pubic and axillary hair, and the onset of menstruation, called menarche. The average time between breast development and menarche is 2.3 years.

Boys experience linear growth spurts; an increase in the size of the external genitals; the appearance of pubic, axillary, and facial hair; deepening of the voice; and nocturnal seminal emissions (called wet dreams) without sexual stimulation. These early seminal emissions do not usually contain mature sperm.

The physical changes of puberty present themselves differently in each person. The age at onset and progress of puberty vary widely, physical changes overlap, and the sequence of events can vary from person to person. This diversity results from each individual's response to hormonal stimulation.

Physiology of Onset

Puberty is initiated by the maturation of the hypothalamic-pituitary-gonad complex (the *gonadostat*) and input from the central nervous system. The process, which begins during fetal life, is sequential and complex.

The central nervous system releases a neurotransmitter that stimulates the hypothalamus to synthesize and release **gonadotropin-releasing hormone (GnRH)** (Ferin, 2003). GnRH is transmitted to the anterior pituitary, where it causes the synthesis and secretion of the gonadotropins **follicle-stimulating hormone (FSH)** and **luteinizing hormone (LH)** (Figure 10–2 ◆).

Although the gonads do produce small amounts of *androgens* (male sex hormones) and *estrogens* (female sex hormones) before the onset of puberty, FSH and LH stimulate increased secretion of these hormones. Androgens and estrogens influence the development of secondary sex characteristics. FSH and LH stimulate the processes of spermatogenesis and maturation of ova.

Other hormones are involved in the onset of puberty. Although less direct, their action is essential. Abnormally high or low levels of adrenocorticotropic hormone (ACTH), thyroid hormone, or growth hormone (GH) can disrupt the onset of normal puberty (Ferin, 2003). The maturation process that begins during fetal life continues through puberty and childbearing years. The external and internal female reproductive organs develop and mature in response to estrogen and progesterone.

FEMALE REPRODUCTIVE SYSTEM

The female reproductive system consists of the external and internal genitals and accessory organs of the breasts. The structure of the bony pelvis is also discussed in this section because of its importance in childbearing.

External Genitals

All the external reproductive organs, except the glandular structures, can be directly inspected. The appearance of the external

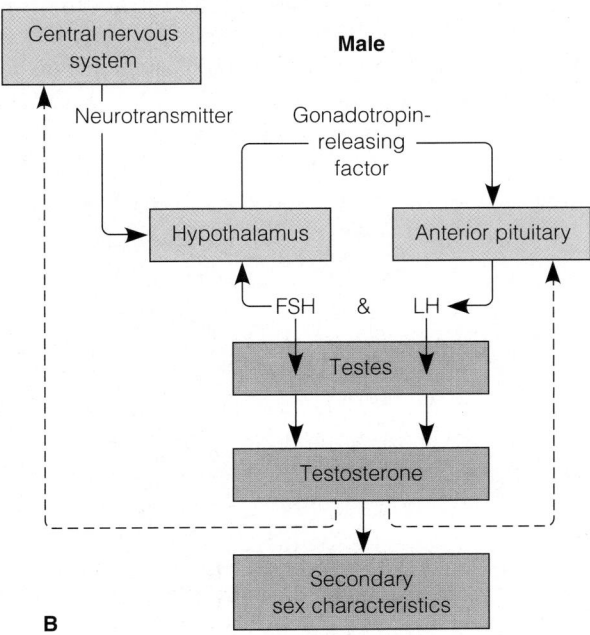

Figure 10–2 ◆ Physiologic changes leading to onset of puberty. *A,* In females; and *B,* in males. Solid lines illustrate stimulation of hormone production, and broken lines illustrate inhibition. Through a neurotransmitter the central nervous system (CNS) stimulates the hypothalamus, which in turn produces a gonadotropin-releasing factor that causes the anterior pituitary to produce gonadotropins (FSH or LH). These hormones stimulate specific structures in the gonads to secrete steroid hormones (estrogen, progesterone, or testosterone). The rise in pituitary hormone production increases hypothalamus activity. Elevated steroid hormone levels stimulate the CNS and pituitary gland to inhibit hormone production.

genitalia varies greatly among women. Heredity, age, race, and the number of children a woman has borne influence the size, color, and shape of her external organs.

The female external genitals, called the **vulva,** include the following structures (Figure 10–3 ◆):

- Mons pubis
- Labia majora
- Labia minora
- Clitoris
- Urethral meatus and opening of the paraurethral (Skene's) glands
- Vaginal vestibule (vaginal orifice, vulvovaginal glands, hymen, and fossa navicularis)
- Perineal body

Although they are not true parts of the female reproductive system, the urethral meatus and perineal body are considered here because of their proximity and relationship to the vulva. The vulva has a generous supply of blood and nerves. As a woman ages, estrogen secretions decrease, causing the vulvar organs to atrophy and become subject to a variety of lesions.

MONS PUBIS

The mons pubis is a softly rounded mound of subcutaneous fatty tissue beginning at the lowest portion of the anterior abdominal wall. Also known as the mons veneris, this structure covers the anterior portion of the symphysis pubis. The mons pubis is covered with pubic hair, typically with the hairline forming a transverse line across the lower abdomen (see Figure 10–3). The hair is short in all women. It can vary from sparse and fine in Asian women to heavy, coarse, and curly in women of African descent. The mons pubis protects the pelvic bones, especially during coitus.

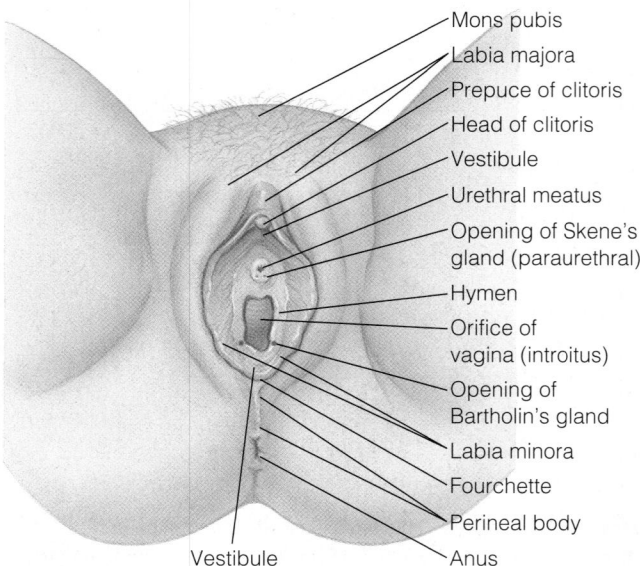

Mons pubis
Labia majora
Prepuce of clitoris
Head of clitoris
Vestibule
Urethral meatus
Opening of Skene's gland (paraurethral)
Hymen
Orifice of vagina (introitus)
Opening of Bartholin's gland
Labia minora
Fourchette
Perineal body
Anus
Vestibule

Figure 10–3 ◆ Female external genitals, longitudinal view.

LABIA MAJORA

The *labia majora* are longitudinal, raised folds of pigmented skin, one on either side of the vulvar cleft (see Figure 10–3). As the pair descend, they narrow, enclosing the vulvar cleft, and merge to form the posterior junction of the perineal skin. Their chief function is to protect the structures lying between them. The labia majora are covered by stratified squamous epithelium containing hair follicles and sebaceous glands with underlying adipose and muscle tissue. The dartos muscle sheath is responsible for the wrinkled appearance of the labia majora as well as for their sensitivity to heat and cold.

The inner surface of the labia majora in women who have not had children is moist and looks like a mucous membrane, but after many births it is more skinlike (Cunningham et al., 2005). With each pregnancy the labia majora become less prominent. Because of the extensive venous network in the labia majora, varicosities may occur during pregnancy, and birth trauma or sexual trauma may cause hematomas. The labia majora share an extensive lymphatic supply with the other structures of the vulva, which can facilitate the spread of cancer in the female reproductive organs. Because nerves from the first lumbar and third sacral segment of the spinal cord supply the labia majora, certain regional anesthesia blocks will affect them and cause numbness.

LABIA MINORA

The *labia minora* are soft folds of skin within the labia majora that converge near the anus, forming the *fourchette* (see Figure 10–3). Each labium minus has the appearance of a shiny mucous membrane, moist and devoid of hair follicles. The labia minora are rich in sebaceous glands, which lubricate and waterproof the vulvar skin and provide bactericidal secretions. Because sebaceous glands do not open into hair follicles but directly onto the surface of the skin, sebaceous cysts commonly occur in this area. The labia minora are composed of erectile tissue and involuntary muscle tissue. Vulvovaginitis in this area is very irritating because of the many tactile nerve endings. The labia minora increase in size at puberty and decrease after menopause because of changes in estrogen levels.

CLITORIS

The *clitoris,* located between the labia minora, is about 5 to 6 mm long and 6 to 8 mm across. Its tissue is essentially erectile (see Figure 10–3). The glans of the clitoris is partly covered by a fold of skin called the *prepuce,* or clitoral hood. This area resembles an opening to an orifice and may be confused with the urethral meatus. Accidental attempts to insert a catheter in this area produce extreme discomfort. The clitoris has very rich blood and nerve supplies and is the primary erogenous organ of women (Cunningham et al., 2005). In addition, it secretes *smegma,* which, along with other vulval secretions, has a unique odor that may be sexually stimulating to the male.

URETHRAL MEATUS AND PARAURETHRAL GLANDS

The *urethral meatus* is located 1 to 2.5 cm beneath the clitoris in the midline of the vestibule; it often appears as a puckered, slitlike opening. At times the meatus is difficult to visualize because of the presence of blind dimples, small mucosal folds.

The paraurethral glands, or *Skene's glands,* open into the posterior wall of the urethra close to its opening (see Figure 10–3). Their secretions help lubricate the vaginal vestibule, facilitating sexual intercourse.

VAGINAL VESTIBULE

The vaginal vestibule is a boat-shaped depression enclosed by the labia majora and visible when they are separated (see Figure 10–3). The vestibule contains the vaginal opening, or *introitus,* which is the border between the external and internal genitals.

The *hymen* is a thin, elastic collar or semicollar of tissue that surrounds the vaginal opening. The appearance of the hymen changes during the woman's lifetime. At birth the hymen is fluffy and full, and the tissue appears to fold back on itself and to cover the vaginal opening. These characteristics are due to exposure to estrogen in utero. With the loss of exposure to estrogen after birth, the hymen's appearance begins to change to a thin membranous tissue that is still in a collar or semicollar shape at approximately 3 years of age (Cunningham et al., 2005). The hymen is without estrogen stimulation and is hypersensitive to touch. At puberty, under the stimulation of the girl's own increasing estrogen levels, the hymen once again becomes more full. The hymen is essentially avascular. For thousands of years, some societies have perpetuated the belief that the hymen covers the vaginal opening and thus that an intact hymen is a sign of virginity. However, modern studies of female genital anatomy have revealed that the hymen surrounds rather than entirely covers the vaginal opening, and can be torn not only through sexual intercourse, but also through strenuous physical activity, masturbation, menstruation, or the use of tampons, thus dispelling old beliefs.

External to the hymen at the base of the vestibule are two small papular elevations containing the openings of the ducts of the *vulvovaginal (Bartholin's) glands.* They lie under the constrictor muscle of the vagina. These glands secrete a clear, thick, alkaline mucus that enhances the viability and motility of sperm deposited in the vaginal vestibule. These gland ducts can harbor *Neisseria gonorrhoeae* and other bacteria, which can cause suppuration and abscesses in the Bartholin's glands.

The vestibular area is innervated mainly by the perineal nerve from the sacral plexus. The area is not sensitive to touch generally; however, the hymen contains numerous free nerve endings as receptors to pain.

PERINEAL BODY

The **perineal body** is a wedge-shaped mass of fibromuscular tissue measuring about 4 × 4 × 4 cm, found between the lower part of the vagina and the anus (see Figure 10–3). The superficial area between the anus and the vagina is referred to as the *perineum.*

The muscles that meet at the perineal body are the external sphincter ani, both levator ani (the superficial and deep transverse perineal), and the bulbocavernosus. These muscles mingle with elastic fibers and connective tissue in an arrangement that allows a remarkable amount of stretching. During the last part of labor, the perineal body thins out until it is just a few centimeters thick. This tissue is often the site of an episiotomy or lacerations during childbirth (see Chapter 27 ∞).

Female Internal Reproductive Organs

The female internal reproductive organs—the vagina, uterus, fallopian tubes, and ovaries—are target organs for estrogenic hormones, and they play a unique part in the reproductive cycle (Figure 10–4 ◆). Certain internal reproductive organs can be palpated during vaginal examination and assessed with various instruments.

VAGINA

The **vagina** is a muscular and membranous tube that connects the external genitals with the uterus (see Figure 10–4). It extends from the vulva to the uterus in a position nearly parallel to the plane of the pelvic brim. The vagina is often referred to as the *birth canal* because it forms the lower part of the axis through which the fetus must pass during birth.

Because the cervix of the uterus projects into the upper part of the anterior wall of the vagina, the anterior wall is approximately 2.5 cm shorter than the posterior wall. Measurements range from 6 to 8 cm for the anterior wall and 7 to 10 cm for the posterior wall.

In the upper part of the vagina, which is called the vaginal vault, there is a recess or hollow around the cervix. This area is called the vaginal fornix. Because the walls of the vaginal vault are very thin, various structures can be palpated through them, including the uterus, a distended bladder, the ovaries, appendix, cecum, colon, and the ureters. The upper fourth of the vagina is separated from the rectum by the pouch of Douglas (sometimes referred to as the cul-de-sac of Douglas). This deep pouch or recess is posterior to the cervix.

When a woman lies on her back after intercourse, the space in the fornix permits the pooling of semen. The collection of a large number of sperm near the cervix at or near the time of ovulation in the woman increases the chances of pregnancy.

The walls of the vagina are covered with ridges, or rugae, crisscrossing each other. These rugae allow the vaginal tissues to stretch enough for the fetus to pass through during childbirth. A rich blood supply is needed to maintain a high glycogen content in the epithelial cells as well as to nourish the underlying musculofascial layer, through which the vaginal vault has strong attachments to the cervix. These muscle layers are continuous with the superficial muscle fibers of the uterus. A thin band of striated muscle, the sphincter vaginae, is found at the lowest extremity of the vagina. However, the levator ani is the principal muscle that closes the vagina.

During a woman's reproductive life, the vaginal environment is normally acidic (pH 4 to 5). Secretion from the vaginal epithelium provides a moist environment. The acidic environment is maintained by a symbiotic relationship between lactic acid-producing bacilli (Döderlein's bacillus or lactobacillus) and the vaginal epithelial cells. These cells contain glycogen, which is broken down by the bacilli into lactic acid. The amount

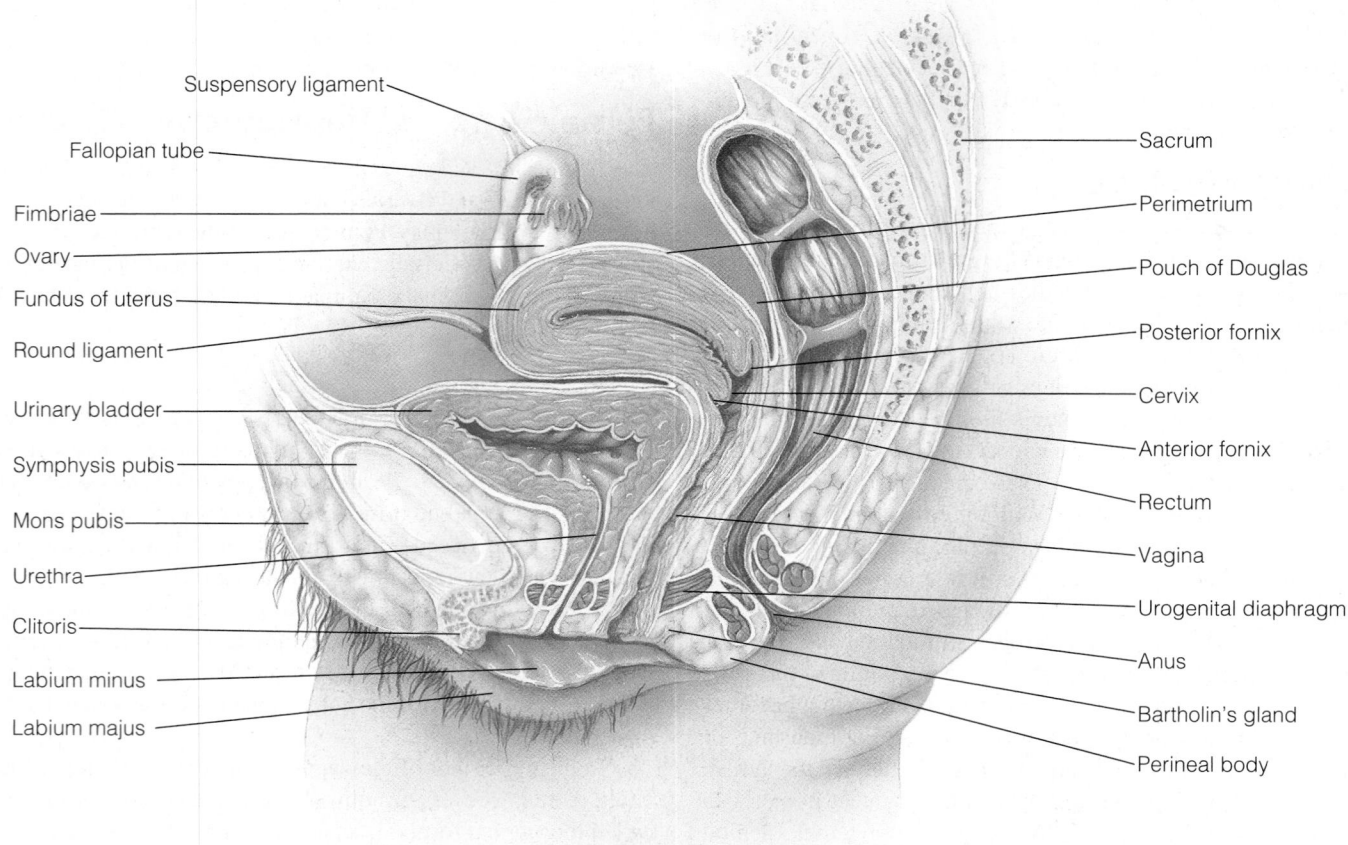

Figure 10–4 ◆ Female internal reproductive organs.

of glycogen is regulated by the ovarian hormones. Any interruption of this process can destroy the normal self-cleansing action of the vagina. Such interruption may be caused by antibiotic therapy, douching, or use of vaginal sprays or deodorants. For further discussion, see Chapter 5. ∞ The acidic vaginal environment is normal only during the mature reproductive years and in the first days of life, when maternal hormones are operating in the infant. A relatively neutral pH of 7.5 is normal from infancy until puberty and after menopause.

Each third of the vagina is supplied by a distinct vascular and lymphatic pattern. Although one would expect venous drainage to go directly to the heart and then the lungs, anastomoses of veins are present and make it possible for a pelvic embolism or carcinoma to bypass the heart and lungs and lodge in the brain, spine, or other remote part of the body.

Vaginal lymphatics drain into the external and internal iliac nodes, the hypogastric nodes, and the inguinal glands. The posterior wall drains into nodes lying in the rectovaginal septum. Any vaginal infection follows these routes.

The pudendal nerve supplies what relatively little somatic innervation there is to the lower third of the vagina. Thus vaginal sensation during sexual excitement and coitus is minimal, as is vaginal pain during the second stage of labor.

The vagina has the following functions:

- To serve as the passageway for sperm and for the fetus during birth
- To provide passage for the menstrual blood flow from the uterine endometrium to the outside of the body
- To protect against infection from pathogenic organisms

UTERUS

As the core of reproduction and hence continuation of the human race, the uterus, or womb, has been endowed with a mystical aura. Numerous customs, taboos, mores, and values have evolved about women and their reproductive function. Although scientific knowledge has replaced much of this folklore, remnants of old ideas and superstitions persist. To provide effective care, nurses must be cognizant of their own attitudes and beliefs, as well as those of their clients.

The **uterus** is a hollow, muscular, thick-walled organ shaped like an upside-down pear. It lies in the center of the pelvic cavity between the base of the bladder and the rectum and above the vagina (Figure 10–5 ◆). It is level with or slightly below the brim of the pelvis, with the external opening of the cervix (the external os) about the level of the ischial spines. The

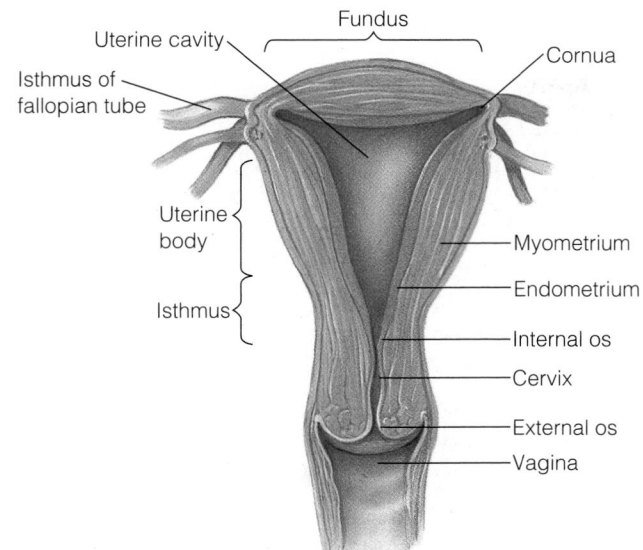

Uterine cavity
Fundus
Cornua
Isthmus of fallopian tube
Uterine body
Myometrium
Endometrium
Isthmus
Internal os
Cervix
External os
Vagina

Figure 10–5 ◆ Structures of the uterus.

mature organ in adult women weighs about 50 to 70 g and is 6 to 8 cm long (Cunningham et al., 2005; Monga & Sanborn, 2004).

Many uterine anomalies are thought to be congenital. A normal uterus requires two symmetric, parallel, equal-sized paramesonephric ducts to meet in the midline. Their ultimate midline fusion gives rise to the fallopian tubes, uterine fundus, cervix, and upper vagina. Anomalies represent the absence of either one or both of the ducts, degrees of failure to fuse, or canalization defects. Uterine malformations such as the uterus bicornuate ("two-horned") and uterus didelphys ("double uterus") are associated with habitual abortion. Because both the urinary and reproductive systems develop from the common urogenital fold in the embryo, anomalies in one system are frequently accompanied by anomalies in the other. Problems of infertility and premature labor and birth are common.

The body of the uterus can move freely forward or backward. Only the cervix is anchored laterally. Thus the position of the uterus can vary, depending on a woman's posture, number of children borne, bladder and rectal fullness, and even normal respiratory patterns. Generally, the uterus bends forward, forming a sharp angle with the vagina. There is a bend in the area of the isthmus of the uterus, and from there the cervix points downward. The uterus is said to be anteverted when it is in this position. The anteverted position is considered normal.

Four pairs of ligaments (i.e., the cardinal, uterosacral, round, and broad) support the uterus. Single anterior and posterior ligaments also support the uterus.

The uterus is divided into two major parts: an upper triangular portion called the **corpus,** or uterine body, and a lower cylindric portion called the cervix. The corpus comprises the upper two thirds of the uterus and is composed mainly of a smooth muscle layer (myometrium). The lower third is the cervix, or neck. The rounded uppermost portion of the corpus that extends above the points of attachment of the fallopian

tubes is called the **fundus.** The elongated portion of the uterus where the fallopian tubes enter is called the **cornua.**

The isthmus is that portion of the uterus between the internal cervical os and the endometrial cavity. The isthmus is about 6 mm above the uterine opening of the cervix (the internal os), and it is in this area that the uterine lining changes into the mucous membrane of the cervix; it joins the corpus to the cervix. The isthmus takes on importance in pregnancy because it becomes the lower uterine segment. With the cervix, it is a passive segment and not part of the contractile uterus. At birth this thin lower segment, situated behind the bladder, is the site for lower-segment cesarean births (see Chapter 27 ∞).

The blood and lymphatic supplies to the uterus are extensive (Figure 10–6 ◆). The uterus is innervated entirely by the autonomic nervous system. Efferent sympathetic motor nerves arise from the ganglia of the 5th to 10th thoracic vertebrae, come together over the sacrum, and reach the uterus through ganglia that lie near the base of the uterosacral ligaments. These sympathetic motor nerves are believed to cause vasoconstriction and muscular contraction. Even without an intact nerve supply, the uterus can contract adequately for birth. Thus, for example, hemiplegic women have adequate uterine contractions.

Pain of uterine contractions is carried to the central nervous system by the 11th and 12th thoracic nerve roots. Pain from the cervix and upper vagina passes through the ilioinguinal and pudendal nerves. The motor fibers to the uterus arise from the 7th and 8th thoracic vertebrae. Because the sensory and motor levels are separate, epidural anesthesia can be used during labor and birth.

The function of the uterus is to provide a safe environment for fetal development. The uterine lining is cyclically prepared by steroid hormones for implantation of the embryo, a process known as **nidation.** Once the embryo is implanted, the developing fetus is protected until it is expelled.

Both the body of the uterus and the cervix are changed permanently by pregnancy. The body never returns to its prepregnant size, and the external os changes from a circular opening of about 3 mm to a transverse slit with irregular edges.

Uterine Corpus

The uterine corpus is made up of three layers. The outermost layer is the *serosal layer,* or **perimetrium,** which is composed of peritoneum. The middle layer is the *muscular uterine layer,* or **myometrium.** This muscular uterine layer is continuous with the muscle layer of the fallopian tubes and with that of the vagina. This characteristic helps the organs present a unified reaction to various stimuli—ovulation, orgasm, or the deposit of sperm in the vagina. These muscle fibers also extend into the ovarian, round, and cardinal ligaments and minimally into the uterosacral ligaments, which helps explain the vague but disturbing pelvic "aches and pains" reported by many pregnant women.

The myometrium has three distinct layers of uterine (smooth) involuntary muscles (Figure 10–7 ◆). The outer layer, found mainly over the fundus, is made up of longitudinal muscles especially suited to expel the fetus during birth. The middle layer is thick and made up of interlacing muscle fibers in figure-eight

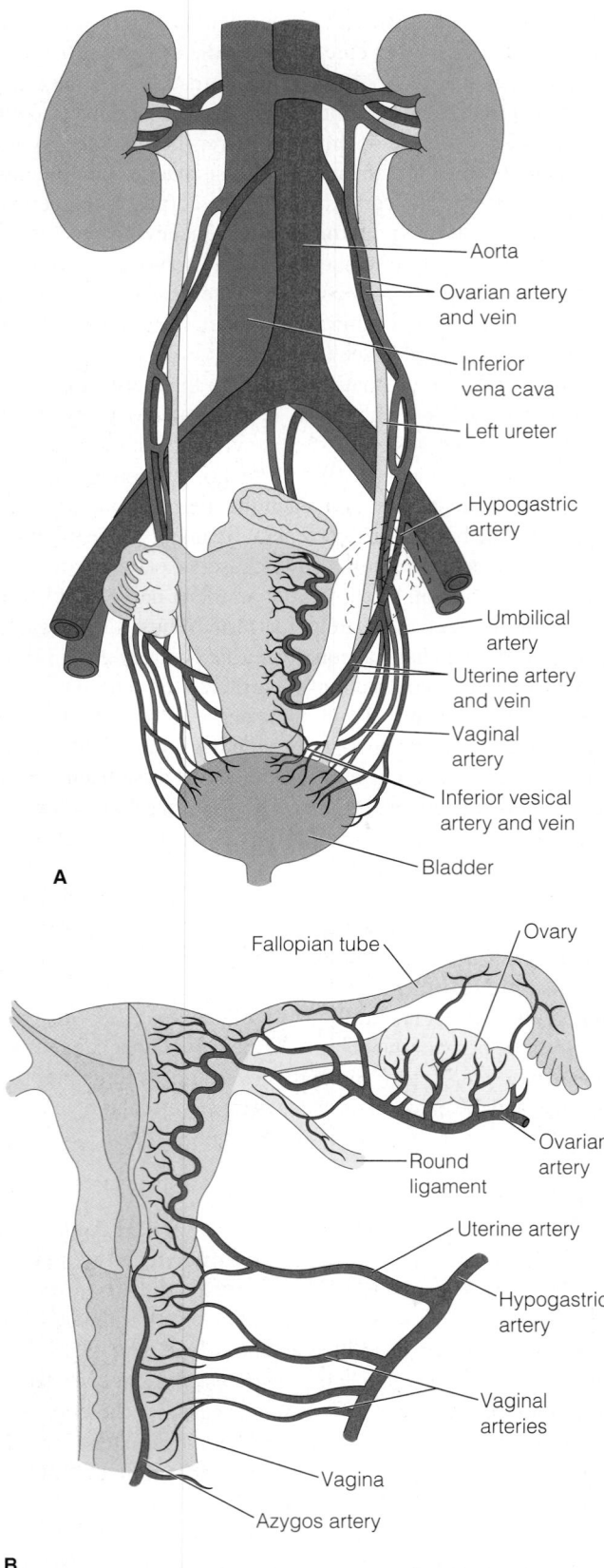

Figure 10–6 ◆ Blood supply to internal reproductive organs: *A,* Pelvic blood supply. *B,* Blood supply to the vagina, ovary, uterus, and fallopian tube.

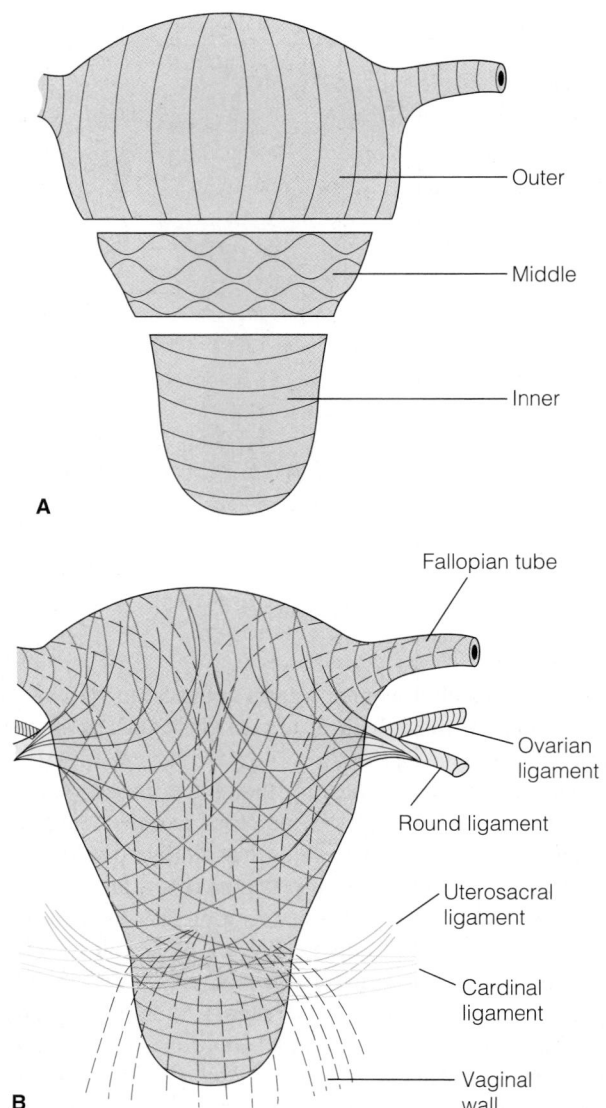

Figure 10–7 ◆ Uterine muscle layers: *A,* Muscle fiber placement. *B,* Interlacing of uterine muscle layers.

patterns. These muscle fibers surround large blood vessels, and their contraction produces a hemostatic action (a tourniquet-like action on blood vessels to stop bleeding after birth). The inner muscle layer is made up of circular fibers, which form sphincters at the fallopian tube attachment sites and at the internal os. The internal os sphincter inhibits the expulsion of the uterine contents during pregnancy but stretches in labor as cervical dilatation occurs. An incompetent cervical os can be caused by a torn, weak, or absent sphincter at the internal os. The sphincters at the fallopian tubes prevent menstrual blood from flowing backward into the fallopian tubes from the uterus.

Although each layer of muscle has been discussed as having a unique function, it must be remembered that the uterine musculature works as a whole. The uterine contractions of labor are responsible for the dilatation of the cervix and provide the major force for the passage of the fetus through the pelvic and vaginal canal at birth.

The innermost layer of the uterine corpus is the *mucosal layer,* or **endometrium,** which is composed of a single layer of columnar epithelium, glands, and stroma. From menarche to menopause, the endometrium undergoes monthly renewal and degeneration in the absence of pregnancy. As it responds to a governing hormonal cycle and prostaglandin influence as well, the endometrium varies in thickness from 0.5 to 5 mm.

The glands of the endometrium produce a thin, watery, alkaline secretion that keeps the uterine cavity moist. This endometrial milk not only helps sperm travel to the fallopian tubes but also nourishes the developing embryo before it implants in the endometrium (see Chapter 11 ∞).

The blood supply to the endometrium is unique. In the myometrium, the radial arteries branch off from the arcuate arteries at right angles. Once inside the endometrium, they become the basal arteries supplying the zona basalis (a layer of the endometrium) and ultimately become the coiled arteries supplying the zona functionalis (also part of the endometrium). The straighter basal arteries are smaller than the coiled arteries and are not sensitive to cyclic hormonal control. Hence the zona basalis portion remains intact and is the site of new endometrial tissue generation. The coiled arteries are extremely sensitive to cyclic hormonal control. Their response is alternate relaxation and constriction during the ischemic, or terminal, phase of the menstrual cycle. This response allows for part of the endometrial tissue to remain intact while other endometrial tissue is shed during menstruation.

When pregnancy occurs and the endometrium is not shed, the reticular stromal cells surrounding the endometrial glands become the decidual cells of pregnancy. The stromal cells are highly vascular, channeling a rich blood supply to the endometrial surface.

The Cervix

The narrow neck of the uterus is the **cervix.** It meets the body of the uterus at the internal os and descends about 2.5 cm to connect with the vagina at the external os (see Figure 10–5). Thus it provides a protective portal for the body of the uterus. The cervix is divided by its line of attachment into the vaginal and supravaginal areas. The vaginal cervix projects into the vagina at an angle from 45 to 90 degrees. The *supravaginal* cervix is surrounded by the attachments that give the uterus its main support: the uterosacral ligaments, the transverse ligaments of the cervix (Mackenrodt's ligaments), and the pubocervical ligaments.

The vaginal cervix appears pink and ends at the external os. The cervical canal appears rosy red and is lined with columnar ciliated epithelium, which contains mucus-secreting glands. Most cervical cancer begins at this *squamocolumnar junction.* The specific location of the junction varies with age and number of pregnancies. Figure 10–8 ◆ shows this junction at various stages of a woman's life.

Elasticity is the chief characteristic of the cervix. Its ability to stretch is due to the high fibrous and collagenous content of the supportive tissues and also to the vast number of folds in the cervical lining.

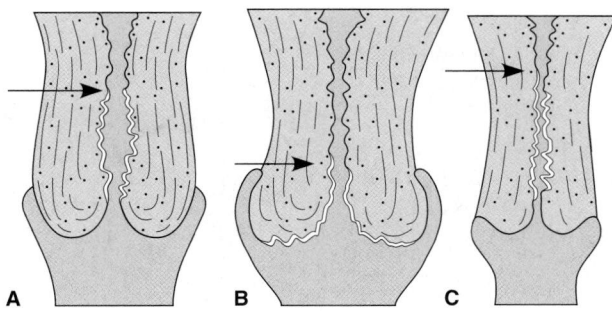

Figure 10–8 ◆ Changes in squamocolumnar junction (arrows) at various stages of life: *A,* Childhood. *B,* Reproductive years. *C,* Postmenopausal years.

The cervical mucosa has three functions:

- To provide lubrication for the vaginal canal
- To act as a bacteriostatic agent
- To provide an alkaline environment to shelter deposited sperm from the acidic vagina

At ovulation, cervical mucus is clearer, thinner, and more alkaline than at other times.

UTERINE LIGAMENTS

The uterine ligaments support and stabilize the various reproductive organs. The ligaments shown in Figure 10–9 ◆ are described in this section.

- The **broad ligament** keeps the uterus centrally placed and provides stability within the pelvic cavity. It is a double layer that is continuous with the abdominal peritoneum. The broad ligament covers the uterus anteriorly and posteriorly and extends outward from the uterus to enfold and stabilize the fallopian tubes. The round and ovarian ligaments are at the upper border of the broad ligament. At its lower border, the broad ligament forms the cardinal ligaments. Between the folds of the broad ligament are connective tissue, involuntary muscle, blood and lymph vessels, and nerves.

- The **round ligaments** keep the uterus in place. The round ligaments arise from the sides of the uterus near the fallopian tube insertions. They extend outward between the folds of the broad ligament, passing through the inguinal ring and canals and eventually fusing with the connective tissue of the labia majora. The round ligaments are made up of longitudinal muscle and enlarge during pregnancy. During labor the round ligaments steady the uterus, pulling downward and forward, so that the presenting part of the fetus is forced into the cervix.

- The **ovarian ligaments** anchor the lower pole of the ovary to the cornua of the uterus. They are composed of muscle fibers, which allow the ligaments to contract. This contractile ability influences the position of the ovary to some extent, thus helping the fimbriae of the fallopian tubes to "catch" the ovum as it is released each month.

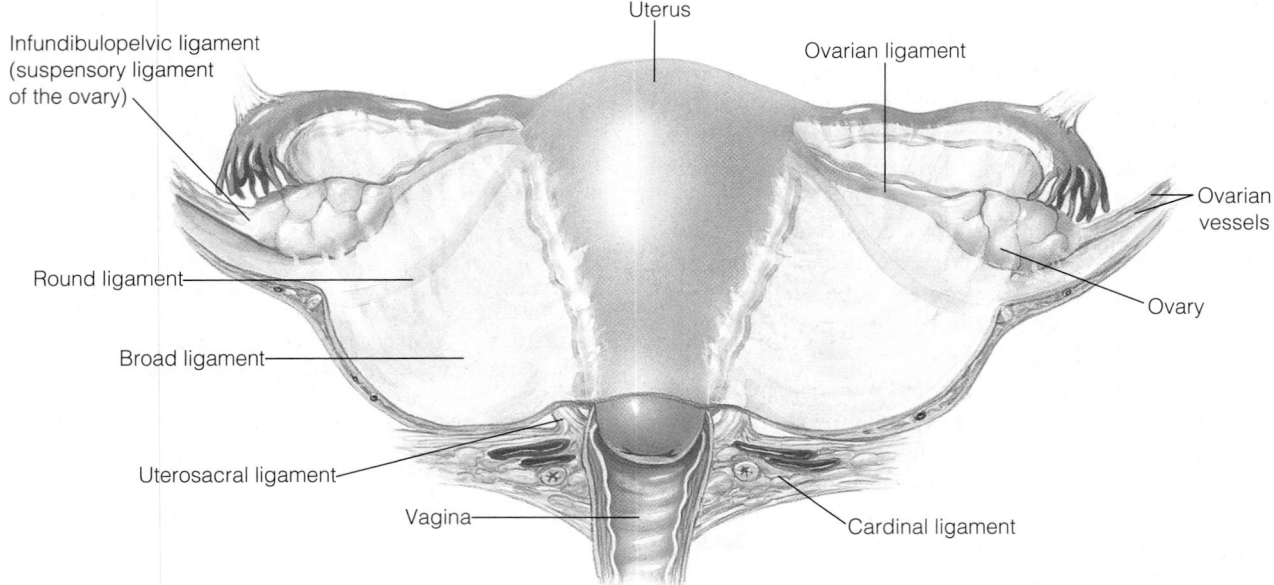

Figure 10–9 ◆ Uterine ligaments.

- The **cardinal ligaments** are the chief uterine supports, suspending the uterus from the side walls of the true pelvis. These ligaments, also known as Mackenrodt's ligaments or transverse cervical ligaments, arise from the sides of the pelvic walls and attach to the cervix in the upper vagina. These ligaments prevent uterine prolapse and also support the upper vagina.

- The **infundibulopelvic ligament** suspends and supports the ovaries. Arising from the outer third of the broad ligament, the infundibulopelvic ligament contains the ovarian vessels and nerves.

- The **uterosacral ligaments** provide support for the uterus and cervix at the level of the ischial spines. Arising on each side of the pelvis from the posterior wall of the uterus, the uterosacral ligaments sweep back around the rectum and insert on the sides of the first and second sacral vertebrae. The uterosacral ligaments contain smooth muscle fibers, connective tissue, blood and lymph vessels, and nerves. Providing support for the uterus and cervix at the level of the ischial spines, they also contain sensory nerve fibers that contribute to dysmenorrhea (painful menstruation; see Chapter 4 ∞).

FALLOPIAN TUBES

The two **fallopian tubes,** also known as *oviducts* or *uterine tubes,* arise from each side of the uterus and reach almost to the side of the pelvis, where they turn toward the ovaries (Figure 10–10 ◆). Each tube is approximately 8 to 13.5 cm long. A short section of each fallopian tube is inside the uterus; its opening into the uterus is 1 mm in diameter. The fallopian tubes link the

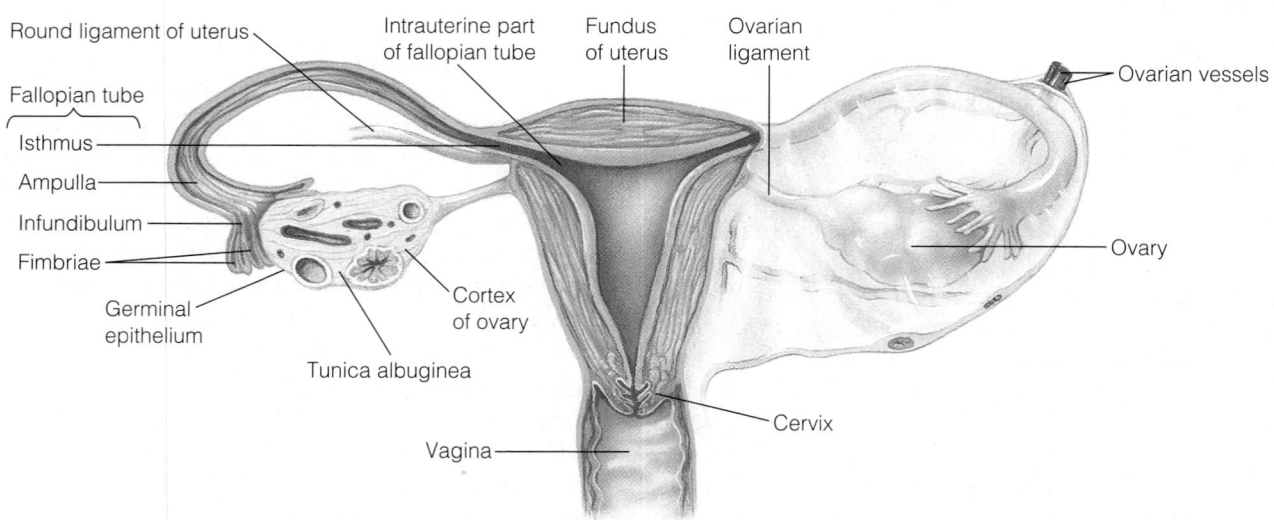

Figure 10–10 ◆ Fallopian tube and ovaries.

peritoneal cavity with the uterus and vagina. This linkage increases a woman's vulnerability to disease processes.

Each fallopian tube may be divided into three parts: the **isthmus,** the ampulla, and the infundibulum or fimbria. The isthmus is straight and narrow, with a thick muscular wall and an opening (lumen) 2 to 3 mm in diameter. It is the site of tubal ligation (a surgical procedure to prevent pregnancy; see Chapter 5 ∞).

Next to the isthmus is the curved **ampulla,** which comprises the outer two thirds of the tube. Fertilization of the secondary oocyte by a spermatozoon usually occurs here. The ampulla ends at the **fimbria,** which is a funnel-like enlargement with many moving fingerlike projections (fimbriae) reaching out to the ovary. The longest of these, the *fimbria ovarica,* is attached to the ovary to increase the chances of intercepting the ovum as it is released.

The wall of the fallopian tube is made up of four layers: peritoneal (serous), subserous (adventitial), muscular, and mucous tissues. The peritoneum covers the tubes. The subserous layer contains the blood and nerve supply, and the muscular layer is responsible for the peristaltic movement of the tube. The mucosal layer, immediately next to the muscular layer, is composed of ciliated and nonciliated cells, with the number of ciliated cells more abundant at the fimbria. Nonciliated cells secrete a protein-rich, serous fluid that nourishes the ovum. The constantly moving tubal cilia propel the ovum toward the uterus. Because the ovum is a large cell, this ciliary action is needed to assist the tube's muscular layer peristalsis. Any malformation or malfunction of the tubes could result in infertility, ectopic pregnancy, or even sterility. A well-functioning tubal transport system involves active fimbriae close to the ovary, peristalsis of the tube created by the muscular layer, ciliated currents beating toward the uterus, and the proximal contraction and distal relaxation of the tube caused by different types of prostaglandins.

A rich blood and lymph supply serves each fallopian tube. Thus the fallopian tubes have an unusual ability to recover from any inflammatory process.

The functions of the fallopian tubes are as follows:

- To provide transport for the ovum from the ovary to the uterus (transport through the fallopian tubes varies from 3 to 4 days)
- To provide a site for fertilization
- To serve as a warm, moist, nourishing environment for the ovum or zygote (a fertilized egg; see also Chapter 11 ∞)

OVARIES

The **ovaries** are two almond-shaped glandular structures just below the pelvic brim. One ovary is located on each side of the pelvic cavity. Their size varies among women and according to the stage of the menstrual cycle. Each ovary weighs 6 to 10 g and is 1.5 to 3 cm wide, 2 to 5 cm long, and 1 to 1.5 cm thick. The ovaries of girls are small, but they become larger after puberty and then decrease in size following menopause. They also change in appearance from smooth-surfaced, dull white organs to pitted gray organs as the woman ages. This pitting is caused by scarring due to ovulation.

It is rare for both ovaries to be at the same level in the pelvic cavity. The ovary is held in place by the ovarian, broad, and infundibulopelvic ligaments (see Figure 10–9), discussed earlier in the chapter. There is no peritoneal covering for the ovaries. Although this lack of covering assists the mature ovum to erupt, it also allows easier spread of malignant cells from cancer of the ovaries. A single layer of cuboidal epithelial cells, called the germinal epithelium, covers the ovaries. The ovaries are composed of three layers: the tunica albuginea, the cortex, and the medulla. The *tunica albuginea* is dense and dull white and serves as a protective layer. The *cortex* is the main functional part, containing ova, graafian follicles, corpora lutea, degenerated corpora lutea (corpora albicantia), and degenerated follicles. The *medulla* is completely surrounded by the cortex and contains the nerves and the blood and lymphatic vessels.

The ovaries are the primary source of two important hormones: the estrogens and progesterone. *Estrogens* are associated with characteristics contributing to femaleness, including breast alveolar lobule growth and duct development. The ovaries secrete large amounts of estrogens; the adrenal cortex (extraglandular sites) produces minute amounts of estrogens in nonpregnant women.

Progesterone is often called the *hormone of pregnancy* because its effects on the uterus allow pregnancy to be maintained. The placenta is the primary source of progesterone during pregnancy. This hormone also inhibits the action of prolactin in α-lactalbumin synthesis, thereby preventing lactation during pregnancy (Lawrence & Lawrence, 2004).

The interplay between the ovarian hormones and other hormones such as follicle-stimulating hormone (FSH) and luteinizing hormone (LH) is responsible for the cyclic changes that allow pregnancy to occur. The hormonal and physical changes that occur during the female reproductive cycle are discussed later in this chapter. Between the ages of 45 and 55 years, the woman's ovaries secrete decreasing amounts of estrogen. Eventually ovulatory activity ceases, and menopause occurs.

Bony Pelvis

The female bony pelvis has two unique functions:

- To support and protect the pelvic contents
- To form the relatively fixed axis of the birth passage

Because the pelvis is so important to childbearing, its structures should be understood clearly.

BONY STRUCTURE

The pelvis is made up of four bones: two innominate bones, the sacrum, and the coccyx (or tailbone) (Figure 10–11 ◆). The pelvis resembles a bowl or basin; its sides are the innominate bones, and its back is composed of the sacrum and coccyx. Lined with fibrocartilage and held tightly together by ligaments, the four bones join at the symphysis pubis, the two sacroiliac joints, and the sacrococcygeal joints.

The *innominate* bones, also known as the hip bones or os coxae, are made up of three separate bones: the ilium, the ischium, and the pubis. These bones fuse to form a circular cavity, the *acetabulum,* which articulates with the femur.

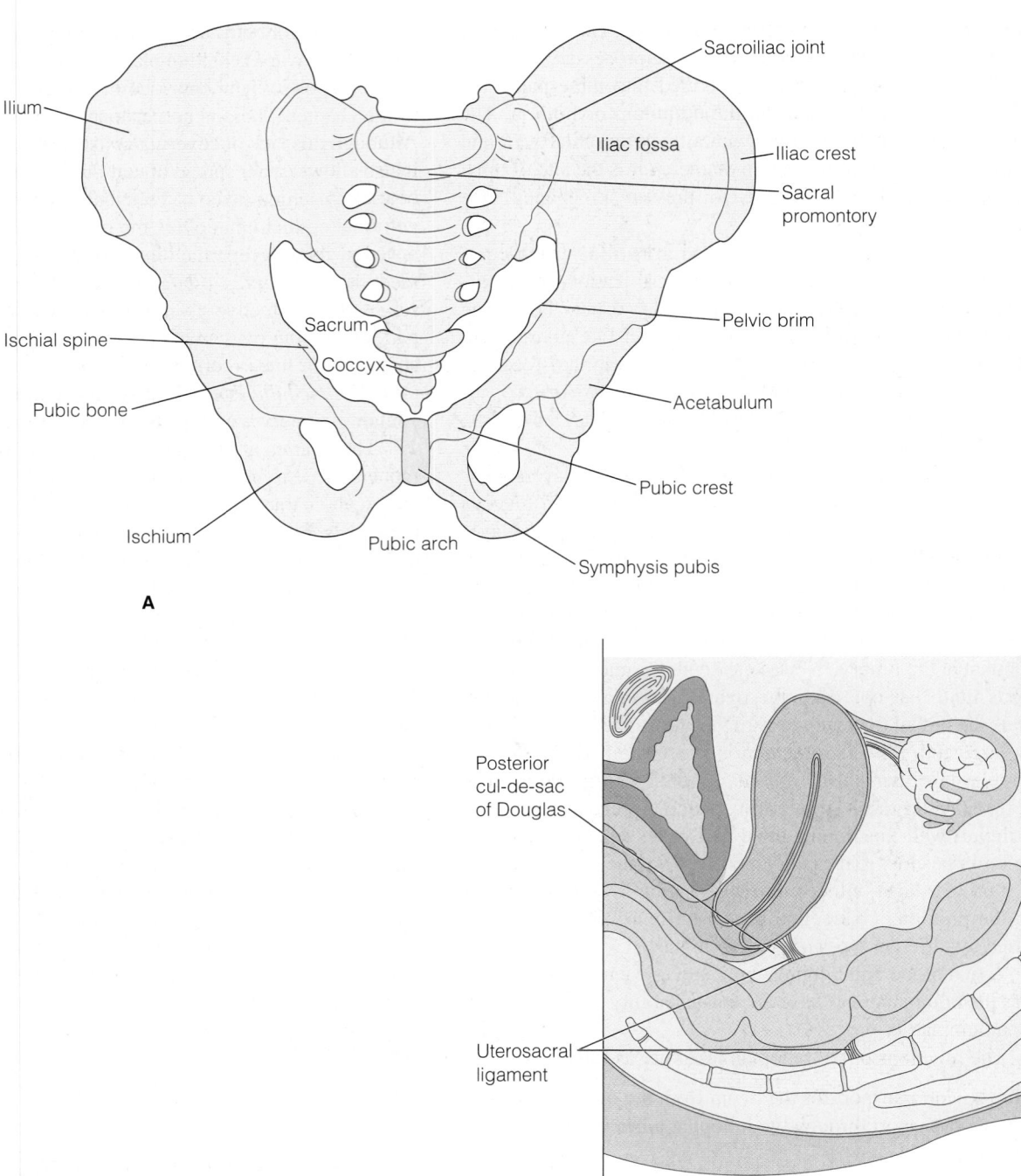

Figure 10–11 ◆ Pelvis: *A,* Pelvic bones. *B,* Midsagittal view in supine position with some ligaments.

The *ilium* is the broad, upper prominence of the hip. The *iliac crest* is the margin of the ilium. The ischial spines, the foremost projections nearest the groin, are the site of attachment for ligaments and muscles.

The *ischium,* the strongest bone, lies under the ilium and below the acetabulum. The L-shaped ischium ends in a marked protuberance, the *ischial tuberosity,* on which the weight of a seated body rests. The **ischial spines** arise near the junction of the ilium and ischium and jut into the pelvic cavity. The shortest diameter of the pelvic cavity is located between the ischial spines. The ischial spines can serve as a reference point during labor to evaluate the descent of the fetal head into the birth canal. (See Chapter 22 ∞ and Figure 22–7).

The **pubis** forms the slightly bowed front portion of the innominate bone. Extending medially from the acetabulum to the midpoint of the bony pelvis, the two pubic bones meet to form a joint, the **symphysis pubis.** The triangular space below this junction is known as the pubic arch. The fetal head passes under this arch during birth. The symphysis pubis is formed by heavy fibrocartilage and the superior and inferior pubic ligaments. The mobility of the inferior ligament increases during the first pregnancy and to a greater extent in subsequent pregnancies.

The sacroiliac joints also have a degree of mobility that increases near the end of pregnancy and results in an upward gliding movement. The pelvic outlet may be increased by 1.5 to 2 cm in the squatting, sitting, and dorsal lithotomy positions. The relaxation of the joints is induced by the hormones of pregnancy.

The *sacrum* is a wedge-shaped bone formed by the fusion of five vertebrae. On the anterior upper portion of the sacrum is a projection into the pelvic cavity known as the **sacral promontory.** This projection is another obstetric guide in determining pelvic measurements. (For discussion of pelvic measurements, see Chapter 15 ∞).

The small triangular bone last on the vertebral column is the coccyx. It articulates with the sacrum at the sacrococcygeal joint. The coccyx usually moves backward during labor to provide more room for the fetus.

PELVIC FLOOR

The muscular *pelvic floor* of the bony pelvis is designed to overcome the force of gravity exerted on the pelvic organs. It acts as a supporting structure to the irregularly shaped pelvic outlet, thereby providing stability and support for surrounding structures.

Deep fascia and the levator ani and coccygeal muscles form the part of the pelvic floor known as the **pelvic diaphragm.** The components of the pelvic diaphragm function as a whole, yet they are able to move over one another. This feature provides an exceptional capacity for dilatation during birth and return to prepregnancy condition following birth. Above the pelvic diaphragm is the **pelvic cavity;** below and behind it is the perineum. The sacrum is located posteriorly.

The levator ani muscle makes up the major portion of the pelvic diaphragm. It consists of four muscles: the iliococcygeus, pubococcygeus, puborectalis, and pubovaginalis muscles. The iliococcygeal muscle, a thin muscular sheet underlying the sacrospinous ligament, helps the levator ani support the pelvic

organs. Muscles of the pelvic floor are shown in Figure 10–12 ◆ and discussed in Table 10–1.

Endopelvic fascia covers the pelvic diaphragm and allows the pelvic diaphragm components to function as a whole, yet allows them to move over one another. This feature provides the pelvic diaphragm with the exceptional capacity for dilatation during birth and facilitates the return to prepregnant condition following birth.

The urogenital triangle (diaphragm) is external to the pelvic diaphragm, in the triangular area between the ischial tuberosities and the hollow of the pubic arch. The most important muscles in this region are the deep transverse perineal muscles, which are flat bands of muscle arising from the ischiopubic rami and intertwining in the midline to form a seam, or raphe. These muscles are modified to encircle both the urinary meatus and the vaginal orifice, forming the urethral and vaginal sphincters.

PELVIC DIVISION

The pelvic cavity is divided into the false pelvis and the true pelvis (Figure 10–13 ◆). The **false pelvis** is the portion above the pelvic brim, or linea terminalis, bounded by the lumbar vertebrae posteriorly, the iliac fossae laterally, and the lower abdominal wall anteriorly. Its primary function is to support the weight of the enlarged pregnant uterus and direct the presenting fetal part into the true pelvis below.

The **true pelvis** is the portion that lies below the pelvic brim. The bony circumference of the true pelvis is made up of the sacrum, coccyx, and innominate bones and represents the bony limits of the birth canal. It measures about 5 cm at its anterior wall at the symphysis pubis and about 10 cm at its posterior wall. When a woman is standing upright, the upper portion

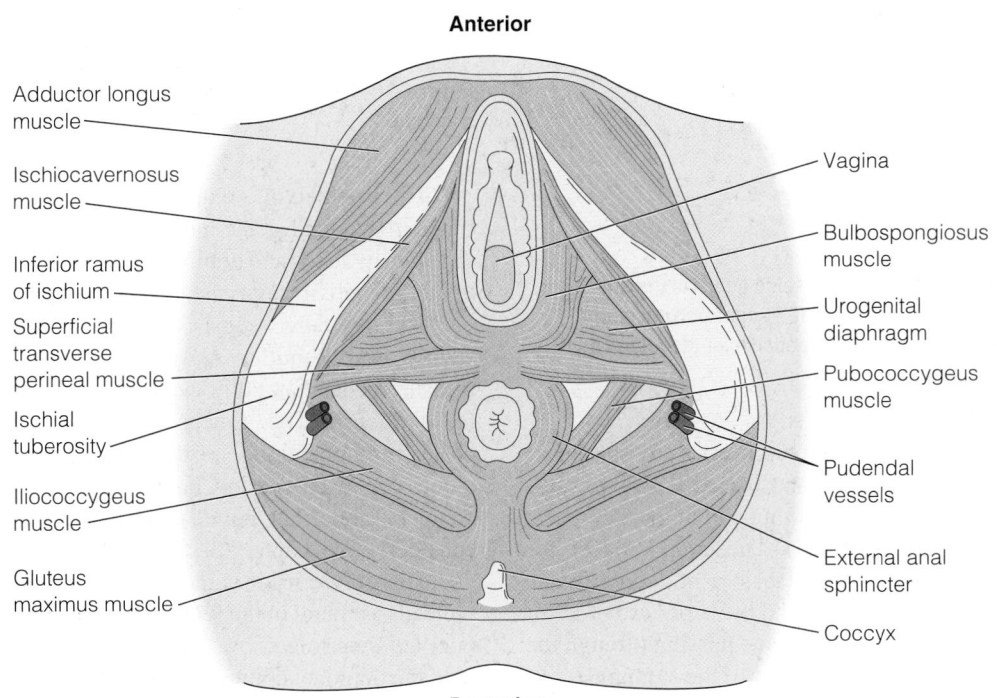

Figure 10–12 ◆ Muscles of the pelvic floor. (The puborectalis, pubovaginalis, and coccygeal muscles cannot be seen from this view.)

Table 10–1		MUSCLES OF THE PELVIC FLOOR		
Muscle	**Origin**	**Insertion**	**Innervation**	**Action**
Levator ani	Pubis, lateral pelvic wall, and ischial spine	Blends with organs in pelvic cavity	Inferior rectal, second and third sacral nerves, plus anterior rami of third and fourth sacral nerves	Supports pelvic viscera; helps form pelvic diaphragm
Iliococcygeus	Pelvic surface of ischial spine and pelvic fascia	Central point of perineum, coccygeal raphe, and coccyx		Assists in supporting abdominal and pelvic viscera
Pubococcygeus	Pubis and pelvic fascia	Coccyx		
Puborectalis	Pubis	Blends with rectum; meets similar fibers from opposite side		Forms sling for rectum, just posterior to it; raises anus
Pubovaginalis	Pubis	Blends into vagina		Supports vagina
Coccygeus	Ischial spine and sacrospinous ligament	Lateral border of lower sacrum and upper coccyx	Third and fourth sacral nerves	Supports pelvic viscera; helps form pelvic diaphragm; flexes and abducts coccyx

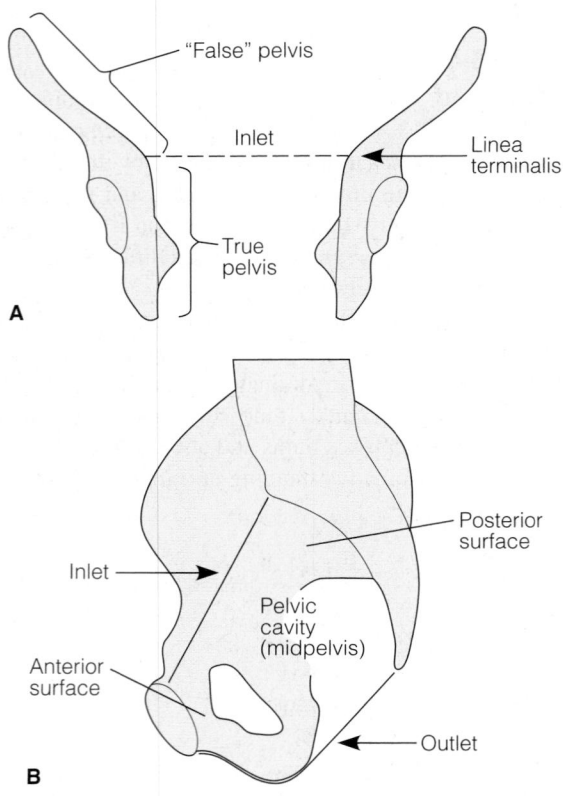

Figure 10–13 ◆ Female pelvis: *A,* The false pelvis is the shallow cavity above the inlet; the true pelvis is the deeper portion of the cavity below the inlet. *B,* The true pelvis consists of the inlet, cavity (midpelvis), and outlet.

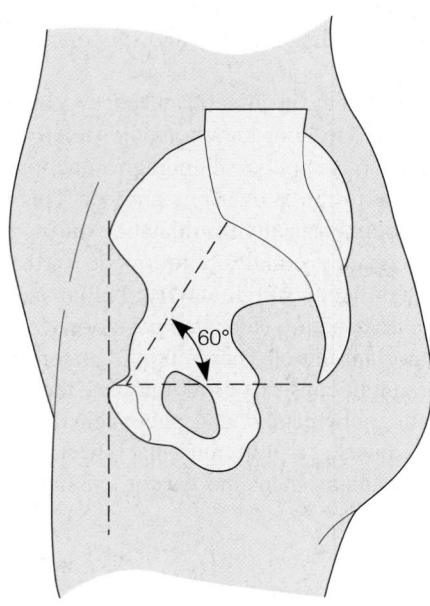

Figure 10–14 ◆ Pelvic angle of inclination while the woman is standing.

of the pelvic cavity or canal is directed downward and backward; its lower portion, downward and forward. This forms a curved canal through which the presenting part of the baby must pass during birth (see Figure 10–13). The inclination of the pelvis is the angle formed by two planes: a horizontal plane passing through the tip of the coccyx and the superior border of the symphysis pubis, and an inclined plane passing through the sacral promontory and the superior border of the symphysis pubis. This pelvic angle of inclination usually measures 50 to 60 degrees (Figure 10–14 ◆).

The true pelvis is extremely important in childbearing because its size and shape must be adequate for normal fetal passage during labor and at birth. The relationship of the fetal head to the true pelvic cavity is of critical importance.

The true pelvis consists of three parts: the inlet, the pelvic cavity, and the outlet. Associated with each part are distinct measurements that aid in evaluating the adequacy of the pelvis for childbirth. The dimensions of the true pelvis and their obstetric implications are described here. Measurement techniques are discussed in Chapter 15. ∞ The effects of inadequate or abnormal pelvic diameters on labor and birth are considered in Chapter 23. ∞

The **pelvic inlet** is the upper border of the true pelvis and typically is round in the female. The size and shape of the pelvic inlet are determined by assessing three anteroposterior diameters: the diagonal conjugate, obstetric conjugate, and conjugate vera. (For an in-depth discussion, see Chapter 15 ∞). The **diagonal conjugate** extends from the subpubic angle to the middle of the sacral promontory and is typically 12.5 cm. The diagonal conjugate can be measured manually during a pelvic examination. The **obstetric conjugate** extends from the middle of the sacral promontory to an area approximately 1 cm below the pubic crest. Its length is estimated by subtracting 1.5 cm from the diagonal conjugate. The fetus passes through the obstetric conjugate, and the size of this diameter determines whether the fetus can move down into the birth canal in order for engagement to occur. The true (anatomic) conjugate, or **conjugate vera,** extends from the middle of the sacral promontory to the middle of the pubic crest (superior surface of the symphysis). One additional measurement, the transverse diameter, helps determine the shape of the inlet. The **transverse diameter** is the largest diameter of the inlet and is measured by using the linea terminalis as the point of reference.

The *pelvic cavity* (canal) is a curved canal with a longer posterior than anterior wall. A change in the lumbar curve can increase or decrease the pelvic inclination and can influence the progress of labor, because the fetus has to adjust itself to this curved path as well as to the different diameters of the true pelvis.

The **pelvic outlet** is at the lower border of the true pelvis. The size of the pelvic outlet can be determined by assessing the *transverse diameter.* The anteroposterior diameter of the pelvic outlet increases during birth as the presenting part pushes the coccyx posteriorly at the mobile sacrococcygeal joint. Decreased mobility, a large fetal head, and/or a forceful birth can cause the coccyx to break. As the infant's head emerges, the long diameter of the head (occipital frontal) parallels the long diameter of the outlet (anteroposterior).

The transverse diameter *(bi-ischial or intertuberous)* extends from the inner surface of one ischial tuberosity to the other. It is the shortest diameter of the pelvic outlet and becomes even shorter if the woman has a narrowed pubic arch. The pubic arch has great importance because the baby must pass under it during birth. If it is narrow, the baby's head may be pushed backward toward the coccyx, making the extension of the head difficult. This situation, known as *outlet dystocia,* may require the use of forceps or a cesarean birth. The shoulders of a large baby may also get stuck under the pubic arch, making birth more difficult. The clinical assessment of each of these obstetric diameters is discussed further in Chapter 15. ∞

PELVIC TYPES

The Caldwell-Moloy classification of pelves (Figure 10–15 ◆) is widely used to differentiate types of bony pelves (Caldwell & Moloy, 1933). *Gynecoid, android, anthropoid,* and *platypelloid* are the four basic types. However, variations in the female pelvis are so great that classic types are not usual.

Each type of pelvis has a characteristic shape, and each shape has implications for labor and birth. The types are described briefly here, and their implications for labor and birth are discussed in detail in Chapter 22. ∞

Gynecoid Pelvis

The most common female pelvis is the gynecoid type. The inlet is rounded, with the anteroposterior diameter a little shorter than the transverse diameter. All of the inlet diameters are at least adequate. The posterior segment is broad, deep, and roomy, and the anterior segment is well rounded. The gynecoid midpelvis has nonprominent ischial spines, straight and parallel side walls, and a wide, deep sacral curve. The sacrum is short and slopes backward. All of the midpelvic diameters are at least adequate. The gynecoid pelvic outlet has a wide and round pubic arch; the inferior pubic rami are short and concave. The anteroposterior diameter is long; the transverse diameter, adequate. The capacity of the outlet is adequate. The bones are of medium structure and weight. Approximately 50% of female pelves are classified as gynecoid.

Android Pelvis

The normal male pelvis is the android type; however, it occasionally is seen in females. The inlet is heart shaped. The anteroposterior and transverse diameters are adequate for birth, but the posterior sagittal diameter is too short, and the anterior sagittal diameter is long. The posterior segment is shallow because the sacral promontory is indented, resulting in a reduced capacity. The anterior segment is narrow, and the forepelvis is sharply angled. The android midpelvis has prominent ischial spines, convergent sidewalls, and a long, heavy sacrum inclining forward. All of the midpelvic diameters are reduced. The distance from the linea terminalis to the ischial tuberosities is long, yet the overall capacity of the midpelvis is reduced. The android outlet has a narrow, sharp, and deep pubic arch; the inferior pubic rami are straight and long. The anteroposterior diameter is short, and the transverse diameter is narrow. The capacity of the outlet is reduced. The bones are of medium to heavy structure and weight.

Approximately 20% of female pelves are classified as android. The influence of an android pelvis on labor is not favorable. Descent into the pelvis is slow. The fetal head usually engages in the transverse or occipital posterior diameter in asynclitism (oblique presentation) with extreme molding. Arrest of labor is frequent, requiring difficult forceps manipulation (rotation and extraction), and the deep, narrow pubic arch may lead to extensive perineal lacerations. Cesarean birth may be required.

Anthropoid Pelvis

The inlet of an anthropoid pelvis is oval, with a long anteroposterior diameter and an adequate but rather short transverse diameter. Both the posterior and anterior segments are deep; the posterior sagittal diameter is extremely long, as is the anterior sagittal diameter. The anthropoid midpelvis has variable ischial spines, straight side walls, and a narrow and long sacrum that inclines backward. The midpelvic diameters are at least adequate, making its capacity adequate. The anthropoid outlet has a normal or moderately narrow pubic arch; the interior pubic rami are long and narrow. The outlet capacity is adequate, and the bones are of medium weight and structure. Approximately 25% of female pelves are classified as anthropoid.

Platypelloid Pelvis

The platypelloid type refers to the flat female pelvis. The inlet is a distinctly transverse oval, with a short anteroposterior and

	Gynecoid	Android	Anthropoid	Platypelloid

Shape

Inlet

Midpelvis

Outlet

Figure 10–15 ◆ Comparison of Caldwell-Moloy pelvic types.

extremely short transverse diameter. The posterior sagittal and anterior sagittal diameters are short. Both the anterior and posterior segments are shallow. The platypelloid midpelvis has variable ischial spines, parallel side walls, and a wide sacrum with a deep curve inward. Only the transverse diameter is adequate; thus the midpelvic capacity is reduced. The platypelloid outlet has an extremely wide pubic arch; the inferior pubic rami are straight and short. The transverse diameter is wide, but the anteroposterior diameter is short. The outlet capacity may be inadequate. The platypelloid bones are similar to the gynecoid type. Only 5% of female pelves are classified as platypelloid.

Breasts

The **breasts,** or *mammary glands,* considered accessories of the reproductive system, are specialized sebaceous glands. They are conical and symmetrically placed on the sides of the chest. The greater pectoral and anterior serratus muscles underlie each breast. Suspending the breasts are fibrous tissues, called *Cooper's ligaments,* which extend from the deep fascia in the chest outward to just under the skin covering the breast. The left breast is frequently larger than the right. In different racial groups breasts develop at slightly different levels in the pectoral region of the chest.

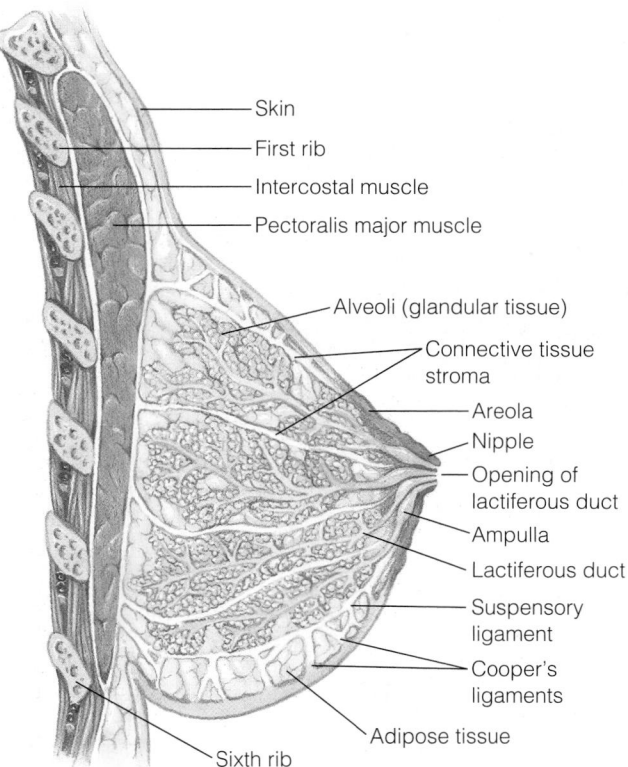

Figure 10–16 ◆ Anatomy of the breast.

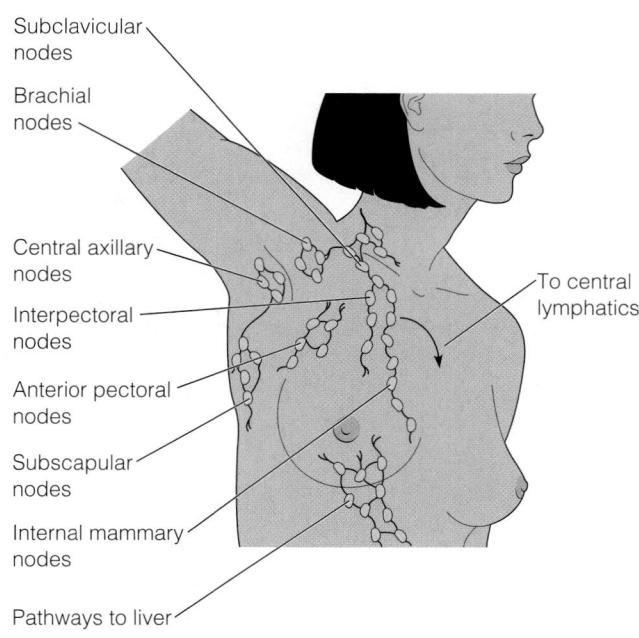

Figure 10–17 ◆ Lymphatic vessels draining the breast.

The arterial, venous, and lymphatic systems communicate medially with the internal mammary vessels and laterally with the axillary vessels. Therefore, in cancer of the breast, metastasis follows the vascular supply both medially and laterally (Figure 10–17 ◆).

The biologic function of the breasts is to provide nourishment and protective maternal antibodies to infants through the lactation process. They are also a source of pleasurable sexual sensation.

FEMALE REPRODUCTIVE CYCLE

The **female reproductive cycle (FRC)** is composed of the ovarian cycle, during which ovulation occurs, and the menstrual cycle, during which menstruation occurs. These two cycles take place simultaneously (Figure 10–18 ◆).

Effects of Female Hormones

After menarche, a woman undergoes a cyclic pattern of ovulation and menstruation, which is disrupted only by pregnancy, for a period of 30 to 40 years. This cycle is an orderly process under neurohormonal control. Each month, one oocyte matures, ruptures from the ovary, and enters the fallopian tube. The ovary, vagina, uterus, and fallopian tubes are major target organs for female hormones.

The ovaries produce mature gametes and secrete hormones. Ovarian hormones include the estrogens, progesterone, and testosterone. The ovary is sensitive to FSH and LH. The uterus is sensitive to estrogen and progesterone. The relative proportions of these hormones control the events of both ovarian and menstrual cycles.

ESTROGENS

Estrogens are hormones that are associated with those characteristics contributing to "femaleness." The major estrogenic

In the center of each mature breast is the **nipple,** a protrusion about 0.5 to 1.3 cm in diameter. The nipple is composed mainly of erectile tissue, which becomes more rigid and prominent during the menstrual cycle, sexual excitement, pregnancy, and lactation. The nipple is surrounded by the heavily pigmented **areola,** 2.5 to 10 cm in diameter. Both the nipple and areola are roughened by small papillae called *tubercles of Montgomery.* As an infant suckles, these tubercles secrete a fatty substance that helps lubricate and protect the breasts.

The breasts are composed of glandular, fibrous, and adipose tissue. The glandular tissue consists of acini, or alveoli (Figure 10–16 ◆), which are arranged in a series of 15 to 24 lobes separated from each other by adipose and fibrous tissue.

Each lobe is made up of several lobules, which are made up of many grapelike clusters of alveoli around tiny ducts. They are lined with a single layer of cuboidal epithelium, which secretes the various components of milk. The ducts from several lobules combine to form larger lactiferous ducts and then join to form the lactiferous sinuses, which serve as reservoirs for milk collection and open on the surface of the nipple. The smooth muscle of the nipple causes erection of the nipple on contraction.

Cyclic hormonal control of the mature breast is complex. Essentially, estrogenic hormones stimulate the growth and development of the ductal epithelium. Progesterone, in association with estrogen, is responsible for the acinar and lobular development during the luteal phase of menstruation. Adrenal corticosteroids, prolactin, somatotropin (growth hormone), and thyroxine are also necessary for estrogen and progesterone to act.

Figure 10–18 ◆ Female reproductive cycle: Interrelationships of hormones, the four phases of the uterine cycle, and the two phases of the ovarian cycle.

effects are due primarily to three estrogens: estrone, β-estradiol, and estriol. β-estradiol is the major estrogen.

Estrogens control the development of the female secondary sex characteristics: breast development, growth of body hair, widening of the hips, and deposits of tissue (fat) in the buttocks and mons pubis. In addition, estrogens assist in the maturation of the ovarian follicles and cause the endometrial mucosa to proliferate following menstruation. The amount of estrogens is greatest during the proliferative (follicular or estrogenic) phase of the menstrual cycle. Estrogens also cause the uterus to increase in size and weight because of increased glycogen, amino acids, electrolytes, and water. Blood supply is expanded as well. Under the influence of estrogens, myometrial contractility increases in both the uterus and the fallopian tubes, and uterine sensitivity to oxytocin increases. Estrogens inhibit FSH production and stimulate LH production.

Estrogens have effects on many hormones and other carrier proteins, such as contributing to the increased amount of protein-bound iodine in pregnant women and women who use oral contraceptives containing estrogen. Estrogens may increase libidinal feelings in humans. They decrease the excitability of the hypothalamus, which may cause an increase in sexual desire.

PROGESTERONE

Progesterone is secreted by the corpus luteum and is found in greatest amounts during the secretory (luteal or progestational) phase of the menstrual cycle. It decreases uterine motility and contractility caused by estrogens, thereby preparing the uterus for implantation after the ovum is fertilized. The endometrial mucosa is in a ready state as a result of estrogenic influence. Progesterone causes the uterine endometrium to increase further its supply of glycogen, arterial blood, secretory glands, amino acids, and water. This hormone is often called the *hormone of pregnancy* because its effects on the uterus allow pregnancy to be maintained. Under the influence of progesterone, the vaginal epithelium proliferates, and the cervix secretes thick, viscous mucus. Breast glandular tissue increases in size and complexity. Progesterone also prepares the breasts for lactation.

The temperature rise of about 0.3C to 0.6C (0.5F to 1F) that accompanies ovulation and persists throughout the secretory phase of the menstrual cycle is due to progesterone.

PROSTAGLANDINS

Prostaglandins (PGs) are oxygenated fatty acids that are produced by the cells of the endometrium and are also classified as hormones. Prostaglandins have varied actions in the body. The two primary types of prostaglandins are group E and F. Generally, PGE relaxes smooth muscles and is a potent vasodilator; PGF is a potent vasoconstrictor and increases the contractility of muscles and arteries. Although their primary actions seem antagonistic, their basic regulatory functions in cells are achieved through an intricate pattern of reciprocal events.

Prostaglandin production increases during follicular maturation, is dependent on gonadotropins, and seems to be critical to follicular rupture (Cunningham et al., 2005). Extrusion of the ovum, resulting from follicular swelling and increased contractility of the smooth muscle in the theca layer of the mature follicle, is thought to be caused by $PGF_{2\alpha}$. Significant amounts of PGs are found in and around the follicle at the time of ovulation.

Although the exact mechanism by which the corpus luteum degenerates in the absence of pregnancy remains obscure, $PGF_{2\alpha}$ is thought to induce progesterone withdrawal, the lowest point of which coincides with the onset of early menses.

During the late secretory phase, the level of $PGF_{2\alpha}$ is higher than that of PGE (Blackburn, 2003). This event increases vasoconstriction and contractility of the myometrium, which contributes to the ischemia preceding menstruation. A high concentration of PGs may also account for the vasoconstriction of the endometrium venous lacunae, allowing for platelet aggregation at vascular rupture points, thereby preventing a rapid blood loss during menstruation. The menstrual flow's high concentration of PGs may also facilitate the process of tissue digestion, which allows for an orderly shedding of the endometrium during menstruation.

Neurohormonal Basis of the Female Reproductive Cycle

The female reproductive cycle is controlled by complex interactions between the nervous and endocrine systems and their target tissues. These interactions involve the hypothalamus, anterior pituitary, and ovaries.

The hypothalamus secretes gonadotropin-releasing hormone (GnRH) to the pituitary gland in response to signals received from the central nervous system. This releasing hormone is often called follicle-stimulating hormone-releasing hormone (FSHRH) or luteinizing hormone-releasing hormone (LHRH) (Blackburn, 2003). This is because, in response to GnRH, the anterior pituitary secretes the gonadotropic hormones *FSH* and *LH*.

FSH is primarily responsible for the maturation of the ovarian follicle. As the follicle matures, it secretes increasing amounts of estrogen, which enhance the development of the follicle (Cunningham et al., 2005). (This estrogen also is responsible for the rebuilding/proliferation phase of the endometrium after it is shed during menstruation.)

Final maturation of the follicle will not come about without the action of LH. The anterior pituitary's production of LH increases sixfold to tenfold as the follicle matures. The peak production of LH can precede ovulation by as much as 12 hours (Cunningham et al., 2005).

LH is also responsible for "luteinizing" the increase in production of progesterone by the granulosa cells of the follicle. As a result, estrogen production declines and progesterone secretion continues. Thus, estrogen levels fall a day before ovulation; tiny amounts of progesterone are in evidence. **Ovulation** takes place following the very rapid growth of the follicle—as the sustained high level of estrogen diminishes and progesterone secretion begins.

The ruptured follicle undergoes rapid change, complete luteinization is accomplished, and the mass of cells becomes the **corpus luteum.** The lutein cells secrete large amounts of progesterone with smaller amounts of estrogen. (Concurrently, the excessive amounts of progesterone are responsible for the secretory phase of the uterine cycle.) On day 7 or 8 following ovulation, the corpus luteum begins to involute, losing its secretory function. The production of both progesterone and estrogen is severely diminished. The anterior pituitary responds with increasingly large amounts of FSH; a few days later, LH production begins. New follicles become responsive to another ovarian cycle and begin maturing.

OVARIAN CYCLE

The ovarian cycle has two phases: the *follicular phase* (days 1 to 14) and the *luteal phase* (days 15 to 28 in a 28-day cycle). Figure 10–19 ◆ depicts the changes that the follicle undergoes

MediaLink

Activity: Ovulation

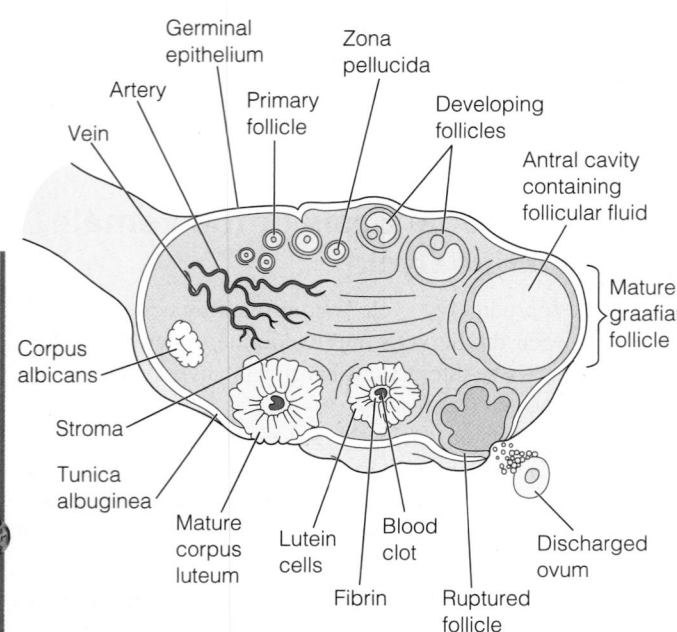

Figure 10–19 ◆ Various stages of development of the ovarian follicles.

during the ovarian cycle. In women whose menstrual cycles vary, usually it is only the length of the follicular phase that varies, because the luteal phase is of fixed length. During the follicular phase, the immature follicle matures as a result of FSH. Within the follicle, the oocyte grows.

A mature **graafian follicle** appears about the 14th day under dual control of FSH and LH. It is a large structure, measuring about 5 to 10 mm, and produces increasing amounts of estrogen. In the mature graafian follicle, the cells surrounding the fluid-filled antral cavity are called granulosa cells. The mass of granulosa cells surrounding the oocyte and follicular fluid is called the *cumulus oophorus*. The stromal elements of the ovary are condensed around the follicle in two layers: the theca interna and the theca externa. The theca interna cells resemble the luteal cells of the corpus luteum. In the fully mature graafian follicle, the zona pellucida (oolemma), a thick, elastic capsule, develops around the oocyte. Just before ovulation, the mature oocyte completes its first meiotic division (see Chapter 11 ∞ for a description of meiosis). As a result of this division, two cells are formed: a small cell called a *polar body,* and a larger cell called the *secondary oocyte.*

As the graafian follicle matures and enlarges, its walls thin and it travels outward to the surface of the ovary. This surface has a blisterlike protrusion 10 to 15 mm in diameter, where the secondary oocyte, polar body, and follicular fluid are pushed out. The ovum is discharged near the fimbria of the fallopian tube and is pulled into the tube to begin its journey toward the uterus. (See Figure 11–5.)

In some women, ovulation is accompanied by midcycle pain, known as *mittelschmerz.* This pain may be caused by a thick tunica albuginea or by a local peritoneal reaction to the expelling of the follicular contents. Vaginal discharge may increase during ovulation, and a small amount of blood (midcycle spotting) may be discharged as well.

The body temperature increases about 0.3C to 0.6C (0.5F to 1F) 24 to 48 hours after the time of ovulation. It remains elevated until the day before menstruation begins. There may be an accompanying sharp basal body temperature drop just before the increase. These temperature changes are useful clinically to determine the approximate time ovulation occurs.

Generally the ovum takes several minutes to travel through the ruptured follicle to the fallopian tube opening. The contractions of the tube's smooth muscle and its ciliary action propel the ovum through the tube. The ovum remains in the ampulla, where it may be fertilized and cleavage can begin. The ovum is thought to be fertile for only 6 to 24 hours. It reaches the uterus 72 to 96 hours after its release from the ovary.

The luteal phase begins when the ovum leaves its follicle. Under the influence of LH, the corpus luteum develops from the ruptured follicle. Within 2 or 3 days the corpus luteum becomes yellowish and spherical and increases in vascularity. If the ovum is fertilized and implants in the endometrium, the fertilized egg begins to secrete **human chorionic gonadotropin (hCG),** which is needed to maintain the corpus luteum. The corpus luteum of pregnancy provides progesterone to maintain the pregnancy until the fourth month of pregnancy. If fertilization does not occur, within about a week after ovulation, the corpus luteum begins to degenerate, eventually becoming a connective tissue scar called the *corpus albicans.* With degeneration comes a decrease in estrogen and progesterone. This allows for an increase in LH and FSH, which triggers the hypothalamus.

Menstrual Cycle

Menstruation is cyclic uterine bleeding in response to cyclic hormonal changes. Menstruation occurs when the ovum is not fertilized and begins about 14 days after ovulation (in an ideal 28-day cycle), in the absence of pregnancy. The menstrual discharge, also referred to as the *menses* or *menstrual flow,* is composed of blood mixed with cervical and vaginal secretions, bacteria, mucus, leukocytes, and other cellular debris. The menstrual discharge is dark red and has a distinctive odor.

Frequently, ovulation does not occur in early menstrual cycles; these are called anovulatory cycles. Early cycles also are often irregular in frequency, amount of flow, and duration. Within several months to 2 to 3 years, a regular cycle becomes established.

Menstrual parameters vary greatly among individuals. Generally, menstruation occurs every 29 days but varies from 21 to 35 days. Some women normally have longer cycles, which can skew standard calculations of the estimated date of birth (EDB). Emotional and physical factors such as illness, excessive fatigue, stress or anxiety, and rigorous exercise programs can alter the cycle interval. The duration of menses is from 2 to 8 days, with the blood loss averaging 25 to 60 mL and the loss of iron averaging 0.5 to 1 mg daily.

A review of the endometrium and its arterial blood supply will provide further understanding of the menstrual process (Figure 10–20 ◆). Blood flow from the spiral arterioles in the superficial endometrium is reduced, leading to a lack of blood and oxygen, which in turn produces tissue death (necrosis) and

Figure 10–20 ◆ Blood supply to the endometrium (cross-sectional view of the uterus).

discharge of the superficial endometrium (menses). At the same time, the straight arterioles provide the basal endometrium with sufficient blood flow to maintain this layer of the endometrium and the endometrial glands (or seeds) that are responsible for the generation of the endometrium in the next female reproductive or menstrual cycle (see Figure 10–18). Bleeding is controlled by vasospasm of the straight basal arterioles, resulting in coagulative necrosis at the vessel tips.

The uterine (menstrual) cycle has four phases: the menstrual phase, proliferative phase, secretory phase, and ischemic phase (Table 10–2). Menstruation occurs during the *menstrual phase*. Some endometrial areas are shed, whereas others remain. Some of the remaining tips of the endometrial glands begin to regenerate. The endometrium is in a resting state following menstruation. Estrogen levels are low, and the endometrium is

1 to 2 mm deep. During this part of the cycle the cervical mucus is scanty, viscous, and opaque.

The *proliferative phase* begins when the endometrial glands enlarge, becoming twisted and longer, in response to increasing amounts of estrogen. The blood vessels become prominent and dilated, and the endometrium increases in thickness sixfold to eightfold. This gradual process reaches its peak just before ovulation. The cervical mucus becomes thin, clear, watery, and more alkaline, making the mucus more favorable to spermatozoa. As ovulation nears, the cervical mucus shows increased elasticity, called *spinnbarkheit*. At ovulation, the mucus will stretch more than 5 cm. The cervical mucosa pH increases from below 7.0 to 7.5 at the time of ovulation. On microscopic examination, the mucus shows a characteristic ferning pattern (see Figure 12–4, *B*). This ferning pattern is a useful aid in

MEDIALINK

Care Plan Activity: Irregular Menses in a Client with Anxiety

Table 10–2	CHARACTERISTICS OF MENSTRUAL CYCLE AND OVULATION
Menstrual phase (days 1–6)	Estrogen levels are low.
	Cervical mucus is scanty, viscous, and opaque.
	Endometrium is shed.
Proliferative phase (days 7–14)	Endometrium and myometrium thickness increases.
	Estrogen peaks just before ovulation.
	Cervical mucus at ovulation:
	Is clear, thin, watery, and alkaline
	Is more favorable to sperm
	Has elasticity (spinnbarkheit) greater than 5 cm
	Shows ferning pattern on microscopic exam
	Just prior to ovulation body temperature drops; then at ovulation basal body temperature increases 0.3C to 0.6C, and mittelschmerz and/or midcycle spotting may occur.
Secretory phase (days 15–26)	Estrogen drops sharply, and progesterone dominates.
	Vascularity of entire uterus increases.
	Tissue glycogen increases, and the uterus is made ready for implantation.
Ischemic phase (days 27–28)	Both estrogen and progesterone levels fall.
	Spiral arteries undergo vasoconstriction.
	Endometrium becomes pale.
	Blood vessels rupture.
	Blood escapes into uterine stromal cells.

Table 10–3	SIGNS OF OVULATION

The cervical mucus changes in the following ways:

- The amount of mucus increases.
- It appears thin, watery, and clear.
- Spinnbarkheit greater than 5 cm is present.
- A ferning pattern appears on microscopic examination.

Basal body temperature increases 0.3C to 0.6C 24 to 48 hours after ovulation.

Mittelschmerz may be present.

Midcycle spotting may occur.

Figure 10–22 ◆ Scanning electron micrograph of the inner lining of the uterus at the time of blastocyst implantation. The blastocyst is an embryo at an early stage of development.
SOURCE: Courtesy of Dr. E.S.E. Hafez, Wayne State University, Detroit, Michigan.

assessment of ovulation time (Table 10–3). For an in-depth discussion, see Chapter 12. ∞

The *secretory phase* follows ovulation. The endometrium, under estrogenic influence, undergoes slight cellular growth. Progesterone, however, causes such marked swelling and growth that the epithelium is warped into folds (Figure 10–21 ◆). The amount of tissue glycogen increases. The glandular epithelial cells begin to fill with cellular debris, and the glands become tortuous and dilate. The glands secrete small quantities of endometrial fluid in preparation for a fertilized ovum. The vascularity of the entire uterus increases greatly, providing a nourishing bed for implantation. If implantation occurs, the endometrium, under the influence of progesterone, continues to develop and becomes even thicker (Figure 10–22 ◆; see Chapter 11 ∞ for an in-depth discussion of implantation).

A

B

Figure 10–21 ◆ Scanning electron micrographs of the uterine lining during different phases of the uterine cycle. *A,* During the luteal phase, some of the cells have cilia, and some are secreting droplets. The secreting cells are covered with microvilli. *B,* In the secretory phase, microvilli are still present on the surface of the secreting cells, but the general surface of the lining has a lumpier appearance than during the proliferative phase, and the cilia appear shorter and less numerous. The named phases refer to the uterine condition at the time the photographs were taken.
SOURCE: Courtesy of Dr. E.S.E. Hafez, Wayne State University, Detroit, Michigan.

Table 10–4   SUMMARY OF FEMALE REPRODUCTIVE CYCLE

Ovarian Cycle

Follicular phase (days 1–14): Primordial follicle matures under influence of FSH and LH up to the time of ovulation.

Luteal phase (days 15–28): Ovum leaves follicle, corpus luteum develops under LH influence and produces high levels of progesterone and low levels of estrogen.

Menstrual Cycle

Menstrual phase (days 1–6): Estrogen levels are low, cervical mucus is scant, viscous, and opaque.

Proliferative phase (days 7–14): Estrogen peaks just prior to ovulation Cervical mucus at ovulation is clear, thin, watery, alkaline, and more favorable to sperm; shows ferning pattern; and has spinnbarkheit greater than 5 cm. At ovulation body temperature drops, then rises sharply and remains elevated under influence of progesterone.

Secretory phase (days 15–26): Estrogen drops sharply, and progesterone dominates.

Ischemic phase (days 27–28): Both estrogen and progesterone levels drop.

If fertilization does not occur, the *ischemic phase* begins. The corpus luteum begins to degenerate, and as a result both estrogen and progesterone levels fall. Areas of necrosis appear under the epithelial lining. Extensive vascular changes also occur. Small blood vessels rupture, and the spiral arteries constrict and retract, causing a deficiency of blood in the endometrium, which becomes pale. This ischemic phase is characterized by the escape of blood into the stromal cells of the uterus. The menstrual flow begins, thus beginning the menstrual cycle again. After menstruation, the basal layer remains so that the tips of the glands can regenerate the new functional endometrial layer. See Table 10–4 for a summary of the female reproductive cycle.

MALE REPRODUCTIVE SYSTEM

The primary reproductive functions of the male genitals are to produce and transport the male sex cells (sperm) through and eventually out of the genital tract into the female genital tract. The male reproductive system consists of the external and internal genitals (Figure 10–23 ◆).

External Genitals

The two external reproductive organs are the penis and the scrotum. The *penis* is an elongated, cylindrical structure consisting of a body, termed the *shaft,* and a cone-shaped end called the *glans.* The penis lies in front of the scrotum.

PENIS

The shaft of the penis is made up of three longitudinal columns of erectile tissue: the paired *corpora cavernosa* and a third, the *corpus spongiosum.* These columns are covered by a dense, fibrous connective tissue and then enclosed by an elastic tissue. The penis is covered by a thin outer layer of skin.

The corpus spongiosum contains the urethra and becomes the glans at the distal end of the penis. The urethra widens within the glans and ends in a slitlike orifice, located in the tip of the glans, called the *urethral meatus.* A circular fold of skin arises just behind the glans and covers it. Known as the *prepuce,* or *foreskin,* it is frequently removed by the surgical procedure of circumcision (see Chapter 30 ∞). If the corpus spongiosum does not surround the urethra completely, the urethral meatus may occur on the ventral aspect of the penile shaft (hypospadias) or on the dorsal aspect (epispadias).

The penis is innervated by the pudendal nerve. Sexual stimulation causes the penis to elongate, thicken, and stiffen, a process called *erection.* The penis becomes erect when its blood vessels become engorged, a consequence of parasympathetic nerve stimulation. If sexual stimulation is intense enough, the forceful and sudden expulsion of semen occurs through the rhythmic contractions of the penile muscles. This phenomenon is called *ejaculation.*

The penis serves both the urinary and reproductive systems. Urine is expelled through the urethral meatus. The primary reproductive function of the penis is to deposit sperm in the female vagina during sexual intercourse so that fertilization of the ovum can occur.

Figure 10–23 ◆ Male reproductive system, sagittal view.

SCROTUM

The *scrotum* is a pouchlike structure that hangs in front of the anus and behind the penis. Composed of skin and the *dartos muscle,* the scrotum shows increased pigmentation and scattered hairs. The sebaceous glands open directly onto the scrotal surface; their secretion has a distinctive odor. Contraction of the dartos and cremasteric muscles shortens the scrotum and draws it closer to the body, thus wrinkling its outer surface. The degree of wrinkling is greatest in young men and at cold temperatures and is least in older men and at warm temperatures.

Inside the scrotum are two lateral compartments. Each compartment contains a testis with its related structures. Because the left spermatic cord grows longer, the left testis and its scrotal sac hang lower than the right. A ridge (raphe) on the external scrotal surface marks the position of the medial septum and continues anteriorly on the urethral surface of the penis but disappears in the perineal area.

The function of the scrotum is to protect the testes and the sperm by maintaining a temperature lower than that of the body. Spermatogenesis will not occur if the testes fail to descend and thus remain at body temperature. Because it is sensitive to touch, pressure, temperature, and pain, the scrotum defends against potential harm to the testes.

Internal Reproductive Organs

The male internal reproductive organs include the gonads (testes or testicles), a system of ducts (epididymis, vas deferens, ejaculatory duct, and urethra), and accessory glands (seminal vesicles, prostate gland, bulbourethral glands, and urethral glands). See Table 10–5 for a summary of male reproductive organ functions.

TESTES

The *testes* are a pair of oval compound glandular organs contained in the scrotum (Figure 10–24 ◆). In the sexually mature male, they are the site of spermatozoa production and the secretion of several male sex hormones.

Each testis is 4 to 6 cm long, 2 to 3 cm wide, and 3 to 4 cm deep and weighs 10 to 15 g. Each testis is covered by a serous membrane and an inner capsule that is tough, white, and fibrous. The connective tissue sends projections inward to form septa, dividing the testis into 250 to 400 lobules. Each lobule contains one to three tightly packed, convoluted *seminiferous tubules* containing sperm cells in all stages of development.

The seminiferous tubules are surrounded by loose connective tissue, which houses abundant blood and lymph vessels and the *interstitial (Leydig's) cells.* The interstitial cells produce testosterone, the primary male sex hormone. The tubules also contain Sertoli's cells, which nourish and protect the spermatocytes. The seminiferous tubules come together to form the 20 or 30 straight tubules, which in turn form an anastomosing network of thin-walled spaces, the rete testis. The rete testis forms 10 to 15 efferent ducts that empty into the duct of the epididymis.

Most of the cells lining the seminiferous tubules undergo *spermatogenesis,* a process of maturation in which spermatocytes become spermatozoa. (See Chapter 11 ∞ for further discussion of spermatogenesis). Sperm production varies among

Table 10–5   SUMMARY OF MALE REPRODUCTIVE ORGAN FUNCTIONS

The testes house seminiferous tubules and gonads.

- Seminiferous tubules contain sperm cells in various stages of development and undergoing meiosis.
- Sertoli's cells nourish and protect spermatocytes (phase between spermatids and spermatozoa).
- Leydig's cells are the main source of testosterone.
- Epididymides provide an area for maturation of sperm and a reservoir for mature spermatozoa.
- The vas deferens connects the epididymis with the prostate gland, then connects with ducts from the seminal vesicle to become an ejaculatory duct.
- Ejaculatory ducts provide a passageway for semen and seminal fluid into the urethra.
- Seminal vesicles secrete yellowish fluid rich in fructose, prostaglandins, and fibrinogen. This provides nutrition that increases motility and fertilizing ability of sperm. Prostaglandins also aid fertilization by making the cervical mucus more receptive to sperm.
- The prostate gland secretes thin, alkaline fluid containing calcium, citric acid, and other substances. Alkalinity counteracts acidity of ductus and seminal vesicle secretions.
- Bulbourethral (Cowper's) glands secrete alkaline, viscous fluid into semen, aiding in neutralization of acidic vaginal secretions.

and within the tubules, with cells in different areas of the same tubule undergoing different stages of spermatogenesis. The sperm are eventually released from the tubules into the epididymis, where they mature further.

Like the female reproductive cycle, the process of spermatogenesis and other functions of the testes are the result of complex neural and hormonal controls. The hypothalamus secretes releasing factors, which stimulate the anterior pituitary to release the gonadotropins—FSH and LH. These hormones cause the testes to produce testosterone, which maintains spermatogenesis, increases sperm production by the seminiferous tubules, and stimulates production of seminal fluid.

Testosterone is the most prevalent and potent of the testicular hormones. It is also responsible for the development of secondary male characteristics and certain behavioral patterns. The effects of testosterone include structural and functional development of the male genital tract, emission and ejaculation of seminal fluid, distribution of body hair, promotion of growth and strength of long bones, increased muscle mass, and enlargement of the vocal cords. The action of testosterone on the central nervous system is thought to produce aggressiveness and sexual drive. The action of testosterone is constant, not cyclic like that of the female hormones. Its production is not limited to a certain number of years but is thought to decrease with age.

The testes have two primary functions:

- To serve as the site of spermatogenesis
- To produce testosterone

EPIDIDYMIS

The *epididymis* (plural, *epididymides*) is a duct about 5.6 m long, although it is convoluted into a compact structure about 3.75 cm long. An epididymis lies behind each testis. It arises

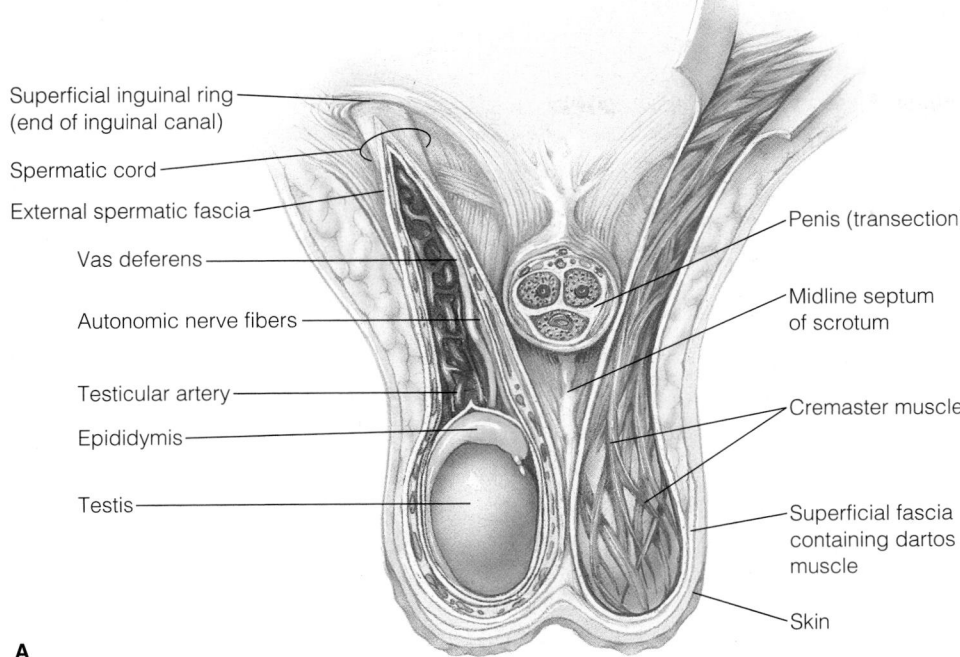

- Superficial inguinal ring (end of inguinal canal)
- Spermatic cord
- External spermatic fascia
- Vas deferens
- Autonomic nerve fibers
- Testicular artery
- Epididymis
- Testis
- Penis (transection)
- Midline septum of scrotum
- Cremaster muscle
- Superficial fascia containing dartos muscle
- Skin

A

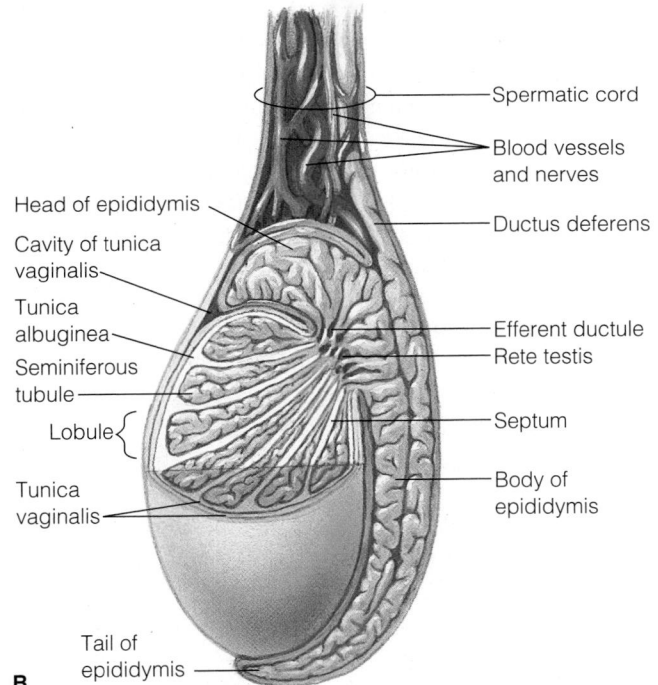

- Spermatic cord
- Blood vessels and nerves
- Head of epididymis
- Cavity of tunica vaginalis
- Tunica albuginea
- Seminiferous tubule
- Lobule
- Tunica vaginalis
- Ductus deferens
- Efferent ductule
- Rete testis
- Septum
- Body of epididymis
- Tail of epididymis

B

Figure 10–24 ◆ The testes: *A,* External view. *B,* Sagittal view showing interior anatomy.

from the top of the testis, extends downward, and then passes upward, where it becomes the vas deferens.

The epididymis provides a reservoir where spermatozoa can survive for a long period. When discharged from the seminiferous tubules into the epididymis, the sperm are immobile and incapable of fertilizing an ovum. The spermatozoa remain in the epididymis for 2 to 10 days. As the sperm are transported along the tortuous course of the epididymis, they become both motile and fertile.

VAS DEFERENS AND EJACULATORY DUCTS

The *vas deferens,* also known as the *ductus deferens,* is about 40 cm long and connects the epididymis with the prostate (see Figure 10–23). One vas deferens arises from the posterior border of each testis. It joins the spermatic cord and weaves over and between several pelvic structures until it meets the vas deferens from the opposite side. Each vas deferens terminus expands to form the *terminal ampulla.* It then unites with the seminal vesicle duct (a gland) to form the ejaculatory duct, which enters the prostate gland and ends in the prostatic urethra. The ejaculatory ducts serve as a passageway for semen and fluid secreted by the seminal vesicles. The main function of the vas deferens is to rapidly squeeze the sperm from their storage sites (the epididymis and distal part of the vas deferens) into the urethra.

Men who choose to take total responsibility for birth control may elect to have a vasectomy. In this procedure, the scrotal portion of the vas deferens is surgically incised or cauterized. Although sperm continue to be produced for the next several years, they can no longer reach the outside of the body. Eventually, the sperm deteriorate and are reabsorbed.

URETHRA

The *male urethra* is a passageway for urine and semen. The urethra begins in the bladder and passes through the prostate gland, where it is called the *prostatic urethra.* The urethra emerges from the prostate gland to become the *membranous urethra.* It terminates in the penis, where it is called the *penile urethra.* In the penile urethra, goblet secretory cells are present, and smooth muscle is replaced by erectile tissue.

ACCESSORY GLANDS

The male accessory glands secrete a unique and essential component of the total seminal fluid in an ordered sequence.

MEDIALINK

Activities: Male Reproductive System

The *seminal vesicles* are two glands composed of many lobes. Each vesicle is about 7.5 cm long. They are situated between the bladder and rectum and immediately above the base of the prostate. The epithelium lining the seminal vesicles secretes an alkaline, viscous, clear fluid rich in high-energy fructose, prostaglandins, fibrinogen, and amino acids. During ejaculation this fluid mixes with sperm in the ejaculatory ducts. This fluid helps provide an environment favorable to sperm motility and metabolism.

The prostate gland encircles the upper part of the urethra and lies below the neck of the bladder. Made up of several lobes, it measures about 4 cm in diameter and weighs 20 to 30 g. The prostate is made up of both glandular and muscular tissue. It secretes a thin, milky, alkaline fluid containing high levels of zinc, calcium, citric acid, and acid phosphatase. This fluid protects the sperm from the acidic environment of the vagina and the male urethra, which could be spermicidal.

The *bulbourethral glands (Cowper's glands)* are a pair of small round structures on either side of the membranous urethra. The glands secrete a clear, thick, alkaline fluid rich in mucoproteins that becomes part of the semen. This secretion also lubricates the penile urethra during sexual excitement and neutralizes the acid in the male urethra and the vagina, thereby enhancing sperm motility.

The *urethral glands (Littre's glands)* are tiny mucus-secreting glands found throughout the membranous lining of the penile urethra. Their secretions add to those of the bulbourethral glands.

SEMEN

The male ejaculate, *semen* or *seminal fluid,* is made up of spermatozoa and the secretions of all the accessory glands. The seminal fluid transports viable and motile sperm to the female reproductive tract. Effective transportation of sperm requires adequate nutrients, an adequate pH (about 7.5), a specific concentration of sperm to fluid, and an optimal osmolarity.

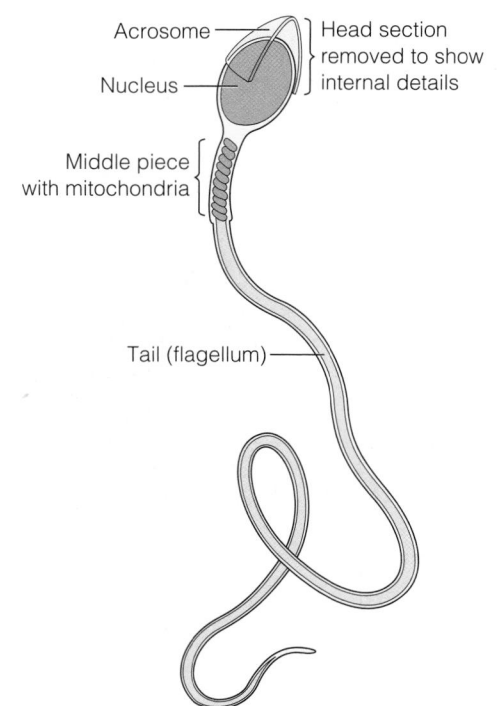

Figure 10–25 ◆ Schematic illustration of a mature spermatozoon.

A spermatozoon is made up of a head and a tail (Figure 10–25 ◆). The head's main components are the acrosome and the nucleus. The head carries the male's haploid number of chromosomes (23), and it is the part that enters the ovum at fertilization (see Chapter 11 ∞). The tail, or *flagellum,* is specialized for motility. The tail is divided into the middle and end piece.

Sperm may be stored in the male genital system up to 42 days, depending primarily on the frequency of ejaculations. The average volume of ejaculate following abstinence for several days is 2 to 5 mL but may vary from 1 to 10 mL. Repeated ejaculation results in decreased volume. Once ejaculated, sperm can live only 2 or 3 days in the female genital tract.

CHAPTER REVIEW

FOCUS YOUR STUDY

- The genetic sex of an embryo is determined at fertilization. The male and female reproductive systems are undifferentiated initially. By the 12th week the external genitals are fully differentiated.

- Reproductive activities require complex interactions between the reproductive structures, the central nervous system, and such endocrine glands as the pituitary, hypothalamus, testes, and ovaries.

- At puberty, an alteration in brain sensitivity leads to an increased release of GnRH, which stimulates LH and FSH, leading in the male to an increase in testosterone and in the female to an increase in estrogen and progesterone.

- Estrogen is the principal cause of the events of puberty in females (maturation of ova, enlargement of the uterus and fallopian tubes, deposition of fat in the breasts and hips, and characteristic hair growth).

- Puberty changes for the male (onset of spermatogenesis; enlargement of the penis, scrotum, and testes; voice changes; and characteristic hair growth) occur as a result of increased testosterone production by the testes.

- The female reproductive system consists of the ovaries, where female germ cells and female sex hormones are formed; the fallopian tubes, which capture the ovum and allow transport to the uterus; the uterus, which is the implantation site for the fertilized ovum (blastocyst); the cervix, which is a protective portal for the body of the uterus and the connection between the vagina and the uterus; and the vagina, which is the passageway from the external genitals to the uterus and provides for discharge of menstrual products to the outside of the body.

- The female reproductive cycle may be described in terms of the ovarian cycle, during which ovulation occurs, and the menstrual cycle, during which menstruation occurs. These two cycles take place simultaneously and are under neurohormonal control.

- The ovarian cycle has two phases: the follicular phase and the luteal phase. During the follicular phase, the primordial follicle matures under the influence of FSH and LH until ovulation occurs. The luteal phase begins when the ovum leaves the follicle and the corpus luteum develops under the influence of LH. The corpus luteum produces high levels of progesterone and low levels of estrogen.

- The menstrual cycle has four phases: menstrual, proliferative, secretory, and ischemic. Menstruation is the actual shedding of the endometrial lining, when estrogen levels are low. The proliferative phase begins when the endometrial glands begin to enlarge under the influence of estrogen and cervical mucosal changes occur; the changes peak at ovulation. The secretory phase follows ovulation, and, influenced primarily by progesterone, the uterus increases its vascularity to make ready for possible implantation. The ischemic phase is characterized by degeneration of the corpus luteum, decreases in both estrogen and progesterone levels, constriction of the spiral arteries, and escape of blood into the stromal cells of the endometrium.

- The male reproductive system consists of the testes, where male germ cells and male sex hormones are formed; a series of continuous ducts through which spermatozoa are transported outside the body; accessory glands that produce secretions important to sperm nutrition, survival, and transport; and the penis, which serves as the reproductive organ of intercourse.

EXPLORE MEDIALINK

http://www.prenhall.com/davidson

NCLEX review questions, case studies, and other interactive resources for this chapter can be found on the Web Site at http://www.prenhall.com/davidson. Click on "Chapter 10" to select the activities for this chapter.

For tutorials including animations and videos, more NCLEX review questions, and an audio glossary, access the accompanying Prentice Hall Nursing MediaLink DVD-ROM in this book.

PRENTICE HALL NURSING MEDIALINK DVD-ROM

Audio Glossary

NCLEX Review

Activities: *Female Reproductive System labeling exercise; Female Reproductive System matching exercise; Male Reproductive System labeling exercise; Male Reproductive System matching exercise*

COMPANION WEBSITE

Additional NCLEX Review

Case Study: *Sex Education for Teens*

Care Plan Activity: *Irregular Menses in a Client with Anxiety*

Applications: *Pelvic Structures; Ovarian Cycle*

Critical Thinking

CRITICAL THINKING IN ACTION

TALKING WITH A TEENAGE GIRL ABOUT MENSTRUATION

View the Critical Thinking in Action video in Chapter 10 of the DVD-ROM. Then answer the questions that follow.

You are working in the OB/GYN clinic when Sally Smith, a 17- year-old teenager, comes in complaining of irregular menses. She believes her periods are really "messed up" and interfering with her active schedule. She wants them to be more regular and asks you for birth control. She tells you that she is a member of the swimming team and is a senior in high school. She says she is planning to start community college next year to obtain an associate degree in computer technology. You assess Sally's history as follows:

menarche began at age 12; periods occur every 28 to 32 days. She usually experiences cramping in the first 2 days and the flow lasts 4 to 5 days. She uses an average of 4 to 5 tampons a day during her period. She has never been hospitalized, has no prior medical problems, and is up-to-date on her immunizations except for meningitis.

1. Based on your knowledge of menstruation, how would you describe Sally's menstrual cycle?
2. What is your primary goal in discussing Sally's menstrual cycle with her?
3. What information would you give Sally relating to her menstrual cycle?
4. What important request does Sally have?
5. Sally expresses problems dealing with the cramping she experiences with the first 2 days of her menses. What would you suggest to Sally to cope with the discomfort?

REFERENCES

Blackburn, S. T. (2003). *Maternal, fetal, & neonatal physiology: A clinical perspective* (2nd ed.). St. Louis, MO: Saunders.

Caldwell, W. E., & Moloy, H. C. (1933). Anatomical variations in the female pelvis and their effect on labor with a suggested classification [Historical article]. *American Journal of Obstetrics & Gynecology, 26,* 479–505.

Cunningham, F. G., Leveno, K. J., Bloom, S. L., Hauth, J. C., Gilstrap, L. C., & Wenstrom, K. D.

(2005). *Williams obstetrics* (22nd ed.). New York: McGraw-Hill.

Ferin, M. (2003). The hypothalamus-hypophyseal-ovarian axis and the menstrual cycle. In J. J. Sciarri (Ed.), *Gynecology and obstetrics* (Vol. 5, chap. 6, pp. 1–21). Philadelphia: Lippincott Williams & Wilkins.

Lawrence, R. M., & Lawrence, R. A. (2004). The breast and the physiology of lactation. In R. K. Creasy & R. Resnik (Eds.), *Maternal-fetal*

medicine: Principles and practice (5th ed.). Philadelphia: Saunders.

Monga, M., & Sanborn, B. M. (2004). Biology and physiology of the reproductive tract and control of myometrial contraction. In R. K. Creasy & R. Resnik (Eds.), *Maternal-fetal medicine: Principles and practice* (5th ed.). Philadelphia: Saunders.

CHAPTER 11
Conception and Fetal Development

My friends tease me when I say this, but I know the moment my daughter was conceived. My husband and I had both been so busy at work, but we finally went away for a long weekend together. It was wonderful—we got back some of the magic as we took long walks and talked and talked. Until that weekend, whenever we discussed having children it was always "maybe someday." On the second night we decided to skip the diaphragm for the first time ever. Our lovemaking seemed so special that evening, a true reflection of the emotional closeness we had recaptured. I never went back to using the diaphragm after that weekend, but I am convinced that Jennifer is the result of that night together!

OBJECTIVES

1. Explain the differences between mitotic cellular division and meiotic cellular division.
2. Compare the processes by which ova and sperm are produced.
3. Describe the process of fertilization.
4. Identify the differing processes by which fraternal (dizygotic) and identical (monozygotic) twins are formed.
5. Describe in order of increasing complexity the structures that form during the cellular multiplication and differentiation stages of intrauterine development.
6. Describe the development, structure, and functions of the placenta during intrauterine life.
7. Summarize the significant changes in growth and development of the fetus at 4, 6, 12, 16, 20, 24, 28, 32, 36, and 38 weeks postconception.
8. Identify the vulnerable periods during which malformations of the various organ systems may occur, and describe the resulting congenital malformations.

KEY TERMS

MEDIALINK

Additional resources for this content can be found on the Prentice Hall Nursing MediaLink DVD-ROM and on the Companion Website at http://www.prenhall.com/davidson. Click on "Chapter 11" to select the activities for this chapter.

Each person is unique. Nonetheless, everyone has many if not all of the same "parts," which usually function similarly. The human genome consists of large amounts of chemical deoxyribonucleic acid (DNA) that contains within its structure the genetic information needed to specify all aspects of embryogenesis, development, growth, metabolism, and reproduction. The genome contains, by current estimates, about 50,000 *genes,* which at this point are defined as units of genetic information (Hamilton & Wynshaw-Boris, 2004). Genes are encoded in the DNA that makes up the chromosomes in the nucleus of each cell. Even chromosomes, those determinants of the structure and function of organ systems and traits, are made of the same biochemical substances. How does each person become unique, then? The answer lies in the physiologic mechanisms of heredity, the processes of cellular division, and the environmental factors that influence development from the moment a person is conceived. This chapter explores the processes involved in conception and fetal development—the basis of human uniqueness.

CHROMOSOMES

Human (body) cells contain within their nuclei threadlike bodies known as **chromosomes,** which are composed of strands of *DNA* and protein. Each chromosome contains two longitudinal halves called *chromatids,* which are joined together at a point called the *centromere* (Figure 11–1 ◆, *A*). Chromosomes are classified according to their length and to the position of their centromere. When the centromere is centrally located, the longitudinal halves are divided into one short arm region and one long arm region, and the chromosome resembles an X. This is the shape of most human chromosomes.

Every body (somatic) cell in the human body contains 46 chromosomes, referred to as the **diploid number of chromosomes.** These are divided into 23 pairs. There are 22 pairs of similar cells in both males and females, called *autosomes,* and one pair of sex chromosomes (XX in females, XY in males). One chromosome of each pair is contributed by the individual's mother, and the other is contributed by the father. The two chromosomes carrying matching genetic information that make up each pair are called *homologous chromosomes* or *homologs.*

Genes are regions in the DNA strands that contain coded information used to determine the unique characteristics—or *traits*—of an individual. Genes in the autosomes determine such traits as hair color or blood type, whereas genes in the sex chromosomes determine the individual's gender. Genes are arranged in linear order on the chromosomes and can be numbered and studied accordingly.

Each homologous chromosome pair carries genes coding for similar traits in identical locations on the chromosomes. Genes that are similar are called *homozygous* genes, whereas dissimilar genes are referred to as *heterozygous* genes (Figure 11–1, *B*). When an individual is homozygous for a particular trait, he or she has inherited similar genes for that trait from each parent. Genetics is discussed in greater detail in Chapter 12. ∞

CELLULAR DIVISION

Each human begins life as a single cell called a fertilized ovum or zygote. This single cell reproduces itself, and in turn each new cell also reproduces itself in a continuing process. The new cells are similar to the cells from which they came. Cells are reproduced either by mitosis or meiosis, two different but related processes.

Mitosis is a process of cell division that results in daughter cells that are exact copies of the original cell. They are identical to the parent cell and to each other. These cells contain a full set of chromosomes or genetic material and are called diploid because of this. Mitosis makes growth and development possible, and in mature individuals it is the process by which the (somatic) body cells continue to divide and replace themselves.

Meiosis is a process of cell division that leads to the development of eggs and sperm needed to produce a new organism. Unlike cells produced during mitosis, the cells produced during meiosis contain only half the genetic material or number of chromosomes (the haploid number).

Mitosis

During mitosis, the cell undergoes several changes, ending in cell division. Although mitosis is a continuous process, it is generally divided into five stages: interphase, prophase, metaphase, anaphase, and telophase (Figure 11–2 ◆).

Before cell division takes place during interphase, the DNA within the chromosomes replicates so that the genes will be

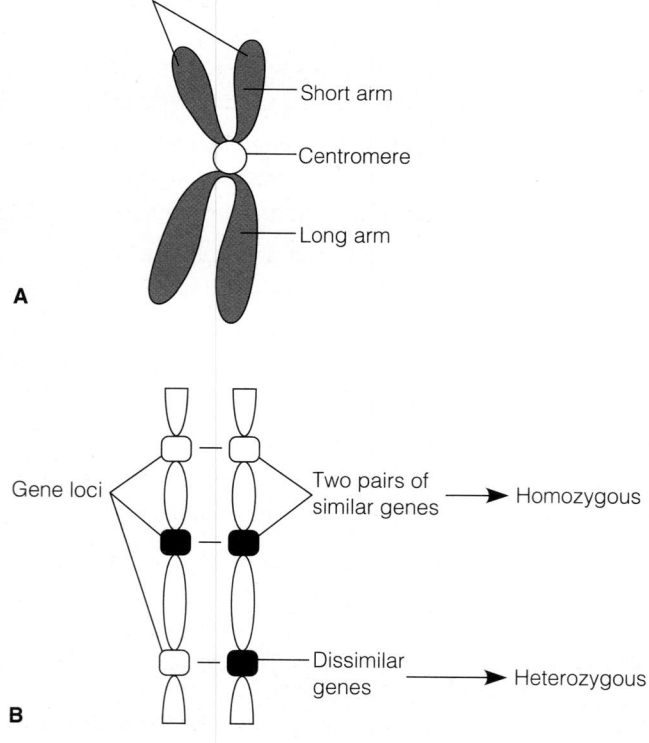

A

B

Figure 11–1 ◆ *A,* Chromosomes contain two longitudinal halves called *chromatids,* which are joined together at a point called the *centromere. B,* One pair of homologous chromosomes with similar (homozygous) genes and dissimilar (heterozygous) genes.

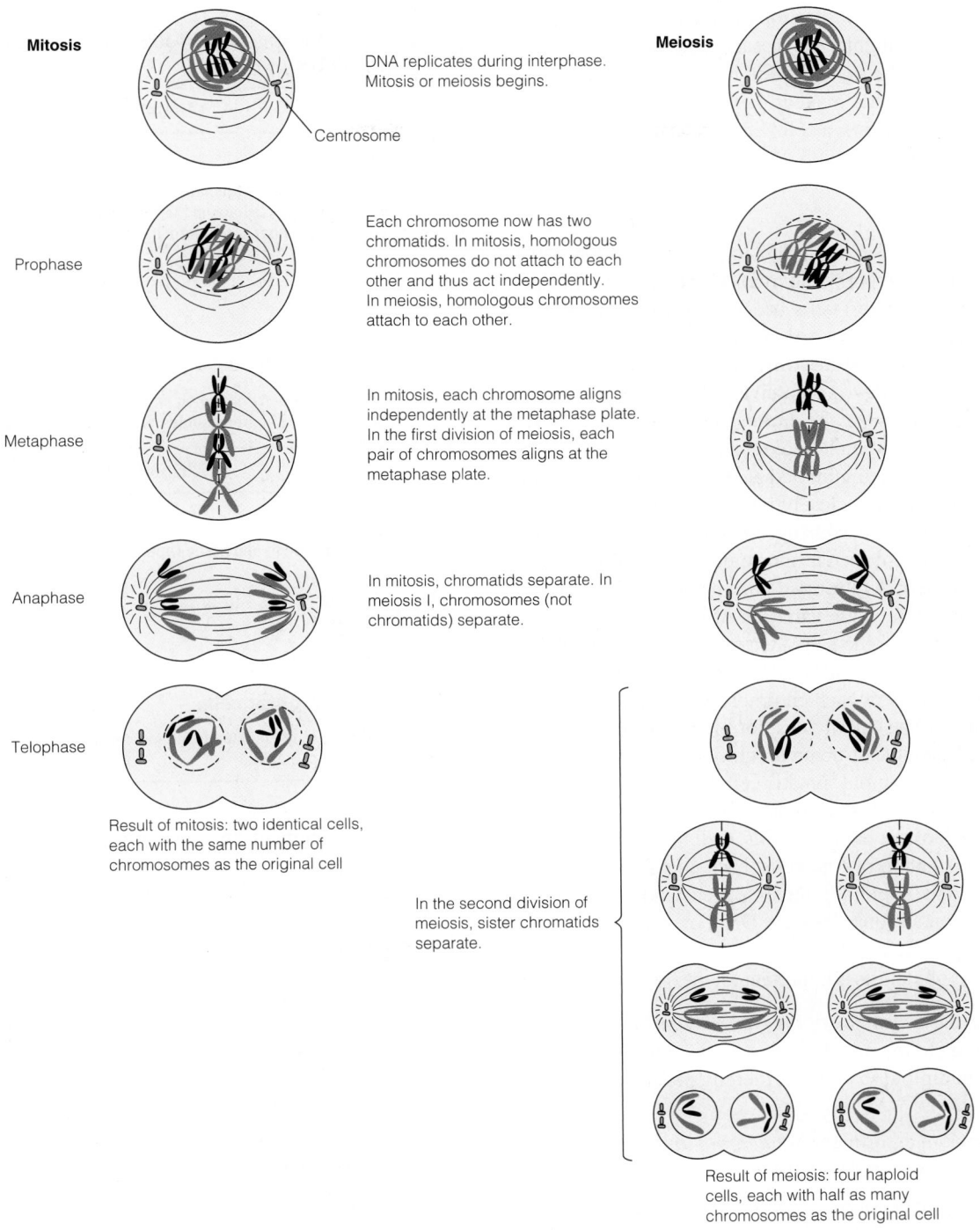

Mitosis

DNA replicates during interphase. Mitosis or meiosis begins.

Centrosome

Meiosis

Prophase

Each chromosome now has two chromatids. In mitosis, homologous chromosomes do not attach to each other and thus act independently. In meiosis, homologous chromosomes attach to each other.

Metaphase

In mitosis, each chromosome aligns independently at the metaphase plate. In the first division of meiosis, each pair of chromosomes aligns at the metaphase plate.

Anaphase

In mitosis, chromatids separate. In meiosis I, chromosomes (not chromatids) separate.

Telophase

Result of mitosis: two identical cells, each with the same number of chromosomes as the original cell

In the second division of meiosis, sister chromatids separate.

Result of meiosis: four haploid cells, each with half as many chromosomes as the original cell

Figure 11–2 ◆ Comparison of mitosis and meiosis.

doubled. Mitosis begins when the cell enters prophase. During prophase, the chromosomes condense and form the shape we usually recognize as a chromosome. Next comes the appearance of a mitotic apparatus known as a spindle, in which fine threads extend from the top and bottom poles of the nucleus. At each pole of the spindle, a body known as the *centrosome* is formed, so the threads of the spindle extend from one centrosome to the other. Next the nuclear membrane, which separates the nucleus from the cytoplasm, disappears, the nucleus as a separate entity disappears, and the cell enters metaphase.

During metaphase, the chromosomes line up at the equator (midway between the poles) of the spindle. Metaphase is followed by anaphase, in which the two chromatids of each chromosome separate and move to opposite ends of the spindle, where they cluster in masses near the two poles of the cell.

Telophase is essentially the opposite of prophase. A new nuclear membrane forms, separating each newly formed nucleus from the cytoplasm. The spindle disappears, and the centrioles relocate outside of each new nucleus. Within the nucleus the chromosomes lengthen and become threadlike. As telophase nears completion, a furrow develops in the cell cytoplasm and divides it into two daughter cells, each with its own nucleus. Daughter cells have the same diploid number of chromosomes (46) and the same genetic makeup as the cell from which they came. At the end of mitosis, a cell with 46 chromosomes results in two identical cells, each with 46 chromosomes.

Meiosis

Meiosis is a special type of cell division by which diploid cells give rise to **gametes** (sperm and ova). These cells are different from other somatic (body) cells because they contain half the genetic material of the parent cell—only 23 chromosomes—the **haploid number of chromosomes.**

Meiosis consists of two successive cell divisions (see Figure 11–2). In the first division, the chromosomes replicate. Next a pairing takes place between homologous chromosomes (Sadler, 2004). Instead of separating immediately, as in mitosis, the similar chromosomes become closely intertwined. At each point of contact, there is a physical exchange of genetic material between the chromatids (arms of the chromosomes). New combinations are provided by the newly formed chromosomes; these combinations account for the wide variation of traits, such as hair or eye color. The chromosome pairs then separate, each member of a pair moving to opposite sides of the cell. (In contrast, during mitosis the chromatids of each chromosome separate and move to opposite poles.) The cell divides, forming two daughter cells, each with 23 double-structured chromosomes—the same amount of DNA as a normal somatic cell. In the second division, the chromatids of each chromosome separate and move to opposite poles of each of the daughter cells. Cell division occurs, resulting in the formation of four cells, each containing 23 single chromosomes, the haploid number of chromosomes. These daughter cells contain only half the DNA of a normal somatic cell (Sadler, 2004) (Table 11–1).

The process of meiosis is important for the following reasons:

- It maintains the *constancy of the chromosome number* from one generation to the next by reducing the chromosome number from diploid to haploid, thereby producing haploid gametes.

- It allows random assortment of *maternal and paternal chromosomes* between the gametes.

- It relocates segments of maternal and paternal chromosomes by *crossing over of chromosome segments,* which "shuffles" the genes and produces a recombination of genetic material.

Mutations may occur during the second meiotic division if two of the chromatids do not move apart rapidly enough when the cell divides. The still-paired chromatids are carried into one of the daughter cells and eventually form an extra chromosome. This condition is referred to as an *autosomal nondisjunction* (chromosomal mutation) and is harmful to the offspring that may result should fertilization occur. The implications of nondisjunction are discussed in Chapter 12. ∞

Another type of chromosomal mutation can occur if chromosomes break during meiosis. If the broken segment is lost, the result is a shorter chromosome; this is known as a *deletion.*

Table 11–1   COMPARISON OF MEIOSIS AND MITOSIS

Meiosis
Purpose Produce reproductive cells (gametes). Reduction of chromosome number by half (from diploid [46] to haploid [23]), so that when fertilization occurs the normal diploid number is restored. Introduces genetic variability.
Cell division Two-stage reduction.
Number of daughter cells Four daughter cells, each containing one half the number of chromosomes as the mother cell, or 23 chromosomes. Nonidentical to original cell.
Mitosis
Purpose Produce cells for growth and tissue repair. Cell division characteristic of all somatic cells.
Cell division One-stage cell division.
Number of daughter cells Two daughter cells identical to the mother cell, each with the diploid number (46 chromosomes).

If the broken segment becomes attached to another chromosome, a harmful mutation called a *translocation* is the result. The effects of translocation are described in Chapter 12. ∞

GAMETOGENESIS

Meiosis occurs during **gametogenesis,** the process by which germ cells, or gametes, are produced. These cells contain only half the genetic material of a typical body cell. The female gamete, called an ovum, and the male gamete, called a sperm, unite during fertilization, resulting in a **zygote** with a complete set of genetic material (46 chromosomes)—half of it from the mother and half from the father.

Oogenesis

Oogenesis is the process that produces the female gamete, called an ovum (egg). As discussed in Chapter 10 ∞, the ovaries begin to develop early in the fetal life of the female. All the ova that the female will produce in her lifetime are present at birth. The ovary gives rise to oogonial cells, which develop into oocytes. Meiosis (cell replication by division) begins in all oocytes before the female infant is born but stops before the first division is complete and remains in this arrested phase until puberty. During puberty the mature primary oocyte continues through the first meiotic division in the graafian follicle of the ovary.

The first meiotic division produces two cells of unequal size with different amounts of cytoplasm, but with the same number of chromosomes. One of these cells is the *secondary*

MediaLink

Animation: Spermatogenesis

MediaLink

Animation: Oogenesis & Spermatogenesis Compared

MediaLink

Activity: Matching Oogenesis and Spermatogenesis

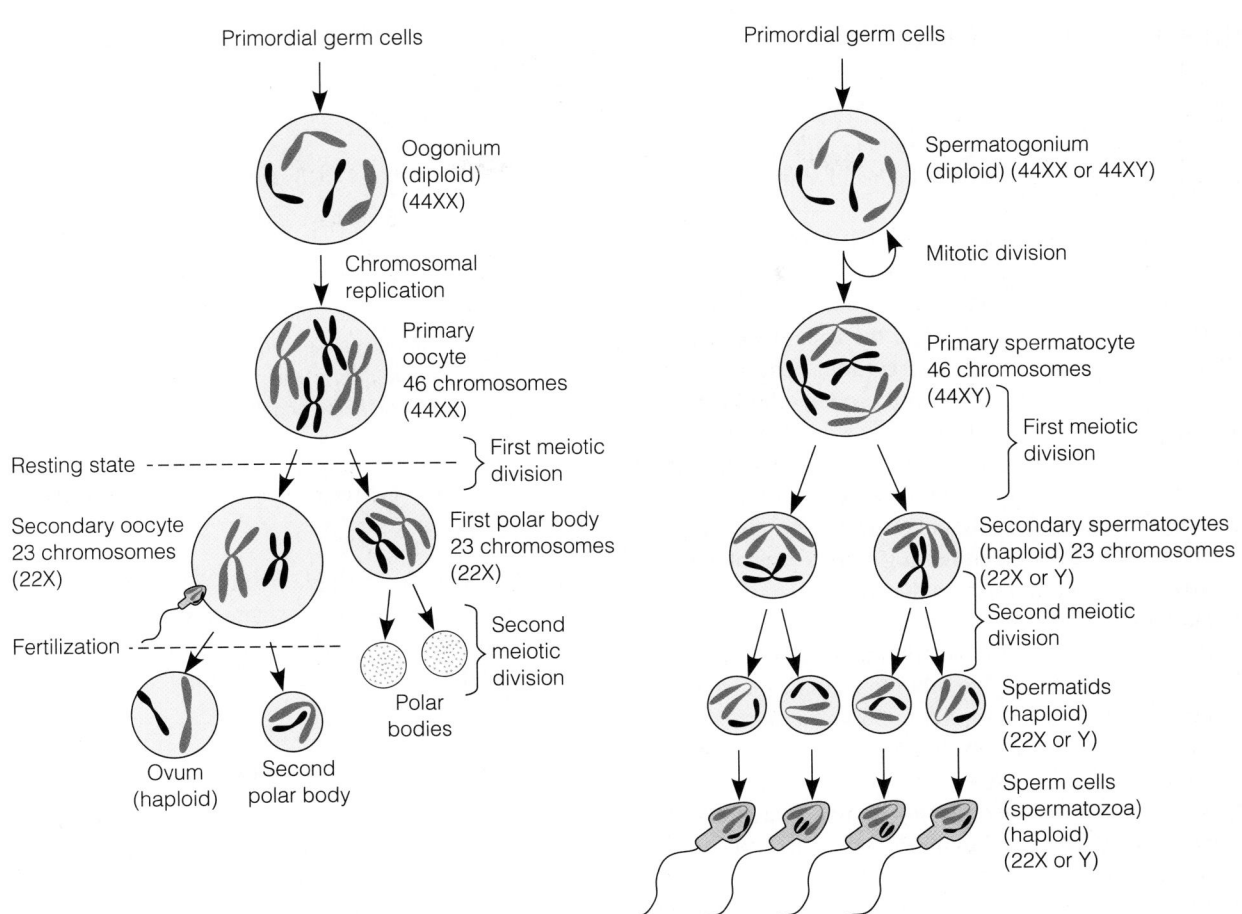

Figure 11–3 ◆ Gametogenesis involves meiosis within the ovary and testis. *A,* During meiosis, each oogonium produces a single haploid ovum once some cytoplasm moves into the polar bodies. *B,* Each spermatogonium, in contrast, produces four haploid spermatozoa.

oocyte and the other is a minute *polar body.* Both the secondary oocyte and the first polar body contain 22 double-structured autosomal chromosomes and one double-structured sex chromosome (X).

At the time of ovulation, the second meiotic division begins immediately and proceeds as the oocyte moves down the fallopian tube. Division is again not equal, and the secondary oocyte moves into the metaphase stage of cell division, where its meiotic division is arrested until and unless the oocyte is fertilized.

When the secondary oocyte completes the second meiotic division after fertilization, the result is a mature ovum with the haploid number of chromosomes and virtually all the cytoplasm. In addition, the second polar body (also haploid) forms at this time (Figure 11–3 ◆). The first polar body has now also divided, producing two additional polar bodies. Thus when meiosis is completed, four haploid cells have been produced: three small polar bodies, which eventually disintegrate, and one ovum (Sadler, 2004).

Spermatogenesis

During puberty, the germinal epithelium in the seminiferous tubules of the testes begins the process of spermatogenesis, which produces the male gametes (sperm). As the (diploid num-

ber) spermatogonium enters the first meiotic division, it is called the *primary spermatocyte.* During this first meiotic division, the spermatogonium replicates and forms two haploid cells termed *secondary spermatocytes,* each of which contains 22 double-structured autosomal chromosomes and either a double-structured X sex chromosome or a double-structured Y sex chromosome. During the second meiotic division they divide to form four spermatids, each with the haploid number of chromosomes (see Figure 11–3).

The spermatids undergo a series of changes during which they lose most of their cytoplasm and become sperm (spermatozoa). The nucleus becomes compacted into the head of the sperm, which is covered by a cap called an acrosome that is, in turn, covered by a plasma membrane. A long tail is produced from one of the centrioles.

THE PROCESS OF FERTILIZATION

When an ovum and a sperm unite, a fertilized ovum, or zygote, is created. This zygote begins life as a single cell with a complete set of genetic material, 23 chromosomes from the mother's ovum and 23 chromosomes from the father's sperm for a total of 46 chromosomes.

Preparation for Fertilization

The mature ovum and spermatozoa have only a brief time to unite. Ova are considered fertile for about 12 to 24 hours after ovulation. Sperm can survive in the female reproductive tract for 48 to 72 hours but are believed to be healthy and highly fertile for only about the first 24 hours.

The ovum's cell membrane is surrounded by two layers of tissue. The layer closest to the cell membrane is called the *zona pellucida*. It is a clear, noncellular layer whose thickness influences the fertilization rate. Surrounding the zona pellucida is a ring of elongated cells, called the *corona radiata*, because they radiate from the ovum like the gaseous corona around the sun. These cells are held together by hyaluronic acid. The ovum has no power of movement of its own. During ovulation, high estrogen levels increase peristalsis within the fallopian tubes, which helps move the ovum through the tube toward the uterus. The high estrogen levels also cause a thinning of the cervical mucus, easing passage of the sperm through the cervix, into the uterus, and up the fallopian tube.

The process of fertilization usually takes place in the ampulla (outer third) of the fallopian tube. In a single ejaculation, the male deposits approximately 200 to 500 million spermatozoa in the vagina, of which only hundreds of sperm actually reach the ampulla (Sadler, 2004). Fructose in the semen, secreted by the seminal vesicles, is the energy source for the sperm. The spermatozoa propel themselves up the female tract by the flagellar movement of their tails. Transit time from the cervix into the fallopian tube can be as short as 5 minutes but usually takes an average of 2 to 7 hours after ejaculation (Sadler, 2004). Prostaglandins in the semen may increase uterine smooth muscle contractions, which help transport the sperm. The fallopian tubes have a dual ciliary action that facilitates movement of the ovum toward the uterus and movement of the sperm from the uterus toward the ovary.

The sperm must undergo two processes before fertilization can occur: capacitation and the acrosomal reaction. **Capacitation** is the removal of the plasma membrane and glycoprotein coat overlying the spermatozoa's acrosomal area and the loss of seminal plasma proteins. If the glycoprotein coat is not removed, the sperm will not be able to fertilize the ovum (Sadler, 2004). Capacitation occurs in the female reproductive tract (aided by uterine enzymes) and is thought to take about 7 hours. Sperm that undergo capacitation take on three characteristics: (1) the ability to undergo the acrosomal reaction, (2) the ability to bind to the zona pellucida, and (3) the acquisition of hypermotility.

The **acrosomal reaction** follows capacitation. The acrosome caps of the sperm surrounding the ovum release their enzymes (hyaluronidase, a protease called acrosin, and trypsin-like substances). These enzymes break down the hyaluronic acid that holds the elongated cells of corona radiata, the outer layer of the ovum, together (Sadler, 2004). Hundreds of acrosomes must rupture to clear enough hyaluronic acid for even a single sperm to penetrate the ovum successfully.

At the moment of penetration by a fertilizing sperm, the zona pellucida undergoes a reaction that prevents additional

DEVELOPING CULTURAL COMPETENCE

IRAQI CHILDBIRTH CUSTOMS

"My sister, she did not have baby for very, very long time, you see. This is very sad where I am from [Iraq]. Her husband's family wanted him to leave her and we so feared he would. Then my sister became pregnant and it was very nice, we all so happy you see. Then I learned my sister birthed a baby girl and I cried and cried for a week. My mother cried too, so sad all this time no baby come and then finally to have a girl. I still feel sad for her."

(Excerpt from author's interview with Iraqi on childbirth customs in Iraq)

sperm from entering a single ovum. This is known as the *block to polyspermy*. This cellular change is mediated by release of materials from the cortical granules, organelles found just below the ovum's surface, and is called the *cortical reaction* (Figure 11–4 ◆).

The Moment of Fertilization

After the sperm enters the ovum, a chemical signal prompts the secondary oocyte to complete the second meiotic division, forming the nucleus of the ovum and ejecting the second polar body. Then the nuclei of the ovum and sperm swell and approach each other. The true moment of **fertilization** occurs as the nuclei unite. Their individual nuclear membranes disappear, and their chromosomes pair up to produce the diploid zygote. Because each nucleus contains a haploid number of chromosomes (23), this union restores the diploid number (46). The zygote contains a new combination of genetic material that results in an individual different from either parent and from anyone else.

It is also at the moment of fertilization that the sex of the zygote is determined. The two chromosomes (the sex chromosomes) of the 23rd pair—either XX or XY—determine the sex of an individual. X chromosomes are larger and bear more genes than Y chromosomes. Females have two X chromosomes, and males have an X and a Y chromosome. The mature ovum produced by oogenesis can have only one type of sex chromosome—an X—while spermatogenesis produces two sperm with an X chromosome and two sperm with a Y chromosome. When each gamete contributes an X chromosome, the resulting zygote is female. When the ovum contributes an X chromosome and the sperm contributes a Y, the resulting zygote is male. As discussed in Chapter 12 ∞, certain traits are termed *sex-linked* because they are controlled by the genes on the X sex chromosome. Two examples of sex-linked traits are color blindness and hemophilia.

PREEMBRYONIC STAGE

The first 14 days of human development, starting on the day the ovum is fertilized (conception), are referred to as the preembryonic stage, or the stage of the ovum. Development after fertil-

B

Figure 11–4 ◆ Sperm penetration of an ovum. *A,* The sequential steps of oocyte penetration by a sperm are depicted moving from top to bottom. *B,* Scanning electron micrograph of human sperm surrounding a human oocyte (750×). The smaller spherical cells are granulosa cells of the corona radiata.
SOURCE: Used with permission from Nilsson, L. (1990). *A child is born.* New York: Dell Publishing.

ization can be divided into two phases: cellular multiplication and cellular differentiation. These phases are characterized by rapid cellular multiplication and differentiation and the establishment of the embryonic membranes and primary germ layers. Development of both the endometrium and embryo must be synchronized for implantation to succeed (Groll & Lessey, 2003). These phases and the process of implantation (nidation), which occurs between them, are discussed next.

Cellular Multiplication

Cellular multiplication begins as the zygote moves through the fallopian tube toward the cavity of the uterus. This transportation takes 3 days or more (Cunningham, Leveno, Bloom et al., 2005) and is accomplished mainly by a very weak fluid current in the fallopian tube resulting from the beating action of the ciliated epithelium that lines the tube.

The zygote now enters a period of rapid mitotic divisions called **cleavage,** during which it divides into two cells, four cells, eight cells, and so on. These cells, called *blastomeres,* are so small that the developing cell mass is only slightly larger than the original zygote. The blastomeres are held together by the zona pellucida, which is under the corona radiata. The blastomeres will eventually form a solid ball of 12 to 16 cells called the **morula.**

As the morula enters the uterus, two things happen: the intracellular fluid in the morula increases, and a central cavity forms within the cell mass. Inside this cavity is an inner solid mass of cells called the **blastocyst.** The outer layer of cells that surround the cavity and have replaced the zona pellucida is the **trophoblast.** Eventually, the trophoblast develops into one of the embryonic membranes, called the chorion. The blastocyst

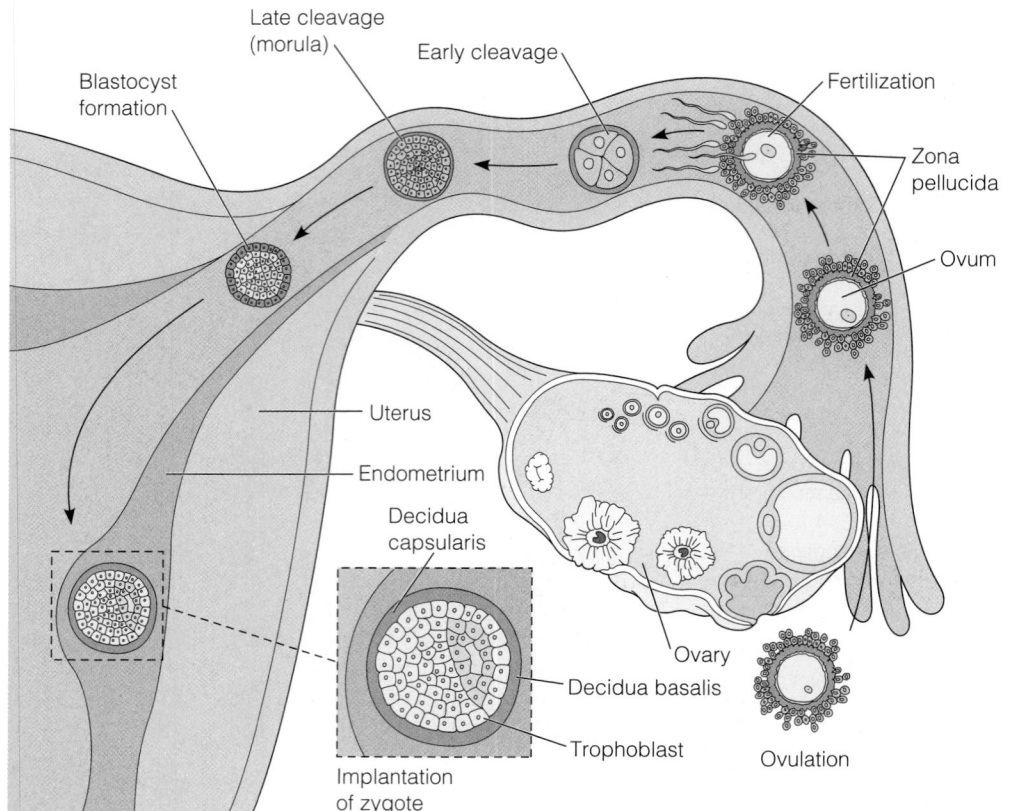

Figure 11–5 ◆ During ovulation, the ovum leaves the ovary and enters the fallopian tube. Fertilization generally occurs in the outer third of the fallopian tube. Subsequent changes in the fertilized ovum from conception to implantation are depicted.

develops into a double layer of cells called the *embryonic disc,* from which the embryo and the amnion (embryonic membrane) will develop. The journey of the fertilized ovum to its destination in the uterus is illustrated in Figure 11–5 ◆.

Early pregnancy factor (EPF), an immunosuppressant, is secreted by the trophoblastic cells. EPF appears in the maternal serum within 24 to 48 hours after fertilization and forms the basis of a pregnancy test during the first 10 days of development (Moore & Persaud, 2003).

Implantation (Nidation)

While floating in the uterine cavity, the blastocyst is nourished by the uterine glands, which secrete a mixture of lipids, mucopolysaccharides, and glycogen. The trophoblast attaches itself to the surface of the endometrium for further nourishment. The most frequent site of attachment is the upper part of the posterior uterine wall (Figure 11–6 ◆). Between days 7 and 10 after fertilization, the zona pellucida disappears, and the blastocyst implants itself by burrowing into the uterine lining and penetrating down toward the maternal capillaries until it is completely covered (Liu, 2004). The lining of the uterus thickens below the implanted blastocyst, and the cells of the trophoblast grow down into the thickened lining, forming processes called chorionic villi.

Under the influence of progesterone, the endometrium increases in thickness and vascularity in preparation for implantation and nourishment of the ovum. After implantation, the endometrium is called the decidua. The portion of the decidua

that covers the blastocyst is called the **decidua capsularis;** the portion directly under the implanted blastocyst is the **decidua basalis;** and the portion that lines the rest of the uterine cavity is the **decidua vera (parietalis)** (see Figure 11–5, inset) (Benirschke, 2004b). The maternal part of the placenta develops from the decidua basalis, which contains large numbers of blood vessels. The chorionic villi (discussed shortly) in contact with the decidua basalis will form the fetal portion of the placenta.

Cellular Differentiation
PRIMARY GERM LAYERS

About 10 to 14 days after conception, the homogenous mass of blastocyst cells differentiates into the primary germ layers. These layers—the **ectoderm, mesoderm,** and **endoderm** (see Figure 11–6)—are formed at the same time as the embryonic membranes. All tissues, organs, and organ systems will develop from these primary germ cell layers (Table 11–2). For example, differentiation of the endoderm results in the formation of the epithelium lining the respiratory and digestive tracts (Figure 11–7 ◆).

EMBRYONIC MEMBRANES

The **embryonic membranes** begin to form at the time of implantation (Figure 11–8 ◆). These membranes protect and support the embryo as it grows and develops inside the uterus. The first and outermost membrane to form is the **chorion.** This thick membrane develops from the trophoblast and has many finger-

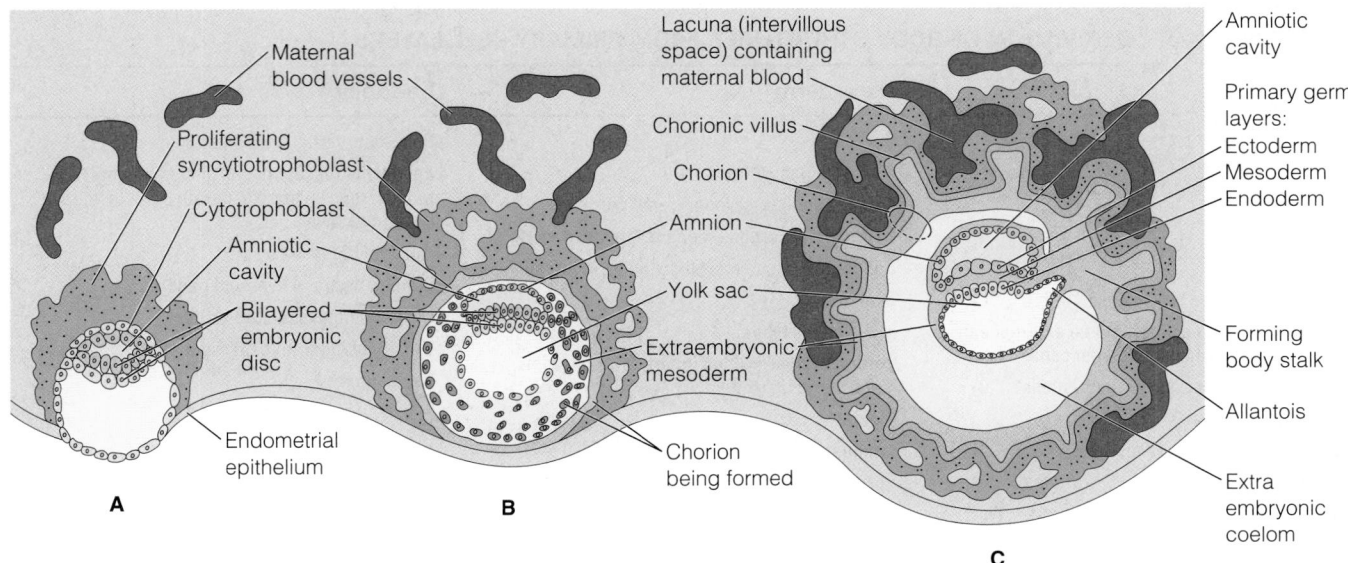

Figure 11–6 ◆ Formation of primary germ layers. *A,* Implantation of a 7 1/2-day blastocyst in which the cells of the embryonic disc are separated from the amnion by a fluid-filled space. The erosion of the endometrium by the syncytiotrophoblast is ongoing. *B,* Implantation is completed by day 9, and extraembryonic mesoderm is beginning to form a discrete layer beneath the cytotrophoblast. *C,* By day 16, the embryo shows all three germ layers, a yolk sac, and an allantois (an outpouching of the yolk sac that forms the structural basis of the body stalk, or umbilical cord). The cytotrophoblast and associated mesoderm has become the chorion, and chorionic villi are developing.

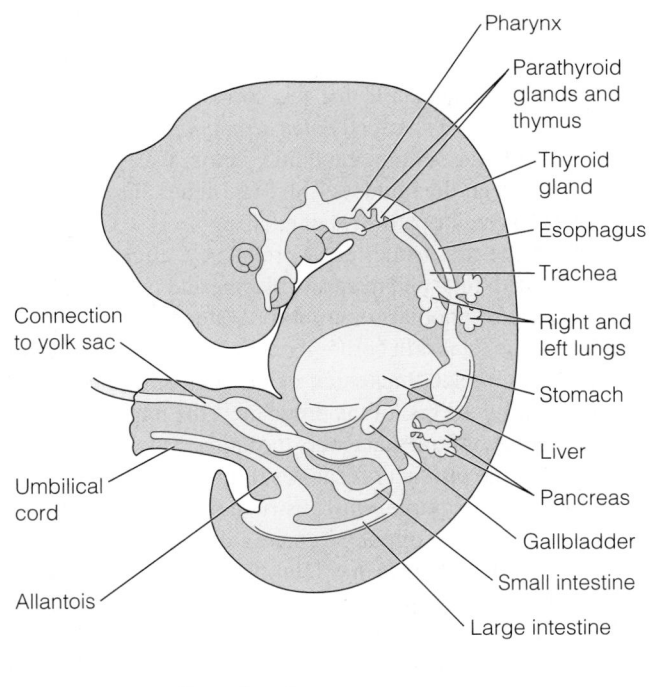

5-week embryo

Figure 11–7 ◆ Endoderm differentiates to form the epithelial lining of the digestive and respiratory tracts and associated glands.

Figure 11–8 ◆ Early development of primary embryonic membranes. At 4 1/2 weeks, the decidua capsularis (placental portion enclosing the embryo on the uterine surface) and decidua basalis (placental portion encompassing the elaborate chorionic villi and maternal endometrium) are well formed. The chorionic villi lie in blood-filled intervillous spaces within the endometrium. The amnion and yolk sac are well developed.

like projections, called *chorionic villi,* on its surface. These chorionic villi can be used for early genetic testing of the embryo at 8 to 11 weeks' gestation by chorionic villi sampling (see Chapter 21 ∞). As the pregnancy progresses, the villi begin to degenerate, except for those just under the embryo, which grow and branch into depressions in the uterine wall, forming the fe-

tal portion of the placenta. By the fourth month of pregnancy, the surface of the chorion is smooth except at the place of attachment to the uterine wall.

The second membrane, the amnion, originates from the ectoderm, a primary germ layer, during the early stages of embryonic development. The **amnion** is a thin protective membrane

Table 11–2	DERIVATION OF BODY STRUCTURES FROM PRIMARY CELL LAYERS	
Ectoderm	**Mesoderm**	**Endoderm**
Epidermis	Dermis	Respiratory tract epithelium
Sweat glands	Wall of digestive tract	Epithelium (except nasal), including pharynx tongue, tonsils, thyroid, parathyroid, thymus tympanic cavity
Sebaceous glands	Kidneys and ureter (suprarenal cortex)	
Nails	Reproductive organs (gonads, genital ducts)	
Hair follicles	Connective tissue (cartilage, bone, joint cavities)	Lining of digestive tract
Lens of eye	Skeleton	Primary tissue of liver and pancreas
Sensory epithelium of internal and external ear, nasal cavity, sinuses, mouth, anal canal	Muscles (all types)	Urethra and associated glands
Central and peripheral nervous systems	Cardiovascular system (heart, arteries, veins, blood, bone marrow)	Urinary bladder (except trigone)
Nasal cavity	Pleura	Vagina (parts)
Oral glands and tooth enamel	Lymphatic tissue and cells	
Pituitary gland	Spleen	
Mammary glands		

that contains amniotic fluid. The space between the amniotic membrane and the embryo is the *amniotic cavity.* This cavity surrounds the embryo and yolk sac, except where the developing embryo (germ layer disc) attaches to the trophoblast via the umbilical cord. As the embryo grows, the amnion expands until it comes in contact with the chorion. These two slightly adherent membranes form the fluid-filled amniotic sac, also called **bag of waters (BOW),** which protects the floating embryo.

AMNIOTIC FLUID

The primary functions of **amniotic fluid** are to:

- Act as a cushion to protect the embryo against mechanical injury
- Help control the embryo's temperature (relies on the mother to release heat)
- Permit symmetric external growth and development of the embryo
- Act as an extension of fetal extracellular space (hydropic infants have increased amniotic fluid)
- Prevent adherence of the embryo-fetus to the amnion (decreases chance of amniotic band syndrome) to allow freedom of movement so that the embryo-fetus can change position (flexion and extension), thus aiding in musculoskeletal development
- Allow the umbilical cord to be relatively free of compression
- Act as a wedge during labor
- Provide fluid for analysis to determine fetal health and maturity

Amniotic fluid is slightly alkaline and contains albumin, urea, uric acid, creatinine, lecithin, sphingomyelin, bilirubin, fat, fructose, leukocytes, proteins, epithelial cells, enzymes, and fine hair called **lanugo.** The amount of amniotic fluid at 10 weeks is about 30 mL and increases to 350 mL at 20 weeks. After 20 weeks the volume ranges from 700 to 1000 mL. The amniotic fluid vol-

ume is constantly changing as the fluid moves back and forth across the placental membrane. As the pregnancy continues, the fetus contributes to the volume of amniotic fluid by excreting urine. The fetus also swallows up to 600 mL of the fluid every 24 hours. Approximately 400 mL of amniotic fluid flows out of the fetal lungs each day. Abnormal variations in amniotic fluid volume are *oligohydramnios* (less than 400 mL of amniotic fluid) and *hydramnios* (more than 2000 mL or amniotic fluid index greater than 97.5 percentile for the corresponding gestational age). Hydramnios is also called *polyhydramnios.* Chapter 27 ∞ discusses alterations in amniotic fluid volume. Water and solutes must pass between the amniotic fluid and fetus. Figure 11–9 ◆ summarizes the major pathways of exchange.

Early in the first trimester of pregnancy, amniotic fluid is iso-osmolar with fetal and maternal plasma and is secreted from the developing trophoblast or embryo. Water and solutes move freely across the fetal skin before the time of skin keratinization. After 23 to 25 weeks, thickening of the fetal skin inhibits this diffusion. During the rest of the pregnancy, the fetal kidneys are the major source of fluid that enters the amniotic sac. Abnormalities of fetal urine production can result in changes in amniotic fluid volume. For example, with obstruction of urine outflow, as in Potter's syndrome, oligohydramnios develops. Conversely, Bartter's syndrome results in a fetal diuresis and hydramnios. The fetal lungs are also significant contributors to amniotic fluid. Fetal breathing movements are associated with the bidirectional flow of fluid through the trachea. Net outflow from the fetal lungs averages 4.3 mL/kg/hr or 10% of body weight per day. This outflow of lung and tracheal fluid is used as the basis for amniotic fluid tests of fetal lung maturity.

The major mechanism by which amniotic fluid is removed in the last half of the pregnancy is fetal swallowing, which occurs mostly during periods of fetal breathing movements. In pregnancy when the fetus does not swallow normal amounts of amniotic fluid (as in esophageal atresia and anencephalus), hydramnios will result. A potential route of amniotic fluid removal is by the transmembranous pathway, that is, the movement of fluid across the amniochorion and into the maternal circulation

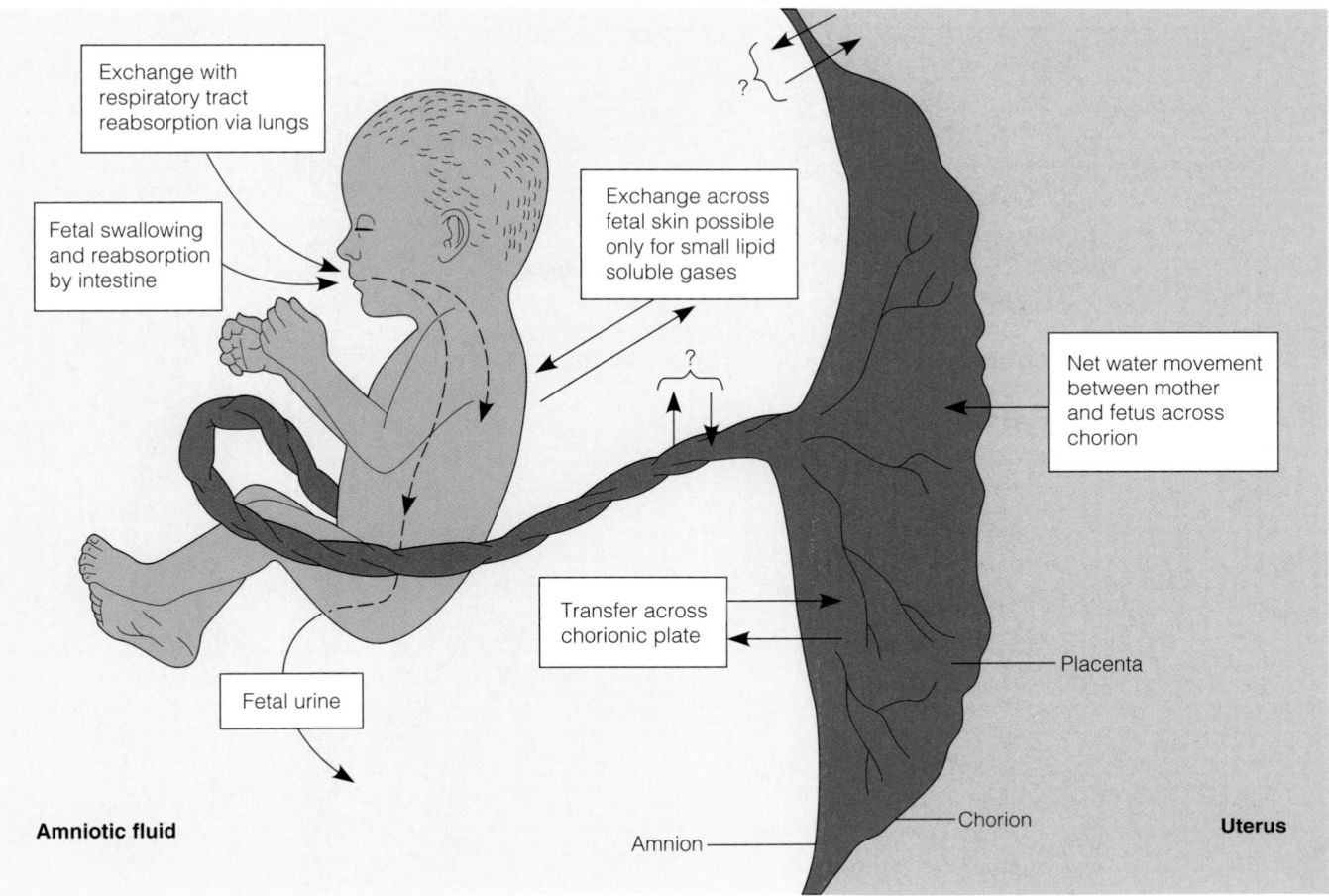

Figure 11–9 ◆ Summary of the significant pathways of water and solute exchange between the amniotic fluid and fetus.
SOURCE: Used with permission from Seeds, A. E. (1980, November). Current concepts of amniotic fluid dynamics. *American Journal of Obstetrics and Gynecology, 138,* 575.

within the uterine wall. Another major regulator of amniotic fluid volume and composition is the intramembranous pathway. This pathway causes amniotic water and/or solutes to be absorbed by the fetal blood that perfuses the fetal surface of the placenta.

YOLK SAC

In humans the yolk sac is small and functions only in early embryonic life. It develops as a second cavity in the blastocyst, about day 8 or 9 after conception, and forms primitive red blood cells during the first 6 weeks of development until the embryo's liver takes over the process. As the embryo develops, the yolk sac is incorporated in the umbilical cord, where it can be identified as a degenerate structure after birth.

UMBILICAL CORD

As the placenta is developing, the **umbilical cord** is also being formed from the amnion. The *body stalk,* which attaches the embryo to the yolk sac, contains blood vessels that extend into the chorionic villi. The body stalk fuses with the embryonic portion of the placenta to provide a circulatory pathway from the chorionic villi to the embryo (see Figure 11–9). As the body stalk elongates to become the umbilical cord, the vessels in the cord decrease to one large vein and two smaller arteries. About 1% of umbilical cords have only two vessels, an artery and a vein;

this condition may be associated with congenital malformations, primarily of the renal, cardiovascular, and gastrointestinal systems. A specialized connective tissue known as **Wharton's jelly** surrounds the blood vessels in the umbilical cord. This tissue, plus the high blood volume pulsating through the vessels, prevents compression of the umbilical cord in utero. The umbilical cord has no sensory or motor innervation, so cutting the cord after birth is not painful. At term (38 to 42 weeks' gestation), the average cord is 2 cm (0.8 in.) across and about 55 cm (22 in.) long. The cord can attach itself to the placenta at various sites. Central insertion into the placenta is considered normal. (Chapter 26 ∞ discusses the various attachment sites).

Umbilical cords appear twisted or spiraled. This is most likely caused by fetal movement. A true knot in the umbilical cord rarely occurs; if it does, the cord is usually long. More common are so-called false knots caused by the folding of cord vessels. A nuchal cord exists when the umbilical cord encircles the fetal neck.

TWINS

Twinning occurs in approximately 1 in 80 pregnancies, and triplets in 1 in 8000 pregnancies. Fraternal (dizygotic) twins have been reported to occur more often among black than among white women and more often among white individuals

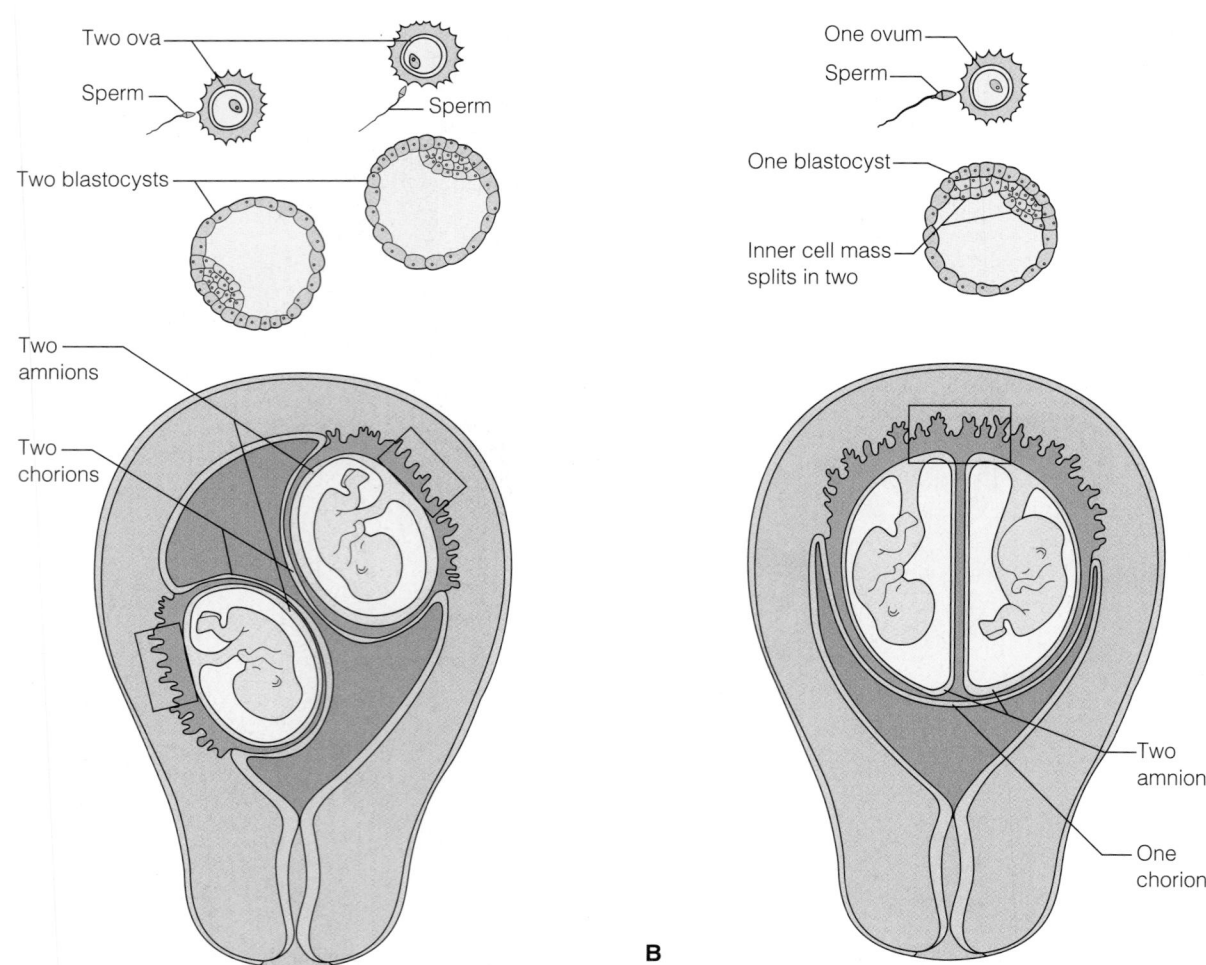

Figure 11–10 ◆ *A,* Formation of fraternal twins. (Note separate placentas.) *B,* Formation of identical twins.

than among women of Asian origin (Moore & Persaud, 2003). Among all groups, as parity (having given birth to a viable infant) increases so does the chance for multiple births.

Twins may be either fraternal or identical (Figure 11–10 ◆). If they are fraternal, they are dizygotic, which means they arise from two separate ova fertilized by two separate spermatozoa. There are two placentas, two chorions, and two amnions; however, the placentas sometimes fuse and look as if they are one. Despite their birth relationship, fraternal twins are no more similar to each other than they would be to siblings born singly. They may be the same or different sex.

Dizygotic twinning increases with maternal age up to about 35 years and then decreases abruptly. The chance of dizygotic twins increases with parity, in conceptions that occur in the first 3 months of a relationship, and with increased coital frequency. The chance of dizygotic twinning decreases during periods of malnutrition and during winter and spring for women living in the Northern hemisphere. Studies indicate that dizygotic twins tend to occur in certain families, perhaps because of genetic factors that result in elevated serum gonadotropin levels leading to double ovulation (Benirschke, 2004a).

Identical, or monozygotic, twins develop from a single fertilized ovum. They are of the same sex and have the same phenotype (appearance). Identical twins usually have a common placenta (see Figure 11–10). Monozygosity is not affected by environment, race, physical characteristics, or fertility.

Monozygotic twins originate from division of the fertilized ovum at different stages of early development, after the zygote consists of thousands of cells. Complete separation of the cellular mass into two parts is necessary for twin formation. The number of amnions and chorions present depends on the timing of the division.

• If division occurs within 3 days of fertilization (before the inner cell mass and chorion are formed), two embryos, two amnions, and two chorions will develop. This dichorionic-diamniotic situation occurs about 20% to 30% of the time, and there may be two distinct placentas or a single fused placenta.

• If division occurs about 5 days after fertilization (when the inner cell mass is formed and the chorion cells have differentiated but those of the amnion have not), two embryos develop with separate amnion sacs. These sacs will eventually be covered by a common chorion; thus there will be a monochorionic-diamniotic placenta.

• If the amnion has already developed approximately 7 to 13 days after fertilization, division results in two embryos with a common amnion sac and a common chorion. This type occurs about 1% of the time (Benirschke, 2004a).

Monozygotic twinning is considered a random event and occurs in approximately 3.5 per 1000 live births (Benirschke, 2004a). The survival rate of monozygotic twins as a group is 10% lower than that of dizygotic twins, and congenital anomalies are more prevalent. Both twins may have the same malformation.

DEVELOPMENT AND FUNCTIONS OF THE PLACENTA

The **placenta** is the means of metabolic and nutrient exchange between the embryonic and maternal circulations. Placental development and circulation does not begin until the third week of embryonic development. The placenta develops at the site where the developing embryo attaches to the uterine wall. Expansion of the placenta continues until about 20 weeks, when it covers about half the inside of the uterus. After 20 weeks' gestation, the placenta becomes thicker but not wider. At 40 weeks' gestation, the placenta is about 15 to 20 cm (5.9 to 7.9 in.) in diameter and 2.5 to 3.0 cm (1 to 1.2 in.) in thickness. It weighs approximately 400 to 600 g (14 to 21 oz).

The placenta has two parts: the maternal portion and the fetal portion. The maternal portion consists of the decidua basalis and its circulation. Its surface is red and fleshlike. The fetal portion consists of the chorionic villi and their circulation. The fetal surface of the placenta is covered by the amnion, which gives it a shiny, gray appearance (Figures 11–11 ◆ and 11–12 ◆).

Development of the placenta begins with the chorionic villi. The trophoblast cells of the chorionic villi form spaces in the tissue of the decidua basalis. These spaces fill with maternal blood, and the chorionic villi grow into these spaces. As the chorionic villi differentiate, two trophoblastic layers appear: an outer layer called the *syncytium* (consisting of syncytiotrophoblasts), and an inner layer known as the *cytotrophoblast* (Figure 11–13 ◆). The cytotrophoblast thins out and disappears about the fifth month, leaving only a single layer of syncytium covering the chorionic villi. The syncytium is in direct contact with the maternal blood

Figure 11–11 ◆ Maternal side of placenta (Dirty Duncan).
SOURCE: Photo courtesy of M. London.

Figure 11–12 ◆ Fetal side of placenta (Shiny Schultz).
SOURCE: Photo courtesy of M. London.

Figure 11–13 ◆ Longitudinal section of placental villus. Spaces formed in the maternal decidua are filled with maternal blood; chorionic villi proliferate into these maternal blood-filled spaces and differentiate into a syncytium layer and a cytotrophoblast layer.

in the intervillous spaces. It is the functional layer of the placenta and secretes the placental hormones of pregnancy.

A third, inner layer of connective mesoderm develops in the chorionic villi, forming *anchoring villi*. These anchoring villi eventually form the *septa* (partitions) of the placenta. These septa divide the mature placenta into 15 to 20 segments called **cotyledons** (subdivisions of the placenta made up of anchoring villi and decidual tissue). In each cotyledon, the *branching villi* form a highly complex vascular system that allows compartmentalization of the uteroplacental circulation. The exchange of gases and nutrients takes place across these vascular systems.

Exchange of substances across the placenta is minimal during the first 3 to 5 months of development because the villous membrane is initially too thick, which limits its permeability. As the villous membrane thins, the placental permeability increases (until about the last month of pregnancy, when permeability begins to decrease as the placenta ages). In the fully developed placenta, fetal blood in the villi and maternal blood in the intervillous spaces are separated by three to four thin layers of tissue.

Placental Circulation

After implantation of the blastocyst, the cells differentiate into fetal cells and trophoblastic cells. The proliferating trophoblast successfully invades the decidua basalis of the endometrium, first opening the uterine capillaries and later opening the larger uterine vessels. The chorionic villi are an outgrowth of the blastocystic tissue. As these villi continue to grow and divide, the fetal vessels begin to form. The intervillous spaces in the decidua basalis develop as the endometrial spiral arteries are opened.

By the fourth week the placenta has begun to function as a means of metabolic exchange between embryo and mother. The

completion of the maternal-placental-fetal circulation occurs about 17 days after conception, when the embryonic heart begins functioning (Moore & Persaud, 2003). By 14 weeks the placenta is a discrete organ. It has grown in thickness as a result of growth in the length and size of the chorionic villi and accompanying expansion of the intervillous space.

The *cotyledons* of the maternal surface contain branches of a single placental mainstream villus, allowing for some compartmentalization of the uteroplacental circulation. Each cotyledon is a vascular unit containing branching vessels that are distributed throughout a particular lobule and partially separated from other lobules by the cotyledon's thin septal partitions.

The capillaries of the villi are lined with an extremely thin endothelium and are surrounded by a layer of mesenchymal (connective) tissue. This connective tissue is covered by chorionic epithelium consisting of cytotrophoblast and syncytiotrophoblast (see Figure 11–13). As previously discussed, the cytotrophoblast thins out and disappears after the fifth month.

In the fully developed placenta's umbilical cord, fetal blood flows through the two umbilical arteries to the capillaries of the villi, and oxygen-enriched blood flows back through the umbilical vein to the fetus (Figure 11–14 ◆). Late in pregnancy, a soft blowing sound (*funic souffle*) can be heard over the area of the umbilical cord of the fetus. The sound is synchronous with the fetal heartbeat and the flow of fetal blood through the umbilical arteries.

Maternal blood, rich in oxygen and nutrients, moves from the arcuate artery to the radial artery to the uterine spiral arteries and then spurts into the intervillous spaces. These spurts are produced by the maternal blood pressure. The spurt of blood is directed toward the chorionic plate, and as the blood flow loses

Figure 11–14 ◆ Vascular arrangement of the placenta. Arrows indicate the direction of blood flow. Maternal blood flows through the uterine arteries to the intervillous spaces of the placenta and returns through the uterine veins to maternal circulation. Fetal blood flows through the umbilical arteries into the villous capillaries of the placenta and returns through the umbilical vein to the fetal circulation.

pressure, it becomes lateral (spreads out). Fresh blood continually enters and exerts pressure on the contents of the intervillous spaces, pushing blood toward the exits in the basal plate. Blood is then drained through the uterine and other pelvic veins. A *uterine souffle* is also heard in the later months of pregnancy. This uterine souffle, which is timed precisely with the mother's pulse and heard just above the mother's symphysis pubis, is caused by the augmented blood flow entering the dilated uterine arteries.

Circulation within the intervillous spaces depends on maternal blood pressure producing a gradient between arterial and venous channels. The lumen of the spiral uterine artery is narrow when it pierces the chorionic plate and enters the intervillous space, resulting in an increased blood pressure. The pressure in the arteries forces the blood into the intervillous spaces and bathes the numerous small villi in oxygenated blood. As the pressure decreases, the blood flows back from the chorionic plate toward the decidua, where it enters the endometrial veins.

Braxton Hicks contractions (see Chapter 14 ∞) are believed to facilitate placental circulation by enhancing the movement of blood from the center of the cotyledon through the intervillous space. Placental blood flow is thought to be enhanced when the woman is lying on her left side, because the vena cava is not compromised. Some evidence exists that lying on either side can enhance blood flow.

Placental Functions

Placental exchange functions occur only in those fetal vessels that are in intimate contact with the covering syncytial membrane. The syncytium villi have brush borders containing many microvilli, which greatly increase the exchange rate between maternal and fetal circulation (Sadler, 2004).

The placental functions, many of which begin soon after implantation, include fetal respiration, nutrition, and excretion. To carry out these functions, the placenta is involved in metabolic and transfer activities. It also has endocrine functions and special immunologic properties.

METABOLIC ACTIVITIES

The placenta produces glycogen, cholesterol, and fatty acids continuously for fetal use and hormone production. The placenta also produces numerous enzymes required for fetoplacental transfer, and it breaks down certain substances, such as epinephrine and histamine. In addition it stores glycogen and iron.

TRANSPORT FUNCTIONS

The placental membranes actively control the transfer of a wide range of substances by four major mechanisms (Bawdon & Hnat, 2003):

1. *Simple diffusion* moves substances from an area of higher concentration to an area of lower concentration. Substances that move across the placenta by simple diffusion include water, oxygen, carbon dioxide, electrolytes (sodium and chloride), anesthetic gases, and drugs. Insulin and steroid hormones originating from the adrenal glands and thyroid hormones also cross the placenta, but at a very slow rate. The rate of oxygen transfer across the placental membrane is greater than that allowed by simple diffusion, indicating that oxygen is also transferred by facilitated diffusion of some type. Unfortunately many substances of abuse, such as cocaine, also cross the placenta via diffusion.

2. *Facilitated transport* involves a carrier system to move molecules from an area of greater concentration to an area of lower concentration. Molecules such as glucose, galactose, and some oxygen are transported by this method. The glucose level in the fetal blood is ordinarily 20% to 30% lower than the glucose level in the maternal blood, because glucose is being metabolized rapidly by the fetus. This lower level, in turn, causes rapid transport of additional glucose from the maternal blood into the fetal blood.

3. *Active transport* can work against a concentration gradient, allowing molecules to move from areas of lower concentration to areas of higher concentration. Amino acids, calcium, iron, iodine, water-soluble vitamins, and glucose are transferred across the placenta this way. The measured amino acid content of fetal blood is greater than that of maternal blood, and calcium and inorganic phosphate occur in greater concentration in fetal blood than in maternal blood (Blackburn, 2003).

Other modes of transport also exist. *Pinocytosis* is important for transferring large molecules, such as albumin and gamma globulin. Materials are engulfed by amoeba-like cells forming plasma droplets. *Hydrostatic and osmotic pressures* allow the bulk flow of water and some solutes. Fetal red blood cells pass into the maternal circulation through breaks in the placental membrane, particularly during labor and birth. Certain cells, such as maternal leukocytes, and microorganisms, such as viruses (e.g., the human immunodeficiency virus [HIV], which causes acquired immunodeficiency syndrome [AIDS]) and the bacterium *Treponema pallidum,* which causes syphilis, can also cross the placental membrane under their own power (Moore & Persaud, 2003). Some bacteria and protozoa infect the placenta by causing lesions and then entering the fetal blood system.

Several factors, including the following, affect transfer rate:

- Molecular size
- Electrical charge
- Lipid solubility
- Placental area
- Diffusion distance
- Maternal-placental-fetal blood flow
- Blood saturation with gases and nutrients
- pK_a of the substance
- Maternal-placental-fetal metabolism of the substance

Substances that have a molecular weight of 1000 daltons or more have difficulty crossing the placenta by simple diffusion. Therefore, heparin, with a molecular weight above 6000, does not cross the placenta, but warfarin sodium (Coumadin), which has a molecular weight in the 300 to 400 range, crosses easily. Electrically charged molecules cross the placenta more slowly. An example is the muscle relaxant succinylcholine. A lipid-soluble substance moves quickly across the placenta into the fetal circulation.

Reduction of the placental surface area, as with abruptio placentae (partial or complete premature separation of a normally implanted placenta), will lessen the area that is functional for exchange. Placental diffusion distance also affects exchange. In conditions such as diabetes and placental infection, edema of the villi increases the diffusion distance, thus increasing the distance the substance has to be transferred.

Changes in blood flow between the fetus and the maternal intervillous space can be influenced by the transfer rate of substances, the ratio of blood on each side of the placenta, and the binding and dissociation abilities of carrier molecules in the blood. Decreased intervillous space blood flow is seen during labor and with certain maternal disease conditions such as hypertension. Mild fetal hypoxia increases the umbilical blood flow, but severe hypoxia results in decreased blood flow.

As the maternal blood picks up fetal waste products and carbon dioxide, it drains back into the maternal circulation through the veins in the basal plate. Fetal blood is hypoxic by comparison; it therefore attracts oxygen from the mother's blood. Affinity for oxygen also increases as the fetal blood gives up its carbon dioxide, which decreases its acidity.

ENDOCRINE FUNCTIONS

The placenta produces hormones that are vital to survival of the fetus. These include human chorionic gonadotropin (hCG); human placental lactogen (hPL); and two steroid hormones, estrogen and progesterone.

The hormone hCG is similar to luteinizing hormone (LH) and prevents the normal involution of the corpus luteum at the end of the menstrual cycle (see Chapter 10 ∞). If the corpus luteum stops functioning before the 11th week of pregnancy, spontaneous abortion occurs. The hCG also causes the corpus luteum to secrete increased amounts of estrogen and progesterone.

After the 11th week, the placenta produces enough progesterone and estrogen to maintain pregnancy. In the male fetus, hCG also exerts an interstitial cell–stimulating effect on the testes, resulting in the production of testosterone. This small secretion of testosterone during embryonic development causes male sex organs to grow. The hormone hCG may play a role in the trophoblast's immunologic capabilities (ability to exempt the placenta and embryo from rejection by the mother's system). This hormone is used as a basis for pregnancy tests (for discussion of pregnancy tests, see Chapter 14 ∞).

The hormone hCG is present in maternal blood serum 8 to 10 days after fertilization, just as soon as implantation has occurred, and is detectable in maternal urine at the time of the missed menses. Chorionic gonadotropin reaches its maximum level at 50 to 70 days' gestation and then begins to decrease as placental hormone production increases.

Progesterone is a hormone essential for pregnancy. It increases the secretions of the fallopian tubes and uterus to provide appropriate nutritive matter for the developing morula and blastocyst. It also appears to aid in ovum transport through the fallopian tube (Liu, 2004). Progesterone causes decidual cells to develop in the uterine endometrium, and it must be present in

high levels for implantation to occur. Progesterone also decreases the contractility of the uterus, thus preventing uterine contractions from causing spontaneous abortion.

Before hCG stimulation, the production of progesterone by the corpus luteum reaches a peak about 7 to 10 days after ovulation. Implantation occurs at about the same time as this peak. At 16 days after ovulation, the production of progesterone reaches a level between 25 and 50 mg per day and continues to rise slowly in subsequent weeks. After 10 weeks, the placenta (specifically, the syncytiotrophoblast) takes over the production of progesterone and secretes it in tremendous quantities, reaching levels of more than 250 mg per day late in pregnancy.

By 7 weeks, the placenta produces more than 50% of the estrogens in the maternal circulation. *Estrogens* serve mainly a proliferative function, causing enlargement of the uterus, breasts, and breast glandular tissue. Estrogens also have a significant role in increasing vascularity and vasodilation, particularly in the villous capillaries, near the end of pregnancy. Placental estrogens increase markedly toward the end of pregnancy, to as much as 30 times the daily production in the middle of a normal monthly menstrual cycle. The primary estrogen secreted by the placenta is different from that secreted by the ovaries. The placenta secretes mainly *estriol*, whereas the ovaries secrete primarily estradiol. The placenta cannot synthesize estriol by itself. Essential precursors are provided by the adrenal glands of the fetus and are transported to the placenta for the final conversion to estriol.

The hormone hPL (human placental lactogen; sometimes referred to as human chorionic somatomammotropin, or hCS) is similar to human pituitary growth hormone; hPL stimulates certain changes in the mother's metabolic processes. These changes ensure that more protein, glucose, and minerals are available for the fetus. Secretion of hPL can be detected by about 4 weeks.

IMMUNOLOGIC PROPERTIES

The placenta and embryo are transplants of living tissue within the same species and are therefore considered *homografts*. Unlike other homografts, the placenta and embryo appear exempt from immunologic reaction by the host. The most recent data suggest that there is a suppression of cellular immunity by the placental hormones (progesterone and hCG) during pregnancy. One theory used to explain this phenomenon suggests that trophoblastic tissue is immunologically inert. It may contain a cell coating that masks transplantation antigens, repels sensitized lymphocytes, and protects against antibody formation.

DEVELOPMENT OF THE FETAL CIRCULATORY SYSTEM

The circulatory system of the fetus has several unique features that, by maintaining the blood flow to the placenta, provide the fetus with oxygen and nutrients while removing carbon dioxide and other waste products.

Most of the blood supply bypasses the fetal lungs because they do not carry out respiratory gas exchange. The placenta assumes the function of the fetal lungs by supplying oxygen and allowing the fetus to excrete carbon dioxide into the maternal

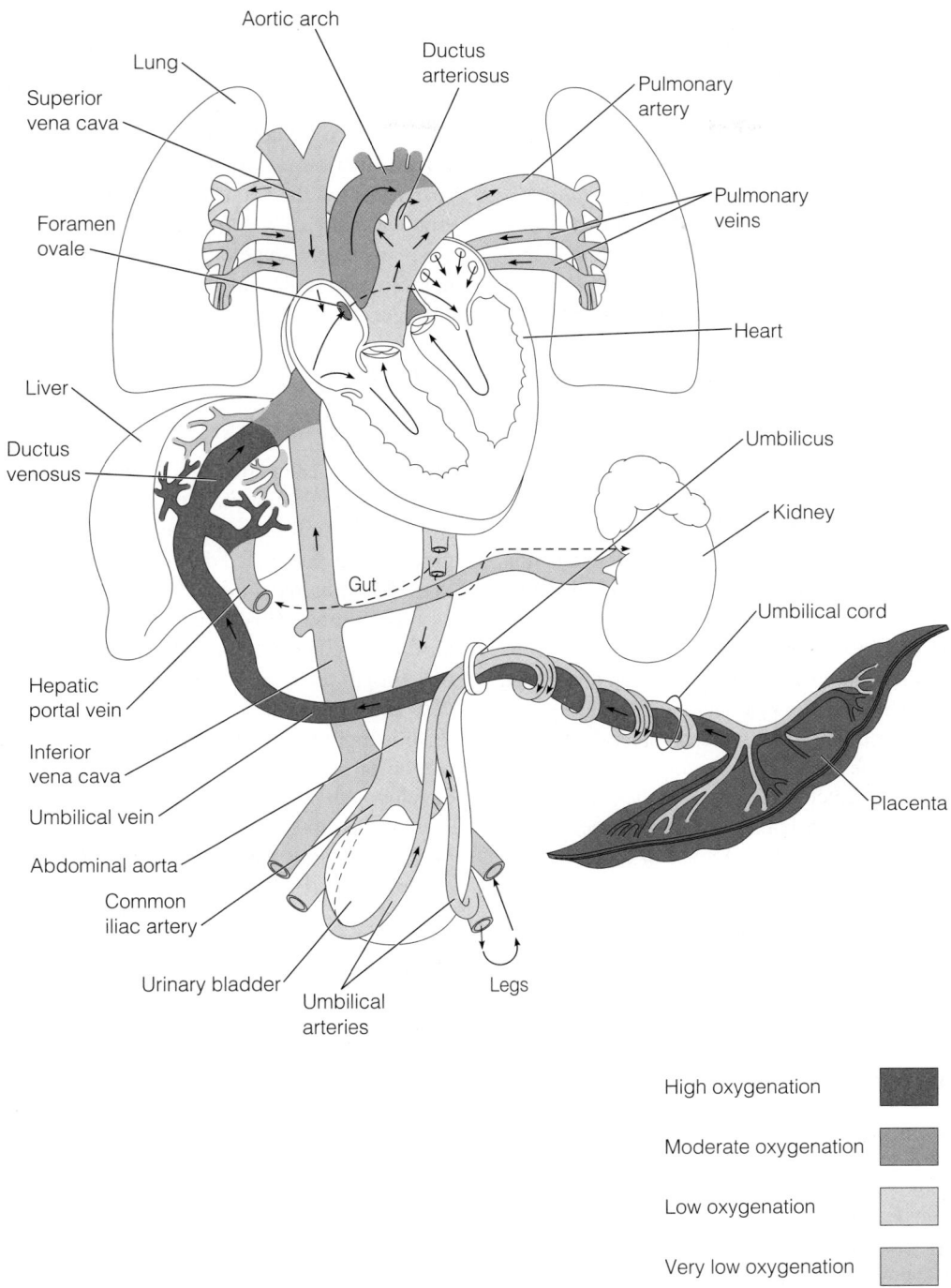

Figure 11–15 ◆ Fetal circulation. Blood leaves the placenta and enters the fetus through the umbilical vein. After circulating through the fetus, the blood returns to the placenta through the umbilical arteries. The ductus venosus, the foramen ovale, and the ductus arteriosus allow the blood to bypass the fetal liver and lungs.

bloodstream. Figure 11–15 ◆ shows the fetal circulatory system. The blood from the placenta flows through the umbilical vein, which enters the abdominal wall of the fetus at the site that, after birth, is the umbilicus (belly button). As umbilical venous blood approaches the liver, a small portion of the blood enters the liver sinusoids, mixes with blood from the portal circulation, and then enters the inferior vena cava via hepatic veins. Most of the umbilical vein's blood flows through the **ductus venosus** directly into the inferior vena cava, bypassing the liver. This blood then enters

the right atrium, passes through the **foramen ovale** into the left atrium, and pours into the left ventricle, which pumps it into the aorta. Some blood returning from the head and upper extremities by way of the superior vena cava is emptied into the right atrium and passes through the tricuspid valve into the right ventricle. This blood is pumped into the pulmonary artery, and a small amount passes to the lungs and provides nourishment only. The larger portion of blood passes from the pulmonary artery through the **ductus arteriosus** into the descending aorta, bypassing the lungs. Finally, blood returns to the placenta through the two umbilical arteries, and the process is repeated.

The fetus receives oxygen via diffusion from the maternal circulation because of the gradient difference of Po_2 of 50 mm Hg in maternal blood in the placenta to a 30 mm Hg Po_2 in the fetus. At term the fetus receives oxygen from the mother's circulation at a rate of 20 to 30 mL/min (Sadler, 2004). Fetal hemoglobin facilitates obtaining oxygen from the maternal circulation because it carries as much as 20% to 30% more oxygen than adult hemoglobin. For further discussion, see Chapter 28. ∞

Fetal circulation delivers the highest available oxygen concentration to the head, neck, brain, and heart (coronary circulation) and a lesser amount of oxygenated blood to the abdominal organs and the lower body. This circulatory pattern leads to cephalocaudal (head-to-tail) development in the fetus.

Fetal Heart

The heart of the fetus, as in the adult, is under the control of its own pacemaker. The sinoatrial (SA) node sets the rate and is supplied by the vagus nerve. Bridging the atrium and the ventricle is the atrioventricular (AV) node, also supplied by the vagus nerve. Baseline changes in the fetal heartbeat have been shown to be under the influence of this nerve. Atropine will block this effect.

When the fetus is stressed, the sympathetic nervous system causes the release of norepinephrine, which increases the fetal heart rate. To counteract the increase in blood pressure, baroreceptors, which respond to stretch, are present in the vessel walls at the junction of the internal and external carotid arteries. When stimulated, these receptors, under the influence of the vagus and glossopharyngeal nerves, cause the heart rate to slow.

Chemoreceptors in the fetal peripheral and central nervous systems respond to decreased oxygen tensions and to increased carbon dioxide tensions, leading to fetal tachycardia and an increase in blood pressure. The central nervous system (CNS) also has control over heart rate. Increased activity of the fetus in a wakeful period is exhibited in an *increase in the beat-to-beat variability* of the fetal heart baseline. Sleep patterns demonstrate a *decrease in the beat-to-beat baseline variability*. In cases of severe hypoxia, increased levels of epinephrine and norepinephrine act on the fetal heart to produce a faster and stronger rate.

EMBRYONIC AND FETAL DEVELOPMENT

Pregnancy is calculated to last an *average* of 10 lunar months: 40 weeks, or 280 days. This period of 280 days is calculated from the beginning of the last normal menstrual period to the time of birth. Estimated date of birth (EDB), sometimes referred to as the *estimated date of delivery (EDD)*, is usually calculated by this method. Most fetuses are born within 10 to 14 days of the calculated date of birth. The fertilization age (or postconception age) of the fetus is calculated to be *about* 2 weeks less, 266 days (38 weeks) or 9 1/2 calendar months. The latter measurement is more accurate because it measures time from the fertilization of the ovum, or conception. The basic events of organ development in the embryo and fetus are outlined in Table 11–3. The time periods used in Table 11–3 are **postconception age periods.** During the period from fertilization to the end of the embryonic period (8 weeks), age is often expressed in days but

---

Table 11–3 SUMMARY OF ORGAN SYSTEM DEVELOPMENT	
Age: 2–3 Weeks	**Age: 5 Weeks**
Length: 2 mm C–R (Crown to rump).	**Length:** 8 mm C–R.
Nervous system: Groove forms along middle back as cells thicken; neural tube forms from closure of neural groove.	**Weight:** Only 0.5% of total body weight is fat (to 20 weeks).
Cardiovascular system: Beginning of blood circulation; tubular heart begins to form during third week.	**Nervous system:** Brain has differentiated and cranial nerves are present.
Gastrointestinal system: Liver begins to function.	**Musculoskeletal system:** Developing muscles have innervation.
Genitourinary system: Formation of kidneys beginning.	**Cardiovascular system:** Atrial division has occurred.
Respiratory system: Nasal pits forming.	
Endocrine system: Thyroid tissue appears.	**Age: 6 Weeks**
Eyes: Optic cup and lens pit have formed; pigment in eyes.	**Length:** 12 mm C–R.
Ears: Auditory pit is now enclosed structure.	**Musculoskeletal system:** Bone rudiments present; primitive skeletal shape forming; muscle mass begins to develop; ossification of skull and jaws begins.
Age: 4 Weeks	**Cardiovascular system:** Chambers present in heart; groups of blood cells can be identified.
Length: 4–6 mm C–R.	**Gastrointestinal system:** Oral and nasal cavities and upper lip formed; liver begins to form red blood cells.
Weight: 0.4 g.	**Respiratory system:** Trachea, bronchi, and lung buds present.
Nervous system: Anterior portion of neural tube closes to form brain; closure of posterior end forms spinal cord.	**Ears:** Formation of external, middle, and inner ear continues.
Musculoskeletal system: Noticeable limb buds.	**Sexual development:** Embryonic sex glands appear.
Cardiovascular system: Tubular heart beats at 28 days, and primitive red blood cells circulate through fetus and chorionic villi.	**Age: 7 Weeks**
Gastrointestinal system: Mouth: formation of oral cavity; primitive jaws present; esophagotracheal septum begins division of esophagus and trachea. Digestive tract: stomach forms; esophagus and intestine become tubular; ducts of pancreas and liver forming.	**Length:** 18 mm C–R.
	Cardiovascular system: Fetal heartbeats can be detected.

Table 11–3   SUMMARY OF ORGAN SYSTEM DEVELOPMENT continued

Gastrointestinal system: Mouth: tongue separates; palate folds. Digestive tract: stomach attains final form.

Genitourinary system: Separation of bladder and urethra from rectum.

Respiratory system: Diaphragm separates abdominal and thoracic cavities.

Eyes: Optic nerve formed; eyelids appear, thickening of lens.

Sexual development: Differentiation of sex glands into ovaries and testes begins.

Age: 8 Weeks

Length: 2.5–3 cm C–R.

Weight: 2 g.

Musculoskeletal system: Digits formed; further differentiation of cells in primitive skeleton; cartilaginous bones show first signs of ossification; development of muscles in trunk, limbs, and head; some movement of fetus now possible.

Cardiovascular system: Development of heart essentially complete; fetal circulation follows two circuits—four extraembryonic and two intraembryonic. Heartbeat can be heard with Doppler at 8–12 weeks.

Gastrointestinal system: Mouth: completion of lip fusion. Digestive tract: rotation in midgut; anal membrane has perforated.

Ears: External, middle, and inner ear assuming final forms.

Sexual development: Male and female external genitals appear similar until end of ninth week.

Age: 10 Weeks

Length: 5–6 cm C–H (crown to heel).

Weight: 14 g.

Nervous system: Neurons appear at caudal end of spinal cord; basic divisions of brain present.

Musculoskeletal system: Fingers and toes begin nail growth.

Gastrointestinal system: Mouth: separation of lips from jaw; fusion of palate folds. Digestive tract: developing intestines enclosed in abdomen.

Genitourinary system: Bladder sac formed.

Endocrine system: Islets of Langerhans differentiated.

Eyes: Eyelids fused closed; development of lacrimal duct.

Sexual development: Males: production of testosterone and physical characteristics between 8 and 12 weeks.

Age: 12 Weeks

Length: 8 cm C–R; 11.5 cm C–H.

Weight: 45 g.

Musculoskeletal system: Clear outlining of miniature bones (12–20 weeks); process of ossification is established throughout fetal body; appearance of involuntary muscles in viscera.

Gastrointestinal system: Mouth: completion of palate. Digestive tract: appearance of muscles in gut; bile secretion begins; liver is major producer of red blood cells.

Respiratory system: Lungs acquire definitive shape.

Skin: Pink and delicate.

Endocrine system: Hormonal secretion from thyroid; insulin present in pancreas.

Immunologic system: Appearance of lymphoid tissue in fetal thymus gland.

Age: 16 Weeks

Length: 13.5 cm C–R; 15 cm C–H.

Weight: 200 g.

Musculoskeletal system: Teeth beginning to form hard tissue that will become central incisors.

Gastrointestinal system: Mouth: differentiation of hard and soft palate. Digestive tract: development of gastric and intestinal glands; intestines begin to collect meconium.

Genitourinary system: Kidneys assume typical shape and organization.

Skin: Appearance of scalp hair; lanugo present on body; transparent skin with visible blood vessels; sweat glands developing.

Eyes, ears, and nose: Formed.

Sexual development: Sex determination possible.

Age: 18 Weeks

Musculoskeletal system: Teeth beginning to form hard tissue (enamel and dentine) that will become lateral incisors.

Cardiovascular system: Fetal heart tones audible with fetoscope at 16–20 weeks.

Age: 20 Weeks

Length: 19 cm C–R; 25 cm C–H.

Weight: 435 g (6% of total body weight is fat).

Nervous system: Myelination of spinal cord begins.

Musculoskeletal system: Teeth beginning to form hard tissue that will become canine and first molar. Lower limbs are of final relative proportions.

Gastrointestinal system: Fetus actively sucks and swallows amniotic fluid; peristaltic movements begin.

Skin: Lanugo covers entire body; brown fat begins to form; vernix caseosa begins to form.

Immunologic system: Detectable levels of fetal antibodies (IgG type).

Blood formation: Iron is stored and bone marrow is increasingly important.

Age: 24 Weeks

Length: 23 cm C–R; 28 cm C–H.

Weight: 780 g.

Nervous system: Brain looks like mature brain.

Musculoskeletal system: Teeth are beginning to form hard tissue that will become the second molars.

Respiratory system: Respiratory movements may occur (24–40 weeks). Nostrils reopen. Alveoli appear in lungs and begin production of surfactant; gas exchange possible.

Skin: Reddish and wrinkled, vernix caseosa present.

Immunologic system: IgG levels reach maternal levels.

Age: 28 Weeks

Length: 27 cm C–R; 35 C–H.

Weight: 1200–1250 g.

Nervous system: Begins regulation of some body functions.

Skin: Adipose tissue accumulates rapidly; nails appear; eyebrows and eyelashes present.

Eyes: Eyelids open (28–32 weeks).

Sexual development: Males: testes descend into inguinal canal and upper scrotum.

Age: 32 Weeks

Length: 31 cm C–R; 38–43 cm C–H.

Weight: 2000 g.

Nervous system: More reflexes present.

(Continued on next page)

Table 11–3 SUMMARY OF ORGAN SYSTEM DEVELOPMENT continued	
Age: 36 Weeks	**Age: 38–40 Weeks**
Length: 35 cm C–R; 42–48 cm C–H.	**Length:** 40 cm C–R; 48–52 cm C–H.
Weight: 2500–2750 g.	**Weight:** 3200 + g (16% of total body weight is fat).
Musculoskeletal system: Distal femoral ossification centers present.	**Respiratory system:** At 38 weeks, lecithin-sphingomyelin (L/S) ratio approaches 2:1 (indicates decreased risk of respiratory distress from inadequate surfactant production if born now).
Skin: Pale; body rounded, lanugo disappearing, hair fuzzy or woolly; few sole creases; sebaceous glands active and helping to produce vernix caseosa (36–40 weeks).	**Skin:** Smooth and pink; vernix present in skin folds; moderate to profuse silky hair; lanugo on shoulders and upper back; nails extend over tips or digits; creases cover sole.
Ears: Earlobes soft with little cartilage.	**Ears:** Earlobes firmer due to increased cartilage.
Sexual development: Males: scrotum small and few rugae present; descent of testes into upper scrotum to stay (36–40 weeks). Females: labia majora and minora equally prominent.	**Sexual development:** Males: rugous scrotum. Females: labia majora well developed and minora small or completely covered.

NOTE: Age refers to postfertilization or postconception age.

SOURCE: Data from Sadler, T. W. (2004). *Langman's medical embryology* (9th ed). Baltimore: Lippincott, Williams & Wilkins.

can be given in weeks. During the fetal period (9th week until birth), age is given in weeks (Moore & Persaud, 2003). For a detailed discussion of each body system's development, see Chapter 28 ∞; the foldout poster at the front of the book summarizes fetal development.

Human development follows three stages. The preembryonic stage just discussed consists of the first 14 days of development after the ovum is fertilized; the embryonic stage covers the period from day 15 until approximately the eighth week; and the fetal stage extends from the end of the eighth week until birth.

Embryonic Stage

The stage of the **embryo** starts on day 15 (beginning of the third week after conception) and continues until approximately 8 weeks or until the embryo reaches a crown-to-rump (C–R) length of 3 cm (1.2 in.). This length is usually reached about 56 days after fertilization (the end of the eighth gestational week). During the embryonic stage, tissue differentiates into essential organs, and the main external features develop (Figure 11–16 ◆). The embryo is most vulnerable to teratogens during this period.

Fertilization
1-week conceptus
2-week conceptus
Embryo
3-week embryo
4-week embryo
5-week embryo
6-week embryo
7-week embryo
8-week embryo
9-week fetus
12-week fetus

Figure 11–16 ◆ The actual size of a human conceptus from fertilization to the early fetal stage. The embryonic stage begins in the third week after fertilization; the fetal stage begins in the ninth week.

THREE WEEKS

In the third week, the embryonic disc becomes elongated and pear-shaped, with a broad cephalic end and a narrow caudal end. The ectoderm has formed a long cylindrical tube called the notochord for brain and spinal cord development. The gastrointestinal tract, created from the endoderm, appears as another tubelike structure communicating with the yolk sac. The most advanced organ is the heart. At 3 weeks, a single tubular heart forms just outside the body cavity of the embryo.

FOUR TO FIVE WEEKS

During days 21 to 32, *somites,* a series of mesodermal blocks, form on either side of the embryo's midline. The vertebrae that form the spinal column will develop from these somites. Before 28 days, arm and leg buds are not visible, but the tail bud is present. The pharyngeal arches—which will form the lower jaw (mandibular arch), hyoid bone, and cartilage of the larynx—develop at this time. The pharyngeal pouches appear now; these pouches will form the eustachian tube and cavity of the middle ear, the tonsils, and the parathyroid and thymus glands. The primordia of the ear and eye are also present (Figure 11–17 ◆). By the end of 28 days, the tubular heart is beating at a regular rhythm and pushing its own primitive blood cells through the main blood vessels.

During the fifth week, the optic cups and lens vesicles of the eye form and the nasal pits develop. Partitioning in the heart occurs with the dividing of the atrium. The embryo has a marked C-shaped body, accentuated by the rudimentary tail and the large head folded over a protuberant trunk (Figure 11–18 ◆). By day 35, the arm and leg buds are well developed, with paddle-shaped hand and foot plates. The heart, circulatory system, and brain show the most advanced development. The brain

has differentiated into five areas, and 10 pairs of cranial nerves are recognizable.

SIX WEEKS

At 6 weeks, the head structures are more highly developed, and the trunk is straighter than in earlier stages. The upper and lower jaws are recognizable, and the external nares are well formed. The trachea has developed, and its caudal end is bifurcated for beginning lung formation. The upper lip has formed, and the palate is developing. The ears are developing rapidly. The arms have begun to extend ventrally across the chest, and both arms and legs have digits, although they may still be webbed. There is a slight elbow bend in the arm, which is more advanced in development than the leg. Beginning at this stage the prominent tail will recede. The heart now has most of its definitive characteristics, and fetal circulation begins to be established. The liver begins to produce blood cells.

SEVEN WEEKS

At 7 weeks, the head of the embryo is rounded and nearly erect (Figure 11–19 ◆). The eyes have shifted from their original lateral position to a forward location, where they are closer together, and the eyelids are beginning to form. The palate is nearing completion, and the tongue is developing in the formed mouth. The gastrointestinal and genitourinary tracts undergo significant changes during the seventh week. Before this time the rectal and urogenital passages formed one tube that ended in a blind pouch; they now separate into two tubular structures. The intestines enter the extraembryonic coelom in the area of the umbilical cord (called umbilical herniation) (Moore & Persaud, 2003). The beginnings of all essential external and internal structures are present.

Figure 11–17 ◆ The embryo at 4 weeks. Pharyngeal arches, pharyngeal pouches, and primordia of the ear and eye are present.
SOURCE: Petit Format/Nestle/Science Source/Photo Researchers, Inc., 60 East 56th Street, New York, NY 10022, www.photoresearchers.com,info@photoresearchers.com.

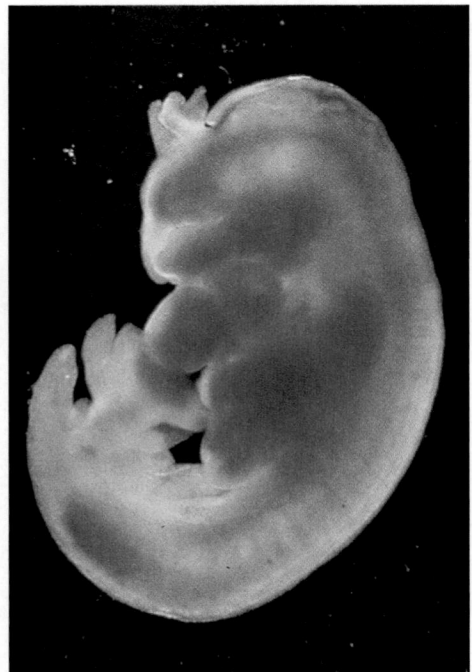

Figure 11–18 ◆ The embryo at 5 weeks. The embryo has a marked C-shaped body and a rudimentary tail.
SOURCE: Petit Format/Nestle/Science Source/Photo Researchers, Inc., 60 East 56th Street, New York, NY 10022, www.photoresearchers.com,info@photoresearchers.com.

Figure 11–19 ◆ The embryo at 7 weeks. The head is rounded and nearly erect. The eyes have shifted forward and are closer together, and the eyelids begin to form.
SOURCE: Petit Format/Nestle/Science Source/Photo Researchers, Inc., 60 East 56th Street, New York, NY 10022, www.photoresearchers.com,info@photoresearchers.com.

EIGHT WEEKS

At 8 weeks, the embryo is approximately 3 cm (1.2 in) C–R and clearly resembles a human being (Figure 11–20 ◆). Facial features continue to develop. The eyelids begin to fuse. Auricles of the external ears begin to assume their final shape, but they are still set low (Moore & Persaud, 2003). External genitals appear, but the embryo's sex is not clearly identifiable. The rectal passage opens with the perforation of the anal membrane. The circulatory system through the umbilical cord is well established. Long bones are beginning to form, and the large muscles are now capable of contracting.

Fetal Stage

By the end of the eighth week, the embryo is sufficiently developed to be called a **fetus.** Every organ system and external

Figure 11–20 ◆ The embryo at 8 weeks. Although only 3 cm in C–R length, the embryo clearly resembles a human being. Facial features continue to develop.
SOURCE: Petit Format/Nestle/Science Source/Photo Researchers, Inc., 60 East 56th Street, New York, NY 10022, www.photoresearchers.com,info@photoresearchers.com.

structure that will be found in the full-term newborn is present. The remainder of gestation is devoted to refining structures and perfecting function.

NINE TO TWELVE WEEKS

By the end of the ninth week, the fetus reaches a C–R length of 5 cm (2 in.) and weighs about 14 g (0.5 oz). The head is large and comprises almost half of the fetus's entire size (Figure 11–21 ◆).

At 12 weeks, the fetus reaches an 8 cm (3.2 in.) C–R length and weighs about 45 g (1.6 oz). The face is well formed, with the nose protruding, the chin small and receding, and the ears acquiring a more adult shape. The eyelids close at about the 10th week and will not begin to reopen until about the 26th week. Some movements of the lips suggestive of the sucking reflex have been observed at 3 months. Tooth buds now appear for all 20 of the child's first teeth (baby teeth). The limbs are long and slender, with well-formed digits. The fetus can curl the fingers toward the palm and make a tiny fist. The legs are still shorter and less developed than the arms. The urogenital tract completes its development, well-differentiated genitals appear, and the kidneys begin to produce urine. Red blood cells are produced primarily by the liver. Spontaneous movements of the

Figure 11–21 ◆ The fetus at 9 weeks. Every organ system and external structure is present.
SOURCE: Used with permission from Nilsson, L. (1990). *A child is born.* New York: Dell Publishing.

Figure 11–22 ◆ The fetus at 14 weeks. During this period of rapid growth, the skin is so transparent that blood vessels are visible beneath it. More muscle tissue and body skeleton have developed, which holds the fetus more erect.
SOURCE: Used with permission from Nilsson, L. (1990). *A child is born.* New York: Dell Publishing.

Figure 11–23 ◆ The fetus at 20 weeks. The fetus weighs approximately 435 to 465 g and measures about 19 cm. Subcutaneous deposits of brown fat make the skin less transparent. "Woolly" hair covers the head, and nails have developed on the fingers and toes.
SOURCE: Used with permission from Nilsson, L. (1990). *A child is born.* New York: Dell Publishing.

fetus occur. Fetal heart tones (the sound of the heartbeat) can be ascertained by electronic devices between 8 and 12 weeks. The heart rate is 120 to 160 beats per minute.

THIRTEEN TO SIXTEEN WEEKS

This is a period of rapid growth. At 13 weeks, the fetus weighs 55 to 60 g (1.9 to 2.1 oz) and is about 9 cm (3.6 in.) in C–R length. Lanugo, or fine hair, begins to develop, especially on the head. Blood vessels are clearly visible beneath transparent skin. More muscle tissue and body skeleton have developed, which holds the fetus more erect (Figure 11–22 ◆). Active movements are present—the fetus stretches and exercises its arms and legs. It makes sucking motions, swallows amniotic fluid, and produces meconium in the intestinal tract. Bronchial tubes are branching out in the primitive lungs, and sweat glands are developing. The liver and pancreas now begin production of their appropriate secretions. By the beginning of week 16, skeletal ossification is clearly identifiable.

TWENTY WEEKS

The fetus doubles its C–R length and now measures about 19 cm (8 in.). Fetal weight is between 435 and 465 g (15.2 and 16.3 oz). Lanugo covers the entire body and is especially prominent on the shoulders. Subcutaneous deposits of brown fat, which has a rich blood supply, make the skin a little less transparent. Nipples now appear over the mammary glands. The head is covered with fine, "woolly" hair, and the eyebrows and eyelashes are beginning to form (Figure 11–23 ◆). Muscles are well developed, and the fetus is active. Fetal movement, known as quickening, is felt by the mother. The fetal heartbeat is audible through the fetoscope. Quickening and fetal heartbeat can help in validating the EDB.

TWENTY-FOUR WEEKS

The fetus at 24 weeks reaches a crown-to-heel (C–H) length of 28 cm (11.2 in.). It weighs about 780 g (1 lb, 10 oz). The hair on the head is growing long, and eyebrows and eyelashes have formed. The eyes are structurally complete and will soon open. The fetus has a reflex hand grip (grasp reflex) and, by the end of 6 months, a startle reflex. Skin covering the body is reddish and wrinkled, with little subcutaneous fat. Skin on the hands and feet has thickened, with skin ridges on palms and soles forming distinct footprints and fingerprints. The skin over the entire body is covered with a protective cheeselike fatty substance, called **vernix caseosa,** secreted by the sebaceous glands. The alveoli in the lungs are just beginning to form.

TWENTY-FIVE TO TWENTY-EIGHT WEEKS

At 6 calendar months, the fetal skin is still red, wrinkled, and covered with vernix caseosa. The brain is developing rapidly, and the nervous system is complete enough to provide some degree of regulation of body functions. The eyelids open and close under neural control. The fetus has nails on both fingers and toes. If the fetus is a male, the testes begin to descend into the scrotal sac. Even though the lungs are still physiologically immature, they are sufficiently developed to provide gas exchange. A fetus born at this time will require immediate and prolonged intensive care in order to survive and to decrease the risk of major handicap. The fetus at 28 weeks is about 35 to 38 cm (14 to 15 in.) long C–H and weighs 1200 to 1250 g (2 lb, 10.5 oz to 2 lb, 12 oz).

TWENTY-NINE TO THIRTY-TWO WEEKS

At 30 weeks, the pupillary light reflex is present (Moore & Persaud, 2003). The fetus is gaining weight from an increase in body muscle and fat and weighs about 2000 g (4 lb, 6.5 oz) with a length of about 38 to 43 cm (15 to 17 in.) by 32 weeks of age. The CNS has matured enough to direct rhythmic breathing movements and partially control body temperature. However, the lungs are not yet fully mature. Bones are now fully developed but are soft and flexible. The fetus begins storing iron, calcium, and phosphorus. In males, the testicles may be located in the scrotal sac but are often still high in the inguinal canals.

THIRTY-FIVE TO THIRTY-SIX WEEKS

The fetus is beginning to get plump with less-wrinkled skin covering the deposits of subcutaneous fat. Lanugo hair is beginning to disappear, and the nails reach the edge of the fingertips. By 35 weeks, the fetus has a firm grasp and exhibits spontaneous orientation to light. By 36 weeks of age, the weight is usually 2500 to 2750 g (5 lb, 12 oz to 6 lb, 11.5 oz), and the C–H length of the fetus is about 42 to 48 cm (16 to 19 in.). An infant born at this time has a good chance of surviving but may require some special care, especially if there is intrauterine growth restriction.

THIRTY-EIGHT TO FORTY WEEKS

The fetus is considered full term at 38 weeks and up to 40 weeks after conception. The C–H length varies from 48 to 52 cm (18 to 21 in.), with males usually longer than females. Males also usually weigh more than females. The weight at term is about 3000 to 3600 g (6 lb, 10 oz to 7 lb, 15 oz) and varies in different ethnic groups. The skin has a smooth polished look. The only lanugo left is on the upper arms and shoulders. The hair on the head is no longer woolly but coarse and about an inch long.

Vernix caseosa is present, with heavier deposits remaining in creases and folds of the skin. The body and extremities are plump, with good skin turgor, and the fingernails extend beyond the fingertips. The chest is prominent but still a little smaller than the head, and mammary glands protrude in both sexes. The testes are in the scrotum or are palpable in the inguinal canals.

As the fetus enlarges, amniotic fluid diminishes to about 500 mL or less, and the fetal body mass fills the uterine cavity. The fetus assumes what is referred to as its *position of comfort,* or lie. The head is generally pointed downward, following the shape of the uterus (and also possibly because the head is heavier than the feet). The extremities and often the head are well flexed. After 5 months, feeding patterns, sleeping patterns, as well as activity patterns become established, so the fetus at term has its own body rhythms and individual style of response. See Table 11–4 Embryonic and Fetal Development: What Parents Want to Know.

FACTORS INFLUENCING EMBRYONIC AND FETAL DEVELOPMENT

Factors that may affect embryonic development include the quality of the sperm or ovum from which the zygote was formed,

Table 11–4	EMBRYONIC AND FETAL DEVELOPMENT: WHAT PARENTS WANT TO KNOW
4 weeks:	The fetal heart begins to beat.
8 weeks:	All body organs are formed.
8–12 weeks:	Fetal heart tones can be heard by Doppler device.
16 weeks:	Baby's sex can be seen. Although thin, the fetus looks like a baby.
20 weeks:	Heartbeat can be heard with fetoscope. Mother feels movement (quickening). Baby develops a regular schedule of sleeping, sucking, and kicking. Hands can grasp. Baby assumes a favorite position in utero. Vernix (lanolin-like covering) protects the body, and lanugo (fine hair) keeps oil on skin. Head hair, eyebrows, and eyelashes present.
24 weeks:	Weighs 1 lb, 10 oz. Activity is increasing. Fetal respiratory movements begin.
28 weeks:	Eyes begin to open and close. Baby can breathe at this time. Surfactant needed for breathing at birth is formed. Baby is two thirds its final size.
32 weeks:	Baby has fingernails and toenails. Subcutaneous fat is being laid down. Baby appears less red and wrinkled.
38+ weeks:	Baby fills total uterus. Baby gets antibodies from mother.

Table 11–5	DEVELOPMENTAL VULNERABILITY TIMETABLE	
Weeks Since Conception	**Potential Teratogen-Induced Malformation**	
3	Ectromelia (congenital absence of one or more limbs)	
	Ectopia cordis (heart lies outside thoracic cavity)	
4	Omphalocele (herniation of abdominal viscera into the umbilical cord)	
	Tracheoesophageal fistula (abnormal connection between trachea and esophagus) (4–5 weeks)	
	Hemivertebra (4–5* weeks)	
5	Nuclear cataract	
	Microphthalmia (abnormally small eyeballs) (5–6* weeks)	
	Facial clefts	
	Carpal or pedal ablation (5–6* weeks)	
6	Gross septal or aortic abnormalities	
	Cleft lip, agnathia (absence of the lower jaw)	
7	Interventricular septal defects	
	Pulmonary stenosis	
	Cleft palate, micrognathia (smallness of the jaw)	
	Epicanthus	
	Brachycephalism (shortness of the head) (7–8* weeks)	
	Mixed sexual characteristics	
8	Persistent ostium primum (persistent opening in atrial septum)	
	Digital stunting (shortening of fingers and toes)	

*May occur in several time periods after conception.

SOURCE: Modified from Danforth, D. N., & Scott. J. R., (1986). *Obstetrics and Gynecology* (5th ed., p. 319). Philadelphia: Lippincott.

the genetic code established at fertilization, and the adequacy of the intrauterine environment. If the environment is unsuitable before cellular differentiation occurs, all the cells of the zygote are affected. The cells may die, which causes spontaneous abortion, or growth may be slowed, depending on the severity of the situation. When differentiation is complete and the fetal membranes have formed, an injurious agent has the greatest effect on those cells undergoing the most rapid growth. Thus the time of injury is critical in the development of anomalies.

Because organs are formed primarily during embryonic development, the growing organism is considered most vulnerable to hazardous agents during the first months of pregnancy. Table 11–5 lists potential malformations related to the time of insult. Any agent, such as a drug, virus, or chemicals, which can cause development of abnormal structures in an embryo is referred to as a **teratogen.** It is important to remember that the effects of teratogens depend on the (1) maternal and fetal genotype, (2) stage of development when exposure occurs, and (3) dose and duration of exposure of the agent. Chapter 14 ∞ discusses the effects of specific teratogenic agents on the developing fetus.

Adequacy of the maternal environment is also important during the periods of rapid embryonic and fetal development.

Maternal nutrition can affect brain development. The period of maximum brain growth and myelination begins with the fifth lunar month before birth and continues during the first 6 months after birth, when there is a twofold increase in myelination (Volpe, 2000). Amino acids, glucose, and fatty acids are considered to be the primary dietary factors in brain growth. A subtle type of damage that affects the associative capacity of the brain, possibly leading to learning disabilities, may be caused by nutritional deficiency at this stage. Vitamins and folic acid supplements taken before conception can reduce the incidence of neural tube defects (Chacko, Anding, Kozinetz et al., 2003). Maternal nutrition may also predispose to the development of adult coronary heart disease, hypertension, and diabetes in babies who were small or disproportionate at birth. Maternal nutrition is discussed in depth in Chapter 18. ∞

Another prenatal influence on the intrauterine environment is maternal hyperthermia associated with sauna baths or hot tub use. Studies of the effects of maternal hyperthermia (temperature over 104F) during the first trimester have raised concern about possible spontaneous abortion, CNS defects, and failure of neural tube closure. The effects of maternal substance abuse on fetal development are discussed in Chapters 19 ∞ and 32. ∞

CHAPTER REVIEW

FOCUS YOUR STUDY

- Humans have 46 chromosomes, which are divided into 23 pairs—22 pairs of autosomes and one pair of sex chromosomes.

- Mitosis is the process by which additional somatic (body) cells are formed. It provides growth and development of the organs and replacement of body cells.

- Meiosis is the process by which gametes (ova and sperm) are formed. It occurs during gametogenesis (oogenesis and spermatogenesis) and consists of two successive cell divisions (reduction division), which produce a gamete with 23 chromosomes (22 chromosomes and 1 sex chromosome)—the haploid number of chromosomes.

- Gametes must have a haploid number (23) of chromosomes so that when the female gamete (ovum) and the male gamete (spermatozoon) unite to form the zygote, the normal human diploid number of chromosomes (46) is reestablished.

- An ovum is considered fertile for about 12 to 24 hours after ovulation, and the sperm is believed to be capable of fertilizing the ovum for about 24 hours after it is deposited in the female reproductive tract.

- Fertilization usually takes place in the ampulla (outer third) of the fallopian tube. Both capacitation and the acrosomal reaction must occur for the sperm to fertilize the ovum. Capacitation is the removal of the plasma membrane, which exposes the acrosomal covering of the sperm head. The acrosomal reaction is the deposit of hyaluronidase in the corona radiata, which allows the sperm head to penetrate the ovum.

- Sex chromosomes are referred to as X and Y. Females have two X chromosomes, and males have an X and a Y chromosome. Y chromosomes are carried only by the sperm. To produce a female child, both the mother and the father contribute an X chromosome. To produce a male child, the mother contributes an X chromosome and the father contributes a Y chromosome.

- Intrauterine development first proceeds via cellular multiplication in which the zygote undergoes rapid mitotic division called cleavage. As a result of cleavage, the zygote divides and multiplies into cell groupings called blastomeres, which are held together by the zona pellucida. The blastomeres will eventually become a solid ball of cells called the morula. When a cavity forms in the morula cell mass, the inner solid cell mass is called the blastocyst.

- Implantation usually occurs in the upper part of the posterior uterine wall when the blastocyst burrows into the uterine lining.

- After implantation, the endometrium is called the decidua. Decidua capsularis is the portion that covers the blastocyst. Decidua basalis is the portion that is directly under the blastocyst. Decidua vera is the portion that lines the rest of the uterine cavity.

- Embryonic membranes are called the amnion and the chorion. The amnion is formed from the ectoderm and is a thin protective membrane that contains the amniotic fluid and the embryo. The chorion is a thick membrane that develops from the trophoblast and encloses the amnion, embryo, and yolk sac.

- Amniotic fluid cushions the fetus against mechanical injury, controls the embryo's temperature, allows symmetric external growth, prevents adherence to the amnion, and permits freedom of movement.

- Primary germ layers will give rise to all tissues, organs, and organ systems. The three primary germ cell layers are ectoderm, endoderm, and mesoderm.

- The umbilical cord contains two umbilical arteries, which carry deoxygenated blood from the fetus to the placenta, and one umbilical vein, which carries oxygenated blood from the placenta to the fetus. The umbilical cord has a central insertion into the placenta. Wharton's jelly, a specialized connective tissue, prevents compression of the umbilical cord in utero.

- Twins are either dizygotic (fraternal) or monozygotic (identical). Dizygotic twins arise from two separate ova fertilized by two separate spermatozoa. Monozygotic twins develop from a single ovum fertilized by a single spermatozoon.

- The placenta, which develops from the chorionic villi and the decidua basalis, has two parts. The maternal portion, consisting of the decidua basalis, is red and flesh-looking; the fetal portion, consisting of chorionic villi, is covered by the amnion and appears shiny and gray. The placenta is made up of 15 to 20 segments called cotyledons.

- The placenta serves metabolic functions, endocrine functions (production of hPL, hCG, estrogen, and progesterone), and immunologic functions. It acts as the fetus's respiratory organ, is an organ of excretion, and aids in the exchange of nutrients.

- Fetal circulation is a specially designed circulatory system that provides for oxygenation of the fetus while bypassing the fetal lungs.

- Stages of fetal development include the preembryonic stage (the first 14 days of human development starting at fertilization), the embryonic stage (from day 15 after fertilization, or the beginning of the third week, until approximately 8 weeks after conception), and the fetal stage (from 8 weeks until birth at approximately 38 weeks postconception).

- Significant events that occur during the embryonic stage are that at 4 weeks the fetal heart begins to beat and at 6 weeks fetal circulation is established.

- The fetal stage is devoted to refining structures and perfecting function. The following are some significant developments during the fetal stage:

  At 8 to 12 weeks, all organ systems are formed and now require maturation.

  At 16 weeks, the sex of the fetus can be determined visually.

  At 20 weeks, fetal heartbeat can be auscultated by a fetoscope, and the mother can feel movement (quickening).

  At 24 weeks, vernix caseosa covers the entire body.

  At 26 to 28 weeks, the eyes reopen.

  At 32 weeks, skin appears less wrinkled and red because subcutaneous fat has been laid down.

  At 35 weeks, fingernails reach the ends of fingers.

  At 38 weeks, vernix caseosa is apparent only in creases and folds of skin, and lanugo remains on upper arms and shoulders only.

- The embryo is particularly vulnerable to teratogenesis during the first 8 weeks of cell differentiation and organ system development.

EXPLORE MediaLink

http://www.prenhall.com/davidson

NCLEX review questions, case studies, and other interactive resources for this chapter can be found on the Web Site at http://www.prenhall.com/davidson. Click on "Chapter 11" to select the activities for this chapter.

   For tutorials including animations and videos, more NCLEX review questions, and an audio glossary, access the accompanying Prentice Hall Nursing MediaLink DVD-ROM in this book.

PRENTICE HALL NURSING MEDIALINK DVD-ROM

Audio Glossary

NCLEX Review

Animations: *Cell Division; Oogenesis; Spermatogenesis; Oogenesis and Spermatogenesis Compared; Conception; Development of Placenta; Fetal Circulation; Embryonic Heart Formation and Circulation*

Activities: *Oogenesis and Spermatogenesis* matching exercise; *Oogenesis and Spermatogenesis* labeling exercise

Video: *Through the Eyes of a Nurse—The First Trimester*

COMPANION WEBSITE

Additional NCLEX Review

Case Study: *Teaching about Pregnancy*

Care Plan Activity: *Client Fearful of Multiple Gestations*

Applications: *Fraternal or Identical Twins; Fetal Development*

Critical Thinking

CRITICAL THINKING IN ACTION

VULNERABILITY OF THE UNBORN CHILD TO MATERNAL ILLNESSES

View the Critical Thinking in Action video in Chapter 11 of the DVD-ROM. Then answer the questions that follow.

You are working at the local clinic when Frances, a 28-year-old G2 P1001 at 11 weeks' gestation, comes into the office. Frances tells you that early in the first trimester, her husband experienced a flulike syndrome and that he was later diagnosed with cytomegalovirus (CMV) pneumonia. She tells you that his physician found an enlarged supraclavicular lymph node and an ul-

cer on one tonsil. Laboratory testing revealed elevated liver enzymes. Further testing led to the discovery of positive CMV IgM levels. She has come today with symptoms including night sweats, persistent sore throat, joint pain, headache, vomiting, and fatigue. You obtain vital signs of temperature 99°F, pulse 90, respirations 14, BP 110/70. Her physical exam is normal; no lymphadenopathy are present. Her weight gain is 2 lb even with nausea and some vomiting. She is worried that her husband's illness could be related to her current symptoms.

1. How would you respond to Frances's concern?

2. Frances asks you if her baby is formed. How would you discuss the three stages of development?

3. Frances asks when her baby is most vulnerable for abnormal growth or structure. How would you answer?

4. Frances asks what stage her baby is in. What would you tell her?

REFERENCES

Bawdon, R. E., & Hnat, M. (2003). Placental transmission of antibiotics. In J. J. Sciarra & T. J. Watkins (Eds.), *Gynecology and obstetrics* (Vol. 3, chap. 34, pp. 1–9). Philadelphia: Lippincott Williams & Wilkins.

Benirschke, K. (2004a). Multiple gestation: The biology of twinning. In R. K. Creasy & R. Resnik (Eds.), *Maternal-fetal medicine: Principles and practice* (5th ed.). Philadelphia: Saunders.

Benirschke, K. (2004b). Normal early development. In R. K. Creasy & R. Resnik (Eds.), *Maternal-fetal medicine: Principles and practice* (5th ed.). Philadelphia: Saunders.

Blackburn, S. T. (2003). *Maternal, fetal, & neonatal physiology: A clinical perspective* (2nd ed.). St. Louis, MO: Saunders.

Chacko, M. R., Anding, R., Kozinetz, C. A., Grover, J. L., & Smith, P. B. (2003). Neural tube defects: Knowledge and preconceptional prevention practices in minority young women. *Pediatrics, 112* (3), 536–542.

Cunningham, F. G., Leveno, K. J., Bloom, S. L., Hauth, J. C., Gilstrap, L. C., & Wenstrom, K. D. (2005). *Williams obstetrics* (22nd ed.). New York: McGraw-Hill.

Groll, J. M., & Lessey, B. A. (2003). Implantation. In J. J. Sciarra & T. J. Watkins (Eds.), *Gynecology and obstetrics* (Vol. 5, chap. 47, pp. 1–23). Philadelphia: Lippincott Williams & Wilkins.

Hamilton, B. A., & Wynshaw-Boris, A. (2004). Basic genetics and patterns of inheritance. In R. K.

Creasy & R. Resnik (Eds.), *Maternal-fetal medicine: Principles and practice* (5th ed.). Philadelphia: Saunders.

Liu, J. H. (2004). Endocrinology of pregnancy. In R. K. Creasy & R. Resnik (Eds.), *Maternal-fetal medicine: Principles and practice* (5th ed.). Philadelphia: Saunders.

Moore, K. L., & Persaud, T. V. N. (2003). *The developing human: Clinical oriented embryology* (7th ed.). Philadelphia: Saunders.

Sadler, T. W. (2004). *Langman's medical embryology* (9th ed.). Philadelphia: Lippincott Williams & Wilkins.

Volpe, J. J. (2000). *Neurology of the newborn* (4th ed.). Philadelphia: Saunders.

Special Reproductive Concerns: Infertility and Genetics

As we sat in the waiting room at the in vitro clinic, I felt great apprehension. For 4 years we had been unable to conceive. I'd been through two surgeries, dozens of blood tests, and hormone drugs that made me irrational and emotional. It was difficult at times—I blamed myself, felt out of control, and had surprisingly painful reactions to seeing mothers with babies. After many long talks we decided that if in vitro didn't work for us, we would adopt. Still, we felt that we wanted to experience childbirth together.

OBJECTIVES

1. Identify the components of fertility.
2. Describe the elements of the preliminary investigation of infertility.
3. Summarize the indications for the tests and associated treatments, including assisted reproductive technologies, that are done in an infertility work-up.
4. Summarize the physiologic and psychologic effects of infertility.
5. Describe the nurse's roles as counselor, educator, and advocate during infertility evaluation and treatment.
6. Discuss the indications for preconceptual genetic counseling and prenatal testing.
7. Identify the characteristics of autosomal dominant, autosomal recessive, and X-linked (sex-linked) recessive disorders.
8. Compare prenatal and postnatal diagnostic procedures used to determine the presence of genetic disorders.
9. Explore the emotional impact on a couple undergoing genetic testing or coping with the birth of a baby with a genetic disorder, and explain the nurse's role in supporting the family undergoing genetic counseling.

KEY TERMS

Autosomes 279
Basal body temperature (BBT) 260
Chromosomes 279
Endometrial biopsy 263
Ferning capacity 264
Gamete intrafallopian transfer (GIFT) 274
Genotype 284
Huhner test 266
Hysterosalpingography (HSG) 267
Infertility 259
In vitro fertilization (IVF) 273
Karyotype 279
Laparoscopy 268
Mendelian (single-gene) inheritance 283
Monosomies 280

Mosaicism 281
Nonmendelian (multifactorial) inheritance 283
Pedigree 284
Phenotype 284
Postcoital test (PCT) or Huhner test 266
Secondary infertility 259
Sonohysterography 268
Spinnbarkheit 264
Subfertility 259
Therapeutic insemination 272
Transvaginal ultrasound 263
Trisomies 280
Tubal embryo transfer (TET) 274
Zygote intrafallopian transfer (ZIFT) 274

MEDIALINK

Additional resources for this content can be found on the Prentice Hall Nursing MediaLink DVD-ROM and on the Companion Website at http://www.prenhall.com/davidson. Click on "Chapter 12" to select the activities for this chapter.

Most couples who want children conceive with little difficulty. Pregnancy and childbirth usually take their normal course, and a healthy baby is born. But some less fortunate couples are unable to fulfill their dream of having a healthy baby because of infertility or genetic problems.

This chapter explores two particularly troubling reproductive problems facing some couples: the inability to conceive, and the risk of bearing babies with genetic problems.

INFERTILITY

Infertility is defined as lack of conception despite unprotected sexual intercourse for at least 12 months (Kakarla & Bradshaw, 2003). It has a profound emotional, psychologic, and economic impact on both the affected couple and society. *Sterility* is a term applied when there is an absolute factor preventing reproduction. **Subfertility** is used to describe a couple having difficulty conceiving because both partners have reduced fertility. The term **secondary infertility** is applied to couples who have been unable to conceive after one or more successful pregnancies. The medical causes are similar to those of primary infertility.

Approximately 16% of couples in their reproductive years are infertile in the United States (Klock, 2004). Public perception is that the incidence of infertility is increasing, but in fact there has been no significant change in the proportion of infertile couples in the United States. What has changed is the composition of the infertile population; the infertility diagnosis has increased in the age group 25 to 44 years because of delayed childbearing and the entry of the baby-boom cohort into this age range in Western society. The mean age for a first birth is now 3.5 years older than that of women three decades ago (Speroff & Fritz, 2005).

The perception that infertility is on the rise may be related to the following factors:

- The deferring of marriage and then the desire to have a family shortly after marriage
- The increase in assisted reproduction techniques
- The increase in availability and use of infertility services
- The increase in insurance coverage of some ethnic groups for diagnosis of and treatment for infertility
- The increased number of childless women over 35 seeking medical attention for infertility

Essential Components of Fertility

Understanding the elements essential for normal fertility can help the nurse identify the many factors that may cause infertility. The components necessary for normal fertility are correlated with possible causes of deviation in Table 12–1. In addition, adequate reproductive hormones must be present.

With the intricacies of timing and environment playing such a crucial role, it is an impressive natural phenomenon that the majority of couples in the United States are able to conceive. The remaining couples experience infertility due to a male factor (40%), a female factor (40%), or either an unknown cause (unexplained infertility) or a problem with both partners (20%) (Klock, 2004). Professional intervention can help approximately 65% of infertile couples achieve pregnancy (Klock, 2004).

Couples should be referred for infertility evaluation if they have been unable to conceive after at least 1 year of attempting to achieve pregnancy. In women over 35 years of age, it may be appropriate to refer the couple after only 6 to 9 months of

MediaLink

Infertility

Table 12–1   POSSIBLE CAUSES OF INFERTILITY

Necessary Norms	Deviations from Normal
Female	
Favorable cervical mucus	Cervicitis, cervical stenosis, use of coital lubricants, antisperm antibodies (immunologic response)
Clear passage between cervix and tubes	Myomas, adhesions, adenomyosis, polyps, endometritis, cervical stenosis, endometriosis, congenital anomalies (e.g., septate uterus, diethylstilbestrol [DES] exposure)
Patent tubes with normal motility	Pelvic inflammatory disease, peritubal adhesions, endometriosis, IUD, salpingitis (e.g., chlamydia, recurrent sexually transmitted infections [STIs]), neoplasm, ectopic pregnancy, tubal ligation
Ovulation and release of ova	Primary ovarian failure, polycystic ovarian disease, hypothyroidism, pituitary tumor, lactation, periovarian adhesions, endometriosis, premature ovarian failure, hyperprolactinemia, Turner syndrome
No obstruction between ovary and tubes	Adhesions, endometriosis, pelvic inflammatory disease
Endometrial preparation	Anovulation, luteal phase defect, malformation, uterine infection, Asherman syndrome
Male	
Normal semen analysis	Abnormalities of sperm or semen, polyspermia, congenital defect in testicular development, mumps after adolescence, cryptorchidism, infections, gonadal exposure to x-rays, chemotherapy, smoking, alcohol abuse, malnutrition, chronic or acute metabolic disease, medications (e.g., morphine, aspirin [ASA], ibuprofen), cocaine, marijuana use, constrictive underclothing, heat
Unobstructed genital tract	Infections, tumors, congenital anomalies, vasectomy, strictures, trauma, varicocele
Normal genital tract secretions	Infections, autoimmunity to semen, tumors
Ejaculate deposited at the cervix	Premature ejaculation, impotence, hypospadias, retrograde ejaculation (e.g., diabetic), neurologic cord lesions, obesity (inhibiting adequate penetration)

unprotected intercourse without conception. At 25 years of age, when couples are the most fertile, the average length of time needed to achieve conception is 5.3 months. In about 20% of cases, conception occurs within the first month of unprotected intercourse (Johnson, 2003).

Initial Investigation: Physical and Psychosocial Issues

The easiest and least intrusive infertility testing approach is used first. Extensive testing is avoided until data confirm that the timing of intercourse and the length of coital exposure have been adequate. The nurse informs the couple of the most fertile times to have intercourse during the menstrual cycle. Teaching the couple factors that influence fertility, the signs and timing of ovulation, and the most effective timing for intercourse within the cycle may solve the problem (Table 12–2). Primary assessment, including a comprehensive history (with a discussion of genetic conditions) and physical examination for any obvious causes of infertility, is done before a costly, time-consuming, and emotionally trying investigation is initiated.

During the first visit for the preliminary investigation, the nurse explains the basic infertility work-up. The basic investigation for the couple depends on the individuals' history and usually includes assessment of ovarian function, cervical mucosal adequacy and receptivity to sperm, sperm adequacy, tubal patency, and the general condition of the pelvic organs. Because about 40% of infertility is related to a male factor, a semen analysis should be one of the first diagnostic tests before moving on to the more invasive diagnostic procedures involving the woman. The initial infertility evaluation offers nurses a unique opportunity to initiate preconception counseling, thereby help-

ing infertile couples maximize their chances of delivering a healthy baby. Prenatal vitamins are often one of the earliest recommendations for women planning to conceive. Studies show that folic acid supplementation of at least 400 micrograms (0.4 mg/day) greatly reduces the incidence of neural tube defects such as anencephaly and spina bifida. Preconception is the optimal time to review the importance of rubella and varicella immunity and the risk of congenital anomalies associated with exposure. It also provides the opportunity to address risks associated with alcohol, tobacco, and medications. Women may warrant a change in medication or stricter management of chronic illnesses.

The mutual desire to have children is a cornerstone of many marriages. A fertility problem is a deeply personal, emotion-laden area in a couple's life. The self-esteem of one or both partners may be threatened if the inability to conceive is seen as a lack of virility or femininity (Klock, 2004). It is never easy to discuss one's sexual activity, especially when potentially irreversible problems with fertility may exist. The nurse can provide comfort to couples by offering a sympathetic ear, a nonjudgmental approach, and appropriate information and instructions throughout the diagnostic and therapeutic process. Because counseling includes discussion of very personal matters, nurses who are comfortable with their own sexuality are more capable of establishing rapport and eliciting relevant information from couples with fertility problems.

The first interview should involve both partners and include a comprehensive history and a physical examination. Table 12–3 lists the items in a complete infertility physical work-up and laboratory evaluation for both partners. Figure 12–1 ◆ outlines the historical database, diagnostic tests usually performed, and healthcare interventions in cases of infertility.

Assessment of the Woman's Fertility

After a thorough history and physical examination, both partners may undergo tests to identify causes of infertility. A thorough evaluation of the woman's fertility includes assessment of the hypothalamic-pituitary axis in terms of ovulatory function, as well as structure and function of the cervix, uterus, fallopian tubes, and ovaries.

EVALUATION OF OVULATORY FACTORS

Ovulation problems account for approximately 15% of couples' infertility. For review of the characteristics of the female reproductive cycle, see Table 12–4 and Figure 12–2 ◆. For an in-depth discussion on female reproductive cycle characteristics, see Chapter 10. ∞

Basal Body Temperature Recording

One basic test of ovulatory function is the **basal body temperature (BBT)** recording, which aids in identifying follicular and luteal phase abnormalities. At the initial visit, the nurse instructs the woman in the technique of recording BBT on a special form. The woman is instructed to begin a new chart on the first day of every monthly cycle. The temperature can be taken with a standard oral or rectal thermometer calibrated by tenths of a degree, making slight temperature changes readily appar-

Table 12–2	SUGGESTIONS FOR IMPROVING FERTILITY

Avoid douching and artificial lubricants (gels, oils, saliva) that can alter sperm mobility. Prevent alteration of pH of vagina and introduction of spermicidal agents.

Promote retention of sperm. The male superior position with the female remaining recumbent for at least 20–30 minutes after intercourse maximizes the number of sperm reaching the cervix.

Avoid leakage of sperm. Elevate the woman's hips with a pillow after intercourse for 20–30 minutes to allow liquefaction of seminal fluid and motility of the sperm toward the egg. Avoid getting up to urinate, shower, or douche for 1 hour after intercourse.

Maximize the potential for fertilization. Instruct the couple that it is optimal if sexual intercourse occurs every other day during the fertile period. Because each woman's menstrual cycle varies in length, the fertile period can extend from cycle day (CD) 7 through CD 17. Note: CD 1 is considered the first day of actual menstrual flow.

Avoid emphasizing conception during sexual encounters to decrease anxiety and potential sexual dysfunction.

Maintain adequate nutrition and reduce stress. Stress reduction techniques and good nutritional habits increase sperm production.

Explore other methods to increase fertility awareness, such as home assessment of cervical mucus and basal body temperature (BBT) recordings.

Seek counsel and advice from a valued friend or family member.

Consider incorporating culturally appropriate methods to enhance fertility.

Table 12–3   INITIAL INFERTILITY PHYSICAL WORK-UP AND LABORATORY EVALUATIONS

Female	Male
Physical Examination	**Physical Examination**
Assessment of height, weight, blood pressure, temperature, and general health status	General health (assessment of height, weight, blood pressure)
Endocrine evalution of thyroid for exophthalmos, lid lag, tremor or palpable gland	Endocrine evaluation (e.g., presence of gynecomastia)
Optic fundi evaluation for presence of increased intracranial pressure, especially in oligomenorrheal or amenorrheal women (possible pituitary tumor)	Visual fields evaluation for bitemporal hemianopia
Reproductive features (including breast and external genital area)	Abnormal hair patterns
Physical ability to tolerate pregnancy	
Pelvic Examination	**Urologic Examination**
Papanicolaou smear	Presence or absence of phimosis
Culture for gonorrhea if indicated and possibly chlamydia or mycoplasma culture (opinions vary)	Location of urethral meatus
Signs of vaginal infections (see Chapter 6 ∞)	Size and consistency of each testis, vas deferens, and epididymis
Shape of escutcheon (e.g., does pubic hair distribution resemble that of a male?)	Presence of varicocele
Size of clitoris (enlargement caused by endocrine disorders)	
Evaluation of cervix: old lacerations, tears, erosion, polyps, condition and shape of os, signs of infections, cervical mucus (evaluate for estrogen effect of spinnbarkheit and cervical ferning)	**Rectal Examination**
	Size and consistency of the prostate with microscopic evaluation of prostate fluid for signs of infection
Bimanual Examination	Size and consistency of seminal vesicles
Size, shape, position, and motility of uterus	
Presence of congenital anomalies	**Laboratory Examination**
Presence of endometriosis	Complete blood count
Evaluation of adnexa: ovarian size, cysts, fixations, or tumors	Sedimentation rate if indicated
	Serology
Rectovaginal Examination	Urinalysis
Presence of retroflexed or retroverted uterus	Rh factor and blood grouping
Presence of rectouterine pouch masses	Semen analysis
Presence of possible endometriosis	If indicated, testicular biopsy, buccal smear
	Hormonal assays, FSH, LH, prolactin
Laboratory Examination	
Complete blood count	
Sedimentation rate if indicated	
Serology	
Urinalysis	
Rh factor and blood grouping	
Rubella IgG	
Follicle-stimulating hormone (FSH) level regardless of age and regularity of menstrual cycles	
If indicated depending on age and regularity of menstrual cycles: thyroid-stimulating hormone (TSH), prolactin levels (PRL), glucose tolerance test, hormonal assays including estradiol (E_2), luteinizing hormone (LH), mid-luteal progesterone (MLP), dehydroepiandrosterone sulfate (DHEAS), androstenedione, testosterone, 17 α-hydroxyprogesterone (17-OHP).	

ent. A special kind of thermometer (BBT) may be used to measure temperature only between 35C and 37.8C (96F and 100F). In addition to traditional or digital thermometers, tympanic thermometry, which provides a reading in only a few seconds, may also be a valid method.

The woman records daily variations on a temperature graph. The temperature graph typically shows a biphasic pattern during ovulatory cycles, whereas in anovulatory cycles it remains monophasic. The woman uses the readings on the temperature graph to detect ovulation and direct the timing of intercourse (Figure 12–3 ◆, A).

Basal temperature for females in the preovulatory (follicular) phase is usually below 36.7C (98F). As ovulation approaches, production of estrogen increases and at its peak may cause a slight drop, then rise, in the basal temperature. The slight drop in temperature before ovulation is often difficult to capture on the BBT chart. After ovulation there is a surge of luteinizing hormone (LH), which stimulates production of progesterone. Because progesterone is thermogenic (produces heat), it causes a 0.3C to 0.6C (0.5F to 1F) sustained rise in basal temperature during the second half of the menstrual cycle (luteal phase). Immediately before or coincident with the onset of

Figure 12–1 ◆ Flow chart for management of the infertile couple.

Table 12–4   FEMALE REPRODUCTIVE CYCLE

Ovarian Cycle	Menstrual Cycle
Follicular phase (days 1–14): Primordial follicle matures under influence of FSH and LH up to the time of ovulation. *Luteal phase* (days 15–28): Ovum leaves follicle, corpus luteum develops under LH influence and produces high levels of progesterone and low levels of estrogen.	*Menstrual phase* (days 1–6): Estrogen levels are low; cervical mucus is scant, viscous, and opaque. *Proliferative phase* (days 7–14): Estrogen peaks just before ovulation. Cervical mucus at ovulation is clear, thin, watery, alkaline, and more favorable to sperm; shows ferning pattern; and has spinnbarkheit greater than 8 cm. At ovulation body temperature drops, then rises sharply and remains elevated under influence of progesterone. *Secretory phase* (days 15–26): Estrogen drops sharply and progesterone dominates. *Ischemic phase* (days 27–28): Both estrogen and progesterone levels drop.

menses, the temperature falls below 98F. These changes in the basal temperature create the typical biphasic pattern. Figure 12–3, *B* shows a biphasic ovulatory BBT chart. Temperature elevation does not predict the day of ovulation but provides supportive evidence of ovulation about a day after it has occurred. Actual release of the ovum probably occurs 24 to 36 hours before the first temperature elevation (estrogen peak).

Although there are other, more reliable methods to detect ovulatory function, BBT offers couples a low-tech, noninvasive, and inexpensive option. Based on serial BBT charts, the clinician might recommend sexual intercourse *every other day* beginning 3 to 4 days before and continuing for 2 to 3 days after the expected time of ovulation. See Client Teaching: Methods of Determining Ovulation on pages 265–266.

Hormonal Assessments of Ovulatory Function

Hormonal assessments of ovulatory function fall into the following categories:

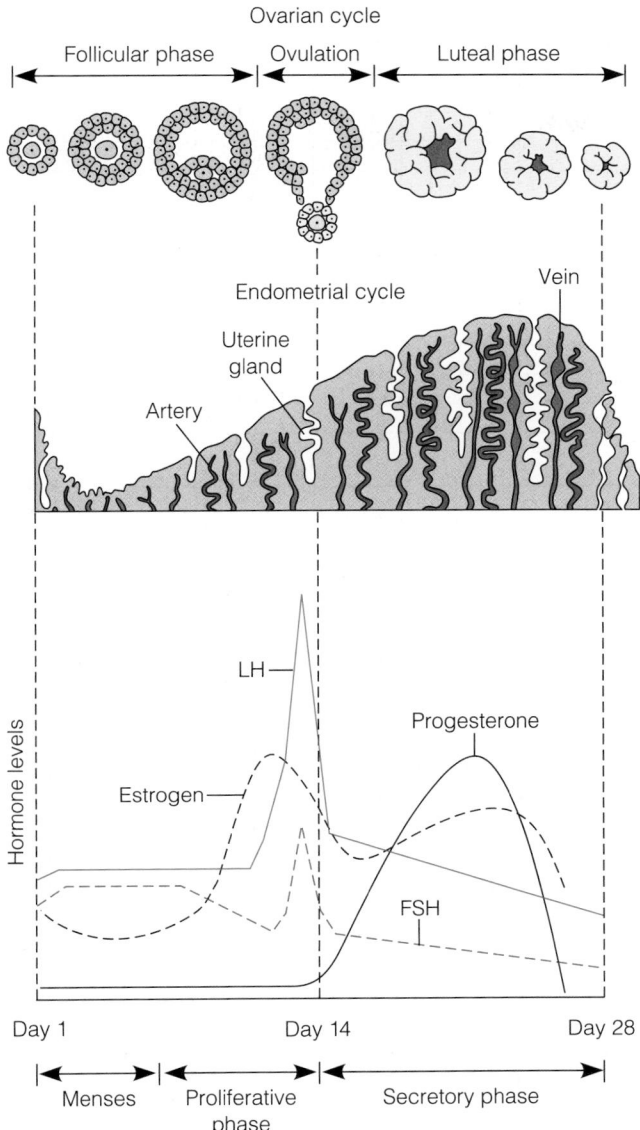

Figure 12–2 ◆ Sequence of events in a normal reproductive cycle showing the relationship of hormone levels to events in the ovarian and endometrial cycles.

1. *Gonadotropin levels (FSH, LH).* Baseline hormonal assessment of follicle-stimulating hormone (FSH) and luteinizing hormone (LH) provides valuable information about normal ovulatory function. Measured on cycle day 3, FSH is the single most valuable test in assessing ovarian reserve and function and should always be measured, particularly in women over 35, to predict the potential for successful treatment with ovulation induction treatment cycles. LH levels may be measured early in the cycle to rule out disorders associated with androgen excess, causing a disruption in normal follicular development and oocyte maturation. Daily sampling of serum LH at midcycle can detect the LH surge. The day of the LH surge is believed to be the time of maximum fertility. Urine and salivary LH ovulation prediction kits are also available for home use to better time postcoital testing, insemination, and coitus (Moghissi, 2003).

2. *Progesterone assays.* Progesterone levels furnish the best evidence of ovulation and corpus luteum function. Serum levels begin to rise with the LH surge and peak about 8 days later. A level of 5 ng/mL 3 days after the LH surge generally confirms ovulation (Johnson, 2003). On day 21 (7 days postovulation) a level of 10 ng/mL or higher generally indicates an adequate luteal phase.

3. *Prolactin.* Elevated levels of the anterior pituitary hormone prolactin are a frequent cause of ovulatory dysfunction, which may range from a luteal phase defect to anovulation to amenorrhea.

4. *Thyroid-stimulating hormone (TSH).* Thyroid hormone is necessary for most body functions, not only metabolism but also specific tissue activities. TSH stimulates prolactin secretion by the pituitary gland. Hypothyroidism may have a dramatic effect on ovulatory function and cause menstrual irregularities and bleeding irregularities.

5. *Androgen levels (testosterone, DHEAS, androstenedione).* Androgen excess can originate from the adrenal glands, ovaries, or peripheral tissue. Despite the origin, it usually results in specific clinical symptoms such as acne, hirsutism, virilization, and ovulatory dysfunction—which can range from oligomenorrhea to anovulation to amenorrhea.

Endometrial Biopsy

Endometrial biopsy provides information about the effects of progesterone produced by the corpus luteum after ovulation and endometrial receptivity. The biopsy is performed not earlier than 10 to 12 days after ovulation (usually day 22 or 23 of a 28-day menstrual cycle) and involves removing a sample of endometrium with a small pipette attached to suction (Varney, Kriebs, & Gegor, 2004). The woman should be informed that some pelvic discomfort, cramping, and vaginal spotting are normal during and following the procedure. The onset of menses following biopsy should be disclosed for accurate interpretation of the biopsy report. A dysfunction may exist if the endometrial lining does not show the expected amount of secretory tissue for that day of the woman's menstrual cycle. A repeat biopsy is indicated to confirm luteal phase dysfunction. Serum progesterone levels may also be used in conjunction with endometrial biopsy to confirm adequate luteal phase function. Although endometrial biopsy was once thought to be a very important tool in the evaluation of luteal phase defect, a recent investigation has concluded that "[h]istologic dating of the endometrium does not discriminate between women of fertile and infertile couples and should not be used in the routine evaluation of infertility" (Coutifaris et al., 2004).

Transvaginal Ultrasound

Transvaginal ultrasound is the method of choice for follicular monitoring of women undergoing ovulation induction cycles, for timing ovulation for insemination and intercourse, for retrieving oocytes for in vitro fertilization (IVF), and for monitoring early pregnancy. The use of transvaginal color flow Doppler to investigate uterine blood flow may in the future help

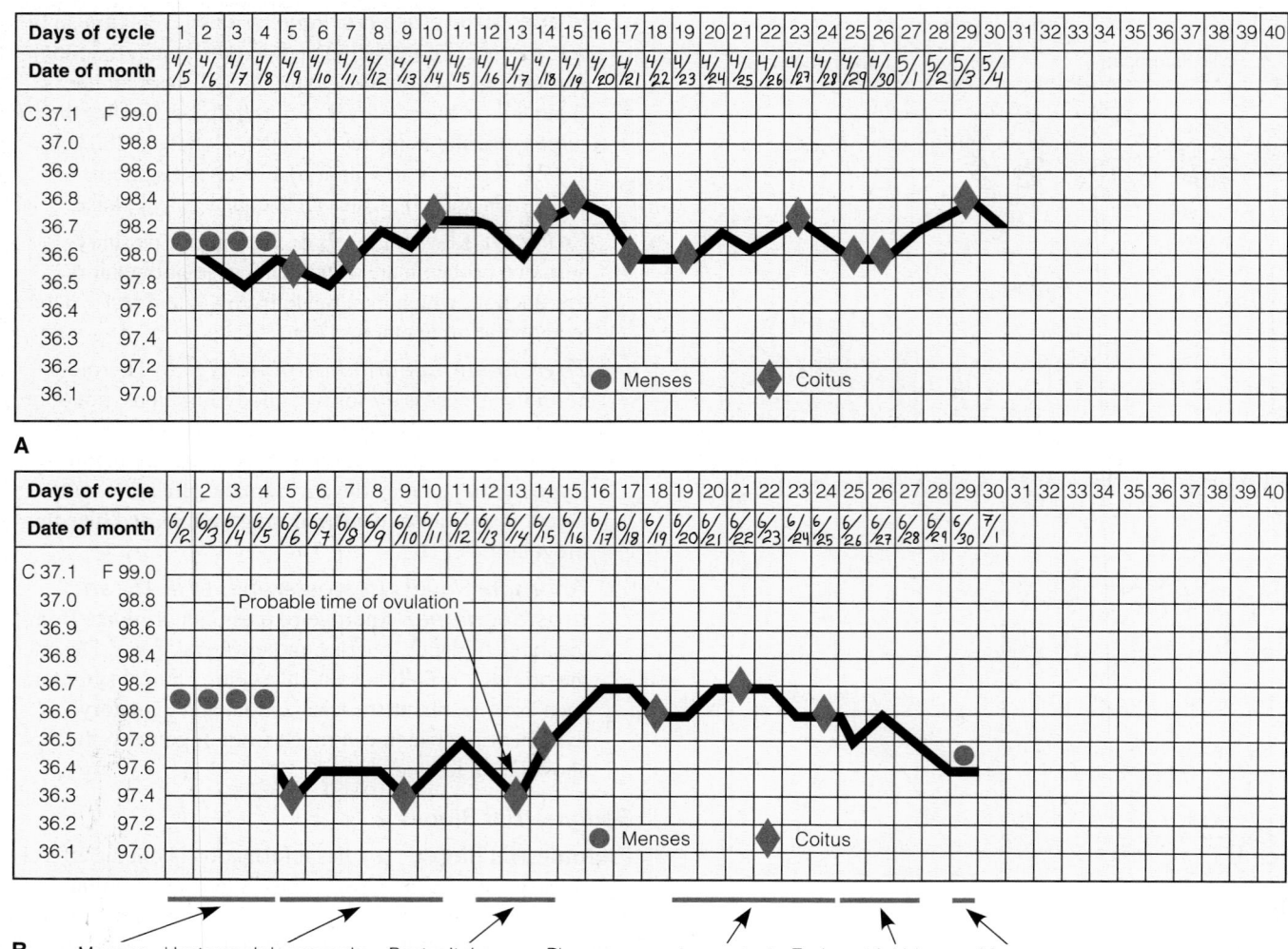

Figure 12–3 ◆ *A,* A monophasic, anovulatory basal body temperature (BBT) chart. *B,* A biphasic BBT chart illustrating probable time of ovulation, the different types of testing, and the time in the cycle that each would be performed.

the endocrinologist evaluate the adequacy of the developing follicle, further assessing oocyte maturity and endometrial development and patterns, and improve the diagnosis of luteal phase defects (Pierson & Olatunbosum, 2004).

EVALUATION OF CERVICAL FACTORS

The mucus cells of the endocervix consist predominantly of water. As ovulation approaches, the ovary increases its secretion of estrogen and produces changes in the cervical mucus. The amount of mucus increases 10-fold, and the water content rises significantly. At ovulation, mucus elasticity, or **spinnbarkheit,** increases, and the viscosity decreases. Excellent spinnbarkheit exists when the mucus can be stretched 8 to 10 cm or longer. Mucus elasticity is determined by using two glass slides (Figure 12–4 ◆, *A*) or by grasping some mucus at the external os and stretching it in the vagina toward the introitus. (See Client Teaching: Methods of Determining Ovulation.)

The **ferning capacity** (crystallization) (Figure 12–4, *B* and *C*) of the cervical mucus also increases as ovulation approaches. Ferning is caused by decreased levels of salt and water interacting with the glycoproteins in the mucus during the

ovulatory period and is thus an indirect indication of estrogen production. To test for ferning, mucus from the cervical os is spread on a glass slide, allowed to air dry, and then examined under the microscope.

Within 24 to 48 hours postovulation, rising levels of progesterone cause a marked decrease in the quantity of cervical mucus and an increase in viscosity and cellularity. The resulting absence of spinnbarkheit and ferning capacity decreases sperm survival.

To be receptive to sperm, cervical mucus must be thin, clear, watery, profuse, alkaline, and acellular. As shown in Figure 12–5 ◆, the mazelike microscopic mucoid strands align in a parallel manner to allow for easy sperm passage. The mucus is termed *inhospitable* if these changes do not occur.

Cervical mucus inhospitable to sperm survival can have several causes, some of which are treatable. For example, estrogen secretion may be inadequate for the development of receptive mucus. Cone biopsy, electrocautery, or cryosurgery of the cervix may remove large numbers of mucus-producing glands, creating a "dry cervix" that decreases sperm survival. Treatment with clomiphene citrate may have deleterious effects on cervical

CLIENT TEACHING Methods of Determining Ovulation

CLIENT GOALS At the completion of the teaching the woman will be able to:

1. Accurately identify cervical mucus changes

2. Accurately take and record BBT

3. Discuss the changes in BBT and cervical mucus that indicate ovulation

4. Discuss alternative methods of ovulation detection

5. Summarize physical symptoms that may indicate ovulation has occurred

TEACHING PLAN

CONTENT	TEACHING METHOD
BASAL BODY TEMPERATURE (BBT) METHOD The basal body temperature (BBT) method relies on assessing the woman's temperature pattern. Describe the expected findings with an ovulatory (biphasic) cycle and stress the need to monitor BBT for 3 to 4 months to establish a pattern. BBT can be used to time intercourse if pregnancy is desired or as a method of natural family planning. Describe the timing of intercourse to achieve or avoid pregnancy. Describe the procedure for measuring BBT: • Using a BBT thermometer, the woman chooses one site (oral, vaginal, or rectal), which she uses consistently. • The woman takes her temperature every day before arising and before starting any activity, including smoking. Note: Read and follow manufacturers' instructions for each type of BBT thermometer in regard to amount of time needed for accurate reading. • The result is then recorded immediately on a BBT chart, and the temperature dots for each day are connected to form a graph. • The woman then shakes the thermometer down in preparation for use the next day. Explain that certain situations can disturb body temperature such as large alcohol intake, sleeplessness, fever, warm climate, jet lag, shift work, or the use of an electric blanket.	Choose a private location, free of distractions for the discussion. Create a supportive, comfortable atmosphere by attitude and communication style. *Briefly* explain how BBT can indicate ovulation. Use pictures or graphs to demonstrate the BBT changes that indicate ovulatory and ovulatory cycles. Break content down into smaller steps to facilitate learning. Show the woman the BBT thermometer and demonstrate its use. *Note:* A tympanic (ear) electric thermometer may also be used. Remind the women to use the same type of thermometer throughout the menstrual cycle. Provide a blank chart. Ask the woman to chart 3 days' findings using temperature results you identify. Remind the woman that BBT charts are not a prediction of ovulation and that the temperature rise is a response to ovulation that has already occurred. Provide the woman with an example of LH testing results for comparison. Provide a handout summarizing the procedure. Provide frequent opportunities for questions and discussion.
CERVICAL MUCUS METHOD Explain that cervical mucus characteristics change throughout a woman's menstrual cycle, and the quality of the mucus can be used to predict ovulation. Describe the various characteristics of the cervical mucus throughout the menstrual cycle. Describe the procedure for assessing cervical mucus changes: • Every day when she uses the bathroom the woman checks her vagina, either by dabbing the vaginal opening with toilet paper or by putting a finger in the opening. • She notes the wetness (presence of mucus), collects some mucus, determines its color and consistency, and records her findings on a chart. For discussion of mucus characteristics, see page 264. • She washes her hands before and after the procedure. Stress that it may take several cycles for the woman to become familiar with the pattern.	Discuss the characteristics of the mucus and the rationale for the changes. Explore the woman's feelings about using the procedure. Show pictures of the mucus changes including spinnbarkheit of different degrees of elasticity. Encourage the woman to ask questions. Stress that the presence and consistency of the mucus are altered by vaginal infection, vaginal medications, spermicides, lubricants, douching, sexual arousal, and semen.

(Continued on next page)

CLIENT TEACHING   Methods of Determining Ovulation   continued

CONTENT	TEACHING METHOD

CONTENT

LH PREDICTOR KIT METHOD

Explain that LH kits are a good predictor of ovulation for woman with a history of regular menstrual cycles.

Describe the procedures for using an LH predictor kit:

- Determine the length of the woman's menstrual cycle. Use a calendar to determine the cycle day the woman will initiate testing.

- The testing must occur the same time daily. The morning is recommended, because the LH concentration is highest upon wakening.

- Begin testing with the first morning urine void and examine the test strips for color changes that indicate if ovulation has occurred or is close to occurring.

MITTELSCHMERZ

Explain that mittelschmerz (midcycle pain) located in the lower pelvis is a common symptom of ovulation.

Encourage the woman to document this occurrence (or absence) on her BBT chart.

EVALUATION

Evaluate the learning by providing time for discussion, questions, and practice using the charts and thermometer. Ask the woman to describe the selected procedure in her own words.

Provide a written handout describing the process and findings so that the woman has information readily available. Review at a follow-up visit the BBT and cervical mucus assessment from the previous cycle(s).

DOCUMENTATION

The nurse should document the information that was given, the type of teaching method used, indicate if the client performed BBT thermometer assessment, if it was demonstrated, or if verbal or written directions were given. Verbalization of understanding and clarification of any information should be documented. Safety issues and instruction were reviewed.

---

mucus because of its antiestrogenic properties. Therapy with supplemental estrogen for approximately 6 days before expected ovulation is sometimes employed to encourage formation of suitable spinnbarkheit. However, intrauterine insemination (IUI) is more often the most appropriate therapy to overcome these obstacles. When mucosal hostility to sperm is due to cervical infection, antimicrobial therapy may be effective.

The cervix can also be the site of secretory immunologic reactions in which antisperm antibodies are produced, causing agglutination or immobilization of sperm. The most widely used serum sperm bioassay to detect specific classes of antibodies in serum and seminal fluid is direct immunobead binding testing (IBT) (Kipersztok et al., 2003). The treatment for antisperm antibodies may include IUI of the male's washed sperm to bypass the cervical factor.

The **postcoital test (PCT),** also called the **Huhner test,** is performed 1 or 2 days before the expected date of ovulation as determined by previous BBT charts, the length of prior cycles, or urinary LH kit. This examination evaluates the cervical mucus, sperm motility, sperm-mucus interaction, and the sperm's ability to negotiate the cervical mucus barrier. The cou-

ple can have intercourse 2 to 8 hours before examination. If the results are abnormal, the test should be repeated at the optimal time of 2 to 3 hours after intercourse. A small plastic catheter attached to a 10-mL syringe is placed in the cervix. Mucus is aspirated from the endocervical canal, measured, and examined microscopically for signs of infection, spinnbarkheit, ferning, number of active spermatozoa per high-power field (HPF), and number of sperm with poor or no motility. The focus of the postcoital examination is on the timing of intercourse with respect to ovulation, and may promote sexual difficulties for some infertile couples. In the last 10 years, research has called into question the usefulness of this test, and its routine use is no longer recommended (Speroff & Fritz, 2005).

EVALUATION OF UTERINE STRUCTURES AND TUBAL PATENCY

Uterine abnormalities are a relatively uncommon cause of infertility but should always be considered. A few tests offer the ability to evaluate the uterine cavity and tubal patency simultaneously. These tests are usually done after BBT evaluation, semen analysis, and the other less invasive tests. Tubal patency

A

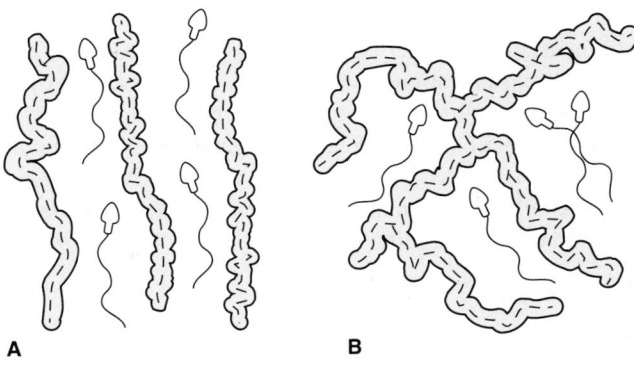

Figure 12–5 ◆ Sperm passage through cervical mucus. *A,* Appearance at the time of ovulation with channels favoring efficient sperm penetration and migration upward. *B,* Unfavorable mazelike configuration found at other times of the menstrual cycle.
SOURCE: Corson, S. (1990). *Conquering infertility* (p. 16). A guide for couples (4th ed.). Vancouver, BC: EMIS-Canada.

B

C

Figure 12–4 ◆ *A,* Spinnbarkheit (elasticity). *B,* Ferning pattern. *C,* Lack of ferning pattern.
SOURCE: (*B*) Courtesy of Lavena Porter OB/GYN NP (*C*) From *Clinical gynecologic endocrinology and infertility,* 5e, by L. Speroff, et al., p. 818. Copyright 1994 Lippincott, Williams & Wilkins. Reprinted with permission. (http://www.com).

and uterine assessment are usually evaluated by hysterosalpingography or laparoscopy. Other invasive tests used to evaluate only the uterine cavity are hysteroscopy and sonohysterography. Hysteroscopy may be performed earlier in the evaluation if the woman's history suggests the potential for adhesive disease or uterine abnormalities.

Hysterosalpingography

Hysterosalpingography (HSG), or hysterogram, involves an instillation of a radiopaque substance into the uterine cavity. In addition the oil-based dye and injection pressure used in HSG may have a therapeutic effect. This effect may be caused by the flushing of debris, breaking of adhesions, or induction of peristalsis produced by the instillation.

The hysterosalpingogram should be performed in the follicular phase of the cycle to avoid interrupting an early pregnancy. This timing also avoids the lush secretory changes in the endometrium that occur after ovulation, which may prevent the passage of the dye through the tubes and present a false picture of cornual obstruction. HSG causes moderate discomfort. The pain is referred from the peritoneum (which is irritated by the subdiaphragmatic collection of gas) to the shoulder. The cramping may be decreased if the radiopaque dye is warmed to body temperature before instillation. Women can take an over-the-counter prostaglandin synthesis inhibitor (such as ibuprofen) 30 minutes before the procedure to decrease the pain, cramping, and discomfort. HSG can also cause serious recurrence of pelvic inflammatory disease, so prophylactic antibiotics are recommended to prevent infection that could be triggered by the procedure (Johnson, 2003).

Hysteroscopy

Hysteroscopy is the definitive method for both diagnosis and treatment of intrauterine pathology (Speroff & Fritz, 2005). Hysteroscopy allows the physician to further evaluate any areas of suspicion within the uterine cavity revealed by HSG. It can be done in conjunction with a laparoscopy or independently in the office and does not require general anesthesia. A fiberoptic instrument called a hysteroscope is placed into the uterus and allows direct visualization of the size, shape, and location of any intrauterine pathology, such as polyps, myomata (fibroids), or structural variations (American College of Obstetricians and Gynecologists [ACOG], 2005a). The newest generation hysteroscope allows for minor operative procedures to be performed in the office setting.

Laparoscopy

Laparoscopy enables direct visualization of the pelvic organs and is usually done 6 to 8 months after HSG unless symptoms or findings suggest the need for earlier evaluation. Diagnostic laparoscopy is an outpatient procedure requiring the use of general anesthesia. Generally a three-puncture approach is used; entry is made through the umbilical area, and supporting instruments are inserted in two suprapubic incisions. The peritoneal cavity is distended with carbon dioxide gas, and the pelvic organs can be directly visualized with a fiberoptic instrument. Tube patency can be assessed by instilling dye into the uterine cavity through the cervix. The pelvis is evaluated for endometriosis, adhesions, organ fixations, pelvic inflammatory disease, tumors, and cysts. The intraperitoneal gas is usually manually expressed at the end of the procedure. In routine preanesthesia instructions, the woman is told that she may have some discomfort from organ displacement and shoulder to chest pain caused by gas in the abdomen. She should be informed that she can resume normal activities as tolerated after 24 hours. Using postoperative pain medication and assuming a supine position may help relieve residual shoulder and chest discomfort caused by any remaining gas.

Sonohysterography

Sonohysterography, involving transvaginal ultrasound during or after the introduction of sterile saline, defines the uterine cavity contour and readily demonstrates even small intrauterine lesions. The use of fluid instillation into the uterus, coupled with high-resolution endovaginal probes, can allow tremendous diagnostic enhancement with an inexpensive, simple, well-tolerated office procedure.

Assessment of the Man's Fertility

Male infertility can be caused by numerous factors and categorized as ductal obstructions or abnormalities of sperm production or sperm function (Speroff & Fritz, 2005). Sperm function abnormalities may be due to problems with sperm binding or penetration of the egg, prostatitis, or varicocele. Varicocele accounts for approximately 40% of male infertility (Speroff & Fritz, 2005). If the man's history indicates the need, he may be referred to a urologist for testing. A semen analysis of sperm quality, quantity, and motility is the single most important diagnostic study of the man. It should be done early in the couple's evaluation, before invasive testing of the woman. Although a postcoital test can provide information about sperm viability, it does not provide sufficient information concerning normal seminal parameters.

To obtain accurate results, the specimen is collected after 2 to 3 days of abstinence and usually by masturbation to avoid contamination or loss of any ejaculate. If the man has difficulty producing sperm by masturbation, special medical grade condoms are available to collect the sperm during intercourse. Regular latex and nonlatex condoms should not be used because they contain agents that impair the mobility of sperm and because sperm can be lost in the condom. Most lubricants also are spermicidal and should not be used unless approved by the andrology laboratory.

Both seasonal and incidental variability may be seen in count and motility in successive semen samples from the same person. Thus a repeat semen analysis may be required to assess the man's fertility potential adequately; a minimum of two separate analyses is recommended for confirmation. In the case in which a known testicular insult has occurred, such as infection, high fevers, or surgery, a repeat analysis may not be done for at least 2.5 months to allow for new sperm maturation.

Semen analysis provides information about sperm motility and morphology as well as a determination of the absolute number of spermatozoa present (Table 12–5). Although it is known that low numbers and motility may indicate compromised fertility, other parameters such as morphology, volume, motion patterns, viscosity, pH, and progression are important prognostic indicators. Values previously thought to indicate subfertility may in fact be compatible with normal fertility when these factors are considered. An infertile specimen is one that reveals fewer than 20 million sperm per milliliter, less than 50% motility at 6 hours, or less than 30% normal sperm forms. Some studies have indicated that the quality of sperm decreases with increased age (Hassan & Killick, 2003). For example, fathers older than 50 years have infants at increased risk for trisomy.

A variety of environmental factors can affect male fertility. Causes of increased scrotal heat, such as jockey shorts, hot tubs, or occupations requiring long hours of sitting, are thought to decrease fertility potential, but there are no clinical studies to substantiate this belief (Honig, 2005). Heavy use of marijuana, alcohol, or cocaine within 2 years of testing can depress sperm count and testosterone levels; cigarette smoking may depress sperm motility (American Society for Reproductive Medicine, 2005). The use of anabolic steroids lowers the ability of the body to make endogenous testosterone, causing low sperm counts, which may not be reversible (Honig, 2005). Neurologic

Table 12–5	NORMAL SEMEN ANALYSIS
Factor	**Value**
Volume	Greater than 2 mL
pH	7 to 8
Total sperm count	Greater than 20 million/mL
Liquefaction	Complete in 1 hour
Motility	50% or greater forward progression
Normal forms	30% or greater
Round cells	Less than 5 million/mL
White cells	Less than 1 million/mL

SOURCE: Courtesy of the World Health Organization. (1999). *WHO Laboratory Manual for the Examination of Human Semen and Sperm-Cervical Mucus Interaction* (4th ed., pp. 9–106). Cambridge, UK: Cambridge University Press.

ejaculatory dysfunction can be caused by alpha blockers, phentolamine, methyldopa, guanethidine, and reserpine. Sperm quality may be affected by medicines such as calcium channel blockers, propranolol, cimetidine, nitrofurantoin, or allopurinol/colchicine (Honig, 2005). Heavy metals (lead), pesticide exposure, and cadmium can also reduce sperm count (Denson, 2006). A low sperm count of at least 10 million/mL may benefit from IUI because an increased concentrated amount of sperm can be deposited directly into the uterine cavity. For a sperm count of less than 5% normal forms, IVF with intracytoplasmic sperm injection (ICSI) is recommended (Speroff & Fritz, 2005).

Spermatozoa have been shown to possess intrinsic antigens that can provoke male immunologic infertility. This is especially apparent following vasectomy reversals or genital trauma, such as testicular torsion, in which autoimmunity to sperm develops (the man produces antibodies to his own sperm). Research indicates that it is the actual presence of antibodies on the spermatozoal surface (not just the presence of antibodies in the serum) that affects sperm function and thus leads to subfertility. Antisperm antibodies can be screened for by the immunobead binding test (Kipersztok et al., 2003). Treatment for antisperm antibodies is directed toward preventing the formation of antibodies or arresting the underlying mechanism that

compromises sperm function. Therapies such as immunosuppression with corticosteroids and IUI have not proved effective. The treatment of choice for clinically significant antisperm antibodies is IVF and ICSI.

Tests such as the hamster sperm penetration assay (SPA), hemizona (HZA), acrosome reaction assay, and sperm density evaluation may be performed, but their usefulness is controversial. If the man's history indicates, he may be referred to a urologist for further testing.

Methods of Managing Infertility

Methods of managing infertility include pharmacologic agents, therapeutic insemination, IVF, and other assisted reproductive techniques. In addition, many couples choose adoption as their preferred response to infertility.

PHARMACOLOGIC AGENTS

This section provides a brief overview of the drugs commonly used for ovarian stimulation in the follicular phase, control of midcycle release, and luteal phase support. The pharmacologic treatment chosen depends on the specific cause of the infertility. Table 12–6 lists some of the drugs commonly used and indications for use.

Table 12–6   DRUGS COMMONLY USED TO TREAT INFERTILITY

Drugs	Women	Men
Clomiphene citrate (Clomid, Serophene)	• PCOS • Hyper-androgenemia • Premature follicle rupture	• Low levels of gonadotropins • Hypothalamic hypogonadism
Human menopausal gonadotropin (hMG) (Repronex, Bravelle)	• Hypothalamic ovulatory dysfunction (after failure of clomiphene) • Hypopituitarism • PCOS (rarely) • Luteinized unruptured follicle syndrome (after failure of hCG alone) • Inadequate cervical mucus • In vitro fertilization, GIFT, ZIFT • Controlled super-ovulation	• Hypothalamic pituitary failure due to Kallmann syndrome or delayed puberty • Hypo-gonadotrophic hypogonadism (deficiency of FSH and LH)
Recombinant follicle-stimulating hormone (rFSH) (Follistim, Gonal-F)	• PCOS • Too long cycles • In vitro fertilization, GIFT, ZIFT	
Human chorionic gonadotropin (hCG) (Pregnyl, Novarel, A.P.L.)	• Induces dominant follicle to release egg • Luteinized unruptured follicle syndrome	
Bromocriptine (Parlodel) Cabergoline (Dostinex)	• Pituitary adenoma • Hyper-pituitarism	• Hyper-prolactinemia (functional or pituitary adenoma)
Gonadotropin releasing hormone (GnRh) (Factrel, Lutre-pulse)	• Hypothalamic ovulatory dysfunction—to ensure a pulsatile release of GnRH by a small pump	• Hypothalamic pituitary failure due to Kallmann syndrome or delayed puberty (pulsed infusion)
GnRh analogs • Leuprolide acetate (Lupron) • Nafarelin acetate (Synarel) • Goserelin acetate (Zoladex)	• Premature follicular rupture • In vitro fertilization, GIFT, ZIFT • Endometriosis	• Hypo-gonadotrophic hypogonadism
GnRH antagonists • Ganirelix acetate (Antagon)	• Same as GnRH analogs	
Progesterone (Crinone, Prometrium, progesterone in oil)	• Luteal phase dysfunction • Luteal phase support	

SOURCE: Adapted from American Society for Reproductive Medicine Booklet. (2006). *Medications for inducing ovulation —A guide for patients.* http://www.asrm.org/Patientbooklets/ovulation_drugs.pdf; Shane, J. (1993). Evaluation and treatment of infertility. Clinical Symposia, *45, 2;* Wilson, B. A., Shannon, M. T., Shields, K. M., & Stang, C. L. (2007). *Prentice Hall nurse's drug guide 2007.* Upper Saddle River, N. J.: Pearson Education.

Clomiphene Citrate

If a woman has normal ovaries, a normal prolactin level, and an intact pituitary gland, *clomiphene citrate* (Clomid, Serophene) is often used as first-line therapy to induce ovulation. See Drug Guide: Clomiphene Citrate. This medication induces ovulation in 80% of women by action at both the hypothalamic and ovarian levels; 40% of these women will become pregnant. Approximately 8% of women develop multiple gestation pregnancies, almost exclusively twins (Johnson, 2003). Clomiphene citrate works by stimulating the hypothalamus to secrete more gonadotropin-releasing hormone (GnRH), which increases the secretion of FSH and LH. These stimulate follicular growth and facilitate the release of ova (Speroff & Fritz, 2005).

The woman is informed that if ovulation occurs, it is expected to occur 5 to 9 days after the last dose. The nurse determines if the couple has been advised to have sexual intercourse every other day for 1 week, beginning 5 days after the last day of medications. Upon a negative pregnancy test, another trial of clomiphene can be initiated. After the first treatment cycle, a pelvic ultrasound should be done to rule out ovarian enlargement, ovarian cysts, or hyperstimulation. The risk of ovarian hyperstimulation is reported to be 10% but is rarely as severe as that reported with gonadotropin therapy (discussed shortly). Ovarian enlargement and abdominal discomfort (bloating) may result from follicular growth and the formation of multiple corpus lutea. Persistence of ovarian cysts is a contraindication for subsequent treatment cycles. Other side effects include hot flashes, abdominal distention, bloating, breast discomfort, nausea and vomiting, vision problems, headache, and dryness or loss of hair. Some women experience severe mood swings (Bambi-Hitler syndrome). Supplemental low-dose estrogen may be given to ensure appropriate quality and quantity of cervical mucus, or IUI may be employed to overcome this obstacle. Women can assess the presence of ovulation and possible response to clomiphene therapy by doing BBT and urinary LH tests. The woman should be knowledgeable about side effects and call her healthcare provider if they occur. When visual disturbances (flashes, blurring, spots) occur, the woman should avoid bright lighting. This side effect disappears within a few days or weeks after discontinuation of therapy. Hot flashes may be due to the antiestrogenic properties of clomiphene citrate. The woman can obtain some relief through increasing intake of fluids and using fans. Fecundability (the ability to become pregnant) declines with advancing age as described earlier; therefore, prolonged treatment with clomiphene is unjustified in women in their later reproductive years. Clomiphene treatment should generally be limited to the minimum effective dose and to no more than six ovulatory cycles. Failure to conceive after clomiphene induction is an indication to expand the diagnostic evaluation or to change the overall treatment plan if evaluation is complete.

Insulin Sensitizing Agents

Insulin resistance and hyperinsulinemia are now recognized as a common feature of polycystic ovary syndrome (PCOS) and a

 DRUG GUIDE   Clomiphene Citrate (Clomid, Milophene, Serophene)
Pregnancy Category: X

Overview of Action

Clomiphene citrate stimulates follicular growth by stimulating the release of FSH and LH. Ovulation is expected to occur 5 to 9 days after the last dose. Used when anovulation is caused by hypothalamic dysfunction, luteal phase dysfunction, or oligo-ovulation, as seen in polycystic ovary syndrome (PCOS).

Route, Dosage, Frequency

Administered orally. Treatment should begin with a low dose, 50 mg/day (one tablet) for 5 days from cycle day 3 to day 7 or cycle day 5 to day 9. In nonresponders, the dose may be increased to 100 mg/day to a maximum of 250 mg/day, although doses in excess of 100 mg/day are not approved by the FDA (Wilson, Shannon, Shields et al., 2007). May need to give estrogen simultaneously if decrease in cervical mucus occurs.

Contraindications

Presence of ovarian enlargement, ovarian cysts, hyperstimulation syndrome, liver disease, visual problems, pregnancy. *Interaction:* Herbal: Black cohosh may antagonize infertility treatments (Wilson et al., 2007).

Side Effects

Antiestrogenic effects may cause decrease in cervical mucus production and endometrial lining development. Other side effects include vasomotor flushes; abdominal distention and ovarian enlargement secondary to follicular growth (bloating) and multiple corpus luteum formation; pain, soreness, breast discomfort; nausea and vomiting; visual symptoms (spots, flashes); headaches, dryness or loss of hair; multiple pregnancies.

Nursing Considerations

- Determine if couple has been advised to have sexual intercourse every other day for 1 week, beginning 5 days after the last day of medications. If insemination is the preferred treatment strategy ascertain that this is appropriately timed within the ovulatory window (24 to 36 hours of an LH surge).

- Instruct the couple on use of the BBT chart to assess whether ovulation has occurred, or instruct on the use of urinary LH kits to predict the onset of LH surge. Also inform couple that plasma progesterone, cervical mucus, and postcoital tests may be done. Remind couples of the need to confirm outcome with a pregnancy test with either a home pregnancy test or a serum blood test. Clomiphene cycle may be cancelled for ovarian hyperstimulation and subsequent risk of a high-order multiple pregnancy.

contributing cause of chronic anovulation. Anovulatory women with PCOS are hyperinsulinemic and subsequently are more resistant to clomiphene treatment. Recently, studies have shown that oral hypoglycemia agents (e.g., metformin and rosiglitazone) can induce ovulation in women with PCOS. Clinical trials are under way to determine the appropriateness of oral hypoglycemic agents with and without clomiphene in the infertility setting.

Gonadotropins

Therapy using *human menopausal gonadotropins (hMG)*, which include menotropins (Repronex and Menopur) and urofollitropin (Bravelle), is indicated as a first line of therapy for the anovulatory infertile woman with low to normal levels of gonadotropins (FSH and LH) and as a second line of therapy in women who fail to ovulate or conceive with clomiphene citrate therapy and in women undergoing controlled ovarian stimulation with assisted reproduction. Menotropin is a mixture of FSH and LH, and urofollitropin is a further purified form and contains mainly FSH with trace amounts of LH. Immediately before injection, the powder is reconstituted with a diluent and injected subcutaneously. More recently, however, recombinant gonadotropins (rFSH and rLH) have been produced through genetic engineering, giving rise to more consistent preparations. They have been approved by the Food and Drug Administration (FDA) for use when ovulation induction therapy is indicated. Recombinant FSH is homogenous and free of contaminants by proteins. It is marketed under the names Gonal-F (follitropin alpha) and Follistim (follitropin beta). Luveris, a recombinant form of LH, is used concomitantly with recombinant FSH in women with profound LH deficiency such as hypogonadotropic hypogonadism. It is thought that the use of recombinant gonadotropins will eventually become the preferred preparation and that the use of urinary preparations will be phased out (Figure 12–6 ◆).

Normal functioning of the pituitary is not necessary with gonadotropins because their mechanisms of action are direct stimulation of follicular development in the ovary, thus totally bypassing the hypothalamic-pituitary axis. However, normal ovarian reserve and functioning are necessary to ensure that follicles can be stimulated by FSH and LH. As previously described, the single most valuable test to assess ovarian reserve and function is the FSH level, with elevated levels being a poor prognostic sign for conception and pregnancy.

Urofollitropin (FSH only) is indicated for women who have excessive androgen production, such as those with polycystic ovary disease (PCO). Clients with PCO have high endogenous LH levels. Urofollitropin, which is predominantly FSH, is used to equalize the hormonal ratio and induce ovulation.

Gonadotropin therapy requires close observation with serum estradiol levels and ultrasound. Follicle development must be monitored to minimize the risk of multiple pregnancy and to avoid ovarian hyperstimulation syndrome. The daily dose of medication given is titrated based on serum estradiol and ultrasound findings. Then once optimal follicle growth has occurred, human chorionic gonadotropin (hCG) may be administered by either intramuscular or subcutaneous injection to in-

A

B

Figure 12–6 ◆ *A,* A selection of commonly prescribed medications for ovulation induction. SOURCE: Courtesy of PENN Fertility Care, Philadelphia, PA. *B,* Derivation of gonadotropin medications. SOURCE: Courtesy of Serono, Inc., Rockland, MA.

duce final follicular maturation and stimulate ovulation. The couple is advised to have intercourse 24 to 36 hours after hCG administration and for the next 2 days. Women who elect to undergo ovarian stimuation with gonadotropins have usually passed through all other forms of management without conceiving. Strong emotional support and thorough education are needed because of the numerous office visits and injections. Often the partner is instructed, with return demonstration, to administer the daily injections.

Bromocriptine

High prolactin levels may impair production of FSH and LH or block their action on the ovaries. When hyperprolactinemia accompanies anovulation, the infertility may be treated with bromocriptine (Parlodel). This medication acts directly on the prolactin-secreting cells in the anterior pituitary. It inhibits the pituitary's secretion of prolactin—thus preventing suppression of the pulsatile secretion of FSH and LH. This restores normal menstrual cycles and induces ovulation by allowing FSH and LH production. If treatment is successful, the tests of ovulatory function will indicate that ovulation is occurring with a normal luteal phase. Bromocriptine should be discontinued if pregnancy is suspected or at the anticipated time of ovulation because of its possible teratogenic effects. Other side effects, which include nausea, diarrhea, dizziness, headache, and fatigue, can be attributed to the dopaminergic action of bromocriptine. To mimimize side effects for women who are extremely sensitive, treatment may be initiated with a dose of 1.25 mg, slowly building tolerance toward the usual dose of 2.5 mg bid. Intravaginal administration also has been shown to decrease the occurrence of side effects (Johnson, 2003).

Danazol

When endometriosis is determined to be the cause of the infertility, *danazol* (Danocrine) may be given to suppress ovulation and menstruation and to effect atrophy of the ectopic endometrial tissue. Temporary suppression has been shown to result in healing of the endometriosis. The treatment regimen may last for 6 to 12 months or longer, depending on the severity of the disease. Other pharmacologic treatments involve use of the oral contraceptives or oral medroxyprogesterone acetate, and GnRH agonists. For in-depth discussion of the management and care needed for endometriosis, see Chapter 7. ∞

OTHER PHARMACOLOGIC AGENTS

GnRH is a therapeutic tool for inducing ovulation, but its use is limited to women who have insufficient endogenous release of GnRH. Administration is usually by continuous intravenous infusion accomplished by a portable infusion pump with a pulsatile mechanism worn on a belt around the waist. The length of treatment varies from 2 to 4 weeks, and hCG is also given to stimulate ovulation. The risk of multiple gestation and hyperstimulation of the ovaries is less than with gonadotropin therapy, and the treatment is also less expensive. Significant client education and support are necessary for effective use of the pump. Some women find the pump cumbersome.

GnRH agonists (Lupron) and antagonists (Cetrotide and Ganirelix) are often used adjunctively with gonadotropin therapy to suppress the pituitary secretion of endogenous LH and FSH. This is often referred to as down-regulation.

Progesterone

Treatment of luteal phase defects may include the use of progesterone to augment luteal phase progesterone levels or the use of ovulation induction agents, such as clomiphene citrate or gonadotropins (discussed previously), which will augment proliferative phase FSH production of the developing follicle. Women with luteal phase defects have been found to have decreased FSH production in the proliferative phase. This is associated with a decline in luteal phase progesterone and estrogen production and is manifested by an out-of-phase endometrial biopsy. It is also common to use progesterone supplementation in conjunction with these ovulation induction agents for luteal phase support, thereby increasing endometrial receptivity for embryonic implantation. The initiation of progesterone (vaginal or rectal suppositories, intramuscular injections, or orally) occurs after the hCG injection in ovulation induction cycles or IVF cycles with gonadotropins; the treatment continues until

COMPLEMENTARY AND ALTERNATIVE THERAPIES

COMMON TREATMENTS FOR INFERTILITY

Couples experiencing infertility may seek out alternative treatments. Some common treatments include acupuncture and herbs.

Acupuncture: Acupuncture is a therapy used in traditional Chinese medicine (TCM), and it has become a popular complementary treatment. Sterile needles are inserted into specific points on the body to control the flow of chi, or life energy. Acupuncture treatment focuses on balancing the flow of chi in the kidneys and adrenal glands. Several clinical studies have shown acupuncture to be effective in treating infertility in both men and women (Paulus, Zhang, Strehler, et al., 2002). In men, acupuncture treatments may increase sperm counts (Gurfinkel, Cedenho, Yamamura et al., 2003). Three studies of acupuncture given to women at various stages of infertility treatment are promising (White, 2003). In one of these studies, two acupuncture sessions before and after embryo transfer resulted in a 42.5% higher pregnancy rate, versus 26.3% in the control groups (Paulus et al., 2002).

Herbal Treatments: Herbs frequently recommended to treat infertility include ginseng and astragalus. Herbalists cite the healing and hormone-balancing effects of these herbs. Ginseng has historically been used in TCM to enhance male virility and fertility. Several studies also cite ginseng, as well as astragalus, in enhancing in vitro sperm motility (Skidmore-Roth, 2006).

The nurse should be alert for signs that the couple is pursuing complementary therapies out of desperation. A sensitive, nonjudgmental approach will go a long way toward comforting a couple and assuring them that many complementary therapies used are helpful and not harmful.

pregnancy testing and may continue further if pregnancy testing is positive. Occasionally, hCG therapy may be used in the luteal phase to stimulate corpus luteum production of progesterone.

THERAPEUTIC INSEMINATION

Therapeutic insemination has replaced the previously used term *artificial insemination* and involves depositing sperm at the cervical os or in the uterus by mechanical means. *Therapeutic donor insemination (TDI)* is the current term for use of donor semen, and *therapeutic husband insemination (THI)* is the current term for use of the husband's semen.

THI is generally indicated for such seminal deficiencies as oligospermia (low sperm count), asthenospermia (decreased motility), and teratospermia (low percentage, abnormal morphology); for anatomic defects that are accompanied by inadequate deposition of sperm, such as hypospadias (a congenital abnormal male urethral opening on the underside of the penis); and for ejaculatory dysfunction, such as retrograde ejaculation

(Kakarla & Bradshaw, 2003). THI is also indicated in unexplained infertility and some cases of female factor infertility, specifically infertility due to cervical factors, such as scant or inhospitable mucus, persistent cervicitis, or cervical stenosis. In such cases, *IUI* would be indicated to bypass the cervical factor. Because the seminal fluid contains high levels of prostaglandins, IUI prevents the violent reaction of nausea, severe cramps, abdominal pain, and diarrhea that can result from the absorption of prostaglandins by the cervical lining. Sperm preparation for IUI involves washing sperm from the seminal plasma. IUI, with or without ovulation induction therapy, is an option for many couples before more aggressive treatments such as IVF are employed.

TDI is considered in cases of azoospermia (absence of sperm), severe oligospermia or asthenospermia, inherited male sex-linked disorders, and autosomal dominant disorders. In the past several years, indications for donor insemination have expanded to include single women or lesbians desirous of pregnancy. Some states have specified the parental rights of the single woman and the donor, but most are silent on this issue.

TDI has become more complicated and expensive in the last decade because of the need for strict screening and processing procedures to prevent transmission of a genetic defect or sexually transmitted infection to the offspring or recipient. Guidelines were established and updated by the American Society for Reproductive Medicine (2002) that include mandatory medical and infectious disease screening of both the donor and recipient, the need for informed consent from all parties, the need to limit the number of pregnancies per donor, and the need to establish an accurate means of record keeping. Finally, because of the risk of transmitting infectious disease, donated sperm must be frozen and quarantined for 6 months from the time of acquisition and the donor must be retested before sperm can be released for use.

Numerous factors must be evaluated before TDI is performed. Has every possible effort been made to diagnose and treat the cause of the male infertility? Do tests indicate normal ovulation and sperm/ovum transport in the woman? Has the couple had an opportunity to discuss this option with an infertility counselor to explore the issues of secrecy, disclosure, and potential feelings of loss that the couple (particularly the male partner) may feel because of their inability to have a genetic child? After making the decision, the couple should allow themselves time to assess their concerns further and explore their feelings individually and together to ensure that this option is acceptable to both.

IN VITRO FERTILIZATION

In vitro fertilization (IVF) is selectively used in cases in which infertility has resulted from tubal factors, mucus abnormalities, male infertility, unexplained infertility, male and female immunologic infertility, and cervical factors. In IVF, a woman's eggs are collected from her ovaries, fertilized in the laboratory, and placed into her uterus after normal embryo development has begun. If the procedure is successful, the embryo continues to develop in the uterus, and pregnancy proceeds naturally.

DEVELOPING CULTURAL COMPETENCE

INFERTILITY TREATMENTS

The acceptance of infertility treatments varies widely around the world. Some belief systems do not allow various treatments, because using a treatment is considered interfering with God's design or because the treatment itself is seen as tainted or sinful. For example, fertility practices in Arab cultures are influenced by traditional Arab Bedouin values that support tribal dominance and beliefs that "God decides family sizes." In Arab cultures, procreation is the purpose of marriage.

If a couple is infertile, the approved methods for treating infertility are limited to use of therapeutic insemination using the husband's sperm and IVF involving the fertilization of the wife's ovum by the husband's sperm because of lineage concerns (Kridli, 2002; Purnell & Paulanka, 2005).

Sterility in a woman can lead to rejection and divorce. Also with the advent of ICSI, male-initiated divorce is becoming more common for aging wives of infertile husbands (Inhorn, 2002). Contemporary Islamic religious opinion forbids any kind of egg, embryo, or semen donation, as well as surrogacy (Inhorn, 2002).

In Jewish cultures, infertile couples are to try all possible means to have children, including egg and sperm donation. However, Orthodox Jewish opinion is virtually unanimous in prohibiting artificial insemination when the semen donor is a Jewish man other than the woman's husband, because it may constitute adultery (Purnell & Paulanka, 2005). If the infertility is because of a male factor, artificial insemination with sperm from a non-Jewish sperm donor is acceptable because "Jewishness" is conferred through the matriline. IVF and embryo transfer (ET) are also acceptable artificial insemination methods because they do not involve putting sperm into another's wife (Kahn, 2002).

The potential for a successful pregnancy with IVF is maximized by replacing three to four embryos (rather than one). For this reason, fertility drugs are used to induce ovulation before the process. Follicular growth is monitored frequently with ultrasound and hormonal assays. Monitoring usually begins around cycle day 5, and medications are titrated according to individual response. When the follicles have grown to an appropriate size, hCG is given to induce final egg maturation and control the induction of ovulation. Egg retrieval is performed approximately 35 hours later, before ovulation occurs.

In the majority of cases, egg retrieval is performed by a transvaginal approach under ultrasound guidance (Figure 12–7 ◆, *A*). It is an outpatient procedure performed with intravenous sedation and a cervical block for anesthesia. A needle guide that helps direct the aspirating needle through the posterior vaginal wall into the follicle is attached to the vaginal ultrasound probe (Figure 12–7, *B*). Many follicles can be aspirated with only one puncture, and the procedure generally lasts no more than 30 minutes. The woman usually tolerates the

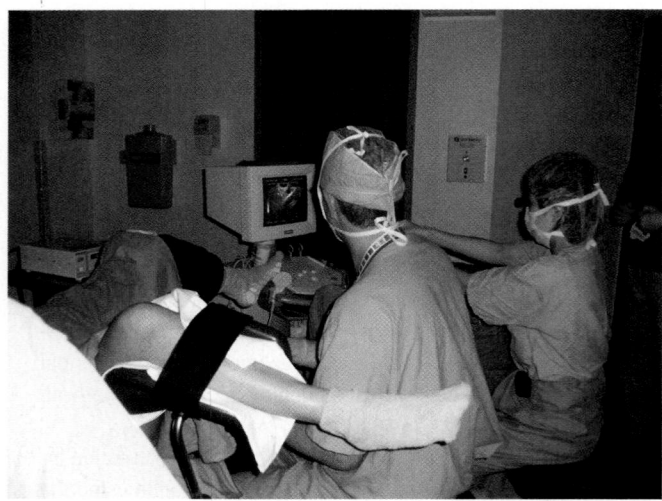

A

B

Figure 12–7 ◆ *A,* Operating room setup for ultrasound-guided oocyte retrieval. SOURCE: Courtesy of PENN Fertility Care, Philadelphia, PA. *B,* Transvaginal ultrasound-guided oocyte retrieval. SOURCE: Courtesy of Serono, Inc., Rockland, MA.

procedure well and is discharged to home within 2 hours with instructions for limited activity for 24 hours.

Once the eggs are fertilized and progress to the embryo stage, the embryos are placed in the uterus. After the procedure, the woman is advised to engage in only minimal activity for 12 to 24 hours, and progesterone supplementation is prescribed. Sperm used to fertilize the eggs in vitro can be obtained naturally or surgically via microsurgical epididymal sperm aspiration (MESA) and testicular sperm aspiration (TESA). These are procedures that address severe male factor infertility. MESA and TESA involve the retrieval of sperm from the gonadal tissue of men who have azoospermia or an ejaculatory disorder. ICSI is a microscopic procedure to inject a single sperm into the outer layer of an ovum so that fertilization will occur.

Success with IVF depends on many factors, the two most important of which are the woman's age and the indication.

Women with an average of three cycles of IVF have a good chance of achieving pregnancy. Many couples find the emotional, physical, and financial costs of going beyond three cycles too great. Clinical birth rates reported by the Society of Assisted Reproductive Technology (SART) in 2002 were 35% per embryo transfer for women regardless of age or indication (Centers for Disease Control and Prevention, 2004). The increase in maternal and neonatal morbidity associated with IVF because of the multiple gestation rates remains an issue. Differences in successful IVF may exist between various ethnic groups (Sharara & McClamrock, 2000).

OTHER ASSISTED REPRODUCTIVE TECHNIQUES

Other assisted reproductive techniques include procedures for transferring gametes, zygotes, or embryos; cryopreservation of embryos; IVF using donor oocytes; micromanipulation techniques; and use of a gestational carrier (Kashyap & Davis, 2003) (Figure 12–8 ◆).

Gamete Intrafallopian Transfer

Gamete intrafallopian transfer (GIFT) involves the retrieval of oocytes by laparoscopy; immediate placement of the oocytes in a catheter with washed, motile sperm; and placement of the gametes into the fimbriated end of the fallopian tube. Fertilization occurs in the fallopian tube as with normal conception (in vivo), rather than in the laboratory (in vitro). The fertilized egg then travels through the fallopian tube to the uterus for implantation as in normal reproduction. This practice is acceptable to the Roman Catholic Church.

GIFT has proven to be a very effective therapy for couples whose infertility results from various seminal deficiencies, unexplained factors, cervical factors, immunologic factors, and endometriosis when less aggressive means of therapy have failed. In cases of male factor infertility, GIFT offers an opportunity for the egg and an adequate concentration of sperm to meet in the fallopian tube; with coitus, in contrast, sperm with low count or motility may never reach the tube. The major prerequisite for GIFT is the presence of at least one normal fallopian tube. It is not an appropriate therapy for any woman with a history of pelvic inflammatory disease, tubal disease, or ectopic gestation because the passage of the fertilized ova to the uterus is slowed, thereby increasing the chance of sustaining an ectopic tubal pregnancy.

From the GIFT technology evolved several other transfer procedures such as **zygote intrafallopian transfer (ZIFT)** and **tubal embryo transfer (TET).** In these procedures eggs are retrieved and incubated with the man's sperm. However, the eggs are transferred back to the woman's body at a much earlier stage of cell division than in IVF and, as in GIFT, are placed in the fallopian tube or tubes and not in the uterus. In TET, the placement is done at the embryo stage. These procedures allow fertilization to be documented, which is not possible with GIFT, and the pregnancy rate is theoretically increased when the fertilized ovum is placed in the fallopian tube.

When considering IVF and the transfer procedures, several factors must be weighed. IVF success rates approximate those

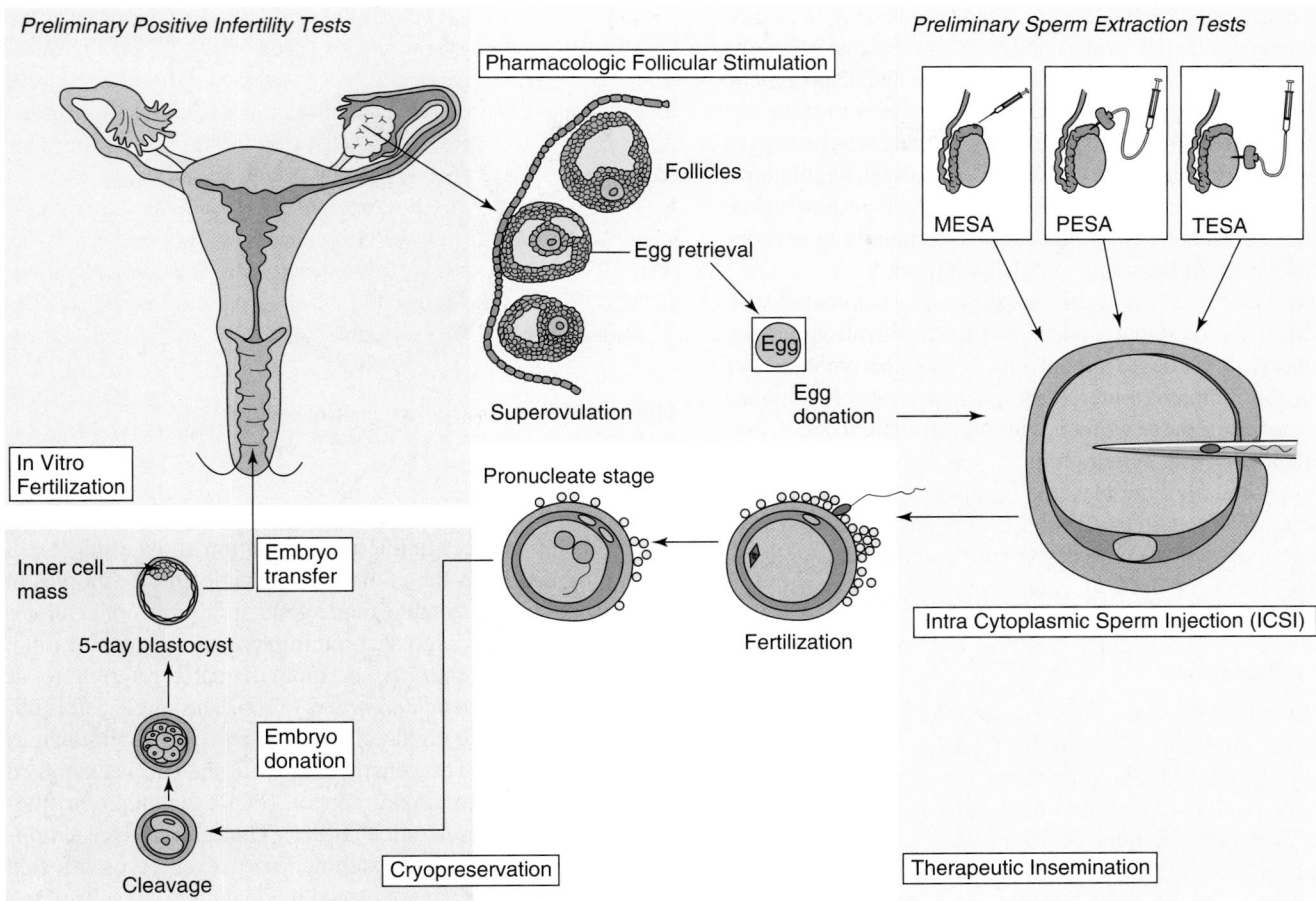

Figure 12–8 ◆ Assisted reproductive techniques.

that have been achieved with the transfer procedures, and IVF is a much less invasive and costly procedure. For these reasons, the transfer procedures have lost some acceptance and IVF techniques are more often used. However, GIFT may be more acceptable to adherents of some religions, because fertilization does not occur outside the woman's body.

Embryo Cryopreservation

Research has shown that replacing three to four embryos in a treatment cycle offers the best chances for pregnancy. Replacing more than four only increases the chance for a multiple pregnancy. To minimize this risk, excess embryos may be stored using freezing, or cryopreservation. Should a pregnancy not ensue, frozen embryos can be thawed. After they are maintained in culture for a short time to confirm resumption of growth, they are replaced in the woman's uterus at the appropriate time in her menstrual cycle. Thus freezing affords the couple another attempt at pregnancy without having to undergo stimulation and egg retrieval again.

Ethical issues to consider in this situation include the following: Who has legal custody of the embryos? How long can they be frozen? What options does the couple have in the event of divorce, if one or both partners die, or if they do not wish to use the embryos at a later date? These issues must be ad-

dressed with all couples so that they may make informed decisions when executing their consent forms and legal statements. Reproductive endocrine nurses need to be involved in establishing standards and guidelines for assisted reproduction technologies. Clinically, the reproductive endocrine nurse is instrumental in providing support, education, and counseling to couples considering assisted reproductive methods. The nurse assesses the couple for personal, marital, and parenting difficulties and initiates interventions that help establish family roles and bonds. Follow-up care mechanisms can be set, thereby aiding in individual growth, marital stability, and family development.

In Vitro Fertilization Using Donor Oocytes

The use of donor eggs, a natural extension of IVF, is reserved for women who do not produce viable eggs because of premature ovarian failure, surgical removal of the ovaries, advanced maternal age, chemotherapy or radiation exposure, or inherent oocyte defects but who do have a functional uterus. Women with normal ovarian function may also benefit from egg donation if they have an autosomal dominant or sex-linked genetic disorder such as hemophilia or Duchenne muscular dystrophy.

Oocyte donors may be either known or anonymous. In either case, both donors and recipients undergo psychologic evaluation and counseling to ensure that all parties have explored and discussed potential issues and are comfortable with the process. The donors are subject to extensive medical and genetic testing. Effective May 2005, the FDA has instituted screening and testing requirements for all tissue donors, which includes donors of oocytes, sperm, and embryos (Code of Federal Regulations, 2005). The nurse functions as a case manager by coordinating the many tests, procedures, and educational and counseling sessions that are involved for the donor and recipient couple.

Once donor eggs are available, they are inseminated with the sperm of the recipient's partner. After fertilization has occurred and embryo development has begun, the embryos are placed in the recipient's uterus. Pregnancies can be achieved and maintained in these women with an estrogen/progesterone replacement protocol. When pregnancy occurs, hormonal support is continued until the placenta is capable of supporting the pregnancy, usually at 10 to 12 weeks. Live birth rates of recipients of donor eggs in 2002 were 44% per embryo transfer as reported by SART in 2002 (Centers for Disease Control and Prevention, 2004).

Embryo Donation

Much like egg donation, embryo donation offers couples another option in creating a family. Couples who have gone through ART (assisted reproductive technology) and have completed their family may choose to donate their cryopreserved embryos to another couple. There are two types of donation, known or directed donation and anonymous donation. Couples interested in being the recipients of these donations include those with severe or untreatable male and female factor infertility, those who have experienced repeated treatment failures or multiple pregnancy losses not due to implantation problems, and those at risk for transmitting genetic diseases to their offspring. Screening and assessment guidelines have been established (ASRM 2004).

Micromanipulation and Blastomere Analysis

Micromanipulation allows individual eggs and sperm to be handled through the use of very fine, specialized instruments. Using the micromanipulators allows the clinician to handle cells under the microscope with magnification of 200 to 400 times and to inject a sperm cell directly into an egg. This procedure, known as *ICSI*, has revolutionized the treatment of severe male factor infertility. The procedure has achieved fertilization in cases of extremely low sperm concentrations, in cases of absence of motility, and in cases where previous IVF therapy failed.

Assisted embryo hatching is another micromanipulation procedure that has proved to be an effective adjunct therapy in IVF. It is indicated for women in whom the normal "hatching" process may be impeded because of a hardening or thickening of the zona pellucida, most commonly seen in women of advanced maternal age. Assisted hatching involves creating a small opening in the zona pellucida of the embryo using micromanipulators (Figure 12–9 ◆). The small opening may facilitate the natural hatching process, allowing the embryo to escape from the zona pellucida and interact with the endometrium for implantation.

"Fragile site" made in zona by: Acidified medium, Pipette or Laser

Injection Pipette

Holding Pipette

Figure 12–9 ◆ Assisted hatching of embryo.
SOURCE: Courtesy of Serono, Inc., Rockland, MA.

Preimplantation Genetic Diagnosis (PGD)

Other recent advances in micromanipulation allow a single cell to be removed from the embryo for genetic study. Couples at risk for having a detectable single gene or chromosomal anomaly may wish to undergo such preimplantation genetic testing, called *blastomere analysis,* or more recently referred to as *preimplantation genetic diagnosis (PGD).* The single cell is obtained from a six- to eight-cell embryo by a process known as blastomere biopsy. The genetic content of the cell is examined using the polymerase chain reaction (PCR) technique or fluorescence in situ hybridization (FISH). The cell's DNA is amplified 1,000,000 times and examined so that embryos affected with genetic disease are not placed in the mother. Results of genetic testing on the preimplantation embryos are available in 4 to 24 hours, so unaffected embryos may still be transferred during the required biologic window of time without the need for cryopreservation.

The diagnosis of genetic disorders before implantation provides couples with the option of forgoing the attempt to establish a pregnancy and thereby avoiding a difficult decision about terminating an affected pregnancy (Simpson, 2002). This technology also raises several ethical issues, including the following:

- Identification of couples at risk. There is a need for criteria that identify couples at risk for diseases that constitute significant hardship and suffering so that "wrongful birth" cases can be avoided.

- Availability of and access to centers providing PGD. Should society provide access for those at risk for genetic transfer of disease but without the financial resources to pay for the services?

- Analysis of blastomeres for sex chromosome testing when a genetic disorder carried on the sex chromosomes is suspected. In X-linked diseases, the only way to prevent the disorder is to select against the blastomere with the Y chromosome.

- Identification of late-onset diseases. The Human Genome Project has aided in the identification of genetic markers for late-onset disease. Couples may wish to choose to implant blastomeres that do not carry these markers.

- Effect on the offspring as a result of removing cells from the embryo.
- Selection for nonmedical reasons and potential concern of eugenics "designer babies."

In Vitro Fertilization Using a Gestational Carrier

A *gestational carrier* is a woman who has contracted with the infertile woman or couple to carry an embryo/fetus that is not genetically her own offspring. This must be distinguished from surrogate motherhood, wherein the surrogate is both gestational carrier and gamete donor. IVF using a gestational carrier is appropriate for the infertile woman who is able to produce her own eggs but unable to carry a pregnancy because of (1) congenital absence or surgical removal of her uterus; (2) a reproductively impaired uterus, myomas, uterine synechiae (adhesion of uterus), or any other congenital abnormalities; or (3) a medical condition that might be life threatening during pregnancy, such as diabetes, immunologic problems, or a severe heart, kidney, or liver disease (Pergament & Fiddler, 2000). Use of a gestational carrier allows a couple with any of these conditions to have a child that is a genetic relation (Pergament & Fiddler, 2000). All participants are required to have medical and psychologic screening as well as legal counsel before acceptance into the program.

ADOPTION

Infertile couples consider various alternatives for resolving their infertility; adoption is one option that will be considered at several points during the treatment process. As couples begin to consider adoption, an important aspect of this exploration is the reading of books, magazines, and informational Web sites such as the National Adoption Information Clearinghouse; attending adoption support groups and conferences; and meeting with adoptive parents to discuss their experiences with adoption.

The adoption of an infant in the United States can be difficult and frustrating, often involving long waiting periods, continual setbacks, and high costs. Thus many couples seek international adoptions or consider adopting older children, children with disabilities, or children of mixed parentage, because the adoption process in such cases is quicker and more children are available. Nurses in the community can assist couples considering adoption by providing information on community resources for adoption as well as by providing support throughout the adoption process. Informational books, Web sites such as Childless by Choice, and support groups such as San Francisco RESOLVE's "Living Without Children" are available to those who remain or choose to be childless.

PREGNANCY AFTER INFERTILITY

The feeling of being infertile does not necessarily disappear with pregnancy. Although there may be initial ecstasy, the couple may also face a whole new arena of fear and anxieties, and the parents-to-be often do not know where they "fit in." They may feel a great sense of loss and isolation because those who have had no trouble conceiving cannot relate to the physical and emotional pain they endured to achieve the pregnancy. Contact

with their past "infertile" support system may vanish when peers learn the couple has resolved their infertility. Although the desperation to become pregnant may have superseded the couple's ability to acknowledge their concerns about undergoing various treatments or procedures, questions about the repeated cycle of fertility drugs or the achievement of pregnancy through IVF technology or cryopreservation may now arise. The expectant couple may be very concerned about the potential of these treatments for adverse effects on the fetus (Johnson, 2003). Couples may need much reassurance throughout the pregnancy to allay these anxieties. The nurse can assist couples who conceive after infertility by acknowledging their past experience of infertility treatment; validating their fears and anxieties as they face childbirth classes, birth, and parenting issues; and providing education and support regarding what to anticipate physically and emotionally throughout the pregnancy. The nurse can also counsel couples that infertility due to nonstructural causes may correct itself following a successful pregnancy and delivery; therefore, postdelivery contraception counseling may be warranted. These interventions will go a long way toward normalizing the experience for the couple.

NURSING CARE MANAGEMENT

Infertility therapy taxes a couple's financial, physical, and emotional resources. Treatment can be costly, and often insurance coverage is limited. Years of effort and numerous evaluations and examinations may take place before a conception occurs, if one occurs at all. In a society that values children and considers them to be the natural result of marriage, infertile couples may face a myriad of tensions and discrimination.

The clinic nurse needs to be constantly aware of the emotional needs of the couple confronting infertility evaluation and treatment. Often an intact marriage will become stressed with the intrusive but necessary infertility procedures and treatments. Constant attention to temperature charts and instructions about their sex life from a person outside the relationship naturally affect the spontaneity of a couple's interactions.

Tests and treatments may heighten feelings of frustration or anger between partners. The need to share this intimate area of a relationship, especially when one or the other is identified as "the cause" of infertility, may precipitate feelings of guilt or shame. Infertility often becomes a central focus for role identity, especially for women (Klock, 2004).

The couple may experience feelings of loss of control, feelings of reduced competency and defectiveness, loss of status and ambiguity as a couple, a sense of social stigma, stress on the marital and sexual relationship, and a strained relationship with healthcare providers. The nurse's roles can be summarized as those of counselor, educator, and advocate.

Tasks of the infertile couple and appropriate nursing interventions are summarized in Table 12–7. Throughout the evaluation process, nurses can play a key role in lessening the stress these couples must endure by providing them with appropriate resources and accurate information about what treatment entails

RESEARCH IN PRACTICE

ASSOCIATIONS OF PSYCHOSOCIAL FACTORS WITH THE STRESS OF INFERTILITY TREATMENT

What is this study about? Infertility rates are expected to increase over the next 20 years. Treatment for infertility involves an indeterminate, often extended, time frame. The process and outcome are ambiguous and may affect self-esteem, health functioning, and psychologic well-being. All of these factors come together to create a time of substantial stress for the infertile couple. This study was an investigation of psychosocial factors that may be associated with perceptions of stress during the course of treatment for infertility. The purpose of the study was to identify which factors are associated with stress, and to discover any associations between the stage of treatment and stress-related factors.

How was this study done? This research involved subjects who answered infertility-related stress questions at three prescribed intervals during treatment. The data were secondary data, meaning they were collected previously for a different, but related, research question. A subset of the data was analyzed for this study. The original data were collected through personal interview; 185 infertile and 90 presumed fertile couples were interviewed. The interview included questions related to treatment; social support; spousal support; self-esteem; perceived health; importance of biologic children; life events; and attribution of responsibility. Couples entered the study at different points in their treatment and were interviewed at entry, after 1 year of treatment, and after 2 years of treatment. Of those recruited into the study, 128 people completed all three measurements and had not become pregnant.

What were the results of the study? At the study baseline period, stress was associated with self-esteem and perceived level of health. After 1 year of treatment, stress was related to personal issues, such as the importance assigned to having a biologic family, and the extent of the husband's supportive behavior. After 2 years of treatment, stress was related to factors that pertain to the treatment itself, including the number of treatments and relationships with healthcare providers. Only one of the factors—self-esteem—was consistently associated with stress regardless of the length of treatment.

What additional questions might I have? Are the factors different for those who are in extended treatment and become pregnant than for those who remain infertile? How long do these factors affect couples once they decide to discontinue infertility treatments? Do these factors change if a couple becomes adoptive parents?

How can I use this study? Families undergoing extended treatments for infertility have unique psychosocial needs. The results of this study can be used to design client counseling plans that recognize the stresses that these couples experience. Interventions designed to help couples maintain emotional balance and self-esteem during treatment can be beneficial. This study can help the nurse design an approach that is appropriate for the stage of treatment and level of stress of the clients.

SOURCE: Schneider, M., & Forthofer, M. (2005). Associations of psychosocial factors with the stress of infertility treatment. *Health and Social Work, 30*(3), 183–191.

Table 12–7   TASKS OF THE INFERTILE COUPLE

Tasks	Nursing Interventions
Recognize how infertility affects their lives and express feelings (may be negative toward self or mate)	Supportive: help to understand and facilitate free expression of feelings
Grieve the loss of potential offspring	Help to recognize feelings
Evaluate reasons for wanting a child	Help to understand motives
Decide about management	Identify alternatives; facilitate partner communication

SOURCE: Sawatzky, M. (1981). Tasks of the infertile couple. *Journal of Obstetric, Gynecologic, and Neonatal Nursing, 10,* 132.

and what physical, emotional, and financial demands they can anticipate throughout the process (Klock, 2004).

The nurse's ability to assess and respond to emotional and educational needs is essential to give infertile couples control and help them negotiate the treatment process. An assessment tool such as an infertility questionnaire (Table 12–8) may be helpful. Extensive and repeated explanations and written instruction may be necessary because the couple's anxiety often overwhelms their ability to retain all the information given. It is important to use a nursing framework that recognizes the multidimensional needs of the infertile individual or couple within physical, social, psychologic, spiritual, and environmental contexts.

Infertility may be perceived as a loss by one or both partners. Affected individuals have described this as loss of their relationship with spouse, family, or friends; their health; their status or prestige; their self-esteem and self-confidence; their security; and the potential child. Any one of these types of losses may lead to depression and, in many cases, the crisis of infertility evokes feelings similar to ones associated with all these losses (Klock, 2004). Each couple passes through several stages, not unlike those identified by Kübler-Ross: surprise, denial, anger, isolation, guilt, grief, and resolution.

The impact of these feelings on the couple and how fast they move into resolution, if ever, may depend on the cause and duration of treatment. Each partner may progress through the stages at different rates (Klock, 2004). Nonjudgmental acceptance and a professional, caring attitude on the nurse's part can go far to dissipate the negative emotions the couple may experience while going through these stages.

Table 12–8	INFERTILITY QUESTIONNAIRE

Self-Image

1. I feel bad about my body because of our inability to have a child.
2. Since our infertility, I feel I can do anything as well as I used to.
3. I feel as attractive as before our infertility.
4. I feel less masculine/feminine because of our inability to have a child.
5. Compared with others, I feel I am a worthwhile person.
6. Lately, I feel I am sexually attractive to my wife/husband.
7. I feel I will be incomplete as a man/woman if we cannot have a child.
8. Having an infertility problem makes me feel physically incompetent.

Guilt/Blame

1. I feel guilty about somehow causing our infertility.
2. I wonder if our infertility problem is due to something I did in the past.
3. My spouse makes me feel guilty about our problem.
4. There are times when I blame my spouse for our infertility.
5. I feel I am being punished because of our infertility.

Sexuality

1. Lately I feel I am able to respond to my spouse sexually.
2. I feel sex is a duty, not a pleasure.
3. Since our infertility problem, I enjoy sexual relations with my spouse.
4. We have sexual relations for the purpose of trying to conceive.
5. Sometimes I feel like a "sex machine," programmed to have sex during the fertile period.
6. Impaired fertility has helped our sexual relationship.
7. Our inability to have a child has increased my desire for sexual relations.
8. Our inability to have a child has decreased my desire for sexual relations.

NOTE: The questionnaire is scored on a Likert scale, with responses ranging from "strongly agree" to "strongly disagree." Each question is scored separately, and the mean score is determined for each section (Self-Image, Guilt/Blame, and Sexuality). The total mean score is then divided by 3. A final mean score of greater than 3 indicates distress.

SOURCE: Reproduced with permission from AWHONN. (1985). Bernstein, J., Potts, N., and Mattox, J. H., Assessment of psychological dysfunction association with infertility. *Journal of Obstetric, Gynecologic, and Neonatal Nursing.* 14 (Suppl.), 64S, Table 1. Washington, DC: Author. © 1985 by the Association of Women's Health, Obstetric and Neonatal Nurses. All rights reserved.

This is also a time when the nurse may assess the quality of the couple's relationship: Are they able and willing to communicate verbally and share feelings? Are they mutually supportive? The answers to these questions may help the nurse identify areas of strength and weakness and construct an appropriate plan of care.

Referral to mental health professionals is helpful when the emotional issues become too disruptive in the couple's relationship or life. Couples should be made aware of infertility support and education organizations such as RESOLVE (National Infertility Association), which may help meet some of these needs and validate their feelings. Finally, individual or group counseling with other infertile couples may help the couple resolve feelings brought about by their own difficult situation.

GENETIC DISORDERS

Even when conception has been achieved, families can have special reproductive concerns. The desired and expected outcome of any pregnancy is the birth of a healthy, "perfect" baby. Parents experience grief, fear, and anger when they discover that their baby has been born with a defect or a genetic disease. Such an abnormality may be evident at birth or may not appear for some time. The baby may have inherited a disorder from one parent or both, creating guilt and strife within the family.

Regardless of the type or scope of the problem, parents will have many questions: "What did I do?" "What caused it?" "How do I cope with it?" "Will it happen again?" The nurse must anticipate the parents' questions and concerns, direct the family to the appropriate resources, and support the family. To do so, the nurse must have a basic knowledge of genetics and genetic counseling. Professional nurses can help expedite this questioning process if they understand the principles involved and can direct the family to the appropriate resources.

Chromosomes and Chromosomal Analysis

All hereditary material is carried on tightly coiled strands of DNA known as **chromosomes.** The chromosomes carry the *genes,* the smallest unit of inheritance, as discussed in greater detail in Chapter 11. ∞ The Human Genome Project has made remarkable advances toward determining the exact DNA sequence of human genes and the precise genes that are associated with certain abnormalities, such as fragile X syndrome and cystic fibrosis, as discussed in greater detail later in this chapter (Prosen & Hogge, 2004).

All *somatic* (*body*) *cells* contain 46 chromosomes, which is the *diploid* number; the sperm and egg contain half as many (23) chromosomes, or the *haploid* number (see Chapter 11 ∞). There are 23 pairs of homologous chromosomes (a matched pair of chromosomes, one inherited from each parent). Twenty-two of the pairs are known as **autosomes** (nonsex chromosomes), and one pair is the sex chromosome, X and Y. A normal female has a 46, XX chromosome constitution, the normal male, 46, XY (Figures 12–10 ◆ and 12–11 ◆).

The **karyotype,** or pictorial analysis of an individual's chromosomes, is usually obtained from specially treated and stained peripheral blood lymphocytes. Placenta tissue taken from a site near the insertion of the cord and deep enough to include chorion can be sent for karyotyping of the fetus.

Chromosome abnormalities can occur in either the autosomes or the sex chromosomes and can be divided into two categories: abnormalities of number and abnormalities of structure. Even small alterations in chromosomes can cause problems, especially those associated with delayed growth and development. Some of these abnormalities can also be passed on to other offspring. Thus in some cases chromosomal analysis is appropriate even if clinical manifestations are mild.

ABNORMALITIES OF CHROMOSOME NUMBER

Abnormalities of chromosome number are most commonly seen as trisomies, monosomies, and as mosaicism. In all three cases,

Figure 12–10 ◆ Normal female karyotype.
SOURCE: Courtesy of David Peakman, Reproductive Genetics Center, Denver, CO.

Figure 12–11 ◆ Normal male karyotype.
SOURCE: Courtesy of David Peakman, Reproductive Genetics Center, Denver, CO.

the abnormality is most often caused by nondisjunction, a failure of paired chromosomes to separate during cell division. If nondisjunction occurs in either the sperm or the egg before fertilization, the resulting zygote (fertilized egg) will have an abnormal chromosome makeup in all of the cells (trisomy or monosomy). If nondisjunction occurs after fertilization, the developing zygote will have cells with two or more different chromosome makeups, evolving into two or more different cell lines (mosaicism).

Trisomies are the product of the union of a normal gamete (egg or sperm) with a gamete that contains an extra chromosome. The individual will have 47 chromosomes and be tri-

Figure 12–12 ◆ Karyotype of a female who has trisomy 21, Down syndrome. Note the extra chromosome 21.
SOURCE: Courtesy of Greenwood Genetics Center. (2002). *Genetic Counseling Aids, Ed. 4.*

Figure 12–13 ◆ A boy with Down syndrome.

somic (have three copies of the same chromosome) for whichever chromosome is extra (Table 12–9). Down syndrome (formerly called mongolism) is the most common trisomy abnormality seen in children (Figure 12–12 ◆). The presence of the extra chromosome 21 produces distinctive clinical features (Figure 12–13 ◆). Although children born with Down syndrome have a variety of physical ailments, advances in medical science have extended their life expectancy.

The other two common trisomies are trisomy 18 and trisomy 13 (see Table 12–9 and Figures 12–14 ◆ and 12–15 ◆). The prognosis for both trisomy 18 or 13 is extremely poor. Most children (70%) die within the first 3 months of life as a result of complications related to respiratory and cardiac abnormalities. However, 10% survive the first year of life; therefore, the family needs to plan for the possibility of long-term care of a severely affected infant and for family support.

Monosomies occur when a normal gamete unites with a gamete that is missing a chromosome. In this case, the individual will have only 45 chromosomes and is said to be monosomic. Monosomy of an entire autosomal chromosome is incompatible with life.

Table 12–9   CHROMOSOMAL SYNDROMES

Altered Chromosome: 21

Genetic defect: trisomy 21 (Down syndrome) (secondary nondisjunction or 14/21 unbalanced translocation) (see Figures 12–12 & 12–13)

Incidence: average 1 in 700 live births, incidence variable with age of woman

Characteristics:

CNS: mental retardation; hypotonia at birth

Head: flattened occiput; depressed nasal bridge; mongoloid slant of eyes; epicanthal folds; white specking of the iris (Brushfield spots); protrusion of the tongue; high, arched palate; low-set ears

Hands: broad, short fingers; abnormalities of finger and foot; dermal ridge patterns (dermatoglyphics); transverse palmar crease (simian line)

Other: congenital heart disease

Altered chromosome: 18

Genetic defect: trisomy 18

Incidence: 1 in 3000 live births

Characteristics:

CNS: mental retardation; severe hypotonia

Head: prominent occiput; low-set ears; corneal opacities; ptosis (drooping of eyelids)

Hands: third and fourth fingers overlapped by second and fifth fingers; abnormal dermatoglyphics; syndactyly (webbing of fingers)

Other: congenital heart defects; renal abnormalities; single umbilical artery; gastrointestinal tract abnormalities; rocker-bottom feet; cryptorchidism; various malformations of other organs

Altered chromosome: 13

Genetic defect: trisomy 13

Incidence: 1 in 5000 live births

Characteristics:

CNS: mental retardation; severe hypotonia; seizures

Head: microcephaly; microphthalmia and/or coloboma (keyhole-shaped pupil); malformed ears; aplasia of external auditory canal; micrognathia (abnormally small lower jaw); cleft lip and palate

Hands: polydactyly (extra digits); abnormal posturing of fingers; abnormal dermatoglyphics

Other: congenital heart defects; hemangiomas; gastrointestinal tract defects; various malformations of other organs

Characteristics:

CNS: severe mental retardation; a catlike cry in infancy

Head: microcephaly; hypertelorism (widely spaced eyes); epicanthal folds; low-set ears

Other: failure to thrive; various organ malformations

Altered Chromosome: 5p

Genetic defect: deletion of short arm of chromosome 5 (cri du chat, or cat cry, syndrome) (see Figure 12–17)

Incidence: 1 in 20,000 live births (see Figure 12–17)

Characteristics:

CNS: no intellectual impairment; some perceptual difficulties

Head: low hairline; webbed neck

Trunk: short stature; cubitus valgus (increased carrying angle of arm); excessive nevi (congenital discoloration of skin due to pigmentation); broad shieldlike chest with widely spaced nipples; puffy feet; no toenails

Other: fibrous streaks in ovaries; underdeveloped secondary sex characteristics; primary amenorrhea; usually infertile; renal anomalies; coarctation of the aorta

Altered chromosome: XO (sex chromosome)

Genetic defect: only one X chromosome in female (Turner syndrome)

Incidence: 1 in 300–7000 live female births (see Figure 12–18)

Characteristics:

CNS: mild mental retardation

Trunk: occasional gynecomastia (abnormally large male breasts); eunuchoid body proportions (lack of male muscular and sexual development)

Other: small, soft testes; underdeveloped secondary sex characteristics; usually sterile

Altered chromosome: XXY (sex chromosome)

Genetic defect extra X chromosome in male (Klinefelter syndrome)

Incidence: 1 in 1000 live male births, approximately 1% to 2% of institutionalized males

---

Mosaicism occurs after fertilization and results in an individual with two different cell lines, each having a different chromosomal number. Mosaicism tends to be more common in the sex chromosomes; when it does occur in the autosomes, it is most common in Down syndrome. An individual with many of the classic signs of Down syndrome but with normal or near-normal intelligence should be investigated for the possibility of mosaicism.

ABNORMALITIES OF CHROMOSOME STRUCTURE

Abnormalities of chromosome structure involve only parts of the chromosome and generally occur in two forms: translocation, and deletions or additions. Some children born with Down syndrome have trisomy 21, whereas others have an abnormal rearrangement of chromosomal material known as *translocation*. Clinically, the two types of Down syndrome are

Trisomy 18 Karyotype - 47,XY,+18

Trisomy 13 Karyotype - 47,XY,+13

Greenwood Genetic Center

Greenwood Genetic Center

Figure 12–14 ◆ Karyotype of a male who has trisomy 18.
SOURCE: Courtesy of Greenwood Genetics Center. (2002). *Genetic Counseling Aids, Ed. 4.*

Figure 12–15 ◆ Karyotype of male with trisomy 13.
SOURCE: Courtesy of Greenwood Genetics Center. (2002). *Genetic Counseling Aids, Ed. 4.*

indistinguishable; the only way to distinguish them is to do a chromosome analysis.

The translocation occurs when the carrier parent has 45 chromosomes, usually with one chromosome fused to another. For example, a common translocation is one in which a particle of chromosome 14 breaks and fuses to chromosome 21. The parent has one normal 14, one normal 21, and one 14/21 chromosome. Because all the chromosomal material is present and

functioning normally, the parent is clinically normal. This individual is known as a *balanced translocation carrier.* When a person who is a balanced translocation carrier has a child with a person who has a structurally normal chromosome constitution, the child can have a normal number of chromosomes, be a carrier, or have an extra chromosome 21 (Figure 12–16 ◆). Such a child has an *unbalanced translocation* and has Down syndrome.

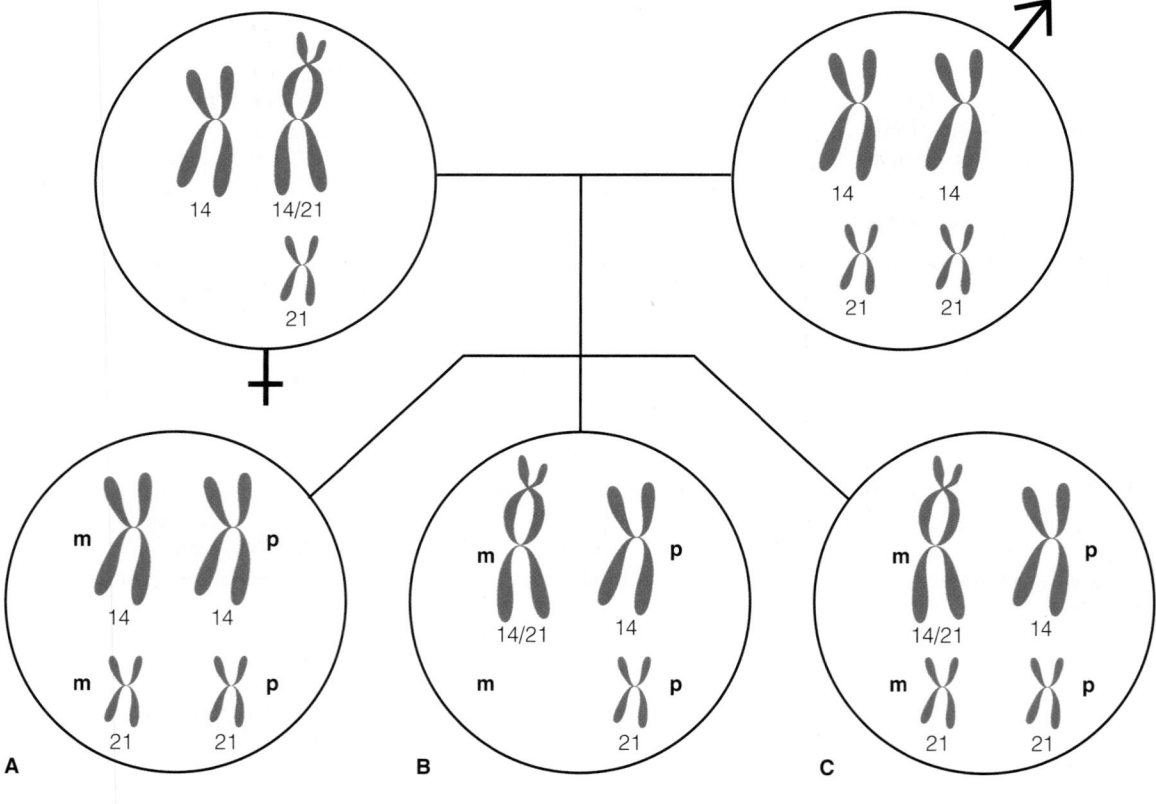

m = maternal origin
p = paternal origin

Figure 12–16 ◆ Diagram of various types of offspring when the mother has a balanced translocation between chromosomes 14 and 21 and the father has a normal arrangement of chromosomal material. *A,* Normal offspring. *B,* Balanced translocation carrier. *C,* Unbalanced translocation. Child has Down syndrome.

Structural abnormality is also caused by *additions* or *deletions* of chromosomal material. Any portion of a chromosome may be lost or added, generally leading to some adverse effect. Depending on how much chromosomal material is involved, the clinical effects may be mild or severe. Many types of additions and deletions have been described, such as a deletion of the short arm of chromosome 5 (cri du chat, or cat cry, syndrome; Figure 12–17 ◆) or the deletion of the long arm of chromosome 18 (Edwards' syndrome). Table 12–9 lists other chromosomal syndromes.

ABNORMALITIES OF THE SEX CHROMOSOME

To better understand abnormalities of the sex chromosomes, the nurse should know that in females, at an early embryonic stage, one of the two normal X chromosomes becomes inactive. The inactive X chromosome forms a dark-staining area known as the *Barr body,* or sex chromatin body. The typical female has one Barr body because one of her two X chromosomes has been inactivated. The typical male has no Barr bodies because he has only one X chromosome.

The most common sex chromosome abnormalities are Turner syndrome in females (45,XO with no Barr bodies present) and Klinefelter syndrome in males (47,XXY with one Barr body present). See Figure 12–18 ◆ and Table 12–9 for clinical descriptions of these abnormalities.

The mosaic form of the XO chromosome is associated with daughters of women who took the drug diethylstilbestrol (DES) during pregnancy. The fertility of women with the mosaic form of the XO chromosome may not be impaired; however, there is a higher percentage of uterine malformation and hormonal difficulty associated with it, and hence a high degree of miscarriage.

There is a concern that children born as a result of ICSI might be at increased risk for chromosomal and other major congenital anomalies, cancer, or infertility, because ICSI may override natural safeguards that serve to prevent fertilization. Therefore it is strongly recommended that karyotyping and Y chromosome deletion analysis be offered to all men with severe male factor infertility who are candidates for IVF with ICSI (Speroff & Fritz, 2005).

Modes of Inheritance

Many inherited diseases are produced by an abnormality in a single gene or pair of genes. In such instances the chromosomes are grossly normal. The defect is at the gene level. Some of these gene defects can be detected by new technologies, including DNA and other biochemical assays.

There are two major categories of inheritance: **mendelian (single-gene) inheritance** and **nonmendelian (multifactorial) inheritance.** Each single-gene trait is determined by a pair of genes working together. These genes are responsible for

Figure 12–17 ◆ Infant with cri du chat syndrome resulting from deletion of part of the short arm of chromosome 5. Note characteristic facies with hypertelorism, epicanthus, and retrognathia.
SOURCE: Reprinted from *Genetics in Medicine,* 5e, by J. S. Thompson & M. W. Thompson, Copyright 1991, with permission from Elsevier.

Figure 12–18 ◆ Infant with Turner syndrome at 1 month of age. Note the prominent ears.
SOURCE: Reprinted from *Journal of Pediatrics, 63,* L. Lemli & D. W. Smith, "The XO Syndrome: A Study of the Differential Phenotype in 25 Patients," p. 577, Copyright 1963, with permission from Elsevier.

the observable expression of the traits (e.g., brown eyes, dark skin), referred to as the **phenotype.** The total genetic makeup of an individual is referred to as the **genotype** (pattern of the genes on the chromosomes).

One of the genes for a trait is inherited from the mother; the other, from the father. Individuals who have two identical genes at a given locus are considered to be *homozygous* for that trait. Individuals are considered to be *heterozygous* for a particular trait when they have two different alleles (alternate forms of the same gene) at a given locus on a pair of homologous chromosomes.

The best known modes of single-gene inheritance are autosomal dominant, autosomal recessive, and X-linked (sex-linked) recessive. There is also a less common, X-linked dominant mode of inheritance, and a new identified mode of inheritance, the fragile X syndrome.

AUTOSOMAL DOMINANT INHERITANCE

A person is said to have an autosomal dominantly inherited disorder if the disease trait is heterozygous; that is, the abnormal gene overshadows the normal gene of the pair to produce the trait. In autosomal dominant inheritance, the following occurs:

- An affected individual generally has an affected parent. The family **pedigree** (graphic representation of a family tree) usually shows multiple generations having the disorder.

- Affected individuals have a 50% chance of passing on the abnormal gene to each of their children (Figure 12–19 ◆).

- Males and females are equally affected, and a father can pass the abnormal gene on to his son. This is an important principle when distinguishing autosomal dominant disorders from X-linked disorders.

- Autosomal dominant inherited disorders have varying degrees of presentation. This is an important factor when counseling families concerning autosomal dominant disorders. Although a parent may have a mild form of the disease, the child may have a more severe form.

Autosomal dominant conditions such as phocomelia (a developmental anomaly characterized by the absence of the upper portion of the limbs) can have very minimal expression in a parent but severe effects in a child. Other common autosomal dominantly inherited disorders are Huntington disease, polycystic kidney disease, neurofibromatosis (von Recklinghausen disease), and achondroplasia dwarfism.

AUTOSOMAL RECESSIVE INHERITANCE

In an autosomal recessively inherited disorder, the individual must have two abnormal genes to be affected. A *carrier* is an individual who is heterozygous for the abnormal gene and clinically normal. It is not until two carriers mate and pass on the same abnormal gene that affected children may appear. In autosomal recessive inheritance, the following occurs:

- An affected individual can have clinically normal parents, but both parents must be carriers of the abnormal gene (Figure 12–20 ◆).

- In the case where both parents are carriers, there is a 25% chance that the abnormal gene will be passed on to any of their offspring. Each pregnancy has a 25% chance of resulting in an affected child.

- If the child of two carrier parents is clinically normal, there is a 50% chance that the child is a carrier of the gene.

- Both males and females are equally affected.

- There is an increased history of consanguineous matings (mating of close relatives).

Some common autosomal recessive inherited disorders are cystic fibrosis, phenylketonuria (PKU), galactosemia, sickle cell anemia, Tay-Sachs disease, and most metabolic disorders.

X-LINKED RECESSIVE INHERITANCE

X-linked, or sex-linked, disorders are those for which the abnormal gene is carried on the X chromosome. Thus an X-linked disorder is manifested in a male who carries the abnormal gene on

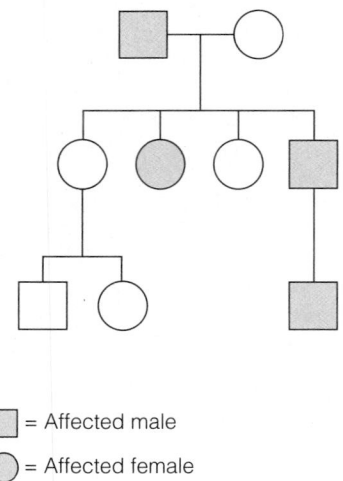

☐ = Affected male

◯ = Affected female

Figure 12–19 ◆ Autosomal dominant pedigree. One parent is affected. Statistically, 50% of offspring will be affected, regardless of sex.

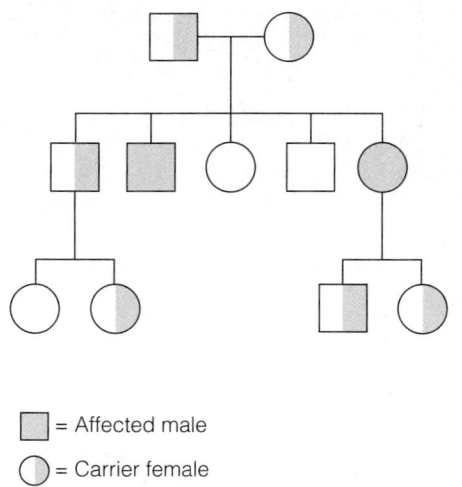

☐ = Affected male

◯ = Carrier female

Figure 12–20 ◆ Autosomal recessive pedigree. Both parents are carriers. Statistically, 25% of offspring will be affected, regardless of sex.

his X chromosome. His mother is considered to be a carrier when the normal gene on one X chromosome overshadows the abnormal gene on the other X chromosome. In X-linked recessive inheritance, the following occurs:

- There is no male-to-male transmission. Affected males are related through the female line (Figure 12–21 ◆).
- There is a 50% chance that a carrier mother will pass the abnormal gene to each of her sons, who will thus be affected.
- There is a 50% chance that a carrier mother will pass the normal gene to each of her sons, who will thus be unaffected.
- There is a 50% chance that a carrier mother will pass the abnormal gene to each of her daughters, who become carriers.
- Fathers affected with an X-linked disorder cannot pass the disorder to their sons, but all their daughters become carriers of the disorder.

Common X-linked recessive disorders are hemophilia, Duchenne muscular dystrophy, and some forms of color blindness.

X-LINKED DOMINANT INHERITANCE

X-linked dominant disorders are extremely rare, the most common being vitamin D-resistant rickets and now the recognized fragile X syndrome. When X-linked dominance does occur, the pattern is similar to X-linked recessive inheritance except that heterozygous females may also be affected. In X-linked dominant inheritance, there is no male-to-male transmission. Affected fathers will have affected daughters, but no affected sons.

FRAGILE X SYNDROME

The fragile X syndrome is a common inherited form of mental retardation second only to Down syndrome among all cases of

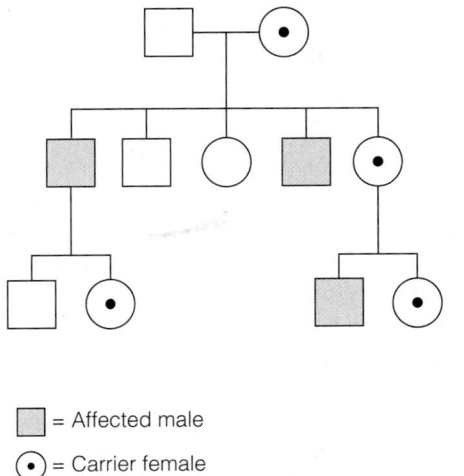

☐ = Affected male

⊙ = Carrier female

Figure 12–21 ◆ X-linked recessive pedigree. The mother is the carrier. Statistically, 50% of male offspring will be affected, and 50% of female offspring will be carriers.

moderate mental retardation in males. Fragile X syndrome is a central nervous system (CNS) disorder linked to a "fragile site" on the X chromosome. It is characterized by moderate mental retardation, large protuberant ears, and large testes after puberty. The carrier females do not have the abnormal features, but about one third are mildly retarded.

MULTIFACTORIAL INHERITANCE

Many common congenital malformations, such as cleft palate, heart defects, spina bifida, dislocated hips, clubfoot, and pyloric stenosis, are caused by an interaction of many genes and environmental factors. They are therefore multifactorial in origin. In multifactorial inheritance, the following occurs:

- The malformations may vary from mild to severe. For example, spina bifida may range in severity from mild, as spina bifida occulta, to more severe, as a myelomeningocele. It is believed that the more severe the defect, the greater the number of genes present for that defect.
- There is often a sex bias. Pyloric stenosis is more common in males, whereas cleft palate is more common among females. When a member of the less commonly affected sex shows the condition, a greater number of genes must usually be present to cause the defect.
- In the presence of environmental factors (such as seasonal changes, altitude, radiation exposure, chemicals in the environment, or exposure to toxic substances) that affect the parents, fewer genes may be needed to manifest the disease in the offspring.
- In contrast to single-gene disorders, there is an additive effect in multifactorial inheritance. The more family members who have the defect, the greater the risk that the next pregnancy will also be affected (Prosen & Hogge, 2004).

Although most congenital malformations are multifactorial, a careful family history should always be taken because occasionally cleft lip and palate, certain congenital heart defects, and other malformations can also be inherited as autosomal dominant or recessive traits. Other disorders thought to be within the multifactorial inheritance group are diabetes, hypertension, some heart diseases, and mental illness.

Prenatal Diagnostic Tests

Parent-child and family-planning counseling have become a major responsibility of professional nurses. To be effective counselors, nurses need to have the most current knowledge available concerning prenatal testing options. Appropriate counseling should occur before prenatal screening is done. It is essential that the couple be completely informed as to the known and potential risks of each of the genetic diagnostic procedures. The prescreening counseling should include the conditions detectable by the screen, diagnostic test available if screen is positive, risk to mother and child of the test performed, accuracy of the test, and limitations of the test (Evans, Bui, & Yaron, 2003). The nurse needs to recognize the emotional impact on the family of a decision to undergo or not to undergo a genetic diagnostic procedure. The ability to diagnose certain genetic diseases by various diagnostic tools has enormous implications for the practice of preventive health care. Several methods are available for prenatal diagnosis, although some are still experimental.

GENETIC ULTRASOUND

Ultrasound may be used to assess the fetus for genetic or congenital problems. With ultrasound, one can visualize the fetal head for abnormalities in size, shape, and structure. (For a detailed discussion of ultrasound technology, see Chapter 21 ∞). Craniospinal defects (anencephaly, microcephaly, hydrocephalus), gastrointestinal malformations (omphalocele, gastroschisis), renal malformations (dysplasia or obstruction), and skeletal malformations (caudal regression, conjoined twins) are only some of the disorders that have been diagnosed in utero by ultrasound. Screening by ultrasound for congenital anomalies is best done at 18 to 20 weeks, when fetal structures have completed development. With the addition of fetal nuchal translucency measurement at 10 to 13 weeks, there is high correlation with fetal chromosome abnormalities (ACOG, 2004). There is no information documenting harm to the fetus or long-term effects with exposure to ultrasound. However, there is no guarantee of complete safety; therefore, the practitioner and the parents must evaluate the risks against the benefits on an individual basis.

GENETIC AMNIOCENTESIS

A major method of prenatal diagnosis is genetic amniocentesis (Figure 12–22 ◆). The procedure is described in Chapter 21. ∞ The indications for genetic amniocentesis include the following:

- *Maternal age 35 or older.* Women 35 or older are at greater risk for having children with chromosome abnormalities. Chromosomal abnormalities due to maternal age are trisomy 21, 13, 18, XXX, or XXY. The risk of having a live-born infant with a chromosome problem is 1 in 200 for a 35-year-old woman; the risk for trisomy 21 is 1 in 365. At age 45 the risks are 1 in 20 and 1 in 40, respectively (Verp, 2004).

- *Previous child born with a chromosomal abnormality.* Young couples who have had a child with trisomy 21, 18, or 13 have approximately a 1% to 2% risk of a future child having a chromosome abnormality.

- *Parent carrying a chromosomal abnormality (balanced translocation).* A woman who carries a balanced 14/21 translocation has a risk of approximately 10% to 15% that her children will be affected with the unbalanced translocation of Down syndrome; if the father is a carrier, there is a 2% to 5% risk.

- *Mother carrying an X-linked disease.* In families in which the woman is a known or possible carrier of an X-linked disorder, such as Duchenne muscular dystrophy or hemophilia A or B, options may include genetic amniocentesis, chorionic villus sampling (CVS), or percutaneous umbilical cord sampling (PUBS). For a known female carrier, the risk of having an affected male

fetus is 50%. DNA testing may make it possible to distinguish affected males from nonaffected males in some disorders. In disorders where female carriers can be distinguished from noncarriers, only the carrier females would be offered prenatal diagnosis.

- *Parents carrying an inborn error of metabolism that can be diagnosed in utero.* Metabolic disorders detectable in utero include argininosuccinicaciduria, cystinosis, Fabry disease, galactosemia, Gaucher disease, homocystinuria, Hunter syndrome, Hurler disease, Krabbe disease, Lesch-Nyhan syndrome, maple syrup urine disease, Niemann-Pick disease, Pompe disease, Sanfilippo syndrome, and Tay-Sachs disease.

- *Both parents carrying an autosomal recessive disease.* When both parents are carriers of an autosomal recessive disease, there is a 25% risk for *each pregnancy* that the fetus will be affected. Diagnosis is made by testing the cultured amniotic fluid cells (enzyme level, substrate level, product level, or DNA) or the fluid itself. Autosomal recessive diseases identified by amniocentesis are hemoglobinopathies such as sickle cell anemia, thalassemia, and cystic fibrosis (ACOG, 2005a).

- *Family history of neural tube defects.* Genetic amniocentesis is available to those couples who have had a child with neural tube defects or who have a family history of these conditions, which include anencephaly, spina bifida, and myelomeningocele. Neural tube defects are usually multifactorial traits.

CHORIONIC VILLUS SAMPLING AND PERCUTANEOUS UMBILICAL BLOOD SAMPLING

Chorionic villus sampling (CVS) is a technique used in selected regional centers. Its diagnostic capability is similar to that of amniocentesis. Its advantages are that diagnostic information is available at 8 to 10 weeks' gestation and that products of conception are tested directly. (For further discussion, see Chapter 21 ∞). *Percutaneous umbilical blood sampling (PUBS)* is a technique used for obtaining blood that allows for more rapid chromosome diagnosis, for genetic studies, or for transfusion for Rh isoimmunization or hydrops fetalis. (For more in-depth discussion, see Chapter 21 ∞).

ALPHA-FETOPROTEIN (AFP AND AFP3)

The maternal circulation or amniotic fluid is tested for alpha-fetoprotein (AFP). Maternal serum AFP (MSAFP) is elevated in infants with open neural tube defect, anencephaly, omphalocele, or gastroschisis, and in multiple gestation (Jenkins & Wapner, 2004). Low MSAFP has been associated with Down syndrome. MSAFP is tested at 15 to 22 weeks' gestation (Jenkins & Wapner, 2004). Ultrasound and amniocentesis are offered with low or high MSAFP. Inaccurate dating is the most common cause for abnormal AFP; therefore, ultrasound dating is very important. With high MSAFP, normal amniotic fluid AFP, and normal ultrasound, there is an increased risk for preterm labor, perinatal death, and intrauterine growth restriction.

A Amniocentesis

Fetus (14–16 weeks)

Amniotic fluid

Placenta

Amniotic fluid withdrawn

Cervix

Centrifugation

Amniotic Fluid

Biochemical studies
Alpha fetoprotein

Cells

Cultured for:
• chromosome analysis
• biochemical studies
• DNA analysis

Several weeks later

Placenta

Fetus (8–10 weeks)

Chorionic villi

B Chorionic villus sampling

Next day

Human karyotype

Figure 12–22 ◆ *A,* Genetic amniocentesis for prenatal diagnosis is done at 14 to 16 weeks' gestation. *B,* Chorionic villus sampling is done at 8 to 10 weeks, and the cells are karyotyped within 48 to 72 hours.

IMPLICATIONS OF PRENATAL DIAGNOSTIC TESTING

It is imperative that counseling precede any procedure for prenatal diagnosis. Many questions and points must be considered if the family is to reach a satisfactory decision. See Table 12–10 and Developing Cultural Competence: Genetic Screening Recommendations for Various Ethnic and Age Groups. With the advent of diagnostic techniques such as amniocentesis and CVS, at-risk couples who would not otherwise have a first child or additional children can decide to conceive. Following prenatal diagnosis a couple can decide not to have a child with a genetic disease. For many couples, prenatal diagnosis is not selected because abortion is not an option for them. The decision whether to use prenatal diagnosis can be made only by the family. Even when termination is not an option, prenatal diagnosis can give parents an opportunity to prepare for the birth of a child with special needs, to contact other families with children with similar problems, or to contact support services before the birth.

Every pregnancy has a 3% to 4% risk of resulting in an infant with a birth defect. When an abnormality is detected or

Table 12–10 COUPLES WHO MAY BENEFIT FROM PRENATAL DIAGNOSIS

Women age 35 or over at time of birth

Couples with a balanced translocation (chromosomal abnormality)

Family history of known or suspected mendelian genetic disorder (e.g., cystic fibrosis, hemophilia A & B; Duchenne muscular dystrophy)

Couples with a previous child with chromosomal abnormality

Couples in which either partner or a previous child is affected with, or in which both partners are carriers for, a diagnosable metabolic disorder

Family history of birth defects and/or mental retardation (e.g., neural tube defects, congenital heart disease, cleft lip and/or palate).

Ethnic groups at increased risk for specific disorders (see Developing Cultural Competence: Genetic Screening Recommendations for Various Ethnic and Age Groups)

Couples with history of two or more first trimester spontaneous abortions

Women with an abnormal maternal serum alpha-fetoprotein (MSAFP or AFP3) test

Women with a teratogenic risk secondary to an exposure or maternal health condition (e.g., diabetes)

DEVELOPING CULTURAL COMPETENCE

GENETIC SCREENING RECOMMENDATIONS FOR VARIOUS ETHNIC AND AGE GROUPS

Background of Population at Risk	Disorder	Screening Test	Definitive Test
Ashkenazic Jewish, French-Canadians, Cajuns	Tay-Sachs disease	Decreased serum hexosaminidase-A	CVS* or amniocentesis for hexosaminidase-A assay
African; Hispanic from Caribbean, Central America, or South America; Arabs, Egyptians; Asian Indians	Sickle cell anemia	Presence of sickle cell hemoglobin; confirmatory hemoglobin electrophoresis	CVS or amniocentesis for genotype determination; direct molecular studies
Greek, Italian	Beta-thalassemia	Mean corpuscular volume less than 80% confirmatory hemoglobin electrophoresis	CVS or amniocentesis for genotype determination (direct molecular studies or indirect RFLP† analysis)
Southeast Asian (Vietnamese, Loation, Cambodian), Filipino	Alpha-thalassemia	Mean corpuscular volume less than 80%; confirmatory hemoglobin electrophoresis	CVS or amniocentesis for genotype determination (direct molecular studies)
Women over age 35 (all ethnic groups)	Chromosomal trisomies	None	CVS or amniocentesis for cytogenetic analysis
Women of any age (all ethnic groups; particularly suggested for women from British Isles, Ireland)	Neural tube defects and selected other anomalies	Maternal serum alpha-fetoprotein (MSAFP).	Amniocentesis for amniotic fluid, alpha-fetoprotein, and acetylcholinesterase assays
Ashkenazic Jewish	Gaucher disease	Decreased glucocerebrosidase	CVS
Caucasians (Northern Europeans, Celtic population), Ashkenazic Jewish	Cystic fibrosis	Transmembrane regulation (CFTR) gene	CVS or amniocentesis for genotype determination; definitive diagnosis for all fetuses not possible

*Chorionic villus sampling.
†Restriction fragment length polymorphism.

suspected, an attempt is made to determine the diagnosis by assessing the family health history (via the pedigree) and the pregnancy history, and by evaluating the fetal anomaly or anomalies via ultrasound. Experts on a specific disorder are consulted, and healthcare professionals can then present the parents with information and options. Treatment of prenatally diagnosed disorders may begin during the pregnancy, thus possibly preventing irreversible damage. For example, a mother carrying a fetus with galactosemia may follow a galactose-free diet. In light of the philosophy of preventive health care, information on what data can be obtained prenatally should be made available to all couples who are expecting a baby or who are contemplating pregnancy.

POSTNATAL DIAGNOSIS

Questions concerning genetic disorders (cause, treatment, and prognosis) are most often first discussed in the newborn nursery or during the infant's first few months of life. When a child is born with anomalies, has a stormy neonatal period, or does not progress as expected, a genetic evaluation may well be warranted. Accurate diagnosis and an optimal treatment plan incorporate the following:

- Complete and detailed histories to determine whether the problem is prenatal (congenital), postnatal, or familial in origin.

- Thorough physical examination, including dermatoglyphic analysis (Figure 12–23 ◆).
- Laboratory analysis, which includes chromosome analysis; enzyme assay for inborn errors of metabolism (see Chapter 32 ∞ for further discussion on these specific tests); DNA studies (both direct and by linkage); and antibody titers for infectious teratogens, such as toxoplasmosis, rubella, cytomegalovirus, and herpes virus (TORCH syndrome) (see Chapter 19 ∞). To make an accurate diagnosis, the geneticist consults with other specialists and reviews the current literature. This lets the geneticist evaluate all the available information before arriving at a diagnosis and plan of action.

The Human Genome Project will have significant implications for the identification and management of inherited disorders. Once genes have been identified, it will be possible to detect their presence in carriers and lead to better genetic counseling. New genetic material might be inserted into cells to provide important missing information (gene transfer) as may be possible in cystic fibrosis, or medications can be specifically designed to target the disease on a molecular level (Hamilton & Wynshaw-Boris, 2004).

However, concerns have been voiced about ethical considerations with genetic research. What guidelines are needed to protect children and families so that genetic testing does not

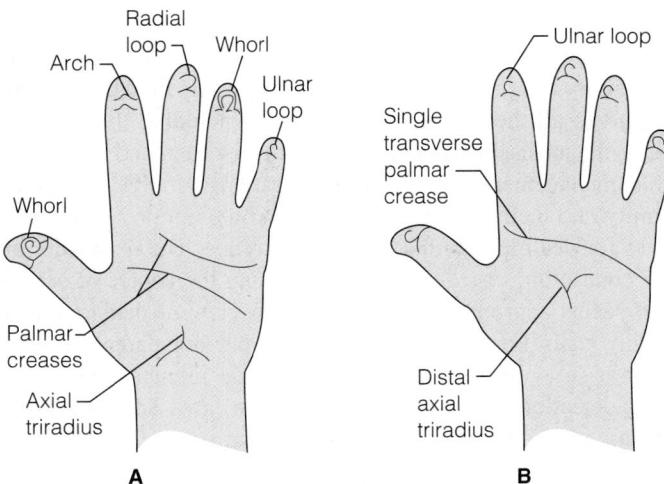

Figure 12–23 ◆ Dermatoglyphic patterns of the hands in *A*, a normal individual and *B*, a child with Down syndrome. Note the single transverse palmar crease, distally placed axial triradius, and increased number of ulnar loops.

lead to discrimination in future employment or health insurance? Who should be tested for genetic diseases, and who should have access to the results? Because children cannot yet give informed consent for genetic testing (see Chapter 1 ∞ for discussion of informed consent), it is recommended that children and adolescents should have genetic testing *only* when medical treatment could help if the disease is identified, or when another family member might benefit from the knowledge for his or her own health and the child will not be harmed by the testing (American Academy of Pediatrics, Committee on Genetics, 2000; Drenkard & Ferguson, 2002). Whenever genetic testing is performed, counseling about the results must be available. Some nurses are choosing special educational programs to enable them to work in the growing field of genetics and health care (Tinkle & Cheek, 2002).

Genetic Counseling

Genetic counseling is a communication process in which the genetic counselor, physician, or specially trained and certified nurse tries to provide a family with the most complete and accurate information on the occurrence or the risk of recurrence of a genetic disease in that family (Pagon, Hanson, Neufeld-Kaiser et al., 2001). Genetic counseling is thus an appropriate course of action for any family wondering, "Will it happen again?"

REFERRAL

Genetic counseling referral is advised for any of the following categories:

- *Congenital abnormalities, including mental retardation.* Any couple who has a child or a relative with a congenital malformation may be at an increased risk and should be so informed. If mental retardation of unidentified cause has occurred in a family, there may be an increased risk of recurrence. In some cases, the genetic counselor will identify the cause of a malformation as a teratogen (see

Chapter 16 ∞). The family should be aware of teratogenic substances so they can avoid exposure during any subsequent pregnancy.

- *Familial disorders.* Families should be told that certain diseases may have a genetic component and that the risk of their occurrence in a particular family may be higher than that for the general population. Such disorders as diabetes, heart disease, cancer, and mental illness fall into this category.

- *Known inherited diseases.* Families may know that a disease is inherited but not know the mechanism or the specific risk for them. An important point to remember is that family members who are not at risk for passing on a disorder should be as well informed as family members who are at risk.

- *Metabolic disorders.* Any families at risk for having a child with a metabolic disorder or biochemical defect should be referred for genetic counseling. Because most inborn errors of metabolism are autosomal recessively inherited ones, a family may not be identified as at risk until the birth of an affected child. Carriers of the sickle cell trait can be identified before pregnancy is begun, and the risk of having an affected child can be determined. Prenatal diagnosis of an affected fetus is available on an experimental basis only.

- *Chromosomal abnormalities.* As discussed previously, any couple who has had a child with a chromosomal abnormality may be at an increased risk of having another child similarly affected. This group includes families in which there is concern for a possible translocation.

After the couple has been referred to the genetic clinic, they are sent a form requesting information on the health status of various family members. This information assists the genetic counselor in creating the family's pedigree. The pedigree and health history facilitate identification of other family members who might also be at risk for the same disorder (Figure 12–24 ◆). The

DEVELOPING CULTURAL COMPETENCE

CONSANGUINEOUS MARRIAGES

In the United States, marriage between related individuals is generally taboo. In Western medicine, there is a concern that a child conceived by people who are related by blood may have an increased risk for birth defects. This has not, however, been supported by recent research unless the relationship is closer than first cousins. In many other cultures, marriage of first cousins and others who are related by blood is acceptable and even common. Egypt has a high rate of consanguineous (blood relationship) marriages. Reasons for consanguineous marriage include: "increase family links," "they knew each other and everything would be clear before marriage," "customs and traditions," and "less cost." The most common type of consanguineous marriage in Egypt is between first cousins.

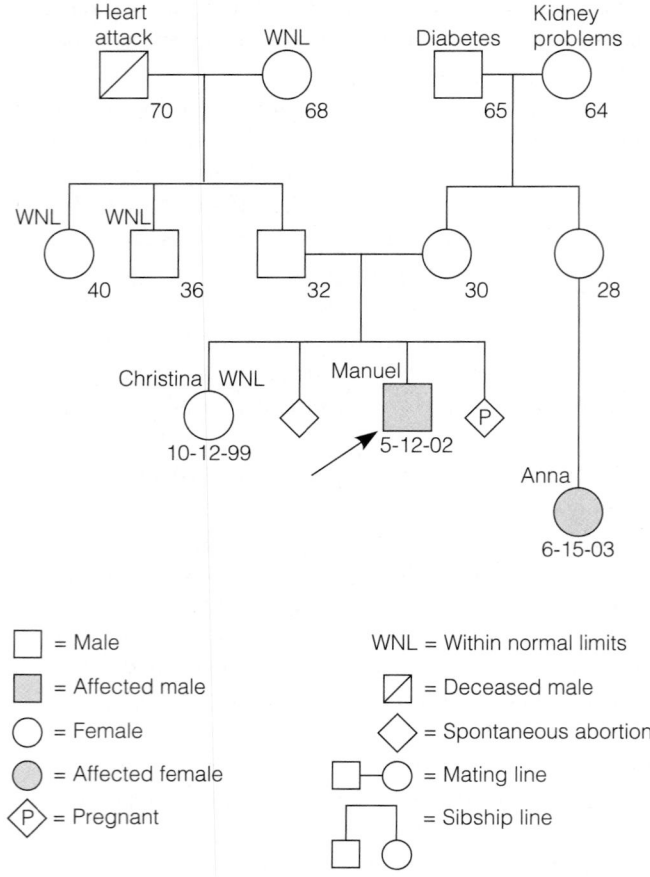

Figure 12–24 ◆ Screening pedigree. Arrow indicates the nearest family member affected with the disorder being investigated. Numbers refer to the ages of family members.

couple being counseled may wish to notify those relatives at risk so that they, too, can be given genetic counseling. When done correctly, the family history and pedigree are two of the most powerful and useful tools for determining a family risk.

INITIAL SESSION

During the initial session, the counselor gathers additional information about the pregnancy, the affected child's growth and development, and the family's understanding of the problem. The counselor also elicits information concerning ethnic background and family origin. Many genetic disorders are more common among certain ethnic groups or in particular geographic areas. For example, families from the British Isles are at higher risk of having children with neural tube defects; Ashkenazi Jews (from eastern Europe) and French Canadians are at higher risk for Tay-Sachs disease; people of African descent for sickle cell anemia; Mennonites for maple syrup urine disease; and people of Mediterranean heritage for thalassemias. (See Developing Cultural Competence: Genetic Screening Recommendations for Various Ethnic and Age Groups.)

Generally the child is given a physical examination. Other family members may also be examined. If any laboratory tests, such as chromosomal analysis, metabolic studies, or viral titers, are indicated, they are performed at this time. The genetic counselor may then give the family some preliminary information based on the data at hand.

FOLLOW-UP COUNSELING

When all the data have been carefully examined and analyzed, the family returns for a follow-up visit. At this time the parents are given all the information available, including the medical facts, diagnosis, probable course of the disorder, and any available management; the inheritance pattern for this particular family and their risk of recurrence; and the options or alternatives for dealing with the risk of recurrence. The remainder of the counseling session is spent discussing the course of action that seems appropriate to the family in view of their risk and family goals. For couples who desire to become parents or who want a subsequent child, options include prenatal diagnosis, early detection and treatment and, in some cases, adoption, therapeutic insemination, or delayed childbearing.

The couple may consider TDI, discussed earlier in this chapter. This alternative is appropriate in several instances; for example, if the man has an autosomal dominant disease, TDI would decrease to zero the risk of having an affected child (if the sperm donor is not at risk) because the child would not inherit any genes from the affected parent. If the man is affected with an X-linked disorder and does not wish to continue the gene in the family (all his daughters will be carriers), TDI would be an alternative to terminating all pregnancies with a female fetus. If the man is a carrier for a balanced translocation and if termination of pregnancy is against family ethics, TDI is an appropriate alternative. If both parents are carriers of an autosomal recessive disorder, TDI lowers the risk to a very low level or to zero if a carrier test is available. Finally, TDI may be appropriate if the family is at high risk for a multifactorial disorder.

Couples who are young and at risk may decide to delay childbearing for a few years. These couples may find in a few years that prenatal diagnosis will be available or that a disease can be detected and treated early to prevent irreversible damage.

When the parents have completed the counseling sessions, the counselor sends them and their physician a letter detailing the contents of the sessions. The family keeps this document for reference. See Table 12–11 for a list of nursing responsibilities in genetic counseling.

NURSING CARE MANAGEMENT

In both prospective and retrospective genetic counseling, timely nursing intervention is a crucial factor. During annual examinations and other clinical appointments, the nurse should interview all women of childbearing age to determine any family history or other risk factors for genetic disorders. If the woman is planning to conceive, genetic counseling should be encouraged before discontinuation of contraception.

The nurse has a key role in preventing recurrence. One cannot expect a couple who has just learned that their child has a birth defect or Down syndrome to take in any information concerning future risks. However, the couple should never be "put off" from genetic counseling for so long that they conceive another affected child because of lack of information. The perinatal nursing team frequently has the first contact with the family who has a newborn with a congenital abnormality. At the birth of an affected child, the nurse can inform the parents that before they attempt having another child, genetic counseling is available. After genetic counseling, the

Table 12–11   NURSING RESPONSIBILITIES IN GENETIC COUNSELING

Identify families at risk for genetic problems.

Determine how the genetic problem is perceived and what information is desired before proceeding.

Assist families in acquiring accurate information about the specific problem.

Act as liaison between family and genetic counselor.

Assist the family in understanding and dealing with information received.

Provide information on support groups.

Aid families in coping with this crisis.

Provide information about known genetic factors.

Assure continuity of nursing care to the family.

nurse with the appropriate knowledge of genetics is in an ideal position to help families review what has been discussed during the sessions and to answer any additional questions they might have. As the family returns to the daily aspects of living, the nurse can provide helpful information on the day-to-day aspects of caring for the child, answer questions as they arise, support parents in their decisions, and refer the family to other health and community agencies.

The family may return to the genetic counselor a number of times to air their questions and concerns, especially if the couple is considering having more children, or if siblings want information about their affected brother or sister. It is most desirable for the nurse working with the family to attend many or all of these counseling sessions. Because the nurse has already established a rapport with the couple, the nurse can act as a liaison between the family and the genetic counselor. Hearing directly what the genetic counselor says helps the nurse clarify issues for the family, which in turn helps them formulate questions. Many genetic centers have found the public health nurse to be the ideal health professional to provide such follow-up care.

Nurses must be careful not to assume a diagnosis, determine carrier status or recurrence risks, or provide genetic counseling without adequate information and training. Inadequate, inappropriate, or inaccurate information may be misleading or harmful. Healthcare professionals need to learn the appropriate referral systems and options for care in their region.

CHAPTER REVIEW

FOCUS YOUR STUDY

- A couple is considered infertile when they do not conceive after 1 year of unprotected coitus.

- At least 8% of couples in the United States are infertile.

- A thorough history and physical of both partners is essential as a basis for infertility investigation.

- General fertility investigations include evaluation of ovarian function, cervical mucus adequacy and receptivity to sperm, sperm number and function, tubal patency, general condition of the pelvic organs, and certain laboratory tests.

- Among cases of infertility, 40% involve male factors, 40% involve female factors, or 20% have no identifiable cause or 35% have multifactorial causes.

- Medications may be prescribed to induce ovulation, facilitate cervical mucus formation, reduce antibody concentration, increase sperm count and motility, and suppress endometriosis.

- The emotional aspect of infertility may be more difficult for the couple than the testing and therapy.

- The nurse needs to be prepared to provide accurate information about infertility and dispel myths.

- The nurse assesses coping responses and initiates counseling referrals as indicated.

- In autosomal dominant disorders, an affected parent has a 50% chance of having an affected child. Such disorders equally affect both males and females. The characteristic presentation will vary in each individual with the gene. Some of the common autosomal dominant inherited disorders are Huntington disease, polycystic kidney disease, and neurofibromatosis (von Recklinghausen disease).

- Autosomal recessive disorders are characterized by both parents being carriers; each offspring has a 25% chance of having the disease, a 25% chance of not being affected, and a 50% chance of being a carrier. Males and females are equally affected. Some common autosomal recessive inheritance disorders are cystic fibrosis, phenylketonuria (PKU), galactosemia, sickle cell anemia, Tay-Sachs disease, and most metabolic disorders.

- X-linked recessive disorders are characterized by no male-to-male transmission; effects limited to males; a 50% chance that a carrier mother will pass the abnormal gene to her sons; a 50% chance that her daughters will be carriers;

and a 100% chance that daughters of affected fathers will be carriers. Common X-linked recessive disorders are hemophilia, some forms of color blindness, and Duchenne muscular dystrophy.

- Multifactorial inheritance disorders include cleft lip and palate, spina bifida, dislocated hips, clubfoot, and pyloric stenosis.

- Some genetic conditions that can currently be diagnosed prenatally are neural tube and cranial defects, renal malformations, hemophilia, fragile X syndrome, thalassemia, cystic fibrosis, and many inborn errors of metabolism such as

Tay-Sachs disease. This list expands daily as new technology allows more conditions to be detected.

- The chief tools of prenatal diagnosis are ultrasound, maternal serum alpha-fetoprotein testing, amniocentesis, chorionic villus sampling, and percutaneous umbilical blood sampling.

- Based on sound knowledge about common genetic problems, the nurse should prepare the family for counseling and act as a resource person during and after the counseling sessions. Many nurses with advanced training are entering the field of genetic counseling.

EXPLORE MediaLink

http://www.prenhall.com/davidson

NCLEX review questions, case studies, and other interactive resources for this chapter can be found on the Web Site at http://www.prenhall.com/davidson. Click on "Chapter 12" to select the activities for this chapter.

For tutorials including animations and videos, more NCLEX review questions, and an audio glossary, access the accompanying Prentice Hall Nursing MediaLink DVD-ROM in this book.

PRENTICE HALL NURSING MEDIALINK DVD-ROM
Audio Glossary
NCLEX Review
Activity: *Ovulation*
Video: *Through the Eyes of a Nurse—The First Trimester*

COMPANION WEBSITE
Additional NCLEX Review
Case Study: *Infertility*
Care Plan Activity: *Infertile Couple*
Applications: *Infertility Testing; In Vitro Fertilization*
Critical Thinking

CRITICAL THINKING IN ACTION

BASAL BODY TEMPERATURE (BBT) METHOD OF FERTILITY AWARENESS

View the Critical Thinking in Action video in Chapter 12 of the DVD-ROM. Then answer the questions that follow.

Marie Neives, age 19, presents while you are working at a Planned Parenthood Clinic. She is there for a GYN exam and tells you that she is sexually active with her boyfriend but doesn't want to become pregnant. Because she lives at home with her parents, she does not want to use "the pill" because her mother might find out. Marie asks you for information concerning fertility awareness. You obtain a menstrual history

as follows: menarche age 12, cycle every 28 days × 5 days, dysmenorrhea the first 2 days with moderate flow. She has had one sexual partner. She states her boyfriend doesn't like to use condoms and that she has been lucky so far in not getting pregnant. You assist the nurse practitioner with a physical and pelvic exam. The results show that Marie is essentially healthy. The nurse practitioner asks you to review with Marie the basal body temperature (BBT) method of fertility awareness.

1. Explore with Marie "natural family planning." How would you explain this to her?

2. Briefly explain why the BBT method can predict ovulation.

3. How would you describe to Marie the procedure for obtaining BBT?

4. After figuring out her menstrual cycle, to avoid conception, when do you tell Marie to abstain from unprotected intercourse?

REFERENCES

American Academy of Pediatrics, Committee on Genetics. (2000). Molecular genetic testing in pediatric practice: A subject review. *Pediatrics, 106*, 1494–1497.

American College of Obstetricians and Gynecologists (ACOG). (2004). First-trimester screening for fetal aneuploidy (Committee Opinion No. 296). *Obstetrics and Gynecology, 104*, 215–217.

American College of Obstetricians and Gynecologists (ACOG). (2005a). Hysteroscopy (Technology Assessment in Obstetrics and Gynecology). *Obstetrics and Gynecology, 106*(4), 439–442.

American College of Obstetricians and Gynecologists (ACOG). (2005b). Update on carrier screening for cystic fibrosis (Committee Opinion No. 325). *Obstetrics and Gynecology, 106*, 1465–1468.

American Society for Reproductive Medicine. (2002). Assisted reproductive technology in the United States: 1999 results generated from the American Society for Reproductive Medicine/Society for Assisted Reproductive Technology Registry. *Fertility and Sterility, 78*(5), 918–931.

American Society for Reproductive Medicine (ASRM). (2004). 2004 compendium of ASRM practice committee and ethics committee reports. *Fertility and Sterility, 82*(Suppl. 1).

American Society for Reproductive Medicine. (2005). *Patient's fact sheet.* Retrieved October 19, 2005, from http://www.asrm.org/patients/faqs.htm

Centers for Disease Control and Prevention. (2004, December). *2002 assisted reproductive technology success rates: National summary and fertility clinic reports.* Retrieved November 30, 2005, from http://www.cdc.gov/reproductivehealth/ART/index.htm

Code of Federal Regulations. (2005). Title 21, Part 1271: Human cells, tissues, and cellular and tissue-based products; donor screening and testing, and related labeling. *Federal Register, 70*(100), 29949–29952.

Coutifaris, C., Myers, E. R., Guzick, D. S., Diamond, M. P., Carson, S. A., Legro, R. S., et al. (2004). Histological dating of timed endometrial biopsy tissue is not related to fertility status. *Fertility and Sterility, 82*(5), 1264–1272.

Denson, V. (2006). Diagnosis and management of infertility. *Journal for Nurse Practitioners, 2*(6), 380–386.

Drenkard, K., & Ferguson, S. (2002). Genetic testing and discrimination: Case example—Virginia. *Pediatric Nursing, 28*(1), 71–73.

Evans, M. I., Bui, T.-H., & Yaron, Y. (2003). Biochemical screening. In J. J. Sciarri (Ed.), *Gynecology and obstetrics* (Vol. 3, chap. 114, pp. 1–8). Hagerstown, MD: Harper & Row.

Gurfinkel, E., Cedenho, A. P., Yamamura, Y., & Srougi, M. (2003). Effects of acupuncture and moxa treatment in patients with semen abnormalities. *Asian Journal of Andrology, 5*, 345–348.

Hamilton, B. A., & Wynshaw-Boris, A. (2004). Basic genetics and patterns of inheritance. In R. K. Creasy & R. Resnik (Eds.), *Maternal-fetal medicine: Principles and practice* (5th ed., pp. 3–36). Philadelphia: Saunders.

Hassan, M. A. M., & Killick, S. R. (2003). Effect of male age on fertility: Evidence for the decline in male fertility with increasing age. *Fertility and Sterility, 79*(3), 1520–1527.

Honig, S. (2005). *Preventive medicine and male factor infertility: Facts & fiction.* Retrieved December 17, 2005, from http://www.resolve.org/site/PageServer?pagename2lrn_jfm_pm

Inhorn, M. C. (2002). "Local" confronts the "Global": Infertile bodies and the new reproductive technology in Egypt. In M. C. Inhorn & F. Van Balen (Eds.), *Infertility around the globe: New thinking on childlessness, gender, and reproductive technologies.* Berkeley and Los Angeles: University of California Press.

Jenkins, T. M., & Wapner, R. J. (2004). Prenatal diagnosis of congenital disorders. In R. K. Creasy & R. Resnik (Eds.), *Maternal-fetal medicine: Principles and practice* (5th ed., pp. 235–280). Philadelphia: Saunders.

Johnson, J. (2003). Infertility. In J. R. Scott, R. S. Gibbs, B. Y. Karlan, & A. F. Haney (Eds.), *Danforth's obstetrics and gynecology* (9th ed., pp. 685–695). Philadelphia: Lippincott Williams & Wilkins.

Kahn, S. M. (2002). Rabbis and reproduction: The uses of new reproductive technologies among Ultraorthodox Jews in Israel. In M. C. Inhorn & F. Van Balen (Eds.), *Infertility around the globe: New thinking on childlessness, gender, and reproductive technologies.* Berkeley and Los Angeles: University of California Press.

Kakarla, N., & Bradshaw, K. (2003). Evaluation and management of the infertile couple. In J. J. Sciarri (Ed.), *Gynecology and obstetrics* (Vol. 5, chap. 50, pp. 1–18). Hagerstown, MD: Harper & Row.

Kashyap, S., & Davis, O. K. (2003). In vitro fertilization. In J. J. Sciarri (Ed.), *Gynecology and obstetrics* (Vol. 5, chap. 97, pp. 1–18). Hagerstown, MD: Harper & Row.

Kipersztok, S., Kim, B. D., Morris, L., Drury, K. C., Williams, R. S., & Rhoton-Viasak, A. (2003). Validity of a rapid assay for antisperm antibodies in semen. *Fertility and Sterility, 79*(3), 522–528.

Klock, S. C. (2004). Psychological issues related to infertility. In J. J. Sciarri (Ed.), *Gynecology and obstetrics* (Vol. 6, chap. 74, pp. 1–8). Philadelphia: Lippincott Williams & Wilkins.

Kridli, S. A. (2002). Health beliefs and practices among Arab women. *American Journal of Maternal Child Nursing, 27*(3), 178–182.

Moghissi, K. S. (2003). Documentation of ovulation. In J. J. Sciarri (Ed.), *Gynecology and obstetrics* (Vol. 5, chap. 54, pp. 1–14). Philadelphia: Lippincott Williams & Wilkins.

Pagon, R. A., Hanson, N. B., Neufeld-Kaiser, W., & Covington, M. L. (2001). Genetic consultation. *Western Journal of Medicine, 174*(6), 397–399.

Paulus, W. E., Zhang, M., Strehler, E., El-Danasouri, I., & Sterzik, K. (2002). Influence of acupuncture on the pregnancy rate in patients who undergo assisted reproduction therapy. *Fertility and Sterility, 77*(4), 721–724.

Pergament, E., & Fiddler, M. (2000). Indications and patient selection for preimplantation-related chromosome abnormalities. In J. J. Sciarri & T. J. Watkins (Eds.), *Gynecology and obstetrics* (Vol. 5, chap. 107, pp. 1–7). Philadelphia: Lippincott Williams & Wilkins.

Pierson, R. A., & Olatunbosum, O. (2004). Transvaginal ultrasonography and the evaluation of female infertility. In J. J. Sciarri (Ed.), *Gynecology and obstetrics* (Vol. 5, chap. 55, pp. 1–12). Philadelphia: Lippincott Williams & Wilkins.

Prosen, T., & Hogge, W. A. (2004). Molecular and mendelian disorders. In J. J. Sciarri (Ed.), *Gynecology and obstetrics* (Vol. 3, chap. 115, pp. 1–13). Philadelphia: Lippincott Williams & Wilkins.

Purnell, L. D., & Paulanka, B. J. (2005). *Guide to culturally competent health care.* Philadelphia: F. A. Davis.

Sharara, F. I., & McClamrock, H. D. (2000). Differences in in-vitro fertilization (IVF) outcome between white and black women in an inner city university-based IVF program. *Fertility and Sterility, 73*(6), 1170–1173.

Simpson, J. L. (2002). Genetic counseling and prenatal diagnosis. In S. G. Gabbe, J. R. Niebyl, & J. L. Simpson (Eds.), *Obstetrics: Normal and problem pregnancies* (4th ed., pp. 187–219). Philadelphia: Churchill Livingstone.

Skidmore-Roth, L. (2006). *Mosby's handbook of herbs & natural supplements.* St. Louis, MO: Elsevier Mosby.

Speroff, L., & Fritz, M. (2005). *Clinical gynecologic endocrinology and infertility.* Philadelphia: Lippincott Williams & Wilkins.

Tinkle, M. B., & Cheek, D. J. (2002). Human genomics: Challenges and opportunities. *Journal of Obstetric, Gynecologic, & Neonatal Nursing, 31*(2), 178–187.

Varney, H., Kriebs, J. M., & Gegor, C. L. (2004). *Varney's midwifery* (4th ed.). Boston: Jones and Bartlett.

Verp, M. S. (2004). Antenatal diagnosis of chromosomal abnormalities. In J. J. Sciarri (Ed.), *Gynecology and obstetrics* (Vol. 3, chap. 113, pp. 1–17). Philadelphia: Lippincott Williams & Wilkins.

White, A. R. (2003). A review of controlled trials of acupuncture for women's reproductive health care. *Journal of Family Planning and Reproductive Health Care, 29*(4), 233–236.

Wilson, B. A., Shannon, M. T., Shields, K. M., & Stang, C. L. (2007). *Prentice Hall nurse's drug guide—2007.* Upper Saddle River, NJ: Pearson Education.

UNIT
4

Pregnancy

CHAPTER 13

Preparation for Parenthood

I couldn't wait to begin our childbirth classes. Attending the classes with the other expectant parents made the pregnancy and upcoming labor seem so much more real. Our childbirth educator helped ease our anxiety and gave us guidance on how to make the most of the birth. I still keep in contact with a few of my classmates and send an annual holiday greeting card with my son's photograph to our instructor.

OBJECTIVES

1. Apply the nursing process to help couples prepare for childbirth.
2. Identify the various issues related to preconception counseling, pregnancy, labor, and birth that require decision making by parents.
3. Discuss the basic goals of childbirth education.
4. Summarize the role of the doula/labor companion during labor and birth.
5. Describe the types of prenatal education programs available to expectant couples and their families.
6. Delineate the childbirth educator's role in promoting relaxation for pregnant women.
7. Compare methods of childbirth preparation.

KEY TERMS

Birth plan 299
Disassociation relaxation 309
Doula 301
Effleurage 310

Prenatal education 302
Progressive relaxation 308
Touch relaxation 309

 MEDIALINK

Additional resources for this content can be found on the Prentice Hall Nursing MediaLink DVD-ROM and on the Companion Website at http://www.prenhall.com/davidson. Click on " Chapter 13" to select the activities for this chapter.

Preparation for parenthood begins with one's own birth into a family. Attitudes, feelings, and fears about pregnancy, birth, and parenthood are molded by numerous factors, including relationships within and outside one's own family, cultural conditioning, personal history, and discussions with healthcare providers, friends, and other women.

A person's experiences with parenting or children may have been pleasant or uncomfortable. A person's information about parenthood and related areas may or may not be accurate. Because people bring their beliefs and fears with them to the childbearing period, the nurse can do much to correct misconceptions and calm fears about pregnancy, childbirth, and early parenting. Although some women may approach labor and birth with great excitement and anticipation, others may view it as a fearful, unpleasant experience. One way that a couple can cope with feelings about impending parenthood is to assume an active, participatory role during the preconception, prenatal, intrapartal, and postpartal periods. This involvement offers them a degree of control over what could otherwise be an overwhelming experience.

Some of the decisions that the childbearing family must consider are presented in this chapter. These include the decision to have a baby, choice of care provider, type of childbirth preparation, place of birth, activities during the birth, method of infant feeding, and choices surrounding the care of the newborn. The chapter also considers the role of the nurse, who provides information that enables the family to make informed decisions.

Throughout this chapter the term "childbearing family" is used to include all family types. In today's society, the childbearing family may be composed of a man and a woman joined by marriage or simply by mutual personal commitment, a single woman living alone or with a friend or family member, or a lesbian couple. No matter what the family structure and configuration, the expectant woman and her support person have similar concerns and educational needs during this time.

Today's professional nurse has many opportunities to help the childbearing family make the decisions that are part of pregnancy and birth. The nurse can help families seek preconceptual counseling, select a healthcare provider, find prenatal classes that meet their needs, and make informed choices. Even more important, as the family works through these decisions, the nurse is able to affirm their decision-making abilities and their ability to take on parenting roles. For first-time parents in particular, the decisions may seem numerous, complicated, and sometimes overwhelming. The nurse has a unique opportunity to help these families establish a pattern of decision making that will serve them well in their years as parents (Figure 13–1 ◆).

PRECONCEPTION COUNSELING

One of the first questions a couple should ask before conception is whether they wish to have children. This involves consideration of each person's goals, expectations of their relationship, and desire to be a parent. At times one individual wishes to have a child whereas the other does not. In such situations, an open discussion is essential to reach a mutually acceptable decision. In some cases, professional counseling for the couple may be necessary.

Couples who wish to have a child face a decision about the timing of pregnancy. At what point in their lives do they believe it would be best to become parents? Pregnancy comes as a surprise even when the decision about timing is made, but at least the couple has some control over it.

For couples who have religious beliefs that do not support contraception or who feel that family planning is unnatural and

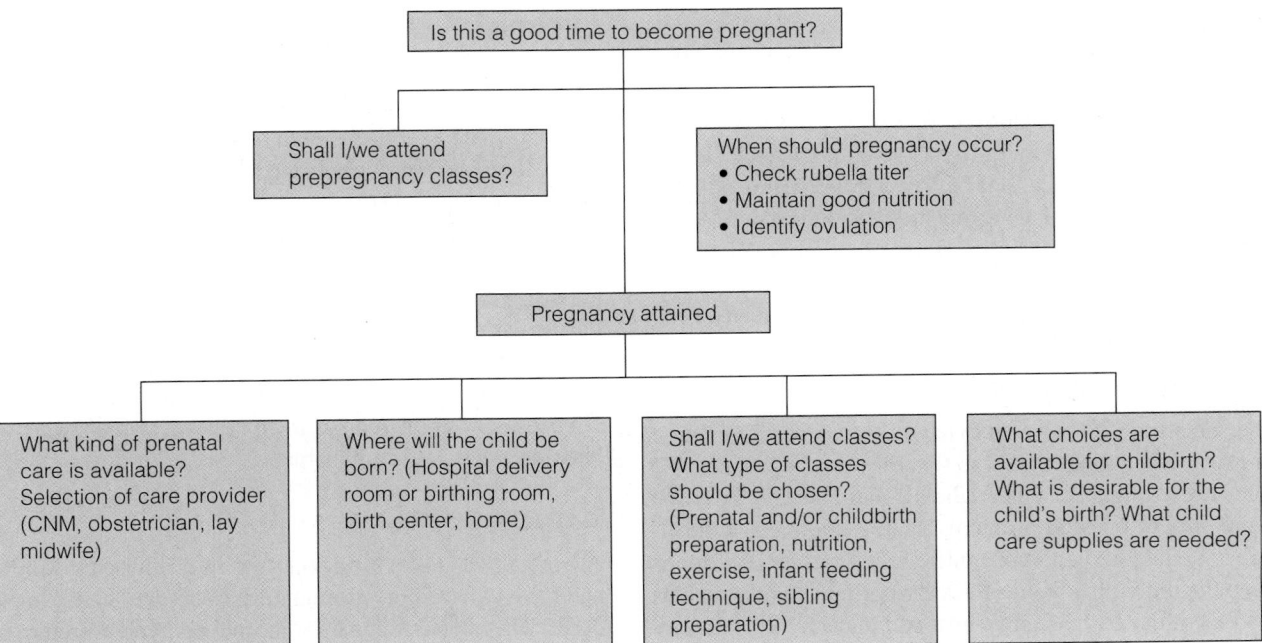

Figure 13–1 ◆ Pregnancy decision tree.

wrong, planning the timing of pregnancy is unacceptable and ir- relevant. These couples can still take steps to ensure that they are in the best possible physical and mental health when preg- nancy occurs.

Ideally, the decision to become pregnant and have a child should be a conscious one; however, this is not always the case. Nearly half of the pregnancies in the United States are unin- tended or unplanned (Cunningham et al., 2005). Couples with unplanned pregnancies may need additional support from the nurse, such as information about community resources avail- able for the couple and their infant. Encouragement and reassur- ance are especially needed for these families.

Preconception Health Measures

The nurse working with a woman or couple during the precon- ception period explains about known or suspected health risks. The nurse advises the woman to cease smoking if possible, or to at least limit her cigarette intake. Placenta previa, abruptio pla- centae, preterm rupture of membranes, and pregnancy loss are factors that are increased in smoking mothers. It is estimated that there would be a 10% reduction in perinatal mortality and an 11% reduction in the incidence of low birth weight if smok- ing during pregnancy were eliminated (American Academy of Pediatrics [AAP] and the American College of Obstetricians and Gynecologists [ACOG], 2002). Secondhand smoke has been found to increase the risk of small-for-gestational-age infants; therefore, partners of pregnant women should refrain from smoking in the woman's presence. Research from the AAP has found that smoking during pregnancy is a significant risk factor in the incidence of sudden infant death syndrome (SIDS) (Barclay & Lie, 2005). (See Chapter 36 ∞ for a detailed dis- cussion on SIDS prevention).

The effects of caffeine are less clearly understood; how- ever, as a precaution the woman is advised to avoid caffeine or limit her intake. Alcohol, social drugs, and street drugs pose a real threat to the fetus. Smoking, alcohol (greater than 2 oz/wk), and heavy coffee (caffeine) consumption are associated with a slight, but statistically significant, increase in absolute risk of re- current abortion (Lebovic, Gordon, & Taylor, 2005). A woman who uses any prescription or over-the-counter medications needs to discuss the implications of their use with her healthcare provider. It is best to avoid using any medication if possible. Be- cause of the possible teratogenic effects of environmental haz- ards in the workplace, the nurse urges the couple contemplating pregnancy to determine whether they are exposed to any envi- ronmental hazards at work or in their community.

PHYSICAL EXAMINATION

It is advisable for both partners to have a physical examination to identify any health problems so that they can be corrected if possible. These might include medical conditions, such as high blood pressure or obesity; problems that pose a threat to fertil- ity, such as certain sexually transmitted infections; or conditions that keep the individual from achieving optimal health, such as anemia or colitis. If the family history indicates previous ge- netic disorders, or if the couple is planning pregnancy when the

woman is over age 35, the healthcare provider may suggest that the couple consider genetic counseling.

In addition to the history and physical exam, the woman may have the following laboratory tests: urinalysis, complete blood count, blood type and Rh factor, venereal disease research laboratory (VDRL) test, Pap smear, gonorrhea culture, chlamy- dia screen, and rubella and hepatitis screens. Women who are nonimmune to rubella should be counseled about the possible effects on the fetus should infection occur during the first trimester of pregnancy. Women may choose to receive the vac- cine and then wait 3 months before conceiving to eliminate the risk of prenatal infection. Women should be counseled to use contraception during the 3-month time period to prevent preg- nancy. Before conception, the woman is also advised to have a dental examination and any necessary dental work to avoid ex- posure to x-rays and the risk of infection.

NUTRITION

Before conception, it is advisable for the woman to be at an average weight for her body build and height. The nurse can dis- cuss nutrition and recommend that the woman follow a nutri- tious diet that contains ample quantities of all the essential nutrients. Some nutritionists advocate emphasizing the follow- ing nutrients: calcium, protein, iron, B complex vitamins, vita- min C, magnesium, and folic acid. Folic acid supplementation should be initiated before conception because it decreases the incidence of neural tube defects in infants. (See discussion in Chapter 18 ∞). Four milligrams of folic acid per day at least 1 month before conception is recommended (Scott, Gibbs, Kar- lan, et al., 2003). Consumption of a balanced diet with the ap- propriate distribution of the basic food pyramid groups is especiallly important during pregnancy. Diet can be affected by food preferences, cultural beliefs, and eating patterns (AAP & ACOG, 2002). Excessive intake of certain vitamins can cause severe fetal problems and should be avoided.

EXERCISE

A woman is advised to establish a regular exercise plan begin- ning at least 3 months before she plans to attempt to become pregnant. The exercise should be one she enjoys and will con- tinue. It needs to provide some aerobic conditioning and some general toning. Exercise improves the woman's circulation and general health and tones her muscles. Once an exercise program is well established, the woman is generally encour- aged to continue it during pregnancy. Prepregnancy obesity, defined as a body mass index of 30 or above, has been associ- ated with severe pregnancy and delivery complications, in- cluding stillbirth (Nohr, Bech, Davies et al., 2005); therefore, advocating weight reduction for obese women who want to become pregnant is advisable.

Contraception

A woman who takes birth control pills is advised to stop the pill and have two or three normal menses before attempting to con- ceive. This allows the natural hormonal cycle to return and fa- cilitates dating the subsequent pregnancy. A woman using an intrauterine device is advised to have it removed and wait 1 month before attempting to conceive. This allows the endometrium to be resterilized. During the waiting period, she can use barrier methods of contraception (condoms, diaphragm, or cervical cap with a spermicide).

Conception

Most preconception recommendations focus on helping the couple attain their best possible health state so that they do not enter pregnancy with unnecessary risks. Conception is a personal and emotional experience and, even if a couple is prepared, they may feel some ambivalence. This is a normal response, but they may require reassurance that the ambivalence will pass. A couple may get so caught up in preparation and in their efforts to "do things right" that they lose sight of the pleasure they derive from each other and their lives together and cease to value the joy of spontaneity in their relationship. It is often helpful for the healthcare provider to remind an overly zealous couple that moderation is always appropriate and that there is value in "taking time to smell the roses."

CHILDBEARING DECISIONS

Parents face several decisions about their childbirth experience. A method that has assisted many couples in making these choices is called a birth plan. In the **birth plan,** prospective parents identify aspects of the childbearing experience that are most important to them. (A sample birth plan is presented in Figure 13–2 ◆). The birth plan helps identify available options and becomes a tool for communication among the expectant parents, the healthcare providers, and the healthcare professionals at the birth setting. The plan can also specify options the couple might wish to avoid.

The birth plan also helps pregnant women and couples set priorities. Using the plan, they identify areas that they want to incorporate in their own birth experience. Then they can take the birth plan to a visit with their certified nurse-midwife or other care provider and use it in discussing and comparing their wishes with the philosophy and beliefs of the provider. It is imperative that the couple discusses their preferences at a prenatal visit before labor. Sometimes couples may include requests that need clarification. For example, if the couple states they do not want any external monitoring, the provider needs to explain that intermittent monitoring could be provided but that eliminating all monitoring during labor could jeopardize both the mother and the fetus. Possible obstetric interventions that may be needed should also be part of the birth plan. They can also take the birth plan to the birth setting and use it as a basis for communicating their wishes during the childbirth experience.

There are many more choices that pregnant women and couples make. Some of these are explored in Table 13–1. Although most birth experiences are close to the desired experience, at times expectations cannot be met. This may be because of unavailability of some choices in the community or unexpected problems during pregnancy or birth. It is impor-

Sample Birth Plan

Choice	Choice
Care provider:	Position during birth:
Certified nurse-midwife	On side
Obstetrician	Hands and knees
Family physician	Kneeling
Lay midwife	Squatting
Birth setting	Birthing chair
Hospital:	Birthing bed
Birthing room	Other:
Delivery room	Family present (sibs)
Birth center	Filming of birth (videotaping)
Home	Photography of birth
Support during labor and birth:	Leboyer
Partner present	Episiotomy
Doula present	No sterile drapes
During labor:	Partner to cut umbilical cord
Ambulate as desired	Hold baby immediately after birth
Shower if desired	Breastfeed immediately after birth
Wear own clothes	No separation after birth
Use hot tub	Save the placenta
Use own rocking chair	Collect cord blood for banking
Have perineal prep	Newborn care:
Have enema	Eye treatment for the baby
Water birth	Vitamin K injection
Electronic fetal monitor	Heptovac injection
Membranes:	Breastfeeding
Rupture naturally	Formula feeding
Amniotomy if needed	Pacifier use
Labor stimulation if needed	Glucose water
Medication:	Circumcision
Identify type desired	Postpartum care:
Fluids or ice as desired	Short stay
Music during labor and birth	48-hour stay after vaginal birth
Massage	Home visits after discharge
Therapeutic touch	Home doula
Healing touch	Other:

Figure 13–2 ◆ Birth plan for childbirth choices. The columns list various choices that the couple may consider during their childbirth experience. Once the couple has considered each of the choices, they may circle the items they desire.

tant for nurses to help expectant parents keep sight of what is realistic for their situation. Maternal satisfaction is obviously important when outcomes of childbirth are considered. However, it must not be seen as separate from, or a greater priority than, the physical safety of both mother and child (de Costa & Robson, 2004).

Care Provider

One of the first decisions facing expectant parents is the selection of a healthcare provider. The nurse assists them by explaining the various options and outlining what can be expected from each. A thorough understanding of the differences of education preparation, skill level, practice style, and general philosophy and characteristics of practice of certified nurse-midwives, obstetricians, family practice physicians, and lay midwives is essential. The nurse can encourage expectant parents to investigate the care provider's credentials, basic and special education and training, fee schedule, and availability to new clients; this is often accomplished by telephoning the provider's office.

MEDIALINK

Childbirth Solutions

Table 13–1	BENEFITS AND RISKS OF SOME CONSUMER DECISIONS DURING PREGNANCY, LABOR, AND BIRTH	
Issue	**Benefits**	**Risks**
Breastfeeding	• No additional expense • Contains maternal antibodies • Decreases incidence of infant otitis media, vomiting, and diarrhea, hospitalizations during the first year of life, and allergies • Easier to digest than formula • Immediately after birth, promotes uterine contractions and decreases incidence of postpartum hemorrhage • Promotes maternal-infant bonding	• Transmission of maternal infections to newborn, such as HIV • Irregular ovulation and menses can cause false sense of security and nonuse of hormonal contraceptives • Increased nutritional requirement in mother
Perineal prep	• May decrease risk of infection • Facilitates episiotomy repair	• Nicks can be portal for bacteria • Discomfort as hair grows back
Enema	• May facilitate labor • Increases space for infant in pelvis • May increase strength of contractions • May prevent contamination of sterile field	• Increases discomfort and anxiety

Ambulation during labor	• Comfort for laboring woman
	• May assist in labor progression by
	  • Stimulating contractions
	  • Allowing gravity to help descent of fetus
	  • Giving sense of independence and control
		• Cord prolapse with rupture of membranes unless engagement has occurred
		• Birth of infant in undesirable locations (hallways, outdoors, waiting area)
		• Inability to monitor fetal heart rate unless telemetry unit available

Electronic fetal monitoring	• Helps evaluate fetal well-being • Helps identify fetal stress • Useful in diagnostic testing • Helps evaluate labor progress	• Supine postural hypotension • Intrauterine perforation (with internal uterine pressure device) • Infection (with internal monitoring) • Decreases personal interaction with mother because of attention paid to the machine • Mother is unable to ambulate or change her position freely
Whirlpool (jet hydrotherapy)	• Increased relaxation • Decreased anxiety • Stimulation of labor • Provides pain relief • Slight decrease in BP • Increased diuresis • Decreased incidence of vacuum and forceps deliveries • Increased pain threshold • Higher satisfaction with birth • Decreased use of pain medication	• May slow contractions if used before active labor is established • Possible risk of infection if membranes are ruptured • Slight increase in maternal temperature and pulse in tub • Hypothermia • Increases FHR by 10–20 BPM (Teschendorf & Evans, 2000)
Analgesia	• Maternal relaxation facilitates labor	• All drugs reach the fetus in varying degrees and with varying effects
Episiotomy	• Decreases irregular tearing of perineum • Easier to repair for practitioner	• Increased pain after birth and for 1–3 months following birth • Dyspareunia • Infection • Increased frequency of 3rd- and 4th-degree lacerations (Low, Seng, Murtland et al., 2000)

NOTE: For additional information regarding these issues, refer to Chapter 26. ∞

The nurse can also help the woman/couple develop a list of interview questions for their first visit to a care provider. These could include the following:

• Who is in practice with you, or who covers for you when you are unavailable?

• At what point after admission do you come to the hospital or birth setting to provide support?

• How do your partners' philosophies compare to yours?

• How do you feel about my partner, other support person, or other children coming to the prenatal visits?

• What weight gain do you recommend and why?

• What are your feelings about (fill in special desires for the birth event, such as different positions assumed during labor, avoidance of an episiotomy, induction of labor, other people present during the birth, pain control measures, breastfeeding immediately after the birth, no separation of infant and parents following birth, and so on)?

• If a cesarean is necessary, can my partner be present?

• What are your feelings regarding complementary treatments during labor (herbs to augment labor, use of acupressure/massage/hypnosis, use of oils for perineal massage, and so on)?

Expectant parents also need to discuss the qualities they want in a care provider for the newborn. They may want to visit several before the birth to select someone who will meet their needs and those of their child.

Birth Setting

The nurse can help expectant parents choose a birth setting by suggesting they tour facilities and talk with nurses there, as well as talk with friends or acquaintances who are recent parents. Questions that may be asked of new parents include the following:

- What kind of support did you receive during labor? Was it what you wanted?
- If the setting has both labor and delivery rooms and birthing rooms, was a birthing room available when you wanted it?
- Were you encouraged to be mobile during labor or to do what you wanted to do (walking, sitting in a rocking chair, remaining in bed, sitting in a hot tub, standing in a shower, and so on)?
- Was your labor partner or coach treated well?
- Were you allowed to take an active role in decision making throughout the birth process?
- If you had a doula, was her role respected? Was she welcome in the birth setting?
- Was your birth plan respected? Did you share it with the facility before the birth? If something did not work, why do you think there were problems?
- Did the nurse offer suggestions regarding comfort measures?
- Did the healthcare team provide emotional support?
- How were medications handled during labor? Were you comfortable with this?
- Were siblings welcomed in the birth setting? At the birth? After the birth?
- Did you feel you were given ample time to spend with your baby immediately after childbirth?
- Was the nursing staff helpful after the baby was born? Did you receive self-care and infant care information? Was it in a usable form? Did you have a choice about what information you got? Did they let you decide what information you needed?
- Did you feel your choice of feeding method was supported?

The nurse helps expectant parents understand the array of choices available to them. The nurse can encourage them to consider options early in the pregnancy to allow time for talking with other parents and touring facilities.

What I've seen time and again is that the technology of the hospital overwhelms patients' natural instincts; they are intimidated, afraid of appearing stupid or clumsy or sentimental in a surrounding that seems too efficient and immaculate and intelligent.

~ A MIDWIFE'S STORY ~

Nurses involved in childbirth education need to include the concept of individuality when providing information to expectant parents about the process of childbirth and their own pattern of coping. The wave of the future in childbirth education is to encourage women to incorporate their natural responses into coping with the pain of labor and birth. Alternative self-care activities should be explored with the expectant couple to identify preferences.

Nurses should encourage expectant women and couples to personalize the birth setting. The woman might plan, for example, to bring items from home to enhance relaxation and comfort, such as warm socks, slippers, bath powder, lotion, or a favorite blanket. She may wish to bring photographs of children, parents, or friends who cannot be there to share the birth experience. Many expectant parents enjoy listening to tapes of favorite music or watching home videotapes or favorite films. Such personalization of the birth setting may give expectant parents feelings of increased serenity and empowerment.

> **CLINICAL TIP**
>
> Call the birthing facilities in your community and inquire about what choices are available in each facility so that you can answer expectant parents' questions.

Labor Support Person

Some of the first formal childbirth preparation classes were patterned after a book entitled *Husband Coached Childbirth* by Dr. Robert Bradley, published in 1965. Since that time, husbands and other partners of expectant women have been very involved in acting as "coaches" or support persons during childbirth classes, labor, and birth. Although some men or support persons welcome the role and look forward to providing emotional and physical support, others do not. Some men may become anxious and fearful. These feelings can be related to past experiences and/or cultural factors. In these situations, the nurse provides encouragement and support to both the woman and her support person. Women who had continuous intrapartum support were less likely to have intrapartum analgesia, operative birth, or to report dissatisfaction with their childbirth experiences (Hodnett, Gates, Hofmeyr et al., 2003). A recent study identified women's satisfaction with childbirth as being directly affected by four key factors: the relationship with the caregiver, the support she received from caregivers, personal expectations, and her involvement with decision making (Hodnett, 2002). Clearly, the role of the nurse cannot be overestimated.

For centuries, women have been serving and assisting other women in childbirth. Out of this need for companionship and special support in the birthing journey, the role of the **doula** has evolved. *Doula* is a Greek word that means "woman's servant." In the birthing environment, a doula is a companion who provides support but does not perform any clinical tasks. The doula provides emotional, physical, and informational support and acts as an advocate for the woman and her family by verbalizing their wishes to the nurses and physicians or certified nurse-midwives. Continuous support facilitates birth, enhances the mother's memory of the experience, strengthens mother-infant bonding, increases breastfeeding success, and significantly reduces many forms of medical intervention, including cesarean delivery and the use of analgesia, anesthesia, vacuum extraction, and forceps (Pascali-Bonaro & Kroeger, 2004). A doula

MEDIALINK   Doulas of North America

MEDIALINK   Application: Benefits of Having a Doula

may also be trained to provide support and care during the postpartum period. Later postpartum benefits include increased bonding/interaction with the infant and decreased symptoms of depression. The doula may accompany the childbearing couple on a volunteer basis or may be paid a fee by the family. Another support person who has been involved in labor and birthing is a monitrice. *Monitrice* is a French word that refers to a specially trained nurse who provides assessment, nursing care, and support. The role of monitrice is not common in the United States.

Siblings at Birth

Some couples decide to have their other children present at the birth. Children who will attend a birth can be prepared through books, audiovisual materials, models, discussion, and sibling classes. Nurses can assist parents with sibling preparation by helping them understand the stresses a child may experience. For example, the child may feel left out when there is a new child to love or disappointed if a brother is born when a sister is expected.

It is imperative that the child has his or her own support person or coach whose sole responsibility is tending to the needs of that child. The support person should be familiar to the child, warm, sensitive, flexible, knowledgeable about the birth process, and comfortable with sexuality and birth. This person must be prepared to interpret what is happening to the child and to intervene when necessary. The support person should not be one who would hesitate to leave the birthing room (such as a maternal grandmother) but should be amenable to the child's desire to leave. The support person for the child should assume responsibility for providing distractions when needed. Trips to the cafeteria, visits to the nursery window, outdoor walks, and other age-appropriate activities should be available for the child.

Children should be given the option of relating to the birth in whatever manner they choose as long as it is not disruptive. Children should understand that it is their own choice to be there and that they may stay or leave the room as they choose. To help children recognize their needs and desires, the nurse may wish to elicit exactly what they expect from the experience. Children need to feel free to ask questions and express feelings.

In general, the presence of siblings at birth engenders feelings of interest and the desire to nurture "our" baby, as opposed to jealousy and rivalry directed at "Mom's" baby. The mother

does not disappear mysteriously into the hospital and return with a demanding outsider. Instead, the family attending the birth together finds a new opportunity for closeness and growth by sharing in the birth of a new member.

CLASSES FOR FAMILY MEMBERS DURING PREGNANCY

Childbirth classes are routinely taught by certified childbirth educators (CBEs or CCEs). These are individuals who have received specific educational preparation related to pregnancy, labor, birth, and postpartum/newborn care and issues. Many CBEs are also registered nurses; however, nursing training is not required. The majority of the certification programs do, however, require witnessing a minimum number of births.

The CBE should consider elements developed by authoritative organizations such as the Coalition for Improving Maternity Services (CIMS) when developing their own Philosophy of Childbirth for their classes. The "Mother-Friendly Childbirth Initiative" was created in 1996 by the CIMS, a national alliance of more than 50 childbirth organizations and many prominent individuals. The coalition's mission is to promote a wellness model of maternity care that will improve birth outcomes and substantially reduce costs. The philosophical cornerstones of mother-friendly care are: (1) normalcy of the birthing process, (2) empowerment, (3) autonomy, (4) do no harm, and (5) responsibility (Amis & Green, 2002).

Prenatal education programs provide important opportunities to share information about pregnancy, childbirth, coping mechanisms, and choices available for the woman and her support person. Studies have shown that prepared childbirth education programs can have a beneficial effect on performance in labor and delivery. The prenatal period should be used to expose the prospective parents to information about labor and delivery, pain relief, obstetric complications and procedures, breastfeeding, normal newborn care, and postpartum adjustment (AAP & ACOG, 2002). The content of each class is generally directed by the overall goals of the program. For example, in classes that aim to provide preconception information, preparations for becoming pregnant would be the major topics. Other classes may be directed toward childbirth choices available today, preparation of the mother for pregnancy and birth, preparation for cesarean birth, preparation for vaginal birth after cesarean, preparation for couples who desire an unmedicated birth, and preparation of specific people such as grandparents or siblings for the birth. The nurse who knows the types of prenatal programs available in the community can direct expectant parents to programs that meet their special needs and learning goals. Childbirth preparation classes usually contain information about changes in the woman and the developing baby (Table 13–2).

From the expectant parents' point of view, class content is best presented in chronology with the pregnancy (Figure 13–3 ◆). It is important that the classes begin by identifying the parents' needs, goals, and learning styles. Although both

DEVELOPING CULTURAL COMPETENCE

FEMALE RELATIVES AS CAREGIVERS

In most Middle Eastern countries, childbirth is exclusively attended to by women. A woman in labor is most commonly surrounded by female relatives and friends. It is customary for the husband to be excluded from the delivery room. In Iran, full segregation is mandated by law. Women can only be cared for by female healthcare providers.

Table 13–2   POSSIBLE CONTENT OF CLASSES FOR CHILDBIRTH PREPARATION

Early Classes (First Trimester)

Early gestational changes

Self-care during pregnancy

Fetal development, environmental dangers for the fetus

Sexuality in pregnancy

Birth settings and types of care providers

Nutrition, rest, and exercise suggestions

Relief measures for common discomforts of pregnancy

Psychologic changes in pregnancy

Information for getting pregnancy off to a good start

Danger signs that warrant immediate medical attention

Feeding choices/benefits of breastfeeding

Later Classes (Second and Third Trimesters)

Preparation for birth process

Postpartum self-care

Birth choices (episiotomy, medications, fetal monitoring, perineal prep, enema, etc.)

Relaxation techniques

Breathing techniques

Infant stimulation

Newborn safety issues, such as car seats and sleeping positions

Alternative therapies in pregnancy and labor

Adolescent Preparation Classes

Stresses specific to adolescents

Newborn care

Health dangers for the baby

Weight gain issues and nutrition

How to recognize when baby is ill

Baby care: Physical and emotional

Sexuality

Peer relationships

Breastfeeding Programs

Advantages and disadvantages

Medical benefits of breastfeeding

Maternal nutrition

Techniques of breastfeeding

Involvement of fathers in feeding process

Cultural considerations

Figure 13–3 ◆ In a group setting with a nurse-instructor, expectant parents share information about pregnancy and childbirth.

be able to make appropriate and informed decisions by participating in a class where information is given in a nonjudgmental, nonthreatening environment. Classes may be divided into early and late classes so specific needs can be addressed.

Early Classes: First Trimester

Early prenatal classes may include prepregnant women and couples as well as those in early pregnancy. In addition to the topics listed in Table 13–2, the classes cover early gestational changes; self-care during pregnancy; fetal development and environmental dangers for the fetus; sexuality in pregnancy; birth settings and types of care providers; nutrition, rest, and exercise suggestions; common discomforts of pregnancy and relief measures; psychologic changes in pregnancy for the woman and man; and getting the pregnancy off to a good start by following a healthful lifestyle, learning methods of coping with stress, and avoiding alcohol and smoking. Early classes should provide information about factors that place the woman at risk for preterm labor and about how to recognize symptoms of preterm labor. Early classes should also present the advantages and disadvantages of formula feeding or breastfeeding. The majority of women (50% to 80%) have made their infant feeding decision before the sixth month of pregnancy.

Later Classes: Second and Third Trimesters

The later classes focus on preparation for the birth, infant care and feeding, postpartum self-care, birth choices (episiotomy, medications, fetal monitoring, perineal prep, enema, and so forth), and newborn safety issues. Many childbirth education programs now provide labor preparation classes that focus on preparation for the birth, birth choices, and postpartum self-care with expectant parents attending separate classes that focus singly on breastfeeding or newborn care. Subjects such as emergency situations or labor and birth complications should be reviewed during the class. This includes information regarding assisting with an unattended birth when the couple fails to reach the hospital in a timely manner.

parents expect to learn breathing and relaxation techniques and infant care, fathers usually expect facts and mothers expect coping strategies. Women's goals commonly include gaining information, reducing anxiety/increasing confidence, having their partner present and involved, and having a positive emotional experience in childbirth. Classes that provide an environment supportive of practicing newly learned techniques and the freedom to ask questions and receive explanations are beneficial in helping class participants obtain these goals. By the end of the class, parents should feel that they will

THROUGH THE EYES OF A NURSE

Childbirth Education

FAMILY EXPERIENCE: "I can't help but be nervous about labor and the pain I will feel. All my friends are asking me what childbirth preparation method I am going to use. I did some research on the Internet; there are a ton of different opinions. It is almost overwhelming!"

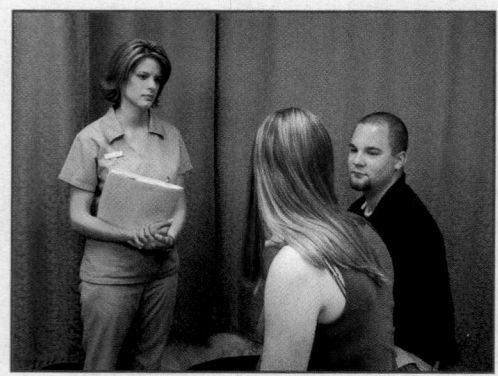

NURSE'S RESPONSE: "Many women are anxious about the labor and birth process. These are normal feelings and your concerns are very common. It is helpful to use a method of childbirth preparation because it will give you some sense of control.

"Many couples, especially first-time parents, enroll in childbirth education courses. I can give you information about the classes offered at the birthing center, the hospital, and the community center. These classes tell you about pregnancy and teach relaxation and breathing techniques that can help you in labor. If you take classes, I encourage you to practice these techniques at home. Some families choose to gain information from instructional videos, books, or the Internet. There are even Web-based specialty programs that address specific needs, such as vaginal birth after cesarean (VBAC), or breastfeeding interventions for women who are having problems with nursing."

NURSE'S ACTIONS AND RATIONALE:

The nurse provides information about educational opportunities such as classes, videos, books, and the Internet. Some couples may not be able to attend classes due to financial restraints, child care issues, or work conflicts. Providing alternatives to traditional classroom instruction enables the family to pursue other educational sources. Recent studies have examined alternative resources and found that they are effective in teaching couples childbirth education information and relaxation practice techniques (Wang, Chung, Sung et al., 2006). The nurse bases advice to the family on evidence-based practice and current research.

As a childbirth educator, I find one of the least favorite topics to discuss in class is unexpected outcomes, a topic that introduces the topic of grief that may be related to various situations. This can apply to patients who feel that they did not experience their envisioned perfect birth, or on a much more serious note, those who have a baby which is ill, has a disability, or those who have experienced a fetal loss. I have found it helpful to share a short story written by Emily Pearl Kingsley, a mother who explains her journey raising a child with special needs. She says it is rather like leaving on a trip to Italy that you have planned in detail for a long time, but instead of landing in Italy, you find yourself in Holland. . . . It is not bad, it is just different. She explains that if you spend the rest of your life mourning the fact you didn't get to Italy, you may never be free to enjoy the very special, the very lovely things about Holland. (Amis & Green, 2002).

Infant stimulation concepts can easily be incorporated into infant care class content. This will aid in the development of parenting skills and enhance prenatal and neonatal bonding. Stimulation methods that can be used include tactile, vestibular, auditory, and visual stimulation. Parents who use these methods may have better parenting skills and higher self-esteem. Infant massage classes are becoming very popular as an instructional series that parents attend after pregnancy with their infants to learn and practice different massage strokes to use on their infant as she or he grows. Vimala McClure, the founder of the International Association of Infant Massage, states that infant massage has physiologic and psychologic benefits for babies and their caregivers, providing colic relief, parent-infant bonding, as well as other benefits. Numerous studies support its use in infants. Infants who receive infant massage have exhibited decreased stress levels, increased weight gain, and improved motor function when compared with nonmassaged controls (Mainous, 2002).

Tactile stimulation can be discussed when maternal physiology is being presented. As the uterine wall thins during the pregnancy, the mother and father are better able to feel the baby, and the fetus can sense the parents' stroking and patting through the abdominal wall. *Effleurage* (a light, stroking movement made with the fingertips) can also be used over the abdominal wall to provide tactile stimulation to the fetus. Vestibular stimulation through movement of the fetus is provided while the expectant woman does the pelvic-tilt exercise. Rocking in a rocking chair is also a comfortable way to provide relaxation for the expectant woman and vestibular stimulation for the fetus. Auditory stimulation can be provided by playing music. Classical music (such as Vivaldi, Mozart, Beethoven, and Bach) is found to be pleasing to the fetus. In the prenatal period, actual visual stimulation for the fetus is not possible.

Adolescent Parenting Classes

Adolescents have special learning needs during pregnancy. Adolescents often need more support and more extensive teaching during pregnancy (Montgomery, 2003). Pregnant teens face a myriad of both psychologic and physical risks throughout pregnancy. Prenatal education and mentoring are essential. The childbirth educator should consider the teenager's need for privacy, acceptance, and respect. For this reason, classes designed specifically for the teenage population are highly desirable be-cause many teenagers may feel that they may not receive this in a standard adult-centered childbirth class (Amis & Green, 2002). Often teenage mothers face pregnancy and childbirth without adequate support from a partner or parents. Prenatal education classes specifically designed for teens can provide a forum for verbalization of fears and concerns. The nurse can also identify community resources for young mothers and their infants.

Breastfeeding Programs

Programs offering information on breastfeeding are increasing. For decades, a primary source of information has been La Leche League. Information can also be obtained from lactation consultants, peer counselors, labor and postpartum nurses, birthing centers, hospitals, and health clinics. Rates of breastfeeding in the United States are well below the *Healthy People 2010* objective of 75%. Breastfeeding education and support is positively correlated to successful breastfeeding. A goal of the surgeon general's national breastfeeding conference is to have 25% of women breastfeeding their infants a minimum of 1 full year by 2010 compared with the current data showing most mothers wean before the recommended 6 months (Atkins & Anderson, 2005). Dennis's (2002) data stated that this was because of perceived difficulties with breastfeeding rather than because of maternal choice. Lack of education and knowledge, both on the part of caregivers and mothers, is the biggest barrier to breastfeeding (Scott et al., 2003).

The father's support and encouragement of the mother is vital, so it is important to include him in the educational program and involve him in the decision making. Some fathers may feel negative and resentful about breastfeeding and need opportunities in the prenatal period for discussion and sharing of information. The decision to breastfeed is strongly related to the father's feeding preference.

Sibling Preparation: Adjustment to a Newborn

The birth of a new sibling is a significant event in a child's life. Positive adjustment can be enhanced by attendance at formal sibling preparation classes (Figure 13–4 ◆). Typically, the classes are attended by children ages 3 to 12 years. Children younger than 3 tend to have shorter attention spans and may have difficulty participating in the class; however, many facilities will allow younger children to attend, especially if an older sibling is enrolled in the class. These classes can assist with decreasing sibling rivalry and reducing children's anxiety. They help children feel that they are part of the birthing process. The classes also enable parents to identify children's concerns related to the new baby. They provide a means to facilitate communication and explore children's feelings. They also provide basic information about pregnancy, childbirth, and the characteristics and behavior of newborns.

Typically, parents and their children attend the class together. Many activities are devised to help each child feel special. Time is usually allotted at the end of the class for talking with parents about coping skills and providing hints about dealing with sibling jealousy. Class content typically includes care and

Figure 13–4 ◆ It is especially important that siblings be well prepared when they are going to be present at the birth. However, even siblings who will not be present at the birth can benefit from information about birth and the new baby ahead of time.

behavior of new babies, a practice session holding anatomically correct dolls, changing diapers, and a tour of the "bedroom" and the nursery where Mom and baby will stay. Many times, a newborn is held up at the nursery window so the children can see a "real baby." Some facilities give the children a special gift for attendance or a trip to the cafeteria for a special treat.

Sibling preparation can be addressed through a formal class like the one just described, or in a less formal way by preparing a booklet for parents that addresses issues affecting both parents and children. Also, several excellent books and videos are available to help children prepare for a new sibling.

Classes for Grandparents

Grandparents are an important source of support and information for prospective and new parents. They are now being included in the birthing process more frequently. Prenatal programs for grandparents can address current roles, transitioning to a new role, beliefs regarding childbirth, and ways to support the new family unit. Grandparents can also benefit from educational information, such as the benefits of breastfeeding, and updates on infant care, such as proper infant sleep positions and when to introduce foods. Grandparents who will be integral members of the labor and birth team need information about being coaches.

EDUCATION OF THE FAMILY HAVING CESAREAN BIRTH

Cesarean birth is an alternative method of birth via an abdominal and uterine incision.

Preparation for Cesarean Birth

Because one out of every four or five births is a cesarean, preparation for this possibility should be an integral part of every childbirth education curriculum. The national cesarean rate has rebounded to 26.1% (Meikle, Steiner, Zhang et al., 2005). The instructor should treat cesarean birth as a normal event and pres-

ent factual information that allows expectant parents to make choices and be full participants in their birth experience. The instructor can emphasize the similarities between cesarean and vaginal births to minimize undertones of "normal" versus "abnormal" birth. This helps diminish the feelings of anger, loss, and grief that often accompany cesarean births.

Cesarean birth classes should cover what the parents can expect to happen during a cesarean birth, what they will feel, and what they can do. All pregnant women and couples should be encouraged to discuss with their certified nurse-midwife/physician what the approach would be in the event of a cesarean. They can also discuss their needs and preferences regarding the following:

• Participating in the choice of anesthetic
• Father (or significant other) being present during the birth
• Planning initial contact with their newborn

As a nurse midwife, I felt extremely disappointed when I learned I would have to have a cesarean birth with my second child. I had great expectations about how much easier my second birth would be, and how I would "do everything different this time." I was amazed at how satisfied and happy I was immediately after the cesarean birth. During the birth, I asked the physician if the baby was almost out and how things were progressing. In the end, I had a beautiful, healthy baby and it turned out to be even a better experience than my first birth. I always try to comfort women who have medically indicated cesarean births by telling them it is still an amazing experience and a wonderful birthday!

Preparation for Repeat Cesarean Birth

When expectant parents are anticipating a repeat cesarean birth, they have time to plan and prepare. Many hospitals or local groups (such as C-Sec, Inc.) provide preparation classes for cesarean birth. Parents who have had previous negative experiences need an opportunity to describe what contributed to their feelings. They should be encouraged to identify what they would like to change and to list interventions that would make the experience more positive. Those who have had positive experiences need reassurance that their needs and desires will be met in the same manner. In addition, all parents are encouraged to air any fears or anxieties.

A specific concern of the woman facing a repeat cesarean is anticipation of pain. She needs reassurance that subsequent cesareans are often less painful than the first. If her first cesarean was preceded by a long or strenuous labor, she will not experience the same fatigue. Giving this information will help her cope more effectively with all stressful stimuli, including pain. The nurse can remind the woman that she has already had experience with how to prevent, cope with, and alleviate painful stimuli.

Preparation for Parents Desiring Vaginal Birth after Cesarean Birth

Parents who are anticipating a vaginal birth after cesarean birth (VBAC) have unique needs. Because they may have unresolved questions and concerns about the last birth, it is helpful to begin the series of classes with an informational session. During this session, they can ask questions, share experiences, and begin to form bonds with one another. The nurse can supply information regarding the criteria necessary to attempt a trial of labor and identify decisions regarding the birth experience. Concerns regarding the complications associated with VBAC can also be discussed. Some women may wish to undergo a repeat cesarean birth to avoid the risk of uterine rupture associated with a trial of labor. Some CBEs find it helpful to have the parents prepare two birth plans: one for vaginal birth and one for cesarean birth. The preparation of the two plans seems to help parents take more control of the birth experience and tends to increase the positive aspects of the experience.

After an informational session, the classes may be divided according to the needs of the expectant parents. Those with recent coached childbirth experiences may need only refresher classes, whereas others may need complete training. Some parents may choose to attend regular classes after participating in the informational session.

METHODS OF CHILDBIRTH PREPARATION

Various methods of childbirth preparation are taught in North America. The most common methods of this type are Lamaze (psychoprophylactic), Kitzinger (sensory memory), Bradley (partner-coached childbirth), and HypnoBirthing. See Table 13–3 for differentiating characteristics of each method.

The programs in prepared childbirth share some similarities. All have an educational component to help eliminate fear and teach coping mechanisms. The classes vary in coverage of subjects related to the maternity cycle, but all teach relaxation techniques and all prepare the participants for what to expect during labor and birth. Most methods also feature exercises to condition muscles and use breathing patterns needed in labor. The greatest differences among the methods lie in the theories of why they work and in the relaxation techniques and breathing patterns they teach.

Table 13–3 SUMMARY OF SELECTED CHILDBIRTH PREPARATION METHODS

Method	Purpose or Philosophy	Goals	Techniques	Class Content
Bradley	To have the best, safest, and most rewarding birth experience possible.	• Natural childbirth. • Active participation of the husband as coach. • Excellent nutrition. • Breastfeeding, beginning at birth.	• Working in harmony with your body using controlled breathing and deep abdomino-pelvic breathing (Bradley, 1974) • Promoting general body relaxation (Bradley,1974)	• Nutrition • Coach's role • Introduction to stages of labor • Birth planning • Variations and complications of labor • Postpartum preparation • Advanced first- and second-stage techniques • Preparation for your new family
Lamaze	Childbirth education empowers women to make informed choices in health care, to assume responsibility for their health, and to trust their inner wisdom.	• Birth is normal, natural, and healthy. • The experience of birth profoundly affects women and their families. • Women's inner wisdom guides them through birth. • Women have the right to give birth free from routine medical interventions.	• Disassociation relaxation • Controlled muscular relaxation • Breathing patterns	• Nutrition • Gestational changes • Labor and birth techniques for easing pain • Breathing techniques • Positioning during labor
Kitzinger	• Sheila Kitzinger campaigns for women to have the information they need to make choices about childbirth. • She is a strong believer in the benefits of home birth for women who are not high risk.	• Uses sensory memory to help the woman understand and work with her body in preparation for birth.	• Uses chest breathing in conjunction with abdominal relaxation. • Incorporates elements of the Stanislavesky method of acting in a way to teach relaxation	• Antenatal care • Birth plans • Therapeutic touch during labor • Post-traumatic stress following childbirth • Breastfeeding
HypnoBirthing	HypnoBirthing is about eliminating fear and experiencing birth in a stress-free, calm, and gentle environment that most resembles nature's own design.	• With both mind and body relaxed, the muscles of the uterus work in complete neuromuscular harmony. • When in a relaxed state, the body releases endorphins, the body's natural anesthesia.	• Relaxation techniques • Deep breathing • Slow breathing • Breathing your baby down • Maintaining comfort and eliminating pain	• HynoBirthing philosophy • Rapid, progressive relaxation/deepening techniques for transition • Visualizations for labor • Composing a birth plan • Early signs of labor • Birthing companion's integral role in labor • Pushing techniques • Postnatal bonding of parents with baby

RESEARCH IN PRACTICE

LACK OF PREPAREDNESS: EXPERIENCES OF FIRST-TIME MOTHERS

What is this study about? The postpartum period has sometimes been called the "fourth trimester" because of the ongoing dramatic adaptations required of the family. The first weeks of motherhood represent a period of increased stress and vulnerability. Identifying and meeting the needs of new mothers in the early postpartum period represents an ongoing challenge for nursing. Mothers with an uncomplicated birth can expect a brief hospital stay, and the time available for in-hospital teaching and support is limited. This qualitative study sought to understand the lived experience of first-time motherhood following hospital discharge.

How was this study done? Mothers were recruited for this study if they were primiparous and had uncomplicated vaginal births. A total of 21 women were interviewed. The mothers were discharged from an urban acute care hospital less than 48 hours after birth and were interviewed within 4 weeks. The researcher followed a semistructured interview guide comprised of open-ended questions. The responses of the mothers were tape-recorded and transcribed in their entirety. The transcripts were analyzed using a constant comparison coding procedure and themes were identified. The analysis was checked with selected members of the sample.

What were the results of the study? The new mothers in this sample reported feeling well prepared for pregnancy, labor, and birth but a clear "lack of preparedness" for the early postpartum period. This lack of preparedness was the over-arching premise but was comprised of multiple themes. The mothers reported a dramatic shift in priorities, with an associated reorganization of both parents' lives. The mothers also experienced an overwhelming sense of responsibility combined with a lack of clarity of the role required of them. Most reported a knowledge deficit, which they addressed by soliciting advice from family and friends. Often feeling frustrated, these mothers were confused by conflicting advice and demands. Many were surprised at how unwell and isolated they felt. Many of the mothers described feeling abandoned by the healthcare system, which was a source of much contact during the pregnancy but was notably absent after the birth.

What additional questions might I have? Do multiparous mothers adapt more easily in the "fourth trimester"? What can nurses do before discharge to help new mothers adapt to postpartum demands?

How can I use this study? This study provides valuable insight in the experiences of new mothers in the early postpartum period. The nurse can use these insights to help prepare the new mother for what she might expect after discharge. New mothers need advice and support during this period of vulnerability. These authors recommend developing a telephone support system for nurses to provide information to new mothers, including breastfeeding knowledge and support.

George, L. (2005). Lack of preparedness: Experiences of first-time mothers. *MCN American Journal of Maternal Child Nursing, 30*(4), 251–255.

There are several advantages to these methods of childbirth preparation. The most important is that the baby may be healthier because of the reduced need for analgesics and anesthetics. Another is the satisfaction of the parents, for whom childbirth becomes a shared and profound emotional experience over which they feel a sense of control. In addition, each method has been shown to shorten labor. All nurses must know how these methods differ, so that they can support each birth experience effectively.

The International Childbirth Education Association (ICEA) is a well-known organization that provides antepartum education. Although this is not a method of preparation, it offers education and resources to the CBE with a philosophy grounded in providing support to the individual couple's choices and decisions. Many couples find ICEA classes appealing because they discuss all alternatives and choices that are available. Many hospital-based childbirth education programs now use this approach.

Body-Conditioning Exercises

Some body-conditioning exercises, such as the pelvic tilt, pelvic rock, and Kegel exercises, are taught in childbirth preparation classes. Other exercises strengthen the abdominal muscles for the expulsive phase of labor. (See Chapter 16 ∞ for a description of recommended exercises.)

Relaxation Exercises

Relaxation during labor allows the woman to conserve energy and allows the uterine muscles to work more efficiently. Without practice it is very difficult to relax the whole body in the midst of intense uterine contractions. However, many people can quickly master one or more of the following exercises.

PROGRESSIVE RELAXATION

In **progressive relaxation** exercises, the woman learns how to tense and then relax one muscle group at a time. An example follows:

- Lie down on your back or side. (The left side position is best for pregnant women.)
- Tighten your muscles in both feet. Hold the tightness for a few seconds, and then relax the muscles completely, letting all the tension drain out.

Table 13–4　TOUCH RELAXATION

Practice is vital to the following exercises, which require that the pregnant woman and her partner work very closely together. Tell the woman, "With practice you will train yourself to release not only in response to your partner's touch but also to the touch of doctors or nurses as they examine you. This technique will also help you to be more comfortable with your own body."

Goals

(For her) To recognize and release tension in response to partner's touch; to be able to do this automatically and spontaneously.

(For partner) To recognize her tension in its very early stages; to learn how to touch in a firm yet sensitive way; to concentrate on her problem areas.

Tools

(For her) Conscious relaxation, comfortable positioning, and trust.

(For partner) Sensitivity, patience, and warm hands!

Procedure

She tenses.

Partner touches.

She immediately releases toward touch.

Partner strokes "drawing" tension from her.

She releases all residual tension.

Sequence

- Contract muscles of the scalp and raise eyebrows. Partner cups hands on either side of the scalp. Immediately release tension in response to the pressure of your partner's touch. Then release any residual tension as your partner strokes your head.
- Frown, wrinkle nose, and squeeze eyes shut. Partner rests hands on brow and then strokes down over temples. Release.
- Grit teeth and clench jaw. Partner rests hands on either side of jaw. Release.
- Press shoulder blades back. Partner rests hands on front of shoulders. Release.
- Pull abdominal wall toward spine. Partner rests hands on sides of abdomen and then strokes down over her hips. Partner might also stroke the lower curve of abdomen across pubic symphysis. Release.
- Press thighs together. Partner touches outside of each leg. Relax and let legs move apart. Partner strokes firmly down outside of leg with light strokes up on inner thigh.
- Press legs outward, still flexed but forcing thighs apart. Partner rests hands with fingers pointing downward, on inner thighs. Firmly strokes down to knees, then lightly strokes upward on outside of leg. Release.
- Tense arm muscles. Partner places hands on the upper arm and shoulder area, one on the inside and one on the outside of the arm. Strokes down to the elbow and then down forearm to wrist, and over fingertips. Release. Repeat with other arm.
- Tighten leg muscles, being careful not to cramp them. Partner touches foot around the instep, firmly without tickling. Release whole leg. Partner moves hands up, placing one on either side of the thigh, stroking down to the knee then down the calf to the foot and over the toes. Release. Repeat with other leg.
- Change to the Sims, lateral, or side-lying position. Raise chin, contracting the muscles at the back of the neck. Partner rests hand on nape of neck and massages. Release.
- Curl into fetal position, drawing shoulders forward. Partner applies pressure to back of shoulders. Strokes upper back. Release.
- Hollow the small of back by arching back. Partner rests hands against either side of spine and follows with stroking down over buttocks. Release.
- Press buttocks together. Partner rests one hand on each buttock. After initial release, strokes down toward thighs.

SOURCE: O'Halloran, S. (1984). *Pregnant and prepared: A guide to preparing for childbirth* (p. 45). Wayne, NJ: Avery Publishing Group.

- Tighten your lower legs, hold for a few seconds, then relax the muscles, letting all the tension drain out.
- Continue tensing and relaxing parts of your body, moving up the body as you do so.

TOUCH RELAXATION

Another type of relaxation exercise, called **touch relaxation,** requires cooperation between the woman and her coach. It is particularly useful in working together during labor. An example is provided in Table 13–4.

DISASSOCIATION RELAXATION

An additional exercise, **disassociation relaxation,** is used in both Lamaze and Bradley methods. The woman is taught to become familiar with the sensation of contracting and relaxing the voluntary muscle groups throughout her body. She then learns to contract a specific muscle group and relax the rest of her body. This process of isolating the action of one group of voluntary muscles from the rest of the body is called *neuromuscular disassociation*. The exercise conditions the woman to relax uninvolved muscles while the uterus contracts, creating an active relaxation pattern (Table 13–5).

Although it is not possible to simulate the pain of uterine contractions, the coach may use one of two methods to induce some discomfort so the woman can practice the relaxation exercises:

1. The coach places both hands in a grasping position firmly on the upper arm and turns them in opposite directions to create a burning sensation. This is begun slowly and gently and increased at the direction of the woman as she continues to practice relaxation breathing techniques (Figure 13–5 ◆).

2. The coach places a hand on the woman's inner thigh just above the knee and pinches the area.

While practicing, the coach checks the woman's neck, shoulders, arms, and legs for relaxation. As tense areas are found, the coach encourages the woman to relax those particular body parts. The woman learns to respond to her own perceptions of tense muscles and also to the suggestion from others. The suggestion can come verbally or from touch. The exercises are usually practiced each day so that they become comfortable and easy to do.

Table 13–5	DISASSOCIATION RELAXATION

The uterus, an involuntary muscle over which you have no control, will work most efficiently and effectively when the rest of your body is free from tension. The following exercises will give you further practice in conscious release. They will also give you and your partner a way to evaluate your progress.

Goals

During pregnancy, disassociation relaxation will teach you consciously to release certain sets of muscles, while contracting others, and to disassociate yourself from voluntary tension. During labor, this technique will release all voluntary muscles of your body at will, while the uterus contracts. This conserves energy and fights fatigue.

Tools

Body awareness, touch release, and concentration.

Procedure

Partner gives consistent suggestions.
Partner checks relaxation using touching.

Example

Partner: "Contraction begins."
Mother: Relaxation breath (following with a comfortable rate of breathing).
Partner: [See suggested patterns.]
Mother: Relaxation breath.

Sequence

"Contract right arm. Hold. Release."
"Contract left arm. Hold. Release."
"Contract right leg. Hold. Release."
"Contract left leg. Hold. Release."
"Contract both arms. Hold. Release."
"Contract both legs. Hold. Release."
"Contract right side (arm and leg). Hold. Release."
"Contract left side (arm and leg). Hold. Release."
"Contract right arm and left leg. Hold. Release."
"Contract left arm and left leg. Hold. Release."

For Variety

"Contract right arm and left leg."
"Release left leg. Contract right leg. Release right arm. Contract left arm."
"Release."

SOURCE: O'Halloran, S. (1984). *Pregnant and prepared: A guide to preparing for childbirth* (pp. 45–46). Wayne, NJ: Avery Publishing Group.

Figure 13–5 ◆ To help the woman practice relaxing in the presence of discomfort, the coach can induce discomfort by "twisting" the skin of her upper arm or by pinching her inner thigh.

OTHER RELAXATION TECHNIQUES

A specific type of cutaneous stimulation called abdominal **effleurage** is used before the transitional phase of labor (Figure 13–6 ◆). This light abdominal stroking effectively relaxes the woman experiencing mild to moderate pain. Deep pressure over the sacrum is more effective for relieving back pain.

Additional modalities that may be used to promote relaxation in labor include guided imagery, hypnosis, meditation, music, massage, aromatherapy, therapeutic touch, biofeedback, transcutaneous electrical nerve stimulation (TENS) unit, acupressure, and acupuncture. In addition to these measures, the nurse can promote relaxation by encouraging and supporting the client's controlled breathing.

Individualization is essential when choosing appropriate relaxation techniques. The nurse should encourage techniques that are comfortable for the woman. Some techniques that may be beneficial are as follows:

- Vocalization or "sounding" to relieve tension in pregnancy and labor.
- Massage (light touch) to facilitate relaxation.
- Breathing in any manner that seems to bring relief. No specific pattern is followed.
- Use of warm water for showers or bathing during labor.
- Visualization (imagery).
- Relaxing music and subdued lighting.

Breathing Techniques

Breathing techniques are a key element of most childbirth preparation programs. They help keep the mother and her unborn baby adequately oxygenated and help the mother relax and focus her attention appropriately (Table 13–6). Breathing techniques are best taught during the final trimester of pregnancy when the expectant mother's attention is focused on the birth experience. The nurse then supports the mother's use of breathing techniques during labor. Breathing techniques are described in detail in Chapter 24. ∞

Figure 13–6 ◆ Effleurage is light stroking of the abdomen with the fingertips. *A,* Starting at the symphysis, the woman lightly moves her fingertips up and around in a circular pattern. *B,* An alternative approach involves using one hand in a figure-eight pattern. This light stroking can also be done by the support person.

Table 13–6   GOALS OF BREATHING TECHNIQUES
• Provide adequate oxygenation of mother and baby, open maternal airways, and avoid inefficient use of muscles.
• Increase physical and mental relaxation.
• Decrease pain and anxiety.
• Provide a means of focusing attention.
• Control inadequate ventilation patterns that are related to pain and stress.
• Provide a sense of control for the mother.

CLINICAL TIP

Practice the techniques for relaxation yourself. This practice will prepare you to help expectant parents and laboring women.

Vocalization Techniques

With the increased use of analgesics and epidural anesthesia, many nurses have become unfamiliar with and may be uncomfortable about natural sounds made by laboring women. Vocalization or *sounding* during uterine contractions can be encouraged to promote relaxation and relieve tension. The nurse should encourage the woman to relax, drop her jaw to her chest, and make low-pitched sounds. Suggesting that the woman try to sound like a man or a mother bear can help her to produce the appropriate pitch. These low, moaning sounds open the glottis, helping the woman to relax, breathe freely, and feel confident and strong. In contrast, high-pitched sounds can promote tension, closure, and a feeling of fear.

CHAPTER REVIEW

FOCUS YOUR STUDY

- Preconception counseling can be used to identify risk factors and unhealthy behaviors before a pregnancy occurs. Healthful lifestyle changes can be employed.
- Childbearing decisions include the care provider, the birth setting, support persons, and whether to include siblings in the birth experience.

- Prenatal education programs vary in their goals, content, leadership techniques, and method of teaching. The major childbirth preparation methods are Lamaze, Kitzinger, Bradley, and HypnoBirthing.
- Prenatal classes may be offered early or late in the pregnancy. The class content varies depending on the type

of class and the individual offering it. Expectant parents tend to want information in chronologic sequence with the pregnancy.

- Breastfeeding programs in the prenatal period offer encouragement, practical instruction, and resources for the breastfeeding family.
- Siblings are now included in the whole birthing process, and classes for them are available from many sources.

- Grandparents have unique information needs that are addressed in grandparents' classes.
- Information regarding cesarean birth is included in antepartal classes to help prepare all parents for this alternative method of birth.
- Most childbirth classes include information on body-toning exercises, relaxation techniques, breathing method, and vocalization techniques.

EXPLORE MediaLink

http://www.prenhall.com/davidson

NCLEX review questions, case studies, and other interactive resources for this chapter can be found on the Web Site at http://www.prenhall.com/davidson. Click on "Chapter 13" to select the activities for this chapter.

For tutorials including animations and videos, more NCLEX review questions, and an audio glossary, access the accompanying Prentice Hall Nursing MediaLink DVD-ROM in this book.

PRENTICE HALL NURSING MEDIALINK DVD-ROM
Audio Glossary
NCLEX Review
Videos: *Through the Eyes of a Nurse—The First Trimester; Through the Eyes of a Nurse—The Third Trimester*

COMPANION WEBSITE
Additional NCLEX Review
Case Study: *Preparing for Pregnancy*
Care Plan Activity: *Preconception Counseling*
Applications: *Benefits of Having a Doula; Lamaze*
Critical Thinking

CRITICAL THINKING IN ACTION

BIRTH PLANS WITH EXPECTANT PARENTS

View the Critical Thinking in Action video in Chapter 13 of the DVD-Rom. Then answer the questions that follow.

Terry Dole, a 38-year-old G1, P0000, at 6 weeks' gestation, presents to you at the OB clinic for her first prenatal visit with the certified nurse-midwife (CNM). One of the first decisions facing Terry is the selection of a healthcare provider. The midwife explains the various options available to Terry at the clinic related to the differences in educational preparation, skill level, practice characteristics, and general philosophy of CNMs and obstetricians. Terry tells you that she has been married for 6 years and works as a massage therapist. You obtain the following data: BP 110/70, temperature 97F, pulse 76, respirations 12, weight 140 lb, height 5′7 less than or equal to. The physical and pelvic exams are essentially normal. The CNM asks you to teach Terry about birth plans.

1. Discuss the advantages of a birth plan.
2. Discuss the disadvantages of a birth plan.
3. Explain the role of a doula.
4. What gender differences are there in moving toward parenthood?

REFERENCES

American Academy of Pediatrics (AAP) and the American College of Obstetricians and Gynecologists (ACOG). (2002). *Guidelines for perinatal care* (5th ed.). Washington, DC: ACOG.

Amis, D., & Green, J. (2002). *Prepared childbirth—The educator's guide.* Plano, TX: The Family Way Publications.

Atkins, K. E., & Anderson, R. J. (2005). Breastfeeding in an urban county hospital. *Obstetrics and Gynecology, 105*(4), 96S.

Barclay, L., & Lie, D. (2005). *American Academy of Pediatrics updates: Guidelines to reduce the incidence of SIDS.* Medscape Medical News. Retrieved January 1, 2006, from http://medgenmed.com/viewarticle/514267

Bradley, R. A. (1965). Husband-coached childbirth. New York: Harper Row.

Bradley, R. A. (1974). Husband-coached childbirth (3rd ed.). New York: Harper Row.

Cunningham, G., Leveno, K. J., Bloom, S. L., Hauth, J. C., Gilstrap, L. C., & Wenstrom, K. D. (2005). *Williams obstetrics* (22th ed.). New York: McGraw-Hill.

de Costa, C. M., & Robson, S. (2004). Throwing out the baby with the spa water? *Medical Journal of Australia,181*(8), 438–440.

Dennis, C. L. (2002). Breastfeeding initiation and duration: A 1990–2000 literature review. *Journal of Obstetric, Gynecologic, & Neonatal Nursing, 31,* 12–32.

Hodnett, E. D. (2002). Pain and women's satisfaction with the experience of childbirth: A systematic review. *American Journal of Obstetrics & Gynecology, 186* (Suppl. 5, Nature), S160–172.

Hodnett, E. D., Gates, S., Hofmeyr, G. J., & Sakala, C. (2003). Continuous support for women during childbirth *The Cochrane Database of Systemic Reviews, 3.* (Article No. CD003766. DOI: 10.1002/14651858.CD003766).

Lebovic, D. I., Gordon, J. D., & Taylor, R. N. (2005). *Reproductive endocrinology & infertility.* Arlington, VA: Scrub Hill Press.

Low, L. K., Seng, J. S., Murtland, T. L., & Oakley, D. (2000). Clinician-specific episiotomy rates: Impact on perinatal outcomes. *Journal of Nurse Midwifery & Women's Health, 45*(2), 87–93.

Mainous, R. O. (2002). Infant massage as a component of developmental care: Past, present, and future. *Holistic Nursing Practice,17*(1), 1–7.

Meikle, S. F., Steiner, C. A., Zhang, J., & Lawrence, W. L. (2005). A national estimate of the elective primary cesarean delivery rate. *Obstetrics and Gynecology, 105*(4), 751–756.

Montgomery, K. S. (2003). Nursing care for pregnant adolescents. *Journal of Obstetric, Gynecologic, & Neonatal Nursing, 32,* 249–257.

Nohr, E. A., Bech, B. H., Davies, M. J., Frydenberg, M., Henriksen, T. B., & Olsen, J. (2005). Prepregnancy obesity and fetal death. *Obstetrics and Gynecology, 106,* 250–259.

Pascali-Bonaro, D., & Kroeger, M. (2004). Continuous female companionship during childbirth: A crucial resource in times of stress or calm. *Journal of Midwifery & Women's Health, 49*(6), 552.

Scott, J. R., Gibbs, R. S., Karlan, B. Y., & Haney, A. F. (2003). *Danforth's obstetrics and gynecology* (9th ed.). Philadelphia: Lippincott Williams & Wilkins.

Teschendorf, M., & Evans, C. P. (2000). Hydrotherapy during labor.: An example of a developing practice policy. *American Journal of Maternal Child Nursing, 25*(4),198–203.

14 Physical and Psychologic Changes of Pregnancy

The atmosphere of approval in which I was bathed—even by strangers on the street, it seemed—was like an aura I carried with me.... This is what women have always done.

~Adrienne Rich, Of Woman Born*~*

OBJECTIVES

1. Identify the anatomic and physiologic changes that occur during pregnancy.

2. Relate the physiologic and anatomic changes that occur in the body systems during pregnancy to the signs and symptoms that develop in the woman.

3. Compare subjective (presumptive), objective (probable), and diagnostic (positive) changes of pregnancy.

4. Contrast the various types of pregnancy tests.

5. Discuss the emotional and psychologic changes that commonly occur in a woman, her partner, and her family during pregnancy.

6. Summarize cultural factors that may influence a family's response to pregnancy.

KEY TERMS

MEDIALINK

Additional resources for this content can be found on the Prentice Hall Nursing MediaLink DVD-ROM and on the Companion Website at http://www.prenhall.com/davidson. Click on "Chapter 14" to select the activities for this chapter.

Through modern technology and highly evolved research methods, we know a great deal about how pregnancy occurs and what happens to the fetus and the woman's body during gestation. Yet no matter how much we learn about this event, it never ceases to amaze us. First, it is nothing short of a miracle that the union of two microscopic entities—an ovum and a sperm—can produce a living being. Second, the woman's body must undergo extraordinary physical changes to sustain a pregnancy. A pregnant woman's body changes in size and shape, and all her organ systems modify their functions to create an environment that protects and nurtures the growing fetus.

Pregnancy is divided into three trimesters, each a 3-month period. Each trimester has its own predictable developments in both the fetus and the mother. This chapter describes both obvious and subtle physical and psychologic changes caused by pregnancy. It also discusses the various cultural factors that can affect a woman's well-being during pregnancy.

ANATOMY AND PHYSIOLOGY OF PREGNANCY

The changes that occur in the pregnant woman's body are caused by several factors. Many changes are the result of hormonal influences, some are caused by the growth of the fetus inside the uterus, and some are a result of the mother's physical adaptation to the changes that are occurring.

Reproductive System

UTERUS

The changes in the uterus during pregnancy are phenomenal. Before pregnancy the uterus is a small, almost solid, pear-shaped organ measuring approximately 7.5 × 5 × 2.5 cm and weighing about 60 g (2 oz). At the end of pregnancy the dimensions are approximately 28 × 24 × 21 cm, with an organ weight of approximately 1100 g (2.5 lb). Its capacity increases from 10 mL to 5000 mL (5 L) or more (Cunningham, Leveno, Bloom et al., 2005).

The enlargement of the uterus is primarily a result of an increase in size (hypertrophy) of the preexisting myometrial cells. Only a limited increase in cell number (hyperplasia) occurs. The amount of fibrous tissue between the muscle bands increases markedly, which adds to the strength and elasticity of the muscle wall.

The uterine walls become considerably thicker during the first few months of pregnancy than during the nonpregnant state. The initial changes are stimulated by increased estrogen and progesterone levels and not by mechanical distention (enlargement) by the fetus, placenta, and amniotic fluid. In general, the uterus enlarges more around the placental insertion site and in the upper portion of the uterus, the *fundus* (Cunningham et al., 2005). After approximately the third month, the uterine contents begin to exert intrauterine pressure. The myometrial hypertrophy continues during the first few months of pregnancy. Then the musculature begins to distend, resulting in a thinning of the muscle wall to a thickness of about 1.5 cm or less at term

(38 through 41 weeks of gestation). The ease of palpating the fetus through the abdominal wall attests to this thinning.

The circulatory requirements of the uterus increase as the uterus enlarges and the fetus and placenta develop. The size and number of the blood and lymphatic vessels within the uterine layers increase greatly. By the end of pregnancy, one sixth of the total maternal blood volume is contained within the vascular system of the uterus.

Braxton Hicks contractions—irregular contractions of the uterus—occur intermittently throughout pregnancy. They may be palpated bimanually beginning about the fourth month of pregnancy. These contractions help stimulate the movement of blood through the intervillous spaces of the placenta. In late pregnancy as these contractions increase in frequency, they can become uncomfortable and may be confused with true labor contractions.

> **CLINICAL TIP**
>
> Beginning early in pregnancy, have the woman feel her uterus periodically so that she becomes familiar with the size and the way it feels. As her pregnancy progresses she then will be more likely to identify Braxton Hicks contractions and preterm labor, should it occur.

CERVIX

The major component of cervical tissue is connective tissue, which is rearranged as pregnancy progresses. At term its strength is 1/12 of its prepregnant strength, facilitating cervical changes during labor (Cunningham et al., 2005).

Estrogen stimulates the glandular tissue of the cervix, which increases in cell number and becomes hyperactive. The endocervical glands occupy about half the mass of the cervix at term, as compared with a small fraction in the nonpregnant state. They secrete a thick, tenacious mucus, which accumulates and thickens to form the **mucous plug** that seals the endocervical canal and prevents the ascent of bacteria or other substances into the uterus. This plug is expelled when cervical dilatation begins. The hyperactive glandular tissue also causes an increase in the normal physiologic mucorrhea, at times resulting in a profuse discharge. Increased vascularization causes both the softening of the cervix (**Goodell's sign**) and a blue-purple discoloration of the cervix (**Chadwick's sign**). Increased vascularization is a result of hypertrophy and engorgement of the vessels below the growing uterus.

OVARIES

The ovaries cease ovum production during pregnancy. Many follicles develop temporarily but never to the point of maturity. The cells lining these follicles, the thecal cells, become active in hormone production and have been called the interstitial glands of pregnancy.

During early pregnancy human chorionic gonadotropin (hCG) maintains the corpus luteum, which persists and produces hormones until about weeks 6 to 8 of pregnancy. The corpus luteum engulfs approximately a third of the ovary at its peak of hypertrophy. By the middle of pregnancy it has regressed to almost complete obliteration. The corpus luteum secretes progesterone to maintain the endometrium until the placenta produces enough progesterone to maintain the pregnancy; then the corpus luteum disintegrates slowly.

VAGINA

The vaginal epithelium undergoes hypertrophy, increased vascularization, and hyperplasia during pregnancy. As with the cervical changes, these changes are estrogen induced and result in a thickening of mucosa, a loosening of connective tissue, and an increase in vaginal secretions. The secretions are thick, white, and acidic (pH 3.5 to 6). The acid pH plays a significant role in preventing infections. However, it also favors the growth of yeast organisms, resulting in moniliasis, a common vaginal infection during pregnancy.

As in the uterus, the smooth muscle cells of the vagina hypertrophy, with an accompanying loosening of the supportive connective tissue. By the end of pregnancy, the vaginal wall and perineal body have become sufficiently relaxed to permit distention of the tissues and passage of the infant.

Because the blood flow to the vagina increases, it may show the same blue-purple color (Chadwick's sign) seen in the cervix.

Breasts

Soon after the woman first misses her menstrual period, estrogen- and progesterone-induced changes occur in the mammary glands. Increases in breast size and nodularity are the result of glandular hyperplasia and hypertrophy in preparation for lactation. By the end of the second month, superficial veins are prominent, nipples are more erectile, and pigmentation of the areola is obvious. Pigmentation tends to be more pronounced in women with dark complexions. Hypertrophy of Montgomery's follicles is noted within the primary areola. **Striae** (purplish stretch marks that slowly turn silver after childbirth) may develop as the pregnancy progresses. Breast changes are often most noticeable in the woman who is pregnant for the first time.

Colostrum, an antibody-rich, yellow secretion, may be expressed manually by the 12th week and may leak from the breasts during the last trimester of pregnancy. Colostrum gradually converts to mature milk during the first few days following childbirth.

Respiratory System

Pulmonary function is modified throughout pregnancy. Pregnancy induces a small degree of hyperventilation as the tidal volume (amount of air breathed with ordinary respiration) increases steadily throughout pregnancy. There is a 30% to 40% rise from nonpregnant values in the volume of air breathed each minute. Between weeks 16 and 40, oxygen consumption increases approximately 15% to 20% to meet the increased needs of the mother as well as those of the fetus and placenta. The vital capacity (maximum amount of air that can be moved in and out of the lungs with forced respiration) increases slightly, while lung compliance (elasticity) and pulmonary diffusion remain constant. Measurements of airway resistance show a marked decrease in pregnancy in response to elevated progesterone levels. The diaphragm is elevated and the subcostal angle is increased as a result of pressure from the enlarging uterus. This change

causes the rib cage to flare, with a decrease in the vertical diameter and increases in the anteroposterior and transverse diameters. The circumference of the chest may increase by as much as 6 cm. The increase compensates for the elevated diaphragm, and there is no significant loss of intrathoracic volume. Breathing changes from abdominal to thoracic as pregnancy progresses. Overall, pulmonary function is not impaired by pregnancy. Many women experience an increased awareness of the need to breathe, however, starting early in pregnancy. This may be perceived as dyspnea and is thought to be due to the increased tidal volume, which causes a slight decrease in blood Pco_2. Actual lung disease may be aggravated by pregnancy because of the increased need for oxygen by the woman and her fetus (Cunningham et al., 2005).

Nasal stuffiness and congestion, referred to as rhinitis of pregnancy, are not uncommon. Epistaxis (nosebleeds) may also occur. They are primarily the result of estrogen-induced edema and vascular congestion of the nasal mucosa.

Cardiovascular System

The growing uterus exerts pressure on the diaphragm, pushing the heart upward and to the left and rotating it forward. This lateral displacement makes the heart appear somewhat enlarged on x-ray examination. A systolic murmur can be heard in 90% of pregnant women, and the first and third heart sounds are louder.

Blood volume progressively increases throughout pregnancy, beginning in the first trimester and peaking near term at about 40% to 45% above nonpregnant levels. This increase is due to increases in both plasma and erythrocytes. No increase occurs in pulmonary capillary wedge pressure or in central venous pressure despite the increase in blood volume. This is due to decreases in both systemic vascular resistance and pulmonary vascular resistance, which enable the circulation to adapt to higher blood volume while maintaining normal vessel pressures. Cardiac output begins to increase early in pregnancy and peaks at 25 to 30 weeks' gestation at 30% to 50% above prepregnant levels. Cardiac output is less predictable in the third trimester—some studies show a slight increase, others show a slight decrease, and still others show no change. It is likely that changes in the third trimester are individually determined (Gordon, 2002).

During pregnancy, organ systems receive additional blood flow according to their increased workload. Thus blood flow to the uterus and kidneys increases, whereas hepatic and cerebral flow remains unchanged.

The pulse rate frequently increases during pregnancy, although the amount varies from almost no increase to an increase of 10 to 15 beats per minute. The blood pressure decreases slightly during pregnancy, reaching its lowest point during the second trimester. The blood pressure then gradually increases during the third trimester and is near prepregnant levels at term (when the baby is due).

The femoral venous pressure slowly rises as the uterus exerts increasing pressure on return blood flow. There is an increased tendency toward stagnation of blood in the lower extremities, with a resulting dependent edema and tendency toward varicose vein formation in the legs, vulva, and rectum late in pregnancy. In addition to the effects of increased femoral venous pressure, a reduction of plasma colloid osmotic pressure resulting from a reduction in plasma albumin further maintains the presence of fluid in the extravascular space. The pregnant woman becomes more prone to develop postural hypotension because of the increased blood volume in the lower extremities.

During pregnancy the enlarging uterus may put pressure on the vena cava when the woman is supine, resulting in **supine hypotensive syndrome,** also called **vena caval syndrome** or **aortocaval compression.** This pressure interferes with returning blood flow and produces a marked decrease in blood pressure with accompanying dizziness, pallor, and clamminess, which can be corrected by having the woman lie on her left side. Research indicates that the enlarging uterus may press on the aorta and its collateral circulation as well (Cunningham et al., 2005) (Figure 14–1 ◆).

The total erythrocyte volume increases by about 30% in women who receive iron supplementation but increases only about 18% without iron supplements (Gordon, 2002). This increase is necessary to transport the additional oxygen required during pregnancy. The increase in plasma volume averages about 50%. Because the plasma volume increase is greater than the erythrocyte increase, however, the hematocrit, which measures the portion of whole blood that is composed of erythrocytes, decreases slightly. This decrease is sometimes referred to as the **physiologic anemia of pregnancy** (pseudoanemia).

Iron is necessary for hemoglobin formation, and hemoglobin is the oxygen-carrying component of erythrocytes. Thus the increase in erythrocyte levels results in an increased need for iron by the pregnant woman. Even though the gastrointestinal absorption of iron is moderately increased during pregnancy, it is usually necessary to add supplemental iron to the diet to meet the expanded red blood cell and fetal needs.

Leukocyte production equals or is slightly greater than the increase in blood volume. The average cell count is 5000 to 12,000/mm^3, with an occasional woman developing a physiologic leukocytosis of 15,000/mm^3. During labor and the early postpartum period, these levels may reach 25,000/mm^3. The reason for this dramatic increase remains unknown, but similar leukocyte changes occur with physiologic stress such as vigorous exercise. It probably represents the return to the circulation of mature leukocytes that had been shunted out of the circulatory system (Cunningham et al., 2005).

The platelet count does not change much in pregnancy, but the plasma fibrinogen has been known to increase by as much as 50%. The increased fibrinogen accounts for the nonpathologic rise of the sedimentation rate. Although the clotting time of the pregnant woman does not differ significantly from that of the nonpregnant woman, blood factors VII, VIII, IX, and X are increased so that pregnancy becomes a somewhat hypercoagulable state. These changes, coupled with venous stasis in late pregnancy, place the pregnant woman at increased risk of developing venous thrombosis.

Gastrointestinal System

Many of the discomforts of pregnancy are attributed to changes in the gastrointestinal system. Nausea and vomiting during the first trimester are sometimes associated with the hCG secreted by the implanted blastocyst and with a change in carbohydrate metabolism that occurs in early pregnancy. Peculiarities of taste and smell are common and can further aggravate gastrointestinal discomfort. Gum tissue may become hyperemic and softened and may bleed when only mildly traumatized. The secretion of saliva may increase or become excessive (*ptyalism*).

During the second half of pregnancy, numerous gastrointestinal symptoms are attributable to the pressure of the growing uterus and smooth muscle relaxation due to elevated progesterone levels. The intestines are displaced laterally and posteriorly and the stomach superiorly. Heartburn (pyrosis) is caused by the reflux of acidic secretions from the stomach into the lower esophagus as a result of relaxation of the cardiac sphincter. Gastric emptying time and intestinal motility are delayed, leading to frequent complaints of bloating and constipation, which can be aggravated by the smooth muscle relaxation and increased electrolyte and water reabsorption in the large intestine. Hemorrhoids frequently develop if constipation is a problem or, in the second half of pregnancy, from pressure on vessels below the level of the uterus.

Only minor liver changes occur with pregnancy. Plasma albumin concentrations and serum cholinesterase activity decrease with normal pregnancy as with certain liver diseases.

The emptying time of the gallbladder is prolonged during pregnancy as a result of smooth muscle relaxation from progesterone. Hypercholesterolemia may follow, and it can predispose the woman to gallstone formation. Pruritus (itching) caused by retained bile salts may also occur (Cunningham et al., 2005).

Urinary Tract

During the first trimester, the growing uterus puts pressure on the bladder, producing urinary frequency until the second trimester, when the uterus becomes an abdominal organ. Near term, when the presenting part engages in the pelvis, pressure is again exerted on the bladder. This pressure can impair the drainage of blood and lymph from the hyperemic bladder, rendering it more susceptible to infection and trauma. The bladder, normally a convex organ, becomes concave from the external pressure, and its capacity is greatly reduced.

Figure 14–1 ◆ Vena caval syndrome. The gravid uterus compresses the vena cava when the woman is supine. This reduces the blood flow returning to the heart and may cause maternal hypotension.

Dilation of the kidneys and ureter may occur, most frequently on the right side above the pelvic brim, because of the lie of the uterus. This dilation is accompanied by elongation and curvature of the ureter. There appears to be no single factor accounting for this anatomic variation; instead a combination of ureteral atonia and hypoperistalsis, probably caused by pressure from the enlarging fetus with some progesterone effects, seems to be involved. The presence of amino acids and glucose in the urine in conjunction with the tendency toward ureteral atonia and stasis of urine in the ureters may increase the risk of urinary tract infection.

The glomerular filtration rate (GFR) and renal plasma flow (RPF) increase early in pregnancy. The GFR rises by as much as 50% by the beginning of the second trimester and remains elevated until birth. The increase in RPF is slightly less and decreases somewhat during the third trimester (Cunningham et al., 2005). The mechanism for these rises remains unclear.

An increased renal tubular reabsorption rate compensates for the increased glomerular activity. Amino acids and water-soluble vitamins are excreted in greater amounts than in the nonpregnant woman. Glycosuria is not uncommon or necessarily pathogenic during pregnancy but is merely a reflection of the kidneys' inability to reabsorb all of the glucose filtered by the glomeruli. However, pregnancy can be diabetogenic, so the possibility of diabetes mellitus cannot be disregarded.

The increased renal function during pregnancy results in an increased clearance of urea and creatinine and in a lowering of the blood urea and nonprotein nitrogen values. Because of this, measurement of creatinine clearance provides an accurate test of renal functioning during pregnancy.

Skin and Hair

Changes in skin pigmentation commonly occur during pregnancy. These changes are thought to be stimulated by increased estrogen, progesterone, and α-melanocyte-stimulating hormone levels.

Pigmentation of the skin increases primarily in areas that are already hyperpigmented: the areolae, the nipples, the vulva, the perianal area, and the linea alba. The linea alba refers to the midline of the abdomen from the pubic area to the umbilicus and above. During pregnancy increased pigmentation may cause this area to darken. It is then referred to as the **linea nigra** (Figure 14–2 ◆). Some women also develop facial **chloasma** (or **melasma gravidarum**), the "mask of pregnancy." This is an irregular pigmentation of the cheeks, forehead, and nose that occurs in many women during pregnancy and is accentuated by sun exposure. Similar changes may occur in women who are taking oral contraceptives. Facial melasma is more prominent in dark-haired women and is occasionally disfiguring. Fortunately, it fades or at least regresses soon after birth when the hormonal influence of pregnancy has stopped.

Striae, or stretch marks, are reddish, wavy, depressed streaks that may occur over the abdomen, breasts, and thighs as pregnancy progresses. They are caused by reduced connective tissue strength due to elevated adrenal steroid levels.

Vascular spider nevi may develop on the chest, neck, face, arms, and legs. They are small, bright-red elevations of the skin

Figure 14–2 ◆ Linea nigra.

radiating from a central body. They may be caused by increased subcutaneous blood flow in response to increased estrogen levels. This condition is of no clinical significance and disappears after pregnancy ends.

The rate of hair growth may decrease during pregnancy, and the number of hair follicles in the resting or dormant phase also decreases. After birth the number of hair follicles in the resting phase increases sharply, and the woman may notice increased shedding of hair for 1 to 4 months. Practically all hair is replaced within 6 to 12 months, however (Cunningham et al., 2005).

Finally, the sweat and sebaceous glands are frequently hyperactive during pregnancy. Some women may notice heavy perspiration, night sweats, and/or the development of acne even if they have never experienced these symptoms before.

Musculoskeletal System

No demonstrable changes occur in the teeth of the pregnant woman. No demineralization takes place. The fairly common occurrence of dental caries during pregnancy has led to the myth "a tooth for every pregnancy." The dental caries that may accompany pregnancy is likely to be caused by inadequate oral hygiene and dental care.

The sacroiliac, sacrococcygeal, and pubic joints of the pelvis relax in the later part of the pregnancy, presumably as a result of hormonal changes. This often causes a waddling gait. A slight separation of the symphysis pubis can often be demonstrated on radiologic examination.

As the pregnant woman's center of gravity gradually changes, the lumbodorsal spinal curve is accentuated, and the woman's posture changes (Figure 14–3 ◆). This posture change compensates for the increased weight of the uterus anteriorly and frequently results in low backache. Late in pregnancy, aches

12 weeks   20 weeks   28 weeks   36 weeks   40 weeks

Figure 14–3 ◆ Postural changes during pregnancy. Note the increasing lordosis of the lumbosacral spine and the increasing curvature of the thoracic area.

in the neck, shoulders, and upper extremities may occur because of shoulder slumping and anterior flexion of the neck accompanying the lumbodorsal lordosis. Paresthesias of the extremities may occur late in pregnancy as a result of pressure on peripheral nerves.

Often pressure of the enlarging uterus on the abdominal muscles causes the rectus abdominis muscle to separate, producing *diastasis recti*. If the separation is severe and muscle tone is not regained postpartally, subsequent pregnancies will not have adequate support, and the woman's abdomen may appear pendulous.

Eyes

Two changes generally occur in the eyes during pregnancy. First, intraocular pressure decreases, probably as a result of increased vitreous outflow. Second, a slight thickening of the cornea occurs, which is generally attributed to fluid retention. Although these changes are not readily perceived, some pregnant women experience difficulty wearing previously comfortable contact lenses (Cunningham et al., 2005). The change in the corneas generally disappears by 6 weeks postpartum.

Central Nervous System

Pregnant women frequently describe decreased attention, concentration, and memory during and shortly after pregnancy, but few studies have explored this phenomenon. One study did compare a group of pregnant women against a control group, finding a decline in memory that could not be attributed to depression, anxiety, sleep deprivation, or other physical changes of pregnancy. This memory loss disappeared soon after childbirth. Another study found that sleep problems are common in pregnancy. These include difficulty going to sleep, frequent awakenings, fewer hours of night sleep, and reduced sleep efficiency (Cunningham et al., 2005).

Metabolism

Most metabolic functions accelerate during pregnancy to support the additional demands of the growing fetus and its support system. The expectant mother must meet her own tissue replacement needs, those of the fetus, and those preparatory for labor and lactation. No other event in life induces such profound metabolic changes.

WEIGHT GAIN

Growth of the uterus and its contents, and of the breasts, and increases in intravascular fluids account for most of the weight gain in pregnancy. In addition, extra water, fat, and protein are stored; these are usually called *maternal reserves.*

The recommended total weight gain during pregnancy for a woman of normal weight before pregnancy is 11.5 to 16 kg (25 to 35 lb); for women who were overweight before becoming pregnant, the recommended gain is 6.8 to 11.5 kg (15 to 25 lb). Underweight women are advised to gain the weight needed to reach their ideal weight plus 11.5 to 16 kg (25 to 35 lb) (Mattson & Smith, 2004). Weight may decrease slightly during the first trimester because of nausea, vomiting, and food intolerances of early pregnancy. The lost weight is soon regained, and an average increase of 1.6 to 2.3 kg (3.5 to 5 lb), 5.5 to 6.8 kg (12 to 15 lb), and 5.5 to 6.8 kg (12 to 15 lb) occurs in the first, second, and third trimesters, respectively.

Adequate nutrition and weight gain are important during pregnancy. Maternal nutrition is discussed in detail in Chapter 18. ∞

WATER METABOLISM

Increased water retention is a basic chemical alteration of pregnancy. Several interrelated factors cause this phenomenon. The increased level of steroid sex hormones affects sodium and fluid retention. The lowered serum protein also influences the fluid balance, as do the increased intracapillary pressure and permeability. The extra water is needed for the products of conception—the fetus, placenta, and amniotic fluid—and the mother's increased blood volume, interstitial fluids, and enlarged organs.

NUTRIENT METABOLISM

The fetus makes its greatest protein and fat demands during the second half of gestation, doubling in weight in the last 6 to 8 weeks. The increased protein retention that begins in early pregnancy is initially used for hyperplasia and hypertrophy of maternal tissues, such as the uterus and breasts. Protein must also be stored during pregnancy to maintain a constant level within the breast milk and to avoid depletion of maternal tissues.

Fats are more completely absorbed during pregnancy, resulting in a marked increase in the serum lipids, lipoproteins, and cholesterol and decreased elimination through the bowel. Fat deposits in the fetus increase from about 2% at midpregnancy to almost 12% at term. The excess nitrogen and lipidemia are considered to be a preparation for lactation. In addition, the woman's body switches from glucose metabolism to lipid metabolism once glucose from food intake has been used up. This leads to an increased tendency to develop ketosis between meals and overnight. The demand for carbohydrate increases, especially during the last two trimesters. Intermittent glycosuria is not uncommon during pregnancy. When it is not accompanied by a rise in blood sugar levels, glycosuria is a physiologic entity secondary to the increased glomerular filtration rate. Fasting blood sugar levels tend to fall slightly, returning to more normal levels by the sixth postpartal month. The oral glucose tolerance test shows no change with pregnancy.

The possibility of diabetes must not be overlooked during pregnancy. Plasma levels of insulin increase during pregnancy (probably because of hormonal changes that cause increased tissue resistance), and rapid destruction of insulin takes place within the placenta. Insulin production must be increased by the mother during the second trimester, and any marginal pancreatic function quickly becomes apparent. The diabetic woman often experiences increased exogenous insulin demands during pregnancy.

The demand for iron during pregnancy is accelerated, and the pregnant woman needs to guard against anemia. Iron is necessary for the increase in erythrocytes, hemoglobin, and blood volume, as well as for the increased tissue demands of both woman and fetus.

Iron transfer takes place at the placenta in only one direction—toward the fetus. It has been demonstrated that approximately five sixths of the iron stored in the fetal liver is assimilated during the last trimester of pregnancy. This stored iron in the fetal liver compensates in the first 4 months of neonatal life for the normal inadequate amounts of iron available in breast milk and non-iron-fortified formulas.

The progressive absorption and retention of calcium during pregnancy has been noted. The maternal plasma concentration of bound calcium decreases as the levels of bindable plasma proteins fall. Approximately 30 g of calcium is retained in maternal bone for fetal deposition late in pregnancy.

Pregnancy produces little change in the metabolism of most other minerals, other than retention of amounts needed for fetal growth.

COMPLEMENTARY AND ALTERNATIVE THERAPIES

HERBS DURING PREGNANCY

Pharmaceutical companies continue to refuse to include children and babies in their studies of drug safety, claiming excessive costs and other research problems. As a result, very few over-the-counter or prescription drugs can claim to be safe for pregnant women and nursing mothers. The same can be said for herbal medicines. Although herbs have been researched extensively in Europe and Asia, there has been little clinical research done in the United States on the use of herbs in pregnancy. Every pregnant or nursing woman must be extremely cautious about everything she ingests—foods, liquids, medications, and herbs. If a problem warrants intervention, she and her primary healthcare provider should discuss the benefits and risks of all treatments, synthetic and natural.

More information about the use of herbs in pregnancy can be found in Chapter 3. ∞

Vitamin metabolism does not change appreciably with pregnancy. (See Chapter 18 ∞ for the mother's requirements of minerals and vitamins).

Endocrine System

THYROID

Pregnancy influences the thyroid gland's size and activity. Often a palpable change is noted, which represents an increase in vascularity and hyperplasia of glandular tissue. Total serum thyroxine (T_4) increases in early pregnancy, and thyroid-stimulating hormone (TSH) decreases. The elevated levels of total T_4 continue until several weeks postpartum, although the level of free serum T_4 returns to normal after the first trimester (Cunningham et al., 2005). Increased thyroxine-binding capacity is evidenced by an increase in serum protein-bound iodine (PBI), probably due to the increased levels of circulating estrogens.

The basal metabolic rate (BMR) increases by as much as 20% to 25% during pregnancy. The increased oxygen consumption is due primarily to fetal metabolic activity.

PARATHYROID

The concentration of the parathyroid hormone and the size of the parathyroid glands increase, paralleling the fetal calcium requirements. Parathyroid hormone concentration reaches its highest level of approximately twofold between 15 and 35 weeks of gestation, returning to a normal or even subnormal level before childbirth.

PITUITARY

During pregnancy, the pituitary gland enlarges somewhat, but it returns to normal size after birth. There is no significant change in the posterior lobe of the gland, although the anterior lobe increases in weight with each successive pregnancy.

Pregnancy is made possible by the hypothalamic stimulation of the anterior pituitary hormones: follicle-stimulating hormone

(FSH), which stimulates follicle growth within the ovary, and luteinizing hormone (LH), which effects ovulation. Pituitary stimulation prolongs the corpus luteal phase of the ovary, which maintains the secretory endometrium for development of the pregnancy.

Two additional pituitary hormones, thyrotropin and adrenotropin, alter maternal metabolism to support the pregnancy. Prolactin, also an anterior pituitary secretion, is responsible for initial lactation. Its levels increase 10-fold during pregnancy and then, somewhat surprisingly, decrease after childbirth, even in breastfeeding women. (Continued lactation depends on the suckling of the infant.)

The posterior pituitary contains the mechanism for the release of oxytocin and vasopressin, which exert oxytocic, vasopressor, and antidiuretic effects. The main effects of oxytocin are the promotion of uterine contractility and the stimulation of milk ejection from the breasts. Vasopressin causes vasoconstriction, which results in increased blood pressure; it also has an antidiuretic effect and plays an important role in the regulation of water balance. Vasopressin secretion is controlled by changes in plasma osmolarity and blood volume.

ADRENALS

Little structural change occurs in the adrenal glands during a normal pregnancy. Estrogen-induced increases in the levels of circulating cortisol result primarily from lowered renal excretion. The circulating cortisol levels regulate carbohydrate and protein metabolism. A normal level resumes 1 to 6 weeks postpartum.

The adrenals secrete increased levels of aldosterone by the early part of the second trimester. The levels of secretion are even more elevated in the woman on a sodium-restricted diet. This increase in aldosterone in a normal pregnancy may be the body's protective response to the increased sodium excretion associated with progesterone (Cunningham et al., 2005).

PANCREAS

The pregnant woman has increased insulin needs. The islets of Langerhans are stressed to meet this increased demand, and a latent deficiency may become apparent during pregnancy, producing symptoms of gestational diabetes (see Chapter 19 ∞).

HORMONES IN PREGNANCY

Several hormones are required to maintain pregnancy. Most of these are produced initially by the corpus luteum; production is then assumed by the placenta. (For an in-depth discussion of placental hormones, see Chapter 11 ∞).

Human Chorionic Gonadotropin

The trophoblast secretes hCG in early pregnancy. This hormone stimulates progesterone and estrogen production by the corpus luteum to maintain the pregnancy until the placenta is developed sufficiently to assume that function.

Human Placental Lactogen

Also called human chorionic somatomammotropin (hCS), human placental lactogen (hPL) is produced by the syncytiotrophoblast. This hormone is an antagonist of insulin; it increases the amount of circulating free fatty acids for maternal metabolic needs and decreases maternal metabolism of glucose to favor fetal growth.

Estrogen

Secreted originally by the corpus luteum, estrogen is produced primarily by the placenta as early as the seventh week of pregnancy. Estrogen stimulates uterine development to provide a suitable environment for the fetus. It also helps to develop the ductal system of the breasts in preparation for lactation.

Progesterone

Progesterone, also produced initially by the corpus luteum and then by the placenta, plays the greatest role in maintaining pregnancy. It maintains the endometrium and also inhibits spontaneous uterine contractility, thus preventing early spontaneous abortion due to uterine activity. In addition, progesterone helps develop the acini and lobules of the breasts in preparation for lactation.

Relaxin

Relaxin is detectable in the serum of a pregnant woman by the time of the first missed menstrual period. Relaxin inhibits uterine activity, diminishes the strength of uterine contractions, aids in the softening of the cervix, and has the long-term effect of remodeling collagen. Its primary source is the corpus luteum, but small amounts are believed to be produced by the placenta and uterine decidua throughout pregnancy.

PROSTAGLANDINS IN PREGNANCY

Prostaglandins (PGs) are lipid substances that can arise from most body tissues but occur in high concentrations in the female reproductive tract and are present in the decidua during pregnancy. The exact functions of PGs during pregnancy are still unknown, although it has been proposed that they are responsible for maintaining reduced placental vascular resistance. Decreased PG levels may contribute to hypertension and preeclampsia. Prostaglandins are also believed to play a role in the complex biochemistry that initiates labor, although their specific functions are still being defined.

SIGNS OF PREGNANCY

Many of the changes women experience during pregnancy are used to diagnose the pregnancy itself. They are called the subjective (or presumptive) changes, the objective (or probable) changes, and the diagnostic (or positive) changes of pregnancy.

Subjective (Presumptive) Changes

The subjective changes of pregnancy are the symptoms the woman experiences and reports. They can be caused by other conditions (Table 14–1) and therefore cannot be considered proof of pregnancy. The following can be diagnostic clues when other signs and symptoms of pregnancy are also present.

Amenorrhea is the earliest symptom of pregnancy. In a healthy woman whose menstrual cycles are regular, missing one or more menstrual periods leads to the consideration of pregnancy.

Nausea and vomiting of pregnancy (NVP) are experienced by almost half of all pregnant women during the first 3 months of pregnancy and may be the result of elevated hCG levels and changed carbohydrate metabolism. Further research is being conducted to determine other causes for nausea and vomiting.

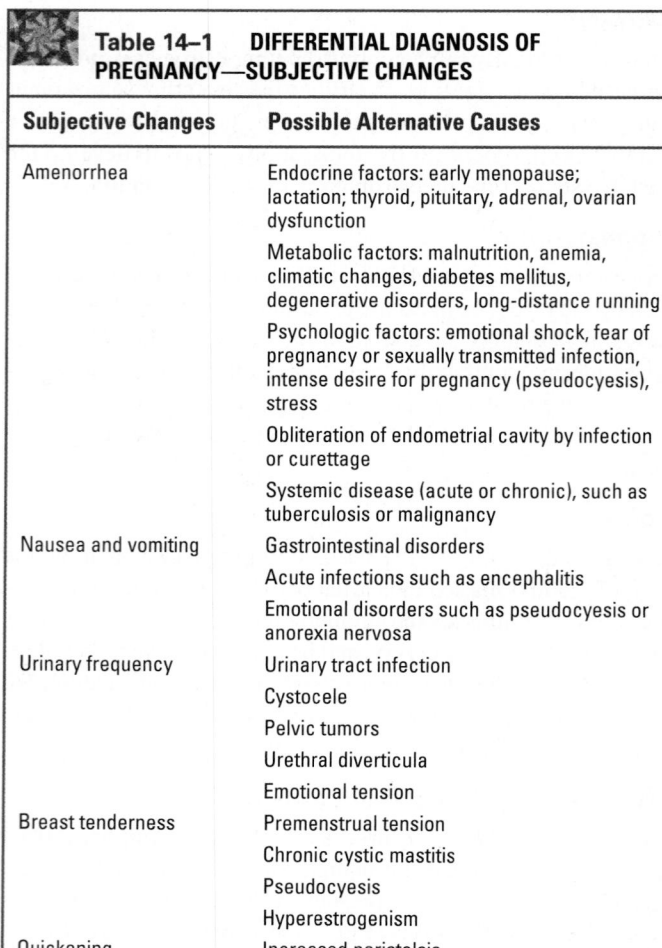

Table 14–1   DIFFERENTIAL DIAGNOSIS OF PREGNANCY—SUBJECTIVE CHANGES

Subjective Changes	Possible Alternative Causes
Amenorrhea	Endocrine factors: early menopause; lactation; thyroid, pituitary, adrenal, ovarian dysfunction
	Metabolic factors: malnutrition, anemia, climatic changes, diabetes mellitus, degenerative disorders, long-distance running
	Psychologic factors: emotional shock, fear of pregnancy or sexually transmitted infection, intense desire for pregnancy (pseudocyesis), stress
	Obliteration of endometrial cavity by infection or curettage
	Systemic disease (acute or chronic), such as tuberculosis or malignancy
Nausea and vomiting	Gastrointestinal disorders
	Acute infections such as encephalitis
	Emotional disorders such as pseudocyesis or anorexia nervosa
Urinary frequency	Urinary tract infection
	Cystocele
	Pelvic tumors
	Urethral diverticula
	Emotional tension
Breast tenderness	Premenstrual tension
	Chronic cystic mastitis
	Pseudocyesis
	Hyperestrogenism
Quickening	Increased peristalsis
	Flatus ("gas")
	Abdominal muscle contractions
	Shifting of abdominal contents

The woman may feel merely a distaste for food or may suffer extreme vomiting, which may be accompanied by dehydration and ketosis. Because these symptoms frequently occur in the early part of the day and disappear within a few hours, they are commonly called **morning sickness.** In reality, symptoms may occur at any time. This gastrointestinal disturbance usually appears about 6 weeks after the first day of the last menstrual period (LMP) and usually disappears spontaneously 6 to 12 weeks later, although it may be prolonged in some instances. Research suggests that women who experience NVP often have a more favorable pregnancy outcome than those who do not.

I believed that the nausea and vomiting would only occur in the morning because everyone called it morning sickness. I soon realized that it could occur at any time of the day or night. I was exhausted all the time and nauseated. Everyone told me the nausea was a sign of a healthy baby, which was reassuring I guess but I was so relieved when I started my second trimester and the nausea ended. The rest of my pregnancy was a breeze.

Excessive fatigue may be noted within a few weeks after the first missed menstrual period and may persist throughout the first trimester.

Table 14–2   DIFFERENTIAL DIAGNOSIS OF PREGNANCY—OBJECTIVE CHANGES

Objective Changes	Possible Alternative Causes
Changes in pelvic organs	Increased vascular congestion
Goodell's sign	Estrogen-progestin oral contraceptives
Chadwick's sign	Vulvar, vaginal, cervical hyperemia
Hegar's sign	Excessively soft walls of nonpregnant uterus
Uterine enlargement	Uterine tumors
Braun von Fernwald's sign	Uterine tumors
Piskacek's sign	Uterine tumors
Enlargement of abdomen	Obesity, ascites, pelvic tumors
Braxton Hicks contractions	Hematometra, pedunculated, submucous, and soft myomas
Uterine souffle	Large uterine myomas, large ovarian tumors, or any condition with greatly increased uterine blood flow
Pigmentation of skin	Estrogen-progestin oral contraceptives
Chloasma (Melasma)	Melanocyte hormonal stimulation
Linea nigra	
Nipples/areola	
Abdominal striae	Obesity, pelvic tumor
Ballottement	Uterine tumors/polyps, ascites
Pregnancy tests	Increased pituitary gonadotropins at menopause, choriocarcinoma, hydatidiform mole
Palpation for fetal outline	Uterine myomas

Urinary frequency is experienced during the first trimester as the enlarging uterus exerts pressure on the bladder. The increased vascularization and pelvic congestion that occur in each pregnancy can also cause frequent voiding. This symptom decreases during the second trimester, when the uterus is an abdominal organ, but reappears during the third trimester, when the presenting part descends into the pelvis.

Changes in the breasts are frequently noted in early pregnancy. Some women report significant breast changes even before missing their first menses. Engorgement of the breasts due to the hormone-induced growth of the secretory ductal system results in the subjective symptoms of tenderness and tingling, especially of the nipple area. The veins also become more visible and form a bluish pattern beneath the skin in fair-skinned women.

Quickening, or the mother's perception of fetal movement, occurs about 18 to 20 weeks after the LMP in a primigravida (a woman who is pregnant for the first time) but may occur as early as 16 weeks in a multigravida (a woman who has been pregnant more than once). Quickening is a fluttering sensation in the abdomen that gradually increases in intensity and frequency.

CLINICAL TIP

Some women suggest that it is easiest to imagine the fluttering associated with quickening by letting the outer tips of the eyelashes brush a finger and then imagining that same sensation deep inside the abdomen.

Objective (Probable) Changes

An examiner can perceive the objective changes that occur in pregnancy. They are more diagnostic than the subjective symptoms. However, their presence does not offer a definite diagnosis of pregnancy (Table 14–2).

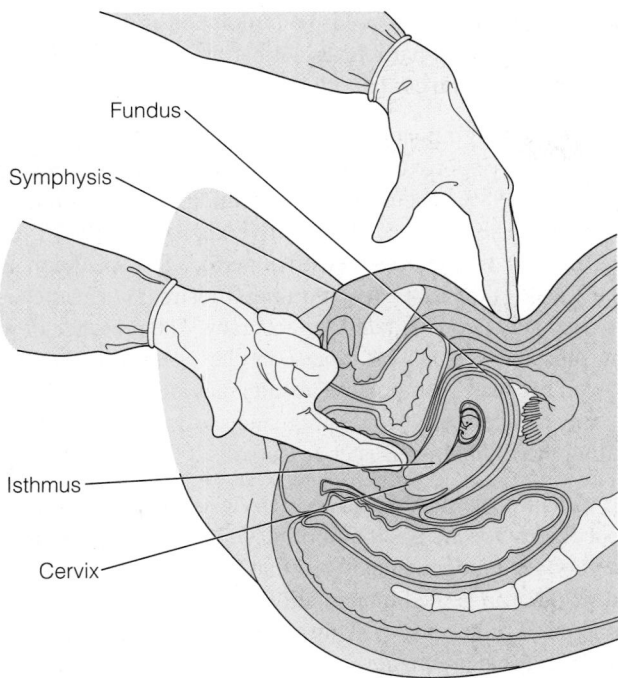

Figure 14–4 ◆ Hegar's sign, a softening of the isthmus of the uterus, can be determined by the examiner during a vaginal examination.

Changes in the pelvic organs caused by increased vascular congestion are the only physical signs detectable within the first 3 months of pregnancy. These changes are noted on pelvic examination. There is a softening of the cervix, called Goodell's sign. Chadwick's sign is the deep red to purple or bluish coloration of the mucous membranes of the cervix, vagina, and vulva due to increased vasocongestion of the pelvic vessels. **Hegar's sign** is a softening of the isthmus of the uterus, the area between the cervix and the body of the uterus, which occurs at 6 to 8 weeks of pregnancy. This area may become so soft that on a bimanual exam there seems to be nothing between the cervix and the body of the uterus (Figure 14–4 ◆).

Ladin's sign is a soft spot anteriorly in the middle of the uterus near the junction of the body of the uterus and cervix (Figure 14–5, *A* ◆). **McDonald's sign** is an ease in flexing the body of the uterus against the cervix.

The uterus assumes an irregular globular shape during the early months of pregnancy. Irregular softening and enlargement at the site of implantation, known as *Braun von Fernwald's sign*, occurs about the fifth week (Figure 14–5, *B*). Occasionally an almost tumorlike, asymmetric enlargement occurs, called *Piskacek's sign* (Figure 14–5, *C*). Generalized enlargement and softening of the body of the uterus are present after the eighth week of pregnancy. The fundus of the uterus is palpable just above the symphysis pubis at approximately 10 to 12 weeks' gestation and at the level of the umbilicus at 20 to 22 weeks' gestation (Figure 14–6 ◆).

Enlargement of the abdomen during the childbearing years is usually regarded as evidence of pregnancy, especially if the enlargement is progressive and is accompanied by a continuing amenorrhea. It is generally more pronounced in a woman whose abdominal musculature has lost some of its tone because of previous childbirth.

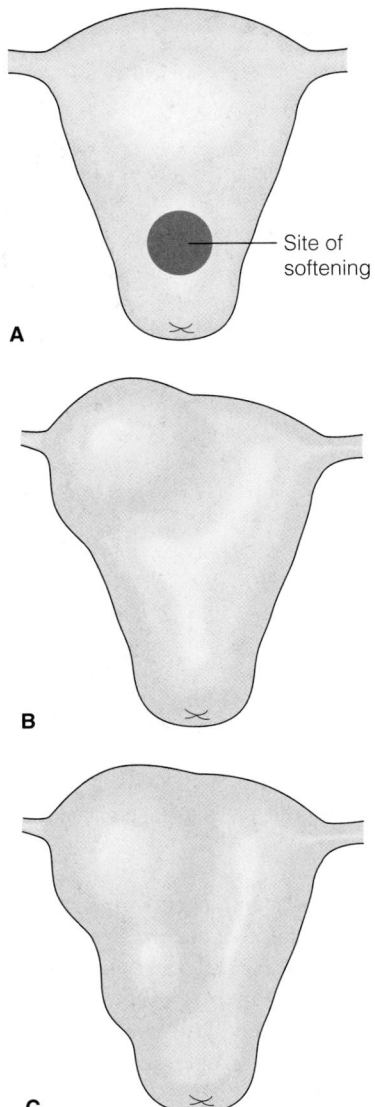

Figure 14–5 ◆ Early uterine changes of pregnancy. *A,* Ladin's sign, a soft spot anteriorly in the middle of the uterus near the junction of the body of the uterus and the cervix. *B,* Braun von Fernwald's sign, irregular softening and enlargement at the site of implantation. *C,* Piskacek's sign, a tumorlike, asymmetric enlargement.

As mentioned earlier, *Braxton Hicks* contractions are irregular, ordinarily painless contractions that occur at irregular intervals throughout pregnancy but are felt with abdominal palpation after week 28. As the woman approaches the end of the pregnancy, these contractions often become more uncomfortable and are then called *false labor.*

Uterine souffle may be heard when auscultating the abdomen over the uterus. It is a soft blowing sound at the same rate as the maternal pulse and is due to the increased uterine vascularization and the blood pulsating through the placenta. It is sometimes confused with the *funic souffle,* which is a soft blowing sound of blood pulsating through the umbilical arteries. The funic souffle is at the same rate as the fetal heart rate.

Changes in pigmentation of the skin and the *appearance of abdominal striae* are common manifestations in pregnancy.

Figure 14–6 ◆ Approximate height of the fundus at various weeks of pregnancy.

Facial melasma (chloasma) occurs in varying degrees after week 16. The pigmentation of the nipple and areola may darken, especially in primigravidas and dark-haired women. The Montgomery glands of the areola may become enlarged. The skin in the midline of the abdomen may develop a pigmented line, the linea nigra. As pregnancy progresses, striae appear on the abdomen and buttocks.

The *fetal outline* may be identified by palpation in many pregnant women after 24 weeks of gestation, becoming easier to distinguish as term approaches. **Ballottement** is the passive fetal movement elicited by pushing up against the cervix with two fingers. This pushes the fetal body up and, as it falls back, the examiner feels a rebound.

Pregnancy tests are based on analysis of maternal blood or urine for the detection of hCG, the hormone secreted by the trophoblast. These tests are not considered positive signs of pregnancy because the similarity of hCG and the pituitary-secreted LH occasionally results in cross-reactions. In addition, certain conditions other than pregnancy can cause elevated levels of hCG.

CLINICAL PREGNANCY TESTS

A variety of assay techniques are available to detect hCG during early pregnancy. Historically, the following two tests were commonly used urine pregnancy tests.

- *Hemagglutination-inhibition test,* an immunoassay, is based on the fact that no clumping of cells occurs when the urine of a pregnant woman is added to the hCG-sensitized red blood cells of sheep.

- *Latex agglutination test,* also an immunoassay, is based on the fact that latex particle agglutination is inhibited in the presence of urine containing hCG.

The hemagglutination-inhibition test and the latex agglutination tests are approximately 95% accurate in diagnosing pregnancy and 98% accurate in determining the absence of pregnancy. The tests become positive approximately 10 to 14 days after the first missed menstrual period. The specimen used for the tests is the first early morning midstream urine because it is adequately concentrated for accuracy. The presence of protein substances (such as blood) in the specimen should be avoided because false-positive results may occur.

Several newer types of pregnancy tests are available, including the following (Buster & Carson, 2002):

- β-*Subunit radioimmunoassay* (RIA) uses an antiserum with specificity for the β-subunit of hCG in blood plasma. This is a very accurate pregnancy test that becomes positive a few days after presumed implantation, thereby permitting earlier diagnosis of pregnancy. This test is also used in the diagnosis of ectopic pregnancy or trophoblastic disease. However, because it requires several hours to perform and has only limited sensitivity, it is being replaced by other, simpler tests such as the immunoradiometric assay.

- *Immunoradiometric assay* (IRMA) uses a radioactive antibody to identify the presence of hCG in the serum. This test can identify very low concentrations of hCG and requires only about 30 minutes to perform. Because this test reguires a gamma counter, many laboratories are switching to the enzyme-linked immunosorbent assays.

- *Enzyme-linked immunosorbent assay* (ELISA) does not use radioisotopes but a substance that results in a color change after binding. A blue color develops, the intensity of which is related to the amount of hCG present. This assay, which may be done on urine or blood, is sensitive and quick. It can detect hCG levels as early as 7 to 9 days after ovulation and conception, which is 5 days before the first missed period.

- *Fluoroimmunoassay* (FIA) uses an antibody tagged with a fluorescent label to detect serum hCG. The test, which takes about 2 to 3 hours to perform, is extremely sensitive and is used primarily to identify and follow hCG concentrations.

OVER-THE-COUNTER PREGNANCY TESTS

Home pregnancy tests (HPTs) are available over the counter at a reasonable cost. These enzyme immunoassay tests are quite sensitive and detect even low levels of hCG in urine. Many physicians and nurse-midwives use them in the office to confirm pregnancy for their clients because they are less expensive and faster than time-consuming clinical pregnancy tests.

HPT instructions are quite explicit and should be followed carefully. The newer HPTs claim to be 97% to 99% accurate at the time of the missed menses. However, that accuracy is being questioned. Research indicates that many variables, such as reading the tests at the wrong time, can impact the results (Cole, Khanlian, Sutton et al., 2004). The false-positive rate of these tests is quite low, but the false-negative results are higher and should be followed up in the presence of pregnancy symptoms. If the results are negative, the woman should repeat the test in 1 week if she has not started her menstrual period. A false-negative result may lead to delays in beginning prenatal care or to the use of drugs that may be harmful to the fetus. It is important that women using the home kits understand that a positive result merely indicates growing trophoblastic tissue and not necessarily a uterine pregnancy. If the woman delays seeking prenatal care after pregnancy is confirmed, an early ectopic pregnancy may be missed.

Diagnostic (Positive) Changes

The positive signs of pregnancy are completely objective, cannot be confused with pathologic states, and offer conclusive proof of pregnancy.

The *fetal heartbeat* can be detected with a fetoscope by approximately weeks 17 to 20 of pregnancy. With the electronic Doppler device it is possible to detect the fetal heartbeat as early as weeks 10 to 12. The fetal heart rate is between 120 and 160 beats per minute and must be counted and compared with the maternal pulse for differentiation. Auscultation of the abdomen may reveal sounds other than that of the fetal heart. The maternal pulse, emanating from the abdominal aorta, may be unusually loud, or a uterine souffle may be heard.

Fetal movement is actively palpable by a trained examiner after about 20 weeks' gestation. The movements vary from a faint flutter in the early months to more vigorous movements late in pregnancy.

Visualization of the fetus by ultrasound confirms a pregnancy. The gestational sac can be observed by 4 to 5 weeks' gestation (2 to 3 weeks after conception). Fetal parts and fetal heart movement can be seen as early as 8 weeks. Recently, ultrasound using a vaginal probe has been used to detect a gestational sac as early as 10 days after implantation (Cunningham et al., 2005).

PSYCHOLOGIC RESPONSE OF THE EXPECTANT FAMILY TO PREGNANCY

Pregnancy is a developmental challenge, a turning point, in a family's life and therefore is accompanied by stress and anxiety whether the pregnancy is desired or not. Pregnancy confirms one's biologic capabilities to reproduce. It is evidence of one's participation in sexual activity and as such is an affirmation of one's sexuality. For beginning families, pregnancy is the transition period from childlessness to parenthood. If the pregnancy terminates in the birth of a child, the couple enters a new stage of their life together, one that is irreversible and characterized by awesome responsibilities.

The expectant couple may be unaware of the physical, emotional, and cognitive states peculiar to pregnancy. The couple may anticipate no problem from such a normal event as pregnancy and therefore may be confused and distressed by new feelings and behaviors that are generally considered normal.

If the expectant woman is married or has a stable partner, she no longer is only a mate but also must assume the role of mother. Her partner will also assume a parenting role. Career goals and mobility may be altered or thwarted for one or both partners. Each partner begins to see the other in a different light. Their relationship takes on a different meaning to them and within the larger family and community. Their lifestyle changes. With each pregnancy, routines and family dynamics are altered, requiring readjustment and realignment.

If a pregnant woman is without a stable partner, she will still experience changes in role identity and psychobiologic maturation. She must deal alone with the role changes, fears, and adjustments of pregnancy or seek support from family and friends. She also faces the reality of planning for the future as a single parent. Even if the pregnant woman plans to relinquish her infant, she must still deal with the adjustments of pregnancy. She is no longer a separate individual; she must consider the needs of another being who depends on her totally, at least during the pregnancy. This adjustment can be especially difficult without a good support system.

In most pregnancies, whether of a mother with a supportive partner, a single mother, or a relinquishing mother, finances are an important consideration. Traditional lore relegates to the father the role of primary breadwinner, and indeed finances are often a very real concern for fathers. However, in today's society even pregnant women with stable partners recognize the financial impact of a child and may feel concern about financial issues. For the single mother, finances may be a major source of concern.

Decisions about financial matters need to be made at this time. Will the woman work during the pregnancy and return to work after the baby is born? Who will provide child care if she works? Decisions may also need to be made about the division of tasks within the home. Any differences of opinion must be discussed openly and resolved so that the family can meet its members' needs.

The couple must face the realities of labor and birth. Many nonparents have little idea what labor entails. Their information is frequently based on contacts with visual or print media and on experiences related to them by family members or friends, and these tales are often fraught with myths and exaggerations. Classes in prepared childbirth can help them address this lack of information or misinformation.

Labor is threatening in many respects. Pain, disfigurement, disruption of bodily function, and even death are potential threats for the woman. The partner faces the threat of the woman's disfigurement, impairment of her health, or her death. Both fear that the baby may be ill or disfigured. The expectant couple is subject to anxiety during this period because no one can provide total reassurance about the outcome.

Pregnancy can be viewed as a developmental stage with its own distinct developmental tasks. It can be a time of support or conflict for a couple, depending on the amount of adjustment each is willing to make to maintain the family's equilibrium. Family dynamics are an important factor in adjusting to pregnancy. Family strengths include the ability of the couple to talk about issues that are important to them, to resolve conflicts and make compromises, and to seek and receive assistance and support from loved ones.

During pregnancy, the couple plans together for the first child's arrival, collecting information on how to be parents. At the same time, each continues to participate in some separate activities with friends or family members. The availability of social support is an important factor in psychosocial well-being during pregnancy. Most pregnant women turn to their partners as their primary source of social support. In particular, a woman needs support from her partner that affirms that she is valued and that her baby will be welcomed and accepted (Logsdon, 2000–2001). The broader social network often is a major source of advice for the pregnant woman. However, evidence indicates that both sound and unsound information is given.

Although individual activities are important, some conflict may arise if the couple's activities become too divergent. Thus they may find it necessary to limit their outside associations.

The expectant mother and her partner both face significant changes during pregnancy and must deal with major psychosocial adjustments (Table 14–3). Other family members, especially other children of the woman or couple, and the grandparents-to-be, must also adjust to the pregnancy.

In late pregnancy, the concerns of expectant fathers tend to focus most on the health of the unborn child and the safety of the mother. The concerns of expectant mothers center on the health of the baby and their ability to handle labor and birth. Couples typically agree on the primary concern, the health of the unborn child. Nurses can use this focus as a springboard for discussing other concerns. Couples can then come to understand the differences between their second most important concerns. A woman worries about how she will handle labor and birth, but has little concern for her own safety; the father's expression of his fear for her safety can be seen as evidence that he cares enough to worry about her. This response may allow the mother to depend on him more during the vulnerable time of late pregnancy and birthing. Sharing his views gives the father a chance to express his love and concern for mother and child, encouraging the development of stronger marital and paternal relationships.

For some couples, pregnancy is more than a developmental stage; it is a crisis. *Crisis* can be defined as a disturbance or conflict in which the individual cannot maintain a state of equilibrium. Pregnancy can be considered a *maturational crisis* because it is a common event in the normal growth and development of the family. During such a crisis, the individual or family is in disequilibrium. Egos weaken, usual defense mech-

Table 14–3   PARENTAL REACTIONS TO PREGNANCY

First Trimester	Second Trimester	Third Trimester
Mother's Reactions	**Mother's Reactions**	**Mother's Reactions**
Informs father secretively or openly.	Remains regressive and introspective, projects all problems with authority figures onto partner, may become angry as if lack of interest is sign of weakness in him.	Experiences more anxiety and tension, with physical awkwardness.
Feels ambivalent toward pregnancy, anxious about labor and responsibility of child.	Continues to deal with feelings as a mother and looks for furniture as something concrete.	Feels much discomfort and insomnia from physical condition.
Is aware of physical changes, daydreams of possible miscarriage.	May have other extreme of anxiety and wait until 9th month to look for furniture and clothes for baby.	Prepares for birth, assembles layette, picks out names.
Develops special feelings for and renewed interest in her own mother, with formation of a personal identity.	Feels movement and is aware of fetus and incorporates it into herself.	Dreams often about misplacing baby or not being able to give birth, fears birth of deformed baby.
	Dreams that partner will be killed, telephones him often for reassurance.	Feels ecstasy and excitement, has spurt of energy during last month.
	Experiences more distinct physical changes; sexual desires may increase or decrease.	
Father's Reactions	**Father's Reactions**	**Father's Reactions**
Differ according to age, parity, desire for child, economic stability.	If he can cope, will give her extra attention she needs; if he cannot cope, will develop a new time-consuming interest outside of home.	Adapts to alternative methods of sexual contact.
Acceptance of pregnant woman's attitude or complete rejection and lack of communication.	May develop a creative feeling and a "closeness to nature."	Becomes concerned over financial responsibility.
Is aware of his own sexual feelings, may develop more or less sexual arousal.	Many become involved in pregnancy and buy or make furniture.	May show new sense of tenderness and concern, treats partner like doll.
Accepts, rejects, or resents mother-in-law.	Feels for movement of baby, listens to heartbeat, or remains aloof, with no physical contact.	Daydreams about child as if older and not newborn, dreams of losing partner.
May develop new hobby outside of family as sign of stress.	May have fears and fantasies about himself being pregnant, may become uneasy with this feminine aspect in himself.	Renewed sexual attraction to partner.
	May react negatively if partner is too demanding, may become jealous of physician and of physician's importance to partner and her pregnancy.	Feels he is ultimately responsible for whatever happens.

anisms lose their effectiveness, unresolved issues from the past reappear, and relationships shift. The period of disequilibrium and disorganization is marked by abortive attempts to solve the perceived problems. If the crisis is unresolved, it will result in maladaptive behaviors in one or more family members and possible disintegration of the family. Families who are able to resolve a maturational crisis successfully will return to normal functioning and can even strengthen the bonds in the family relationship.

Mother

Pregnancy is a condition that alters body image and also necessitates a reordering of social relationships and changes in roles of family members. The way a particular woman meets the stresses of pregnancy is influenced by her emotional makeup, her sociologic and cultural background, and her acceptance or rejection of the pregnancy. However, many women manifest similar psychologic and emotional responses during pregnancy, including ambivalence, acceptance, introversion, mood swings, and changes in body image.

INTENDEDNESS

Large-scale surveys have included questions about whether women's pregnancies have been intended and have revealed that many pregnancies are not intended. An unintended pregnancy is a risk factor for depression. Women with an unintended pregnancy may also perceive life events as being more stressful than women with an intended pregnancy—another contributor to depression. Depression, in turn, can negatively impact a pregnant woman's health choices and behaviors (Messer, Dole, Kaufman et al., 2005).

Interest in the large number of unintended pregnancies and their impact has resulted in the Institute of Medicine reports and objectives listed in *Healthy People 2010* to decrease unintended pregnancies. However, researchers have not considered the nuances among such terms as *intended* and *unintended, planned* and *unplanned*, and *wanted, unwanted*, or *mistimed*. This makes the data hard to interpret. For example, a pregnancy can be mistimed, unintended, and wanted all at the same time, with prospective parents who are happy to find themselves expecting. In addition, contraceptive failure does not always lead to the report of unintended pregnancy. Current research is exploring definitions and terms to clarify the many dimensions of the intendedness of pregnancy (Aquilino & Losch, 2005).

AMBIVALENCE

Initially, even if the pregnancy is planned, the mother may experience a sense of surprise that conception has actually occurred. This may be coupled with a feeling that pregnancy is desirable "some day" but "not now." Such ambivalence may be related to feelings that the timing is somehow "wrong," worries about the need to modify existing relationships or career plans, fears about assuming a new role, unresolved emotional conflicts with the woman's own mother, and fears about pregnancy, labor, and birth. Indirect evidence of ambivalence includes complaints about prolonged or frequent depression, considerable physical discomfort, significant dissatisfaction with body shape,

excessive mood swings, and difficulty accepting the life changes resulting from the pregnancy (Lederman, 1996).

Such feelings may be even more pronounced if the pregnancy is unintended or unwanted. Women who view their pregnancy as unwanted are more likely to delay prenatal care and to experience complications. The support and opinion of the woman's current partner, even if he is not the father of the child, have a major impact on pregnancy wantedness. Financial and emotional support from the partner are essential to the woman's positive attitude. Involving the partner in the prenatal care may help promote a supportive attitude. During the early months, the pregnant woman may consider the possibility of a therapeutic abortion if the pregnancy is unwanted. In the event of religious conflicts about induced abortion, the woman may experience guilt feelings about her thoughts or may tend to focus on the possibility of spontaneous abortion (miscarriage). Even when the pregnancy is planned, thoughts of abortion and miscarriage arise. Concurrently, the pregnant woman may feel guilty for having such negative thoughts and may worry that in some way these thoughts will harm the baby.

ACCEPTANCE

Acceptance of pregnancy is influenced by many factors. Lower acceptance tends to be related to an unplanned pregnancy and greater evidence of fear and conflict. The woman carrying an unplanned pregnancy tends to experience more physical discomfort and depression. When a pregnancy is well accepted, the woman demonstrates feelings of happiness and pleasure in the pregnancy. She experiences less physical discomfort and shows a high degree of tolerance for the discomforts associated with the third trimester (Lederman, 1996).

Conflicts about adapting to pregnancy are no more pronounced for older pregnant women (age 35 and older) than for younger ones. Moreover, older pregnant women tend to be less concerned about the normal physical changes of pregnancy and are confident about handling issues that arise during pregnancy and parenting. This may be because mature pregnant women have more experience with problem solving. However, mature pregnant women may have fewer pregnant peers and thus may have fewer people with whom to share concerns and expectations.

For some women, an unintended pregnancy has more psychologic and social advantages than disadvantages. It provides purpose and direction to life and allows a woman to test the devotion and love of her partner and family.

> *I didn't expect to get pregnant, but my baby seems like a gift from God. Suddenly I feel like I have a purpose in life. I know I have to do the right things so the baby will be okay. Being pregnant made me grow up in a hurry, but I don't regret it–not at all.*

During the *first trimester*, evidence of pregnancy is often limited to amenorrhea and to the word of the caregiver that the pregnancy test was positive. Unless the woman has the opportunity to see the gestational sac during an ultrasound, her baby may not seem real. Consequently, she may tend to focus on herself and her pregnancy. In an effort to verify her condition, a woman may become minutely conscious of changes in her body that could validate the pregnancy.

The *second trimester* is relatively tranquil. Morning sickness generally passes, the threat of spontaneous abortion diminishes, and the woman begins to accept the reality of her pregnancy. It is not unusual for an enthusiastic primigravida to don maternity clothes at the beginning of this trimester even when it is not truly necessary. The clothing serves as a verification of her pregnant state.

The highlight of the second trimester is quickening, which generally occurs about week 20—midway through the pregnancy. Actual perception of fetal movement frequently produces dramatic changes in the woman. She now perceives her baby as a real person and generally becomes excited about the pregnancy even if she hasn't been before this time.

As quickening and her altered physical appearance confirm her pregnant state, the woman adjusts to the idea of change and begins to prepare for her new role and her new set of relationships—with her partner and family, the child-to-be and other children, friends, and loved ones. When the pregnancy is well accepted, the woman takes pleasure in the sensations of pregnancy and attempts to picture her baby in order to know him or her better. She may seek out other women who are pregnant or have recently given birth. She feels well, is excited, and may exhibit the "glow" so often attributed to pregnant women.

The *third trimester* combines a sense of pride with anxiety about what is to come in order for the child to be born. During this time, the special prerogatives of pregnancy may be most marked. As her protruding abdomen proclaims her advanced pregnancy, the woman may find that others become more solicitous, that a chair may be offered in a crowded room, that others may carry her parcels. The woman may actually need this help, she may simply enjoy the attention as a privilege of pregnancy, or she may reject it if she fears that such gestures indicate she is helpless.

During the final trimester, physical discomforts again increase, and adequate rest becomes a necessity. The woman makes final preparation for the baby and may spend long periods considering names for the child. During this time she worries more about the health and safety of her unborn child and may have concerns that she will not behave well during childbirth.

The woman may feel vulnerable to rejection, loss, or insult. She may worry about a variety of things and may withdraw into the security and quiet of her home. Toward the end of this period many women report bursts of energy in which they vigorously clean and organize their homes ("nesting").

INTROVERSION

Introversion, or turning in on oneself, is a common occurrence in pregnancy. An active, outgoing woman may become less interested in previous activities and more concerned with needs for rest and time alone. This concentration of attention permits the woman to plan, adjust, adapt, build, and draw strength in preparation for her child's birth. As she becomes more aware of herself, her partner may feel she is being overly sensitive. Her partner may perceive her introversion and passivity as exclusionary and may in turn become unable to interact with her,

either verbally or physically, or to provide the affection, support, and consideration she requires. This change may result in disequilibrium and stress for the entire family. It is essential that the couple work together to establish new, mutually acceptable patterns of response to overcome these blocks to communication.

Fantasies about the unborn child are quite common among pregnant women. However, the themes of the fantasies (baby's appearance, gender, traits, impact on parents, and so forth) vary by trimester and also differ between women pregnant for the first time and women who already have children.

MOOD SWINGS

Throughout pregnancy, the emotions of many women are characterized by mood swings, from great joy to deep despair. Frequently, the woman will become tearful with little apparent cause. When asked why she is crying, she may find it difficult or impossible to give a reason. The situation may be extremely unsettling for the partner, causing him to feel confused and inadequate. Because the man may feel unable to handle the woman's tears, he often reacts by withdrawing and ignoring the problem. Because the pregnant woman needs increased love and affection, she may perceive his reaction as unloving and nonsupportive. Once the couple understands that this behavior is characteristic of pregnancy, it becomes easier for them to deal with it more effectively—although it will be a source of stress to some extent throughout pregnancy.

CHANGES IN BODY IMAGE

Pregnancy produces marked changes in a woman's body within a relatively short period of time. With these changes, women also experience changes in body image. The degree of this change is related to a certain extent to personality factors, social network responses, and attitudes toward pregnancy. Changes in body image are normal but can be very stressful for the pregnant woman. Explanation and discussion of the changes may help both the woman and her partner deal with the stress associated with this aspect of pregnancy.

I'm due in 2 weeks and I can't wait. These last few weeks have been hard on my self-image. I can't see my feet anymore and I feel awkward and lumbering, not graceful at all.

PSYCHOLOGIC TASKS OF THE MOTHER

Rubin (1984) identified four major tasks that the pregnant woman undertakes to maintain her intactness and that of her family and at the same time incorporate her new child into the family system. These tasks form the basis for a mutually gratifying relationship with her baby:

1. *Ensuring safe passage through pregnancy, labor, and birth.* The pregnant woman feels concern for both her unborn child and herself. She seeks competent maternity care to provide a sense of control. She may also seek knowledge from literature, observation of other pregnant women and new mothers, and discussion with others. The pregnant woman also seeks to ensure safe passage by engaging

THROUGH THE EYES OF A NURSE

Psychologic Changes in Pregnancy

FAMILY'S EXPERIENCE: "I am dealing with a lot of shifting emotions right now. One minute I feel happy and elated, and then suddenly I am so blue. I feel like I am on an emotional roller coaster! I find myself tearful for no reason and can't even explain to my husband why I am crying. When he doesn't act supportive, I feel unloved and angry like I am the one dealing with all of these changes while my family stands by, unaffected."

NURSE'S RESPONSE: "Even though each woman is different in her reactions to pregnancy and every pregnancy is different, mood swings with extremes in emotions are common. So what you are describing is pretty typical but it can be hard to handle, and you may feel overwhelmed at times.

"During pregnancy, women experience a wide variety of responses such as ambivalence, mood swings, and changes in body image. Because your emotional well-being is so important during pregnancy, we will assess your adjustment to pregnancy at each visit, much like we routinely monitor your blood pressure, the baby's movements, and the size of your uterus.

"It might help if you express your feelings to your family and ask them for additional support when you are sad, overwhelmed, or ambivalent about the pregnancy. Also, I would be glad to talk to your husband about these changes and suggest ways for him to be supportive if you feel that would help."

NURSE'S ACTIONS AND RATIONALE:

The nurse validates the woman's feelings and provides reassurance that the feelings she is experiencing are normal. The nurse also takes the opportunity to provide teaching about the common emotional responses that occur during pregnancy. The father's actions can be a positive influence during a woman's pregnancy and postpartum so it is important to seek opportunities to provide him with interventions to ease the adjustment process for his partner (Tiedje & Darling-Fisher, 2003).

in self-care activities related to diet, exercise, alcohol consumption, and so forth. In the third trimester, as her movements slow and her body mass increases, she becomes aware of external threats in the environment—a toy on a stair, the awkwardness of an escalator—that pose a threat to her intactness and represent hazards to be overcome. She may worry if her partner is late or if she is home alone. Sleep becomes difficult, and she begins to long for the baby's birth, even though it, too, is frightening.

2. *Seeking of acceptance of this child by others.* The birth of a child alters a woman's primary support group, her family, and her secondary affiliative groups. The family generally makes the transition, and the woman slowly and subtly alters her secondary network to meet the needs of her pregnancy. In this adjustment the woman's partner is the most important figure. The partner's support and acceptance influence her completion of her maternal tasks and the formation of her maternal identity. If there are other children in the home, the mother also works to ensure their acceptance of the coming child. Accepting the coming change in exclusive relationships—woman and partner or mother and first child—can be stressful, and the woman will often work to maintain some special time with her partner or older child. Achieving social acceptance of the child and of herself as mother may be more difficult for the adolescent mother or single woman. The child to come is not always wanted, and the woman often must direct her energies to changing this situation.

3. *Seeking of commitment and acceptance of self as mother to the infant (binding-in).* During the first trimester, the child remains a rather abstract concept. With quickening, however, the child begins to become a real person, and the mother begins to develop bonds of attachment. The mother experiences the movement of the child within her in an intimate, exclusive way, and out of this experience bonds of love form. The mother develops a fantasy image of her ideal child. This binding-in process, characterized by its strong emotional component, motivates the pregnant woman to become competent in her role and provides satisfaction for her in her role of mother (Mercer, 2004). This possessive love increases her maternal commitment to protect her fetus now and her child after she or he is born.

4. *Learning to give of oneself on behalf of one's child.* Childbirth involves many acts of giving. The man "gives" a child to a woman; she in turn "gives" a child to the man. Life is given to an infant; a sibling is given to older children of the family. The woman begins to develop a capacity for self-denial and learns to delay immediate personal gratification to meet the needs of another. Baby showers and baby gifts are acts of giving that help the mother's self-esteem while also helping her acknowledge the separateness and needs of the coming baby.

Accomplishment of these tasks helps the expectant woman develop her self-concept as mother. The expectant mother who was well nurtured by her own mother may view her mother as a role model and emulate her; the woman who views her own mother as a "poor mother" may worry that she will make similar mistakes (Lederman, 1996). A woman's self-concept as mother expands with actual experience and continues to grow through subsequent childbearing and childrearing. Occasionally, a woman never accepts the mother role but plays the role of babysitter or older sister.

Father

Until fairly recently, the expectant father was often viewed as a "bystander" or observer of his partner's pregnancy. He was necessary for conception, for bill paying, and for providing male guidance as his child matured. This view has changed, and the father of today is expected to fulfill the role of nurturing, caring, involved parent as well as provider. In response to societal pressures, the influence of the feminist movement, and the economic pressures that result in more women employed outside the home, shared parenting and breadwinning have become more commonplace. Many men have actively sought to be more involved in the experience of childbirth and parenting.

Expectant fathers experience many of the same feelings and conflicts experienced by expectant mothers when the pregnancy has been confirmed. Initially, expectant fathers may feel pride in their virility, which pregnancy confirms, but also have ambivalent feelings. The extent of ambivalence depends on many factors, including the father's relationship with his partner, his previous experience with pregnancy, his age, his economic stability, and whether the pregnancy was planned. The expectant father must first deal with the reality of the pregnancy and then struggle to gain recognition as a parent from his partner, family, friends, coworkers, society—and from his baby as well. The expectant mother can help her partner be a participant and not merely a helpmate to her if she has a definite sense of the experience as their pregnancy and their infant and not her pregnancy and her infant.

Men whose partners are pregnant following a previous pregnancy loss may experience a variety of emotions attributable to the loss. These emotions might include an increased sense of risk, feelings of increased concern about the outcome of the current pregnancy, the recognition that something could go wrong again, and the sense that increased vigilance is essential (Armstrong, 2001). These fathers may call home more often to check on the mother's condition and the baby and may also feel an increased need to be involved more actively in the current pregnancy. They wish to be acknowledged as more than just a support person; they want their important role as family protector recognized (O'Leary & Thorwick, 2006).

In general, the expectant father faces psychologic stress as he makes the transition from nonparent to parent or from parent of one to parent of two or more. Sources of stress include financial issues, unexpected events during pregnancy, concern that the baby will not be healthy and normal, worry about the pain the partner will experience in childbirth, and his role during labor and birth. Other sources of stress for expectant fathers include concern over the changing relationship with their partner, diminished sexual responsiveness in their partner or in themselves, change in relationships with their family or male friends, and their ability to parent.

The expectant father must establish a fatherhood role just as the woman develops a motherhood role. The mother experiences biological changes of pregnancy that aid in the transition to motherhood. Fathers may feel left out because they are unable to experience what their partner is experiencing. Fathers who are most successful at developing a fatherhood role generally like children, are excited about the prospect of fatherhood, are eager to nurture a child, have confidence in their ability to be a parent, and share the experiences of pregnancy and childbirth with their partners (Lederman, 1996).

FIRST TRIMESTER

After the initial excitement of the announcement of the pregnancy to friends and relatives and receipt of their congratulations, an expectant father may begin to feel left out of the pregnancy. He is also often confused by his partner's mood changes and perhaps bewildered by his responses to her changing body. He may resent the attention given to the woman and the need to change their relationship as she experiences fatigue and a decreased interest in sex.

During this time, his child is a "potential baby." Fathers often picture interacting with a child of 5 or 6 rather than a newborn. Even the pregnancy itself may seem unreal until the woman shows more physical signs.

SECOND TRIMESTER

The father's role in the pregnancy is still vague in the second trimester, but his involvement can be increased by his watching and feeling fetal movement. It is helpful if the father, as well as the mother, has the opportunity to hear the fetal heartbeat. That requires a visit to the nurse-midwife's or physician's office. Involvement of fathers in antepartal care is increasing and may even be an expectation of their partner. For many men, seeing the infant on ultrasound is an important experience in accepting the reality of the pregnancy.

Like expectant mothers, expectant fathers need to confront and resolve some of their own conflicts about the fathering they received. A father needs to sort out those behaviors in his own fathering that he wants to imitate and those he wishes to avoid. This process usually occurs gradually as the pregnancy progresses.

> I was excited about the chance to be the kind of father who was involved and available. However, I also wanted to provide adequately for my child, support my wife, and still have time to do the things I loved to do. I was surprised by how excited my father was about becoming a grandfather. He even talked to me about the regrets he had about not being around as I was growing up. I think the experience will help to bring my dad and me closer as he tries to be a great grandfather and I understand more about his struggles as a father.

Evidence suggests that the father-to-be's anxiety is lessened if both parents agree on the support role the man is to assume during pregnancy and on his projected paternal role. For example, if both see his role as that of breadwinner, the man's stress is low. However, if the man views his role as that of breadwinner and the woman expects him to be actively involved in

preparations and child care, his stress increases. An open and honest discussion about the expectations each parent has about their roles will help the father-to-be to determine his transition to fatherhood (Goodman, 2005).

The woman's appearance begins to alter at this time too, and men react differently to the physical change. For some it decreases sexual interest; for others it may have the opposite effect. Both partners experience a multitude of emotions, and it continues to be important for them to communicate and accept each other's feelings and concerns. In situations in which the expectant mother's demands dominate the relationship, the expectant father's resentment may increase to the point that he is spending more time at work, involved in a hobby, or with his friends. The behavior is even more likely if the expectant father did not want the pregnancy and/or if the relationship was not a good one before the pregnancy.

THIRD TRIMESTER

If the couple have communicated their concerns and feelings to one another and grown in their relationship, the third trimester is a special and rewarding time. A more clearly defined role evolves at this time for the expectant father, and it becomes more obvious how the couple can prepare together for the coming event. They may become involved in childbirth education classes and make concrete preparations for the arrival of the baby, such as shopping for a crib, car seat, and other equipment. If the expectant father has developed a detached attitude about the pregnancy before this time, however, it is unlikely that he will become a willing participant even though his role becomes more obvious.

Concerns and fears may recur. Many men are afraid of hurting the unborn baby during intercourse. The father may also begin to have anxiety and fantasies about what could happen to his partner and the unborn baby during labor and birth and feels a great sense of responsibility. The questions asked earlier in pregnancy emerge again. What kind of parents will he and his partner be? Will he really be able to help his partner in labor? Can they afford to have a baby?

COUVADE

The term **couvade** traditionally referred to the observance of certain rituals and taboos by the male to signify the transition to fatherhood. This observance affirms his psychosocial and biophysical relationship to the woman and child. These taboos may have taken specific form—for example, the man may have been forbidden to eat certain foods or carry certain weapons before and immediately after the birth. More recently, the term has been used to describe the unintentional development of physical symptoms, such as fatigue, increased appetite, difficulty sleeping, depression, headache, or backache by the partner of the pregnant woman. Men who demonstrate couvade syndrome tend to have a higher degree of paternal role preparation and be involved in more activities related to this preparation.

Siblings

The introduction of a new baby into the family is often the beginning of sibling rivalry. Sibling rivalry results from children's fear of change in the security of their relationships with their parents. Some of the behaviors demonstrating feelings of

RESEARCH IN PRACTICE

FATHERS MASSAGING AND RELAXING THEIR PREGNANT WIVES LOWERED ANXIETY AND FACILITATED MARITAL ADJUSTMENT

What is this study about? A father's feelings of anxiety, marital adjustment, and attachment to the fetus are all important factors that can be expected to affect the quality of a pregnancy experience. Paternal-fetal attachments are processes that are based on an enduring affectionate bond that deepens over time. The time of pregnancy also deeply affects the marital relationship. The quality of this relationship has demonstrated an association with both partners' attachment to the infant. Massage therapy has been shown to improve intimacy and decrease anxiety, improving the marital relationship. Various relaxation methods have been shown to have similar effects. These researchers studied whether massage and/or relaxation techniques would reduce a pregnant couple's anxiety, enhance marital adjustment, and increase paternal fetal attachment.

How was this study done? The sample included 175 adult expectant fathers married to pregnant women with singleton pregnancies. The couples were recruited from Lamaze classes in southern California. The subject couples were randomly assigned to two treatment groups and a control. The treatment groups received instruction in either massage therapy or relaxation techniques. The massage therapy fathers received training by a licensed massage therapist and were asked to massage the mothers for 20 minutes at least two times a week. In the relaxation group, the couple was taught a 20-minute relaxation program and was asked to practice the techniques at home two times a week. The couples began the study at between 24 and 32 weeks of gestation. Outcomes were measured by paternal self-report on the *Paternal Fetal Attachment Scale*, the *Dyadic Adjustment Scale*, and the *State-Trait Anxiety Inventory*. The instruments were administered at the beginning and end of the 5-week study period.

What were the results of the study? Both massage therapy and relaxation training were associated with improved marital adjustment, so both interventions were effective in this population. Paternal anxiety levels decreased over time in the massage therapy group. Neither massage nor relaxation training had an effect on paternal fetal attachment. However, fathers who experienced high levels of marital adjustment also had high levels of paternal fetal attachment.

What additional questions might I have? Were these fathers who were highly involved in the prenatal process representative of the majority of fathers? Are there any gestational conditions in which massage therapy is contraindicated?

How can I use this study? Couples can use massage therapy and relaxation techniques to deepen their sense of intimacy and marital adjustment during the stressful prenatal period. Fathers who massage their pregnant wives have less anxiety, and so this intervention benefits both partners. Fathers can be directed to licensed massage therapists who can help them learn techniques that will relax their spouse and enhance their relationship.

Latifses, V., Estroff, D., Field, T., & Bush. J. (2005). Fathers massaging and relaxing their pregnant wives lowered anxiety and facilitated marital adjustment. *Journal of Bodywork and Movement Therapies, 9,* 277–282.

sibling rivalry may even be directed toward the mother during the pregnancy as she experiences more fatigue and less patience with her toddler, for example. Parents who recognize the situation early in pregnancy and begin constructive actions can help minimize the problems of sibling rivalry.

Preparation of the young child begins several weeks before the anticipated birth and is designed according to the age and experience of the child. Because they do not have a clear concept of time, young children should not be told too early about the pregnancy. From the toddler's point of view "several weeks" is an extremely long time. The mother may let the child feel the baby moving in her uterus, explaining that this is "a special place where babies grow." The child can help the parents put the baby clothes in drawers or prepare the baby's room.

The concept of consistency is important in dealing with young children. They need reassurance that certain people, special things, and familiar places will continue to exist after the new baby arrives. The crib is an important though transient object in a child's life. If it is to be given to the new baby, the parents should thoughtfully help the child adjust to this change. Any move from crib to bed or from one room to another should precede the baby's birth by at least several weeks. If the new baby must share a room with siblings, the parents must discuss this with the siblings.

Some parents advocate cosleeping or bed sharing (one or both parents sleeping with their baby or young child), and so the crib is less of an issue. Cosleeping, which is common in many non-Western cultures, is on the increase in the United States. In fact a recent study reports that approximately 12.8% of infants regularly share an adult bed at night, and almost 50% of the infants in the study had spent at least some time sleeping in an adult bed at night in the preceding 2 weeks. Among the group studied, African American infants were four times more likely to cosleep than white infants and Asian or other infants were three times more likely to do so than white infants (National Institute of Child Health and Human Development, 2003). However, the practice has sparked controversy in the United States. In its recommendations for ways to reduce the incidence of sudden infant death syndrome (SIDS), the American Academy of Pediatrics (AAP) (2005) recommends against cosleeping. The AAP stresses that the infant can be brought to the bed to be comforted or for breastfeeding but should be placed supine in a separate bed ("back to bed") to sleep. (See the discussion in Chapter 36 ∞). Parents who choose to cosleep must make decisions about the sleeping arrangements of other siblings following the birth of the baby.

If the child is ready for toilet training, it is most effectively done several months before or after the baby's arrival. Parents should know that the older, toilet-trained child may regress to wetting or soiling because he or she sees the new baby getting attention for such behavior. The older, weaned child may want to drink from the breast or bottle again after the new baby comes. If the new mother anticipates these behaviors, they will be less frustrating during her early postpartum days.

During the pregnancy, older children should be introduced to a new baby for short periods to get an idea of what a new baby is like. This introduction dispels fantasies that the new arrival will be big enough to be a playmate. Pregnant women may also find it helpful to bring their children to a prenatal visit after they have been told about the expected baby. The children are encouraged to become involved in prenatal care and to ask any questions they may have. They are also given the opportunity to hear the baby's heartbeat, either with a stethoscope or with the Doppler. This helps make the baby more real to them.

If siblings are school-age children, the pregnancy should be viewed as a family affair. Teaching about the pregnancy should be based on the child's level of understanding and interest. Overeager parents may go into lengthier and more in-depth responses than the child is able to understand. Some children are more curious than others. Books at their level of understanding can be made available in the home. Involvement in family discussions, attendance at sibling preparation classes, encouragement to feel fetal movement, and an opportunity to listen to the fetal heart supplement the learning process and help make the school-age child feel part of the pregnancy. Sibling preparation classes assist in the transition process for both parents and children. After attending the classes, children often exhibit less anxiety and increased ability to express their feelings.

Older children or adolescents may appear to have a sophisticated knowledge base, but it may be intermingled with many misconceptions. Thus the parents should make opportunities to discuss their concerns and should involve the children in preparation for the new baby.

Even after the birth, siblings need to feel that they are part of a family affair. Changes in hospital regulations allowing siblings to be present at the birth or to visit their mother and the new baby facilitate this process. Participation in special programs for siblings may help in this process. On arrival at home, siblings can share in "showing off" the new baby.

Sibling preparation for the arrival of a new baby is essential, but other factors are equally important. These include the amount of parental attention focused on the new arrival, the amount of parental attention given the older child after the birth of the new arrival, and parental skill in dealing effectively with regressive and/or aggressive behavior.

Grandparents

The first relatives told about a pregnancy are usually the grandparents. Although relationships with parents can be very complex, this period in a family's life most often promotes a closer relationship between the expectant couple and their parents. Usually the expectant grandparents become increasingly supportive of the expectant couple, even if conflicts previously existed.

Grandparents may be unsure about the amount of involvement they are "allowed" during the pregnancy and childbearing

process. Most want to be helpful; some may bestow advice and/or gifts unsparingly. Because grandparenting can occur over a wide span of years, people's response to this role can vary considerably. For some, this new role may occur at a relatively young age, and the connotation of aging that accompanies the role may affect their response to the pregnancy. The younger grandparent may also be involved in work and other activities and may not demonstrate as much interest as the young couple would like.

It can be difficult for even sensitive grandparents to know how much involvement the couple wants. Expectant couples want to feel in control of their new situation, which may be initially difficult in their changing roles. Grandparents find that this factor, as well as changing roles in their own lives (e.g., retirement, financial concerns, menopause of the expectant grandmother, death of a friend), may contribute to conflicts in the changing family structure. Some parents of expectant couples may already be grandparents and have already developed their own style of grandparenting, which will be an important factor in how they respond to the pregnancy.

Childbearing and childrearing practices are very different for today's childbearing couple. It helps family cohesiveness for young couples to share with interested grandparents what today's practices are and why they feel they are effective. At the same time, it is important for young couples to listen to any differences expectant grandparents want to explain. When grandparents give advice, it helps to remember that they care. When their recommendations seem effective, it is significant to grandparents that young couples do listen and follow their advice.

Occasionally young couples feel they are receiving more advice than they can tolerate. Too often they perceive parents' suggestions as criticizing their ability to prepare adequately for the childbearing process—and later as criticizing their care of the newborn. It is useful for the young couple to discuss the problem and agree on a plan of action. The role of the helping grandparents when the new baby is brought home needs to be clarified before the event to ensure a comfortable situation for all.

In some areas, classes for grandparents provide information about changes in birthing and parenting practices. These classes help familiarize grandparents with new parents' needs and may offer suggestions for ways in which the grandparents can support the childbearing woman or couple.

CULTURAL VALUES AND PREGNANCY

A universal tendency exists to create ceremonial rituals and rites around important life events. Thus pregnancy, childbirth, marriage, and death are often tied to ritual (Spector, 2003). The rituals, customs, and practices of a group are a reflection of the group's values. Consequently the identification of cultural values is useful in planning and providing culturally sensitive care.

Generalizations about cultural characteristics or cultural values are difficult because not every individual in a culture may display these characteristics. Just as variations are seen among cultures, variations are also seen within cultures. These variations are often related to social and economic factors such as

DEVELOPING CULTURAL COMPETENCE

PROVIDING CULTURALLY SENSITIVE CARE

Nurses who are interacting with expectant families from a different culture or ethnic group can provide more effective, culturally sensitive nursing care by:

- Critically examining their own cultural beliefs

- Identifying personal biases, attitudes, stereotypes, and prejudices

- Making a conscious commitment to respect and study the values and beliefs of others

- Using sensitive, current language when describing others' cultures

- Learning the rituals, customs, and practices of the major cultural and ethnic groups with whom they have contact

- Including cultural assessment and assessment of the family's expectations of the healthcare system as a routine part of prenatal nursing care

- Incorporating the family's cultural practices into prenatal care as much as possible

- Fostering an attitude of respect for and cooperation with alternative healers and caregivers whenever possible

- Providing for the services of an interpreter if language barriers exist

- Learning the language (or at least several key phrases) of at least one of the cultural groups with whom they interact

- Recognizing that ultimately it is the woman's right to make her own healthcare choices

- Evaluating whether the client's healthcare beliefs have any potential negative consequences for her health

class, income, and education. For example, because of their exposure to the American culture, a third-generation Chinese American family might have very different values and beliefs from those of a traditional Chinese family who has recently immigrated to America. For this reason, the nurse needs to supplement a general knowledge of cultural values and practices with a complete assessment of the individual's values and practices. The Developing Cultural Competence box summarizes the key actions a nurse can take to become more culturally aware.

Cultural assessment is an important aspect of prenatal care (see Figure 2–8 ∞). Healthcare professionals are becoming increasingly aware of the importance of addressing cultural,

physiologic, and psychologic needs in the prenatal assessment in order to provide culture-specific health care during pregnancy. The nurse needs to identify the main beliefs, values, and behaviors that relate to pregnancy and childbearing. This includes information about ethnic background, amount of affiliation with the ethnic group, patterns of decision making, religious preferences, language, communication style, and common etiquette practices. The nurse can also explore the woman's (or family's) expectations of the healthcare system. Once this information is gathered, the nurse can then plan and provide care that is appropriate and responsive to the family's needs. These topics are discussed in detail in Chapter 2. ∞

CHAPTER REVIEW

FOCUS YOUR STUDY

- Virtually all systems of a woman's body are altered in some way during pregnancy. Blood pressure decreases slightly during pregnancy. It reaches its lowest point in the second trimester and gradually increases to near normal levels in the third trimester. The enlarging uterus may exert pressure on the vena cava when the woman lies supine, causing a

drop in blood pressure. This is called the vena caval syndrome or supine hypotension.

- A physiologic anemia may occur during pregnancy because the total plasma volume increases more than the total number of erythrocytes. This produces a drop in the hematocrit.

- The glomerular filtration rate increases during pregnancy. Glycosuria may be caused by the body's inability to reabsorb all the glucose filtered by the glomeruli.

- Changes in the skin include the development of chloasma; linea nigra; darkened nipples, areolae, and vulva; striae; and spider nevi.

- Insulin needs increase during pregnancy. A woman with a latent deficiency state may respond to the increased stress on the islets of Langerhans by developing gestational diabetes mellitus.

- The subjective (presumptive) signs of pregnancy are those symptoms experienced and reported by the woman, such as amenorrhea, nausea and vomiting, fatigue, urinary frequency, breast changes, and quickening.

- The objective (probable) signs of pregnancy can be perceived by the examiner but may be caused by conditions other than pregnancy.

- The diagnostic (positive) signs of pregnancy can be perceived by the examiner and can be caused only by pregnancy.

- During pregnancy the expectant woman may experience ambivalence, acceptance, introversion, emotional lability, and changes in body image.

- Rubin (1984) identified four developmental tasks for the pregnant woman: (1) ensuring safe passage through pregnancy, labor, and birth; (2) seeking acceptance of this child by others; (3) seeking commitment and acceptance of self as mother to the infant; and (4) learning to give of oneself on behalf of one's child.

- Fathers also face a series of adjustments as they accept their new role.

- Siblings of all ages require assistance in dealing with the birth of a new baby.

- Cultural values, beliefs, and behaviors influence a couple's response to childbearing and the healthcare system.

- A cultural assessment should focus on factors that will influence the practices of the childbearing family with regard to their health needs.

EXPLORE MediaLink

http://www.prenhall.com/davidson

NCLEX review questions, case studies, and other interactive resources for this chapter can be found on the Web Site at http://www.prenhall.com/davidson. Click on "Chapter 14" to select the activities for this chapter.

For tutorials including animations and videos, more NCLEX review questions, and an audio glossary, access the accompanying Prentice Hall Nursing MediaLink DVD-ROM in this book.

PRENTICE HALL NURSING MEDIALINK DVD-ROM

Audio Glossary

NCLEX Review

Videos: *Through the Eyes of a Nurse— The First Trimester; Through the Eyes of a Nurse— The Second Trimester; Through the Eyes of a Nurse— The Third Trimester; Through the Eyes of a Nurse— Welcoming the New Arrival at the Postpartum Visit*

COMPANION WEBSITE

Additional NCLEX Review

Case Study: *Prenatal Education*

Care Plan Activity: *Preparing Siblings for New Baby*

Applications: *Endocrine Hormones; Internet Pregnancy Information*

Critical Thinking

CRITICAL THINKING IN ACTION

PRENATAL EDUCATION: NAUSEA, URINARY FREQUENCY, AND EXERCISE SAFETY

View the Critical Thinking in Action video in Chapter 14 of the DVD-ROM. Then answer the questions that follow.

Twenty-two-year-old Jean Simmons is an aerobic instructor, G0, P0000 in her first trimester of pregnancy. She presents to you at the local clinic complaining of frequent nausea, urinary frequency, and fatigue. You obtain her vital signs as: BP 108/60, temperature 97F, pulse 68, respirations 12, weight 125 lb, height 64 inches. Her urine tests negative for ketones, albumin, leukocytes, and sugar. You note that Jean has lost 3 lb since her last visit. You assist the certified nurse-midwife with a physical exam, the findings of which are essentially normal. Jean says that while she knows it could become an issue, she would like to continue working as an aerobic instructor for as long as she possibly can during the pregnancy. You identify Jean's complaints as normal discomforts of pregnancy, and proceed with prenatal education.

1. What advice would you suggest to cope with the nausea of pregnancy?
2. What advice might you suggest to cope with urinary frequency?
3. What teaching would be important relating to exercise in pregnancy?
4. What symptoms related to exercise should Jean report to her physician?

REFERENCES

American Academy of Pediatrics (AAP). (2005). Policy statement: The changing concept of sudden infant death syndrome: Diagnostic coding shifts, controversies regarding the sleeping environment, and new variables to consider in reducing risk. *Pediatrics, 116*(5), 1245–1255.

Aquilino, M. L., & Losch, M. E. (2005). Across the fertility lifespan: Desire for pregnancy at conception. *American Journal of Maternal-Child Nursing, (30)*4, 256–262.

Armstrong, D. (2001). Exploring fathers' experiences of pregnancy after a prior perinatal loss. *American Journal of Maternal-Child Nursing, 26*(1), 147–153.

Buster, J. E., & Carson, S. A. (2002). Endocrinology and diagnosis of pregnancy. In S. G. Gabbe, J. R. Niebyl, & J. L. Simpson (Eds.), *Obstetrics: Normal and problem pregnancies* (4th ed.). New York: Churchill Livingstone.

Cole, L. A., Khanlian, S. A., Sutton, J. M., Davies, S., & Rayburn, W. F. (2004). Accuracy of home pregnancy tests at the time of missed menses. *American Journal of Obstetrics & Gynecology, 190,* 100–105.

Cunningham, F. G., Leveno, K. J., Bloom, S. L., Hauth, J. C., Gilstrap, L. C., III, & Wenstrom, K. D. (2005). *Williams obstetrics* (22nd ed.). New York: McGraw-Hill.

Goodman, J. H. (2005). Becoming an involved father of an infant. *Journal of Obstetric, Gynecologic, & Neonatal Nursing, 34*(2), 190–200.

Gordon, M. C. (2002). Maternal physiology in pregnancy. In S. G. Gabbe, J. R. Niebyl, & J. L. Simpson (Eds.), *Obstetrics: Normal and problem pregnancies* (4th ed.). New York: Churchill Livingstone.

Lederman, R. P. (1996). *Psychosocial adaptation in pregnancy* (2nd ed.). New York: Springer.

Logsdon, M. C. (2000–2001). Helping hands: Exploring the cultural implications of social support during pregnancy. *AWHONN Lifelines, 4*(6), 29–32.

Mattson, S., & Smith, J. E. (2004). *Core curriculum for maternal-newborn nursing* (3rd ed.). Philadelphia: Saunders.

Mercer, R. T. (2004). Becoming a mother versus maternal role attainment. *Journal of Nursing Scholarship, 36*(3), 226–232.

Messer, L. C., Dole, N., Kaufman, J. S., & Savitz, D. A. (2005). Pregnany intendedness, maternal psychosocial factors and preterm birth. *Maternal and Child Health Journal, 9*(4), 403–412.

National Institute of Child Health and Human Development. (2003, January 13). *NIH news release.* Retrieved on January 19, 2003, from http://www.nih.gov/new/releases/bed_shaving.cfm

O'Leary, J., & Thorwick, C. (2006). Fathers' perspectives during pregnancy, postperinatal loss. *Journal of Obstetric, Gynecologic, & Neonatal Nursing, 35*(1), 78–86.

Rubin, R. (1984). *Maternal identity and the maternal experience.* New York: Springer.

Spector, R. E. (2003). *Cultural diversity in health and illness* (6th ed.). Upper Saddle River, NJ: Prentice Hall.

CHAPTER
15 Antepartal Nursing Assessment

My daughter, one of the authors of this book, invited me to write a few paragraphs. What would I write about? How about comparing the father's role at childbirth when she was born to the role of today's father? The father of the 1940s. . . . Main objective: Get your wife to the hospital on time. Check her in and find the father's waiting lounge. You won't be needed until the baby is born. Fathers are really useless at this time. Try not to be nervous. Coffee is available. Lots of coffee. This hospital is very considerate.

Delivery may take anywhere from 20 minutes to 20 hours. Hope it's not 20 hours.

More coffee, pacing, no sleep, waiting for word. What a drain on the father. . . . The baby finally comes. "It's a beautiful, healthy baby girl. Mother and baby are doing fine. You can see them now, but only for 5 minutes." What a relief. The pressure is finally off. Isn't nature wonderful?

Today's father, my grandson. Attends most of the prenatal visits. Schooled in Lamaze. Drives his wife to the hospital. Coaches her through her labor. Helps her push. His digital camera is ready. The baby is born. He cuts the cord. He sends e-mail & pictures of the baby to everyone. Isn't nature wonderful?

OBJECTIVES

1. Summarize the essential components of a prenatal history.
2. Define common obstetric terminology found in the history of maternity clients.
3. Identify factors related to the father's health that should be recorded on the prenatal record.
4. Describe the normal physiologic changes one would expect to find when performing a physical assessment on a pregnant woman.
5. Explain the use of Nägele's rule to determine the estimated date of birth.
6. Develop an outline of the essential measurements that can be determined by clinical pelvimetry.
7. Describe areas that should be evaluated as part of the initial assessment of psychosocial factors related to a woman's pregnancy.
8. Relate the danger signs of pregnancy to their possible causes.

KEY TERMS

Abortion 338	Nullipara 338
Antepartum 338	Obstetric conjugate 353
Diagonal conjugate 353	Para 338
Estimated date of birth (EDB) 344	Postpartum 338
	Postterm labor 338
Gestation 338	Preterm or premature labor 338
Gravida 338	Primigravida 338
Intrapartum 338	Primipara 338
Multigravida 338	Risk factors 340
Multipara 338	Stillbirth 338
Nägele's rule 344	Term 338
Nulligravida 338	

 MEDIALINK

Additional resources for this content can be found on the Prentice Hall Nursing MediaLink DVD-ROM and on the Companion Website at http://www.prenhall.com/davidson. Click on "Chapter 15" to select the activities for this chapter.

Today nurses are assuming a more important role in prenatal care, particularly in the area of assessment. The certified nurse-midwife has the education and skill to perform in-depth prenatal assessments. The nurse practitioner may share the assessment responsibilities with a physician. An office nurse, whose primary role may be to counsel and meet the psychologic needs of the expectant family, performs assessments in those areas.

The nurse needs to establish an environment of comfort and open communication with each prenatal visit, conveying concern for the woman as an individual and being available to listen and discuss the woman's concerns and desires. A supportive atmosphere coupled with the information found in the prenatal assessment guides in this chapter will enable the nurse to identify needed areas of education and counseling.

INITIAL CLIENT HISTORY

The course of a pregnancy depends on a number of factors, including the past pregnancy history (if this is not a first pregnancy), prepregnancy health of the woman, presence of disease states, emotional status, and past health care. Ideally, health care before the advent of pregnancy has been adequate, and antenatal care will be a continuation of that established care. One important method of determining the adequacy of a woman's prepregnancy care is a thorough history.

Definition of Terms

The following terms are used in recording the obstetric history of maternity clients:

- **Antepartum:** Time between conception and onset of labor, usually used to describe the period during which a woman is pregnant; used interchangeably with *prenatal*.
- **Intrapartum:** Time from onset of labor until the birth of the infant and placenta.
- **Postpartum:** Time from birth until the woman's body returns to an essentially prepregnant condition.
- **Gestation:** The number of weeks since the first day of the last menstrual period (LMP).
- **Abortion:** Birth that occurs before 20 weeks' gestation or the birth of a fetus-newborn who weighs less than 500 g (Cunningham, Levino, Bloom et al., 2005).
- **Term:** The normal duration of pregnancy (38 to 42 weeks' gestation).
- **Preterm or premature labor:** Labor that occurs after 20 weeks but before the completion of 37 weeks of gestation.
- **Postterm labor:** Labor that occurs after 42 weeks of gestation.
- **Gravida:** Any pregnancy, regardless of duration, including present pregnancy.
- **Nulligravida:** A woman who has never been pregnant.
- **Primigravida:** A woman who is pregnant for the first time.
- **Multigravida:** A woman who is in her second or any subsequent pregnancy.

- **Para:** Birth after 20 weeks' gestation, regardless of whether the infant is born alive or dead.
- **Nullipara:** A woman who has not given birth at more than 20 weeks' gestation.
- **Primipara:** A woman who has had one birth at more than 20 weeks' gestation, regardless of whether the infant is born alive or dead.
- **Multipara:** A woman who has had two or more births at more than 20 weeks' gestation.
- **Stillbirth:** A fetus born dead after 20 weeks' gestation.

The terms *gravida* and *para* refer to pregnancies, not to the fetus. Thus, traditionally, twins, triplets, and other multiple fetuses counted as one pregnancy and one birth. This approach is confusing, however, precisely because it fails to identify the number of children a woman might have. Consequently, to provide more comprehensive data, a more detailed approach is now used by many facilities. Using the detailed system, *gravida* keeps the same meaning but the use of *para* changes because the detailed system counts *each infant born* rather than the number of pregnancies carried to viability (Cunningham et al, 2005; Varney, Kriebs, & Gegor, 2004). Thus, for example, in the traditional approach, twins would count as *one* pregnancy and *one* birth. In the detailed system, twins count as *one* pregnancy but *two* babies. A useful acronym for remembering the system is TPAL.

T: number of *term* infants born; that is, the number of infants born at the completion of 37 weeks' gestation or beyond

P: number of *preterm* infants born; that is, the number of infants born after 20 weeks' but before the completion of 37 weeks' gestation, whether living or stillborn

A: number of pregnancies ending in either spontaneous or therapeutic *abortion*

L: number of currently *living* children to whom the woman has given birth.

The following examples delineate the differences between the two systems.

1. Jean Sanchez has one child born at 38 weeks' gestation and became pregnant for a second time. The second pregnancy ended in a miscarriage at 15 weeks' gestation. Using the *traditional approach* her obstetric history would be recorded as "gravida 2 para 1 ab 1." Using the *detailed approach,* her obstetric history would be recorded as "gravida 2 para 1011."

2. Tracy Hopkins is pregnant for the fourth time. At home she has a child who was born at term. Her second pregnancy ended at 10 weeks' gestation. She then gave birth to twins at 35 weeks. One of the twins died soon after birth. Using the *traditional approach* her obstetric history would be recorded as gravida 4 para 2 ab 1. Using the *detailed approach* her obstetric history would be recorded as "gravida 4 para 1212.

Occasionally a fifth digit is added to indicate the number of pregnancies that ended in multiple births (Varney et al., 2004).

Name	Gravida	Term	Preterm	Abortions	Living Children
Jean Sanchez	2	1	0	1	1
Tracy Hopkins	4	1	2	1	2

Figure 15–1 ◆ The TPAL approach provides more detailed information about the woman's pregnancy history.

Thus, using the five-digit system, Tracy Hopkins would be gravida 4 para 12121.

Some practice settings seem to have adopted variations of these two approaches. Consequently, to avoid confusion, it is best for practicing nurses to clarify the recording system used at their facilities. (Figure 15–1 ◆)

Client Profile

The history is essentially a screening tool that identifies the factors that may detrimentally affect the course of a pregnancy. For optimal prenatal care, the nurse should obtain the following information for each maternity client at the first prenatal assessment:

1. Current pregnancy
   - First day of last normal menstrual period (LMP). Is she sure of date or uncertain? Do her cycles normally occur every 28 days, or do her cycles tend to be longer?
   - Presence of cramping, bleeding, or spotting since LMP
   - Woman's opinion about time when conception occurred and when infant is due
   - Woman's attitude toward pregnancy (Is pregnancy planned? Wanted?)
   - Results of pregnancy test, if completed
   - Any discomforts since LMP, such as nausea, vomiting, urinary frequency, fatigue, breast tenderness

2. Past pregnancies
   - Number of pregnancies
   - Number of abortions, spontaneous or therapeutic
   - Number of living children
   - History of previous pregnancies: length of pregnancy, length of labor and birth, type of birth (vaginal, forceps or vacuum-assisted birth, cesarean), type of anesthesia used (if any), woman's perception of the experience, complications (antepartal, intrapartal, postpartal)
   - Neonatal status of previous children: Apgar scores, birth weights, general development, complications, feeding patterns (breast or formula)
   - Loss of a child (miscarriage, elective or medically indicated abortion, stillbirth, neonatal death, relinquishment, death after the neonatal period). What was the experience like for her? What coping skills helped? How did her partner, if involved, respond?
   - Blood type and Rh factor (If Rh negative, was medication received after birth to prevent sensitization?)
   - Prenatal education classes, resources (books)

3. Gynecologic history
   - Date of last Pap smear; any history of abnormal Pap results?
   - Previous infections: vaginal, cervical, tubal, sexually transmitted
   - Previous surgery
   - Age of menarche
   - Regularity, frequency, and duration of menstrual flow
   - History of dysmenorrhea
   - Sexual history
   - Contraceptive history (If birth control pills were used, did pregnancy immediately follow cessation of pills? If not, how long after?)

4. Current medical history
   - Weight (prepregnant and current)
   - Blood type and Rh factor, if known
   - General health, including nutrition (dietary practices such as vegetarianism; if so, which kind of vegetarian? Vegan?), regular exercise program (type, frequency, duration)
   - Any medications being taken currently (including nonprescription, homeopathic, or herbal medications) or taken since the onset of pregnancy
   - Previous or present use of alcohol, tobacco, or caffeine (Ask specifically about the amounts of alcohol, cigarettes, and caffeine [specify coffee, tea, colas, chocolate] consumed each day.)
   - Illicit drug use or abuse (Ask about specific drugs such as cocaine, crack, marijuana, methamphetamines.)
   - Drug allergies and other allergies (Ask about latex allergies or sensitivities.)
   - Potential teratogenic insults to this pregnancy, such as viral infections, medications, x-ray examinations, surgery, or cats in home (possible source of toxoplasmosis)
   - Presence of disease conditions, such as diabetes, hypertension, asthma, cardiovascular disease, renal problems, or thyroid disorders
   - Record of immunizations (especially rubella)
   - Presence of any abnormal symptoms

5. Past medical history
   - Childhood diseases
   - Past treatment for any disease condition: Any hospitalizations? History of hepatitis? Rheumatic fever? Pyelonephritis? Cancer?

- Surgical procedures
- Presence of bleeding disorders or tendencies (Has she received blood transfusions?)

6. Family medical history

- Presence of diabetes, cardiovascular disease, hypertension, hematologic disorders, tuberculosis, preeclampsia-eclampsia
- Occurrence of multiple births
- History of congenital diseases or deformities
- History of mental illness
- Occurrence of cesarean births and cause, if known
- Cause of death of deceased parents or siblings

7. Religious/cultural history

- Does the woman wish to specify a religious preference on her chart? Does she have any spiritual beliefs or practices that might influence her health care or that of her child, such as prohibition against receiving blood products, dietary considerations, circumcision rites, or other practices?
- What practices are important to maintain her spiritual well-being?
- Are there practices in her culture or that of her partner that might influence her care or that of her child?

8. Occupational history

- Occupation
- Physical demands (Does she stand all day, or are there opportunities to sit and elevate her legs? Does she do any heavy lifting?)
- Exposure to lead, chemicals, or other harmful substances
- Opportunity for regular meals and breaks for nutritious snacks
- Provision for maternity or family leave

9. Partner's history

- Presence of genetic conditions or diseases in him or in his family history
- Age
- Significant health problems
- Previous or present alcohol intake, drug use, or tobacco use
- Blood type and Rh factor
- Occupation
- Educational level; methods by which he learns best
- Attitude toward the pregnancy

10. Personal information

- Age
- Educational level; methods by which she learns best
- Race or ethnic group (to identify need for prenatal genetic screening or counseling)
- Housing; stability of living conditions

- Economic level
- Any history of emotional or physical deprivation or abuse of herself or children (Does she experience any abuse in her current relationship? Ask specifically whether she has been hit, slapped, kicked, or hurt within the past year or since she has been pregnant. Ask whether she is afraid of her partner or anyone else. If yes, of whom is she afraid?)
- History of emotional problems (Ask specifically about depression in general, postpartum depression, anxiety, and so forth.)
- Support systems
- Overuse or underuse of healthcare system
- Acceptance of pregnancy—intended or unintended
- Personal preferences about the birth (expectations of both the woman and her partner, presence of others, and so on) (See Chapter 13 ∞).
- Plans for care of child following birth
- Feeding preference for the baby (breast milk or formula)

Obtaining Data

In many instances, nurses use a questionnaire like the one shown in Figure 15–2 ◆ to obtain information. The woman should complete the questionnaire in a quiet place with a minimum of distractions.

The nurse can obtain further information in a direct interview, which allows the pregnant woman to expand or clarify her responses to questions and gives the nurse and client the opportunity to begin developing a good relationship. The expectant father or partner should be encouraged to attend the initial and subsequent prenatal assessments. He or she is often able to contribute information to the history and may use the opportunity to ask questions and express concerns that may be of particular importance to him or her.

I didn't know what to expect when I went for my first prenatal visit. I'm clean now and wanted to be honest, but I was afraid they would yell if I told them about some of the really dumb things I did in high school—the drinking, the marijuana, the sex and stuff. I really liked the nurse-midwife who was taking care of me, so I decided to be straight with her—for the baby's sake, you know. She was great about everything and really made me feel okay.

Prenatal High-Risk Screening

A highly significant part of the prenatal assessment is the screening for high-risk factors. **Risk factors** are any findings that have been shown to have a negative effect on pregnancy outcome, either for the woman or her unborn child. Many risk factors can be identified during the initial prenatal assessment; others may be detected during subsequent prenatal visits. It is important that high-risk pregnancies be identified early so that appropriate interventions can be instituted immediately.

All risk factors do not threaten the pregnancy to the same degree. Thus many agencies use a risk-scoring sheet to deter-

Name _____   Age _____

Address _____Home Phone _____

What was the last year of schooling completed? _____

How old were you when your menstrual periods started? _____

How many days does a normal period last? _____

How many days are there between periods? _____

Do you have cramping with your periods? yes _____ no _____

Is the pain: minimal _____

             moderate _____

             severe _____

What was the date of your last normal menstrual period? _____

Have you had bleeding or spotting

since your last menstrual period? yes _____ no _____

Have you been on birth control pills? yes _____ no _____

   If yes, when did you stop taking them? _____

How many previous pregnancies have you had? _____

How many living children do you have? _____

Have you had any abortions or stillbirths? yes _____ no _____

   If yes, how many? _____

Were any of your previous babies born prematurely?

yes _____ no _____

List the birth weight of all previous children.

1. _____   3. _____

2. _____   4. _____

Did any of your children have problems immediately after birth?

yes _____ no _____

   If yes, check the problems that occurred:

     _____ Respiratory   _____ Feeding

     _____ Jaundice   _____ Heart

     _____ Bleeding

Did you have any problems with:

   previous pregnancies? yes _____ no _____

     If yes, what was the problem? _____

   previous labors? yes _____ no _____

     If yes, what was the problem? _____

   previous postpartal periods: yes _____ no _____

     If yes, what was the problem? _____

Are you Rh negative? yes _____ no _____

Did you receive Rh immune globulin after each pregnancy? yes _____ no _____

What is your present weight?_____

Are you presently taking any prescription or nonprescription drugs?

yes _____ no _____

   If yes, please list the medications:

1. _____   3. _____

2. _____   4. _____

Do you smoke? yes _____ no _____

   If yes, how many cigarettes per day? _____

How much alcohol do you consume each day? _____

   each week? _____

How much caffeine do you consume each day? _____

If you have had any of the following diseases,
place a check beside it.

_____ Chickenpox   _____ High blood pressure

_____ Mumps   _____ Heart disease

_____ Measles (3 day)   _____ Respiratory disease

_____ Measles (2 week)   _____ Kidney disease

_____ Asthma   _____ Frequent bladder

_____ Hepatitis   infections

If any of the following are present in your family,
place a check beside the item.

_____ Diabetes   _____ Preeclampsia-eclampsia

_____ Cardiovascular disease _____ Multiple pregnancies

_____ High blood pressure   _____ Congenital disorder

_____ Breast cancer

The following questions pertain to the father of this child.

What is the father's age? _____

Does he smoke? yes _____ no _____

   If yes, how many cigarettes per day? _____

Does he take prescription or nonprescription drugs?

yes _____ no _____

   If yes, please list the medications:

1. _____   3. _____

2. _____   4. _____

What is his alcohol intake each day? _____

   each week?_____

Figure 15–2 ◆ Sample prenatal questionnaire.

mine the degree of risk. The sheet is initiated at the first visit and becomes a permanent part of the woman's record. Information may be updated throughout the pregnancy as necessary. It is always possible that a pregnancy may begin as low risk and change to high risk because of complications. Risk is also assessed intrapartally and postpartally.

Table 15–1 identifies one risk-scoring protocol. Table 15–2 identifies the major prenatal risk factors currently recognized.

The table describes maternal and fetal/neonatal implications should the risk be present in the pregnancy. In addition to the factors listed, the perinatal health team also needs to evaluate such psychosocial factors as ethnic background; occupation and education; financial status; environment, including living arrangements and location; and the woman's and her family's or significant other's concept of health, which might influence her attitude toward seeking health care.

Table 15–1 SYSTEM FOR DETERMINING RISK OF SPONTANEOUS PRETERM BIRTH

Points Assigned	Socioeconomic Factors	Previous Medical History	Daily Habits	Aspects of Current Pregnancy
1	Two children at home Low socioeconomic status	Abortion × 1 Less than 1 year since last birth	Works outside home	Unusual fatigue
2	Maternal age 18–20 years or greater than 40 years Single parent	Abortion × 2	Smokes more than 10 cigarettes per day	Gain of less than 5 kg by 32 weeks
3	Very low socioeconomic status Height less than 150 cm Weight less than 45 kg	Abortion × 3	Heavy or stressful work, Long, tiring trip	Breech at 32 weeks Weight loss of 2 kg Head engaged at 32 weeks Febrile illness
4	Maternal age less than 18 years	Pyelonephritis		Bleeding after 12 weeks Effacement Dilatation Uterine irritability
5		Uterine anomaly Second trimester abortion DES exposure Cone biopsy		Placenta previa Hydramnios
10		Preterm birth Repeated second trimester abortion		Twins Abdominal surgery

NOTE: The score is computed by adding the number of points given any item. The score is computed at the first visit and again at 22 to 26 weeks' gestation. A total score of 10 or more places the woman at high risk of spontaneous preterm birth.

SOURCE: Adapted from Creasy, R. K., Gummer, B. A., & Liggins, G. C. (1980). A system of predicting spontaneous preterm birth. *Obstetrics & Gynecology, 55,* 692.

Table 15–2 PRENATAL HIGH-RISK FACTORS

Factor	Maternal Implications	Fetal/Neonatal Implications
Social-Personal		
Low income level/or low educational level	Poor antenatal care or late antenatal care Poor nutrition ↑ risk of preeclampsia	Low birth weight Intrauterine growth restriction (IUGR)
Poor diet	Inadequate nutrition/inadequate weight gain ↑ risk anemia ↑ risk preeclampsia	Fetal malnutrition Prematurity Small for gestational age
Living at high altitude	↑ hemoglobin	Prematurity IUGR ↑ hemoglobin (polycythemia)
Multiparity greater than 3	↑ risk antepartum or postpartum hemorrhage	Anemia Fetal death
Weight less than 45.5 kg (100 lb)	Poor nutrition Cephalopelvic disproportion Prolonged labor	IUGR Hypoxia associated with difficult labor and birth
Weight greater than 91 kg (200 lb)	↑ risk hypertension ↑ risk cephalopelvic disproportion ↑ risk diabetes	↓ fetal nutrition ↑ risk macrosomia
Age less than 16	Poor nutrition Poor antenatal care ↑ risk preeclampsia ↑ risk cephalopelvic disproportion	Low birth weight ↑ fetal demise
Age greater than 35	↑ risk preeclampsia ↑ risk cesarean birth Psychosocial issues	↑ risk congenital anomalies ↑ chromosomal aberrations
Smoking one pack/day or more	↑ risk hypertension ↑ risk cancer	↓ placental perfusion → ↓ O$_2$ and nutrients available Low birth weight IUGR Preterm birth
Use of addicting drugs	↑ risk poor nutrition ↑ risk of infection with IV drugs ↑ risk HIV, hepatitis C ↑ risk abruptio placentae	↑ risk congenital anomalies ↑ risk low birth weight Neonatal withdrawal Lower serum bilirubin
Excessive alcohol consumption	↑ risk poor nutrition Possible hepatic effects with long-term consumption	↑ risk fetal alcohol syndrome

Table 15–2   PRENATAL HIGH-RISK FACTORS continued

Factor	Maternal Implications	Fetal/Neonatal Implications
Preexisting Medical Disorders		
Diabetes mellitus	↑ risk preeclampsia, hypertension Episodes of hypoglycemia and hyperglycemia ↑ risk cesarean birth	Low birth weight Macrosomia Neonatal hypoglycemia ↑ risk congenital anomalies ↑ risk respiratory distress syndrome
Cardiac disease	Cardiac decompensation Further strain on mother's body ↑ maternal death rate	↑ risk fetal demise ↑ perinatal mortality
Anemia: hemoglobin less than 11 g/dL less than 32% hematocrit	Iron deficiency anemia Low energy level Decreased oxygen-carrying capacity	Fetal death Prematurity Low birth weight
Hypertension	↑ vasospasm ↑ risk CNS irritability → convulsions ↑ risk CVA ↑ risk renal damage	↓ placental perfusion → low birth weight Preterm birth

Thyroid disorder
    Hypothyroidism
    Hyperthyroidism
	↑ infertility
	↓ BMR, goiter, myxedema
	↑ risk postpartum hemorrhage
	↑ risk preeclampsia
	Danger of thyroid storm
		↑ spontaneous abortion
		↑ risk congenital goiter
		Mental retardation → cretinism
		↑ incidence congenital anomalies
		↑ incidence preterm birth
		↑ tendency to thyrotoxicosis

Renal disease (moderate to severe)	↑ risk renal failure	↑ risk IUGR ↑ risk preterm birth
DES exposure	↑ infertility, spontaneous abortion ↑ cervical incompetence ↑ risk breech presentation	↑ spontaneous abortion ↑ risk preterm birth
Obstetric Considerations		
Previous Pregnancy Stillborn	↑ emotional/psychologic distress	↑ risk IUGR ↑ risk preterm birth
Habitual abortion	↑ emotional/psychologic distress ↑ possibility diagnostic work-up	↑ risk abortion
Cesarean birth	↑ possibility repeat cesarean birth Risk of uterine rupture	↑ risk preterm birth ↑ risk respiratory distress
Rh or blood group sensitization	↑ financial expenditure for testing	Hydrops fetalis Icterus gravis Neonatal anemia Kernicterus Hypoglycemia
Large baby	↑ risk cesarean birth ↑ risk gestational diabetes ↑ risk instrument-assisted birth	Birth injury Hypoglycemia
Current Pregnancy Rubella (first trimester)		Congenital heart disease Cataracts Nerve deafness Bone lesions Prolonged virus shedding
Rubella (second trimester)		Hepatitis Thrombocytopenia
Cytomegalovirus		IUGR Encephalopathy
Herpesvirus type 2	Severe discomfort Concern about possibility of cesarean birth, fetal infection	Neonatal herpesvirus type 2 Hepatitis with jaundice Neurological abnormalities
Syphilis	↑ incidence abortion	↑ fetal demise Congenital syphilis
Urinary tract infection	↑ risk preterm labor Uterine irritability	↑ risk preterm birth
Abruptio placentae and placenta previa	↑ risk hemorrhage Bed rest Extended hospitalization	Fetal/neonatal anemia Intrauterine hemorrhage ↑ fetal demise
Preeclampsia/eclampsia	See hypertension	↓ placental perfusion → low birth weight
Multiple gestation	↑ risk postpartum hemorrhage	↑ risk preterm birth ↑ risk fetal demise
Elevated hematocrit (greater than 41%)	Increased viscosity of blood	Fetal death rate 5 times normal rate
Spontaneous premature rupture of membranes	↑ uterine infection	↑ risk preterm birth ↑ fetal demise

INITIAL PRENATAL ASSESSMENT

The assessment focuses on the woman holistically by considering physical, cultural, and psychosocial factors that influence her health. At the initial visit the woman may be concerned with the diagnosis of pregnancy. However, during this visit she and her primary support person are also evaluating the health team that she has chosen. The establishment of the nurse-client relationship will help the woman evaluate the health team and also provide the nurse with a basis for developing an atmosphere that is conducive to interviewing, support, and education. Because many women are excited and anxious at the first antepartal visit, the initial psychosocial-cultural assessment is general.

As part of the initial psychosocial-cultural assessment the nurse discusses with the woman any religious, cultural, or socioeconomic factors that influence the woman's expectations of the childbearing experience. It is especially helpful if the nurse is familiar with common practices of various religious and cultural groups who reside in the community. Gathering these data in a tactful, caring way can help make the childbearing woman's experience a positive one.

After the history is obtained, the nurse prepares the woman for the physical examination. The physical examination begins with assessment of vital signs; then the woman's body is examined. The pelvic examination is performed last.

Before the examination, the woman should provide a clean urine specimen. When her bladder is empty, the woman is more comfortable during the pelvic examination, and the examiner can palpate the pelvic organs more easily. After the woman has emptied her bladder, the nurse asks her to disrobe and gives her a gown and sheet or some other protective covering.

CLINICAL TIP

In a clinic or office setting, gowns and goggles for the healthcare provider are not usually necessary because splashing of body fluids is unlikely. Gloves are worn for procedures that involve contact with body fluids such as drawing blood for lab work, handling urine specimens, and conducting pelvic examinations. Because of the increased incidence of latex allergies, it is becoming more common for nonlatex gloves to be used.

Increasing numbers of nurses, such as certified nurse-midwives and other nurses in advanced practice, are prepared to perform physical examinations. The nurse who has not yet fully developed these specific assessment skills assesses the woman's vital

DEVELOPING CULTURAL COMPETENCE

USING CULTURAL INFORMATION EFFECTIVELY

During prenatal assessment, it is important for nurses to avoid stereotyping women based on race or ethnicity. However, race and ethnicity may provide valuable information about cultural, behavioral, environmental, and medical factors that might affect a pregnant woman's health (American College of Obstetricians and Gynecologists [ACOG], 2005a).

signs, explains the procedures to allay apprehension, positions her for examination, and assists the examiner as necessary. Each nurse is responsible for operating at the expected standard for a professional with that individual nurse's skill and knowledge base.

Thoroughness and a systematic procedure are the most important considerations when performing the physical portion of an antepartal examination (see the Initial Prenatal Assessment Guide). To promote completeness, the Initial Prenatal Assessment Guide is organized into three columns that address the areas to be assessed, the variations or alterations that may be observed, and nursing responses to the data. The nurse should be aware that certain organs and systems are assessed concurrently with other systems during the physical portion of the examination.

Nursing interventions based on assessment of the normal physical and psychosocial changes, as well as the cultural influences associated with pregnancy and client teaching and counseling needs that have been mutually defined, are discussed further in Chapter 16. ∞

Determination of Due Date

Childbearing families generally want to know the "due date," or the date around which childbirth will occur. Historically, the due date has been called the *estimated date of confinement (EDC)*. The concept of confinement is, however, rather negative, and there is a trend among caregivers to avoid it by referring to the birth date as the *estimated date of delivery (EDD)*. However, childbirth educators often stress that babies are not "delivered" like a package; they are *born*. In keeping with a view that emphasizes the normality of the process, we have chosen to refer to the due date as the **estimated date of birth (EDB)** throughout this text.

To calculate the EDB, it is helpful to know the first day of the woman's LMP. However, some women have episodes of irregular bleeding or fail to keep track of menstrual cycles. Thus other techniques also help determine how far along a woman is in her pregnancy, that is, at how many weeks' gestation she is. Other techniques that can be used include evaluating uterine size, determining when quickening occurs, using ultrasound, and auscultating the fetal heart rate.

NÄGELE'S RULE

The most common method of determining the EDB is **Nägele's rule.** To use this method, begin with the first day of the LMP, subtract 3 months, and add 7 days. For example,

First day of LMP	July 20
Subtract 3 months	− 3 months
	April 20
Add 7 days	+ 7 days
EDB	April 27 (of the next year)

It is simpler to change the months to numeric terms:

July 20 becomes	07 − 20
Subtract 3 months	− 3
	04 − 20
Add 7 days	+ 7
EDB	04 − 27 (of next year)

(Text continues on p. 351)

ASSESSMENT GUIDE Initial Prenatal Assessment

PHYSICAL ASSESSMENT/ NORMAL FINDINGS	ALTERATIONS AND POSSIBLE CAUSES*	NURSING RESPONSES TO DATA†
VITAL SIGNS		
Blood Pressure (BP): Less than or equal to 135/85 mm Hg	High BP (essential hypertension; renal disease; pregestational hypertension, apprehension or anxiety associated with pregnancy diagnosis, exam, or other crises; preeclampsia if initial assessment not done until after 20 weeks' gestation)	BP greater than 140/90 requires immediate consideration; establish woman's BP; refer to healthcare provider if necessary. Assess woman's knowledge about high BP; counsel on self-care and medical management
Pulse: 60–90 beats/min; rate may increase 10 beats/min during pregnancy	Increased pulse rate (excitement or anxiety, cardiac disorders)	Count for 1 full minute; note irregularities.
Respirations: 12–22 breaths/min (or pulse rate divided by four); pregnancy may induce a degree of hyperventilation; thoracic breathing predominant	Marked tachypnea or abnormal patterns	Assess for respiratory disease.
Temperature: 36.2–37.6C (97–99.6F)	Elevated temperature (infection)	Assess for infection process of disease state if temperature is elevated; refer to healthcare provider.
WEIGHT		
Depends on body build	Weight less than 45 kg (100 lb) or greater than 91 kg (200 lb); rapid, sudden weight gain (preeclampsia)	Evaluate need for nutritional counselling; obtain information on eating habits, cooking practices, food regularly eaten, income limitations, need for food supplements, pica and other abnormal food habits. Note initial weight to establish baseline for weight gain throughout pregnancy.
SKIN		
Color: Consistent with racial background; pink nail beds	Pallor (anemia); bronze, yellow (hepatic disease; other causes of jaundice)	The following tests should be performed: complete blood count (CBC), bilirubin level, urinalysis, and blood urea nitrogen (BUN).
	Bluish, reddish, mottled; dusky appearance or pallor of palms and nail beds in dark-skinned women (anemia)	If abnormal, refer to healthcare provider.
Condition: Absence of edema (slight edema of lower extremities is normal during pregnancy)	Edema (preeclampsia); rashes, dermatitis (allergic response)	Counsel on relief measures for slight edema. Initiate preeclampsia assessment; refer to healthcare provider.
Lesions: Absence of lesions	Ulceration (varicose veins, decreased circulation)	Futher assess circulatory status; refer to healthcare provider if lesion is severe.
Spider nevi common in pregnancy	Petechiae, multiple bruises, ecchymosis (hemorrhagic disorders; abuse)	Evaluate for bleeding or clotting disorder, Provide opportunities to discuss abuse if suspected.
	Change in size or color (carcinoma)	Refer to healthcare provider.
Moles		
Pigmentation: Pigmentation changes of pregnancy include linea nigra, striae gravidarum, melasma		Assure woman that these are normal manifestations of pregnancy and explain the physiologic basis for the changes.
Café-au-lait spots	Six or more (Albright syndrome or neurofibromatosis)	Consult with healthcare provider.
NOSE		
Character of mucosa: Redder than oral mucosa; in pregnancy nasal mucosa is edematous in response to increased estrogen, resulting in nasal stuffiness (rhinitis of pregnancy) and nosebleeds	Olfactory loss (first cranial nerve deficit)	Counsel woman about possible relief measures for nasal stuffiness and nosebleeds (epistaxis); refer to healthcare provider for olfactory loss.
	*Possible causes of alterations are identified in parentheses.	†This column provides guidelines for further assessment and initial intervention.

(Continued on next page)

ASSESSMENT GUIDE Initial Prenatal Assessment continued

PHYSICAL ASSESSMENT/ NORMAL FINDINGS	ALTERATIONS AND POSSIBLE CAUSES*	NURSING RESPONSES TO DATA†
MOUTH		
May note hypertrophy of gingival tissue because of estrogen	Edema, inflammation (infection); pale in color (anemia)	Assess hematocrit for anemia; counsel regarding dental hygiene habits. Refer to healthcare provider or dentist if necessary. Routine dental care appropriate during pregnancy (no x-ray studies, no nitrous anesthesia).
NECK		
Nodes: Small, mobile, nontender nodes	Tender, hard, fixed, or prominent nodes (infection, carcinoma)	Examine for local infection; refer to healthcare provider.
Thyroid: Small, smooth, lateral lobes palpable on either side of trachea; slight hyperplasia by third month of pregnancy	Enlargement or nodule tenderness (hyperthyroidism)	Listen over thyroid for bruits, which may indicate hyperthyroidism. Question woman about dietary habits (iodine intake). Ascertain history of thyroid problems; refer to healthcare provider.
CHEST AND LUNGS		
Chest: Symmetric, elliptic, smaller anteroposterior (AP) than transverse diameter	Increased AP diameter, funnel chest, pigeon chest (emphysema, asthma, chronic obstructive pulmonary disease [COPD])	Evaluate for emphysema, asthma, pulmonary disease (COPD).
Ribs: Slope downward from nipple line	More horizontal (COPD) Angular bumps Rachitic rosary (vitamin C deficiency)	Evaluate for COPD. Evaluate for fractures. Consult healthcare provider. Consult nutritionist.
Inspection and palpation: No retraction or bulging of intercostal spaces (ICS) during inspiration or expiration; symmetric expansion.	ICS retractions with inspirations, bulging with expiration; unequal expansion (respiratory disease)	Do thorough initial assessment. Refer to healthcare provider.
Tactile fremitus	Tachypnea, hyperpnea, Cheyne-Stokes respirations (respiratory disease)	Refer to healthcare provider.
Percussion: Bilateral symmetry in tone	Flatness of percussion, which may be affected by chest wall thinckness	Evaluate for pleural effusions, consolidations, or tumor.
Low-pitched resonance of moderate intensity	High diaphragm (atelectasis or paralysis), pleural effusion	Refer to healthcare provider.
Auscultation: Upper lobes—bronchovesicular sounds above sternum and scapulas; equal expiratory and inspiratory phases	Abnormal if heard over any other area of chest	Refer to healthcare provider.
Remainder of chest: Vesicular breath sounds heard; inspiratory phase longer (3:1)	Rales, rhonchi, wheezes; pleural friction rub; absence of breath sounds; bronchophony, egophony, whispered pectoriloquy	Refer to healthcare provider.
BREASTS		
Supple: Symmetric in size and contour; darker pigmentation of nipple and areola; may have supernumerary nipples, usually 5–6 cm below normal nipple line	"Pigskin" or orange-peel appearance, nipple retractions, swelling, hardness (carcinoma); redness, heat, tenderness, cracked or fissured nipple (infection)	Encourage monthly self-examination; instruct woman how to examine her own breasts.
Axillary nodes unpalpable or pellet sized	Tenderness, enlargement, hard node (carcinoma); may be visible bump (infection)	Refer to healthcare provider if evidence of inflammation.
Pregnancy changes: 1. Size increase noted primarily in first 20 weeks. 2. Become nodular. 3. Tingling sensation may be felt during first and third trimester; woman may report feeling of heaviness. 4. Pigmentation of nipples and areolae darkens. 5. Superficial veins dilate and become more prominent.		Discuss normalcy of changes and their meaning with the woman. Teach and/or institute appropriate relief measures. Encourage use of supportive, well-fitting brassiere.
	*Possible causes of alterations are identified in parentheses.	†This column provides guidelines for further assessment and initial intervention.

ASSESSMENT GUIDE   Initial Prenatal Assessment continued

PHYSICAL ASSESSMENT/ NORMAL FINDINGS	ALTERATIONS AND POSSIBLE CAUSES*	NURSING RESPONSES TO DATA†
BREASTS (continued) 6. Striae seen in multiparas. 7. Tubercles of Montgomery enlarge. 8. Colostrum may be present after 12th week. 9. Secondary areola appears at 20 weeks, characterized by series of washed-out spots surrounding primary areola. 10. Breasts less firm, old striae may be present in multiparas.		
HEART Normal rate, rhythm, and heart sounds ***Pregnancy changes:*** 1. Palpitations may occur due to sympathetic nervous system disturbance. 2. Short systolic murmurs that increase in held expiration are normal due to increased volume.	Enlargement, thrills, thrusts, gross irregularity or skipped beats, gallop rhythm or extra sounds (cardiac disease)	Complete an initial assessment. Explain normalcy pregnancy-induced changes. Refer to healthcare provider if indicated.
ABDOMEN Normal appearance, skin texture, and hair distribution; liver nonpalpable; abdomen nontender ***Pregnancy changes:*** 1. Purple striae may be present (or silver striae on a multipara) as well as linea nigra. 2. Diastasis of the rectus muscles late in pregnancy. 3. Size: Flat or rotund abdomen; progressive enlargement of uterus due to pregnancy. 10–12 weeks: Fundus slightly above symphysis pubis. 16 weeks: Fundus halfway between symphysis and umbilicus. 20–22 weeks: Fundus at umbilicus. 28 weeks: Fundus three finger breadths above umbilicus. 36 weeks: Fundus just below ensiform cartilage. 4. Fetal heart rate: 110–160 beats/min may be heard with Doppler at 10–12 weeks' gestation; may be heard with fetoscope at 17–20 weeks. 5. Fetal movement palpable by a trained examiner after the 18th week. 6. Ballottement: During fourth to fifth month fetus rises and then rebounds to original position when uterus is tapped sharply.	Muscle guarding (anxiety, acute tenderness); tenderness, mass (ectopic pregnancy, inflammation, carcinoma) Size of uterus inconsistent with length of gestation (intrauterine growth restriction [IUGR], multiple pregnancy, fetal demise, hydatidiform mole) Failure to hear fetal heartbeat with Doppler (fetal demise, hydatidiform mole) Failure to feel fetal movements after 20 weeks' gestation (fetal demise, hydatidiform mole) No ballottement (oligohydramnios)	Assure woman of normalcy of diastasis. Provide initial information about appropriate prenatal and postpartum exercises. Evaluate woman's anxiety level. Refer to healthcare provider if indicated. Reassess menstrual history regarding pregnancy dating. Evaluate increase in size using McDonald's method. Use ultrasound to establish diagnosis. Refer to healthcare provider. Administer pregnancy tests. Use ultrasound to establish diagnosis. Refer to healthcare provider for evaluation of fetal status. Refer to healthcare provider for evaluation of fetal status.
EXTREMITIES Skin warm, pulses palpable, full range of motion; may be some edema of hands and ankles in late pregnancy; varicose veins may become more pronounced; palmar erythema may be present	Unpalpable or diminished pulses (arterial insufficiency); marked edema (preeclampsia)	Evaluate for other symptoms of heart disease; initiate follow-up if woman mentions that her rings feel tight. Discuss prevention and self-treatment measures for varicose veins; refer to healthcare provider if indicated.
	*Possible causes of alterations are identified in parentheses.	†This column provides guidelines for further assessment and initial intervention.

(Continued on next page)

ASSESSMENT GUIDE   Initial Prenatal Assessment continued

PHYSICAL ASSESSMENT/ NORMAL FINDINGS	ALTERATIONS AND POSSIBLE CAUSES*	NURSING RESPONSES TO DATA†
SPINE		
Normal spinal curves: Concave cervical, convex thoracic, concave lumbar	Abnormal spinal curves; flatness, kyphosis, lordosis	Refer to healthcare provider for assessment of cephalopelvic disproportion (CPD).
In pregnancy, lumbar spinal curve may be accentuated	Backache	May have implications for administration of spinal anesthetics; see Chapter 25 ∞ for relief measures.
Shoulders and iliac crests should be even	Uneven shoulders and iliac crests (scoliosis)	Refer very young women to healthcare provider; discuss back-stretching exercise with older women.
REFLEXES		
Normal and symmetric	Hyperactivity, clonus (preeclampsia)	Evaluate for other symptoms of preeclampsia.
PELVIC AREA		
External female genitals: Normally formed with female hair distribution; in multiparas, labia majora loose and pigmented; urinary and vaginal orifices visible and appropriately located	Lesions, hematomas, varicosities, inflammation of Bartholin's glands; clitoral hypertrophy (masculinization)	Explain pelvic examination procedure. Encourage woman to minimize her discomfort by relaxing her hips. Provide privacy.
Vagina: Pink or dark pink, vaginal discharge odorless, nonirritating; in multiparas, vaginal folds smooth and flattened; may have episiotomy scar	Abnormal discharge associated with vaginal infections	Obtain vaginal smear. Provide understandable verbal and written instructions about treatment for woman and partner, if indicated.
Cervix: Pink color; os closed except in multiparas, in whom os admits fingertip	Eversion, reddish erosin, nabothian or retention cysts, cervical polyp; granular area that bleeds (carcinoma of cervix); lesions (herpes, human papilloma virus [HPV]); presence of string or plastic tip from cervix (intrauterine device [IUD] in uterus)	Provide woman with a hand mirror and identify genital structures for her; encourage her to view her cervix if she wishes. Refer to healthcare provider if indicated. Advise woman of potential serious risks of leaving an IUD in place during pregnancy; refer to healthcare provider for removal.
Pregnancy changes:		
1–4 weeks' gestation: Enlargement in anteroposterior diameter		
4–6 weeks' gestation: Softening of cervix (Goodell's sign). softening of isthmus of uterus (Hegar's sign); cervix takes on bluish coloring (Chadwick's sign)	Absence of Goodell's sign (inflammatory conditions, carcinoma)	Refer to healthcare provider.
8–12 weeks' gestation: Vagina and cervix appear bluish violet in color (Chadwick's sign)	Fixed (pelvic inflammatory disease [PID]); nodular surface (fibromas)	Refer to healthcare provider.
Uterus: Pear shaped, mobile; smooth surface		
Ovaries: Small, walnut shaped, nontender (ovaries and Fallopian tubes are located in the adnexal areas)	Pain on movement of cervix (PID); enlarged or nodular ovaries (cyst, tumor, tubal pregnancy, corpus luteum of pregnancy)	Evaluate adnexal areas; refer to healthcare provider.
PELVIC MEASUREMENTS		
Internal measurements:	Measurement below normal	Vaginal birth may not be possible if deviations are present.
1. Diagonal conjugate at least 11.5 cm (Figure 15–7)		
2. Obstetric conjugate estimated by subtracing 1.5–2 cm from diagonal conjugate	Disproportion of pubic arch	
3. Inclination of sacrum	Abnormal curvature of sacrum	
4. Motility of coccyx; external intertuberosity diameter greater than 8 cm	Fixed or malposition of coccyx	
	*Possible causes of alterations are identified in parentheses.	†This column provides guidelines for further assessment and initial intervention.

ASSESSMENT GUIDE   Initial Prenatal Assessment continued

PHYSICAL ASSESSMENT/ NORMAL FINDINGS	ALTERATIONS AND POSSIBLE CAUSES*	NURSING RESPONSES TO DATA†
ANUS AND RECTUM		
No lumps, rashes, excoriation, tenderness; cervix may be felt through rectal wall	Hemorrhoids, rectal prolapse; nodular lesion (carcinoma)	Counsel about appropriate prevention and relief measures; refer to healthcare provider for further evaluation.
LABORATORY EVALUATION		
Hemoglobin: 12–16 g/dL; women residing in areas of high altitude may have higher levels of hemoglobin	Less than 11 g/dL (anemia)	Note: Wear nonlatex gloves when drawing blood. Hemoglobin less than 12 g/dL requires nutritional counseling; less than 11 g/dL requires iron supplementation.
ABO and Rh typing: Normal distribution of blood types	Rh negative	If Rh negative, check for presence of anti-Rh antibodies. Check partner's blood type; if partner is Rh positive, discuss with woman the need for antibody titers during pregnancy, management during the intrapartal period, and possible need for Rh immune globulin. (See Chapter 20 ∞).
Complete blood count (CBC)		
Hematocrit: 38%–47% physiologic anemia (pseudoanemia) may occur	Marked anemia or blood dyscrasias	Perform CBC and Schilling differential cell count.
Red blood cells (RBC): 4.2–5.4 million/microliter		
White blood cells (WBC): 5000–12,000/microliter	Presence of infection; may be elevated in pregnancy and with labor	Evaluate for other signs of infection.
Differential		
Neutrophils: 40%–60%		
Bands: up to 5%		
Eosinophils: 1%–3%		
Basophils: up to 1%		
Lymphocytes: 20%–40%		
Monocytes: 4%–8%		
Syphilis tests: Serologic tests for syphilis (STS), complement fixation test, veneral disease research laboratory (VDRL) test—nonreactive	Positive reaction STS—tests may have 25%–45% incidence of biologic false-positive results; false results may occur in individuals who have acute viral or bacterial infections, hypersensitivity reactions, recent vaccinations, collagen disease, malaria, or tuberculosis	Positive results may be confirmed with the fluorescent treponemal antibody-absorption (FTA-ABS) test; all tests for syphilis give positive results in the secondary stage of the disease; antibiotic tests may cause negative test results.
Gonorrhea culture: Negative	Positive	Refer for treatment.
Urinalysis (u/a): Normal color, specific gravity; pH 4.6–8	Abnormal color (porphyria, hemoglobinuria, bilirubinemia): alkaline urine (metabolic alkalemia, *Proteus* infection, old specimen)	Repeat u/a; refer to healthcare provider.
Negative for protein, red blood cells, white blood cells, casts	Positive findings (contaminated speciman, kidney disease)	Repeat u/a; refer to healthcare provider.
Glucose: Negative (small degree of glycosuria may occur in pregnancy)	Glycosuria (low renal threshold for glucose, diabetes mellitus)	Assess blood glucose level; test urine for ketones.
Rubella titer: Hemagglutination-inhibition (HAI) test–1:10 or above indicates woman is immune	HAI titer less than 1:10	Immunization will be given on postpartum or within 6 weeks after childbirth. Instruct woman whose titers are less than 1:10 to avoid children who have rubella.
Hepatitis B screen for hepatitis B surface antigen (HbsAg): negative	Positive	If negative, consider referral for hepatitis B vaccine. If positive, refer to physician. Infants born to women who test positive are given hepatitis B immune globulin soon after birth followed by first dose of hepatitis B vaccine.
	*Possible causes of alterations are identified in parentheses.	†This column provides guidelines for further assessment and initial intervention.

(Continued on next page)

ASSESSMENT GUIDE   Initial Prenatal Assessment continued

PHYSICAL ASSESSMENT/ NORMAL FINDINGS	ALTERATIONS AND POSSIBLE CAUSES*	NURSING RESPONSES TO DATA†
LABORATORY EVALUATION (continued)		
HIV screen: Offered to all women; encouraged for those at risk; negative	Positive	Refer to healthcare provider.
Illicit drug screen: Offered to all women; negative	Positive	Refer to healthcare provider.
Sickle-cell screen for clients of African descent: Negative	Positive; test results would include a description of cells	Refer to healthcare provider.
Pap smear: Negative	Test results that show atypical cells	Refer to healthcare provider. Discuss with the woman the meaning of the findings and the importance of follow-up.

CULTURAL ASSESSMENT	VARIATIONS TO CONSIDER*	NURSING RESPONSES TO DATA†
Determine the woman's fluency in written and oral English.	Woman may be fluent in language other than English.	Work with a knowledgeable translator to provide information and answer questions.
Ask the woman how she prefers to be addressed.	Some women prefer informality; others prefer to use titles.	Address the woman according to her preference. Maintain formality in introducing oneself if that seems preferred.
Determine customs and practices regarding prenatal care:	Practices are influenced by individual preference, cultural expectations, or religious beliefs.	Honor a woman's practices and provide for specific preferences unless they are contraindicated because of safety.
• Ask the woman if there are certain practices she expects to follow when she is pregnant.	Some women believe that they should perform certain acts related to sleep, activity, or clothing.	Have information printed in the language of different cultural groups that live in the area.
• Ask the woman if there are any activities she cannot do while she is pregnant.	Some women have restrictions or taboos they follow related to work, activity, sexual, environmental, or emotional factors.	
• Ask the woman whether there are certain foods she is expected to eat or avoid while she is pregnant. Determine whether she has lactose intolerance.	Foods are an important cultural factor. Some women may have certain foods they must eat or avoid; many women have lactose intolerance and have difficulty consuming sufficient calcium.	Respect the woman's food preferences, help her plan an adequate prenatal diet within the framework of her preferences, and refer to a dietitian if necessary.
• Ask the woman whether the gender of her caregiver is of concern.	Some women are comfortable only with a female caregiver.	Arrange for a female caregiver if it is the woman's preference.
• Ask the woman about the degree of involvement in her pregnancy that she expects or wants from her support person, mother, and other significant people.	A woman may not want her partner involved in the pregnancy. For some the role falls to the woman's mother or a female relative or friend.	Respect the woman's preferences about her partner or husband's involvement; avoid imposing personal values or expectations.
• Ask the woman about her sources of support and counseling during pregnancy.	Some women seek advice from a family member, *curandera,* tribal healer, and so forth.	Respect and honor the woman's sources of support.
PSYCHOLOGIC STATUS		
Excitement and/or apprehension, ambivalence	Marked anxiety (fear of pregnancy diagnosis, fear of medical facility)	Establish lines of communication. Active listening is useful. Establish trusting relationship. Encourage woman to take active part in her care.
	Apathy; display of anger with pregnancy diagnosis	Establish communication and begin counseling. Use active listening techniques.
EDUCATIONAL NEEDS		
May have questions about pregnancy or may need time to adjust to reality of pregnancy		Establish educational, supporting environment that can be expanded throughout pregnancy.
	*Possible causes of alterations are identified in parentheses.	†This column provides guidelines for further assessment and initial intervention.

ASSESSMENT GUIDE   Initial Prenatal Assessment continued

CULTURAL ASSESSMENT	VARIATIONS TO CONSIDER*	NURSING RESPONSES TO DATA†
SUPPORT SYSTEM Can identify at least two or three individuals with whom woman is emotionally intimate (partner, parent, sibling, friend)	Isolated (no telephone, unlisted number); cannot name a neighbor or friend whom she can call upon in an emergency; does not perceive parents as part of her support system	Institute support system through community groups. Help woman to develop trusting relationship with healthcare professionals.
FAMILY FUNCTIONING Emotionally supportive Communications adequate Mutually satisfying Cohesiveness in times of trouble	Long-term problems or specific problems related to this pregnancy, potential stressors within the family, pessimistic attitudes, unilateral decision making, unrealistic expectations of this pregnancy or child	Help identify the problems and stressors, encourage communication, and discuss role changes and adaptations.
ECONOMIC STATUS Source of income is stable and sufficient to meet basic needs of daily living and medical needs	Limited prenatal care; poor physical health; limited use of healthcare system; unstable economic status	Discuss available resources for health maintenance and the birth. Institute appropriate referral for meeting expanding family's needs—food stamps and so forth.
STABILITY OF LIVING CONDITIONS Adequate, stable housing for expanding family's needs	Crowded living conditions; questionable supportive environment for newborn	Refer to appropriate community agency. Work with family on self-help ways to improve situation.
	*Possible causes of alterations are identified in parentheses.	†This column provides guidelines for further assessment and initial intervention.

A gestation calculator or "wheel" permits the caregiver to calculate the EDB even more quickly (Figure 15–3 ◆).

If a woman with a history of menses every 28 days remembers her LMP and was not taking oral contraceptives before becoming pregnant, Nägele's rule may be a fairly accurate determiner of her predicted birth date. However, if her cycle is irregular or 35 to 40 days in length, the time of ovulation may be delayed by several days. Ovulation usually occurs 14 days before the onset of the next menses, not 14 days after the previous menses. In such cases a sonogram is done to visualize the gestational sac and obtain measurements of the embryo/fetus. (See discussion of ultrasound in Chapter 21 ∞).

Thus Nägele's rule, although helpful, is not foolproof. It is of no use in calculating EDB for (1) women with markedly irregular periods that include one or more months of amenorrhea, (2) women who are amenorrheic but ovulating and conceive while breastfeeding, or (3) women who conceive before regular menstruation is established following discontinuation of oral contraceptives or termination of a pregnancy (Varney et al., 2004).

Uterine Assessment

PHYSICAL EXAMINATION

When a woman is examined in the first 10 to 12 weeks of her pregnancy and the nurse practitioner, certified nurse-midwife, or physician thinks that her uterine size is compatible with her menstrual history, uterine size may be the single most important

Figure 15–3 ◆ The EDB wheel can be used to calculate the due date. To use it, place the arrow labeled "first day of last period" on the date of the woman's LMP. Then read the EDB at the arrow labeled 40. In this case, the LMP is September 8th and the EDB is June 17th.

clinical method for dating her pregnancy. In many cases, however, women do not seek obstetric care until well into their second trimester, when it becomes much more difficult to evaluate specific uterine size. In the case of the obese woman, it is most difficult to determine uterine size early in pregnancy because the uterus is more difficult to palpate.

FUNDAL HEIGHT

Fundal height may be used as an indicator of uterine size, although this method cannot be used late in pregnancy. A centimeter tape measure is used to measure the distance from the top of the symphysis pubis over the curve of the abdomen to the top of the uterine fundus (McDonald's method) (Figure 15–4 ◆).

Fundal height in centimeters correlates well with weeks of gestation between 22 to 24 weeks and 34 weeks. At 26 weeks' gestation, for example, fundal height is probably about 26 cm. Typically ±2 cm is considered normal. To be most accurate, fundal height should be measured by the same examiner each time. The woman should empty her bladder before the examiner takes the measurement (Cunningham et al., 2005). Maternal position (trunk elevation, knee flexion) also influences fundal height measurement. If the woman is very tall or very short, fundal height will differ. In the third trimester, variations in fetal weight decrease the accuracy of fundal height measurements. Unfortunately, this method of dating a pregnancy can be quite inaccurate in the following situations:

- Obese women (because of difficulty palpating the fundus accurately)

- Women with uterine fibroids (because uterine size may be distorted)
- Women who develop hydramnios (because the excess fluid increases uterine size, leading the examiner to conclude the fetus is larger than it is)

Measurements of fundal height from month to month and week to week may yield other information as well. For example, a lag in the progression of fundal height may indicate intrauterine growth restriction (IUGR); a sudden increase in height may indicate the presence of twins or hydramnios.

Assessment of Fetal Development
QUICKENING

Fetal movements felt by the mother—*quickening*—may give some indications that the fetus is nearing 20 weeks' gestation. However, quickening may be experienced between 16 and 22 weeks' gestation, so this is not a completely accurate method. Because multiparous women have experienced quickening before, they often report it earlier than a primigravida does.

FETAL HEARTBEAT

The ultrasonic Doppler device (Figure 15–5 ◆) is the primary tool for assessing fetal heartbeat. It may detect fetal heartbeat at about 10 to 12 weeks' gestation. If an ultrasonic Doppler is not available, a special type of stethoscope called a *fetoscope* may be used. The fetal heartbeat can be detected by fetoscope as early as week 16 and almost always by 19 or 20 weeks of ges-

Figure 15–4 ◆ A cross-sectional view of fetal position when McDonald's method is used to assess fundal height.

Figure 15–5 ◆ Listening to the fetal heartbeat with a Doppler device.

tation. In the case of twins or the obese woman, it may be later before the fetal heartbeat can be detected.

> *I went with my daughter to her prenatal visit, which included an ultrasound. I was not only able to hear the heartbeat of my first grandchild, I was also able to see the baby. What a blessing to be part of this experience! It was a special moment for me as a soon-to-be grandfather.*

ULTRASOUND

In the first trimester, ultrasound scanning can detect a gestational sac as early as 5 to 6 weeks after the LMP, fetal heart activity by 6 to 7 weeks, and fetal breathing movement by 10 to 11 weeks of pregnancy. Crown-to-rump measurements can be made for assessment of fetal age until the fetal head can be defined. Biparietal diameter measurements can be made by approximately 12 to 13 weeks and are most accurate between 20 and 30 weeks, when rapid growth in biparietal diameter occurs. (See Chapter 21 ∞ for an in-depth discussion of ultrasound scanning of the fetus).

Assessment of Pelvic Adequacy

By performing a series of assessments and measurements, the examiner assesses the pelvis vaginally to determine whether the size and shape are adequate for a vaginal birth. This procedure, *clinical pelvimetry,* is performed by physicians and by advanced practice nurses such as certified nurse-midwives or nurse practitioners. For a detailed description of clinical pelvimetry, refer to a nurse-midwifery text. This section provides general information about the assessment of the inlet, midpelvis, and outlet. These terms are defined in Chapter 10. ∞

PELVIC INLET

The important anteroposterior diameters of the inlet for childbearing are the diagonal conjugate, the obstetric conjugate, and

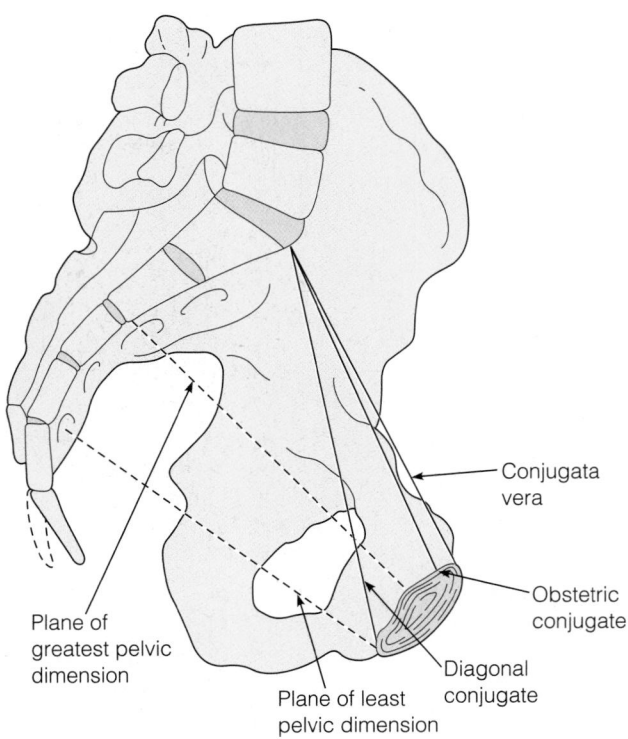

Figure 15–6 ◆ Anteroposterior diameters of the pelvic inlet and their relationship to the pelvic planes.

the conjugata vera, or true conjugate (Figure 15–6 ◆). Other diameters are the transverse (approximately 13.5 cm) and the oblique (averages 12.75 cm).

The anteroposterior diameters of the pelvic inlet may be assessed. To measure the **diagonal conjugate,** the distance from the lower border of the symphysis pubis to the sacral promontory, the examiner inserts a gloved hand into the vagina with index and middle finger extended. The thumb remains extended outside the vagina. The examiner then attempts to reach from the lower border of the symphysis pubis to the sacral promontory with the middle finger. The clinician should determine the length of the finger before attempting this. The diagonal conjugate can then be measured by marking the place where the proximal part of the hand makes contact with the pubis (Figure 15–7 ◆, *A*). Then the examiner measures the distance (which normally measures at least 11.5 cm). The **obstetric conjugate** is the smallest and thus the most important anteroposterior diameter through which the fetus must pass. It extends from the middle of the sacral promontory to the upper inner point on the symphysis. Because it cannot be measured manually (but only by x-ray examination), it is estimated by subtracting 1.5 to 2 cm from the length of the diagonal conjugate. It should measure 10 cm or more in order for an average size baby (7.5 to 8 lb) to pass through without difficulty. The true conjugate extends from the upper border of the symphysis pubis to the middle of the sacral promontory. It can be determined by subtracting 1 cm from the diagonal conjugate.

PELVIC CAVITY (MIDPELVIS)

Important midpelvic measurements include the plane of least dimension, or midplane (anteroposterior diameter, normally

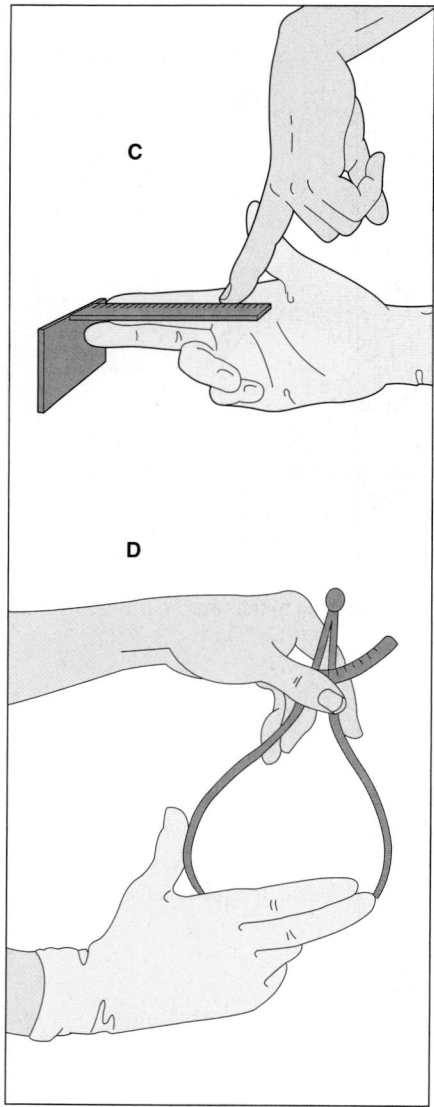

Figure 15–7 ◆ Manual measurement of inlet and outlet. *A,* Estimation of the diagonal conjugate, which extends from the lower border of the symphysis pubis to the sacral promontory. *B,* Estimation of the anteroposterior diameter of the outlet, which extends from the lower border of the symphysis pubis to the tip of the sacrum. *C* and *D,* Methods that may be used to check the manual estimation of anteroposterior measurements.

11.5 to 12 cm; posterior sagittal diameter, 4.5 to 5 cm; and transverse diameter [interspinous], 10 cm). It is shown in Figure 15–6. The planes of the midpelvis cannot be accurately measured by clinical examination. An evaluation of adequacy is made based on the prominence of the ischial spines and degree of convergence of the side walls.

Location of the sacrospinous ligament, a firm ridge of tissue, makes location of the ischial spines easier. When this ligament is located, the examiner should run the fingers along it laterally toward the anterior portion of the pelvis. The spines may range from a small, firm bump like the knuckle of a finger (termed *not encroaching*) to a very prominent bone (called *encroaching*).

The sacrosciatic notch should admit two fingers. A wide notch means that the sacrum curves posteriorly, giving the anteroposterior diameter of the midpelvis a greater length. A narrow notch indicates a decreased diameter. The width of the sacrosciatic notch is more accurately evaluated through x-ray examination but can be estimated through vaginal examination.

The length of the sacrospinous ligament is measured by tracing the ligament from its origin on the ischial spines to its insertion on the sacrum. It is usually 4 cm, or two to three finger breadths long.

The capacity of the cavity can be assessed by sweeping the fingers down the side walls bilaterally to evaluate the shape of the pelvic side walls. They may be termed *convergent* (closer together at the outlet than the inlet, like a funnel), *divergent* (side walls farther apart at the outlet, which typically means the pubic arch will have a wide angle), or *straight* (normal finding). The curvature, inclination, and hollowness of the sacrum help indicate the capacity of the posterior pelvis. It is estimated digitally by palpating the sacrococcygeal junction and by inching up toward the promontory. The examiner then estimates the hollowness of the sacrum. A flat or shallow sacrum has less room; a hollow sacrum is considered normal.

The plane of greatest pelvic dimensions represents the largest portion of the pelvic cavity and has no obstetric significance.

PELVIC OUTLET

The anteroposterior diameter of the pelvic outlet (9.5 to 11.5 cm), which extends from the lower border of the symphysis pubis to the tip of the sacrum, can be measured digitally (Figure 15–7, B). The transverse diameter of the outlet is measured by placing the fist between the ischial tuberosities. It usually measures 8 to 10 cm (Figure 15–8 ◆). The posterior sagittal diameter, the third important outlet diameter, normally measures at least 7.5 cm.

The mobility of the coccyx is determined by pressing down on it with the forefinger and middle finger during the initial vaginal examination. An immobile coccyx can decrease the diameter of the outlet.

The subpubic angle is estimated by palpating the bony structure externally with two fingers placed side by side at the border of the symphysis (Figure 15–9 ◆). It should be 85 to 90 degrees. The angle is probably less if the examiner cannot separate his or her fingers.

The length and shape of the pubic rami affect the transverse diameter of the outlet. The pubic ramus is expected to be short and concave inward, as opposed to straight and long.

The height and inclination of the symphysis pubis are measured, and the contour of the pubic arch is estimated. Excessively long or angulated bone structure shortens the diameter of

Figure 15–8 ◆ Use of a closed fist to measure the outlet. Most examiners know the distance between their first and last proximal knuckles. If they do not, they can use a measuring device.

Figure 15–9 ◆ Evaluation of the outlet. *A,* Estimation of the subpubic angle. *B,* Estimation of the length of the pubic ramus. *C,* Estimation of the depth and inclination of the pubis. *D,* Estimation of the contour of the subpubic angle.

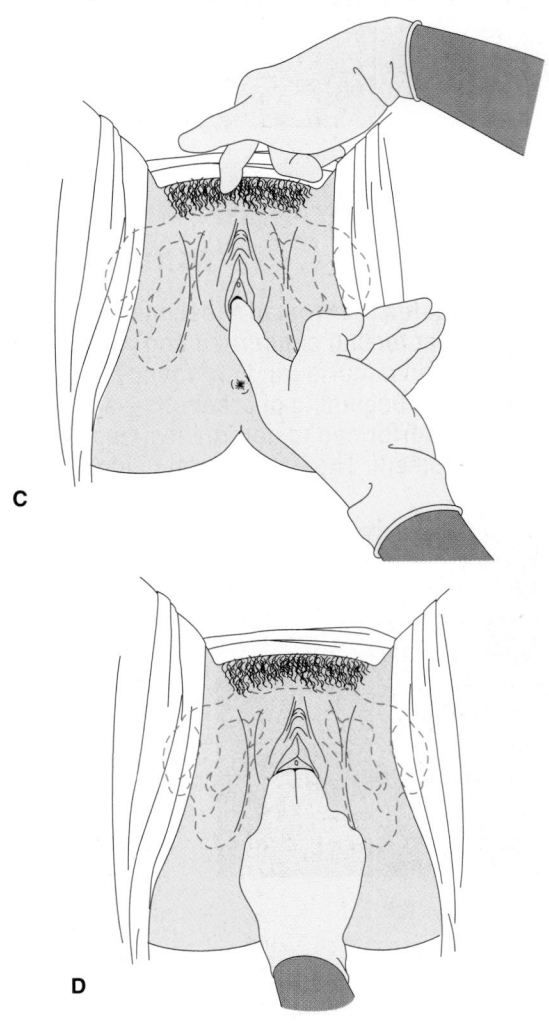

THROUGH THE EYES OF A NURSE

Prenatal Testing in Pregnancy

FAMILY'S EXPERIENCE: "I know there are things that can go wrong in pregnancy. Maybe I have just read too much, but I am really scared something is going to go wrong. How will you know if there is a problem?"

NURSE'S RESPONSE: "It is not uncommon to be nervous or scared about the baby and yourself. At your first visit, you remember that we asked you a lot of medical information and questions about your medical history, the medical history of the father of the baby, and questions about your social situation and environmental factors in your everyday life. This provides us with information to determine if there are problems that you may be at risk for developing.

"The physical exam and lab tests you have had done also allow us to look for underlying or developing complications. So far, all of your test results have been normal. We will continue monitoring you and the baby throughout the pregnancy to make sure things are progressing normally and that there are no concerns."

NURSE'S ACTIONS AND RATIONALE:

The nurse validates the woman's feelings and provides reassurance that feeling concerned and worried about problems that can occur during pregnancy are normal responses. In the beginning of pregnancy, a physical examination is performed to determine a baseline physical assessment. The assessment guide in this chapter reviews the physical examination, along with laboratory tests that are commonly performed. The nurse should also assess for cultural, educational, psychologic, and financial needs or concerns. A family assessment (discussed in Chapter 2 ∞) should also be performed during the pregnancy.

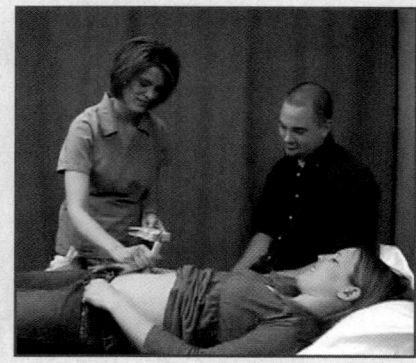

the obstetric conjugate. Height can be determined by placing the index finger of the gloved hand up to the superior border of the symphysis. The examiner should measure the length of the first phalanx of the index finger (normally about 2.5 cm). Inclination can be determined by externally placing one finger on the top of the symphysis while the internal finger palpates the internal margin. An imaginary line is drawn between the fingers, and the angle is estimated.

A posterior inclination with the lower border of the pubis slanting inward decreases the anteroposterior diameter. The anteroposterior sagittal diameter is the most significant diameter of the outlet because it is the shortest diameter through which the infant must pass. Estimating the contour of the pubic arch provides information on the width of the angle at which these bones come together. The pubic arch has obstetric importance; if it is narrow, the infant's head may be pushed backward toward the coccyx, making extension of the fetal head difficult, which may lengthen the second stage of labor.

Screening Tests

Many screening tests are routinely performed during pregnancy, either at the initial prenatal visit or at specified times during pregnancy. These include a Pap smear, a complete blood count, hemoglobin, rubella titer, ABO and Rh typing, and a hepatitis B screen as well as testing for sexually transmitted infections such as syphilis and gonorrhea. A sickle cell screen is provided for all women of African or Latino descent.

The urine is screened for abnormal findings initially and at each prenatal visit. In addition, a urine culture at 12 to 16 weeks of pregnancy is recommended for all pregnant women to detect asymptomatic bacteriuria (US Preventive Services Task Force, 2004). Other tests such as HIV screen and a drug screen are offered to all women.

Prenatal screening for cystic fibrosis is available. Originally the screening was offered before conception or in early pregnancy to Caucasian couples (including Ashkenazi Jews) because the condition is most common in those populations. However, ACOG (2005b) now recommends that cystic fibrosis carrier screening be offered to all couples regardless of ethnicity or race.

Multiple marker screening tests are available to help identify women at increased risk for certain genetic conditions. The *quadruple screen* (quad screen) is a safe, useful screening test performed on the mother's serum between weeks 15 and 20 of pregnancy. The test is used to detect levels of specific serum markers—alpha-fetoprotein (AFP), human chorionic gonadotropin (hCG), unconjugated estriol (UE), and inhibin-A (a placental hormone). (The quad test has replaced the triple screen, which did not include inhibin-A testing.) Test results that reveal higher than normal AFP levels might indicate a fetal neural tube defect, a multiple gestation, or a pregnancy that is farther along than believed. Lower than normal AFP could indicate that the woman is at risk for having a baby with Down syndrome or trisomy 18. Higher than normal levels of hCG and inhibin-A and lower than normal UE may also indicate that a woman is at increased risk of having a baby with Down syndrome. If the screening results are not in the normal range, follow-up testing

using ultrasound and amniocentesis is often indicated (Cleveland Clinic, 2004).

First trimester ultrasound assessment of the thickness of the fetal nuchal fold (called *nuchal translucency* [NT]) combined with a serum screen of pregnancy-associated plasma protein A (PAPP-A) is useful in detecting Down syndrome, trisomy 18, a variety of heart defects, and other abnormalities. Completed between 10 and 14 weeks' gestation, an NT measurement greater than 3 mm is abnormal (Lemon, 2004–2005). These tests are generally combined with second trimester quad screening. The combined protocol is more effective in identifying Down syndrome than the quad test alone and allows for first trimester detection, but the NT evaluation requires a skilled ultrasonographer and specialized training (Dolan, 2004). Some caregivers do not recommend a quad screen to women who have a negative NT and PAPP-A in the first trimester. Instead they are simply offered a test for maternal serum AFP to detect the risk of neural tube defects.

It is important for healthcare professionals to provide parents with factual information about the results of tests that detect chromosomal defects or fetal anomalies including the false-positive and detection rates and the implications of the findings (Nicolaides, 2005). Parents then need to decide on any course of action based on their own spiritual and cultural beliefs.

Between 24 and 28 weeks' gestation a 50-g 1-hour glucose screen is completed to detect gestational diabetes mellitus. Additional testing is indicated if abnormal results are obtained (see Chapter 19 ∞). Group B streptococcus (GBS) can cause serious problems for a newborn. Consequently rectal and vaginal swabs of the mother are obtained at 35 to 37 weeks' gestation to screen for the infection.

SUBSEQUENT CLIENT HISTORY

At subsequent prenatal visits, the nurse continues to gather data about the family's adjustment to the pregnancy and the course of the pregnancy to date. The nurse asks the pregnant woman how she thinks the pregnancy is progressing. In what ways is it the same as her expectations, and how is it different? The nurse also asks about the adjustment of the support person and expectations of the support person and other children, if any, in the family. As the pregnancy progresses, the nurse asks about preparations the family has made for the new baby. Taking time to address psychosocial issues is necessary in helping the nurse assess the family's success in meeting their developmental tasks.

The nurse also asks specifically whether the woman has experienced any discomfort, especially the kinds of discomfort that are often seen at specific times during a pregnancy. The nurse inquires about physical changes that relate directly to the pregnancy, such as the woman's perception of fetal movement. Other pertinent information includes any exposure to contagious illnesses, medical treatment and therapy prescribed for nonpregnancy problems since the last visit, and any prescription, over-the-counter medications, or herbal supplements that were not prescribed as part of the woman's prenatal care.

RESEARCH IN PRACTICE

PRENATALLY DIAGNOSED DOWN SYNDROME: MOTHERS WHO CONTINUED THEIR PREGNANCIES EVALUATE THEIR HEALTHCARE PROVIDER

What is this study about? A diagnosis of Down syndrome can now be confirmed in a fetus in the first trimester of pregnancy. There is inconsistency, though, about how this diagnosis should be communicated to the pregnant mother. One study showed that doctors tend to emphasize the negative in communicating that a fetus is affected by Down syndrome; fewer than 15% of physicians emphasized the positive so that parents would be more likely to continue the pregnancy. The mother who decides to continue the pregnancy after prenatal identification of Down syndrome may find it difficult to find support for her decision. The purpose of this study was to examine the way that a prenatal diagnosis of Down syndrome is communicated, and how this communication could be improved.

How was this study done? This study was part of a larger epidemiological study of prenatal and postnatal support for mothers who have children with Down syndrome in the United States and in Spain. Participants were recruited from five organized family support groups, selected because of their size and geographic distribution. Survey packets were sent to the members of the support groups; the packets included a questionnaire developed for this specific study. The survey instrument gathered both quantitative and qualitative data directly from mothers only, using scales and open-ended questions.

What were the results of the study? A total of 1250 responses were received, which represented a 42.4% response rate. The majority reported feeling anxious and scared about the results of the antenatal testing. Many indicated that their physician did not explain Down syndrome adequately, either before or after the testing. About half felt rushed or pressured into making a decision about continuing the pregnancy. Analysis revealed that the level of a mother's fear was related to the amount of pressure she perceived. A minority of mothers felt positive about the experience, but for these, satisfaction was associated with providers who explained the results in an understandable manner and who presented a discussion that balanced positive aspects of Down syndrome with negative ones. Nearly all mothers strongly agreed that physicians should give their personal opinions about what to do in a similar situation. A mother's conscience was the primary influence on continuing the pregnancy, followed by religious influence and influence of her partner's opinion. Overall, most mothers found printed material about Down syndrome to be helpful. Mothers agreed that their physician was supportive of their decision once it had been made and communicated. Respondents recommended that the experience would be improved if physicians would clearly explain the screening tests, deliver the results in person, and provide balanced information about Down syndrome. These mothers recalled that contact information about local Down syndrome support groups was helpful. The use of consistent, sensitive language was also suggested; these respondents noted that beginning the conversation with "I'm sorry . . . " or "I have bad news . . . " reinforces negative aspects of Down syndrome.

What additional questions might I have? These results were limited to the mothers of Down syndrome babies; would other family members have different opinions? How would these suggestions differ for women who elected to terminate the pregnancy after the antenatal diagnosis?

How can I use this study? Receiving an antenatal diagnosis of fetal Down syndrome is a dramatic event for a woman, and the nurse can be instrumental in counseling mothers about their options. The nurse should focus on giving information in a way that is sensitive, balanced, and honest and that incorporates printed materials that can be used later for reference. Once the mother has made a decision to continue the pregnancy, the nurse's role becomes one of support for the decision and help in finding support groups or other resources.

Skotko, B. (2005) Prenatally diagnosed Down syndrome: Mothers who continued their pregnancies evaluate their health care providers. *American Journal of Obstetrics and Gynecology, 192,* 670–677.

The danger signs that a woman should report immediately are generally discussed during the initial prenatal visit and reviewed when she comes for her second prenatal visit. Many caregivers also provide printed information on the subject written in lay terms. Table 15–3 identifies the danger signs of pregnancy and possible causes for each.

Periodic prenatal examinations offer the nurse an opportunity to assess the childbearing woman's psychologic needs and emotional status. If the woman's partner attends the prenatal visits, his or her needs and concerns can also be identified.

The interchange between the nurse and woman will be facilitated if it takes place in a friendly, trusting environment. The nurse should give the woman sufficient time to ask questions and to air concerns. If the nurse provides the time and demonstrates genuine interest, the woman will feel more at ease bringing up questions that she may believe are silly or concerns that she has been afraid to verbalize. The nurse who has an accurate understanding of all the changes of pregnancy is most able to answer questions and provide information. See the foldout color chart, "Maternal-Fetal Development," for vivid illustrations of some of this information.

The nurse should also be sensitive to religious, spiritual, cultural, and socioeconomic factors that may influence a family's response to pregnancy, as well as to the woman's expectations of the healthcare system. The nurse can avoid stereotyping clients simply by asking each woman about her expectations for the antepartal period. Although many women's responses may reflect what are thought to be traditional norms, other women will have decidedly different views or may have expectations that represent a blending of beliefs or cultures.

Table 15–3 DANGER SIGNS IN PREGNANCY

The woman should report the following danger signs in pregnancy immediately.

Danger Sign	Possible Cause
Sudden gush of fluid from vagina	Premature rupture of membranes
Vaginal bleeding	Abruptio placentae, placenta previa
	Lesions of cervix or vagina
	"Bloody show"
Abdominal pain	Premature labor, abruptio placentae
Temperature above 38.3C (101F) and chills	Infection
Dizziness, blurring of vision, double vision, spots before eyes	Hypertension, preeclampsia
Persistent vomiting	Hyperemesis gravidarum
Severe headache	Hypertension, preeclampsia
Edema of hands, face, legs, and feet	Preeclampsia
Muscular irritability, convulsions	Preeclampsia, eclampsia
Epigastric pain	Preeclampsia, ischemia in major abdominal vessel
Oliguria	Renal impairment, decreased fluid intake
Dysuria	Urinary tract infection
Absence of fetal movement	Maternal medication, obesity, fetal death

COMPLEMENTARY AND ALTERNATIVE THERAPIES

YOGA DURING PREGNANCY

The following advice is important for women who practice yoga during pregnancy (Fontaine, 2005):

- During pregnancy, some yoga poses or positions are contraindicated. In particular pregnant women should avoid those poses that put pressure on the uterus as well as any extreme stretching positions.
- Because of the changed center of gravity that occurs as pregnancy progresses, women need to be especially careful to maintain balance when doing stretching.
- Pregnant women should avoid stomach-lying for any poses. After 20 weeks' gestation, women should lie on their left side rather than their back for floor positions.
- Pregnant women should immediately stop any pose that is uncomfortable.
- Warning signs that indicate the need to contact the physician or certified nurse-midwife immediately include the following: dizziness, extreme shortness of breath, sudden swelling, vaginal bleeding.

During the prenatal period, it is essential that the nurse begin assessing the developing readiness of the woman (and her partner, if possible) to take on the responsibilities of parenthood successfully. Table 15–4 identifies areas for assessment and provides some sample questions the nurse might use to obtain necessary information. If the woman's responses are primarily negative, the nurse can plan interventions for the prenatal and postpartal periods.

SUBSEQUENT PRENATAL ASSESSMENT

The Subsequent Prenatal Assessment Guide, which begins on page 361, provides a systematic approach to the regular physical examinations the pregnant woman should undergo for optimal prenatal care and a model for evaluating both the pregnant woman and the expectant father, if he is involved in the pregnancy.

CLINICAL TIP

When assessing blood pressure, have the pregnant woman sit up with her arm resting on a table so that her arm is at the level of her heart. Expect a decrease in her blood pressure from baseline during the second trimester because of normal physiologic changes. If this decrease does not occur, evaluate further for signs of preeclampsia.

The woman's individual needs and the assessment of her risks should determine the frequency of subsequent visits. Generally, the recommended frequency of prenatal visits is as follows:

- Every 4 weeks for the first 28 weeks of gestation
- Every 2 weeks until 36 weeks' gestation
- After week 36, every week until childbirth

During the subsequent antepartal assessments, most women demonstrate ongoing psychologic adjustment to pregnancy and ever-improving coping skills. However, some women may exhibit signs of psychologic problems. These signs may include one or more of the following:

- Increasing anxiety
- Depression or feelings of sadness
- Inability to establish communication
- Inappropriate responses or actions
- Denial of pregnancy
- Inability to cope with stress
- Intense preoccupation with the sex of the baby
- Failure to acknowledge quickening
- Failure to plan and prepare for the baby (for example, living arrangements, clothing, feeding methods)
- Indications of substance abuse

If the woman's behavior indicates possible psychologic problems, the nurse should provide ongoing support and counseling and also refer the woman to appropriate professionals.

Table 15–4   GUIDE TO PRENATAL ASSESSMENT OF PARENTING

Areas Assessed	Sample Questions
I. Perception of complexities of mothering A. Desires baby for itself Positive: 1. Feels positive about pregnancy Negative: 1. Wants baby to meet own needs such as someone to love her, someone to get her out of unhappy home	1. Did you plan on getting pregnant? 2. How do you feel about being pregnant? 3. Why do you want this baby?
B. Expresses concern about impact of mothering role on other roles (wife, career, school) Positive: 1. Realistic expectations of how baby will affect job, career, school, and personal goals 2. Interested in learning about child care Negative: 1. Feels pregnancy and baby will make no emotional, physical, or social demands on self 2. Has no insight that mothering role will affect other roles or lifestyle	1. What do you think it will be like to take care of a baby? 2. How do you think your life will be different after you have your baby? 3. How do you feel this baby will affect your job, career, school, and personal goals? 4. How will the baby affect your relationship with your boyfriend or husband? 5. Have you done any reading, baby-sitting, or made any things for a baby?
C. Gives up routine habits because "not good for baby" (e.g., quits smoking, adjusts time schedule) Positive: 1. Gives up routines not good for baby (quits smoking, adjusts eating habits)	
II. Attachment A. Strong feelings regarding sex of baby. Why? Positive: 1. Verbalizes positive thoughts about the baby Negative: 1. Baby will be like negative aspects of self and partner	1. Why do you prefer a certain sex? (Is reason inappropriate for a baby?) 2. Note comments client makes about baby not being normal and why client feels this way.
B. Interested in data regarding fetus (e.g., growth and development, heart tones) Positive: 1. As above Negative: 1. Shows no interest in fetal growth and development, quickening, and fetal heart tones 2. Expresses negative feelings about fetus by rejecting counseling regarding nutrition, rest, hygiene	
C. Fantasies about baby Positive: 1. Follows cultural norms regarding preparation 2. Time of attachment behaviors appropriate to her history of pregnancy loss Negative: 1. Bonding conditional depending on sex, age of baby, and/or labor and birth experience 2. Woman considers only own needs when making plans for baby 3. Exhibits no attachment behaviors after critical period of previous pregnancy 4. Failure to follow cultural norms regarding preparation	1. What did you think or feel when you first felt the baby move? 2. Have you started preparing for the baby? 3. What do you think your baby will look like—what age do you see your baby at? 4. How would you like your new baby to look?
III. Acceptance of child by significant others A. Acknowledges acceptance by significant other of the new responsibility inherent in child Positive: 1. Acknowledges unconditional acceptance of pregnancy and baby by significant others 2. Partner accepts new responsibility inherent with child 3. Timely sharing of experience of pregnancy with significant others	1. How does your partner feel about this pregnancy? 2. How do your parents feel? 3. What do your friends think? 4. Does your partner have a preference regarding the baby's sex? Why? 5. How does your partner feel about being a father? 6. What do you think he'll be like as a father?

Table 15–4   GUIDE TO PRENATAL ASSESSMENT OF PARENTING continued

Areas Assessed	Sample Questions
Negative:	7. What do you think he'll do to help you with child care?
1. Significant others not supportively involved with pregnancy	8. Have you and your partner talked about how the baby might change your lives?
2. Conditional acceptance of pregnancy depending on sex, race, age of baby	9. Who have you told about your pregnancy?
3. Decision making does not take in needs of fetus (e.g., spends food money on new car)	
4. Takes no/little responsibility for needs of pregnancy, woman/fetus	
B. Concrete demonstration of acceptance of pregnancy/baby by significant others (e.g., baby shower, significant other involved prenatal education)	
Positive:	1. Note if partner attends clinic with client (degree of interest; e.g., listens to heart tones). Significant other plans to be with client during labor and birth.
1. Baby shower	2. Is your partner contributing financially?
2. Significant other attends prenatal class with client	
IV. Ensures physical well-being	
A. Concerns about having normal pregnancy, labor and birth, and baby	
1. Preparing for labor and birth, attends prenatal classes, interested in labor and birth	1. What have you heard about labor and birth?
2. Aware of danger signs of pregnancy	2. Note data about client's reaction to prenatal class.
3. Seeks and uses appropriate health care (e.g., time of initial visit, keeps appointments, follows through on recommendations)	
Negative:	
1. Denies signs and symptoms that might suggest complications of pregnancy	
2. Verbalizes extreme fear of labor and birth—refuses to talk about labor and birth	
3. Misses appointments, fails to follow instructions, refuses to attend prenatal classes	
B. Family/client decisions reflect concern for health of mother and baby (e.g., use of finances, time)	
Positive:	
1. As above	

NOTE: When "Negative" is not listed in a section, the reader may assume that negative is the absence of positive responses.

SOURCE: Modified and used with permission of the Minneapolis Health Dept., Minneapolis, MN.

ASSESSMENT GUIDE   Subsequent Prenatal Assessment

PHYSICAL ASSESSMENT/ NORMAL FINDINGS	ALTERATIONS AND POSSIBLE CAUSES*	NURSING RESPONSES TO DATA†
VITAL SIGNS		
Temperature: 36.2–37.6C (97–99.6F)	Elevated temperature (infection)	Evaluate for signs of infection. Refer to healthcare provider.
Pulse: 60–90/min Rate may increase 10 beats/min during pregnancy	Increased pulse rate (anxiety, cardiac disorders)	Note irregularities. Assess for anxiety and stress.
Respiration: 12–22/min	Marked tachypnea or abnormal patterns (respiratory disease)	Refer to healthcare provider.
Blood pressure: Less than or equal to 135/85 (falls in second trimester)	Greater than 140/90 or increase of 30 mm systolic and 15 mm diastolic (preeclampsia)	Assess for edema, proteinuria, and hyperreflexia. Refer to healthcare provider. Schedule appointments more frequently.
	*Possible causes of alterations are identified in parentheses.	†This column provides guidelines for further nursing assessment and initial intervention.

(Continued on next page)

ASSESSMENT GUIDE   Subsequent Prenatal Assessment continued

Physical Assessment/ Normal Findings	Alterations and Possible Causes*	Nursing Responses to Data†
WEIGHT GAIN *First trimester:* 1.6–2.3 kg (3.5–5 lb) *Second trimester:* 5.5–6.8 kg (12–15 lb) *Third trimester:* 5.5–6.8 kg (12–15 lb)	Inadequate weight gain (poor nutrition, nausea, IUGR) Excessive weight gain (excessive caloric intake, edema, preeclampsia)	Discuss appropriate weight gain. Provide nutritional counseling. Assess for presence of edema or anemia.
EDEMA Small amount of dependent edema, especially in last weeks of pregnancy	Edema in hands, face, legs, and feet (preeclampsia)	Identify any correlation between edema and activities, blood pressure, or proteinuria: Refer to healthcare provider if indicated.
UTERINE SIZE See "Assessment Guide: Initial Prenatal Assessment" for normal changes during pregnancy	Unusually rapid growth (multiple gestation, hydatidiform mole, hydramnios, miscalculation of EDB)	Evaluate fetal status. Determine height of fundus (page 352). Use diagnostic ultrasound.
FETAL HEARTBEAT 120–160/min Funic souffle	Absence of fetal heartbeat after 20 weeks' gestation (maternal obesity, fetal demise)	Evaluate fetal status.
LABORATORY EVALUATION *Hemoglobin:* 12–16 g/dL Pseudoanemia of pregnancy	Greater than 11 g/dL (anemia)	Provide nutritional counseling. Hemoglobin is repeated at 7 months' gestation. Women of Mediterranean heritage need a close check on hemoglobin because of possibility of thalassemia.
Quad marker screen: Blood test performed at 15–20 weeks' gestation. Evaluates four factors—maternal serum alpha-fetoprotein (MSAFP), unconjugated estriol (UE), hCG, and inhibin-A: normal levels	Elevated MSAFP (neural tube defect, underestimated gestational age, multiple gestation). Lower than normal MSAFP (Down syndrome, trisomy 18). Higher than normal hCG and inhibin-A (Down syndrome). Lower than normal UE (Down syndrome).	Recommended for all pregnant women; especially indicated for women with any of the following risk factors: age 35 and over, family history of birth defects, previous child with a birth defect; insulin-dependent diabetes prior to pregnancy (Cleveland Clinic, 2004). If quad screen abnormal further testing such as ultrasound or amniocentesis may be indicated.
Indirect Coombs test done on Rh negative women: Negative (done at 28 weeks' gestation)	Rh antibodies present (maternal sensitization has occurred)	If Rh negative and unsensitized, Rh immune globulin given (see Chapter 20 ∞). If Rh antibodies present, Rh immune globulin not given; fetus monitored closely for isoimmune hemolytic disease. Discuss implications of GDM. Refer for a diagnostic 100 g oral glucose tolerance test.
50-g 1-hour glucose screen (done between 24 and 28 weeks' gestation)	Plasma glucose level greater than 140 mg/dL (gestational diabetes mellitus [GDM]) *Note:* Some facilities use level greater than 130 mg/dL, which identifies 90% of women with GDM (American Diabetes Association, 2004)	
Urinalysis: See "Assessment Guide: Initial Prenatal Assessment" for normal findings *Protein:* Negative	See "Assessment Guide: Initial Prenatal Assessment" for deviations Proteinuria, albuminuria (contamination by vaginal discharge, urinary tract infection, preeclampsia)	Repeat urinalysis at 7 months' gestation. Repeat dipstick test at each visit. Obtain dipstick urine sample. Refer to healthcare provider if deviations are present.
	*Possible causes of alterations are identified in parentheses.	†This column provides guidelines for further nursing assessment and initial intervention.

ASSESSMENT GUIDE   Subsequent Prenatal Assessment continued

PHYSICAL ASSESSMENT/ NORMAL FINDINGS	ALTERATIONS AND POSSIBLE CAUSES*	NURSING RESPONSES TO DATA†
LABORATORY EVALUATION (continued)		
Glucose: Negative	Persistent glycosuria (diabetes mellitus)	Refer to healthcare provider.
Note: Glycosuria may be present due to physiologic alterations in glomerular filtration rate and renal threshold		
Screening for Group B streptococcus (GBS):	Positive culture (maternal infection)	Explain maternal and fetal/neonatal risks (see Chapter 20 ∞).
Rectal and vaginal swabs obtained at 35–37 weeks' gestation for all pregnant women (Centers for Disease Control and Prevention [CDC], 2002).		Refer to healthcare provider for therapy.

CULTURAL ASSESSMENT	VARIATIONS TO CONSIDER*	NURSING RESPONSES TO DATA†
Determine the mother's (and family's) attitudes about the sex of the unborn child.	Some women have no preference about the sex of the child; others do. In many cultures, boys are especially valued as firstborn children.	Provide opportunities to discuss preferences and expectations; avoid a judgmental attitude to the response.
Ask about the woman's expectations of childbirth. Will she want someone with her for the birth? Whom does she choose? What is the role of her partner?	Some women want their partner present for labor and birth; others prefer a female relative or friend. Some women expect to be separated from their partner once cervical dilation has occured.	Provide information on birth options but accept the woman's decision about who will attend.
Ask about preparations for the baby. Determine what is customary for the woman.	Some women may have a fully prepared nursery; others may not have a separate room for the baby.	Explore reasons for not preparing for the baby. Support the mother's preferences and provide information about possible sources of assistance if the decision is related to a lack of resources.

EXPECTANT MOTHER		
Psychologic Status	Increased stress and anxiety	Encourage woman to take an active part in her care.
First trimester: Incorporates idea of pregnancy; may feel ambivalent, especially if she must give up desired role; usually looks for signs of verification of pregnancy, such as increase in abdominal size or fetal movement	Inability to establish communication; inability to accept pregnancy; inappropriate response or actions; denial of pregnancy; inability to cope	Establish lines of communication. Establish a trusting relationship. Counsel as necessary. Refer to appropriate professional as needed.
Second trimester: Baby becomes more real to woman as abdominal size increases and she feels movement; she begins to turn inward, becoming more introspective		
Third trimester: Begins to think of baby as separate being; may feel restless and may feel that time of labor will never come; remains self-centered and concentrates on preparing place for baby		
Educational needs **Self-care measures and knowledge about the following:**	Inadequate information	Provide information and counseling.
Health promotion		
Breast care		
Hygiene		
Rest		
	*Possible causes of alterations are identified in parentheses.	†This column provides guidelines for further nursing assessment and initial intervention.

(Continued on next page)

ASSESSMENT GUIDE   Subsequent Prenatal Assessment continued

CULTURAL ASSESSMENT	VARIATIONS TO CONSIDER*	NURSING RESPONSES TO DATA†
EXPECTANT MOTHER (continued)		
Exercise		
Nutrition		
Relief measures for common discomforts of pregnancy		
Danger signs in pregnancy (see Table 15–3)		
Sexual activity: Woman knows how pregnancy affects sexual activity	Lack of information about effects of pregnancy and/or alternative positions during sexual intercourse	Provide counseling.
Preparation for parenting: Appropriate preparation	Lack of preparation (denial, failure to adjust to baby, unwanted child)	Counsel. If lack of preparation is due to inadequacy of information, provide information.
Preparation for childbirth *Client aware of the following:*		If couple chooses particular technique refer to classes (see page 303 in Chapter 13 ∞ for description of childbirth preparation techniques).
1. Prepared childbirth techniques		
2. Normal processes and changes during childbirth		Encourage prenatal class attendance. Educate woman during visits based on current physical status. Provide reading list for more specific information.
3. Problems that may occur as a result of drug and alcohol use and of smoking	Continued abuse of drugs and alcohol; denial of possible effect on self and baby	Review danger signs that were presented on initial visit.
Woman has met other physician or nurse-midwife who may be attending her birth in the absence of primary caregiver	Introduction of new individual at birth may increase stress and anxiety for woman and partner	Introduce woman to all members of group practice.
Impending labor *Client knows signs of impending labor:*	Lack of information	Provide appropriate teaching, stressing importance of seeking appropriate medical assistance.
1. Uterine contractions that increase in frequency, duration, and intensity		
2. Bloody show		
3. Expulsion of mucous plug		
4. Rupture of membranes		
EXPECTANT FATHER		
Psychologic status		
First trimester: May express excitement over confirmation of pregnancy and of his virility; concerns move toward providing for financial needs; energetic, may identify with some discomforts of pregnancy and may even exhibit symptoms	Increasing stress and anxiety; inability to establish communication; inability to accept pregnancy diagnosis; withdrawal of support; abandonment of the mother	Encourage expectant father to come to prenatal visits. Establish line of communication. Establish trusting relationship.
Second trimester: May feel more confident and be less concerned with financial matters; may have concerns about wife's changing size and shape, her increasing introspection		Counsel. Let expectant father know that it is normal for him to experience these feelings.
Third trimester: May have feelings of rivalry with fetus, especially during sexual activity; may make changes in his physical appearance and exhibit more interest in himself; may become more energetic; fantasizes about child but usually imagines older child; fears mutilation and death of woman and child		Include expectant father in pregnancy activities as he desires. Provide education, information, and support. Increasing numbers of expectant fathers are demonstrating desire to be involved in many or all aspects of prenatal care, education, and preparation.
	*Possible causes of alterations are identified in parentheses.	† This column provides guidelines for further nursing assessment and initial intervention.

CHAPTER REVIEW

FOCUS YOUR STUDY

- A complete history forms the basis of prenatal care and is reevaluated and updated as necessary throughout the pregnancy.

- The initial prenatal assessment is a careful and thorough physical examination and cultural and psychosocial assessment designed to identify variations and potential risk factors.

- Laboratory tests completed at the initial visit, such as a complete blood count, ABO and Rh typing, urinalysis, Pap smear, chlamydia culture, gonorrhea culture, rubella titer, and various blood screens (such as rapid plasma reagin [RPR], HIV, and hepatitis B), provide information about the woman's health during early pregnancy and also help detect potential problems.

- The estimated date of birth (EDB) can be calculated using Nägele's rule. Using this approach, one begins with the first day of the last menstrual period, subtracts 3 months, and adds 7 days. A "wheel" may also be used to calculate the EDB.

- Accuracy of the EDB may be evaluated by physical examination to assess uterine size, measurement of fundal height, and ultrasound. Perception of quickening and auscultation of fetal heartbeat are also useful tools in confirming the gestation of a pregnancy.

- The diagonal conjugate is the distance from the lower posterior border of the symphysis pubis to the sacral promontory. The obstetric conjugate is estimated by subtracting 1.5 to 2 cm from the length of the diagonal conjugate.

- As part of the assessment of the pelvic cavity (midpelvis), the prominence of the ischial spines is assessed, the sacrosciatic notch and the length of the sacrospinous ligament are measured, and the shape of the pelvic side walls is evaluated. Finally, the hollowness of the sacrum is determined.

- The anteroposterior diameter of the pelvic outlet is determined, the mobility of the coccyx is assessed, the suprapubic angle is estimated, and the contour of the pubic arch is evaluated to assess the adequacy of the pelvic outlet.

- The nurse begins evaluating the woman psychosocially during the initial prenatal assessment. This assessment continues and is modified throughout the pregnancy.

- Cultural and ethnic beliefs may strongly influence the woman's attitudes and apparent cooperation with care during pregnancy.

EXPLORE MEDIALINK

 http://www.prenhall.com/davidson

NCLEX review questions, case studies, and other interactive resources for this chapter can be found on the Web Site at http://www.prenhall.com/davidson. Click on "Chapter 15" to select the activities for this chapter.

For tutorials including animations and videos, more NCLEX review questions, and an audio glossary, access the accompanying Prentice Hall Nursing MediaLink DVD-ROM in this book.

 PRENTICE HALL NURSING MEDIALINK DVD-ROM

Audio Glossary

NCLEX Review

Videos: *Through the Eyes of a Nurse—The First Trimester; Through the Eyes of a Nurse—The Second Trimester; Through the Eyes of a Nurse—The Third Trimester*

 COMPANION WEBSITE

Additional NCLEX Review

Case Study: *Initial Prenatal Assessment*

Care Plan Activity: *Initial Assessment of Primigravida*

Application: *Ovulation Calculator*

Critical Thinking

CRITICAL THINKING IN ACTION

HEALTHY PREGNANCY SIGNS

View the Critical Thinking in Action video in Chapter 15 of the DVD-ROM. Then answer the questions that follow.

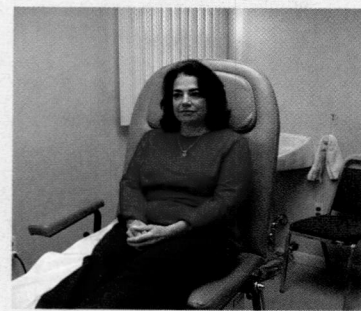
Wendy Stodard, age 40, G3, P0020 comes to the obstetrician's office where you are working for a prenatal visit. Wendy has experienced two spontaneous abortions followed by a D&C at 14 and 15 weeks' gestation during the previous year. She has a history of *Chlamydia trachomatis* infection 3 years ago, which was treated with azithromycin. She is at 10 weeks' gestation. Wendy tells you that she is afraid of losing this pregnancy as she did previously. She says that she has been experiencing some mild nausea, breast tenderness, and fatigue, which did not occur with her other pregnancies. You assist the obstetrician with an ultrasound. The gestational sac is clearly seen, fetal heartbeat is observed, and crown-to-rump measurements are consistent with gestational age of 10 weeks. The pelvic exam demonstrates a closed cervix, and positive Goodell's, Hegar's, and Chadwick's signs. You discuss with Wendy the signs of a healthy pregnancy.

1. What signs are reassuring with this pregnancy?
2. What symptoms should be reported to the obstetrician immediately?
3. What is the frequency of antepartal visits?

REFERENCES

American College of Obstetricians and Gynecologists. (2005a). *Racial and ethnic disparities in women's health* (ACOG Committee Opinion No. 317). Washington, DC: Author.

American College of Obstetricians and Gynecologists. (2005b). Update on carrier screening for cystic fibrosis (ACOG Committee Opinion No. 325). Washington, DC: Author.

American Diabetes Association. (2004). Position statement: Gestational diabetes mellitus. *Diabetes Care, 27*(Suppl. 1), 80–91.

Centers for Disease Control and Prevention. (2002). Prevention of perinatal group B streptococcal disease: Revised guidelines from the CDC. *Morbidity and Mortality Weekly Reports, 51*(RR-11), 1–22.

Cleveland Clinic. (2004). *Quad marker screen.* Retrieved April 10, 2004, from http://www.cchs.net/health/health-info/docs/0300/0386.asp?index54698

Cunningham, F. G., Leveno, K. J., Bloom, S. L., Hauth, J. C., Gilstrap, L. C., III, & Wenstrom, K. D. (2005). *Williams obstetrics* (22nd ed.). New York: McGraw-Hill.

Dolan, S. (2004). New approaches to screening for Down syndrome. *Medscape Ob/Gyn and Women's Health, 9*(1). Retrieved April 2, 2004, from http://www.medscape.com/viewarticle/469782_print

Fontaine, K. L. (2005). *Healing practices: Alternative therapies for nursing* (2nd ed.). Upper Saddle River, NJ: Prentice Hall Health.

Lemon, B. S. (2004–2005). Nuchal translucency for prenatal screening? What nurses need to know about this tool. *AWHONN Lifelines, 8*(6), 520–526.

Nicolaides, K. H. (2005). First-trimester screening for chromosomal abnormalities. *Seminars in Perinatology, 29,* 190–194.

US Preventive Services Task Force. (2004). *Recommendation statement: Screening for asymptomatic bacteriuria.* Retrieved February 20, 2006, from http://www.ahrq.gov/clinic/3rduspstf/asymbac/ asymbacrs.htm

Varney, H., Kriebs, J. M., & Gegor, C. L. (2004). *Varney's midwifery* (4th ed.). Sudbury, MA: Jones & Bartlett.

16 The Expectant Family: Needs and Care

I don't know how I timed it, but my nursing program OB rotation finishes up right about my due date. Watching all the births during my clinicals has been really exciting. The labor and delivery nurses laugh and say my hormones should be hopping now, but I think this baby is subliminally telling me that we won't "hatch" until I take my final exam!

OBJECTIVES

1. Describe the significance of using the nursing process to promote health in the woman and her family during pregnancy.

2. Describe actions the nurse can take to help maintain the well-being of the expectant father and siblings during a family's pregnancy.

3. Discuss the significance of cultural considerations in managing nursing care during pregnancy.

4. Explain the causes of the common discomforts of pregnancy.

5. Summarize appropriate measures to alleviate the common discomforts of pregnancy.

6. Delineate self-care actions a pregnant woman and her family can take to maintain and promote well-being during each trimester of pregnancy.

7. Identify some of the concerns that an expectant couple may have about sexual activity.

8. Describe factors that have contributed to the increased incidence of pregnancy in women over age 35.

9. Compare similarities and differences in the needs of expectant women in various age groups.

KEY TERMS

Fetal alcohol syndrome (FAS) 396

Fetal movement record (FMR) 383

Kegel exercises 390

Leukorrhea 378

Lightening 382

Pelvic tilt 389

Ptyalism 379

Teratogens 392

MEDIALINK

Additional resources for this content can be found on the Prentice Hall Nursing MediaLink DVD-ROM and on the Companion Website at http//www.prenhall.com/davidson. Click on "Chapter 16" to select the activities for this chapter.

From the moment a woman finds out that she is pregnant, she faces a future marked by dramatic changes. Her appearance will be altered. Her relationships will change. She will experience a variety of unique physical changes throughout the pregnancy. Even her psychologic state will be affected. In coping with these changes she needs to make adjustments in her daily life.

Her family must also adjust to the pregnancy. Roles and responsibilities of family members will change as the woman's ability to perform certain activities changes. They too must adapt psychologically to the situation.

The expectant woman and her family will probably have many questions about the pregnancy and its impact on her and the other members of the family. In addition, the daily activities and healthcare practices of the woman become of concern when she and her family realize that what she does can affect the well-being of the unborn child.

Nurses caring for pregnant women need a clear understanding of pregnancy and the changes it brings if they are to be effective in managing nursing care. With this in mind, Chapter 14 provides a database for the nurse by presenting material related to the normal physical, psychologic, social, and cultural changes of pregnancy. Chapter 15 then uses that database to begin a discussion of nursing care management by focusing on client assessment. This chapter further addresses nursing care management as it relates to the needs of the expectant woman and her loved ones.

NURSING CARE DURING THE PRENATAL PERIOD

Nursing Diagnosis

The nurse may see a pregnant woman only once every 4 to 6 weeks during the first several months of her pregnancy. To ensure continuity of care, therefore, a written care plan that incorporates assessment data, nursing diagnoses, and client goals is essential.

The nurse can anticipate that, for many women with a low-risk pregnancy, certain nursing diagnoses will be made more frequently than others will. Nursing diagnoses will, of course, vary from woman to woman and according to the time in the pregnancy. Examples of common nursing diagnoses include the following:

- *Constipation* related to the physiologic effects of pregnancy
- *Ineffective Sexuality Patterns* related to discomfort during late pregnancy

After formulating an appropriate diagnosis, the nurse establishes related goals to guide the nursing plan and interventions.

Nursing Plan and Implementation

Once nursing diagnoses have been identified, the next step is to establish priorities of nursing care. Sometimes priorities of care are based on the most immediate needs or concerns perceived by the woman. For example, during the first trimester, a woman is probably not ready to hear about labor and birth because she is likely to have more immediate concerns, such as nausea or concerns about sexual intimacy with her partner.

At other times priorities may develop as a result of findings during a prenatal visit. For example, the nurse may stress the need for frequent rest periods for a woman who is showing signs of preeclampsia (a pregnancy complication discussed in Chapter 20 ∞). However, the woman may feel well physically and find it difficult to accept the nurse's emphasis on rest. It is the responsibility of medical and nursing professionals to help the woman and her family understand the significance of a problem and to plan appropriate interventions to deal with it.

The intervention methods most used by nurses in caring for the expectant woman and her family are communication techniques and teaching-learning strategies. These intervention methods are often used in groups, such as early pregnancy classes and childbirth education classes, but the nurse in the prenatal setting also applies these techniques with individuals.

COMMUNITY-BASED NURSING CARE

Prenatal care, especially for women with low-risk pregnancies, is community based, typically in a clinic or private office. The healthcare community recognizes the value of providing a primary care nurse in these settings to coordinate care for each childbearing family. The nurse in a clinic or health maintenance organization (HMO) may be the only source of continuity for the woman, who may see a different physician or certified nurse-midwife at each visit. The nurse can be extremely effective in working with the expectant family by answering their questions; providing them with complete information about pregnancy, appropriate prenatal self-care measures, and community resources or referral agencies; and supporting the healthcare activities of the woman and her family. Communities often have a wealth of services and educational opportunities available for pregnant women and their families, and the knowledgeable nurse can help the woman access these services. This allows the family to assume equal responsibility with healthcare providers in working toward their common goal of a positive childbearing experience.

Home Care

Home care can be of benefit to any pregnant woman, but it is especially effective in removing barriers for women who have difficulty accessing health care. These barriers may include lack of locally available healthcare facilities, problems with transportation to the facility, or schedule conflicts with available appointment times because of employment hours or family responsibilities.

In-home nursing assessments vary according to the scope of practice of the nurse and include current history and those screening procedures typically completed in an office or clinic: vital signs, weight, urine screen, physical activity, and dietary intake. Advanced practice nurses can also assess reflexes, perform tests of fetal well-being, and even do cervical examinations. Once the assessments are completed, the nurse can determine the level of follow-up home care or telephone contact needed.

A prenatal home care visit or phone contact can also be useful for women who anticipate a short inpatient stay after childbirth. At the prenatal contact, the nurse explains the postpartum program and answers any questions the woman or her family has.

Although the use of home care for women with uncomplicated pregnancies is growing, it is most often used for women with prenatal complications that can be managed without hospitalization if effective nursing assessment and care are provided in the home (see Chapters 19 ∞ and 20 ∞).

TEACHING FOR SELF-CARE

Throughout the prenatal period the nurse provides informal and formal teaching to the childbearing family designed to help the family carry out self-care when appropriate and to report changes that may indicate a possible health problem. The teaching is most effective if timed to coincide with the woman's (couple's) readiness and needs (Table 16–1). The nurse also provides anticipatory guidance to help the family plan for changes that will occur following childbirth. The expectant couple should discuss issues that could be possible sources of postpartal stress.

Table 16–1	TOPICS FOR CLIENT TEACHING DURING PREGNANCY

All Three Trimesters

Discomforts of pregnancy (see Table 16–3)
Nutrition and weight gain
Sexual activity
Sibling preparation

First Trimester

Attitude toward pregnancy
Exercise and rest
Smoking; use of alcohol and other drugs
Traveling
Fetal growth and development
Danger signals associated with spontaneous abortion
Employment
Early pregnancy classes

Second Trimester

Concerns related to changes in body
Fetal growth and development
Fetal movement
Clothing
Care of skin and breasts
Beginning preparation for care of the infant (equipment and room)
Decisions about infant feeding

Third Trimester

Exercise and rest
Traveling
Danger signals
Preparation for labor and birth
Completion of preparation in home for new baby
Decisions about the infant (circumcision, method of feeding, and so forth)
Decision making for the early postpartum period
Education about psychologic and physical expectations in the early postpartum period

Issues to be resolved beforehand may include the sharing of infant and household chores, help in the first few days, reapportionment of family finances, options for baby-sitting to allow the mother (and couple) some free time, the mother's return to work after the baby's birth, and sibling rivalry.

CARE OF THE PREGNANT WOMAN'S FAMILY

Relieving the expectant woman's discomforts, maintaining her physical health, and providing anticipatory guidance are important parts of nursing care management. In addition, the nurse helps meet the needs of the woman's family to better maintain the harmony and integrity of the family unit. The nurse does this by providing support and prenatal education. If the nurse is effective, family members may gain greater problem-solving ability, self-esteem, self-confidence, and ability to participate in health care.

Care of the Father

Although the father of the baby is generally present, his presence cannot be assumed. If he is not a part of the family structure, it is important to assess the woman's support system to determine what significant persons in her life will play a major role during this childbearing experience.

When the father is part of the family or support system, providing anticipatory guidance to him is a necessary part of any plan of care. He may need information about the anatomic, physiologic, and emotional changes that occur during pregnancy and postpartum, the couple's sexuality and sexual response, and the reactions that he may experience. He may wish to express his feelings about breastfeeding versus formula-feeding, the sex of the child, and other topics. If it is culturally acceptable to the couple and personally acceptable to him, the nurse refers the couple to expectant parents' classes. These classes provide valuable information about pregnancy and childbirth using a variety of teaching strategies such as discussion, films, demonstrations with educational models, and written handouts. Some classes even give fathers the opportunity to get a "feel" for pregnancy by wearing a pregnancy simulator (Figure 16–1 ◆).

The nurse assesses the father's intended degree of participation during labor and birth and his knowledge of what to expect. If the couple prefers that his participation be minimal or restricted, the nurse supports their decision and does not try to impose personal values. Research indicates that increased focus on the father's needs during prenatal care aids his transition to fatherhood and also improves the mother's emotional status in the postpartum period (Buist, Morse, & Durkin, 2003). With this type of consideration and collaboration, the father is less apt to develop feelings of alienation, helplessness, and guilt during the pregnancy. The relationship between the couple may be strengthened and his self-esteem raised.

Care of Siblings and Other Family Members

In the plan for prenatal care, the nurse considers the effect of the pregnancy on any other children the couple may have. For example, the nurse may initiate a discussion about the ambivalence that

Figure 16–1 ◆ The Empathy Belly is a pregnancy simulator that allows males and females to experience some of the symptoms of pregnancy. The "belly," which weighs 33 lb, produces symptoms such as shortness of breath, bladder pressure, shift in the center of gravity with resulting waddling gait, increased lordosis and backache, and fatigue. It can also simulate fetal kicking movements.
SOURCE: Photograph courtesy of Birthways, Inc. at empathybelly.org.

older children may feel about the pregnancy. Parents who are unprepared for the older child's feelings of anger, jealousy, and rejection may respond inappropriately in their confusion and surprise. The nurse emphasizes that open communication between parents and children (or acting out feelings with a doll if the child is too young to verbalize) helps children master their feelings and may prevent them from hurting the baby when they are unsupervised. Children may feel less neglected and more secure if they know that their parents are willing to listen to their expressions of sadness or to help with their anger and aggressiveness.

Parents may be encouraged to bring their children to antepartal visits. Seeing what is involved and listening to the fetal heartbeat may make the pregnancy more real to siblings. Many agencies also provide sibling classes geared to different ages and levels of understanding. Relationship changes with in-laws should be addressed as well as the woman's or couple's expectations of the grandparents. Although some grandparents are eager to assist with child care by baby-sitting, others are not. The parents should also give some thought to the best ways of dealing with possible conflicts with the grandparents over childrearing approaches. Couples resolve these issues in different ways; however, postpartal adjustment is easier for a couple who agrees on the issues beforehand than for a couple who does not confront and resolve these issues.

CULTURAL CONSIDERATIONS IN PREGNANCY

As discussed in Chapter 2 ∞, culturally competent nursing care is critical to the provision of quality health care. In the United States, the Caucasian population is decreasing while the population of other ethnic or minority groups, such as the Latino population, is increasing. Moreover, in many countries throughout the world diversity is increasing as more stable or prosper-

DEVELOPING CULTURAL COMPETENCE

PREGNANT WOMEN OF AFRICAN AMERICAN HERITAGE

In caring for pregnant women of African American heritage, it is helpful to consider the following general points (Purnell & Paulanka, 2005):

- African American pregnant women may be guided by their extended family into common practices such as geophagia, the ingestion of dirt or clay, which is believed to reduce mineral deficiencies. This practice has implications for the focus of teaching a nurse offers.

- Many African American families are matriarchal. Women are respected and heeded in decision making and often stress good behavior and firm parenting with their children, especially to keep them safe in dangerous situations.

- Three-generation extended families are common, and the grandmother is often highly respected for her wisdom. She may play a critical role in the care of the children.

- Certain taboos may exist, such as the belief in the necessity to avoid taking pictures during pregnancy to prevent stillbirths. Some women of African American descent may also believe that the purchase of infant clothing or supplies can result in a stillbirth. Thus they may appear to be unprepared for the arrival of the baby.

ous areas experience an influx of immigrants seeking a more secure life. Consequently, prenatal care should always include a cultural assessment. This assessment helps the nurse better understand the client's health beliefs and practices.

Based on the cultural assessment, the nurse can adapt to the specific healthcare needs of each perinatal client. Using the nursing process, the nurse can then formulate a transcultural nursing diagnosis that is focused on the cultural needs of the specific woman. The nursing diagnosis should reflect cultural sensitivity and build on the strengths of the client, such as "*Anxiety* related to culturally unusual expectations for behavior and treatment" (Mattson, 2004).

A major goal of transcultural nursing is to understand and assist people of diverse cultural groups with their healthcare needs. Culturally competent nurses recognize that each childbearing family, shaped by culture and life experience, has expectations of both its members and the healthcare system during pregnancy and birth.

Pregnancy and childbirth are recognized as special or transitional events in virtually all cultures (Mattson, 2004). Additionally, specific actions during pregnancy are often determined by cultural beliefs. According to Mattson (2004), these beliefs can be divided into three types:

- Prescriptive beliefs or requirements that describe expected behaviors

Table 16–2   CULTURAL BELIEFS AND PRACTICES DURING PREGNANCY

Here are a few examples of cultural beliefs and practices related to pregnancy. It is important not to make assumptions about a client's beliefs, because cultural norms vary greatly within a culture and from generation to generation. The nurse should observe the client carefully and take the time to ask questions. Clients will benefit greatly from the nurse's increased awareness of their cultural beliefs and practices.

Belief or Practice	Nursing Consideration
Home Remedies Pregnant women of Native American background may use herbal remedies. An example is the dandelion, which contains a milky juice in its stem believed to increase breast milk flow in mothers who choose to breastfeed (Spector, 2004). Clients of Chinese descent may drink ginseng tea for faintness after childbirth or as a sedative when mixed with bamboo leaves. Some people of African heritage may use self-medication for pregnancy discomforts—for example, laxatives to prevent or treat constipation (Spector, 2004).	Find out what medications and home remedies your client is using, and counsel your client regarding overall effects. It is common for individuals to avoid telling healthcare workers about home remedies; the client may feel this will be judged unfavorably. Phrase your questions in a sensitive, accepting way.
Nutrition Some women of Italian background may believe that it is necessary to satisfy desires for certain foods in order to prevent congenital anomalies. Also, they may believe that they must eat food that they smell, or else the fetus will move "inside," which will result in a miscarriage. Pregnant women of African descent may continue the tradition of eating clay, dirt, or starch, which they believe will benefit the mother and fetus (Spector, 2004).	Discuss the client's beliefs and practices in regard to nutrition during pregnancy. Obtain a diet history from the client. Discuss the importance of a well-balanced diet during pregnancy, with consideration of the client's cultural beliefs and practices. In some cases, you might want to suggest remedies that may be more effective—for example, eating high-fiber foods to reduce constipation. If the home remedy is not harmful, there is no reason to ask a client to discontinue this practice.
Alternative Healthcare Providers Pregnant women of Mexican background may choose to seek out the care of a *partera* (midwife) for prenatal and intrapartal care. A partera speaks their language, shares a similar culture, and can care for pregnant women at home or in a birthing center instead of a hospital. Some people in Hispanic-American communities may use the *curandero,* the folk healer. The *curandero* frequently uses herbs, massage, and religious artifacts for treatment (Spector, 2004).	Discuss the variety of choices of healthcare providers available to the pregnant woman. Contrast the benefits and risks of different settings for prenatal care and birth. Provide reassurance that the goal of health care during pregnancy and birth is a healthy outcome for mother and baby, with respect for the specific cultural beliefs and practices of the client.
Exercise Pregnant women of Italian descent may fear changing their body position in certain ways because they believe this may cause the fetus to develop abnormally (Spector, 2004). Some people of European, African, and Mexican descent believe that reaching over the head during pregnancy can harm the baby.	Ask your client whether there are any activities she is afraid to do because of the pregnancy. Assure her that reaching over her head will not harm the baby, and evaluate other activities to their effect on the pregnancy.
Spirituality Navajo Indians are aware of the mind-soul connection and may try to follow certain practices to have a healthy pregnancy and birth. Practices could include focus on peace and positive thoughts as well as certain types of prayers and ceremonies. A traditional healer may assist them (Purnell & Paulanka, 2005). Some people of European background may tend to pay more attention to spirituality in their life to alleviate fears and ensure a safe birth.	Encourage the use of support systems and spiritual aids that provide comfort for the mother.

- Restrictive beliefs, which are stated negatively and limit behaviors
- Taboo beliefs, which refer to specific supernatural consequences

These activities are viewed as having the potential to impact the outcome of the pregnancy either positively or negatively. Table 16–2 describes activities that are encouraged (prescriptive) or forbidden (restrictive) or taboo by specific cultures. The table is not meant to be all-inclusive but rather to offer a few examples of cultural activities that may be important to some clients during the prenatal period.

In working with clients of another culture, the healthcare professional should be as open as possible to other beliefs. If certain activities are not harmful, there is no need to impose one's beliefs and practices upon a person of another culture. If the activities are proving to be harmful, the nurse can consult or work with someone within the culture or someone aware of the cultural beliefs and values to see whether the client's behavior can be modified (Figure 16–2 ◆).

In providing effective, culturally sensitive care, nurses can use the following strategies (Mattson, 2004):

- Take actions that help break down language barriers.
- Explain the reasons for suggestions made to the woman or couple.
- Integrate folk treatments and Western medicine as much as possible.

Figure 16–2 ◆ The culturally competent nurse respects the culture and values of the pregnant woman.

- Enlist the family caretaker and others as needed.
- Get permission or consent to act from the right person.
- Provide printed materials in the client's language.

See the Nursing Care Plan: Language Barriers at First Prenatal Visit on page 373.

RELIEF OF THE COMMON DISCOMFORTS OF PREGNANCY

Healthcare professionals often refer to the common discomforts of pregnancy as minor discomforts. These discomforts, however, are not minor to the pregnant woman.

Most of the discomforts of pregnancy are a result of physiologic and anatomic changes and are fairly specific to either the first trimester or to the second and third trimesters. Table 16–3 identifies the common discomforts of pregnancy, their possible causes, and the self-care measures that might relieve the discomfort.

CLINICAL TIP

At each prenatal visit, focus your teaching on changes or possible discomforts the woman might encounter during the coming month and the next trimester. If the pregnancy is progressing normally, spend a few minutes describing her baby at this stage of development.

First Trimester

The dramatic hormonal changes of the first trimester account for many of the discomforts experienced in this period. These discomforts tend to abate by the beginning of the fourth month of pregnancy.

NAUSEA AND VOMITING

Nausea and vomiting of pregnancy (NVP) are early, very common symptoms. These symptoms appear sometime after the first missed menstrual period and usually cease by the fourth missed menstrual period. Research indicates that approximately 70% to 85% of pregnant women experience NVP (American College of Obstetricians and Gynecologists [ACOG], 2004). Of these women, approximately 50% actually experience vomiting (Jewell & Young, 2003). Some women develop an aversion only to specific foods. Many experience nausea on arising in the morning, and others experience nausea only in the evening.

The exact cause of NVP is unknown but is believed to be multifactorial. Research has identified possible hormonal, metabolic, neurologic, and psychosomatic factors contributing to its development. Human chorionic gonadotropin (hCG) is often cited as a major factor because it begins to be present in the body at about the time symptoms of morning sickness usually begin, and hCG levels are subsiding when the discomfort of nausea and vomiting usually ends. Evidence also suggests that nausea is linked to rising estrogen levels, which are similar to rising hCG levels (Cunningham, Leveno, Bloom et al., 2005). Changes in carbohydrate metabolism, fatigue, and emotional factors may also play a role in the development of NVP.

Teaching for Self-Care

Treatment of nausea and vomiting is not always successful, but the symptoms can be reduced. To decrease the potential for development of hyperemesis gravidarum, ACOG (2004) recommends the initiation of prompt treatment for nausea and vomiting. Risk factors for NVP include a previous history of motion sickness or migraine headaches, female fetus, young age, first pregnancy, obesity, stress, and being a nonsmoker. If a woman has had nausea and vomiting in a previous pregnancy or when taking combined oral contraceptives, she is also more likely to have nausea and vomiting (Davis, 2004).

The nurse needs to assess the onset, frequency, and duration of symptoms and actual nutritional intake to be helpful in suggesting methods of relief. Physical assessment of the woman should include particular attention to skin color, texture, and turgor as well as vital signs and bowel sounds. For some women, simply avoiding the odor of certain foods or other conditions that precipitate the problem may relieve nausea. If nausea occurs most frequently during early morning, the woman may find it helpful to eat dry crackers or toast before arising and to rise from bed slowly. Rising slowly and avoiding sudden position changes throughout the day may also help prevent nausea due to hypotensive episodes. In addition, the nurse can suggest that the woman avoid brushing her teeth right after eating, because this, too, may trigger vomiting. Evidence suggests that a pregnant woman should start a multivitamin before reaching 6 weeks' gestation to reduce the effects of nausea and vomiting (ACOG, 2004; Davis, 2004).

Generally, it is helpful to eat small meals every 2 to 3 hours during the day and to avoid greasy or highly seasoned foods. Food may be salted to taste. The salt increases the palatability of the food and replaces any chloride lost when the woman vomits hydrochloric acid from the stomach. Eating dry meals and taking all liquids, including soups, between meals may help some women by avoiding overdistention of the stomach. Sudden changes in blood sugar levels can be avoided if the small meals are high in low-fat protein or complex carbohydrates.

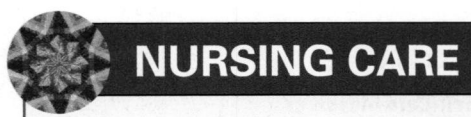

NURSING CARE PLAN

Language Barriers at First Prenatal Visit

INTERVENTION	RATIONALE	EXPECTED OUTCOME
1. Nursing diagnosis: Ineffective Health Maintenance related to alteration in verbal and written communication skils		
Goal: Client will demonstrate understanding of health information received during prenatal visits.		
• If no interpreter is available, refer to posters with pictures to explain routine care and procedures during the prenatal examination.	• Posters put words into verbal images and are helpful in communicating information.	• *Effective communication occurs. The client will gain an understanding of basic prenatal information as evidenced by using hand gestures, by pointing to pictures on posters and translated phrases on handouts, and through an interpreter, if one is available.*
• Provide handouts and brochures about prenatal care in the woman's native language.	• Translated handouts provide information that the client can refer to at home. This reinforces information discussed during the visit and helps the family understand what the woman will experience during the pregnancy and at each visit.	
• Use teaching models to demonstrate procedures. Teaching models may include plastic pelvis, knitted uterus, fetal model, breast model, birth control devices, ultrasound equipment, and so forth.	• Visual aids help to communicate information during the examination.	
• Schedule an interpreter for subsequent prenatal visits.	• If a family member cannot translate the health information to the client, an independent translator is essential to ensure that information is accurately provided. When an interpreter is used (especially a family member), the nurse should be sure that the interpreter is translating information received from the woman and not simply answering the questions for her.	
• Refer the woman to prenatal classes taught in her own language, if available.	• Prenatal classes taught in the woman's language enable her to receive health information that is easily understood, which will prove a better understanding of what she should expect during pregnancy, birth, and postpartum. Prenatal classes may also provide a social outlet for clients.	
• Involve other members of the healthcare team in planning and providing care.	• Cultures vary in language, nonverbal expression, dietary habits, use of time, spatial expectations, and so forth. Use of medication and blood products may also be influenced by cultural beliefs. Social workers who are familier with the client's cultural beliefs, for example, may help the client adjust to different healthcare practices while providing suggestions to ensure prenatal care that is more in line with the woman's cultural beliefs. Dietitians may help the woman plan meals that are aligned with her cultural practices while meeting the nutritional needs of pregnancy.	

Table 16–3   SELF-CARE MEASURES FOR COMMON DISCOMFORTS OF PREGNANCY

Discomfort	Influencing Factors	Self-Care Measures
First Trimester		
Nausea and vomiting	Increased levels of human chorionic gonadotropin Changes in carbohydrate metabolism Emotional factors Fatigue	Avoid odors or causative factors. Eat dry crackers or toast before arising in morning. Have small but frequent meals. Avoid greasy or highly seasoned foods. Take dry meals with fluids between meals. Drink carbonated beverages.
Urinary frequency	Pressure of uterus on bladder in both first and third trimesters	Void when urge is felt. Increase fluid intake during the day. Decrease fluid intake *only* in the evening to decrease nocturia.
Fatigue	Specific causative factors unknown May be aggravated by nocturia due to urinary frequency	Plan time for a nap or rest period daily. Go to bed earlier. Seek family support and assistance with responsibilities so that more time is available to rest.
Breast tenderness	Increased levels of estrogen and progesterone	Wear well-fitting, supportive bra.
Increased vaginal discharge	Hyperplasia of vaginal mucosa and increased production of mucus by the endocervical glands due to the increase in estrogen levels	Promote cleanliness by daily bathing. Avoid douching, nylon underpants, and pantyhose; cotton underpants are more absorbent; powder can be used to maintain dryness if not allowed to cake.
Nasal stuffiness and nosebleed (epistaxis)	Elevated estrogen levels	May be unresponsive, but cool-air vaporizer may help; avoid use of nasal sprays and decongestants.
Ptyalism (excessive, often bitter salivation)	Specific causative factors unknown	Use astringent mouthwashes, chew gum, or suck hard candy.
Second and Third Trimesters		
Heartburn (pyrosis)	Increased production of progesterone, decreasing gastrointestinal motility and increasing relaxation of cardiac sphincter, displacement of stomach by enlarging uterus, thus regurgitation of acidic gastric contents into the esophagus	Eat small and more frequent meals. Use low-sodium antacids. Avoid overeating, fatty and fried foods, lying down after eating, and sodium bicarbonate.
Ankle edema	Prolonged standing or sitting Increased levels of sodium due to hormonal influences Circulatory congestion of lower extremities Increased capillary permeability Varicose veins	Practice frequent dorsiflexion of feet when prolonged sitting or standing is necessary. Elevate legs when sitting or resting. Avoid tight garters or restrictive bands around legs.
Varicose veins	Venous congestion in the lower veins that increases with pregnancy Hereditary factors (weakening of walls of veins, faulty valves) Increased age and weight gain	Elevate legs frequently. Wear supportive hose. Avoid crossing legs at the knees, standing for long periods, garters, and hosiery with constrictive bands.
Hemorrhoids	Constipation (see following discussion) Increased pressure from gravid uterus on hemorrhoidal veins	Avoid constipation Apply ice packs, topical ointments, anesthetic agents, warm soaks, or sitz baths; gently reinsert into rectum as necessary.
Constipation	Increased levels of progesterone, which cause general bowel sluggishness Pressure of enlarging uterus on intestine Iron supplements Diet, lack of exercise, and decreased fluids	Increase fluid intake, fiber in the diet, and exercise. Develop regular bowel habits. Use stool softeners as recommended by physician.
Backache	Increased curvature of the lumbosacral vertebrae as the uterus enlarges Increased levels of hormones, which cause softening of cartilage in body joints Fatigue Poor body mechanics	Use proper body mechanics. Practice the pelvic-tilt exercise. Avoid uncomfortable working heights, high-heeled shoes, lifting heavy loads, and fatigue.
Leg cramps	Imbalance of calcium/phosphorus ratio Increased pressure of uterus on nerves Fatigue Poor circulation to lower extremities Pointing the toes	Practice dorsiflexion of feet to stretch affected muscle. Evaluate diet. Apply heat to affected muscles. Arise slowly from resting position.

Table 16–3   SELF-CARE MEASURES FOR COMMON DISCOMFORTS OF PREGNANCY continued

Discomfort	Influencing Factors	Self-Care Measures
Second and Third Trimesters		
Faintness	Postural hypotension Sudden change of position causing venous pooling in dependent veins Standing for long periods in warm area Anemia	Avoid prolonged standing in warm or stuffy environments. Evaluate hematocrit and hemoglobin.
Dyspnea	Decreased vital capacity from pressure of enlarging uterus on the diaphragm	Use proper posture when sitting and standing. Sleep propped up with pillows for relief if problem occurs at night.
Flatulence	Decreased gastointestinal motility leading to delayed emptying time Pressure of growing uterus on large intestine Air swallowing	Avoid gas-forming foods. Chew food thoroughly. Get regular daily exercise. Maintain normal bowel habits.
Carpal tunnel syndrome	Compression of median nerve in carpal tunnel of wrist Aggravated by repetitive hand movements	Avoid aggravating hand movements. Use splint as prescribed. Elevate affected arm.

EVIDENCE-BASED PRACTICE

RELIEF OF NAUSEA AND VOMITING IN PREGNANCY

Clinical Question

What interventions are safe and effective for relieving nausea and vomiting in pregnancy?

The Evidence

One evidence-based review involved a single appraiser who critically evaluated 90 qualitative and quantitative research studies for an integrative review. That review investigated both the effectiveness of interventions and the lived experience of nausea and vomiting of pregnancy. A second review summarized results from a systematic appraisal of 28 randomized trials. The latter studies were independently assessed by two reviewers. The interventions that were assessed included dietary and lifestyle changes; antiemetic medications; vitamin B_6 (pyridoxine) 10 mg; P6 acupressure and an associated elastic pressure wristband; and consumption of "natural" substances, primarily gingerroot. The antiemetic medications included diphenhydramine (Benadryl), dimenhydrinate (Dramamine) and the combination tablet Debendox (Bendectin). The authors note that Bendectin was voluntarily withdrawn from the US market in 1983 amid concerns about its potential teratogenic effects (which were not supported by any randomized controlled trials). The drug was included in these reviews because it is chemically still available by combining one half a tablet of the over-the-counter sleep aid Unasom with 10 mg of B_6. Outcomes that were evaluated were the frequency and severity of nausea and vomiting and the incidence of maternal/fetal adverse effects.

What Is Effective?

All of the antiemetics reduced the frequency of nausea but tended to cause sleepiness. There was very little information from the randomized controlled trials about fetal effects, but no teratogenic effects were detected in these studies. Vitamin B_6 was effective in reducing the severity of nausea and had the lowest rate of side effects. Early results for the use of gingerroot are encouraging. Two studies demonstrated its effectiveness, resulting in a decreased frequency and severity of nausea when compared with placebo. No major adverse effects or fetal effects were detected. The use of the organic substance raspberry leaf is *contraindicated,* because it increases the risk of uterine contractions and may lead to preterm labor.

What Is Unclear?

The effects of P6 acupressure and the associated pressure wristband did not consistently demonstrate better effects than sham acupressure. There were no clinical trials that supported any clear dietary interventions, although there was a great deal of anecdotal information to support the usefulness of small, frequent, high-protein meals. Studies of treatments for nausea and vomiting of pregnancy are hampered by several inherent characteristics. There is a lack of clarity about the etiology of nausea and vomiting in pregnancy, so treatment is symptomatic. Ethically, it is not possible to test drugs in a classic experimental sense because of a concern for teratogenic effects. As a result, many studies of interventions for nausea and vomiting of pregnancy are based on anecdotal information or expert opinion and so are not subjected to the rigorous standards for randomized controlled trials. Drawing definitive conclusions about effectiveness are rarely clear and compelling, but rather focus on what works for individual mothers through trial and error.

Best Practice

Interventions should begin with early prevention. Vitamin supplementation in very early pregnancy (less than 6 weeks) has been associated with a lower risk of nausea and vomiting. The nurse should assess the presence and severity of nausea and vomiting in all

(Continued on next page)

EVIDENCE-BASED PRACTICE   continued

pregnant women in order to plan targeted interventions. This assessment is especially needed to detect the presence of hyperemesis gravidarum. This condition is a complication of pregnancy involving severe symptoms that are not amenable to conservative treatment, and may cause serious morbidity and even mortality in the mother and fetus. Anecdotal information supports a recommendation for small, high-protein meals; there is no support for the common advice to eat carbohydrate foods before rising in the morning. Behavioral interventions may also be helpful. These involve slow deep breathing and the use of positive imagery. The nurse may help the mother identify triggers for nausea and vomiting, which may include odors or environmental stimuli. Identifying ways to avoid these triggers may reduce the incidence of symptoms. Gingerroot or B_6 may reduce the severity of symptoms without resorting to pharmacologic therapy. A cautionary note to mothers is recommended, though, because these substances are not controlled by the Food and Drug Administration and so composition may vary

widely among commercially available tablets. Drug therapy should be considered only if conservative dietary and lifestyle changes are not effective and symptoms are interfering with quality of life in a substantive way.

Critical Thinking

What assessment questions will help the nurse determine if nausea and vomiting is exceeding that which is normally expected for the pregnant woman? What plan of care will help the nurse best address nausea and vomiting of pregnancy with the lowest risk of adverse effects?

REFERENCES: Davis, M. (2004). Nausea and vomiting of pregnancy: An evidence-based review. *Journal of Perinatal and Neonatal Nursing, 18*(4), 312–328.

Jewell, D., & Young, G. (2003). Interventions for nausea and vomiting in early pregnancy: A review. *The Cochrane Database of Systematic Reviews,* 4. (Article No. CD000145).

Some women find that slowly sipping herbal tea (peppermint, chamomile, or spearmint) or a carbonated beverage helps reduce nausea.

In addition to common self-care measures, certain complementary therapies may be useful. For example, many women find that acupressure applied to pressure points in the wrists is helpful (Figure 16–3 ◆). Ginger may also relieve NVP. (See the accompanying Complementary and Alternative Therapies boxed discussion.) Pyridoxine (vitamin B_6) or vitamin B_6 plus doxylamine (Unisom), an over-the-counter antihistamine, is considered a first-line treatment. Antihistamine H_1 receptor blockers, benzamines, and phenothiazines are considered safe and effective for treating refractory cases. In very severe cases, methylprednisolone, a steroid, may be used,

but as a last resort because it poses a potential risk to the fetus (ACOG, 2004).

Although some nausea is common, the woman who suffers from extreme nausea coupled with vomiting requires further assessment. She should be advised to contact her care provider if she vomits more than once per day or shows signs of dehydration, such as dry mouth, decreased amounts of highly concentrated urine, and the like. In such cases, the physician or certified nurse-midwife (CNM) may order antiemetics. However, antiemetics should be avoided if at all possible during the first trimester because of the danger of teratogenic effects on embryo development.

Nausea and vomiting generally cease by the fourth month of pregnancy. If they do not, hyperemesis gravidarum, which occurs in 0.5% to 2% of pregnancies (a complication of pregnancy discussed in Chapter 20 ∞), must be considered (Davis, 2004).

URINARY FREQUENCY

Urinary frequency is a common discomfort of pregnancy. It occurs early in pregnancy and again during the third trimester because of the pressure of the enlarging uterus on the bladder. Coughing or sneezing in the last month may even cause leakage of urine. Although the glomerular filtration rate increases in pregnancy, it does not cause a significant increase in urine output. Urinary frequency is considered normal during the first and third trimesters; however, the nurse should advise the woman to contact her healthcare provider if she experiences any signs of bladder infection such as painful urination (dysuria), burning with voiding, or blood in the urine (hematuria).

Teaching for Self-Care

There are no methods of decreasing the frequency of urination in pregnancy. Fluid intake should never be decreased to prevent frequency. The woman should be encouraged to maintain an ad-

Figure 16–3 ◆ Acupressure wristbands are sometimes used to help relieve nausea during early pregnancy.

THROUGH THE EYES OF A NURSE

Physical Symptoms in the First Trimester of Pregnancy

FAMILY'S EXPERIENCE: "I know that each pregnancy is different and some women have nausea and some don't but I feel so sick! I have a lot of nausea and feel awful most of the time. I am not really worried because I haven't lost weight and I only throw up occasionally but I would like to find better ways of handling this. I eat dry crackers in the morning and during the day but that only helps a little."

NURSE'S RESPONSE: "Nausea and vomiting frequently occur in the first trimester of pregnancy as a result of changes in the gastrointestinal system as well as changes in carbohydrate metabolism. The nausea and vomiting commonly begin at 6 weeks and can continue another 6 to 12 weeks. Try small frequent meals, avoiding hot and spicy foods. The use of antiemetic medication has been shown to reduce nausea. You might want to discuss that with your nurse-midwife. Some studies have also shown that vitamin B_6 reduces the severity of vomiting. Other studies have shown that ginger reduces nausea and vomiting, so you may want to consider taking that. We have also found that some women have found relief with acupressure bands. You can purchase these bands at any pharmacy. I would try these things and see if they help.

"We are monitoring your weight at each visit and checking your urine for ketones. You actually gained a pound and your urine is negative for ketones, so those are both good signs. Please let us know if the nausea and vomiting become so severe that you are unable to keep anything down within a 24-hour period. If you have questions or concerns, you can call us."

NURSE'S ACTIONS AND RATIONALE:

The nurse explains the physiologic process that leads to nausea and provides evidence-based information on ways of relieving or reducing nausea and vomiting (ACOG, 2004; Davis, 2004; Jewell & Young, 2003). As discussed in this chapter and in Table 16–3, interventions such as ginger, acupressure wrist bands, and vitamin B_6 are often helpful. The nurse also provides reassurance and explains how the woman will be monitored to ease the family's anxiety. Finally the nurse reassures the woman that she can call if questions arise and reviews the parameters for the woman to follow as to when to call the healthcare provider.

COMPLEMENTARY AND ALTERNATIVE THERAPIES

GINGER AND ACUPRESSURE FOR MORNING SICKNESS

Ginger and acupressure are among the most frequently used alternative therapies for the nausea and vomiting of morning sickness.

Ginger: Ginger is widely used in traditional Chinese medicine and has been used throughout history to treat nausea and vomiting of pregnancy. Although other medications or herbs are contraindicated in the first trimester of pregnancy, the safety of ginger has been demonstrated in clinical trials (ACOG, 2004; Born & Barron, 2005; Borrelli, Capasso, Aviello et al., 2005). One study reported that ginger is similar to vitamin B_6 in reducing the nausea and vomiting symptoms of early pregnancy (Smith, Crowther, Willson et al., 2004). Once a woman has decided to try ginger for relief of nausea and vomiting, it is important to find the correct product and dose to decrease her symptoms. Ginger is available in a variety of forms, including the fresh root, capsules, tea, candy, cookies, crystals, inhaled powdered ginger, and sugared ginger (Lie, 2004). In the first trimester, the daily dosage should not exceed 2 g of dried ginger or 1 g of ginger syrup (Born & Barron, 2005).

Acupressure: Acupressure, like acupuncture, is a therapy based on the ancient philosophy of traditional Chinese medicine. Acupressure involves the application of pressure using fingers or thumbs to stimulate and balance the body's healing energy known by the Chinese as chi. A specific acupressure point that relieves nausea is located on the forearm, three finger widths above the wrist closest to the palm, toward the elbow. The point is pressed firmly for 5 minutes every 4 hours (Davis, 2004). A motion sickness elasticized wristband (brand names include Sea-Band and Acuband) can be purchased that puts gentle pressure on this acupressure point. ACOG (2004) reports that the evidence supporting or refuting the use of acupressure for nausea and vomiting of pregnancy is unclear.

equate fluid intake: at least 2000 mL per day. She should also be encouraged to empty her bladder frequently (approximately every 2 hours while awake).

Frequent bladder emptying helps decrease the incidence of leakage of urine. Because frequency often results in several trips to the bathroom each night, it is important to remind the woman to consider safety factors in the home, such as a clear path to the bathroom, the use of a night-light, and the like. The woman who leaks urine may choose to wear pantyliners during the day. If she does, she should change them as soon as they become damp to avoid perineal excoriation and to avoid contamination of the perineum from the rectal area if the pads move back and forth as she walks. Tightening of the pubococcygeus muscle, which supports internal organs and controls voiding, can help maintain good perineal tone. This procedure, known as Kegel exercise, is discussed later in this chapter.

FATIGUE

Marked fatigue, often out of proportion to the woman's normal pattern, is so common in early pregnancy that it is considered a presumptive sign of pregnancy. The sleep-inducing effects of progesterone may play a role in the development of this sign (Cunningham et al., 2005). It is aggravated if the woman has to arise several times each night because of urinary frequency. Typically, it resolves soon after the end of the first trimester.

Teaching for Self-Care

Scheduling activities to allow for napping is helpful. Women should be encouraged to use every opportunity available to rest, including going to bed earlier in the evening. The woman's partner, if he is involved in the pregnancy, needs to understand that the fatigue is normal and will subside. He can be encouraged to assume more home responsibilities to support the woman and enable her to rest.

BREAST TENDERNESS

Sensitivity of the breasts occurs early and continues throughout the pregnancy. Increased levels of estrogen and progesterone contribute to the soreness and tingling felt in the breasts and to the increased sensitivity of the nipples.

Teaching for Self-Care

A well-fitting, supportive brassiere gives the most relief for this discomfort. The qualities of a properly supportive brassiere are discussed in Breast Care, later in this chapter.

INCREASED VAGINAL DISCHARGE

Increased whitish vaginal discharge, called **leukorrhea,** is common in pregnancy. It occurs as the result of hyperplasia of vaginal mucosa and increased production of mucus by the endocervical glands. In addition, the increased acidity of the secretions encourages the growth of *Candida albicans,* and the woman is thus more susceptible to monilial vaginitis.

Teaching for Self-Care

Cleanliness is important in preventing excoriation and vaginal infections. Daily bathing is adequate; douching is generally avoided during pregnancy. The woman should avoid nylon underpants and pantyhose because they retain heat and moisture in the genital area; absorbent cotton underpants should be worn to help prevent problems. The nurse can advise the pregnant woman to report any change in vaginal discharge, any irritation in the perineal area, and intense vaginal itching. These changes frequently indicate vaginal infections.

NASAL STUFFINESS AND EPISTAXIS

Once pregnancy is well established, elevated estrogen levels may produce edema of the nasal mucosa, resulting in nasal stuffiness, nasal discharge, and obstruction (rhinitis of pregnancy). *Epistaxis* (nosebleed) may also result.

Teaching for Self-Care

Cool air vaporizers and normal saline nose drops may be helpful. However, the problem is often unresponsive to treatment. Women experiencing these problems find it difficult to sleep and may resort to medicated nasal sprays and decongestants to relieve the problem. Such interventions may provide relief initially but can actually increase the nasal stuffiness over time. The use of any medication in pregnancy should be avoided if possible.

PTYALISM

Ptyalism is a rare discomfort of pregnancy in which excessive, often bitter, saliva is produced. Its cause has not been established, although stimulation of the salivary glands by the ingestion of starch has been suggested as a possible cause (Cunningham et al., 2005). Effective treatments are limited.

Teaching for Self-Care

Using astringent mouthwashes, chewing gum, or sucking on hard candy may minimize the problem of ptyalism. It may also be helpful to reduce or limit starch intake.

Second and Third Trimesters

It is difficult to classify discomforts as specifically occurring in the second or third trimester because their timing varies because of individual variations in women. The symptoms discussed in this section usually do not appear until the third trimester in primigravidas but may occur earlier with each succeeding pregnancy.

HEARTBURN (PYROSIS)

Heartburn is the regurgitation of acidic gastric contents into the esophagus. It creates a burning or irritating sensation in the esophagus and radiates upward, sometimes leaving a bad taste in the mouth. Heartburn appears to be primarily a result of the displacement of the stomach by the enlarging uterus. The increased production of progesterone in pregnancy, decreases in gastrointestinal motility, and relaxation of the cardiac (esophageal) sphincter also contribute to heartburn.

Teaching for Self-Care

Heartburn is aggravated by overeating, ingesting fatty and fried foods, and lying down soon after eating. The woman should therefore avoid these situations. The woman should be encouraged to drink an adequate amount of fluid (8 to 10 8-oz glasses) each day and to eat smaller, more frequent meals to accommodate the decreased size of her stomach. Good posture is important because it allows more room for the stomach to function. Some women choose complementary approaches to relieving their heartburn. See Complementary and Alternative Therapies: Meadowsweet for Heartburn.

The caregiver may recommend a low-sodium antacid, such as aluminum hydroxide (Amphojel) or a combination of aluminum hydroxide and magnesium hydroxide (Maalox). Because aluminum alone tends to cause constipation, and magnesium alone is associated with diarrhea, the combined approach is more desirable. Sodium bicarbonate (baking soda) and Alka-Seltzer should be avoided because of the potential for electrolyte imbalance.

If maternal heartburn is severe, not relieved by antacids, and accompanied by gastrointestinal reflux, an antisecretory agent (H₂-blocker) such as ranitidine (Zantac), cimetidine (Tagamet), or omeprazole (Losec) may be necessary. Research

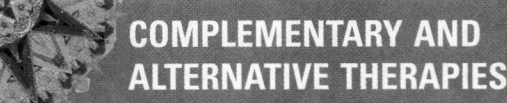

MEADOWSWEET FOR HEARTBURN

Meadowsweet has traditionally been used as a pain reliever (the analgesic substance *salicin* was first isolated from meadowsweet leaves in 1827); it also provides relief for heartburn (Blumenthal, 2003). However, because it contains salicylates, a woman with a sensitivity to aspirin should not take meadowsweet. See Complementary and Alternative Therapies later in this chapter for more information on the use of herbs during pregnancy.

to date has not linked these medications with an excessive risk of birth defects, preterm birth, or intrauterine growth restriction.

ANKLE EDEMA

Most women experience ankle edema in the last part of pregnancy because of the increasing difficulty of venous return from the lower extremities. Prolonged standing or sitting and warm weather increase the edema. It is also associated with varicose veins. Ankle edema becomes a concern only when accompanied by hypertension or proteinuria or when the edema is not postural in origin.

Teaching for Self-Care

The aggravating conditions just mentioned should be avoided. If the woman has to sit or stand for long periods, frequent dorsiflexion of her feet will help contract muscles, thereby squeezing the fluid back into circulation. The pregnant woman should not wear tight garters or other restrictive bands around her legs. During rest periods, the woman should elevate her legs and hips as described in the following section on varicose veins.

VARICOSE VEINS

Varicose veins are a result of weakening of the walls of veins or faulty functioning of the valves. Poor circulation in the lower extremities predisposes the woman to varicose veins in the legs and thighs, as does prolonged standing or sitting. The weight of the gravid uterus on the pelvic veins aggravates the development of varicosities in the legs and pelvic area by preventing good venous return. Increased maternal age, excessive weight gain, a large fetus, heredity, and multiple pregnancy can all contribute to the problem.

Vulvar varicosities may also be a problem in pregnancy, although they are less common. Varicosities in the vulva and perineum cause aching and a sense of heaviness.

Treatment of varicose veins by surgery or by the injection method is not recommended during pregnancy (Cunningham et al., 2005). The woman should be aware that treatment might be needed after pregnancy because the problem will be aggravated by a succeeding pregnancy.

Teaching for Self-Care

Regular exercise, such as swimming, cycling, or walking, promotes venous return, which helps prevent varicosities. Avoiding factors that contribute to venous stasis is also helpful. The pregnant woman should avoid standing or sitting for prolonged periods. She should also avoid crossing her legs at the knees because of the pressure on her veins. She should not wear garters or hosiery with constricting bands, such as knee-high hose. However, supportive hose or elastic stockings may be extremely helpful. Supportive hose should be put on in the morning and should be washed daily with soap and warm water to help retain elasticity. In addition, some women advocate the use of complementary care in relieving varicose veins.

The pregnant woman should be encouraged to elevate her legs level with her hips when she sits. She can enhance comfort by supporting the entire leg rather than simply propping her feet up on a stool, which may lead to hyperextension of the knees. The woman who sits or stands for long periods should walk around frequently to promote venous return to the heart. She can also be encouraged to dorsiflex her feet, hold the position for 3 seconds, then release, with 8 to 10 repetitions several times each day. Venous return is most effectively promoted if the woman lies down with her feet elevated several times a day. To avoid difficulty related to pressure of the uterus on the vena cava, the woman can lie with her legs elevated on pillows and a pillow placed under one hip to displace the uterus to one side (Figure 16–4 ◆).

Wearing one of the foam rubber commercial products that is placed across the perineum and held in place by a sanitary pad type belt can provide support for vulvar varicosities (Cunningham et al., 2005). Elevation of only the legs aggravates vulvar varicosities by creating stasis of blood in the pelvic area. Therefore, it is important that the pelvic area also be elevated to promote venous drainage into the trunk of the body. More than one firm pillow under the hips may be needed to accomplish this elevation. Near the end of pregnancy, this position may be extremely awkward; the woman may best relieve uterine pressure on the pelvic veins by resting on her side. Blocks may also be placed under the foot of her bed to elevate it slightly.

FLATULENCE

Flatulence results from decreased gastrointestinal motility, leading to delayed emptying, and from pressure upon the large intestine by the growing uterus. Air swallowing may also contribute to the problem.

Figure 16–4 ◆ Swelling and discomfort from varicosities can be decreased by lying down with the legs and one hip elevated (to avoid compression of the vena cava).

Teaching for Self-Care

The woman should be advised to avoid gas-forming foods and to chew her food thoroughly. Regular bowel habits and exercise can also decrease flatulence.

HEMORRHOIDS

Hemorrhoids are varicosities of the veins in the lower end of the rectum and anus. During pregnancy, the gravid uterus presses on the veins and interferes with venous circulation. As the pregnancy progresses, the straining that accompanies constipation can contribute to the development of hemorrhoids.

Hemorrhoids may not bother some women until the second stage of labor, when the hemorrhoids appear as they push just before birth. Hemorrhoids that occur in pregnancy or at birth usually become asymptomatic after the early postpartal period.

Symptoms of hemorrhoids include itching, swelling, pain, and bleeding. Internal hemorrhoids are located above the anal sphincter and are responsible for bleeding, usually with defecation. They are not usually painful unless they protrude from the anus. External hemorrhoids are located outside the anal sphincter. They are not usually the source of bleeding or pain; however, thrombosis of the hemorrhoids can occur, and in that case they become extremely painful. The thrombosis may resolve itself in 24 hours, or the physician can treat it by incising and evacuating the blood clot. Women who have hemorrhoids before pregnancy frequently experience more difficulties with them during pregnancy.

Teaching for Self-Care

Relief can be achieved by gently and carefully reinserting the hemorrhoids. The woman lies on her side or in the knee to chest position. She places some lubricant on her finger and presses against the hemorrhoids, pushing them inside. She holds them in place for 1 to 2 minutes and then gently withdraws her finger. The anal sphincter should then hold them inside the rectum. The woman will find it especially helpful if she can then maintain a side-lying (Sims') position for a time, so this procedure is best done before bed or before a daily rest period.

Avoiding constipation is important in preventing or relieving the discomfort of hemorrhoids. Relief measures for existing hemorrhoid symptoms include ice packs, use of topical ointments and anesthetic agents, and warm soaks. In consultation with a healthcare provider, the woman may decide to try complementary therapies, such as abdominal massage, reflexology, and herbal remedies, as additional self-help measures to treat hemorrhoids (Tiran, 2003).

The woman should contact her healthcare provider if the hemorrhoids become hardened and noticeably tender to touch. Rectal bleeding that is more than spotting following defecation should also be reported.

CONSTIPATION

Conditions in pregnancy that predispose the woman to constipation include general bowel sluggishness caused by increased progesterone and steroid metabolism; displacement of the intestines, which increases with the growth of the fetus; and oral iron supplements, which most pregnant women need.

Teaching for Self-Care

Increased fluid intake (at least 2000 mL/day), adequate roughage or bulk in the diet, regular bowel habits, and adequate daily exercise can often maintain good bowel function in women who have not had previous problems. Some women find it helpful to drink a warm beverage or glass of prune juice in the morning. Women should leave sufficient time following breakfast so that the natural action of the body will produce defecation.

In severe or preexisting cases of constipation, the woman may need a mild laxative, stool softeners, or suppositories as recommended by her caregiver.

BACKACHE

Many pregnant women experience backache due primarily to the increased curvature of the lumbosacral vertebrae that occurs as the uterus enlarges and becomes heavier. Circulating steroid hormones cause a softening and relaxation of pelvic joints, contributing to the problem. If the woman does not learn how to correct this curvature, the strain on the muscles and ligaments will cause backache. Low backache can occur at any point during pregnancy. Risk factors include increased maternal age, previous history of back pain during menstruation or a previous pregnancy, and a general history of back pain (Wang et al., 2004).

Teaching for Self-Care

An exercise called the pelvic tilt (discussed later in this chapter) can help restore proper body alignment. As the anterior pelvis is tilted upward, the curvature of the back is automatically decreased, relieving much of the discomfort. If proper body alignment is maintained throughout pregnancy, backaches can be relieved or even prevented. Other measures to prevent backache include good posture, avoidance of fatigue, use of aquatic exercise, use of extension exercises, use of lumbar support devices when standing or sitting, and use of pillows for support when lying supine (Lile, Perkins, Hammer et al., 2003). See Exercises to Prepare for Childbirth, later in this chapter.

The use of proper posture and good body mechanics throughout pregnancy is important. The pregnant woman should avoid bending over to lift or pick up items from the floor. The strain is felt in the muscles of the back. Leg muscles should be used to do the work instead. The woman can keep her back straight by bending her knees to lower her body into the squatting position (Figure 16–5 ◆). She should place her feet 12 to 18 inches apart to maintain body balance. When lifting a heavy object, such as a child, she should place one foot flat on the floor, slightly in front of the other foot, and lower herself to the other knee. The object is held close to her body for lifting. This same principle of keeping the back straight and bending the knees applies when the woman sits down or gets out of a chair. Work heights that require constant bending can contribute to backache and should be adjusted as necessary. See Complementary and Alternative Therapies: Physical Modalities for Relief of Backache and Other Pregnancy-Related Muscular Pain for information on other relief measures.

A pendulous abdomen contributes to backache by increasing the curvature of the spine. The use of a supportive maternity

Figure 16–5 ◆ When picking up objects from floor level or lifting objects, the pregnant woman must use proper body mechanics.

girdle is discussed later in this chapter, as is the role of high-heeled shoes in increasing the lumbosacral curvature.

LEG CRAMPS

Leg cramps are painful muscle spasms in the gastrocnemius muscles. They occur most frequently at night after the woman has gone to bed but may occur at other times. Extension of the foot can often cause leg cramps. The nurse should warn the pregnant woman not to extend the foot during childbirth preparation exercises or during rest periods.

The exact cause of leg cramps is not known, but pressure of the enlarged uterus on pelvic nerves or blood vessels leading to the legs may be a contributing factor (Varney, Kriebs, & Gregor, 2004), especially during the third trimester.

Teaching for Self-Care

The woman can achieve immediate relief of the muscle spasm by stretching the muscle. With the woman lying on her back, another person can press the woman's knee down to straighten her leg while pushing her foot toward her leg (Figure 16–6 ◆). The woman may also stand and put her foot flat on the floor. Massage and warm packs can be used to alleviate discomfort from leg cramps. Stretching exercises before bedtime may help prevent leg cramps. The caregiver may recommend that the woman drink no more than a pint of milk daily and take calcium carbonate or that she drink a quart of milk daily and take aluminum hydroxide gel. The gel absorbs phosphorus and eliminates it directly through the intestinal tract. The treatment recommendations depend on the frequency of the leg cramps.

FAINTNESS

Many pregnant women occasionally feel faint, especially in warm, crowded areas. Faintness is caused by a combination of changes in the blood volume and postural hypotension due to venous pooling of blood in the dependent veins. Sudden change

COMPLEMENTARY AND ALTERNATIVE THERAPIES

PHYSICAL MODALITIES FOR RELIEF OF BACKACHE AND OTHER PREGNANCY-RELATED MUSCULAR PAIN

The following are some modalities that have been used successfully in clients with backache and other muscular pain.

Massage Therapy for Low Back Pain: Massage often helps relieve low back pain associated with pregnancy. During the first 4 months of pregnancy, the body should be massaged with a gentle, soft touch. The best position for lumbar massage is with the woman sitting on a stool, resting her arms on a table, and leaning her forehead against her arms. The person doing the massage kneels on the floor behind her, which enhances the ability to apply an effective amount of pressure to the back muscles.

Yoga: Many women find that the regular practice of yoga builds and tones muscles, increases flexibility, improves endurance, and promotes a state of relaxation. One of the many applications of yoga is in pregnancy and childbirth. In fact, many of the techniques taught in childbirth classes, such as focus, relaxation, and systematic breathing, have their roots in yoga. The gentle stretching of the poses helps ease the muscle aches of pregnancy and strengthens the muscles that are used during childbirth. The breathing techniques may lessen the shortness of breath that often accompanies advanced pregnancy.

Yoga practiced while pregnant is slightly different from regular yoga in that some poses are contraindicated. These poses are the extreme stretching positions and any position that puts pressure on the uterus. Full forward bends will probably be uncomfortable for both woman and baby. A woman's center of balance has shifted, and thus she must be careful with balance poses. Pregnant women should never lie on the stomach for any pose. If any pose feels uncomfortable, the woman should stop at once. If she experiences dizziness, sudden swelling, extreme shortness of breath, or vaginal bleeding, she should see her certified nurse-midwife or doctor immediately.

Reflexology for Sciatica: Reflexology is a field of therapy that uses specific touch techniques to stimulate "reflex points and areas" on the feet, hands, and ears. Reflexologists believe that each of these points corresponds to a specific part of the body. The growing baby can put pressure on the large sciatic nerve. The pressure inflames the nerve, causing severe lower back pain that radiates into the legs. Reflexology may help this condition. The reflex points for the sciatic nerve are on the heel. A woman in her second or third trimester can press gently and release with her thumbs to stimulate first one whole heel, then the other. Each heel can be worked for a minute or two twice a day until the pain is gone.

Women who are in the first trimester of pregnancy should not have reflexology that stimulates the uterine points on the hands, feet, or ears. In general, it is best for pregnant women to receive reflexology that uses light, gentle pressure.

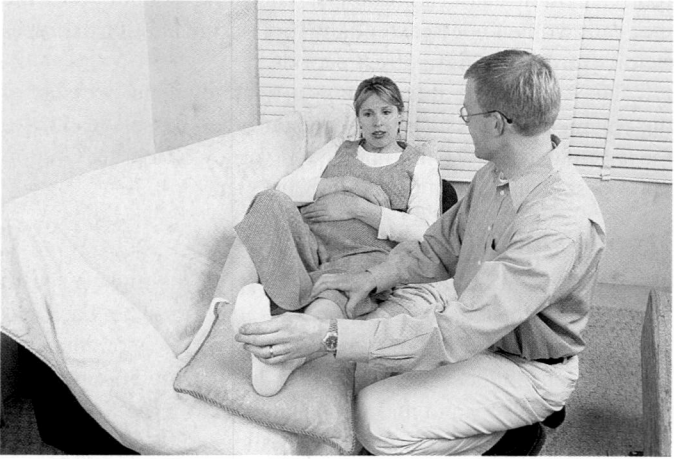

Figure 16–6 ◆ The expectant father can help relieve the woman's painful leg cramps by flexing her foot and straightening her leg.

of position or standing for prolonged periods can cause this sensation, and fainting can occur.

Teaching for Self-Care

The nurse should first be certain that the pregnant woman understands the symptoms of faintness. These include slight dizziness, a "swirling" or "floating" sensation, and a decreased ability to hear or focus attention. If a woman feels faint from prolonged standing or from being in a warm,

crowded room, she should sit down and lower her head between her knees. If this procedure does not help, the woman should be assisted to an area where she can lie down and get fresh air. When arising from a resting position, she should move slowly. Women whose jobs require standing in one place for long periods should march in place regularly to increase venous return from the legs.

SHORTNESS OF BREATH

Shortness of breath occurs as the uterus rises into the abdomen and causes pressure on the diaphragm. This problem worsens in the last trimester as the enlarged uterus presses directly on the diaphragm, decreasing vital capacity. The primigravida experiences considerable relief from shortness of breath in the last few weeks of pregnancy, when **lightening** occurs, and the fetus and uterus move down in the pelvis. Because the multigravida does not usually experience lightening until labor, shortness of breath will continue throughout her pregnancy.

Teaching for Self-Care

During the day, sitting straight in a chair and using proper posture when standing help provide relief. If distress is great at night, the woman can sleep propped up in bed with several pillows behind her head and shoulders.

DIFFICULTY SLEEPING

From 12 weeks of pregnancy into the postpartum period, sleep disturbances are common. The pregnant woman may have difficulty falling asleep or wake up throughout the night, resulting in fewer overall hours of sleep (Cunningham et al., 2005). Although the pregnant woman may experience difficulty sleeping for many of the same psychologic reasons as the nonpregnant woman, many physical factors also contribute to this problem. The enlarged uterus may make it difficult to find a comfortable position for sleep, and an active fetus may aggravate the problem. The other discomforts of pregnancy such as urinary frequency, shortness of breath, and leg cramps may also be contributing factors.

Teaching for Self-Care

The nurse should conduct a thorough assessment of the sleep habits of the pregnant woman and offer information about habits and activities that help promote restful sleep. The pregnant woman may find it helpful to drink a warm (caffeine-free) beverage before bed and may benefit from a soothing backrub given by her partner or a family member. Pillows may be used to provide support for her back, between her legs, or for her upper arm when she lies on her side. Relaxation techniques may also help. The woman should avoid caffeine products, stimulating activity, and sleeping medication.

ROUND LIGAMENT PAIN

As the uterus enlarges during pregnancy, the round ligaments stretch, hypertrophy, and lengthen as the uterus rises up in the abdomen. Round ligament pain is attributed to this stretching.

Teaching for Self-Care

The woman may feel concern when she first experiences round ligament pain because it is often intense and causes a "grabbing" sensation in the lower abdomen and inguinal area. The nurse should warn women of this possible discomfort. Few treatment measures really alleviate this discomfort, but understanding the cause will help decrease anxiety. Once the caregiver has ascertained that the cause of the discomfort is not related to a medical complication such as appendicitis or gallbladder disease, the woman may find that a heating pad applied to the abdomen brings some relief. She may also benefit from bringing her knees up on her abdomen.

CARPAL TUNNEL SYNDROME

Carpal tunnel syndrome (CTS) results from compression of the median nerve in the carpal tunnel of the wrist. The syndrome is commonly bilateral but may be more pronounced in the dominant hand and is characterized by numbness, tingling, or burning in the fleshy part of the palm near the thumb. The syndrome is aggravated by repetitive hand movements, such as typing, and may disappear following birth. Treatment involves splinting, avoiding aggravating movements, and in some cases injecting steroids into the carpal tunnel. Surgery is indicated in severe cases (Cunningham et al., 2005).

Teaching for Self-Care

Although the condition is not preventable, the woman should be advised to avoid aggravating activities and use her splint as directed.

PROMOTION OF SELF-CARE DURING PREGNANCY

The pregnant woman is faced with the important responsibility of maintaining her health not only for her sake but also for the sake of her fetus. Nurses can help promote maternal and fetal well-being by providing expectant couples with accurate and complete information about health behaviors that can affect pregnancy and childbirth. Some women prefer to gather their own information. The nurse can refer these women to a variety of sources, including the National Women's Health Information Center, which is sponsored by the US Public Health Service's Office on Women's Health.

Fetal Activity Monitoring

Many caregivers encourage pregnant women to monitor their unborn child's well-being by regularly assessing fetal activity beginning at 28 weeks' gestation. Research has documented a good positive correlation between maternal perception of fetal movement and fetal movement confirmed by ultrasound monitoring (Cunningham et al., 2005). Vigorous fetal activity generally provides reassurance of fetal well-being, whereas a marked decrease in activity or cessation of movement may indicate possible fetal compromise requiring immediate evaluation. Sound, drugs, cigarette smoking, fetal sleep state, and time of day affect fetal activity. At times, a healthy fetus may be minimally active or inactive.

A variety of methods for assessing fetal activity have been developed. They focus on having the woman keep a **fetal movement record (FMR)**, such as the Cardiff Count-to-Ten Method (Figure 16–7 ◆). An FMR is a noninvasive technique that enables the pregnant woman to monitor and record fetal well-being easily and without expense. The woman's perceptions of fetal movements and her commitment to completing a movement record may vary. Ideally, when the woman understands the purpose of the assessment, how to complete the form, whom to call with questions, and what to report, and has the opportunity for follow-up during each visit, she will see this as an important activity. See Client Teaching: What to Tell the Pregnant Woman About Assessing Fetal Activity.

I like doing the fetal movement counts each day. It gives me a "time out," when I can focus on my baby and really enjoy this special time in my life.

Breast Care

Whether the pregnant woman plans to formula-feed or breast-feed her infant, proper support of the breasts is important to promote comfort, retain breast shape, and prevent back strain, particularly if the breasts become large and pendulous. The sensitivity of the breasts in pregnancy is also relieved by good support.

A well-fitting, supportive brassiere has the following qualities:

- The straps are wide and do not stretch (elastic straps soon lose their tautness because of the weight of the breasts and frequent washing).

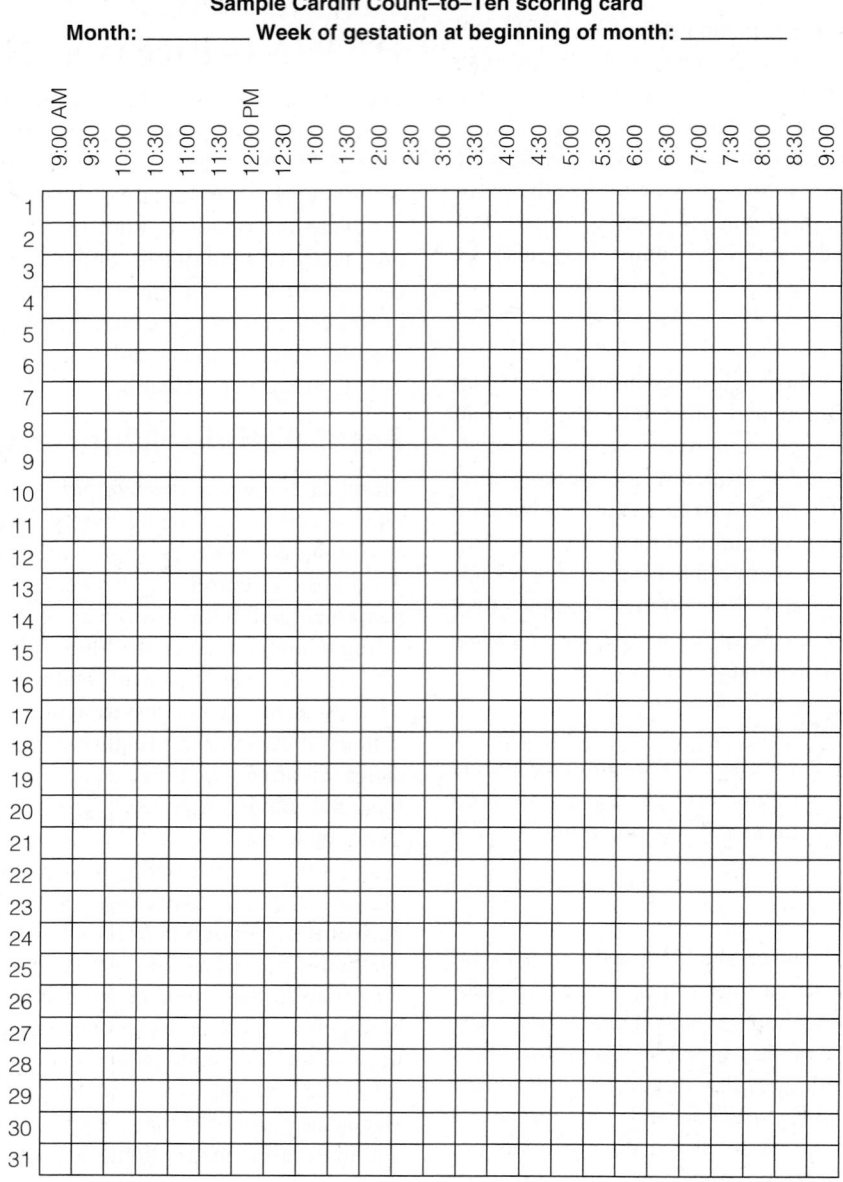

Figure 16–7 ◆ An adaptation of the Cardiff Count-to-Ten scoring card for fetal movement assessment.

- The cup holds all breast tissue comfortably.
- The brassiere has tucks or other devices that allow it to expand, thus accommodating the enlarging chest circumference.
- The brassiere supports the nipple line approximately midway between the elbow and shoulder. At the same time, the brassiere is not pulled up in the back by the weight of the breasts.

Cleanliness of the breasts is important, especially as the woman begins producing colostrum. Colostrum that crusts on the nipples should be removed with warm water. The woman planning to breastfeed should not use soap on her nipples because of its drying effect.

Some women have flat or inverted nipples. True nipple inversion, which is rare, is usually diagnosed during the initial an-

tepartal assessment. Occasionally, a nipple appears inverted at all times. In other cases, the nipple appears normal initially, but pressure on the areola with the examiner's thumb and finger causes the nipple to retract. The normal or flat nipple protrudes when this is done (Figure 16–8 ◆).

Some women with truly inverted nipples may benefit from wearing special breast shields for the last 3 months of pregnancy (Figure 16–9 ◆). Others gain no benefit from them (Chez & Friedmann, 2000). These shields tend to absorb moisture and can cause a rash, so they should not be worn more than a few hours at a time. Alternatively, women with flat or inverted nipples who wish to breastfeed may find it helpful to stimulate the nipple or nipples postpartally by using an electric breast pump before having the baby latch on (Chez & Friedmann, 2000).

Table 16–4 provides a list of Web sites available for women who want more information on breastfeeding.

CLIENT TEACHING   What to Tell the Pregnant Woman About Assessing Fetal Activity

CLIENT GOALS   At the completion of the teaching session the woman will:

1. Discuss the types of fetal assessment methods, reasons for assessment, how to accomplish the assessment, and methods of record keeping

2. Demonstrate the use of a fetal movement record

3. Identify resources to call if questions arise

4. Agree to bring the fetal movement record to each prenatal visit

TEACHING PLAN

CONTENT

Explain that fetal movements are first around 18 weeks' gestation. From that time the fetal movements get stronger and easier to detect.

A slowing or stopping of fetal movement may be an indication that the fetus needs some attention and evaluation.

Explain procedure for Cardiff Count-to-Ten method or for the Daily Fetal Movement Record (DFMR). For both methods, advise the woman to:

- Beginning at about 27 weeks' gestation, keep a daily record of fetal movement

- Try to begin counting at about the same time each day, about 1 hour after a meal if possible

- Lie quietly in a side-lying position

Using the Cardiff card, have the woman place an X for each fetal movement until she has recorded 10. Movement varies considerably, but most women feel fetal movement at least 10 times in 3 hours (see Figure 16–7).

Using the DFMR have the woman count three times a day for 20 to 30 minutes each session. If there are fewer than three movements in a session, have the woman count for 1 hour or more.

Explain when to contact the care provider:

- If there are fewer than 10 movements in 3 hours

- If overall the fetus's movement are slowing, and it takes much longer each day to note 10 movements

- If there are no movements in the morning

- If there are fewer than 3 movements in 8 hours

TEACHING METHOD

Describe procedures and demonstrate how to assess fetal movement.

Sit beside the woman and show her how to place her hand on the fundus to feel fetal movement.

Provide a written teaching sheet for the woman's use at home.

Demonstrate how to record fetal movements on Cardiff Count-to-Ten scoring card or on DFMR.

Watch woman fill out record as examples are provided. Encourage her to complete the record each day and bring it with her to each prenatal visit. Assure her that the record will be discussed at each prenatal visit, and questions may be addressed at the time if desired.

Provide the woman with a name and phone number in case she has further questions.

EVALUTION

Evaluate learning by having the woman explain the method and by asking the woman to fill the card in using a fictitious situation. At each prenatal visit review the expectant woman's record. Review of the record provides opportunities for questions and clarification.

DOCUMENTATION

Document the information given to the woman, including specifics on when to contact her healthcare provider (specify if written instructions were provided in addition to verbal ones) and the type of teaching method used. Indicate if the woman practiced counting fetal movements. Document the woman's verbalization of understanding and your clarification of any information.

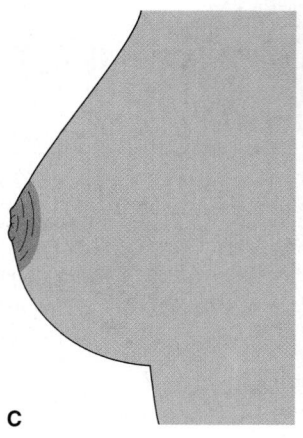

A   B   C

Figure 16–8 ◆ *A,* When not stimulated, normal and inverted nipples often look alike. *B,* When stimulated, the normal nipple protrudes. *C,* When stimulated, the inverted nipple retracts. However, great variation exists; in some women, for example, one or both nipples always appear inverted, even when not stimulated.

Figure 16–9 ◆ This breast shield is designed to increase the protractility of inverted nipples. Worn the last 3 to 4 months of pregnancy, they exert gentle pulling pressure at the edge of the areola, gradually forcing the nipple through the center of the shield. They may be used after birth if necessary.
SOURCE: Photographer, Elena Dorfman.

Table 16–4	WEB SITES FOR INFORMATION ABOUT BREASTFEEDING
Site	**Usefulness**
http://www.lalecheleague.org	Home page of the LaLeche League. Offers useful information on all aspects of breastfeeding.
http://www.aap.org	Home page of the American Academy of Pediatrics. Offers information on a variety of issues related to infant care. Also provides information about medications that will pass into breast milk.
http://www.nomotc.org	Home page of the National Organization of Mothers of Twins Club. Provides useful information about caring for multiple births, including successful breastfeeding.
http://www.breastfeeding.com	Contains a wide range of information such as choosing nursing bras and breast pumps, getting started breastfeeding, and frequently asked questions. Also contains a link to video clips about breastfeeding.
http://www.babyfriendly.org	Home page of UNICEF UK Baby Friendly Initiative. Contains information for practitioners and for parents with a British focus.

Clothing

Traditionally, maternity clothes have been constructed with fuller lines to allow for the increase in abdominal size during pregnancy. Skirts and slacks have soft elastic waistbands and a stretchable panel over the abdominal area. However, maternity wear has changed in recent years and now also includes clothes that are more fitted, with little attempt to hide the pregnant abdomen. Maternity clothing is expensive, however, and is worn for a relatively short time. Women can economize by sharing clothes with friends, sewing their own garments, or buying used maternity clothing.

Clothing should be loose and nonconstricting. Women with large, pendulous abdomens may benefit from a well-fitting, supportive girdle. Without this support, the pendulous abdomen increases the curvature of the spine and is a source of backache and general discomfort. Tight leg bands on girdles should be avoided.

High-heeled shoes aggravate back discomfort by increasing the curvature of the spine. They should not be worn if the woman experiences backache or problems with her balance. Shoes should fit properly and feel comfortable.

Bathing

Daily bathing is important because of the increased perspiration and mucoid vaginal discharge that occurs during pregnancy. The woman may take either a shower or a tub bath, according to her preference. Caution is needed during tub baths because balance becomes a problem as pregnancy advances. Rubber tub mats and handgrips are valuable safety devices. Moreover, vasodilation due to the warm water may cause the woman to experience some faintness when she attempts to get out of the tub. Thus she may require assistance, especially in the third trimester. To avoid introducing infection, tub baths are contraindicated in the presence of vaginal bleeding or when the membranes are ruptured. During the first trimester, pregnant women should avoid hyperthermia associated with the use of a hot tub or Jacuzzi because it may increase the risk for miscarriage or neural tube defects (Cunningham et al., 2005).

Employment

Because increasing numbers of women of childbearing age are part of the workforce, it is important to be aware of the effects of occupation on pregnancy. General guidelines recommend that pregnant women who have no complications can continue to work until they go into labor (American Academy of Pediatrics & ACOG, 2002). Pregnant women who are employed in jobs that require prolonged standing do have a higher incidence of preterm birth but no effect on fetal growth (Cunningham et al., 2005). However, women who engage in strenuous physical activity during pregnancy tend to have babies with lower birth weight, possibly because of decreased placental flow (Rao, Kanade, Margetts et al., 2003).

Major deterrents to employment during pregnancy include fetotoxic hazards in the environment, excessive physical strain, overfatigue, and medical or pregnancy-related complications. In the last half of pregnancy, occupations involving balance should be adjusted to protect the mother.

Fetotoxic hazards in the environment are always a concern to the expectant couple. If the pregnant woman or the woman contemplating pregnancy is working in industry, she should contact her company physician or nurse about possible hazards in her work environment and should do her own reading and research on environmental hazards as well.

Travel

If medical or pregnancy complications are not present, there are no restrictions on travel. Pregnant women should avoid travel if there is a history of bleeding or preeclampsia or if multiple births are anticipated.

Travel by automobile can be especially fatiguing, aggravating many of the discomforts of pregnancy. The pregnant woman needs frequent opportunities to get out of the car and walk. (A good pattern to follow is to stop every 2 hours and walk around for approximately 10 minutes.) A pregnant woman should use a seat belt, specifically a properly positioned three-point restraint. She should wear both lap and shoulder belts. The lap belt should fit snugly and be positioned under the abdomen and across the upper thighs. The shoulder belt should be positioned snugly between the breasts. Seat belts play an important role in preventing fetal and maternal mortality and morbidity (Cunningham et al., 2005; Hyde, Cook, Olson et al., 2003). Fetal loss in car accidents is also caused by placental separation as a result of uterine distortion. Use of the shoulder belt decreases the risk of traumatic flexion of the woman's body, thereby decreasing the risk of placental separation. Thus, although it clearly is important for nurses to provide information about car safety early in the prenatal period, not all women are receiving this important information. A recent study reported that in the 19 states with data from a population-based survey, approximately 48.2% of pregnant women received prenatal counseling about the importance of the use of seat belts; more encouraging, however, 83.8% of pregnant women actually used seat belts during pregnancy (Beck, Gilbert, & Shults, 2005).

As pregnancy progresses, travel by airplane or train is generally recommended for long distances. However, those women who have medical or obstetric complications such as poorly controlled diabetes, sickle cell disease, or preeclampsia, and those women with placental abnormalities or who are at risk for preterm birth are advised to avoid flying during pregnancy. Before flying, the pregnant woman should check with her particular airline to see if it has any travel restrictions. Currently, flying is considered safe up to 36 weeks' gestation in the absence of any obstetric or medical complications (ACOG, 2004). To avoid the development of phlebitis or blood clots, pregnant women should drink plenty of fluid to avoid dehydration and hemoconcentration; avoid caffeinated beverages, which act as diuretics, and smoking, which causes vasoconstriction; and wear support hose while flying. They should also be advised to request an aisle seat and walk about the plane at regular intervals. The availability of medical care at her destination is an important consideration for the near-term woman who travels.

Activity and Rest

Exercise during pregnancy helps maintain maternal fitness and muscle tone, leads to improved self-image, increases energy, improves sleep, relieves tension, helps control weight gain, promotes regular bowel function, and is associated with improved postpartum recovery. Regular aerobic exercise maintains or improves a pregnant woman's general physical fitness and body image (Kramer, 2006). Normal participation in regular exercise can continue and in fact is encouraged throughout an uncomplicated pregnancy. Like the nonpregnant woman, the pregnant woman should focus her efforts on aerobic exercise that improves cardiorespiratory status and on resistance and flexibility exercises that improve musculoskeletal status (Artal & O'Toole, 2003).

Exercise may play a role in the prevention of certain complications. Research suggests that regular physical exercise before and during the first 20 weeks of pregnancy may aid in the prevention of preeclampsia (Sorenson, Williams, Lee et al., 2003; Weissgerber, Wolfe, & Davies, 2004). For women who are morbidly obese, exercise may assist in the prevention of gestational diabetes. Exercise is also recommended by the American Diabetes Association to assist in glycemic control for gestational diabetics (ACOG, 2002).

Before beginning an exercise program, a pregnant woman should be examined by her certified nurse-midwife or physician. A pregnant woman who is already in an exercise program can discuss her degree of participation with her caregiver. If a woman has not been physically active before her pregnancy, she should gradually increase her exercise period. However, maximum benefit of exercise for pregnant women is derived for those who have been physically fit before conception. As pregnancy progresses walking tends to be the most popular form of exercise for women (Mottola & Campbell, 2003).

Women should seek the opinion of their healthcare provider about taking part in strenuous sports, such as skiing and horseback riding. In general, the skilled sportswoman is no longer discouraged from participating in these activities if her pregnancy is uncomplicated. Pregnancy is not the time, however, to learn a new or strenuous sport. High-risk activities requiring balance and coordination, such as skydiving, mountain climbing, ice skating, surfing, and racquetball, should be avoided. In addition, women who are or may become pregnant should be advised not to scuba dive because the fetus is at risk for decompression illness (Artal & O'Toole, 2003). Certain conditions do contraindicate exercise. Absolute contraindications to exercise include the following (ACOG, 2002):

- Rupture of the membranes
- Preeclampsia-eclampsia
- Incompetent cervix (cerclage)
- Persistent vaginal bleeding in the second or third trimesters
- Multiple gestation at risk for preterm labor
- History of preterm labor in the prior or current pregnancy
- Placenta previa after 26 weeks' gestation
- Chronic medical conditions that might be negatively impacted by vigorous exercise such as significant heart disease or restrictive lung disease

Research related to the effects of maternal exercise on the fetus is varied and contradictory. Exercise can lead to increased maternal core temperature and hyperthermia. However, research suggests that the incidence of neural tube defects or other birth defects is not increased in the pregnancies of women who continue to exercise, even vigorously, during early pregnancy (Kelly, 2005).

Uterine blood flow is reduced during exercise as blood is shunted from visceral organs to muscles. The fetus does seem able to withstand this stress, however, without developing hypoxia. For most healthy pregnant women with no additional risk factors for preterm labor, exercise does not increase the incidence of preterm labor and birth or baseline uterine activity (Kelly, 2005). Benefits to the fetus of a sustained maternal program of moderate weight-bearing exercise include improved fetoplacental growth and a decreased incidence of nonreassuring fetal status during labor. Research indicates that the children of mothers who exercised regularly during pregnancy have a decrease in fat mass and improved neurologic development through the fifth year of life (Clapp, 2001).

The following guidelines are helpful in counseling pregnant women about exercise:

- Even mild to moderate exercise is beneficial during pregnancy. Regular exercise—at least 30 minutes of moderate exercise daily or at least most days of the week—is preferred (ACOG, 2002).

- After the first trimester, women should avoid exercising in the supine position. In most pregnant women, the supine position is associated with decreased cardiac output. Because uterine blood flow is reduced during exercise as blood is shunted from the visceral organs to the muscles, the remaining cardiac output is further decreased. Similarly, women should avoid standing motionless for prolonged periods (ACOG, 2002).

- Because decreased oxygen is available for aerobic exercise during pregnancy, women should modify the intensity of their exercise based on their symptoms, should stop when they become fatigued, and should avoid exercising to the point of exhaustion. Non-weight-bearing exercises, such as swimming or cycling, are recommended because they decrease the risk of injury and provide fitness with comfort (Artal & O'Toole, 2003).

- As pregnancy progresses and the center of gravity changes, especially in the third trimester, exercises in which the loss of balance or falling could pose a risk to mother or fetus (e.g., gymnastics, downhill skiing, horseback riding) are best avoided. Similarly, the woman should avoid any type of exercise that has a high potential for physical contact such as basketball, soccer, and ice hockey because it could result in trauma to the woman or her fetus.

- A normal pregnancy requires an additional 300 kcal per day. Women who exercise regularly during pregnancy should be careful to ensure that they consume an adequate diet.

- To augment heat dissipation, especially during the first trimester, pregnant women who exercise should wear appropriate clothing, ensure adequate hydration, and avoid the prolonged overheating associated with vigorous exercise in hot, humid weather because of the possible teratogenic effects of hyperthermia on the fetus (Berk, 2004). For the same reason, they should avoid hot tubs and saunas. Swimming may be suggested as a beneficial exercise during pregnancy, without concern for hyperthermia (Katz, 2003).

• As a result of the cardiovascular changes of pregnancy, heart rate is not an accurate indicator of the intensity of exercise for pregnant women (Wolfe & Weissgerber, 2003). To judge intensity of the exercise, the Borg relative ratings of perceived exertion has been found to be a more reliable technique. On a scale of 6–20, moderate exercise should be rated as 12–14 by the mother (Artal & O'Toole, 2003; Berk, 2004). If a pregnant woman is unable to talk or feels unable to breathe, then the exercise effort is too high.

In addition, the nurse may suggest that the woman wear a supportive bra and appropriate shoes when exercising. She should be advised to warm up and stretch to help prepare the joints for activity and cool down with a period of mild activity to help restore circulation and avoid pooling of blood. A moderate, rhythmic exercise routine involving large muscle groups such as swimming, cycling, walking, or cross-country skiing is best. Jogging or running is acceptable for women already conditioned to these activities as long as they avoid exercising at maximum effort and overheating.

Warning signs include the following: pain of any kind, vaginal bleeding, uterine contractions, decreased or absent fetal movement, fluid loss from the vagina, dizziness, headache, dyspnea before exertion, and muscle weakness (ACOG, 2002). The woman should stop exercising if any of these symptoms occur and contact her caregiver.

Adequate rest in pregnancy is important for both physical and emotional health. Women need more sleep throughout pregnancy, particularly in the first and last trimesters, when they tire easily. Without adequate rest, pregnant women have less resilience.

Finding time to rest during the day may be difficult for women who work outside the home or have small children. The nurse can help the expectant mother examine her daily schedule to develop a realistic plan for short periods of rest and relaxation.

Sleeping becomes more difficult during the last trimester because of the enlarged abdomen, increased frequency of urination, and greater activity of the fetus. Finding a comfortable position becomes difficult for the pregnant woman. Figure 16–10 ◆ shows a position most pregnant women find comfortable. Progressive relaxation techniques similar to those taught in prepared childbirth classes can help prepare the woman for sleep.

Exercises to Prepare for Childbirth

Certain exercises help strengthen muscle tone in preparation for birth and promote more rapid restoration of muscle tone after birth. The woman can reduce some physical changes of pregnancy considerably by faithfully practicing prescribed body-conditioning exercises. Many body-conditioning exercises for pregnancy are taught; a few of the more common ones are discussed here.

The **pelvic tilt,** or pelvic rocking, helps prevent or reduce back strain and strengthens abdominal muscle tone. To do the

Figure 16–10 ◆ Position for relaxation and rest as pregnancy progresses.
SOURCE: Photographer, Elena Dorfman.

pelvic tilt, the pregnant woman lies on her back and puts her feet flat on the floor. This bent position of the knees helps prevent strain and discomfort. She decreases the curvature in her back by pressing her spine toward the floor. With her back pressed to the floor, the woman tightens her buttocks and abdominal muscles as she tucks in her buttocks. The pelvic tilt can also be performed on hands and knees (Figure 16–11 ◆), while sitting in a chair, or while standing with the back against a wall. The body alignment achieved when the pelvic tilt is correctly done should be maintained as much as possible throughout the day.

> **CLINICAL TIP**
>
> Doing the pelvic tilt on hands and knees may aggravate back strain. Teach women with a history of minor back problems to do the pelvic tilt only in the standing position.

ABDOMINAL EXERCISES

A basic exercise to increase abdominal muscle tone is tightening abdominal muscles with each breath. It can be done in any position, but it is best learned while the woman lies supine. With knees flexed and feet flat on the floor, the woman expands her abdomen and slowly takes a deep breath. As she slowly exhales, she gradually pulls in her abdominal muscles until they are fully contracted. She relaxes for a few seconds and then repeats the exercise.

Partial sit-ups strengthen abdominal muscle tone and are done according to individual comfort levels. When doing a partial sit-up, the woman lies on the floor as just described (Figure 16–12 ◆). This exercise is done with the knees bent and the feet flat on the floor to avoid undue strain on the lower back. She stretches her arms toward her knees as she slowly pulls her head and shoulders off the floor to a comfortable level. (If she has poor abdominal muscle tone, she may not be able to pull up very far.) She then slowly returns to the starting position, takes a deep breath, and repeats the exercise. To strengthen the oblique abdominal muscles, she repeats the process but stretches the left arm to the side of her right knee, returns to the floor, takes a deep breath, and then reaches with the right arm to the left knee.

A

B

C

D

Figure 16–11 ◆ *A,* Starting position when the pelvic tilt is done on hands and knees. The back is flat and parallel to the floor, the hands are under the head, and the knees are directly under the buttocks. *B,* A prenatal yoga instructor offers pointers for proper positioning for the first part of the tilt: head up, neck long and separated from the shoulders, buttocks up, and pelvis thrust back, allowing the back to drop and release on an inhaled breath. *C,* The instructor helps the woman assume the correct position for the next part of the tilt. It is done on a long exhalation, allowing the pregnant woman to arch her back, drop her head loosely, push away from her hands, and draw in the muscles of her abdomen to strengthen them. Note that in this position the pelvis and buttocks are tucked under, and the buttock muscles are tightened. *D,* Proper posture. The knees are slightly bent but not locked, the pelvis and buttocks are tucked under, thereby lengthening the spine and helping support the weighty abdomen. With her chin tucked in, this woman's neck, shoulders, hips, knees, and feet are all in a straight line perpendicular to the floor. Her feet are parallel. This is also the starting position for doing the pelvic tilt while standing.
SOURCE: Photographer, Elena Dorfman.

These exercises can be done approximately five times in a sequence, and the sequence can be repeated several times during the day as desired. It is important that the woman do the exercises slowly to prevent muscle strain and overtiring.

PERINEAL EXERCISES

Perineal muscle tightening, also referred to as **Kegel exercises,** strengthens the pubococcygeus muscle and increases its elasticity (Figure 16–13 ◆). This muscle helps support the pelvic organs, including the uterus and bladder. A strong pubococcygeus muscle helps prevent stress incontinence, cystocele, rectocele, and uterine prolapse in women following childbirth.

The woman can feel the specific muscle group to be exercised by stopping urination midstream. However, doing Kegel exercises while urinating is discouraged because this practice has been associated with urinary stasis and urinary tract infection.

Figure 16–12 ◆ The pregnant woman can strengthen her abdominal muscles by doing partial sit-ups.
SOURCE: Photographer, Elena Dorfman.

Pubococcygeus muscle with good tone

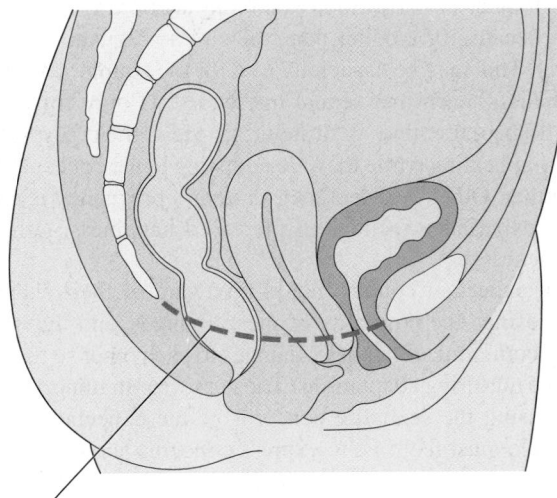

Pubococcygeus muscle with poor tone

Figure 16–13 ◆ Kegel exercises. The woman tightens the pubococcygeus muscle to improve support to the pelvic organs.

Childbirth educators sometimes use the following technique to teach Kegel exercises. They tell the woman to think of her perineal muscles as an elevator. When she relaxes, the elevator is on the first floor. To do the exercises, she contracts, bringing the elevator to the second, third, and fourth floors. She keeps the elevator on the fourth floor for a few seconds, and then gradually relaxes the area. If the exercise is properly done, the woman does not contract the muscles of the buttocks and thighs.

Kegel exercises can be done at almost any time. Some women use ordinary events—for instance, stopping at a red light—as a cue to remember to do the exercise. Others do Kegel exercises while waiting in a checkout line, talking on the telephone, or watching television.

INNER THIGH EXERCISES

The pregnant woman should assume a cross-legged sitting position whenever possible. This "tailor sit" stretches the muscles of the inner thighs in preparation for labor and birth.

Sexual Activity

As a result of the physiologic, anatomic, and emotional changes of pregnancy, the couple usually have many questions and concerns about sexual activity during pregnancy. Often these questions are about possible injury to the baby or the woman during intercourse and about changes in the desire each partner feels for the other.

In the past, couples were frequently warned to avoid sexual intercourse during the last 6 to 8 weeks of pregnancy to prevent complications such as infection or premature rupture of the membranes. However, these fears seem to be unfounded. In a healthy pregnancy, there is no medical reason to limit sexual activity. Intercourse is contraindicated for medical reasons such as threatened spontaneous abortion or risk of preterm labor (Cunningham et al., 2005).

The expectant mother may experience changes in sexual desire and response. Often these are related to the various discomforts that occur throughout pregnancy. For instance, during the first trimester, fatigue or nausea and vomiting may decrease desire, and breast tenderness may make the woman less responsive to fondling of her breasts. During the second trimester, many of the discomforts have lessened, and with the vascular congestion of the pelvis the woman may experience even greater sexual satisfaction than she experienced before pregnancy.

During the third trimester, interest in coitus may again decrease as the woman becomes more uncomfortable and fatigued. In addition, shortness of breath, painful pelvic ligaments, urinary frequency, and decreased mobility may lessen sexual desire and activity. If they are not already using them, the couple should consider coital positions other than male superior, such as side-by-side, female superior, and vaginal rear entry.

Sexual activity does not have to include intercourse. Cuddling, kissing, and being held can satisfy many of the nurturing and sexual needs of the pregnant woman. The warm, sensual feelings that accompany these activities can be an end in themselves. Her partner, however, may need to masturbate more frequently than before.

The sexual desires of men are also affected by many factors in pregnancy. These include the previous relationship with the partner, acceptance of the pregnancy, attitudes toward the partner's change of appearance, and concern about hurting the expectant mother or baby. Some men may withdraw from sexual contact because of a belief that sex with a pregnant woman is immoral. This may be especially true for the couple whose religious beliefs teach that sexual intercourse is only for procreation. Some men find it difficult to view their partners as sexually appealing while they are adjusting to the concept of her as a mother. Other men feel their partner's pregnancy is arousing and experience feelings of increased happiness, intimacy, and closeness.

The expectant couple should be aware of their changing sexual desires, the normality of these changes, and the importance of communicating these changes to each other so that they can make nurturing adaptations. The nurse has an important role in addressing the sexuality concerns of the expectant couple. The couple must feel free to express concerns about sexual activity, and the nurse must be able to respond and give anticipatory guidance in a comfortable manner. See Client Teaching: Sexual Activity During Pregnancy.

Dental Care

No evidence suggests that pregnancy causes or accelerates the development of dental caries. Nevertheless, in spite of such discomforts as nausea and vomiting, gum hypertrophy and tenderness, possible ptyalism, and heartburn, it is important for pregnant women to maintain regular oral hygiene.

Ensuring a healthy oral environment is essential to overall health. Women should be advised to do the following:

- Have extensive dental work done before becoming pregnant if possible.
- Eat a healthy diet including foods high in protein, calcium, phosphorus, and vitamins C, A, and D.
- Take prenatal vitamins daily.
- Maintain good oral hygiene by brushing at least twice a day and flossing daily.
- Use an antibacterial fluoride mouth rinse.
- If morning sickness occurs, brush teeth following vomiting to prevent tooth erosion caused by stomach acids.
- Have teeth cleaned every 6 months.

The pregnant woman is encouraged to have a dental checkup early in her pregnancy. The woman should inform her dentist of her pregnancy so that she is not exposed to teratogenic substances. The second trimester is considered the most appropriate time for minor dental treatments such as general repairs and extractions, preferably under local anesthetic. Dental x-ray examinations and extensive dental work should be delayed when possible until after birth. Extensive dental care during pregnancy requires consultation between the dentist and the woman's healthcare professional.

Immunizations

All women of childbearing age need to be fully aware of the risks of receiving specific immunizations if pregnancy is possible. Expectant women, especially those who intend to travel internationally, should be aware of the immunizations that are contraindicated during pregnancy. Immunizations with attenuated live viruses, such as rubella vaccine, should not be given in pregnancy because of the possible teratogenic effect of the live viruses on the developing embryo. The most current recommendations on vaccines related to pregnancy should be obtained from the Centers for Disease Control and Prevention Web site (Cunningham et al., 2005). Recommendations for immunizations during pregnancy are summarized in Table 16–5.

Complementary and Alternative Therapy

As discussed in Chapter 3 ∞, many women are electing to use complementary and alternative medicine (CAM), such as homeopathy, herbal medicine, acupressure, acupuncture, biofeedback, therapeutic touch, massage, and chiropractic, as part of a holistic approach to their healthcare regimens. The nurse should inquire about the use of CAM as part of a routine antepartal assessment. It is important that nurses working with pregnant women and their families develop a general understanding of the more commonly used therapies to be able to answer questions and provide resources as needed.

It is important for the pregnant woman to understand that herbs are considered dietary supplements and are not regulated as prescription or over-the-counter drugs through the FDA. Herbal products have not been studied for potential harmful effect on the fetus during pregnancy and therefore should be avoided, particularly in the first trimester (Born & Barron, 2005). See Complementary and Alternative Therapies: Homeopathy and Herbal Medicine. Table 16–6 identifies common herbs that pregnant women should avoid or use with caution.

Teratogenic Substances

Substances that adversely affect the normal growth and development of the fetus are called **teratogens.** Many of these effects are readily apparent at birth, but others may not be identified for years. A well-known example is the development of cervical cancer in adolescent females whose mothers took diethylstilbestrol (DES) during pregnancy.

Known teratogens include chemicals, viruses, environmental factors, physical factors, and drugs (Cunningham et al.,

CLIENT TEACHING Sexual Activity During Pregnancy

CLIENT GOALS   At the completion of the teaching the woman will be able to:

1. Relate the changes in sexuality and sexual response that may occur during pregnancy to changes in technique, frequency, and response that may be indicated

2. Explore personal attitudes, beliefs, and expectations about sexual activity during pregnancy

3. Cite maternal factors that would contraindicate sexual intercourse

TEACHING PLAN

CONTENT

Begin by explaining that the pregnant woman may experience changes in desire during the course of pregnancy. During the first trimester, discomforts such as nausea, fatigue, and breast tenderness may make intercourse less desirable for many women.

In the second trimester, as symptoms decrease, desire may increase. In the third trimester, discomfort and fatigue may lead to decreased desire in the woman.

Explain that men may notice changes in their level of desire, too. Among other things, this change may be related to feelings about their partner's changing appearance, their belief about the acceptability of sexual activity with a pregnant woman, or concern about hurting the woman or fetus. Some men find the changes of pregnancy erotic; others must adjust to the notion of their partners as mothers.

Explain that the woman may notice that orgasms are much more intense during the last weeks of pregnancy and may be followed by cramping. Because of the pressure of the enlarging uterus on the vena cava, the woman should not lie flat on her back for intercourse after about the fourth month. If the couple prefer that position, a pillow should be placed under her right hip to displace the uterus. Alternate positions such as side-by-side, female superior, or vaginal rear entry may become necessary as her uterus enlarges.

Stress that sexual activities that both partners enjoy are generally acceptable. It is not advisable for couples who favor anal sex to go from anal penetration to vaginal penetration because of the risk of introducing *Escherichia coli* into the vagina.

Suggest that alternative methods of expressing intimacy and affection such as cuddling, holding and stroking each other, and kissing may help maintain the couple's feelings of warmth and closeness. If the man feels desire for further sexual release, his partner may help him masturbate to ejaculation, or he may prefer to masturbate in private.

Advise the woman who is interested in masturbation as a form of gratification that the orgasmic contractions may be especially intense in later pregnancy.

Stress that sexual intercourse in contraindicated once the membranes are ruptured or if bleeding is present. Women with a history of preterm labor may be advised to avoid intercourse because the oxytocin that is released with orgasm stimulates uterine contractions and may trigger preterm labor. Because oxytocin is also released with nipple stimulation, fondling the breasts may also be containdicated in those cases.

TEACHING METHOD

Universal statements that give permission, such as "Many couples experience changes in sexual desire during pregnancy. What kind of changes have you experienced?" are often effective in starting discussion. Depending on the woman's (or couple's) level of knowledge and sophistication, part or all of this discussion may be necessary.

If the partner is present, approach him in the same nonjudgmental way used above. If not, ask the woman if she has noticed any changes in her partner or if he has expressed any concerns.

Deal with any specific questions about the physical and psychologic changes that the couple may have.

Discussion about various sexual activities requires that you be comfortable with your sexuality and that you be tactful.

The couple may be content with these approaches to meeting their sexual needs, or they may require assurance that such approaches are indeed "normal."

An explanation of the contraindications accompanied by their rationale provides specific guidelines that most couples find helpful.

(Continued on next page)

CLIENT TEACHING   Sexual Activity During Pregnancy   continued

CONTENT

A discussion of sexuality and sexual activity should stress the importance of open communication so that the couple feel comfortable expressing their feelings, preferences, and concerns.

TEACHING METHOD

Some couples are skilled at expressing their feelings about sexual activity. Others find it difficult and can benefit from specific suggestions. The nurse should provide opportunities for discussion throughout the talk.

Specific handouts on sexual activity are also helpful for couples and may address topics that were not discussed.

EVALUATION

Evaluate the learning by assessing the woman's (or couple's) response to information throughout the discussion. Ask the woman to express information such as the contraindications to intercourse in her own words. Follow-up sessions and questions from the woman also provide information about teaching effectiveness.

DOCUMENTATION

Document the information given to the woman, including specifics on contraindications to sexual activity (specify if written instructions were provided in addition to verbal ones) and the type of teaching method used. Document the woman's verbalization of understanding and your clarification of any information.

Table 16–5   RECOMMENDATIONS FOR IMMUNIZATION DURING PREGNANCY

Live Attenuated Virus Vaccines	Inactivated bacterial vaccines	Hyperimmune globulins
Measles—contraindicated	Pneumococcal—same as nonpregnant	Hepatitis B—postexposure prophylaxis: give along with
Mumps—contraindicated	Meningococcal—same as nonpregnant	hepatitis B vaccine initially, then vaccine alone at 1 and 6 mo
Rubella—contraindicated	Typhoid—not recommended	Rabies—postexposure prophylaxis
Varicella-zoster—contraindicated		Tetanus—postexposure prophylaxis
Poliomyelitis—no longer recommended		Varicella—consider for postexposure within 96 h
Yellow fever—high-risk areas only		
Smallpox—contraindicated		
Inactivated virus vaccines	**Toxoids**	**Pooled immune serum globulins**
Influenza—after first trimester request	Tetanus-diptheria—same as nonpregnant	Hepatitis A—postexposure prophylaxis
Rabies—same as nonpregnant		Measles—postexposure prophylaxis
Hepatitis A and B—same as nonpregnant		
Enhanced poliomyelitis (IPV-e)—risk of exposure		

SOURCE: Cunningham, T. G., Grant, N. F., & Leveno, K. J. (2001). *Williams obstetrics,* 21st ed. New York: McGraw-Hill. Reproduced with permission of The McGraw-Hill Companies.

Table 16–6   COMMON HERBS TO AVOID IN PREGNANCY*

Blue cohosh	Goldenseal
Black cohosh	Gingko
Chamomile, Valeria	Ginseng
Comfrey	Horehound
Dong quai	Horseradish (fresh)
Ephedra	

Use with caution:

Garlic

Ginger

Turmeric

*Avoid excessive consumption relative to usual and customary food use.

SOURCE: Hardy, M. (2000). Herbs of special interest to women. *Journal of the American Pharmaceutical Association, 40*(2), 234–242.

2005). Medications are perhaps the most likely documented teratogens, but other factors can also harm the fetus, including certain infections such as rubella, syphilis, herpesvirus type 2, toxoplasmosis, and cytomegalovirus (CMV). During pregnancy, women need to have adequate information available and a realistic perspective on potential environmental hazards. Factors that are suspected to be hazardous to the general population should obviously be avoided if possible.

MEDICATIONS

The use of medications during pregnancy, including prescriptions, over-the-counter drugs, and herbal remedies, is of great concern because maternal drug exposure is thought to account for at least 10% of birth defects (Black & Hill, 2003). Statistics indicate that the use of prescription and over-the-counter medications by pregnant women is more widespread than might be expected (McCarter-Spaulding, 2005). Many pregnant women

COMPLEMENTARY AND ALTERNATIVE THERAPIES

HOMEOPATHY AND HERBAL MEDICINE

Homeopathy and herbal medicine are alternative therapies for pregnancy-related symptoms.

Homeopathy: Homeopathy means "like suffering." Homeopathic medicine is based on the theory that a miniscule amount of a substance can cure symptoms in a sick person that are similar to the symptoms the substance causes in healthy people. Thus, for example, ipecac, which induces vomiting, may be used to treat a person who is vomiting, such as a pregnant woman with severe nausea and vomiting. Currently, homeopathic practitioners have more than 2000 plant, animal, and mineral remedies available for their use (Fontaine, 2005).

Homeopathic therapies are available for pregnancy-related symptoms such as musculoskeletal disorders, anemia, nausea, ptyalism, pica, threatened miscarriage, and preterm labor. According to homeopathic theory, homeopathic remedies either help an individual or have no effect. However, a healing crisis or aggravation of symptoms can occur if the remedy is given in too high a potency or repeated too frequently. More information about homeopathy can be found on our Companion Web Site.

Herbal Medicine: Herbal medicine uses therapies derived from plants. Many have been used for centuries in different parts of the world and are well recognized. In fact, countries such as Germany, Canada, England, and France recognize the benefits of scores of herbs and include information about their use as part of formal educational programs for physicians and pharmacists.

In the United States, herbs are categorized as dietary supplements rather than drugs and may be used by pregnant women. In general, it is best to advise pregnant women not to ingest any herbs, except ginger, during the first trimester of pregnancy (Born & Barron, 2005). Pregnant women need to avoid certain categories of herbs such as abortifacient (abortion-inducing) herbs, herbs that induce menstruation, nervous system stimulants, stimulant laxatives, and so forth. Lists identifying common herbs that women are advised to avoid or use with caution during pregnancy and lactation are available; an example is shown in Table 16–6.

For a reliable source of information about herbs, homeopathic therapies, and other alternative options, consumers or healthcare providers can access the National Center for Complementary and Alternative Medicine Web site and the Office of Dietary Supplements Web site.

---

need medication for therapeutic purposes, such as the treatment of infections, allergies, or other pathologic processes. In these situations, the problem can be extremely complex. Known teratogenic agents are not prescribed and usually can be replaced by medications considered safe. Even when a woman is highly motivated to avoid taking any medications, she may have taken potentially teratogenic medications before her pregnancy was diagnosed, especially if she had an irregular menstrual cycle.

The greatest potential for gross abnormalities in the fetus occurs during the first trimester of pregnancy, when fetal organs are first developing. Many factors influence teratogenic effects, including the specific identity and dose of the teratogen, the state of embryo development, and the genetic sensitivity of the mother and fetus. For example, the commonly prescribed acne medication isotretinoin (Accutane) is associated with a high incidence of spontaneous abortion and congenital malformations if taken early in pregnancy. Valproic acid, an anticonvulsant, is associated with an increased risk of neural tube defects (Cunningham et al., 2005).

To provide information for caregivers and clients, the Food and Drug Administration (FDA) has developed the following classification system for medications administered during pregnancy:

Category A. Controlled studies in women have demonstrated no associated fetal risk. Few drugs fall into this category. Vitamin C is cited as a category A drug as long as its use does not exceed the recommended dietary allowance.

Category B. Either animal studies show no risk, but there are no controlled studies in women; or animal studies indicate a risk, but controlled human studies fail to demonstrate a risk. The penicillins fall into this category.

Category C. Either (1) no adequate studies, either in animals or women, are available; or (2) animal studies show teratogenic effects, but no controlled studies in women are available. Many drugs fall into this category, and the lack of information poses a problem for caregivers. Zidovudine, a drug used to decrease perinatal transmission of human immunodeficiency virus (HIV), falls into this category.

Category D. Evidence of human fetal risk does exist, but the benefits of the drug in certain situations are thought to outweigh the risks. Examples in this category include tetracycline, vincristine, lithium, and hydrochlorothiazide.

Category X. The demonstrated fetal risks clearly outweigh any possible benefit. An example of a drug in this category is isotretinoin (Accutane), the acne medication, which can cause multiple central nervous system (CNS), facial, and cardiovascular anomalies.

If a woman has taken a drug in category D or X, she should be informed of the risks associated with that drug and of her alternatives. Similarly, a woman who has taken a drug in the safer categories can be reassured. For up-to-date information on the risks associated with specific drugs, women can contact drug information centers, either by telephone or by using online databases.

The FDA system, although useful, has been criticized because the letter system suggests a risk grading that is not necessarily accurate. More important, not all drugs in a category have the same risk level. Currently the FDA is working to develop a new evidence-based system (Cunningham et al., 2005).

Although the first trimester is the critical period for teratogenesis, some medications are known to have teratogenic effect when taken in the second and third trimesters. For example, tetracycline taken in late pregnancy is commonly associated with staining of teeth in children and has been shown to depress skeletal growth, especially in preterm infants. Warfarin (Coumadin), a commonly prescribed anticoagulant, is associated with CNS defects following fetal exposure during the second and third trimesters (Cunningham et al., 2005). Because heparin does not cross the placenta, it is safer for the fetus than warfarin and other anticoagulants.

Pregnant women should avoid all medication—prescribed, homeopathic, or over-the-counter—if possible. If a medication is necessary during pregnancy, the benefits must clearly outweigh the risks. If no alternative exists, it is wisest to select a well-known medication rather than a newer drug whose potential teratogenic effects may not be known. When possible, the oral form of the drug should be used, and it should be prescribed in the lowest possible therapeutic dose for the shortest time possible. Finally, the caregiver should carefully consider the multiple components of the medication.

A woman clearly has a right to the most comprehensive information available concerning medications. The nurse can assist her by suggesting appropriate references and helping her research information. Some excellent reference books on drugs and pregnancy are currently available and should be part of the library of every office and clinic that provides prenatal care. In addition, several online databases that provide information on teratogens are available for convenient reference.

The nurse should remind the woman of the need to check with her caregiver about medications she was taking when pregnancy occurred and about any nonprescription drugs she is contemplating using. Any medication with possible teratogenic effects must be avoided.

TOBACCO

In the United States, smoking during pregnancy is one of the most significant, modifiable causes of poor pregnancy outcomes. Smoking during pregnancy has a strong association with low-birth-weight infants. In addition, mothers who smoke have an increased risk of infertility, spontaneous abortion, intrauterine growth restriction (IUGR), placentae previa, abruptio placentae, premature rupture of membranes, and preterm birth (ACOG, 2005; Kuczkowski, 2003; Magee, Hattis, & Kivel, 2004). Pregnant women who smoke as well as participate in other unhealthy behaviors, such as alcohol use, further increase their risk for low-birth-weight infants (Okah, Cai, & Hoff, 2005). Smoking has also been linked to an increased risk of cleft lip and palate in the newborn (Cunningham et al., 2005; Little, Cardy, & Munger, 2004). Research also links maternal smoking, both during pregnancy and afterward, with an increased risk of sudden infant death syndrome (SIDS). Maternal smoking exposes young children to other risks of secondhand smoke including middle ear infections, acute and chronic respiratory tract illnesses, and behavioral and learning disabilities (Albrecht et al., 2004).

The specific mechanism by which smoking affects the fetus is not known. However, the ingredients in cigarette smoke, such as carbon monoxide, nicotine, lead, and cotinine, are toxic to the fetus and decrease the availability of oxygen to maternal and fetal tissue (Cunningham et al., 2005).

In response to public health education campaigns in the United States, smoking during pregnancy has decreased significantly. In fact, approximately 46% of women who smoke quit during pregnancy. Unfortunately, 60% to 80% of women who quit smoking during their pregnancy resume smoking within a year after birth (ACOG, 2005). This finding suggests that although women are aware of the potential impact of smoking on the fetus, they may be less knowledgeable about the effects of passive smoke on the baby.

Smoking cessation programs decrease the number of women who smoke in pregnancy and the incidence of low-birth-weight infants and preterm births (Lumley, Oliver, Chamberlain et al., 2005). Studies demonstrate that any decrease in smoking during pregnancy improves fetal outcome, and researchers continue to explore approaches designed to help women quit smoking. ACOG (2005) suggests a 5- to 15-minute intervention, with women who smoke fewer than 20 cigarettes a day, to be most effective. This program and other programs encourage healthcare providers to use the five As:

- *Ask* about tobacco use.
- *Advise* to quit smoking.
- *Assess* willingness to quit.
- *Assist* in attempt to quit.
- *Arrange* for follow-up care.

The nurse can play an important role in counseling women about the importance of smoking cessation during pregnancy, and can be actively involved in offering smoking cessation programs.

If smoking cessation efforts are not successful, the healthcare provider might consider the pharmacologic approaches of nicotine gum (FDA category C) or a transdermal system (FDA category D). However, these approaches are somewhat controversial. They should be offered only if the pregnant woman has failed at prior attempts to quit smoking and continues to smoke 10 to 15 cigarettes per day. In this case, the potential benefit of stopping smoking outweighs the unknown risk of nicotine replacement (ACOG, 2005; Cunningham et al., 2005).

Many educational resources are available for healthcare providers and consumers on smoking cessation programs. Organizations that might be helpful include the following:

- American Lung Association
- March of Dimes
- American Cancer Society
- Healthy Mothers, Healthy Babies

ALCOHOL

Alcohol is now considered one of the primary teratogens in the Western world. Fetuses of women who are heavy drinkers are at increased risk for developing **fetal alcohol syndrome (FAS),** which is characterized by growth restriction, behavioral distur- bances, craniofacial abnormalities, and brain, cardiac, and spinal defects. FAS is also the major cause of mental retardation in the United States (Cunningham et al., 2005). The Centers for Disease Control and Prevention (CDC) analysis of the 2002 Behavioral Risk Factor Surveillance System (BRFSS) survey revealed that 10% of pregnant women used alcohol and approx- imately 2% engaged in binge drinking (CDC, 2004). Approxi- mately 12,000 children are born with FAS each year in the United States, somewhere between 1 in 500 to 1 in 2000 live births (Harvard Medical School, 2004).

The effects of moderate consumption of alcohol during pregnancy are not clearly known, but research suggests there is an increased incidence of lower birth weight and of some neu- rologic effects, such as attention deficit disorder. Evidence suggests that the risk of teratogenic effects increases propor- tionately with increased average daily intake of alcohol. Al- though an occasional drink during pregnancy does not carry any known risk, no safe level of drinking during pregnancy has been identified, and caregivers should recommend that pregnant women abstain from all alcohol during pregnancy (CDC, 2005a). In 2005, the US surgeon general issued an advisory on alcohol use in pregnancy to increase public awareness about this serious health concern (CDC, 2005b).

Alcohol passes the placental barrier within minutes after consumption, with fetal blood alcohol levels becoming equiv- alent to maternal blood alcohol levels. The effects of alcohol consumption vary according to the stage of fetal development. During the first trimester, alcohol probably alters embryonic development; throughout pregnancy, alcohol may interfere with cell division and growth; in the third trimester, the time of most rapid brain growth, alcohol may alter CNS development and contribute to growth retardation (Cunningham et al., 2005). The risk of neurologic damage is lessened if heavy drinking ceases in the third trimester. Decreased consumption of alcohol in midpregnancy is associated with a lower inci- dence of growth retardation.

Assessment of alcohol intake should be a chief part of each woman's medical history, with questions asked in a direct, non- judgmental manner. All women should be counseled about the role of alcohol in pregnancy. When pregnant women become aware of the risk of alcohol to the fetus, most usually attempt to modify their alcohol consumption. For example, in a study by Chang et al. (2005), pregnant women with a positive alcohol screening assessment who received an educational intervention for them and for their partners had decreased alcohol use during pregnancy. If heavy consumption is involved, women should be referred early to an alcoholic treatment program. Because the drug disulfiram (Antabuse), which is often used in the treatment of alcoholism, is a suspected teratogen, a woman in such a pro- gram should inform her counselor if she becomes pregnant.

Counseling pregnant women about the effects of alcohol during pregnancy has been effective in reducing drinking among pregnant women and it should, of course, continue. Be- cause the most profound impact of alcohol occurs in the first weeks after conception, however, nurses and other healthcare providers will see the most dramatic decrease in the effects of alcohol during pregnancy by increasing their teaching efforts in the period before conception. All women of childbearing age who are sexually active and not using an effective method of birth control should be advised of the tetratogenic effect of al- cohol (CDC, 2005b).

CAFFEINE

Current research reveals no evidence that moderate levels of caffeine are linked to birth defects. However, caffeine ingestion at high levels may increase the risk of spontaneous abortion (Cunningham et al., 2005). An increased risk of decreased birth weight has been found in infants of mothers who consume at least 600 mg of caffeine daily (Bracken, Triche, Belanger et al., 2003; Vika, Bakketeiga, Trygg et al., 2003). The American Dietetic Association (2002) has recommended that pregnant women limit their caffeine intake to 300 mg per day. The aver- age cup of brewed coffee has 100 mg, a cup of tea has 50 mg, a regular cola drink has up to 40 mg, and a normal-sized choco- late bar has up to 50 mg. Until more definitive data are available, nurses should advise women of common sources of caffeine, in- cluding coffee, tea, colas, and chocolate, and suggest they use good judgment in moderating their caffeine intake.

MARIJUANA

Research reveals that approximately 15% of pregnant women use marijuana. The prevalence of marijuana use in our society raises concerns about its effect on the fetus, but to date no ter- atogenic effects of marijuana use during pregnancy have been documented (Cunningham et al., 2005). Research on marijuana use in pregnancy is difficult, however, because it is an illegal drug. Unreliability of reporting, lack of a representative popu- lation, inability to determine strength or composition of the marijuana used, presence of herbicides, and use of other drugs at the same time are major factors complicating the research be- ing done.

COCAINE

Research indicates that 2.8% of pregnant women use illicit sub- stances, with marijuana use at 75% and cocaine use at 10% (Ebrahim & Gfroerer, 2003). A woman who uses cocaine is at increased risk for acute myocardial infarction, cardiac arrhyth- mias, ruptured ascending aorta, seizures, cerebrovascular accidents, hypertension, bowel ischemia, and sudden death (Cunningham et al., 2005). During pregnancy, cocaine use has been related to abruptio placentae, preterm birth, nonreassuring fetal status, meconium-stained amniotic fluid, low birth weight, neonatal irritability, and SIDS (King, 2003; Vidaeff & Mastro- battista, 2003). In particular, preschool children can have detri- mental cognitive outcomes as a result of prenatal cocaine exposure (King, 2003; Singer, Arendt, Minnes et al., 2002). Sev- eral congenital anomalies in the newborn have been linked to maternal cocaine use, including genitourinary anomalies, con- genital heart defects, limb reduction defects, CNS anomalies, prune belly syndrome (congenital absence of abdominal mus- cles), and segmental intestinal atresia (Cunningham et al., 2005).

As cocaine becomes more widely used by women of child- bearing age, healthcare providers need to be alert to early signs of cocaine use. The pregnant woman who uses cocaine may have risk factors such as tobacco and alcohol use, lower socioeconomic status, and poor prenatal care. All these factors can affect maternal and fetal health (King, 2003; Vidaeff & Mastrobattista, 2003).

It is often difficult for a healthcare provider to face the fact that a client may be using cocaine, but ongoing alertness and an open, nonjudgmental approach are important in early detection. Maternal urine screening for cocaine is valuable, but because cocaine is metabolized rapidly, the drug screen is negative within 24 to 48 hours after cocaine use. Thus it is probable that many abusers are missed. However, the newborn may also be screened to document maternal cocaine use. It is important for the nurse to promote early detection of fetal exposure to cocaine in order to provide appropriate newborn care.

Evaluation

Throughout the antepartal period, evaluation is an essential part of effective nursing care. As nurses ask questions of the pregnant woman and her family or make observations of physical changes, they are evaluating the results of previous interventions. In evaluating the effectiveness of the interventions, the nurse should not be afraid to try creative solutions if they are logical and carefully thought out. This is especially important in dealing with families from other cultures. If a practice is important to a woman and not harmful, the culturally competent nurse will not discourage it.

In completing an evaluation, the nurse must also recognize situations that require referral for further evaluation. For example, a woman who has gained 4 lb in 1 week probably does not require counseling about nutrition; she needs further assessment for preeclampsia. The nurse who has a sound knowledge of theory will recognize this and act immediately.

The ongoing and cyclic nature of the nursing process is especially evident in the prenatal setting. However, throughout the course of pregnancy nurses can use certain criteria to determine the quality of care provided. In essence, nursing care has been effective if the following have been met:

- The common discomforts of pregnancy are quickly identified and are relieved or lessened effectively.
- The woman is able to discuss the physiologic and psychologic changes of pregnancy.
- The woman implements appropriate self-care measures, if they are indicated, during pregnancy.
- The woman avoids substances and situations that pose a risk to her well-being or that of her child.
- The woman seeks regular prenatal care.

CARE OF THE EXPECTANT COUPLE OVER 35

Today an increasing number of women are choosing to have their first baby after age 35 (Table 16–7). In fact, in 2004, over 14% of pregnancies occurred in women who were age 35 or

Table 16–7   PREGNANCY IN WOMEN OVER AGE 35
• Couples who choose pregnancy at a later age are usually financially secure and have made a thoughtful, planned choice.
• If the woman has no existing health problems, her risk during pregnancy is not appreciably higher than that of the general population.
• The decreased fertility of women over age 35 may make conception more difficult.
• The incidence of Down syndrome increases somewhat in women over age 35 and significantly in those over age 40.
• The couple may choose to have amniocentesis or chorionic villus sampling to gain information about the health of their fetus.

older (Hamilton, Ventura, Martin et al., 2005). Many factors contribute to this trend, including the following:

- The availability of effective birth control methods
- The expanded roles and career options available for women
- The increased number of women obtaining advanced education, pursuing careers, and delaying parenthood until they are established professionally
- The increased incidence of later marriage and second marriage
- The high cost of living, which causes some young couples to delay childbearing until they are more secure financially
- The increased number of women in this older reproductive age group because of the baby boom between 1946 and 1964
- The increased availability of specialized fertilization procedures, which offers opportunities for women who had previously been considered infertile

There are advantages to having a first baby after the age of 35. Single women or couples who delay childbearing until they are older tend to be well educated and financially secure. Usually their decision to have a baby was deliberately and thoughtfully made (Figure 16–14 ◆). Because of their greater life experiences, they are also more aware of the realities of having a child than younger women, and they recognize what it means

Figure 16–14 ◆ For many older couples, the decision to have a child may be a very rewarding one.
SOURCE: Photographer, Elena Dorfman.

to have a baby at their age. Many of the women have experienced fulfillment in their careers and feel secure enough to take on the added responsibility of a child (Neumann & Graf, 2003). Some women are ready to make a change in their lives, desiring to stay home with a new baby. Those who plan to continue working tend to be more able to afford good child care.

Medical Risks

Historically, medical professionals considered women who were over 30 at the time of their first pregnancy, and especially those who were 35 or older, at higher risk for maternal or fetal complications. This age-related concern began to change during the 1980s, when studies comparing healthy pregnant women over 35 years of age with healthy younger women did not confirm these beliefs. In addition, adverse pregnancy outcomes in this age group have been linked to socioeconomic status, which can, in turn, influence a woman's health status and her access to care (Cunningham et al., 2005). However, the current medical literature does report some adverse pregnancy outcomes associated with advanced maternal age.

In the United States and Canada over the past 30 years, the risk of death has declined dramatically for women of all ages as a result of advances in maternal health and obstetric practice. However, the risk for maternal death is significantly higher for women over age 35, and even higher for women age 40 and older. This is true regardless of a woman's parity, the time at which she begins prenatal care, and her level of education (Callan & Berg, 2003). Women over age 35, and even more, women over age 40, are more likely to have chronic medical conditions. Preexisting medical conditions, such as hypertension or diabetes, probably play a more significant role than age in maternal well-being and the outcome of pregnancy. The incidence of low-birth-weight infants and preterm births is higher among women age 35 or older (Newburn-Cook & Onyskiw, 2005). In addition, the rate of miscarriage is significantly higher in older women. Women over age 35 who become pregnant also have an increased risk for gestational diabetes mellitus, hypertension, placenta previa, difficult labor, and newborn complications (March of Dimes [MOD], 2006).

The cesarean birth rate is also increased in pregnant women over 35. This practice may be related to increased concern by the woman and physician about the pregnancy outcome (MOD, 2006).

The risk of conceiving a child with Down syndrome does increase with age, especially over 35. Amniocentesis is routinely offered to all women over age 35 to permit the early detection of several chromosomal abnormalities, including Down syndrome. Research has also focused on the use of quadruple screening to detect Down syndrome and trisomy 18 (see Chapter 15 ∞). If the screening results are not in the normal range, follow-up testing using ultrasound and amniocentesis is often indicated (Cleveland Clinic, 2004).

Routine genetic testing has not been offered to couples in which the only risk is advanced paternal age, because there is no sufficient evidence to determine a specific paternal age at which to start genetic testing. However, advanced paternal age increases the risk of spontaneous new mutations, which can affect autosomal dominant diseases, such as neurofibromatosis, achondroplasia, and Marfan syndrome. Early pregnancy loss can be increased as a result of these mutations (Cunningham et al., 2005). Additionally, advanced paternal age increases the risk for late fetal death, especially if the father is 50 or older at the time of conception (Andersen, Hansen, Andersen, et al., 2004).

Special Concerns of the Expectant Couple Over 35

No matter what their age, most expectant couples have concerns regarding the well-being of the fetus and their ability to parent. The older couple has additional concerns related to their age, especially the closer they are to 40 or more. Some couples are concerned about whether they will have enough energy to care for a new baby. Of greater concern is their ability to deal with the needs of the older child when they, too, are older.

I didn't really think I would get married but then I met Antonio and fell hard. I was 35 and he was 43, a widower with no children. We both really wanted a baby, so here I am 36 and pregnant. How I pray that this baby will be healthy.

The financial concerns of an older couple are usually different from those of a younger couple. The older couple is generally more financially secure than the younger couple. However, when their "baby" is ready for college, the older couple may be near retirement and might not have the means to provide for their child.

While considering their financial future and future retirement, the older couple may be forced to face their own mortality. Certainly this is not uncommon in midlife, but instead of confronting this issue at 40 to 45 years of age or later, the older expectant couple may confront the issue several years earlier as they consider what will happen as their child grows.

The older couple facing pregnancy following a late or second marriage or after therapy for infertility may find themselves somewhat isolated socially. They may feel "different" because they are often the only couple in their peer group expecting their first baby. In fact, many of their peers are likely to be parents of adolescents or young adults and may be grandparents as well.

The response of older couples who already have children to learning that the woman is pregnant may vary greatly depending on whether the pregnancy was planned or unexpected. Other factors influencing their response include the attitudes of their children, family, and friends to the pregnancy; the impact on their lifestyle; and the financial implications of having another child. Sometimes couples who had previously been married to other mates will choose to have a child together. The concept of blended family applies to situations in which "her" children, "his" children, and "their" children come together as a new family group.

Healthcare professionals may treat the older expectant couple differently from the way they would a younger couple. Older women may be asked to submit to more medical procedures, such as amniocentesis and ultrasound, than younger women. An older woman may be prevented from using a birthing room or birthing center even if she is healthy because her age is considered to put her at risk.

The woman who has delayed pregnancy may be concerned about the limited amount of time that she has to bear children. When pregnancy does not occur as quickly as she hoped, the older woman may become increasingly anxious as time slips away on her "biological clock." When an older woman becomes pregnant but experiences a spontaneous abortion, her grief for the loss of her unborn child is exacerbated by her anxiety about her ability to conceive again in the time remaining to her.

NURSING CARE MANAGEMENT
Nursing Assessment and Diagnosis

In working with a woman in her 30s or 40s who is pregnant, the nurse makes the same assessments as are appropriate in caring for any woman who is pregnant. These include assessing physical status, the woman's understanding of pregnancy and the changes that accompany it, any health teaching needs that exist, the degree of support the woman has available to her, and her knowledge of infant care. In addition, the nurse explores the woman's and her partner's attitudes about the pregnancy and their expectations of the impact a baby will have on their lives.

The nursing diagnoses that are applicable to any pregnant woman apply to the pregnant woman who is over the age of 35. Examples of other nursing diagnoses that may apply include the following:

- *Decisional Conflict* related to unexpected pregnancy
- *Impaired Social Interaction* related to changes associated with pregnancy

Nursing Plan and Implementation

Once an older couple has decided to have a child, it is the nurse's responsibility to respect and support them in this decision. As with any client, the nurse needs to discuss risks, identify concerns, and promote strengths. The woman's age should not be made an issue. To promote a sense of well-being, the nurse should treat the pregnancy as "normal" unless specific health risks are identified.

As the pregnancy continues, the nurse should identify and discuss concerns the woman may have related to her age or to specific health problems. The older woman who has made a conscious decision to become pregnant often has carefully thought through potential problems and may actually have fewer concerns than a younger woman or one with an unplanned pregnancy.

Childbirth education classes are important in promoting adaptation to the event of childbirth for expectant couples of any age. However, older expectant couples, who are still in the minority, often feel uncomfortable in classes where the majority of participants are much younger. Because of the differences in age and life experiences, many of the needs of the older couple may

not be met in the class. The nurse teaching a childbirth education class should try to anticipate the informational needs of the older couple. At the same time, the nurse should not make the couple feel uncomfortable by drawing attention to their age. Fortunately, classes for expectant parents over age 35 are now available in many communities. Women who are over 35 years of age and having their first baby tend to be better educated than other healthcare consumers. These clients frequently know the kind of care and services they want and are assertive in their interactions with the healthcare system. The nurse should neither be intimidated by these clients nor assume that they do not need anticipatory guidance and support. Instead, the nurse should support the couple's strengths and be sensitive to their individual needs.

A particularly difficult issue older expectant couples face is the possibility of bearing an unhealthy child. Because of the risk of Down syndrome in these families, amniocentesis is encouraged. Chorionic villus sampling may also be suggested if available in the area. The decision to have amniocentesis can be difficult to make merely on the basis of its possible risks to the fetus. But that becomes almost a minor concern when the couple thinks of the implications of the possible findings of Down syndrome or other chromosomal abnormalities. The finding of abnormalities means that the couple may be faced with an even more difficult decision about continuing the pregnancy.

A couple's decision to have amniocentesis is usually related to their beliefs and attitudes about abortion. Generally, amniocentesis is not even considered by couples who are strongly opposed to abortion for any reason. Health professionals must respect the couple's decision, take a nonjudgmental approach, and provide them with emotional support throughout the pregnancy.

The decision to have an abortion is a painful one even when couples are not opposed to abortion on political or philosophic grounds. Even though the couple may believe that terminating a high-risk pregnancy is right for their family, they may feel a great deal of ambivalence about amniocentesis. If the results are such that the couple elects to have an abortion, they will usually feel much grief for their loss.

Many health professionals assume that the couple who agrees to amniocentesis will also elect to have an abortion if Down syndrome or another condition is diagnosed. This is not necessarily the case. Some couples choose not to have an abortion after being informed that their unborn child has genetic abnormalities.

For the couple who agrees to amniocentesis, the first few months of pregnancy are a difficult time. Amniocentesis cannot be done until 14 weeks of pregnancy, and the chromosomal studies take roughly 2 weeks to complete. Their fear that the fetus is at risk may delay the successful completion of the psychologic tasks of early pregnancy.

The nurse can support couples who decide to have amniocentesis in several ways:

- The nurse should make sure that the couple is aware of the risks of amniocentesis and why it is being performed.
- The nurse who is present during the amniocentesis procedure can offer comfort and emotional support to the

expectant woman. The nurse can also provide information about the procedure as it is being performed.

- The nurse can facilitate a support group for women during the difficult waiting period between the procedure and the results.

- If the results indicate that the fetus has Down syndrome or another genetic abnormality, the nurse can ensure that the couple has complete information about the condition, its range of possible manifestations, and its developmental implications.

- The nurse can support the couple in their decision about continuing or terminating the pregnancy. It is essential that the nurse and other health professionals involved with the couple not impose their philosophic or political beliefs about abortion on the couple. The decision is the couple's, and it should be based on their belief system and a nonbiased presentation of risks and choices from caregivers.

Amniocentesis is discussed further in Chapter 21. ∞

Evaluation

Expected outcomes of nursing care include the following:

- The woman and her partner are knowledgeable about the pregnancy and make appropriate healthcare choices.

- The expectant couple is able to cope successfully with the pregnancy and its implications for the future.

- The woman receives effective health care throughout her pregnancy and during birth and the postpartum period.

- The woman and her partner develop skills in child care and parenting as necessary.

CHAPTER REVIEW

FOCUS YOUR STUDY

- Providing anticipatory guidance about childbirth, the postpartum period, and childrearing is a primary responsibility of the nurse caring for women in an antepartal setting.

- The nurse assesses the expectant father's knowledge level and intended degree of participation and then works with the couple to help ensure a satisfying experience.

- Culturally based practices and forbidden activities may have a major impact on the childbearing family.

- The common discomforts of pregnancy occur as a result of physiologic and anatomic changes. The nurse provides the woman with information about self-care activities aimed at reducing or relieving discomfort.

- To make appropriate self-care choices and ensure healthful habits, a pregnant woman requires accurate information about a range of subjects from exercise to sexual activity, from bathing to immunization.

- Maternal assessment of fetal activity keeps the woman "in touch" with her fetus and provides ongoing assessment of fetal status.

- Teratogenic substances are substances that adversely affect the normal growth and development of the fetus.

- A pregnant woman should avoid taking nonessential medications or using over-the-counter preparations during pregnancy.

- Evidence confirms that smoking, consuming alcohol, or using social drugs during pregnancy may be harmful to the fetus.

- Childbirth among women over 35 is becoming increasingly common. It poses fewer health risks than previously believed and offers advantages for the woman or couple who make the choice.

- A major risk for the older expectant couple relates to the increased incidence of Down syndrome in children born to women over age 35. Amniocentesis can provide information as to whether the fetus has Down syndrome. The couple can then decide whether they wish to continue the pregnancy.

EXPLORE MediaLink

http://www.prenhall.com/davidson

NCLEX review questions, case studies, and other interactive resources for this chapter can be found on the Web Site at http://www.prenhall.com/davidson. Click on "Chapter 16" to select the activities for this chapter.

For tutorials including animations and videos, more NCLEX review questions, and an audio glossary, access the accompanying Prentice Hall Nursing MediaLink DVD-ROM in this book.

PRENTICE HALL NURSING MEDIALINK DVD-ROM

Audio Glossary

NCLEX Review

Videos: *Through the Eyes of a Nurse—The First Trimester; Through the Eyes of a Nurse—The Second Trimester; Through the Eyes of a Nurse—The Third Trimester*

COMPANION WEBSITE

Additional NCLEX Review

Case Study: *First Trimester Client*

Care Plan Activity: *Common Discomforts of Pregnancy*

Applications: *Teaching Resouces for Pregnant Couples; Exercise During Pregnancy; Smoking Cessation Plan; Fetal Alcohol Syndrome*

Critical Thinking

CRITICAL THINKING IN ACTION

THIRD TRIMESTER PREGNANCY DISCOMFORTS

View the Critical Thinking in Action video in Chapter 16 of the DVD-ROM. Then answer the questions that follow.

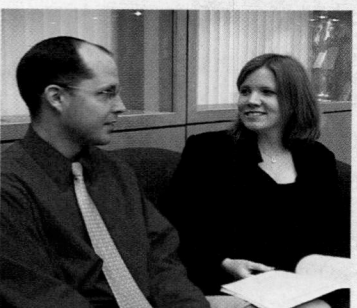

Thirty-seven-year-old Cathy Sommers, G1, P0000, presents to you, with her husband, at the OB physician's office at 32 weeks' gestation. Cathy tells you that she and her husband are practicing lawyers with their own firm. The couple delayed starting a family because it has been important to them to advance their careers and establish their firm. Cathy had an amniocentesis at 18 weeks' gestation because of her advanced maternal age, and the results ruled out chromosomal abnormalities. The couple knows that the baby is a boy and are anticipating a vaginal birth. Cathy tells you that she is experiencing more fatigue, leg cramps, and shortness of breath when climbing stairs. The physical exam including a negative Homans' sign is within normal limits with the exception of slight ankle edema. Her weight is 150 lb, temperature 98.6F, pulse 88, respirations 16, BP 126/70. You discuss pregnancy discomforts in the third trimester with Cathy and her husband.

1. What measures can you suggest to cope with fatigue?
2. Discuss measures to decrease leg cramps.
3. Discuss the physiologic changes underlying dyspnea.
4. Review Braxton Hicks contractions.

REFERENCES

Albrecht, S. A., Maloni, J. A., Thomas, K. K., Jones, R., Halleran, J., & Osborne, J. (2004). Smoking cessation for pregnant women who smoke: Scientific basis for practice:AWHONN's SUCCESS Project. *Journal of Obstetric, Gynecologic, & Neonatal Nursing, 33*(3), 298–305.

American Academy of Pediatrics and the American College of Obstetricians and Gynecologists (ACOG). (2002). *Guidelines for perinatal care* (5th ed.). Washington, DC: Author.

American College of Obstetricians and Gynecologists (ACOG). (2001, Reaffirmed 2004). *Air travel during pregnancy* (Committee Opinion No. 264). Washington, DC: Author.

American College of Obstetricians and Gynecologists (ACOG). (2002). *Exercise during pregnancy and the postpartum period* (Technical Bulletin No. 267). Washington, DC: Author.

American College of Obstetricians and Gynecologists (ACOG). (2004). *Diagnosis and treatment of nausea and vomiting of pregnancy* (Practice Bulletin No. 52). Washington, DC: Author.

American College of Obstetricians and Gynecologists (ACOG). (2005). *Smoking cessation during pregnancy* (Committee Opinion No. 316). Washington, DC: Author.

American Dietetic Association. (2002). Position of the American Dietetic Association: Nutrition and lifestyle for a healthy pregnancy outcome. *Journal of the American Dietetic Association, 102*, 479.

Andersen, A. N., Hansen, K. D., Andersen, P. K., & Smith, G. D. (2004). Advanced paternal age and risk of fetal death: A cohort study. *American Journal of Epidemiology, 160*(12), 1214–1222.

Artal, R., & O'Toole, M. (2003). Guidelines of the American College of Obstetricians and Gynecologists for exercise during pregnancy and the postpartum period. *British Journal of Sports Medicine, 37*(7), 6–13.

Beck, L. F., Gilbert, B. C., & Shults, R. A. (2005). Prevalence of seat belt use among reproductive-aged women and prenatal counseling to wear seat belts. *American Journal of Obstetrics & Gynecology, 192,* 580–585.

Berk, B. (2004). Recommending exercise during and after pregnancy: What the evidence says. *The International Journal of Childbirth Education, 19*(2), 18–22.

Black, R. A., & Hill, D. A. (2003). Over-the-counter medications in pregnancy. *American Family Physician, 67*(12), 2517–2524.

Blumenthal, M. (2003). Ginger as an antiemetic during pregnancy. *Alternative Therapies in Health and Medicine, 9,* 19–21.

Born, D., & Barron, M. L. (2005). Herb use in pregnancy. *American Journal of Maternal/Child Nursing, 30*(3), 201–206.

Borrelli, F., Capasso, R., Aviello, G., Pittler, M., & Izzo, A. A. (2005). *Obstetrics and Gynecology, 105,* 849–856.

Bracken, M. B., Triche, E. W., Belanger, K., Hollenbrand, K., & Leaderer, B. P. (2003). Association of maternal caffeine consumption with decrements in fetal growth. *American Journal of Epidemiology, 157*(5), 456–466.

Buist, A., Morse, C. A., & Durkin, S. (2003). Men's adjustment to fatherhood: Implications for obstetric health care. *Journal of Obstetric, Gynecologic, & Neonatal Nursing, 32*(2), 172–180.

Callan, W. M., & Berg, C. J. (2003). Pregnancy-related mortality among women aged 35 years and older, United States, 1991–1997. *Obstetrics and Gynecology, 102*(5, Pt. 1), 1015–1021.

Centers for Disease Control and Prevention (CDC). (2004). Alcohol use among women who are pregnant or might become pregnant—United States. *Morbidity and Mortality Weekly Report, 53,* 1178–1181.

Centers for Disease Control and Prevention (CDC). (2005a). Guidelines for identifying and referring persons with fetal alcohol syndrome. *Morbidity and Mortality Weekly Report, 54* (RR-11), 1–15.

Centers for Disease Control and Prevention (CDC). (2005b). Surgeon general's advisory on alcohol use in pregnancy. *Morbidity and Mortality Weekly Report, 54,* 229.

Chang, G., McNamara, T. K., Orav, J., Koby, D., Lavigne, A., Ludman, B., et al. (2005). Brief intervention for prenatal alcohol use: A randomized trial. *Obstetrics and Gynecology, 105*(5), 991–998.

Chez, R. A., & Friedmann, A. K. (2000). Offering effective breastfeeding advice. *Contemporary OB/GYN, 45*(8), 32–50.

Clapp, J. F., III. (2001). Recommending exercise during pregnancy. *Contemporary OB/GYN, 46*(1), 30–50.

Cleveland Clinic. (2004). Quad marker screen. Retrieved April 10, 2004, from www.cchs.net/health_health-info/docs/0300/0386.asp?index=4698

Cunningham, F. G., Leveno, K. J., Bloom, S. L., Hauth, J. C., Gilstrap, L. C., III, & Wenstrom,

K. D. (2005). *Williams obstetrics* (22nd ed.). New York: McGraw-Hill.

Davis, M. (2004). Nausea and vomiting of pregnancy: An evidence-based review. *Journal of Perinatal and Neonatal Nursing, 18*(4), 312–328.

Ebrahim, S. H., & Gfroerer, J. (2003). Pregnancy-related substance use in the United States during 1996–1998. *Obstetrics and Gynecology, 101,* 374.

Fontaine, K. L. (2005). *Complementary and alternative therapies for nursing practice* (2nd ed.). Upper Saddle River, NJ: Prentice-Hall.

Hamilton, B. E., Ventura, S. J., Martin, J. A., & Sutton, P. D. (2005). *Preliminary births for 2004.* Health-E stats. Hyattsville, MD: National Center for Health Statistics. Retrieved March 8, 2006, from http://www.cdc.gov/nchs

Harvard Medical School. (2004). Alcohol before birth. *Harvard Mental Health Letter, 21*(3), 1–3.

Hyde, L. K., Cook, L. J, Olson, L. M., Weiss, H. B., & Dean, J. M. (2003). Effect of motor vehicle crash on adverse fetal outcomes. *Obstetrics and Gynecology, 102,* 279–286.

Jewell, D., & Young, G. (2003). Interventions for nausea and vomiting in early pregnancy: A review. *The Cochrane Database of Systematic Reviews, 4* (Article No. CD000145. DOI: 10,1002/14651858. CD000145).

Katz, V. L. (2003). Exercise in water during pregnancy. *Clinical Obstetrics and Gynecology, 46*(2), 432–441.

Kelly, A. K. (2005). Practical advice during pregnancy. *Sportsmedicine, 33*(6), 1–8.

King, D. E. (2003). Statistics: Cocaine use and infant development. *The International Journal of Childbirth Education, 18*(2), 15.

Kramer, M. S. (2006). Aerobic exercise for women during pregnancy. *Cochrane Library* (1). (Article 2006 No.CD 000180).

Kuczkowski, K. M. (2003). Tobacco and ethanol use in pregnancy: Implications for obstetric and anesthetic management. *The Female Patient, 28*(4), 16–22.

Lie, D. (2004). *Ginger helpful for nausea and vomiting of pregnancy.* Medscape CME offering. Retrieved January 13, 2004, from http://www.medscape.com/viewarticle/466746_print

Lile, J., Perkins, J., Hammer, R. L., & Loubert, P. V. (2003). Diagnostic and management strategies for pregnant women with back pain: Once a serious cause is ruled out, conservative measures may help to relieve the discomfort. *Journal of the American Academy of Physicians Assistants, 16*(12), 31–39.

Little, J., Cardy, A., & Munger, R. G. (2004). Tobacco smoking and oral clefts: A meta-analysis. *Bulletin of the World Health Organization, 82,* 213–218.

Lumley, J., Oliver, S. S., Chamberlain, C., & Oakley, L. (2005). Interventions for promoting smoking cessation during pregnancy (Review). *The Cochrane Database of Systematic Review* (3) (Article No. CD001055).

Magee, D., Hattis, D., & Kivel, N. M. (2004). Role of smoking in low birth weight. *Journal of Reproductive Medicine, 49*(1), 23–27.

March of Dimes (MOD). (2006). Pregnancy after 35. Retrieved January 16, 2006, from http://www.marchofdimes.com/printableArticles/14332_1155.asp

Mattson, S. (2004). Ethnocultural considerations in the childbearing period. In S. Mattson & J. E. Smith (Eds.), *Core curriculum for maternal-

newborn nursing* (3rd ed.). St. Louis, MO: Elsevier Saunders.

McCarter-Spaulding, D. E. (2005). Medications in pregnancy and lactation. *American Journal of Maternal/Child Nursing, 30*(1), 10–17.

Mottola, M. F., & Campbell, M. K. (2003). Activity patterns during pregnancy. *Canadian Journal of Applied Physiology, 28*(4), 642–653.

Neumann, M., & Graf, C. (2003). Pregnancy after 35: Are these women at high risk? *AWHONN Lifelines, 7*(5), 422–430.

Newburn-Cook, C. V., & Onyskiw, J. E. (2005). Is older maternal age a risk factor for preterm birth and fetal growth restriction? A systematic review. *Health Care for Women International, 26,* 852–875.

Okah, F. A., Cai, J., & Hoff, G. L. (2005). Term gestation low birth weight and health compromising behaviors during pregnancy. *Obstetrics and Gynecology, 105*(3), 543–550.

Purnell, L. D., & Paulanka, B. J. (2005). *Guide to culturally competent health care.* Philadelphia: F. A. Davis.

Rao, S., Kanade, A., Margetts, B. M., Yajnik, C. S., Lubree, H., Rege, S. et al. (2003). Maternal activity in relation to birth size in rural India. The Pune Maternal Nutrition Study. *European Journal of Clinical Nutrition, 57*(4), 531–542.

Singer, L. T., Arendt, R., Minnes, S., Farkas, K., Salvator, A., Kirchner, H. L., et al. (2002). Cognitive and motor outcomes of cocaine exposed infants. *Journal of the American Medical Association, 287*(15), 1952–1960.

Smith, C., Crowther, C., Willson, K., Hotham, N., & McMillian, V. (2004). A randomized controlled trial of ginger to treat nausea and vomiting of pregnancy. *Obstetrics and Gynecology, 103,* 639–645.

Sorenson, T. K., Williams, M. A., Lee, I. M., Dashow, E. E., Thompson, M. L., & Luthy, D. A. (2003). Recreational physical activity during pregnancy and the risk of preeclampsia. *Hypertension, 41,* 1273–1280.

Spector, R. E. (2004). *Cultural diversity in health and illness* (6th ed.). Upper Saddle River, NJ: Prentice-Hall Health.

Tiran, D. (2003). Self help for constipation and haemorrhoids in pregnancy. *British Journal of Midwifery, 11*(9), 579–581.

Varney, H., Kriebs, J. M., & Gregor, C. L. (2004). *Varney's midwifery* (4th ed.). Sudbury, MA: Jones and Bartlett.

Vidaeff, A. C., & Mastrobattista, J. M. (2003). In utero cocaine exposure: A thorny mix of science and mythology. *American Journal of Perinatology, 20*(4), 165–172.

Vika, T., Bakketeiga, L. S., Trygg, K. U., Lund-Larsen, K., & Jacobsen, G. (2003). High caffeine consumption in the third trimester of pregnancy: Gender specific effects on fetal growth. *Paediatric and Perinatal Epidemiology, 17*(4), 324.

Wang, S. M., Dezinno, P., Maranets, Berman, M. R., Caldwell-Andrews, A. A., & Kain, Z. N. (2004). Low back pain during pregnancy: Prevalence, risk factors and outcomes. *Obstetrics and Gynecology, 104*(1), 65–70.

Weissgerber, T. L., Wolfe, L. A., & Davies, G. A. (2004). The role of regular physical activity in preeclampsia prevention. *Medicine & Science in Sports & Exercise, 36*(12), 2024–2031.

Wolfe, L. A., & Weissgerber, T. L. (2003). Clinical physiology of exercise in pregnancy: A literature review. *Journal of Obstetrics and Gynaecology Canada, 25*(6), 473–483.

CHAPTER
17 Adolescent Pregnancy

I am a freshman in college, and so is my daughter. I had her when I was 15, and that forced me to grow up in a hurry. For years I've thought about being a nurse, and now is my chance. Please understand, my daughter is very precious to me, but a part of me knows that if I had it to do over, I would change so much of my life—if only I had known!

KEY TERMS

Early adolescence 406	Late adolescence 406
Emancipated minors 413	Middle adolescence 406

OBJECTIVES

1. Briefly discuss the physical and psychosocial changes of adolescence.

2. Compare the three stages of adolescence: early adolescence, middle adolescence, and late adolescence.

3. Summarize the developmental tasks of adolescence and the impact that pregnancy superimposes on these tasks.

4. Describe the major factors that contribute to teenage pregnancy.

5. Identify the impact of cultural factors on the desirability of early pregnancy.

6. Identify the physical, psychologic, and sociologic risks faced by an adolescent who is pregnant.

7. Delineate characteristics of the fathers of children of adolescent mothers.

8. Discuss the reactions of the adolescent's family and social support groups to her pregnancy.

9. Formulate a plan of care to meet the needs of a pregnant adolescent.

10. Describe successful community approaches to adolescent pregnancy prevention.

MEDIALINK

Additional resources for this content can be found on the Prentice Hall Nursing MediaLink DVD-ROM and on the Companion Website at http://www.prenhall.com/davidson. Click on "Chapter 17" to select the activities for this chapter.

Adolescent pregnancy is a health and social issue with no single cause or cure. For a teen, pregnancy comes at a time when her physical development and the developmental tasks of adolescence are incomplete. She may not be prepared physically, psychologically, or economically for parenthood. Thus both she and her child are at high risk. Compared with women of similar socio-economic status who postpone childbearing, teen mothers are less likely to finish high school, more likely to end up on welfare and to have babies who are born prematurely and with low birth weight. In addition, children of teen mothers are at increased risk for mental retardation, poverty, welfare dependency, and poor school performance. They are also more likely to grow up without a father. In addition, they suffer higher rates of abuse and neglect than would occur if their mothers had delayed childbearing (National Campaign to Prevent Teen Pregnancy [NCPTP], 2004b).

Approximately 820,000 teenage girls (ages 15 to 19) in the United States become pregnant each year, and most of these pregnancies (78%) are unplanned (NCPTP, 2004b). Of these pregnancies, about one third are terminated by therapeutic abortion, and about 14% end in miscarriage. More than half the teens who become pregnant give birth and keep their babies.

The US birth rate (number of births per 1000 women) for adolescents ages 15 to 19 has dropped steadily over the past years, from 61.8 per 1000 females in 1991 to 41.2 in 2004, a 33% decline (Figure 17–1 ◆) (Hamilton, Ventura, Martin, et al., 2005). This continuing decline is extremely encouraging. However, the US teenage birth rate remains the highest of any industrialized nation (NCPTP, 2004a). The incidence of sexual activity among teens in other countries is as high as in the United States. These countries may have lower adolescent pregnancy rates because of family influences, a greater openness about sexuality, better access to contraceptives, and a more comprehensive approach to sex education.

This chapter explores the incidence, risk factors, and consequences of adolescent pregnancy. It then presents the role of the nurse in meeting the special needs and concerns of pregnant adolescents and their families and concludes with a discussion of efforts to prevent adolescent pregnancy.

Figure 17–1 ◆ Birth rates for teenagers by age: United States, 1990–2004.
SOURCE: Hamilton, B. E., et al. (2005). *Preliminary births for 2004*. Health E-Stats. National Center for Health Statistics.

OVERVIEW OF ADOLESCENCE
Physical Changes

Adolescence is the period of development during which an individual makes the psychologic and physiologic transition from childhood to young adulthood, usually between 13 and 20 years of age. Puberty, the period during which an individual becomes capable of reproduction, is a maturational process that can last from 1.5 to 6 years and generally coincides with adolescence. The major physical changes of puberty include a growth spurt, weight change, and the appearance of secondary sexual characteristics. *Menarche,* or the time of the first menstrual period, usually occurs in the last half of this maturational process, with the average age between 12 and 13.

The initial menstrual cycles are usually irregular and often anovulatory for the first 12 to 18 months; however, this is not true for all females. Some adolescents do not use contraception during this time because they falsely assume that they cannot get pregnant. Even if their initial menstrual cycles are anovulatory, there is no certainty about when the first ovulatory cycle will occur; thus, contraception is important during this time for all adolescents who are sexually active.

Psychosocial Development

Although it is well documented that the onset of puberty now occurs at a younger age than it did 50 years ago, there are no data to indicate that psychosocial development, particularly cognitive development, occurs at an earlier age. Developmental tasks of adolescence have been described by many writers and are based on a variety of classic theories. These tasks are issues that individuals may struggle with at other times in their lives, but they are especially significant during adolescence to help ensure a successful transition from childhood to adulthood. The following are major developmental tasks of this period (Steinberg, 2002):

- Developing an identity
- Gaining autonomy and independence
- Developing intimacy in a relationship
- Developing comfort with one's own sexuality
- Developing a sense of achievement

Resolving these tasks is a developmental process that occurs over time. This developmental process is reflected in the behaviors of youths during early, middle, and late adolescence.

During adolescence, there is a need to "try on" various roles in a process of experimentation and exploration as adolescents grapple with ideas about who they want to be and how they want to live. This developmental process occurs in youths during all stages of adolescence and is affected by many factors, including culture, religion, and socioeconomic status.

Teens work to separate themselves from their parents to establish their own identity and they begin to express themselves with music, clothing, and hairstyles. Some choose peer-identity behaviors such as body modifications (body piercing) and body art (tattoos). Although these forms of peer identity have been around for thousands of years, they are gaining popularity, especially among teens and preteens. See discussion in Chapter 4. ∞

During **early adolescence** (age 14 and under), psychosocial development is marked by rapid physical changes that engender self-centeredness and initiate the struggle for independence. The teen at this age still sees authority as resting with the parents. She perceives her locus of control as external; that is, her destiny is controlled by others, such as parents and school authorities. However, she begins the process of "leaving the family" by spending more time with friends, especially friends of the same sex. Conformity to peer group standards is reflected in her behavior and her clothing. She may lack impulse control, which can result in risk-taking behaviors. During this phase, the adolescent has a rich fantasy life. She is also struggling to become comfortable with her changing body and body image and to fit this image with her fantasy life. Much time is spent in front of the mirror. The adolescent in this phase is very egocentric and is a concrete thinker. She has only minimal ability to see herself in the future or foresee the consequences of her behavior.

Middle adolescence (15 to 17 years) is the time for challenging authority. Experimentation with drugs, alcohol, and sex is a common method of rebellion. As the middle adolescent seeks independence, she turns increasingly to her peer group,

identifying with and conforming to them in her choice of dress, makeup, hairstyle, and music. These years are often a time of great turmoil for the family as the adolescent struggles for independence and challenges the family's values and expectations.

The middle adolescent wants to be treated as an adult. However, fear of adult responsibility may cause fluctuation in behavior. At times she seems like a child; at other times she is surprisingly mature. She is beginning to move from concrete thinking to formal operational thought but is not yet able to anticipate the long-term implications of all her actions. She may even believe that she is invincible and will not suffer negative consequences from risk-taking behaviors.

In **late adolescence** (18 to 19 years), the young woman is more at ease with her individuality and decision-making ability. She can think abstractly and anticipate consequences. During this time, she becomes more confident of her personal identity. The late adolescent is capable of formal operational thought. She is learning to solve problems, to conceptualize, and to make decisions. These abilities help her see herself as having control, which leads to the ability to understand and accept the consequences of her behavior.

Table 17–1 describes successful resolution of each of the developmental tasks of adolescence and identifies high-risk factors for adolescent pregnancy.

Table 17–1   DEVELOPMENTAL TASKS OF ADOLESCENCE

Tasks	Description of Successful Resolution	High-Risk Factors for Teen Pregnancy
Developing an identity	As individuals enter puberty, their physical appearance begins to change, and others begin to respond differently to them. The media present idealized images of the teenage female. Self-esteem may fluctuate, and hormonal changes create awareness of sexual desire. Adolescents experience confusion about their self-image. This is a time of experimentation until they become comfortable with who they are.	If the young adolescent feels she cannot live up to parents' expectations or is in a dysfunctional family situation, she may adopt a negative identity. She may become rebellious and actively involved in risk-taking behaviors, such as substance abuse and early sexual activity.
Gaining independence	Adolescents gradually move away from parental control and are influenced by peers. Eventually, they develop values that help govern their behavior responsibly without extrinsic control of peers or parents.	Peer pressure is highest during early and middle adolescence. If peers are involved in antisocial behavior, this influences their behavior and all other developmental tasks. Substance abuse and sexual activity are common in these groups.
Developing emotional intimacy in relationships	Adolescents begin to develop a close emotional attachment with another individual. They can share innermost feelings and have empathy for the other. This usually begins with a friend of the same sex and eventually develops into a trusting and loving relationship with someone of the opposite sex.	Sexual activity may be an attempt to meet needs for intimacy. This is a problem for victims of neglect or abuse. Although sexual intercourse has become a common adolescent experience, emotional intimacy is not associated with the majority of dating relationships, and most teenage marriages end in divorce.
Developing comfort with their sexuality	Puberty causes a new awareness of sexual desire and new meaning about physical contact with others. Adolescents learn to express sexual feelings appropriately and comfortably in a relationship.	Many young adolescent females who become sexually involved at an early age do so for a variety of reasons that do not lead to comfort with their own sexuality peer pressure, pressure from an older male partner, rebellion against parents, sexual abuse and its consequences.
Gaining a sense of achievement	Adolescents begin to look toward the future and compare talents, work skills, and/or academic achievement with reality in preparing for adult working roles.	Those who drop out of school prematurely tend to be from economically disadvantaged backgrounds. Data show that early sexual experimentation by adolescents correlates with poor school performance whatever their background. Use of contraception is more likely among adolescent females who are high academic achievers and have a future orientation (Alan Guttmacher Institute, 2002).

SOURCE: Adapted from Steinberg, L. (2002). *Adolescence* (6th ed.). New York: McGraw-Hill.

FACTORS CONTRIBUTING TO ADOLESCENT PREGNANCY

Teenagers rarely plan pregnancy. *Pregnancy risk taking* (sexual activity without use of pregnancy prevention measures) is believed to stem from a complex variety of factors, the most important of which are discussed next.

Socioeconomic and Cultural Factors

Poverty is a major risk factor for adolescent pregnancy. Adolescents who do not have access to middle-class opportunities tend to maintain their pregnancies, because they see pregnancy as their only option for adult status; 85% of births to unmarried teens occur to those from poor or low-income families (Alan Guttmacher Institute, 2002). Not surprisingly, research indicates that the more time high-school students spend without adult supervision, the greater their level of sexual activity.

In the United States, the adolescent birth rate is higher among African American and Hispanic teens than among white teens. However, pregnancy rates in these groups are declining steadily (Hamilton et al. 2005). To some degree, the higher teenage pregnancy rate in these groups reflects the impact of poverty, because a disproportionately higher number of African American and Hispanic youths live in poverty.

Low educational achievement is another major risk factor for adolescent pregnancy. Teenaged girls who participate in after-school activities are less likely to be sexually experienced than girls who do not participate (Cohen, Farley, Taylor et al., 2002). Similarly, compared with other teens, teens with future goals (i.e., college or job) tend to use birth control more consistently; if they become pregnant, they are also more likely to have abortions.

The younger the teen when she first gets pregnant, the more likely she is to have another pregnancy in her teens. Moreover, the likelihood of repeat pregnancies increases when the teen is living with her sexual partner and has dropped out of school. Daughters and sisters of women who had a baby in their early teens tend to have intercourse earlier and are at higher risk for teen pregnancy themselves (Short & Rosenthal, 2003).

High-Risk Behaviors

Among American adolescents there is tremendous peer pressure to become sexually active during the teen years. Premarital sexual activity is commonplace, and teenage pregnancy is more socially acceptable today than it was in the past although the incidence is decreasing. Statistics indicate that 46.8% of high school students have had sexual intercourse, which is down from 54.1% in 1991. The percentage of students who have had intercourse with four or more people (14.3%) has also decreased since 1991 (18.7%) (Eaton, Kann, Kincher et al., 2006).

Sexual innuendo permeates every aspect of the popular media, including music, music videos, television, and movies. The Internet, too, provides teens with unlimited access to information about sex as well as a steady supply of people willing to discuss it with them. These experiences and images feed the adolescent's rich fantasy life and may glamorize unprotected intercourse as proof of "true love." At the same time, media aimed at teens largely ignore issues of sexual responsibility and fail to convey the physical, emotional, financial, and social costs of pregnancy risk-taking behaviors.

In addition to vaginal intercourse, many adolescents engage in other sexual behaviors. The incidence of oral sex is increasing. The increase has occurred, especially among young and early-middle adolescents, because of the pressure to have sex coupled with the fear of pregnancy. The question of whether "oral sex" is really "sex" has led adolescents to perceive that they are still virgins if they have not had vaginal-penile sexual activity. Adolescents believe that they are less likely to get a bad reputation, get into trouble, or feel bad about themselves if they have oral rather than vaginal sex. However, they typically underestimate the risks of contracting chlamydia, human immunodeficiency virus (HIV), and other sexually transmitted infections (STIs).

High-risk sexual behaviors, including, for example, multiple partners and lack of contraceptive use, are of concern. Research indicates that young people aged 15 to 24 constitute 25% of the sexually experienced population in the United States. However, they account for 48% of the new cases of STIs. This is particularly worrisome because many STIs, including HIV, are asymptomatic. Thus, apparently healthy young people who are infected may not seek health care (Weinstock, Berman, & Cates, 2004).

Statistics have demonstrated an increased use of condoms among the adolescent population, probably because of widespread educational efforts related to HIV. Among currently sexually active students, 62.8% report using a condom during their last sexual intercourse (Eaton et al., 2006). Nevertheless, adolescents remain inconsistent contraceptive users. Contraceptive use is more consistent in situations in which teens discuss contraception before having sex, when they have waited a longer time after starting a relationship to have sex with that person, and when they use dual methods of contraception (Manlove, Ryan, & Franzetta, 2003).

Many teens lack accurate and adequate knowledge about contraceptive options. This is a common topic of sex education programs; however, debate continues about the appropriateness of such programs in schools. Proponents advocate early sex education to provide teens with the knowledge they need to avoid unwanted pregnancy and the risk of STIs. Opponents feel that sex education is the responsibility of parents and worry that sex education in the schools will promote sexual activity. However, a review of research on sex education reveals that it does not increase initiation of sexual activity at an earlier age (Doniger, Adams, Utter et al., 2001). Other factors affecting the use of contraception include access or availability, cost of supplies, and concern regarding confidentiality.

Adolescent sexuality is not pathologic but a part of normal development as a human being. Emphasizing sexual health rather than discussing sex exclusively as a behavior that has only bad consequences results in more effective work with adolescents (Kelly, Lesser, & Smoots, 2005).

RESEARCH IN PRACTICE

ADOLESCENT PREGNANCY: DO EXPECTATIONS AFFECT INTERVENTIONS?

What is this study about? Adolescent pregnancy is a complex problem with biologic, psychologic, and social aspects. It is a serious public health threat because teens have babies who are smaller and have more physical problems, and the teenage mothers are at risk for health problems themselves. Persuading teens to postpone pregnancy gives both them and their babies an advantage. It is unclear why teens who say they want to postpone pregnancy simultaneously use inadequate contraception methods. It has been hypothesized that teens who do not fully understand the effects of a pregnancy in the teen years do not adequately protect themselves from conception. This study sought to establish the relationship between expectations about the effects of childbearing and the strength of the desire to remain nonpregnant during adolescence.

How was this study done? The researchers recruited 351 nulligravida teens from three urban teen health clinics. The teens were ethnically diverse, and the primary inclusion criterion was the use of no or unreliable contraceptive methods. The teens responded to 60 items on an author-developed questionnaire; the questionnaire was acceptably reliable and valid. The survey asked the teens about their expectations of childbearing and the advantages and disadvantages of getting pregnant. A third of the teenagers were asked to complete the study questionnaire for a second time 4 to 6 months after enrollment and to participate in a face-to-face interview at that time. The interviewer used a standardized question set to clarify whether the teens thought the effects of childbearing they anticipated in their written survey would have a positive or negative effect on their lives. Data collected by the interviewer were consistent with the written survey results. Six items on a separate questionnaire asked for the teen's strength of desire to avoid conception. A statistical technique was used to find the underlying belief systems associated with the desire to remain nonpregnant.

What were the results of the study? Most participants in the study did not anticipate that having a child would have a specifically positive or negative impact on their lives. However, negative expectations were more common than positive ones. The responses were statistically grouped into nine groups of expectations: future plans, self-esteem, autonomy, boyfriend relations, peer relations, family relations, norming relations, like babies, need babies. These teens felt most strongly that pregnancy would negatively affect their future plans, but there were also concerns for self-esteem and interpersonal relationships. Among the social influences measured, boyfriends were more influential than peers or family members. All of the childbearing expectations were related to the strength of the desire to remain nonpregnant. However, the strength of this relationship varied significantly among the groups of expectations. The larger the number of negative expectation groups a teen reported, the stronger the desire of the teen to remain nonpregnant. Strongly negative perceptions of pregnancy were more protective than were ambivalent or positive ones.

What additional questions might I have? These data were all generated from urban areas; would teens in rural or suburban areas exhibit the same associations? All of these subjects were using no or unreliable contraception. Would the results be different if compared with those of teens who are using reliable contraception methods?

How can I use this study? Helping teens understand realistic expectations of pregnancy can help them find more reliable methods of preventing pregnancy. These authors generated an eight-item screening tool from this study that is published in full in the article. Nurses could use this screening tool to identify teens who may have positive or ambivalent feelings about pregnancy and counsel them appropriately to delay pregnancy. Delay of pregnancy in teens improves outcomes for both baby and mother, and so attention should be paid to both expectations and actions of teens.

Stevens-Simon, C., Sheeder, J., Beach, R., & Harter, S. (2005). Adolescent pregnancy: Do expectations affect interventions? *Journal of Adolescent Health, 37,* 243.e15–243.e22.

Psychosocial Factors

Family dysfunction and poor self-esteem are also major risk factors for adolescent pregnancy. Some young teenagers deliberately plan to get pregnant. The adolescent girl may use pregnancy for various subconscious or conscious reasons: to punish her father and/or mother, to escape from an undesirable home situation, to gain attention, or to feel that she has someone to love and to love her. In these cases, pregnancy may in a sense be the young woman's form of delinquency. Like delinquent males, pregnant adolescents often have a history of troubled family relationships, poor school achievement, and drug abuse. For others, however, pregnancy marks an important milestone that leads to positive lifestyle changes and healthier behaviors (Klima, 2003).

More teens who become pregnant, compared with teens who have not been pregnant, have been physically, emotionally, or sexually abused. In fact, maltreatment of any kind is a high-risk contributor to early teen pregnancy (Montgomery, 2003).

Teenage pregnancy can result from an incestuous relationship. In the very young adolescent, incest or sexual abuse should be suspected as a possible cause of pregnancy. Teenage pregnancy could also be caused by other nonvoluntary sexual experiences such as acquaintance rape.

International Perspective

Worldwide the average birth rate (births per 1000 females) is 65 for girls aged 15 to 19 but that rate varies dramatically from country to country. The highest birth rates are found in sub-

Saharan Africa (average birth rate of 143) and in some parts of Latin America and south Asia. Intermediate birth rates are found in areas such as the Middle East and North Africa (56) and central Asia (59). The lowest teen birth rates are found in Scandinavia, the Netherlands, Switzerland, Japan, Korea, and China (World Health Organization [WHO], 2004). Age at marriage is an important consideration. Early marriage tends to be more common in developing countries and is usually followed by immediate childbearing as proof of the fertility of the couple.

Cultural factors often play a significant role in the desirability of early pregnancy. Specifically, adolescent women are more likely to welcome a pregnancy in a country where Islam is the predominant religion, where large families are desired, where social change is slow in coming, and where most childbearing occurs within marriage. Early pregnancy is less desired in countries where the reverse is true.

Information on pregnancy rates is not always available. In general pregnancy rates tend to be lower in countries where contraception is more readily available. Among industrialized countries, adolescent pregnancy rates for girls ages 15 to 19 years vary from a low of 12 pregnancies per 1000 adolescents in the Netherlands to a high of 102 pregnancies per 1000 in the Russian Federation. Most western European countries and Japan have low rates (fewer than 40 per 1000), whereas the United States joins four other countries—Belarus, Bulgaria, Romania, and the Russian Federation—that have pregnancy rates of greater than 70 per 1000 adolescents (Alan Guttmacher Institute, 2002).

Despite these seemingly high rates, the trend toward lower adolescent birth rates and pregnancy rates over the past 25 years is widespread and occurs in most industrialized countries. The reasons for this decrease may be related to the increased recognition of the importance of education along with an ever-increasing desire in many young people to attain education. In addition, in many parts of the world, young women now have goals in their life beyond marriage and motherhood (WHO, 2004).

Growing evidence suggests a significant number of girls in developing countries have experienced coercive (forced) sex. Although the actual magnitude of the problem and its implications for women's health are not well known, several negative consequences have been identified. These include unintended pregnancy and abortion, increased incidence of STIs including HIV, low self-esteem, depression, and substance abuse (Population Council, 2004).

RISKS TO THE ADOLESCENT MOTHER

Physiologic Risks

Adolescents over age 15 who receive early, thorough prenatal care are at no greater risk during pregnancy than women over 20 years. Unfortunately, many adolescents fail to seek early prenatal care. Those who do seek care may fail to cooperate with recommendations. In addition, teenage mothers are more likely to

DEVELOPING CULTURAL COMPETENCE

EDUCATIONAL LEVEL AND CHILDBEARING
Throughout the world, the higher a woman's educational level, the more likely she is to delay marriage and childbirth.

smoke than older pregnant women and less likely to gain sufficient weight during their pregnancy. Thus risks for pregnant adolescents include preterm births, low-birth-weight (LBW) infants, preeclampsia-eclampsia and its sequelae, iron deficiency anemia, and cephalopelvic disproportion (CPD). In the adolescent age group, prenatal care is the critical factor that most influences pregnancy outcome.

Iron deficiency anemia is a problem in all pregnant women. The adolescent who begins her pregnancy already anemic, however, is at increased risk and must be followed closely and counseled carefully regarding nutrition during pregnancy. The increased risk of CPD is a concern in adolescent pregnancy, especially with the early adolescent, because of a lack of pelvic maturity.

Teenagers 15 to 19 years old have a high incidence of STIs including herpesvirus, syphilis, and gonorrhea. The incidence of chlamydial infection is also increased in this age group. The presence of such infections during a pregnancy greatly increases the risk to the fetus (refer to Chapter 20 ∞). Other problems seen in adolescents are alcohol and drug use. By the time pregnancy is confirmed in young women, the fetus may already be harmed by these substances.

Psychologic Risks

The most profound psychologic risk to the adolescent who maintains her pregnancy is the interruption of progress in her developmental tasks. Although adolescents have become sexually active at an earlier age and the incidence of adolescent pregnancy has decreased, the developmental tasks of this age group remain the same. Add to this the tasks of pregnancy, and the young woman has an overwhelming amount of psychologic work to do, the success of which will affect her own and her newborn's future.

Table 17–2 identifies typical behaviors of the early, middle, and late adolescent when she becomes aware of her pregnancy. In reviewing these behaviors, the nurse should realize that other factors may influence the age at which the behaviors are seen.

Table 17–3 identifies the early adolescent's response to the developmental tasks of pregnancy. The early adolescent's response reflects her level of development, with pregnancy as an interruption of the normal process of development. The middle and late adolescents respond differently, reflecting their maturational progress through the developmental tasks. In addition to her maturational level, the amount of nurturing the pregnant adolescent receives is also a critical factor in the way she handles pregnancy and motherhood.

MEDIALINK Application: Preeclampsia in an Adolescent Client

Table 17-2   INITIAL REACTION TO AWARENESS OF PREGNANCY

Age	Adolescent Behavior	Nursing Implications
Early adolescent (14 and under)	Fears rejection by family and peers. Enters healthcare system with an adult, most likely mother (parents still seen as locus of control). Value system still closely reflects that of parents, so still turns to parents for decision or approval of decision. Pregnancy probably not result of intimate relationship. Is self-conscious about normal adolescent changes in body. Self-consciousness and low self-esteem likely to increase with rapid breast enlargement and abdominal enlargement of pregnancy.	Be nonjudgmental in approach to care. Focus on needs and concerns of adolescent, but if parent accompanies daughter, include parent in plan of care. Encourage both to express concerns and feelings regarding pregnancy and options: abortion, maintaining pregnancy, adoption. Be realistic and concrete in discussing implications of each option. During physical exam of adolescent, respect increased sense of modesty. Explain in simple and concrete terms physical changes that are produced by pregnancy versus puberty. Explain each step of physical exam in simple and concrete terms.
Middle adolescent (15–17 years)	Fears rejection by peers and parents. Unsure in whom to confide. May seek confirmation of pregnancy on own with increased awareness of options and services, such as over-the-counter pregnancy kits and Planned Parenthood. If in an ongoing, caring relationship with partner (peer), may choose him as confidant. Economic dependence on parents may determine if and when parents are told. Future educational plans and perception of parental support or lack of support are significant factors in decision regarding termination or maintenance of the pregnancy. Possible conflict in parental and own developing value system.	Be nonjudgmental in approach to care. Reassure the adolescent that confidentiality will be maintained. Help adolescent identify significant individuals in whom she can confide to help make a decision about the pregnancy. Be aware of state laws regarding requirement of parental notification if abortion intended. Also be aware of state laws regarding requirements for marriage: usually, minimum age for both parties is 18; 16- and 17-year-olds are, in most states, allowed to marry only with consent of parents. Encourage adolescent to be realistic about parental response to pregnancy.
Late adolescent (18–19 years)	Most likely to confirm pregnancy on own and at an earlier date due to increased acceptance and awareness of consequences of behavior. Likely to use pregnancy kit for confirmation. Relationship with father of baby, future educational plans, and own value system are among significant determinants of decision about pregnancy.	Be nonjudgmental in approach to care. Reassure the adolescent that confidentiality will be maintained. Encourage adolescent to identify significant individuals in whom she can confide. Refer to counseling as appropriate. Encourage adolescent to be realistic about parental response to pregnancy.

Table 17-3   THE EARLY ADOLESCENT'S RESPONSE TO THE DEVELOPMENTAL TASKS OF PREGNANCY

Stage	Developmental Tasks of Pregnancy	Early Adolescent's Response to Pregnancy	Nursing Implications
First trimester	Pregnancy confirmation. Seeking early prenatal care as a confirmation tool. Begins to evaluate her diet and general health habits. Initial ambivalence common. Usually supportive partner.	May delay confirmation of pregnancy until late part of first trimester or later. Reasons for delay may include lack of awareness that she is pregnant, fear of confiding in anyone, or denial. Rapid enlargement and sensitivity of breasts are embarrassing and frightening to early adolescent—may be perceived as changes of puberty. If confiding in mother, may be experiencing family turmoil in response to pregnancy.	Explain physiologic changes of pregnancy versus those associated with puberty. Explain that ambivalence is normal with any pregnancy, but recognize it as a much greater concern with adolescent pregnancy. Emphasize need for good nutrition as important for her well-being as much as infant's (prevention of preeclampsia and anemia). Use simple explanations and lots of audiovisuals. Have adolescent listen to fetal heart rate (FHR) with Doppler.
Second trimester	Changes in physical appearance begin, and fetal movement is experienced, causing pregnancy to be experienced as a reality. Begins wearing maternity clothes to accommodate the physical changes. As a result of quickening she perceives her fetus as a real baby and begins preparing for the maternal role and new relationships with her partner and members of her family.	Some teenagers may delay validation of pregnancy until now, with family turmoil occurring at this time. Abdominal enlargement and quickening may be perceived as loss of control over body image. May try to maintain prepregnant weight and wear restrictive clothing to control and conceal changing body. Becomes dependent on her own mother for support. Egocentric; unable to develop a maternal role at this time.	Continue to discuss importance of good nutrition and adequate weight gain as noted above. Discuss ways of utilizing common teenage clothing (large sweatshirts, blouses) to promote comfort but preserve adolescent image to some degree. Discuss plans being made for baby, continued educational plans, and role of teen's parents.
Third trimester	At end of second trimester begins to view fetus as separate from self. Buys baby clothes and supplies. Prepares a place for the baby. Realistic about what baby is like. Prepares to give birth to infant. Anxiety increases as labor and birth approach and has concerns about well-being of fetus.	May focus on "wanting it to be over." May have trouble individuating fetus. May have fantasies, dreams, or nightmares about childbirth. Natural fears of labor and birth greater than with older primigravida. Probably has not been in a hospital, and may associate this with negative experiences.	Assess whether adolescent is preparing for baby by buying supplies and preparing a place in the home. Childbirth education important. Provide hospital tour. Assess for discomforts of pregnancy, such as heartburn and constipation. Adolescent may be uncomfortable mentioning these and other problems.

Sociologic Risks

A substantial body of research indicates that the adolescent mother is at higher risk for social and economic disadvantages than her teenage counterpart who is not pregnant and lives in the same social environment. Being forced into adult roles before completing adolescent developmental tasks causes a series of events that affects the adolescent's entire life. These events may result in a prolonged dependence on parents, lack of stable relationships with the opposite sex, and lack of economic and social stability.

Many teen mothers drop out of school during their pregnancy. This tendency may have as much to do with low academic achievement and low academic commitment as it does with the pregnancy. Many never complete their education. Lack of education reduces the quality of jobs available to these women. Childbearing at an early age is a strong predictor of need for public assistance, especially in lower socioeconomic groups and when the pregnant adolescent's family will not support her. Adolescent mothers frequently fail to establish a stable family, especially if they have a second child while still an adolescent. Their family structure tends to be a single-parent, matriarchal family structure, often the same type in which the adolescent herself was raised.

Some pregnant adolescents choose to marry the father of the baby, who may also be a teen. Unfortunately, the majority of adolescent marriages end in divorce. This fact is not surprising because pregnancy and marriage interrupt the partners' "childhood" and basic education. Failure to be self-supporting logically follows lack of education and lost career goals. Lack of maturity in dealing with an intimate relationship also contributes to marital breakdown in this age group.

Studies suggest that 16% to 37% of pregnant teens experience domestic violence. This rate is higher than that estimated for pregnant adults and suggests that teens are more susceptible to such victimization than pregnant adults (Scheiman & Zeoli, 2003). Dating violence is often an issue for teens, especially for younger girls dating older boys. These younger teens may interpret such actions as hitting, pushing, and making verbal threats as signs of love, caring, and a deep commitment to the relationship that will ultimately produce long-term positive results (Glass, Freeland, Campbell et al., 2003).

In the United States, the results of teenage childbearing cost taxpayers $7 billion each year (NCPTP, 2004a). Simply delaying these births could result in significant savings because of the improvement in both education and occupational status of these young women.

The increased incidence of maternal complications, premature birth, and LBW babies among adolescent mothers also has an impact on society because many of these mothers are on welfare. The need for increased financial support for good prenatal care and nutritional programs remains critical.

Risks for Her Child

Children of adolescent parents are at a disadvantage in many ways because teens are not developmentally or economically prepared to be parents. In general, children of teenage mothers are at a developmental disadvantage compared with children whose mothers were older at the time of their birth. Many factors contribute to these differences, especially the adverse social and economic conditions many teenage mothers face. These factors result in high rates of family instability, disadvantaged neighborhoods, and high rates of behavior problems. In addition, often these children do not do as well in school and are less likely to complete high school. Children born to adolescent mothers also have higher rates of abuse and neglect (NCPTP, 2004a).

PARTNERS OF ADOLESCENT MOTHERS

Statistics indicate that approximately two thirds of the male partners of adolescent mothers are not teens themselves but are 20 years of age or older. In particular, teens in poorer, recently immigrant populations have considerably older partners (Males, 2004).

Adolescent males tend to become sexually active at an earlier age than females, and they have more sexual partners in their teenage years (Marcell, Raine, & Eyre, 2003). When the father is an adolescent, he, too, generally has not yet completed the developmental tasks of his age group and is no better prepared psychologically to deal with the consequences of pregnancy than the adolescent mother. Consequently, the adolescent who attempts to assume his responsibility as a father faces many of the same psychologic and sociologic risks as the adolescent mother. The mother and father are generally from similar socioeconomic backgrounds and have similar educational levels.

Although not married, many adolescent couples are involved in meaningful relationships. Adolescent fathers may be very involved in the pregnancy and may be present for the birth. Although relationships among fathers, teenage mothers, and their infants appear prone to deterioration over time, research suggests that many young fathers genuinely want to be involved with their children and would have more contact and input if they could. Issues such as conflicts with the teen mother or maternal grandparents and a lack of financial resources may act as additional barriers for the young father (Bunting & McAuley, 2004).

The lack of responsibility shown by some unwed fathers has caused a shift in cultural and community attitudes. Fathers are being included on birth certificates far more frequently today than in the past. This helps ensure the father's rights and encourages him to meet his responsibilities to his child. In addition, legal paternity gives children access to military and social security benefits and to medical information about their fathers.

In some situations, the pregnant adolescent may not want to identify or contact the father of the baby, and the father may not readily acknowledge paternity. Those situations include rape, exploitative sexual relations, incest, and casual sexual relations. If healthcare providers suspect any of the first three causes, further investigation into the situation is important for the well-being of the pregnant adolescent, and referral to other resources should be made as appropriate.

In situations in which the adolescent father wants to assume some responsibility, healthcare providers should support him in his decision. It is important, however, that the pregnant adolescent have the opportunity to decide whether she wants the father to participate in her health care.

If the adolescents perceive that they have a caring relationship, the adolescent father may want to be supportive and protective but probably does not understand the physical and psychologic changes that his partner is experiencing. The young man will need education regarding pregnancy, childbirth, child care, and parenting.

Although the adolescent father may have been included in the health care of the young woman throughout the pregnancy, it is not unusual for her to want her mother as her primary support person during labor and birth. This is especially true with younger adolescents. It is important both to support her wishes and also to acknowledge and support the adolescent father's wishes as appropriate.

As a part of counseling, the nurse should assess the young man's stressors, his support systems, his plans for involvement in the pregnancy and childbearing, and his future plans. He should be referred to social services for an opportunity to be counseled regarding his educational and vocational future. When the father is involved in the pregnancy, the young mother feels less deserted, more confident in her decision making, and better able to discuss her future.

REACTIONS OF FAMILY AND SOCIAL SUPPORTS TO ADOLESCENT PREGNANCY

The reactions of family members and social supports to adolescent pregnancy are as varied as the motivation and cause of the pregnancy. In families who foster educational and career goals for their children, adolescent pregnancy is often a shock. Anger, shame, and sorrow are common reactions. The majority of pregnant adolescents from these families are most likely to use contraception or choose abortion, with the exception of those teens whose cultural and religious beliefs prevent them from seeking an abortion.

Some adolescent fathers also face negative reactions from people, including their own families and the families of their young partners. They may experience others' anger, shame, and disappointment. Their relationships with their peers may be altered as well.

In populations in which adolescent pregnancy is more prevalent and more socially acceptable, family and friends may be more supportive of the adolescent parents. In many cases, friends as well as the teen's mother are present at the birth. The expectant couple may also have friends who are already teen parents. For some male partners of these adolescent mothers, pregnancy and the birth of a baby are seen as a sign of adult status and increased sexual prowess—a sense of pride.

The mother of the pregnant adolescent is usually among the first to be told about the pregnancy. She typically becomes involved with decision making, especially with the younger adolescent, about issues such as maintaining the pregnancy, abortion, and dealing with the father-to-be and his family. As discussed previously, the pregnant adolescent may not want to identify or contact the father of the baby, especially in situations where rape or other exploitative sex was involved, or with casual sexual relationships. Family input in these matters is important in the adolescent's decision making.

Once the decision about the pregnancy has been made, it is usually the mother who helps the teen access health care and accompanies her to her first visit. If the pregnancy is maintained, the mother may participate in prenatal care classes and can be an excellent support system for her daughter. She should be encouraged to participate if the mother-daughter relationship is positive. If the baby's father is involved in the pregnancy, he and the pregnant teen's mother may be able to work together to support the teenage mother. The nurse can update the pregnant teen's mother on childbearing practices to clarify any misconceptions she might have. During labor and birth, the mother may be a key figure for her daughter, offering reassurance and instilling confidence in the teen.

The younger the adolescent when she gives birth, the more she needs her mother's support. Children of adolescent parents experience more negative outcomes, including more aggressive behavior at a young age, when the adolescent is in constant conflict with her mother and becomes less involved in parenting.

> *Miranda left for college back East in September. She was just 18 and I thought she had the world in front of her. At Thanksgiving she came home to tell us she was 4 months pregnant and planned to keep the baby even though she and Tony had broken up and he wanted no part of fatherhood. She finished the semester, then moved back home and transferred to a state college near us. Tina was born 2 days after her mom finished the spring semester. Now Miranda's life is a juggling act—part-time job, part-time school, full-time mom. We help all we can. I am so sorry that my child has lost out on so much but I am so proud of the woman she has become.*

NURSING CARE MANAGEMENT

In working with adolescents, the nurse should remember that they often think differently than adults. Adolescents, especially younger adolescents, tend to be more concrete thinkers and may not plan ahead for more than a few days. As a result, nurses need to recognize that missed appointments are not unusual. Missed appointments may also be caused by other factors such as a lack of transportation, especially for those teens who are not old enough to drive. Teens may avoid health care because they are underinsured, uninsured, or lack the funds to pay for care. Many adolescents have never before accessed health care without a parent. They may fear that using their healthcare insurance for reproductive health visits will be discovered by their parents. If they are unable to share their concerns with a parent, they must be highly motivated to seek health care independently for purposes of contraception, treatment of STIs, diagnosis of pregnancy, or prenatal care.

Nursing Assessment and Diagnosis

The nurse begins her care of the pregnant adolescent by establishing a database to plan interventions for the adolescent mother and family. Areas of assessment include history of family health and personal physical health, developmental level and impact of pregnancy, and emotional and financial support. The nurse also assesses the family and social support network and the father's degree of involvement in the pregnancy. It is important for the nurse to demonstrate a sincere sense of caring for the young woman and the outcome of her pregnancy during early prenatal visits.

As with all pregnant women, it is important that the caregiver have information on the teen's general physical health. This may be the first time many adolescents have ever provided a health history. The nurse may find it helpful to ask very specific questions and give examples if the young woman appears confused about a question. The nurse may find that the teen's mother is best able to answer questions about family history because the adolescent is often unaware of this information.

The following areas should be assessed:

- Family and personal health history
- Medical history
- Menstrual history
- Obstetric and gynecologic history
- Substance abuse history

It is important to assess the maturational level of each individual. The adolescent's development level and the impact of pregnancy are reflected in the degree to which the teen recognizes the realities and responsibilities involved in pregnancy and parenting. The mother's self-concept (including body image), her relationship with the significant adults in her life, her attitude toward her pregnancy, and her coping methods in the situation are just a few of the significant factors that need to be assessed.

The socioeconomic status of the pregnant teen often places the baby at risk throughout life, beginning with conception. It is essential that the nurse assess family and social support as well as the extent of financial support.

Adolescent lifestyles and support systems vary greatly. It is imperative that the interdisciplinary health team have information about the expectant adolescents' feelings and perceptions about themselves, their sexuality, and the coming baby; their knowledge of, attitude toward, and anticipated ability to care for and support the infant; and their maturational level and needs.

The nursing diagnoses that are applicable to any pregnant woman apply to the pregnant adolescent. Other nursing diagnoses are influenced by the adolescent's age, support systems, socioeconomic situation, health, and maturity. Examples of nursing diagnoses more specific to the pregnant adolescent may include the following:

- ***Imbalanced Nutrition: Less than Body Requirements*** related to poor eating habits
- ***Risk for Situational Low Self-Esteem*** related to unanticipated pregnancy

Nursing Plan and Implementation

Early, thorough prenatal care is the strongest and most critical determinant for reducing risk for the adolescent mother and her newborn. When an adolescent presents for health care, her needs must be met and she must be treated as an individual who can make decisions about her own health care. Excessive wait times and inappropriate staff behaviors toward the young woman can contribute to delays in seeking prenatal care (Montgomery, 2003).

COMMUNITY-BASED NURSING CARE

Many new and innovative community-based agencies have evolved to provide care for high-risk clients throughout the childbearing experience and beyond. Nurses in all community-based agencies can help adolescents access the healthcare system as well as social services and other support services (i.e., food banks and the Special Supplemental Food Program for Women, Infants, and Children [WIC]). Community programs providing educational materials and group classes can be an important adjunct to routine prenatal care. Helping pregnant adolescents understand the importance of finding a healthcare provider they are comfortable with, maintaining scheduled appointments, childbirth and labor preparation, and other health-promoting content may be included. Many adolescents prefer group activities and these may be helpful forums to exchange ideas and help them cope with the demands of pregnancy and adolescence (Montgomery, 2003).

Nurses working with pregnant adolescents are also involved extensively in counseling and client teaching. During their interactions, several challenges typically arise, including safeguarding the client's confidentiality, winning her trust, and helping to build her sense of self-esteem. These and other challenges of adolescent prenatal care are discussed here.

Issues of Confidentiality and Consent to Care

Most states in the United States have passed legislation that confirms the right of some minors to assume the rights of adults. These adolescents are referred to as **emancipated minors.** An adolescent may be considered emancipated if he or she is self-supporting and living away from home, married, pregnant, a parent, or in the military. Even if a minor has not become formally emancipated, all 50 states have passed legislation that enables teens to consent to care without a parent's knowledge for certain "medically emancipated" conditions. These conditions vary from state to state. For example, all 50 states permit confidential testing for STIs but only about half (27) of states explicitly permit minors to consent to contraception without a parent's knowledge or consent (Anderson, Schaechter, & Brosco, 2006). The pregnant adolescent, even if very young, is considered emancipated and has the right and responsibility to consent to health care for herself and later for her child. She is entitled to respect and confidentiality in her dealings with healthcare providers. Only with her consent can other adults, including her parents, be included in communication.

Development of a Trusting Relationship with the Pregnant Adolescent

The first visit to the clinic or office may cause anxiety for the young woman. She may be nervous not only because of her situation, but also because this may well be her first exposure to the healthcare system since early childhood. Making this experience as positive as possible for the young woman will encourage a favorable attitude toward health care and increase the likelihood that she will return for follow-up visits, whether she chooses to terminate or maintain the pregnancy.

Depending on how young the adolescent is, this may be her first pelvic examination, an anxiety-provoking experience for any woman. The nurse can help provide a thorough explanation of the procedure. A gentle and thoughtful examination technique will help the young woman to relax.

CLINICAL TIP

During the initial pelvic examination, with the consent of the examiner, offer the teen the opportunity to visualize her external genitalia and cervix with a handheld mirror. A mirror is helpful in enabling the young woman to see her cervix, thus educating her about her anatomy. It also gives her an active role in the exam if she so desires.

Developing a trusting relationship with the pregnant adolescent is essential. Honesty and respect for the individual and a caring attitude promote self-esteem. As the nurse develops a trusting relationship with the young woman, the nurse's attitudes about self-care and responsibility affect the adolescent's maturation process. When adolescents are treated positively, they value the experience and respond by asking more questions and seeking more assistance (Low, Martin, Sampselle et al., 2003).

Promotion of Self-Esteem and Problem-Solving Skills

The nurse assists the adolescent in her decision-making and problem-solving skills so that she can proceed with her developmental tasks and begin to assume responsibility for her own as well as her newborn's life. An overview of what the young woman will experience over the prenatal course, along with thorough explanations and rationale for each procedure as it occurs, will foster the adolescent's understanding and give her some measure of control. Actively involving the young woman in her care gives her a sense of participation and responsibility (Figure 17–2 ◆).

Adolescents tend to be egocentric, and even if they realize that their health-related behaviors affect their fetus, they might not feel that this is important. In light of this fact, it is often more helpful to emphasize the effects of these practices on the client *herself.* Because of their immature cognitive development, they also need help in problem solving, in visualizing themselves in the future, and in imagining what the consequences of their actions might be.

Promotion of Physical Well-Being

Baseline weight and blood pressure measurements will be valuable in assessing weight gain and predisposition to preeclampsia-eclampsia. The adolescent may be encouraged to take part in her care by measuring and recording her weight. The nurse may use

Figure 17–2 ◆ The nurse gives a young mother an opportunity to listen to her baby's heartbeat.
SOURCE: Photographer, Elena Dorfman.

this time as an opportunity for assisting the young woman in problem solving: "Have I gained too much or too little weight?" "What influence does my diet have on my weight?" "How can I change my eating habits?"

The nurse can also introduce the subject of nutrition during measurement of baseline and subsequent hemoglobin and hematocrit values. Because the adolescent is at risk for anemia, she will need education regarding the importance of iron in her diet. Indeed, basic education about nutrition is a critical component of care for pregnant teens.

Preeclampsia-eclampsia is one of the most common, serious complications of pregnancy in general. It also represents the most prevalent medical complication of pregnant adolescents. Preeclampsia-eclampsia is typically characterized by high blood pressure, proteinuria, and edema. In adult women, a blood pressure reading of 140/90 is often used as evidence of hypertension. However, it is sometimes difficult to recognize hypertension in adolescent females. Women ages 14 to 20 years without evidence of high blood pressure usually have diastolic readings between 50 and 66 mm Hg. Gradual increases from the prepregnant diastolic readings, along with excessive weight gain, proteinuria, and sudden edema, must be evaluated as precursors to preeclampsia. Blood pressure readings of 140/90 mm Hg are not acceptable as the determinant of preeclampsia in teens. This is one reason why early prenatal care is vital to the effective management of the adolescent.

Adolescents have an increased incidence of STIs. The initial prenatal examination should include gonococcal and chlamydial cultures and wet prep for *Candida, Trichomonas,* and *Gardnerella.* Tests for syphilis should also be done. Education about STIs is important, as is careful observation for herpetic lesions or other symptoms throughout the young woman's pregnancy. Although today's teens are knowledgeable about acquired immunodeficiency syndrome (AIDS), they know much less about other STIs, especially with regard to symptoms and risk reduction. If the adolescent's history indicates that she is at increased risk for HIV, she should be given information about it and offered HIV screening.

The nurse should also discuss substance abuse with adolescents. It is important to review the risks associated with the use of tobacco, caffeine, drugs, and alcohol. The young woman should be aware of the effects of these substances on her development as well as on the development of the fetus.

Ongoing care includes the same assessments that the older woman receives. Special attention should be paid to evaluating fetal growth by determining when quickening occurs and by measuring fundal height, fetal heart tones, and fetal movement. Comparing the dates of auscultating fetal heart tones with the date of the last menstrual period and quickening can be helpful in determining correct estimates of time of birth. If, when measuring fundal height, there is a question of size-date discrepancy by 2 cm either way, an ultrasound is warranted to establish fetal age so that instances of intrauterine growth restriction (IUGR) may be diagnosed and treated early. To ensure the most accurate dating possible, an ultrasound is also warranted early in pregnancy if the date of the last menstrual period is not known.

Promotion of Family Adaptation

The nurse assesses the family situation during the first prenatal visit and ascertains the level of involvement the adolescent desires from each of her family members and the father of the child, as well as her perception of their present support. A sensitive approach to daughter-mother relationships helps motivate their communication. If the mother and daughter agree, the mother should be included in the client's care. Pregnancy may change a teen's relationship with her mother from one of antagonism to one of understanding and empathy. The opportunity to renew or establish a positive relationship with their mothers is welcomed by most teens. It symbolizes approval, acceptance, and support from the individual who would serve as her role model for mothering.

The nurse should also help the mother assess her daughter's needs and assist her in meeting them. Some adolescents become more dependent during pregnancy, and some become more independent. The mother can ease and encourage her daughter's self-growth by understanding how best to respond and support the adolescent.

Finally, the father of the adolescent's infant can be included to promote the family's successful adaptation to the pregnancy. He may be asked to attend prenatal visits, classes, and health teaching and to be present at the birth itself and involved to the extent that he wishes and that is acceptable to the teenage mother. He should also have the opportunity to express his feelings and concerns and to have his questions answered.

Facilitation of Prenatal Education

Some school systems are currently attempting to meet prenatal education needs in a variety of ways. The most effective method appears to be mainstreaming the pregnant adolescent in academic classes with her peers and adding classes appropriate to her needs during pregnancy and initial parenting experiences. Classes about growth and development, beginning with the newborn and early infancy, can help teenage parents have more realistic expectations of their infants and may help decrease child abuse. Mainstreaming pregnant adolescents in school is also an ideal way to help them complete their education while learning the skills they need to cope with childbearing and parenting. Vocational guidance in this setting is also most beneficial to their future. Some schools provide infant and toddler child care facilities on their premises, which may allow the mother to continue her education without the added difficulty of finding appropriate child care.

As stated previously, early adolescents especially tend to be oriented to the present and to be concrete thinkers. As a result, teaching needs to be simple, direct, and responsive to their more immediate needs. For example, teaching about preparation for birth is most effective in the last weeks of pregnancy when this topic is of greater concern and teens are more motivated to practice breathing and relaxation techniques for labor.

Although some childbirth educators believe that older couples can be role models for pregnant adolescents, most believe that prenatal classes with other teens are generally preferable even though these classes can be challenging to teach (Figure 17–3 ◆). Attendance may be sporadic. The pregnant teen may be accompanied by her mother, her boyfriend, or her girlfriends. Those who bring girlfriends may bring a different one each time. In such cases, giggling and side conversations may occur. Such activity reflects the short attention span of the teen and is fairly typical. Thus, to keep the attention of the participants, it is important to use a variety of teaching strategies, including age-appropriate audiovisual aids, demonstrations, and games.

Goals for prenatal classes may include some or all of the following:

- Providing anticipatory guidance about pregnancy
- Preparing the participants for labor and birth
- Helping participants identify the problems and conflicts of teenage pregnancy and parenting
- Increasing self-esteem
- Providing information about available community resources
- Helping participants develop more adaptive coping skills

During prenatal classes, nurses can also share information on breastfeeding, which has significant health benefits for both

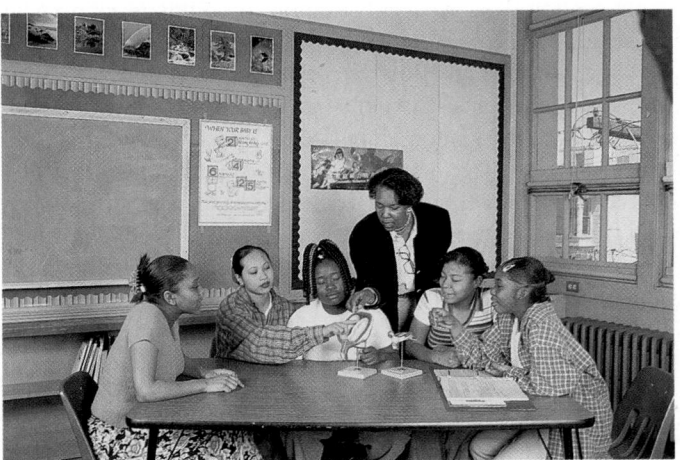

Figure 17–3 ◆ Young adolescents may benefit from prenatal classes designed specifically for them.
SOURCE: Photographer, Jenny Thomas.

the adolescent mother and her infant. Adolescents often do not choose a feeding method until later in pregnancy, so early education can help ensure success for the adolescent who chooses to breastfeed her infant. Peer groups can be an important source of information for the young mother considering breastfeeding, especially for the adolescent who has not been around other breastfeeding women (Montgomery, 2003).

Topics on parenting, although sometimes included in prenatal classes for adolescents, tend to be less effective, again because adolescents tend to be oriented to the present. Parenting skills are crucial, but adolescents generally are not ready to learn about these skills until birth makes the newborn a reality.

HOSPITAL-BASED NURSING CARE

The adolescent in labor has the same care needs as any pregnant woman. However, the importance of a sustained presence for her cannot be overemphasized. Adolescents want their care provider to be respectful, caring, and supportive. The nurse must be readily available and should answer questions simply and honestly, using lay terminology. Adolescents need their caregiver to provide education to guide their choices. The nurse can also help the adolescent's support people understand their roles in assisting the teen. If the father is involved, the nurse can encourage him to work within his own level of comfort to play an active role in all phases of the birth process, perhaps by feeding ice chips to the mother, timing her contractions, and coaching her with her breathing. The nurse can also let the couple know that holding hands, backrubs, and supportive touching are acceptable and therapeutic. Chapter 24 ∞ provides further information on care of the adolescent during labor and birth.

During the postpartum period, most teens do not foresee that they will become sexually active in the near future and are often adamant about the fact that they will not become pregnant again for an extended period. However, the statistics demonstrate a different reality. Thus, contraception remains a critical part of the national effort to decrease adolescent pregnancy. Before discharge, it is important for the nurse to provide information about the resumption of ovulation and the importance of contraception. It is especially helpful to do this teaching with the sexual partner present.

Several safe and effective contraceptive options are available for adolescents. Condoms are by far the most common method of contraception among teens and, when used consistently and correctly, they offer the added advantage of protection against STIs. Increasingly, experts are recommending a dual approach to prevent pregnancy and STIs—a condom combined with a second method of contraception, typically a hormonal method such as a combined oral contraceptive (Hillard, 2005; WHO, 2004).

As part of discharge planning, the nurse should ensure that the teen is aware of community resources available to assist her and her family. Postpartum classes and new-mother support groups, especially with peers, can be extremely beneficial. Such classes address a variety of topics, including postpartum adaptation, infant and child development, and parenting skills.

Evaluation

Expected outcomes of nursing care include the following:

- A trusting relationship is established with the pregnant adolescent.

- The adolescent is able to use her problem-solving abilities to make appropriate choices.

- The adolescent follows the recommendations of the healthcare team and receives effective health care throughout her pregnancy, the birth, and the postpartum period.

- The adolescent, her partner (if he is involved), and their families are able to cope successfully with the effects of the pregnancy.

- The adolescent is able to discuss pregnancy, prenatal care, and childbirth.

- The adolescent demonstrates developmental and pregnancy progression within established normal parameters.

- The adolescent develops skill in child care and parenting.

PREVENTION OF ADOLESCENT PREGNANCY

Beginning in the 1980s, the federal government allocated millions of dollars for abstinence-only sex education programs because of the belief of some legislators that abstinence was the only method of prevention that would work or would be accepted by the general public. These programs have had little impact on teenage pregnancy rates in the United States (Hillard, 2005). Research indicates that countries that give their young people balanced and comprehensive information about sexual activity have low rates of STIs and pregnancy (Nadeau, 2005).

A national effort to prevent teen pregnancy was initiated in 1996 with the establishment of the National Campaign to Prevent Teen Pregnancy. Its purpose is to reduce teenage pregnancy by one third between 2006 and 2015 (NCPTP, 2006). The National Campaign is a private, nonprofit organization made up of a broad spectrum of religious, political, social, human services, health, and academic organizations. The Association of Women's Health, Obstetric, and Neonatal Nurses (AWHONN) is one of the professional organizations that joined this group and made a commitment to focus on adolescent pregnancy prevention.

One of the first actions of the National Campaign was to commission a task force to do a comprehensive review of the incidence of adolescent pregnancy and its impact on the nation. At the same time, another task force was commissioned to review the research on the effectiveness of pregnancy prevention programs. The purpose of these task forces was to provide accurate information based on fact and research. In the first year, the National Campaign summarized the results in several publications. Not surprisingly, they have found that adolescent pregnancy is a multifaceted problem with no easy answers. The best approach in local areas needs to be based on strong, community-wide involvement, with a variety of programs directed at multiple causes of the problem. Three interventions that have shown promising results are accurate, balanced, and realistic sexuality education; youth development programs that build on the assets and strengths of young people; and confidential and low-cost access to contraceptive services (Advocates for Youth, 2005). The NCPTP publishes a regular newsletter and maintains an active Web site to communicate its work and disseminate information.

One of the major problems in local communities continues to be intense conflict among different groups about how to approach adolescent pregnancy prevention. Many parents advocate an "abstinence-plus" approach that stresses abstinence as the best approach but includes information on condoms and contraception for those teens who do not abstain.

Interestingly, recent research suggests that only 7% of people in the United States believe that sex education should not be provided in schools. Moreover, controversy about the type of sex education offered in schools seems to have decreased. Nearly three fourths (74%) of principals surveyed state that they have not had any recent discussions or debate (in school board, PTA, or other public meetings) about what should be taught (National Public Radio [NPR], Kaiser Family Foundation, & John F. Kennedy School of Government, 2004).

Research indicates that balanced, realistic sexuality education, which includes information on both abstinence and contraception, can delay teens' onset of sexual activity, increase the use of contraception by sexually active teens, and reduce the number of their sexual partners. Most Americans support providing education in junior and senior high schools with information about protection against unplanned pregnancy and STIs. Youth development programs that focus on meeting the needs of adolescents by building on young people's capacities, assisting them to cultivate their own talent and to increase their feelings of self-worth, ease their transition into adulthood and can reduce sexual risk behaviors and unintended teen pregnancy (Advocates for Youth, 2005).

The National Campaign's task forces have identified characteristics shared by all successful programs, regardless of the type of offering or community. Effective adolescent pregnancy prevention programs are long term and intensive. They also involve adolescents in program planning, include good role models from the same cultural and racial backgrounds, and focus on the adolescent male. Survey data from a representative sample of teens and adults provide some additional interesting insights (NCPTP, 2004b):

- Parents tend to underestimate their influence on their adolescents. Teens report that their parents, and not their friends, have the most influence on the teens' decisions about sex. However, a preponderance of teens also report that it would be easier to deal with issues related to sexuality and teen pregnancy if they could have more honest, open conversations with their parents.

- Teens' expressed attitudes about sexual activity reflect more cautious values and attitudes than generally believed. Teens report that their values, morals, and religious beliefs, and concern for their future influence their decisions about sex more than concerns about becoming pregnant or developing an STI.

- Almost all the adults and teens surveyed said that society should give teens a strong message that they should not have sex until they are at least out of high school.

- The majority of both groups advocate a message stressing abstinence while also providing information about contraception. They rejected the notion that such an approach sends a "mixed message."

- Teens want more information about sexuality, abstinence, and contraception.

- Teens tend to overestimate the percentage of their classmates and peers who have had sex.

MediaLink

National Campaign to Prevent Teen Pregnancy

CHAPTER REVIEW

FOCUS YOUR STUDY

- Birth rates for teens ages 15 to 19 have decreased from 61.8 per 1000 females in 1991 to 41.2 in 2004, a 33% decline. Although this is a significant improvement, the US teenage pregnancy rate is the highest of any industrialized nation.

- Many factors contribute to the high teenage pregnancy rate, including earlier age of first sexual intercourse, lack of knowledge about conception, lack of easy access to contraception, lessened stigma associated with adolescent pregnancy in some populations, poverty, early school failure, and early childhood sexual abuse.

- The major psychologic risk the pregnant adolescent faces is the interruption of her own developmental tasks.

- Physical risks of adolescent pregnancies include preterm births, low-birth-weight infants, cephalopelvic disproportion, iron deficiency anemia, and preeclampsia and its sequelae.

- Almost half of the fathers of infants of adolescent mothers are age 20 or older, but they are often similar to adolescent fathers psychosocially and are no more likely to be able to support the mother.

- Factors affecting an adolescent's response to pregnancy include her degree of achievement of the developmental tasks of adolescence (which can be closely associated with age), as well as cultural, religious, and socioeconomic factors.

- Nurses working with pregnant adolescents face many challenges, including safeguarding the client's confidentiality, winning her trust, and helping to build her sense of self-esteem.

- Often the adolescent has little understanding of pregnancy, childbirth, or parenting. Consequently, education is a primary responsibility of the nurse.

- Adolescent pregnancy prevention programs should be multifaceted, target males as well as females, and involve community-wide approaches.

EXPLORE MediaLink

http://www.prenhall.com/davidson

NCLEX review questions, case studies, and other interactive resources for this chapter can be found on the Web Site at http://www.prenhall.com/davidson. Click on "Chapter 17" to select the activities for this chapter.

For tutorials including animations and videos, more NCLEX review questions, and an audio glossary, access the accompanying Prentice Hall Nursing MediaLink DVD-ROM in this book.

PRENTICE HALL NURSING MEDIALINK DVD-ROM
Audio Glossary
NCLEX Review

COMPANION WEBSITE
Additional NCLEX Review
Case Study: *Late Detection of Adolescent Pregnancy*
Care Plan Activity: *Adolescent's Response to Pregnancy*
Applications: *Teen Pregnancy; Preeclampsia in an Adolescent Client*
Critical Thinking

CRITICAL THINKING IN ACTION

PSYCHOLOGIC AND CULTURAL FACTORS IN TEENAGE PREGNANCY

View the Critical Thinking in Action video in Chapter 17 of the DVD-ROM. Then answer the questions that follow.

Sixteen-year-old Linda Perez and her mother present to you at the OB clinic for Linda's first prenatal visit. You determine that Linda is 20 weeks pregnant. Her weight is 135 lb, height 5'4", T 98°F, P 80, R 14, BP 100/64. You assess that Linda's mother has type 2 diabetes, and that her siblings are healthy. Linda admits to having one sexual partner and says she has never been hospitalized. Her immunizations are up to date and she's never used tobacco or recreational drugs. To date, the father of the baby is not involved. Mrs. Perez is clearly upset over the fact that Linda's pregnancy is so far advanced without her knowledge. Linda is very quiet and speaks only when questioned directly. You do your best to try to establish a trusting relationship with Linda and her mother by providing an atmosphere where issues can be discussed.

1. What psychologic factors contribute to teenage pregnancy?

2. Explore reasons why teenagers delay prenatal care.

3. Linda's mother asks you what factors facilitate adolescent pregnancies.

4. You assess that Linda has some anxiety concerning the birth process. She states she is not interested in prenatal classes because she is single and does not want to have natural childbirth. How would you respond to her?

REFERENCES

Advocates for Youth. (2005). *Teenage pregnancy, the case for prevention: An updated analysis of recent trends and federal expenditures associated with teenage pregnancy.* Retrieved October 7, 2005, from http://www.advocatesforyouth.org

Alan Guttmacher Institute. (2002). *Facts in brief: Teenagers' sexual and reproductive health.* Retrieved September 21, 2002, from http://www.agi-usa.org/pubs/fb_teens.html

Anderson, S. L., Schaechter, J., & Brosco, J. P. (2006). Adolescent patients and their confidentiality: Staying within legal bounds. *Contemporary OB/GYN, 51*(5), 53–64.

Bunting, L., & McAuley, C. (2004). Research review: Teenage pregnancy and parenthood: The role of fathers. *Child and Family Social Work* (9), 295–303

Cohen, D. A., Farley, T. A., Taylor, S. N., Martin, D. H, & Schuster, M. A. (2002). When and where do youths have sex? The potential role of adult supervision. *Pediatrics, 110*(6), 66.

Doniger, A., Adams, E., Utter, C., & Riley, J. (2001). Impact evaluation of the "not me, not now" abstinence-oriented, adolescent pregnancy prevention communications program, Monroe County, New York. *Journal of Health Communication, 6*(1), 45–60.

Eaton, D. K., Kann, L., Kinchen, S., Ross, J., Hawkins, M. A., Harris, W. A., et al. (2006, June 9). Youth risk behavior surveillance—United States, 2005. *Morbidity and Mortality Weekly Report, 55*(SS05), 1–108.

Glass, N., Fredland, N., Campbell, J., Yonas, M., Sharps, P., & Kub, J. (2003). Adolescent dating violence: Prevalence, risk factors, health outcomes, and implications for clinical practice. *Journal of Obstetric, Gynecologic, & Neonatal Nursing, 32*(2), 227–238.

Hamilton, B. E., Ventura, S. J., Martin, J. A., & Sutton, P. D. (2005). *Preliminary births for 2004.* Health E-Stats. National Center for Health Statistics. Retrieved July 3, 2006, from http://www.cdc.gov/nchs

Hillard, P. J. A. (2005). Contraceptive behaviors in adolescents. *Pediatric Annals, 34*(10), 794–802.

Kelly, P. J., Lesser, J., & Smoots, A. (2005). Tailoring STI & HIV prevention programs for teens. The American Journal of Maternal-Child Nursing, *30* (4), 237–244.

Klima, C. S. (2003). Centering pregnancy: A model for pregnant adolescents. *Journal of Midwifery & Women's Health, 48*(3), 220–225.

Low, L. K., Martin, K., Sampselle, C., Guthrie, B., & Oakley, D. (2003), Adolescents' experiences of childbirth: Contrasts with adults. *Journal of Midwifery & Women's Health, 48*(3), 192–198.

Males, M. (2004). *Teens and older partners.* Resource Center for Adolescent Pregnancy Prevention (ReCAPP). Retrieved October 11, 2005, from http://www.etr.org/recap/research/AuthoredPapOlderPrtnrs0504.htm

Manlove, J., Ryan, S., & Franzetta, K. (2003). Patterns of contraceptive use within teenagers' first sexual relationships. *Perspectives on Sexual and Reproductive Health, 35*(6), 246–255.

Marcell, A. V., Raine, T., & Eyre, S. L. (2003). Where does reproductive health fit into the lives of adolescent males? *Perspectives on Sexual and Reproductive Health, 35*(4), 180–186.

Montgomery, K. (2003). Health promotion for pregnant adolescents. *AWHONN Lifelines, 7*(5), 433–444.

Nadeau, J. (2005). *News release: Teen sex is common worldwide.* The Alan Guttmacher Institute. Retrieved May 29, 2006, from http://www.guttmacher.org/media/nr/2005/11/08/index.html

National Campaign to Prevent Teen Pregnancy (NCPTP). (2004b). *Survey slices: Highlights from the National Campaign's 2003 annual survey.* Retrieved January 22, 2004, from http://www.teenpregnancy.org

National Campaign to Prevent Teen Pregnancy (NCPTP). (2004a). *Recent trends in teen pregnancy, sexual activity, and contraceptive use* (Fact Sheet). Retrieved June 30, 2006, from http://www.teenpregnancy.org

National Campaign to Prevent Teen Pregnancy (NCPTP). (2006). *Home page goal statement.* Retrieved July 5, 2006, from http://www.teenpregnancy.org

National Public Radio [NPR], Kaiser Family Foundation, & John F. Kennedy School of Government. (2004). *NPR/Kaiser/Kennedy School poll: Sex education in America.* Retrieved April 18, 2004, from http://www.kff.org

Population Council. (2004). *The adverse health and social outcomes of sexual coercion: Experiences of young women in developing countries.* Retrieved July 3, 2006, from http://www.popcouncil.org

Scheiman, L., & Zeoli, A. M. (2003). Adolescents' experiences of dating and intimate partner violence: "Once is not enough." *Journal of Midwifery & Women's Health, 48*(3), 226–228.

Short, M. B., & Rosenthal, S. (2003). Helping teenaged girls make wise sexual decisions. *Contemporary OB/GYN, 48*(5), 84–95.

Steinberg, L. (2002). *Adolescence* (6th ed.). New York: McGraw-Hill.

Weinstock, H., Berman, S., & Cates, W. (2004). Sexually transmitted diseases among American youth: Incidence and prevalence estimates, 2000. *Perspectives on Sexual and Reproductive Health, 36*(1), 6–10.

World Health Organization (WHO). (2004). *Adolescent pregnancy: Issues in adolescent health and development.* Geneva, Switzerland: Author.

18 Maternal Nutrition

I'm trying to be very careful about what I eat. I've had more salads and fresh fruit than I can remember. Sometimes, though, I get a "cookie attack" and indulge myself. My husband says I should eat oatmeal cookies so I could feel that my cravings were nutritionally sound!

OBJECTIVES

1. Identify the role of specific nutrients in the diet of the pregnant woman.
2. Compare nutritional needs during pregnancy, postpartum, and lactation with nonpregnant requirements.
3. Discuss effects of maternal nutrition on fetal outcomes.
4. Evaluate adequacy and pattern of weight gain during different stages of pregnancy.
5. Plan adequate prenatal vegetarian diets based on nutritional requirements of pregnancy.
6. Describe ways in which various physical, psychosocial, and cultural factors can affect nutritional intake and status.
7. Compare recommendations for weight gain and nutrient intakes in the pregnant adolescent with those for the mature pregnant adult.
8. Describe basic factors a nurse should consider when offering nutritional counseling to a pregnant adolescent.
9. Compare nutritional counseling issues for breastfeeding and formula-feeding mothers.
10. Formulate a nutritional care plan for pregnant women based on a diagnosis of nutritional problems.

KEY TERMS

Adequate intake (AI)   421
Calorie   424
Dietary reference intake (DRIs)   421
Folic acid   430
Kilocalorie   424
Lactase deficiency (lactose intolerance)   433
Lacto-ovovegetarians   431
Lactovegetarians   431
Pica   435
Recommended dietary allowance (RDA)   421
Vegans   431

MEDIALINK

Additional resources for this content can be found on the Prentice Hall Nursing MediaLink DVD-ROM and on the Companion Website at http://www.prenhall.com/davidson. Click on "Chapter 18" to select the activities for this chapter.

A woman's nutritional status before and during pregnancy can significantly influence her own health and that of her unborn child. In most prenatal clinics and offices, nurses provide nutritional counseling directly or work closely with dietitians in providing any necessary nutritional assessment and teaching.

This chapter focuses on the nutritional needs of a normal pregnant woman. Special sections consider the nutritional needs of the pregnant adolescent and the woman after birth.

Many factors influence a woman's ability to achieve good prenatal nutrition, including the following:

- *General nutritional status before pregnancy.* Good prenatal nutrition is the result of proper eating throughout life, not just during pregnancy, although pregnancy may motivate a woman to improve poor eating habits. Nutritional deficits at conception and during the early prenatal period may influence the outcome of the pregnancy.

- *Maternal age.* An expectant adolescent must meet the nutritional needs for her own growth in addition to the nutritional needs of pregnancy.

- *Maternal parity.* A mother's nutritional needs and the outcome of her pregnancy are influenced by the number of pregnancies she has had and by the intervals between them.

A mother's nutritional status does affect her fetus. Factors influencing fetal well-being are interrelated, but nutrient deficiencies alone can produce measurable effects on cell and organ growth of the developing fetus. Fetal growth occurs in three overlapping stages: (1) growth by increase in cell number, (2) growth by increase in cell number and cell size, and (3) growth by increase in cell size alone. The nutritional problems that interfere with cell division may have permanent consequences. If the nutritional insult occurs when cells are mainly enlarging, the changes are usually reversible when normal nutrition resumes.

Growth of fetal and maternal tissues requires increased quantities of nutrients. These are listed in the **dietary reference intakes (DRIs)** as specific allowances for pregnant and lactating women (Table 18–1). The DRIs distinguish between pregnant women and pregnant adolescents because of the greater nutrient needs of the adolescent. The DRIs are subdivided into the **recommended dietary allowance (RDA)** and **adequate intake (AI).** An RDA is the daily dietary intake that is considered sufficient to meet the nutritional requirements of nearly all individuals in a specific life stage and gender group. An AI is a value cited for a nutrient when there is not sufficient data to calculate an estimated average requirement.

MATERNAL WEIGHT
Prepregnancy Weight

Prepregnancy weight is an important factor for both mothers and their babies. Women who are underweight before pregnancy, especially younger adolescents, have a higher risk of giving birth to a low-birth-weight infant than women who begin pregnancy at normal weight for height. On the other hand, women who are obese before pregnancy have an increased risk of pregnancy-related complications such as gestational diabetes mellitus, high blood pressure, and hospitalization. Their babies are at increased risk for prematurity and congenital malformations. Moreover, as these babies grow up they are more likely to be obese and have obesity-related health problems such as cardiovascular disease, hypertension, and diabetes (March of Dimes, 2002).

Maternal Weight Gain

Maternal weight gain is an important factor in fetal growth and in infant birth weight. An adequate weight gain over time indicates an adequate caloric intake. It does not, however, ensure that the woman has a sufficient nutrient intake. The diet may not be of high enough nutritional quality even though its caloric content supports the recommended weight gain. The pregnant woman must maintain the nutritional quality of her diet as her weight gain progresses.

Weight gain, even in women with a healthy pregnancy outcome, tends to be quite variable. Optimal weight gain depends on the woman's weight for height (body mass index [BMI]) and her prepregnant nutritional state. The Institute of Medicine (IOM, 1992) recommends weight gain in terms of optimum ranges based on prepregnant BMI (Table 18–2). Studies examining these recommendations have demonstrated that women who fail to reach the lower end of the IOM recommended weight gain ranges have a higher risk of having a low-birth-weight infant, whereas women who gained above the IOM recommended upper limit are more likely to retain the weight 10 to 18 months postpartum (Salzberg, 2002).

The pattern of weight gain during pregnancy is also important. For example, inadequate prenatal weight gain during the second trimester is closely associated with reduced birth weight in the newborn. For women of normal weight, the recommended pattern consists of a gain of 1.6 to 2.3 kg (3.5 to 5 lb) during the first trimester, followed by an average gain of 0.5 kg (1 lb) per week during the last two trimesters. The rate of weight gain in the second and third trimesters needs to be slightly higher for underweight women and slightly lower (0.7 lb per week) for overweight women (IOM, 1990). A maternal weight gain of 1.5 lb per week has been suggested for normal-weight women during the second half of a twin pregnancy. Underweight women should strive for a gain of 1.75 lb per week after 20 weeks' gestation.

The average maternal weight gain is distributed as follows:

5 kg (11 lb)	Fetus, placenta, amniotic fluid
0.9 kg (2 lb)	Uterus
1.8 kg (4 lb)	Increased blood volume
1.4 kg (3 lb)	Breast tissue
2.3 to 4.5 kg (5 to 10 lb)	Maternal stores

Adequate maternal weight gain contributes to the tissue expansion and growth of both the mother and the developing fetus. Inadequate weight gain has been associated with preterm birth and its related problems for the newborn (Salzberg, 2002).

Obesity is becoming increasingly prevalent in the United States and in many developed countries. Pregnant women who

Table 18–1   DIETARY REFERENCE INTAKES (DRIs) FOR NONPREGNANT FEMALES AND FOR PREGNANT AND LACTATING FEMALES

	Age	Vitamin A (mcg/d)	Vitamin D (mcg/d)	Vitamin E (mg/d α-tocopherol)	Vitamin K (mcg/d)	Vitamin C (mg/d)	Thiamine (mg/d)	Riboflavin (mg/d)
Females	9–13 y	600	5*	11	60*	45	0.9	0.9
	14–18 y	700	5*	15	75*	65	1.0	1.0
	19–30 y	700	5*	15	90*	75	1.1	1.1
	31–50 y	700	5*	15	90*	75	1.1	1.1
	50–70 y	700	10*	15	90*	75	1.1	1.1
	Greater than 70 y	700	15*	15	90*	75	1.1	1.1
Pregnancy	Less than or equal to 18 y	750	5*	15	75*	80	1.4	1.4
	19–30 y	770	5*	15	90*	85	1.4	1.4
	31–50 y	770	5*	15	90*	85	1.4	1.4
Lactation	Less than or equal to 18 y	1200	5*	19	75*	115	1.4	1.6
	19–30 y	1300	5*	19	90*	120	1.4	1.6
	31–50 y	1300	5*	19	90*	120	1.4	1.6

*Values are adequate intakes (AIs) rather than recommended dietary allowances (RDAs). All other values on chart are RDAs.

SOURCE: All data from the Institute of Medicine (1997–2001). Dietary reference intakes, Washington, DC: National Academy Press. Also available at http://www.nap.edu.

Table 18–2   RECOMMENDED TOTAL WEIGHT GAIN RANGES FOR PREGNANT WOMEN

Pregnancy Weight-for-Height Category	Recommended Total Gain	
	lb	kg
Low (BMI less than 19.8)	28–40	12.5–18
Normal (BMI 19.8–26)	25–35	11.5–16
High (BMI greater than 26–29)	15–25	7–11.5
Obese (BMI greater than 29)	Equal to or more than 15	Equal to or more than 7

NOTE: For singleton pregnancies: The range for women carrying twins is 16–20 kg (35–45 lb); Young adolescents (less than 2 years after menarche) and African American women should strive for gains at the upper end of the range. Short women (less than 157 cm or less than 62 in) should strive for gains at the lower end of the range.

SOURCE: Institute of Medicine Subcommittee for a Clinical Application Guide (1992). *Nutrition during pregnancy and lactation: An implementation guide* (p. 44). Washington, DC: National Academy Press.

Figure 18–1 ◆ It is important to monitor a pregnant woman's weight over time.
SOURCE: Michael Newman/Photo Edit.

are obese are at increased risk for many pregnancy complications including prematurity, neural tube defect, stillbirth, and macrosomia. They also are at increased risk of cesarean birth. Moreover, obese women who have a cesarean are at increased risk for wound breakdowns and infections. Consequently, it is important that, when possible, obese women receive preconception counseling about the risks and the importance of weight reduction before conceiving (American College of Obstetricians and Gynecologists [ACOG], 2005).

Because of the association between maternal weight gain and pregnancy outcome, most caregivers pay close attention to weight gain during pregnancy (Figure 18–1 ◆). Weight gain charts can be useful in monitoring the rate of weight gain over time. If a significant deviation from the anticipated pattern occurs, the cause should be determined and appropriate interventions planned with the woman.

As mentioned earlier, weight gain alone does not guarantee adequate nutrition. A diet may be high in energy (calories) but low in vitamins, minerals, or complex carbohydrates and protein. Pregnancy is not a time to diet, and severe caloric restric-

Niacin (mg/d)	Vitamin B$_6$ (mg/d)	Folate (mcg/d)	Vitamin B$_{12}$ (mcg/d)	Calcium (mg/d)	Phosphorus (mg/d)	Magnesium (mg/d)	Iron (mg/d)	Zinc (mg/d)	Iodine (mcg/d)	Selenium (mcg/d)
12	1	300	1.8	1300*	1250	240	8	8	120	40
14	1.2	400	2.4	1300*	1250	360	15	9	150	55
14	1.3	400	2.4	1000*	700	310	18	8	150	55
14	1.3	400	2.4	1000*	700	320	18	8	150	55
14	1.5	400	2.4	1200*	700	320	8	8	150	55
14	1.5	400	2.4	1200*	700	320	8	8	150	55
18	1.9	600	2.6	1300*	1250	400	27	12	220	60
18	1.9	600	2.6	1000*	700	350	27	11	220	60
18	1.9	600	2.6	1000*	700	360	27	11	220	60
17	2	500	2.8	1300*	1250	360	10	13	290	70
17	2	500	2.8	1000*	700	310	9	12	290	70
17	2	500	2.8	1000*	700	320	9	12	290	70

tion during pregnancy can result in maternal ketosis. Counseling the pregnant woman to eat a variety of nutrients from each of the food groups places less emphasis on the amount of her weight gain and more on the quality of her intake. The newly designed food group pyramid, renamed MyPyramid in 2005, offers users a colorful plan that emphasizes variety, proportionality, moderation, and physical activity and is designed to help guide individuals to healthier choices (Figure 18–2 ◆).

The pregnant woman can obtain most of the recommended nutrients by eating a well-balanced diet each day. The basic food groups and recommended amounts during pregnancy and lactation are presented in Table 18–3.

CLINICAL TIP

Weight varies with time of day, amount of clothing, inaccurate scale adjustment, or weighing error. Do not overemphasize a single weight but pay attention to the pattern of weight gain.

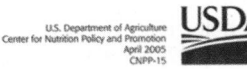

Figure 18–2 ◆ MyPyramid: Steps to a Healthier You identifies the basic food groups and provides guidance about healthful eating. Grains, vegetables, fruits, and dairy products are emphasized with slightly less emphasis on protein. The narrow yellow bar is designated for fats, sugar, and salt. People are encouraged to have most of their fat intake come from fish, nuts, and vegetable oils while limiting solid fats like butter, margarine, shortening, and lard. The emphasis is also placed on limiting added sugars, which contribute calories but few, if any, nutrients.
SOURCE: US Department of Agriculture; US Department of Health and Human Services.

Table 18–3   DAILY FOOD PLAN FOR PREGNANCY AND LACTATION

Food Group	Nutrients Provided	Food Source	Recommended Daily Amount During Pregnancy	Recommended Daily Amount During Lactation
Dairy products	Protein; riboflavin; vitamins A, D, and others; calcium; phosphorus; zinc; magnesium	Milk—whole, 2%, low-fat, skim, dry, buttermilk Cheeses—hard, semisoft, cottage Yogurt—plain, low-fat Soybean milk—canned, dry	Four (8 oz) cups (five for teenagers) used plain or with flavoring, in shakes, soups, puddings, custards, cocoa Calcium in 1 cup milk equivalent to 1½ cups cottage cheese, 1½ oz hard or semisoft cheese, 1 cup yogurt, 1½ cups ice cream (high in fat and sugar)	Four (8 oz) cups (five for teenagers); equivalent amount of cheese, yogurt, and so forth
Meat and meat alternatives	Protein; iron; thiamine, niacin, and other vitamins; minerals	Beef, pork, veal, lamb, poultry, animal organ meats, fish, tofu; eggs; legumes; nuts, seeds, peanut butter, grains in proper vegetarian combination (vitamin B_{12} supplement needed)	Three servings (one serving = 2 oz), combination in amounts necessary for same nutrient equivalent (varies greatly)	Two servings
Grain products, whole grain or enriched	B vitamins; iron; whole grain also has zinc, magnesium, and other trace elements; provides fiber	Breads and bread products such as cornbread, muffins, waffles, hotcakes, biscuits, dumplings, cereals, pastas, rice	Six to 11 servings daily: one serving = one slice bread, ¾ cup or 1 oz dry cereal, ½ cup rice or pasta	Same as for pregnancy
Fruits and fruit juices	Vitamins A and C; minerals; raw fruits for roughage	Citrus fruits and juices, melons, berries, all other fruits and juices	Two to four servings (one serving for vitamin C): one serving = one medium fruit, ½–1 cup fruit, 4 oz orange or grapefruit juice	Same as for pregnancy
Vegetables and vegetable juices	Vitamins A and C; minerals; provides roughage	Leafy green vegetables; deep yellow or orange vegetables such as carrots, sweet potatoes, squash, tomatoes; green vegetables such as peas, green beans, broccoli; other vegetables such as beets, cabbage, potatoes, corn, lima beans	Three to five servings (one serving of dark green or deep yellow vegetable for vitamin A): one serving = ½–1 cup vegetable, two tomatoes, one medium potato	Same as for pregnancy
Fats	Vitamins A and D; linoleic acid	Butter, cream cheese, fortified table spreads; cream, whipped cream, whipped toppings; avocado, mayonnaise, oil, nuts	As desired in moderation (high in calories): one serving = 1 tbsp butter or enriched margarine	Same as for pregnancy
Sugar and sweets		Sugar, brown sugar, honey, molasses	Occasionally, if desired	Same as for pregnancy
Desserts		Nutritious desserts such as puddings, custards, fruit whips, and crisps; other rich, sweet desserts and pastries	Occasionally, if desired	Same as for pregnancy
Beverages		Coffee, decaffeinated beverages, tea, bouillon, carbonated drinks	As desired, in moderation	Same as for pregnancy
Miscellaneous		Iodized salt, herbs, spices, condiments	As desired	Same as for pregnancy

NOTE: The pregnant woman should eat regularly, three meals a day, with nutritious snacks of fruit, cheese, milk, or other foods between meals if desired. (More frequent but smaller meals are also recommended.) Four to 6 (8 oz) glasses of water and a total of 8 to 10 (8 oz) cups total fluid intake should be consumed daily. Water is an essential nutrient.

NUTRITIONAL REQUIREMENTS

The requirements for calories and almost all nutrients increase during pregnancy, although the amount of increase varies with each nutrient. These increases reflect the additional requirements of both the mother and the developing fetus (see Table 18–1).

Calories

The term **calorie** (cal) stands for the amount of heat required to raise the temperature of 1 gram of water 1 degree centigrade. The **kilocalorie** (kcal) is equivalent to 1000 cal and is the unit used to express the energy value of food.

Energy requirements remain the same during the first trimester but increase by 300 kcal per day during the second and third trimesters. Women with a twin pregnancy should add an additional 300 kcal, for a total of 600 kcal above nonpregnant levels. Weight gains should be monitored regularly, and dietary recommendations should be individualized to help the pregnant woman meet her caloric needs. Prepregnant weight, height, maternal age, activity, and health status all affect caloric requirements.

See Client Teaching: Helping the Pregnant Woman Add 300 kcal to Her Diet for basic nutritional information and suggestions for increasing caloric intake.

CLIENT TEACHING Helping the Pregnant Woman Add 300 kcal to Her Diet

CLIENT GOALS At the completion of the teaching the woman will be able to:

1. Identify the MyPyramid categories and the foods included in each

2. Cite the increase in kilocalories indicated during pregnancy

3. Discuss the most nutritionally sound way to use the additional calories

4. Use the information she has gained to plan a nutritionally sound sample menu

TEACHING PLAN

CONTENT

Describe the basic food groups, which include the following:

Grains: 6 to 11 servings (one serving = 1 slice bread, ½ hamburger roll, 1 oz dry cereal, 1 tortilla, ½ cup pasta, rice, grits)

Fruits: Two to four servings; one should be a good source of vitamin C (one serving = 1 medium-sized piece of fruit, ½ cup juice).

Vegetables: Three to five servings (one serving = 1 cup raw vegetable, 1 cup green leafy vegetable, ½ cup cooked vegetable)

Dairy: Two to three servings (one serving = 1 cup milk or yogurt, 1.5 oz hard cheese, 2 cups cottage cheese, 1 cup pudding made with milk)

Meats and alternatives: Two to three servings (one serving = 2 oz cooked lean meat, poultry, or fish; 2 eggs, ½ cup cottage cheese; 1 cup cooked legumes [kidney, lima, garbanzo, or soybeans, split peas]; 6 oz tofu; 2 oz nuts or seeds; 4 tbsp peanut butter)

Point out that not all foods that are nutritionally equivalent have the same number of calories; it is important to consider that when making food choices.

Explain the design of MyPyramid.

MyPyramid is designed to represent the food groups needed to make a balanced diet. The grain, fruit, vegetable, and dairy groups are the widest color bands of the pyramid and should account for the majority of the food selections. Fewer servings of meat or meat alternatives are required in the diet. Fats, oils, sweets, and sodium do not have a high nutritional value and should be used sparingly.

Emphasize that a woman only has to add 300 kcal/day during pregnancy. This can be achieved by adding two milk servings and one serving of meat or alternative. Because of the varying caloric value, a woman needs to consider the advisability of using low-fat milk, lean cuts of meat, or fish broiled or baked instead of fried.

Foods can be combined. For example, 1 cup spaghetti with a 2 oz meatball would count as 1 serving meat, ¾ cup spaghetti = 1 grain, and ¼ cup tomato sauce = ½ serving vegetable.

TEACHING METHOD

Ask woman if she has received nutritional information using this approach before. Discuss her understanding of it. Use that information to plan the amount of detail you will use.

Use a chart or colorful handout to explain the basic food groups and to give examples of equivalent foods.

Use a calorie-counting guide to compare the calories in a variety of foods that are equivalent, such as 2 oz beef and 2 oz fish or 1 cup low-fat milk and 1 cup whole milk.

Use a similar approach to evaluate the calories in fats, oils, and sweets, but also evaluate their nutrient content, especially levels of nutrients such as vitamin C, iron, and calcium.
Discuss the MyPyramid recommendations about the importance of regular exercise in controlling weight gain and maintaining good health.

In planning the woman's diet to get optimum nutrition without too many additional calories, it is often helpful to ask her to plan and evaluate a sample menu.

Provide handouts on which the woman can list the foods she has eaten and check off the corresponding nutrient categories. Have her bring her completed handouts to a subsequent visit.

(Continued on next page)

CLIENT TEACHING   Helping the Pregnant Woman Add 300 kcal to Her Diet   continued

EVALUATION

Evaluate the learning by providing time for discussion, questions, and practice using the calorie-counting guide.

Teaching has been effective if all the identified goals are achieved and if the woman seems comfortable planning her diet to provide for the best nutrition possible.

DOCUMENTATION

Document the information given to the woman, including specifics on food groups, foods, and portion size. Specify if written instructions were provided in addition to verbal ones and describe the type of teaching method used. Document woman's verbalization of understanding and your clarification of any information.

Carbohydrates

Carbohydrates provide the body's primary source of energy as well as fiber necessary for proper bowel functioning. If the carbohydrate intake is not adequate, the body uses protein for energy. Protein then becomes unavailable for growth needs. In addition, protein breakdown leads to ketosis. Ketosis can be a problem, especially in diabetic women, because of glycosuria, reduced alkaline reserves, and lipidemia.

The carbohydrate and caloric needs of the pregnant woman increase, especially during the last two trimesters. Carbohydrate intake promotes weight gain and growth of the fetus, placenta, and other maternal tissues. Dairy products, fruits, vegetables, and whole grain cereals and breads all contain carbohydrates.

Protein

During pregnancy, the woman needs increased amounts of protein to provide amino acids for fetal development, blood volume expansion, and growth of other maternal tissues, such as the breasts and uterus. Protein also contributes to the body's overall energy metabolism. The recommendation for protein during pregnancy is 60 g, an increase of about 14 g over nonpregnant levels. The quality of dietary protein is as important as the total amount consumed. The quality is determined by the complex of amino acids that makes up the protein. Proteins are said to be *complete* when they are made up of all the amino acids necessary to sustain growth and are considered *incomplete* when they lack some of the necessary amino acids. The two terms exaggerate the differences in quality between plant and animal proteins because plant proteins contain all amino acids necessary for growth (Messina, Mangels, & Messina, 2004). Plant proteins can meet a woman's protein needs; however, more of a given protein may be needed as animal proteins are of higher quality.

To obtain high-quality protein in the diet, it is best to eat a variety of foods. Animal products, such as lean meats, fish, poultry, and eggs, are sources of high-quality, complete protein. Dairy products are also important protein sources. A quart of milk supplies 32 g of protein, more than half the average daily protein requirement. Milk can be incorporated into the diet in a variety of dishes, including soups, puddings, custards, sauces, yogurt, and beverages such as hot chocolate and fruited milk drinks. Various kinds of hard and soft cheeses and cottage cheese are also excellent protein sources, although cream cheese is categorized as a fat source only. Table 18–4 provides information on the protein content of common foods.

Table 18–4   AMOUNT OF PROTEIN IN COMMON FOODS

Food	Protein (g)
Dairy Products	
Milk, 8 oz	8
Cheese: cheddar, Swiss, and so forth, 1 oz	7
Cottage cheese ¼ cup	7
Meat and Meat Alternatives	
Meat, fish, poultry, 1 oz	7
Egg, 1	7
Cooked dry beans and peas, ½ cup	7
Cooked soybeans, ½ cup	11
Tofu, raw ½ cup	10
Peanut butter, 2 tbsp	7
Peanuts (3 tbsp), cashews/almonds (5 tbsp)	7
Breads and Cereals	
Bread, 1 slice	2
Buns, biscuits, muffins, 1	2
Cooked cereals and grains, ½ cup	2
Breakfast cereal, 1 oz	2
Vegetables and Fruits	
Vegetables, ½ cup	0.5–1
Fruits and juices, ½ cup	0.5
Miscellaneous	
Soy milk, 8 oz	6.6

Women who have allergies to milk, who have lactose intolerance, or who practice vegetarianism may find soy milk acceptable. It can be used in cooked dishes or as a beverage. Soy cheeses are also available.

Fat

Fats are valuable sources of energy for the body. Fats are more completely absorbed during pregnancy, resulting in a marked increase in serum lipids, lipoproteins, and cholesterol and decreased elimination of fat through the bowel. Fat deposits in the fetus increase from about 2% at midpregnancy to almost 12% at term. However, fat requirements are unchanged during preg-

COMPLEMENTARY AND ALTERNATIVE THERAPIES

ESSENTIAL FATTY ACIDS

The essential fatty acids (EFAs) are important for the development of the central nervous system of the fetus. The omega-3 fatty acids are of particular importance in the American diet, including their derivative, docosahexaenoic acid (DHA). Maternal dietary intake of DHA during pregnancy and breastfeeding enhances infant attention and visual development (Agostoni & Verduci, 2003; Smuts, Borod, Peeples et al., 2003). Studies have also shown that an intake of omega-3 fatty acids during pregnancy may lower the risk of preterm birth (Smuts et al., 2003; Villar, Merialdi, Gulmezoglu et al., 2003).

The best sources of omega-3 fatty acids are flaxseeds and their oil and fish oil (but see information on fish consumption under "Mercury in Fish" later in this chapter). Another source includes eggs that have been enriched with omega-3 fatty acids, which can now be purchased in some grocery stores.

Table 18–5	FOODS THAT PROVIDE COMPARABLE AMOUNTS OF CALCIUM
Food	**Amount**
Dairy Products	
Milk	8 oz
Cheese, cheddar	1½ oz
Pudding, vanilla	1 cup
Dairy Alternatives	
Soy milk*	8 oz
Fruits	
Figs	10
Raisins	2 cups
Vegetables	
Broccoli	2½ cups
Collards	1 cup
Kale	3 cups
Mustard greens	3½ cups
Turnip greens	1½ cups
Fish	
Salmon, canned, with bones	2/3 cup
Sardines	6
Nuts	
Almonds	4 oz
Brazil nuts	¼ cup
Miscellaneous	
Molasses, blackstrap	2 tbsp

SOURCE: Data from Pennington, J. A. T. (1989). *Bowes and Church's food values of portions commonly used* (15th ed.). Philadelphia: Lippincott.
*Amounts may vary with brand; be sure to check label.

nancy and should account for about 30% of the total daily caloric intake (Salzberg, 2002). US dietary guidelines recommend that less than 10% of fat calories should be saturated fat (US Department of Health and Human Services & US Department of Agriculture, 2005).

When dairy products are used as a regular part of the diet, it may be helpful to select items that have a reduced fat content. Selecting lean cuts of meats, fish, and poultry will also help decrease dietary fat.

Minerals

The woman can increase minerals needed for the growth of new tissue during pregnancy by improving mineral absorption and increasing mineral intake.

CALCIUM AND PHOSPHORUS

Calcium and phosphorus are involved in the mineralization of fetal bones and teeth, energy and cell production, and acid-base buffering. Calcium is absorbed and used more efficiently during pregnancy. Some additional calcium and phosphorus are required early in pregnancy, but most of the fetus's bone calcification occurs during the last 2 or 3 months. Teeth begin to form at about 8 weeks' gestation and are formed by birth. The 6-year molars begin to calcify just before birth. Additional calcium is stored in the maternal skeleton as a reserve for lactation.

The identified adequate intake for calcium for the pregnant or lactating woman 19 years of age or older is 1000 mg per day. It is 1300 mg/day for pregnant women under 19. If calcium intake is not adequate, fetal needs will be met at the mother's expense by demineralization of maternal bone. Food is the preferred source of calcium because food provides other nutrients as well. A diet that includes 4 cups of milk or an equivalent dairy alternative (see Table 18–2) and a variety of other foods will provide sufficient calcium. Smaller amounts of calcium are

supplied by legumes, nuts, dried fruits, and dark green leafy vegetables (such as kale, broccoli, collard greens, and beet greens). It is important to remember that some of the calcium in beet greens, spinach, and Swiss chard is bound with oxalic acid, which makes it less available to the body. Larger amounts of these foods need to be consumed if they are substituted for dairy sources of calcium (Table 18–5).

The RDA for phosphorus does not change from that of a nonpregnant woman age 19 or older: 700 mg per day. Similarly, for females age 18 and younger it remains stable at 1250 mg per day. Phosphorus is readily supplied through calcium- and protein-rich foods, especially milk, eggs, and meat.

IODINE

Iodine is an essential part of the thyroid hormone thyroxine. Inorganic iodine is excreted in the urine during pregnancy. Enlargement of the thyroid gland may occur if iodine is not replaced by adequate dietary intake or additional supplement. Iodine deficiency is the most widespread nutritional cause of impaired brain development. This can result in cretinism and lesser degrees of retardation.

A woman can meet the iodine requirement of 220 mcg per day by using iodized salt. Seafood is also a good source of iodine. Plant sources vary because they reflect the iodine content of the soil in which they grow. When sodium is restricted, the physician may prescribe an iodine supplement.

SODIUM

The sodium ion is essential for proper metabolism and the regulation of fluid balance. Sodium intake in the form of salt is never entirely curtailed during pregnancy, even when hypertension or preeclampsia is present. The woman can obtain moderate sodium intake (2 to 3 g) by using fresh food lightly seasoned to taste during cooking. The use of extra salt at the table should be avoided. Salty foods, such as potato chips, ham, sausages, and sodium-based seasonings, can be eliminated to avoid excessive intake.

ZINC

Zinc is a part of numerous enzymes and is involved in protein metabolism and the synthesis of DNA and RNA. It is essential for normal fetal growth and development as well as milk production during lactation. The RDA during pregnancy for women age 19 and older is 11 mg per day. This increases to 12 mg during lactation. Best sources of zinc are meats, shellfish, and poultry. Good sources include whole grains and legumes.

MAGNESIUM

Magnesium is essential for cellular metabolism and structural growth. The RDA for pregnancy is 320 mg. Good sources include milk, whole grains, dark green vegetables, nuts, and legumes.

IRON

Iron requirements increase during pregnancy because of the growth of the fetus and placenta and the expansion of maternal blood volume. Anemia in pregnancy is mainly caused by low iron stores, although it may also result from inadequate intake of other nutrients, such as vitamins B_6 and B_{12}, folic acid, ascorbic acid, copper, and zinc. Women with poor diet histories, frequent conceptions, or records of prior iron depletion are particularly at risk.

Iron deficiency anemia is generally defined as a decrease in the oxygen-carrying capacity of the blood. This significantly reduces the hemoglobin per deciliter of blood, the volume of packed red cells per deciliter of blood (hematocrit), or the number of erythrocytes. Iron deficiency anemia is associated with a higher incidence of low-birth-weight infants and preterm birth (Cunningham, Leveno, Bloom et al., 2005).

The normal hematocrit in the nonpregnant woman is 38% to 47%. In the pregnant woman, the level may drop to as low as 34%, even when nutrition is adequate. This condition is called the *physiologic anemia of pregnancy* (see Chapter 14 ∞). Fetal demands for iron further contribute to symptoms of anemia in the pregnant woman. The fetal liver stores iron, especially during the third trimester. The infant will need this stored iron during the first 4 months of life to compensate for the normally inadequate levels of iron in breast milk and non-iron-fortified formulas. To prevent anemia, the woman must balance iron re-

quirements and intake. Doing so is a problem for nonpregnant women and a greater one for pregnant women. Although the rate of absorption increases during pregnancy, it is still important to select foods high in iron to increase the daily intake. Lean meats, dark green leafy vegetables, eggs, and whole grain and enriched breads and cereals are the foods usually depended on for their iron content. Other iron sources include dried fruits, legumes, shellfish, and molasses.

Iron absorption is generally higher for animal products than for vegetable products. However, the woman may enhance absorption of iron from nonmeat sources by combining them with meat or a food rich in vitamin C. In addition, the use of iron-fortified foods is a cost-effective and efficient way to increase iron intake.

The most iron that can reasonably be obtained from the average diet is about 15 to 18 mg per day. However, the recommended intake for iron during pregnancy is 27 mg per day. Thus during pregnancy a supplement of simple iron salt, such as ferrous gluconate, ferrous fumarate, or ferrous sulfate, is needed. This amount is available in most prenatal vitamins. Unfortunately iron supplements often cause gastrointestinal discomfort, especially if taken on an empty stomach. Consequently caregivers often begin iron supplementation in the second trimester after the incidence of nausea and vomiting subsides. Once the woman begins taking an iron supplement, absorption is increased if she takes it with a source of vitamin C such as orange juice. In addition, iron is often constipating, so it is important for the woman to consume sufficient fluids and roughage in her diet to combat this effect.

Vitamins

Vitamins are organic substances necessary for life and growth. They are found in small amounts in specific foods and generally cannot be synthesized by the body in adequate amounts.

Vitamins are grouped according to their solubility. Those that dissolve in fat are A, D, E, and K; those soluble in water include vitamin C and the B complex vitamins. An adequate intake of all vitamins is essential during pregnancy; however, several are required in larger than normal amounts to fulfill specific needs.

A balanced diet generally provides necessary vitamins without the need for supplementation. Despite this, many people who are concerned about nutrition have become involved in the practice of taking exceptionally large doses—megadoses—of vitamins. However, in vitamin therapy, more is not necessarily better. Megadoses of vitamins, especially vitamins A, D, C, and B_6, have been documented to have a negative effect on the fetus. Furthermore, excessive intake of one vitamin may interfere with the body's use of another vitamin. For example, excessive intake of vitamin C may block the body's use of vitamin B_{12}. Consequently, although it is important to meet the recommended dietary allowances of vitamins during pregnancy, megadoses are best avoided.

FAT-SOLUBLE VITAMINS

The fat-soluble vitamins A, D, E, and K are stored in the liver and thus are available should the dietary intake become inadequate. They are not excreted in the urine, so excessive consumption of these vitamins, particularly vitamins A and D, can lead to toxicity. Symptoms of fat-soluble vitamin toxicity include nausea, gastrointestinal upset, dryness and cracking of the skin, and loss of hair.

Vitamin A

Vitamin A is involved in the growth of epithelial cells, which line the entire gastrointestinal tract and compose the skin. Vitamin A plays a role in the metabolism of carbohydrates and fats. The body cannot synthesize glycogen in the absence of vitamin A, and the body's ability to handle cholesterol is also affected. In addition, the protective layer of tissue surrounding nerve fibers does not form properly if vitamin A is lacking. Probably the best known function of vitamin A is its effect on vision in dim light. A person's ability to see in the dark depends on the eye's supply of retinol, a form of vitamin A. In this manner, vitamin A prevents night blindness. Vitamin A is associated with the formation and development of healthy eyes in the fetus.

If maternal stores of vitamin A are adequate, the overall effects of pregnancy on the woman's vitamin A requirements are not remarkable. The blood serum level of vitamin A decreases slightly in early pregnancy, rises in late pregnancy, and falls before the onset of labor. Thus the RDA for vitamin A is 770 mcg per day for pregnant women age 19 and older.

Deficiencies of vitamin A are not common. However, an inadequate maternal intake has been associated with preterm birth, intrauterine growth restriction, and decreased birth weight (IOM, 1990). Although routine supplementation with vitamin A is not recommended, supplementation with 5000 international units is indicated for women whose dietary intake may be inadequate, specifically strict vegetarians and recent emigrants from countries where deficiency of vitamin A is endemic.

Rich plant sources of vitamin A include deep green and yellow or deep orange vegetables and some fruits; animal sources include liver, egg yolk, cream, butter, fortified margarine, and milk.

Vitamin D

Vitamin D is best known for its role in the absorption and utilization of calcium and phosphorus in skeletal development. To supply the needs of the developing fetus, the pregnant woman should have a vitamin D intake of 5 mcg per day.

Main food sources of vitamin D include fortified milk, margarine, butter, liver, and egg yolks. Drinking a quart of vitamin D–fortified milk daily provides the vitamin D needed during pregnancy. Exposure to the ultraviolet rays of sunlight is also an important source of vitamin D. However, season, time of day, latitude, smog, cloud cover, and sunscreens affect ultraviolet (UV) ray exposure. (Note: It is still important to use sunscreens routinely.) For example, the average amount of sunlight in Boston and in points further north is insufficient to produce significant synthesis of vitamin D from November through February. Thus it is vital for people with limited sun exposure to consume a diet that contains good sources of vitamin D (National Institutes of Health, 2002).

Excessive intake of vitamin D is not usually a result of eating but of taking high-potency vitamin preparations. Overdoses during pregnancy can cause hypercalcemia or high blood calcium levels because of withdrawal of calcium from the skeletal tissue. Symptoms of toxicity include excessive thirst, loss of appetite, vomiting, weight loss, irritability, and high blood calcium levels.

Vitamin E

The major function of vitamin E, or tocopherol, is as an antioxidant. Vitamin E takes on oxygen, thus preventing other nutrients from undergoing chemical changes. For example, vitamin E helps spare vitamin A by preventing its oxidation in the intestinal tract and the tissues. It decreases the oxidation of polyunsaturated fats, thus helping to retain the flexibility and health of the cell membrane. In protecting the cell membrane, vitamin E affects the health of all cells in the body.

Vitamin E is also involved in certain enzymatic and metabolic reactions. It is an essential nutrient for the synthesis of nucleic acids required in the formation of red blood cells in the bone marrow. Vitamin E is beneficial in treating certain types of muscular pain and intermittent claudication, in surface healing of wounds and burns, and in protecting lung tissue from the damaging effects of smog. These functions may help explain the abundant claims and cures attributed to vitamin E, many of which have not been scientifically proved.

The newborn's need for vitamin E has been widely recognized. Human milk provides adequate vitamin E, whereas cow's milk is lower in vitamin E content. Deficiency symptoms of vitamin E are related to long-term inability to absorb fats. In humans, malabsorption problems exist in cases of cystic fibrosis, liver cirrhosis, postgastrectomy, obstructive jaundice, pancreatic problems, and sprue.

The recommended intake of vitamin E is unchanged at 15 mg per day. Vitamin E is widely distributed in foodstuffs, especially vegetable fats and oils, whole grains, greens, and eggs.

Some pregnant women massage vitamin E oil on the abdominal skin to make it supple and possibly prevent permanent stretch marks. It is questionable whether taking high doses orally will accomplish this goal or satisfy any other claims related to vitamin E's role in reproduction or virility. In addition, excessive intake of vitamin E has been associated with abnormal coagulation in the newborn.

Vitamin K

Vitamin K, or menadione as used synthetically in medicine, is an essential factor for the synthesis of prothrombin; its function is thus related to normal blood clotting. Synthesis occurs in the intestinal tract by the *Escherichia coli* normally inhabiting the large intestine. However, the body's need for vitamin K is not totally met through synthesis. Green leafy vegetables and liver are excellent sources. The requirement for vitamin K does not increase during pregnancy. It is 90 mcg per day.

Intake of vitamin K is usually adequate in a well-balanced prenatal diet. Secondary problems may arise if an illness results in malabsorption of fats or if antibiotics are used for an extended period. Antibiotics inhibit vitamin K synthesis by destroying intestinal *E. coli*.

WATER-SOLUBLE VITAMINS

Water-soluble vitamins are excreted in the urine. Only small amounts are stored, so there is little protection from dietary inadequacies. Thus adequate amounts must be ingested daily. During pregnancy, the concentration of water-soluble vitamins in the maternal serum falls, whereas high concentrations are found in the fetus.

Vitamin C

The requirement for vitamin C (ascorbic acid) is increased in pregnancy from 75 to 85 mg per day. The major function of vitamin C is to aid the formation and development of connective tissue and the vascular system. Ascorbic acid is essential to the formation of collagen. Collagen is like a cement that binds cells together, just as mortar holds bricks together. If the collagen begins to disintegrate because of lack of ascorbic acid, cell functioning is disturbed, and cell structure breaks down, causing muscular weakness, capillary hemorrhage, and eventual death. These are symptoms of scurvy, the disease caused by vitamin C deficiency. Newborns of women who have taken megadoses of vitamin C may experience a rebound form of scurvy.

Maternal plasma levels of vitamin C progressively decline throughout pregnancy, with values at term being about half those at midpregnancy. It appears that ascorbic acid concentrates in the placenta; levels in the fetus are 50% or more above maternal levels.

A nutritious diet should meet the pregnant woman's needs for vitamin C without additional supplementation. Common food sources of vitamin C include citrus fruit, tomatoes, cantaloupe, strawberries, potatoes, broccoli, and other leafy green vegetables. Ascorbic acid is readily destroyed by water and oxidation. Therefore, foods containing vitamin C should have limited exposure to air, heat, and water during storage and cooking.

The B Vitamins

The B vitamins include thiamine (B_1), riboflavin (B_2), niacin, folic acid, pantothenic acid, vitamin B_6, and vitamin B_{12}. These vitamins serve as vital coenzyme factors in many reactions, such as cell respiration, glucose oxidation, and energy metabolism. Consequently, the quantities needed invariably increase as caloric intake increases to meet the metabolic and growth needs of the pregnant woman.

The *thiamine* requirement increases from the prepregnant level of 1.1 mg per day to 1.4 mg per day. Sources include pork, liver, milk, potatoes, enriched breads, and cereals.

Riboflavin deficiency is manifested by *cheilosis* (fissures and cracks of the lips and the corners of the mouth) and other skin lesions. During pregnancy, women may excrete less riboflavin and still require more because of increased energy and protein needs. Thus the recommended intake of riboflavin increases by 0.3 mg per day, to 1.4 mg per day for pregnant women age 19 and older. Sources include milk, liver, eggs, enriched breads, and cereals.

Niacin requirements increase by 4 mg per day during pregnancy to 18 mg. Sources of niacin include meat, fish, poultry, liver, whole grains, enriched breads, cereals, and peanuts.

Folic acid, or folate, is required for normal growth, reproduction, and lactation and prevents the macrocytic, megaloblastic anemia of pregnancy. Megaloblastic anemia due to folic acid deficiency is seldom found in the United States, but those caring for pregnant women must be aware that it does occur.

Even more significantly, an inadequate intake of folic acid has been associated with neural tube defects (NTDs) (spina bifida, anencephaly). Although these defects are considered multifactorial (see Chapter 12 ∞), research indicates that 50% to 70% of spina bifida and anencephaly could be prevented by adequate intake of folic acid (Centers for Disease Control and Prevention [CDC] and the Pan American Health Organization, 2003). Consequently experts recommend that all women of childbearing age (15 to 45 years) consume 400 mcg of folic acid daily, because half of all US pregnancies are unplanned and NTDs occur very early in pregnancy (3 to 4 weeks after conception), before most women realize they are pregnant (National Center on Birth Defects and Developmental Disabilities, 2004).

The best food sources of folates are fresh green leafy vegetables, liver, peanuts, and whole-grain breads and cereals. Folic acid can be made inactive by oxidation, UV light, and heating. It can easily be lost during improper storage and cooking. To prevent unnecessary loss, foods should be stored covered to protect them from light, cooked with only a small amount of water, and not overcooked.

No allowance has been set for *pantothenic acid* in pregnancy but 5 mg per day is considered an adequate intake. Sources include meats, egg yolk, legumes, and whole grain cereals and breads.

Vitamin B_6 (pyridoxine) is associated with amino acid metabolism; thus a higher-than-average protein intake requires increased pyridoxine intake. The RDA for vitamin B_6 during pregnancy is 1.9 mg per day, an increase of 0.6 mg over the allowance for nonpregnant women. Generally the slightly increased need can be supplied by dietary sources, which include wheat germ, yeast, fish, liver, pork, potatoes, and lentils.

Vitamin B_{12}, or *cobalamin*, is the cobalt-containing vitamin found only in animal sources. Rarely is B_{12} deficiency found in women of reproductive age. Vegans (see later discussion of vegetarian diets) can develop a deficiency, however, so it is essential that their dietary intake be supplemented with this vitamin. A deficiency may also be due to a congenital inability to absorb vitamin B_{12}, resulting in pernicious anemia; however, infertility is a complication of this type of anemia.

Occasionally, vitamin B_{12} levels decrease during pregnancy but increase again after birth. The RDA during pregnancy is 2.6 mcg per day, an increase of 0.2 mcg.

Folic acid and iron are the only nutritional supplements generally recommended during pregnancy. The increased need for other vitamins and minerals can usually be met with an adequate diet. To avoid possible deficiencies, however, many healthcare professionals still recommend a daily vitamin supplement.

CLINICAL TIP

More women are consuming over-the-counter vitamin, mineral, and food supplements today than in the past. Ask about the use of any over-the-counter supplements to help avoid potentially harmful excess intakes.

Fluid

The nutrient water is essential for life and is found in all body tissues. It is necessary for many biochemical reactions. It also serves as a lubricant, acts as a medium of transport for carrying substances in and out of the body, and aids in the regulation of body temperature. A pregnant woman should consume at least 8 to 10 (8 oz) glasses of fluid each day, of which 4 to 6 glasses should be water. Other beverages such as juices and milk can contribute water as well as other nutrients to the diet. Sodas and diet sodas should be used in moderation because they do not contribute to the nutritional value of the diet.

Caffeine is found in beverages, foods, and medications. Its use during pregnancy remains controversial. Caffeinated beverages also have a diuretic effect, which may be counterproductive to increasing fluid intake. Caffeine readily crosses the placenta and can affect fetal heart rate and breathing (American Dietetic Association [ADA], 2002). However, no conclusive evidence has been found linking caffeine consumption to birth defects or spontaneous abortion. At this time, most healthcare providers advise pregnant women to limit their daily intake of caffeine to moderate amounts (see Chapter 16 ∞).

VEGETARIANISM

Vegetarianism is the dietary choice of many people for religious, health, ethical, and economic reasons. There are several types of vegetarians. **Lacto-ovovegetarians** include milk, dairy products, and eggs in their diet. **Lactovegetarians** include dairy products but no eggs. **Vegans** are strict vegetarians who will not eat any food from animal sources.

In their position statement on vegetarian diets, the American Dietetic Association stated that "appropriately planned vegetarian diets are healthful, are nutritionally adequate, and provide health benefits in the prevention and treatment of certain diseases" (ADA, 2003). People following vegetarian diets tend to have lower blood pressure; a lower incidence of coronary artery disease, lung cancer, and colorectal cancer; and lower morbidity and mortality rates from chronic degenerative diseases than do nonvegetarians (ADA, 2003).

The expectant woman who is lacto-ovovegetarian can obtain ample and complete proteins from dairy products and eggs. Plant protein quality may be improved if consumed with these animal proteins. If the diet contains fewer than four servings of milk and dairy products, calcium supplementation may be necessary.

If the woman follows a vegan diet, careful planning is necessary to obtain complete proteins and sufficient calories. Protein needs increase slightly for vegans because of the lower quality protein sources provided through the exclusion of animal proteins. Adequate dietary protein can be obtained by consuming a varied diet with adequate caloric intake and complementary amino acids. Complete proteins may be obtained by eating different types of plant-based proteins such as beans and rice, peanut butter on whole grain bread, and whole grain cereal with soy milk, either in the same meal or over the course of a day. Protein and amino acid supplements are not recommended. Obtaining sufficient calories to achieve adequate weight gains can be difficult because vegan diets tend to be higher in fiber and therefore filling. Low prepregnancy weight and optimum pregnancy weight gains are often a problem. Supplementation with energy-dense foods helps provide increased energy intake to prevent the body from using protein for caloric needs.

Because vegans use no animal products, a daily supplement of 4 mg of vitamin B_{12} is necessary. If soy milk is used, only partial supplementation may be needed. If no soy milk is taken, daily supplements of 1200 mg of calcium and 10 mg of vitamin D are needed.

A vegan diet may be low in iron and zinc because the best sources of these minerals are found in animal products. In addition, a high-fiber intake may reduce mineral (calcium, iron, and zinc) bioavailability. The nurse should emphasize the use of foods containing these nutrients.

Figure 18–3 ◆ depicts the vegetarian food pyramid. A guide to vegetarian food groups is provided in Table 18–6.

FACTORS INFLUENCING NUTRITION

It is important to consider the many factors that affect a client's nutrition. What are the age, lifestyle, dietary practices, and culture of the pregnant woman? What food beliefs and habits does she have? What a person eats is also determined by availability, economics, and symbolism. These and other factors influence the expectant mother's acceptance of the nurse's intervention.

Table 18–6	**VEGETARIAN FOOD GROUPS**			
Food Group	**Mixed Diet**	**Lacto-ovovegetarian**	**Lacto-vegetarian**	**Vegan**
Grain	Bread, cereal, rice, pasta	Bread, cereal, rice, pasta	Bread, cereal, rice, pasta	Bread, cereal, rice, pasta
Fruit	Fruit, fruit juices	Fruit, fruit juices	Fruit, fruit juices	Fruit, fruit juices
Vegetable	Vegetables, vegetable juices	Vegetables, vegetable juices	Vegetables, vegetable juices	Vegetables, vegetable juices
Dairy and dairy alternatives	Milk, yogurt, cheese	Milk, yogurt, cheese	Milk, yogurt, cheese	Fortified soy milk, rice milk
Meat and meat alternatives	Meat, fish, poultry, eggs, legumes, tofu, nuts, nut butters	Eggs, legumes, tofu, nuts, nut butters	Legumes, tofu, nuts, nut butters	Legumes, tofu, nuts, nut butters

Figure 18–3 ◆ The vegetarian food pyramid.
SOURCE: Adapted from The Health Connection, 55 West Oak Ridge Drive, Hagerstown, MD 21740-7390.

COMPLEMENTARY AND ALTERNATIVE THERAPIES

NUTRITIONAL CONTENT OF HERBS

Several herbs are good sources of various vitamins and minerals. Like other "whole" foods, herbs contain all the necessary nutrients and enzymes to increase bioavailability versus isolated substances (such as in vitamin and mineral supplements).

Dandelion root and herb: Contains high concentrations of vitamins A and C, beta carotene, and potassium (Blumenthal, 2000).

Oat straw: Rich in calcium and magnesium, plus iron, manganese, and zinc (Blumenthal, 2000; Skidmore-Roth, 2004). Note that this is the same plant from which we derive oatmeal.

Raspberry leaf: Contains vitamin C and naturally chelated iron (Skidmore-Roth, 2004).

Common Discomforts of Pregnancy

Gastrointestinal functioning can be altered at times during pregnancy, resulting in discomforts such as nausea, vomiting, heartburn, and constipation. Although these changes can be uncomfortable for the woman, they are seldom a major problem. These discomforts and dietary modifications that may provide relief are discussed in Chapter 16. ∞

Use of Artificial Sweeteners

Foods and beverages that contain artificial sweeteners are increasingly available. Sweeteners classified as Generally Recognized as Safe (GRAS) by the Food and Drug Administration (FDA) are acceptable for use during pregnancy. As with other foods, moderation should be exercised in using artificial sweeteners, as saccharin can cross the placenta and may remain in fetal tissues. Aspartame also appears to be safe if taken within FDA guidelines. Women affected by phenylketonuria (PKU) should avoid aspartame, as phenylalanine intake needs to be monitored. Splenda, or sucralose, is the newest artificial sweetener to become available to the public. Tests have shown Splenda to have no effects on fetal or neonatal development and support the safety of sucralose for use in pregnant or lactating women.

Mercury in Fish

Fish and shellfish are important parts of a healthy diet but nearly all contain traces of mercury. Although this is not a concern for most people, some fish and shellfish contain higher levels of mercury than others, and mercury can pose a threat to the unborn baby or a young child. The developing fetal brain is quite susceptible to the neurotoxic effects of mercury, which crosses the placenta and the blood-brain barrier. Mercury exposure can have a negative effect on cognitive functioning, resulting in deficiencies in language, attention, motor function, memory, and visual-spatial abilities (Huffling, 2006). Because of this, the US government has issued the following guidelines for women who are pregnant or who may become pregnant, breastfeeding mothers, and young children (US Department of Health and Human Services & US Environmental Protection Agency, 2004):

- Do not eat swordfish, shark, tilefish, or king mackerel, because these fish contain high levels of mercury.

- Eat up to 12 oz/week (two average meals) of a variety of shellfish and fish that are lower in mercury. (Commonly eaten fish that are lower in mercury include canned light tuna, shrimp, salmon, catfish, and pollack. Albacore [white] tuna has more mercury than canned light tuna, so only 6 ounces/week of albacore tuna is recommended.)

- Check local advisories about the mercury content of fish caught locally by family and friends. If no information is available, limit fish caught in local areas to 6 oz/week and avoid consuming additional fish that week.

Salmonella and Listeria Infection

The pregnant woman's immune system is somewhat weakened during pregnancy, As a result, pregnant women and their fetuses are at high risk for foodborne illnesses, which can cause miscarriage, serious health problems, or even maternal death.

Because of the risk of *Salmonella* contamination in raw eggs, pregnant women are advised to avoid eating or tasting foods that may contain raw or lightly cooked eggs. These foods include, for example, cake batter, cookie dough made with raw eggs, homemade eggnog, sauces made with raw eggs such as Caesar salad dressing and hollandaise sauce, and homemade ice cream (FDA, 2005).

Listeria monocytogenes is another bacterium that poses a threat to an expectant mother and her fetus. Listeria is especially challenging because the organism can be found in refrigerated, ready-to-eat foods such as unpasteurized milk and dairy products, meat, poultry, and seafood. To prevent listeriosis, pregnant women should be advised to do the following (FDA, 2005):

- Maintain refrigerator temperature at 40F (4C) or below and the freezer at 0F (−18C).

- Refrigerate or freeze prepared foods, leftovers, and perishables within 2 hours after eating or preparation.

- Do not eat hot dogs and luncheon meats unless they are reheated until they are steaming hot.

- Avoid soft cheeses such as feta, brie, Camembert, blue veined cheeses, queso fresco, or queso blanco (a soft cheese often used by Hispanic women in their cooking) unless the label clearly states that they are made with pasteurized milk.

- Do not eat refrigerated pates or meat spreads or foods that contain raw (unpasteurized) milk or drink unpasteurized milk.

- Avoid eating refrigerated smoked seafood such as salmon, trout, cod, tuna, or mackerel unless it is in a cooked dish such as a casserole. Canned or shelf-stable pates, meat spreads, and smoked seafood are considered safe to eat.

Lactase Deficiency (Lactose Intolerance)

Some individuals have difficulty digesting milk and dairy products. This condition, known as **lactase deficiency,** or **lactose intolerance,** results from an inadequate amount of the enzyme lactase, which breaks down the milk sugar lactose into smaller digestible substances.

Lactase deficiency is found primarily in many people of African, Mexican, Native American, Ashkenazic Jewish, and Asian descent although it is found in other cultural groups as well. In the United States, 30 to 50 million people have lactose intolerance. Furthermore up to 80% of African Americans, 80% to 100% of Native Americans, and 90% to 100% of Asian Americans are lactose intolerant (National Digestive Diseases Information Clearinghouse, 2006). People who are not affected are mainly of Northern European heritage. Symptoms may include abdominal distention, discomfort, nausea, vomiting, loose stools, and cramps. When counseling pregnant women who might be intolerant of milk and milk products, the nurse should be aware that tolerances vary between individuals and even a partial serving of milk or dairy products can produce symptoms. Lactase deficiency need not be a problem for pregnant women, as the enzyme is available over the counter in tablets or drops. In addition, specially treated cow's milk is now available in most large grocery stores.

Cultural, Ethnic, and Religious Influences

Cultural, ethnic, and, occasionally, religious backgrounds determine one's experiences with food and influence food preferences and habits (Figure 18–4 ◆). People of different nationalities are accustomed to eating foodstuffs available in their country of origin and prepared in a manner consistent with the customs and traditions of their ethnic and cultural group. In addition, the laws of certain religions allow particular foods, prohibit others, and direct the preparation and serving of meals. (See Developing Cultural Competence: The Kosher Diet.)

In each culture, certain foods have symbolic significance. Generally, these symbolic foods are related to major life experiences such as birth, death, or developmental milestones. Although generalizations have been made about the food practices of ethnic and religious groups, there are many variations. Food customs will differ among groups in various regions of the same country, among families within local regions, and among individuals within the same family. The extent to which the use of traditional ethnic foods and customs is continued is affected by the recency of immigration, the extent of exposure to other cultures, and the availability, quality, and cost of the traditional foods.

When working with a pregnant woman from any ethnic background, the nurse needs to understand the cultural influences on the woman's eating habits and to identify beliefs she may have about foods and pregnancy. Talking with the client

Figure 18–4 ◆ Cultural factors affect food preferences and habits.
SOURCE: Photographer, Elena Dorfman.

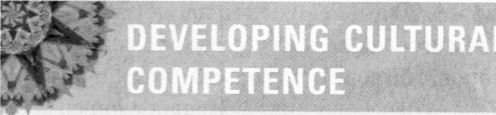

DEVELOPING CULTURAL COMPETENCE

THE KOSHER DIET

The kosher diet followed by many Jewish people forbids the eating of pig products and shellfish. Certain cuts of meat from sheep and cattle are allowed as are fish with fins and scales. In addition, many Jews believe that meat and milk should not be mixed and eaten at the same meal.

can enable the nurse to determine the level of influence that traditional food customs exert. Only then can the nurse provide dietary advice in a manner that is meaningful to the client.

Psychosocial Factors

The sharing of food has long been a symbol of friendliness, warmth, and social acceptance in many cultures. Food is also symbolic of motherliness; that is, taking care of the family and feeding them well is a part of the traditional mothering role. Some foods and food-related practices are associated with status. Certain items may be prepared "just for company." Other foods are served only on special occasions—holidays such as Thanksgiving, for example.

Socioeconomic level may be a determinant of nutritional status. Poverty-level families are unable to afford the same foods that higher income families can. Thus, pregnant women with low incomes are frequently at risk for inadequate intake of nutrients.

Knowledge about the basic components of a balanced diet is essential. Often educational level is related to economic status, but even people on very limited incomes can prepare well-balanced meals if their knowledge of nutrition is adequate.

The expectant woman's attitudes and feelings about her pregnancy may influence her nutritional status. For example, food may be used as a substitute for the expression of emotions such as anger or frustration, or as a way of expressing feelings of joy. The woman who is depressed or who does not wish to be pregnant may manifest these feelings by loss of appetite or by an overindulgence of certain foods.

Eating Disorders

Millions of men and women are affected by eating disorders each year, but eating disorders are most common in adolescent girls and young women. These psychologic disorders can have a major impact on a pregnant client's physiologic and emotional well-being.

Anorexia nervosa is an eating disorder that is characterized by an extreme fear of weight gain and fat. People with this problem have distorted body images and perceive themselves as fat even when they are extremely underweight. Their dietary intake is very restrictive in both variety and quantity. They may also engage in excessive exercise to prevent weight gain.

Bulimia nervosa, another eating disorder, is characterized by bingeing (secretly consuming large quantities of food in a

short period of time) and purging. Self-induced vomiting is the most common method of purging; laxatives and/or diuretics may also be used. Individuals with bulimia often maintain normal or near-normal weight for their height, so it is often difficult to know whether bingeing and purging occur.

Although pregnancies occur most often in women of normal weight, the underweight woman can conceive. The presence of an eating disorder can be difficult to detect because of the secretive nature of the behaviors. Many women will decrease or discontinue their eating disorder behaviors during pregnancy, only to resume them postpartum. Table 18–7 identifies abnormalities that may indicate an eating disorder.

Women with eating disorders who become pregnant are at risk for a variety of complications. The consequences of the restricting, bingeing, and purging behaviors characteristic of eating disorders can result in a lack of nutrients available for the fetus. Women with eating disorders are at increased risk for miscarriage, hyperemesis gravidarum, preeclampsia, and birth complications, whereas their infants have an increased incidence of preterm birth, low birth weight, low Apgar scores, and intrauterine death (Martos-Ordonez, 2005).

Pregnancy can be an especially difficult time for the woman with an eating disorder, even if she has long desired a child. For someone who already struggles with eating and body image, the consumption of additional food and the expectations that she will gain additional weight can result in feelings of fear, anxiety, depression, and guilt. Women with eating disorders also have

Table 18–7   ABNORMALITIES THAT MAY INDICATE AN UNDISCLOSED EATING DISORDER

Somatic

Arrested growth

Marked change or frequent fluctuation in weight

Inability to gain weight

Fatigue

Constipation or diarrhea

Susceptibility to fractures

Delayed menarche

Hypokalemia, hyperphosphatemia, metabolic acidosis or alkalosis, or high serum amylase levels

Behavioral

Change in eating habits

Difficulty eating in social settings

Reluctance to be weighed

Depression

Social withdrawal

Absence from school or work

Deceptive or secretive behavior

Stealing (e.g., to obtain food)

Substance abuse

Excessive exercise

SOURCE: Becker, A. E., Grinspoon, S. K., Klibanski, A., & Herzog, D. B. (1999). Eating disorders. *New England Journal of Medicine, 340,* 1092–1098. Copyright © 1999 Massachusetts Medical Society. All rights reserved.

high rates of depression postpartally (Martos-Ordonez, 2005). When working with a pregnant woman with an eating disorder, education and individualized meal plans can help the woman increase her dietary intake while maintaining a sense of control.

The treatment needs of a woman with an eating disorder can best be met by a team approach that includes medical, nutritional, and psychiatric practitioners who are familiar with eating disorders. The pregnant woman with an eating disorder needs to be closely monitored and supported throughout her pregnancy to help ensure the best possible outcome.

I developed anorexia during my sophomore year in college. My parents were shocked when they saw me at Thanksgiving and, fortunately, they got me some help. For the past several years I have maintained my weight in the low normal range and feel OK about it. Now I am expecting my first child. It is so hard to think of gaining 25 to 30 pounds but I am working very hard to eat properly for my baby. I have reconnected with my therapist so that I can be sure I keep my head on straight about the importance of good nutrition. I don't think people realize how tough eating disorders are to overcome but I will NOT jeopardize my child, I just won't!

Pica

Pica is the persistent craving and eating of substances such as ice, freezer frost, cornstarch, laundry starch, baby powder, clay, dirt, and other nonnutritive substances. Most women who eat such substances do so only during pregnancy. In the United States, pica is more common among economically disadvantaged women, women of African American descent, women who practiced pica before pregnancy, women whose culture encourages pica as important for fertility, and women who have family members who also practice pica (Corbett, Ryan, & Weinrich, 2003).

Iron deficiency anemia is the most common concern with pica. The ingestion of laundry starch or certain types of clay may contribute to iron deficiency by replacing iron-containing foods from the diet or by interfering with iron absorption. Women with pica that involves eating ice or freezer frost often have poor weight gain because of lack of appetite, whereas the ingestion of starch may be associated with excessive weight gain. The ingestion of large quantities of clay could fill the intestine and cause fecal impaction.

Assessment for pica is an important part of a nutritional history. However, women may be embarrassed about their cravings or reluctant to discuss them for fear of criticism. It is helpful if the nurse uses a nonjudgmental approach and explains the possible harmful effects. Some women are able to switch to eating nonfat powdered milk instead of laundry starch and frozen fruit pops instead of ice. Others find that sucking on hard lemon or mint candies helps decrease the craving (Salzberg, 2002).

NUTRITIONAL CARE OF THE PREGNANT ADOLESCENT

Nutritional care of the pregnant adolescent is of particular concern to healthcare professionals. Many adolescents are nutritionally at risk because of a variety of complex and interrelated emotional, social, and economic factors that may adversely affect dietary intake. Nutritional status is an important, modifiable variable in any pregnancy, but especially in adolescent pregnancy because teens are more likely than older women to be underweight at the onset of pregnancy and to gain less weight during pregnancy. For women who are underweight when they become pregnant, the greater the weight gain, the lower the incidence of perinatal mortality. Conversely, more adolescents are overweight or obese today than in the past. Overweight and obese teens are at increased risk for adult obesity and for developing diabetes and risk factors for coronary heart disease (Groth, 2006). Important nutrition-related factors to assess in pregnant adolescents include low prepregnant weight, low weight gain during pregnancy, younger age with regard to menarche, smoking, excessive prepregnant weight, anemia, unhealthy lifestyle (drugs, alcohol use), chronic disease, and history of an eating disorder.

Adolescent women generally are considered physiologically mature about 4 years after menarche because linear growth is usually completed by this time. Their nutritional needs would be similar to those of other "adult" women. Adolescents who become pregnant fewer than 4 years after menarche, however, are at a high biologic risk because of their physiologic and anatomic immaturity. They are most likely to be growing, which can impact the fetus's development. Nutritional needs for these young women will be higher than for those whose growth has been completed.

The nutritional needs of pregnant adolescents are generally estimated by using the DRI for nonpregnant teenagers (ages 11 to 14 or 15 to 18) and adding nutrient amounts recommended for all pregnant women (see Table 18–1). If she is mature (more than 4 years since menarche), the pregnant adolescent has nutritional needs approaching those reported for pregnant adults. However, adolescents who become pregnant less than 4 years after menarche are at risk because of their physiologic and anatomic immaturity. They are more likely than older adolescents to still be growing, which can affect the fetus's development. Thus young adolescents (13 to 15 years) need to gain more weight than older adolescents (16 years or older) to produce babies of equal size. In determining the optimum weight gain for a pregnant adolescent, the nurse needs to add the recommended weight gain for a normal adult pregnancy to the amount of weight gain expected during the postmenarcheal year during which the pregnancy occurs. Young adolescents (2 years after menarche) should strive for a weight gain at the upper end of the range of weight gain for adults (see Table 18–3).

Specific Nutrient Concerns

Caloric needs of pregnant adolescents vary widely. Major factors in determining caloric needs include whether growth has been completed and the physical activity level of the individual. Figures as high as 50 kcal/kg have been suggested for young, growing teens who are very active physically. A satisfactory weight gain will confirm adequacy of caloric intake in most cases.

An inadequate iron intake is a major concern with the adolescent diet. Iron needs are high for the pregnant teen because of

DIETARY SUPPLEMENTS AND PREVENTION OF PREECLAMPSIA

Clinical Question

What dietary restrictions and/or supplements may safely reduce the risk of preeclampsia in pregnancy?

The Evidence

Four systematic reviews were conducted to study the effects of dietary salt restriction and specific supplements on the incidence of preeclampsia of pregnancy. Dietary salt restriction was compared to advice to "continue a normal diet." The supplements reviewed included calcium, magnesium, and three antioxidants (vitamins C and E and beta-carotene) and were compared to placebo. In each case, two reviewers appraised selected studies and extracted data independently. There were two salt restriction studies involving 603 women; both were multicenter trials, and the women were healthy and nulliparous. Eleven studies of calcium were reviewed, with a total sample size of 6634 women. Antioxidants and magnesium were studied via seven trials each, the former involving 6082 women and the latter 2689 women.

What Is Effective?

Dietary supplementation with at least 1 gram of calcium daily was associated with a lower risk of both gestational hypertension and preeclampsia. This effect was greater if the mother was at high risk for hypertension or if the mother had low baseline calcium intake. Any antioxidant supplementation during pregnancy, when compared with a placebo, was associated with a 39% reduction in risk of preeclampsia. No side effects were recorded for either calcium or antioxidant supplementation. Reducing salt intake had no effect on the incidence of preeclampsia. Insufficient evidence was found to conclude that magnesium had any therapeutic effect.

What Is Unclear?

There was little information in these studies about the potential long-term effects of dietary supplements on the infant's health. The reviewers were unanimous, though, in assuming that dietary supplementation was unlikely to have negative effects on the fetus. The

lowest dosage of calcium tested was 1 gram, and it is possible that lower doses might have protective effects. The antioxidant vitamin C is water soluble, and so an excess is excreted. Vitamin E and beta-carotene are not, though, and may accumulate in the body. The exact effective dosage of these antioxidants is not clear, and there is a potential for harm with high doses. None of the studies determined if purely dietary increases in foods rich in these substances would have the same effect as dietary supplements.

Best Practice

Pregnant women should be advised that salt intake during pregnancy is a matter of personal preference and will have no effect on subsequent hypertension or preeclampsia. Supplementation of the daily diet with 1 gram of calcium appears to reduce the risk of gestational hypertension and preeclampsia. This is particularly true if the mother is at high risk or begins her pregnancy with low calcium intake. The protection is modest, though, if the mother is low risk, and so a recommendation may be dependent upon the mother's risk level. A variety of antioxidant supplements also appear to reduce the risk of preeclampsia. Vitamin C is the preferred antioxidant because any excess intake is excreted. Mothers can be reassured that there is no evidence that these dietary supplements will have a negative effect on the fetus.

Critical Thinking

What risk factors will help the nurse determine if dietary supplements should be recommended for a pregnant woman? What foods can be recommended to the mother who does not want to take supplements but wants to increase the consumption of these protective substances?

REFERENCES: Duley, L., Henderson-Smart, D., & Meher. S. (2005). Altered dietary salt for preventing pre-eclampsia and its complications. *The Cochrane Database of Systematic Reviews* (4) (Article No.: CD005548).

Hofmeyr, G., Atallah, A., & Duley, L. (2004). Calcium supplementation during pregnancy for preventing hypertensive disorders and related problems. *The Cochrane Database of Systematic Reviews* (1) (Article No.: CD001059).

Makrides, M., & Crowther, C. (2003). Magnesium supplementation in pregnancy. *The Cochrane Database of Systematic Reviews* (4) (Article No.: CD000937).

Rumbold, A., Duley, L., Crowther, C., & Haslam, R. (2005). Antioxidants for preventing pre-eclampsia. *The Cochrane Database of Systematic Reviews* (4) (Article No.: CD004227).

the requirement for iron by the enlarging maternal muscle mass and blood volume. Iron supplements—providing 30 to 60 mg of elemental iron—are indicated.

Calcium is another nutrient that demands special attention from pregnant adolescents. Inadequate intake of calcium is frequently a problem in this age group. Adequate calcium intake is needed to support normal growth and development of the fetus as well as growth and maintenance of calcium stores in the adolescent. Inadequate calcium has been associated with maternal hypertension and preeclampsia. Pregnant adolescents who consume adequate calcium have a lower incidence of hypertension, preterm, birth, and low-birth-weight infants (Stang, Story, & Feldman, 2005). An extra serving of dairy products is usually

recommended for teenagers. Calcium supplementation is indicated for teens with an aversion to or intolerance of milk unless other dairy products or significant calcium sources are consumed in sufficient amounts.

Because folic acid plays a role in cell reproduction, it is also an important nutrient for pregnant teens. As previously indicated, a supplement is often suggested for pregnant females, whether adult or adolescent.

Other nutrients and vitamins must be considered when evaluating the overall nutritional quality of the teenager's diet. Nutrients that have frequently been found to be deficient in this age group include zinc and vitamins A, D, E, and B_6. Eating a wide variety of foods—especially fresh and lightly processed foods—is helpful in obtaining adequate amounts of trace minerals, fiber, and other vitamins.

Dietary Patterns

Healthy adolescents often have irregular eating patterns. Many skip breakfast, and most tend to be frequent snackers. Teens rarely follow the traditional three-meals-a-day pattern; their day-to-day intake often varies drastically; and they eat food combinations that may seem bizarre to adults. Despite this, adolescents usually achieve a better nutritional balance than most adults would expect.

My mom is so cool. She has hung in with me throughout this pregnancy even though I know she feels bad about it—she thinks my life will be harder and I guess she is right. She is really working to make sure that I eat right so that I have a healthy baby but instead of nagging, she has turned this into something we are doing together. We have taken a couple of cooking classes and experimented with different recipes. Last week we made some great but healthy snacks and I brought them to my friend Cary's birthday party. Those snacks just disappeared!

In assessing the diet of the pregnant adolescent, the nurse should consider the eating pattern over time, not simply a single day's intake. This pattern is critical because of the irregularity of most adolescent eating patterns. Once the pattern is identified, counseling can be directed toward correcting deficiencies.

Counseling Issues

A positive approach to nutritional counseling for the pregnant adolescent is more effective than a negative one. The nurse must be ready to suggest nutrient-dense foods that pregnant teens can choose in many places and at any time. If an adolescent's family member does most of the meal preparation, it may be useful to include that person in the discussion if the adolescent agrees. Involving the expectant father in counseling may be beneficial. The pregnant teenager will soon become a parent, and her understanding of nutrition will influence not only her well-being but also that of her child. However, teens tend to live in the present, and counseling that stresses long-term changes may be less effective than more concrete approaches. Messages should emphasize that the pregnant teen is eating for her own health and that of the baby and should focus on foods themselves rather than on nutrients. In many cases, classes with other teens are effective. In a group atmosphere, adolescents often work together to plan adequate meals including foods that are their special favorites.

POSTPARTUM NUTRITION

Nutritional needs will change following the birth. Nutrient requirements will vary depending on whether the mother decides to breastfeed. An assessment of postpartal nutritional status is necessary before the nurse provides nutritional guidance.

Postpartal Nutritional Status

Postpartal nutritional status is determined primarily by assessing the new mother's weight, hemoglobin and hematocrit levels, clinical signs, and dietary history.

As previously discussed, an ideal weight gain for the normal-weight woman during pregnancy is between 11.5 and 16 kg (25 and 35 lb). After birth, there is a weight loss of approximately 10 to 12 lb. Additional weight loss will be most rapid during the first few weeks after birth as the uterus returns to normal size, tissue fluids are released, and maternal blood volume returns to normal. The mother's weight will then begin to stabilize. Weight loss may also be affected by lactation. Individual weight loss of women who breastfeed will vary but tends to be greater than that of women who do not if breastfeeding continues for at least 6 months.

The rate of postpartum weight loss is influenced by many factors. Some women approach their prepregnancy weight several weeks after birth; most approach this weight about 6 months later. The amount of weight gained during pregnancy is a major determinant of weight loss after childbirth. Generally, women who gain excessive weight during pregnancy are more likely to sustain a weight gain 1 year following childbirth, putting them at increased risk of long-term overweight or obesity (Johnson, Gerstein, Evans et al., 2006).

It is important to evaluate the mother's current weight, ideal weight for her height, weight before pregnancy, and weight before the birth. Women who are interested in weight reduction should be referred to a dietitian. Hemoglobin and erythrocyte values vary after birth, but they should return to normal levels within 2 to 6 weeks. Hematocrit levels should rise gradually because of hemoconcentration as extracellular fluid is excreted. The hematocrit is usually checked at the postpartum visit to detect any anemia. Mothers can be encouraged to eat a diet high in iron. Iron supplements are generally prescribed for 2 to 3 months following birth to replenish supplies depleted by pregnancy.

The nurse assesses any clinical symptoms the new mother may be experiencing. Food cravings and aversions typically drop significantly during the postpartal period and do not usually pose a problem. However, constipation is a common problem following birth. The nurse can encourage the woman to maintain a high fluid intake to keep the stool soft. Dietary sources of fiber and physical exercise are also helpful in preventing constipation.

The nurse obtains specific information on diet and eating habits directly from the woman. Visiting the mother during mealtimes provides an opportunity for unobtrusive nutritional assessment. Which foods has a woman selected? Has she avoided fruits and vegetables? Is her diet nutritionally sound? A comment focusing on a positive aspect of her meal selection may initiate a discussion of nutrition.

The dietitian should be informed about any woman whose cultural or religious beliefs require specific foods. Appropriate meals can then be prepared for her. The nurse may also refer women with unusual eating habits or numerous questions about food or nutrition to a dietitian. In all cases, the nurse should provide literature on nutrition so that the woman will have a source of appropriate information at home.

Nutritional Care of Formula-Feeding Mothers

After birth, the formula-feeding mother's dietary requirements return to prepregnancy levels (see Table 18–1). If the mother has a good understanding of nutritional principles, it is sufficient to advise her to reduce her daily caloric intake by about 300 kcal and to return to prepregnancy levels for other nutrients.

If the mother has a poor understanding of nutrition, this is an opportunity to teach her the basic principles and the importance of a well-balanced diet. Her eating habits and dietary practices will eventually be reflected in the diet of her child.

If the mother has gained excessive weight during pregnancy (or perhaps was overweight before pregnancy), referral to a dietitian is appropriate. The dietitian can design weight reduction diets to meet nutritional needs and food preferences. Weight loss goals of 1 to 2 lb per week are usually suggested.

In addition to learning how to meet her own nutritional needs, the new mother will usually be interested in learning how to provide for her infant's nutritional needs. A discussion of infant feeding, which includes topics such as selecting infant formulas, formula preparation, and vitamin and mineral supplementation, is appropriate and generally well received.

Nutritional Care of Breastfeeding Mothers

Nutrient needs increase during breastfeeding. Table 18–1 lists the DRIs during breastfeeding for specific nutrients. Table 18–2 includes a sample daily food guide for lactating women. A few key nutrients need further discussion.

CALORIES

One of the most important factors in the breastfeeding woman's diet is calories. An inadequate caloric intake can reduce milk volume. However, milk quality generally remains unaffected. The breastfeeding mother should increase her caloric intake by 200 kcal over the pregnancy requirements (that is, a 500-kcal increase from her prepregnancy requirement). This results in a total of about 2500 to 2700 kcal per day for most women.

Depending on her own dietary preferences, the breastfeeding mother can use the MyPyramid food guide or the vegetarian food pyramid to assess her dietary intake. She should strive to include a variety of foods from each food group. Her caloric intake needs to provide enough energy to sustain lactation. After her weight stabilizes several weeks following childbirth, weight loss should not exceed more than 1 lb per week.

PROTEIN

An adequate protein intake is essential while breastfeeding because protein is an important component of breast milk. An intake of 65 g per day during the first 6 months of breastfeeding and 62 g per day thereafter is recommended. As in pregnancy, it is important that the woman consume adequate nonprotein calories to prevent the use of protein as an energy source.

CALCIUM

Calcium is also an important nutrient in milk production, and increases over nonpregnancy needs are expected. Requirements during breastfeeding remain the same as requirements during pregnancy: 1000 mg per day. An inadequate intake of calcium from food sources necessitates the use of calcium supplements.

IRON

Iron needs during lactation are not substantially different from those of nonpregnant women because iron is not a principal component of breast milk. However, as previously mentioned, continued supplementation of the mother for 2 to 3 months after parturition is advisable to replenish maternal stores depleted by pregnancy.

FLUIDS

Liquids are especially important during lactation because inadequate fluid intake may decrease milk volume. The recommended fluid intake of 8 to 10 (8 oz) glasses daily can be met by the consumption of water, juices, milk, and soups.

For me, the hardest part of breastfeeding was drinking enough fluid. I am not a big water person and they told me to go easy on caffeine beverages. Once I started adding a slice of lemon to my water, I found it a lot easier. My baby is 13 months old now and I have stopped breastfeeding, but I still drink the water with lemon. I think I have developed a good new habit!

Counseling Issues

In addition to counseling mothers on how to meet their increased nutrient needs during breastfeeding, nurses should discuss a few issues related to infant feeding. For example, many mothers are concerned about how specific foods they eat will affect their babies during breastfeeding. Generally, there are no foods the nursing mother must avoid except those to which she might be allergic. Occasionally, however, some breastfeeding mothers find that their babies are affected by certain foods. Onions, turnips, cabbage, chocolate, spices, and seasonings are commonly listed as offenders. The best advice to give the breastfeeding mother is to avoid those foods she suspects cause distress in her infant. For the most part, however, she should be able to eat any nourishing food she wants without fear that her baby will be affected. For further discussion of successful infant feeding, see Chapter 31. ∞

NURSING CARE MANAGEMENT
Nursing Assessment and Diagnosis

The nurse needs to assess nutritional status in order to plan an optimal diet with each woman. The nurse may gather data by consulting the woman's chart and by interviewing her. Information is obtained about the following:

- The woman's height and weight and her weight gain during pregnancy
- Pertinent laboratory values, especially hemoglobin and hematocrit
- Clinical signs that have possible nutritional implications, such as constipation, anorexia, or heartburn
- Diet history to determine the woman's views on nutrition as well as her specific nutrient intake

The nurse can obtain a diet history by asking the woman to complete a 24-hour diet recall, in which she lists everything consumed in the previous 24 hours, including foods, fluids, and any supplements. At least 3 days of diet recalls should be done to compensate for daily variations. Diet may also be evaluated using a food frequency questionnaire. The questionnaire lists common categories of foods and asks the woman how frequently in a day (or week) she consumes foods from the list. Common categories include vegetables, fruits, milk or cheese, meat or poultry, fish, desserts or sweets, coffee or tea, and alcoholic beverages. This method may be less reliable because it requires the individual to be accurate about her intake.

CLINICAL TIP

When completing a diet history it is as important to identify the foods a woman avoids as it is to determine which foods she eats.

During the data-gathering process, the nurse has an opportunity to discuss important aspects of nutrition in the context of the family's needs and lifestyle. The nurse also seeks information about psychologic, cultural, and socioeconomic factors that may influence food intake.

The nurse can use a nutritional questionnaire to gather and record important facts. This information provides a database the nurse can use to develop an intervention plan to fit the woman's individual needs. The sample questionnaire shown in Figure 18–5 ◆ has been filled in to demonstrate this process.

Once the data are obtained, the nurse begins to analyze the information, formulate appropriate nursing diagnoses, and develop client goals. For a woman during the first trimester, for example, the diagnosis may be *Imbalanced Nutrition: Less than Body Requirements* related to nausea and vomiting. In many cases the diagnosis may be related to excessive weight gain. In such cases the diagnosis might be *Imbalanced Nutrition: More than Body Requirements* related to excessive calorie intake. Although these diagnoses are broad, the nurse must be specific in addressing issues such as inadequate intake of nutrients such as iron, calcium, or folic acid; problems with nutrition because of a limited food budget; problems related to physiologic alterations, such as anorexia, heartburn, or nausea; and behavioral problems related to excessive dieting, anorexia nervosa, or bulimia. In some instances, the diagnosis *Health-Seeking Behavior* may seem most appropriate, especially if the woman asks for information about nutrition.

Nursing Plan and Implementation

After the nursing diagnosis is made, the nurse can plan an approach to correct any nutritional deficiencies or improve the overall quality of the diet.

TEACHING FOR SELF-CARE

In counseling the pregnant woman, the nurse needs to avoid "talking down" to her or "preaching" to her. The nurse should present information in a clear, logical way, using appropriate language but avoiding jargon. Examples are often helpful in clarifying material. The nurse should also answer all questions appropriately and clearly.

When a person requires nutritional counseling, a dietary change usually is necessary. Change is often difficult, however. Counseling will be more effective if the nurse understands the client's values and explains the needed change in a way that is meaningful to the client. Because the pregnant woman must follow the plan, it should be developed in cooperation with her, be suitable for her financial level and background, and be based on reasonable, achievable goals.

The following example demonstrates one way a nurse can implement a plan with a client based on the nursing diagnosis.

Diagnosis: *Imbalanced Nutrition: Less than Body Requirements* related to low intake of calcium

Client goal: The woman will increase her intake of calcium to the DRI level.

Implementation:
1. Plan with the woman additional milk or dairy products that she can reasonably add to the diet (specify amounts).
2. Encourage the use of other calcium sources, such as leafy green vegetables and legumes.
3. Plan for the addition of powdered milk in cooking and baking.
4. If none of the above are realistic or acceptable, consider the use of calcium supplements.

Most families can benefit from guidance about food purchasing and preparation. The nurse should advise women to plan food purchases thoughtfully by preparing menus and a grocery list before shopping. It is also helpful to advise clients to monitor sales, compare brands, and be selective when purchasing "convenience" foods, which tend to be expensive. Other techniques for keeping food costs down without jeopardizing quality include buying food in season, using bulk foods when appropriate, using whole grain or enriched products, buying lower grade eggs (grading has no relation to the egg's nutritional value but indicates color of the shell and delicacy of flavor), and avoiding fancy grades of food and foods in elaborate packaging.

COMMUNITY-BASED NURSING CARE

Food is a significant portion of a family's budget, and meeting nutritional needs may be a challenge for families on limited incomes. Community-based services offered through clinics, local agencies, schools, and volunteer organizations are effective in addressing these needs. Increasingly, nurses play an important role in managing such community-based services, especially those services focusing on client education. In addition, most communities offer special assistance to qualifying families to meet their nutritional needs. The Food Stamp Program provides stamps or coupons for participating households whose net monthly income is below a specified level. These stamps can be used to purchase food for the household each month.

The Special Supplemental Nutrition Program for Women, Infants, and Children (WIC) is designed to assist low-income pregnant, postpartum, or breastfeeding women and their children under 5 years of age. To be eligible, applicants must meet income guidelines (income at or below 185% of the US poverty

NUTRITIONAL QUESTIONNAIRE

Name __Susan Longmont__   Date __8-15-08__

Age __20__

Ethnic group __Caucasian__

Religion __Protestant__

Gravida __1__   Para __0__   EDB __3-21-09__

Age of youngest child? __NA__

Birth weights of previous children? __NA__

Usual nonpregnant weight __115__   Present weight __125__

Weight gain during last pregnancy? __NA__

Vitamin supplements? __none__

Current medications? __aspirin for headache__

Do you smoke? __yes__   How much per day? __1-1½ packs__

Eating patterns:

1. How many meals per day? __2__   when __12:30 pm 6:30 pm__

2. How many snacks per day? __3__   when __10:30 am 4:00 pm 10:00 pm__

3. What other foods are important to your usual diet? __chocolate and candy bars__

4. Amount per day __4 bars/week__

5. Do you have any different food preferences now? __no__

6. Do you eat nonfoods such as:

		Amount
laundry starch	no	NA
ice	yes	10 cubes/day
other (name)	no	NA

7. What foods do you dislike or do not eat? __spinach and dried beans__

8. For added information complete a typical daily intake (24-hour recall is suggested).

Do you have special problems in food preparation such as:

1. Physical disability   yes ____   no ✓ ____   Explain ____

2. Cooking appliances   yes ____   no ✓ ____   Explain ____

3. Refrigeration of food   yes ____   no ✓ ____   Explain ____

Who does the meal planning? __I do.__   shopping? __We both do.__

cooking? __I do most of the time but my husband likes to help.__

Are there transportation problems? __We have only one car but we go in the evening.__

Financial situation: __My husband is working and going to school.__
__I am not working.__   Food stamps __yes__   WIC __no__

Do you have any previous nutritional problems? __No. I have never paid much attention__
__to food before, but now I have lots of questions.__

Are there any problems with this pregnancy? Nausea __Yes, in the morning.__

Constipation __No__   Other __NA__

Assessment by the nurse following the completion of the questionnaire.

Basic estimated nutrient and caloric value of typical daily intake.

Please circle one of the following:

Protein intake was	low	adequate (circled)	high
Caloric intake was	low	adequate	high (circled)
Calcium intake was	low (circled)	adequate	high
Iron intake was	low (circled)	adequate	high
Vitamin C intake was	low	adequate (circled)	high

Figure 18–5 ◆ Sample nutritional questionnaire used in nursing management of a pregnant woman.

level, which currently is $35,798 for a family of four), state residency requirements, and be individually determined to be nutritionally at risk by a healthcare professional (Food and Nutrition Service, 2006). The program provides food assistance, nutrition education, and referrals to healthcare providers. The food distributed, including dried beans and peas, peanut butter, eggs, cheese, milk, fortified adult and infant cereals, juice, and iron-fortified infant formula, is designed to provide good sources of iron, protein, and certain vitamins for individuals with an inadequate diet. Participation in the WIC program during pregnancy and infancy is associated with a reduced risk of infant death. In addition, the WIC program is credited with helping reduce the incidence of low birth weight in infants and in decreasing the incidence of anemia in the infants and young children of low-income families.

Evaluation

Once a plan has been developed and implemented, the nurse and client may wish to identify ways of evaluating its effectiveness. Evaluation may involve keeping a food journal, writing out weekly menus, returning weekly for weighing, and the like. If anemia is a special problem, periodic hematocrit assessments are also indicated.

Women with serious nutritional deficiencies are referred to a dietitian. The nurse can then work closely with the dietitian and the client to improve the pregnant woman's health by modifying her diet.

CHAPTER REVIEW

FOCUS YOUR STUDY

- Maternal weight gains averaging 11.5 to 16 kg (25 to 35 lb) for a normal-weight woman are associated with the best reproductive outcomes.

- If the diet is adequate, folic acid and iron are the only supplements generally recommended during pregnancy.

- Women should not restrict caloric intake to reduce weight during pregnancy.

- Pregnant women should be encouraged to eat regularly and to eat a wide variety of foods, especially fresh and lightly processed foods.

- Taking megadoses of vitamins during pregnancy is unnecessary and potentially dangerous.

- Pregnant women who eat vegetarian diets should place special emphasis on obtaining ample complete proteins, calories, calcium, iron, vitamin D, vitamin B_{12}, and zinc through food sources or supplementation if necessary.

- Pregnant women should avoid eating fish such as swordfish, shark, tilefish, or king mackerel, which contain high levels of mercury, and should limit their intake of fish that are lower in mercury.

- Food safety and sanitation should be a priority when preparing and storing food; foods that are known to cause foodborne illness should be avoided during pregnancy.

- Evaluation of physical, psychosocial, and cultural factors that affect food intake is essential before the nurse can determine nutritional status and plan nutritional counseling.

- Adolescents who become pregnant less than 4 years after menarche have higher nutritional needs and are considered to be at high biologic risk.

- Weight gains during adolescent pregnancy must accommodate recommended gains for a normal pregnancy plus necessary gains due to growth.

- After childbirth, the formula-feeding mother's dietary requirements return to prepregnancy levels.

- Breastfeeding mothers require an additional 200 calories above pregnancy intake and increased fluid intake to maintain ample milk volume.

EXPLORE MediaLink

http://www.prenhall.com/davidson

NCLEX review questions, case studies, and other interactive resources for this chapter can be found on the Web Site at http://www.prenhall.com/davidson. Click on "Chapter 18" to select the activities for this chapter.

For tutorials including animations and videos, more NCLEX review questions, and an audio glossary, access the accompanying Prentice Hall Nursing MediaLink DVD-ROM in this book.

 PRENTICE HALL NURSING MEDIALINK DVD-ROM

Audio Glossary

NCLEX Review

Video: *Through the Eyes of a Nurse—The First Trimester*

 COMPANION WEBSITE

Additional NCLEX Review

Case Study: *Maternal Weight Gain*

Care Plan Activity: *Maternal Nutritional Requirements*

Applications: *Nutritional Needs During Pregnancy; Pica*

Critical Thinking

CRITICAL THINKING IN ACTION

NUTRITIONAL NEEDS OF MOTHER AND FETUS DURING PREGNANCY

View the Critical Thinking in Action video in Chapter 18 of the DVD-ROM. Then answer the questions that follow.

Sandra Hill is a 17-year-old at 19 weeks' gestation with her first pregnancy. She presents to you accompanied by her mother. Her mother tells you that Sandra is an active teenager who plays sports and has been taking dance lessons for 5 years. She maintains a B average in school. Sandra voices concern about potential weight gain during pregnancy. She tells you that this was not a planned pregnancy, and she has ambivalent feelings about it. You become concerned as she tells you that she has reduced her caloric intake over the last few months to try to keep her weight down and camouflage her pregnancy. You do a nutritional assessment and find that she is deficient in calcium, iron, and protein. Sandra seems to have irregular eating patterns and she admits to often skipping breakfast. She asks why she has to gain so much weight when you explain the nutritional needs of her baby during the pregnancy.

1. Discuss weight distribution in pregnancy.

2. Discuss foods that will increase calcium, protein, and iron in her diet.

3. Explain why folate supplementation is important.

4. What criteria will measure adequate caloric intake during pregnancy?

REFERENCES

Agostoni, C., & Verduci, E. (2003). DHA in pregnancy benefits child development. *Pediatric Research, 54*(3), 292–293.

American College of Obstetricians and Gynecologists (ACOG). (2005). Obesity in pregnancy (Committee Opinion No. 315). Washington, DC: Author.

American Dietetic Association (ADA). (2002). Position of ADA: Nutrition and lifestyle for a healthy pregnancy outcome. *Journal of the American Dietetic Association, 102,* 1479–1490.

American Dietetic Association (ADA). (2003). Position of ADA and Dietitians of Canada: Vegetarian diets. *Journal of the American Dietetic Association, 103,* 748–765.

Centers for Disease Control and Prevention and the Pan American Health Organization. (2003). *The prevention of neural tube defects with folic acid.* Retrieved April 26, 2004, from http://www.cdc.gov/Images_-_Video_and_Audio/Images/Birth_Defects/Folic_Acid/ntd_dave.pdf

Corbett, R. W., Ryan, C., & Weinrich, S. P. (2003). Pica in pregnancy. *American Journal of Maternal-Child Nursing, 28*(3), 183–189.

Cunningham, F. G., Leveno, K. J., Bloom, S. L., Hauth, J. C., Gilstrap III, L. C., & Wenstrom, K. D. (2005). *Williams Obstetrics*, ed. 22. New York: McGraw-Hill.

Food and Drug Administration (FDA). (2005). *Food safety for mothers-to-be: Educator's resources guide*. College Park, MD: Center for Food Safety and Applied Nutrition.

Food and Nutrition Service. (2006). *WIC: The special supplemental nutrition program for women, infants, and children*. Retrieved March 31, 2006, from http://www.fns.usda.gov.wic/

Groth, S. (2006). Adolescent gestational weight gain: Does it contribute to obesity? *American Journal of Maternal-Child Nursing, 31*(2), 101–105.

Huffling, K. (2006). The effects of environmental contaminants in food on women's health. *Journal of Midwifery & Women's Health, 51*(1), 19–25.

Institute of Medicine (IOM), Subcommittee for a Clinical Application Guide. (1992). *Nutrition during pregnancy and lactation: An implementation guide*. Washington, DC: National Academy Press.

Institute of Medicine (IOM), Subcommittee on Dietary Intake and Nutrient Supplements During Pregnancy, Committee on Nutrition Status During Pregnancy and Lactation, Food and Nutrition Board. (1990). *Nutrition during pregnancy: Weight gain and nutrient supplements*. Washington, DC: National Academy Press.

Johnson, D. B., Gerstein, D. E., Evans, A. E., & Woodward-Lopez, G. (2006). Preventing obesity: A life cycle perspective. *Journal of the American Dietetic Association, 106*(1), 97–102.

March of Dimes. (2002). *Nutrition today matters tomorrow: A report from the March of Dimes task force on nutrition and optimal human development*. Washington, DC: Author.

Martos-Ordonez, C. (2005). Pregnancy in women with eating disorders: A review. *British Journal of Midwifery, 13*(7), 446–448.

Messina, V., Mangels, R., & Messina, M. J. (2004). *The dietitian's guide to vegetarian diets: Issues and applications* (2nd ed.). Sudbury, MA: Jones and Bartlett.

National Center on Birth Defects and Developmental Disabilities. (2004). *Birth defects*. Retrieved April 26, 2004, from http://www.cdc.gov/ncbddd/bd/mp.htm.

National Digestive Diseases Information Clearinghouse. (2006). *Lactose intolerance*. Retrieved May 1, 2006, from http://www.niddk.nih.gov

National Institutes of Health. (2002). *Facts about dietary supplements: Vitamin D*. Retrieved April 24, 2004, from http://www.cc.nih.gov.

Salzberg, H. S. (2002). Nutrition in pregnancy. In J. J. Sciarra (Ed.), *Gynecology and obstetrics* (Vol. 2, chap. 7). Philadelphia: Lippincott Williams & Wilkins.

Skidmore-Roth, L. (2004). *Mosby's handbook of herbs & natural supplements* (2nd ed.). St. Louis, MO: Mosby.

Smuts, C. M., Borod, E., Peeples, J. M., & Carlson, S. E. (2003). High-DHA eggs: Feasibility as a means to enhance circulating DHA in mother and infant. *Lipids, 38*(4), 407–414.

Stang, J., Story, M., & Feldman, S. (2005). Nutrition in adolescent pregnancy. *International Journal of Childbirth Education, 20*(2), 4–11.

US Department of Health and Human Services and US Department of Agriculture. (2005). *Dietary guidelines for Americans 2005*. Retrieved January 1, 2007, from http://www.healthierus.gov/dietaryguidelines.

US Department of Health and Human Services & US Environmental Protection Agency. (2004). *What you need to know about mercury in fish and shellfish*. Retrieved April 24, 2004, from http://www.cfsan.fda.gov/-dms/admchg3.html.

Villar, J., Merialdi, M., Gulmezoglu, A. M., Abalos, E., Carroli, G., Kulier, R., et al. (2003). Nutritional interventions during pregnancy for the prevention or treatment of maternal morbidity and preterm delivery: An overview of randomized, controlled trials. *Journal of Nutrition, 133*(5, Suppl. 2), 1606S–1625S.

CHAPTER 19

Pregnancy at Risk: Pregestational Problems

Today is the anniversary of my Julie's death. She died of a heroin overdose. During the years before her death, we tried everything to help her, but nothing worked. She would disappear, sometimes for weeks, and then reappear filled with good intentions to kick her habit—but she never could. She was 29 when I lost her, and 3 months pregnant with our grandchild. I miss her so. I don't know if my heart will ever mend.

OBJECTIVES

1. Summarize the effects of alcohol and illicit drugs on the childbearing woman and her fetus/newborn.

2. Discuss the pathology, treatment, and nursing care of pregnant women with diabetes.

3. Discriminate among the four major types of anemia associated with pregnancy with regard to signs, treatment, and implications for pregnancy.

4. Discuss acquired immunodeficiency syndrome (AIDS), including care of the pregnant woman with HIV/AIDS, neonatal implications, and ramifications for the childbearing family.

5. Describe the effects of various heart disorders on pregnancy, including their implications for nursing care.

6. Compare the effects of selected gestational medical conditions on pregnancy.

KEY TERMS

Acquired immunodeficiency syndrome (AIDS)   465

Crack   447

Gestational diabetes mellitus (GDM)   451

Human immunodeficiency virus (HIV)   465

Macrosomia   450

MEDIALINK

Additional resources for this content can be found on the Prentice Hall Nursing MediaLink DVD-ROM and on the Companion Website at http://www.prenhall.com/davidson. Click on "Chapter 19" to select the activities for this chapter.

Pregnancy is biologically, physiologically, and psychologically stressful, even for healthy women. For women with preexisting (pregestational) conditions such as substance abuse, diabetes, human immunodeficiency virus (HIV) infection, and cardiac disease it may be life threatening. For these women, pregestational counseling is especially important to identify early interventions designed to diminish the adverse effects of pregnancy on both the mother and fetus. In some cases, interventions before conception may be critical.

Prenatal care is aimed toward identification, assessment, and care management of women whose pregnancies are at risk because of potential or existing complications. This chapter focuses on women with pregestational medical disorders and their possible effects on the outcome of pregnancy. Chapter 20 ∞, in turn, focuses on medical disorders that develop during pregnancy.

CARE OF THE WOMAN PRACTICING SUBSTANCE ABUSE

Substance abuse occurs when an individual experiences difficulties with work, family, social relations, and/or health as a result of alcohol or drug use. National survey data indicate that approximately 7.9% of people in the United States used illicit drugs in the month before the survey (Substance Abuse and Mental Health Services Administration [SAMHSA], 2005). In general, the rate of illicit drug use among pregnant women is less than half the rate as among nonpregnant women (10.2%). Specifically, 4.6% of pregnant women reported using an illicit drug during pregnancy. However, illicit drug usage varies greatly by age, peaking at 21.7% of users in the 18- to 20-year-old age group for both males and females (SAMHSA, 2005). See Figure 19–1 ◆.

Because women of childbearing age (15 to 44 years) make up a substantial proportion of the drug-using population, the problem has major significance for women and children. In testimony to these statistics is the increasing number of drug-exposed infants being born throughout the United States. Indiscriminate use of drugs during pregnancy, particularly in the first trimester, may adversely affect the health of the woman and the growth and development of her fetus. Drugs that are commonly misused include tobacco, alcohol, cocaine, marijuana, amphetamines, barbiturates, hallucinogens, club drugs, heroin, and other narcotics. Tobacco is discussed in Chapter 16 ∞ as a teratogenic substance. Table 19–1 identifies common addictive drugs and their effects on the fetus and newborn.

Drug use during pregnancy may be the most frequently missed diagnosis in all of maternity care. Substance-abusing women typically do not seek prenatal care until late in their pregnancy. They may be noncompliant or they may present in labor with no history of prenatal care. Even when they do seek care early, physicians and nurses may fail to ask the woman about drug and alcohol use because of their own lack of knowl-

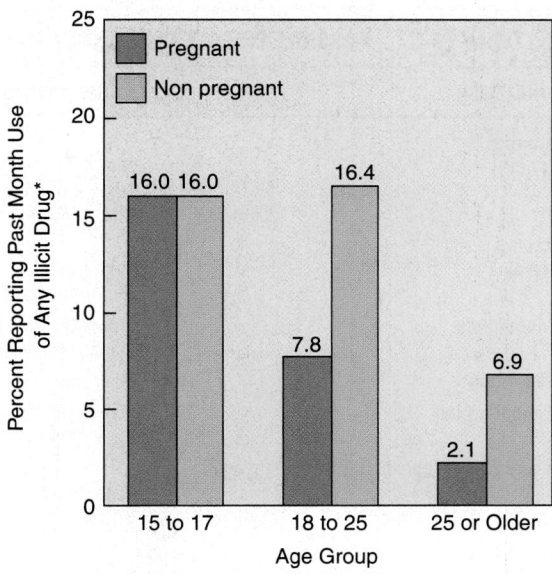

*Refers to marijuana/hashish, cocaine (including crack), inhalants, hallucinogens, heroin, or perscription-type drugs used nonmedically.

Figure 19–1 ◆ Percentages of females ages 15 to 44 reporting past month use of any illicit drugs, by pregnancy status and age, 2003–2004.
SOURCE: Substance Abuse and Mental Health Services Administration (SAMHSA). (2005). *Results from the 2004 National Survey on Drug Use and Health: National Findings.* Office of Applied Science Studies, NSDUH Series H-28 DHHS Publication No. SMA 05-4062. Rockville, MD.

edge, discomfort, or biases. When asked, women may deny use of illegal substances out of fear or shame. Although some clinics perform routine or random drug screens, consent from the client is required.

> **CLINICAL TIP**
>
> Keep in mind that approximately 1 of 10 women in the United States, regardless of socioeconomic status or ethnic background, is currently abusing a substance. If you consider that possibility with every woman, you will ask the important questions about drug use and be alert for signs of substance abuse.

Providing prenatal care to chemically dependent women presents multiple dilemmas and challenges to clinicians. However, pregnancy represents a period in most women's lives when they recognize the need for and are receptive to caring and responsive interventions. By optimizing the prenatal experience of chemically dependent women, maternal-fetal outcomes can be improved and the groundwork laid for the ongoing therapeutic services that are needed to maintain the health and well-being of the mother and child (Chasnoff, McGourty, Bailey et al., 2005).

The substance-abusing woman who seeks prenatal care may not voluntarily reveal her addiction, so caregivers should be alert for a history or physical signs that suggest substance abuse (Table 19–2). Because substance abuse has increased rapidly in the past decade, it is helpful to discuss the specific substances that are abused to increase understanding of this serious problem.

Table 19–1	POSSIBLE EFFECTS OF SELECTED DRUGS OF ABUSE/ADDICTION ON FETUS AND NEWBORN
Maternal Drug	**Effect on Fetus/Newborn**
Depressants	
Alcohol	Mental retardation, microcephaly, midfacial hypoplasia, cardiac anomalies, intrauterine growth restriction (IUGR), potential teratogenic effects, fetal alcohol syndrome (FAS), fetal alcohol effects (FAE)
Narcotics	
Heroin	Withdrawal symptoms, convulsions, IUGR, tremors, irritability, sneezing, vomiting, fever, diarrhea, and abnormal respiratory function
Methadone	Nonreassuring fetal status, meconium aspiration; with abrupt termination of the drug, severe withdrawal symptoms, preterm labor, rapid labor, abruption
Barbiturates	Withdrawal symptoms
Phenobarbital	Withdrawal symptoms Fetal growth restriction
"T's and Blues" (combination of the following)	
Talwin (narcotic)	Safe for use in pregnancy; depresses respiration if taken close to time of birth
Amytal (barbiturate)	See barbiturates
Tranquilizers	
Phenothiazine derivatives	Withdrawal, extrapyramidal dysfunction, delayed respiratory onset, hyperbilirubinemia, hypotonia or hyperactivity, decreased platelet count
Diazepam (Valium)	Hypotonia, hypothermia, low Apgar score, respiratory depression, poor sucking reflex, possible cleft lip
Antianxiety drugs	
Lithium	Congenital anomalies
Stimulants	
Amphetamines	
Amphetamines sulfate (Benzedrine)	Generalized arthritis, learning disabilities, poor motor coordination, transposition of the great vessels, cleft palate
Dextroamphetamine sulfate (Dexedrine)	Congenital heart defects, biliary atresia, limb reduction defects
Cocaine	Cerebral infarctions, microcephaly, learning disabilities, poor state organization, decreased interactive behavior, central nervous system (CNS) anomalies, cardiac anomalies, genitourinary anomalies, sudden infant death syndrome (SIDS)
Nicotine (half to one pack cigarettes/day)	Increased rate of spontaneous abortion, increased incidence of placental abruption, small for gestational age (SGA), small head circumference, decreased length, SIDS, attention deficit hyperactivity disorder (ADHD) in school-age children
Psychotropics	
PCP ("angel dust")	Withdrawal symptoms Newborn behavioral and developmental abnormalities
LSD	Chromosomal breakage?
Marijuana	IUGR?

Substances Commonly Abused During Pregnancy

The substances most commonly abused during pregnancy are alcohol, cocaine/crack, marijuana, phencyclidine, MDMA (Ecstasy), and heroin. In this section, we also discuss the prescription drug methadone, which can have negative effects on pregnancy outcome.

ALCOHOL

Alcohol abuse has increased dramatically among women in the United States. The incidence is highest among women 20 to 40 years old; alcoholism is also seen in teenagers. An estimated 11% of pregnant women use alcohol in a given month (SAMHSA, 2005). This figure is of concern because birth defects that are related to prenatal fetal exposure to alcohol can occur in the first 3 to 8 weeks' gestation, often before the woman even knows that she is pregnant. Figure 19–2 ◆ identifies alcohol use by trimester.

Chronic abuse of alcohol can undermine maternal health by causing malnutrition (especially folic acid and thiamine deficiencies), bone marrow suppression, increased incidence of infections, and liver disease. As a result of alcohol dependence, the woman may have withdrawal seizures in the intrapartal period as early as 12 to 48 hours after she stops drinking. Delirium tremens may occur in the postpartal period, and the newborn may suffer withdrawal syndrome.

The effects of alcohol on the fetus may result in a group of signs referred to as fetal alcohol spectrum disorders (FASD). The syndrome has characteristic physical and mental abnormalities that vary in severity and combination. (See discussion in Chapter 32 ∞).There is no definitive answer as to how much alcohol a woman can safely consume during pregnancy. Consequently, the expectant woman should "play it safe" by avoiding alcohol completely. Even low levels of alcohol cannot be recommended (Food and Drug Administration [FDA], 2005).

The nursing staff in the maternal-newborn unit must be aware of the manifestations of alcohol abuse so that they can

Table 19–2 POSSIBLE SIGNS OF SUBSTANCE ABUSE

History

- History of vague or unusual medical complaints
- Family history of alcoholism or other addiction
- History of childhood physical, sexual, or emotional abuse
- History of cirrhosis, pancreatitis, hepatitis, gastritis, sexually transmitted infections, or unusual infections such as cellulitis or endocarditis
- History of high-risk sexual behavior
- Psychiatric history of treatment and/or hospitalization

Physical Signs

- Dilated or constricted pupils
- Inflamed nasal mucosa
- Evidence of needle "track marks" or abscesses
- Poor nutritional status
- Slurred speech or staggering gait
- Odor of alcohol on breath

Behavioral Signs

- Memory lapses, mood swings, hallucinations
- Pattern of frequently missed appointments
- Frequent accidents, falls
- Signs of depression, agitation, euphoria
- Suicidal gestures

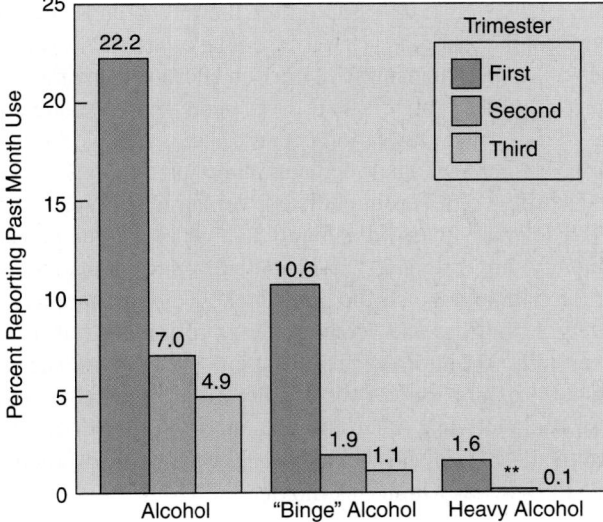

Binge alcohol use is defined as drinking 5 or more drinks on the same occasion (i.e., at the same time or within a couple of hours of each other) on at least 1 day in the past 30 days. Heavy alcohol use is defined as drinking 5 or more drinks on the same occasion on each of 5 or more days in the past 30 days; all heavy alcohol users are also binge alcohol users.

Figure 19–2 ◆ Percentages of pregnant females ages 15 to 44 reporting past month alcohol use, by trimester, 2003–2004.
SOURCE: Substance Abuse and Mental Health Services Administration (SAMHSA). (2005). *Results from the 2004 National Survey on Drug Use and Health: National Findings.* Office of Applied Science Studies, NSDUH Series H-28 DHHS Publication No. SMA 05-4062. Rockville, MD: Author.

prepare for the client's special needs. The care regimen includes sedation to decrease irritability and tremors, seizure precautions, intravenous fluid therapy for hydration, and preparation for an addicted newborn. Although high doses of sedatives and analgesics may be necessary for the woman, caution is advised because these can cause fetal depression.

Breastfeeding generally is not contraindicated, although alcohol is excreted in breast milk. Excessive alcohol consumption may intoxicate the infant and inhibit maternal let-down reflex. Discharge planning for the alcohol-addicted mother and newborn should be correlated with the social service department of the hospital.

COCAINE/CRACK

Cocaine use appears to have reached its peak during the 1990s, but it continues to be of concern for the childbearing family (Bauer, Langer, Shankaran et al., 2005). Cocaine acts at the nerve terminals to prevent the reuptake of dopamine and norepinephrine, which in turn results in vasoconstriction, tachycardia, and hypertension. Placental vasoconstriction decreases blood flow to the fetus.

Cocaine is usually taken in three ways: snorting, smoking, and intravenous (IV) injection. **Crack** is a form of freebase cocaine that is made up of baking soda, water, and cocaine mixed into a paste and microwaved to form a rock. The rock can then be smoked. Many women, especially those in low-income areas, favor this form of the drug over other forms because it is cheaper and readily available. In addition, smoking crack leads to a quicker, more intense high because the drug is absorbed through the large surface area of the lungs.

The onset of effects of cocaine occurs rapidly, but the euphoria lasts only about 30 minutes. Irritability, depression, pessimism, fatigue, and a strong desire for more cocaine usually follow this profound euphoria and excitement. This pattern often leads the user to take repeated doses to sustain the effect. Cocaine metabolites may be present in the urine of a pregnant woman for up to 4 to 7 days following use.

The cocaine user is difficult to identify prenatally. Because cocaine is an illegal substance, many women are reluctant to volunteer information about their drug use. The nurse who is familiar with the woman may recognize subtle signs of cocaine use, including mood swings and appetite changes, and withdrawal symptoms such as depression, irritability, nausea, lack of motivation, and psychomotor changes.

Major adverse maternal effects of cocaine use include seizures and hallucinations, pulmonary edema, respiratory failure, and cardiac problems. Women who use cocaine have an increased incidence of spontaneous first trimester abortion, abruptio placentae, intrauterine growth restriction (IUGR), preterm birth, and stillbirth (Ogunyemi & Hernandez-Loera, 2004).

Exposure of the fetus to cocaine in utero seems to be associated with increased incidence of neonatal complications, especially decreased birth weight and head circumference (Shankaran, Das, Bauer et al., 2004). A recent large, prospective randomized study demonstrated more autonomic nervous system dysfunction (irritability, jitteriness, tremors, high-pitched cry, and excessive suck) in exposed newborns (Bauer et al., 2005). The study's authors note that often these women also use alcohol, tobacco, and marijuana as well as other drugs, so fetal exposure to multiple drugs may contribute to an increased incidence of congenital anomalies.

Exposed infants are found to have more feeding difficulties than nonexposed infants. These difficulties may be related to some extent to the infant's behaviors but have also been found to be related to maternal behaviors. Cocaine-using mothers were found to be less flexible, less engaged, and less responsive to their infants' feeding cues (LaGasse, Messinger, Lester et al., 2003). Nursing interventions that help mothers interpret infant feeding cues and optimize the mother-infant relationship should be emphasized (Coyer, 2003).

Cocaine does cross into the breast milk and may cause such symptoms in the breastfeeding infant as extreme irritability, vomiting, diarrhea, dilated pupils, and apnea. Thus women who continue to use cocaine following childbirth should avoid breastfeeding.

MARIJUANA

Typically, pregnant women use marijuana in conjunction with alcohol and tobacco. Men who smoke marijuana may have decreased sperm counts and may develop gynecomastia (enlarged breasts); women may experience menstrual cycle irregularities. To date, however, there is no evidence that marijuana has any teratogenic effects on the fetus. The impact of heavy marijuana use on pregnancy is difficult to evaluate because of the variety of social factors that may influence the results (Shankaran et al., 2004).

PHENCYCLIDINE (PCP)

Phencyclidine (PCP) is a popular hallucinogen that can be smoked, taken orally, or injected intravenously. The onset of effects occurs in 2 to 4 minutes and lasts about 4 to 6 hours, with no withdrawal state. The drug causes confusion, delirium, and hallucinations and may produce feelings of euphoria. Signs of PCP use include constricted pupils, ataxia, nystagmus, double vision (diplopia), dizziness, and diaphoresis. The greatest risk for the pregnant woman is overdose or a psychotic response. Signs of overdose include hypertension, hyperthermia, diaphoresis, and possible coma, which may jeopardize fetal well-being (Rayburn & Bogenschutz, 2004).

MDMA (ECSTASY)

MDMA (methylenedioxymethamphetamine), better known as Ecstasy, is the most commonly used of a group of drugs referred to as *club drugs,* so called because they have become popular among adolescents and young adults who frequent dance clubs and "raves." Other club drugs include flunitrazepam (Rohypnol), gamma hydroxybutyrate (GHB), and ketamine hydrochloride. PCPs and LSD are sometimes classified as club drugs as well. MDMA is the third most widely used illicit drug after marijuana and amphetamines.

Ecstasy has been widely perceived as "safe" because of a relatively low incidence of adverse reactions. However, adverse responses are very unpredictable and the incidence is growing (Gamma, Jerome, Liechti et al., 2005).

MDMA is taken by mouth usually in tablet form. Its effects last for about 4 to 6 hours. MDMA use is appealing because it produces euphoria and feelings of empathy for others (thus it is also called the "hug drug"). The most common significant side effects include hyperthermia (elevated body temperature) and hyponatremia (low blood sodium). Other side effects include hypertension and heart or kidney failure. Deaths have occurred among users. Repeated use of Ecstasy is associated with mood, sleep, and anxiety disorders, memory deficits, increased impulsiveness, and attention problems, which may last for up to 2 years following cessation of use. In addition, because MDMA may deplete levels of serotonin, users may increase their risk of neurologic and psychiatric problems (O'Malley, 2005).

Little is yet known about the effects of MDMA on pregnancy. Preliminary research using rats suggests that prenatal use of MDMA may be associated with long-term impaired memory and learning. However, the impact of the timing of Ecstasy exposure during brain development may be a critical issue (Koprich, Chen, Kanaan et al., 2003).

HEROIN

Heroin is an illicit central nervous system (CNS) depressant narcotic that alters perception and produces euphoria. It is an addictive drug that is generally administered intravenously. Pregnancy in women who use heroin is considered high risk because of the associated increased incidence of poor nutrition, iron deficiency anemia, and preeclampsia-eclampsia (see Chapter 20 ∞). There is also an increased rate of breech position, abnormal placental implantation, abruptio placentae, preterm labor, premature rupture of the membranes (PROM), and meconium staining. Heroin users also have a higher incidence of sexually transmitted infection because many must rely on prostitution to support their drug habit. They also are at increased risk of HIV infection because they may use nonsterile needles or share needles when administering the drug.

The fetus of a heroin-addicted woman is at increased risk for IUGR and withdrawal symptoms after birth. The newborn frequently shows signs of heroin addiction, such as restlessness; lack of habituation; shrill, high-pitched cry; irritability; fist sucking; vomiting; and seizures. Signs of withdrawal usually appear within 72 hours and may last for several days. The newborn may exhibit poor consolability for 3 months or more. These behaviors may interfere with successful maternal-infant attachment and increase the potential for parenting problems or abuse in an already high-risk mother.

METHADONE

Methadone is the most commonly used drug in the treatment of women who are dependent on opioids such as heroin. Methadone blocks withdrawal symptoms and the craving for street drugs. Dosage should be individualized to achieve the most therapeutic level for the mother during pregnancy. Methadone does cross the placenta, but various studies have demonstrated inconsistent effects on the newborn. There currently does not seem to be as much of a dose-related effect on the newborn as previously felt (Jansson, DiPietro, & Elko, 2005; McCarthy, Leamon, Parr et al., 2005). The most important goal is to help the mother recover from illicit drug abuse to optimize the long-term health of both the mother and baby.

Clinical Therapy

Antepartal care of the substance-abusing woman involves medical, socioeconomic, and legal considerations. The use of a team approach allows for the comprehensive management necessary to provide safe labor and childbirth for the woman and her fetus.

The management of drug addiction may include hospitalization as necessary to initiate detoxification. "Cold turkey" withdrawal is not advisable during pregnancy because of potential risk to the fetus. Maintenance and support therapy are best individualized to the woman's history and condition.

Urine screening may also be done regularly throughout pregnancy if the woman is known or suspected to be abusing drugs. This testing is helpful in identifying the type and amount of drug being abused and in providing objective feedback to the woman. Screening strategies should include maternal informed consent before screening. Healthcare providers need to stay abreast of their state laws requiring consent for screening in pregnancy to ensure they are in compliance (Hulsey, 2005; Welch & Poulin, 2003).

NURSING CARE MANAGEMENT
Nursing Assessment and Diagnosis

Nurses and other healthcare providers should make it a practice to screen all pregnant women for substance abuse. Because illicit drug users seldom use only one drug, it is necessary to complete a thorough drug and alcohol abuse history (Chasnoff et al., 2005). Several simple screening tools are available. In addition, the nurse should be alert for clues in the history or appearance of the woman that suggest substance abuse (refer to Table 19–2). If abuse is suspected, the nurse needs to ask direct questions, beginning with less threatening questions about the use of tobacco, caffeine, and over-the-counter medications. The nurse can then progress to questions about alcohol consumption and finally to questions focusing on past and current use of illicit drugs. The nurse who is matter-of-fact and nonjudgmental in approach is more likely to elicit honest responses.

Nursing assessment of the woman who is known to abuse substances focuses on her general health status, with specific attention to nutritional status, susceptibility to infections, and evaluation of all body systems. The nurse also assesses the woman's understanding of the impact of substance abuse on herself and her pregnancy. Some women are reluctant to discuss their substance abuse; others are quite open about it. Once the nurse establishes a relationship of trust, the nurse can gain information to use in planning the woman's ongoing care.

Nursing diagnoses that may apply to the woman practicing substance abuse include the following:

- *Imbalanced Nutrition: Less than Body Requirements* related to inadequate food intake secondary to substance abuse
- *Risk for Infection* related to use of inadequately cleaned syringes and needles secondary to IV drug use
- *Risk for Ineffective Health Maintenance* related to a lack of information about the impact of substance abuse on the fetus

Nursing Plan and Implementation

Preventing substance abuse during pregnancy is the ideal nursing goal and is best accomplished through education. Unfortunately, many women who abuse substances do not receive regular health care and may not seek care until far along in their pregnancy or at the onset of labor.

The nurse's role in providing prenatal care for the woman who is practicing substance abuse focuses on ongoing assessment and client teaching. Unfortunately, some maternal-newborn nurses have only limited knowledge about substance abuse and may be negative and punitive rather than positive and supportive toward women who abuse substances during pregnancy. It is essential that nurses caring for childbearing families develop the knowledge and skill necessary to identify pregnant women who abuse substances. To provide care that is truly effective, it is equally important that nurses develop and maintain a nonjudgmental, nonpunitive, positive attitude when caring for these women.

When the nurse encounters a pregnant woman who screens positive for substance abuse, the nurse should review with the woman what the screen revealed and express concern for the health of the mother and infant. The nurse can then go on to state the belief that the mother is concerned about the baby's health and stress the need for the woman to stop using drugs or alcohol during pregnancy. The nurse can then discuss possible strategies to help the woman quit (addiction treatment programs, 12-step programs, individual counseling) and suggest a referral for more in-depth assessment by a specialist. If feasible, the nurse can make an appointment while the woman is in the office or clinic. Nurses should also be aware of treatment options available for women who lack financial resources. Finally the nurse should make a follow-up appointment to see the woman again after her drug or alcohol assessment. The knowledgeable nurse can provide information about the relationship between substance abuse and existing health problems and the implications for the woman's unborn child. By establishing a relationship of trust and support, the nurse may foster the woman's cooperation.

Preparation for labor and birth should be part of the prenatal planning. Fear, tension, or discomfort may be relieved through nonnarcotic psychologic support and careful explanation of the labor process. If pain medication is necessary, it should not be withheld, however, because the notion that it will contribute to further addiction is not correct. Preferred methods of pain relief include the use of psychoprophylaxis and regional or local anesthetics, such as pudendal block and local infiltration. These techniques decrease the risk of additional fetal respiratory depression. Immediate intensive care should be available for the newborn, who may have respiratory depression, be small for gestational age (SGA), and be premature. For care of the addicted newborn, see Chapter 32. ∞

Evaluation

Expected outcomes of nursing care include the following:

- The woman is able to describe the impact of substance abuse on herself and her unborn child.

- The woman successfully gives birth to a healthy infant.
- The woman agrees to cooperate with referral to social services (or other appropriate community agency) for follow-up care after discharge.

CARE OF THE WOMAN WITH DIABETES MELLITUS

Diabetes mellitus, an endocrine disorder of carbohydrate metabolism, results from inadequate production or utilization of insulin.

Normal Glucose Homeostasis

After consumption of a meal, the body metabolizes carbohydrates into glucose. Insulin, produced by the beta cells of the islets of Langerhans in the pancreas, lowers blood glucose levels by enabling the glucose to move from the blood into muscle and liver cells, where it is stored as glycogen. When several hours have passed since a meal, falling blood glucose levels stimulate the pancreas to release glucagon, which in turn stimulates breakdown of liver glycogen stores into glucose, which is returned to the bloodstream. Glucagon can also stimulate the synthesis of glucose directly from amino acids in stored body proteins.

Carbohydrate Metabolism in Normal Pregnancy

Carbohydrate metabolism is affected early in pregnancy by a rise in serum levels of estrogen, progesterone, and other hormones. These hormones stimulate maternal insulin production and increase tissue response to insulin; therefore, anabolism (building up) of glycogen stores in the liver and other tissues occurs.

In the second half of pregnancy, the woman demonstrates prolonged hyperglycemia and hyperinsulinemia (increased secretion of insulin) following a meal. Although the mother is producing more insulin, placental secretion of human placental lactogen (hPL) and prolactin (from the decidua), as well as elevated levels of cortisol (an adrenal hormone) and glycogen, cause increased maternal peripheral resistance to insulin. This resistance helps ensure that there is a sustained supply of glucose available for the fetus. This glucose is transported across the placenta to the fetus, who uses it as a major source of fuel. Maternal amino acids are also actively transported by the placenta from the mother to her fetus. These amino acids are used by the fetus for protein synthesis and as a source of energy. In addition to ensuring that glucose is available to the fetus, the increased maternal resistance to insulin also means that the pregnant woman has a lower peripheral uptake of glucose to meet her own needs. This results in a catabolic (destructive) state during fasting periods (e.g., during the night and after meal absorption). Because increasing amounts of circulating maternal glucose are being diverted to the fetus, maternal fat is metabolized (lipolysis) during fasting periods much more read-

ily than in a nonpregnant person. This process is called *accelerated starvation.* Ketones may be present in the urine as a result of lipolysis.

The delicate system of checks and balances that exists between glucose production and glucose use is stressed by the growing fetus, who derives energy from glucose taken from the mother and by maternal resistance to the insulin her body produces. This stress is referred to as the diabetogenic effect of pregnancy. Thus any preexisting disruption in carbohydrate metabolism is augmented by pregnancy, and any diabetic potential may precipitate gestational diabetes mellitus.

Pathophysiology of Diabetes Mellitus

In diabetes mellitus, the pancreas does not produce sufficient amounts of insulin to allow necessary carbohydrate metabolism. With inadequate amounts of insulin, glucose cannot enter the cells but remains circulating in the blood. The body cells become energy depleted while the blood glucose level remains elevated. Fats and proteins in the body tissues are then oxidized by the cells as a source of energy. This results in wasting of fat and muscle tissue of the body, negative nitrogen balance due to protein breakdown, and ketosis due to fat metabolism. The strong osmotic force of the glucose concentration in the blood pulls water from the cells into the blood, which results in cellular dehydration. The high level of glucose in the blood eventually spills over into the urine, producing glycosuria. Osmotic pressure of the glucose in the urine prevents reabsorption of water into the kidney tubules, causing extracellular dehydration.

These pathologic developments cause the four cardinal signs and symptoms of diabetes mellitus: polyuria, polydipsia, weight loss, and polyphagia. *Polyuria* (frequent urination) results because water is not reabsorbed by the renal tubules because of the osmotic activity of glucose. *Polydipsia* (excessive thirst) is caused by dehydration from polyuria. *Weight loss* (seen in insulin-dependent diabetes, also called type 1 diabetes) is due to the use of fat and muscle tissue for energy. *Polyphagia* (excessive hunger) is caused by tissue loss and a state of starvation, which results from the inability of the cells to utilize the blood glucose. Diagnosis of diabetes is based on the presence of clinical symptoms and laboratory tests showing elevated glucose levels in the blood, glycosuria, and ketoacidosis.

Classification of Diabetes Mellitus

States of altered carbohydrate metabolism have been classified several different ways. Table 19–3 shows the classification of diabetes mellitus based on its cause. This classification contains four main categories: type 1 diabetes, type 2 diabetes, other specific types, and gestational diabetes mellitus. Type 1 diabetes develops because of β-cell destruction and generally results in an absolute insulin deficiency. Type 2 diabetes, which is the most common form, results from a combination of an insulin secretory defect and insulin resistance (American Diabetes Association [ADA], 2004).

Table 19–4 shows White's classification of diabetes in pregnancy. This classification is useful for describing the extent of the disease.

Table 19–3 ETIOLOGIC CLASSIFICATION OF DIABETES MELLITUS

I. Type 1 diabetes* (β-cell destruction, usually leading to absolute insulin deficiency)
  A. Immune mediated
  B. Idiopathic
II. Type 2 diabetes* (may range from predominantly insulin resistance with relative insulin deficiency to a predominantly secretory defect with insulin resistance)
III. Other specific types†
IV. Gestational diabetes mellitus

Individuals with any form of diabetes may require insulin treatment at some stage of their disease. Such use of insulin does not classify the person.

†The more detailed classification, which can be found in medical-surgical texts and the original source, provides eight subcategories of type.

SOURCE: Adapted from American Diabetes Association. (2006). Position statement. Diagnosis and classification of diabetes mellitus. *Diabetes Care, 29*(1), 543–549.

Table 19–4 WHITE'S CLASSIFICATION OF DIABETES IN PREGNANCY

Class	Criterion
A	Chemical diabetes
B	Maturity onset (age over 20 years), duration under 10 years, no vascular lesions
C_1	Age 10 to 19 years at onset
C_2	10 to 19 years' duration
D_1	Under 10 years at onset
D_2	Over 20 years' duration
D_3	Benign retinopathy
D_4	Calcified vessels of legs
D_5	Hypertension
E	No longer sought
F	Nephropathy
G	Many failures
H	Cardiopathy
R	Proliferating retinopathy
T	Renal transplant (added by Tagatz and colleagues of the University of Minnesota)

SOURCE: Reprinted from White, P. (1978). Classification of obstetric diabetes. *American Journal of Obstetrics and Gynecology, 130*, 228. Copyright © 1978, with permission from Elsevier.

Gestational diabetes mellitus (GDM) is defined as carbohydrate intolerance of variable severity with onset or first recognition during pregnancy. It results from (1) an unidentified preexistent disease, (2) the unmasking of a compensated metabolic abnormality by the added stress of pregnancy, or (3) a direct consequence of the altered maternal metabolism stemming from changing hormonal levels. When GDM is diagnosed, the goal of treatment is to decrease the likelihood of fetal macrosomia, shoulder dystocia, birth trauma, and cesarean birth (American College of Obstetricians and Gynecologists [ACOG], 2001). (See discussion in Fetal-Neonatal Risks.) Although GDM incidence rates vary, many of these individuals progress to overt type 2 diabetes mellitus with time (ACOG, 2001).

Influence of Pregnancy on Diabetes

Pregnancy can affect diabetes significantly. First, the physiologic changes of pregnancy can drastically alter insulin requirements. Second, pregnancy may accelerate the progress of vascular disease secondary to diabetes.

The disease may be more difficult to control during pregnancy because insulin requirements are changeable. Insulin need frequently decreases early in the first trimester. Levels of hPL, an insulin antagonist, are low; energy demands of the embryo are minimal; and the woman may be consuming less food because of nausea and vomiting. Nausea and vomiting may also cause dietary fluctuations, which can increase the risk of hypoglycemia or insulin shock. Insulin requirements usually begin to rise late in the first trimester as glucose use and glycogen storage by the woman and fetus increase. As a result of placental maturation and production of hPL and other hormones, insulin requirements may double or quadruple by the end of pregnancy.

Increased energy needs during labor may require more insulin to balance intravenous glucose. After delivery of the placenta, insulin requirements usually decrease abruptly with loss of hPL in the maternal circulation.

Other factors contribute to the difficulty in controlling the disease. As pregnancy progresses, the renal threshold for glucose decreases. There is an increased risk of ketoacidosis, which may occur at lower serum glucose levels in the pregnant woman with diabetes than in the nonpregnant woman with diabetes. The vascular disease that accompanies diabetes may progress during pregnancy. Hypertension may occur. Nephropathy may result from renal blood vessel impairment, and retinopathy may develop (from occlusion of the microscopic blood vessels of the eye).

The primary concern for the pregnant woman who has diabetes is control of circulating blood glucose levels. If control can be achieved and maintained, diabetes generally does not worsen during pregnancy. The woman's health status may even improve because of close medical supervision.

Influence of Diabetes on Pregnancy Outcome

The pregnancy of a woman who has diabetes carries a higher risk of complications, especially perinatal mortality and congenital anomalies. The risk has been reduced by the recent recognition of the importance of tight metabolic control (fasting blood glucose less than 95 mg/dL and 2-hour postprandial less than 120 mg/dL). New techniques for monitoring blood glucose, delivering insulin, and monitoring the fetus have also reduced perinatal mortality (ACOG, 2005).

MATERNAL RISKS

Maternal health problems in diabetic pregnancy have been greatly reduced by the team approach to preconception planning and early prenatal care and by the increased emphasis on maintaining tight control of blood glucose levels. The prognosis for the pregnant woman with gestational, type 1, or type 2 diabetes that has not resulted in significant vascular damage is positive.

However, diabetic pregnancy still carries higher risks for complications than normal pregnancy.

Hydramnios, or an increase in the volume of amniotic fluid, occurs in 10% to 20% of pregnant women with diabetes. It is thought to be a result of excessive fetal urination because of fetal hyperglycemia (Forsbach-Sanchez, Tamez-Perez, & Vazquez-Lara, 2005). *Preeclampsia-eclampsia* occurs more often in diabetic pregnancies, especially when diabetes-related vascular changes already exist.

Hyperglycemia due to insufficient amounts of insulin can lead to *ketoacidosis* as a result of the increase in ketone bodies (which are acidic) in the blood released when fatty acids are metabolized. Ketoacidosis usually develops slowly, but it may develop more rapidly in the pregnant woman because of the hyperketonemia associated with accelerated starvation in the fasting state. The tendency for higher postprandial glucose levels because of decreased gastric motility and the contrainsulin effects of hPL also predispose the woman to ketoacidosis. If the ketoacidosis is not treated, it can lead to coma and death of both mother and fetus.

Another risk to the pregnant woman with diabetes is a difficult labor (*dystocia*), caused by fetopelvic disproportion if fetal macrosomia exists. The pregnant woman with diabetes is also at increased risk for recurrent monilial vaginitis and urinary tract infections because of increased glycosuria, which contributes to a favorable environment for bacterial growth. If untreated, asymptomatic bacteriuria can lead to pyelonephritis, a serious kidney infection.

Several studies have demonstrated that pregnancy worsens *retinopathy* in women with diabetes. Most investigators agree that during diabetic pregnancy, good control of blood glucose levels and the use of laser photocoagulation (a treatment used to prevent retinal hemorrhage when the retina shows changes in the blood vessels) when indicated minimize the risk of the negative effects of pregnancy. Hence, women with preexisting diabetes should be referred to an ophthalmologist for evaluation during pregnancy (ACOG, 2005).

FETAL-NEONATAL RISKS

Many of the problems of the newborn result directly from high maternal plasma glucose levels. In the presence of severe maternal ketoacidosis, the risk of fetal death has ranged from 35% to a decrease more recently of 10% (ACOG, 2005). Fetal enzyme systems cease functioning in an acidic environment.

The incidence of *congenital anomalies* in diabetic pregnancies is 5% to 10% and is the major cause of death for infants of diabetic mothers. Research suggests that this increased incidence of congenital anomalies is related to multiple factors including high glucose levels in early pregnancy (Wyatt, Frias, Hoyme et al., 2005). The anomalies often involve the heart, CNS, and skeletal system. Septal defects, coarctation of the aorta, and transposition of the great vessels are the most common heart lesions seen. CNS anomalies include hydrocephalus, meningomyelocele, and anencephaly. One anomaly, *sacral agenesis,* appears only in infants of diabetic mothers. In sacral agenesis, the sacrum and lumbar spine fail to develop and the lower extremities develop incompletely. To reduce the incidence of congenital anomalies, preconception counseling and strict diabetes control before conception and in the early weeks of pregnancy are indicated.

Characteristically, infants of diabetic mothers in White's classes A, B, and C (see Table 19–4) are large for gestational age (LGA) as a result of high levels of fetal insulin production stimulated by the high levels of glucose crossing the placenta from the mother. Sustained fetal hyperinsulinism and hyperglycemia ultimately lead to excessive growth, called **macrosomia,** and deposition of fat. If born vaginally, the macrosomic infant is at increased risk for birth trauma such as fractured clavicle or brachial plexus injuries due to shoulder dystocia. To prevent such injuries, cesarean birth may be indicated if birth weight is expected to exceed 4500 g (ACOG, 2005).

After birth, the umbilical cord is severed, and thus the generous maternal blood glucose supply is eliminated. However, continued islet cell hyperactivity leads to excessive insulin levels and depleted blood glucose (hypoglycemia) in 2 to 4 hours. Macrosomia can be significantly reduced by tight maternal blood glucose control.

Infants of diabetic mothers with vascular involvement may demonstrate *IUGR.* This occurs because vascular changes in the mother decrease the efficiency of placental perfusion, and the fetus is not as well sustained in utero.

Respiratory distress syndrome appears to result from inhibition, by high levels of fetal insulin, of some fetal enzymes necessary for surfactant production. Polycythemia in the newborn is due primarily to the diminished ability of glycosylated hemoglobin in the mother's blood to release oxygen. *Hyperbilirubinemia* is a result of the inability of immature liver enzymes to metabolize the increased bilirubin resulting from the polycythemia. Hypocalcemia, characterized by signs of irritability or even tetany, may occur. The cause of these low calcium levels in infants of diabetic mothers is not known.

Clinical Therapy
DETECTION AND DIAGNOSIS OF GESTATIONAL DIABETES

Gestational diabetes is more common than pregestational diabetes. It is estimated to range from 1% to 14% of pregnancies, depending on the population studied (ADA, 2004). Therefore, screening for its detection is a standard part of prenatal care. If diabetes is suspected, further testing is undertaken for diagnosis.

All pregnant women, regardless of risk factors, should have their risk assessed at the first prenatal visit. Those at low risk should be tested toward the end of the second trimester (24 to 28 weeks) using a 1-hour, 50-g oral glucose tolerance test. Women with risk factors (age over 40; family history of diabetes in a first-degree relative; a prior macrosomic, malformed, or stillborn infant; obesity; hypertension; or glucosuria) should be tested as soon as feasible early in pregnancy (ADA, 2004). The oral glucose load is administered without regard to time of day or time of last meal, and venous plasma glucose is measured 1 hour later. A plasma level that is equal to or greater than 130 to 140 mg/dL (depending on the lab used) indicates a need for further diagnostic testing.

During pregnancy, if the 1-hour oral glucose screen indicates that a woman might have gestational diabetes, diagnosis is

RESEARCH IN PRACTICE

MATERNAL OBESITY AND DIABETES AS RISK FACTORS FOR ADVERSE PREGNANCY OUTCOMES: DIFFERENCES AMONG FOUR RACIAL/ETHNIC GROUPS

What is this study about? The prevalence of diabetes and obesity continues to rise among American women. The association between pregestational or gestational diabetes and complications of pregnancy are well known. Obesity is similarly associated with negative outcomes for both the mother and infant. There are established differences in the prevalence of these conditions across diverse ethnic groups. The purpose of this study was to determine the association between diabetes, obesity, and three adverse pregnancy and birth outcomes in women of four different ethnic groups.

How was this study done? The source of information for this study was a large, population-based database from New York City. Data obtained from birth certificates for all babies born in 1999, 2000, and 2001 were included in the study. This large sample size—nearly 330,000 records—allowed for the in-depth subgroup analysis described in the purpose statement. Specific maternal variables were collected from the records, including prepregnancy weight, maternal weight gain during the pregnancy, maternal diabetes, chronic and pregestational hypertension, and eclampsia. The outcomes that were measured included primary cesarean birth, preterm birth (defined as less than 37 weeks' gestation), and low birth weight (defined as 2500 grams or less). The four racial/ethnic groups used for subgroup comparison were non-Hispanic black (black), non-Hispanic white (white), Asian, and Hispanic. The authors analyzed the data for correlations between specific maternal problems and outcomes, and for differences between the groups on these relationships.

What were the results of the study? Virtually all of the key risk factors and pregnancy outcomes varied by race/ethnic group. Black women were significantly more likely to be in the heaviest weight groups, and were also more likely to have excessive weight gain during the pregnancy. Black women also had the highest rates of both chronic hypertension and gestational hypertension. This group also had the highest percentages of primary cesarean births, preterm births, and low birth weight. Asian women had the highest

rate of gestational diabetes. Obesity contributed the most to eclampsia for white women, whereas excess weight gain was a more important predictor of eclampsia for Asians. The risk for preeclampsia and eclampsia increased as weight increased for women in all groups and was highest among the heaviest mothers. All of the risk factors significantly increased the likelihood of a primary cesarean birth, with the heaviest of the women at the most risk. Women with chronic diabetes and preeclampsia were more than twice as likely to have a cesarean birth than women without these conditions. Preeclampsia and eclampsia presented the greatest risk for a preterm birth, although both chronic diabetes and chronic hypertension were also associated with high rates. The hypertensive variables were the strongest contributors to an increased likelihood of a low-birth-weight infant, whereas obese women were most at risk of having a macrosomic infant (one weighing more than 4000 grams).

What additional questions might I have? The data did not allow for the calculation of body mass index, which is thought to have a greater impact on morbidity than simple weight. Would the results be different if this more sensitive standard were used? Would analysis of data from mothers who experienced a stillbirth differ from these, which were collected from birth certificates from live births only?

How can I use this study? Pregnancy and the postpartum period can be seen as a "teachable moment" in the life of a mother, during which women may be more open to counseling about the risks of being obese. This may be an opportunity for the nurse to present health teaching at a time when the mother will be most receptive and may lead to significant personal change. The longer-term public health approach should be aimed at efforts to prevent gestational diabetes by controlling women's weight over their lifetimes. This is particularly needed for the most at-risk group, non-Hispanic black women. Understanding these risk factors can help the nurse in an inpatient unit design assessments and interventions that can detect and respond to maternal and infant complications.

Rosenberg T., Garbers, S., Lipkind, H., & Chiasson, M. (2005). Maternal obesity and diabetes as risk factors for adverse pregnancy outcomes: Differences among four racial/ethnic groups. *American Journal of Public Health, 95*(9), 1545–1551.

made using a 3-hour, 100-g oral glucose tolerance test (OGTT). To do this test, the woman eats an unrestricted diet, consuming at least 150 g of carbohydrates per day for at least 3 days before her scheduled test. She then ingests 100-g oral glucose solution in the morning after an overnight fast. Plasma glucose is measured fasting and at 1, 2, and 3 hours. The woman should remain seated and not smoke throughout the test. Gestational diabetes is diagnosed if two or more of the following values are met or exceeded:

Fasting	95 mg/dL
1 hour	180 mg/dL
2 hours	155 mg/dL
3 hours	140 mg/dL

If only one value is elevated, many clinicians recommend exercise and nutrition counseling and then either repeat the 3-hour OGTT in 1 month or perform periodic glucose monitoring (ACOG, 2001). In cases of borderline values and the presence of risk factors, some clinicians repeat the testing at 32 weeks' gestation.

LABORATORY ASSESSMENT OF LONG-TERM GLUCOSE CONTROL

Glycosylated hemoglobin (HbA_{1c}) is a laboratory test that loosely reflects glucose control over the previous 4 to 8 weeks. It measures the percentage of glycohemoglobin in the blood. Glycohemoglobin, or HbA_{1c}, is the hemoglobin to which a glucose molecule is attached. The test is not reliable for screening for gestational diabetes and is not recommended at this time (ADA, 2004). However, in women with known pregestational diabetes, abnormal HbA_{1c} values correlate directly with the frequency of fetal congenital anomalies. A value greater than 10% is associated with a fetal anomaly rate of 20% to 25% (ACOG, 2005).

Antepartal Management of Diabetes

The major goals of medical care for a pregnant woman with diabetes—whether gestational or pregestational—are (1) to maintain a physiologic equilibrium of insulin availability and glucose utilization during pregnancy and (2) to ensure an optimally healthy mother and newborn. To achieve these goals, good prenatal care using a team approach is a top priority. The team consists of an obstetrician, an endocrinologist, a perinatologist, a diabetes nurse-educator, a perinatal nurse, a nutritionist, a social worker, and, most important, the diabetic woman and her partner if he is involved in the pregnancy. Education of the couple and their active involvement in managing her care are essential for a good outcome.

For the woman with gestational diabetes, the diagnosis may be a shock, leaving her frightened and anxious. This anxiety may lead to an inability to adhere to important treatment regimens (Kendrick, Wilson, Elder et al., 2005). She needs clear explanation and teaching to enlist her participation in ensuring a good outcome. The diabetes nurse-educator plays a major role in this counseling.

Diet therapy and regular exercise form the cornerstone of intervention for GDM. Insulin therapy is indicated when dietary management is unable to achieve a 1-hour postprandial blood glucose value less than 130 to 140 mg/dL, a 2-hour postprandial level less than 120 mg/dL, or a fasting glucose less than 95 mg/dL. In most instances, the overt diabetic manifestation disappears postpartum, though subtle manifestations of impaired insulin secretory capacity may remain.

The woman with pregestational diabetes needs to understand changes she can expect during pregnancy; thus she should receive such teaching in preconception counseling. At the initial prenatal visit, height, weight, and vital signs are assessed along with a thorough assessment of thyroid and cardiac function. Special attention is given to dating the pregnancy. Laboratory data are obtained, and the diabetes is classified using White's criteria. Women should be screened for diabetic neuropathy, and a funduscopic examination is done to detect any retinopathy. In some cases, the woman may be referred to an ophthalmologist for further evaluation (ACOG, 2005).

DIETARY REGULATION

The pregnant woman requires about 300 kilocalories (kcal) per day more than she does when she is not pregnant to meet increased metabolic demands. In general, women need approximately 30 kcal/kg of ideal body weight (IBW) during the first trimester and 35 to 36 kcal/kg IBW during the second and third trimesters. If ketonuria develops or the woman complains of hunger, the number of calories may be increased. Dietary guidelines are similar for women with gestational and pregestational diabetes. Approximately 40% to 50% of the kcal should come

from complex carbohydrates, 15% to 20% from protein, and 20% to 30% from fats (Fowles, 2004).

This caloric intake is divided among three meals and three snacks. The prebedtime snack is the most important and must include both protein and complex carbohydrates to prevent hypoglycemia at night. Because it is so important that the pregnant woman follow these guidelines, a nutritionist works out meal plans based on the woman's lifestyle, culture, and food preferences and teaches her food exchanges so she can vary and plan her own meals. Cookbooks for people with diabetes are available and can be a great help.

GLUCOSE MONITORING

Glucose monitoring is an essential part of diabetes management for determining the need for insulin and assessing glucose control. Many physicians have the woman come in for a weekly assessment of her fasting glucose levels and one or two postprandial levels. In addition, frequent self-monitoring of glucose levels is paramount in maintaining good glucose control. Self-monitoring is discussed on page 460.

INSULIN ADMINISTRATION

Whether the woman with gestational diabetes needs additional insulin (over her own body production) depends on how well her blood glucose levels can be maintained by diet alone. Individuals with pregestational diabetes usually have type 1 diabetes, requiring insulin administration. Whether the client has gestational or pregestational diabetes, human insulin should be used because it is the least likely to cause an allergic response. If the woman has previously used bovine or porcine insulin, she may require smaller doses of human insulin to achieve the same pharmacologic effect. Insulin is given either in multiple injections or by continuous subcutaneous infusion. Multiple injections are used more commonly and with excellent results. Most women will need a mixture of intermediate and regular insulin. Some clinicians have moved away from the use of regular insulin, replacing it with a fast-acting human analog called lispro. Lispro is associated with better glucose control (ACOG, 2005). Often a four-dose approach is used, with regular insulin or lispro taken before each meal and NPH or Lente insulin added at bedtime (ACOG, 2005). Other clinicians vary the NPH and regular insulin patterns slightly but still prefer a four-dose approach. It is important to remember that the amount of insulin needed usually increases during each trimester of pregnancy.

Oral hypoglycemics are rarely used during pregnancy because they cross the placenta and have not been well studied. However, glyburide, a second-generation sulfonylurea, does not cross the placenta and has been found to be comparable to insulin without evidence of adverse effects in the mother or fetus (Jacobson, Ramos, Ching et al, 2005; Langer, Yogev, Xenakis et al., 2005). This oral agent is now being used to treat women with gestational diabetes mellitus (ACOG, 2005).

EVALUATION OF FETAL STATUS

Information about the well-being, maturation, and size of the fetus is important for planning the course of the pregnancy and the timing of birth. Because pregnancies complicated by diabetes are at increased risk of neural tube defects, maternal serum α-*fetoprotein (AFP)* screening is offered at weeks 16 to 20 of gestation (see Chapter 21 ∞).

Daily maternal evaluation of *fetal activity,* begun at about 28 weeks, is effective and simple to do. The woman is taught a particular method for counting fetal movements (see Chapter 16 ∞). She records the results on a special card, and brings the card to each subsequent office visit.

Nonstress testing (NST) is usually begun weekly at about 28 weeks. If evidence of IUGR, preeclampsia, oligohydramnios, or poorly controlled blood glucose exists, testing may begin as early as 26 weeks and may be done more often. NSTs are increased to twice weekly at 32 weeks' gestation. If the NST is nonreactive, a fetal biophysical profile or *contraction stress test* is performed (ACOG, 2001). If the woman requires hospitalization (for example, to control glycemia or for complications), NSTs may be done daily.

Ultrasound at 18 weeks establishes gestational age and diagnoses multiple pregnancy or congenital anomalies. It is repeated at 28 weeks to monitor fetal growth for IUGR or macrosomia. Some physicians order *fetal biophysical profiles* (ultrasound evaluation of fetal well-being in which fetal breathing movements, fetal activity, reactivity, muscle tone, and amniotic fluid volume are assessed) as part of an ongoing evaluation of fetal status.

Intrapartal Management of Diabetes Mellitus

During the intrapartal period, medical therapy includes the following:

- *Timing of birth.* Most diabetic pregnancies are allowed to go to term, with spontaneous labor, thereby decreasing the risk of respiratory distress in the newborn. Some clinicians do opt to induce labor in a woman at term to avoid problems related to an aging placenta. Cesarean birth may be indicated if evidence of nonreassuring fetal status exists. Birth before term may be indicated for diabetic women with vascular changes and worsening hypertension or if evidence of IUGR exists (ACOG, 2005). In pregnancies in which there is evidence of fetal macrosomia, fetal compromise, or elevated maternal HbA$_{1c}$, amniocentesis is done for lecithin/sphingomyelin (L/S) ratio and the presence of phosphatidylglycerol (PG). Whereas levels of 2:1 for the L/S ratio indicate fetal lung maturity in the nondiabetic pregnancy, levels of up to 3.5:1 L/S ratio have been found necessary at some centers before low risk of respiratory distress syndrome (RDS) is achieved. The presence of phosphatidylglycerol seems to enhance lecithin activity, and its presence is considered favorable for lung maturity. Fetal lung maturity must be weighed against other considerations when deciding time of childbirth. If preterm labor occurs, tocolytic therapy (use of medications in an attempt to halt preterm labor) (see Chapter 20 ∞) and β-sympathomimetic drugs should not be administered because they may worsen maternal glucose control (ACOG, 2003a).

- *Labor management.* The degree of prenatal maintenance of normal maternal glucose levels (euglycemia) and the

Figure 19–3 ◆ During labor the nurse closely monitors the blood glucose levels of the woman with diabetes mellitus.

maintenance of maternal euglycemia during labor are important in preventing neonatal hypoglycemia. Maternal insulin requirements often decrease dramatically during labor. Consequently, maternal glucose levels are measured hourly to determine insulin need. (See Figure 19–3 ◆.) The primary goal in controlling maternal glucose levels intrapartally is to prevent neonatal hypoglycemia (ACOG, 2005). During active labor, insulin may not be needed. Long-acting insulin should be reduced or stopped and regular insulin should be used to meet most or all of the woman's identified needs. Often two intravenous lines are used, one with a 5% dextrose solution and one with a saline solution. The saline solution is then available if a bolus is needed or for piggybacking insulin. Insulin clings to the plastic intravenous bag and tubing. To ensure that the woman receives the desired dose, the intravenous tubing must be flushed with insulin before the prescribed amount is added. During the second stage of labor and the immediate postpartum period, the woman may not need additional insulin. The intravenous insulin is discontinued with the completion of the third stage of labor.

Postpartal Management of Diabetes Mellitus

Maternal insulin requirements fall significantly postpartally because the levels of hPL, progesterone, and estrogen fall after placental separation, and their anti-insulin effect ceases, resulting in decreased blood glucose levels. The diabetic mother may require no insulin for the first 24 hours or only one fourth to one half her previous dose. Then, reestablishment of insulin needs based on blood glucose testing is necessary. Diet and exercise levels must also be redetermined. Consequently, the woman with diabetes that is not controlled by diet alone may need insulin for a time (ACOG, 2005).

Women with GDM who did not require insulin during pregnancy generally do not need it during the postpartum period. Clinicians routinely discontinue insulin for women with GDM following childbirth and then monitor blood glucose levels. If elevated glucose levels develop, oral antihyperglycemic agents may be tried if the woman is not breastfeeding (ACOG, 2005). Antihyperglycemics are contraindicated during breastfeeding. The woman should be reassessed 6 weeks postpartum to determine whether her glucose levels are normal. If her levels are normal, she should be reassessed at a minimum of 3-year intervals (ADA, 2004).

Diabetic control and the establishment of parent-child relationships in light of neonatal needs are the priorities of this period. If her newborn must be cared for in a special care nursery, the mother needs support and information about the baby's condition. Every effort must be made to provide as much contact as possible between the parents and their newborn.

Breastfeeding is encouraged as beneficial to both mother and baby. The composition of breast milk is not altered by diabetes, and infants of mothers with diabetes gain weight appropriately. The lactating mother with diabetes often has a sense of well-being and diminished insulin needs even while increasing caloric intake. Blood glucose levels may be lower because glucose is transferred from serum to breast to be converted to lactose, and energy is expended in milk production. Caloric needs increase during lactation to 500 to 800 kcal above prepregnant requirements. Insulin must be adjusted according to individual needs. Home blood glucose monitoring should continue for the insulin-dependent diabetic.

The woman and her partner, if he is involved, should receive information on family planning. Barrier methods of contraception (diaphragm and condom) used with spermicide are safe, effective, and inexpensive and are the method of choice for insulin-dependent diabetic women. The use of combined oral contraceptives (COCs) by women with diabetes is controversial. Some evidence suggests that women with diabetes may be at greater risk for COC complications such as myocardial infarction and thrombophlebitis. Many physicians who prescribe low-dose COCs to women with diabetes restrict them to women who have no vascular disease and who do not smoke. The progesterone-only pill may also be used as may Depo-Provera. Many couples who have completed their families choose elective sterilization.

It's hard to realize that I have gestational diabetes and to know that it increases my chances of getting diabetes later. My grandmother had diabetes, so I always thought of it as an old person's disease. All the finger sticks, watching my diet, and keeping track has taken some getting used to. I'll be glad when our baby is born and I can put this behind me, at least for now.

NURSING CARE MANAGEMENT

The Nursing Care Plan on pages 457–459 for a woman with diabetes mellitus summarizes nursing management.

Nursing Assessment and Diagnosis

Whether diabetes has been diagnosed before pregnancy occurs or the diagnosis is made during pregnancy (GDM), careful assessment of the disease process and the woman's understanding of diabetes is important. Thorough physical examination, including assessment for vascular complications, any signs of infectious conditions, and urine and blood testing for glucose, is essential at the first prenatal visit. Follow-up visits are usually scheduled twice a month during the first two trimesters and weekly during the last trimester.

Assessment also yields vital information about the woman's ability to cope with the combined stress of pregnancy and diabetes and her ability to follow a recommended regimen of care. It is necessary to determine the woman's knowledge about diabetes and self-care before formulating a teaching plan.

Nursing diagnoses that may apply to the pregnant woman with diabetes mellitus include the following:

- **Risk for Imbalanced Nutrition: More than Body Requirements** related to imbalance between intake and available insulin
- **Risk for Injury** related to possible complications secondary to hypoglycemia or hyperglycemia
- **Interrupted Family Processes** related to the need for hospitalization secondary to GDM

Nursing Plan and Implementation

Prepregnancy counseling may be provided by a nurse and a physician, using a team approach. Ideally, the couple is seen before pregnancy so that the diabetes can be assessed by ophthalmologic evaluation, electrocardiographic study, and a 24-hour urine collection for creatinine clearance and protein excretion. Prepregnancy counseling about the importance of tight glucose control is cost-effective in preventing congenital anomalies. If the diabetes is of recent onset without vascular complications, the outcome of pregnancy should be good, provided that glucose levels are controlled.

COMMUNITY-BASED NURSING CARE

In many cases, women with GDM are stabilized in the hospital, and necessary teaching for self-care is begun. Women with preexisting diabetes may also require hospitalization for stabilization of their diabetes. In either case, the majority of ongoing teaching and supervision of pregnant women with diabetes is then carried out by nurses in clinics, community agencies, and the women's homes.

Effective Insulin Use

The nurse ensures that the couple understands the purpose of the insulin, the types of insulin the woman is to use, the number of

NURSING CARE PLAN

The Woman with Diabetes Mellitus

INTERVENTION	RATIONALE	EXPECTED OUTCOME
1. Nursing Diagnosis: Risk for Altered Nutrition: Less than Body Requirements related to poor carbohydrate metabolism		
Goal: Client will maintain adequate nutrition throughout pregnancy.		
• Emphasize importance of regular prenatal visits for assessment of weight gain, blood sugar levels, fetal heart tones, urine ketones, and fundal height measurement. • Coordinate care with a dietitian to assist client in meal planning and educate client on the daily caloric needs of pregnancy. • Instruct client on signs and symptoms of hyperglycemia: polyphagia, nausea, hot flushes, polydipsia, polyuria, fruity breath, abdominal cramps, rapid deep breathing, headache, weakness, drowsiness, and general malaise. Instruct client on signs and symptoms of hypoglycemia: hunger, clammy skin, irritability, slurred speech, seizures, tachycardia, headache, pallor, sweating, disorientation, shakiness, blurred vision, and, if untreated, coma or convulsions. • Instruct client on management of hyperglycemia and hypoglycemia. • Include family members in meal planning.	• Regular follow-up and assessment of weight, blood sugar levels, fetal heart tones, urine ketones, and fundal height will promote a healthy pregnancy and outcome, as well as allow for modifications in the treatment regimen if necessary. • A daily intake of high-quality foods promotes fetal growth and controls maternal glucose levels. • Maintaining a euglycemic state throughout pregnancy aids in preventing diabetic complications and promotes a positive pregnancy outcome. • Gives the family member a sense of involvement and an understanding of the importance of adequate nutrition in pregnancy.	• *The client will maintain adequate nutrition as evidenced by adequate weight gain, controlled blood sugar levels, verbalization of understanding of personal treatment regimen, and appropriate fetal growth and development during pregnancy.* • *Client will recognize signs and intervene appropriately.*
2. Nursing Diagnosis: Risk for Fetal Injury related to possible complications associated with altered tissue perfusion secondary to maternal diagnosis of diabetes mellitus		
Goal: Uncomplicated birth of a healthy newborn.		
• Assess fetal heart tones for reassuring variability and accelerations.	• Reassuring fetal heart rate variability and accelerations are interpreted as adequate placental oxygenation.	• *The fetus will not exhibit signs and symptoms of altered tissue perfusion as evidenced by positive fetal activity, reassuring fetal heart rate patterns, a biophysical profile score between 8 and 10, negative CST, L/S ratio indicating fetal lung maturity, and a reactive nonstress test.*

(Continued on next page)

NURSING CARE PLAN

The Woman with Diabetes Mellitus continued

INTERVENTION	RATIONALE	EXPECTED OUTCOME
• Instruct mother on how to lie in a left recumbent position after eating and record how many fetal movements she feels in an hour.	• More than five fetal kicks in an hour are indicative of fetal well-being.	
Collaborative: Perform oxytocin challenge test (OCT)/contraction stress test (CST) and nonstress tests as determined by physician.	• Fetal surveillance testing assesses fetal well-being and adequate placental perfusion.	
• Prepare client for frequent ultrasound assessments.	• Ultrasonography is indicated at 8, 12, 18, 28, and 36–38 weeks per physician's orders to confirm gestational age and fetal well-being.	
• Prepare client for amniocentesis procedure.	• A sample of amniotic fluid contains two phospholipids (lecithin/sphingomyelin) that can be used to detect fetal lung maturity and enables medical personnel to prepare for a potential preterm birth.	
• Assist physician with biophysical profile assessment.	• Helps ensure fetal well-being and a positive fetal outcome.	

3. Nursing Diagnosis: Health-Seeking Behaviors: Information About the Effects of Blood Sugar on Pregnancy related to an expressed desire to maintain stable blood glucose levels

Goal: The client and her family will verbalize the importance of maintaining blood sugar within prescribed ranges during pregnancy.

INTERVENTION	RATIONALE	EXPECTED OUTCOME
• Assess the client and family's cognitive level and develop a teaching strategy that will facilitate learning at that level.	• Behavior changes occur when teaching strategies are appropriate for the client and family's cognitive level.	• *The client and family members will verbalize understanding of the effects of blood sugar fluctuations on pregnancy as evidenced by asking questions and seeking health information when necessary. The client adheres to personal treatment regimen throughout pregnancy.*
• Teach blood glucose monitoring, insulin administration, and predicted insulin needs throughout pregnancy, and then have client and family members repeat the discussion.	• Basic understanding of the relationship between blood sugar levels and how insulin needs change throughout pregnancy will foster compliance with prescribed regimen.	
• Emphasize the importance of maintaining a healthy diet and exercise program during pregnancy. Encourage client and family to develop a sample diabetic diet and exercise regimen that is appropriate for pregnancy while present in the clinic or hospital and evaluate for appropriateness.	• Involves the client and her family members in her care, and the evaluation method promotes positive reinforcement and a time for modifications of regimen if necessary.	
• Emphasize the importance of prenatal care for the purpose of maternal and fetal surveillance.	• Frequent prenatal visits allow for modifications in regimen and promote a healthy pregnancy outcome.	

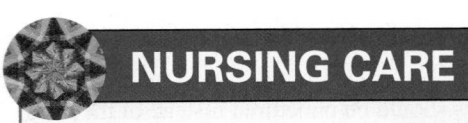

NURSING CARE PLAN

The Woman with Diabetes Mellitus continued

INTERVENTION	RATIONALE	EXPECTED OUTCOME
4. Nursing Diagnosis: Risk for Infection related to increased levels of glucose in urine		
Goal: The client will have no urinary tract infections (UTIs) during pregnancy.		
• Encourage client to utilize preventive measures to prevent UTIs: increasing intake of water and cranberry juice, wearing cotton underwear, wiping perineum from front to back, voiding frequently, and voiding before and immediately after sexual intercourse.	• Utilizing preventive measures decreases the likelihood of client acquiring a UTI.	• *Client will remain free of UTIs during pregnancy as evidenced by verbalizing and complying with appropriate preventive measures, increasing fluid intake, and identifying negative urine samples during prenatal visits.*
• Instruct client on the signs and symptoms of UTIs: urinary frequency, dysuria, cloudy urine, hematuria, lower back pain, and foul-smelling urine.	• Client will be aware of signs and symptoms of UTIs and report to physician for immediate intervention.	
Collaborative:		
• Instruct client on how to obtain a clean-catch urine sample and send to lab for culture and sensitivity per physician's orders.	• A clean-catch urine sample will contain bacteria if a UTI is present.	
• Administer prescribed antibiotic therapy and teach client about medication, adverse effects, and appropriate dosage.	• Antibiotic therapy is the appropriate treatment for a UTI. Compliance increases when a client fully understands medication regimen.	
• Encourage client to drink 8–10 glasses of water each day.	• Increased fluid intake assists in flushing bacteria out of the urinary tract system.	
5. Nursing Diagnosis: Anxiety related to unfamiliarity with diagnosis		
Goal: The client expresses less anxiety.		
• Assess client's level of anxiety (mild-1, moderate-2, or severe-3) and have client verbalize causes of anxiety.	• Verbalization of anxiety provokers encourages expression of feelings and questions.	• *The client demonstrates appropriate coping strategies as evidenced by utilizing resources efficiently and verbalizing feelings of anxiety and the ways to deal with them.*
• Share information on diabetes care such as nutrition, exercise, and glucose control in a clear and concise manner.	• Accurate information gives the client a sense of control and comfort.	
• Instruct client on anxiety-reducing techniques such as imagery, breathing exercises, and massage used in pregnancy.	• Gives client the tools necessary for decreasing anxiety.	
• Refer client to a diabetes support group.	• A support group allows clients with similar problems to express concerns and share information with each other.	

Figure 19–4 ◆ The nurse teaches the pregnant woman with gestational diabetes mellitus how to do home glucose monitoring. SOURCE: Photographer, Jenny Thomas.

doses she is to receive daily, and the correct procedure for its administration. The woman's partner is also instructed about insulin administration in case it should be necessary for him to give it. For some highly motivated women whose glucose levels are not well controlled with multiple injections, the continuous insulin infusion pump may improve glucose control.

The nurse teaches the client how and when to monitor her blood sugar, the desired range of blood sugar levels, and the importance of good control (Figure 19–4 ◆). Most women use a glucose meter because it provides a more accurate reading. The nurse teaches the client to follow the manufacturer's directions exactly, to wash hands thoroughly before puncturing her finger, and to touch the blood droplet, not her finger, to the test pad on the strip.

With a blood glucose meter, an electronic eye measures the blood sugar, and a digital reading is given. The blood droplet should cover the test pad because uncovered portions are read as low sugar. The glucose meter is a portable pocket-sized device that is more accurate than the visual, color comparison method. Some meters are able to store and recall a specified number of readings, which helps ensure the accuracy of recorded results.

CLINICAL TIP

When teaching a pregnant woman to do her own blood glucose testing, have gloves available and put them on if it becomes necessary to help the woman obtain a blood sample. The woman does not need to wear gloves during the procedure.

Also be sure to wear gloves when doing finger sticks for blood glucose levels, when testing the urine for ketones, when starting an IV for insulin therapy, or when drawing blood for other laboratory tests.

The nurse may offer the client the following tips about finger puncture:

- Various spring-loaded devices are available that make puncturing easier.
- Hanging the arm down for 30 seconds increases blood flow to the fingers.
- Warming the hands under running water increases blood flow to them.
- The sides of fingers should be punctured instead of the ends because the ends contain more pain-sensitive nerves.

Clients with diabetes need to keep a record of each blood sugar reading as a guide for management. Specific record sheets are available for this purpose and should be brought to each visit.

Planned Exercise Program

Exercise is encouraged for the woman's overall well-being. If she is used to a regular exercise program, she is encouraged to continue. She is advised to exercise after meals (when blood sugar levels are high), to wear diabetic identification, to carry a simple sugar such as hard candy (because of the possibility of exercise-induced hypoglycemia), to monitor her blood glucose levels regularly, and to avoid injecting insulin into an extremity that will soon be used during exercise.

If she has not been following a regular exercise plan, she is encouraged to begin gradually. Because exercise can alter metabolism, the woman's blood glucose should be well controlled before she begins an exercise program. Women with GDM should not use unusual, strenuous, and excessive exercise in an attempt to reduce glucose levels (ACOG, 2001).

Teaching for Self-Care

Using the information gained during the nursing assessment of the pregnant woman with diabetes, the nurse provides appropriate teaching to the woman and her family so that the woman can meet her own healthcare needs as much as possible.

- *Glucose monitoring.* Home blood glucose monitoring is the most accurate and convenient way to determine insulin dose and assess control. It should be taught at the first visit after the diagnosis of gestational diabetes has been established. The woman with pregestational diabetes may already be monitoring her own blood sugar. Women are taught to perform the procedure four to six times per day—generally at least a fasting blood sugar before breakfast, then a postprandial test 2 hours after each meal. Women are encouraged to maintain blood sugars in the normal ranges as follows: fasting (before eating or taking insulin), less than 95 mg/dL; 2 hours after each meal less than 120 mg/dL (ACOG, 2005). New technology that is capable of automatically and painlessly monitoring blood glucose levels is currently being investigated and shows great promise.

- *Symptoms of abnormal blood glucose levels.* The pregnant diabetic woman must recognize symptoms of changing glucose levels—whether hypoglycemia or hyperglycemia accompanied by ketoacidosis—and take appropriate action by immediately checking her capillary blood glucose level. Hypoglycemia may develop fairly rapidly. Symptoms include sweating, periodic tingling, disorientation, shakiness, pallor, clammy skin, irritability, hunger, headache, and blurred vision. If the pregnant woman is hypoglycemic with a blood glucose level less than 65 to 70 mg/dL, she is advised to take 20 g of carbohydrate, wait 20 minutes, and then retest her glucose level. She can obtain the necessary carbohydrate by drinking 1 cup of skim milk, 1/2 cup orange or apple juice, or 1/2 cup cola or by eating 1 tbsp honey or brown sugar (Cleveland Clinic, 2003). Many people overtreat their symptoms by continuing to eat. This can cause a rebound hyperglycemia. The woman should carry a snack at all times and should have other fast sources of glucose (simple carbohydrates such as hard candy) at hand so that she can treat an insulin reaction when milk is not available. Family members are also taught how to inject glucagon in the event that food does not work or is not feasible, for instance, in the presence of severe morning sickness.

Hyperglycemia and ketoacidosis typically develop more slowly and tend to occur more commonly during the second half of pregnancy. Because most problems for the fetus are related to maternal hyperglycemia, this is a serious situation. Symptoms include polyuria, polydipsia, dry mouth, fatigue, nausea, hot flushed skin, rapid deep breathing, abdominal cramps, acetone breath, headache, drowsiness, depressed reflexes, oliguria or anuria, stupor, or coma. Hyperglycemia is treated with insulin.

- *Smoking.* Smoking has harmful effects on the maternal vascular system and the developing fetus and is contraindicated for both pregnancy and diabetes.

- *Travel.* Insulin can be kept at room temperature while traveling. Insulin supplies should be kept with the traveler and not packed in the baggage. Most airlines can supply special meals if notified a few days before departure. The woman should wear a diabetic identification bracelet or necklace. In addition, the woman should check with her physician for any instructions or advice before leaving.

- *Support groups.* Many communities have diabetes support groups or education classes, which can be helpful to women with newly diagnosed diabetes.

- *Cesarean birth.* Chances for a cesarean birth increase if the pregnant woman is diabetic because of the risk of fetal macrosomia and shoulder dystocia. This possibility should be anticipated—enrollment in cesarean birth preparation classes may be suggested. Many hospitals offer classes, and information is available through other organizations. The couple may prefer simply to discuss cesarean birth with the nurse and their obstetrician and read some books on the topic.

HOSPITAL-BASED NURSING CARE

Hospitalization may become necessary during the pregnancy to evaluate blood glucose levels and adjust insulin dosages. In such cases, nurses monitor the woman's status and continue to provide teaching so that the woman is knowledgeable about her condition and its management. During the intrapartal period, the nurse must have a clear understanding about the impact of labor on the condition. The nurse carefully monitors the woman's status, maintains her intravenous fluids, is alert for signs of hypoglycemia, and provides the care indicated for any woman in labor. If a cesarean birth is indicated, the nurse provides appropriate care as described in Chapter 27. ∞

Evaluation

Expected outcomes of nursing care include the following:

- The woman is able to discuss her condition and its possible impact on her pregnancy, labor and birth, and postpartal period.

- The woman participates in developing a healthcare regimen to meet her needs and follows it throughout her pregnancy.

- The woman avoids developing hypoglycemia or hyperglycemia.

- The woman gives birth to a healthy newborn.

- The woman is able to care for her newborn.

CARE OF THE WOMAN WITH ANEMIA

Anemia indicates inadequate levels of hemoglobin (Hb) in the blood. *Anemia* is defined as hemoglobin less than 12 g/dL in nonpregnant women and less than 11 g/dL in pregnant women (Cuervo & Mahomed, 2005). Race, altitude, smoking, nutrition, and medications can affect the normal limits of hemoglobin. The lower limit of normal tends to be higher for women who smoke and those who live at higher altitudes because their bodies require a greater quantity of red blood cells to maintain their tissue oxygen levels. For example, a pregnant woman who lives in Denver, Colorado (elevation 5280 feet), would be considered anemic if her hemoglobin dropped below 10.5 g/dL. Similarly, the lower limit of normal for a pregnant woman who smokes 1/2 to 1 pack of cigarettes per day would increase by 0.3 g/dL to 10.3 g/dL (Varney, Kriebs, & Gegor, 2004). Reference tables are available that indicate these adjustments in the lower level of normal hemoglobin.

The common anemias of pregnancy are due either to insufficient hemoglobin production related to nutritional deficiency in iron or folic acid during pregnancy, or to hemoglobin destruction in inherited disorders, specifically sickle cell anemia and thalassemia.

Iron Deficiency Anemia

Dietary iron is needed to synthesize hemoglobin. Because hemoglobin is necessary to transport oxygen, a deficiency of iron may affect the body's transport of oxygen.

Iron deficiency anemia is the most common medical complication of pregnancy, primarily as a consequence of expansion of plasma volume without normal expansion of maternal hemoglobin mass (Cuervo & Mahomed, 2005). Approximately 200 mg of iron will be conserved because of the functional amenorrhea of pregnancy, but a pregnant woman needs approximately 1000 mg more iron intake during the pregnancy. Between 300 and 400 mg of iron is transferred to the fetus; 500 mg is needed for the increased red blood cell mass in the woman's own increased circulating blood volume; another 100 mg is needed for the placenta; and about 280 mg is needed to replace the 1 mg of iron lost daily through feces, urine, and sweat.

The greatest need for increased iron intake occurs in the second half of pregnancy. When the iron needs of pregnancy are not met, maternal hemoglobin falls below 11 g/dL. Serum ferritin levels, indicating iron stores, are below 12 mg/L.

Many women begin pregnancy in a slightly anemic state. In pregnancy, mild anemia can rapidly become more severe; therefore, it needs immediate treatment.

MATERNAL RISKS

The woman with iron deficiency anemia may be asymptomatic, but she is more susceptible to infection, may tire easily, has an increased chance of preeclampsia and postpartal hemorrhage, and tolerates poorly even minimal blood loss during birth. Healing of an episiotomy or an incision may be delayed. If the anemia is severe (Hb less than 6 g/dL), cardiac failure may ensue.

FETAL-NEONATAL RISKS

There is evidence of increased risk of low birth weight, prematurity, stillbirth, and neonatal death in infants of women with severe iron deficiency (maternal Hb less than 6 g/dL). The infant is not iron deficient at birth because of active transport of iron across the placenta, even when maternal iron stores are low. However, these babies do have lower iron stores and are at increased risk for developing iron deficiency during infancy.

CLINICAL THERAPY

The first goal of health care is to prevent iron deficiency anemia. If it occurs, the goal is to return low iron and hemoglobin levels to normal. To prevent anemia, the American Academy of Pediatrics and the American College of Obstetricians and Gynecologists (2002) recommend that pregnant women take at least 27 mg supplements of iron daily. This amount is contained in most prenatal vitamins. In addition, the woman should be encouraged to eat an iron-rich diet. To prevent constipation, the most common side effect of iron supplementation, a stool softener may be necessary.

If anemia is diagnosed, the dosage should be increased to 60 to 120 mg per day of iron. If the woman remains anemic after 1 month of therapy, further evaluation is indicated. With a twin pregnancy, a larger dose is needed. If a large dose of oral iron causes vomiting, diarrhea, or constipation, or if the anemia is discovered late in pregnancy, parenteral iron may be needed.

NURSING CARE MANAGEMENT
Nursing Assessment and Diagnosis

The main presenting symptom of iron deficiency anemia may be fatigue. Nutritional history usually gives evidence of poor dietary intake of iron. Physical examination reveals pallor of skin and conjunctiva. Laboratory studies show hemoglobin values below 10 g/dL, serum ferritin levels below 12 mg/L, and possibly microcytic and hypochromic red blood cells (a late finding).

Nursing diagnoses that may apply to a pregnant woman with iron deficiency anemia include the following:

- **Risk for Imbalanced Nutrition: Less than Body Requirements** related to inadequate intake of iron-containing foods
- **Constipation** related to daily intake of iron supplements

Nursing Plan and Implementation

The nurse stresses the importance of an iron-rich diet and of iron supplements during pregnancy. Supplements are indicated because dietary sources cannot meet the extra requirements. The woman is taught to take iron tablets with vitamin C (e.g., orange juice) to increase absorption. Iron absorption is reduced by 40% to 50% if the tablets are taken with meals. However, gastrointestinal upset is more likely if they are taken on an empty stomach. The client may tolerate the iron better if she starts with small doses and gradually increases the dosage over several days. She is informed that her stool will turn black and may be more formed. She is also advised to keep the tablets out of the reach of children because ingestion may be fatal to a young child.

Evaluation

Expected outcomes of nursing care include the following:

- The woman is able to identify the risks associated with iron deficiency anemia during pregnancy.
- The woman takes her iron supplements as recommended.
- The woman's Hb levels remain normal or return to normal during her pregnancy.

Folic Acid Deficiency Anemia

Folate deficiency is the most common cause of megaloblastic anemia during pregnancy, affecting between 1% and 4% of pregnant women in the United States. It is more prevalent with twin pregnancies.

Folic acid is needed for DNA and RNA synthesis and cell duplication. In its absence, immature red blood cells fail to divide, become enlarged (megaloblastic), and are fewer in number. Even more significantly, an inadequate intake of folic acid has been associated with neural tube defects (NTDs) (spina bifida, anencephaly, meningomyelocele) in the fetus or newborn. With the tremendous cell multiplication that occurs in pregnancy, an adequate amount of folic acid is crucial. However, increased urinary excretion of folic acid and fetal uptake can rapidly result in folic acid deficiency.

CLINICAL THERAPY

Diagnosis of folic acid deficiency anemia may be difficult, and it is usually not detected until late in pregnancy or the early puerperium. This is because serum folate levels normally fall as pregnancy progresses. Even though folate levels are lower with deficiency, they will fluctuate with diet. Measurement of erythrocyte folate status is more reliable but indicates folate status of several weeks previously. Women with true folic acid deficiency anemia often present with nausea, vomiting, and anorexia. Hemoglobin levels as low as 3 to 5 g/dL may be found. Typically the blood smear reveals that the newly formed erythrocytes are macrocytic.

Folic acid deficiency during pregnancy is prevented by a daily supplement of 0.4 mg of folate. Treatment of deficiency consists of 1-mg folic acid supplement. Because iron deficiency anemia almost always coexists with folic acid deficiency, the woman also needs iron supplements.

NURSING CARE MANAGEMENT

The nurse can help the pregnant woman avoid folate deficiency by teaching her food sources of folic acid and cooking methods for preserving folic acid. The best sources are fresh leafy green vegetables, orange juice, other citrus fruits and juices, red meats, fish, poultry, and legumes. As much as 50% to 90% of folic acid can be lost by cooking in large volumes of water. Microwave cooking destroys more folic acid than conventional cooking.

The FDA requires the addition of folic acid for all foods labeled "enriched." Even with this addition, the US Public Health Service recommends that all women of childbearing age (15 to 45 years) consume 0.4 mg of folic acid daily. This recommendation is important because half of all US pregnancies are unplanned and NTDs occur very early in pregnancy (3 to 4 weeks after conception), before most women realize they are pregnant (CDC, 2004). Nurses can play a crucial role in helping young women become aware of this important recommendation.

Sickle Cell Anemia

Sickle cell anemia (HbSS) is a recessive autosomal disorder in which the normal adult hemoglobin, hemoglobin A (HbA), is abnormally formed. It occurs primarily in people of African descent and occasionally in people of Southeast Asian or Mediterranean origin (i.e., Greeks, Italians, Arabs, and Turks) (Buchanan, DeBaun, Quinn et al., 2004). The anemia is characterized by acute, recurring episodes of tissue, abdominal, and joint pain. Individuals with the disorder are homozygous for the sickle cell gene. They inherit from each parent an allele causing an amino acid substitution in the two beta protein chains in the hemoglobin molecule. This abnormal hemoglobin is called hemoglobin S (HbS). Heterozygous individuals are carriers for sickle cell anemia but are usually asymptomatic. This condition is called sickle cell trait (HbSA). One of the beta protein chains formed in their hemoglobin is normal; the other has the amino acid substitution. Sickle cell trait occurs in 1 out of 12 African Americans; sickle cell anemia is found in 1 out of 576 (Cunningham, Leveno, Bloom et al., 2005).

HbS causes the red blood cells to be sickle or crescent shaped. In conditions of low oxygenation, normal hemoglobin is soluble, but HbS becomes semisolid and distorts the red blood cell shape. These erythrocytes easily interlock and clog capillaries, particularly in organs characterized by slow flow and high oxygen extraction, such as the spleen, bone marrow, and pla-

centa. This phenomenon, called *sickling,* varies in frequency depending on the amount of the HbS in the red blood cells (there is seldom a crisis with levels below 40%) and other hemoglobin factors. Diagnosis is confirmed by hemoglobin electrophoresis or a test to induce sickling in a blood sample. Prenatal diagnosis of sickle cell disease is also available now (ACOG, 2000a).

MATERNAL RISKS

Women with sickle cell trait have a good prognosis for pregnancy if they have adequate nutrition and prenatal care. They are, however, at increased risk for nephritis, bacteriuria, and hematuria, and tend to become anemic.

Women with sickle cell anemia have considerably more risk during pregnancy. Low oxygen pressure—caused by high temperature, dehydration, infection, or acidosis, for example—may precipitate a vaso-occlusive crisis. The crisis produces sudden attacks of pain that may be general or localized in bones or joints, lungs, abdominal organs, or the spinal cord. The pain is due to ischemia in the tissues from occluded capillaries. Vaso-occlusive crises occur more often in the second half of pregnancy.

Maternal mortality due to sickle cell anemia is rare. However, 50% to 67% of pregnant women with sickle cell anemia develop infections, often urinary tract infections or pulmonary infections, because of impaired immune functioning (Serjeant, Loy, Crowther et al., 2004). Congestive heart failure or acute renal failure may also occur.

FETAL-NEONATAL RISKS

The incidence of fetal death during and immediately following an attack has decreased greatly in recent years but is still high. Perinatal mortality is estimated to be 18% (Serjeant et al., 2004). Prematurity and IUGR are also associated with sickle cell anemia. Fetal death is believed to be due to sickling attacks in the placenta.

CLINICAL THERAPY

Because the woman with sickle cell anemia maintains her hemoglobin levels by intense erythropoiesis, additional folic acid supplements (1 mg/day) are required. Maternal infection should be treated promptly because dehydration and fever can trigger sickling and crisis. Vaso-occlusive crisis is best treated by a perinatal team in a medical center. Proper management requires close observation and evaluation of all symptoms. The term *sickle cell crisis* should be applied only after all other possible causes for the pain are excluded (Serjeant et al., 2004).

Rehydration with intravenous fluids; administration of oxygen, antibiotics, and analgesics; and monitoring of fetal heart rate are important aspects of therapy. Antiembolism stockings are used postpartally.

If vaso-occlusive crisis occurs during labor, the previous therapies are instituted and the woman is kept in a left lateral position. Oxytocics may be used if needed to promote labor. Episiotomy and outlet forceps are recommended to shorten the second stage of labor.

Several antisickling agents are being researched, and in the future sickle cell crisis may be prevented.

NURSING CARE MANAGEMENT
Nursing Assessment and Diagnosis

The woman with sickle cell anemia usually relates a history of frequent illnesses and recurrent abdominal and joint pains and is found to be extremely anemic. The woman may appear undernourished and have long, thin extremities. Ulcers are often present on her ankles. Anemia may be severe.

A diagnosis of sickle cell anemia is confirmed by hemoglobin electrophoresis or a test to induce sickling in a blood sample. The woman is assessed for infection, which is associated with one third of sickle cell crises in adults. Infections most often seen during pregnancy or postpartum are pneumonia, urinary tract infections, puerperal endomyometritis, and osteomyelitis.

Fetal status is assessed during a crisis by electronic fetal monitoring. During labor, the woman's vital signs are assessed frequently and continuous fetal heart rate monitoring is initiated. Compatible blood should be available for transfusion. Oxygen is administered if necessary. The woman is assessed for joint pains and other signs of sickle cell crisis.

Nursing diagnoses that might apply to the pregnant woman with sickle cell anemia include the following:

- *Acute Pain* related to the effects of sickle cell crisis
- *Risk for Ineffective Health Maintenance* related to lack of understanding of the need to avoid exposure to infection secondary to the risk of a sickle cell crisis

Nursing Plan and Implementation

The nursing goal for a pregnant woman with sickle cell disease is to provide effective health teaching to help prevent a sickle cell crisis, improve the anemia, and prevent infection. The nurse teaches the woman to increase hydration, use good hygiene, avoid people with infections, seek immediate treatment for infection, and take folic acid supplements (Figure 19–5 ◆). As stated earlier, folic acid is important because of its role in red

Figure 19–5 ◆ Health teaching is an important part of nursing care for the pregnant woman with sickle cell anemia.
SOURCE: Mark Richards/Photo Edit

blood cell production; therefore, folic acid supplements are essential. Bed rest is sometimes recommended to decrease the chance of preterm labor. Other nursing interventions are aimed at facilitating the medical therapy and alleviating anxiety through support and education.

Partners should be screened to evaluate their sickle cell status. If both partners have either sickle cell trait or sickle cell disease, genetic counseling is warranted.

Evaluation

Expected outcomes of nursing care include the following:

- The woman is able to describe her condition and identify its possible impact on her pregnancy, labor and childbirth, and postpartal period.
- The woman takes appropriate healthcare measures to avoid a sickle cell crisis.
- The woman gives birth to a healthy infant.
- The woman and her caregivers quickly identify and successfully manage any complications that arise.

Thalassemia

The thalassemias are a group of autosomal recessive disorders characterized by a defect in the synthesis of the alpha or beta chains in the hemoglobin molecule. The one most frequently encountered in the United States is β-thalassemia. Symptoms are caused by the shortened lifespan of the red blood cells, which result in active erythropoiesis in the liver, spleen, and bones. This produces hepatosplenomegaly and sometimes bony malformations. The thalassemias are seen most often in persons from Greece, Italy, or southern China and are also known as Mediterranean anemia and Cooley anemia. Early identification of thalassemia and preventive management avoids missed diagnosis and unnecessary treatment for iron deficiency anemia (ACOG, 2000a). Prenatal genetic diagnosis is now available for this disorder.

If the woman is heterozygous for β-thalassemia, half of the beta chains are formed normally. This is β-thalassemia minor, or β-thalassemia trait. Mild anemia is usually the only symptom.

Persons born homozygous for the disease have β-thalassemia major. Because newborns have fetal hemoglobin (HbF), which does not have beta chains, no symptoms are present for several months. Once infants with β-thalassemia major start producing adult type hemoglobin (HbA), they develop severe anemia and are dependent on transfusions, from which they eventually develop iron overload. Iron chelation therapy must be instituted soon after chronic transfusions are begun because excess iron damages the liver and heart. Without chelation therapy, these children do not live past the second or third decade, and those who reach puberty are often amenorrheic and infertile.

MATERNAL-FETAL-NEONATAL RISKS

The woman with β-thalassemia minor has mild anemia with small (microcytic) red cells. This mild anemia must be distinguished from iron deficiency anemia because a woman with β-thalassemia minor should not receive iron therapy unless she is also deficient in iron. A woman with iron deficiency anemia typically has low serum iron and serum ferritin levels, whereas the woman with β-thalassemia minor has normal levels. β-thalassemia minor varies in degree of severity from extremely mild (minima) anemia, which results in a relatively smooth pregnancy, to a more symptomatic form (intermedia). Pregnancy is rare in women with β-thalassemia major. If it does occur, the woman generally has severe anemia, needs transfusion therapy, and is at risk for congestive heart failure. These women are generally cared for by a perinatologist in a facility that can accommodate high-risk pregnancies.

CLINICAL THERAPY

Folic acid supplements are indicated for women with thalassemia, but iron supplements are not given. Those with thalassemia intermedia and thalassemia major may need transfusion and chelation therapy. They should avoid exposure to infections and seek treatment promptly if an infection develops. Their care is similar to that of women with sickle cell anemia.

NURSING CARE MANAGEMENT

The woman with thalassemia needs to understand her disease and the possibility of transmitting it to her offspring. These clients have lived with thalassemia since childhood but may have questions about its effect on pregnancy outcome and their own prognosis.

CARE OF THE WOMAN WITH ACQUIRED IMMUNODEFICIENCY SYNDROME (AIDS)

Acquired immunodeficiency syndrome (AIDS), caused by the **human immunodeficiency virus (HIV),** is one of today's major health concerns. By the end of 2003, an estimated 1,039,000 to 1,185,000 persons in the United States were living with HIV/AIDS, with 24% to 27% undiagnosed and unaware of their HIV infection (Glynn & Rhodes, 2005). In 2004, 38,730 new cases of HIV/AIDS were diagnosed in 35 reporting areas (33 states, US Virgin Islands, and Guam). Between 2000 and 2004, the number of persons in the United States living with AIDS increased by 30% (from 320,177 to 415,193), primarily because of better treatment options (CDC, 2005).

Adult and adolescent males are still the largest group of infected individuals (73%). Of this group, infection occurred as follows: homosexual contact (60%), IV drug use (19%), heterosexual contact (13%), and homosexual IV drug users (7%). Among females with HIV/AIDS, 71% were infected through heterosexual contact, whereas 27% were infected because of IV drug use (CDC, 2005).

DEVELOPING CULTURAL COMPETENCE

VARIATIONS IN THE RATE OF HIV/AIDS

The rate of HIV/AIDS–infected individuals varies significantly among races and ethnic groups: 56.4 per 100,000 in the black population, 18.6 per 100,000 in the Hispanic population, and 6 per 100,000 in the white population (CDC, 2005).

In 2004, the cumulative estimated pediatric total of AIDS cases was 9443 including both males and females under the age of 13. Of these pediatric cases, the vast majority were infants who became infected perinatally (CDC, 2005). Fortunately the number of new pediatric AIDS cases is declining rapidly. The decline is associated with (1) the implementation of universal counseling about the risks of transmission from mother to fetus, (2) voluntary testing of pregnant women for the presence of HIV, and (3) the use of zidovudine therapy for infected pregnant women and their infants.

Pathophysiology of HIV/AIDS

HIV found in blood, semen, vaginal fluid, and breast milk has been implicated in disease transmission, although the virus has been isolated in urine, tears, cerebrospinal fluid, lymph nodes, brain tissue, and bone marrow. HIV shedding has also been detected in the genital tract of women.

Once infected with the virus, the individual develops antibodies that can be detected with enzyme-linked immunosorbent assay (ELISA) and confirmed with the Western blot test. Antibodies can be detected in most individuals within 6 months after exposure, but in rare circumstances the latent period is longer. An asymptomatic period lasting from a few months to as long as 17 years (with a median length of 10 years) follows seroconversion. The majority of infected pregnant women fall into this category.

The diagnosis of AIDS is made when an individual is HIV positive and is identified as having one of several specific opportunistic infections. AIDS can also be diagnosed without laboratory evidence of HIV infection when one of the opportunistic infections is definitively diagnosed and there is no other known cause for the immune deficiency.

Maternal Risks

AIDS-defining diseases that are more common in women than men include wasting syndrome, esophageal candidiasis, and herpes simplex virus disease. Kaposi's sarcoma is rare in women. Non-AIDS-defining gynecologic conditions, such as vaginal *Candida* infections and cervical pathology, are prevalent among women at all stages of HIV infection.

Many women who are HIV positive choose to avoid pregnancy because of the risk of infecting the fetus and the likelihood of dying before the child is raised. Women who are asymptomatic and who do become pregnant should be advised that pregnancy is not believed to accelerate the progression of

HIV/AIDS. In contrast, women with low $CD4^+$ counts who are symptomatic have been reported to have accelerated progression of the disease during pregnancy (Ibrahim, Moodley, & Doorasamy, 2004). The use of zidovudine (ZDV), formerly called azidothymidine (AZT), during pregnancy significantly reduces the risk of transmitting HIV to the fetus, and most medications used to treat HIV can be taken safely during pregnancy.

Fetal-Neonatal Risks

HIV transmission can occur during pregnancy and through breast milk; however, it is believed that at least half of all infection occurs during labor and birth. Beginning in the early 1990s, rates of mother-to-child transmission of HIV began to decrease in Europe and the United States, possibly because of changes in clinical management. For HIV-infected pregnant women who receive no prophylactic medication, the rate of transmission to the newborn is about 15% to 25%. However, for HIV-infected pregnant women who receive prophylactic therapy with ZDV, give birth by elective cesarean at 38 weeks (before rupture of membranes), and avoid breastfeeding, the rate of transmission drops to less than 2% (Public Health Service Task Force, 2005). These decreases in transmission are dramatic and impressive.

Following birth, infants will often have a positive antibody titer, which reflects the passive transfer of maternal antibodies and does not indicate HIV infection. Although infected infants are usually asymptomatic at birth, they are likely to be premature, low birth weight, and SGA. However, these findings are associated with several socioeconomic factors and may not be unique to HIV infection (Wei, Msamanga, Spiegelman et al., 2004). The signs of AIDS in infants may include failure to thrive, hepatosplenomegaly, interstitial lymphocytic pneumonia, recurrent infections, cell-mediated immunodeficiency, evidence of Epstein-Barr virus, and neurologic abnormalities. Recurrent bacterial infections are common in children with AIDS; Kaposi's sarcoma is rare. Encephalopathy, characterized by delayed developmental milestones or the loss of acquired skills, including cognitive abilities, is found in 50% to 90% of children with AIDS. Treatments that prevent the CNS effects of HIV have yet to be identified. The prognosis for an infected child remains poor.

Clinical Therapy

Early knowledge of a woman's HIV status is important for her well-being and that of her child. Thus the revised CDC screening guidelines for pregnant women state that HIV screening should be emphasized as a routine part of all prenatal care. To this end, the recommendation that all pregnant women should be tested for HIV has been strengthened while continuing to ensure that testing of pregnant women and their infants is voluntary and informed (Public Health Service Task Force, 2005). Initial testing is done using ELISA, followed by a confirmatory Western blot assay. Women who test positive should be counseled about the implications of the diagnosis for themselves and their fetus to ensure an informed reproductive choice. The care of the woman who chooses to continue her pregnancy should focus on stabilizing the disease, preventing opportunistic infections and transmission of the virus from mother to fetus, and providing psychosocial and educational support.

Antiretroviral therapy should be recommended to all infected pregnant women to reduce the rate of perinatal transmission. A triple therapy approach is recommended during the prenatal period. It includes ZDV, a nucleoside analog, plus a second nucleoside analog such as zalcitabine, didanosine, or lamivudine combined with a protease inhibitor such as indinavir, ritonavir, or saquinavir. Alternatively, the ZDV and second nucleoside analog can be combined with a nonnucleoside analog such as nevirapine or delavirdine (Public Health Service Task Force, 2005). Treatment recommendations have also been developed for the mother and infant for the intrapartum and postpartum periods. The decision about which regimen is most appropriate should be determined following discussion with the woman about the risks and benefits based on her individual HIV status.

HIV-infected women should be evaluated and treated for other sexually transmitted infections and for conditions occurring more commonly in women with HIV, such as tuberculosis, cytomegalovirus, toxoplasmosis, and cervical dysplasia. HIV-infected women with no history of hepatitis B should receive the hepatitis vaccine, which is not contraindicated prenatally, as well as the pneumococcal vaccine and an annual flu shot. In addition to routine prenatal laboratory tests, a platelet count and a complete blood count with differential should be obtained at the first prenatal visit and repeated each trimester to identify anemia, thrombocytopenia, and leukopenia, which are associated both with HIV infection and with antiviral therapy.

COMPLEMENTARY AND ALTERNATIVE THERAPIES

GARLIC SUPPLEMENTS INTERFERE WITH HIV MEDICATION

Garlic has been well regarded as a natural way of combating elevated cholesterol levels. This has made it attractive to many HIV-positive individuals on combination drug therapy because increased cholesterol is a side effect of treatment. However, research has revealed that garlic supplements may actually interfere with the effectiveness of the HIV medication saquinavir, a protease inhibitor, which is usually prescribed in combination with other HIV medications.

The study was conducted with nine healthy, HIV-negative volunteers. Blood analysis revealed that the blood concentrations of saquinavir decreased by over 50% when the volunteers took garlic caplets twice daily for 3 weeks. Moreover, even after a 10-day period with no garlic, the participants' blood levels were about 35% lower than the expected baseline.

At present, researchers do not know what impact the garlic supplements would have on a combined medication regimen but they do recommend that individuals on saquinavir *avoid* taking garlic supplements.

SOURCES: National Institutes of Health News Release. (2001, December 5). Retrieved November 17, 2002, from http://www.nih.gov/news; Piscitelli, S. C., et al. (2001, December 3). The effect of garlic supplements on the pharmacokinetics of saquinavir [Electronic edition]. *Clinical Infectious Diseases*.

The woman with HIV also should be assessed regularly for serologic changes that indicate the disease is progressing. This is determined by the absolute CD4$^+$ T-lymphocyte count, which provides the number of helper T4 cells. When CD4$^+$ counts fall to 200/mm^3 or lower, opportunistic infections such as *Pneumocystis carinii* pneumonia are more likely to develop, and prophylaxis may need to be instituted (Public Health Service Task Force, 2005).

At each prenatal visit, asymptomatic HIV-infected women are monitored for early signs of complications, such as weight loss in the second or third trimester or fever. The woman is asked about signs of vaginal infection. Her mouth is inspected for signs of infections such as thrush (candidiasis) or hairy leukoplakia; her lungs are auscultated for signs of pneumonia; and her lymph nodes, liver, and spleen are palpated for signs of enlargement. Each trimester the woman should have a visual examination and a funduscopic examination to detect such complications as toxoplasmosis retinitis. Further discussion of therapy for the pregnant woman who is HIV positive or who has AIDS may be found in journal articles and specialty texts.

A pregnancy complicated by HIV infection, even if asymptomatic, is considered high risk, and the fetus is monitored closely. Weekly NST is begun at 32 weeks' gestation, and serial ultrasounds are done to detect IUGR. Biophysical profiles are also indicated (see Chapter 21 ∞). Invasive procedures such as amniocentesis are avoided when possible to prevent the contamination of a noninfected infant.

ACOG (2000b) recommends that scheduled cesarean birth should be discussed with HIV-positive pregnant women. This procedure may be done as early as 38 weeks' gestation to decrease the risk of rupture of the membranes. Other authorities have expressed concern that cesarean birth may increase the HIV-infected woman's risk of complications following surgery. They suggest that the use of combined antiretroviral therapy reduces the risk of vertical transmission of infection significantly (Public Health Service Task Force, 2005).

Intrapartal care is similar to that for all pregnant women, although strict adherence to universal precautions is crucial to avoid nosocomial infection. To prevent exposure of an uninfected infant to HIV during labor and birth, invasive procedures such as vaginal examinations following rupture of the membranes, fetal scalp electrode monitoring, fetal scalp sampling, and vacuum extraction should be done only after carefully evaluating the risks and benefits (ACOG, 2000b).

Women who are HIV positive are at increased risk for complications such as intrapartal or postpartal hemorrhage, postpartal infection, poor wound healing, and infections of the genitourinary tract. Thus they need careful monitoring and appropriate therapy as indicated.

Following childbirth, the HIV-positive woman should be referred to a physician knowledgeable about treating individuals with HIV infection. Because of the profound implications of HIV infection for the woman, her family, the fetus/newborn, and her healthcare providers, screening is recommended for all pregnant women, but especially those at increased risk, including the following: prostitutes; women with multiple sexual partners; women whose current or previous sex partners have been bisexual, have abused IV drugs, had hemophilia, or tested positive for HIV; women who are or have been IV drug users; and women from countries where heterosexual transmission is common. In addition, clinics located in areas with a large HIV-positive population may require routine HIV screening of all prenatal clients.

NURSING CARE MANAGEMENT
Nursing Assessment and Diagnosis

A woman who tests positive for HIV may be asymptomatic or may present with any of the following signs or symptoms: fatigue, anemia, malaise, progressive weight loss, lymphadenopathy, night sweats, diarrhea, fever, neurologic dysfunction, cell-mediated immunodeficiency, or evidence of Kaposi's sarcoma (purplish, reddish brown lesions, either externally or internally).

If a woman tests HIV positive or is involved in a relationship or an activity that places her at high risk, the nurse should assess the woman's knowledge level about the disease, its implications for her and her fetus, and self-care measures the woman can take.

Examples of nursing diagnoses that might apply for an HIV-positive pregnant woman include the following:

- *Risk for Ineffective Health Maintenance* related to lack of information about HIV/AIDS and its long-term implications for the woman and her unborn child
- *Risk for Infection* related to altered immunity secondary to HIV/AIDS
- *Compromised Family Coping* related to the implications of a positive HIV test in one of the family members

I've been a nurse for 35 years now, and I've never seen anything change nursing practice more than HIV/AIDS has. Nursing students today will take universal precautions for granted because they won't know any other way, but I can remember when we could touch more freely. I remember drying a newly born infant and stroking him—my hands warm against his skin. I remember a time when people didn't think twice before trying to stop bleeding or give other first aid at an accident scene. I know this way is safer, but a part of me mourns what we have lost.

Nursing Plan and Implementation
COMMUNITY-BASED NURSING CARE

Nurses need to help women understand that HIV/AIDS is a fatal disease. HIV infection can be avoided if women avoid sharing IV drug needles and practice safe sex, including insisting that their sex partners wear a latex condom for each act of intercourse.

Women at risk for AIDS should be offered premarital and prepregnancy screening for HIV antibodies (ACOG, 2004). They should be given clear information about the implications of a diagnosis of HIV, including societal attitudes. Access to information about the disease and about the test results empowers women by enabling them to make informed decisions about their sexual activities and about becoming pregnant.

A detailed drug and sexual history of each prenatal client is the first step in perinatal HIV/AIDS prevention. All women should be offered HIV counseling. The following are counseling guidelines for HIV testing:

- The nurse should discuss HIV testing during the normal prenatal assessment.

- The nurse should assure the woman of confidentiality, explaining the difference between anonymity and confidentiality.

- The nurse should provide an environment that is private, comfortable, and nonjudgmental.

- The nurse should provide the woman with information about AIDS, including pathophysiology, mode of transmission of HIV, high-risk behaviors, and methods of decreasing transmission, such as practicing safe sex and not sharing needles.

- If the woman chooses to have an antibody test for HIV (ELISA, Western blot), written consent should be obtained.

- Posttest counseling should be provided. A negative test means that no HIV antibodies were found; it does not ensure that the woman has not been infected with the virus, because antibodies may not be detected for 6 weeks to 6 months after exposure.

- If test results are positive, supportive follow-up is necessary. This includes an explanation of the implications for the woman and her unborn child as well as the value of ZDV therapy, recommended medical therapy, follow-up of sex partners, transmission prevention, discussion of immediate posttest plans, and referral to appropriate psychologic and educational services. The nurse should tell the woman not to donate blood or blood products and not to share toothbrushes, razors, and other implements that could be contaminated with blood.

This information can be overwhelming to the woman who is HIV positive and should be provided orally and in writing. She will need more than one counseling session to absorb the information. The initial reaction may be one of shock or denial, so it is important for the nurse to allow her a little time to think and to give her empathy and support. The nurse needs to stress that being HIV positive does not mean that the woman has AIDS but that she can transmit the virus to others (by sexual contact, sharing IV drug needles, and donating blood) and to her fetus during pregnancy or childbirth or by breastfeeding. Most people develop AIDS within 10 years of being infected with HIV. It is currently impossible to prevent AIDS from developing in people who are HIV positive or to predict when they will develop the disease.

In monitoring the asymptomatic HIV-positive pregnant woman, the nurse should be alert for nonspecific symptoms such as fever, weight loss, fatigue, persistent candidiasis, diarrhea, cough, skin lesions, and behavior changes. Laboratory findings—such as decreased hemoglobin, hematocrit, and T4 lymphocytes; elevated erythrocyte sedimentation rate (ESR); and abnormal complete blood count, differential, and platelets—may indicate complications or progression of the disease.

Education about optimal nutrition and maintenance of wellness are important and should be reviewed frequently with the woman.

HOSPITAL-BASED NURSING CARE

The Nursing Care Plan for the Woman with HIV Infection beginning on page 469 summarizes essential nursing management during the antepartum, intrapartum, and postpartum periods.

In community and hospital settings, the nurse faces the important task of taking the precautions necessary to protect staff, other clients, and families from exposure to HIV while meeting the needs of the childbearing woman with this infection.

In 1987 the CDC stated that the prevalence of AIDS and the risk of exposure faced by healthcare workers is significant enough that *precautions should be taken with all clients* (not only those with known HIV infection), especially in dealing with blood and body fluids. These practices are now called *standard precautions.*

Nurses who deal with childbearing families are exposed to blood and body fluids and should pay careful attention to the CDC guidelines, which are addressed in introductory nursing courses in preparation for clinical practice. Protocols have been established for postexposure treatment of caregivers who experience a needle stick or exposure to the body fluids of a person with HIV or a person whose HIV status is not known. The effectiveness of such therapy, using a combined drug approach, depends on starting therapy rapidly. Thus such exposure should be reported immediately.

TEACHING FOR SELF-CARE

The psychologic implications of HIV/AIDS for the childbearing family are staggering. The woman is faced with the knowledge that she and her newborn, if infected, have a decreased life expectancy. If her infant is not infected, she must face the probability that others will raise her child. She may have feelings of fear, helplessness, anger, and isolation. If she shares her diagnosis with others, she may face rejection and condemnation. The couple must deal with the impact of the illness on the partner, who may or may not be infected, and on other children. Dealing with the tasks and responsibilities of a newborn may be especially difficult if the woman is physically depleted or if she is trying to come to grips with the long-term implications of her condition.

The nonjudgmental, supportive nurse plays an essential role in preserving confidentiality and the client's right to privacy. In addition, the nurse can help ensure that the woman receives complete, accurate information about her condition and ways she might cope. This usually involves a referral to social services for follow-up care.

Evaluation

Expected outcomes of nursing care include the following:

- The woman discusses the implications of her positive HIV antibody screen (or diagnosis of AIDS), its implications for herself and her unborn child, the method of transmission, and treatment options.

NURSING CARE PLAN

The Woman with HIV Infection

INTERVENTION	RATIONALE	EXPECTED OUTCOME
1. Nursing Diagnosis: Risk for Infection related to inadequate defenses (leukopenia, suppressed inflammatory response) secondary to HIV-positive status		
Goal: Client will remain free of opportunistic infection during the course of pregnancy.		
• Obtain a complete health history and physical examination during first prenatal visit.	• A complete health history will help determine risk factors for the development of opportunistic infections, and a physical examination will assist in identifying any underlying problem symptoms or illnesses that may compromise the pregnancy or complicate the treatment of HIV.	• *Client will remain free of opportunistic infection as evidenced by CD4$^+$ T-lymphocyte count within normal limits; no complaints of chills, fever, or sore throat; normal weight gain throughout pregnancy.*
• Educate the woman as to the signs and symptoms of infection.	• Early recognition of signs and symptoms of infection will allow for immediate treatment, which may decrease the severity of the infection. Signs and symptoms of infections include fever, weight loss, fatigue, persistent candidiasis, diarrhea, cough, and skin lesions (Kaposi's sarcoma and hairy leukoplakia in the mouth).	
• Obtain nutritional history and monitor weight gain at each prenatal visit.	• The HIV-infected woman needs to maintain optimal nutritional intake. A compromised nutritional status may affect maternal and fetal well-being. Depleted reserves of protein and iron may decrease the client's ability to fight infection, thereby making her more susceptible to opportunistic infections.	
Collaborative: Monitor the absolute CD4$^+$ T-lymphocyte count, erythrocyte sedimentation rate (ESR), complete blood count (CBC) with differential, and hemoglobin and hematocrit (H & H) at each prenatal visit.	• Lab results provide information about the woman's immune system and the potential for disease progression. Opportunistic infections are more likely to occur when the CD4$^+$ T-lymphocyte count drops below a level of 200/mm^3. ESR can rise above 20 mm/hr with anemia and with acute and chronic inflammation. CBC with differential and platelet count helps identify anemia, thrombocytopenia, and leukopenia. H & H can also identify anemia.	
2. Nursing Diagnosis: Risk for Ineffective Health Maintenance related to lack of information about HIV/AIDS and its long-term implications for the woman, her unborn child, and her family		
Goal: The client and her family will verbalize the importance of following her medication regimen and of regular prenatal care.		
• Assess the client's and family's level of understanding of HIV infection, its methods of spread, and the long-term implications.	• Knowledge of the woman's (and her family's) level of understanding about her HIV infection forms a starting point for further health teaching.	• *Woman will actively seek information about her condition, her treatment regimen, and her pregnancy and will cooperate with her caregivers.*

(Continued on next page)

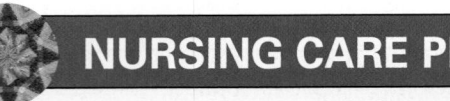

NURSING CARE PLAN

The Woman with HIV Infection continued

INTERVENTION	RATIONALE	EXPECTED OUTCOME
• Explain the risks of mother-to-child transmission of HIV infection.	• In untreated women the risk of transmission is 21%. That risk has been reduced dramatically because of the availability of antiretroviral therapy, the use of cesarean birth when indicated, and formula-feeding rather than breastfeeding.	
• Describe antiretroviral therapy. Include the regimen prescribed, its purposes, and the procedures for taking it.	• ARV therapy approaches vary based on the health status of the individual woman and whether she is currently on ARV therapy. Generally it includes oral ZDV daily, IV ZDV during labor and until birth, and ZDV therapy for the infant for 6 weeks following birth.	
• Discuss signs the woman should be alert for, including fever, fatigue, weight loss, persistent candidiasis, diarrhea, cough, skin lesions, and behavior changes.	• These symptoms may indicate that the woman is developing symptomatic HIV infection.	

3. Nursing Diagnosis: Compromised Family Coping related to the implications of positive maternal HIV status on fetal/neonatal well-being and long-term family functioning

Goal: Family is able to manage stressors related to the maternal diagnosis.

INTERVENTION	RATIONALE	EXPECTED OUTCOME
• Assess ability and readiness of family to learn about HIV and its long-term implications.	• Readiness is a key element in the teaching-learning process.	*Family members actively participate in the treatment plan, are involved in planning for labor and birth in light of a positive HIV status, and are able to express unresolved feelings about the diagnosis.*
• Provide woman and her family with accurate, reliable information about her diagnosis, its prognosis for her and for her baby, and the immediate and long-term implications for her care.	• Fear and anxiety will lessen when the woman and her family understand her health status and the implications of the HIV diagnosis and can then plan for the future.	
• Assess interactions between the woman and her family. Be alert for potentially destructive behaviors.	• If the HIV diagnosis was not expected, the couple may have to deal with issues of blame, concerns about mortality, and worries about the status of the baby. If the HIV diagnosis was known, concerns may focus on fetal/neonatal well-being. In either case, negative responses can lead to destructive behaviors.	
• Assist family in realistically identifying the needs of the woman and family unit.	• Once needs are identified realistically, it is possible to plan interventions to meet the needs.	
Collaborative: Explore available community resources and family support systems.	• Because HIV is a long-term condition, the family may require ongoing assistance.	

- The woman uses information about referral to social services (or other agency) for follow-up assistance and counseling.
- The woman begins to verbalize her feelings about her condition and its implications in an atmosphere she finds supportive.

CARE OF THE WOMAN WITH HEART DISEASE

A healthy woman with a normal heart has adequate cardiac reserve to adjust easily to the demands of pregnancy. The woman with heart disease, however, has decreased cardiac reserve, making it more difficult for her heart to accommodate the higher workload of pregnancy.

Heart disease ranks fourth after hypertension, hemorrhage, and infection as a cause of maternal mortality. Currently, cardiac disease complicates about 1% of pregnancies. Although rheumatic heart disease used to predominate, at least half of all cases of heart disease currently encountered during pregnancy are caused by congenital heart defects (Klein & Galan, 2004). Other less common causes of heart disease in pregnancy include Marfan syndrome, peripartum cardiomyopathy, and Eisenmenger syndrome. All can cause significant maternal mortality. Mitral valve prolapse is usually asymptomatic but is addressed here because of its frequent occurrence during pregnancy.

Congenital Heart Defects

Congenital heart defects have become a more common finding in pregnant women as improved surgical techniques enable females born with heart defects to live to childbearing age. The exact pathology depends on the specific defect. Congenital defects most often seen in pregnant women include tetralogy of Fallot, atrial septal defect, ventricular septal defect, patent ductus arteriosus, and coarctation of the aorta. When surgical repair can be accomplished with no remaining evidence of organic heart disease, pregnancy may be undertaken with confidence. In such cases, antibiotic prophylaxis is recommended to prevent subacute bacterial endocarditis at the time of birth. When congenital heart disease is associated with cyanosis, whether the defect was originally uncorrected or the correction failed to relieve the cyanosis, the woman should be counseled that the risk to both her and the fetus would be higher than in the general population. She also needs to know that there is an increased risk that the baby will inherit the disorder.

Rheumatic Heart Disease

Rheumatic heart disease has declined rapidly in the last four decades, because of prompt identification of pharyngeal infections caused by group A β-hemolytic streptococcus and the availability of penicillin for treatment. Rheumatic fever, which may develop in untreated streptococcal infections, is an inflammatory connective tissue disease that can involve the heart, joints, CNS, skin, and subcutaneous tissue. When the heart is affected, mitral valve stenosis is the most common and serious lesion. Aortic valve involvement, manifested by aortic insufficiency, is the second most common problem. The tricuspid and pulmonic valves are rarely affected.

The increased blood volume of pregnancy, coupled with the pregnant woman's need for increased cardiac output, stresses the heart of a woman with mitral valve stenosis. She may develop dyspnea, orthopnea, and pulmonary edema and is at increased risk for congestive heart failure (CHF). Even the woman who has no symptoms at the onset of pregnancy is at risk for CHF.

Marfan Syndrome

Marfan syndrome is an autosomal dominant disorder of connective tissue in which there may be serious cardiovascular involvement—usually dissection or rupture of the aorta. Because maternal mortality rate may be as high as 25% to 50%, a pregnant woman with Marfan syndrome needs very careful cardiovascular assessment and counseling about her prognosis for pregnancy (Klein & Galan, 2004). Because of its inheritance pattern, there is a 50% chance that the disease will be passed on to offspring.

Peripartum Cardiomyopathy

Peripartum cardiomyopathy is a dysfunction of the left ventricle that occurs in the last month of pregnancy or the first 5 months postpartum in a woman with no previous history of heart disease. This is a relatively rare but serious condition, which occurs in 1 in 3000 to 4000 live births. Mortality rates range from 18% to 56% (Klein & Galan, 2004). The symptoms are related to CHF: dyspnea, orthopnea, chest pain, palpitations, weakness, and edema. The cause is unknown, although symptoms are often attributable to chronic hypertension, mitral stenosis, obesity, or viral myocarditis. The condition usually presents with anemia and infection; consequently, treatment focuses on underlying abnormalities. Digitalis, diuretics, vasodilators, anticoagulants, sodium restriction, and strict bed rest are often part of the treatment. Peripartum cardiomyopathy may resolve with bed rest as the heart gradually returns to normal size. Subsequent pregnancy is strongly discouraged because the disease tends to recur during pregnancy.

Eisenmenger Syndrome

Eisenmenger syndrome is not a single congenital defect, but a complication that can develop as a result of other cardiac lesions causing left-to-right shunting (as with atrial septal defects or ventricular septal defects). This shunting can result in progressive pulmonary hypertension. As pulmonary vascular resistance increases, the shunting becomes bidirectional or reverses to right-to-left shunting. This condition cannot be corrected surgically and is associated with maternal mortality rates of 30% to 50% (Klein & Galan, 2004).

Mitral Valve Prolapse

Mitral valve prolapse (MVP) is usually an asymptomatic condition that is found in as many as 12% to 17% of women of childbearing age (Klein & Galan, 2004). The condition is more common in women than in men and seems to be inherited. In MVP, the mitral valve leaflets tend to prolapse into the left atrium during ventricular systole because the chordae tendineae that support them are long and thin. As a result, some mitral regurgitation may occur. On auscultation a midsystolic click and a late systolic murmur are heard.

Women with MVP usually tolerate pregnancy well, and the prognosis is excellent. Most women require assurance that they can continue with normal activities. A few women experience symptoms such as palpitations, chest pain, and dyspnea, which are usually due to arrhythmias. They are often treated with propranolol hydrochloride (Inderal). Limiting caffeine intake also helps decrease palpitations. Antibiotic prophylaxis is no longer recommended (ACOG, 2003b).

Clinical Therapy

The primary goal of medical management is early diagnosis and ongoing treatment of the woman with cardiac disease. Echocardiogram, chest x-ray, electrocardiogram, auscultation of heart sounds, and sometimes cardiac catheterization are essential for establishing the type and severity of the heart disease. The severity of heart disease can also be determined by the individual's ability to perform ordinary physical activity. The following classification of functional capacity for those with cardiac disease has been standardized by the Criteria Committee of the New York Heart Association (1994):

- *Class I.* Individuals with cardiac disease but with no resulting limitation of physical activity and no symptoms of cardiac insufficiency. Ordinary physical activity causes no undue fatigue, dyspnea, or palpitations; anginal pain is not present.

- *Class II.* Individuals with cardiac disease that results in slight limitation of physical activity. They are comfortable at rest but ordinary physical activity causes fatigue, dyspnea, palpitation, or anginal pain.

- *Class III.* Individuals with cardiac disease that results in marked limitation of physical activity. They are comfortable at rest but less than ordinary physical activity results in fatigue, dyspnea, palpitation, or anginal pain.

- *Class IV.* Individuals with cardiac disease that results in the inability to carry on any physical activity without experiencing discomfort. Even at rest, they may experience symptoms of cardiac insufficiency or anginal pain; discomfort increases with any physical activity.

Women in classes I and II usually experience a normal pregnancy and have few complications, whereas those in classes III and IV are at risk for more severe complications, which may affect both maternal and fetal outcomes. Preconception counseling is important for these women to optimize maternal and fetal outcomes.

Because anemia increases the work of the heart, it should be diagnosed early and treated. Infection also increases the cardiac workload, so even minor infections should be treated thor-

oughly. To reduce the risk of pyelonephritis, monthly screening for asymptomatic bacteriuria is indicated, with antibiotic therapy as needed.

As pregnancy progresses, it is important to minimize cardiac workload and promote tissue perfusion. Depending on the specific lesion, the woman's activity, weight gain, and sodium intake may need to be limited (Klein & Galan, 2004).

DRUG THERAPY

Besides the iron and vitamin supplements prescribed during pregnancy, the pregnant woman with heart disease may need additional drug therapy to maintain health. Antibiotics, usually penicillin if not contraindicated by allergy, are used to prevent recurrent bouts of rheumatic fever and subsequent heart valve damage. Depending on the specific lesion, antibiotics may also be recommended during labor and the early postpartum period for either acquired or congenital disease to prevent bacterial endocarditis. If the woman develops coagulation problems, the anticoagulant heparin may be used. Heparin offers the greatest safety to the fetus because it does not cross the placenta. The thiazide diuretics and furosemide (Lasix) may be used to treat congestive heart failure if it develops. Digitalis glycosides and common antiarrhythmic drugs may be used to treat cardiac failure and arrhythmias. These agents do cross the placenta but have no reported teratogenic effect; however, they have not been adequately studied to establish their safety in pregnancy (Klein & Galan, 2004).

LABOR AND CHILDBIRTH

Spontaneous natural labor with adequate pain relief is usually recommended for clients in classes I and II. Special attention should be given to the prompt recognition and treatment of any signs of heart failure (Figure 19–6 ◆). Those in classes III and IV may need to be hospitalized before onset of labor for cardiovascular stabilization. They may also require invasive cardiac monitoring during labor.

Use of low forceps or vacuum assistance provides the safest method of birth, with lumbar epidural anesthesia to reduce the stress of pushing. Cesarean birth is used only if fetal or maternal indications exist, not on the basis of heart disease alone.

NURSING CARE MANAGEMENT
Nursing Assessment and Diagnosis

The nurse assesses the stress of pregnancy on the functional capacity of the heart during every antepartal visit. The nurse notes the category of functional capacity assigned to the woman; takes the woman's pulse, respirations, and blood pressure; and compares them to the normal values expected during pregnancy and to the woman's previous values. The nurse then determines the woman's activity level, including rest, and any changes in the pulse and respirations that have occurred since previous visits. The nurse also identifies and evaluates other factors that would increase strain on the heart. These might include anemia,

Figure 19–6 ◆ When a woman with heart disease begins labor, the nursing students and instructor caring for her monitor her closely for signs of congestive heart failure.

infection, anxiety, lack of support system, and household and career demands.

The following symptoms, if they are progressive, are indicative of CHF, the heart's signal of its decreased ability to meet the demands of pregnancy:

- Cough (frequent, with or without hemoptysis)
- Dyspnea (progressive, upon exertion)
- Edema (progressive, generalized, including extremities, face, eyelids)
- Heart murmurs (heard on auscultation)
- Palpitations
- Rales (auscultated in lung bases)

Progressiveness of the cycle is the critical factor, because some of these same symptoms are seen to a minor degree in a pregnancy without cardiac problems.

Nursing diagnoses that might apply to the pregnant woman with heart disease include the following:

- *Decreased Cardiac Output:* Easy fatigability
- *Impaired Gas Exchange* related to pulmonary edema secondary to cardiac decompensation
- *Fear* related to the effects of the maternal cardiac condition on fetal well-being

Nursing Plan and Implementation

Nursing care is directed toward maintaining a balance between cardiac reserve and cardiac workload.

ANTEPARTAL PERIOD

Nursing actions are designed to meet the physiologic and psychosocial needs of the pregnant woman with heart disease. The priority of nursing actions varies according to the severity of the disease process and the individual needs of the woman as determined by nursing assessment.

The woman and her family should thoroughly understand her condition and its management and should recognize signs of potential complications. This will increase their understanding and decrease anxiety. When the nurse provides explanations, uses printed material, and offers frequent opportunities to ask questions and discuss concerns, the woman is better able to meet her own healthcare needs and seek assistance appropriately.

As part of health teaching, the nurse explains the purposes of the dietary and activity changes that are required. A diet is instituted that is high in iron, protein, and essential nutrients but low in sodium, with adequate calories to ensure normal weight gain. Such a diet best meets the nutrition needs of the client with cardiac disease. Excessive weight gain is avoided because it taxes the heart. To help preserve her cardiac reserves, the woman may need to restrict her activities. In addition, 8 to 10 hours of sleep and frequent daily rest periods are essential. The nurse can encourage the woman to rest in the side-lying position to promote optimal placental perfusion. Because upper respiratory infections may tax the heart and lead to decompensation, the woman must avoid contact with sources of infection and report symptoms of infection immediately.

During the first half of pregnancy, the woman is seen approximately every 2 weeks to assess cardiac status. During the second half of pregnancy, the woman is seen weekly. These assessments are especially important between weeks 28 and 30, when the blood volume reaches maximum amounts. If symptoms of cardiac decompensation occur, prompt medical intervention is indicated to correct the cardiac problem.

INTRAPARTAL PERIOD

Labor and birth exert tremendous stress on the woman and her fetus. This stress could be fatal to the fetus of a woman with cardiac disease because the fetus may be receiving an inadequate oxygen and blood supply. Thus the intrapartal care of a woman with cardiac disease is aimed at reducing the amount of physical exertion and accompanying fatigue.

The nurse evaluates maternal vital signs frequently to determine the woman's response to labor. A pulse rate greater than 100 beats per minute or respirations greater than 24 per minute may indicate beginning cardiac decompensation, especially if accompanied by dyspnea, and require further evaluation. The nurse also auscultates the woman's lungs frequently for rales and carefully observes for other signs of developing decompensation.

To ensure cardiac emptying and adequate oxygenation, the nurse encourages the laboring woman to assume either a semi-Fowler's position with lateral tilt or side-lying position with her head and shoulders elevated. Oxygen by mask, diuretics to reduce fluid retention, sedatives and analgesics, prophylactic antibiotics, and digitalis may also be used as indicated by the woman's status.

The nurse remains with the woman to support her. It is essential that the nurse keep the woman and her family informed of labor progress and management plans, collaborating with them to fulfill their wishes for the birth experience as much as possible. The nurse needs to maintain an atmosphere of calm to lessen the anxiety of the woman and her family.

Continuous electronic fetal monitoring is used to provide ongoing assessment of the fetus's response to labor. To prevent overexertion and the accompanying fatigue, the nurse encourages the woman to sleep and relax between contractions and provides her with emotional support and encouragement. During pushing, the nurse encourages the woman to use shorter, more moderate open glottis pushing (see Chapter 24 ∞), with complete relaxation between pushes. The nurse monitors vital signs closely during the second stage.

POSTPARTAL PERIOD

The postpartal period is a significant time for the woman with cardiac disease. After birth, the intra-abdominal pressure and the venous pressure are reduced, the splanchnic vessels engorge, and blood flow to the heart increases. As extravascular fluid returns to the bloodstream for excretion, cardiac output and blood volume increase. This physiologic adaptation places great strain on the heart and may lead to decompensation, especially in the first 48 hours postpartum.

So that the healthcare team can detect any possible problems, the woman may remain in the hospital longer than the low-risk woman postpartally. Her vital signs are monitored frequently, and she is assessed for signs of decompensation. She stays in the semi-Fowler's or side-lying position, with her head and shoulders elevated, and begins a gradual, progressive activity program. Appropriate diet and stool softeners facilitate bowel movement without undue strain.

The postpartum nurse gives the woman opportunities to discuss her birth experience and helps her deal with any feelings or concerns that cause her distress. The nurse also encourages maternal-infant attachment by providing frequent opportunities for the mother to interact with her child.

Because there is no evidence that cardiac output is compromised during lactation, the only concern about breastfeeding for women with cardiovascular disease is related to medications that the mother may be taking. These must be evaluated for their ability to pass into the milk and for any effect of the drug on lactation. The nurse can assist the breastfeeding mother to a comfortable side-lying position with her head moderately elevated

or to a semi-Fowler's position. To conserve the mother's energy, the nurse should position the newborn at the breast and be available to burp the baby and reposition him or her at the other breast. The nurse can also encourage family members to provide the new mother with support and assistance as needed to help her avoid becoming fatigued.

In addition to providing the normal postpartum discharge teaching, the nurse stresses that follow-up for the new mother is imperative. Moreover, the nurse should ensure that the woman and her family understand the signs of possible problems resulting from her heart disease or from other postpartal complications. For women with heart disease, postpartum complications such as hemorrhage, thromboembolism, anemia, and infection pose a real threat and may even precipitate heart failure.

The nurse plans with the woman an activity schedule that is gradual, progressive, and appropriate to her needs and home environment. The nurse provides appropriate health teaching, including information about resumption of sexual activity and contraception. Visiting nurse or homemaker assistance referrals may be necessary, depending on the woman's status.

Evaluation

Expected outcomes of nursing care include the following:

- The woman is able to discuss her condition and its possible impact on her pregnancy, labor and birth, and the postpartal period.
- The woman participates in developing an appropriate healthcare regimen and follows it throughout her pregnancy.
- The woman gives birth to a healthy infant.
- The woman does not develop CHF, thromboembolism, or infection.
- The woman is able to identify signs and symptoms of possible postpartum complications.
- The woman is able to care effectively for her newborn infant.

OTHER MEDICAL CONDITIONS AND PREGNANCY

A woman with a preexisting medical condition should be aware of the possible impact of pregnancy on her condition, as well as the impact of her condition on the outcome of her pregnancy. Table 19–5 discusses some of the less common medical conditions vis-à-vis pregnancy.

Table 19–5   LESS COMMON MEDICAL CONDITIONS AND PREGNANCY

Condition	Brief Description	Maternal Implications	Fetal/Neonatal Implications
Asthma	Asthma, an obstructive lung condition, is the most common respiratory disease found in pregnancy, complicating 1% to 4% of all pregnancies (Davidson, Doyle, & Ramin, 2005). Typical symptoms include wheezing, dyspnea, and episodic coughing. A severe asthmatic attack often requires hospitalization. It is managed by long-term comprehensive drug therapy to prevent airway inflammation, combined with drug treatment to manage attacks or exacerbations and client education about triggers (such as cold air, dust, smoke, exercise, food additives), methods of prevention, and treatment options.	During pregnancy, in approximately one third of women, their asthma improves, in one third it remains unchanged, and in one third the condition worsens. The highest incidence of exacerbation occurs between 24 and 36 weeks' gestation. Asthma is often quiescent during labor and birth but peak expiratory flow rate should be monitored to detect changes in maternal respiratory status (Davidson et al., 2005).	Prematurity and low birth weight are more common among the infants of women who have asthma (Dombrowski, 2006). Asthma has also been linked with higher rates of hyperemesis gravidarum, preeclampsia, uterine hemorrhage, and perinatal mortality. The goal of therapy is to prevent maternal exacerbations because even a mild exacerbation can cause severe hypoxia-related complications in the fetus. If an exacerbation occurs, it should be managed in the same way as for a nonpregnant woman because the asthma drugs used are less of a threat to the fetus than a serious asthma attack (Davidson et al., 2005).
Epilepsy	Chronic disorder characterized by seizures; may be idiopathic or secondary to other conditions, such as head injury, metabolic and nutritional disorders such as PKU or vitamin B_6 deficiency, encephalitis, neoplasms, or circulatory interferences. Treated with anticonvulsants.	Vast majority of pregnancies in women with seizure disorders are uneventful and have an excellent outcome. Women with more frequent seizures before pregnancy may have exacerbations during pregnancy, but this may be related to nausea and vomiting, lack of cooperation with drug regimen, or sleep deprivation. During pregnancy the woman should continue to be treated with the medication that best controls her seizures. Folic acid therapy should be started prior to conception if possible. Folic acid and vitamin D are indicated throughout pregnancy (AAFP, 2004).	Certain anticonvulsant medications are associated with increased incidence of congenital anomalies, especially cleft lip and heart defects, although the incidence has decreased in recent years. This may be due to the fact that the current ability to determine blood levels of medications has led to more accurate dosages and the resultant use of a single medication; consequently multiple medications are used less often (AAFP, 2004).
Hepatitis B	Hepatitis B, caused by the hepatitis B virus (HBV), is a major, growing health problem. Groups at risk include those from areas with a high incidence (primarily developing countries), illegal IV drug users, prostitutes, homosexuals, those with multiple sex partners, or occupational exposure to blood, although many infected people have no identifiable source of infection. HBV transmission is blood borne, primarily sexually and perinatally transmitted. Because of the dramatic increase and the difficulty of vaccinating high-risk individuals before they become infected, the CDC now recommends (1) testing all pregnant women for the presence of hepatitis B surface antigen and prophylactic treatment for all infants born to women who are HBsAG-positive or whose status is unknown; (2) routine infant vaccination; (3) vaccination of children and adolescents through age 18 years who have not been vaccinated; (4) vaccination of unvaccinated adults who are at risk for hepatitis B (CDC, 2006).	Hepatitis B does not usually affect the course of pregnancy. However, chronic HBV carriers have a great potential for infecting others when exposure to blood and body fluids occurs. In addition, chronic carriers may develop long-term sequelae, such as chronic liver disease and liver cancer. Approximately 4000 to 5000 deaths are caused annually by liver disease associated with chronic HBV infection. It is now recommended that all pregnant women be tested for the presence of hepatitis B surface antigen (HBsAg). A woman who is negative may be given the hepatitis vaccine.	Perinatal transmission most often occurs at or near the time of childbirth. More important, the risk of becoming a chronic carrier of the HBV is inversely related to the age of the individual at the time of initial infection. Therefore infants infected perinatally have the highest risk of becoming chronically infected if not treated. Recommendations now include routine vaccination of all neonates born to HBsAg-negative women and immunoprophylaxis to all newborns of HBsAg-positive women (CDC, 2006).
Hyperthyroidism (thyrotoxicosis)	Enlarged, overactive thyroid gland; increased T_4: TBG ratio and increased BMR. Symptoms include muscle wasting, tachycardia, excessive sweating, and exophthalmos. Treatment by antithyroid drug propylthiouracil (PTU) while monitoring free T_4 levels. Surgery used only if drug intolerance exists.	Mild hyperthyroidism is not dangerous. Increased incidence of preeclampsia and postpartum hemorrhage if not well controlled. Serious risk related to thyroid storm characterized by high fever, tachycardia, sweating, and congestive heart failure. Now occurs rarely. When diagnosed during pregnancy, may be transient or permanent.	Neonatal thyrotoxicosis is rare. Even low doses of antithyroid drug in mother may produce a mild fetal/neonatal hypothyroidism; higher dose may produce a goiter or mental deficiencies. Fetal loss not increased in euthyroid women. If untreated, rates of abortion, intrauterine death, and stillbirth increase. Breast-feeding contraindicated for women on antithyroid medication because it is excreted in the milk (may be tried by woman on low dose if neonatal T_4 levels are monitored).

(Continued on next page)

Table 19–5   LESS COMMON MEDICAL CONDITIONS AND PREGNANCY continued

Condition	Brief Description	Maternal Implications	Fetal/Neonatal Implications
Hypothyroidism	Characterized by inadequate thyroid secretions (decreased T_4: TBG ratio), elevated TSH, lowered BMR, and enlarged thyroid gland (goiter). Symptoms include lack of energy, excessive weight gain, cold intolerance, dry skin, and constipation. Treated by thyroxine replacement therapy.	Long-term replacement therapy usually continues at same dosage during pregnancy as before. Weekly nonstress test (NST) after 35 weeks' gestation.	If mother untreated, fetal loss 50%; high risk of congenital goiter or true cretinism. Therefore newborns are screened for T_4 level. Mild TSH elevations present little risk because TSH does not cross the placenta.
Maternal phenylketonuria (PKU) (hyperphenylalaninemia)	Inherited recessive single gene anomaly causing a deficiency of the liver enzyme needed to convert the amino acid phenylalanine to tyrosine, resulting in high serum levels of phenylalanine. Brain damage and mental retardation occur if not treated early.	Low phenylalanine diet is mandatory before conception and during pregnancy. The woman should be counseled that her children will either inherit the disease or be carriers, depending on the zygosity of the father for the disease. Treatment at a PKU center is recommended.	Risk to fetus if maternal treatment not begun preconception. In untreated women increased incidence of fetal mental retardation, microcephaly, congenital heart defects, and growth retardation. Fetal phenylalanine levels are approximately 50% higher than maternal levels.
Multiple sclerosis	Neurologic disorder characterized by destruction of the myelin sheath of nerve fibers. The condition occurs primarily in young adults, more commonly in females, and is marked by periods of remission; progresses to marked physical disability in 10 to 20 years.	Associated with remission during pregnancy, but with slightly increased relapse rate postpartum (Haas, 2000). Rest is important; help with child care should be planned. Uterine contraction strength is not diminished, but because sensation is frequently lessened, labor may be almost painless.	Increased evidence of a genetic predisposition. Therefore reproductive counseling is recommended.
Rheumatoid arthritis	Chronic inflammatory disease believed to be caused by a genetically influenced antigen-antibody reaction. Symptoms include fatigue, low-grade fever, pain and swelling of joints, morning stiffness, pain on movement. Treated with salicylates, physical therapy, and rest. Corticosteroids used cautiously if not responsive to above.	Usually there is remission of rheumatoid arthritis symptoms during pregnancy, often with a relapse postpartum. Anemia may be present due to blood loss from salicylate therapy. Mother needs extra rest, particularly to relieve weight-bearing joints, but needs to continue range-of-motion exercises. If in remission, may stop medication during pregnancy.	Possibility of prolonged gestation and longer labor with heavy salicylate use. Possible teratogenic effects of salicylates.
Systemic lupus erythematosus (SLE)	Chronic autoimmune collagen disease, characterized by exacerbations and remissions; symptoms range from characteristic rash to inflammation and pain in joints, fever, nephritis, depression, cranial nerve disorders, and peripheral neuropathies.	Women who conceive when the disease is in remission appear to have little risk for adverse outcomes, whereas those with active disease have less favorable outcomes. Pregnancy does not appear to alter the long-term prognosis of women with SLE (Molad, Berkowski, Monselise, et al., 2005).	Increased incidence of spontaneous abortion, stillbirth, prematurity, and IUGR. Infants born to women with SLE may have characteristic skin rash, which usually disappears by 12 months. Infants are at increased risk for complete congenital heart block, a condition that can be diagnosed prenatally. Fetal echocardiography is then performed to rule out other cardiac defects (Buyon & Clancy, 2005). No known treatment exists although various therapies have been tried. The prognosis for the fetus varies but, because the heart damage is permanent, a pacemaker may be necessary if the newborn is to survive (Porter, Peltier, & Branch, 2003).
Tuberculosis (TB)	Infection caused by *Mycobacterium tuberculosis;* inflammatory process causes destruction of lung tissue, increased sputum, and coughing. Associated primarily with poverty and malnutrition and may be found among refugees from countries where TB is prevalent. Treated with isoniazid and either ethambutol or rifampin, or both.	The incidence of tuberculosis has begun to increase significantly since the late 1980s, and it is increasingly associated with HIV infection (Laibl & Sheffield, 2005). If TB inactive due to prior treatment, relapse rate no greater than for nonpregnant women. When isoniazid is used during pregnancy, the woman should take supplemental pyridoxine (vitamin B_6). Extra rest and limited contact with others is required until disease becomes inactive.	If maternal TB is inactive, mother may breastfeed and care for her infant. If TB is active, newborn should not have direct contact with mother until she is noninfectious. Isoniazid crosses the placenta, but most studies show no teratogenic effects. Rifampin crosses the placenta. Possibility of harmful effects still being studied.

CHAPTER REVIEW

FOCUS YOUR STUDY

- Almost any health problem that a person can have when not pregnant can coexist with pregnancy. Some problems, such as anemias, may be exacerbated by pregnancy. Others, such as collagen disease, may go into temporary remission with pregnancy. Regardless of the health problem, careful health care is needed throughout pregnancy to improve the outcome for mother and fetus.

- The diagnosis of high-risk pregnancy can shock an expectant couple. Providing emotional support, teaching about the condition and prognosis, and educating for self-care are important nursing measures that help the client cope.

- Substance abuse (either drugs or alcohol) not only is detrimental to the mother's health but also may have profound lasting effects on the fetus.

- The key point in the care of the pregnant woman with diabetes is scrupulous maternal plasma glucose control. This is best achieved by home blood glucose monitoring, multiple daily insulin injections, regular exercise, and a careful diet. To reduce incidence of congenital anomalies and other problems in the newborn, the woman should be euglycemic (have a normal blood glucose) throughout the pregnancy. Women with diabetes, even more than most other clients, need to be educated about their conditions and involved with their own care.

- Anemia indicates inadequate levels of hemoglobin (Hb) in the blood. Anemia is defined as hemoglobin less than 12 g/dL in nonpregnant women and less than 11 g/dL in pregnant and postpartum women. Iron deficiency anemia is the most common form of anemia. Other anemias include folic acid deficiency, sickle cell anemia, and thalassemia.

- HIV infection, which is transmitted via blood and body fluids, may also be transmitted transplacentally to the fetus. Currently, there is no definitive therapy for HIV/AIDS. Nurses should employ blood and body fluid precautions (standard precautions) in caring for all women to avoid potential spread of infection.

- Cardiac disease during pregnancy requires careful assessment, limitation of activity, and knowing and reporting signs of impending cardiac decompensation by both client and nurse.

EXPLORE MEDIALINK

http://www.prenhall.com/davidson

NCLEX review questions, case studies, and other interactive resources for this chapter can be found on the Web Site at http://www.prenhall.com/davidson. Click on "Chapter 19" to select the activities for this chapter.

For tutortials including animations and videos, more NCLEX review questions, and an audio glossary, access the accompanying Prentice Hall Nursing MediaLink DVD-ROM in this book.

PRENTICE HALL NURSING MEDIALINK DVD-ROM
Audio Glossary
NCLEX Review

COMPANION WEBSITE
Additional NCLEX Review
Case Study: *Client with Gestational Diabetes*
Care Plan Activity: *Antepartal Client at Risk*
Applications: *Gestational Diabetes; Iron Deficiency Anemia*
Critical Thinking

CRITICAL THINKING IN ACTION

HIV TRANSMISSION TO THE FETUS DURING LABOR: PREVENTION

View the Critical Thinking in Action video in Chapter 19 of the DVD-ROM. Then answer the questions that follow.

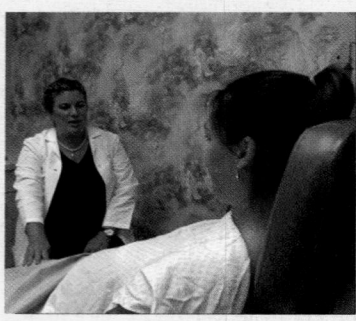

Jane Adams, a 23-year-old, G3 P2, at 37 weeks' gestation, presents to you in the birthing unit complaining of "vaginal pressure" but no contractions. You assess her and find that her history includes being HIV positive for 2 years, second trimester cocaine and marijuana use, a pattern of missed appointments, anemia (Hct 28%), and a positive syphilis serology. Jane tells you that she has other children and that they are being cared for by her mother, who has legal custody of them. You admit Jane to the labor suite and place her on the fetal monitor for evaluation of fetal well-being and contraction patterns. The monitor shows you that the fetal heart rate baseline is 120 to 130 with no decelerations; contractions are mild and irregular, lasting 20 to 30 seconds. You obtain vital signs of BP 130/88, temperature 97F P 88 R 14. Vital signs are normal. A vaginal exam determines that Jane is 7 cm dilated at +1 station with intact membranes. She asks you if being HIV positive will affect her labor.

1. Discuss the prophylactic regimen for the prevention of HIV transmission to the fetus during labor.

2. Discuss the transmission of HIV to the fetus during pregnancy and birth.

3. Identify the emotional impact of HIV infection or other STIs on the woman.

4. On postpartum day 2, you inform Jane that her infant is HIV antibody positive. How would you clarify the results?

REFERENCES

American Academy of Family Physicians (AAFP). (2004, September). *Epilepsy and pregnancy: What you should know.* Retrieved December 11, 2005, from http://familydoctor.org/243.xml

American Academy of Pediatrics (AAP) & American College of Obstetricians and Gynecologists (ACOG). (2002). *Guidelines for prenatal care* (5th ed.). Elk Grove Village, IL: Author.

American College of Obstetricians and Gynecologists (ACOG). (2000a). *Genetic screening for hemoglobinopathies* (ACOG Committee Opinion No. 238). Washington, DC: Author.

American College of Obstetricians and Gynecologists (ACOG). (2000b). *Scheduled cesarean delivery and the prevention of vertical transmission of HIV infection* (ACOG Committee Opinion No. 234). Washington, DC: Author.

American College of Obstetricians and Gynecologists (ACOG). (2001). *Gestational diabetes* (ACOG Practice Bulletin No. 30). Washington, DC: Author.

American College of Obstetricians and Gynecologists (ACOG). (2003a). *Management of preterm labor* (ACOG Practice Bulletin No. 43). Washington, DC: Author.

American College of Obstetricians and Gynecologists (ACOG). (2003b). *Prophylactic antibiotics in labor and delivery* (ACOG Practice Bulletin No. 47). Washington, DC: Author.

American College of Obstetricians and Gynecologists (ACOG). (2004). *Prenatal and perinatal human immunodeficiency virus testing: Expanded recommendations* (ACOG Committee Opinions No. 304). Washington, DC: Author.

American College of Obstetricians and Gynecologists (ACOG). (2005). *Pregestational diabetes mellitus* (ACOG Practice Bulletin No. 60). Washington, DC: Author.

American Diabetes Association. (2004, January). Diagnosis and classification of diabetes mellitus. *Diabetes Care, 27* (Suppl. 1), S5–S10.

Bauer, C. R., Langer, J. C., Shankaran, S., Bada, H. S., Lester, B., Wright L. L., et al. (2005). Acute neonatal effects of cocaine exposure during pregnancy. *Archives of Pediatrics & Adolescent Medicine, 159*(9), 824–834.

Buchanan, G. R., DeBaun, M. R., Quinn, C. T., & Steinberg, M. H. (2004). Sickle cell disease. *American Society of Hematology Education Program. Pub Med Citation Number 1556167,* 85–87.

Buyon, J. P., & Clancy, R. M. (2005). Neonatal lupus: Basic research and clinical perspectives. *Rheumatic Diseases Clinics of North America, 31*(2), 299–313.

Centers for Disease Control and Prevention. (2004). Use of vitamins containing folic acid among women of childbearing age—United States, 2004. *Morbidity and Mortality Weekly Report, 53*(36), 847–850.

Centers for Disease Control and Prevention (CDC). (2005). *HIV/AIDS surveillance report, 2004.* US Department of Health and Human Services (Vol. 16, pp. 1–46). Retrieved July 19, 2006, from http://www.cdc.gov/hiv/stats/hasrlink.htm

Centers for Disease Control and Prevention (CDC). (2006, August 4). Sexually transmitted disease guidelines, 2006. *Morbidity and Mortality Weekly Report, 55,* (RR-11), 1–93.

Chasnoff, I. D., McGourty, R. F., Bailey, G. W., Hutchins, E., Lightfoot, S. O., Pawson, L. L., et al. (2005). The 4P's plus(C) screen for substance use in pregnancy: Clinical application and outcomes. *Journal of Perinatology, 25*(6), 368–374.

Cleveland Clinic. (2003). Hypoglycemia. Retrieved February 3, 2003, from http://www.clevelandclinic.org/ health/health-info/docs/0000/0098.asp

Coyer, S. (2003). Women in recovery discuss parenting while addicted to cocaine. *American Journal of Maternal-Child Nursing, 28*(1), 45–49.

Criteria Committee of the New York Heart Association. (1994). *Nomenclature and criteria for diagnosis of diseases of the heart and great vessels* (9th ed.). Dallas, TX: American Heart Association.

Cuervo, L. G., & Mahomed, K. (2005). Treatments for iron deficiency anaemia in pregnancy. *The Cochrane Library (Oxford)(3)* (ID #CD003094).

Cunningham, F. G., Leveno, K. J., Bloom, S. L., Hauth, J. C., Gilstrap, L. C., III, & Wenstrom, K. D. (2005). *Williams obstetrics* (22nd ed.). New York: McGraw-Hill.

Davidson, C. M., Doyle, N. M., & Ramin, S. M. (2005). Don't undertreat asthma in pregnancy. *Contemporary OB/GYN, 50*(8), 34–41.

Dombrowski, M. P. (2006). Asthma and pregnancy. *Obstetrics and Gynecology, 108,* 667–681.

Food and Drug Administration (FDA). (2005). Alcohol warning for pregnant women. *FDA Consumer 39*(3), 4.

Forsbach-Sanchez, G., Tamez-Perez, H. E., & Vazquez-Lara, J. (2005). Diabetes and pregnancy. *Archives of Medical Research, 36*(3), 291–299.

Fowles, E. R. (2004). Clinical issues. Prenatal nutrition and birth outcomes. *Journal of Obstetric, Gynecologic, & Neonatal Nursing, 33*(6), 809–822.

Gamma, A., Jerome, L., Liechti, M. E., & Sumnall, H. R. (2005). Is ecstasy perceived to be safe? A critical survey. *Drug and Alcohol Dependence, 77*(2), 185–193.

Glynn, M., & Rhodes, P. (2005, June). *Estimated HIV prevalence in the United States at the end of 2003* [Abstract 595]. National HIV Prevention Conference, Atlanta.

Haas, J. (2000). High dose IVIG in the post partum period for prevention of exacerbations in MS. *Multiple Sclerosis, 6* (Suppl. 2), S18–20.

Hulsey, T. (2005). Prenatal drug use: The ethics of testing and incarcerating pregnant women. *Newborn and Infant Nursing Reviews, 5*(2), 93–96.

Ibrahim, T., Moodley, J., & Doorasamy, T. (2004). Lymphocyte changes in pregnancy: A comparison of the human immunodeficiency virus in infected and non-infected women. *Journal of Obstetrics and Gynaecology, 24*(5), 498–503.

Jacobson, G. F., Ramos, G. A., Ching, J. Y., Kirby, R. S., Ferrara, A., & Field, D. R. (2005). Comparison of glyburide and insulin for the management of gestational diabetes in a large managed care organization. *American Journal of Obstetrics & Gynecology, 193*(1), 118–124.

Jansson, L. M., DiPietro, J., & Elko, A. (2005). Fetal response to maternal methadone administration. *American Journal of Obstetrics & Gynecology, 193*(3, Pt. 1), 611–617.

Kendrick, J. M., Wilson, C., Elder, R. F., & Smith, C. S. (2005). Reliability of reporting of self-monitoring of blood glucose in pregnant women. *Journal of Obstetric, Gynecologic, & Neonatal Nursing, 34*(3), 329–334.

Klein, L. L., & Galan, H. L. (2004). Cardiac disease in pregnancy. *Obstetrics and Gynecology Clinics of North America, 31*(2), 429–459.

Koprich, J. S., Chen, E.-R., Kanaan, N. M., Campbell, N. C., Kordower, J. H., & Lipton, J. W. (2003). Prenatal 3,4-methylenedioxymeth-amphetamine (ecstasy) alters exploratory behavior, reduces monoamine metabolism, and increases forebrain tyrosine hydroxylase fiber density of juvenile rats. *Neurotoxicology and Teratology, 25*(5), 509–517.

LaGasse, L. L., Messinger, D., Lester, B. M., Seifer, R., Tronick, E. Z., Bauer, C. R., et al. (2003). Prenatal drug exposure and maternal and infant feeding behaviour. *Archives of Disease in Childhood Fetal & Neonatal Edition, 88*(5), F391–399.

Laibl, V. R., & Sheffield, J. S. (2005). Tuberculosis in pregnancy. *Clinics in Perinatology, 32*(3), 739–747.

Langer, O., Yogev, Y., Xenakis, E. M., & Rosenn, B. (2005). Insulin and glyburide therapy: Dosage, severity level of gestational diabetes, and pregnancy outcome. *American Journal of Obstetrics & Gynecology, 192*(1), 134–139.

McCarthy, J. J., Leamon, M. H., Parr, M. S., & Anania, B. (2005). High-dose methadone maintenance in pregnancy: Maternal and neonatal outcomes. *American Journal of Obstetrics & Gynecology, 193*(3, Pt. 1), 606–610.

Molad, Y., Borkowski, T., Monselise, A., Ben-Haroush, A., Sulkes, J., Hod, M., et al. (2005). Maternal and fetal outcome of lupus pregnancy: A prospective study of 29 pregnancies. *Lupus, 14*(2), 145–151.

Ogunyemi, D., & Hernandez-Loera, G. E. (2004). The impact of antenatal cocaine use on maternal characteristics and neonatal outcomes. *Journal of Maternal-Fetal and Neonatal Medicine, 15*(4), 253–259.

O'Malley, P. (2005). Ecstasy for intimacy: Potentially fatal choices for adolescents and young adults: Update for the clinical nurse specialist. *Clinical Nurse Specialist, 19*(2), 63–64.

Porter, T. F., Peltier, M., & Branch, D. W. (2003). Immunologic disorders in pregnancy. In J. R. Scott, R. S. Gibbs, B. Y. Karlan, & A. F. Haney (Eds.), *Danforth's obstetrics and gynecology* (9th ed.). Philadelphia: Lippincott Williams & Wilkins.

Public Health Service Task Force. (2005, February 24). Recommendations for use of antiretroviral drugs in pregnant HIV-1-infected women for maternal health and interventions to reduce perinatal HIV-1 transmission in the United States. Retrieved November 3, 2005, from http://aidsinfo.nih.gov/guidelines/perinatal/PER_022405.pdf

Rayburn, W. F., & Bogenschutz, M. P. (2004). Pharmacotherapy for pregnant women with addictions. *American Journal of Obstetrics & Gynecology, 191*(6), 1885–1897.

Serjeant, G. R., Loy, L. L., Crowther, M., Hambleton, I. R., & Thame, M. (2004). Outcome of pregnancy in homozygous sickle cell disease. *Obstetrics and Gynecology, 103*(6), 1278–1285.

Shankaran, S., Das, A., Bauer, C. R., Bada, H. S., Lester, B., Wright, L. L., et al. (2004). Association between patterns of maternal substance use and infant birth weight, length, and head circumference. *Pediatrics, 114*(2), e226–234.

Substance Abuse and Mental Health Services Administration. (2005). *Results from the 2004 national survey on drug use and health: National findings* (Office of Applied Studies, NSDUH Series H-28, DHHS Publication No. SMA 05-4062). Rockville, MD: Author.

Varney, H., Kriebs, J. M., & Gegor, C. L. (2004). *Varney's midwifery* (4th ed.). Sudbury, MA: Jones and Bartlett.

Wei, R., Msamanga, G. I., Spiegelman, D., Hertzmark, E., Baylin, A., Manji, K., et al. (2004). Association between low birth weight and infant mortality in children born to human immunodeficiency virus 1-infected mothers in Tanzania. *Pediatric Infectious Disease Journal, 23*(6), 530–536.

Welch, R. A., & Poulin, V. (2003). Specific roles of the obstetrician-gynecologist. *Obstetrics and Gynecology Clinics of North America, 30*(3), 601–615.

Wyatt, J. W., Frias, J. L., Hoyme, H. E., Jovanovic, L., Kaaja, R., Brown, F., et al. (2005). Congenital anomaly rate in offspring of mothers with diabetes treated with insulin lispro during pregnancy. *Diabetic Medicine, 22*(6), 803–807.

I had taken more than a year to conceive and was so excited when my home pregnancy test turned positive. My husband was with me when I called my family. I could hardly breathe with the excitement of the moment. Five weeks later, I was in an ambulance speeding to a medical center equipped to save my life. My ectopic pregnancy had not yet been diagnosed when it ruptured at home. I underwent surgery to remove my tube and the pregnancy that was contained within. Afterward, I was dazed and debilitated. For weeks I focused on my recovery rather than my loss. How ironic that I was fully confronted with the reality of my loss on what would have been my due date when in the mail I received a package of samples congratulating me on the birth of my new baby.

~Kristin, R.N.~

OBJECTIVES

1. Contrast the etiology, medical therapy, and nursing interventions for the various bleeding problems associated with pregnancy.
2. Identify the medical therapy and nursing interventions indicated in caring for a woman with an incompetent cervix.
3. Discuss the medical therapy and nursing care of a woman with hyperemesis gravidarum.
4. Discuss the nursing care for a woman experiencing premature rupture of the membranes or preterm labor.
5. Describe the development and course of hypertensive disorders associated with pregnancy.
6. Explain the cause and prevention of hemolytic disease of the newborn secondary to Rh incompatibility.
7. Compare Rh incompatibility to ABO incompatibility with regard to occurrence, treatment, and implications for the fetus/newborn.
8. Summarize the effects of surgical procedures on pregnancy, and explain ways in which pregnancy may complicate diagnosis of conditions that require surgery.
9. Discuss the implications of trauma due to accidents or battering for the pregnant woman and her fetus.
10. Describe the effects of infections on the woman and her unborn child.

KEY TERMS

MEDIALINK

Additional resources for this content can be found on the Prentice Hall Nursing MediaLink DVD-ROM and on the Companion Website at http://www.prenhall.com/davidson. Click on "Chapter 20" to select the activities for this chapter.

Pregnancy is usually a normal, uncomplicated experience. In some cases, however, problems arise during the pregnancy that place the woman and her unborn child at risk. Regular prenatal care serves to detect these potential complications quickly so that effective care can be provided. This chapter focuses on problems that primarily occur during pregnancy, those with a gestational onset.

CARE OF THE WOMAN AT RISK BECAUSE OF BLEEDING DURING PREGNANCY

During the first and second trimesters of pregnancy the major cause of bleeding is **abortion.** This is the expulsion of the fetus before viability, which is considered 20 weeks' gestation or weight of less than 500 g. Abortions are either spontaneous, occurring naturally, or induced, occurring as a result of artificial or mechanical interruption. **Miscarriage** is a lay term applied to spontaneous abortion.

Other complications that can cause bleeding in the first half of pregnancy are ectopic pregnancy and gestational trophoblastic disease. In the second half of pregnancy, particularly in the third trimester, the two major causes of bleeding are placenta previa and abruptio placentae.

General Principles of Nursing Intervention

Spotting is relatively common during pregnancy and can occur following sexual intercourse or exercise as a result of trauma to the highly vascular cervix. However, the woman is advised to report any spotting or bleeding that occurs during pregnancy so that it can be evaluated.

It is often the nurse's responsibility to make the initial assessment of bleeding. In general, the following nursing measures should be implemented for pregnant women being evaluated for bleeding during pregnancy:

- Monitor blood pressure and pulse frequently.
- Observe the woman for indications of shock, such as pallor, clammy skin, perspiration, dyspnea, or restlessness.
- Count and weigh pads to assess amount of bleeding over a given time period; save any tissue or clots expelled.
- If pregnancy is of 12 weeks' gestation or beyond, assess fetal heart tones with a Doppler.
- Prepare for intravenous (IV) therapy. There may be standing orders to start IV therapy on bleeding clients.
- Prepare equipment for examination.
- Have oxygen therapy available.
- Collect and organize all data, including antepartal history, onset of bleeding episode, laboratory studies (hemoglobin, hematocrit, Rh status, and hormonal assays).
- Obtain an order to type and cross-match for blood if there is evidence of significant blood loss.

- Assess coping mechanisms and support system of the woman in crisis. Give emotional support to enhance her coping abilities by continuous, sustained presence, by clear explanation of procedures, and by communicating her status to her family. Most important, prepare the woman for possible fetal loss. Assess her expressions of anger, denial, guilt, depression, or self-blame.
- Assess the family's response to the situation.

Spontaneous Abortion (Miscarriage)

Many pregnancies end in the first trimester as a result of spontaneous abortion. Statistics are inaccurate because some women abort without being aware that they were pregnant during the early weeks of gestation, when the bleeding may be seen as a heavy menstrual period. If these very early abortions are included, the actual incidence of spontaneous abortion may be as high as 60%. However, when only clinically recognized pregnancies are considered, the incidence falls to approximately 10% to 15% (Schieve, Tatham, Peterson et al., 2003). About 0.5% to 1% of childbearing couples have experienced three or more previous miscarriages (Carrell, Wilcox, Lowy et al., 2004).

Sixty percent of first trimester spontaneous abortions are related to chromosomal abnormalities (Hill, 2004). Other causes include inherited thrombophilias such as factor V Leiden mutation, activated protein C resistance, and the prothrombin G20210A mutation (Krabbendam & Dekker, 2004). Teratogenic drugs, faulty implantation due to abnormalities of the female reproductive tract, a weakened cervix, placental abnormalities, chronic maternal diseases, endocrine imbalances, and maternal infections are also implicated in pregnancy loss. Women who use hot tubs or jacuzzis are twice as likely to have miscarriages as nonusers (Li, Janevic, Odouli et al., 2003). The pathophysiology of spontaneous abortion differs according to the cause. In most cases, embryonic death occurs, which results in loss of human chorionic gonadotropin (hCG) and decreased progesterone and estrogen levels. The uterine decidua is then sloughed off (vaginal bleeding), and the uterus becomes irritable, contracts, and usually expels the embryo/fetus. In late spontaneous abortion, the cause is usually a maternal factor, for example, incompetent cervix or maternal disease, and fetal death may not precede the onset of abortion.

Spontaneous abortion can be extremely distressing to the couple desiring a child. Chances for carrying the next pregnancy to term after one spontaneous abortion are as good as they are for the general population. Thereafter, however, chances of successful pregnancy decrease with each succeeding abortion. Following two to three consecutive losses, a woman and her partner should be evaluated and are candidates for genetic counseling.

CLASSIFICATION

Spontaneous abortions are subdivided into the following categories so that they can be differentiated clinically:

- *Threatened abortion* (Figure 20–1, A ◆). Unexplained bleeding, cramping, or backache indicate that the fetus may be in jeopardy. Bleeding may persist for days. The cervix is

Figure 20–1 ◆ Types of spontaneous abortion. *A,* Threatened. The cervix is not dilated, and the placenta is still attached to the uterine wall, but some bleeding occurs. *B,* Imminent. The placenta has separated from the uterine wall, the cervix has dilated, and the amount of bleeding has increased. *C,* Incomplete. The embryo/fetus has passed out of the uterus; however, the placenta remains.

closed. It may be followed by partial or complete expulsion of pregnancy, or it may resolve without threatening the fetus. Evaluation for hydatidiform mole or ectopic pregnancy (discussed shortly) is advisable.

- *Imminent abortion* (Figure 20–1, *B* ◆). Bleeding and cramping increase. The internal cervical os dilates. Membranes may rupture. The term *inevitable abortion* also applies.

- *Incomplete abortion* (Figure 20–1, *C* ◆). Part of the products of conception are retained, most often the placenta. The internal cervical os is dilated.

- *Complete abortion.* All the products of conception are expelled. The uterus is contracted and the cervical os may be closed.

- *Missed abortion.* The fetus dies in utero but is not expelled. Uterine growth ceases, breast changes regress, and the woman may report a brownish vaginal discharge. The cervix is closed. Diagnosis is made based on history, pelvic examination, and a drop in hCG levels or a negative pregnancy test and may be confirmed by ultrasound if necessary. If the fetus is retained beyond 4 weeks, fetal autolysis (breakdown of cells or tissue) results in the release of thromboplastin, and disseminated intravascular coagulation (DIC) may develop.

- *Recurrent pregnancy loss, formerly called habitual abortion.* Abortion occurs consecutively in three or more pregnancies.

- *Septic abortion.* Presence of infection. Septic abortion is less common since the availability of legal abortion. May occur with prolonged, unrecognized rupture of the membranes, pregnancy with intrauterine device (IUD) in utero, or attempts by inadequately prepared individuals to terminate a pregnancy.

ETIOLOGY

Numerous factors have been implicated as possible causes for recurrent pregnancy loss. They include genetic factors such as a trisomy or a balanced translocation in one of the parents (see Chapter 12 ∞), polycystic ovary syndrome, maternal metabolic abnormalities, uterine anatomic abnormalities, and problems with maternal antibody responses (American College of Obstetricians and Gynecologists [ACOG], 2001). Other possible causes include thyroid abnormalities; severe maternal illness such as poorly controlled diabetes mellitus, cyanotic heart disease, inflammatory bowel disease, and phenylketonuria; incompetent cervix (discussed later); maternal infections; environmental chemicals such as benzene, formaldehyde, pesticides, and anesthetic gases; exposure to radiation; chemotherapy; presence of an IUD; and trauma. In approximately 50% of couples, after a thorough evaluation, the cause of recurrent pregnancy loss remains unexplained.

CLINICAL THERAPY

One of the more reliable indicators of potential spontaneous abortion is the presence of pelvic cramping and backache. These symptoms are usually absent in bleeding caused by polyps, ruptured cervical blood vessels, or cervical erosion.

Vaginal bleeding occurs in up to 25% of first trimester pregnancies (Harville, Wilcox, Bird, et al., 2004; Schauberger, Mathiason, & Rooney, 2005). Evaluations to help determine the cause of vaginal bleeding include speculum examination to determine the presence of cervical polyps or cervical erosion, ultrasound scanning for the presence of cardiac activity and a ges-tational sac, or crown-rump length that is small for gestational age. Presence of a fetal heart beat on ultrasound provides a high likelihood (86%) of the pregnancy's continuing (Schauberger et al., 2005). Laboratory determination of hCG level can confirm a pregnancy, but because the hCG level falls slowly after fetal death, it cannot confirm a live embryo/fetus. Hemoglobin and hematocrit levels are obtained to assess blood loss. Blood is typed and cross-matched for possible replacement needs.

Although there is no evidence that supports the value of re-stricting physical activity, the therapy prescribed for the preg-nant woman with bleeding often includes bed rest, abstinence from coitus, and, perhaps, sedation. If bleeding persists and abortion is imminent or incomplete, the woman may be hospi-talized, IV therapy or blood transfusions may be started to re-place fluid, and dilation and curettage (D&C) or suction evacuation is performed to remove the remainder of the prod-ucts of conception. If the woman is Rh negative and not sensi-tized, and there has been prior ultrasound documentation of fetal cardiac activity, Rh immune globulin (RhoGAM) is given within 72 hours (Jabara & Barnhart, 2003). (See discussion on Rh sensitization later in this chapter.)

In missed abortions, the products of conception eventu-ally are expelled spontaneously. If this does not occur within 1 month to 6 weeks after fetal death, hospitalization is neces-sary. Suction evacuation, or D&C, is done if the pregnancy is in the first trimester. Beyond 12 weeks' gestation, induction of labor by IV oxytocin and intra-amniotic prostaglandin $F_{2\alpha}$, intravaginal prostaglandin E_2, or intravaginal misoprostol (a synthetic prostaglandin E_1 analog) may be used to expel the dead fetus.

Recent studies have indicated that dysfunctional folate me-tabolism is linked to failed pregnancies. The current recommen-dation is for periconceptual supplementation with folic acid. (See discussion of folate supplementation in Chapter 18 ∞).

NURSING CARE MANAGEMENT
Nursing Assessment and Diagnosis

The nurse assesses the amount and appearance of any vaginal bleeding and monitors the woman's vital signs and degree of discomfort. The woman's blood type and antibody status should be identified to determine the need for Rh immune globulin (see page 525). If the pregnancy is 10 to 12 weeks or more, fetal heart rate should be assessed by Doppler. The nurse also as-sesses the responses of the woman and her family to this crisis and evaluates their coping mechanisms and ability to comfort each other.

Nursing diagnoses that may apply include the following:

- *Fear* related to the risk of pregnancy loss
- *Acute Pain* related to abdominal cramping secondary to threatened abortion
- *Anticipatory Grieving* related to expected loss of unborn child

CULTURE AND RESPONSE TO FETAL LOSS

Remember that individual responses to fetal loss following miscarriage may vary greatly and may be influenced by ethnic or cultural norms.

- Miscarriage may be viewed in many ways. For example, it may be seen as a punishment from God, as the result of the evil eye or of a hex or curse by an enemy, or as a natural part of life.

- When grieving over a pregnancy loss, women from some cultures and ethnic groups may show their emotions freely, crying and wailing, whereas other women may hide their feelings behind a mask of stoicism.

- In some cultures the woman's partner is her primary source of support and comfort. In others, the woman turns to her mother or close female relatives for comfort.

- Avoid falling into the trap of stereotyping women according to culture. Individual responses are influenced by many factors, including the degree of assimilation into the dominant culture.

Nursing Plan and Implementation
COMMUNITY-BASED NURSING CARE

If a woman in her first trimester of pregnancy begins cramping or spotting, she may be evaluated on an outpatient basis if the bleeding is not heavy. Providing emotional support is an impor-tant task for nurses caring for women who have spontaneously aborted. Couples who approached the pregnancy with feelings of joy and a sense of expectancy now feel grief, sadness, and possibly anger.

Because many women, even with planned pregnancies, feel some ambivalence initially, guilt is a common emotion. The woman may harbor negative feelings about herself, ranging from lowered self-esteem resulting from a belief that she is lacking or abnormal in some way, to a notion that the abortion may be a punishment for some wrongdoing.

The nurse can offer invaluable psychologic support to the woman and her family by encouraging them to verbalize their feelings. Reflective listening gives the woman an opportunity to express and explore her feelings. The nurse can take cues from questions the woman asks, discuss the grief cycle, and provide resources. Referrals can help the woman and her family find ways to deal with their loss. If the woman has older children, she may need guidance in how to help them understand and cope with what has occurred. Commemorating the pregnancy and baby is helpful in validating the significance of the loss (Easter-wood, 2004). The grieving period following a spontaneous abortion usually lasts 6 to 24 months. Many couples can be helped during this period by an organization or support group established for parents who have lost a fetus or newborn. Nurses may benefit from education to help them understand the impact of early pregnancy loss through programs such as "Facilitating Healing in Families Who Experience Miscarriage." This is a scripted slide presentation available through Bereavement Services of LaCrosse, WI (Easterwood, 2004). See Chapter 37 ∞ for further discussion.

> *I was stunned by the depth of loss I felt following my miscarriage when I was 2½ months along. It didn't seem possible that I had already become so emotionally attached to the baby I carried. Afterward I was surprised by the number of women I knew who shared stories of their own miscarriages and confirmed that the emotions I was feeling were normal, if painful.*

The physical pain of the cramps and the amount of bleeding may be more severe than a couple anticipates, even when they are prepared for the possibility of an abortion. Nurses need to be aware that couples feel unprepared for their first experience of spontaneous abortion. Nurses should offer support in dealing with the physical experience by explaining why the discomfort is occurring and by offering analgesics for pain relief.

HOSPITAL-BASED NURSING CARE

A suction D&C is performed if the woman experiences an incomplete or missed abortion. This can be performed on an outpatient basis, and, barring any complications, the woman can return home a few hours after the procedure with instructions for self-care. An Rh-negative woman with a negative antibody screen should be given Rh immune globulin before discharge.

Throughout the procedure the nurse monitors the woman's physical status and provides emotional support. The nurse also answers any questions the woman or her partner may have and provides referrals to community agencies as needed.

TEACHING FOR SELF-CARE

If the woman had a D&C, someone should remain with her for the first 12 to 24 hours. The pregnant woman is instructed to report all episodes of heavy bleeding, fever, chills, foul-smelling vaginal discharge, or abdominal tenderness to her healthcare provider. The woman who experiences a pregnancy loss requires information about possible causes of the loss and the chances of recurrence with a future pregnancy. She may also require information about the grief process so she is prepared for it when she goes home. In addition, she should receive information about available resources, including support groups to help her cope with her feelings related to the loss of the pregnancy. The woman's partner or a family member should be included in the educational process when possible to assist him or her in personal grief work as well as to provide tools to help support the woman through the loss.

Evaluation

Expected outcomes of nursing care include the following:

- The woman is able to explain spontaneous abortion, the treatment measures employed in her care, and long-term implications for future pregnancies.

COMPLEMENTARY AND ALTERNATIVE THERAPIES

HERBS USED FOR PREVENTION OF MISCARRIAGE

Three herbs are frequently used by herbalists for the prevention of miscarriage: black haw, cramp bark, and false unicorn root. (Note that black haw and cramp bark are sometimes considered synonymous, because they are part of the same family: black haw is *Viburnum prunifolium* and cramp bark is *Viburnum opulus*.)

Black Haw: This herb is administered in tincture, tea, or capsule/tablet form. It has a uterine relaxant effect.

Cramp Bark: A "cousin" plant to black haw, cramp bark is reported to also have a relaxant effect on the uterine muscles. The use of black haw or cramp bark is not recommended in pregnancy (Rice, 2002).

False Unicorn Root: Considered a uterine tonic, this root is administered in tincture or dried root form. These three herbs are frequently combined in formulas. They should only be administered by a qualified herbalist.

- The woman suffers no complications.

- The woman and her partner are able to begin verbalizing their grief and to recognize that the grieving process usually lasts several months.

Ectopic Pregnancy

Ectopic pregnancy is an implantation of a fertilized ovum in a site other than the endometrial lining of the uterus. It may result from a number of different causes. Risk factors for ectopic pregnancy include tubal damage caused by pelvic inflammatory disease; previous pelvic or tubal surgery; endometriosis; previous ectopic pregnancy; presence of an IUD; high levels of progesterone, which can alter the motility of the egg in the fallopian tube; congenital anomalies of the tube; use of ovulation-inducing drugs; primary infertility; smoking; and advanced maternal age.

The incidence of ectopic pregnancy in the United States has risen dramatically from 4.5 per 1000 pregnancies in 1970 to 19.7 per 1000 pregnancies in 2000 (Van Den Eeden, Shan, Bruce et al., 2005). In spite of the increasing incidence of ectopic pregnancies, the mortality rate has declined almost 90%. This decrease can be credited to better diagnostic methods, which allow detection before tubal rupture.

The actual pathogenesis of ectopic pregnancy occurs when the fertilized ovum is prevented or slowed in its progress down the tube. The fertilized ovum implants in either the fallopian tube or the ovary, peritoneal cavity, cervix, or uterine cornua (Figure 20–2 ◆). The most common location for implantation of an ectopic pregnancy is the ampulla of the tube. The occurrence of ectopic pregnancy in women who have used assisted reproductive technology is 4%. A heterotopic pregnancy (one conceptus is ectopic and one is intrauterine) is extremely rare in

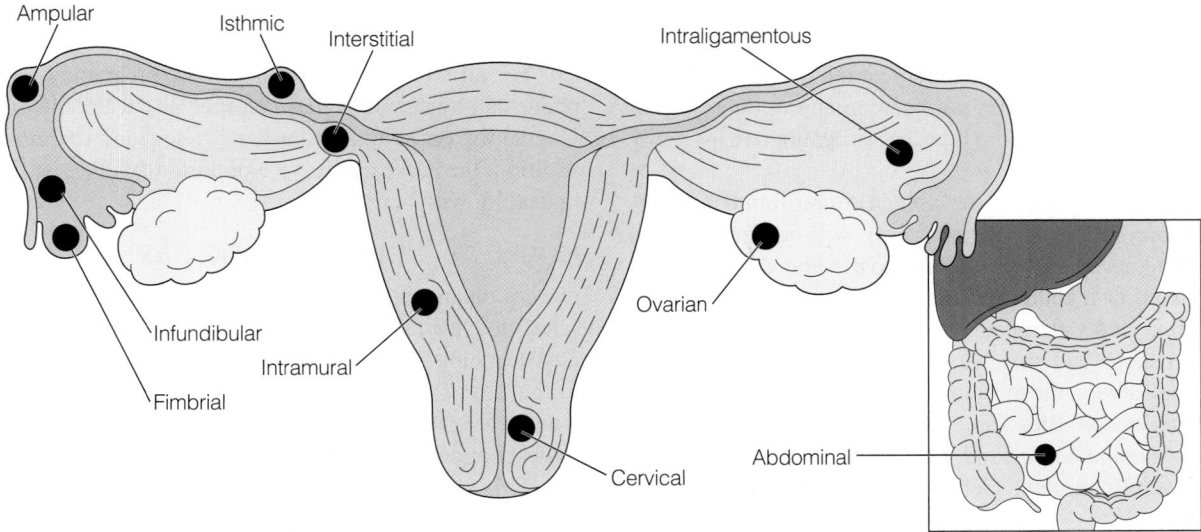

Figure 20–2 ◆ Various implantation sites in ectopic pregnancy. The most common site is within the fallopian tube, hence the name "tubal pregnancy."

spontaneously occurring pregnancies but may be as high as 1% in assisted conception (Braude & Rowell, 2003).

Initially, the normal symptoms of pregnancy may be present, specifically, amenorrhea, breast tenderness, and nausea. The normal clinical signs of early pregnancy such as the bluish discoloration of the cervix (Chadwick's sign) and the softening of the isthmus (Hegar's sign) may be noted on physical exam. The hormone hCG is present in the blood and urine. With an ectopic implantation, the trophoblastic cells grow into the adjacent tissue, often the tubal wall, and arterial vessels. This results in internal hemorrhage. The faulty implantation of the placenta causes fluctuation of hormone levels. Hormones first stimulate the endometrial lining of the uterus to grow, but fluctuation in levels cannot support the endometrium, and vaginal bleeding ensues. The implanted ovum quickly begins to rupture the fallopian tube if it is implanted there. The woman may experience one-sided lower abdominal pain or diffuse lower abdominal pain and vasomotor disturbances such as fainting or dizziness. In about 50% of cases, referred right shoulder pain occurs from blood irritating the subdiaphragmatic phrenic nerve.

In many instances, the symptoms are not obvious. One fourth of ectopic pregnancies may involve uterine enlargement. Physical examination usually reveals adnexal tenderness; an adnexal mass is palpable in approximately one half of the cases.

If internal hemorrhage is profuse, the woman rapidly develops signs of hypovolemic shock. More commonly, the bleeding is slow (chronic), and the abdomen gradually becomes rigid and very tender. If bleeding into the pelvic cavity has been extensive, vaginal examination causes extreme pain, and a mass of blood may be palpated in the cul-de-sac of Douglas.

Laboratory tests may reveal low hemoglobin and hematocrit levels and rising leukocyte levels. In a normal pregnancy β-hCG titers double every 48 hours from 3 to 6 weeks' gestation. Ectopic pregnancies are associated with β-hCG titers that increase more slowly.

CLINICAL THERAPY

It is important to differentiate an ectopic pregnancy from other disorders with similar clinical presenting pictures. Consideration must be given to possible spontaneous abortion, ruptured corpus luteum cyst, appendicitis, salpingitis, torsion of the ovary, ovarian cysts, and urinary tract infection.

The following measures are used to establish the diagnosis of ectopic pregnancy and assess the woman's status:

- A careful assessment of menstrual history, particularly the last menstrual period (LMP).

- Careful pelvic exam to identify any abnormal pelvic masses and tenderness.

- Laboratory testing as described previously.

- Ultrasonography. In a normal pregnancy, transvaginal ultrasound should detect an intrauterine gestational sac when the β-hCG is greater than 1500 milli–International Unit/mL. By transabdominal scan, an intrauterine sac may not be identified until the β-hCG levels reach 6500 milli–International Unit/mL. Confirming an intrauterine pregnancy nearly eliminates the diagnosis of ectopic pregnancy.

- Laparoscopy. If the presence or absence of an ectopic pregnancy cannot be confirmed by other measures, laparoscopic intervention may be necessary for both diagnosis and treatment.

Once an ectopic pregnancy is confirmed, therapy options are reviewed with the woman. Medical management using methotrexate is indicated for the woman who desires future pregnancy if her ectopic pregnancy is unruptured and of 3.5 cm size or less and if her condition is stable. In addition, there must be no fetal cardiac motion and no evidence of maternal thrombocytopenia, leukopenia, kidney disease, or liver disease. The medication is administered intramuscularly. As an outpatient, the woman is monitored for increasing abdominal pain. β-hCG titers are monitored regularly. β-hCG titers increase for 1 to 4 days and then decrease. A single-dose regimen of methotrexate is gaining favor among clinicians. Repeat injections are considered every 7 days if there has not been an appropriate drop in hCG. They are needed in more than 20% of women (Lipscomb, Givens, Meyer et al., 2005).

If surgery is indicated and the woman desires future pregnancies, a laparoscopic linear salpingostomy will be performed to evacuate the ectopic pregnancy gently and preserve the tube. If the tube is ruptured or if future childbearing is not an issue, laparoscopic salpingectomy (removal of the tube) is performed. If the woman is in shock and unstable, an abdominal incision will be made. During surgery, the most important risk to be considered is potential hemorrhage. Bleeding must be controlled, and replacement therapy should be on hand. The Rh-negative nonsensitized woman is given Rh immune globulin to prevent sensitization.

NURSING CARE MANAGEMENT
Nursing Assessment and Diagnosis

When the woman with a suspected ectopic pregnancy is admitted to the hospital, the nurse assesses the appearance and amount of vaginal bleeding. The nurse monitors vital signs, particularly blood pressure and pulse, for evidence of developing shock.

It is also the nurse's responsibility to assess the woman's emotional status and coping abilities and to evaluate the couple's informational needs. If surgery is necessary, the nurse performs the ongoing assessments appropriate for any client postoperatively.

Nursing diagnoses that may apply for a woman with an ectopic pregnancy include the following:

- *Anticipatory Grieving* related to the loss of the pregnancy
- *Pain* related to abdominal bleeding secondary to tubal rupture
- *Health-Seeking Behavior: Information About the Treatment of Ectopic Pregnancy* related to an expressed desire to gain better understanding of the condition and its long-term implications

Nursing Plan and Implementation
COMMUNITY-BASED NURSING CARE

Women with ectopic pregnancy are often seen initially in a clinic or office setting. Nurses need to be alert to the possibility of ectopic pregnancy if a woman presents with complaints of abdominal pain and lack of menses for 1 to 2 months. Once an initial evaluation is complete, if no ultrasound is available, the woman should be referred to another facility where ultrasound is available. The nurse plays an important role in monitoring the woman's condition and in providing her with information.

A woman with a confirmed ectopic pregnancy who meets the criteria for methotrexate administration is followed as an outpatient. The nurse should advise the woman that some abdominal pain is common following the injection but it is generally mild and lasts only 24 to 48 hours. More severe pain might indicate treatment failure and should be evaluated. The woman should also report heavy vaginal bleeding, dizziness, or tachy-

cardia. In addition, the nurse should stress the need to return for follow-up β-hCG testing.

For all women treated for ectopic pregnancy, a follow-up phone call by the nurse may be especially welcome. It gives the woman the opportunity to ask any questions she may have. In addition, the nurse can use the opportunity to assist the woman in dealing with her grief.

HOSPITAL-BASED NURSING CARE

Once a diagnosis of ectopic pregnancy is made and surgery is scheduled, the nurse starts an IV as ordered and begins preoperative teaching. The nurse should report signs of developing shock to the physician immediately and initiate interventions. If the woman is experiencing severe abdominal pain, the nurse can administer appropriate analgesics and evaluate their effectiveness.

TEACHING FOR SELF-CARE

Teaching is an important part of nursing care. The woman may want her condition and various procedures explained. She may need instruction about measures to prevent infection, symptoms to report (pain, bleeding, fever, chills), and her follow-up visit.

The woman and her family will need emotional support during this difficult time. Their feelings and responses to this crisis will probably be similar to those that occur in cases of spontaneous abortion. As a result, similar nursing actions are required.

Evaluation

Expected outcomes of nursing care include the following:

- The woman is able to explain ectopic pregnancy, treatment alternatives, and implications for future childbearing.
- The woman and her caregivers detect possible complications early and manage them appropriately.
- The woman and her partner are able to begin verbalizing their loss and recognize that the grieving process usually lasts several months.

Gestational Trophoblastic Disease

As discussed in Chapter 11 ∞, the trophoblast is the outermost layer of embryonic cells and gives rise to the chorion. **Gestational trophoblastic disease (GTD)** is the pathologic proliferation of trophoblastic cells, and includes partial or complete hydatidiform mole, invasive mole (chorioadenoma destruens), and choriocarcinoma.

Hydatidiform mole (molar pregnancy) is a condition in which a proliferation of trophoblastic cells results in the formation of a placenta characterized by *hydropic* (fluid-filled) grapelike clusters. The significance of this disease for the woman who has it is the loss of the pregnancy and the possibility, though remote, of developing choriocarcinoma, a form of cancer, from the trophoblastic tissue. Molar pregnancies are classified into two types, complete and partial, both of which meet the preceding criteria. Little is known about the cause of either type, but some of the pathophysiology has been clarified. The *complete mole* develops from an anuclear ovum that contains no maternal genetic material, an "empty" egg. In most cases, a haploid sperm, 23X, fertilizes this anuclear egg and duplicates before the first cell division (diandric diploidy). The conceptus then contains in its cells a 46XX chromosomal set of totally paternal origin. In 4% to 10% of the cases, fertilization of an empty egg by two sperm occurs (diandric dispermy), resulting in a 46XY conceptus (Hurteau, 2003; Smith, 2003). The YX karyotype may be associated with a higher incidence of malignancy (Hurteau, 2003). The hydropic vesicles that form from the chorionic villi are avascular in the complete mole. No embryonic or fetal tissue or membranes are found. Choriocarcinoma seems to be associated primarily with the complete mole.

In contrast to the complete mole, the *partial mole* usually has a triploid karyotype, that is, 69 chromosomes. Most often, a normal ovum with 23 chromosomes is fertilized by two sperm (dispermy) or by a sperm that has failed to undergo the first meiosis and therefore contains 46 chromosomes (Smith, 2003). In partial molar pregnancy, the villi are often vascularized and may be hydropic only in sections of the placenta rather than universally as with a complete mole. Often partial moles are recognized only after spontaneous abortion, or they may go unnoticed. Unlike the complete mole, the fetus usually survives to 8 or 9 weeks' gestation and occasionally longer. Twin pregnancies in which a normal fetus coexists with a molar pregnancy have been reported. Because fetal development is not seen in complete moles, this can present a diagnostic pitfall leading to an erroneous diagnosis of a partial mole (Bentley, 2003).

Hydatidiform mole occurs in about 1 in 1500 pregnancies in the United States (Berkowitz & Goldstein, 2005) (see Developing Cultural Competence: Incidence of Complications). The incidence of molar pregnancy increases with extremes in maternal age and has higher rates in certain populations, including Indonesia, Taiwan, the Philippines, and the Far East (Berman, Di Saia, & Tewari, 2004; Smith, 2003). The risk of repeat molar pregnancy has been reported as 1% after one molar pregnancy (Berman et al., 2004).

Invasive mole (chorioadenoma destruens) is similar to a complete mole but involves the uterine myometrium. Treatment is the same as for a complete mole.

Choriocarcinoma is invasive, malignant trophoblastic disease that is usually metastatic and can be fatal. It is discussed in more detail shortly.

CLINICAL THERAPY

Diagnosis of hydatidiform mole is often suspected in the presence of the following signs:

- Vaginal bleeding is almost universal with molar pregnancies and may occur as early as the fourth week or as late as the second trimester. It is often brownish, "like prune juice," because of liquefaction of the uterine clot, but it may be bright red.

- Anemia occurs frequently because of the loss of blood.

- Hydropic vesicles may be passed and, if so, are diagnostic (Figure 20–3 ◆). With a partial mole, the vesicles are often smaller and may not be noticed by the woman.

- Uterine enlargement greater than expected for gestational age is a classic sign, present in about 50% of cases. In the remainder of cases, the uterus is appropriate or small for the gestational stage. Enlargement is due to the proliferating trophoblastic tissue and to a large amount of clotted blood.

- Absence of fetal heart sounds in the presence of other signs of pregnancy is a classic sign of molar pregnancy. (Only rarely has a viable fetus been born in a partial molar pregnancy.)

- Markedly elevated serum hCG may be present because of continued secretion by the proliferating trophoblastic tissue. (Normally hCG levels increase from the time of implantation, peak at 60 to 70 days, and then decline slowly, reaching a low point at 100 to 130 days.)

- Very low levels of maternal serum α-fetoprotein (MSAFP) are found.

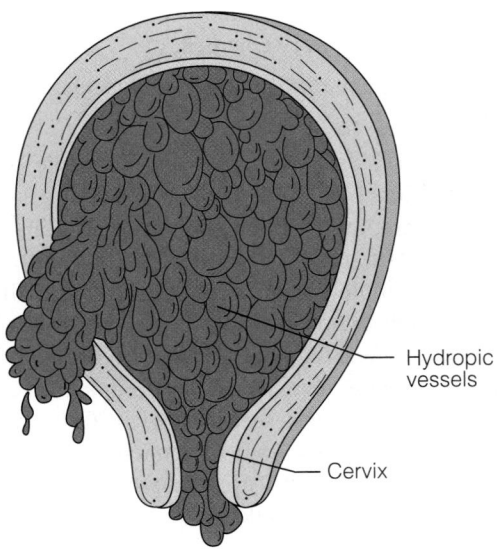

Figure 20–3 ◆ Hydatidiform mole. A common sign is vaginal bleeding, often brownish (the characteristic "prune juice" appearance) but sometimes bright red. In this figure, some of the hydropic vesicles are being passed. This occurrence is diagnostic for hydatidiform mole.

DEVELOPING CULTURAL COMPETENCE

INCIDENCE OF COMPLICATIONS

- The incidence of ectopic pregnancy is higher for nonwhite women than for whites in every age category.

- The incidence of preeclampsia is also related to genetic predisposition. Women of African American descent are at higher risk.

- Hydatidiform mole is seen more frequently in early teens and perimenopausal women. The occurrence rate is significantly higher in the Far East and the tropics, reported at 1 in 120 pregnancies (Berman et al., 2004).

- Hyperemesis gravidarum may occur, probably as a result of the high levels of hCG.

- Preeclampsia (discussed shortly) may be seen, especially if the molar pregnancy continues into the second trimester. Because preeclampsia is a disease of late pregnancy, if symptoms occur in the first half of pregnancy, molar pregnancy must be considered as the first diagnosis.

- Rarely, hyperthyroidism results from production of thyrotropin by molar tissue. It produces thyrotoxicosis, which may precipitate a clinical emergency.

Ultrasound is the primary means of diagnosing a molar pregnancy, usually after 6 to 8 weeks, when the vesicular enlargement of the villi can be identified.

Therapy begins with suction evacuation of the mole and curettage of the uterus to remove all fragments of the placenta. Early evacuation decreases the possibility of other complications. If the woman is older and has completed her childbearing, or if there is excessive bleeding, hysterectomy may be the treatment of choice to reduce the incidence of malignant sequelae. Uterine contractions can cause trophoblastic tissue to be engulfed in the large venous sinusoids of the uterus. Therefore, stimulation of uterine contractions is avoided until the uterus is evacuated to prevent embolization of trophoblastic tissue to the lungs (Berman et al., 2004).

Complications associated with hydatidiform mole that require medical recognition and therapy include the following:

- Anemia

- Hyperthyroidism

- Infection, usually seen with late diagnosis and spontaneous abortion of the mole

- DIC

- Trophoblastic embolization of the lung, usually seen after molar evacuation of a significantly enlarged uterus (this creates a cardiorespiratory emergency)

- Ovarian cysts, which may be small or large enough to displace the uterus

Malignant GTD, usually choriocarcinoma, develops following evacuation of a mole in 20% of women (ACOG, 2004a). To detect this serious problem early and initiate treatment, follow-up care is essential. Follow-up for women who have had a mole evacuated consists of baseline chest x-ray examination to detect metastasis and a repeat x-ray if chemotherapy is necessary. Continued high or rising hCG levels in women who have had molar pregnancy but are not currently pregnant suggest secretion of hCG by metastatic trophoblastic cells. Thus, radioimmunoassay hCG values should be determined every 1 to 2 weeks until negative two consecutive times, then should be monitored every 1 to 2 months for 1 year. If hCG plateaus or rises during this time or metastases are detected, chemotherapy is started immediately. In addition, the woman has physical exams with a pelvic exam every 4 weeks until remission and then every 3 months for 1 year (Berman et al., 2004). If hCG levels plateau for 3 to 6 consecutive weeks or rise more than 50%,

evaluation for metastatic disease should be undertaken and prompt chemotherapy initiated (Berman et al., 2004).

Effective contraception is needed during this time to prevent pregnancy and the resulting confusion about the cause of changes in hCG levels. In addition, pregnancy could mask an hCG rise associated with malignant GTD.

Several systems have been proposed for classifying clients with metastatic gestational neoplasms. The World Health Organization (WHO) system is used most widely and categorizes clients as low risk, intermediate risk, or high risk. Treatment at a center specializing in GTD is advised. Once pregnancy has been ruled out, full physical examination, chest x-ray, abdominopelvic computed tomography (CT) scan, and brain CT scan are done to rule out metastatic spread. Chemotherapy is then begun using methotrexate alone or in combination with other chemotherapy agents.

After treatment, careful follow-up monitoring of hCG levels is important. Malignant GTD is curable if diagnosed early and treated appropriately. Malignant sequelae appear to be increased with repetitive moles.

Currently research is underway to identify risk factors for GTD and to examine the role of genetics in its development. In addition, efforts are underway to develop better, more sensitive ways to detect minimal levels of hCG and clinical trials are focusing on the effectiveness of established chemotherapy approaches in treating malignant GTD (Bess & Wood, 2006).

NURSING CARE MANAGEMENT
Nursing Assessment and Diagnosis

It is important for nurses involved in antepartal care to be aware of symptoms of hydatidiform mole and observe for them at each antepartal visit. The classic symptoms used to diagnose molar pregnancy are found more frequently with the complete than with the partial mole. The partial mole may be difficult to distinguish from a missed abortion before evacuation.

When the woman is hospitalized for evacuation of the mole, the nurse should monitor vital signs and vaginal bleeding for evidence of hemorrhage. In addition, the nurse determines whether abdominal pain is present and assesses the woman's emotional state and coping ability.

Nursing diagnoses that may apply to a woman with a hydatidiform mole include the following:

- *Fear* related to the possible development of choriocarcinoma

- *Health-Seeking Behavior: Information About the Need for Regular Monitoring of hCG Levels* related to an expressed desire to understand the long-term implications of the disease

- *Anticipatory Grieving* related to the loss of the pregnancy

Nursing Plan and Implementation
COMMUNITY-BASED NURSING CARE

When molar pregnancy is suspected, the woman needs emotional support. The nurse can relieve some of the woman's anxiety by answering questions about the disease process and explaining what ultrasound and other diagnostic procedures will entail. If a molar pregnancy is diagnosed, the nurse supports the childbearing family as they deal with their grief about the lost pregnancy. Healthcare counselors, the hospital chaplain, or their own clergy may be of assistance in helping them deal with this loss.

HOSPITAL-BASED NURSING CARE

When the woman is hospitalized for evacuation of the mole, explanation of the curettage procedure is necessary. Although the physician is responsible for providing this explanation, the woman and her partner may have many questions and concerns that the nurse can discuss with them. The nurse may also clarify areas of confusion or misunderstanding.

Typed and cross-matched blood must be available for surgery because of previous blood loss and the potential for hemorrhage. Oxytocin is administered to keep the uterus contracted and prevent hemorrhage. In addition, acute renal failure, a syndrome of rapid onset, may occur when significant hemorrhage results in absolute loss of fluid volume. Following surgery, the nurse carefully observes the woman's urinary output, watches for further signs of bleeding, and assesses for any signs of infection.

If the woman is Rh negative and not sensitized, she is given Rh immune globulin to prevent antibody formation. (See discussion on Rh sensitization later in this chapter.)

TEACHING FOR SELF-CARE

The woman needs to know the importance of the follow-up visits. She is advised to use contraception to delay becoming pregnant again until after the follow-up program is completed.

Evaluation

Expected outcomes of nursing care include the following:

- The woman has a smooth recovery following successful evacuation of the mole.
- The woman is able to explain GTD, its treatment, follow-up, and long-term implications for pregnancy.
- The woman and her partner are able to begin verbalizing their grief at the loss of their anticipated child.
- The woman is able to discuss the importance of follow-up assessment and indicates her willingness to cooperate with the regimen.

Placenta Previa

In *placenta previa,* the placenta is improperly implanted in the lower uterine segment, sometimes over the internal os. As the lower uterine segment contracts and the cervix dilates in the later weeks of pregnancy, the placental villi are torn from the uterine wall, thus exposing the uterine sinuses at the placental site. Bleeding begins, but because its amount depends on the number of sinuses exposed, it may initially be either scanty or profuse. The classic symptom is painless vaginal bleeding usually occurring after 20 weeks' gestation. See Chapter 26 ∞ for an in-depth discussion of placenta previa.

Abruptio Placentae

Abruptio placentae is the premature separation of a normally implanted placenta from the uterine wall. It occurs before birth, usually during the labor process. It is characterized by maternal pain disproportionate to the strength of uterine contractions and may or may not be accompanied by obvious bleeding. See Chapter 26 ∞ for an in-depth description of abruptio placentae.

CARE OF THE WOMAN WITH AN INCOMPETENT CERVIX

Many questions remain unanswered about cervical insufficiency (**incompetent cervix**). The classic definition presents cervical insufficiency or cervical incompetence as painless dilatation of the cervix without contractions because of a structural or functional defect of the cervix. The woman is usually unaware of contractions and presents with advanced effacement and dilatation and, possibly, bulging membranes. The emerging view is that cervical incompetence and cervical resistance to labor occur as a continuum from complete incompetence through, perhaps, excessive competence demonstrated by those women who have prolonged labors (Iams, 2004). It is difficult to determine the incidence because of the inconsistency in definition and lack of clear diagnostic criteria (ACOG, 2003a; Williams & Iams, 2004).

The origin of cervical incompetence is multifactorial (Weiner, Lee, Buhimschi et al., 2005; Williams & Iams, 2004). Factors that may contribute to the tendency for the cervix to dilate prematurely can be divided into three categories: congenital factors, acquired factors, and biochemical (hormonal) factors. Congenitally incompetent cervix may be found in women exposed to diethylstilbestrol (DES) or those with a bicornuate uterus. Acquired cervical incompetence may be related to inflammation, infection, subclinical uterine activity, cervical trauma, cone biopsy or late second trimester elective abortions, or increased uterine volume (as with a multiple gestation). The hormone relaxin may be an endocrine cause of cervical incompetence. Researchers suggest that the increased relaxin levels related to ovulation induction may contribute to connective tissue changes in the cervix (Iams, 2004).

A woman's obstetric history may give her healthcare provider an indication of increased risk for incompetent cervix. Factors include multiple gestations, repetitive second trimester losses, previous preterm birth, progressively earlier births with each subsequent pregnancy, short labors, previous elective abortion or cervical manipulation, DES exposure, or other uterine anomaly. These women will benefit from close surveillance of cervical length with transvaginal ultrasound beginning between 16 and 24 weeks' gestation (Iams, 2004). Cervical effacement occurs from the internal os out and can be seen on ultrasound as "funneling." Alteration is apparent in transvaginal scan when fundal pressure is applied or the woman assumes a standing position. In addition, women at risk for incompetent cervix need to be informed early in pregnancy of warning signs of impending birth, such as lower back pain, pelvic pressure, and changes in vaginal discharge.

Figure 20–4 ◆ A cerclage or purse-string suture is inserted in the cervix to prevent preterm cervical dilatation and pregnancy loss. After placement, the string is tightened and secured anteriorly.

A number of contemporary studies have concluded that endovaginal ultrasound measurements of cervical length between 22 and 24 weeks' gestation identify groups at risk for preterm birth. However, the placement of a cervical cerclage (see the following discussion) does not substantially reduce the risk of prematurity (Meekai, Alfirevic, Health et al., 2004; Williams & Iams, 2004). This has led to a reconsideration of both medical and surgical treatment options for women with a history of midtrimester losses. Medical therapies used are serial cervical ultrasound assessments, bed rest, progesterone supplementation, antibiotics, and anti-inflammatory drugs.

Surgical options include the various types of cerclage procedures. An elective cervical cerclage may be placed late in the first trimester or early in the second trimester (Figure 20–4 ◆). A cervical cerclage involves using a heavy suture to reinforce the cervix at the level of the internal os. The McDonald cerclage utilizes a purse-string technique high up on the cervix to tie it closed. The Shirodkar method uses a submucosal band placed at the level of the internal os.

Abdominal cerclage approach may be required for women with a congenitally short or amputated cervix, cervical defects, a cervix previously scarred, or unhealed lacerations or subacute cervicitis (ACOG, 2003a; Iams, 2004). Figure 20–5 ◆ compares a cervix of normal length with one indicative of cervical shortening. A cerclage is in place.

In cases in which cervical dilatation is discovered unexpectedly, an attempt may be made to "rescue" the pregnancy by placing a cerclage after cervical dilatation is advanced. In some instances, decompression of a bulging amniotic sac must be accomplished immediately before the cerclage placement. In this situation, a preoperative evaluation for infection, ruptured membranes, and uterine activity may be prudent. Tocolytics

A

B

C

Figure 20–5 ◆ Endovaginal ultrasound of the cervix. *A,* Normal cervix measuring 47.2 mm. *B,* Woman at 24 weeks' gestation with chorioamnionitis and preterm labor. Cervix is fully effaced and dilated 2 cm. *C,* Arrow indicates stitch placement of McDonald cerclage. Cervix is 18.5 cm in length.
SOURCE: Courtesy of Debbie McGee, MSN, PNNP, RDMS.

(drugs that stop labor), broad-spectrum antibiotics, and anti-inflammatory agents are given perioperatively and for ongoing treatment. Exposure of the amniotic membranes increases the chance of cerclage failure when compared with an elective placement of a cerclage (Weiner et al., 2005).

An uncomplicated elective cerclage may be done on an outpatient basis or the woman may be hospitalized and discharged after 24 to 48 hours. An emergency cerclage, however, requires hospitalization for 5 to 7 days or longer. After 37 completed weeks' gestation, the suture may be cut and vaginal birth permitted, or the suture may be left in place and a cesarean birth performed to avoid repeating the procedure in subsequent pregnancies.

CARE OF THE WOMAN WITH HYPEREMESIS GRAVIDARUM

Nausea and vomiting of mild to moderate intensity are common during early pregnancy, affecting between 66% and 90% of pregnant women (Scott & Abu-Hamda, 2004; Steinlauf, Chang, & Traube, 2004). It most commonly occurs between 5 and 12 weeks and usually subsides by the end of the first trimester or early second trimester (Steinlauf et al., 2004). **Hyperemesis gravidarum** is a relatively rare condition, occurring in about 0.5% to 2% of all pregnancies, in which nausea and vomiting are so severe that they affect hydration and nutritional status (ACOG, 2004b; Lagiou, Tamimi, Mucci et al., 2003). Dehydration, electrolyte imbalances, acidosis, weight loss, ketonuria, and, possibly, hepatic and renal damage are attributable to hyperemesis.

Hyperemesis can be a temporarily disabling condition in which affected women may need multiple hospitalizations and face disruption of work, family, or social routines. In rare instances, the psychologic impact is so extreme that a woman may request pregnancy termination. It occurs more frequently in nulliparous women, adolescents, women with a multiple gestation, women with increased body weight, certain ethnic groups, pregnancies complicated by GTD, or fetal abnormalities, and women with a mother or sister who experienced hyperemesis or personal history of hyperemesis in a previous pregnancy (ACOG, 2004b; Scott & Abu-Hamda, 2004).

The cause of hyperemesis during pregnancy is still unclear, but it has been suggested that hCG plays a role. An argument against this mechanism is that nausea and vomiting are not common in women with choriocarcinoma, which is characterized by high levels of hCG (Lagiou et al., 2003). Higher levels of estradiol as well as lower levels of prolactin have been implicated as well (Lagiou et al., 2003). Other mechanisms that may relate to hyperemesis are displacement of the gastrointestinal tract, hypofunction of the anterior pituitary gland and adrenal cortex, abnormalities of the corpus luteum, *Helicobacter pylori* infection, and psychologic factors (Scott & Abu-Hamda, 2004). Interestingly, hyperemesis is rare in populations of developing countries. In severe cases, the pathology of hyperemesis begins with dehydration. This leads to fluid-electrolyte imbalance and alkalosis from the loss of hydrochloric acid. More prolonged vomiting can result in loss of predominantly alkaline intestinal

juices and the occurrence of acidosis. Hypovolemia from dehydration leads to hypotension and increased pulse rate, with increased hematocrit and blood urea nitrogen levels and decreased urine output. Severe potassium loss (hypokalemia) interferes with the ability of the kidneys to concentrate urine and disrupts cardiac functioning. Starvation causes muscle wasting and severe protein and vitamin deficiencies. Jaundice, hyperpyrexia, and peripheral neuritis may develop. If inadequately or incorrectly treated, complications such as Wernicke encephalopathy, esophageal rupture, or even maternal death may occur.

The diagnostic criteria for hyperemesis include a history of intractable vomiting in the first half of pregnancy, dehydration, ketonuria, and a weight loss of 5% of prepregnancy weight.

Clinical Therapy

The goals of treatment include controlling vomiting, correcting dehydration, restoring electrolyte balance, and maintaining adequate nutrition. If the woman with intractable nausea and vomiting does not respond to frequent small meals of simple carbohydrates and the occasional use of antiemetics, she may require IV fluids on an outpatient basis. If the woman's symptoms do not improve, hospitalization may be necessary.

The initial work-up should include an ultrasound to exclude the possibility of molar pregnancy. Initially the woman is given nothing by mouth; IV fluids are administered to correct dehydration. Potassium chloride is typically added to the IV infusion to prevent hypokalemia. Replacement of thiamine (vitamin B_1) and pyroxidine (vitamin B_6) is important to correct deficiencies of these vitamins and prevent peripheral neuropathy. Administration of dextrose solution before the correction of thiamine deficiency could lead to Wernicke encephalopathy (loss of memory, confusion). Desired urine output is a minimum of 1000 mL/24 hours.

Corticosteroids are a logical choice for the treatment of hyperemesis because they have been used to treat nausea in oncology patients. Recent studies, however, suggest that steroids have no appreciable effect in the treatment of severe hyperemesis gravidarum or on pregnancy outcomes (Yost, McIntire, Wians et al., 2003). Complementary therapies have also been tried in treating hyperemesis because they may offer relief for nausea and vomiting of pregnancy. Ginger has been used for its beneficial effects on motion sickness, and ginger syrup has been shown to provide significant relief of nausea (Born & Barron, 2005).

The use of acupuncture or acupressure to stimulate the median nerve at the P6 or Neiguan acupuncture point may also cause a reduction in the severity of symptoms (ACOG, 2004b; Rosen, deVeciana, Miller et al., 2003).

If the woman does not respond to this management, total parenteral nutrition may be used to meet the caloric and nutritional needs of the woman and her fetus. When the woman's condition has improved, oral feedings are started. Six small dry feedings followed by clear liquids is one suggested treatment. Another method is 1 oz of water offered each hour, followed as tolerated by clear, then nourishing liquids, progressing on succeeding days to low-fat soft and regular diets.

NURSING CARE MANAGEMENT
Nursing Assessment and Diagnosis

When a woman is hospitalized for control of vomiting, the nurse must regularly assess the amount and character of further emesis, intake and output, fetal heart rate, maternal vital signs, initial weight, evidence of jaundice or bleeding, and the woman's emotional state.

Nursing diagnoses that may apply to the woman with hyperemesis gravidarum include the following:

- *Imbalanced Nutrition: Less than Body Requirements* related to persistent vomiting secondary to hyperemesis
- *Fear* related to the effects of hyperemesis or its treatment on fetal well-being

Nursing Plan and Implementation
COMMUNITY-BASED NURSING CARE

The initial evaluation of the woman is designed to distinguish between morning sickness, which is amenable to self-care, and real nutritional risk. The nurse should take this opportunity to evaluate possible family and lifestyle stressors. It is wise to include both the woman and her family in the discussion of strategies to reduce nausea and vomiting she can try at home, including such tactics as small carbohydrate meals, high-protein snacks, total avoidance of fatty foods, resting with her feet up and head elevated, or slowly sipping carbonated beverages when nauseated. Herbal tea, such as spearmint, peppermint, raspberry, chamomile, or ginger root, may be helpful. Odors, exposure to fresh air, very hot or cold liquids, ice, and straws should be avoided. If the nausea and vomiting progress to a point where oral intake is not tolerated and dehydration is evident, medical intervention is required.

Home Care

Parenteral therapy provided at home in collaboration with a physician and registered dietitian is sometimes used to allow the woman to remain in her home and help decrease healthcare costs. It also gives the nurse an opportunity to observe family interactions and evaluate the home environment. This assessment is often useful in determining the pregnant woman's level of support, any significant stressors in her life, her understanding of nutrition and self-care measures, and so forth.

HOSPITAL-BASED CARE

Nursing care should be supportive and directed at maintaining a relaxed, quiet environment away from food odors or offensive smells. Once oral feedings are started, food should be attractively served. Oral hygiene is important because the mouth is dry and may be irritated from vomitus. Weight gain or loss should be monitored regularly. Because emotional factors have been found to play a major role in this condition, psychotherapy may be recommended. With proper treatment, the prognosis is favorable.

TEACHING FOR SELF-CARE

As part of client teaching, the nurse should review actions the woman can take to prevent or decrease nausea. These are discussed in Chapter 16. ∞

Evaluation

Expected outcomes of nursing care include the following:

- The woman is able to explain hyperemesis gravidarum, its therapy, and its possible effects on her pregnancy.
- The woman's condition is corrected, and possible complications are avoided.

CARE OF THE WOMAN WITH PREMATURE RUPTURE OF MEMBRANES

Spontaneous rupture of the membranes before the onset of labor is known as **premature rupture of membranes (PROM).** Some authorities define PROM as the rupture of the bag of waters any time after 37 weeks but before the onset of labor (Garite, 2004; Mercer, 2003); some have further defined PROM as a specific period elapse without labor, generally between 1 and 12 hours. *Preterm* PROM (PPROM) has been described as rupture before 37 weeks' gestation. Prolonged rupture of the membranes is rupture more than 24 hours before birth. In the United States, PPROM complicates more than 3% (or 120,000) of pregnancies each year and is associated with more than one third of the preterm births (Canavan, Simhan, & Caritis, 2004a; Mercer, 2003).

Whereas preterm labor tends to be the cause of preterm birth in more educated and affluent women, PPROM is seen more frequently in less educated women of lower economic status (Newton, 2005). Although the cause of PPROM is unknown, it is thought that PPROM occurs because of multiple, interrelated factors. The most significant risk factors for PPROM are previous preterm birth and previous PPROM; hence, incompetent cervix may be the cause of second trimester PPROM. Cervicitis, urinary tract infection (UTI), amniocentesis, placenta previa, abruptio placentae, hydramnios, history of laser conization or LEEP procedure, multiple pregnancy, and maternal genital tract anomalies may also result in PPROM. It has been suggested that nulliparous women who work outside the home are at increased risk as well. Other risk factors include smoking, substance abuse, connective tissue disorders, fetal anomalies, and lower socioeconomic status; however, in most cases the cause is undefined (Mercer, 2003). Once membranes have ruptured, labor may occur within a relatively short time. The latency period, the period of time between rupture of membranes and the onset of labor, decreases with increasing gestational age. When PPROM occurs before 26 weeks, approximately 50% of women will begin labor within 1 week (Garite, 2004; Mercer, 2003). Between 80% and 90% of those women who rupture membranes between 28 and 34 weeks will give birth within 7 days.

Maternal Risks

Maternal risk is related to infection, specifically *chorioamnionitis* (intra-amniotic infection resulting from bacterial invasion and inflammation of the membranes before birth) and *endometritis* (infection of the endometrium postpartally that may be related to chorioamnionitis or may occur independently).

Chorioamnionitis occurs in about 3% to 15% of all cases of PROM, but in 15% to 25% of cases of preterm PROM (Garite, 2004). Collection of amniotic fluid by amniocentesis permits analysis of the fluid for subclinical chorioamnionitis. Gram stain, white cell count, glucose concentration, and culture of the fluid are useful in determining treatment; however, the results of the amniotic fluid culture could take as long as 48 hours. Interleukin-6 concentrations appear to be the best biomarker for infection but most hospitals do not yet have the ability to measure them (Canavan et al., 2004a). In addition, fluid gathered either by amniocentesis or from fluid that has pooled in the vagina can be analyzed for fetal lung maturity. When the fetal lungs are mature, the risk of serious pulmonary complication in newborns is minimal and labor is allowed to progress naturally.

Abruptio placentae occurs more frequently in women with PPROM. It is not clear whether infection causes inflammation of the decidua, which facilitates premature separation, or whether the bleeding episode contributes to a weakening of the membranes, which eventually leads to rupture. Childbirth may be complicated by malpresentation and reduced amniotic fluid volume (Mercer, 2003).

Fetal-Neonatal Risks

The most significant cause of neonatal morbidity and mortality is prematurity and its associated complications such as respiratory distress syndrome, necrotizing enterocolitis, and intraventricular hemorrhage (see Chapter 32 ∞). Neonatal infection (sepsis) occurs in 2% to 4% of newborns, but the preterm infant is much more likely to develop sepsis and die than a baby born at term. Fetal hypoxia may occur from cord prolapse or cord compression. In cases of early, prolonged PPROM, the oligohydramnios that occurs may result in fetal pulmonary hypoplasia, facial anomalies, limb position defects, and fetal growth restriction (Garite, 2004).

Clinical Therapy

Any time a woman complains of watery vaginal discharge or a sudden gush of fluid, rupture of the membranes must be considered. The woman should be questioned about the time of initial loss of fluid; if continuous leaking is occurring; the color, consistency, and amount of the fluid; and any odor noted. These questions not only help to determine whether there is blood, meconium, or vernix present, but also may help to differentiate PROM/PPROM from increased vaginal secretions associated with infection or preterm labor, urinary incontinence, normal leukorrhea of pregnancy, or the passage of the mucous plug.

During the initial physical inspection, any fluid leaking from the vaginal introitus can be checked with nitrazine paper. This test relies on the fact that amniotic fluid is more alkaline (pH 7 to 7.5) than normal vaginal secretions (pH 4.5 to 5.5). A color change in the paper to blue-green or blue is highly suggestive of ruptured membranes. Factors that can yield a false-positive result are contamination of the fluid with semen, urine, 50% or more blood in the specimen, or antiseptic cleansers and soap. The elevated pH associated with bacterial vaginosis can also lead to misleading results (Canavan et al., 2004a). If there is copious fluid leaking from the vaginal introitus, the diagnosis of PROM/PPROM is considered confirmed.

If further evaluation is required, a sterile speculum exam is done. Unless the woman is in active labor, direct digital exam of the cervix or vagina is avoided until PPROM is ruled out or a management plan has been determined. Speculum exam relies on gross pooling of amniotic fluid in the vaginal vault. The woman can be asked to "bear down," performing a Valsalva maneuver, if fluid is not visualized in the vagina. The woman may also remain in a supine position for several hours to allow collection of fluid to occur; the exam is then repeated. In addition to performing a nitrazine test on the fluid, a fern test can be performed by applying a thin sample of secretions onto a clean slide and looking for microscopic evidence of a fernlike pattern (see Chapter 21 ∞). When combined with client history, positive Nitrazine testing and positive ferning have been shown to have an accuracy of 93.1% (Canavan et al., 2004a). Vaginal cultures for group B streptococcus, chlamydia, and gonorrhea may be obtained at this time. Ultrasound can be used in conjunction with other tests to look for reduced amniotic fluid.

In situations in which the diagnosis of PPROM cannot be made with any certainty, an amniocentesis may be performed to instill either indigo carmine or Evan's blue dye. A tampon is inserted in the vagina for several hours and then is inspected for blue tinged fluid. The woman should be warned that as the dye is absorbed, it will temporarily change her urine to a green color.

Concurrently, fetal well-being should be assessed through a fetal heart rate tracing or biophysical profile. In addition, the gestational age of the fetus must be calculated to decide on a management plan (Table 20–1). At greater than 36 weeks' gestation, labor will begin in 50% of women within 12 hours. Labor induction may be delayed for 12 to 24 hours unless a situation exists that would preclude expectant management.

Management of PPROM in the absence of infection and gestation of less than 37 weeks is usually conservative. Amniocentesis may be done to evaluate for intra-amniotic infection. Fetal lung maturity studies will also be done if the fetus is nearing 34 weeks' gestation. The woman is hospitalized on bed rest. An admission, complete blood count (CBC), and urinalysis are obtained. Regular nonstress tests (NSTs) or biophysical profiles are used to monitor fetal well-being. Maternal blood pressure, pulse, and temperature are assessed every 4 hours. Regular laboratory evaluations should be performed to detect maternal infection. After initial treatment and observation, if the fetus has not reached viability or if leaking of fluid ceases, some women may be followed at home (Garite, 2004). The woman is advised to continue bed rest (with bathroom privileges); monitor her temperature four times a day; keep a fetal movement record; and avoid intercourse, douches, and tampons ("pelvic rest"). The woman is advised to contact her physician and return to the hospital if she has fever, uterine tenderness or contractions, increased leakage of fluid, decreased fetal movement, or a foul

Table 20–1   CURRENTLY USED PLANS FOR WOMEN WITH PREMATURE RUPTURE OF MEMBRANES

Preterm

Expectant management (observation); birth when labor or clinical infection develops

Fetal pulmonary status determined by amniotic fluid testing; birth if fetus is mature

Risk of infection determined by amniotic fluid Gram stain; white cell count, glucose and culture; maternal white cell count, and assessment for maternal fever or uterine tenderness; assessment for fetal well-being through electronic fetal monitoring or ultrasound for biophysical profile scoring; birth if infection develops

Penicillin G or ampicillin for treatment of group B streptococcus (GBS), or antibiotic prophylaxis if GBS status unknown

Adjunctive antibiotic therapy with Erythromycin or Azithromycin for 7 days to increase latency period from PPROM to birth

Administration of corticosteroids, with or without birth in 48 hours after first dose; tocolytics as needed

Birth after an arbitary latent period (e.g., 16–72 hours)

Assess for group B streptococci, chlamydia, or *Neisseria gonorrhoeae*; treatment indicated if positive

Combinations of the above

Term

Induction if spontaneous labor does not begin in approximately 12 hours, or if cervix is ripe, or if there are other complications (e.g., preeclampsia)

Expectant management for women with uncomplicated pregnancies and cervix unfavorable for induction

vaginal discharge. During this time, twice weekly NSTs and CBCs and weekly ultrasound and cervical visualization may be completed. Research indicates no significant difference in latency periods, gestational age at birth, infection, or perinatal outcomes between home care and hospitalization when this regimen is followed (Canavan et al., 2004b).

Authorities disagree regarding the ideal management of preterm PROM. Prophylactic antibiotics are administered to any woman with an unknown group B streptococcal (GBS) status or a history of a positive culture during the present pregnancy (Canavan et al., 2004b; Mercer, 2003). The goal of antibiotic use for preterm PROM is to treat or prevent ascending infection to prolong the interval from rupture of membranes to childbirth. Antibiotic use also may allow sufficient time for corticosteroids used to enhance fetal lung maturity to take effect. In addition, the neonatal mortality rate is significantly lower in newborns whose mothers received antibiotics (Canavan et al., 2004b; Kenyon, Boulvain, & Neilson, 2004; Mercer, 2003). If vaginal cultures are positive, antibiotics will be continued for at least 7 days. If amniotic fluid studies indicate a low glucose level, high white blood cell (WBC) count, a positive Gram stain, or organisms in the fluid, immediate birth is indicated. Results of studies about the potential benefits versus the risks of cervical cerclage retention after PPROM are conflicting (Garite, 2004; Mercer, 2003). Current practice includes early cerclage removal after PPROM; a multicentered randomized trial to answer this question is needed.

Betamethasone, a corticosteroid, decreases the likelihood of neonatal respiratory distress syndrome, necrotizing entero-

colitis, intraventricular hemorrhage, and perinatal death in infants who are born prematurely. Administration of single-course betamethasone (12 mg IM with a second dose in 24 hours or dexamethasone 6 mg IM every 12 hours for 4 doses) is the current recommendation (Canavan et al., 2004b). Corticosteroids have been associated with increased maternal and neonatal infection, decreased neonatal birth weight, reduction of brain size, maternal and fetal adrenal suppression, and psychomotor delay and behavioral problems. Data on these effects are not conclusive, but until there are additional data from clinical trials, the recommendation is that repeat courses of corticosteroids should not be used routinely (National Institutes of Health Consensus Development Panel [NIHCDP] 2001). See "Drug Guide: Betamethasone."

Use of tocolytics is generally not indicated in the woman who has ruptured membranes. Short-term use of tocolytics may be considered, however, to allow a course of steroids to be given.

NURSING CARE MANAGEMENT
Nursing Assessment and Diagnosis

Determining the duration of the rupture of membranes is a significant component of the antepartal assessment. The nurse asks the woman when her membranes ruptured and when contractions began because the risk of infection may be directly related to the time involved. Gestational age is determined to prepare for the possibility of a preterm birth. The nurse observes the mother for signs and symptoms of infection, especially by reviewing her WBC count, temperature, and pulse rate, and the character of her amniotic fluid. If the mother has a fever, the nurse checks hydration status. Fetal heart rate tracings should be watched for tachycardia, loss of variability, or decelerations. When a preterm or cesarean birth is anticipated, the nurse evaluates the childbirth preparation and coping abilities of the woman and her partner.

Nursing diagnoses that may be used for the woman with PPROM include the following:

- *Risk for Infection* related to premature preterm rupture of membranes
- *Impaired Gas Exchange in the Fetus* related to compression of the umbilical cord secondary to prolapse of the cord
- *Risk for Ineffective Individual Coping* related to unknown outcome of the pregnancy

Nursing Plan and Implementation

Nursing actions should focus on the woman, her partner, and the fetus. Uterine activity and fetal response to the labor are evaluated, but vaginal exams are not done unless absolutely necessary. The woman is encouraged to rest on her right or left side to promote optimal uteroplacental perfusion. Comfort measures may help promote rest and relaxation. The nurse must also ensure that hydration is maintained, particularly if the woman's temperature is elevated.

DRUG GUIDE   Betamethasone (Celestone Soluspan)

Overview of Maternal-Fetal Action

Studies have provided ample evidence that glucocorticoids such as betamethasone are capable of inducing pulmonary maturation and decreasing the incidence of respiratory distress syndrome in preterm infants. The mechanism by which corticosteroids accelerate fetal lung maturity is unclear, but it is related to the stimulation of enzyme activity by the drug. The enzyme is required for biosynthesis of surfactant by the type II pneumocytes. Surfactant is of major importance to the proper functioning of the lung in that it decreases the surface tension of the alveoli. Glucocorticoids also increase the rate of glycogen depletion, which leads to thinning of the interalveolar septa and increases the size of the alveoli. The thinning of the epithelium brings the capillaries into closer proximity with the air spaces and improves oxygen exchange.

Route, Dosage, Frequency

Prenatal maternal intramuscular injections of 12 mg of betamethasone are given once a day for 2 days. Dexamethasone may also be given in doses of 6 mg every 12 hours for four doses (NIH Consensus Development Panel, 2001). To obtain maximum results, birth should be delayed for at least 24 hours after completing the first round of treatment. The effect of corticosteroids may be transient. Currently, it is suggested that repeat courses of corticosteroids should not be used routinely.

Contraindications

Inability to delay birth

Adequate L/S ratio

Presence of a condition that necessitates immediate birth (e.g., maternal bleeding)

Presence of maternal infection, diabetes mellitus (relative contraindication)

Gestational age greater than 34 completed weeks

Maternal Side Effects

Increased risk for infection has not been supported in large studies. There may, however, be some increase in the incidence of infection in women with premature rupture of the membranes. Maternal hyperglycemia may occur during corticosteroid administration. Insulin-dependent diabetics may require insulin infusions for several days to prevent ketoacidosis. Corticosteroids possibly may increase the risk of pulmonary edema, especially when used concurrently with tocolytics (Briggs, Freeman, & Yaffee, 2005).

Effects on Fetus/Newborn

Lowered cortisol levels at birth, but rebound occurs by 2 hours of age

Hypoglycemia

Increased risk of neonatal sepsis

Animal studies have shown serious fetal side effects such as reduced head circumference, reduced weight of the fetal adrenal and thymus glands, and decreased placental weight. Human studies have not shown these effects, however (Briggs et al., 2005).

Nursing Considerations

1. Assess for presence of contraindications.
2. Provide education regarding possible side effects.
3. Administer betamethasone deep into gluteal muscle, avoiding injection into deltoid (high incidence of local atrophy) (Dexamethasone may be administered IM or IV.)
4. Periodically evaluate BP, pulse, weight, and edema.
5. Assess lab data for electrolytes and blood glucose.

Although concomitant use of betamethasone and tocolytic agents has been implicated in increased risk of pulmonary edema, the betamethasone has little mineral corticoid activity; therefore, it probably doesn't add significantly to the salt and water retention effects of beta-adrenergic agonists. Other causes of noncardiogenic pulmonary edema should also be investigated if pulmonary edema develops during administration of betamethasone to a woman in preterm labor.

TEACHING FOR SELF-CARE

Education is another important aspect of nursing care. The couple needs to understand the implications of PROM and all treatment methods. It is important to address side effects and alternative treatments. The couple needs to know that although the membranes are ruptured, amniotic fluid continues to be produced. Accurate information about neonatal outcomes for the given gestational age will help the woman and those she looks to for support have a more realistic view of the situation. This is often done by a care provider experienced in the care of high-risk newborns such as a neonatologist or a neonatal nurse practitioner. Providing psychologic support for the couple is critical. The nurse may reduce anxiety by listening empathetically, relaying accurate information, and providing explanations of procedures. It may be necessary to prepare the couple for a cesarean birth, a preterm newborn, and the possibility of fetal or neonatal demise.

Evaluation

Expected outcomes of nursing care include the following:

- The woman's risk of infection and cord prolapse are decreased.
- The couple is able to discuss the implications of PPROM and all treatment options.
- The pregnancy is maintained without trauma to the mother or fetus.

CARE OF THE WOMAN AT RISK DUE TO PRETERM LABOR

Labor that occurs between 20 and 37 completed weeks of pregnancy is referred to as **preterm labor (PTL).** Prematurity continues to be the number one cause of neonatal mortality in the United States today—preterm births are preceded by preterm labor 40% to 50% of the time (ACOG, 2003b; Hollier, 2005). An additional 30% to 35% are a result of PROM and approximately 20% to 25% are due to medical or obstetric conditions unrelated to PTL/PROM (Hollier, 2005; Iams, 2003).

In the 10 years between 1992 and 2002, the preterm birth rate jumped 13%, reaching a record high of 480,812 (Cockey, 2004; Moos, 2004). In the United States, preterm birth occurs in 11% to 12% of births, amounting to a staggering cost of nearly $6 billion annually (Hollier, 2005). Moreover, 15% of births from socioeconomically underprivileged populations occur before 37 weeks' gestation (AAP & ACOG, 2002). In the United States, African American women experience preterm birth and have low-birth-weight infants at twice the rate of white women (Meis, 2005). In 2001, regardless of gestational age or birth weight, black infants were less likely than white infants to survive (Hogue & Bremner, 2005). Despite new diagnostic and therapeutic technologies, efforts to prevent preterm birth have been largely ineffective. Table 20–2 presents a list of risk factors for spontaneous preterm birth.

Maternal Risks

The initial cause of preterm labor—for example, antepartum hemorrhage, trauma, or maternal infection—may pose a risk to

Table 20–2   RISK FACTORS FOR SPONTANEOUS PRETERM LABOR

Multiple gestation	Uterine irritability
DES exposure	Age (less than 18 or more than 35)
Known cervical incompetence	Low socioeconomic status
Polyhydramnios	Cigarettes—more than 10/day
Uterine anomaly	Substance abuse
Cervix dilated more than 1 cm at 32 weeks	Low maternal weight
	Poor weight gain
Second trimester abortion	More than two first trimester abortions
Fetal abnormality	
Febrile illness	Non-white race
Bleeding after 12 weeks	Cervical cerclage in situ
History of pyelonephritis or other maternal infection	In vitro fertilization (singleton or multiple gestation)
Maternal medical disease	Sexually transmitted infection (STI) (trichomoniasis, chlamydia)
Previous preterm birth	
Previous preterm labor with term birth	Anemia
	Abdominal trauma
Abdominal surgery during 2nd or 3rd trimester	Foreign body (IUD)
	Bacterial vaginosis, *E. coli* (ascending intrauterine infection)
History of cone biopsy	
Uteroplacental ischemia	Periodontal disease
Stress	Domestic violence
Inadequate prenatal care	

the pregnant woman. In addition, the treatment itself is another area of significant risk. Beta-sympathomimetic drugs cause a myriad of maternal side effects including pulmonary edema, especially in women with multiple gestations or chorioamnionitis. Diabetes, cardiac disease, and thyrotoxicosis may contribute to maternal risk with the administration of this class of drugs. Other widely used drugs such as magnesium sulfate, prostaglandin synthesis inhibitors, and calcium channel blockers also may have severe maternal consequence.

Bed rest is frequently prescribed for women having preterm contractions, although there is no evidence to support or refute its use to prevent PTL (Sosa, Althabe, Belizán et al., 2005). Bed rest in general is associated with adverse physiologic effects including maternal thromboembolism and decreased muscle mass. It is also linked with psychologic effects that extend to the entire family. Financial loss, child care issues, disruption of routines, depression, anxiety, and family/marital stress are among the problems that the woman and her family face. Hospitalization of those women with threatened preterm birth for enforced bed rest has an even greater impact on these issues. The social and financial blow to families who face a long-term hospitalization far from home, either because they had traveled away from their usual site of residence on holiday or have been transported to a hospital that provides a higher level of care, adds to the stress of a high-risk pregnancy and the ability of the patient and her partner to cope (Fry, Cartwright, Huang et al., 2004).

Fetal-Neonatal Risks

Mortality increases for newborns born before 37 weeks' gestation. In fact, preterm birth accounts for 75% of neonatal morbidity and mortality in infants who are born without congenital anomalies (Iams, 2003). Although the preterm infant is faced with many maturational deficiencies (fat storage, heat regulation, immaturity of organ systems), the most critical factor is the lack of development of the respiratory system—to the extent that life cannot be supported. In some instances, such as severe maternal diabetes or serious isoimmunization, continuation of the pregnancy may be more life threatening to the fetus than the hazards of prematurity. See Chapter 32 ∞ for in-depth consideration of the preterm newborn.

Clinical Therapy

The prevention and treatment of PTL has been widely studied. In the 1970s, the focus on prevention of preterm birth was on the use of tocolytic drug therapy (Meis, 2005). It has been found that these agents have limited effectiveness and may only delay birth for 2 to 7 days (ACOG, 2003b; Iams, 2003). Preterm birth prevention programs, which were implemented in the 1980s and early 1990s, focused on identifying women who were at high risk for PTL. Once identified, those women were educated about signs and symptoms of PTL and had weekly contact with a nurse or other healthcare provider. However, these educational programs did not significantly prevent preterm birth. One contributing factor is that risk assessment screenings have poor ability to predict those women who will eventually develop PTL and give birth early. Up to 60% of preterm births occur in women who would initially be scored at low risk. Nevertheless,

EVIDENCE-BASED PRACTICE

BED REST FOR PREVENTION OF GESTATIONAL PROBLEMS

Clinical Question

Is some degree of bed rest effective in preventing gestational hypertension or gestational problems leading to miscarriage or preterm birth?

The Evidence

Three systematic reviews appraised the evidence related to bed rest as a preventive intervention for miscarriage, preterm birth, and gestational hypertension. One review assessed two studies that compared complete bed rest against alternative or no treatments. The outcome measured was miscarriage, defined as pregnancy loss prior to 23 weeks' gestation. These studies involved 84 women. A second review evaluated the literature regarding bed rest in the hospital or at home for preventing preterm birth in pregnant women at high risk of preterm birth. Only one study met the inclusion criteria, but it was a multisite study with 1266 women subjects; 432 of the women were prescribed bed rest at home. The third review focused on four trials that tested the effects of strict bed rest, "some rest," and normal activity; 449 women were subjects in these studies. The outcomes in this review were maternal blood pressure and the presence of proteinuria.

What Is Effective?

Bed rest did not demonstrate effectiveness in preventing any of these gestational problems. The reviewers note that these findings are based on a relatively small number of studies. However, none of the studies detected a benefit of strict bed rest. One study found that mothers asked to get "some rest" had a reduced risk of severe hypertension and a borderline reduction in the risk of preterm birth, when compared with normal activity.

What Is Unclear?

Important information about side effects of restricted activity or strict bed rest is missing from these reviews. No data are provided about the costs of bed rest, either financially or emotionally. Only one study compared reduced activity (defined as "some rest") with normal activity. This study showed the most promise as the basis for a successful intervention. Additional randomized trials are needed to determine if reduced activity can be beneficial, given that strict bed rest gives no evidence of being a therapeutic treatment.

Best Practice

Mothers who are concerned about miscarriage, preterm birth, or gestational hypertension do not need to undergo strict bed rest to prevent these complications. More importantly, these mothers need to be reassured that their activity level will not affect their baby's health. Given that strict bed rest puts undue strain on a family, its application should be based on clear evidence of benefit. There is no evidence that strict bed rest is beneficial for either the baby or the mother. In these studies, mothers reported that they would not opt for strict bed rest as a treatment again, given a choice. Mothers need information about the risks and benefits of restricted activity during pregnancy.

Critical Thinking

Under what conditions would restricted activity be a potential intervention during pregnancy? What level of activity is acceptable for mothers during each trimester of pregnancy?

REFERENCES: Aleman, A., Althabe, F., Belizan, J., & Bergel, E. (2005). Bed rest during pregnancy for preventing miscarriage. *The Cochrane Database of Systematic Reviews* (2).

Meher, S., Abalos, E., & Carroli, G. (2005). Bed rest with or without hospitalization for hypertension during pregnancy. *The Cochrane Database of Systematic Reviews* (2).

Sosa, C., Althabe, F., Belizán, J., & Bergel, E. (2004). Bed rest in singleton pregnancies for preventing preterm birth. *The Cochrane Database of Systematic Reviews* (3).

---

the screening tests currently used, such as fetal fibronectin (fFN), cervical length, and Bishop's score, have not been recommended for use in asymptomatic, low-risk women. Screening might be helpful in women with a history of preterm birth and those with symptoms of PTL (Bernhardt & Dorman, 2004).

Nonpharmacologic treatments that historically have been used to prevent preterm births, specifically bed rest, pelvic rest, and hydration, do not appear to aid in PTL prevention and should not be routinely recommended (ACOG, 2003b).

Prompt diagnosis of PTL is difficult because many of its symptoms are also common in normal pregnancy. These include the following:

- Abdominal pain
- Back pain
- Pelvic pain
- Menstrual-like cramps
- Vaginal bleeding

- Increased vaginal discharge (may be pinkish stained or mucus-like in consistency)
- Pelvic pressure
- Urinary frequency
- Diarrhea

Some women have frequent contractions without changes in the cervix. In these women, a clinical assay for fFN obtained between 22 weeks' and 34 weeks' gestation may aid in diagnosis. fFN is an extracellular matrix protein that is an adhesive "glue" produced by the fetal membranes and binds the membranes and placenta to the decidua.

The presence of fFN in the cervicovaginal fluid is normal in the first half of pregnancy as the gestational sac attaches to the inside of the uterus. After 20 weeks' gestation, its presence is abnormal and can signal inflammatory or mechanical disruption of the fused membranes. fFN is also found in the amniotic fluid, and a positive test can indicate ruptured membranes. Near term, it is normal for fFN to once again appear in vaginal secretions (Tekesin, Marek, Hellmeyer et al., 2005). The negative predictive value of the fFN test is 99.2%. This means that a negative fFN in a woman with preterm contractions is associated with a very low risk (less than 1 in 100 chance) of birth within 14 days (Jeavons, 2005). A positive test is associated with recent sexual intercourse, vaginal examination, bacterial vaginosis, and vaginal bleeding. With a positive predictive value of 15% to 25%, fFN does not give a good indication of those women who will give birth in the next 14 days (Tekesin et al., 2005).

Contraction frequency alone is not enough to establish a diagnosis of preterm labor. A woman suspected of being in PTL should have a digital cervical examination once rupture of the membranes has been ruled out. If she is a candidate for fFN testing, this should be performed before a digital or endovaginal ultrasound exam. Electronic fetal monitoring should take place for a minimum of 1 to 2 hours to detect uterine contractions.

Assessing cervical length by endovaginal ultrasonography is another diagnostic tool. In symptomatic women, a cervical length of at least 30 mm (3 cm) is good evidence that the woman is not in PTL (Iams, 2003). However, only 30% to 40% of women with a shortened cervix will give birth prematurely (Bernhardt & Dorman, 2004). Care should be taken when performing an endovaginal ultrasound for cervical length, as excessive pressure on the vaginal probe or a full maternal bladder are associated with falsely long measurements (Bernhardt & Dorman, 2004; Iams, 2003). A cervical length of less than 20 mm in the presence of regular contractions, or a digital exam that identifies the cervix to be 3 cm or more dilated or 80% or more effaced in the presence of regular contractions, establishes the diagnosis of PTL (Iams, 2003). fFN testing is useful when the digital or ultrasound information is equivocal (Iams, 2003).

Intervention to reduce preterm birth can be divided into primary prevention and secondary prevention. Primary prevention includes diagnosis and treatment of infections, cervical cerclage, and progesterone administration. Secondary prevention strategies are antibiotic treatment and tocolysis (Hollier, 2005).

Maternal bacterial infection has been implicated as a causative factor of PTL with microbial invasion of the amniotic cavity being present in approximately 10% of women with PTL (Gomez et al., 2005). The microbial colonization may even precede conception and ascend from the cervix and vagina into the uterus. If a sexually transmitted infection occurs during pregnancy, the risk of preterm birth is increased 50% to 400% regardless of treatment (Newton, 2005). Lower genital tract infections that are associated with preterm birth include bacterial vaginosis (BV), *Trichomonas vaginalis, Chlamydia trachomatis,* urinary GBS, mycoplasmas, high concentration of anaerobes, or aerobic gram-negative rods. It is hypothesized that there may be an association with the ability of a species of bacteria to stimulate prostaglandin production. Hydrogen peroxide-producing lactobacilli, which help to maintain an acidic vaginal environment, are associated with a significant decrease in preterm birth (Newton, 2005).

BV is the most common lower genital tract infection among women of reproductive age and has consistently been associated with increased risks of PTL, PPROM, miscarriage, chorio-amnionitis, endometritis, and cesarean section wound infections. In spite of this, it remains unclear whether screening and treatment of BV will reduce the frequency of these complications (Yudin, 2005). Treatment of BV in low-risk populations has not been shown to improve obstetric outcomes, but some studies have shown that women with a history of preterm birth who received oral treatment with metronidazole or clindamycin had a reduction in preterm birth or PROM. Treatment with vaginal antibiotics, however, did not have any measurable effect on preterm birth (Okun, Gronau, & Hannah, 2005; Yudin, 2005).

An estimated 20% to 30% of all women are GBS carriers (Gibbs, Schrag, & Schuchat, 2004; Savoia, 2004). Neonatal infection from GBS is a potentially severe consequence of maternal GBS infection; nevertheless, there is no association of preterm birth and vaginal GBS colonization (Klein & Gibbs, 2005; Newton, 2005). GBS is discussed more fully on page 533.

PTL is also associated with urinary tract infections (UTIs), so it is prudent to obtain a clean-catch or catheterized urine specimen to identify and treat the infection. If untreated, asymptomatic bacteriuria is associated with a 30% incidence of pyelonephritis later in pregnancy and an up to 50% increase in preterm birth (Klein & Gibbs, 2005; Newton, 2005). Even asymptomatic bacteriuria alone increases the risk of preterm birth; therefore, screening and treatment of all pregnant women at the first prenatal visit are important components of care. Women with a positive culture should be retested following therapy to ensure that the infection is resolved. Because asymptomatic bacteriuria is common during pregnancy, women with frequent UTIs can be given low-dose suppression therapy with daily antibiotics.

A link has been identified between preterm, low-birth-weight infants, and gum disease, and it suggests that periodontal treatment during pregnancy reduces preterm birth (Klein & Gibbs, 2005; Offenbacher, 2004).

As early as the 1950s, progesterone had been investigated for its ability to improve pregnancy outcome. Progesterone's importance related to pregnancy lies in its ability to promote uterine relaxation, suppressing contractions, and to prevent fetal rejection by the mother through suppression of the immune system (Meis & Connor, 2004). It is produced by the corpus luteum and the placenta and is essential for the maintenance of early pregnancy.

When given to women at high risk for preterm births, studies have shown a significant improvement in preterm birth rates (Meis, 2005). Trials examining the use of progesterone for the treatment of PTL have not demonstrated effectiveness in halting labor or as an adjunct to the use of other tocolytic drugs to halt labor (Meis, 2005; Meis & Connor, 2004).

If the efficacy of progesterone is a result of immune suppression, this may explain why progestogens can be effective if given prophylactically, but not once labor has started. Currently the evidence points to treatment for prevention of preterm birth in women with singleton pregnancies at high risk for labor with 17-alpha-hydroxyprogesterone caproate (17P) 250 mg/week. This is administered intramuscularly beginning at 16 weeks and continuing to 36 weeks (Meis, 2005). At this time, 17P has not been approved by the Food and Drug Administration (FDA) for

Table 20–3   CRITERIA FOR DIAGNOSIS OF PRETERM LABOR

Gestation 20–37 weeks

and

Documented uterine contractions (4/20 minute, 8/60 minute)

and

Documented cervical change

or

Cervical effacement of 80%

or

Cervical dilatation 1 cm

SOURCES: From *Guidelines for Perinatal Care*, 5th ed. Copyright © 2002 American Academy of Pediatrics. Used with permission of the American Academy of Pediatrics. American Academy of Pediatrics, American College of Obstetricians and Gynecologists. Guidelines for Perinatal Care, 5th ed. Elk Grove Village (IL): AAP, Washington, DC: ACOG; 2002.

use in the prevention of preterm birth. Moreover, the drug is not readily available and must be obtained from a compounding pharmacy (Petrini, Callaghan, Klebanoff et al., 2005).

Table 20–3 summarizes common criteria for diagnosing PTL.

No attempt is made to stop labor if any of the following conditions exists (Iams & Creasy, 2004):

- Fetal demise
- Lethal fetal anomaly
- Severe preeclampsia/eclampsia
- Hemorrhage/abruptio placentae
- Chorioamnionitis
- Severe fetal growth restriction
- Fetal maturity
- Acute nonreassuring fetal status

Tocolysis is the use of medications in an attempt to stop labor. These medications may delay birth for 2 to 7 days (ACOG, 2003b). Although the delay of childbirth in itself may not improve neonatal outcome, it may permit the administration of betamethasone for fetal surfactant induction or allow for the transport of the mother to a tertiary care facility. Such a facility can generally provide better equipment and services and more experienced, highly trained staff. If the cervix is dilated more than 4 to 5 cm or if there is subclinical amnionitis, the effect of tocolytics on labor is reduced. If labor cannot be arrested, the priority becomes successful preterm birth and management of its psychologic effect on the woman and her partner.

Ritodrine hydrochloride (Yutopar) remains the only drug approved by the FDA for use as a tocolytic (Rideout, 2005). However, drugs currently used for tocolysis include beta-adrenergic agonists (also called β-mimetics or β-agonists), magnesium sulfate, calcium channel blockers (nifedipine), and prostaglandin synthetase inhibitors (celecoxib, sulindac, indomethacin, ketorolac). There is no clear choice for a tocolytic (ACOG, 2003b); however, β-mimetics are often chosen as the first-line agent. The use of β-mimetics does pose a significant risk to the mother in PTL. β-mimetics, which may be adminis-

tered intravenously, intramuscularly, subcutaneously, or orally, can significantly affect maternal cardiovascular and metabolic physiology. The most serious effects include hypotension, cardiac arrhythmia, tachycardia, palpitations, myocardial ischemia, pulmonary edema, and maternal hyperglycemia.

Magnesium sulfate, long used in the treatment of preeclampsia, has gained favor in the treatment of PTL because it is effective and has fewer side effects than beta-adrenergic agonists. The usual recommended loading dose is 4 to 6 g intravenously in 100 mL of IV fluid over 20 minutes. The maintenance dose is then 1 to 4 g/hour titrated to deep tendon reflexes and serum magnesium levels. The therapy is maintained for 12 hours at the lowest rate to significantly diminish contractions (Iams & Creasy, 2004). The maternal serum level that is usually necessary for tocolysis seems to be 5.5 to 7.5 mg/dL.

Side effects with the loading dose may include flushing, a feeling of warmth, headache, nystagmus, nausea, dry mouth, and dizziness. Other side effects include lethargy and sluggishness and a risk of pulmonary edema if the woman has predisposing conditions such as multiple gestation or infection; has had excessive IV fluid administration; or has concurrent β-sympathomimetic therapy (Samol & Lambers, 2005). See Drug Guide: Magnesium Sulfate for other side effects. Fetal side effects may include hypotonia and lethargy that persist for 1 or 2 days following birth, hypoglycemia, and hypocalcemia.

Of the calcium channel blockers approved for use in the United States, nifedipine is frequently used as a tocolytic. Nifedipine acts by reducing the flow of extracellular calcium ions into the intracellular space of the myometrial smooth muscle cells, thereby inhibiting contractile activity. Nifedipine is well absorbed either orally or sublingually, has fewer side effects than comparative agents, and is at least as effective (Rideout, 2005). The most common side effects are related to arterial vasodilation, that is, hypotension, tachycardia, facial flushing, and headache. Because the mechanism of action of nifedipine is different from the beta-adrenergic drugs, coadministration of nifedipine and terbutaline or ritodrine may prove beneficial in the treatment of PTL. Because both magnesium sulfate and nifedipine block calcium, however, coadministration of them has been implicated in serious maternal side effects related to low calcium levels and has resulted in maternal cardiovascular collapse (ACOG, 2003b).

Prostaglandins enhance the formation of myometrial gap junctions and stimulate the influx of intracellular calcium ions needed for muscle contraction. Prostaglandin synthetase inhibitors, therefore, are a logical choice for tocolysis. Indomethacin, sulindac, or celecoxib are the prostaglandin synthetase inhibitors most often used to suppress labor. Maternal side effects are few. Dyspepsia, nausea, vomiting, depression, and dizzy spells may occur. On rare occasions, psychosis or renal failure may result. These drugs are best administered with an antacid or taken with meals to reduce the chance of gastrointestinal (GI) upset. Prostaglandin synthetase inhibitors are generally not used in women with drug-induced asthma, coagulation disorders, hepatic or renal insufficiency, or peptic ulcer disease.

Indomethacin crosses the placenta readily, and oligohydramnios and premature closure of the fetal ductus arteriosus may occur with long-term use. Consequently the drug, which is

DRUG GUIDE   Magnesium Sulfate

Pregnancy Risk Category: B

Overview of Obstetric Action

Magnesium sulfate acts as a CNS depressant by decreasing the quantity of acetylcholine released by motor nerve impulses and thereby blocking neuromuscular transmission. This action reduces the possibility of convulsion, which is why magnesium sulfate is used in the treatment of preeclampsia. Because magnesium sulfate secondarily relaxes smooth muscle, it may decrease the blood pressure, although it is not considered an antihypertensive. Magnesium sulfate may also decrease the frequency and intensity of uterine contractions; as a result it is also used as a tocolytic in the treatment of preterm labor.

Route, Dosage, Frequency

Magnesium sulfate is generally given intravenously to control dosage more accurately and prevent overdosage. An occasional physician still prescribes intramuscular administration. However, it is painful and irritating to the tissues and does not permit the close control that IV administration does. The IV route allows for immediate onset of action. It must be given by infusion pump for accurate dosage.

For Treatment of Preterm Labor

Loading dose: 4–6 g magnesium sulfate administered over a 20-minute period (ACOG, 2003b).

Maintenance dose: 1–4 g/hour via infusion pump.

For Treatment of Preeclampsia

Loading dose: 4–6 g magnesium sulfate is administered over a 15- to 20-minute period.

Maintenance dose: 2 g/hour via infusion pump (Sabai, 2005).

NOTE: Magnesium sulfate is excreted via the kidneys. Because women in preterm labor typically have normal renal function, they generally require higher levels of magnesium to achieve a therapeutic range than women who have preeclampsia and may have compromised renal function. Maintenance dose may need to be adjusted based on serum magnesium levels.

Maternal Contraindications

Diagnosed maternal myasthenia gravis is the only absolute contraindication to the administration of magnesium sulfate (ACOG, 2003b). A history of myocardial damage or heart block is a relative contraindication to use of the drug because of the effects on nerve transmission and muscle contractility. Extreme care is necessary in administration to women with impaired renal function because the drug is eliminated by the kidneys, and toxic magnesium levels may develop quickly.

Maternal Side Effects

Most maternal side effects are dose related. Lethargy and weakness related to neuromuscular blockade are common. Sweating, a feeling of warmth, flushing, and nasal congestion may be related to peripheral vasodilation. Other common side effects include nausea and vomiting, constipation, visual blurring, headache, slurred speech, and pulmonary edema. Signs of developing toxicity include depression or absence of reflexes, oliguria, confusion, respiratory depression, circulatory collapse, and respiratory paralysis. Rapid administration of large doses may cause cardiac arrest.

Effects on Fetus/Newborn

The drug readily crosses the placenta. Some authorities suggest that transient decrease in fetal heart rate (FHR) variability may occur; others report that no change occurred. In general, magnesium sulfate therapy does not pose a risk to the fetus. Ill effects in the newborn may actually be related to fetal growth retardation, prematurity, or perinatal asphyxia.

Nursing Considerations

1. Monitor the blood pressure closely during administration.
2. Monitor maternal serum magnesium levels as ordered (usually every 6–8 hours). Therapeutic levels are in the range of 4–8 mg/dL. Reflexes often disappear at serum magnesium levels of 9–13 mg/dL; respiratory depression may occur at levels of 14 mg/dL; cardiac arrest occurs at levels above 30 mg/dL (Rideout, 2005).
3. Monitor respirations closely. If the rate is less than 12/minute, magnesium toxicity may be developing, and further assessments are indicated. Many protocols require stopping the medication if the respiratory rate falls below 12/minute.
4. Assess knee jerk (patellar tendon reflex) for evidence of diminished or absent reflexes. Loss of reflexes is often the first sign of developing toxicity. Also note marked lethargy or decreased level of consciousness and hypotension.
5. Determine urinary output. Output less than 30 mL/hour may result in the accumulation of toxic levels of magnesium.
6. If the respirations or urinary output fall below specified levels or if the reflexes are diminished or absent, no further magnesium should be administered until these factors return to normal.
7. The antagonist of magnesium sulfate is calcium. Consequently, an ampule of calcium gluconate should be available at the bedside. The usual dose is 1 g given IV over a period of about 3 minutes.
8. Monitor fetal heart tones continuously with IV administration.
9. Continue magnesium sulfate infusion for approximately 24 hours after birth as prophylaxis against postpartum seizures if given for preeclampsia.
10. If the mother has received magnesium sulfate close to birth, the newborn should be closely observed for signs of magnesium toxicity for 24–48 hours.

NOTE: Protocols for magnesium sulfate administration may vary somewhat according to agency policy. Consequently, individuals are referred to their own agency protocols for specific guidelines.

no longer widely used, is not recommended after 32 weeks' gestation or for a course of therapy longer than 48 hours (Iams & Creasy, 2004). Indomethacin has been associated with necrotizing enterocolitis and grades III and IV intravascular hemorrhage (IVH) in the newborn. The risk for IVH increases with decreasing gestational age at birth. Chorioamnionitis is associated with an increased risk of intraventricular hemorrhage in the newborn and may be the cause of IVH rather than the therapy itself.

The NIHCDP (2001) and ACOG (2003b) recommend that corticosteroids (typically betamethasone or dexamethasone) be administered antenatally to women at risk of preterm birth because of their beneficial effect on fetal lung maturation. Any women who are candidates for tocolysis are candidates for antenatal corticosteroids, regardless of fetal gender, race, or availability of surfactant therapy for the newborn, especially between 24 and 34 weeks' gestation.

NURSING CARE MANAGEMENT
Nursing Assessment and Diagnosis

During the antepartal period, the nurse identifies the woman at risk for PTL by noting the presence of predisposing factors. The primary areas for ongoing assessment are change in risk status for PTL, educational needs of the woman and her loved ones, and the woman's responses to medical and nursing interventions.

Nursing diagnoses that may apply to the woman with PTL include the following:

*   ***Health-Seeking Behavior: Information About the Causes, Identification, and Treatment of PTL*** related to an expressed desire to understand the condition and its implications
*   ***Fear*** related to early labor and birth
*   ***Ineffective Individual Coping*** related to need for constant attention to pregnancy

Nursing Plan and Implementation
COMMUNITY-BASED NURSING CARE

Once uterine activity stops, the woman is sometimes placed on oral tocolysis. She may then be discharged and followed by home care nurses or as part of a specialized prematurity prevention program.

Home Care

Once thought to be a potentially effective tool for home management of PTL, more recent studies have cast doubt on the value of home uterine activity monitoring (ACOG, 2003b). Outpatient management of a woman at risk for preterm birth includes frequent office visits to assess symptoms and cervical length and in-depth client education about the signs and symptoms of PTL.

Consideration of the woman's ability to care for herself, the impact of the changes in relationships that will occur, and care of any young children in the home are among the issues that affect the woman's ability to cope effectively with this situation.

Care providers need to be alert to any signs that the woman is failing to achieve the emotional and developmental tasks of pregnancy, such as lack of maternal attachment. An individualized nursing management plan helps focus on each woman's specific needs. Although current evidence does not show that increased social support or home uterine activity monitoring are effective in preventing preterm birth (National Institute of Child Health and Human Development [NICHHD], 2002), these therapies continue to be widely used.

TEACHING FOR SELF-CARE

Once the woman at risk for PTL has been identified, she needs to be taught about the importance of recognizing the onset of labor. Increasing the woman's awareness of the subtle symptoms of PTL is one of the most important teaching objectives of the nurse (see Client Teaching: Preterm Labor).

Signs and symptoms of preterm labor include the following:

*   Uterine contractions that occur every 10 minutes or less with or without pain
*   Mild menstrual-like cramps felt low in the abdomen
*   Constant or intermittent feelings of pelvic pressure that may feel like the baby pressing down
*   Rupture of membranes
*   Low, dull backache, which may be constant or intermittent
*   A change in the vaginal discharge (an increase in amount, a change to more clear and watery, or a pinkish tinge)
*   Abdominal cramping with or without diarrhea

The woman is also taught to evaluate contraction activity once or twice a day. She does so by lying down tilted to one side with a pillow behind her back for support. The woman places her fingertips on the fundus of the uterus (which is above the umbilicus after 20 weeks' gestation). She checks for contractions (hardening or tightening in the uterus) for about 1 hour. It is important for the pregnant woman to know that uterine contractions occur occasionally throughout the pregnancy. If they occur every 10 minutes for 1 hour, however, the cervix could begin to dilate, and labor could continue.

The nurse ensures that the woman knows when to report signs and symptoms. If contractions occur every 10 minutes (or less) for 1 hour, if any of the other signs and symptoms are present for 1 hour, or if clear fluid begins leaking from the vagina, she should telephone her physician or nurse-midwife, clinic, or hospital birthing unit and make arrangements to be checked for ongoing labor. If the woman experiences any PTL symptoms for more than 15 minutes while physically active, she should be instructed to do the following:

*   Empty her bladder.
*   Lie down tilted toward her side.
*   Drink 3 to 4 (8 oz) cups of fluid.
*   Palpate for uterine contractions, and if contractions occur 10 minutes apart or less for 1 hour, notify the healthcare provider.
*   Soak in a warm tub bath with the uterus completely submerged.

THROUGH THE EYES OF A NURSE

Preterm Labor

FAMILY'S EXPERIENCE: "I am getting some contractions throughout the day. I am not sure if I should be concerned or not. I wouldn't say they are painful, but I can definitely feel them. I don't want to be overly concerned, but I don't want to ignore them and end up having the baby early. I read the signs on the sheet the other nurse gave me at my last appointment, but I am still unsure if this is normal or something to be worried about."

Her husband is also concerned about her. "She seems to feel them more at the end of the day. When I get home and see her having contractions, I don't know whether to panic or assume it is normal."

NURSE'S RESPONSE: "Many women experience Braxton-Hicks contractions during the third trimester. This type of contraction is normal. It feels like tightening but is not really painful. Typically, they are irregular, not in a regular pattern. They also occur infrequently compared with preterm labor contractions. It is not uncommon to get them at the end of the day when you have been on your feet all day. When you feel them, get off your feet, rest, and drink several glasses of water. If they continue, you need to time them and call us if they are occurring regularly or if there are more than eight contractions in 1 hour.

"Preterm labor is diagnosed when there are at least eight contractions in 1 hour and cervical change occurs. In order to diagnose preterm labor, you need to call us if you are having frequent contractions and come to the hospital for an examination to see if your cervix has changed."

NURSE'S ACTIONS AND RATIONALE:

The nurse reviews preterm labor symptoms with the couple. The woman should be assessed for possible risk factors. Risk factors are included in Table 20–2. Since Braxton-Hicks contractions are quite common, the differences between preterm labor and these types of contractions should be thoroughly explained. The nurse provides written instructions and provides the couple with a telephone number to call should preterm labor occur.

CLIENT TEACHING Preterm Labor

CLIENT GOALS   At the completion of teaching the woman will be able to:

1. Discuss the risks of preterm labor.
2. Describe the purpose of home monitoring.
3. Demonstrate the correct procedures for doing home monitoring.
4. Explain self-care measures that help decrease the risk of preterm labor.

TEACHING PLAN

CONTENT

- Describe the dangers of preterm labor, especially the risk of prematurity in the infant, and all the potential problems.

  Emphasize that many of the early symptoms of labor, such as backache and increased bloody show, may be subtle initially.

  Be prepared to reinforce the information provided and answer questions that may arise.

- Summarize self-care measures, such as maintaining generous fluid intake (2 to 3 quarts daily), voiding every 2 hours, avoiding lifting and overexertion, avoiding nipple stimulation or orgasm, limiting sexual activity, and cooperating with activity restrictions and bed rest requirements. (See Table 20–4.)

TEACHING METHOD

Discuss the risks specifically. Many people understand in a general way that prematurity can be dangerous, but they fail to understand how the baby is affected.

Use handouts during the discussion. Help the woman clearly understand the value of the program because, to be successful, it requires a real commitment on her part.

Teach the woman how to palpate for uterine contractions. Do a demonstration and ask for a return demonstration.

Use a handout during the discussion. Provide opportunities for discussion. If the woman has concerns about certain recommendations, try to modify the approach to best meet her needs.

EVALUATION

At the end of the teaching session the woman will be able to discuss the risks of preterm labor, demonstrate home monitoring techniques and explain their rationale, and implement self-care activities to decrease the risks of preterm labor.

DOCUMENTATION

Document the information given to the woman including specifics on risk factors, early symptoms, and self-care measures. Specify if written instructions were provided in addition to verbal ones and describe the type of teaching method used. Document the woman's verbalization of understanding and your clarification of any information.

- Rest for 30 minutes after the symptoms have subsided, and gradually resume activity.
- Call her healthcare provider if symptoms persist, even if uterine contractions are not palpable.

Caregivers need to be aware that the woman is knowledgeable and attuned to changes in her body and to take her call seriously. When a woman is at risk for PTL, she may have many episodes of contractions and other signs or symptoms. If she is treated positively, she will feel freer to report problems as they arise. Other preventive measures the woman might follow are presented in Table 20–4.

HOSPITAL-BASED NURSING CARE

Providing supportive nursing care to the woman in PTL is important during hospitalization. This care consists of promoting bed rest, monitoring vital signs, measuring intake and output, and continuously monitoring fetal heart rate (FHR) and uterine contractions. Placing the woman on her left side facilitates maternal-fetal circulation. Vaginal examinations are kept to a minimum. If tocolytic agents are being administered, the mother and fetus are monitored closely for any adverse effects.

Table 20–4   SELF-CARE MEASURES TO PREVENT PRETERM LABOR

Rest two or three times a day lying on your left side.

Drink 2 to 3 quarts of water or fruit juice each day. Avoid caffeine drinks. Filling a quart container and drinking from it will eliminate the need to keep track of numerous glasses of fluid.

Empty your bladder at least every 2 hours during waking hours.

Avoid lifting heavy objects. If small children are in the home, work out alternatives for picking them up, such as sitting on a chair and having them climb on your lap.

Avoid prenatal breast preparation such as nipple rolling or rubbing nipples with a towel. This is not meant to discourage breastfeeding but to avoid the potential increase in uterine irritability.

Pace necessary activities to avoid overexertion.

Sexual activity may need to be curtailed or eliminated.

Find pleasurable ways to help compensate for limitations of activities and boost the spirits.

Try to focus on 1 day or 1 week at a time rather than on longer periods of time.

If on bed rest, get dressed each day and rest on a couch rather than becoming isolated in the bedroom.

SOURCE: Prepared in consultation with Susan Bennett, RN, ACCE, Coordinator of the Prematurity Prevention Program.

Whether PTL is arrested or proceeds, the woman and her partner, if one is involved, experience intense psychologic stress. Decreasing the anxiety associated with the unknown and the risk of a preterm newborn is a primary aim of the nurse. The nurse also recognizes the stress of prolonged bed rest and of lack of sexual contact and helps the couple find satisfactory ways of dealing with these stresses. With empathetic communication, the nurse can facilitate the couple's expression of their feelings, which commonly include guilt and anxiety, thereby helping the couple identify and implement coping mechanisms. The nurse also keeps the couple informed about the labor progress, the treatment regimen, and the status of the fetus so that their full cooperation can be elicited. In the event of imminent vaginal or cesarean birth, the couple should be offered brief but ongoing explanations to prepare them for the actual birth process and the events following the birth. The nurse may also offer to arrange consultation for the woman and her support person with the neonatologist, social worker, or hospital chaplain if requested.

Evaluation

Expected outcomes of nursing care include the following:

- The woman can discuss the cause, diagnosis, and treatment of PTL.
- The woman affirms that her fears about early labor are decreased.
- The woman states that she feels comfortable in her ability to cope with her situation and has resources to call on if needed.
- The woman can identify signs and symptoms of PTL that need to be reported to her caregiver.
- The woman can describe appropriate self-care measures to initiate in the event that she experiences any symptoms of PTL.
- The woman successfully gives birth to a healthy infant.

CARE OF THE WOMAN WITH A HYPERTENSIVE DISORDER

Hypertension is the most common medical disorder in pregnancy, accounting for up to 15% of prenatal hospitalizations. The incidence of hypertension among pregnant women ranges from 12% to 22%, and hypertension is directly responsible for 17.6% of maternal deaths in the United States (ACOG, 2002).

The classification of hypertension in pregnancy is as follows (August, 2004):

- Preeclampsia-eclampsia
- Chronic hypertension
- Chronic hypertension with superimposed preeclampsia
- Gestational hypertension

The pathophysiology and collaborative care of women with these disorders are quite different; thus, each is discussed separately.

Preeclampsia and Eclampsia

Preeclampsia occurs in 5% to 8% of all pregnancies and is the most common hypertensive disorder in pregnancy (Farag, Hassan, & Ledger, 2004). It is estimated that 50,000 women die from preeclampsia each year worldwide. In the United States, it is the second leading cause of maternal death (Baxter & Weinstein, 2004). Although only 3% to 5% of healthy women have preeclampsia during their first pregnancy, 25% of those with chronic hypertension will develop this complication (August, Helseth, Cook et al., 2004; Zeeman, Alexander, McIntire et al., 2003).

Preeclampsia, a syndrome that affects both mother and fetus, is clinically defined as an increase in blood pressure after 20 weeks' gestation accompanied by proteinuria (August, 2004). Edema is no longer included in the definition because it is a common feature in normal pregnancy. However, sudden onset of severe edema warrants close evaluation to rule out preeclampsia or other pathologic processes such as renal disease. In contrast, severe preeclampsia can occur without edema (August, 2004).

Eclampsia is the occurrence of a seizure in a woman with preeclampsia who has no other cause for seizure. Women who are going to develop preeclampsia usually become hypertensive before they develop proteinuria. In any event, the onset of hypertension in pregnancy warrants close observation.

PATHOPHYSIOLOGY OF PREECLAMPSIA

Preeclampsia has been called a "disease of theories" because the true mechanisms behind the pathogenesis are unknown. The only cure for this disease is birth of the fetus and removal of the placenta. Key features of preeclampsia involve the failure of the uterine spiral arteries to transform from thick-walled muscular vessels to saclike flaccid vessels, exaggerated inflammatory response, and inappropriate endothelial-cell activation (Sabai, 2003). Characteristics of preeclampsia include maternal vasospasm resulting in decreased perfusion to virtually all organs, including the placenta (Figure 20–6 ◆), a decrease in plasma volume, activation of the coagulation cascade, and alterations in glomerular capillary endothelium. The increased platelet activation and markers of endothelial activation can predate clinically evident preeclampsia by weeks or even months. In preeclampsia, a greater degree of placental infarction may be seen than occurs in normal pregnancy.

Women who develop preeclampsia become more sensitive to pressor agents (substances that increase blood pressure) rather than less sensitive to them, as in normal pregnancy. This response has been linked to the ratio between the prostaglandins prostacyclin and thromboxane. Prostacyclin, a vasodilator produced by endothelial cells, decreases blood pressure, prevents platelet aggregation, and promotes uterine blood flow. Thromboxane, produced by platelets, causes vessels to constrict and platelets to clump together. Prostacyclin is decreased in preeclampsia, allowing the potent vasoconstrictor and platelet-aggregating effects of thromboxane to dominate. These hormones are produced partially by the placenta, which would help explain the reversal of the condition when the placenta is re-

Figure 20–6 ◆ Clinical manifestations and possible pathophysiology of preeclampsia-eclampsia.

moved and why the incidence is increased when there is a larger than normal placental mass, such as in hydrops, multiple pregnancy, or hydatidiform mole. There also seems to be an increased risk of preeclampsia in women with preexisting vascular disease. The role of prostacyclin-thromboxane imbalance in preeclampsia has prompted several randomized trials designed to evaluate the effect of low-dose aspirin, which suppresses thromboxane, to prevent preeclampsia. Most trials have not been able to demonstrate any beneficial effect (August, 2004).

With increasing use of assisted reproductive techniques to achieve pregnancy, potential obstetric risks have begun to be explored. Because these pregnancies also are distinct for a greater likelihood of advanced maternal age, multiple gestation, and nulliparity, which may potentially lead to pregnancy complica-

tions, it is difficult to separate the contribution of foreign genetic material (donor egg) from these other confounding variables. A recent study of well-matched women concluded that in both singleton and multiple gestations, the use of donor eggs is associated with a significant increase in gestational hypertension and preeclampsia. Published outcomes conclude that pregnancies resulting from donor egg in vitro fertilization have a 20% to 50% of gestational hypertension (Wiggens & Elliott, 2005).

Recently, attention has been directed to another theory, which postulates that uteroplacental ischemia acts as a trigger for preeclampsia, with other factors playing contributory roles. Although the prostacyclin-thromboxane imbalance may provide an explanation for the clinical features of preeclampsia, this theory is now being challenged as the primary cause. In the woman with preeclampsia, in addition to a reduced production of the vasoactive substance prostacyclin, there is also a decreased production of nitric oxide. Nitric oxide is a potent vasodilator and important regulator of maternal blood pressure. Nitric oxide synthesis in the placenta may play a meaningful role in maintaining a low-pressure, high-flow placental system and also may prevent intervillous thrombosis. The loss of normal vasodilatation of uterine arterioles results in decreased placental perfusion (Figure 20–7 ◆), potentially leading to fetal growth restriction and chronic hypoxia or distress.

Hyperhomocysteinemia may play a role in the etiology or pathophysiology of preeclampsia through oxidative stress and endothelial dysfunction. Mild elevations of homocysteine have been found in normotensive women who go on to develop preeclampsia. Once preeclampsia is established, homocysteine levels are considerably increased. It is unclear whether the circulating levels of homocysteine have caused preeclampsia or if they reflect metabolic alterations resulting from the disease process. In the presence of regulatory gene mutations, deficiencies of vitamins B_6, B_{12}, or folic acid may cause a rise in homocysteine. If a causal link can be demon-

strated, this might lead to strategies for preventing preeclampsia (Mignini, Pallavi, Villar et al., 2005).

Decreased renal perfusion is associated with preeclampsia. With a reduction in glomerular filtration rate (GFR), serum levels of creatinine, blood urea nitrogen (BUN), and uric acid begin to rise from normal pregnant levels, whereas urine output diminishes. For each 50% decrease in GFR, serum creatinine and BUN plasma levels double, whereas sodium is retained in increased amounts. Sodium retention results in increased extracellular volume and increased sensitivity to angiotensin II. The typical kidney lesion of preeclampsia involves swollen glomerular capillary endothelial cells containing fibrin deposits. Stretching of the capillary walls allows the large protein molecules, primarily albumin, to escape into the urine, decreasing serum albumin.

Edema is usually more profound in preeclampsia than in normal pregnancy although some of the most severe forms of the disease may occur without edema. The pathologic basis of edema is twofold:

1. The higher salt retention draws out intravascular fluid.
2. Plasma colloid osmotic pressure decreases because of serum albumin loss through edematous renal glomeruli and damaged vascular endothelium. This causes fluid movement to extracellular spaces.

The decreased intravascular volume causes increased viscosity of the blood and a corresponding rise in hematocrit.

HELLP SYNDROME

HELLP syndrome (*h*emolysis, *e*levated *l*iver enzymes, and *l*ow *p*latelet count) is associated with severe preeclampsia, although it may occur in women with normal or minimally elevated blood pressure and no proteinuria (Baxter & Weinstein, 2004). Ninety percent of women with HELLP syndrome present with symptoms before 36 weeks' gestation. In women with severe preeclampsia-eclampsia, the incidence of HELLP syndrome is 10% to 20%. Twenty-five percent first demonstrate the disease in the postpartum period (Baxter & Weinstein, 2004).

The hemolysis that occurs is termed *microangiopathic hemolytic anemia*. It is thought that red blood cells are distorted or fragmented during passage through small, damaged blood vessels. Vascular damage is associated with vasospasm, and platelets aggregate at sites of damage, resulting in low platelet count (less than $100,000/mm^3$) (Baxter & Weinstein, 2004). Elevated liver enzymes occur from blood flow that is obstructed because of fibrin deposits. Deposits of fibrin-like material found in the hepatic sinusoids cause obstruction and hepatocellular injury. This necrosis is the classic hepatic lesion associated with HELLP. Increase in intrahepatic pressure causes swelling of the liver. Liver distention causes epigastric pain and may ultimately result in rupture (Baxter & Weinstein, 2004). Hyperbilirubinemia and jaundice may also be seen.

Symptoms may include nausea, vomiting, malaise, flulike symptoms, or epigastric pain (Baxter & Weinstein, 2004). This may lead to misdiagnoses of gastroenteritis, hepatitis, gallbladder disease, pyelonephritis, renal disease, or thrombocytopenia purpura. Regardless of their blood pressure or the presence of protein in their urine, women presenting with the preceding

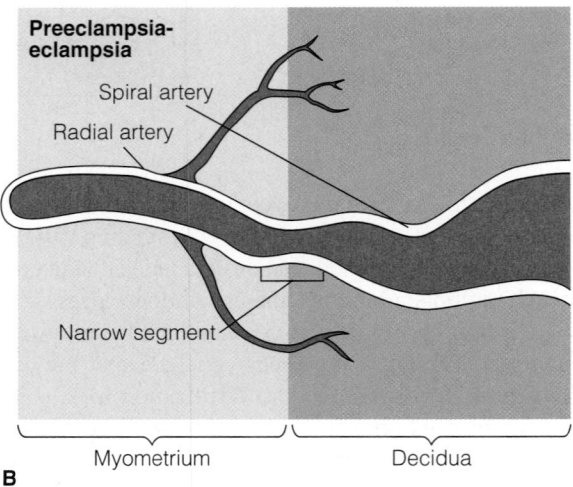

Figure 20–7 ◆ *A,* In a normal pregnancy, the passive quality of the spiral arteries permits increased blood flow to the placenta. *B,* In preeclampsia, vasoconstriction of the myometrial segment of the spiral arteries occurs.

symptoms should have a CBC with platelet count and liver enzymes drawn. Perinatal morbidity and mortality with HELLP syndrome are high; therefore, the possibility of HELLP should be considered carefully.

Women with HELLP syndrome are best cared for in a tertiary care center. Initially, the mother's condition should be assessed and stabilized, especially if her platelets are very low. The fetus is also assessed using a nonstress test and biophysical profile. All women with true HELLP syndrome should give birth regardless of gestational age.

MATERNAL RISKS

Preeclampsia can impact most organ systems, causing serious complications. Central nervous system (CNS) changes include hyperreflexia, headache, and eclamptic seizure. The mechanisms for the seizures is not known. Once thought to be from cerebral edema, there is some controversy as to whether cerebral edema is a feature of eclampsia or a postmortem phenomenon. Also under question is the possible causal relationship of excess administration of IV fluids in women with hypoalbuminemia and thus low oncotic pressure is contributing to cerebral edema (August, 2004). Seizures of eclampsia occur in 1% of all affected women.

Intracerebral hemorrhage is a rare complication but the most common cause of death in women with severe preeclampsia and eclampsia, particularly when systolic hypertension more than 160 mm Hg develops (Martin, Thigpen, Moore et al., 2005). An estimated 8% to 15% of women who sustain a stroke during pregnancy die and those who survive may suffer permanent disability. Risk factors for pregnancy-related stroke include hypertension, cardiac disease, infection, hyperemesis gravidarum, fluid and electrolyte imbalances, anemia/hemorrhage, sickle cell anemia, history of migraine headaches, sickle cell anemia, smoking, drug abuse, thrombocytopenia, age greater than 35, and African American race (James, Bushnell, Jamison et al., 2005).

Increased intraocular pressure can cause retinal detachment, but spontaneous reattachment usually occurs with reduction in blood pressure and diuresis.

Acute tubular necrosis may result from underperfusion of the kidneys. This is associated with hypovolemia and renal vasoconstriction. Although many women with preeclampsia will have oliguria, most do not develop acute tubular necrosis. One of the more common problems related to preeclampsia is pulmonary edema due to increased capillary permeability.

Thrombocytopenia complicates severe preeclampsia in about 7% to 11% of women (Ghulmiyyah & Sabai, 2006). The exact mechanism is not fully understood, but platelet consumption is believed to be related to endothelial damage and activation of thrombin. Abruptio placentae is a risk associated with preeclampsia. The release of procoagulants, such as thromboplastin, can result in acute DIC.

Subcapsular hematoma of the liver is a rare but important occurrence in women with preeclampsia and HELLP syndrome. In addition to the signs of preeclampsia, physical examination may reveal hepatomegaly and peritoneal irritation. Rupture of a subcapsular hematoma is a life-threatening event. The woman may complain of right shoulder pain or severe epigastric pain

persisting for several hours before circulatory collapse is evident. This is a surgical emergency requiring a multidisciplinary approach to management. Maternal and fetal mortality is over 50%, and women who survive are at risk for adult pulmonary distress syndrome, pulmonary edema, and acute renal failure in the postoperative period.

Vaginal birth is preferable to cesarean birth in women with preeclampsia or HELLP syndrome. Aggressive induction of labor should take place regardless of the favorability of the cervix. Cesarean birth is considered if vaginal birth does not take place within a reasonable amount of time, usually 24 hours, or for the usual obstetric indications (NIH, 2000).

FETAL-NEONATAL RISKS

Preeclampsia occurs before 34 weeks of gestational age in approximately 10% of women. Fifteen percent of preterm births in the United States are a result of preeclampsia (Farag et al., 2004). Perinatal mortality associated with preeclampsia is approximately 10%, and that associated with eclampsia is 20%. When preeclampsia is superimposed on chronic hypertension, perinatal mortality may be higher. Stillbirth rates with HELLP syndrome are reported to be approximately 10%, with neonatal death occurring within the first week in another 10% (Baxter & Weinstein, 2004).

Infants of women with preeclampsia during pregnancy tend to be small for gestational age (SGA) because of intrauterine growth restriction. The cause is related specifically to maternal vasospasm and hypovolemia, which result in fetal hypoxia and malnutrition. Placental abruption secondary to hypertension may result in fetal hypoxia or even death. In addition, the newborn may be premature because the treatment for the maternal condition may require early childbirth. Neonatal morbidity and mortality in women with severe preeclampsia is mainly related to the gestational age at birth rather than the effect of the disease process (Baxter & Weinstein, 2004). The concept that severe preeclampsia hastens fetal neurologic and physical development has been challenged in recent reports. Growth restricted preterm newborns do not appear to have accelerated lung maturity compared with appropriately grown newborns of the same gestational age (Shear, Rinfret, & Leduc, 2005).

At birth, the newborn may be oversedated because of medications administered to the woman. The newborn may also have hypermagnesemia caused by treatment of the woman with large doses of magnesium sulfate.

CLINICAL MANIFESTATIONS AND DIAGNOSIS

The most commonly occurring clinical manifestations and diagnoses are discussed here.

Mild Preeclampsia

The diagnosis of mild preeclampsia is made based on the presence of hypertension and proteinuria. Previously, it had been recommended that an increase in blood pressure of 30 mm Hg systolic and 15 mm Hg diastolic be used as a diagnostic criterion. However, it has been found that, in the absence of other symptoms, women in this group are not likely to suffer adverse outcome. Therefore, after 20 weeks' gestation, 140/90 mm Hg on at least two occasions 6 hours apart in a woman who was previously normotensive before pregnancy is used for diagnosis (AAP & ACOG, 2002; Sabai, 2003).

With mild preeclampsia, proteinuria is generally between 300 mg/L (11 dipstick) and 1 g/L (2+ dipstick). This is measured in a midstream clean-catch or catheter-derived urine specimen.

The gold standard for the measurement of proteinuria is the 24-hour urine. Excretion of more than 300 mg of protein in a 24-hour period is considered abnormal. This correlates approximately with a dipstick protein reading of 11 (30 mg/dL) or greater if specific gravity is less than 1.030 or 21 if the specific gravity is higher. Protein measurement may vary throughout the 24-hour period, partly related to urine concentration. This can be adjusted for with the use of a protein/creatinine ratio rather than the simple protein concentration alone. Also, protein concentrations may be elevated in women with UTIs.

Although edema is no longer considered a diagnostic criterion, generalized edema, seen as puffy face, hands, and dependent areas such as the ankles and lower legs, may be present. Edema is identified by a weight gain of more than 1.5 kg/month (3.3 lb) in the second trimester or more than 0.5 kg/week (1.1 lb) in the third trimester. Edema is assessed on a 1+ to 4+ scale.

Severe Preeclampsia

Severe preeclampsia may develop suddenly. The following clinical signs are often present (AAP & ACOG, 2002):

- Blood pressure of 180/110 mm Hg or higher on two occasions at least 6 hours apart while the woman is on bed rest
- Proteinuria 5 g/L or higher in 24 hours or 3+ or greater on two random urine samples collected at least 4 hours apart
- Oliguria: urine output less than or equal to 500 mL in 24 hours
- Cerebral or visual disturbances
- Pulmonary edema or cyanosis
- Epigastric or right upper quadrant pain
- Impaired liver function (elevated hepatic enzymes–alanine aminotransferase (ALT) or aspartate aminotransferase (AST)
- Thrombocytopenia
- Fetal growth restriction

Other signs or symptoms that may be present include headache, blurred vision or scotomata (spots before the eyes), narrowed segments on the retinal arterioles when examined with an ophthalmoscope, retinal edema (retinas appear wet and glistening) on funduscopy, dyspnea due to pulmonary edema, moist breath sounds on auscultation, pitting edema of lower extremities while on bed rest, epigastric pain, hyperreflexia, nausea and vomiting, irritability, and emotional tension.

Eclampsia

Eclampsia, characterized by convulsion or coma, may occur before the onset of labor, during labor, or early in the postpartal period. Late postpartal eclampsia (convulsions occurring more than 48 hours following birth) occurs rarely but has been documented. Some women experience only one convulsion, especially if it occurs late in labor or during the postpartal period. Others may have from 2 to 20 or more. Unless they occur extremely frequently, the woman often regains consciousness between convulsions.

CLINICAL THERAPY

The goals of medical management are prevention of cerebral hemorrhage, convulsion, hematologic complications, and renal and hepatic diseases, and birth of an uncompromised newborn as close to term as possible. Reduction of elevated blood pressure is essential in accomplishing these goals.

Antepartal Management

The only known cure for preeclampsia is birth of the infant. Recent research has focused on preventing preeclampsia in at-risk women through the use of low-dose (50 to 150 mg daily) aspirin begun between 12 and 18 weeks' gestation. Aspirin is known to block the action of an enzyme, cyclooxygenase, essential to the production of prostaglandins. This results in lowered levels of thromboxane, the vasoconstrictor. At the same time, levels of the vasodilator prostacyclin are not significantly affected. However, research has failed to show significant reduction in preeclampsia in women treated with low-dose aspirin therapy. The most likely explanation is that the prostacyclin-thromboxane imbalance is not the only pathogenic biochemical pathway. It is unclear whether low-dose aspirin used before conception or very early in pregnancy might have a more beneficial effect (Yu, Papageorghiou, Parra et al., 2004).

Several dietary approaches have been suggested, including supplementation with calcium, zinc, magnesium, fish oil, and vitamins C and E. Results of trials have either been conflicting or have revealed minimal or no benefit from nutritional supplementation. Based on available data, neither vitamin supplementation nor low-dose aspirin should be prescribed routinely for prevention of preeclampsia in nulliparous women (Sabai, 2003).

Home Care of Gestational Hypertension and Mild Preeclampsia. In general, women with proteinuric preeclampsia should be admitted to the hospital. However, with changes in health care, more attention has been given to decreasing inpatient hospital days for women whose symptoms allow.

A woman should be considered for management at home if she meets the following criteria: blood pressure less than or equal to 150/100 mm Hg, proteinuria less than 1 g/24 hours or 3+ dipstick, platelet count greater than 120,000 mm^3, and normal fetal growth if not at term or showing signs of complicating factors such as vaginal bleeding. She must have a basic understanding of her condition, be able to recognize the signs and symptoms of worsening preeclampsia (Table 20–5), be able to accurately count fetal movements, be cooperative, and know when to call the doctor. She is not restricted to bed rest but is encouraged to rest frequently, especially in the left lateral position.

The woman monitors her blood pressure, weight, and urine protein daily. Weight gains of 1.4 kg (3 lb) in 24 hours or 1.8 kg (4 lb) in a 3-day period are generally cause for concern. Remote NSTs are performed on a daily to biweekly basis. Companies that provide this service have equipment that allows phone transmission of blood pressure readings as well as fetal monitor tracings. This eliminates concerns about inaccurate reporting on the part of the woman. Nursing contact varies from daily to

Table 20–5   SIGNS AND SYMPTOMS OF WORSENING PREECLAMPSIA

Increasing edema, especially of hands and face (If on bed rest, observe for sacral edema.)

Worsening headache

Epigastric pain

Visual disturbances

Decreasing urinary output

Nausea/vomiting

Bleeding gums

Disorientation

Generalized complaints of not feeling well

weekly, depending on physician request. Laboratory testing regularly evaluates platelet counts, uric acid and BUN, liver enzymes, and 24-hour urine specimens for creatinine clearance and total protein. Estimates of fetal growth and amniotic fluid volume should be made at the time preeclampsia is diagnosed and repeated every 3 weeks if normal. Any woman with worsening symptoms or severe preeclampsia should be hospitalized.

Hospital Care of Mild Preeclampsia.   The woman is placed on bed rest, primarily in the left lateral recumbent position, to decrease pressure on the vena cava, thereby increasing venous return, circulatory volume, and placental and renal perfusion. Improved renal blood flow helps decrease angiotensin II levels, promotes diuresis, and lowers blood pressure.

Her diet should be well balanced and nutritious. Sodium intake should be moderate, not to exceed 6 g/day. Excessively salty foods should be avoided, but strict sodium restriction and diuretics are no longer used in treating preeclampsia (Sabai, 2003).

Tests to evaluate fetal status are done more frequently as a pregnant woman's preeclampsia progresses. These tests are described in detail in Chapter 21. ∞ Monitoring fetal well-being is essential to achieving a safe outcome for the fetus. The following tests are used:

- Fetal movement record
- NST
- Ultrasonography at least every 3 to 4 weeks for serial determination of growth
- Biophysical profile
- Amniocentesis to determine fetal lung maturity
- Doppler velocimetry beginning at 30 to 32 weeks to screen for fetal compromise

Maternal well-being is monitored by the following:

- Blood pressure four times daily
- Daily weight and daily evaluation for worsening edema, persistent headache, visual changes, or epigastric pain
- Daily urine dipstick for protein
- Periodic assessment of laboratory values to include CBC with platelet count, liver function tests (AST, ALT), lactic dehydrogenase (LDH), uric acid, serum creatinine, bilirubin, and 24-hour urine for protein and creatinine clearance

Severe Preeclampsia.   Expectant management of severe preeclampsia should be undertaken only in a tertiary care center. If the uterine environment is considered detrimental to fetal growth and maturation, birth may be the treatment of choice for both mother and fetus even if the fetus is immature. Fetal growth restriction has been shown to decrease survival. Other medical therapies for severe preeclampsia include the following:

- *Bed rest.* Bed rest must be complete. Stimuli that may bring on a convulsion should be reduced.

- *Diet.* A high-protein, moderate-sodium diet is given as long as the woman is alert and has no nausea or indication of impending convulsion.

- *Anticonvulsants.* Magnesium sulfate is the treatment of choice for convulsions because of its CNS-depressant action (Sabai, 2003). In fact, research indicates that the use of magnesium sulfate in the treatment of women with preeclampsia cuts the risk of eclampsia and possible maternal death by 50%. It is more effective and has fewer risks than phenytoin and diazepam. Blood levels of magnesium sulfate should be maintained at therapeutic levels (levels vary according to laboratory). Excessive blood levels may produce respiratory paralysis or cardiac arrest. (See Drug Guide: Magnesium Sulfate on page 500.)

- *Corticosteroids.* Betamethasone or dexamethasone is often administered to the woman whose fetus has an immature lung profile. Dexamethasone, which has the potency 1.25 times that of betamethasone, is often chosen for use with HELLP syndrome. Dexamethasone may be administered intravascularly, which may also influence its effectiveness. The benefits of corticosteroids in women with HELLP syndrome were first recognized when the drugs were given for fetal lung maturity enhancement to women with preterm gestations. Antepartum platelet counts stabilized or increased, whereas hepatic enzymes and LDH stabilized or decreased and mean arterial pressure and urinary output improved. A Cochrane review summarized the results of five randomized trials, which concluded that there is insufficient evidence to determine whether the use of corticosteroids in HELLP syndrome decreases maternal and perinatal morbidity and mortality (Matchaba & Moodley, 2005).

- *Fluid and electrolyte replacement.* The goal of fluid intake is to achieve a balance between correcting hypovolemia and preventing circulatory overload. Fluid intake may be oral or supplemented with IV therapy. IV fluids may be started "to keep lines open" in case they are needed for drug therapy, even when oral intake is adequate. Criteria vary for determining appropriate fluid intake. Electrolytes are replaced as indicated by daily serum electrolyte levels. Women with preeclampsia are at risk for hyponatremia (low blood sodium), which is indicative of low serum osmolality. A rapid decrease in serum osmolality can cause seizures as a result of cerebral dysfunction. It is imperative that serum sodium levels be evaluated to assess the need for fluid restriction and the switch from IV administration to an isotonic sodium chloride administration.

• *Antihypertensives.* In general, antihypertensive therapy is given for sustained systolic blood pressure of at least 160 to 180 mm Hg or diastolic blood pressures of 105 to 110 or above (Sabai, 2003). As indicated by a recent study (Martin et al., 2005), women with severe systolic hypertension greater than 160 mm Hg are at special risk for hemorrhagic stroke regardless of their diastolic pressures. To reduce their risk of stroke, immediate treatment with antihypertensives is recommended.

The therapeutic goal is to maintain the diastolic blood pressure between 90 and 100 mm Hg. Decreasing the diastolic below 90 mm Hg may decrease uterine blood flow, causing fetal compromise. Methyldopa is often used for long-term control of mild to moderate hypertension in pregnancy because it is effective and has a well-documented fetal and maternal safety record. However, its slow onset of action does not make it an option for treatment of elevated blood pressure in severe preeclampsia. Hydralazine is the most commonly used drug for the treatment of acute hypertension in pregnancy and is generally administered by IV boluses (Sabai, 2003). Labetalol is used as a second-line IV drug, but should be avoided in women with asthma or congestive heart failure. Oral nifedipine acts rapidly and has favorable hemodynamic effects and fewer side effects than IV hydralazine (Sabai, 2003). Some guidelines recommend against using any calcium channel blocker with magnesium sulfate because of a potential drug interaction resulting in a neuromuscular blockade and hypotension. Based on the Magnesium Sulfate for Prevention of Preeclampsia Trial as well as a retrospective look at concurrent use of nifedipine and magnesium sulfate, there appears to be no clinically significant interaction between the two drugs (Magee, Miremade, Li et al., 2005). If these medications are not successful in controlling blood pressure, sodium nitroprusside may be indicated for an acute emergency (NIH, 2000).

Eclampsia. Eclampsia is defined as the occurrence of either seizure or coma associated with pregnancy and not caused by other neurologic disease. The overall incidence is about 1 in 2000 to 1 in 3448 pregnancies, but it becomes much more common as term approaches (Ghulmiyyah & Sabai, 2006). Seizures may be focal, multifocal, or generalized. The possible etiology of the seizure is likely related to cerebral vasospasm, edema, hemorrhage, ischemia, and hypertensive or metabolic encephalopathy, but no mechanism has been proven conclusively. Many women experience an increase in deep tendon reflexes (DTRs) before seizure, but seizures may also occur without hyperreflexia. The woman with preeclampsia should be monitored for signs and symptoms of impending eclampsia: scotomata, which can appear as dark spots or flashing lights in the field of vision, blurred vision, epigastric pain, vomiting, persistent or severe headache, generally frontal in location, neurologic hyperactivity, pulmonary edema, or cyanosis. If a seizure occurs, nursing assessment should include time of onset, progress of the seizure, body involvement, duration, presence of incontinence, status of the fetus, and signs of placental abruption. The airway should be main-

tained and oxygen administered during the seizure. The woman is positioned on her side to avoid aspiration. Suctioning may be necessary to keep the airway clear; a tongue blade should not be inserted into the back of the throat because it may stimulate the gag reflex. To prevent injury, side rails should be up and padded, but the woman should not be restrained.

A bolus of 6 g magnesium sulfate is administered intravenously over 15 to 20 minutes followed by 2 g/hour IV infusion (ACOG, 2002; Ghulmiyyah & Sabai, 2006). In 10% of cases, an eclamptic woman will experience a second seizure. An additional bolus of 2 g of magnesium sulfate can be administered intravenously over 3 to 5 minutes. If seizures are recurrent in a woman receiving adequate doses of magnesium sulfate, sodium amobarbital 250 mg may be administered intravenously over 3 to 5 minutes (Ghulmiyyah & Sabai, 2006). Antihypertensive agents are used to keep the diastolic blood pressure between 90 and 100 mm Hg, thus avoiding a potential reduction in uteroplacental blood flow or cerebral perfusion. The drugs used to achieve this goal are 5 to 10 mg bolus of hydralazine or 20 to 40 mg bolus of labetalol intravenously every 15 minutes as needed. Nifedipine 10 to 20 mg may be given orally every 30 minutes up to a maximum of 50 mg in 1 hour (Sabai, 2005).

During a seizure, fetal bradycardia, transient late decelerations, decreased variability, or compensatory tachycardia may occur. If possible, the fetus is allowed to recover before birth. The seizure increases uterine irritability and may cause a precipitous birth. Therefore a minimum ratio of one nurse to one client is imperative to assess fetal and maternal status. Although she is still unconscious, the woman should be observed for onset of labor. The woman is also observed for signs of placental separation (see Chapter 25 ∞). She should be checked every 15 minutes for vaginal bleeding, which may or may not be present with abruptio placentae. The abdomen is palpated for uterine rigidity.

Following a seizure, frequent auscultation of maternal lungs is required to assess for complications from aspiration and to rule out pulmonary edema, which is common in eclamptic clients. The woman is watched for circulatory and renal failure and for signs of cerebral hemorrhage. Furosemide (Lasix) may be given in low doses for pulmonary edema; digitalis may be given for circulatory failure. An indwelling Foley catheter is often inserted and intake and output are monitored hourly.

A woman may have a single convulsion or many convulsions, usually followed by a period of coma. She may be combative and confused as she awakens, but having a family member at her side helps to reduce her agitation. Also, it is important to avoid bright light, noises, and frequent disturbances. The most serious complication, cerebral hemorrhage, arises from uncontrolled hypertension. Loss of vision, which is usually temporary, is a sign of impending hemorrhage. IV options for the treatment of hypertension are hydralazine, labetalol, or nitroprusside. Nitroprusside has been restricted to hypertensive crises when childbirth is imminent and other medications have not worked. Fetal cyanide poisoning may occur if the drug is continued and birth is delayed. Use of nitroprusside requires an arterial line because of its quick action and profound effects on blood pressure.

Intrapartum Management

Preeclampsia. Labor may be induced by IV oxytocin when there is evidence of fetal maturity and cervical readiness. In very severe cases, cesarean birth may be necessary regardless of fetal maturity.

The woman may receive both IV oxytocin and magnesium sulfate simultaneously. Because magnesium sulfate has a depressant action on smooth muscle, uterine contractions may diminish, and labor may be augmented with oxytocin. Equipment and IV lines for both fluids must be checked frequently to ensure that they are being administered at the proper rate. Infusion pumps should be used to guarantee accuracy. Bags and tubing must be labeled carefully.

Meperidine (Demerol) or fentanyl may be given intravenously for pain relief in labor. An epidural, spinal, or combined spinal-epidural can be safely administered to the woman with preeclampsia. Hypotension can be avoided by careful attention to technique and careful volume expansion. Spinal or epidural anesthesia is contraindicated in the presence of coagulopathy or a platelet count less than 50,000/mm (Sabai, 2005). Childbirth in the Sims' position should be considered. If the lithotomy position is used, a wedge should be placed under the right buttock to displace the uterus. The wedge should also be used if birth is by cesarean. Oxygen is administered to the woman during labor if the need is indicated by fetal response to the contractions.

Eclampsia. If not in a tertiary care center, the woman with eclampsia is cared for in an intensive care unit until labor begins or is induced. Invasive hemodynamic monitoring of either central venous pressure (CVP) or pulmonary artery wedge pressure (PAWP) may be instituted using a Swan-Ganz catheter. Both these procedures carry risk to the woman, and the decision to use them should be made judiciously. Invasive hemodynamic monitoring may be indicated for the woman with the following (ACOG, 2002):

- Oliguria
- Severe cardiac disease
- Severe renal disease
- Pulmonary edema resulting in impaired maternal oxygenation
- Refractory hypertension with administration of a vasoactive drug, such as nitroprusside or dopamine

When the woman's vital signs have stabilized, urinary output is good, and the maternal and fetal hypoxic and acidotic states are alleviated, birth of the fetus should be considered. Birth is the only known cure for preeclampsia-eclampsia. If the newborn will be preterm, it may be necessary to transfer the woman to a tertiary center for childbirth. The woman and her partner deserve careful explanation about the status of the fetus and woman and the treatment they are receiving. Plans for childbirth and further treatment must be discussed with them.

A pediatrician, neonatologist, or neonatal nurse practitioner must be available to care for the newborn at birth. This caregiver must be aware of all amounts and times of medication the woman has received during labor.

Postpartum Management

The woman with preeclampsia usually improves rapidly after childbirth, although seizures can still occur during the first 48 hours postpartum. A woman who has required magnesium sulfate antepartally will continue to receive the infusion for about 24 hours postpartum. Antihypertensive medication may also be required for a time.

Postpartum nurses should be acutely aware of the possibility of a worsening of the maternal condition in the immediate postpartum period. The potential for HELLP syndrome, liver rupture, or seizure continues. There have been several reports of late postpartum eclampsia occurring more than 48 hours after birth and within 4 weeks postpartum (Sabai, 2005).

When a woman's blood pressure remains above 150/100 mm Hg for 2 to 3 days postpartum, antihypertensive therapy should be used. Blood pressure should then be monitored at least weekly during the postpartum period. If blood pressure fails to return to normal by 12 weeks' postpartum, further evaluation is indicated to rule out underlying causes for hypertension (August, 2004).

In general, the recurrence rate of preeclampsia is 18% to 25% in subsequent pregnancies, but the risk of recurrence depends upon several factors. The rate is substantially higher in women with multiple gestations, early-onset preeclampsia-eclampsia, previous HELLP syndrome, or underlying vascular disease (Sabai, 2003; Sabai, 2005). Women who have had a normotensive previous pregnancy are at increased risk when they conceive with a new partner. Also, in vitro fertilization using donor eggs and/or donor sperm has a higher incidence of preeclampsia (Wiggens & Elliott, 2005).

Selective screening should be done for inherited coagulopathies (clotting disorders) in women who have had early-onset preeclampsia or a poor pregnancy history related to repeated miscarriages, intrauterine growth restriction, fetal demise, or prior history of a thrombotic event (Paidas, Ku, Langhoff-Roos et al., 2005). This information is important in client counseling and management not only related to future pregnancies, but also to assess their risk for thrombotic episodes outside of pregnancy.

NURSING CARE MANAGEMENT

See the Nursing Care Plan: A Woman with Preeclampsia for information on nursing care.

Nursing Assessment and Diagnosis

An essential part of nursing assessment is to obtain a baseline blood pressure early in pregnancy. Arterial blood pressure varies with position and is highest when the woman is sitting, intermediate when she is supine, and lowest when she is in the left lateral recumbent position. Therefore it is important that the woman be in the same position when the blood pressure is measured each visit.

NURSING CARE PLAN

The Woman with Preeclampsia

INTERVENTION	RATIONALE	EXPECTED OUTCOME
1. Nursing Diagnosis: Deficient Fluid Volume related to fluid shift from intravascular to extravascular space secondary to vasospasm		
Goal: Client is restored to normal fluid volume levels.		
• Encourage woman to lie in the left lateral recumbent position.	• The left lateral recumbent position decreases pressure on the vena cava, thereby increasing venous return, circulatory volume, and placental and renal perfusion. Angiotensin II levels are decreased when there is improved renal blood flow, which helps to promote diuresis and lower blood pressure.	• The signs and symptoms of preeclampsia will diminish as evidenced by decreased blood pressure, urine protein levels of zero, and a return of the deep tendon reflexes to normal.
• Assess blood pressure every 1 to 4 hours as necessary.	• Frequent monitoring will assess for progression of the disorder and allow for early intervention to ensure maternal and fetal health and well-being.	
• Monitor urine for volume and proteinuria every shift or every hour per agency protocol.	• Monitoring provides information to assess renal perfusion. Proteinuria is the last cardinal sign of preeclampsia to appear. As the disorder worsens, the capillary walls of the glomerular endothelial cells stretch, allowing protein molecules to pass into the urine. Normally urine does not contain protein. Reading of 3+ and 4+ indicate loss of 5 g or more protein in 24 hours. Urinary output decreases when there is a reduction of the glomerular filtration rate. Urinary output that falls below 30 mL per hour or less than 700 mL in a 24-hour period should be reported.	
• Assess deep tendon reflexes and clonus.	• Hyperreflexia may occur as preeclampsia worsens. Eliciting deep tendon reflexes provides information about CNS status and is also used to assess for magnesium sulfate toxicity. Reflexes are graded on a scale of 0 to 4+ using the Deep Tendon Reflex Rating Scale. A rating of 4+ is abnormal and indicates hyperreflexia. A rating of 0 or no response is also abnormal and is seen with high maternal serum magnesium levels. Clonus, an abnormal finding, is present if the foot "jerks" or taps the examiner's hand, at which time the examiner counts the number of taps or beats. The presence of clonus indicates a more pronounced hyperreflexia and is indicative of CNS irritabillity.	

NURSING CARE PLAN

The Woman with Preeclampsia continued

INTERVENTION	RATIONALE	EXPECTED OUTCOME
• Assess for edema.	• Edema develops as fluid shifts from the intravascular to the extravascular spaces. Edema is assessed either by weight gain (more than 3.3 16/month in the second trimester or more than 1.1 16/week in the third trimester) or by assessing for pitting edema (assessed by using finger pressure to a swollen area, usually the lower extremties, and grading on a scale of 1+ to 4+).	
• Administer magnesium sulfate per infusion pump as ordered.	• As preeclampsia worsens, the risk of an eclamptic seizure increases. Magnesium sulfate is the treatment of choice for seizures because of its CNS depressant action. As a secondary effect, magnesium sulfate relaxes smooth muscles and may therefore decrease the blood pressure.	
• Assess for magnesium sulfate toxicity.	• Side effects of magnesium sulfate are dose related. Therapeutic levels are in the range of 4.8–9.6 mg/dL. As maternal serum magnesium levels increase, toxicity may occur. Signs of toxicity include decreased or absent DTRs, urine output below 30 mL/hr, respirations below 12, and confusion.	
• Provide a balanced diet that includes 80–100 g/day or 1.5 g/kg/day of protein.	• A diet rich in protein is necessary to replace protein that is excreted in the urine.	

2. Nursing Diagnosis: Risk for Injury to the Fetus related to uteroplacental insufficiency secondary to vasospasm

Goal: The fetus avoids complications related to uteroplacental insufficiency.

INTERVENTION	RATIONALE	EXPECTED OUTCOME
• Instruct client to count fetal movements 3 times a day for 20 to 30 minutes.	• Fetal activity provides reassurance of fetal well-being. Decrease in fetal movement or cessation of movement may indicate fetal compromise.	• *The fetus will have an adequate supply of oxygen and nutrients as evidenced by absence of signs of nonreassuring fetal status and fetal diagnostic test results within normal limits.*
• Encourage client to rest in the left lateral recumbent position.	• Lying in the left lateral recumbent position decreases pressure on the vena cava, which increases venous return, circulatory volume, and placental and renal perfusion. Blood flow to the fetus is increased, thereby reducing the risk of fetal hypoxia and malnutrition.	
• **Collaborative:** Assist with serial ultrasounds.	• Maternal vasospasm and hypovolemia result from preeclampsia, which may lead to SGA newborns. Ultrasound provides assessment of fetal growth by measuring the biparietal diameter of the fetal head or the fetal femur length.	

(Continued on next page)

NURSING CARE PLAN

The Woman with Preeclampsia continued

INTERVENTION	RATIONALE	EXPECTED OUTCOME
• Perform nonstress test as ordered.	• A nonstress test is performed to assess the fetal heart rate in response to fetal movement. Accelerations of fetal heart rate with fetal movement may indicate the fetus has adequate oxygenation and an intact central nervous system. (Refer to Chapter 21 ∞ for interpretation of NST results).	
• Describe for the woman the purposes of a biophysical profile (BPP).	• Preeclampsia or eclampsia places the woman at risk for uteroplacental insufficiency due to the loss of normal vasodilation of uterine arterioles and maternal vasospasm. This results in decreased uteroplacental perfusion, which may lead to fetal hypoxia. A BPP is one assessment tool used to evaluate fetal well-being. Providing explanation of the diagnostic test helps relieve anxiety and ensures the woman understands what the test evaluates and what the results mean.	
• Assist with amniocentesis to obtain lecithin/sphingomyelin (L/S) ratio.	• Women with preeclampsia may give birth before term. Amniotic fluid may be analyzed to determine the maturity of the fetal lungs. An L/S ratio of 2:1 or greater indicates fetal lung maturity and is usually achieved by 35 weeks' gestation.	
• Explain the purpose of Doppler flow studies.	• Doppler flow studies (umbilical velocimetry) help to assess placental function and sufficiency. Uteroplacental insufficiency is a risk for a woman with preeclampsia.	

3. Nursing Diagnosis: Risk for Ineffective Health Maintenance related to deficient knowledge about new diagnosis (preeclampsia)

Goal: The woman will describe the condition and treatment regimen.

• Assess the woman and family's understanding of preeclampsia and its implications for pregnancy.	• This assessment provides information about the woman's cognitive level and her understanding of her diagnosis. Behavior changes occur when teaching strategies are appropriate for the woman and family's cognitive level.	• *Woman will demonstrate understanding of preeclampsia and its implications as evidenced by verbalization of basic condition, signs and symptoms of progression, importance of sufficient rest in side-lying position, and need to follow prescribed diet.*

NURSING CARE PLAN

The Woman with Preeclampsia continued

INTERVENTION	RATIONALE	EXPECTED OUTCOME
• Provide information about the disease process, impact on maternal well-being, risks of progression, implications for the fetus, and dangers of eclampsia.	• Basic understanding of the condition and its implications is necessary for the woman to understand the treatment plan. A woman who shows signs of early preeclampsia often feels well and may have difficulty accepting the need to rest.	
• Emphasize the importance of self-monitoring for signs that her condition is worsening and the importance of regular prenatal care for the purpose of maternal and fetal surveillance.	• The woman should be able to identify signs of disease progression, including evidence of increasing edema, decreased urine output, signs of cerebral disturbance (frontal headache, blurred vision, scotomata), epigastric or right upper quadrant pain, nausea or vomiting, and increased irritability.	

Blood pressure is taken and recorded at each antepartal visit. If the blood pressure rises or if the normal slight decrease in blood pressure expected between 8 and 28 weeks of pregnancy does not occur, the woman should be followed closely.

Blood pressure elevations should be based on at least two determinations not more than 1 week apart. To minimize errors in blood pressure measurements and improve reproducibility, the following precautions should be taken when measuring blood pressure:

- Take blood pressure measurements while the woman is seated, with feet supported and her arm at the level of the heart.
- Use Korotkoff phase V (sound disappearance) to measure the diastolic pressure.
- Calibrate the mercury sphygmomanometer and use the nearest 2 mm measurement.
- If using an electronic device, use one that has been validated for pregnancy.

When blood pressure and other signs indicate that the preeclampsia is worsening, hospitalization is necessary to monitor the woman's condition closely. The nurse then assesses the following:

- *Blood pressure.* Blood pressure should be determined every 1 to 4 hours, more frequently if indicated by medication or other changes in the woman's status.
- *Temperature.* Temperature should be determined every 4 hours, every 2 hours if elevated or if PROM has occurred.
- *Pulse and respirations.* Pulse rate and respirations should be determined along with blood pressure.

- *Fetal heart rate.* The FHR should be determined with the blood pressure or monitored continuously with the electronic fetal monitor if the situation indicates.
- *Urinary output.* Every voiding should be measured. Frequently, the woman will have an indwelling catheter. In this case, hourly urine output can be assessed. Output should be 700 mL or greater in 24 hours or at least 30 mL per hour.
- *Urine protein.* Urinary protein is determined hourly if an indwelling catheter is in place or with each voiding. Readings of 3+ or 4+ indicate loss of 5 g or more protein in 24 hours.
- *Urine specific gravity.* Specific gravity of the urine should be determined hourly or with each voiding. Readings over 1.040 correlate with oliguria and proteinuria.
- *Edema.* The face (especially eyelids and cheekbone area), fingers, hands, arms (ulnar surface and wrist), legs (tibial surface), ankles, feet, and sacral area are inspected and palpated for edema. The degree of pitting is determined by pressing over bony areas.
- *Weight.* The woman is weighed daily at the same time, wearing the same robe or gown and slippers. Weighing may be omitted if the woman is to maintain strict bed rest, or a bed scale may be used.
- *Pulmonary edema.* The woman is observed for coughing. The lungs are auscultated for moist respirations.
- *Deep tendon reflexes.* The woman is assessed for evidence of hyperreflexia in the brachial, wrist, patellar, or Achilles tendons (Table 20–6). The patellar reflex is the easiest to assess. (See Procedure 20–1: Assessing Deep Tendon Reflexes and Clonus.)

PROCEDURE 20–1 Assessing Deep Tendon Reflexes and Clonus

NURSING ACTION	RATIONALE

Preparation

- Explain the procedure, indications for its use, and information that will be obtained.
- Check the patellar reflex and one other such as the biceps, triceps, or brachioradialis.

DTRs are assessed to gain information about CNS irritability secondary to preeclampsia and to assess the effects of magnesium sulfate if the woman is receiving it.

Equipment and Supplies

- Percussion hammer

Procedure

1. Elicit reflexes.
   - Patellar reflex. Position the woman with her legs hanging over the edge of the bed (feet should not be touching the floor). (See Figure 20–8 ◆.) Briskly strike the patellar tendon, which is located just below the patella. Normal response is extension or a thrusting forward of the foot.
     Note: In an inpatient setting the patellar reflex is often assessed while the woman lies supine. Flex her knees slightly and support them.
   - Biceps reflex. Flex the woman's arm 45 degrees at the elbow and place your thumb on the biceps tendon. Allow your fingers to hold the biceps muscle. Strike your thumb in a slightly downward motion and assess the response. Normal response is flexion of the arm.
   - Triceps reflex. Flex the woman's arm up to 90 degrees and allow her hand to hang against the side of her body. Using the percussion hammer, strike the triceps tendon just above the elbow. Normal response is contraction of the muscle, which causes extension of the arm.
   - Brachioradialis reflex. Flex the woman's arm slightly and lay it on your forearm with her hand slightly pronated. Using the percussion hammer, strike the brachioradialis tendon, which is found about 1 to 2 inches above the wrist. Normal response is pronation of the forearm and flexion of the elbow.

The correct position causes the muscle to be slightly stretched. Then when the tendon is stretched, with a tap the muscle should contract. Correct positioning and technique are essential to elicit the reflex.

CLINICAL TIP

If a percussion hammer is not available, you may use the side of your hand to elicit DTRs.

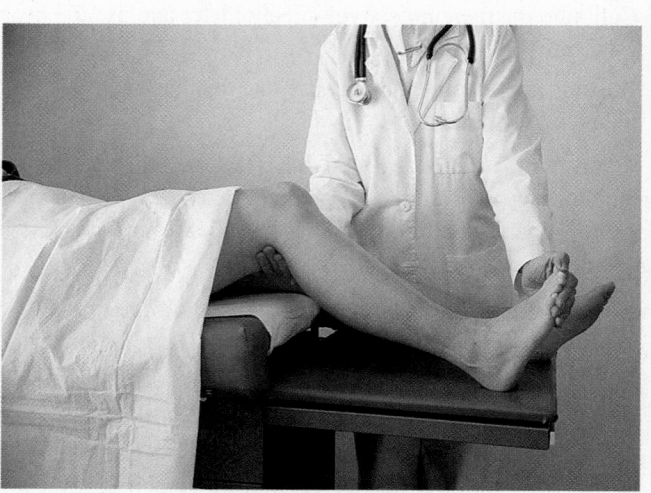

Figure 20–8 ◆ Correct position for eliciting patellar reflex: sitting.
SOURCE: Photographer, Elena Dorfman.

Figure 20–9 ◆ To elicit clonus, sharply dorsiflex the foot.
SOURCE: Photographer, Elena Dorfman.

PROCEDURE 20–1 Assessing Deep Tendon Reflexes and Clonus continued

NURSING ACTION	RATIONALE
2. Grade reflexes. Reflexes are graded on a scale of 0 to 4+, as follows: 4+ Hyperactive; very brisk, jerky, or clonic response; abnormal 3+ Brisker than average; may not be abnormal 2+ Average response; normal 1+ Diminished response; low normal 0 No response; abnormal	*Normally reflexes are 1+ or 2+. With CNS irritation, hyperreflexia may be present; with high magnesium levels, reflexes may be diminished or absent.*
3. Assess for clonus. With the woman's knee flexed and the leg supported, vigorously dorsiflex the foot, maintain the dorsiflexion momentarily, and then release (Figure 20–9 ◆). With a normal response, the foot returns to its normal position of plantar flexion. Clonus is present if the foot "jerks" or taps against the examiner's hand. If so, record the number of taps or beats of clonus.	*Clonus occurs with more pronounced hyperreflexia and indicates CNS irritability.*
4. Report and record findings. For example: DTRs 2+, no clonus or DTRs 4+, 2 beats clonus.	

Table 20–6 DEEP TENDON REFLEX RATING SCALE

Rating	Assessment
4+	Hyperactive; very brisk, jerky, or clonic response; abnormal
3+	Brisker than average; may not be abnormal
2+	Average response; normal
1+	Diminished response; low normal
0	No response; abnormal

CLINICAL TIP

Common errors in measuring blood pressure include the following:

- Incorrect cuff size—a cuff that is too small results in a falsely elevated BP, whereas one that is too large falsely lowers BP.
- Elevating the arm above the level of the heart, such as occurs when a woman lies on her left side using her right arm for a BP measurement, will falsely lower the BP 10 to 20 mm Hg.
- Korotkoff's phase—when BP is checked during pregnancy, the disappearance of the sound (phase V) is the preferred indicator rather than the muffling of the sound (phase IV).
- Anxiety, exercise, and smoking can elevate BP. Wait 10 minutes after the woman's arrival to check a resting BP.

- *Clonus.* Clonus should also be assessed by vigorously dorsiflexing the woman's foot while her knee is held in a flexed position. Normally no clonus is present. If it is present, it is measured as one to four beats, or sustained, and is recorded as such.
- *Placental separation.* The woman should be assessed hourly for vaginal bleeding and/or uterine rigidity.

- *Headache.* The woman should be questioned about the existence and location of any headache.
- *Visual disturbance.* The woman should be questioned about any visual blurring or changes, including scotomata. The results of the daily funduscopic exam should be recorded on the chart.
- *Epigastric pain.* The woman should be asked about any epigastric pain. It is important to differentiate it from simple heartburn, which tends to be familiar and less intense. *Nausea and vomiting or right upper quadrant pain,* occasionally radiating to the back, are also of concern.
- *Laboratory blood tests.* Daily tests of hematocrit to measure hemoconcentration; BUN, creatinine, and uric acid levels to assess kidney function; clotting studies for any indication of thrombocytopenia or DIC; liver enzymes; and electrolyte levels for deficiencies are all indicated.
- *Level of consciousness.* The woman is observed for alertness, mood changes, and any signs of impending convulsion or coma.
- *Emotional response and level of understanding.* The woman's emotional response should be carefully assessed so that support and teaching can be planned accordingly.

In addition, the nurse continues to assess the effects of any medications administered. Because the administration of prescribed medications is an important aspect of care, the nurse is, of course, familiar with the more commonly used medications, their purpose, implications, and associated untoward or toxic effects.

Examples of nursing diagnoses that may apply for the pregnant woman with preeclampsia-eclampsia include the following:

- **Deficient Fluid Volume** related to fluid shift from the intravascular to extravascular space secondary to vasospasm and endothelial injury
- **Risk of Injury to the Woman** related to convulsion secondary to cerebral edema
- **Anxiety** related to uncertain maternal and fetal status

Nursing Plan and Implementation
COMMUNITY-BASED NURSING CARE

A woman with preeclampsia has several major concerns. She may fear losing the fetus. She may worry about her personal relationship with her other children and her personal and sexual relationship with her partner. She may be concerned about finances—health insurance does not always cover all the tests, prolonged hospitalization, and other expenses that may be associated with complications during pregnancy. Finally, the woman may be depressed or resentful about being left alone or may feel bored. If she has small children, she may have difficulty providing for their care. The woman who does not have children may worry that she never will.

The nurse should identify and discuss each of these areas with the woman and her partner. It is necessary to explain to them the reasons for bed rest. A woman with mild preeclampsia may feel very well and be unable to see the need for resting even a few hours a day. The nurse can refer the couple to many community resources, such as homemaking services, a support group for the partner, or a hotline. Arrangements may be made for the partner to attend childbirth classes if both are not able to, or a nurse may be found to teach the classes privately. In addition, childbirth classes can be accessed over the Internet, thereby enabling the couple to participate together even if the woman is limited to bed rest at home.

The woman needs to know which symptoms are significant and should be reported at once. Usually, the woman with mild preeclampsia is seen once or twice a week, but she may need to come in earlier if symptoms indicate the condition is progressing. She must understand her diet plan, which must match her culture, finances, and lifestyle.

HOSPITAL-BASED NURSING CARE

The development of worsening preeclampsia is a cause for increased concern to the woman and her family. The most immediate concerns of the woman and her partner usually are about the prognosis for herself and the fetus. The nurse can offer honest, hopeful information. The nurse can also explain the plan of therapy and the reasons for procedures to the extent that the woman or her partner is interested. The nurse should keep the couple informed of the fetal status and should also take the time to discuss other concerns the couple may express. The nurse provides as much information as possible and seeks other sources of information or aid for the family as needed. Nurses can offer to contact a member of the clergy or counselor for additional support if the couple so chooses. In addition, the nurse

can provide educational videos that help address the couple's educational needs and access other support services including social services, a nutritionist, and even a lactation consultant if the woman is hospitalized for an extended period of time.

The nurse should maintain a quiet, low-stimulus environment for the woman. The woman should be placed in a private room in a quiet location where she can be watched closely. Visitors are limited to close family or main support persons. The woman should maintain the left lateral recumbent position most of the time, with side rails up for her protection. Unlimited phone calls are avoided because the phone ringing unexpectedly may be too jarring. To avoid a sense of isolation, however, some women find it preferable to limit calls to a certain time of the day rather than refusing all calls.

Nursing Management of Eclampsia

The occurrence of a convulsion is frightening to any family member who may be present, although the woman will not be able to recall it when she becomes conscious. Therefore, offering explanations to family members, and to the woman herself later, is essential.

CLINICAL TIP

When caring for a woman with preeclampsia who is receiving IV magnesium sulfate, it is imperative that you follow protocols for monitoring blood levels of magnesium. You are probably already aware of the common signs of increasing magnesium levels, such as diminished reflexes and decreased respiratory rate. However, there are some subtle clues you can also watch for that may suggest either the therapeutic or toxic range. When a woman's magnesium level is in the therapeutic range, she usually has some slurring of speech, awkwardness of movement, and decreased appetite. If the woman begins to have difficulty swallowing and begins to drool, she may be approaching the toxic range.

When the tonic phase of the convulsion begins, the woman should be turned to her side (if she is not already in that position) to aid circulation to the placenta. Her head should be turned face down to allow saliva to drain from her mouth. Attempting to insert a padded tongue blade has been questioned, and in many facilities it is no longer advocated. In others, it is used if it can be done without force because it may prevent injury to the woman's mouth. The side rails should be padded or a pillow put between the woman and each side rail. After 15 to 20 seconds, the clonic phase starts. When the thrashing subsides, intensive monitoring and therapy begin. An oral airway is inserted, the woman's nasopharynx is suctioned, and oxygen administration is begun by nasal catheter. The attending physician and the anesthesiologist should be notified immediately. Fetal heart tones are monitored continuously. Maternal vital signs are monitored every 5 minutes until they are stable, then every 15 minutes.

Nursing Management During Labor and Birth

The plan of care for the woman with preeclampsia in labor depends on both maternal and fetal condition. The woman may have mild or severe preeclampsia, may become eclamptic during labor, or may have been eclamptic before the onset of labor. Therefore, careful monitoring of blood pressure and checking for edema and proteinuria are necessary for all women in labor.

The prenatal record should be obtained so that current blood pressure readings may be compared with the baseline reading.

The woman with preeclampsia in labor is kept positioned on her side as much as possible. Both woman and fetus are monitored carefully throughout labor. Signs of progressing labor are noted. In addition, the nurse must be alert for indications of worsening preeclampsia, placental separation, pulmonary edema, circulatory renal failure, and nonreassuring fetal status.

During the second stage of labor the woman is encouraged to push while lying on her side. If she is unable to do so comfortably or effectively, she can be helped to a semisitting position for pushing and resume the lateral position between each contraction. Birth is in the side-lying position if possible. If the lithotomy position is used, a wedge is placed under the woman's hip.

A family member is encouraged to stay with the woman as long as possible throughout labor and childbirth. This is especially needed if the woman has been transferred to a high-risk center from another facility. The woman in labor and the family member or support person should be oriented to the new surroundings and kept informed of progress and plan of care. When possible the woman should be cared for by the same nurses throughout her hospital stay.

Nursing Management During the Postpartal Period

The amount of postpartal vaginal bleeding should be noted carefully. Because the woman with preeclampsia is hypovolemic, even normal blood loss can be serious. Rising pulse rate and falling urine output are indications of excessive blood loss. The uterus should be palpated frequently and massaged when needed to keep it contracted.

Blood pressure and pulse are checked every 4 hours for 48 hours. Hematocrit, platelets, AST, and ALT may be measured daily. The woman is instructed to report any headache, visual disturbance, or epigastric pain. No ergot preparations, such as Methergine, are given because they have a hypertensive effect. Intake and output recordings are continued for 48 hours postpartum. Increased urinary output within 48 hours after birth is a highly favorable sign. With the diuresis, edema recedes and blood pressure returns to normal.

Postpartal depression can develop after the long ordeal of a difficult pregnancy. Family members are urged to visit, and as much mother-infant contact as possible should be allowed. There may be fears about a future pregnancy. The couple needs information about the chance of preeclampsia occurring again. They also should be given family-planning information. Combined oral contraceptives may be used if the woman's blood pressure has returned to normal by the time they are prescribed (usually 4 to 6 weeks postpartum). Progesterone-only pills may be prescribed regardless of hypertension and may be a good alternative for women with chronic hypertension or for those women who are breastfeeding.

Evaluation

Expected outcomes of nursing care include the following:

- The woman is able to explain preeclampsia, its implications for her pregnancy, the treatment regimen, and possible complications.

- The woman suffers no eclamptic seizures.

- The woman and her caregivers detect signs of increasing severity of the preeclampsia or possible complications early so that appropriate treatment measures can be instituted.

- The woman gives birth to a healthy newborn.

Chronic Hypertension

Chronic hypertension exists when the blood pressure is 140/90 or higher before pregnancy or before the 20th week of gestation or persists 42 days following childbirth. If the diastolic blood pressure is greater than 80 mm Hg during the second trimester, chronic hypertension should be suspected. For the majority of chronic hypertensive women, the disease is mild. One of the challenges the healthcare team faces is differentiating chronic hypertension from preeclampsia. This is even more difficult if a woman arrives for her first prenatal visit during the second trimester when blood pressure is generally lower and preexisting hypertension is more difficult to recognize.

Early prenatal care is important to determine accurately the gestational age and the severity of hypertension. At the time of the first visit, the woman should be counseled on several aspects of her pregnancy:

- *Nutrition.* Sodium is limited to about 2.4 g per day; the woman is advised about recommended weight gain.

- *Bed rest.* Frequent rest periods are advisable. At a minimum, the woman should rest twice a day for 1-hour periods of time.

- *Medication.* Studies have shown that women with mild chronic hypertension have outcomes similar to the general maternity population. Therefore, unless the blood pressure is over 150–160/100–110 mm Hg, antihypertensive medications are not used during pregnancy. Methyldopa is generally the first choice for use in pregnancy when medication is required.

- *Prenatal visits.* Counseling regarding the importance of frequent prenatal visits to reduce the incidence of adverse outcomes for mother or fetus is stressed.

- *Blood pressure monitoring.* The woman and her partner can be taught how to monitor blood pressure at home and maintain a record to be brought to each prenatal visit. Home monitoring is often more accurate because the woman is in a familiar environment and relaxed.

- *Fetal surveillance.* Starting at about 24 weeks, the woman should begin to keep fetal movement records and notify her care provider of any significant decrease in fetal movement. Serial ultrasonography to assess fetal growth and amniotic fluid volume is indicated. Antepartum fetal testing may begin as early as 26 weeks.

During the first prenatal visit, the woman should have a thorough physical examination, which includes a funduscopic examination, blood pressure and pulses in all four extremities, and auscultation of chest and flanks. Laboratory work includes a urinalysis and culture; 24-hour urine for protein, creatinine clearance, sodium, and potassium; CBC; serum electrolytes; and a glucose tolerance test. The usual prenatal laboratory assessments and an ultrasound for confirming gestational age are also done if the woman is currently pregnant. Although essential hypertension is the most likely explanation for hypertension in early pregnancy, a thorough evaluation can rule out rare but serious causes of secondary hypertension such as pheochromocytoma or coarctation of the aorta.

A woman with chronic hypertension generally has more frequent prenatal visits. She should be seen every 2 to 3 weeks in the first two trimesters and then more frequently in the third trimester, depending on how she and the fetus are progressing. Twenty-four-hour urines, serum creatinine, uric acid, hematocrit, and ultrasound examinations are repeated at least once in the second and third trimesters.

Chronic Hypertension with Superimposed Preeclampsia

Preeclampsia develops in approximately 25% of women previously found to have chronic hypertension (NIH, 2000). When elevations of systolic blood pressure 30 mm Hg above the baseline or of diastolic blood pressure 15 mm Hg above the baseline are discovered on two occasions at least 6 hours apart, when proteinuria develops, or when edema occurs in the upper half of the body, the woman needs close monitoring and careful management. If the woman has underlying renal disease, it may be very difficult to confirm the diagnosis of superimposed preeclampsia. A rise in serum uric acid is helpful in identifying preeclampsia, which frequently occurs late in the second trimester or early in the third.

Gestational Hypertension

Gestational hypertension (also called *transient hypertension*) exists when transient elevation of blood pressure occurs for the first time after midpregnancy without proteinuria (August, 2004). The final determination that the woman has gestational hypertension is made in the postpartum period. If preeclampsia does not develop and blood pressure returns to normal by 12 weeks' postpartum, the diagnosis of gestational hypertension may be assigned. If the blood pressure elevation persists after 12 weeks' postpartum, the woman is diagnosed with chronic hypertension.

CARE OF THE WOMAN AT RISK FOR RH ALLOIMMUNIZATION

The Rh blood group is present on the surface of erythrocytes of most of the population. When it is present a person is said to be Rh positive. Those without the factor are Rh negative. If an Rh-negative person is exposed to Rh-positive blood, an antigen-antibody response occurs, antibodies are formed, and the person is said to be *sensitized*. Subsequent exposure to Rh-positive blood can then cause a serious reaction that results in agglutination and hemolysis of red blood cells (RBCs). Rh *alloimmunization* (sensitization), also called *isoimmunization,* most often occurs when an Rh-negative woman carries an Rh-positive fetus either to term

or to termination by miscarriage or induced abortion. It can also occur if an Rh-negative nonpregnant woman receives an Rh-positive blood transfusion, experiences an Rh-positive tubal pregnancy, has an amniocentesis, or experiences any traumatic event that might allow Rh-positive fetal cells to enter the circulation of the Rh-negative woman.

A number of known RBC antigens are involved in the Rh system, all of which are controlled by three pairs of genes: Cc, Dd, and Ee. Antigens in the D group are usually involved with incompatibility between the mother and fetus, although there are 270 other "atypical" RBC antigens that have the potential to cause hemolytic disease of the fetus or newborn (Joy, Rossi, Krugh et al., 2005).

In the United States, approximately 2.5 of 1000 births will be complicated by maternal sensitization to one of these red cell antigens (McLean, Hedrianna, Lanouette et al., 2004). Approximately 85% of white Americans, 92% to 95% of African Americans, and 98% to 99% of Asian and Native Americans are Rh positive (ACOG, 2006).

During a normal pregnancy, small amounts of fetal blood may cross the placenta. An Rh-negative mother whose fetus is Rh positive may develop anti-D antibodies in response to this exposure. During delivery of the placenta or as a result of trauma, even larger quantities of fetal blood can enter maternal circulation. After exposure to the Rh-positive antigen, the primary immune response is development of immunoglobulin M (IgM) antibodies. This primary response develops slowly over several weeks or months with a detectable titer developing 5 to 16 weeks after the sensitizing event (Moise, 2004). IgM antibodies are large and do not cross the placenta (Shaver, 2004). Once a woman develops these antibodies, she is immunized for life.

Fetal RBCs express the Rh D antigen at 38 days after conception. Although the risk is very low, in theory it is possible for Rh D sensitization to occur during the first trimester. Fetal-maternal hemorrhage can occur with elective pregnancy termination, hemorrhage from an early threatened or spontaneous abortion, chorionic villi sampling, or ectopic pregnancy. Although the risk of sensitization is low and the evidence to support the use of RhoGAM in the first trimester is sparce, the reproductive implications of sensitization and the safety of RhoGAM makes it reasonable to treat Rh-negative women if the partner's blood type is not confirmed to be Rh negative (Harkness & Spinnato, 2004; Jabara & Barnhart, 2003). Following the primary response, a subsequent exposure to the Rh (D) cells results in a more rapid production of immunoglobulin G (IgG) anti-D antibodies, developing as quickly as a few days after exposure. IgG is capable of crossing the placenta and coating the fetal Rh (D) positive red cells, causing hemolysis. This secondary immune response may occur with exposure to a very small amount of Rh (D) positive cells and produce a response stronger than the primary response (Figure 20–10 ◆). Thus, although hemolysis is not generally a problem for the fetus during a first pregnancy, it may create problems during subsequent pregnancies. There also may be an increased risk for fetal anemia when multiple maternal antibodies to other red cell antigen groups (collectively referred to as "irregular antibodies") are present as compared with anti-D antibodies alone (Moise, 2004).

Figure 20–10 ◆ Rh alloimmunization sequence. *A*, Rh-positive father and Rh-negative mother. *B*, Pregnancy with Rh-positive fetus. Some Rh-positive blood enters the mother's blood. *C*, As the placenta separates, the mother is further exposed to the Rh-positive blood. *D*, The mother is sensitized to the Rh-positive blood; anti-Rh-positive antibodies (triangles) are formed. *E*, In subsequent pregnancies with an Rh-positive fetus, Rh-positive red blood cells are attacked by the anti-Rh-positive maternal antibodies, causing hemolysis of red blood cells in the fetus.

The possibility also exists that an Rh-negative female fetus carried by an Rh-positive mother may become sensitized in utero. This female would not demonstrate signs of hemolytic disease, but because she would be sensitized before even becoming pregnant, she would have a positive antibody screen when receiving prenatal care with her first Rh-positive fetus.

Needle sharing among addicts poses a risk of sensitization, because addicts draw some of their own blood up into the needle before injecting. Mismatched blood transfusion of Rh-positive blood to an Rh-negative person results in immunization in 55% to 80% of cases. A standard dose of RhoGAM (300 mcg) can prevent sensitization after exposure of up to 30 mL of Rh(D) positive blood or 15 mL of red cells. Whether sensitization is the result of a blood transfusion or maternal-fetal hemorrhage, a Kleihauer-Betke or rosette test can be performed to determine the amount of Rh(D) positive blood present in the maternal circulation and to calculate the amount of RhoGAM needed. Up to five doses may be administered at one time. If additional doses are necessary, they are administered every 12 hours in alternating sites until the appropriate amount has been given (Shaver, 2004).

Fetal-Neonatal Risks

The hemolysis caused by the maternal IgG antibodies in the fetus creates fetal anemia. The fetus responds by increasing RBC production. The presence of nucleated RBCs (erythroblasts) is why the term **erythroblastosis fetalis** was coined for this severe hemolytic disease of the fetus and newborn. If treatment is not initiated, this anemia can also cause marked fetal edema, called **hydrops fetalis.** Congestive heart failure may result. Although maternal sensitization can now be prevented by appropriate administration of Rh immune globulin, infants still die of hemolytic disease secondary to Rh incompatibility.

RBC destruction also leads to hyperbilirubinemia and jaundice (called *icterus gravis*), which can lead to neurologic damage (kernicterus).

Rh sensitization and the resultant hemolytic disease of the newborn are less common today because of the development of RhIgG. See Chapter 33 ∞ for further discussion of kernicterus and of treatment of the newborn affected by Rh sensitization.

SCREENING FOR RH INCOMPATIBILITY AND SENSITIZATION

At the first prenatal visit, (1) a history is taken of past pregnancies, previous sensitization, abortions, blood transfusions, or children who developed jaundice or anemia during the neonatal period; (2) maternal blood type (ABO) and Rh factor are determined, and a routine Rh antibody screen is done; and (3) other medical complications, such as diabetes, infections, or hypertension, are identified. An antibody screen (*indirect Coombs' test*) is done to determine whether an Rh-negative woman is sensitized (has developed isoimmunity) to the Rh antigen. The indirect Coombs' test measures the number of antibodies in the maternal blood. If the Rh-negative woman is not D-isoimmunized, a repeat D antibody determination should be made at 28 weeks' gestation, and the expectant woman should receive 300 mcg of Rh immune globulin. Rh immune globulin is also administered after any amniocentesis, regardless of gestational age; after chorionic villi sampling, if there is an episode of bleeding during pregnancy; or if there has been maternal trauma such as injury resulting from a motor vehicle accident or from domestic violence. In addition, Rh immune globulin must be administered to any Rh-negative woman who experiences a first trimester spontaneous or induced abortion, or an ectopic pregnancy. If the woman is Rh negative (dd), the father of the unborn child is asked to come into the clinic or physician's office to be assessed for his Rh factor and blood type. If he is homozygous for

Rh positive (DD), all his offspring will be Rh positive. If he is heterozygous (Dd), 50% of his offspring will be Rh negative and 50% heterozygous for Rh positive. If the father is Rh negative, all their children will be Rh negative, and no Rh incompatibility with the mother will occur. If the father is Rh positive or the mother is known to have previously carried an Rh-positive fetus, further testing and careful management are needed.

In women who are alloimmunized, anti-D antibody titers should be determined every 2 to 4 weeks beginning at 16 to 18 weeks, biweekly during the third trimester, and the week before the due date. Traditionally, if the test shows a maternal antibody titer of 1:16 or greater, a delta optical density (ΔOD) analysis of the amniotic fluid is performed. (See later discussion.) If the titer is 1:16 or less late in pregnancy, birth at 38 weeks or spontaneous labor at term can be anticipated.

Negative antibody titers can consistently identify the fetus not at risk. However, the titers cannot reliably point out the fetus in danger because the level of the titer does not correlate with the severity of the disease. For instance, in a severely sensitized woman antibody titers may be moderately high and remain at the same level although the fetus is being more and more severely affected. Conversely, a woman sensitized by previous Rh-positive fetuses may show a high fixed antibody titer during a pregnancy in which the fetus is Rh negative. Fetal assessment includes percutaneous umbilical cord blood sampling (PUBS), amniocentesis, amniotic fluid analysis, and ultrasound. Previously, PUBS was the only direct method of assessing the Rh status of a fetus. This procedure requires a highly skilled physician and places the fetus at greater risk than does amniocentesis. It is now possible, however, to determine fetal Rh status from an amniotic fluid specimen using polymerase chain reaction (PCR). Although not yet commercially available, fetal RhD typing through analysis of fetal DNA circulating in maternal plasma shows great promise (Gautier, Benachi, Giovangrandi et al., 2005; Moise, 2005). Ideally, an early ultrasound should be done to determine gestational age. Thereafter serial ultrasounds and amniotic fluid analysis should be done to follow fetal progress.

The presence of ascites and subcutaneous edema are signs of severe fetal involvement (fetal hydrops). Other indicators of the fetal condition include an increase in fetal heart size, hydramnios, and placental thickness and texture. Ultrasound evaluation cannot distinguish mild from severe fetal anemia unless hydropic changes are present. When RBCs are hemolyzed, bilirubin is a breakdown product. If fetal RBCs are being hemolyzed because of isoimmunization, the fetus may excrete bilirubin in the amniotic fluid with voiding. Thus ΔOD analysis is done to determine the amount of bilirubin pigment found in the amniotic fluid. Normally the concentration of bilirubin pigments in the amniotic fluid declines during pregnancy. Elevated bilirubin levels are significant. Because the amount of bilirubin found in the amniotic fluid correlates roughly with the extent of the hemolysis, the ΔOD analysis serves as an indirect predictor of the severity of the fetal anemia. To determine the ΔOD level, amniotic fluid, obtained by transabdominal amniocentesis, is separated from its cellular components by centrifuge. The amount of bilirubin pigment from the degradation of RBCs can then be measured by spectrophotometric analysis and plotted on a special chart called a Liley graph.

Readings within zone III (the highest zone) indicate a severely affected fetus who may require intrauterine transfusion every 1 to 2 weeks between weeks 26 and 32 until viability is reached, followed by birth, usually by cesarean. Neonatal exchange transfusion is anticipated. Prognosis is guarded. Fetal monitoring may identify the very ill fetus by documenting less movement or lack of movement. The appearance of sinusoidal pattern suggests fetal anemia and a deteriorating fetal condition (see Chapter 23 ∞).

Currently, a new approach is replacing the use of the traditional technique of serial amniocentesis and ΔOD in the management of alloimmunized pregnancies (Kumar & Regan, 2005). It is the use of velocimetry of the fetal middle cerebral artery (MCA) to monitor affected pregnancies for the detection of fetal anemia (ACOG, 2006; Kumar & Regan, 2005). The noninvasive method of using Doppler ultrasonography to monitor fetal anemia via the measurement of the peak systolic velocities of the middle cerebral artery (PSV of MCA) has been shown to be accurate and much safer than amniocentesis for detecting fetal anemia (Dongen, Klumper, Sikkel et al., 2005). PSVs correlate well with increasing levels of bilirubin in the amniotic fluid and should be monitored weekly (Figure 20–11 ◆).

Clinical Therapy

The goal of medical management is the birth of a mature fetus who has not developed severe hemolysis in utero. This requires early identification and treatment of maternal conditions that

Figure 20–11 ◆ Ultrasound measurement of peak systolic velocity (PSV) of the middle cerebral artery. The fetal middle cerebral arteries can be seen as major lateral branches of the circle of Willis and may be used during pregnancy to detect either fetal anemia or a fetal response to hypoxia as redistribution of cardiac output in favor of the brain, myocardium, and adrenal glands. This image demonstrates a flow velocity wave form and displays the normal continuous foward blood flow in the fetal cerebral arteries throughout the cardiac cycle. Normal peak systolic velocity values change throughout gestation, increasing with advancing gestational age. In the case of fetal anemia, the velocity of blood will be increased above the norms for gestational age. The PSV in the middle cerebral artery of this fetus is 32.81 cm/s, which is appropriate for this gestational age.
SOURCE: Courtesy of Debbie McGee, MSN, PNNP, RDMS.

predispose the infant to hemolytic disease, coordinated obstetric-pediatric treatment for the seriously affected newborn, and prevention of Rh sensitization if none is present.

ANTEPARTUM MANAGEMENT

Two primary interventions are used by the physician to aid the fetus whose blood cells are being destroyed by maternal antibodies: early birth of the fetus and intrauterine transfusion, both of which carry risks. Ideally, birth should be delayed until fetal pulmonary maturity is confirmed at about 36 to 37 weeks. This is possible for most pregnancies with ΔOD readings in zones I and II. Severely sensitized fetuses may require birth at 32 to 34 weeks. ΔOD readings are not used in the management of a pregnancy complicated by one of the "irregular antibodies." In those cases, the use of Doppler ultrasonography of the PSV of the MCA, when properly performed, is a more accurate predictor of fetal anemia (Dongen et al., 2005; Harkness & Spinnato, 2004).

Intrauterine transfusion is done to correct the anemia produced by the RBC hemolysis and thereby improve fetal oxygenation. This may be done either intravascularly through PUBS or intraperitoneally as early as 18 weeks. In a fetus who shows no signs of hydrops, a fetal blood sample should be used to check for significant anemia (hematocrit greater than 30%) before starting transfusion therapy.

Intravascular transfusion has greatly improved the outcome for severely affected fetuses. Under ultrasound visualization, the umbilical vein is entered, and the fetus is temporarily paralyzed with 0.1 mg/kg estimated fetal weight of pancuronium bromide. A fetal hematocrit is obtained; then leukocyte-poor Rh-negative packed red blood cells (PRBCs) are transfused. The volume of PRBCs is determined by a formula based on estimated normal blood volume, the pretransfusion hematocrit, the hematocrit of the blood to be transfused, and the desired hematocrit. Repeat transfusions can be scheduled as necessary until the fetus is sufficiently mature to tolerate birth. If access to the umbilical vein is problematic, intrauterine transfusions can be performed by introducing the needle into the fetal abdomen and peritoneal cavity. Blood is transfused through a catheter into the peritoneal cavity, where diaphragmatic lymphatics absorbed the RBCs into fetal circulation.

About 80% to 90% of transfused fetuses survive. The procedure is hazardous to the fetus, however. Complications include nonreassuring fetal status, fetal hematoma, fetal-maternal hemorrhage, fetal death, and chorioamnionitis. Birth is delayed until at least 32 weeks' gestation if possible. Premature newborns are generally more susceptible to damage from hemolytic disease. They often require exchange transfusion and usually require intensive nursery care.

POSTPARTUM MANAGEMENT

The goals of postpartum care are to prevent sensitization in the as-yet-unsensitized pregnant woman and to treat the isoimmune hemolytic disease in the newborn.

The Rh-negative mother who has no titer (indirect Coombs' negative, nonsensitized) and who has given birth to an Rh-positive fetus (direct Coombs' negative) is given an intramuscular injection of 300 mcg RhIgG globulin—that is, **Rh immune globulin (RhoGAM,** HypRho-D)—within 72 hours so that she

does not have time to produce antibodies to fetal cells that entered her bloodstream when the placenta separated. This protocol reduces the incidence of antenatal sensitization dramatically. Rh immune globulin works to destroy the fetal cells in the maternal circulation before sensitization occurs, thereby blocking maternal antibody production. This provides temporary passive immunity for the mother, which prevents the development of permanent active immunity (antibody formation).

The normal dose of Rh immune globulin should suppress the immune response to approximately 30 mL Rh-positive whole blood. However, if a larger fetomaternal bleed may have occurred, a Kleihauer-Betke test can be performed to obtain an estimate of its extent. Based on the findings, the appropriate amount of Rh immune globulin is given. When the woman is Rh negative and not sensitized and the father is Rh positive or unknown, Rh immune globulin is also given after each spontaneous or induced abortion, ectopic pregnancy, chorionic villus sampling, multifetal pregnancy reduction, partial molar pregnancy, amniocentesis, PUBS, antepartum hemorrhage, or external version. After any maternal trauma, a Kleihauer-Betke test can be performed to identify the need for Rh immune globulin administration. If abortion or ectopic pregnancy occurs in the first trimester, a smaller (50 mcg) dose of Rh immune globulin (MICRhoGAM or Mini-Gamulin Rh) is used. Most hospitals and offices do not stock this dose; therefore, the standard full dose of 300 mcg Rh immune globulin is given (Moise, 2004). A full dose is used following second trimester amniocentesis. Occasionally, sensitization can occur antepartally because of small transplacental bleeds. To prevent this from occurring, an antibody screen is performed on an Rh-negative woman at 28 weeks' gestation. If it is negative, 300 mcg Rh immune globulin is administered prophylactically.

Rh immune globulin is not given to the newborn or the father. It is not effective for and should not be given to a previously sensitized woman. However, sometimes after childbirth or an abortion, the results of the blood test do not clearly show whether the mother is already sensitized to the Rh antigen. In such cases, Rh immune globulin should be given because it will cause no harm.

NURSING CARE MANAGEMENT
Nursing Assessment and Diagnosis

As part of the initial prenatal history the nurse asks the mother whether she knows her blood type and Rh factor. Many women are aware that they are Rh negative and that this status has implications for pregnancy. If the woman knows she is Rh negative, the nurse can assess the woman's knowledge of what that means. The nurse can also ask the woman whether she ever received Rh immune globulin, whether she has had any previous pregnancies and their outcome, and whether she knows her partner's Rh factor. Should the partner be Rh negative, there is no risk to the fetus, who will also be Rh negative. Uncertain paternity is an awkward situation; nevertheless, it is essential for the physician to have this information. Nurses often have a more intimate relationship with pregnant women, allowing them to obtain sensitive information that is vital in the management of pregnancy. When paternity is uncertain or the father is unavailable for testing, the fetus in assumed to be antigen positive until proven otherwise.

If the woman does not know what Rh immune type she is, intervention cannot begin until the initial laboratory data are obtained. If the woman is Rh negative, the father's blood type and zygosity, if he is Rh positive, are obtained. Once that is complete, the nurse plans intervention based on the findings.

If the woman becomes sensitized during her pregnancy, nursing assessment focuses on the knowledge level and coping skills of the woman and her family. The nurse also provides ongoing assessment during procedures to evaluate fetal well-being, such as ultrasound and amniocentesis.

Postpartally, the nurse reviews data about the Rh type of the fetus. If the fetus is Rh positive, the mother is Rh negative, and no sensitization has occurred, nursing assessment reveals the need to administer Rh immune globulin within 72 hours of birth. If inadvertently the dose of RhIgG is not given within the 72-hour window, some protection has been documented with administration within 13 days. The recommendation is to administer the dose up to 28 days after birth (Moise, 2004).

Nursing diagnoses that might apply to the pregnant woman at risk for Rh sensitization include the following:

- **Health-Seeking Behavior: Information About the Purpose of RhIgG** related to an expressed desire to understand the treatment of Rh incompatibility
- **Ineffective Individual Coping** related to depression secondary to the development of indications of the need for fetal exchange transfusion

I've been a nurse for almost 40 years now. I remember when RhoGAM first started to be used—what a difference it made in the lives of so many women. Young women who are Rh negative today will hopefully never know the pain and tragedy the simple absence of a blood factor can mean. It is nothing short of miraculous!

Nursing Plan and Implementation

During the antepartal period, the nurse explains the mechanisms involved in isoimmunization and answers any questions the woman and her partner may have. It is imperative that the woman understand the importance of receiving Rh immune globulin after every spontaneous or therapeutic abortion or ectopic pregnancy if she is not already sensitized. The nurse also explains the purpose of the Rh immune globulin administered at 28 weeks if the woman is not sensitized.

If the woman is sensitized to the Rh factor, it poses a threat to any Rh-positive fetus she carries. The nurse provides emotional support to the family to help them deal with their grief and any feelings of guilt about the infant's condition. Should an intrauterine transfusion become necessary, the nurse continues to provide emotional support while also assuming responsibilities as part of the healthcare team.

During labor, the nurse caring for an Rh-negative woman who has not been sensitized ensures that the woman's blood is

Table 20–7   RH SENSITIZATION

When trying to work through Rh problems, the nurse should remember the following:

- A potential problem exists when an Rh-negative mother and an Rh-positive father conceive a child who is Rh positive.
- In this situation, the mother may become sensitized or produce antibodies to her fetus's Rh-positive blood.

The following tests are used to detect sensitization:

- Indirect Coombs' tests—done on the mother's blood to measure the number of Rh-positive antibodies.
- Direct Coombs' test—done on the infant's blood to detect antibody-coated Rh-positive RBCs.

Based on the results of these tests, the following may be done:

- If the mother's indirect Coombs' test is negative and the infant's direct Coombs' test is negative (confirming that sensitization has not occurred), the mother is given Rh immune globulin within 72 hours of birth.
- If the mother's indirect Coombs' test is positive and her Rh-positive infant has a positive direct Coombs' test, Rh immune globulin is *not* given, in this case, the infant is carefully monitored for hemolytic disease.
- It is recommended that Rh immune globulin be given at 28 weeks antenatally to decrease possible transplacental bleeding concerns.
- Rh immune globulin is also administered after each abortion (spontaneous or therapeutic), antepartum hemorrhage mismatched blood transfusion, ectopic pregnancy, amniocentesis, chorionic villi sampling (CVS), percutaneous umbilical blood sampling (PUBS), fetal cephalic version, or maternal trauma.

assessed for any antibodies and also has been cross-matched for Rh immune globulin. On the postpartum unit, the nurse generally is responsible for administering the Rh immune globulin (see Procedure 20–2: Administration of Rh Immune Globulin [RhoGAM, HypRho-D]).

Table 20–7 summarizes the major considerations in caring for an Rh-negative woman. The treatment of the newborn with isoimmune hemolytic disease is discussed in Chapter 33. ∞

Evaluation

Expected outcomes of nursing care include the following:

- The woman is able to explain the process of Rh sensitization and its implications for her unborn child and for subsequent pregnancies.
- If the woman has not been sensitized, she is able to explain the importance of receiving Rh immune globulin when necessary and cooperates with the recommended dosage schedule.
- The woman gives birth to a healthy newborn.
- If complications develop for the fetus (or newborn), they are detected quickly, and therapy is instituted.

CARE OF THE WOMAN AT RISK DUE TO ABO INCOMPATIBILITY

ABO incompatibility is rather common (occurring in 20% to 25% of pregnancies) but rarely causes significant hemolysis. In

PROCEDURE 20–2 Administration of Rh Immune Globulin (RhoGAM, HypRho-D)

NURSING ACTION	RATIONALE
Preparation • Confirm that Rh immune globulin is indicated by checking the woman's prenatal or intrapartal record to verify that she is Rh negative. Then confirm that sensitization has not occurred—maternal indirect Coombs' negative. Postpartally, confirm that the baby is Rh positive but not sensitized (direct Coombs' negative) and that the mother's indirect Coombs' is negative. Rh immune globulin is *not* indicated if the infant is Rh negative, too. • Confirm that the woman does not have a history of allergies to immune globulin preparations by checking entries on medication allergies in her chart and by asking her whether she has ever had any allergic reactions to medications, globulins, or blood products. • Explain purpose and procedure. Have consent form signed if required by agency policy. **Equipment and Supplies** • Rh immune globulin, which is obtained from the blood bank or pharmacy according to agency protocol. Lot numbers for the drug and the cross-match should be the same. • Syringe and IM needle **Procedure** 1. Confirm the woman's identity and administer one vial of 300 mcg Rh immune globulin IM in the deltoid muscle. 2. An immune globulin microdose is used after miscarriage, elective abortion, ectopic pregnancy, or molar pregnancy occurring within the first 12 weeks' gestation. Antepartally, the Rh immune globulin is generally given within 3 hours but not longer than 72 hours of the event. 3. If a larger bleed is suspected at birth (as in cases of severe abruptio placentae), additional doses may be administered at one time using multiple sites at regular intervals as long as all doses are given within 72 hours of childbirth. 4. Provide opportunities for the woman to ask questions and express concerns. 5. Chart according to agency policy. Most agencies chart lot number, route, dose, and client education.	*Rh immune globulin is only indicated for Rh-negative, unsensitized women.* *Rh immune globulin is made from the plasma portion of blood. Allergic reactions are possible.* *Many agencies require separate consent for the administration of Rh immune globulin because it is a blood product. The woman should clearly understand the purpose of the Rh immune globulin, its rationale, the administration procedure, and any related risks. Generally the primary side effects are redness and tenderness at the injection site and allergic responses.* *The normal 300-mcg dose provides passive immunity following exposure to 15 mL of transfused RBCs or 30 mL of fetal blood.* *Many women, especially primigravidas, are not aware of the risks for an Rh-positive fetus of a sensitized Rh-negative mother. They need to understand the importance of receiving Rh immune globulin for each pregnancy to ensure continued protection.*

CLINICAL TIP

In most cases, Rh immune globulin is administered in the deltoid muscle. However, in an extremely thin woman, or in the cases of a larger-than-normal dose, consider administering the medication in the ventrogluteal or posterior gluteal site. You may also divide the dose into multiple injections.

most cases, ABO incompatibility is limited to type O mothers with a type A or B fetus. The group B fetus of a group A mother and the group A fetus of a group B mother are only occasionally affected. Group O infants, because they have no antigenic sites on the RBCs, are never affected regardless of the mother's blood type. The incompatibility occurs as a result of the maternal antibodies present in her serum and interaction between the antigen sites on the fetal RBCs.

Anti-A and anti-B antibodies are naturally occurring; that is, women are naturally exposed to the A and B antigens through the foods they eat and through exposure to infection by gram-negative bacteria. As a result, some women have high serum anti-A and anti-B titers before they become pregnant. Once the woman becomes pregnant, the maternal serum anti-A and anti-B antibodies cross the placenta and produce hemolysis of the fetal RBCs. With ABO incompatibility, the first infant is frequently involved, and no relationship exists between the appearance of the disease and repeated sensitization from one pregnancy to the next.

Unlike the case of Rh incompatibility, treatment is never warranted antepartally. As part of the initial assessment, however, the nurse should note whether the potential for an ABO incompatibility exists. This alerts caregivers so that following birth the newborn can be assessed carefully for the development of hyperbilirubinemia (see Chapter 33 ∞).

CARE OF THE WOMAN REQUIRING SURGERY DURING PREGNANCY

Although elective surgery should be delayed until the postpartal period, essential surgery can generally be undertaken during pregnancy. Surgery does pose some risks. The incidence of spontaneous abortion is increased for women who have surgery in the first trimester. The risks to the pregnancy can be significantly reduced when surgery can be delayed until the second trimester or to the postpartum period. Surgery during the third trimester is difficult because of the enlarging uterus and an increased risk of preterm labor.

Clinical Therapy

The most common nonpregnancy-related indications for surgical treatment are appendicitis, cholecystitis, and GI obstruction. Although general preoperative and postoperative care are similar for pregnant and nonpregnant women, special considerations must be kept in mind whenever the surgical client is pregnant. The early second trimester is the best time to operate because there is less risk of causing spontaneous abortion or early labor, and the uterus is not so large as to impinge on the abdominal field.

The preoperative chest radiograph and electrocardiogram, which are routine for persons over age 40, should be done on the same basis for the pregnant woman. If a chest radiograph is done, the fetus should be shielded from the radiation. Because of decreased intestinal motility and decreased free gastric acid secretion during pregnancy, stomach emptying time is delayed, which increases risk of vomiting during induction of anesthesia and during the postoperative period. Therefore, a nasogastric tube is recommended before major surgery. An indwelling urinary catheter prevents bladder distention, decreases risk of injury to the bladder, and promotes ease of monitoring output. Support stockings during and after surgery help prevent venous stasis and the development of thrombophlebitis. Fetal heart tones must be monitored before, during, and after surgery.

Pregnancy causes increased secretions of the respiratory tract and engorgement of the nasal mucous membrane, often making breathing through the nose difficult. Because of this, pregnant women often need an endotracheal tube for respiratory support during surgery. Caregivers must guard against maternal hypoxia during surgery because uterine circulation will be decreased and fetal oxygenation can decline very quickly. During surgery and the recovery period, the woman is positioned to allow optimal uteroplacental-fetal circulation. A wedge is placed under her hip to tip the uterus and thereby avoid pressure by the fetus on the maternal vena cava.

Spinal or epidural anesthesia is preferred because local anesthetics are not associated with birth defects. Caution must be exercised because this type of anesthesia may produce hypotension and respiratory apnea in the pregnant woman. The frequency and degree of the hypotension increase with higher anesthetic levels. This can be prevented in many cases with a preanesthetic infusion of 900 to 1000 mL of fluid.

Blood loss during surgery is monitored carefully. Measurement of fetal heart tones gives the best indication of blood loss. Because of the normal increased blood volume of pregnancy, uterine blood flow may be reduced significantly before the maternal blood pressure begins to fall. Fluid replacement should be done with balanced electrolyte solution and, if needed, with whole blood.

NURSING CARE MANAGEMENT
Nursing Assessment and Diagnosis

During the preoperative period, the nurse assesses the pregnant woman's health status in the same way that any preoperative client is assessed. Is there any sign of respiratory infection, fever, urinary tract infection, or anemia? Are laboratory values all within normal limits for surgery (except in the case of emergency surgery, which may, of necessity, be done even with abnormal laboratory values)? Do the woman and her family understand the surgical procedure? Do they know what to expect postoperatively? Do they have any questions or concerns?

The nurse also considers the impact of surgery on the woman's pregnancy. Is the fetal heart rate normal? Does the woman understand the implications of surgery with regard to her pregnancy? How is she coping?

Intraoperatively, fetal heart rate is assessed if at all possible. Postoperatively, the nurse completes all necessary postoperative assessments and also continues to assess fetal status, primarily by monitoring the fetal heart rate.

Nursing diagnoses that might apply to the pregnant woman who requires surgery include the following:

- **Altered Tissue Perfusion** (fetal) related to the effects of general anesthesia on fetal oxygenation
- **Anxiety** related to lack of knowledge of preoperative and postoperative procedures
- **Fear** related to the possible effect of surgery on fetal outcome

Nursing Plan and Implementation

Much of the nurse's care during the preoperative period is directed toward the educational needs of the woman and her family. The nurse plans time to review the procedure and answer any questions the family may have. The nurse recognizes that the need for surgery during the woman's pregnancy is probably very distressing for the family. The nurse works to help decrease their anxiety by providing information and emotional support.

Postoperatively, the nurse is caring for two clients: the mother and her unborn child. In addition to monitoring the status of both, the nurse considers both in providing care. If surgery is done in the first trimester, the nurse should be aware of the potential teratogenic effect of any medications prescribed and should discuss the implications with the surgeon and obstetrician. During the third trimester, the nurse, recognizing the potential for vena caval syndrome if the woman lies flat on her back, helps the woman maintain a side-lying position. To avoid inadequate oxygenation, the nurse encourages the woman to turn, breathe deeply, and cough regularly and also to use any ventilation therapy, such as incentive spirometry, to avoid developing pneumonia. The pregnant woman is also at increased risk for thrombophlebitis, so the nurse applies antiembolism stockings, encourages leg exercises while the woman is confined to bed, and begins ambulation as soon as possible. In addition, the nurse encourages the woman to maintain or resume an adequate diet as soon as possible. If cultural factors influence the woman's dietary practices, the nurse and dietitian should work together to meet the woman's needs.

Discharge teaching is especially important. The woman and her family should have a clear understanding of what to expect regarding activity level, discomfort, diet, medications, and any special considerations. In addition, they ought to know any warning signs that they should report to their physician immediately.

Evaluation

Expected outcomes of nursing care include the following:

- The woman is able to explain the surgical procedure, its risks and benefits, and its implications for her pregnancy.
- Caregivers maintain adequate maternal oxygenation throughout surgery and postoperatively.
- Potential complications are avoided or detected early and treated successfully.
- The woman is able to describe any necessary postdischarge activities, limitations, and follow-up and agrees to cooperate with the recommended regimen.
- The woman maintains her pregnancy successfully.

CARE OF THE WOMAN SUFFERING TRAUMA FROM AN ACCIDENT

Accidents and injury are the leading causes of death in women of reproductive age. Estimates suggest that accidental injury complicates 6% to 7% of all pregnancies (Gonik & Foley, 2004). When the woman is critically injured, fetal death occurs at least 40% of the time (ACOG, 1998). Approximately two thirds of all trauma during pregnancy is the result of motor vehicle accidents (ACOG, 1998), and these accidents are the leading cause of fetal and maternal death (Gonik & Foley, 2004; Hyde, Cook, Olson, et al., 2003). Falls and assault—including domestic violence—are the next most common causes of injury.

In early pregnancy, body changes increase the potential for injury through fatigue, fainting spells, and hyperventilation. Late in pregnancy, the woman has less balance and coordination and may fall. Her protruding abdomen is vulnerable to a variety of minor injuries. The fetus is usually well protected by the amniotic fluid, which distributes the force of a blow equally in all directions, and by the muscle layers of the uterus and abdominal wall. In early pregnancy, while the uterus is still in the pelvis, it

is shielded from blows by the surrounding pelvic organs, muscles, and bony structures. Trauma that causes concern includes blunt trauma, from an automobile accident, for example; penetrating abdominal injuries, such as knife or gunshot wounds; and the complications that commonly accompany maternal trauma, such as shock, premature labor, and spontaneous abortion.

The normal physiologic changes of pregnancy have clinical implications for victims of trauma. Blood volume increases up to 50% and cardiac output increases about 40%. Generally, the pregnant woman has a greater volume of blood loss compared with a nonpregnant woman before evidence of shock is seen. The pregnant woman with significant volume loss is able to maintain hemodynamic stability temporarily by decreasing uteroplacental perfusion, thereby compromising fetal status. In the second and third trimesters, supine positioning can decrease blood return to the heart and cause overt hypotension and even loss of consciousness. During pregnancy, minute ventilation and oxygen consumption increase. This makes the gravid woman more susceptible to hypoxemia with apnea. Clotting factors normally increase in pregnancy, making it a hypercoagulable state. Thus, the risk of thrombosis after injury is increased. DIC occurs commonly with severe trauma. Because the normal fibrinogen level in pregnancy is increased to between 350 and 400 mg/dL, normal nonpregnant values may indicate early DIC.

Maternal mortality most often occurs from head trauma or hemorrhage. Uterine rupture results from strong deceleration forces in an automobile accident in only 0.1% to 1% of pregnant women (ACOG, 1998). All automobile passengers should wear seat belts. The small risk of uterine or placental injury from seat belt use is far outweighed by the fact that maternal death is the most common cause of fetal death. The use of seat belts by pregnant women has been shown to decrease morbidity and mortality of the mother. Between 31 and 38 weeks, there is a sharp increase in fetal death in unbelted mothers (Hyde et al., 2003). Traumatic separation of the placenta can occur even if the site of injury is remote from the abdomen. It results in a high rate of fetal mortality. Premature labor is another serious hazard to the fetus, often following rupture of membranes during an accident. Premature labor can ensue even if the woman is not injured.

Fractures of the pelvis can result in significant retroperitoneal hemorrhage. If there is an unstable or dislocated fracture of the pelvis, cesarean birth will probably be necessary, but with a slightly displaced pelvic fracture, vaginal birth may be attempted. Hematuria or difficulty placing a urinary catheter may be associated with injuries to the bladder or urethra.

Penetrating trauma includes gunshot wounds and stab wounds. The mother generally fares better than the fetus if the penetrating trauma involves the abdomen as the enlarged uterus is likely to protect the mother's bowel from injury. Unfortunately, the fetal injury rate is 59% to 80% (Gonik & Foley, 2004).

Clinical Therapy

The goals of clinical therapy are to stabilize the injury and promote well-being for both mother and fetus. Thus clinical therapy initially focuses on ensuring airway adequacy, maintaining ventilation and adequate circulatory volume, controlling acute bleeding, and splinting fractures to prevent vascular or tissue injury. The Glascow Coma Scale is useful in evaluating for neurologic deficit. Once the mother is stabilized, fetal status is assessed.

Care must be taken at the scene of the injury to avoid the development of supine hypotensive syndrome. A wedge is generally placed under the woman's right hip. A neck brace is used if a neck injury is suspected, or the woman is placed on a backboard and the entire board is tilted to displace the uterus. Prompt treatment of maternal hypotension or hypovolemia also averts poor fetal oxygenation. Obstetric consultation is necessary to ensure that the needs of both mother and fetus are met.

In cases of noncatastrophic trauma, that is, where the mother's life is not directly threatened, fetal monitoring for 4 hours should be sufficient if there is no vaginal bleeding, uterine tenderness, contractions, or leaking amniotic fluid. Abruptio placentae may occur following a blow to the abdomen as the flexible myometrium of the uterus sustains a contour-changing impact that the relatively inelastic placenta cannot match. The increased intrauterine pressure during the blow further shears the placenta from the underlying decidua basalis. Abruptio placentae may occur in up to 5% of women who sustain minor injuries and in up to 35% of women who sustain major abdominal trauma. Increased uterine irritability in the first few hours following trauma helps identify women who may be at high risk for this potentially catastrophic complication. Of those women who contract every 10 minutes or more, 20% will have placental abruption. Ultrasonography does not seem to be as sensitive as fetal monitoring for diagnosing abruptio placentae. In women who have experienced significant maternal trauma, most cases of placental abruption evolve within 24 hours (Clark, 2004). If the woman is bleeding, contracting, or has uterine tenderness or a nonreassuring fetal heart rate tracing, a 24- to 48-hour observation is recommended. If uterine contractions and bleeding are not present, with a reassuring fetal heart rate tracing, monitoring for 4 to 6 hours is probably sufficient (Clark, 2004).

Fetomaternal hemorrhage occurs four to five times more often in pregnant women who have experienced trauma. A Kleihauer-Betke test may be useful in helping identify unsensitized Rh-negative women who have experienced fetal-maternal bleeds due to trauma. Rh immune globulin should be given to any unsensitized Rh-negative woman to be certain she is covered for small fetal hemorrhages that may be below the sensitivity of the Kleihauer-Betke test.

There has been controversy regarding the use of beta-adrenergic tocolytics in pregnant women following trauma because of the concerns regarding hemodynamic instability and the potential for masking uterine irritability or contractions that forewarn of abruptio placentae. Radiographic studies should be performed as needed to evaluate injuries regardless of fetal exposure.

When cardiopulmonary resuscitation (CPR) is performed on the pregnant woman late in gestation, perimortem cesarean birth is advocated if CPR is unsuccessful in the first 4 minutes. Chest compressions are less effective in the third trimester because of compression of the inferior vena cava by the gravid uterus. Cesarean birth alleviates this compression and improves resuscitation efforts in both the fetus and the mother (Gonik & Foley, 2004; Katz, Balderston, & DeFreest, 2005).

NURSING CARE MANAGEMENT
Nursing Assessment and Diagnosis

Each individual must be assessed according to the type and extent of her injuries. As with all trauma victims, initial assessments focus on adequacy of the airway, evidence of breathing, existence of cardiovascular stability, extent of injury, and a brief neurologic assessment. When an injured woman is pregnant, it is necessary to assess fetal status as well to avoid fetal hypoxia. Frequent maternal blood gas determinations are indicated if respiratory function is compromised.

Ongoing assessments include evaluation of uterine tone, contractions and tenderness, fundal height, fetal heart rate, intake and output and other indicators of shock, normal postoperative evaluation in those women requiring surgery, determination of neurologic status, and assessment of mental outlook and anxiety level.

Nursing diagnoses that might apply to the pregnant woman suffering trauma include the following:

* *Pain* related to the effects of the trauma experienced
* *Constipation* related to immobility secondary to the effects of the accident
* *Fear* related to the effects of the trauma on fetal well-being

Nursing Plan and Implementation

As a member of the healthcare team the nurse is actively involved in the ongoing assessment of the status of the woman and fetus. The nurse also has a primary responsibility to assess the childbearing woman's emotional state. The trauma victim must be oriented to her situation and receive explanation and reinforcement as necessary to help her understand any interventions. Family members should be involved as appropriate. The nurse also gives the pregnant woman an opportunity to discuss her feelings and concerns.

Evaluation

Expected outcomes of nursing care include the following:

* The woman and her family are able to understand the effects of the trauma on her and on her unborn child.
* Adequate maternal oxygenation is maintained to ensure fetal well-being.
* The woman's pain is adequately relieved, and her trauma is treated.
* Potential complications are quickly identified, and appropriate interventions are instituted.
* The woman gives birth to a healthy newborn.
* If the trauma results in fetal demise, the woman is able to verbalize her feelings and begin working through the grief process.

CARE OF THE BATTERED PREGNANT WOMAN

The true extent of domestic violence during pregnancy is difficult to determine. Estimates suggest that violence during pregnancy affects up to 20% of women, roughly 335,000 pregnant women and their fetuses (AAP & ACOG, 2002; Kady, Gilbert, Xing, et al., 2005); however, these statistics are most likely understated because many victims are unwilling to disclose their experiences

Battering may result in psychologic distress, loss of pregnancy, preterm labor, low-birth-weight infants, injury to the fetus, and fetal death. Complications such as poor maternal weight gain, infection, anemia, and second and third trimester bleeding are also seen more frequently among pregnant women who are abused. Women who are battered may also experience sexual abuse and are at increased risk of contracting sexually transmitted infections from their partner. This pattern of violence may escalate during pregnancy and may occur even more frequently in the postpartum period (ACOG, 1999a). The first step toward helping the battered woman is to identify her. She needs support, confidence in her decision making, and the recognition that she can help herself.

Chronic psychosomatic symptoms can be an indicator of abuse. The woman may have nonspecific or vague complaints. It is important to assess old scars around the head, chest, arms, abdomen, and genitalia. Any bruising or evidence of pain is also evaluated. The nurse should be especially alert for signs of bruising or injury to the woman's breasts, abdomen, or genitals because these areas are common targets of violence during pregnancy. Other indicators include a decrease in eye contact, silence when the partner is in the room, and a history of nervousness, insomnia, drug overdose, or alcohol problems. Frequent visits to the emergency department and a history of accidents without understandable causes are possible indicators of abuse.

The goals of treatment are to identify the woman at risk, increase her decision-making abilities to decrease the potential for further abuse, and provide a safe environment for her and her unborn child. In a prospective observational study, investigators found that women who declined to be interviewed about domestic violence were found to be at greater risk for adverse pregnancy outcomes when compared with women who experienced verbal or physical abuse (Yost, Bloom, McIntire et al., 2005). Twenty-seven percent of women who are abused and living in a violent environment will demonstrate abusive behaviors toward the children in that home (AAP & ACOG, 2002).

Screening must be done in a private setting and by using direct questions. ACOG recommends that *all* women be screened for intimate partner violence. During pregnancy, women should be screened multiple times because they may not disclose abuse if they are asked only one time, or the abuse may begin later in pregnancy. The suggested schedule for screening is at the first prenatal visit, at least once per trimester, and at the postpartum visit. See Chapter 9 ∞ for discussion of specific screening questions.

Once domestic violence is identified, the next step is to determine the immediate safety of the woman. She needs to be aware of community resources available to her, such as emergency shelters; police, legal, and social services; and counseling. It is important to establish an exit plan in situations of ongoing violence. Pocket cards and resource materials can be handed to women or left in restrooms for them to pick up. Nurses need to recognize that, ultimately, it is the woman's decision either to seek assistance or to return to old patterns. For further information, see Chapter 9. ∞

CARE OF THE WOMAN WITH A PERINATAL INFECTION AFFECTING THE FETUS

Fetal infection may develop at any time during pregnancy. In general, perinatal infections are most likely to cause harm when the embryo is exposed during first trimester organ development. Infections later in pregnancy create various concerns such as growth restriction, nonimmune hydrops, and neurologic disturbances. The most commonly occurring viral and parasitic infections that may have an impact on the fetus if acquired during pregnancy include toxoplasmosis, rubella, cytomegalovirus, herpes simplex virus, group B streptococcus, and parvovirus B19.

Toxoplasmosis

Toxoplasmosis is caused by the protozoan *Toxoplasma gondii (T. gondii)*. It is innocuous in most adults but can be devastating to the immunosuppressed person. For example, in a woman with systemic lupus erythematosus or acquired immunodeficiency syndrome (AIDS) who has had a previous infection with *T. gondii*, the latent infection may reactivate, increasing the risk of perinatal transmission (Chen, Eskild, Bresnahan et al., 2005; Montoya & Rosso, 2005). A primary infection contracted shortly before or during pregnancy can profoundly affect the fetus and create long-term sequelae for those children and adults. The pregnant woman may contract the organism by eating raw or poorly cooked meat, by drinking unpasteurized goat's milk, or by contact with the feces of infected cats, either through the cat litter box or by gardening in areas frequented by cats. The most infectious organisms can live in warm, moist soil for up to a year (Savoia, 2004).

The percentage of childbearing women in North America who are seropositive for toxoplasmosis varies. In the United States, approximately 38% of pregnant women and approximately 40% to 50% of all adults have antibodies to this organism (ACOG, 2000; Gibbs, Sweet, & Duff, 2004). When a pregnant woman becomes infected with *T. gondii*, there is a 40% chance that her fetus will develop congenital toxoplasmosis (Gibbs et al., 2004; Savoia, 2004). Estimates suggest that about 1 out of every 1000 pregnant women becomes infected by toxoplasmosis, resulting in about 400 to 4000 cases of congenital toxoplasmosis each year (Savoia, 2004). Toxoplasmosis is common in Western Europe (Gibbs et al., 2004). In Paris, for example, more than 80% of women of childbearing age have antibodies to this organism.

FETAL-NEONATAL RISKS

Maternal infection during the first trimester is associated with the lowest incidence of fetal infection, but when it occurs, first trimester infection typically results in more severe fetal damage and often ends in a spontaneous abortion. The highest rate of fetal infection (65%) occurs when the mother contracts the infection in the third trimester, but most infants are born without clinical signs of infection (Gibbs et al., 2004). Up to 85% of these infants will develop signs and symptoms if left untreated (Montoya & Rosso, 2005).

In very mild cases, retinochoroiditis (inflammation of the retina and choroid layer of the eye) may be the only recognizable damage, and it and other manifestations may not appear until adolescence or young adulthood. Severe neonatal disorders associated with congenital infection include convulsions, coma, microcephaly, and hydrocephalus. The infant with a severe infection may die soon after birth. Survivors are often blind, deaf, and severely retarded. Treatment of the mother can reduce the incidence of fetal infection by 60% (ACOG, 2000).

CLINICAL THERAPY

The goal of medical treatment is to identify the woman at risk for toxoplasmosis and to treat the disease promptly if diagnosed. Diagnosis can be made by serologic testing, including the IgM and IgG fluorescent antibody tests. Elevated IgM titers are detectable 5 days after infection and may remain elevated for 1 year or more (ACOG, 2000). Therefore, it is not a reliable test for diagnosing recent infection; a positive IgG and negative IgM in the third trimester or any positive IgM result should be followed by confirmatory testing at a toxoplasma reference lab (Toxoplasma Serology Laboratory at Palo Alto Medical Foundation [PAMF-TSL], Palo Alto, California) (Montoya & Rosso, 2005). Ultrasound can reveal findings suggestive of severe fetal infection such as ascites, ventriculomegaly, microcephaly, and growth restriction (ACOG, 2000). PCR testing of amniotic fluid is used in diagnosing congenital toxoplasmosis.

Women in whom maternal infection is established should receive spiramycin to decreases the frequency of vertical transmission, particularly in the first trimester. It does not reliably cross the placenta, and monotherapy should be avoided in cases of suspected fetal infection. Spiramycin needs to be continued throughout pregnancy, even in women whose amniotic fluid PCR is negative. Spiramycin does not reliably cross the placenta. Thus, if fetal infection is suspected, spiramycin should be replaced with pyrimethamine/sulfadiazine/folinic acid after the 18th week of pregnancy. Spiramycin is not commercially available in the United States, but after consultation with a toxoplasma reference laboratory (PAMF-TSL), the drug will be provided free of charge through the FDA (Montoya & Rosso, 2005).

NURSING CARE MANAGEMENT
Nursing Assessment and Diagnosis

The incubation period for the disease is 10 days. The woman with acute toxoplasmosis may be asymptomatic, or she may develop myalgia, malaise, rash, splenomegaly, fever, headache, and enlarged posterior cervical lymph nodes. Symptoms usually disappear in a few days or weeks.

Nursing diagnoses that might apply to the pregnant woman with toxoplasmosis include the following:

- ***Risk for Ineffective Health Maintenance*** related to lack of knowledge about ways in which a pregnant woman can contract toxoplasmosis
- ***Anticipatory Grieving*** related to potential effects on infant of maternal toxoplasmosis

Nursing Plan and Implementation

The nurse caring for women during the antepartal period has the primary opportunity to discuss methods of prevention of toxoplasmosis with the childbearing woman. The woman must understand the importance of avoiding poorly cooked or raw meat, especially pork, beef, lamb, and, in the arctic region, caribou. Ten percent to 70% of lamb, 25% of pork, and 10% of beef samples have been reported to have *T. gondii* cysts (Savoia, 2004). Fruits and vegetables should be washed. She should avoid contact with the cat litter box by having someone else clean it. In addition, because it takes approximately 48 hours for a cat's feces to become infectious, the litter should be cleaned frequently. The nurse should also discuss the importance of the woman's wearing gloves when gardening and of avoiding garden areas frequented by cats.

Evaluation

Expected outcomes of nursing care include the following:

- The woman is able to discuss toxoplasmosis, its method of transmission, the implications for her fetus, and measures she can take to avoid contracting it.
- The woman implements health measures to avoid contracting toxoplasmosis.
- The woman gives birth to a healthy newborn.

Rubella

Rubella is a mild illness in children and adults. In fact, up to 60% of the cases are subclinical. On the other hand, rubella infection in the fetus can have overwhelming consequences. In 1969, live, attenuated vaccines were licensed for use in the United States. In the following 20 years there was a 99.6% decrease in rubella and a 97.4% decrease in congenital rubella syndrome. Still, today there are pockets of unvaccinated people. Approximately 10% to 20% of the women in the United States remain susceptible (Gibbs et al., 2004). Most countries in the world do not require rubella immunizations, and 100,000 to 200,000 cases of congenital rubella syndrome occur annually internationally (Landry, 2004). These figures emphasize the need for routine immunization programs. Prepubertal girls and nonpregnant women of childbearing age who do not have antirubella antibodies should be immunized with the live, attenuated rubella vaccine. Although no fetal infection has resulted from immunization of a pregnant woman, pregnancy should be avoided for

3 months after immunization. Nurses need to be aware of the importance of postpartum immunization of the nonimmune woman to decrease unnecessary perinatal transmission.

FETAL-NEONATAL RISKS

The period of greatest risk for the teratogenic effects of rubella on the fetus is during the first 10 weeks of pregnancy, when 90% of the fetuses exposed will be affected. The risk drops to 50% of fetuses who acquire the infection between 11 and 12 weeks of gestation (Landry, 2004). The most common clinical signs of rubella syndrome are congenital cataracts, sensorineural deafness, and congenital heart defects (particularly patent ductus arteriosus). Other abnormalities, such as mental retardation or cerebral palsy, may become evident in infancy. Diagnosis in the newborn can be conclusively made in the presence of these conditions and with an elevated rubella IgM antibody titer at birth.

Infants born with congenital rubella syndrome are infectious and should be isolated. These infants may continue to shed the virus for up to 12 months (Landry, 2004).

CLINICAL THERAPY

The best therapy for rubella is prevention. Live, attenuated vaccine is available and should be given to all children. Women of childbearing age should be tested for immunity and vaccinated if susceptible and if it is established that they are not pregnant. Health counseling in high school and in premarital clinic visits can stress the importance of screening before planning a pregnancy. As part of the prenatal laboratory screen the woman is evaluated for rubella using hemagglutination inhibition (HAI), a serology test. The presence of a 1:18 titer or greater is evidence of immunity. A titer less than 1:8 indicates susceptibility to rubella.

Because the vaccine is made with attenuated virus, pregnant women are not vaccinated. However, it is considered safe for newly vaccinated children to have contact with pregnant women.

If a woman who is pregnant becomes infected during the first trimester, therapeutic abortion may be an alternative.

NURSING CARE MANAGEMENT
Nursing Assessment and Diagnosis

A woman who develops rubella during pregnancy may be asymptomatic or may show signs of a mild infection, including a maculopapular rash, lymphadenopathy, muscular achiness, and joint pain. The presence of IgM antirubella antibody is diagnostic of a recent infection. These titers remain elevated for approximately 1 month following infection.

Nursing diagnoses that may apply to the woman who develops rubella early in her pregnancy include:

* *Ineffective Family Coping* due to an inability to accept the possibility of fetal anomalies secondary to maternal rubella exposure
* *Risk for Ineffective Health Maintenance* related to lack of knowledge about the importance of rubella immunization before becoming pregnant

Nursing Plan and Implementation

Nursing support and understanding are vital for the couple contemplating abortion because of a diagnosis of rubella. Such a decision may initiate a crisis for the couple who have planned their pregnancy. They need objective data to understand the possible effects on their fetus and the prognosis for the offspring.

Evaluation

Expected outcomes of nursing care include the following:

* The woman is able to describe the implications of rubella exposure during the first trimester of pregnancy.
* If exposure occurs in a woman who is not immune, she is able to identify her options and make a decision about continuing her pregnancy that is acceptable to her and her partner.
* The nonimmune woman receives the rubella vaccine during the early postpartal period.
* The woman gives birth to a healthy infant.

Cytomegalovirus

Cytomegalovirus (CMV) belongs to the herpes simplex virus group and causes both congenital and acquired disorders. The significance of this virus in pregnancy is related to its ability to be transmitted by asymptomatic women across the placenta to the fetus or by the cervical route during birth.

CMV is the most common viral cause of intrauterine infection (Hollier & Grissom, 2005). In the United States, 50% to 60% of middle-class women are seropositive; this increases to 70% to 80% in lower socioeconomic groups. The virus can be found in urine, saliva, cervical mucus, semen, and breast milk. It can be passed between humans by any close contact such as kissing, breastfeeding, and sexual intercourse. Asymptomatic CMV infection is particularly common in children and gravid women. Transmission in day care centers, especially among toddlers, is very high (Landry, 2004). It is a chronic, persistent infection in that the individual may shed the virus continually over many years. The cervix can harbor the virus, and an ascending infection can develop after birth. Although the virus is usually innocuous in adults and children, it may be fatal to the fetus.

Accurate diagnosis in the pregnant woman is best documented by seroconversion. Shedding of the virus in urine and saliva can be intermittent and does not distinguish primary infection from recurrent infection (Landry, 2004). Identification of the virus in amniotic fluid by PCR or culture is the most sensitive and specific way of diagnosing congenital infection. This is even superior to fetal blood sampling and can be done earlier in pregnancy and with less risk to the fetus (Gibbs et al., 2004). Ultrasound findings may include fetal hydrops, growth restriction, hydramnios, cardiomegaly, and fetal ascites. At present no treatment exists for maternal CMV or for the congenital disease in the newborn.

FETAL-NEONATAL RISKS

CMV is the most frequent agent of viral infection in the human fetus. It infects 0.5% to 2% of newborns (Hollier & Grissom,

2005). Although 85% to 90% of infected fetuses will be asymptomatic at birth, the remaining 10% to 15% will have abnormalities of varying severity. There is a 20% to 30% mortality rate among the symptomatic infants, and 90% of the survivors have significant neurologic complications (Hollier & Grissom, 2005). Subclinical infections in the newborn are capable of producing mental retardation and auditory deficits, sometimes not recognized for several months, or learning disabilities not seen until childhood. CMV may be the most common cause of mental retardation.

For the fetus, this infection can result in extensive intrauterine tissue damage that leads to fetal death; in survival with microcephaly, hydrocephaly, cerebral palsy, or mental retardation; or in survival with no damage at all.

The infected newborn is often SGA. The principal tissues and organs affected are the blood, brain, and liver. However, virtually all organs are potentially at risk. Hemolysis leads to anemia and hyperbilirubinemia. Thrombocytopenia and hepatosplenomegaly may also develop.

Currently no effective therapy exists to manage this infection.

Herpes Simplex Virus

It has been estimated that more than 50 million people are infected with genital herpes in the United States (Centers for Disease Control and Prevention [CDC], 2006). Herpes simplex virus (HSV-I or HSV-II) infection can cause painful lesions in the genital area. Lesions may also develop on the cervix. This condition and its implications for nonpregnant women are discussed in Chapter 6. ∞ However, because the presence of herpes lesions in the genital tract may profoundly affect the fetus, herpes infection as it relates to a pregnant woman is discussed here.

FETAL-NEONATAL RISKS

A primary herpes simplex infection can increase the risk of spontaneous abortion when infection occurs in the first trimester. PTL, intrauterine growth restriction, and neonatal infection are greater risks if the primary infection occurs late in the second trimester or early in the third trimester. Recurrent infections during pregnancy do not appear to increase the risk for abortion or low-birth-weight infants (Gibbs et al., 2004). Following a primary infection with HSV-II, symptomatic and subclinical viral shedding from the lower genital tract occurs during the first 3 months after the lesions have healed (ACOG, 1999b). A local outbreak may occur weeks or months later. When the offending virus is HSV-II, recurrences occur more frequently than when the virus is HSV-I.

The risk to the fetus varies with the route of birth and whether the lesion that is present at the time of birth is primary or recurrent. If HSV-1 or HSV-2 is acquired close to the time of labor, the risk of transmission is 50% for a vaginal birth. Exposure of the newborn to a *recurrent* lesion drops the risk of transmission to between 1% and 5% (Hill & Roberts, 2005). For a woman with either a primary or a secondary outbreak of genital herpes during labor, or symptoms that may indicate an impending outbreak, the preferred method of childbirth is cesarean birth. Although fetal transmission with recurrent outbreaks is

low, a cesarean birth is warranted because of the serious nature of the disease in the newborn. An estimated 1500 to 2000 newborns contract herpes each year, with 85% of neonatal herpes resulting from viral transmission near the time of birth (Hill & Roberts, 2005). Vaginal birth is appropriate for women with a history of HSV but no evidence of active genital disease at the time of childbirth (ACOG, 1999b).

The infected infant is often asymptomatic at birth but after an incubation period of 2 to 12 days develops symptoms of fever (or hypothermia), jaundice, seizures, and poor feeding. Approximately one half of infected infants develop the characteristic vesicular skin lesions. All infants who have neonatal herpes should be evaluated promptly and treated with acyclovir (CDC, 2006).

CLINICAL THERAPY

In women of reproductive age, only 5% to 10% have a history of genital herpes. However, 25% to 30% have HSV-2 antibodies (Sheffield, Hollier, Hill et al., 2003). Of the 5% to 10% of women in whom symptomatic outbreaks occur during pregnancy, 25% will occur in the last month. Seventy percent of neonatal herpes infections occur in asymptomatic women (Sheffield et al., 2003). Viral shedding, which leads to the potential for transmission, may occur during asymptomatic periods. Some women may shed as few as 4% of days, whereas some will shed detectable virus 75% of the time (Cory et al., 2004). Oral antiviral therapies are available, including acyclovir (Zovirax), famciclovir, and valacyclovir. Famciclovir and valacyclovir have an advantage of better absorption and a longer half-life than acyclovir (Gibbs et al., 2004). Currently, there is no evidence that there are any adverse fetal effects related to exposure to any of these drugs during any trimester. Acyclovir has a Category C pregnancy classification, whereas valacyclovir and famciclovir both have a Category B pregnancy classification (Hill & Roberts, 2005). The CDC (2006) does not recommend the routine use of acyclovir for recurrent infection during pregnancy but recognizes that the use of acyclovir near term may reduce the need for cesarean birth. The dosage is unchanged during pregnancy.

NURSING CARE MANAGEMENT
Nursing Assessment and Diagnosis

During the initial prenatal visit, it is important to learn whether the woman or her partner have had previous herpes infections. If so, ongoing assessment is indicated as pregnancy progresses.

Nursing diagnoses that may apply to the pregnant woman with HSV include the following:

- *Pain* related to the presence of lesions secondary to herpes infection

- *Sexual Dysfunction* related to unwillingness to engage in sexual intercourse secondary to the presence of active herpes lesions

- *Ineffective Individual Coping* related to depression secondary to the risk to the fetus if herpes lesions are present at birth

Nursing Plan and Implementation

Nurses need to be particularly concerned with client education about this fast-spreading disease. Women should be informed about what herpes is, how it is spread, and preventive measures. Women should also receive information about the association of genital herpes with spontaneous abortion, neonatal mortality and morbidity, and the possibility of cesarean birth. A woman needs to inform her future healthcare providers of her infection. She also should know of the possible association of genital herpes with cervical cancer and the importance of a yearly Pap smear.

The woman who acquired HSV as an adolescent may be concerned by the possible risks as a mature young adult who wants to have a family. Clients may be helped by counseling that allows expression of the anger, shame, and depression so often experienced by women with herpes. Literature may be helpful and is available from many public health agencies. The American Social Health Association has established the HELP program to provide information and the latest research results on genital herpes. The association has a quarterly journal, *The Helper,* for nurses and herpes clients.

Evaluation

Expected outcomes of nursing care include the following:

- The woman is able to describe her infection with regard to its method of spread, expected medical therapy, comfort measures, implications for her pregnancy, and long-term implications.
- The woman has appropriate cultures done as recommended throughout her pregnancy.
- The woman gives birth to a healthy infant.

Group B Streptococcal Infection

Group B streptococcus (GBS) infection is a bacterial infection found in the lower GI or urogenital tract. Women may transmit GBS to their fetus in utero or during childbirth. During the 1970s, GBS was recognized as the leading infectious cause of neonatal sepsis and mortality and remains so today (Platt & O'Brien, 2003). Fortunately, improved recognition and rapid treatment of infected infants has reduced morbidity and mortality rates considerably. Currently fewer than 10% of neonatal cases of GBS are fatal.

An estimated 20% to 30% of pregnant women are carriers of GBS. Women who are carriers of GBS are asymptomatic between 10% and 30% of the time (Savoia, 2004). GBS is the cause of 1% to 29% of the UTIs that occur during pregnancy (Gibbs et al., 2004; Savoia, 2004). Colonization may be intermittent, transient, or chronic, and it is likely that nearly every woman is GBS colonized at some time. The reservoir for GBS is thought to be the intestinal tract (Gibbs et al., 2004). GBS can be recovered from the vagina or cervix in 10% to 40% of preg-

nant women at some time during gestation depending on population and culture technique. In symptomatic women, GBS is also responsible for considerable maternal morbidity from infections such as pyelonephritis, chorioamnionitis, postpartum endometritis, sepsis, and wound infections (Gibbs et al., 2004; Savoia, 2004).

FETAL-NEONATAL RISKS

Newborns become infected either by vertical transmission from the mother as the fetus passes through the birth canal or from horizontal transmission from colonized nursery personnel or colonized infants. Between 60% and 75% of newborns who are born to colonized mothers will become colonized (Gibbs et al., 2004; Savoia, 2004). The transmission rate is influenced by how heavily the mother is colonized, whether or not she is persistently culture positive, and the site of colonization (rectal versus vaginal).

Risk factors for GBS neonatal sepsis include the following:

- Prematurity
- Maternal intrapartum fever
- Membranes ruptured for longer than 12 to 18 hours
- A previously infected infant with GBS disease
- GBS bacteriuria in the current pregnancy

GBS causes severe, invasive disease in infants. In newborns, the majority of cases occur within the first week of life and are thus designated as early-onset disease. Late-onset disease occurs 1 week or more after birth. Early-onset GBS is often characterized by signs of serious illness including respiratory distress or pneumonia, apnea, and shock. Infants with late-onset GBS often develop meningitis. Long-term neurologic complications are common in survivors of both types of GBS.

CLINICAL THERAPY

Guidelines for the detection of carriers and preventive treatment of newborns at risk include the following (Schrag, Gorwitz, Fultz-Butts, & Schuchat, 2002):

- All pregnant women should be screened for both vaginal and rectal GBS colonization at 35 to 37 weeks' gestation. Treatment should be based on these results, even if cultures were done earlier in pregnancy.
- Women identified as GBS carriers should receive antibiotic prophylaxis at the onset of labor or the rupture of membranes.
- Women with GBS in their urine in any concentration should receive antibiotic prophylaxis intrapartally because such women typically have heavy colonization with GBS and thus have an increased risk of giving birth to a newborn with early-onset disease. These women do not need vaginal and rectal cultures at 35 to 37 weeks because therapy is already indicated.
- Women who have already given birth to a newborn with invasive GBS disease should receive intrapartum antibiotic prophylaxis. Culture-based screening is not necessary for them.

Vaginal and rectal GBS screening cultures at 35–37 weeks' gestation for ALL pregnant women (unless client had GBS bacteriuria during the current pregnancy or a previous infant with invasive GBS disease)

Intrapartum prophylaxis indicated
- Previous infant with invasive GBS disease
- GBS bacteriuria during current pregnancy
- Positive GBS screening culture during current pregnancy (unless a planned cesarean birth, in the absence of labor or amniotic membrane rupture, is performed)
- Unknown GBS status (culture not done, incomplete, or results unknown) and any of the following:
  - Birth at greater than 37 weeks' gestation*
  - Amniotic membrane rupture less than or equal to 18 hours†
  - Intrapartum temperature less than or equal to 100.4F (less than or equal to 38C)†

Intrapartum prophylaxis not indicated
- Previous pregnancy with a positive GBS screening culture (unless a culture was also positive during the current pregnancy)
- Planned cesarean birth performed in the absence of labor or membrane rupture (regardless of maternal GBS culture status)
- Negative vaginal and rectal GBS screening culture in late gestation during the current pregnancy, regardless of intrapartum risk factors

* If onset of labor or rupture of amniotic membrane occurs at greater than 37 weeks' gestation and there is a significant risk for preterm birth (as assessed by the clinician).
† If amnionitis is suspected, broad-spectrum antibiotic therapy that includes an agent known to be active against GBS should replace GBS prophylaxis.

Figure 20–12 ◆ Indications for intrapartum antibiotic prophylaxis to prevent perinatal GBS disease under a universal prenatal screening strategy based on combined vaginal and rectal cultures collected at 35 to 37 weeks' gestation from all pregnant women. SOURCE: Centers for Disease Control and Prevention (CDC).

- If the results of GBS screening are not known when labor begins, prophylaxis is indicated for women with any of the following risk factors: gestation less than 37 weeks, membranes ruptured equal to or longer than 16 hours, temperature greater than 100.4F (38C).
- Women who undergo a cesarean birth and have not been in labor do not require GBS prophylaxis regardless of their GBS status (Platt & O'Brien, 2003).

Figure 20–12 ◆ provides an algorithm for assessing the need for intrapartum antibiotic prophylaxis.

Intrapartum antibiotic therapy is recommended as follows: initial dose of penicillin G 5 million units IV followed by 2.5 million units IV every 4 hours until childbirth. Alternately, ampicillin 2 g initial dose IV followed by 1 g IV every 4 hours until childbirth may be used. Women at high risk for an anaphylactic reaction to penicillin because of marked allergy may be treated with clindamycin or erythromycin.

Human B19 Parvovirus

Human B19 parvovirus causes erythema infectiosum or fifth disease in children. It is a mild disease in adults that produces a characteristic "slapped cheek" rash. Women with school-aged children are more likely to acquire parvovirus, and serologic evaluation should be performed if the pregnant woman has been exposed to a child diagnosed with fifth disease.

Although there is a low risk of fetal morbidity, transplacental transmission is reported to be as high as 33% with a fetal loss rate of 9% (Wilkins, 2004). Fetal infection is associated with sponta-

neous abortion, fetal hydrops, and stillbirth (Landry, 2004). Severe effects occur most frequently with maternal infection before 20 weeks' gestation. The major fetal concern is fetal anemia, which, if left untreated, may result in death (Ramirez & Mastrobattista, 2005). Weekly measurements of peak systolic velocity of the MCA are indicated. Values of greater than 1.5 multiples of the median (MoM) for gestational age have been associated with fetal anemia. Hydrops may be seen up to 8 weeks after maternal infection; however, they may not always occur even in the face of marked anemia. In up to one third of fetuses, there may be spontaneous resolution of hydrops (Ramirez & Mastrobattista, 2005). Fetal transfusion may be required to treat severe anemia.

Fetal death may occur 4 to 12 weeks' postinfection; therefore, fetal surveillance should be maintained for 8 to 12 weeks. In fetuses who survive the infection, long-term development appears to be normal.

OTHER INFECTIONS IN PREGNANCY

Table 20–8 summarizes other urinary tract, vaginal, and sexually transmitted infections that put pregnancy at risk. (These are described in detail in Chapter 6 ∞). Spontaneous abortion is frequently the result of a severe maternal infection, and research links infection with prematurity. In addition, if the pregnancy is carried to term in the presence of infection, the risk of maternal and fetal morbidity and mortality increases. Thus it is essential to maternal and fetal health that infection be diagnosed and treated promptly.

Table 20–8   INFECTIONS THAT PUT PREGNANCY AT RISK

Condition and Causative Organism	Signs and Symptoms	Treatment	Implications for Pregnancy
Urinary Tract Infections (UTI)			
Asymptomatic bacteriuria (ASB): *Escherichia, Klebsiella, Proteus* most common	Bacteria present in urine on culture with no accompanying symptoms.	Oral suffonamides early in pregnancy, ampicillin and nitrofurantoin (Furadantin) in late pregnancy. Antibody sensitivity results will guide the selection of an appropriate antibiotic.	Women with ASB in early pregnancy may go on to develop cystitis or acute pyelonephritis by third trimester if not treated. Oral sulfonamides taken in the last few weeks of pregnancy may lead to neonatal hyperbilirubinemia and kernicterus.
Cystitis (lower UTI): Causative organisms same as for ASB	Dysuria, urgency, frequency, low-grade fever, and hematuria may occur. Urine culture (clean catch) shows ≠ leukocytes. Presence of 10^5 (100,000) or more colonies bacteria per mL urine.	Same	If not treated, infection may ascend and lead to acute pyelonephritis.
Acute pyelonephritis: Causative organisms same as for ASB	Sudden onset. Chills, high fever, flank pain. Nausea, vomiting, malaise. May have decreased urine output, severe colicky pain, dehydration. Increased diastolic BP, positive fluorescent antibody (FA) test, low creatinine clearance. Marked bacteremia in urine culture, pyuria, WBC casts.	Hospitalization; IV antibiotic therapy. Other antibiotics safe during pregnancy include carbenicillin, methenamine, cephalosporins. Catheterization if output is Ø. Supportive therapy for comfort. Follow-up urine cultures are necessary.	Increased risk of premature birth and intrauterine growth restriction (IUGR). These antibiotics interfere with urinary estriol levels and can cause false interpretations of estriol levels during pregnancy.
Vaginal Infections			
Vulvovaginal candidiasis (yeast infections): *Candida albicans*	Often thick, white, curdy discharge, severe itching, dysuria, dyspareunia. Diagnosis based on presence of hyphae and spores in a wet-mount preparation of vaginal secretions.	Intravaginal insertion of miconazole butoconazole, or other topical azole preparation, or clotrimazol vaginal tablets at bedtime for 1 week. Cream may be prescribed for topical application to the vulva if necessary (CDC, 2006).	If the infection is present at birth and the fetus is born vaginally, the fetus may contract thrush.
Bacterial vaginosis: *Gardnerella vaginalis*	Thin, watery, yellow gray discharge with foul odor often described as "fishy." Wet-mount preparation reveals "clue cells." Application of potassium hydroxide (KOH) to a specimen of vaginal secretions produces a pronounced fishy odor.	Metronidazole 250 mg PO TID × 7 days or metronidazole 500 mg PO BID × 7 days or clindamycin 300 mg PO BID × 7 days (CDC, 2006).	CDC (2006) reports that multiple studies have failed to demonstrate a teratogenic effect from metronidazole. BV during pregnancy is associated with PROM, PTL, intra-amniotic infection, and endometritis postpartally (CDC, 2006).
Trichomoniasis: *Trichomonas vaginalis*	Occasionally asymptomatic. May have frothy greenish gray vaginal discharge, pruritus, urinary symptoms. Strawberry patches may be visible on vaginal walls or cervix. Wet-mount preparation of vaginal secretions shows motile flagellated trichomonads.	Single 2-g dose of metronidazole orally (CDC, 2006).	Increased risk for PROM, preterm birth, and low birth weight.
Chlamydial infection: *Chlamydia trachomatis*	Women are often asymptomatic. Symptoms may include thin or purulent discharge, urinary burning and frequency, or lower abdominal pain. Lab test available to detect monoclonal antibodies specific for *Chlamydia*.	Doxycycline, ofloxacin, and levofloxacin are contraindicated during pregnancy. Thus, pregnant women are treated with azithromycin or amoxicillin followed by repeat culture in 3 weeks (CDC, 2006).	Infant of woman with untreated chlamydial infection may develop newborn conjunctivitis, which can be treated with erythromycin eye ointment (but not silver nitrate). Infant may also develop chlamydial pneumonia. May be responsible for premature labor and fetal death.
Syphilis: *Treponema pallidum*, a spirochete	Primary stage: chancre, slight fever, malaise. Chancre lasts about 4 weeks, then disappears. Secondary stage occurs 6 weeks to 6 months after infection. Skin eruptions (condyloma latal) also symptoms of acute arthritis, liver enlargement, iritis, chronic sore throat with hoarseness. Diagnosed by blood tests such as VDRL, RPR, FTA, ABS. Dark-field examination or spirochetes may also be done.	Treatment for pregnant women follows the regimen recommended for the general population and is based on the stage of syphilis. For early latent syphilis (less than 1 year duration), 2.4 million units benzathine penicillin G IM. For late latent syphilis (more than 1 year duration) or latent syphilis of unknown duration, 2.4 million units benzathine penicillin G IM once a week for 3 weeks. Pregnant women who are allergic to penicillin should be desensitized and then treated with penicillin. Sexual partners should also be screened and treated (CDC, 2006).	Syphilis can be passed transplacentally to the fetus. If untreated, one of the following can occur: second trimester abortion, stillborn infant at term, congenitally infected infant, uninfected live infant.

(Continued on next page)

Table 20–8	INFECTIONS THAT PUT PREGNANCY AT RISK continued		
Condition and Causative Organism	**Signs and Symptoms**	**Treatment**	**Implications for Pregnancy**
Vaginal Infections continued			
Gonorrhea: *Neisseria gonorrhoeae*	Majority of women asymptomatic; disease often diagnosed during routine prenatal cervical culture. If symptoms are present they may include purulent vaginal discharge, dysuria, urinary frequency, inflammation, and swelling of the vulva. Cervix may appear eroded.	Nonpregnant women are treated with a single dose of ceftriaxone IM or a single dose of cefixime, ciprofloxacin, ofloxacin, or levofloxacin by mouth. They are also treated for chlamydia using azithromycin or doxycycline. Quinolones (ofloxacin, levofloxacin) and tetracyclines are not used to treat pregnant women. They should be treated with a cephalosporin (ceftriaxone, cefixime); if they cannot tolerate a cephalosporin, they should receive spectinomycin. The chlamydia is treated with azithromycin or amoxicillin (CDC, 2006).	Infection at time of birth may cause ophthalmia neonatorum in the newborn.
Condylomia acuminata: caused by a papovavirus	Soft, grayish pink lesions on the vulva, vagina, cervix, or anus.	Podophyllin, podofilox, and imiquimod are contraindicated during pregnancy. Some caregivers recommend removing warts by surgical methods or laser because the warts can proliferate and become friable (bleed easily) during pregnancy.	Possible teratogenic effect of podophyllin. Large doses have been associated with fetal death.

CHAPTER REVIEW

FOCUS YOUR STUDY

- Several health problems associated with bleeding arise from the pregnancy itself, such as spontaneous abortion, ectopic pregnancy, and gestational trophoblastic disease. The nurse needs to be alert to early signs of these situations, to guard the woman against heavy bleeding and shock, to facilitate the medical treatment, and to provide educational and emotional support.

- Incompetent cervix, the premature dilatation of the cervix, is the most common cause of second trimester abortion. It is treated surgically with a Shirodkar or McDonald cerclage, which involves placing a suture in the cervix to keep it closed.

- Hyperemesis gravidarum, excessive vomiting during pregnancy, may cause fluid and electrolyte imbalance, dehydration, and signs of starvation in the mother and, if severe enough, death of the fetus. Treatment is aimed at controlling the vomiting, correcting fluid and electrolyte imbalance, correcting dehydration, and improving nutritional status.

- Premature rupture of the membranes (PROM) and preterm labor both place the fetus at risk. Women with PROM and no signs of infection are managed conservatively with bed

rest and careful monitoring of fetal well-being. If preterm labor develops, tocolytics are often effective in delaying labor for 2 to 7 days but do have associated side effects.

- Hypertension may exist before pregnancy or, more often, may develop during pregnancy. Preeclampsia can lead to growth retardation for the fetus and, if untreated, may lead to convulsions (eclampsia) and even death for the mother and fetus. A woman's understanding of the disease process helps motivate her to maintain the required rest periods in the left lateral position. Antihypertensive or anticonvulsive drugs may be part of the therapy.

- Rh incompatibility can exist when an Rh-negative woman and an Rh-positive partner conceive a child who is Rh positive. The use of Rh immune globulin has greatly decreased the incidence of severe sequelae due to Rh incompatibility because the drug "tricks" the body into thinking antibodies have been produced in response to the Rh antigen.

- The impact of surgery or trauma on the pregnant woman and her fetus is related to timing in the pregnancy, seriousness of the situation, and other factors influencing the situation.

- Physical violence often begins or continues during pregnancy. The nurse needs to be alert for signs of abuse, including bruising or injury to the breasts, abdomen, and genitals. The nurse should provide the woman information about violence and about community resources available to assist her.

- Toxoplasmosis, rubella, cytomegalovirus, herpes, GBS, and other perinatal infections all pose a grave threat to the fetus. Prevention is the best therapy. There is no known treatment for rubella or CMV, but antimicrobial drugs are available for toxoplasmosis, herpes, and GBS.

- Universal screening for GBS is now recommended for all pregnant women at 35 to 37 weeks' gestation.

EXPLORE MediaLink

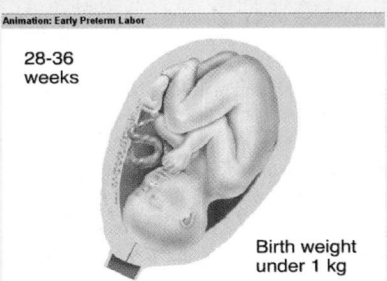

Animation: Early Preterm Labor

28-36 weeks

Birth weight under 1 kg

http://www.prenhall.com/davidson

NCLEX review questions, case studies, and other interactive resources for this chapter can be found on the Web Site at http://www.prenhall.com/davidson. Click on "Chapter 20" to select the activities for this chapter.

For tutorials including animations and videos, more NCLEX review questions, and an audio glossary, access the accompanying Prentice Hall Nursing MediaLink DVD-ROM in this book.

PRENTICE HALL NURSING MEDIALINK DVD-ROM
Audio Glossary
NCLEX Review
Animation: *Early Preterm Labor*

COMPANION WEBSITE
Additional NCLEX Review
Case Study: *Client with Preeclampsia*
Care Plan Activity: *Client at Risk for Preterm Labor*
Applications: *Potential Pregnancy Complications; Preeclampsia and HELLP*
Critical Thinking

CRITICAL THINKING IN ACTION

BED REST AND THE LEFT-SIDE LYING POSITION

View the Critical Thinking in Action video in Chapter 20 of the DVD-Rom. Then answer the questions that follow.

Carol Smith, a 40-year-old, single, G2, P1, whose first pregnancy was a therapeutic abortion presents to you while you are working in the birthing unit. She is 32 weeks pregnant. Her chief complaint is severe headache, nausea, and trouble seeing. She describes "blackened areas" in her visual fields bilaterally. Her prenatal record reveals long-term substance abuse, depression, and hypertension currently treated with nifedipine 60 mg by mouth once in the morning. You note that she has had two prenatal visits with this pregnancy. You determine her blood pressure to be 170/110; deep tendon reflexes are 3+, clonus negative. She has general edema and 3+ proteinuria. You place

Carol on the external fetal monitor to observe for fetal well-being and any contractions. You position her on her left side with her head elevated and use pillows for comfort. You observe that the fetal heart rate is 143–148 with decreased variability. No fetal heart rate decelerations or accelerations are noted. The uterus is soft, and no contractions are palpated or noted on the fetal monitor. Carol asks you why she should stay on her left side.

1. How would you explain the importance of the left side-lying position when on bed rest?

2. You administer nifedipine 10 mg sublingually and a loading dose of magnesium sulfate 4 gm IV piggyback to the main IV line of Ringer's lactate. What findings would indicate that Carol has therapeutic levels of magnesium?

3. What signs of magnesium toxicity should you monitor Carol for?

4. Carol asks if magnesium sulfate will affect her infant. How would you answer her?

5. Which signs of premature labor would you ask Carol to notify you of if she experiences any?

REFERENCES

American Academy of Pediatrics (AAP) & American College of Obstetricians and Gynecologists (ACOG). (2002). Obstetric and medical complications. In *Guidelines for perinatal care*. Elk Grove Village, IL: Author.

American College of Obstetricians and Gynecologists (ACOG). (1998). *Obstetric aspects of trauma management* (ACOG Educational Bulletin No. 251). Washington, DC: Author.

American College of Obstetricians and Gynecologists (ACOG). (1999a). *Domestic violence* (ACOG Educational Bulletin No. 257). Washington, DC: Author.

American College of Obstetricians and Gynecologists (ACOG). (1999b). *Management of herpes in pregnancy* (ACOG Practice Bulletin No. 8). Washington, DC: Author.

American College of Obstetricians and Gynecologists (ACOG). (2000). *Perinatal viral and parasitic infections* (ACOG Practice Bulletin No. 20). Washington, DC: Author.

American College of Obstetricians and Gynecologists (ACOG). (2001). *Management of recurrent early pregnancy loss* (ACOG Practice Bulletin No. 24). Washington, DC: Author.

American College of Obstetricians and Gynecologists (ACOG). (2002). *Diagnosis and management of preeclampsia and eclampsia* (ACOG Practice Bulletin No. 33). Washington, DC: Author.

American College of Obstetricians and Gynecologists (ACOG). (2003a). *Cervical insufficiency* (ACOG Practice Bulletin No. 48). Washington, DC: Author.

American College of Obstetricians and Gynecologists (ACOG). (2003b). *Management of preterm labor* (ACOG Practice Bulletin No. 43). Washington, DC: Author.

American College of Obstetricians and Gynecologists (ACOG). (2004a). *Diagnosis and treatment of gestational trophoblastic disease* (ACOG Practice Bulletin No. 53). Washington, DC: Author.

American College of Obstetricians and Gynecologists (ACOG). (2004b). *Nausea and vomiting of pregnancy* (ACOG Practice Bulletin No. 52). Washington, DC: Author.

American College of Obstetricians and Gynecologists (ACOG). (2006). *Management of alloimmunization during pregnancy* (ACOG Practice Bulletin No. 75). Washington, DC: Author.

August, P. (2004) Hypertensive disorders in pregnancy. In G. N. Burrow, T. P. Duffy, & J. A. Copel (Eds.), *Medical complications during pregnancy* (6th ed.). Philadelphia: Elsevier Saunders.

August, P., Helseth, G., Cook, E. F., & Sison, C. (2004). A prediction model for superimposed preeclampsia in women with chronic hypertension during pregnancy. *American Journal of Obstetrics & Gynecology, 191*(5), 1666–1672.

Baxter, J. K., & Weinstein, L. (2004). HELLP syndrome: The state of the art. *Obstetrical & Gynecological Survey, 59*(12), 838–845.

Bentley, R. C. (2003). Pathology of gestational trophoblastic disease. *Clinical Obstetrics and Gynecology, 46*(3), 513–522.

Berkowitz, R. S., & Goldstein, D. P. (2005). Gestational trophoblastic diseases. In W. J. Hoskins, C. A. Perex, R. C. Young, R. R. Barakat, M. Markman, & M. E. Randall (Eds.), *Principles and practice of gynecologic oncology*. Philadelphia: Lippincott Williams & Wilkins.

Berman, M. L., Di Saia, M. J., & Tewari, K. S. (2004). Pelvic malignancies, gestational trophoblastic neoplasia, and nonpelvic malignancies. In R. K. Creasy, R. Resnik, & J. Iams (Eds.), *Maternal fetal medicine* (5th ed.). Philadelphia: W. B. Saunders.

Bernhardt, J., & Dorman, K. (2004). Pre-term birth risk assessment tools: Exploring fetal fibronectin and cervical length for validating risk. *AWHONN Lifelines, 8*(1), 38–44.

Bess, K. A., & Wood, T. L. (2006). Understanding gestational trophoblastic disease: How nurses can help those dealing with a diagnosis. *AWHONN Lifelines, 10*(4), 321–326.

Born, D., & Barron, M. L. (2005). Herb use in pregnancy: What nurses should know. *American Journal of Maternal/Child Nursing, 30*(3), 201–206.

Braude, P., & Rowell, P. (2003, October). Assisted conception III—problems with assisted conception. *British Medical Journal, 327*, 920–923.

Briggs, G. G., Freeman, R. K., & Yaffee, S. J. (2005). Betamethasone. In G. G. Briggs, R. K. Freeman, & S. J. Yaffee (Eds.), *Drugs in pregnancy and lactation* (7th ed.). Philadelphia: Lippincott Williams & Wilkins.

Canavan, T. P., Simhan, H. N., & Caritis, S. (2004a). An evidence-based approach to the evaluation and treatment of premature rupture of the membranes: Part I. *Obstetrical & Gynecological Survey, 59*(9), 669–677.

Canavan, T. P., Simhan, H. N., & Caritis, S. (2004b). An evidence-based approach to the evaluation and treatment of premature rupture of the membranes: Part II. *Obstetrical & Gynecological Survey, 59*(9), 678–689.

Carrell, D. T., Wilcox, A. L., Lowy, L., Peterson, C. M., Jones, K. P., Erickson, L., et al. (2004). Elevated sperm chromosome aneuploidy and apoptosis in patients with unexplained recurrent pregnancy loss. *Obstetrics and Gynecology, 101*(6), 1229–1235.

Centers for Disease Control and Prevention (CDC). (2006). Sexually transmitted diseases treatment guidelines, 2006. *Morbidity and Mortality Weekly Report, 55*(RR-11), 1–93.

Chen, K. T., Eskild, A., Bresnahan, M., Stray-Pedersen, B., & Jenum, P. A. (2005). Previous maternal infection with *Toxoplasma gondii* and the

risk of fetal death. *American Journal of Obstetrics & Gynecology 193*(2), 443–449.

Clark, S. L. (2004). Placenta previa and abruptio placentae. In R. K. Creasy, R. Resnik, & J. Iams (Eds.), *Maternal fetal medicine* (5th ed.). Philadelphia: W. B. Saunders.

Cockey, C. D. (2004). Prematurity hits record high: More babies born at risk for lifetime disabilities. *AWHONN Lifelines, 8*(2), 104–111.

Corey, L., Wald, A., Patel, R., Sacks, S. L., Tyring, S. K., Warren, T., et al. (2004). Once-daily valacyclovir to reduce the risk of transmission of genital herpes. *New England Journal of Medicine, 350*(1), 11–20.

Dongen, H. V., Klumper, J. J. C. M., Sikkel, E., Vandenbussche, F. P. H. A., & Oepkes, D. (2005). Non-invasive tests to predict fetal anemia in Kell-alloimmunized pregnancies. *Obstetrical & Gynecological Survey, 60*(9), 567–568.

Easterwood, B. (2004). Silent lullabies: Helping parents cope with early pregnancy loss. *AWHONN Lifelines, 8*(4), 356–360.

Farag, K., Hassan, I., & Ledger, W. (2004). Prediction of preeclampsia: Can it be achieved? *Obstetrical & Gynecological Survey, 59*(6), 464–482.

Fry, M. J., Cartwright, D. W., Huang, R. C., & Davies, M. W. (2004). Preterm birth a long distance from home and its significant social and financial stress. *Obstetrical & Gynecological Survey, 59*(2), 86–87.

Garite, T. J. (2004). Premature rupture of the membranes. In R. K. Creasy, R. Resnik, & J. Iams (Eds.), *Maternal fetal medicine* (5th ed.). Philadelphia: W. B. Saunders.

Gautier, E., Benachi, A., Giovangrandi, Y., Ernault, P., Olivi, M., Gaillon, T., et al. (2005). Fetal RhD genotyping by maternal serum analysis: A two-year experience. *American Journal of Obstetrics & Gynecology, 192*(3), 666–669.

Ghulmiyyah, L. M., & Sabai, B. M. (2006). Managing an eclamptic seizure and its aftermath. *Contemporary OB/GYN, 51*(3), 54–66.

Gibbs, R. S., Schrag, S., & Schuchat, A. (2004). Perinatal infections due to group B streptococci. *Obstetrics and Gynecology, 104*(5, Pt 1), 1062–1076.

Gibbs, R. S., Sweet, R. L., & Duff, W. P. (2004). Maternal and fetal infectous disorders. In R. K. Creasy, R. Resnik, & J. Iams (Eds.), *Maternal fetal medicine* (5th ed.). Philadelphia: W. B. Saunders.

Gomez, R., Romero, R., Nien, J. K., Chaiworapongsa, T., Medina, L., Kim, Y. M., et al. (2005). A short cervix in women with preterm labor and intact membranes: A risk factor for microbial invasion of the amniotic cavity. *American Journal of Obstetrics & Gynecology, 192*(3), 678–689.

Gonik, B., & Foley, M. R. (2004). Intensive care monitoring of the critically ill pregnant patient. In R. K. Creasy, R. Resnik, & J. Iams (Eds.), *Maternal fetal medicine* (5th ed.). Philadelphia: W. B. Saunders.

Harkness, U. F., & Spinnato, J. A. (2004). Prevention and management of RhD isoimmunization. *Clinics in Perinatology, 31,* 721–742.

Harville, E. W., Wilcox, A. J., Bird, D. D., & Weinberg, C. R. (2004). Vaginal bleeding in very early pregnancy. *Obstetrical & Gynecological Survey, 59*(3), 172–173.

Hill, J. A. (2004). Recurrent pregnancy loss. In R. K. Creasy, R. Resnik, & J. Iams (Eds.), *Maternal fetal medicine* (5th ed.). Philadelphia: W. B. Saunders.

Hill, J., & Roberts, S. (2005). Herpes simplex virus in pregnancy: New concepts in prevention and management. *Clinics in Perinatology, 32*(3), 657–670.

Hogue, C. J. R., & Bremner, J. D. (2005). Stress model for research into preterm delivery among black women. *American Journal of Obstetrics & Gynecology, 192*(5), S47–S55.

Hollier, L. M. (2005). Preventing preterm birth: What works, what doesn't. *Obstetrical & Gynecological Survey, 60*(2), 124–131.

Hollier, L. M., & Grissom, H. (2005). Human herpes viruses in pregnancy: Cytomegalovirus, Epstein-Barr virus, and varicella zoster virus. *Clinics in Perinatology, 32*(3), 671–696.

Hurteau, J. A. (2003). Gestational trophoblastic disease: Management of hydatidiform mole. *Clinical Obstetrics and Gynecology, 46*(3), 557–569.

Hyde, L. K., Cook, L. J., Olson, L. M., Weiss, H. B., & Dean, J. M. (2003). Effect of motor vehicle crash on adverse fetal outcomes. *Obstetrics and Gynecology, 102*(2), 279–286.

Iams, J. D. (2003). Prediction and early detection of preterm birth. *Obstetrics and Gynecology, 101*(2), 402–412.

Iams, J. D. (2004). Abnormal cervical competence. In R. K. Creasy, R. Resnik, & J. D. Iams (Eds.), *Maternal fetal medicine* (5th ed.). Philadelphia: W. B. Saunders.

Iams, J. D., & Creasy, R. K. (2004). Preterm labor and delivery. In R. K. Creasy, R. Resnik, & J. D. Iams (Eds.), *Maternal fetal medicine* (5th ed.). Philadelphia: W. B. Saunders.

Jabara, S., & Barnhart, K. T. (2003). Is Rh immune globulin needed in early first-trimester abortion? A review. *American Journal of Obstetrics & Gynecology, 188*(3), 623–627.

James, A. H., Bushnell, C. D., Jamison, M. G., & Myers, E. R. (2005). Incidence and risk factors for stroke in pregnancy and the puerperium. *Obstetrics and Gynecology, 106*(3), 509–516.

Jeavons, W. (2005). Sterile speculum exams & fFN collection: How one triage program is helping nurses identify high-risk women. *AWHONN Lifelines, 9*(3), 237–240.

Joy, S. D., Rossi, K. Q., Krugh, D., & O'Shaughnessy, R. W. (2005). Management of pregnancies complicated by anti-E alloimmunization. *Obstetrics and Gynecology, 105*(1), 24–28.

Kady, D. E., Gilbert, W. M., Xing, G., & Smith, L. H. (2005). Maternal and neonatal outcomes of assaults during pregnancy. *Obstetrics and Gynecology, 105*(2), 357–363.

Katz, V., Balderston, K., & DeFreest, M. (2005). Perimortem cesarean delivery: Were our assumptions correct? *American Journal of Obstetrics & Gynecology, 192*(6), 1916–1921.

Kenyon, S., Boulvain, M., & Neilson, J. (2004). Antibiotics for preterm rupture of the membranes: A systematic review. *Obstetrics and Gynecology, 104*(5, Pt.1), 1051–1057.

Klein, L. L., & Gibbs, R. S. (2005). Infection and preterm birth. *Obstetrics and Gynecology Clinics of North America, 32,* 397–410.

Krabbendam, I., & Dekker, G. A. (2004). Pregnancy outcome in patients with a history of recurrent spontaneous miscarriages and documented thrombophilias. *Obstetrical & Gynecological Survey, 59*(9), 651–652.

Kumar, S., & Regan, F. (2005). Management of pregnancies with RhD alloimmunisation. *British Medical Journal, 330,* 1255–1258.

Lagiou, P., Tamimi, R., Mucci, L. A., Trichopoulos, D., Adami, H-O., & Shieh, C. C. (2003). Nausea and vomiting in pregnancy in relation to prolactin, estrogen, and progesterone: A prospective study. *Obstetrics and Gynecology, 101*(4), 639–644.

Landry, M. L. (2004). Viral infections. In G. N. Burrow, T. P. Duffy, & J. A. Copel (Eds.), *Medical complications during pregnancy* (6th ed.). Philadelphia: Elsevier Saunders.

Li, D., Janevic, T., Odouli, R., & Liyan, L. (2003). Hot tub use during pregnancy and the risk of miscarriage. *American Journal of Epidemiology, 158,* 931–937.

Lipscomb, G. H., Givens, V. M., Meyer, N. L., & Bran, D. (2005). Comparison of multidose and single-dose methotrexate protocols for the treatment of ectopic pregnancy. *American Journal of Obstetrics & Gynecology, 192*(6), 1844–1848.

Magee, L. A., Miremade, S., Li, J., Cheng, C., Ensom, M. H. H., Carleton, B., et al. (2005). Therapy with both magnesium sulfate and nifedipine does not increase the risk of serious magnesium-related maternal side effects in women with preeclampsia. *American Journal of Obstetrics & Gynecology, 193*(1), 153–163.

Martin, J. N., Jr., Thigpen, B. D., Moore, R. C., Rose, C. H., Cushman, J., & May, W. (2005). Stroke and severe preeclampsia: A paradigm shift focusing on systolic blood pressure. *Obstetrics and Gynecology, 105*(2), 246–254.

Matchaba, P., & Moodley, J. (2005). Corticosteroids for HELLP syndrome in pregnancy. *The Cochrane Library* (3).

McLean, L. K., Hedrianna, H. L., Lanouette, J. M., & Haesslein, H. C. (2004). A retrospective review of isoimmunized pregnancies managed by middle cerebral artery peak systolic velocity. *American Journal of Obstetrics & Gynecology, 190*(6), 1732–1738.

Meekai, S., Alfirevic, Z., Health, V. C. F., Cicero, S., Cacho, A. M., Williamson, P. R., et al. (2004). Cervical cerclage for prevention of preterm delivery in women with a short cervix: A randomized, controlled trial. *Lancet, 363*(9424), 1849–1853.

Meis, P. J. (2005). 17-Hydroxyprogesterone for the prevention of preterm delivery. *Obstetrics and Gynecology, 105*(5), 1228–1235.

Meis, P. J., & Connor, N. (2004). Progesterone treatment to prevent preterm birth. *Clinical Obstetric and Gynecology, 47*(4), 784–795.

Mercer, B. (2003). Preterm premature rupture of the membranes. *Obstetrics and Gynecology, 101*(1), 178–193.

Mignini, L. E., Pallavi, M. L., Villar, J., Kilby, M. D., Carroli, G., & Khan, K. S. (2005). Mapping the theories of preeclampsia: The role of homocysteine. *Obstetrics and Gynecology, 105*(2), 411–425.

Moise, K. J. (2004). Hemolytic disease of the fetus and newborn. In R. K. Creasy, R. Resnik, & J. Iams (Eds.), *Maternal fetal medicine* (5th ed.). Philadelphia: W. B. Saunders.

Moise, K. J. (2005). Fetal RhD typing with free DNA in maternal plasma. *American Journal of Obstetrics & Gynecology, 192*(3), 663–665.

Montoya, J. G., & Rosso, F. (2005). Diagnosis and management of toxoplasmosis. *Clinics in Perinatology, 32*(3), 705–726.

Moos, M.-K. (2004). Understanding prematurity: Sorting fact from fiction. *AWHONN Lifelines, 8*(1), 32–37.

National Institute of Child Health and Human Development (NICHHD). (2002). *Home uterine monitors not useful for predicting premature birth.* Retrieved September 9, 2005, from http://www.nichd.nih.gov/new/releases/uterine.cfm

National Institutes of Health (NIH). (2000). *Working group report on high blood pressure in pregnancy.* Retrieved December 8, 2002, from www.nhibi.nih.gov/health/prof/heart/hbp/hbp-preg.htm

National Institutes of Health Consensus Development Panel (NIHCDP). (2001). Antenatal corticosteroids revisited: Repeat courses—National Institutes of Health Consensus Development Conference Statement, August 17–18, 2000. *Obstetrics and Gynecology, 98*(1), 144–150.

Newton, E. R. (2005). Preterm labor, preterm premature rupture of membranes, and chorioamnionitis. *Clinics in Perinatology, 32,* 571–600.

Offenbacher, S. (2004). Maternal periodontal infections, prematurity, and growth restriction. *Clinical Obstetrics and Gynecology, 47*(4), 808–821.

Okun, N., Gronau, K. A., & Hannah, M. E. (2005). Antibiotics for bacterial vaginosis or *Trichomonas vaginalis* in pregnancy: A systematic review. *Obstetrics and Gynecology, 105*(4), 857–868.

Paidas, M. J., Ku, D. H., Langhoff-Roos, J., & Arkel, Y. S. (2005). Inherited thrombophilias and adverse pregnancy outcomes: Screening and management. *Seminars in Perinatology, 29*(3), 150–163.

Petrini, J. R., Callaghan, W. M., Klebanoff, M., Green, N. S., Lackritz, E. M., Howse, J. L., et al. (2005). Estimated effect of 17-alpha-hydroxyprogesterone caproate on preterm birth in the United States. *Obstetrics and Gynecology, 105*(2), 267–272.

Platt, J. S., & O'Brien, W. F. (2003). Group B streptococcus: Prevention of early-onset neonatal sepsis. *Obstetrical & Gynecological Survey, 53*(3), 191–196.

Ramirez, M. M., & Mastrobattista, J. M. (2005). Diagnosis and management of human parvovirus B19 infection. *Clinics in Perinatology, 32*(3), 697–704.

Rice, L. (2002). Herbal medicine in pregnancy. Retrieved September 10, 2005, from http://altmed.creighton.edu/preg/supplement_list.htm

Rideout, S. L. (2005). Tocolytics for pre-term labor: What nurses need to know. *AWHONN Lifelines, 9*(1), 56–61.

Rosen, T., de Veciana, M., Miller, H. S., Stewart, L., Rebarber, A., & Slotnick, R. N. (2003). A randomized controlled trial of nerve stimulation for relief of nausea and vomiting of pregnancy. *Obstetrics and Gynecology, 102*(1), 129–135.

Sabai, B. M. (2003). Diagnosis and management of gestational hypertension and preeclampsia. *Obstetrics and Gynecology, 102*(1), 181–192.

Sabai, B. M. (2005). Diagnosis, prevention, and management of eclampsia. *Obstetrics and Gynecology, 105*(2), 402–410.

Samol, J. M., & Lambers, D. S. (2005). Magnesium sulfate tocolysis and pulmonary edema: The drug or the vehicle? *American Journal of Obstetrics & Gynecology, 192*(5), 1430–1432.

Savoia, M. C. (2004). Bacterial, fungal, and parasitic disease. In G. N. Burrow, T. P. Duffy, & J. A. Copel (Eds.), *Medical complications during pregnancy* (6th ed.). Philadelphia: Elsevier Saunders.

Schauberger, C. W., Mathiason, M. A., & Rooney, B. L. (2005). Ultrasound assessment of first-trimester bleeding. *Obstetrics and Gynecology, 105*(2), 333–338.

Schieve, L. A., Tatham, L., Peterson, H. B., Toner, J., & Jeng, G. (2003). Spontaneous abortion among pregnancies conceived using assisted reproductive technology in the United States. *Obstetrics and Gynecology, 101*(5 Pt.1), 959–967.

Schrag, S., Gorwitz, R., Fultz-Butts, K., & Schuchat, A. (2002). Prevention of perinatal group B streptococcus. Revised guidelines from CDC. *Morbidlty and Mortality Weekly Report, 51:* (RR-11), 1–22.

Scott, L. D., & Abu-Hamda, E. (2004). Gastrointestinal disease in pregnancy. In R. K. Creasy, R. Resnik, & J. Iams (Eds.), *Maternal fetal medicine* (5th ed.). Philadelphia: W. B. Saunders.

Shaver, S. M. (2004). Isoimmunization in pregnancy. *Critical Care Nursing Clinics of North America, 16,* 205–209.

Shear, R. M., Rinfret, D., & Leduc, L. (2005). Should we offer expectant management in cases of severe preterm preeclampsia with fetal growth restriction? *American Journal of Obstetrics & Gynecology, 192*(4), 1119–1125.

Sheffield, J. S., Hollier, L. M., Hill, J. B., Stuart, G. S., & Wendel, G. D. (2003). Acyclovir prophylaxis to prevent herpes simplex virus recurrence at delivery: A systematic review. *Obstetrics and Gynecology, 102*(6), 1396–1403.

Smith, H. O. (2003). Gestational trophoblastic disease epidemiology and trends. *Clinical Obstetrics and Gynecology, 46*(3), 541–556.

Sosa, C., Althabe, F., Belizán, J., & Bergel, E. (2005). Bed rest in singleton pregnancies for prevention of preterm birth. *The Cochrane Database for Systemic Reviews* (4). (Article No.: CD003581. DOI: 10.1002/14651858. CD003581.pub2).

Steinlauf, A. F., Chang, P. K., & Traube, M. (2004). Gastrointestinal complications. In G. N. Burrow, T. P. Duffy, & J. A. Copel (Eds.), *Medical complications during pregnancy* (6th ed.). Philadelphia: Elsevier Saunders.

Tekesin, I., Marek, S., Hellmeyer, L., Reits, D., & Schmidt, S. (2005). Assessment of rapid fetal fibronectin in predicting preterm delivery. *Obstetrics and Gynecology, 105*(2), 280–284.

Van Den Eeden, S. K., Shan, J., Bruce, C., & Glasser, M. (2005). Ectopic pregnancy rate and treatment utilization in a large managed care organization. *Obstetrics and Gynecology, 105*(5, Pt. 1), 1052–1057.

Weiner, C. P., Lee, K.-Y., Buhimschi, C. S., Christner, R., & Buhimschi, I. A. (2005). Proetomic biomarkers that predict the clincial success of rescue cerclage. *American Journal of Obstetrics & Gynecology, 192*(3), 710–718.

Wiggens, D. A., & Elliott, M. (2005). Outcomes of pregnancies achieved by donor egg in vitro fertilization—a comparison with standard in vitro fertilization pregnancies. *American Journal of Obstetrics & Gynecology, 192*(6), 2002–2008.

Wilkins, I. (2004). Nonimmune hydrops. In R. K. Creasy, R. Resnik, & J. Iams (Eds.), *Maternal fetal medicine* (5th ed.). Philadelphia: W. B. Saunders.

Williams, M., & Iams, J. D. (2004). Cervical length measurement and cervical cerclage to prevent preterm birth. *Clinical Obstetrics and Gynecology, 47*(4), 775–783.

Yost, N. P., Bloom, S. L., McIntire, D. D., & Leveno, K. J. (2005). A prospective observational study of domestic violence during pregnancy. *Obstetrics and Gynecology, 106*(1), 61–65.

Yost, N. P., McIntire, D. D., Wians, F. H., Ramin, S. M., Balko, J. A., & Leveno, K. J. (2003). A randomized, placebo-controlled trial of corticosteroids for hyperemesis due to pregnancy. *Obstetrics and Gynecology, 102*(6), 1250–1254.

Yu, C. K. H., Papageorghiou, A. T., Parra, M., Dias, R. P., & Nicolaides, K. H. (2004). Randomized, controlled trial using low-dose aspirin in the prevention of preeclampsia in women with abnormal uterine artery Dopplers at 23 weeks' gestation. *Obstetrical & Gynecological Survey, 59*(3), 174–175.

Yudin, M. H. (2005). Bacterial vaginosis in pregnancy: Diagnosis, screening, and management. *Clinics in Perinatology, 32,* 617–627.

Zeeman, G. G., Alexander, J. M., McIntire, D. D., Devaraj, S., & Leveno, K. J. (2003). Homocysteine plasma concentration levels for the prediction of preeclampsia in women with chronic hypertension. *American Journal of Obstetrics & Gynecology, 189*(2), 574–576.

CHAPTER
21
Assessment of Fetal Well-Being

My first pregnancy was so tenuous that I didn't know from one moment to the next how it would end. I hoped for our baby's safety, but in the end, our baby died. When I became pregnant again, I was very nervous. Being able to see the baby on ultrasound helped me so much. I knew our baby was alive and growing.

OBJECTIVES

1. Describe the various psychologic responses to antenatal testing.
2. Identify indications and interpret findings for ultrasound examinations performed in the first trimester.
3. Describe the procedures used in the first trimester to confirm fetal viability.
4. Delineate the use of ultrasound in the second trimester to assess fetal life, number, presentation, anatomy, age, and growth.
5. Compare the indications and procedures for fetal movement awareness, the nonstress test, vibroacoustic stimulation, the contraction stress test, biophysical profile, and amniotic fluid index.
6. Explain the purpose of maternal serum alpha-fetoprotein testing and the implications of abnormal values.
7. Contrast the use of amniocentesis and chorionic villus sampling in detecting a fetus with a chromosomal disorder.
8. Discuss fetal fibronectin and transvaginal measurement of cervical length as predictors of preterm labor.
9. Discuss how the lecithin/sphingomyelin ratio of the amniotic fluid and phosphatidylglycerol (PG) can be used to assess fetal lung maturity.

KEY TERMS

Alpha-fetoprotein (AFP) 564
Amniocentesis 564
Amniotic fluid index (AFI) 550
Beta human chorionic gonadotropin (beta hCG) 546
Biophysical profile (BPP) 560
Birth defects 563
Cervical funneling 544
Chorionic villus sampling (CVS) 568
Contraction stress test (CST) 556
Cordocentesis 570
Fetal fibronectin (fFN) 571
Intrauterine growth restriction (IUGR) 562
Late decelerations 558

Lecithin/sphingomyelin (L/S) ratio 571
Macrosomia 562
Maternal serum alpha-fetoprotein (MSAFP) 564
Nonstress test (NST) 552
Nuchal folds 548
Nuchal translucency testing 548
Oligohydramnios 560
Phosphatidylglycerol (PG) 572
Surfactant 571
Ultrasound 543
Viability 546
Vibroacoustic stimulation (VAS) 555

 MEDIALINK

Additional resources for this content can be found on the Prentice Hall Nursing MediaLink DVD-ROM and on the Companion Website at http://www.prenhall.com/davidson. Click on "Chapter 21" to select the activities for this chapter.

Every parent dreams of a perfectly healthy baby and indeed the vast majority of babies are born healthy. However, maternal conditions, genetics, and environmental influences continue to adversely affect a small percentage of babies. Although the antenatal fetal assessment techniques discussed in this chapter are designed to maximize the chances of identifying a fetus at risk, a perfect pregnancy outcome can never be predicted or guaranteed.

Although the United States spends a greater percentage of its gross national product on health care than any other country, it continues to have a higher infant mortality rate than many other industrialized countries (United States National Center for Health Statistics, 2005). Reproductive technologies significantly raise the cost of health care. These technologic advances are not without risks; therefore, prevention of perinatal morbidity must always be a primary goal. The decision to use the tests discussed in this chapter is made by the childbearing family only after a careful analysis of their risks and costs compared with their possible benefit to the mother or her fetus. The nurse articulates the value of a particular test as well as its possible limitations at any point in pregnancy.

PSYCHOLOGIC REACTIONS TO ANTENATAL TESTING

Little has been written about the psychologic impact of antenatal diagnostic testing on childbearing families; however, several studies indicate that the need for testing usually provokes fear (Hedrick, 2005). Nurses often play a key role not only in teaching families about various testing procedures, but also in providing clarity and emotional support to the woman and her family undergoing antenatal testing. To decrease anxiety and alleviate fear for the woman and her partner, the nurse provides clear, concise explanations of the information expected to be obtained from the test and potential options after the testing has been completed. See Table 21–1 for sample nursing approaches to pretest teaching. Although the family may approach antenatal testing with a great deal of anxiety, the testing itself may assist in alleviating fears and decreasing anxiety.

Some tests, such as ultrasound, have become almost routine, and many couples view this antepartum test as an expected part of the prenatal care. The ultrasound may provide confirmation of a viable pregnancy through visualization of the fetal heartbeat, may identify the sex of the fetus, and may promote psychologic preparation for attachment after birth (Farquharson, Jauniaux, & Exalto, 2005). However, when more invasive testing is recommended, it may evoke fear and anxiety in the woman and her partner as they consider the reason for the test, the risk to the fetus and woman during the test, and the implications of the test results.

NURSING CARE MANAGEMENT

Nurses in a variety of settings have an opportunity to provide care to families undergoing antenatal testing. Antenatal assessment tests are performed by perinatal nurse practitioners and/or

Table 21–1   SAMPLE NURSING APPROACHES TO PRETEST TEACHING

Assess whether the woman knows the reason the screening or diagnostic test is being recommended.
  Examples:
    "What has your doctor/nurse-midwife told you about this test?"
    "Sometimes tests are done for many different reasons. Can you tell me why you are having this test?"
    "What is your understanding about what the test will show?"
Provide an opportunity for questions.
  Examples:
    "What questions do you have about the test?"
    "What things about the test are unclear to you?"
Explain the test procedure, paying particular attention to any preparation the woman needs to do prior to the test.
  Example:
    "The test that has been ordered for you is designed to . . ." (Add specific information about the particular test. Give the explanation in simple language.)
Validate the woman's understanding of the preparation.
  Example:
    "Tell me what you will have to do to get ready for this test."
Give permission for the woman to continue to ask questions if needed.
  Example:
    "I'll be with you during the test. If you have any questions at any time, please don't hesitate to ask."

nurses who have received additional specialized perinatal education and practice. The nurse, whatever the role, is a vital link between the woman and the physician or certified nurse-midwife. Nurses also need to provide easy to understand information to the mother and family. The nurse can encourage the family to ask questions, voice concerns and fears, and become actively involved in the antenatal testing process. Nurses are often responsible for the follow-up care that is needed as a result of test findings, such as arranging for additional testing, interpreting results, and answering questions the woman or her family may have.

Nursing Assessment and Diagnosis

Nursing assessment begins with a history of the present prenatal course and identifying possible indications for a particular diagnostic test. Examples may include identifying possible testing related to advanced maternal age, previous history of a child with a birth defect, or the presence of a particular maternal medical condition. The nurse assesses the woman and her partner's knowledge about the reason the test is being advised, the information that the woman and her support person have about the test, their questions and concerns, and the presence of any psychosociocultural factors that may influence the teaching or learning process. During the test and afterward, the nurse completes needed assessments to monitor the status of the woman and her fetus.

The primary nursing diagnoses are directed toward providing information about the diagnostic test and minimizing any risks to the woman and her unborn child. Examples of nursing diagnoses that may be applicable include:

- *Health-Seeking Behavior: Information About the Fetal Assessment Test* related to an expressed desire to understand its purpose, benefits, risks, and alternatives

- *Fear* related to the risks of a specific test or possible unfavorable test results

- *Risk for Impaired Infant Attachment* because of high-risk label attached to the pregnancy

Nursing Plan and Implementation

The nursing plan of care is directed toward each specific nursing diagnosis. The nurse generally plays a vital role in providing needed and desired information about the diagnostic test. The nurse also functions as an advocate for the expectant woman by helping her clarify question areas and obtain needed information. The nurse frequently knows the areas of greatest concern for women and can anticipate many of their fears. When the woman is not able to verbalize questions, the nurse can assist by providing information that answers questions that other women have had. For example, many women undergoing an amniocentesis fear pain during the procedure. The nurse can inform the woman that she will feel pressure during the insertion of the needle and may feel subsequent cramping, which can last for several hours. The nurse can provide information about the procedure itself and follow-up monitoring to ensure fetal well-being.

It is important for the nurse to realize that women react differently to pregnancy. The nurse's role is to remain nonjudgmental and to offer support when needed. Establishing a trusting relationship increases the possibility that a woman will talk to the nurse and share her concerns and emotional needs. The nurse is often the one to coordinate services the woman may need such as community resources for financial, psychologic, or social support.

Nurses working in community clinics have an integral role in performing fetal surveillance tests throughout the antepartum period. Nurses may find themselves not only performing some of these tests, such as nonstress tests, but also performing comprehensive assessments of the woman's health, her family dynamics, and her living situation. Community health nurses often have a more accurate understanding of the woman's physical resources, such as the adequacy of living conditions, proximity to healthcare resources, and availability of public transportation. It is often the nurse who has the most contact with the pregnant woman. Because of this, the nurse is in an excellent position to provide anticipatory guidance, reiterate teaching provided by the woman's healthcare provider, and monitor her current plan of care. It is important for the nurse to be cognizant of the potential for any fetal surveillance testing to be emotionally charged for the pregnant woman and her family (Sandelowski & Barroso, 2005). The nurse should approach each encounter with calmness, compassion, and warranted reassurance.

Evaluation

The nurse evaluates the woman and her family's understanding of antepartum testing procedures. Determining if the family understands the need for follow-up testing is imperative. The nurse should also assess whether the teaching methods used are effec-

tive for that family. Evaluation should include both physical and psychologic factors. In addition, the nurse determines if adequate resources, such as social support and physical resources, are available for the pregnant woman. Women from different cultures may need additional support because they may encounter language and other cultural barriers.

ULTRASOUND

Ultrasound has become one of the most commonly used diagnostic and screening tools in pregnancy (Cunningham, Leveno, Bloom et al., 2005). For the last 20 years, it has played a critical role in the practice of obstetrics. Because ultrasound is used widely to assess fetal well-being in all three trimesters, it also is discussed within this framework later in the chapter.

Ultrasound is a diagnostic procedure that uses high-frequency sound waves exceeding 20,000 cycles per second to produce an image that varies based on the density of the structure under the transducer. The reflected energy creates a small electrical voltage that is displayed on the screen. Very dense components, such as bone, appear white on the screen, whereas soft tissues appear gray and fluid appears black (Cunningham et al., 2005). Instruments used in ultrasonography operate at 2 to 10 megahertz (MHz). The higher the frequency of the sound, the shallower the depth of penetration but the better the resolution of the image produced. Ultrasound uses a device called a *transducer* to turn the sound waves into electrical signals. Transducers can be used either transabdominally (Figure 21–1 ◆), operating at 3.5 MHz, or transvaginally (Figure 21–2 ◆), operating at 5 to 7 MHz. These transducers and their use are described fully later in the chapter.

Ultrasound can be used to produce images called *sonograms* in several different ways. In motion mode (M mode), the reflected echo generates a moving display. This is how fetal cardiac activity is seen. Brightness modulation (B mode) converts the signals into varying degrees of brightness and produces a two-dimensional image. Three-dimensional ultrasound uses algorithms to vary opacity, transparency, and depth to project an image. This allows curved structures such as the fetal face to be viewed (Figure 21–3 ◆).

Figure 21–1 ◆ Ultrasound scanning permits visualization of the fetus in utero.
SOURCE: Photographer, Elena Dorfman.

Ultrasound in Obstetrics

MEDIALINK

Figure 21–2 ◆ Transvaginal ultrasound transducer.
SOURCE: Photographer, Elena Dorfman.

Figure 21–3 ◆ Ultrasound of the fetal face.

Extent of Ultrasound Exams

According to the American College of Obstetricians and Gynecologists (ACOG)(2004), ultrasound examinations are classified as standard, limited (identifying only certain components), or specialized (sometimes referred to as comprehensive). A *limited sonogram* may be used to address a specific question, or determine specific information. A limited ultrasound should not take the place of a complete ultrasound evaluation (ACOG, 2004). Following are examples of information that can be obtained by a limited ultrasound:

• Determine fetal presentation before or during labor.

• Locate the placenta.

• Confirm fetal viability.

• Determine the amniotic fluid index (AFI).

• Diagnose multiple gestation.

• Guide amniocentesis.

A *standard ultrasound examination* is performed during the second or third trimester. It includes an evaluation of fetal presentation, amniotic fluid volume, placenta placement, cardiac activity, fetal biometry, and anatomic survey. A specialized examination (also referred to as a detailed or targeted sonogram) is performed when an anomaly is suspected. The ultrasound may include fetal Doppler, biophysical profile, fetal echocardiogram, or additional biometric studies (ACOG, 2004).

Methods of Ultrasound Scanning

The two most common methods of ultrasound scanning are *transabdominal* and *transvaginal* scanning.

TRANSABDOMINAL ULTRASOUND

In the transabdominal approach, a transducer is moved across the abdomen (see Figure 21–1). The woman is usually scanned with a full bladder, except when ultrasound is used to localize the placenta before amniocentesis. When the bladder is full, the examiner can assess other structures, especially the vagina and cervix, in relation to the bladder. This is particularly important when vaginal bleeding is noted and placenta previa is the suspected cause. It can also determine if vaginal bleeding is being caused by premature dilatation of the cervix. The woman is advised to drink 1 to 1.5 quarts of water approximately 2 hours before the examination, and she is asked to refrain from emptying her bladder. If the bladder is not sufficiently filled, she is asked to drink 3 to 4 (8 oz) glasses of water and is rescanned 30 to 45 minutes later.

Mineral oil or a transmission gel is generously spread over the woman's abdomen, and the sonographer slowly moves a transducer over the abdomen to obtain a picture of the contents of the uterus. Testing takes 20 to 30 minutes. The woman may feel discomfort from pressure applied over a full bladder. In some instances, the sonographer may advise the woman to urinate a small amount to relieve the discomfort. In addition, if the woman lies on her back during the test, shortness of breath can develop. This may be relieved by elevating her upper body during the test.

TRANSVAGINAL ULTRASOUND

The transvaginal (or endovaginal) method uses a probe inserted into the vagina (see Figure 21–2). Once inserted, the transvaginal probe is close to the structures being imaged and so produces a better, clearer image. The improved images obtained by transvaginal ultrasound have enabled sonographers to identify structures and fetal characteristics earlier in pregnancy (McAuliffe, Fong, Toi et al., 2005). Transvaginal ultrasound also allows better assessment of the cervix. It can identify potential preterm labor, shortened cervical length, and **cervical funneling** (a cone-shaped indentation in the cervical os), which is common in cases of cervical incompetence (Bayramoglu, Arslan, Yazici et al., 2005).

After the procedure is fully explained to the woman, she is prepared in the same manner as for a pelvic examination: in lithotomy position, with appropriate drapes to provide privacy, and a female attendant in the room. It is important that the woman's buttocks are at the end of the table so that, once inserted, the probe can be moved in various directions. The small, lightweight vaginal transducer is covered with a specially fitted sterile sheath, a condom, or one finger of a latex or vinyl glove. Ultrasound coupling gel is then applied to the covering, making insertion into the vagina easier and providing a medium for enhancing the ultrasound image. In addition to providing a clearer image than the transabdominal method, the transvaginal procedure can be accomplished with an empty bladder. Most women do not feel discomfort during the exam. The probe is smaller than a speculum, so insertion is usually completed with ease. The woman may feel some movement of the probe during the exam as various structures are imaged. Some women may want to insert the probe themselves to enhance their comfort; others may feel embarrassed even to be asked. The certified nurse-midwife, physician, or ultrasonographer offers the choice based on the clinician's comfort level and the rapport the clinician has established with the woman.

Safety of Ultrasound

In the last 20 years, the use of ultrasound as a diagnostic tool in pregnancy has increased exponentially. To date, studies show that infants exposed to ultrasound in utero have no significant differences in birth weight or length, childhood growth, cognitive function, acoustic or visual ability, or rates of neurologic deficits (Singh & Malhotra, 2004). Experimental observations from animal studies suggest that high-intensity ultrasound, which is not used in obstetric ultrasounds, has definite and biologically harmful effects. Nevertheless, the Food and Drug Administration (FDA) has stated that obstetric sonograms fall within an acceptable level of safety because they use low-intensity ultrasound.

Is there such a category as "routine ultrasound" in pregnancy? Not necessarily, according to the ACOG. In large studies, researchers compared several outcomes between a group of women who had ultrasound examinations performed and a group of women who did not. Outcomes included perinatal mortality, Apgar score, birth weight, maternal outcome, detections of multiple gestation and abnormalities, as well as cost-effectiveness (Sylvan, Ryding, & Rydhstroem, 2005). The group that had had ultrasound examinations had higher rates of detection of multiple gestations and abnormalities. There were no significant differences in outcomes related to the other factors. The National Institutes of Health (NIH), rather than suggesting routine use of sonograms in pregnancy, has established the following recommended indications for ultrasound. These indications have since been endorsed by ACOG:

- Estimation of gestational age for women with uncertain dates of conception
- Verification of dates for women who are to undergo scheduled elective repeat cesarean birth, indicated induction of labor, or elective termination of pregnancy
- Evaluation of fetal growth
- Evaluation of vaginal bleeding of undetermined cause in pregnancy
- Determination of fetal presentation
- Suspected multiple gestation
- Adjunct to amniocentesis
- Significant discrepancy between uterine size and date of conception

- Pelvic mass
- Suspected hydatidiform mole
- Adjunct to special procedures
- Adjunct to cervical cerclage placement
- Suspected fetal death
- Suspected ectopic pregnancy
- Suspected uterine anomaly
- Intrauterine device localization
- Biophysical profile for fetal well-being
- Observation of intrapartum events
- Suspected hydramnios or oligohydramnios
- Suspected abruptio placentae
- Adjunct to external version from breech to vertex presentation
- Estimation of fetal weight or presentation in premature rupture of membranes or premature labor
- Abnormal serum alpha-fetoprotein value to assess for neural tube defects or trisomy 18 or 21
- Follow-up observation of identified fetal anomaly
- Follow-up observation of placental location for identified "placenta previa"
- History of previous congenital anomaly
- Serial evaluation of fetal growth in multiple gestation
- Evaluation of fetal condition in late registrants for prenatal care

Who Should Perform Ultrasound Examinations?

The accuracy of ultrasound as a diagnostic tool is highly dependent on the knowledge, skills, and judgment of the person performing the exam. The risk of false-positive and false-negative results when performed by inexperienced or unprepared examiners must be considered as an important safety issue (ACOG, 2004). Ultrasound is often used by members of the healthcare team to provide rapid assessment of the well-being of a pregnancy or fetus. However, it has been demonstrated that potential problems may be overlooked or false-positives may necessitate follow-up exams and cause anxiety to the mother and family. The Association of Women's Health, Obstetric and Neonatal Nurses (AWHONN) has set guidelines and nursing practice competencies for experienced maternal-newborn nurses to perform limited ultrasound exams. The guidelines indicate that the nurse must complete an educational program that includes didactic presentations and a clinical practicum (Snelglove-Clarke & Scott-Finlay, 2005).

Although ultrasound is considered safe, the use of pregnancy ultrasound to obtain "keepsake" fetal videos has led to heated debate in the healthcare community. Recently, entrepreneurs have begun business services through which a pregnant women can obtain a videotape as a keepsake of her pregnancy. The FDA views this practice as an unapproved use of a medical device. In some jurisdictions, the use of ultrasound without a practitioner's order can be a violation of state law (ACOG, 2004).

NURSING CARE MANAGEMENT

The nurse plays a key role in providing the mother and family with information related to the ultrasound procedure itself and expected outcomes. The nurse answers questions and helps clarify ultrasound findings. Some women, especially those who lack insurance coverage, may worry about the cost of the test itself. The nurse can discuss the rationale for obtaining an ultrasound and what will be done with the information once it is obtained. The nurse provides support for the woman and her family, recognizing that some women may feel anxious or fearful.

ASSESSMENT OF FETAL WELL-BEING IN THE FIRST TRIMESTER

The first trimester represents a crucial time for establishing fetal viability and determining an accurate gestational age. First trimester ultrasound can now be used to help determine if certain chromosomal disorders may be present. There are a variety of methods that the practitioner can use to determine fetal well-being in early pregnancy.

Viability

Viability, or the potential for the pregnancy to result in a live infant, is the first issue to consider in pregnancy. A positive urine pregnancy test does not confirm viability, only the presence of beta human chorionic gonadotropin (hCG) hormone. The developing embryo implants into the uterus approximately 14 days after conception has occurred (Sciarra, 2004). Although about one third of pregnant women experience bleeding associated with this normal process, bleeding can also be associated with a nonviable pregnancy with an ultimate spontaneous abortion (miscarriage) or ectopic (tubal) pregnancy. Serial quantitative beta hCG testing, progesterone-level testing, and ultrasound can be used to distinguish a normally developing fetus from an ectopic pregnancy, which if undiagnosed carries a high maternal morbidity.

QUANTITATIVE BETA HCG TESTING

Beta human chorionic gonadotropin (beta hCG) is a product of the trophoblast or placenta and is a very accurate marker of the presence of pregnancy and placental health. Beta hCG is detectable in the blood serum of approximately 5% of pregnant women by 8 days after conception, and in virtually all pregnancies by 11 days. The level in the serum approximately doubles every 2 days in the first 10 days of pregnancy, peaking at 60 to 90 days after conception (Cunningham et al., 2005) (Table 21–2). In early pregnancy, two quantitative beta hCG levels drawn 48 hours apart serve as an excellent test of the vi-

Table 21–2 APPROXIMATE BETA hCG VALUES IN PREGNANCY

Gestational Age (Weeks)	Beta hCG Values (milli–International Units/mL)
1–2	16–156
2–3	101–4870
3–4	1110–31,500
4–5	2560–82,300
5–6	23,100–151,000
6–7	27,300–233,000
7–11	20,900–291,000
11–16	6140–103,000
16–21	4720–80,100
21–39	2700–78,100

ability of the pregnancy. Conversely, if the beta hCG level remains stable or falls over 48 hours, a miscarriage or ectopic pregnancy should be suspected.

Although not routine in all pregnancies, serologic evaluation is indicated in women with a history of spontaneous abortion, ectopic pregnancy, or risk of ectopic pregnancy (intrauterine device in place, previous pelvic inflammatory disease, or reversal of a tubal sterilization). Women who are spotting should also have a beta hCG level drawn to ensure adequate levels. Many women who have conceived through assisted reproductive methods also have their beta hCG levels monitored to ensure the pregnancy is developing normally.

The 48 hours between the beta hCG tests can be an extremely anxious time for the couple. To offer effective counseling, the nurse must understand the information these tests provide, as well as their limitations. For example, the woman may not know why she must wait 48 hours for a repeat blood test. The nurse needs to allow time for the woman and her partner, if present, to express their anxiety and fears. False reassurances should not be offered. Instead, attention is directed toward helping them cope with the inherent uncertainty that occurs while the exams are being completed and until a definitive diagnosis can be made.

PROGESTERONE LEVEL TESTING

Progesterone is secreted in early pregnancy by the corpus luteum until approximately 8 weeks' gestation at which point the placenta begins to manufacture its own progesterone. Low levels of progesterone are associated with spontaneous abortions and ectopic pregnancies. Although progesterone levels are not routinely tested in early pregnancy, they can be assessed by performing a simple blood test when there is a history of spontaneous abortions or spotting in early pregnancy. Progesterone levels above 25 ng/mL are typically associated with normally developing intrauterine pregnancies. Progesterone levels that are below 5 ng/mL typically indicate a nonviable fetus. Levels between 5 ng/mL and 25 ng/mL are inconclusive. Approximately 10% of women have progesterone levels below 25 ng/mL. The nurse notifies the physician or certified nurse-midwife if levels are low. The physician or certified nurse-midwife bases the decision of whether or not to supplement progesterone during early pregnancy on current progesterone levels, past history of spontaneous abortions, and presence of spotting or vaginal bleeding. Low progesterone levels can be treated by giving the woman progesterone either orally or via vaginal suppositories. This supplementation is warranted throughout the first trimester. After 12 gestational weeks, supplements are not needed because the placenta will make adequate progesterone levels.

ULTRASOUND

The sonographic landmarks (presence of gestational sac, cardiac motion, embryo development) of normal early pregnancy, detected by transvaginal ultrasound, are very predictable. Up to about 4½ to 5 weeks of gestation, before the appearance of a gestational sac, nothing can be seen in the uterus. The gestational sac at first appears empty and may be confused with the pseudogestational sac of ectopic pregnancy. A true gestational sac is associated with beta hCG levels of 1800 milli–International Units/mL if the sonogram is being done transvaginally and 6500 milli–International Units/mL if the sonogram is being done transabdominally. At approximately 5½ weeks the yolk sac, a small round structure sometimes resembling a "double ring," is visible within the gestational sac. It is an embryonic structure, so its appearance provides strong evidence supporting the presence of an intrauterine pregnancy (Sciarra, 2004). At 6 to 6½ weeks, the embryo itself becomes visible, and shortly thereafter cardiac activity is detectable (Sciarra, 2004). During the ultrasound examination, the gestational sac and embryo are measured to determine gestational age (Figure 21–4 ◆).

Gestational Age

Determination of an accurate expected date of birth (EDB) early in pregnancy is essential for evaluating well-being throughout the pregnancy. Labor contractions that may be perfectly normal at 37 weeks could be a problem if they occur at 34 weeks. Conversely, a 40-week pregnancy inadvertently thought to be 42 weeks may result in an unnecessary and risk-laden induction of labor. Much of the obstetrician or midwife's efforts are aimed at determining the most accurate EDB possible. Traditional means

of establishing an EDB are documenting a reliable last menstrual period (LMP) from the woman, measuring uterine size, noting the date of the first audible fetal heart tones, and noting the date of quickening (the first recognized fetal movement). An accurate LMP established early in pregnancy is considered the most reliable indicator of an EDB (Bennett, Crane, O'Shea et al., 2004). Problems occur if the woman cannot recall her LMP, if her menstrual cycles were extremely irregular, or if she had bleeding in early pregnancy.

An early transvaginal or abdominal sonogram is indicated when there is a need to establish an accurate gestational age. The crown-rump length is considered the most accurate sonographic measurement for gestational age if performed between 6 and 10 weeks' gestation. It is accurate to within plus or minus 3 to 5 days of the EDB based on the crown-rump length (Figure 21–5 ◆). This means that an ultrasound performed at 6 weeks would be accurate in predicting the EDB within either 3 to 5 days before or 3 to 5 days after the predicted EDB. Beyond 12 weeks, the fetus begins to curve and the crown-rump length loses its accuracy. For example, if an EDB based on a 10-week sonogram is September 9, it is reasonable to expect that date is accurate from September 4 through September 14. After the first trimester, gestational age is obtained by a combination of measurements of femur length, abdominal circumference, and biparietal diameter (Figure 21–6 ◆). Gestational age is reliable in the second trimester to plus or minus 7 to 14 days. For example, if a due date of October 1 is given by a second trimester sonogram, the reasonable date of birth can be from September 16 through October 14. Although practice may vary, most obstetricians and midwives do not change a due date based on the second trimester sonogram unless there is a discrepancy of greater than 11 to 14 days from the LMP. After 26 weeks, fetal growth rates are less uniform, making ultrasound an inappropriate means of determining gestational age. Specifically, during the third trimester, ultrasound can estimate an EDB with plus or minus 14 to 21 days of accuracy. See Table 21–3.

Determining an accurate EDB can be extremely important later in pregnancy if there is inadequate uterine or fetal growth.

Figure 21–4 ◆ Measurement of the gestational sac. The ultrasound shows the uterus; the blackened oval area is the gestational sac. The fluid in the gestational sac does not generate echoes from the ultrasound and thus appears dark in contrast to the uterine tissue surrounding it. The lines through the gestational sac represent measurements that are taken.
SOURCE: Reprinted from *Ultrasonography in obstetrics and gynecology,* 2nd ed., by P. W. Cullen, p. 49. Copyright © 1998, with permission from Elsevier.

Figure 21–5 ◆ Measurement of the crown-rump length. *A,* Schematic diagram. Dotted line shows the measurement from the top of the fetal crown (head) to the bottom of the rump (buttocks). *B,* Ultrasound scan of the pregnant uterus, showing the longest length of a 9-week fetus. The head (h) can be differentiated from the body (b), but the internal anatomy cannot be clearly distinguished.
SOURCE: Reprinted from *Ultrasonography in obstetrics and gynecology,* 2nd ed., by P. W. Cullen, p. 50. Copyright © 1998, with permission from Elsevier.

Figure 21–6 ◆ Measurement of the biparietal diameter. *A,* Ultrasound transaxial image of the fetal head, taken with the thalami (T) imaged in the midline, equidistant from the temporoparietal tables of the calvarium. *B,* Diagram and image showing the leading edge (outer) to the leading edge (inner) measurements of the fetal head, taken at the level of the thalami.
SOURCE: Reproduced with permission from *Ultrasonography in obstetrics and gynecology,* 2nd ed., by P. W. Cullen, p. 51. Copyright © 1998, with permission from Elsevier.

Table 21–3 PARAMETERS FOR ESTIMATING GESTATIONAL AGE		
Source of Evidence	**When Obtained**	**Estimated Accuracy**
In vitro fertilization	At conception	Less than 1 day
Ultrasound measurement of crown-rump length	6–10 weeks	3 days
Clinical measurement of normal uterus	Less than 12 weeks	7 days
Ultrasound measurement of biparietal diameter	Less than 20 weeks	7 days
Ultrasound measurement of biparietal diameter	20–26 weeks	10 days
Ultrasound measurement of biparietal diameter	26–30 weeks	14–21 days
Ultrasound measurement of biparietal diameter	Greater than 30 weeks	21–28 days

An accurate EDB based on a first trimester ultrasound can assist the physician or certified nurse-midwife in diagnosing intrauterine growth restriction (to be discussed later in this chapter).

Nuchal Translucency Testing

Nuchal translucency testing is a combination of an ultrasound and a maternal serum test that is used to screen fetuses between 11 weeks and 1 day and 13 weeks and 6 days to determine if a fetus is at risk for a chromosomal disorder, such as Down syndrome (trisomy 21) and trisomy 13, 18. An ultrasound assesses the presence of the fetal nasal bone during the first trimester. The absence of a fetal nasal bone is found in 70% of Down syndrome fetuses in the first trimester, whereas an absent nasal bone is found in only 0.5% of normal fetuses (Sciarra, 2004). The ultrasound then assesses the accumulation of fluid between the posterior cervical spine and the overlying skin in the fetal neck, known as **nuchal folds.** If the nuchal folds are greater than 3 mm, the incidence of Down's syndrome is increased (Sciarra, 2004). The test is performed in conjunction with a maternal serum blood test in which biochemical markers PAPP-A and free beta hCG are obtained to calculate the risk of having an affected fetus. The combination of blood testing and the ultrasound screening test is 90% accurate for detecting Down syndrome and 98% accurate in detecting trisomy 18 (Wenstrom, 2005). Because the screening is noninvasive, there are no maternal or fetal risks. If an abnormal test result is obtained, the mother is referred for diagnostic testing, such as a chorionic villi sampling (CVS) or amniocentesis.

ASSESSMENT OF FETAL WELL-BEING IN THE SECOND TRIMESTER

The second trimester is considered by many to be the most advantageous time for basic obstetric ultrasound for several reasons. First, the relative uniformity of fetal growth during the first 20 weeks allows biometric measurements that continue to provide an accurate estimation of gestational age. Second, the large volume of amniotic fluid relative to the fetal size allows for excellent images of fetal anatomy. Finally, fetal anatomy can be visualized in extreme detail, allowing confirmation of normal anatomy. The ideal time for the second trimester basic sonogram is 18 to 24 weeks. There is some evidence that sonograms done at 20 to 22 weeks may be easier to perform and less likely to require an additional scan than one done at 18 weeks.

A standard (comprehensive) second trimester sonogram provides the following information about the fetus, placenta, and uterine conditions (ACOG, 2004):

- Fetal life
- Fetal number
- Fetal presentation
- Presence of abnormal heart rate or rhythm
- Evaluation of fetal anatomy
- Gestational age and growth
- Amniotic fluid volume
- Placental localization, including relationship to cervical os
- Umbilical cord, including the number of vessels present
- Uterine anatomy

In addition, multiple gestations should be assessed for chorionicity, amnionicity, comparision of fetal sizes, the amount of amniotic fluid on each side of the membrane, and fetal genitalia if visible (ACOG, 2004).

Fetal Life

Presence of cardiac motion confirms fetal life. If gestational age has already been established and fetal heart tones have been visualized with an ultrasound or heard with a Doppler, then absence of cardiac motion in the second trimester is consistent with fetal demise.

Fetal Number

The second trimester is an ideal time to identify multiple gestation or the number of fetuses in the uterus. The number of placentas and their location can also be noted at this point.

Fetal Presentation

Although an ultrasound in the second trimester can determine whether a fetus is in the breech, transverse, or vertex position, the large amount of amniotic fluid relative to the fetal size along with the lack of fetal engagement makes it highly likely that the noted presentation will change repeatedly before birth. Fetal presentation is commonly documented on a second trimester ultrasound, but it is not usually of any clinical significance.

Fetal Anatomy Survey

A systematic examination of the fetal parts is conducted to identify possible abnormalities. Components of this examination include the fetal parts discussed in the following sections.

HEAD

The skull should be symmetrical with the cranium ossified and intact. The ventricular system (passageways within the brain) is evaluated. The choroids should appear symmetrical. The choroid plexus are found within the ventricles of the brain and in the subarachnoid space around the brain and spinal cord. They produce cerebral spinal fluid. Choroid cysts, if noted, are usually benign but have been associated with chromosomal abnormalities in 1% of fetuses. The nuchal fold thickness should be measured because thickening of the nuchal fold, the skin at the base of the fetal skull, has also been associated with certain chromosomal abnormalities.

The most dramatic abnormality diagnosed by ultrasound is anencephaly (a neural tube defect in which a portion of the fetal brain is missing). It is abnormal not to see the bony structures of the skull above the orbits of the eye after 14 weeks' gestation. The skull is brightly echogenic (appearing white because of its increased density) and is easily visualized. Failure to see the skull should alert the experienced examiner to the possibility of anencephaly.

SPINE

The spine is examined both sagittally and coronally for the presence of a sac or an outward splaying of the vertebrae laminae. Either of these conditions may suggest a possible spinal cord defect such as spina bifida.

THORAX AND HEART

A transverse plane of the fetal thorax provides valuable information about the size, shape, and symmetry of the chest. The size, location, and axis of the heart are also evaluated. A four-chambered view of the heart should demonstrate ventricles and atria of approximately equal size and an intact intraventricular septum. The heart occupies one quarter to one third of the chest cavity on transverse image. The lungs should have a homogenous appearance. The diaphragm should be imaged. Chest size is correlated with lung size.

ABDOMEN

The bladder, stomach, and kidneys should all be visualized. The fetal stomach and bladder can be seen on ultrasound by 14 weeks. Persistent failure to visualize the fetal stomach can be due to various fetal abnormalities, the most common being esophageal atresia. Mild dilation of the renal pelvis of less than 10 mm is rarely progressive and usually physiologic. The abdominal wall should be visualized to be intact. A transverse image of the umbilical cord should reveal a three-vessel cord. Insertion site of the umbilical cord is also carefully inspected.

EXTREMITIES

The femur is the only bone routinely measured on the basic ultrasound. If length seems abnormal, a more comprehensive exam is performed to compare it with the lengths of the other long bones. The upper extremities and the presence of hands and feet are also documented.

Gestational Age and Growth

The Hadlock method uses an average of measures of the biparietal diameter, head circumference, abdominal circumference, and femur length to estimate gestational age (Figures 21–7 ◆ to 21–10 ◆). Comparison of measures made at intervals to standardized measures can be used to estimate fetal growth.

Amniotic Fluid Volume

Amniotic fluid volume changes with gestational age. In general, a subjective assessment of amniotic fluid volume as decreased, normal, or increased is adequate during the second trimester examination. However, the **amniotic fluid index (AFI)** is another method of reporting fluid volume. The AFI is calculated by dividing the maternal abdomen into four quadrants with the umbilicus as the reference point. Then, the deepest vertical pocket of fluid in each quadrant is measured, and these four measurements are summed to calculate the AFI.

Placenta Location

The placenta's appearance, location, and relationship to the cervical os should be evaluated. Placental position that is noted by sonogram in early pregnancy may not correlate well with the location at the time of birth. Factors such as the woman's position or overdistention of the bladder may give a false-positive diagnosis of placenta previa. Therefore, a possible low-lying placenta or placenta previa that is identified on a second trimester ultrasound must be confirmed by a follow-up sonogram in the third trimester.

Figure 21–7 ◆ Measurement of the head circumference.
A, Diagram showing a dotted line outlining the head, which indicates the correct place to make a circumference measurement.
B, Ultrasound transaxial scan showing the thalami (arrowheads), positioned in midline. A dotted line created by the digitizer outlines the correct parameter, just outside of the hyperechoic calvarium to obtain a circumference measurement.
SOURCE: Reproduced with permission from *Ultrasonography in obstetrics and gynecology,* 2nd ed., by P. W. Cullen, p. 55. Copyright © 1998, with permission from Elsevier.

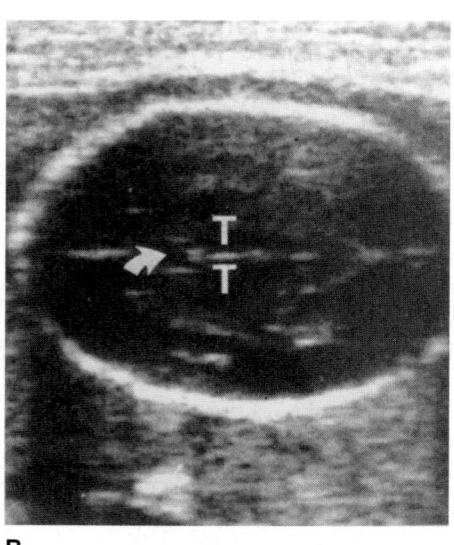

Figure 21–8 ◆ Measurement of the cephalic index. *A,* The biparietal diameter (double arrows) and fronto-occipital diameter (single arrows) are both taken outer edge to outer edge. A ratio of the two gives the cephalic index. *B,* Ultrasound transaxial scan of the fetal head of the thalami (T) and cavum septi pellucidi (curved arrow).
SOURCE: Reprinted from *Ultrasonography in obstetrics and gynecology,* 2nd ed., by P. W. Cullen, p. 53. Copyright © 1998, with permission from Elsevier.

Figure 21–9 ◆ Measurement of the femur length. *A,* Schematic diagram. *B,* Ultrasound image. The hyperechoic line is in the ossified lateral margin of the femoral diaphysis. The ends of the bone are the epiphyseal cartilages that have not yet calcified and are therefore hypoechoic. *C,* The hyperechoic diaphysis is measured from one end to the other, denoted by the cursors and a dotted line. The "distal femoral point" (* and arrow) is a nonossified extension of the distal epiphyseal cartilage. It should be included in the measurement.
SOURCE: Reprinted from *Ultrasonography in obstetrics and gynecology,* 2nd ed., by P. W. Cullen, p. 58. Copyright © 1998, with permission from Elsevier.

Figure 21–10 ◆ Measurement of the abdominal circumference. *A,* Diagram showing the abdominal circumference as a dotted line traced at the outer margin of the abdomen. *B,* Ultrasound transaxial image showing the umbilical portion of the left portal vein (arrowheads) correctly positioned within the liver and equidistant from the lateral walls. (S, spine; L, liver; ST, stomach.) A dotted line, created by a digitizer, outlines the outer margins of the abdomen, the correct place to obtain an abdominal circumference measurement. SOURCE: Reprinted from *Ultrasonography in obstetrics and gynecology,* 2nd ed., by P. W. Cullen, p. 57. Copyright © 1998, with permission from Elsevier.

Survey of Uterine Anatomy

The uterus is assessed to examine maternal anatomy and identify any uterine defects or abnormalities. Adnexal (ovarian) masses may be noted. Uterine myomas (fibroids) are common and must be noted and monitored because they may grow more quickly in pregnancy, affecting the growth and well-being of the fetus or causing overdistention of the uterus, leading to preterm labor or birth. Ultrasound may also be used to measure both cervical length and dilatation of the internal cervical os. A shortened cervix and a dilated internal os noted by ultrasound have been used to predict preterm birth. However, false-positive results using this technique may be common. Some obstetricians will schedule weekly transvaginal ultrasound to measure cervical length beginning at 20 weeks for their clients who have a history of preterm labor or cervical incompetence, and for women with cervical cerclage (a suture placed in the cervix) (see Chapter 20 ∞).

ASSESSMENT OF FETAL WELL-BEING IN THE THIRD TRIMESTER

Various maternal and prenatal conditions warrant antenatal testing during the third trimester. The type of testing performed is determined by the specific condition and the choice of the physician or certified nurse-midwife.

Conditions Warranting Fetal Surveillance

There are several indications for surveillance of fetal well-being in the third trimester. The following maternal and prenatal conditions require regular assessment (Cunningham et al., 2005):

Maternal conditions:

- Hypertensive disorders
- Type 1 diabetes mellitus

- Chronic renal disease
- Cyanotic heart disease
- Systemic lupus erythematosus
- Hyperthyroidism (poorly controlled)
- Antiphospholipid syndrome
- Hemoglobinopathies

Prenatal conditions:

- Preeclampsia
- Decreased fetal movement
- Oligohydramnios
- Hydramnios
- Intrauterine growth restriction
- Postterm pregnancy
- Isoimmunization (moderate to severe)
- Previous fetal demise
- Multiple gestation
- Known fetal anomaly
- Abnormal biochemical test results

Fetal Movement Assessment

Fetal movement assessment is considered an acceptable, noninvasive, cost-effective method of fetal surveillance in both high- and low-risk pregnancies. Monitoring fetal movement serves as an indirect measure of fetal central nervous system integrity and function. The coordination of whole-body movement in the fetus requires complex neurologic control. For this reason, clinicians generally agree that vigorous fetal movement provides reassurance of fetal well-being. A reduction in activity is often associated with complications of chronic rather than acute nonreassuring fetal status as the compromised fetus decreases its oxygen requirements by reducing activity. Documented cessation of activity warns of preterm birth, asphyxia, intrauterine growth restriction, and fetal death (Froen, 2005). It is these observations that provide the rationale for utilizing fetal movement counting as a means of antepartum fetal surveillance.

There is considerable variation in fetal movement that depends on the individual and the gestational age of the fetus. Fetal movement first begins to occur as early as 7 weeks, although the movements are too fine to be perceived until approximately 16 weeks (and later in primigravida women). Muscle tone is limited before 28 weeks (Blackburn, 2003). Certain substances such as tobacco smoke, drugs, alcohol, and caffeine have been shown to affect fetal movements. Altered fetal movements will usually reverse after drug clearance. There have been conflicting reports on whether carbohydrate intake increases fetal movement. One study that examined 14- to 16-week fetuses after maternal oral consumption of 110 grams of glucose found significant increases in fetal movements (Goldstein, 2003).

Several methods are used to assess fetal movement perceived by the pregnant woman. The woman should be clearly instructed regarding the specific technique used and the importance of recognizing decreased fetal activity. Instruction is usually started at 28 weeks' gestation. Fetal movements peak at

26 to 32 weeks and then start to decrease because of the constraints of the uterine environment (Blackburn, 2003). Continued encouragement, education, and support by nurses within the office of the physician, midwife, or community clinic is important. The expectant woman should also be instructed to call the office if at any time she is concerned about a decrease in fetal movement from the fetus's usual daily pattern. The procedure for fetal movement assessment is discussed in Chapter 16. ∞

Pregnant women need to understand that fetal movements are significant and that they change during pregnancy, both in number and strength. The expectant woman should be reassured that there are fetal rest-sleep states during which minimal or no movement may occur for an hour or so as the fetus rests. If less than the expected movements are perceived by the pregnant woman, further fetal surveillance tests, such as the nonstress test, may be used to assess fetal well-being. See Client Teaching: What to Tell the Pregnant Woman about Assessing Fetal Activity in Chapter 16. ∞

In 1981, I visited the First International Peace Hospital in Shanghai. At the prenatal clinic, the mothers and fathers were given a jar that contained many small black stones. The couple was instructed to complete a fetal movement count each day by starting at a similar time and then placing a stone in the jar each time they felt the baby move. Toward the end of the pregnancy, the father was encouraged to place his hand on the expectant mother's abdomen and feel the movements. Then he was responsible for placing the stones in the jar. The mothers and fathers seemed so proud when they brought their recording of the movements back to the clinic for review.

Since that visit, I have often wondered what it would have been like to hold my newborn in my arms and look at the jar of stones. A simple jar but so special.

~SALLY

Nonstress Test

The **nonstress test (NST)** has become a widely accepted method of evaluating fetal status. (See Procedure 21–1.) This test involves using an electronic fetal monitor to obtain a tracing of the fetal heart rate (FHR) and observation of acceleration of the FHR with fetal movement. The test is based on the knowledge that the fetus is normally active throughout pregnancy and that fetal activity will result in acceleration of the FHR when the normal fetus moves. Accelerations of the FHR imply an intact central and autonomic nervous system that is not being affected by intrauterine hypoxia. FHR acceleration in response to fetal movement is, therefore, an accepted sign of fetal health. It must be noted, however, that a nonreactive NST is not diagnostic of fetal compromise. In other words, failure to provide evidence of fetal health does not indicate that the fetus is in trouble.

The advantages of the NST are that it is relatively quick, inexpensive, and easy to interpret; it can be done in an outpatient setting and there are no known side effects. The disadvantages are that it is sometimes difficult to obtain a suitable tracing because the woman has to recline and be relatively still for 20 to 30 minutes, and the fetus may be in a sleep cycle at the time the test is performed, resulting in a nonreactive test result.

Fetal age must be considered in the use and evaluation of NSTs. The central nervous system (parasympathetic and sympathetic nervous systems) of the fetus is not sufficiently mature to allow frequent accelerations of the heart rate when fetal movement occurs until 30 to 32 weeks of gestation. Acceleration patterns are directly affected by gestational age. The acme of acceleration is 15 beats per minute or more above the baseline rate. The acceleration lasts 15 seconds or longer for less than 2 minutes in fetuses at or beyond 32 weeks (Figure 21–11 ◆).

Figure 21–11 ◆ Example of a reactive nonstress test (NST). Accelerations of 15 bpm lasting 15 seconds with each fetal movement (FM). Top of strip shows fetal heart rate (FHR); bottom of strip shows uterine activity tracing. Note that FHR increases (above the baseline) at least 15 beats and remains at that rate for at least 15 seconds before returning to the former baseline.

PROCEDURE 21–1 Performing a Nonstress Test (NST)

NURSING ACTION	RATIONALE

Preparation

- Explain the procedure, the information it provides, and the process for completing the test.
- Ask the woman if she has recently eaten or smoked cigarettes.

The test should be performed after the woman has eaten. Cigarette smoking can adversely affect the test results, so the woman should be counseled to avoid smoking prior to testing.

- Ask the woman to void.

The procedure will take at least 20 minutes to complete and the woman will need to remain in semi-Fowler's or a side-lying position and will be unable to void without interrupting the testing procedure.

Equipment and Supplies

External fetal monitor with a monitoring strip
Blood pressure cuff

Procedure

1. Place the woman in a semi-Fowler's position with a small pillow or towel placed under her right hip after she has voided.
2. Place the ultrasound transducer from the external fetal monitor on the woman's abdomen over the FHR (typically over the fetal back or chest) so a tracing can be obtained on the monitoring strip.
3. If the FHR is not consistently recorded on the monitoring strip, adjust the ultrasound transducer until an adequate reading is obtained.

Fetal or maternal movement can cause an inconsistency in the FHR on the monitoring strip. Multiple adjustments may be needed to obtain consistency in recording the FHR.

4. Place the tocodynamometer (pressure transducer) on the woman's abdomen over the uterine fundus.

Contractions are best detected when the device is directly placed on the uterine fundus.

5. Obtain baseline measurements, including blood pressure, fetal activity, variations in the FHR during fetal movement, and contractions, for 20 minutes.

Baseline measurements provide a reference for normal maternal and fetal assessment parameters.

6. Perform the test for 20 minutes but it may be extended up to 40 minutes.

Testing may be extended for the additional 20 minutes if the fetus is in a sleep cycle.

7. Give the woman a handheld marker to indicate when she feels fetal movement.

Fetal movement is accompanied by an increase in the FHR in the healthy fetus. Lack of FHR accelerations may be an indication of uteroplacental perfusion problems.

8. Interrupt the results as reactive or nonreactive.

A reactive NST has two or more fetal heart accelerations within a 20-minute period. The FHR acceleration must be at least 15 beats per minute above baseline for at least 15 seconds from baseline to baseline. A nonreactive NST is one that lacks sufficient FHR accelerations over a 40-minute period.

(Continued on next page)

PROCEDURE 21–1   Performing a Nonstress Test (NST)   continued

NURSING ACTION	RATIONALE
9. Explain the results to the woman and relate information from the healthcare provider regarding further management needs or additional follow-up that is needed.	*The nurse is the key communicator in providing information regarding the test results and their meaning to the woman.*

Documentation	Document baseline maternal and fetal assessment information that was obtained before and during the test. The results of the test should be documented along with information regarding how the information was reported to the healthcare provider. The specific name of the healthcare provider and date and time should be recorded. Any additional orders and instructions to the client should be documented. Verbalization of understanding of the test results by the woman should be documented along with her understanding follow-up instructions and future appointments.

There must be at least two accelerations within a 20-minute period. Before 32 weeks, accelerations are defined as having an acme of 10 beats per minute or more for 10 seconds or longer (Cunningham et al., 2005). One study examined FHR pattern changes that occurred with advancing gestational age. Mean baseline FHR, signal loss, and fetal movement all decreased in advancing gestational age (Park, Hwang, Cha et al., 2005).

The NST can be used as an assessment tool in any pregnancy but is especially useful in the presence of diabetes, preeclampsia, intrauterine growth restriction, spontaneous rupture of membranes, multiple gestation, postdates, and other high-risk pregnancy conditions. These conditions can lead to a decline in uteroplacental functioning, which can result in decreased oxygenation to the fetus and eventual asphyxia. Testing intervals may vary, depending on the condition of the mother and fetus and recommendations of various experts. Most clinicians test twice weekly for high-risk clients and once a week for other conditions (Cunningham et al., 2005).

PROCEDURE FOR PERFORMING AN NST

The NST is usually scheduled during daytime hours. It may be performed either in the office or hospital setting. Women are requested to be nonfasting and to have refrained from recent cigarette smoking because this can adversely affect test results. The NST is typically performed with the woman in the semi-Fowler's position with a small pillow or blanket under the right hip to displace the uterus to the left. The FHR is monitored by the placement of an electronic fetal monitor (see discussion in Chapter 23 ∞). Either one or two belts are placed around the woman's abdomen. One belt holds the ultrasound transducer to record the FHR and the other holds a tocodynamometer that detects uterine or fetal movement. The FHR is usually monitored for 20 minutes, but monitoring may be extended to 40 minutes if it appears the fetus is in a sleep cycle. The woman is often requested to record each fetal movement by the use of self-operated markers. Under ideal conditions, a correlation of more

than 90% between maternal perceived and actual fetal movements can be achieved; however, typically more than 40% of actual movements remain undetected by pregnant women (Froen, 2005). Recent studies have examined NST administration in alternative positions, such as walking or in a sitting position. These studies found maternal perceptions of fetal movements was highest in the reclining position, but the walking and sitting positions resulted in a shortened time period to obtain three accelerations (Cito, 2005).

INTERPRETATION OF THE NST

NSTs are categorized as either reactive or nonreactive. The most common definition of a reactive (normal) test is that there are two or more fetal heart accelerations within a 20-minute period, with or without fetal movement discernible by the woman. The FHR acceleration must be at least 15 beats per minute above the baseline and last 15 seconds from baseline to baseline. A nonreactive (abnormal) NST is one that lacks sufficient FHR accelerations over a 40-minute period (Figure 21–12 ◆). Again, it is important to take into account the gestational age of the fetus. Both fetal movement and the amplitude of the FHR accelerations increase with gestational age.

Spontaneous decelerations of the FHR during the testing period must also be noted. Variable decelerations may be observed in up to 50% of NSTs. Variable decelerations, if nonrepetitive and brief (less than 30 seconds), do not indicate fetal compromise nor the need for obstetric intervention (Gearhart & Sehdev, 2005). In contrast, repetitive variable decelerations (at least three in 20 minutes), even if mild, have been associated with an increased risk of cesarean birth for nonreassuring intrapartum FHR pattern. The prognosis for decelerations lasting 1 minute or longer is even more ominous (Cunningham et al., 2005). It is the responsibility of the nurse performing this test to consult the physician or nurse-midwife for further evaluation of fetal status if there is any question concerning the reactivity of the test or the presence of repetitive decelerations.

Figure 21–12 ◆ Example of a nonreactive NST. There are no accelerations of FHR with fetal movement (FM). Baseline FHR is 130 bpm. The tracing of uterine activity is on the bottom of the strip.

CLINICAL MANAGEMENT

The clinical management of a woman following an NST may vary. If the NST is reactive after 20 minutes, the test is concluded and the woman is rescheduled for further testing as indicated by the condition of, or risk factors present for, the mother and/or fetus. The interval between testing is typically 1 week if the maternal medical condition is stable. Testing may be performed twice weekly if warranted by maternal or fetal risk factors. Any significant deterioration in the maternal medical status requires fetal reevaluation regardless of the amount of time that has elapsed since the last test (Gearhart & Sehdev, 2005).

NURSING CARE MANAGEMENT

The nurse first must ascertain the woman's understanding of the NST. The nurse then reviews the indications for the NST, the equipment being used, and the procedure before beginning the test. The nurse positions the woman and applies the electronic fetal monitor. Maternal blood pressure is monitored during the NST to determine whether hypotension is present. The nurse administers the NST, may or may not interpret the results, and reports the findings to the obstetrician or certified nurse-midwife and the client. The nurse uses this opportunity to assess learning needs concerning the importance of fetal movement and provides information and teaching.

Vibroacoustic Stimulation

Vibroacoustic stimulation (VAS), also called FAST for fetal acoustic stimulation test or VST for vibroacoustic stimulation test, is an application of sound and vibration to the mother's abdomen to stimulate movement in the fetus (Figure 21–13 ◆). A device is used that delivers 90 dB of sound for 1 to 3 seconds to

Figure 21–13 ◆ Fetal acoustic stimulation testing.
SOURCE: Photographer, Elena Dorfman.

the fetus with the purpose of changing the fetal behavioral state, thereby accelerating the FHR.

NSTs that are interpreted as nonreactive often depict the normal state of quiet sleep by the fetus, which can last for up to 70 minutes. In these cases, VAS can be used to facilitate the timely interpretation of the NST. The typical VAS response of a healthy term fetus shows a rise of at least 10 beats per minute in baseline, occurring within 10 seconds and lasting from 5 to 10 minutes. Gestational age influences the reliability and reproducibility of the fetal response. The purpose of the VAS is to improve the specificity and efficiency of interpretation of FHR monitoring patterns. Although many obstetricians and certified nurse-midwives are enthusiastic about the VAS test because of its potential to minimize the need for more invasive follow-up testing, concerns for fetal hearing loss prevent universal use of this exam. Hearing loss has been demonstrated in newborns whose mothers were exposed to chronic levels of sound at 90 dB or more. Although there are no documented cases of newborn hearing loss related to VAS, some advocate judicious use of this exam. Others have advocated simply rescheduling the NST in 1 to 2 hours when the fetus is likely to have moved from the quiet sleep state that may have resulted in the first nonreactive test as an alternative to VAS.

Contraction Stress Test

The **contraction stress test (CST)** is a means of evaluating the respiratory function (oxygen and carbon dioxide exchange) of the placenta (i.e., uteroplacental function). (See Procedure 21–2). It enables the healthcare team to identify the fetus at risk for intrauterine asphyxia by observing the response of the FHR to the stress of uterine contractions (spontaneous or induced). During contractions, intrauterine pressure increases. Blood flow to the intervillous space of the placenta is reduced momentarily, thereby decreasing oxygen transport to the fetus. A healthy fetus usually tolerates this reduction well. If the placental reserve is insufficient, fetal hypoxia, depression of the myocardium, and a decrease in FHR occur.

INDICATIONS AND CONTRAINDICATIONS

The CST is indicated for pregnancies at risk for placental insufficiency or fetal compromise because of any of the following:

- Intrauterine growth restriction
- Diabetes mellitus
- Postdates (42 or more weeks' gestation)
- Nonreactive NST
- Abnormal or suspicious biophysical profile

  Contraindications for the CST are the following:

- Third trimester bleeding (placenta previa, marginal abruptio placentae, or unexplained vaginal bleeding)
- Previous cesarean birth with classical uterine incision
- Instances in which the risk of possible preterm labor outweighs the advantage of the CST, including:
  a. Premature rupture of the membranes
  b. Incompetent cervix or Shirodkar-Barter operation (cerclage—surgical procedure in which an incompetent cervix is encircled with suture to prevent it from dilating before term) (See Chapter 20 ∞).
  c. Multiple gestation

CST PROCEDURE

A necessary component of the CST is the presence of three uterine contractions of at least 40 seconds' duration in 10 minutes. The response of the FHR when contractions occur provides data on the fetal status. The contractions may occur spontaneously, or they may be induced by oxytocin or nipple stimulation. The most common method of stimulating uterine contractions for a CST has been intravenous administration of oxytocin (Pitocin), but many facilities now use breast self-stimulation to obtain a CST (see later discussion) (Cunningham et al., 2005). This method is based on the fact that endogenous oxytocin is produced in response to stimulation of the breasts or nipples.

The CST is performed on an outpatient basis by qualified maternity nurses well acquainted with fetal monitoring and the interpretation of various FHR patterns. Most facilities require that the test be administered in or near the labor and birth unit so that treatment is available in the event that adverse reactions to oxytocin stimulation occur. The procedure, reasons for administering the test, equipment, and normal variations in monitoring that occur during the test should be clearly explained before the test to alleviate the woman's apprehension. A consent form may be signed.

During the test, the woman assumes a semi-Fowler's or side-lying position to avoid supine hypotension. The ultrasonic transducer (from the electronic fetal monitor) is placed on the woman's abdomen over the area of the fetal back or chest so that the FHR can be accurately recorded on the monitoring strip. (See Chapter 23 ∞ for further discussion of fetal monitoring). To record uterine contractions, the tocodynamometer (pressure transducer) is placed over the area of the uterine fundus. For the first 15 to 20 minutes, the nurse records baseline measurements, including blood pressure, fetal activity, variations of the FHR during fetal movement, and spontaneous contractions. In addition, pertinent medical and obstetric information may be obtained from the woman to aid in her further management.

After the baseline recording is done, an intravenous oxytocin contraction stress test or breast self-stimulation test (BSST) is done.

Intravenous Oxytocin CST

In a CST using intravenous oxytocin, an electrolyte solution such as lactated Ringer's solution is started as a primary infusion. A piggyback infusion of oxytocin in a similar solution is attached. An infusion pump is used so that the amount of oxytocin being infused can be measured accurately. The administration procedure is the same as that for inducing labor through oxytocin administration (see Chapter 27 ∞). Oxytocin is administered until three uterine contractions lasting 40 to 60 seconds occur in a 10-minute period (called the 10-minute window). If late decelerations occur with all three contractions, the oxytocin infusion is discontinued. The woman's blood pressure and pulse are assessed every 15 minutes and recorded on the tracing.

CST with Breast Self-Stimulation Test (BSST)

A woman receiving a BSST is instructed to stimulate her nipples with her fingers, palms, or a warm, moist face cloth, either directly or through her clothing, for 2 minutes or until a contraction begins. Stimulation may also be done mechanically by the use of a breast pump. Once the contraction begins, the woman is instructed to stop the stimulation, waiting to restart if another contraction has not followed by 5 minutes. It is important to monitor the frequency of contractions to avoid uterine hyperstimulation.

INTERPRETATION AND CLINICAL MANAGEMENT

A CST is usually not done before 28 weeks' gestation, primarily for two reasons. First, in light of a positive test, birth and extrauterine survival would be questionable at such an early gestational age. Second, sufficient research has not been done to

PROCEDURE 21–2 Performing a Contraction Stress Test (CST)

NURSING ACTION	RATIONALE

Preparation

- Explain the procedure, the information it provides, and the process for completing the test.
- Ask the woman to void.

The procedure will take at least 10 minutes to complete and the woman will need to remain in semi-Fowler's or a side-lying position and will be unable to void without interrupting the testing procedure.

- Advise the woman if uterine contractions are not occurring spontaneously that intravenous oxytocin or breast stimulation may be needed to perform the test.

The test requires three contractions lasting at least 40 seconds in duration in a 10-minute period in order to be performed.

Equipment and Supplies

External fetal monitor with a monitoring strip
Blood pressure cuff

Procedure

1. Place the woman in a semi-Fowler's or side-lying position after she has voided.
2. Place the ultrasound transducer from the external fetal monitor on the woman's abdomen over the FHR (typically over the fetal back or chest) so a tracing can be obtained on the monitoring strip.
3. If the FHR is not consistently recorded on the monitoring strip, adjust the ultrasound transducer until an adequate reading is obtained.

Fetal or maternal movement can cause an inconsistency in the FHR on the monitoring strip. Multiple adjustments may be needed to obtain consistency in recording the FHR.

4. Place the tocodynamometer (pressure transducer) on the woman's abdomen over the uterine fundus.
5. Obtain baseline measurements, including blood pressure, fetal activity, variations in the FHR during fetal movement, and contractions, for 15 to 20 minutes.
6. If less than three contractions lasting at least 40 seconds are occurring within a 10-minute period, administer intravenous oxytocin or instruct the woman in the breast stimulation technique until three contractions in a 10-minute period are occurring. The method chosen is based on the healthcare provider's orders and the woman's preference.
7. If using intravenous oxytocin, start an electrolyte solution as a primary infusion and attach a piggyback infusion of oxytocin in a similar solution using an infusion pump.

Contractions are best detected when the device is directly placed on the uterine fundus.
Baseline measurements provide a reference for normal maternal and fetal assessment parameters.
If the woman has a preference over one method or another, the healthcare provider should be made aware of that preference.

Intravenous oxytocin is always infused using a piggyback line because a small quantity is infusing. An infusion pump should be used to ensure accuracy.

8. Administer oxytocin and increase at regular intervals per agency protocol until three contractions lasting 40 to 60 seconds occur in a 10-minute period.

Because there are several formulas used to mix oxytocin and several different protocols to increase the dosage, specific agency protocol should be consulted regarding the preparation of the oxytocin solution and the dosage and interval increases used within the facility.

9. If using breast self-stimulation (BSST), instruct the woman to stimulate her breasts with her fingers, palms, or a warm, moist washcloth, either directly or through her clothing for 2 minutes or until a contraction begins.

Breast stimulation will facilitate the natural release of oxytocin by the woman's body. Some women may prefer a more natural method of testing and may prefer BSST over intravenous oxytocin.

(Continued on next page)

PROCEDURE 21–2　Performing a Contraction Stress Test (CST)　continued

NURSING ACTION	RATIONALE
10. Instruct the woman to stop the stimulation once the contraction occurs and to restart the stimulation if a contraction has not occurred within 5 minutes.	*Continuous breast stimulation can result in uterine hyperstimulation, which can lead to a uterine rupture.*
11. Advise the woman to increase the frequency of stimulation as needed to obtain three contractions within a 10-minute period.	
12. Interrupt the test as negative, positive, equivocal-suspicious, equivocal-hyperstimulatory, or unsatisfactory and report the findings to the healthcare provider immediately.	*The CST interpretations are based on specific criteria and should be reported to the healthcare provider as soon as the results are obtained. The results provide data regarding uteroplacental perfusion and indicate whether the fetus can withstand the stress of uterine contractions.*
13. Explain the results to the woman and relate information from the healthcare provider regarding further management needs or additional follow-up that is needed.	*The nurse is the key communicator in providing information regarding the test results and their meaning to the woman.*

Documentation	Document baseline maternal and fetal assessment information that was obtained before and during the test. The results of the test should be documented along with information regarding how the information was reported to the healthcare provider. The specific name of the healthcare provider and date and time should be recorded. Any additional orders and instructions to the client should be documented. Verbalization of understanding of the test results by the woman should be documented along with her understanding follow-up instructions and future appointments.

determine whether the same test results apply to a fetus of this gestation. CST is usually done at 32 to 34 weeks' gestation.

Interpretation of CST Results

A CST can be interpreted once three moderately strong contractions of 40 to 60 seconds' duration have been noted in a 10-minute window of time. A CST can be interpreted as negative, positive, equivocal, or unsatisfactory (Table 21–4). Cunningham et al. (2005) offered the following CST interpretations:

Negative —The absence of late or significant variable decelerations (the most common deceleration pattern noted during labor; attributed to umbilical cord compression or occlusion) is considered a reassuring sign that the fetus is receiving sufficient transfer of oxygen through the placenta (Figure 21–14 ◆).

Positive —The presence of **late decelerations** (a symmetrical decrease in FHR beginning at or after the peak of the contraction and returning to baseline only after the contraction has ended following 50% or more of contractions, even if the contraction frequency is fewer than three in 10 minutes) is a sign of uteroplacental insufficiency and may indicate that the fetus is not receiving adequate oxygenation (Figure 21–15 ◆).

Equivocal-suspicious —The presence of intermittent late decelerations or significant variable decelerations

Table 21–4　INTERPRETATION OF THE CONTRACTION STRESS TEST

Result	Interpretation
Negative	No late or significant variable decelerations.
Positive	Late decelerations following 50% or more of contractions (even if the contraction frequency is fewer than three in 10 minutes).
Equivocal	
Suspicious	Intermittent late decelerations or significant variable decelerations.
Hyperstimulatory	Fetal heart rate decelerations that occur in the presence of contractions more frequent than every 2 minutes or lasting longer than 90 seconds.
Unsatisfactory	Fewer than three contractions in 10 minutes or an uninterpretable tracing.

SOURCE: ACOG Practice Bulletin No. 9, October 1999. *Clinical Management Guidelines for Obstetrician-Gynecologists,* pp. 2–3.

should be viewed as a suspicious finding that merits follow-up testing.

Equivocal-hyperstimulatory —FHR decelerations may occur in the presence of contractions that occur more frequently than every 2 minutes or that last longer than 90 seconds. This test should be repeated after

Figure 21–14 ◆ Example of a negative CST (and reactive NST). The baseline FHR is 130 bpm with acceleration of FHR of at least 15 bpm lasting 15 seconds with each fetal movement (FM). Uterine contractions recorded on the bottom half of the strip indicate three contractions in 8 minutes.

Figure 21–15 ◆ Example of a positive contraction stress test (CST). Repetitive late decelerations occur with each contraction. Note that there are no accelerations of FHR with three fetal movements (FM). The baseline FHR is 120 bpm. Uterine contractions (bottom half of strip) occurred four times in 12 minutes.

hyperstimulation has been rectified and the client has been hydrated and allowed to rest.

Unsatisfactory —The CST cannot be interpreted if fewer than three contractions lasting 40 to 60 seconds occur in a 10-minute window of time.

CST results are also evaluated for the presence of accelerations that would meet the criteria of the NST. Combining the CST assessment with NST results showing characteristics such as variability of the FHR baseline and the presence of other types of decelerations helps the clinician determine the best management plan for the fetus.

Clinical Management Based on CST Results

In most cases, a negative CST with a reactive NST is the desired result. The uteroplacental perfusion is sufficient at present to al-

low the fetus to withstand the stress of uterine contractions. Retesting would most likely be scheduled in 7 days. If the pregnant woman is diabetic, the CST schedule would remain the same, except an NST would be done in 3 to 4 days (Rudra, Williams, Lee et al., 2006). A negative CST with a nonreactive NST is more difficult. It should be assessed very carefully for subtle late decelerations. If there are none, a CST would be repeated in 7 days.

All equivocal tests should be repeated in 24 hours, especially in the presence of a postterm pregnancy (Rudra et al., 2006). If the gestation is less than 37 weeks, then other surveillance methods should be added.

A positive CST with a nonreactive NST presents evidence that the fetus would probably not withstand the stress of labor. If the gestation is 32 weeks or over, a cesarean birth should be scheduled (Rudra et al., 2006).

MEDIALINK

Case Study: Client Undergoing Contraction Stress Test

NURSING CARE MANAGEMENT

The nurse ascertains the woman's or couple's understanding of the CST before the procedure and the possible results. The nurse reviews the reasons for the CST and the procedure before beginning the test. The nurse then applies the external fetal monitor to the maternal abdomen. If oxytocin is to be used, the nurse inserts an intravenous line and begins the medication. If a BSST is being conducted, the nurse instructs the woman on self-stimulation of the breast or on the appropriate use of the breast pump. Continuous monitoring of the contraction pattern is warranted to ensure that hyperstimulation of the uterus or fetal compromise does not occur. The nurse then reports the findings to the physician or certified nurse-midwife and explains the results to the woman.

Amniotic Fluid Index

Assessment of amniotic fluid volume is based on the rationale that decreased uteroplacental perfusion may lead to diminished fetal renal blood flow, decreased urination, and, ultimately, **oligohydramnios** (decreased amniotic fluid volume). Fetal urine output and fetal swallowing are the major determinants of amniotic fluid volume. Oligohydramnios may be the result of diminished urinary output caused by fetal hypoxemia. The resulting placental insufficiency may cause hypoxia and hence oligohydramnios. Therefore, assessment of long-term uteroplacental function may be performed by evaluating amniotic fluid volume (Voxman, Tran, & Wing, 2002). Poor pregnancy outcomes, such as intrauterine growth restriction, postterm pregnancy, and nonreassuring fetal status in labor, have been associated with abnormalities of amniotic fluid volume. The procedure for performing an amniotic fluid index (AFI) was discussed previously on p. 550.

An AFI value of 5 or less serves as a red flag that requires some type of further assessment or management decision (Gearhart & Sehdev, 2005). The gestational age of the fetus and the composite maternal condition may influence management decisions, leading to additional testing, induction of labor, or cesarean birth.

Biophysical Profile

The **biophysical profile (BPP)** represents an assessment of five fetal biophysical variables:

- FHR acceleration
- Fetal breathing
- Fetal movements
- Fetal tone
- Amniotic fluid volume

The first criterion is assessed with the NST. The other variables are assessed by ultrasound scanning. By combining these five assessments, the BPP helps to identify the compromised fetus and confirm the healthy fetus. Average testing time is usually less than 8 minutes, with 90% of normal testing completed within the first 4 minutes (Pinette, 2005). A time period of 30 minutes is selected for BPP testing (ultrasound components) to account for the average duration of sleep-wake cycles in the normal fetus, which are approximately 20 minutes.

Indications for the biophysical profile include those situations in which the NST and CST would be done. Assessment of these fetal biophysical activities is most useful in the evaluation of women who experience decreased fetal movement (who might subsequently have a nonreactive NST) and in the management of intrauterine growth restriction, preterm labor, gestational diabetes, postterm pregnancies, and premature rupture of the membranes (PROM) (Pinette, 2005).

The two most important components of the BPP are the NST and the amniotic fluid volume index. The NST reflects the intactness of the nervous system and the AFI reflects kidney perfusion. A normal AFI indicates that shunting has not occurred and that the fetal kidneys are adequately functioning. Reactive NST and normal fluid therefore reflect fetal well-being.

Specific criteria for normal and abnormal assessments are delineated in Table 21–5. Normal variables are assigned a score of 2 each and abnormal variables a score of 0 (zero). Thus, the highest score possible for a normal fetus is 10.

Clinicians suggest that management not be based solely on BPP scores. Biophysical activities of the fetus that develop first are the last to disappear when all activities are arrested because of asphyxia (Fahey, 2005). Those that are the last to develop are the most sensitive to hypoxia, and their disappearance can be noted

Table 21–5	**CRITERIA FOR NORMAL AND ABNORMAL ASSESSMENTS**	
Component	**Normal (score = 2)**	**Abnormal (score = 0)**
Fetal breathing movements	Greater than or equal to episode of rhythmic breathing lasting greater than or equal to 30 sec within 30 min	Less than or equal to 30 sec of breathing in 30 min
Gross body movements	Greater than or equal to discrete body or limb movements in 30 min (episodes of active continuous movement considered as single movement)	Less than or equal to movements in 30 min
Fetal tone	Greater than or equal to episode of extension of a fetal extremity with return to flexion, or opening or closing of hand	No movements or extension/flexion
Reactive fetal heart rate Nonstress test	Greater than or equal to 2 accelerations of greater than or equal to 15 bpm for greater than or equal to 15 sec in 20–40 min	0 or 1 acceleration in 20–40 min
Amniotic fluid volume	Single vertical pocket less than 2 cm AFI greater than 5 cm	Largest single vertical pocket less than or equal to 2 cm AFI less than 5 cm

Table 21–6 BPP TEST INTERPRETATION AND RECOMMENDED MANAGEMENT

Test Score	Interpretation	Perinatal Mortality Within 1 Week Without Intervention	Management
10/10	Normal nonasphyxiated fetus	Less than 1/1000	No fetal indication for intervention; repeat test weekly except in client with diabetes and pregnancies that are postterm (twice weekly)
8/10 (normal fluid) 8/8 if no NST done	Risk of fetal asphyxia extremely rare	Less than 1/1000	Same as above
8/10 (abnormal fluid)	Chronic fetal asphyxia suspected	89/1000	Induce birth
6/10	Possible fetal asphyxia	89/1000	If amniotic fluid volume abnormal, deliver
			If normal fluid at greater than 36 weeks with favorable cervix, induce birth
			If repeat test less than or equal to 6, induce birth
			If repeat test greater than 6, observe and repeat per protocol
4/10	Probable fetal asphyxia	91/1000	Repeat testing same day; if BPP score less than or equal to 6, deliver
2/10	Almost certain fetal asphyxia	125/1000	Induce birth
0/10	Certain fetal asphyxia	600/1000	Induce birth

first. For example, fetal tone (exhibited by flexion of the extremities) is the first to develop and the last activity to cease during asphyxia. Other activities in the normal developmental sequence are fetal movement, followed by fetal breathing, and then reactivity of the FHR. Therefore, FHR reactivity is the most sensitive to hypoxia. One of the first indications of fetal compromise is a nonreactive NST. Table 21–6 outlines BPP test interpretation and the recommended management (Cunningham et al., 2005).

Modified Biophysical Profile

The biophysical profile is labor intensive and expensive. It requires a trained person in ultrasonic visualization of the fetus. In addition, studies have shown that when the four dynamic ultrasound variables are normal, the probability of encountering an abnormal (nonreactive) NST is exceedingly small (Chauhan, 2004). For these reasons, a modified BPP has been developed. This test consists of an NST and a measurement of the AFI, which reflects long-term uteroplacental function. The functioning of the placenta is important because a poorly functioning placenta (placental dysfunction) may result in diminished fetal renal perfusion, leading to oligohydramnios. The amniotic fluid volume assessment can therefore be used to evaluate long-term uteroplacental function. A modified BPP is considered normal if the amniotic fluid volume is greater than 5 cm and if the NST is reactive. The test is abnormal if either the NST is nonreactive or the AFI is 5 or less. The frequency of this test is the same as with the standard BPP.

Doppler Flow Studies

Recent advances in ultrasound technology have made it possible to study noninvasively blood flow changes that occur in maternal and fetal circulations to assess placental function. An ultrasound beam, like that provided by the pocket Doppler (a handheld ultrasound device), is directed at the umbilical artery. The signal is reflected off the red blood cells moving within the vessels, and the subsequent "picture" (waveform) that is received looks like a series of waves. The highest velocity peak of the waves is the systolic measurement, and the lowest point is the diastolic velocity. The umbilical artery waveform can then be analyzed to provide information about velocity of blood flow in the vessel (Gojnic, 2004). Examples of these waveforms are displayed in Figures 21–16 ◆ and 21–17 ◆.

The most common evaluation of blood flow velocity is the systolic to diastolic (S/D) ratio. The S/D ratio normally decreases as the fetus nears term. This phenomenon reflects the decreasing resistance of placental and umbilical vasculature to allow for greater umbilical blood flow to meet the needs of a growing fetus. The S/D ratio is considered abnormal if elevated above the 95th percentile for gestational age or reversed after 18 to 20 weeks of gestation (Vergani, Roncaglia, Andreotti et al., 2002). Absent or reversed end-diastolic flow signifies increased impedance and is uniquely associated with intrauterine growth restriction. It is also associated with a high perinatal mortality rate (Seyam, Al-Mahmeid, & Al-Tamimi, 2002; Vergani et al., 2002).

A decrease in fetal cardiac output or an increase in resistance of placental vessels will reduce umbilical artery blood flow. Doppler velocimetry is best used when intrauterine growth restriction is diagnosed, whether it occurs as an idiopathic process (cause unknown) or in the presence of hypertension or preeclampsia (Seyam et al., 2002). No benefit has been demonstrated for umbilical artery velocimetry for other conditions such as postterm pregnancy, diabetes, systemic lupus erythematosus, or antiphospholipid antibody syndrome. Also, it has not been shown to be of value as a screening test for detecting fetal compromise in the general obstetric population (Cunningham et al., 2005).

Evaluation of Placental Maturity

Placental maturity is evaluated by a grading process that uses ultrasound to measure the changes in the basal layer, chorionic plate, and intervening placental substance. A grade of 0 through III is assigned (grade III as the most mature, showing extensive calcifications) (Figure 21–18 ◆). Placentas with multiple calcifications are less likely to function as adequately as those with

Figure 21–16 ◆ Serial studies of the umbilical artery velocity waveforms in a normal pregnancy from one client.

Figure 21–17 ◆ Two examples of abnormal umbilical artery velocity waveforms taken from a client with intrauterine growth restriction.

lower grades. Certain factors can cause a placenta to mature, including maternal smoking, postterm pregnancy, and certain maternal conditions, such as preeclampsia and gestational diabetes. Placental grade may be used to correlate with other findings; however, placental grade alone does not dictate management of a pregnancy.

Estimation of Fetal Weight

Estimating the fetal weight in the third trimester of pregnancy is an important aspect of fetal assessment. Particularly, findings of the fetal weight at either end of the spectrum—inadequate fetal growth or excessive fetal growth—are critical risk factors for alterations in fetal well-being.

Intrauterine growth restriction (IUGR) is a term used to describe any fetus that falls below the 10th percentile in ultrasonic estimation of weight at a given gestational age. Other terms to describe the small fetus include *low birth weight, small for gestational age,* and *intrauterine growth retardation.* IUGR may or may not be associated with prematurity.

The etiology of IUGR can be separated into either fetoplacental or maternal origin. Fetoplacental etiologies would include infections, genetic abnormalities, and placental abnormalities. Maternal etiologies stem from reduced uteroplacental blood flow associated with hypertension, poor maternal weight gain, poor nutrition, substance use such as tobacco or medications, anemia, or chronic illness.

If a fetus is suspected to have IUGR, the management includes careful surveillance of the fetus with NSTs and BPPs and continuous assessment of growth through sonographic assessment. In addition to regular fetal surveillance, women with IUGR are instructed to do daily fetal movement assessments (previously discussed in this chapter) and to maintain bed rest. If growth ceases altogether or if other nonreassuring fetal factors occur (nonreassuring FHR patterns), delivery may be warranted.

Macrosomia is defined by ACOG as weight greater than 4000 to 4500 g (8 lb 13 oz to 9 lb 4 oz). If a fetus is suspected

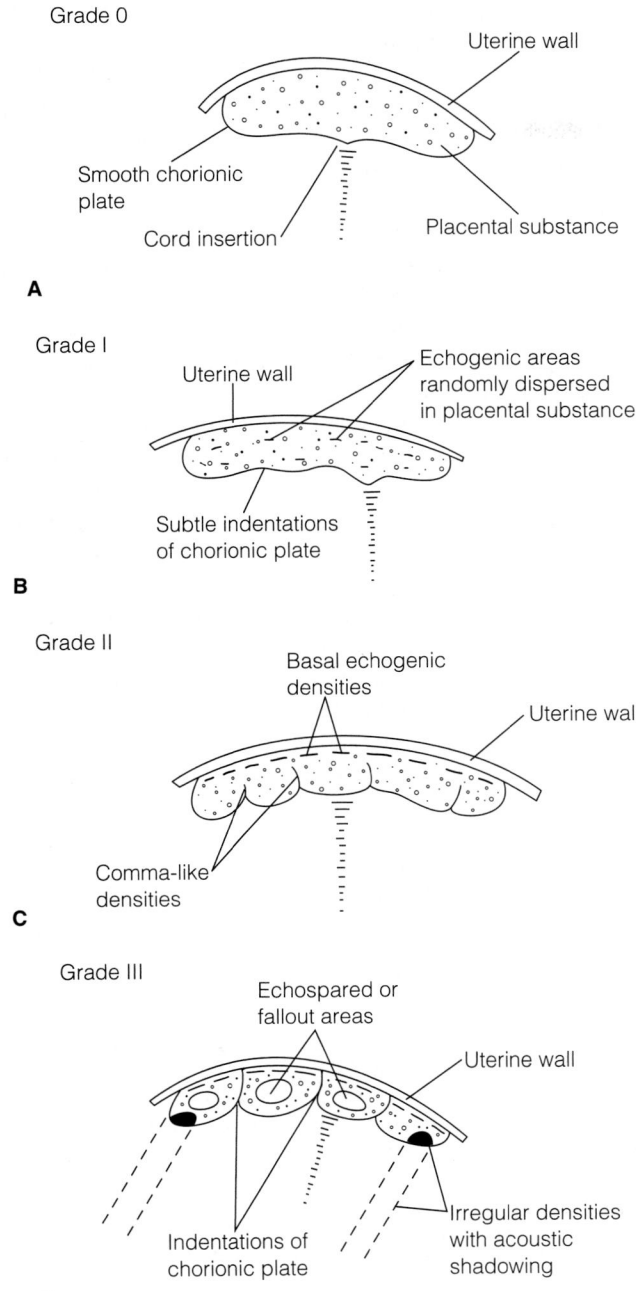

Grade 0

Uterine wall

Smooth chorionic plate

Cord insertion

Placental substance

A

Grade I

Uterine wall

Echogenic areas randomly dispersed in placental substance

Subtle indentations of chorionic plate

B

Grade II

Basal echogenic densities

Uterine wall

Comma-like densities

C

Grade III

Echospared or fallout areas

Uterine wall

Indentations of chorionic plate

Irregular densities with acoustic shadowing

D

Figure 21–18 ◆ Placental grading. *A*, Diagram showing the ultrasonic appearance of a grade 0 placenta. *B*, Diagram showing the ultrasonic appearance of a grade I placenta. *C*, Diagram showing the ultrasonic appearance of a grade II placenta. *D*, Diagram showing the ultrasonic appearance of a grade III placenta.

to be macrosomic, the management of the labor and birth is carefully evaluated to prevent birth-related complications such as *shoulder dystocia* (an intrapartum event that occurs when the infant's head has been delivered, but the shoulders remain wedged behind the mother's pubic bone, causing a difficult birth of the infant with potential for maternal or fetal injury).

The diagnosis of fetal macrosomia is imprecise. The accuracy of estimated fetal weight using ultrasound biometry and that obtained with clinical palpation by the obstetrician or certi-

fied nurse-midwife has yielded similar results (Weiner, Ben-Shoomo, Beck-Fruchter et al., 2002). One study determined the accuracy of obstetric sonography for weight prediction to have an accuracy rate of 15% to 79%, whereas a weight prediction based on clinical palpation had an accuracy rate of 40% to 52% (Chauhan, 2005). This clinical palpation of the fetus through the fetal abdomen by Leopold's maneuvers is done by placing two hands at the fundus of the uterus and moving the hands along the sides of the fetus to estimate the fetal size and position (see Chapter 23 ∞). The fundal height (measured in centimeters with a tape measure from the symphysis pubis to the fundus of the uterus) is another tool in estimating fetal growth. According to ACOG, these two primary methods for the clinical estimation of fetal weight should be combined to produce a more accurate measurement. Experienced providers may also ask the woman to provide her own estimate of the fetal weight if she has had a previous birth.

The greatest risk factor for macrosomic infants is birth trauma due to a shoulder dystocia. When macrosomia is present, a potential shoulder dystocia should be anticipated if the woman is giving birth vaginally. The woman should be positioned in McRobert's position (legs flexed and pulled back toward the woman's shoulders) with the head of the bed lowered. A stool should be readily available in the event that suprapubic pressure is needed. If the physician or certified nurse-midwife requests suprapubic pressure, the nurse applies pressure directly over the symphysis pubis to aid in dislodging the fetal shoulder (see Chapter 26 ∞).

Women who are undergoing a trial of labor after a previous cesarean birth should be counseled on the risks of a shoulder dystocia when macrosomia is suspected. In addition, a macrosomic fetus may decrease the likelihood of a successful vaginal birth after cesarean (VBAC), especially if the previous cesarean birth was performed for cephalopelvic disproportion (see Chapter 26 ∞). Although macrosomia is not a contraindication to a trial of labor, a trial of labor without a previous vaginal birth when the fetus is macrosomic increases the risk of uterine rupture (ACOG, 2004).

OTHER DIAGNOSTIC TESTS

Birth defects, defined as structural abnormalities present at birth, are the leading cause of infant mortality and a major contributor to infant morbidity in the United States. Birth defects affect 8 million children worldwide and affect 6% of all infants born each year (March of Dimes, 2006). Infant mortality due to birth defects has not declined as rapidly as overall infant mortality. It has been estimated that approximately 20% of all birth defects are due to gene mutations, and 5% to 10% are due to exposure to a teratogen such as drugs, chemicals, or radiation. About half of all birth defects remain unexplained (March of Dimes, 2006).

Rapidly developing technologies of biochemical markers and ultrasonography aid in the prenatal diagnosis of fetal anomalies and genetic disorders. As discussed in Chapter 12 ∞, conditions that can be diagnosed prenatally include trisomies 21, 18, and 13, spina bifida and anencephaly, cystic fibrosis, and some familial conditions.

Maternal Serum Alpha-Fetoprotein (MSAFP)

Alpha-fetoprotein (AFP) is a fetal protein that is excreted from the fetal yolk sac during the first 6 weeks of pregnancy. The production of AFP is then taken over by the fetal liver as the pregnancy progresses. If the fetus has a neural tube defect (NTD), AFP levels are elevated. The incidence of NTDs is 1 per 2000 births and is the most commonly occurring birth defect in the United States (March of Dimes, 2006). NTDs can range from *anencephaly* (absence of a portion of the fetal brain that is incompatible with extrauterine life) to *spina bifida* (a lesion on the spinal cord that is associated with lower extremity paralysis, incontinence, and developmental delay).

QUADRUPLE CHECK

Maternal serum alpha-fetoprotein (MSAFP) is a component of the screening test, the *"quadruple check"* that utilizes the multiple markers, including AFP, hCG, diameric inhibin-A, and estriol to screen pregnancies for NTD, trisomy 21 (Down syndrome), and trisomy 18. Screening can be performed between 15 and 22 weeks' gestation (15 to 16 yields the most accurate results). ACOG recommends that all pregnant women be offered MSAFP testing during pregnancy (Norem, Edgar, Schoen et al., 2005). Recent studies have shown that second trimester ultrasound along with MSAFP testing had a higher detection rate than MSAFP testing alone. For that reason, many practitioners perform both ultrasound testing and serologic screening (Norem et al., 2005).

Universal screening should be offered to all women, because 90% of NTD cases occur in women with no risk factors. MSAFP screening detects approximately 85% of open neural tube defects. Most cases of NTDs are unknown; however, risk factors include a previous fetus with an NTD, maternal age less than 20 or greater than 35 years, primiparity or grandmultiparity, low socioeconomic status with nutritional deficiencies, English or Irish ancestry, and inadequate folate intake.

The MSAFP is the first marker used in the quadruple check. Most laboratories use a cutoff of 2 to 2.5 multiples of the mean (MoM) of AFP to define a test as abnormally high. The lower the cutoff, the greater the detection rate but also the higher the false-positive rate. Levels of 2.5 to 3.5 MoM are considered indiscriminate because both normal and abnormal fetuses typically test within this zone. Levels greater than 3.5 MoM are outside the normal distribution and are at high risk for a neural tube defect. Using a cutoff of 2 to 2.5 MoM would yield a 90% detection rate, resulting in 3% to 5% of positive screens with a 2% to 6% false-positive rate (Reddy & Mennuti, 2006). The majority of women with an elevated MSAFP do not have affected fetuses. In 90% to 95% of the group with an elevated MSAFP, the elevation is caused from other variables, such as incorrect gestational age, more than one fetus, other fetal anomalies such as gastroschisis (a hole in the abdominal wall that allows the abdominal contents to protrude outside the body), and fetal death (Cunningham et al., 2005).

The quadruple screen has also been used to screen for trisomy 21 (Down syndrome), which is the most common chromosomal abnormality found in live births, and for trisomy 18, which is less common, but usually results in death of the infant within the first year of life (see Chapter 12 ∞). Unlike NTDs, the risk of Down syndrome and trisomy 18 increases with increasing maternal age; thus genetic counseling and tests are usually offered to women who will be 35 years of age or older at their EDB.

Abnormal test results are generally defined as a calculated Down syndrome risk of 1 in 270 or 1 in 200 (depending on the laboratory). Women who have abnormal results are counseled about these risks and offered an amniocentesis. Unlike the MSAFP, which is considered a screening test, the amniocentesis is a diagnostic test and considered to be greater than 99% accurate in the diagnosis of chromosomal anomalies.

Screening tests require client education and counseling to avoid confusion and undue stress. A key point for the nurse to understand and reinforce to the client is that the MSAFP and the triple check are screening tests, and are **not** diagnostic. The nurse has an important role in educating the woman about various aspects of these tests. The importance of an accurate gestational age determination before taking the test cannot be overstated. A miscalculated gestational age may result in the incorrect interpretation of the MSAFP level, causing extreme stress to the woman and her family. In addition, further testing is required. An elevation of the MSAFP requires recalculation with an accurate gestational age and repeat test, and a low MSAFP may require an amniocentesis. The nurse also educates the client on the importance of proper timing of the MSAFP. As stated earlier, the ideal time for screening is between 15 and 18 weeks. False-positives can occur with tests done either before or after this window in the gestation.

All healthcare providers should be sensitive to the ethical issues these screening tests present to the childbearing family. What benefit would knowing the results of an abnormal MSAFP provide? If the fetus has an NTD, the family and healthcare provider can use this information before the birth to choose the appropriate birth site or birth type. (An infant with an NTD would need to be born in a tertiary care center should immediate care need to be given to the infant.) Knowing an infant has Down syndrome would not necessarily change an obstetric decision about birth method or site, but it would give the family time for psychologic preparation, a chance to talk with social services and support groups, or the opportunity to opt for termination of the pregnancy.

Amniocentesis

Amniocentesis is a procedure used for genetic diagnosis. A sterile needle is inserted into the uterine cavity through the maternal abdomen so a small amount of amniotic fluid can be removed, and genetic testing is performed. Amniocentesis is performed between 15 and 20 weeks' gestation. Two large studies in the United States and Canada have confirmed the safety and the 99% diagnostic accuracy of this procedure (Cunningham et al., 2005).

Amniocentesis can make chromosomal and biochemical determinations (enzyme analysis, AFP measurement for neural tube defects, blood typing, or cytogenetic, metabolic, or other

RESEARCH IN PRACTICE

RACIAL ETHNIC DIFFERENCES IN GENETIC AMNIOCENTESIS UPTAKE

What is this study about? Amniocentesis is performed during the second trimester of pregnancy, and most commonly is indicated by advanced maternal age, abnormal serum screening, and abnormal fetal ultrasound. The procedure is usually preceded by detailed genetic counseling that outlines the potential risks and benefits of the test. There is a range of motives behind a woman's decision to utilize this invasive prenatal diagnostic test. Factors such as costs, knowledge, personal values, and health beliefs may influence the decision. The objective of this study was to determine the role of health beliefs in the decision to undergo amniocentesis among a population of ethnically diverse pregnant women.

How was this study done? All women who were referred for genetic amniocentesis at a single university hospital setting were invited to participate. One hundred fifty seven women agreed and completed a validated questionnaire that examined the decision making of these women and their health beliefs. The questionnaire was administered after the mother had been referred for amniocentesis but before the decision and actual procedure occurred. Three categories of responses were captured by the instrument, including demographic information, health beliefs, and knowledge about amniocentesis. Individual questions measured the mother's perception of susceptibility, seriousness of the condition, benefits of the procedure, and barriers to amniocentesis. The data from these subjects were compared with the overall genetics population at the medical center. Statistical analysis was used to determine associations between amniocentesis decision rates, knowledge level, health beliefs, and demographics.

What were the results of the study? The most common indication for the procedure was advanced maternal age, except in the African American group, where abnormal serum screening was the most common. Of the participants, 73.9% ultimately had an amniocentesis. Women who accepted amniocentesis were more likely to have a college education than the group that declined. There was no significant difference in religious affiliation or parity between women who accepted or declined. Participants who ultimately had the procedure scored higher on perceived seriousness, susceptibility, benefits, and knowledge than those who declined. Although Hispanic women were less likely to accept amniocentesis than Caucasian, African American, or Asian women, this was not in the group of predictors that best explained the final decision to undergo amniocentesis. The most significant predictors of the amniocentesis decision were perceived benefits, knowledge, and perceived seriousness of the potential condition. Perceived susceptibility and ethnicity were significant, but weak, predictors. Individual health beliefs and knowledge about the procedure play a greater role in genetic amniocentesis acceptance than do demographic factors such as ethnicity.

What additional questions might I have? Could these findings be applied to other prenatal procedures that are recommended to women? Does education about the procedure change acceptance rates?

How can I use this study? The nurse should provide information to mothers about the potential benefits and risks of amniocentesis so that she can make an informed decision. The mother's health beliefs will play a major role in her decision to undergo the procedure, and the nurse is in a position to ensure that the mother has accurate information with which to make the decision. The health belief model is more important in the final decision than demographic characteristics such as ethnicity.

Saucier, J., Johnston, D., Wicklund, C., Robbins-Furman, P., Hecht, J., & Monga, M. (2005). Racial-ethnic differences in genetic amniocentesis uptake. *Journal of Genetic Counseling, 14*(3), 189–195.

DNA testing) and can validate abnormalities detected by ultrasound. Later in pregnancy, from about 30 to 35 weeks' gestation, amniocentesis may be done for lung maturity studies, such as lecithin/sphingomyelin ratio and the presence of phosphatidylglycerol and phosphatidylcholine (see discussion on p. 571).

INDICATIONS FOR AMNIOCENTESIS

The following conditions are commonly considered indications for amniocentesis:

- Pregnant women who will be 35 or older on their due date. The risk of having an infant with a chromosomal problem such as Down syndrome increases with the age of the woman (see Chapter 12 ∞).
- Couples who already have had a child with a birth defect or have a family history of certain birth defects.
- Pregnant women with other abnormal genetic test results.

Procedure for Performing Amniocentesis

Amniocentesis is done on an outpatient basis but needs to be performed near a birthing area in case acute nonreassuring fetal status is encountered. The pregnant woman should have a left lateral tilt to prevent hypotension during the procedure.

The abdomen is scanned by ultrasound to locate the placenta, the fetus, and an adequate pocket of fluid. The needle insertion site is of the utmost importance because the fetus, placenta, umbilical cord, bladder, and uterine arteries must all be avoided (Figure 21–19 ◆). The importance of locating the placenta cannot be stressed enough, especially in cases of Rh isoimmunization, in which trauma to the placenta increases fetal–maternal transfusion and worsens the isoimmunization (see Chapter 20 ∞). If the amniocentesis is being performed in the last few weeks of pregnancy, the fetus may occupy what appears to be all the available space in the uterus, and there is a

Figure 21–19 ◆ Amniocentesis. The woman is usually scanned by ultrasound to determine the placental site and to locate a pocket of fluid. As the needle is inserted, three levels of resistance are felt when the needle penetrates the skin, fascia, and uterine wall. When the needle is placed within the amniotic cavity, amniotic fluid is withdrawn.

normal decrease in the amount of amniotic fluid; however, with the aid of ultrasound, fluid can be located. The amniocentesis, or "tap," is then done before the fetus has the opportunity to move.

After the abdomen is scanned, the abdominal skin is cleansed with povidone-iodine (Betadine). The woman is given the option of a local anesthetic for the insertion site. A 22-gauge spinal needle is inserted into the uterine cavity. Generally, fluid immediately flows into the needle. The first few drops are discarded; a syringe is then attached to the needle, and the fluid is aspirated (Figure 21–20 ◆). From 15 to 20 mL of amniotic fluid are withdrawn, placed in brown-tinted test tubes (to shield the fluid from light to prevent breakdown of bilirubin and other pigments), and sent to the laboratory for analysis. The needle is withdrawn using ultrasound, and the insertion site is evaluated for streaming (movement of fluid), which would indicate bleeding into the amniotic fluid. The FHR is monitored to assess fetal well-being. If the woman's vital signs and the FHR are normal, she is allowed to leave (see Procedure 21–3).

If the collected amniotic fluid is contaminated with blood, the fluid should be centrifuged immediately. The woman is observed for alterations in the FHR. The blood should be tested to determine whether it is maternal or fetal.

Rh-negative women are given Rh immune globulin after amniocentesis, provided that they are not already sensitized. If the amniotic fluid from these women is contaminated with blood, the sample should be tested to identify fetal cells. In this situation a larger dose of immune globulin is required.

Figure 21–20 ◆ During amniocentesis, amniotic fluid is aspirated into a syringe.
SOURCE: © John Watney/Photo Researchers.

PROCEDURE 21–3 Assisting During Amniocentesis

NURSING ACTION	RATIONALE

Preparation

- Explain the procedure and the indications for it and reassure the woman.
- Determine whether an informed consent form has been signed. If not, verify that the woman's doctor has explained the procedure and ask her to sign a consent form.

It is the physician's responsibility to obtain informed consent. The woman's signature indicates her awareness of the risks and gives her consent to the procedure.

Equipment and Supplies

22-gauge spinal needle with stylet
10- and 20-mL syringes
1% lidocaine (Xylocaine)
Povidone-iodine (Betadine)
Three 10-mL test tubes with tops (amber colored or covered with tape)

Amniotic fluid must be protected from light to prevent breakdown of bilirubin.

Procedure: Sterile Gloves

1. Obtain baseline vital signs including maternal blood pressure (BP), pulse, respirations, temperature, and fetal heart rate (FHR) before procedure begins.
2. Monitor BP, pulse, respirations, and FHR every 15 minutes during procedure.

Baseline information is essential to detect any changes in maternal or fetal status that might be related to the procedure.

3. The physician uses real-time ultrasound to determine the location of the placenta and to locate a pocket of amniotic fluid. Provide gel for the ultrasound and assist with the procedure as needed.
4. Cleanse the woman's abdomen.
5. The physician dons gloves, inserts the needle into the identified pocket of fluid (See Figure 21–19), and withdraws a sample.

Cleansing the abdomen before needle insertion helps decrease the risk of infection.

6. Obtain the test tubes from the physician. Label the tubes with the woman's correct identification and send to the lab with the appropriate lab slips.
7. Monitor the woman and reassess her vital signs.
   - Determine the woman's BP, pulse, respirations, and the FHR.
   - Palpate the woman's fundus to assess for uterine contractions.
   - Monitor her using an external fetal monitor for 20 to 30 minutes after the amniocentesis.
   - Determine a treatment course to counteract any supine hypotension and to increase venous return and cardiac output.

Monitoring maternal and fetal status postprocedure provides information about response to the procedure and helps detect any complications such as inadvertent fetal puncture.

8. Assess the woman's blood type and determine any need for Rh immune globulin.
9. Administer Rh immune globulin if indicated (see Procedure 20-2 ∞).

To prevent Rh sensitization in an Rh-negative woman, Rh immune globulin is administered prophylactically involving amniocentesis.

10. Instruct the woman to report any of the following changes or symptoms to her primary caregiver:
    - Unusual fetal hyperactivity or, conversely, any lack of fetal movement
    - Vaginal discharge—either clear drainage or bleeding
    - Uterine contractions or abdominal pain
    - Fever or chills

These are signs of potential complications and require further evaluation.

11. Encourage the woman to engage only in light activities for 24 hours and to increase her fluid intake.

Decreased maternal activity helps decrease uterine irritability and increase uteroplacental circulation. Increased fluid intake helps replace amniotic fluid through the uteroplacental circulation.

(Continued on next page)

PROCEDURE 21–3 Assisting During Amniocentesis   *continued*

NURSING ACTION	RATIONALE
12. Complete the client record. Record the type of procedure, the date and time, and the name of the physician who performed the procedure. Also record the maternal-fetal response, disposition of the specimen, and discharge teaching.	

Documentation	The nurse documents maternal and fetal responses to the procedure. Maternal vital signs, including level of discomfort, should be recorded. The FHR, presence of contractions, bleeding, and fluid leakage should be documented. Discharge instructions and abnormal symptoms that need to be reported to the physician should also be documented.

RISKS/SIDE EFFECTS

Minor complications are infrequent and may include transient vaginal spotting, cramping, or amniotic fluid leakage in 1% to 2% of cases performed. Chorioamnionitis may occur in fewer than 1 in 1000 cases. Needle injuries to the fetus are rare when ultrasound guidance is used. Fetal loss rate is less than 0.5% (1 in 200). When early amniocentesis is performed (11 to 14 weeks) there is a higher pregnancy loss and complication rate than with traditional amniocentesis (Cunningham et al., 2005). This is due to the lack of membrane fusion to the uterine wall, which makes the puncture of the sac difficult, and to the fact that there is less fluid to withdraw.

> **CLINICAL TIP**
>
> Have the woman lie on her left side to ensure adequate placental perfusion.

NURSING CARE MANAGEMENT

The nurse assists the physician during the amniocentesis (see Procedure 21–3: Assisting During Amniocentesis). In addition, the nurse supports the woman undergoing amniocentesis. Women are usually apprehensive about the procedure as well as about the information that will be obtained. The physician explains the procedure before the woman signs the consent form. As it is being performed, the woman may need additional emotional support. She may become anxious during the procedure. She may also become lightheaded, nauseated, and diaphoretic from lying on her back with a heavy uterus compressing the abdominal vessels, so it is important to have her in a lateral tilt with a wedge placed under her right hip. The nurse can provide support to the woman by further clarifying the physician's instructions or explanations, by relieving the woman's physical discomfort when possible, and by responding verbally and physically to the woman's need for reassurance.

Chorionic Villus Sampling

Much like amniocentesis, **chorionic villus sampling (CVS)** is a procedure that is used to detect genetic, metabolic, and DNA abnormalities. CVS involves obtaining a small sample (5 to 40 mg) of chorionic villi from the edge of the developing placenta. CVS is performed in some medical centers for first trimester diagnosis. Villi in the chorion frondosum, present from 8 to 12 weeks' gestation, are believed to reflect fetal chromosome, enzyme, and DNA content, thereby permitting earlier diagnosis than can be obtained by amniocentesis. CVS cannot detect neural tube defects, however.

RISKS AND BENEFITS OF CVS

The woman should be aware of the risks and benefits of CVS. An increased risk of spontaneous abortion is associated with CVS, and the pregnancy loss rate reported with CVS is twice as high than that associated with amniocentesis. There is also an incidence of 1 in 3000 births of fetal limb reduction defects (a portion of a finger or a toe is missing), especially when the CVS is performed before 9 1/2 weeks' gestation. It is not recommended that CVS be performed before 10 weeks' gestation (Phillip, Silver, Wilson et al., 2004).

Additional risks of CVS include failure to obtain tissue, rupture of membranes, leakage of amniotic fluid, bleeding, intrauterine infection, maternal tissue contamination of the specimen, oromandibular defects, and Rh isoimmunization. Rh-negative women are given Rh immune globulin to cover the risk of immunization from the procedure (Phillip et al., 2004).

Like amniocentesis, CVS can detect fetal karyotype, hemoglobinopathies (e.g., sickle cell anemia and alpha and some beta thalassemias), phenylketonuria, alpha antitrypsin deficiency, Down syndrome, Duchenne muscular dystrophy, and factor IX deficiency. Early sex determination can be made so that pregnancies with a male fetus who would be affected in X-linked disorders can be identified. Because NTDs are not diagnosed by this test, all mothers undergoing CVS should be offered MSAFP screening at 15 to 20 weeks' gestation. A major disadvantage of the earlier testing (CVS) is that if a woman later has an abnormal MSAFP test indicating an increased risk of NTDs, she may

THROUGH THE EYES OF A NURSE

Genetic Testing Options in Pregnancy

FAMILY'S EXPERIENCE: "There seems like there are so many tests available, we are really confused about what to do. We don't feel like we have any risk factors, but we want to make sure our baby is healthy. What tests should we get? Which ones do we really need?"

NURSE'S RESPONSE: "There are various testing options. I can explain your options and help you weigh the pros and cons of each test. Because of your age and the fact that you do not have any risk factors identified in your medical or family history, you would not be a candidate for the amniocentesis or chorionic villus sampling tests. You may want to consider the other optional tests though, such as the quadruple screen, nuchal translucency test, and cystic fibrosis testing.

"The quadruple screen is a test that screens for neural tube defects and trisomy 18 and 21. This test is only a screening tool, which means it does not tell you if your baby *definitely* has one of these problems. It could help us know if your baby is at risk though. The test is not perfect and you can get false-positives or false-negatives. If the test did come back abnormal, you have other testing options such as a more detailed sonogram or an amniocentesis.

"The nuchal translucency test is a blood test and sonogram combined that screens for trisomy 18 and 21. The test is more accurate than the quadruple screen and is done earlier. Some insurance may not cover the test though, so you will need to call your insurance company to see if it is covered.

"The cystic fibrosis test screens for known gene mutations that cause cystic fibrosis. If your screen is positive, we will then have the father of the baby tested to determine if he is also a carrier. If you are both carriers, there is a 25% chance that the baby could have the disease. If only one of you is a carrier, there would be a chance the baby would also be a carrier, but the baby could not inherit the disease."

NURSE'S ACTIONS AND RATIONALE:

The nurse's role is to explain all testing options and to answer questions related to the various tests. The nurse presents the information in an objective manner without expressing a personal opinion. The couple must weigh each choice carefully and determine what tests are right for them. The nurse can also provide written resource material to the couple. The couple should be allowed to discuss the information and make an informed decision.

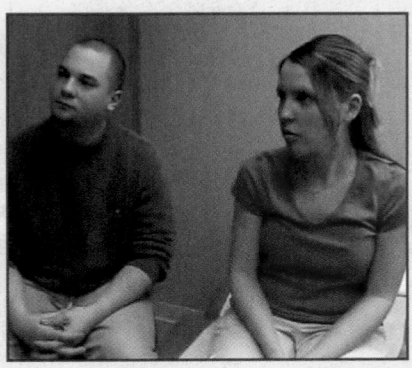

then have to undergo an amniocentesis, thus again putting the fetus at risk with an additional invasive procedure.

One of the greatest advantages to a woman undergoing this procedure is earlier diagnosis and decreased waiting time for results. Whereas amniocentesis is not done until at least 16 weeks' gestation, CVS is performed between 10 and 12 weeks. The CVS results are obtained in 24 hours if the direct preparation method is used and in 7 to 10 days when tissue culture is used. Earlier diagnosis may relieve many of the personal, social, and psychologic concerns of families, particularly if therapeutic abortion is being considered. There may be less emotional stress involved with having an abortion at an earlier stage of gestation. First trimester abortions are also easier to perform, require less time, and are less costly.

PROCEDURE FOR CVS

Before CVS, an ultrasound is done to determine placental location, uterine position (retroverted or anteverted), and presence of intervening structures (i.e., bowel, blood vessels). Various equipment can be used to aspirate chorionic villi from the placenta.

After counseling regarding diagnosis and procedure techniques, preliminary blood work may be obtained. The morning of the procedure, the woman is asked to drink fluids to fill her bladder because displacement of an anteverted uterus by a full bladder may aid in positioning the uterus for catheter insertion. Ultrasound is used to determine uterine position, cervical position, gestational sac size, and crown-rump length measurement and to identify the area of placental formation and cord insertion.

For the transcervical CVS the woman is placed in lithotomy position, the vulva is cleansed with povidone-iodine solution (Betadine), and a sterile speculum is inserted into the vagina. The vaginal vault and cervix are cleansed with the same solution to decrease contamination from the vagina into the uterus. The anterior lip of the cervix is sometimes grasped with a tenaculum to aid in straightening anteflexion of the uterus. The catheter (or cannula) is slowly inserted under ultrasound guidance through the endocervix to the sampling site at the extra-amniotic placental edge (outside the gestational sac). The obturator is withdrawn from the catheter. A 30-mL syringe, containing 3 to 4 mL of tissue culture medium with heparin, is attached, and a sample of villi is aspirated by using a pressure of 20 to 30 mL. The contents of the syringe are flushed into a petri dish containing nutrient medium, and the villi are inspected microscopically and prepared for cell culture.

For the transabdominal sampling, the woman is placed in the supine position. After the skin is cleansed with Betadine and local anesthesia is given, an 18- or 20-gauge needle is inserted percutaneously through the maternal abdominal wall and uterine myometrium. The tip of the needle is advanced into the long axis of the chorion frondosum under ultrasound guidance. Chorionic villi are obtained by repeated, rapid aspirations of the syringe containing tissue culture medium and heparin.

A normal CVS in the first trimester does not ensure a healthy infant. Routine prenatal care and appropriate follow-up are needed. Follow-up ultrasound and lab evaluation of each pregnancy must be done after performance of this procedure to evaluate fetal status. Further neonatal follow-up studies are necessary to evaluate the long-term effects of this technique.

NURSING CARE MANAGEMENT

Before the test, the nurse ascertains the woman's understanding of the CVS, its uses, the procedure, and the possible results. The nurse provides opportunities for questions and acts as an advocate when additional questions or concerns are raised. The nurse completes assessments following the procedure, including monitoring for vaginal bleeding or fluid leakage, excessive cramping, and basic maternal vital signs.

The nurse supports the woman or couple and encourages them to express any feelings and fears regarding the procedure and also regarding the decision-making process if abortion is being considered. That supportive role continues if abortion is chosen, even though the nurse may not be present for the procedure. It is important that support be provided following the procedure by the nurse who established a relationship with the couple previously.

Cordocentesis

Cordocentesis (also called percutaneous umbilical blood sampling [PUBS]) is a technique used to obtain pure fetal blood from the umbilical cord while the fetus is in utero. This procedure has been used for diagnosis of hemophilias, hemoglobinopathies, fetal infections, chromosome abnormalities, nonimmune hydrops, and isoimmune hemolytic disorders, as well as assessment of fetal hemoglobin and hematocrit for calculation of transfusion requirements in the second and third trimesters (Saju, Joy, Rossi et al., 2005). During the 1990s, PUBS was used more frequently; however, its use is now more limited to the diagnosis of anemia and for treatment of fetal anemia when hemoglobin levels fall below 10 g/dL or hematocrit is less than 30%. Although now less commonly used, cordiocentesis can also be used for the following:

- Rapid fetal karyotyping and genotyping
- Diagnosis of fetal infection (cytomegalovirus, toxoplasmosis, parvovirus, rubella)
- Platelet disorders
- Fetal blood grouping
- Diagnosis and treatment of isoimmunization
- Assessment of fetal well-being (pH, Po_2)
- Fetal metabolic disorders

The woman is scanned with an ultrasound transducer with sterile probe cover. A 25-gauge spinal needle is inserted into her abdomen through the skin alongside the transducer and into the fetal umbilical vein approximately 1 to 2 cm from the insertion of the cord into the placenta. The stylet is removed from the needle, and fetal blood is aspirated into a syringe containing an anticoagulant. Red blood cell size is determined to distinguish fetal from maternal cells. A paralytic agent, such as pancuronium bromide (Pavulon), may be given to prevent fetal movement during the procedure. If the mother is given a medication to help her relax, care must be taken to avoid oversedating her and causing deep breathing. Deep chest/diaphragmatic respirations can interfere with accurate puncture of the umbilical vein.

Within the last 10 years, improvements in ultrasonographic technique have made PUBS a relatively safe procedure with overall fetal loss rate less than 2%. The complication rate after PUBS is less than 0.5%. Complications include failure to obtain a sample, bleeding from the sampling site, premature rupture of membranes, chorioamnionitis, and fetal bradycardia (Saju et al., 2005). PUBS is used with less and less frequency because newer tests have replaced the need for a direct fetal sample.

NURSING CARE MANAGEMENT

The nurse collaborates with other members of the healthcare team to provide care for the woman for whom PUBS is recommended. Although a genetic counselor and/or obstetrician will have explained the risk for genetic defects and other disorders, the woman and her partner may need help to understand the procedure and its risks. They may need anticipatory guidance to help lessen their anxiety, as well as emotional support during the procedure and follow-up evaluation and testing. Support can come in many forms, including encouraging relaxation, providing reassurance, and giving the woman information throughout the procedure. The nurse may need to assist with coordination of financial and social service resources. The nurse can help promote relaxation during the procedure by instructing the woman in shallow breathing techniques. The nurse completes assessments during and immediately following the procedure and in some cases performs an NST test following the procedure.

Fetal Fibronectin

Fetal fibronectin (fFN) is a glycoprotein produced by the trophoblast and other fetal tissues. The presence of cervicovaginal fFN between 20 and 34 weeks' gestation has been shown to be a strong predictor of preterm delivery due to spontaneous preterm labor or premature rupture of membranes. fFN levels can be measured with an enzyme immunoassay.

Evaluation of Fetal Lung Maturity

In managing the woman and fetus at risk, the physician is constantly faced with the possibility of having to induce the birth of an infant before term and before the onset of labor. There are many indications for early termination of pregnancy, including repeat cesarean birth, premature rupture of membranes, diabetes, hypertensive conditions in the pregnant woman, and placental insufficiency. Unfortunately, the most common cause of perinatal mortality is prematurity, especially in infants weighing 1500 g or less and with particular complications arising from pulmonary immaturity (Cunningham et al., 2005). Birth of an infant with immature pulmonary function frequently results in

respiratory distress syndrome (RDS), also known as hyaline membrane disease (see Chapter 33 ∞).

Because gestational age, birth weight, and the rate of development of organ systems do not necessarily correspond, it may be necessary to determine the lung maturation of the fetus by amniotic fluid analysis before elective childbirth. In these cases, amniocentesis is performed, and concentrations of certain phospholipids in the amniotic fluid are measured. In many cases, birth of the infant can be delayed until the lungs show maturity.

L/S RATIO

The alveoli of the lungs are lined by a substance called **surfactant,** which is composed of phospholipids. Surfactant lowers the surface tension of the alveoli during extrauterine respiratory exhalation. By lowering the alveolar surface tension, surfactant stabilizes the alveoli, and a certain amount of air always remains in the alveoli during expiration. When a newborn with mature pulmonary function takes his or her first breath, a tremendously high pressure is needed to open the lungs. Upon breathing out, the lungs do not collapse, and about half the air in the alveoli is retained. An infant born too early, when synthesis of surfactant is incomplete, is unable to maintain lung stability, resulting in underinflation of the lungs and development of RDS.

Fetal lung maturity can be assessed by determining the ratio of two components of surfactant—lecithin and sphingomyelin. Early in pregnancy the lecithin concentration in amniotic fluid is less than that of sphingomyelin (0.5:1 at 20 weeks), resulting in a low **lecithin/sphingomyelin (L/S) ratio.** At about 30 to 32 weeks' gestation, the amounts of the two substances become equal (1:1). The concentration of lecithin begins to exceed that of sphingomyelin, and at 35 weeks the L/S ratio is 2:1. When at least two times as much lecithin as sphingomyelin is found in the amniotic fluid, RDS is very unlikely. Clinical outcomes, including respiratory distress and other respiratory disorders, should be correlated in individual institutions before specific ratios indicating pulmonary maturity are accepted. Infants of diabetic mothers (IDMs) are an exception to this finding and have a high incidence of false-positive results (i.e., the L/S ratio is thought to indicate lung maturity, but after birth the baby develops RDS). Although the same ratios are used, it is important to remember that even when IDMs are term (greater than 37 weeks' gestational age), delayed lung maturation can occur because the high blood sugars interfere with biochemical development. A delay in lung maturation has also been found in babies whose mothers have nonhypertensive renal disease and isoimmunization (Baha, 2004).

Some types of chronic intrauterine fetal stress cause an acceleration of lung maturation in the fetus. Prolonged rupture of membranes (over 24 hours) results in acceleration of lung maturation by approximately 1 week and therefore has a protective effect. Although the L/S ratio is the most universally used test for evaluating pulmonary maturity, the results are not accurate when blood or meconium contaminates the amniotic fluid.

The L/S ratio remains a cumbersome and labor-intensive test despite numerous changes to the original technique. Moreover, improper handling can affect results. For these reasons, many institutions are looking to other fetal lung maturity tests that are being developed.

PHOSPHATIDYLGLYCEROL

Phosphatidylglycerol (PG) is the second most abundant phospholipid in surfactant. PG appears at about 36 weeks' gestation and increases in amount until term. In instances of diabetes complicated by premature rupture of membranes, vascular disease, or severe preeclampsia, PG may be present before 35 weeks' gestation. PG is not measured in specific concentrations; rather, the mere presence of this substance is associated with very low risk of RDS, and the absence of PG is associated with the development of RDS.

PG determination is also useful in blood-contaminated specimens. Because PG is not present in blood or vaginal fluids, its presence in a vaginal specimen is reliable for indicating lung maturity.

In recent years lung maturity has been most frequently assessed by a combination of L/S ratio and PG. Lung maturity apparently can be confirmed in most pregnancies if PG is present in conjunction with an L/S ratio of 2:1.

NURSING CARE MANAGEMENT

In women whose amniotic membranes are prematurely ruptured, a vaginal specimen is obtained for analysis. The nurse assists the certified nurse-midwife or physician by gathering appropriate supplies. Typically, a sterile speculum, a light source, a syringe, and appropriate collection tubes are needed. The nurse positions the woman for the speculum exam while providing information about the collection process. The nurse places the woman in a lithotomy position and places her legs in stirrups. If stirrups are not available, the nurse can place a bedpan upside down and position the woman with her buttocks on the bedpan to facilitate collection of the vaginal fluid. The certified nurse-midwife or physician gathers vaginal secretions with a syringe and places the specimen in a collection tube.

In women undergoing early birth for medical indications (uncontrolled preeclampsia or eclampsia or uncontrolled diabetes) when the amniotic membranes are intact, evaluation of fetal lung maturity may be obtained through amniocentesis. See previous discussion on page 568 regarding nursing care management for the woman undergoing amniocentesis.

CHAPTER REVIEW

FOCUS YOUR STUDY

- Nurses often play a key role not only in teaching families about various testing procedures, but also in providing clarity and emotional support to the woman and her family undergoing antenatal testing.

- Ultrasound offers a valuable means of assessing intrauterine fetal growth because the growth can be followed over a period of time. It is noninvasive and painless, allows the physician to study the gestation serially, is nonradiating to both the woman and her fetus, and to date has shown no known harmful effects.

- Using ultrasound, the gestational sac may be detected as early as 5 or 6 weeks after the last menstrual period. Measurement of the crown-rump length in early pregnancy is most useful for accurate dating of a pregnancy. The most important and frequently used ultrasound measurements are biparietal diameter, head circumference, abdominal circumference, and femur length.

- Maternal assessment of fetal activity is very useful as a screening procedure in evaluation of fetal status.

- A nonstress test (NST) measures fetal heart rate (FHR) during fetal activity; FHR normally increases in response to fetal activity. The desired result is a reactive test.

- A contraction stress test (CST) provides a method for observing the response of the FHR to the stress of uterine contractions. The desired result is a negative test.

- A fetal biophysical profile (BPP) includes five fetal variables (breathing movement, body movement, tone, amniotic fluid volume, and FHR reactivity). It assesses the fetus at risk for intrauterine compromise.

- Quadruple screening of AFP, hCG, diameric inhibin-A, and estriol in maternal serum provides information about the possibility of open neural tube defects and chromosome abnormalities (trisomy 18 or 21) in the fetus.

- Amniocentesis can be used to obtain amniotic fluid for testing. A variety of tests is available to evaluate the presence of disease, genetic conditions, and fetal maturity.

- Chorionic villus sampling is a procedure that obtains fetal karyotype in the first trimester. It is used to diagnose hemoglobinopathies (e.g., sickle cell anemia and alpha and some beta thalassemias), phenylketonuria, alpha antitrypsin deficiency, Down syndrome, Duchenne muscular dystrophy, and factor IX deficiency.

- Percutaneous umbilical blood sampling (PUBS) is a technique used in the second and third trimesters for fetal diagnosis, assessment, and therapy.

- The L/S ratio of the amniotic fluid can be used to assess fetal lung maturity. The presence of phosphatidylglycerol may also provide information about fetal lung maturity.

EXPLORE MediaLink

http://www.prenhall.com/davidson

NCLEX review questions, case studies, and other interactive resources for this chapter can be found on the Web Site at http://www.prenhall.com/davidson. Click on "Chapter 21" to select the activities for this chapter.

For tutorials including animations and videos, more NCLEX review questions, and an audio glossary, access the accompanying Prentice Hall Nursing MediaLink DVD-ROM in this book.

PRENTICE HALL NURSING MEDIALINK DVD-ROM
Audio Glossary
NCLEX Review
Video: *Through the Eyes of a Nurse—The Third Trimester*

COMPANION WEBSITE
Additional NCLEX Review
Case Study: *Client Undergoing Contraction Stress Test*
Care Plan Activity: *Monitoring Well-Being of a Slow-Developing Fetus*
Applications: *Fetal Assessment; Fetal Lung Maturity*
Critical Thinking

CRITICAL THINKING IN ACTION

BIOPHYSICAL PROFILE (BPP) FOR FETAL WELL-BEING

View the Critical Thinking in Action video in Chapter 21 of the DVD-ROM. Then answer the questions that follow.

Patricia Adams is a 20-year-old, married, G1, Para 0 at 36 weeks' gestation with gestational diabetes. She presents to you during her prenatal visit with a complaint of decreased fetal movement for the "last day or so." Her OB history includes a 13 lb weight gain, hematocrit of 29%, diastolic BP ranging 80–96 mm Hg, and 1+ proteinuria. A 19-week ultrasound demonstrated no fetal anatomic defects. A hemoglobin A1c at 23 weeks was normal. Patricia has had weekly NST since 28 weeks' gestation. You place Patricia on the fetal monitor for a NST. Her TPR is normal, her BP slightly elevated at 130/88. After 30 minutes you observe that the fetal heart rate baseline is 160–165, variability is decreased, and repetitive variable decelerations are occurring. No contractions are noted. The fetus is very active. You notify the physician of the fetal heart rate baseline and unsatisfactory NST. The physician orders a biophysical profile (BPP) for fetal well-being. You describe and explain the biophysical profile test to Patricia.

1. How would you describe and explain the biophysical profile test?

2. To heighten Patricia's awareness of fetal movement, how would you instruct her to do a daily fetal movement record (FMR)?

3. Explain when Patricia should contact her care provider.

4. Discuss the significance of fetal movement.

5. Explore factors that decrease fetal movements.

REFERENCES

American College of Obstetricians and Gynecologists (ACOG). (2004). *Vaginal birth after previous cesarean delivery* (ACOG Practice Bulletin No. 54). Washington, DC: Author.

Baha, M. S. (2004). Diagnosis, controversies, and management of the syndrome of hemolysis, elevated liver enzymes, and low platelet count. *Obstetrics and Gynecology, 103,* 981–991.

Bayramoglu, O., Arslan, M., Yazici, F. G., Erdem, A., Erdem, M., Bayramoglu, K., et al. (2005). Prediction of spontaneous onset of labor at term: The role of cervical length measurement and funneling of internal cervical os detected by transvaginal ultrasonography. *American Journal of Perinatology, 22*(1), 35–39.

Bennett, K. A., Crane, J. M., O'Shea, P., Lacelle, J., Hutchens, D., & Copel, J. A. (2004). First trimester ultrasound screening is effective in reducing postterm labor induction rates: A randomized controlled trial. *American Journal of Obstetrics & Gynecology, 190,* 1077–1081.

Blackburn, S. T. (2003). *Maternal, fetal, & neonatal physiology: A clinical perspective* (2nd ed.). St. Louis, MO: Saunders.

Chauhan, S. P. (2004). Amniotic fluid index vs single deepest pocket technique during modified biophysical profile: A randomized clinical trial. *American Journal of Obstetrics & Gynecology, 191*(2), 661–667.

Chauhan, S. P. (2005). Suspicion and treatment of the macrosomic fetus: A review. *American Journal of Obstetrics & Gynecology, 193*(2), 332–346.

Cito, G. (2005). Maternal position during non-stress test and fetal heart rate patterns. *Acta Obstetricia et Gynecologica Scandinavica, 84*(4), 335–338.

Cunningham, F. G., Leveno, K. J., Bloom, S. L., Hauth, J. C., Gilstrap, L. C., & Wenstrom, K. D. (2005). *Williams obstetrics* (22nd ed.). New York: McGraw-Hill.

Fahey, J. (2005). Intrauterine asphyxia: Clinical implications for providers of intrapartum care. *Journal of Midwifery & Women's Health, 50*(6), 498–506.

Farquharson, R. G., Jauniaux, E., & Exalto, N. (2005). On behalf of the ESHRE Special Interest Group for Early Pregnancy (SIGEP) updated and revised nomenclature for description of early pregnancy events. *Human Reproduction, 20*(11), 3008–3011.

Froen, J. F. (2005). Clinical practice variation in reduced fetal movements. *Tidsskr Nor Laegeforen, 125*(19), 2631–2634.

Gearhart, P. A., & Sehdev, H. M. (2005). Biophysical profile ultrasound. Retrieved May 5,
2006, from http://www.emedicine.com/radio/topic758.htm

Gojnic, M. (2004). The importance of Doppler ultrasound in delivery planning. *Clinical Experiences in Obstetrics & Gynecology, 31*(4), 282–284.

Goldstein, I. (2003). Influence of maternal carbohydrate intake on fetal movements at 14 to 16 weeks of gestation. *Prenatal Diagnosis, 23*(2), 95–97.

Hedrick, J. (2005). The lived experience of pregnancy while carrying a child with a known, nonlethal congenital abnormality. *Journal of Obstetric, Gynecologic, & Neonatal Nursing, 34*(6), 732–740.

March of Dimes. (2006). Birth defects: 8 million worldwide. Retrieved February 1, 2006, from http://www.marchofdimes.com/aboutus/15796_18678.asp

McAuliffe, F. M., Fong, K. W., Toi, A., Chitayat, D., Keating, S., & Johnson, J. (2005, September). Ultrasound detection of fetal anomalies in conjunction with first-trimester nuchal translucency screening: A feasibility study. *American Journal of Obstetrics & Gynecology, 193*(3, Pt. 2), 1260–1265.

Norem, C. T., Edgar, J., Schoen, D. L., Walton, R. C., Krieger, J., O'Keefe, T. T., et al. (2005). Routine ultrasonography compared with maternal serum alpha-fetoprotein for neural tube defect screening. *Obstetrics and Gynecology, 106,* 747–752.

Park, M. I., Hwang, J. H., Cha, K. J., Park, Y. S., & Koh, S. K (2005). Computerized analysis of fetal heart rate parameters by gestational age. *International Journal of Obstetrics & Gynecology, 74*(2),157–164.

Philip, J., Silver, R. K., Wilson, R. D., Thom, E. A., Zachary, J. M., Mohide, P., et al. (2004). Late first-trimester invasive prenatal diagnosis: Results of an international randomized trial. *Obstetrics and Gynecology, 103,* 1164–1173.

Pinette, M. G. (2005). Using fetal acoustic stimulation to shorten the biophysical profile. *Journal of Clinical Ultrasound, 33*(5), 223–225.

Reddy, U. M., & Mennuti, M. T. (2006). Incorporating first-trimester Down syndrome studies into prenatal screening: Executive summary of the National Institute of Child Health and Human Development workshop. *Obstetrics and Gynecology, 107*(1), 167–173.

Rudra, C. B., Williams, M. A., Lee, I. M., Miller, R. S., & Sorensen, T. K. (2006). Perceived exertion in physical activity and risk of gestational diabetes mellitus. *Epidemiology, 17*(1), 31–37.

Saju, D., Joy, K. Q., Rossi, D., Krugh, R., & O'Shaughnessy, W. (2005). Management of pregnancies complicated by anti-E alloimmunization. *Obstetrics and Gynecology, 105,* 24–28.

Sandelowski, M., & Barroso, J. (2005). The travesty of choosing after positive prenatal diagnosis. *Journal of Obstetric, Gynecologic, & Neonatal Nursing, 34*(3), 307–318.

Sciarra, J. J. (2004). *Gynecology & obstetrics* (Vol. 2). Philadelphia: Lippincott, Williams & Wilkins.

Seyam, Y. S., Al-Mahmeid, M. S., & Al-Tamimi, H. K. (2002). Umbilical artery Doppler flow velocimetry in intrauterine growth restriction and its relation to perinatal outcome. *International Journal of Gynaecology & Obstetrics, 77*(2), 131–137.

Singh, K., & Malhotra, N. (2004). *Step-by-step ultrasound in obstetrics.* New Delhi, India: Jaypee Brothers Medical.

Snelglove-Clarke, E., & Scott-Finlay, S. (2005). Fetal health surveillance: The use of research evidence in practice. *Lifelines, 9*(5), 400–404.

Sylvan, K., Ryding, E. L., & Rydhstroem, H. (2005). Routine ultrasound screening in the third trimester: A population-based study. *Acta Obstetricia et Gynecologica Scandinavica, 84*(12), 1154–1158.

United States National Center for Health Statistics. (2005). *Statistical abstract of the United States.* Washington, DC: Author.

Vergani, P., Roncaglia, N., Andreotti, C., Andreotti, A., Teruzzi, M., Pezzullo, J. C., et al. (2002). Prognostic value of uterine Doppler velocimetry in growth-restricted fetuses delivered near term. *American Journal of Obstetrics and Gynecology, 187*(4), 932–936.

Voxman, E. G., Tran, S., & Wing, D. A. (2002). Low amniotic fluid index as a predictor of adverse perinatal outcome. *Journal of Perinatology, 22*(4), 282–285.

Weiner, Z., Ben-Shoomo, I., Beck-Fruchter, R., Goldberg, Y., & Shaley, E. (2002). Clinical and ultrasonographic weight estimation in large for gestational age fetus. *European Journal of Obstetrics, Gynecology, & Reproductive Biology, 105*(1), 20.

Wenstrom, K. D. (2005). First-trimester Down syndrome screening: Component analysis and timing for optimal performance. *Seminars in Perinatology, 29*(4), 195–202.

UNIT
5

Birth

CHAPTER 22

Processes and Stages of Labor and Birth

Birth usually feels like a steamy kitchen—similar to holiday preparations, except the smells are different. The smell of sweat is more acrid, there are some fetid odors, there is the smell and steam rising from blood. The air is thick, pungent, fertile. It is hard not to be reminded of fresh straw and night stars. There is near and heady promise.

~Penny Armstrong & Sheryl Feldman,
A Midwife's Story~

OBJECTIVES

1. Examine the five critical factors that affect the labor process.
2. Describe the physiology of labor.
3. Discuss premonitory signs of labor.
4. Differentiate between false and true labor.
5. Describe the characteristics of the four stages of labor and their accompanying phases.
6. Describe the physiologic and psychosocial changes that are indicative of the maternal progress during each of the stages of labor.
7. Summarize maternal systemic responses to labor.
8. Describe fetal adaptations to labor.

KEY TERMS

Bloody show   586
Cardinal movements   590
Cervical dilatation   586
Crowning   590
Duration   584
Effacement   586
Engagement   581
Fetal attitude   579
Fetal lie   579
Fetal position   582
Fetal presentation   579
Fontanelle   578

Frequency   584
Intensity   584
Lightening   586
Malpresentations   579
Molding   577
Presenting part   579
Rupture of membranes
 (ROM)   587
Spontaneous rupture of
 membranes (SROM)   587
Station   581
Sutures   577

MEDIALINK

Additional resources for this content can be found on the Prentice Hall Nursing MediaLink DVD-ROM and on the Companion Website at http://www.prenhall.com/davidson. Click on "Chapter 22" to select the activities for this chapter.

In the final weeks of pregnancy, both mother and baby begin to prepare for birth. The fetus develops and grows in readiness for life outside the womb. The expectant woman undergoes various physiologic and psychosocial changes that gradually prepare her for childbirth and for the role of mother. The onset of labor begins a remarkable change in the relationship between the woman and her baby. During labor, particularly at the end, a woman instinctively knows she is engaging in one of the most important tasks she will ever do. A precious life is about to emerge. In those hours and moments the birth process may seem to carry all the power in the universe. The mother-to-be and her partner may be stretched beyond all of their normal limits of concentration, purpose, endurance, and pain. The dynamic nature of this experience is what makes the birth of a baby both a physiologic and a psychosocial transition into parenthood.

CRITICAL FACTORS IN LABOR

Five factors are important in the process of labor and birth: the birth passageway (birth canal), the passenger (fetus), the physiologic forces of labor, the position of the mother, and the woman's psychosocial considerations (Table 22–1). The progress of labor is critically dependent on the complementary relationship of these five factors. Abnormalities that af-

fect any component of these critical forces can alter the outcome of labor and jeopardize both the expectant woman and her baby. Complications during labor and birth are discussed in Chapter 26. ∞

Birth Passageway

The true pelvis and soft tissues of the cervix, vagina, and the pelvic floor form the birth passageway. The true pelvis is the critical factor of the passageway because the fetus must progress through this bony canal during the vaginal birth process. The true pelvis is divided into three sections: the inlet, the pelvic cavity (midpelvis), and the outlet. (See Chapter 10 ∞ for a discussion of each part of the pelvis, and Chapter 15 ∞ for techniques to assess the size and shape of the pelvis.)

The four classic types of pelvises are *gynecoid, android, anthropoid,* and *platypelloid.* Implications of each type for childbirth are described in Table 22–2.

Birth Passenger (Fetus)

Several aspects of the fetus's body and the way the fetus moves through the mother's birth canal are considered critical factors of the passenger that affect the outcome of labor. These interacting factors are: the fetal head, fetal attitude, fetal lie, fetal presentation, and fetal position. The placenta must also pass through the birth canal but rarely impedes the labor process, except in cases of placenta previa (see Chapter 26 ∞ for placental complications).

FETAL HEAD

The fetal head is composed of bony parts, which can either hinder childbirth or make it easier. Once the head (the least compressible and largest part of the fetus) has been born, the birth of the rest of the body is rarely delayed.

The fetal skull has three major parts: the face, the base of the skull (cranium), and the vault of the cranium (roof). The bones of the face and cranial base are well fused and essentially fixed. The base of the cranium is composed of the two temporal bones, each with a sphenoid bone and an ethmoid bone. The bones composing the vault are the two frontal bones, the two parietal bones, and the occipital bone (Figure 22–1 ◆). These bones are not fused, allowing this portion of the head to adjust as it passes through the narrow portions of the maternal pelvis. The cranial bones overlap under pressure of the powers of labor and the demands of the unyielding pelvis. This overlapping is called **molding.**

The **sutures** of the fetal skull are membranous joints that unite the cranial bones. Sutures allow for molding of the fetal head and help the clinician identify the position of the fetal head during vaginal examination. The important sutures of the cranial vault are as follows (see Figure 22–1).

- *Frontal (mitotic) suture:* Located between the two frontal bones; becomes the anterior continuation of the sagittal suture
- *Sagittal suture:* Located between the parietal bones; divides the skull into left and right halves; runs anteroposteriorly, connecting the two fontanelles

Table 22–1   CRITICAL FACTORS IN LABOR

1. Birth passage
   a. Size of the maternal pelvis (diameters of the pelvic inlet, midpelvis, and outlet)
   b. Type of maternal pelvis (gynecoid, android, anthropoid, platypelloid, or a combination)
   c. Ability of the cervix to dilate and efface and ability of the vaginal canal and the external opening of the vagina (the introitus) to distend

2. Fetus
   a. Fetal head (size and presence of molding)
   b. Fetal attitude (flexion or extension of the fetal body and extremities)
   c. Fetal lie
   d. Fetal presentation (the body part of the fetus entering the pelvis in a single or multiple pregnancy)

3. The relationship between the passage and the fetus
   a. Engagement of the fetal presenting part
   b. Station (location of fetal presenting part in the maternal pelvis)
   c. Fetal position (relationship of the presenting part to one of the four quadrants of the maternal pelvis)

4. Physiologic forces of labor
   a. Frequency, duration, and intensity of uterine contractions as the fetus moves through the passage
   b. Effectiveness of the maternal pushing effort

5. Psychosocial considerations
   a. Mental and physical preparation for childbirth
   b. Sociocultural values and beliefs
   c. Previous childbirth experience
   d. Support from significant others
   e. Emotional status

Table 22–2	IMPLICATIONS OF PELVIC TYPE FOR LABOR AND BIRTH	
Pelvic Type	**Pertinent Characteristics**	**Implications for Birth**
Gynecoid	Inlet rounded with all inlet diameters adequate Midpelvis diameters adequate with parallel side walls Outlet adequate	Favorable for vaginal birth
Android	Inlet heart-shaped with short posterior sagittal diameter Midpelvis diameters reduced Outlet capacity reduced	Not favorable for vaginal birth Descent into pelvis is slow Fetal head enters pelvis in transverse or posterior position with arrest of labor frequent
Anthropoid	Inlet oval in shape, with long anteroposterior diameter Midpelvis diameters adequate Outlet adequate	Favorable for vaginal birth
Platypelloid	Inlet oval in shape, with long transverse diameters Midpelvis diameters reduced Outlet capacity inadequate	Not favorable for vaginal birth Fetal head engages in transverse position Difficult descent through midpelvis Frequent delay of progress at outlet of pelvis

Note: Description of pelvic shape is exaggerated for easier comprehension.

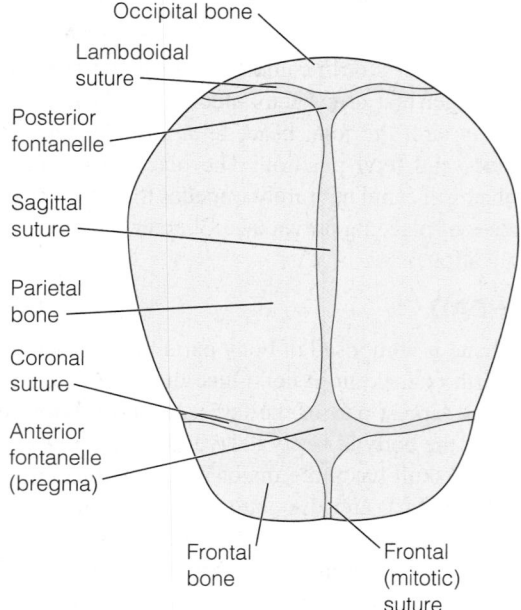

Figure 22–1 ◆ Superior view of the fetal skull.

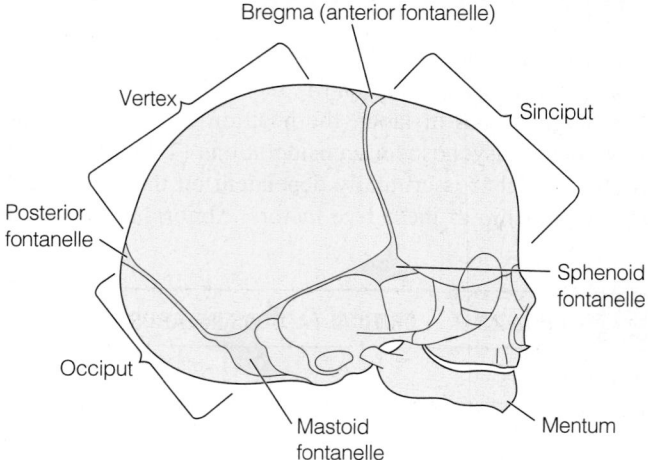

Figure 22–2 ◆ Lateral view of the fetal skull identifying the landmarks that have significance during birth.

- *Coronal sutures:* Located between the frontal and parietal bones; extend transversely left and right from the anterior fontanelle (bregma)

- *Lambdoidal suture:* Located between the two parietal bones and the occipital bone; extends transversely left and right from the posterior fontanelle

The intersection of several cranial sutures forms an irregular space that is enclosed by a membrane and called a **fontanelle.** The anterior and posterior fontanelles are clinically useful in identifying the position of the fetal head in the pelvis and in assessing the status of the newborn after birth. The greater, or anterior, fontanelle (bregma) is diamond shaped, measures 2 to 3 cm, and is situated at the junction of the sagittal, coronal, and frontal sutures. It permits growth of the brain by remaining unossified for as long as 18 months. The lesser, or pos-

terior, fontanelle is shaped like a small triangle, measures about 1 to 2 cm, and is situated at the intersection of the sagittal and lambdoidal sutures. It closes within 8 to 12 weeks after birth.

Following are several other important landmarks of the fetal skull (Figure 22–2 ◆):

- *Mentum:* The fetal chin

- *Sinciput:* The anterior area known as the brow

- *Vertex:* The area between the anterior and posterior fontanelles

- *Occiput:* The area of the fetal skull occupied by the occipital bone, beneath the posterior fontanelle

The diameters of the fetal skull vary considerably within normal limits. Some diameters shorten and others lengthen as the head is molded during labor. Fetal head diameters are measured between the various landmarks on the skull (Figure 22–3 ◆). For example, the suboccipitobregmatic diameter is the distance from the undersurface of the occiput to the center of the bregma (anterior fontanelle).

Figure 22–3 ◆ *A*, Anteroposterior diameters of the fetal skull. When the vertex of the fetus presents and the fetal head is flexed with the chin on the chest, the smallest anteroposterior diameter (suboccipitobregmatic) enters the birth canal. *B*, Transverse diameters of the fetal skull.

FETAL ATTITUDE

Fetal attitude refers to the relation of the fetal body parts to one another. Fetal attitude describes the posture the fetus assumes as it conforms to the shape of the uterine cavity. The normal attitude of the fetus is termed *general flexion*, where the head is flexed so that the chin is on the chest with the arms crossed over the chest, and the legs flexed at the knees with the thighs on the abdomen.

Changes in fetal attitude, particularly in the position of the head, cause the fetus to present larger diameters of the fetal head to the maternal pelvis. These deviations from a normal fetal attitude often contribute to a longer, more difficult labor (Figure 22–4 ◆).

FETAL LIE

Fetal lie refers to the relationship of the long, or cephalocaudal, axis (spinal column) of the fetus to the long, or cephalocaudal, axis of the mother. The fetus may assume either a longitudinal (vertical) or a transverse (horizontal) lie. A *longitudinal lie* occurs when the cephalocaudal axis of the fetus is parallel to the woman's spine. A *transverse lie* occurs when the cephalocaudal axis of the fetal spine is at a right angle to the woman's spine. A transverse lie is associated with a shoulder presentation and can lead to complications in the later stages of labor. This is discussed in detail in Chapter 26. ∞ Table 22–3 identifies the characteristics associated with a longitudinal versus a transverse fetal lie.

FETAL PRESENTATION

Fetal presentation is determined by fetal lie and refers to the body part of the fetus that enters the maternal pelvis first and leads through the birth canal during labor. The **presenting part** or the portion of the fetus that is felt through the cervix on vaginal examination determines the presentation. Fetal presentation may be cephalic (head first), breech (buttocks or feet first), or shoulder.

The most common presentation is cephalic. When this presentation occurs, labor and birth are more likely to proceed normally. Breech and shoulder presentations are associated with difficulties during labor and do not proceed as normal; there-

Figure 22–4 ◆ Fetal attitude. *A*, The attitude (or relationship of body parts) of this fetus is normal. The head is flexed forward with the chin almost resting on the chest. The arms and legs are flexed. *B*, In this view, the head is tilted to the right. Although the arms are flexed, the legs are extended.

fore, they are called **malpresentations.** (See Chapter 26 ∞ for discussion of malpresentations.)

Cephalic Presentation

The fetal head presents to the birth passage in approximately 97% of term births. The cephalic presentation can be further classified according to the degree of flexion or extension of the fetal head (attitude).

Vertex Presentation   When the presenting part is the occiput, the presentation is noted as vertex.

- Vertex is the most common type of presentation.
- The fetal head is completely flexed onto the chest.
- The smallest diameter of the fetal head (suboccipitobregmatic) presents to the maternal pelvis (Figure 22–5, A ◆).

Sinciput Presentation

- The fetal head is partially flexed.
- The occipitofrontal diameter presents to the maternal pelvis (Figure 22–5, B).
- The top of the head is the presenting part.

Table 22–3	CHARACTERISTICS ASSOCIATED WITH LONGITUDINAL VERSUS TRANSVERSE FETAL LIE		
Fetal Lie	**Attitude**	**Presenting Part**	**Landmark**
Longitudinal lie (99.5%)			
Cephalic presentation (96% to 97%)	Flexion of fetal head onto chest	Vertex (posterior part—occiput)	Occiput (O)
	Military (no flexion, no extension)	Vertex (median part)	Occiput (O)
	Partial extension	Brow	Forehead (frontum) (Fr)
	Complete extension of the head	Face	Chin (mentum) (M)
Breech presentation (3% to 4%)			
Complete	Flexed hips and knees	Buttocks	Sacrum (S)
Frank	Flexed hips, extended knees with legs against abdomen and chest	Buttocks	Sacrum (S)
Footling: single, double	Extended hips and at least one knee extended with foot in cervical canal	Feet (one or two)	Sacrum (S)
Kneeling: single, double	Extended hips, flexed knees	Knees	Sacrum (S)
Transverse or oblique lie (0.5%)			
Shoulder presentation	Variable	Shoulder, arm	Scapula (Sc or A)

Brow Presentation

- The fetal head is partially extended.
- The occipitomental diameter, the largest anteroposterior diameter, is presented to the maternal pelvis (Figure 22–5, *C* ◆).

Face Presentation

- The fetal head is hyperextended (complete extension).
- The submentobregmatic diameter presents to the maternal pelvis (Figure 22–5, *D* ◆).
- The face is the presenting part.

Breech Presentation

A breech presentation indicates that the presenting part is the lower extremities or buttocks. Breech presentations occur in 3% of all term births (Cunningham, Leveno, Bloom et al., 2005). These presentations are classified according to the attitude of the fetus's hips and knees. In all variations of the breech presentation the sacrum (the bone on the buttocks that is felt when palpating) is the landmark.

Complete Breech

- The fetal knees and hips are both flexed, the thighs are on the abdomen, and the calves are on the posterior aspect of the thighs.
- The buttocks and feet of the fetus present to the maternal pelvis.

Frank Breech

- The fetal hips are flexed, and the knees are extended.
- The buttocks of the fetus present to the maternal pelvis.

Footling Breech

- The fetal hips and legs are extended.
- The feet of the fetus present to the maternal pelvis.
- In a single footling one foot presents; in a double footling both feet present.

A Suboccipitobregmatic diameter

B Occipitofrontal diameter

C Occipitomental diameter

D Submentobregmatic diameter

Figure 22–5 ◆ Cephalic presentation. *A,* Vertex presentation. Complete flexion of the head allows the suboccipitobregmatic diameter to present to the pelvis. *B,* Military (median vertex) presentation with no flexion or extension. The occipitofrontal diameter presents to the pelvis. *C,* Brow presentation. The fetal head is in partial (halfway) extension. The occipitomental diameter, which is the largest diameter of the fetal head, presents to the pelvis. *D,* Face presentation. The fetal head is in complete extension, and the submentobregmatic diameter presents to the pelvis.

Shoulder Presentation

When the fetal shoulder is the presenting part, the fetus is in a transverse lie and the acromion process of the scapula is the landmark.

Relationship of Maternal Pelvis and Presenting Part

The third critical factor, in addition to the birth passage and fetus, is the relationship between these two factors. When assessing the relationship of the maternal pelvis and the presenting part of the fetal body, the nurse considers fetal position, station, and engagement.

ENGAGEMENT

Engagement of the presenting part occurs when the largest diameter of the presenting part reaches or passes through the pelvic inlet (Figure 22–6 *C* ◆). When the fetal head is flexed, the biparietal diameter is the largest dimension of the fetal skull to pass through the pelvic inlet in a cephalic presentation. The intertrochanteric diameter (transverse diameter between the right and left trochanter) is the largest to pass through the inlet in a breech presentation.

Engagement can be determined by vaginal examination. In primigravidas, engagement usually occurs 2 weeks before term.

Multiparas, however, may experience engagement several weeks before the onset of labor or during the process of labor.

The presenting part is said to be *floating* (or *ballottable*) when it is freely movable above the inlet (see Figure 22–6 *A* ◆). When the presenting part begins to descend into the inlet, before engagement has truly occurred, it is said to be dipping into the pelvis (see Figure 22–6 *B* ◆).

STATION

Station refers to the relationship of the presenting part to an imaginary line drawn between the ischial spines of the maternal pelvis. In a normal pelvis the ischial spines mark the narrowest diameter through which the fetus must pass. These spines are not sharp protrusions but rather blunted prominences at the midpelvis. The ischial spines as a landmark have been designated as zero station (Figure 22–7 ◆). If the presenting part is higher than the ischial spines, a negative number is assigned, noting centimeters above zero station. Station −5 is at the inlet, and station +4 is at the outlet. If the presenting part can be seen at the woman's perineum, birth will occur momentarily. During labor the presenting part should move progressively from the negative stations to the midpelvis at zero station and into the positive stations. Failure of the presenting part to descend in the presence of strong contractions may be due to disproportion between the maternal pelvis and fetal presenting part.

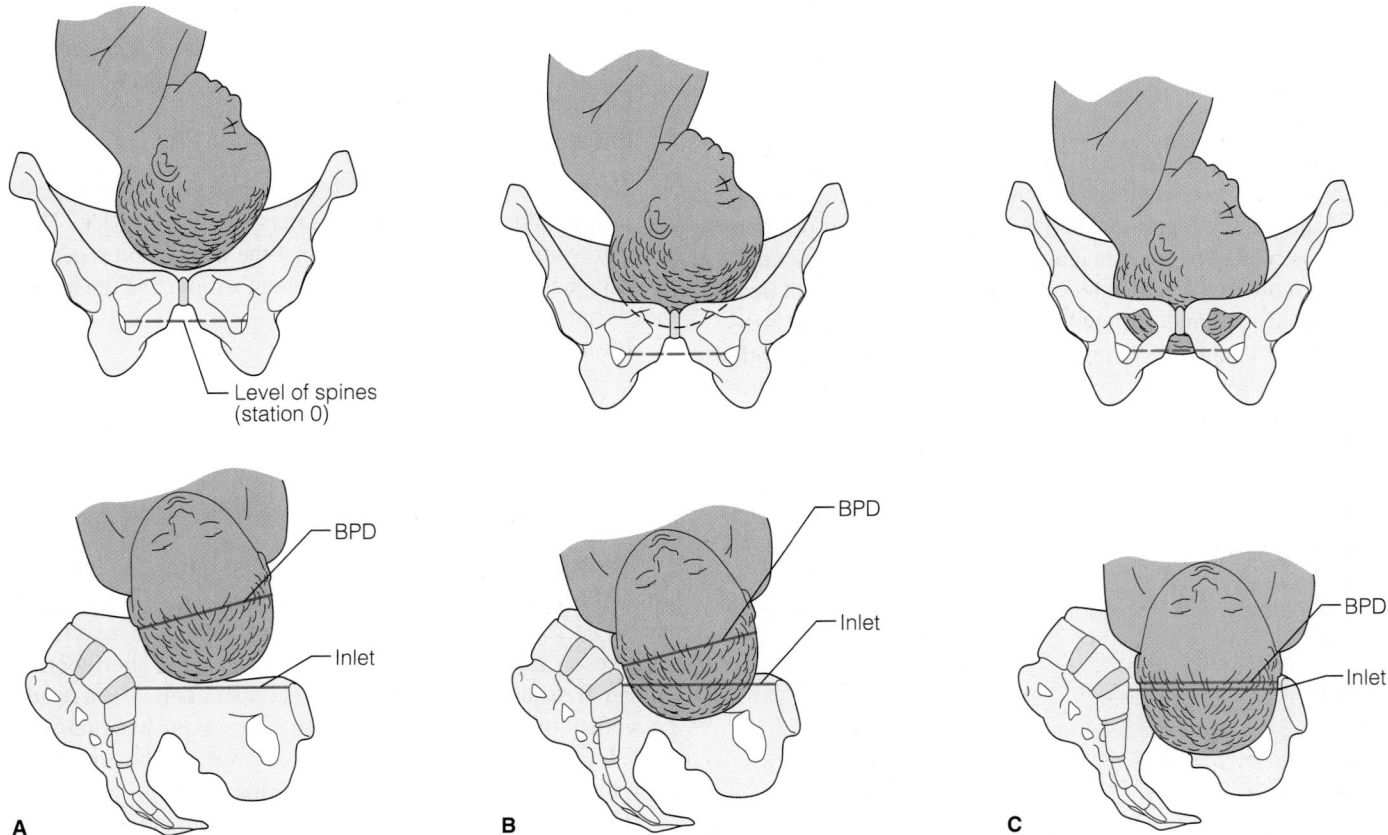

Level of spines (station 0)

BPD

Inlet

BPD

Inlet

BPD

Inlet

A   B   C

Figure 22–6 ◆ Process of engagement in cephalic presentation. *A,* Floating. The fetal head is directed down toward the pelvis but can still easily move away from the inlet. *B,* Dipping. The fetal head dips into the inlet but can be moved away by exerting pressure on the fetus. *C,* Engaged. The biparietal diameter (BPD) of the fetal head is in the inlet of the pelvis. In most instances, the presenting part (occiput) will be at the level of the ischial spines (0 station).

cm
−5
−4
−3
−2
−1
0   ←— Spine —→
+1
+2
+3
+4
+5

Figure 22–7 ◆ Measuring the station of the fetal head while it is descending. In this view the station is 22/23.

FETAL POSITION

Fetal position refers to the relationship of the landmark on the presenting fetal part to the anterior, posterior, or sides (right or left) of the maternal pelvis. The landmark on the fetal presenting part is related to four imaginary quadrants of the maternal pelvis: left anterior, right anterior, left posterior, and right posterior. These quadrants designate where the presenting part is directed. If the landmark is directed toward the center of the side of the pelvis, fetal position is designated as transverse, rather than anterior or posterior.

The landmark chosen for vertex presentations is the occiput, and the landmark for face presentations is the mentum. In breech presentations the sacrum is the designated landmark, and the acromion process on the scapula is the landmark in shoulder presentations.

In summary, three notations are used to describe the fetal position:

1. Right (R) or left (L) side of the maternal pelvis

2. The landmark of the fetal presenting part: occiput (O), mentum (M), sacrum (S), or acromion (scapula[Sc]) process (A)

3. Anterior (A), posterior (P), or transverse (T), depending on whether the landmark is in the front, back, or side of the pelvis

The abbreviations of these notations help the healthcare team communicate the fetal position. Thus, when the fetal oc-

ciput is directed toward the back and to the left of the passage, the abbreviation used is LOP (left-occiput-posterior). The following is a list of positions for various fetal presentations, some of which are illustrated in Figure 22–8 ◆.

Positions in vertex presentation:

ROA Right-occiput-anterior

ROT Right-occiput-transverse

ROP Right-occiput-posterior

LOA Left-occiput-anterior

LOT Left-occiput-transverse

LOP Left-occiput-posterior

Positions in face presentation:

RMA Right-mentum-anterior

RMT Right-mentum-transverse

RMP Right-mentum-posterior

LMA Left-mentum-anterior

LMT Left-mentum-transverse

LMP Left-mentum-posterior

Positions in breech presentation:

RSA Right-sacrum-anterior

RST Right-sacrum-transverse

RSP Right-sacrum-posterior

LSA Left-sacrum-anterior

LST Left-sacrum-transverse

LSP Left-sacrum-posterior

The term *dorsal* (D) is added when denoting the fetal position in a shoulder presentation; it refers to the fetal back. Thus the abbreviation RADA indicates that the acromion process of the scapula is directed toward the woman's right, and the fetus's back is anterior.

Positions in shoulder presentation:

RADA Right-acromion-dorsal-anterior

RADP Right-acromion-dorsal-posterior

LADA Left-acromion-dorsal-anterior

LADP Left-acromion-dorsal-posterior

The fetal position influences labor and birth. For example, the fetal head presents a larger diameter in a posterior position than in an anterior position. A posterior position increases the pressure on the maternal sacral nerves, causing the laboring woman to experience backache and pelvic pressure. As a result, the woman may bear down or feel the urge to push earlier than needed. In addition, the second stage of labor may be prolonged when the fetal head remains in a posterior position.

The most common fetal position is occiput anterior. When this position occurs, the labor and birth are more likely to proceed normally. Positions other than occiput anterior are more frequently associated with problems during labor; therefore, they are called malpositions. (See Chapter 26 ∞ for discussion of malpositions and their management).

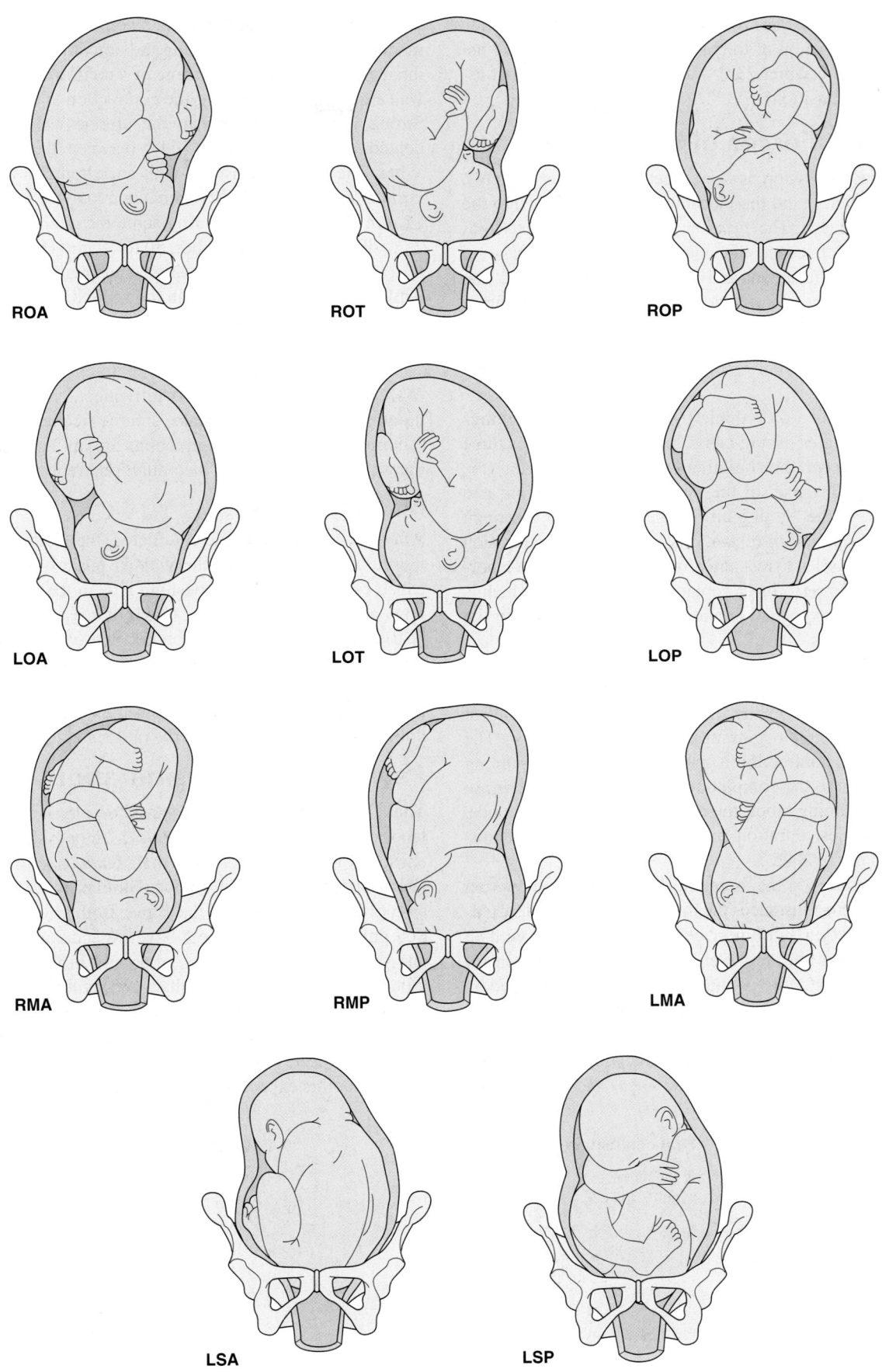

ROA   ROT   ROP

LOA   LOT   LOP

RMA   RMP   LMA

LSA   LSP

Figure 22–8 ◆ Categories of presentation.
SOURCE: Courtesy of Ross Laboratories, Columbus, OH.

Assessment techniques to determine fetal position include inspection and palpation of the maternal abdomen and vaginal examination. (See Chapter 23 ∞ for further discussion of assessment of fetal position).

Physiologic Forces of Labor

Primary and secondary forces work together to deliver the fetus, the fetal membranes, and the placenta from the uterus into the external environment. The *primary force* is uterine muscular contractions, which cause the changes of the first stage of labor—complete effacement and dilatation of the cervix. The *secondary force* is the use of abdominal muscles to push during the second stage of labor. The pushing adds to the primary power after full dilatation.

CONTRACTIONS

Uterine contractions are rhythmic tightenings and shortenings of the uterine muscles during labor. Each contraction has three phases: (1) *increment,* the "building up" of the contraction (the longest phase); (2) *acme,* or the peak of the contraction; and (3) *decrement,* or the "letting up" of the contraction. Between contractions is a period of relaxation. This period of relaxation allows uterine muscles to rest and provides respite for the laboring woman. It also restores uteroplacental circulation, which is important to fetal oxygenation and adequate circulation in the uterine blood vessels.

When describing uterine contractions during labor, caregivers use the terms *frequency, duration,* and *intensity.*

Frequency refers to the time between the beginning of one contraction and the beginning of the next contraction. The **duration** of each contraction is measured from the beginning of the contraction to the completion of the contraction (Figure 22–9 ◆). In beginning labor, the duration is 30 to 40 seconds. As labor continues, duration increases to 30 to 90 seconds (Cunningham et al., 2005).

Intensity refers to the strength of the uterine contraction during acme. In most instances the intensity is estimated by palpating the contraction, but it may be measured directly with an intrauterine catheter attached to an electronic fetal monitor. Intensity of uterine contractions cannot be accurately measured by external monitoring with an electronic fetal monitor, because several variables affect the external monitor, including maternal weight, specifically the amount of adipose tissue, and positioning of the monitor on the maternal abdomen. When estimating

intensity by palpation, the nurse determines whether it is mild, moderate, or strong by judging the amount of indentability of the uterine wall during the acme of a contraction. If the uterine wall can be indented easily, the contraction is considered mild. Strong intensity exists when the uterine wall cannot be indented. Moderate intensity falls between these two ranges. When intensity is measured with an intrauterine catheter, the normal resting tonus (between contractions) is about 10 to 12 mm Hg of pressure. During acme the intensity ranges from 25 to 40 mm Hg in early labor, 50 to 70 mm Hg in active labor, 80 to 100 mm Hg during transition, and greater than 100 mm Hg while the woman is pushing in the second stage (Cunningham et al., 2005). (See Chapter 23 ∞ for further discussion of assessment techniques).

At the beginning of labor the contractions are usually mild, of short duration, and relatively infrequent. As labor progresses, duration and intensity increase, and the frequency is every 2 to 3 minutes. Because the contractions are involuntary, the laboring woman cannot control their duration, frequency, or intensity.

BEARING DOWN

After the cervix is completely dilated, the maternal abdominal musculature contracts as the woman pushes. This pushing is called *bearing down.* The pushing aids in the expulsion of the fetus and the placenta. If the cervix is not completely dilated, bearing down can cause cervical edema (which retards dilatation), possible tearing and bruising of the cervix, and maternal exhaustion. The combined involuntary pressure of the uterine contractions and the voluntary muscle contractions of the abdomen force the fetus toward the outlet so birth can occur.

Psychosocial Considerations

Thus far, the discussion has focused on physical influences on labor outcomes. But the final critical factor is the parents' psychosocial readiness, including their fears, anxieties, birth fantasies, and level of social support. Similar psychosocial factors affect both the mother and the father. Both are making a transition into a new role, and both have expectations of themselves and their partner during the labor and birth experience. Although many prospective mothers and fathers attend childbirth preparation classes, they still tend to be concerned about what labor will be like, whether they will each be able to perform the way they expect, whether the discomfort and pain will be more than the mother expects or can cope with, whether the father can

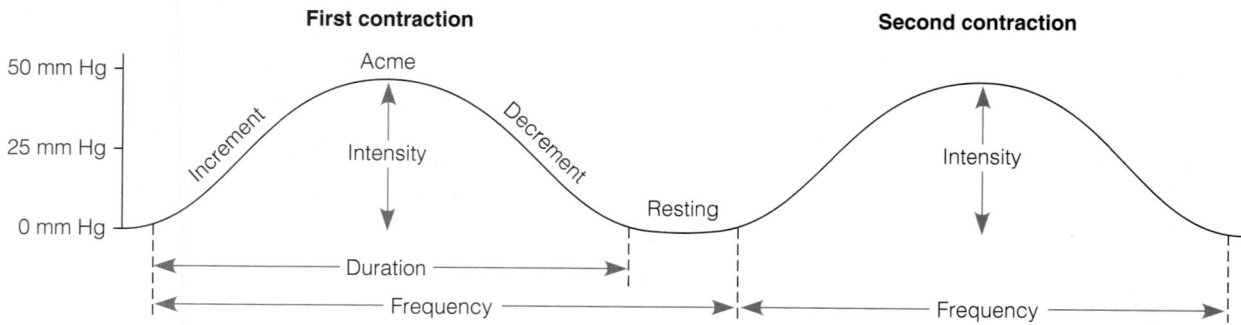

Figure 22–9 ◆ Characteristics of uterine contractions.

provide helpful support, and whether they can maintain a sense of control and be advocates for themselves (Goodman, 2005). In addition, both partners face an irrevocable event—the birth of a new family member—and, consequently, disruption of lifestyle, relationships, and self-image.

Many women have preconceived ideas about what birth should be like and some fear "losing control" of their body functions, emotions, or ability to handle the pain associated with labor. Women whose birth experiences do not meet their preconceived ideas may feel loss and disappointment. They may also feel that they have failed to live up to the expectations of friends, family, and peers.

Various factors influence a woman's reaction to labor and contribute to a positive birth experience (Table 22–4). Her accomplishment of the tasks of pregnancy, usual coping mechanisms in response to stressful life events, previous experiences, support system, preparation for childbirth, and cultural influences are all significant factors (Mullaly, 2004).

Many women have dreams about their birth, their infant, and their early parenting experiences. Dreaming and fantasizing about the unborn baby is a developmental process of pregnancy (Ross, Murray, & Steiner, 2005). The nurse can encourage the woman to share her dreams and fantasies and use them as a tool to examine the woman's expectations, fears, and coping mechanisms. This can assist the woman in forming a maternal role and facilitate bonding with her fetus.

When a woman is facing labor, especially for the first time, she may worry about her ability to withstand the pain of contractions. Some women may place great emphasis on withstanding the pain of childbirth "stoically" without medication, crying, moaning, or making other sounds. The nurse's role is to help the childbearing family explore options and identify interventions to help each woman cope with the discomfort of labor in a way that is acceptable to her.

The laboring woman's support system may also influence the course of labor and birth. Although some women may prefer not to have a support person or family member with them, for many women the presence of the father and other significant persons (especially the nurse) tends to have a positive effect. A labor partner's presence at the bedside provides a means to enhance communication and to demonstrate feelings of love. Communication needs may include talking and the use of affectionate and understanding words from the partner. Showing love may take the form of holding hands, hugging, or touching (Goodman, 2005).

How the woman views the birth experience in hindsight may have implications for mothering behaviors. A significant relationship exists between the birth experience and mothering behaviors. It appears that any activities by the expectant woman or by healthcare providers that enhance the birth experience will be beneficial to the mother-baby connection. The father's experience of childbirth and his opportunities for bonding may have important implications for fathering as well (Goodman, 2005).

PHYSIOLOGY OF LABOR

In addition to considering the five critical factors affecting the progress of labor and birth, it is essential to explore the physiology of the normal labor experience.

Possible Causes of Labor Onset

Labor usually begins between the 38th and the 42nd week of gestation, when the fetus is mature and ready for birth. Despite medical advances, there is still no full understanding of the biochemical substances and interactions that stimulate labor and birth. Some important aspects have been identified. For example, estrogen is known to stimulate uterine muscle contractions to permit softening, stretching, and eventual thinning of the cervix. Collagen fibers in the cervix are broken down by the action of enzymes such as collagenase and elastase. As the collagen fibers change, their ability to bind is decreased because of increasing amounts of hyaluronic acid (which loosely binds collagen fibrils) and decreasing amounts of dermatan sulfate (which tightly binds collagen fibrils). There is also an increase in the water content of the cervix. All these changes result in a weakening and softening of the cervix, which facilitates cervical stretching and effacement.

Hypotheses have also been formed about the roles of progesterone withdrawal, of prostaglandin, and of corticotropin-releasing hormone.

PROGESTERONE WITHDRAWAL HYPOTHESIS

Progesterone produced by the placenta relaxes uterine smooth muscle by interfering with conduction of impulses from one cell to the next. For this reason, the uterus is usually without coordinated contractions during pregnancy. Biochemical changes toward the end of gestation result in decreased availability of progesterone to myometrial cells. The decrease in availability may be associated with a yet-unknown antiprogestin that inhibits the relaxant effect on the uterus but allows other progesterone actions such as lactogenesis (Challis, 2004).

PROSTAGLANDIN HYPOTHESIS

Although the exact relationship between prostaglandin and the onset of labor is not yet established, the effect is clinically demonstrated by the successful induction of labor after vaginal

Table 22–4   FACTORS ASSOCIATED WITH A POSITIVE BIRTH EXPERIENCE

Motivation for the pregnancy

Attendance at childbirth education classes

A sense of competence or mastery

Self-confidence and self-esteem

Positive relationship with mate

Maintaining control during labor

Support from mate or other person during labor

Not being left alone in labor

Trust in the medical/nursing staff

Having personal control of breathing patterns, comfort measures

Choosing a physician/certified nurse-midwife who has a similar philosophy of care

Receiving clear information regarding procedures

MEDIALINK   Physiology of Labor

application of prostaglandin E. In addition, preterm labor may be stopped by using an inhibitor of prostaglandin synthesis such as indomethacin (Challis, 2004).

The amnion and decidua are the focus of research on the source of prostaglandins. Once prostaglandin is produced, stimuli for its synthesis may include rising levels of estrogen, decreased availability of progesterone, increased levels of oxytocin or response to oxytocin, platelet-activating factor, and endothelin-1 (Challis, 2004).

CORTICOTROPIN-RELEASING HORMONE HYPOTHESIS

Corticotropin-releasing hormone (CRH) is also a focus for researchers. Its possible role in onset of labor is suggested by the fact that CRH concentration increases throughout pregnancy, with a sharp increase at term. Also, there is an increase in plasma CRH before preterm labor, and CRH levels are elevated in multiple gestations. Finally, CRH is known to stimulate the synthesis of prostaglandin F and prostaglandin E by amnion cells (Vogel, Thorsen, Currey et al., 2005).

Myometrial Activity

In true labor the uterus divides into two portions. This division is known as the *physiologic retraction ring.* The upper portion, which is the contractile segment, becomes progressively thicker as labor advances. The lower portion, which includes the lower uterine segment and cervix, is passive. As labor continues, the lower uterine segment expands and thins out.

With each contraction, the muscles of the upper uterine segment shorten and exert a longitudinal traction on the cervix, causing effacement. **Effacement** is the taking up (or drawing up) of the internal os and the cervical canal into the uterine side walls. The cervix changes progressively from a long, thick structure to a structure that is tissue-paper thin (Figure 22–10 ◆). In primigravidas effacement usually precedes dilatation. The uterine muscle remains shorter and thicker and does not return to its original length. This phenomenon is known as *brachystasis.* The space in the uterine cavity decreases as a result of brachystasis, and this places downward pressure on the fetus (Cunningham et al., 2005).

The uterus elongates with each contraction, decreasing the horizontal diameter. This elongation causes a straightening of the fetal body, pressing the part of the fetus in the upper portion of the uterus against the fundus and thrusting the presenting part down toward the lower uterine segment and the cervix. The pressure exerted by the fetus is called *fetal axis pressure.* As the uterus elongates, the longitudinal muscle fibers are pulled upward over the presenting part. This action and the hydrostatic pressure of the fetal membranes cause **cervical dilatation.** The cervical os and cervical canal widen from less than 1 cm to approximately 10 cm, allowing birth of the fetus. When the cervix is completely dilated and retracted up into the lower uterine segment, it can no longer be palpated.

The round ligament pulls the fundus forward, aligning the fetus with the bony pelvis. This facilitates engagement of the presenting part. Pressure exerted on the cervix by the presenting part aids in both effacement and cervical dilatation (Simkin & Ancheta, 2005).

Musculature Changes in the Pelvic Floor

The levator ani muscle and fascia of the pelvic floor draw the rectum and vagina upward and forward with each contraction, along the curve of the pelvic floor. As the fetal head descends to the pelvic floor, the pressure of the presenting part causes the perineal structure, which was once 5 cm in thickness, to change to a structure less than 1 cm thick. A normal physiologic anesthesia is produced as a result of the decreased blood supply to the area. The anus everts, exposing the interior rectal wall as the fetal head descends forward (Cunningham et al., 2005).

Premonitory Signs of Labor

Most primigravidas and many multiparas experience one or more of the following signs and symptoms of impending labor.

LIGHTENING

Lightening describes the effects that occur when the fetus begins to settle into the pelvic inlet (engagement). With fetal descent, the uterus moves downward, and the fundus no longer presses on the diaphragm, which eases breathing.

However, with increased downward pressure of the presenting part, the woman may notice the following (Wheeler, 2002):

- Leg cramps or pains due to pressure on the nerves that course through the obturator foramen in the pelvis
- Increased pelvic pressure
- Increased venous stasis, leading to edema in the lower extremities
- Increased urinary frequency
- Increased vaginal secretions resulting from congestion of the vaginal mucous membranes

BRAXTON HICKS CONTRACTIONS

Before the onset of labor, *Braxton Hicks contractions*—the irregular, intermittent contractions that have been occurring throughout the pregnancy—may become uncomfortable. The pain seems to be in the abdomen and groin but may feel like the "drawing" sensations experienced by some women with dysmenorrhea. When these contractions are strong enough for the woman to believe she is in labor, she is said to be in false labor.

CERVICAL CHANGES

Considerable change occurs in the cervix during the prenatal and intrapartal period. At the beginning of pregnancy the cervix is rigid and firm, and it must soften so that it can stretch and dilate to allow fetal passage. This softening of the cervix, called *ripening,* is under the influence of hormonal factors discussed shortly.

BLOODY SHOW

During pregnancy, cervical secretions accumulate in the cervical canal to form a barrier called a *mucous plug.* With softening and effacement of the cervix, the mucous plug is often expelled, resulting in a small amount of blood loss from the exposed cervical capillaries. The resulting pink-tinged secretions are called **bloody show.**

Amniotic fluid
Amniotic sac
Internal os
Cavity of cervix
External os
A

Internal os
Amniotic fluid
External os
B

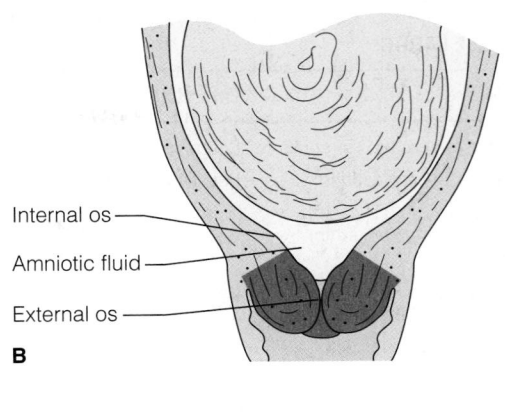

Internal os
Amniotic fluid
External os
C

Internal os
External os
Amniotic fluid
D

Figure 22–10 ◆ Effacement of the cervix in the primigravida. *A,* At the beginning of labor, there is no cervical effacement or dilatation. The fetal head is cushioned by amniotic fluid. *B,* Beginning cervical effacement. As the cervix begins to efface, more amniotic fluid collects below the fetal head. *C,* Cervix is about one-half (50%) effaced and slightly dilated. The increasing amount of amniotic fluid below the fetal head exerts hydrostatic pressure on the cervix. *D,* Complete effacement and dilatation.

Bloody show is considered a sign of impending labor, usually within 24 to 48 hours. Vaginal examination that includes manipulation of the cervix may also result in a blood-tinged discharge, which is sometimes confused with bloody show. However, this discharge is typically brownish in color and is not accompanied by the mucous plug.

RUPTURE OF MEMBRANES

In approximately 12% of women, the amniotic membranes rupture before the onset of labor. This is called **rupture of membranes (ROM).** After membranes rupture, 80% of women will experience spontaneous labor within 24 hours. If membranes rupture and labor does not begin spontaneously within 12 to 24 hours, labor may be induced to avoid infection (once the membranes have ruptured there is an open pathway into the uterine cavity). An induction of labor is done only if the pregnancy is near term.

At the beginning of labor, the amniotic membranes bulge through the cervix in the shape of a cone. When the membranes rupture, the amniotic fluid may be expelled in large amounts. **Spontaneous rupture of membranes (SROM)** generally occurs at the height of an intense contraction with a gush of the fluid out of the vagina. If engagement has not occurred, the danger exists that the umbilical cord may be expelled with the fluid (prolapsed cord). In addition, because of these potential problems, the woman is advised to notify her certified nurse-midwife or physician and proceed to the hospital or birthing center. In some instances the fluid is expelled in small amounts and may be confused with episodes of urinary incontinence associated with urinary urgency, coughing, or sneezing. The discharge should be checked to ascertain its source and to determine further action. (See Chapter 23 ∞ for assessment techniques). In some instances, the membranes are ruptured by the certified nurse-midwife or physician, using an instrument called an amniohook. This procedure is called *amniotomy* or *artificial rupture of membranes (AROM)* and is discussed in Chapter 27. ∞

SUDDEN BURST OF ENERGY

Some women report a sudden burst of energy approximately 24 to 48 hours before labor. The cause of the energy spurt is unknown. In prenatal teaching the nurse should warn prospective mothers not to overexert themselves during this energy burst so that they will not be excessively tired when labor begins.

OTHER SIGNS

Other premonitory signs include the following:

- Weight loss of 2.2 to 6.6 kg (1 to 3 lb) resulting from fluid loss and electrolyte shifts produced by changes in estrogen and progesterone levels

- Increased backache and sacroiliac pressure from the influence of relaxin hormone on the pelvic joints

- Diarrhea, indigestion, or nausea and vomiting just before the onset of labor

The causes of these signs are unknown.

Table 22–5   COMPARISON OF TRUE LABOR AND FALSE LABOR

True Labor	False Labor
Contractions are at regular intervals.	Contractions are irregular.
Intervals between contractions gradually shorten.	Usually no change.
Contractions increase in duration and intensity.	Usually no change.
Discomfort begins in back and radiates around to abdomen.	Discomfort is usually in abdomen.
Intensity usually increases with walking.	Walking has no effect on or lessens contractions.
Cervical dilatation and effacement are progressive.	No change.
Contractions do not decrease with rest or warm tub bath.	Rest and warm tub baths lessen contractions.

Differences Between True Labor and False Labor

The contractions of true labor produce progressive dilatation and effacement of the cervix. They occur regularly and increase in frequency, duration, and intensity. The discomfort of true labor contractions usually starts in the back and radiates around to the abdomen. The pain is not relieved by ambulation (in fact, walking may intensify the pain) or by resting.

The contractions of false labor do not produce progressive cervical effacement and dilatation. Classically, they are irregular and do not increase in frequency, duration, and intensity. The contractions may be perceived as a hardening or "balling up" without discomfort, or discomfort may occur mainly in the lower abdomen and groin. The discomfort may be relieved by ambulation, changes of position, resting, or a hot bath or shower (King, 2002). A comparison between true labor and false labor is provided in Table 22–5.

NURSE'S RESPONSE TO FALSE LABOR

During the third trimester, the woman will find it helpful to learn the characteristics of true labor contractions as well as the premonitory signs of ensuing labor. The nurse informs the woman that false labor is common and many times cannot be distinguished from true labor except by vaginal examination. She must feel free to come in for accurate assessment of labor and should be counseled not to feel foolish if the labor is false.

In addition, false labor can last for several hours and can be exhausting. The nurse can suggest interventions to decrease the anxiety and physical discomforts associated with false labor.

STAGES OF LABOR AND BIRTH

To assist caregivers, common terms have been developed as benchmarks to subdivide the process of labor into *stages* and *phases* of labor. It is important to note, however, that these represent theoretic separations in the process. A laboring woman will not usually experience distinct differences from one to the other. The first stage begins with the beginning of true labor and ends when the cervix is completely dilated at 10 cm. The second stage begins with complete dilatation and ends with the birth of the infant. The third stage begins with the birth of the infant and ends with the expulsion of the placenta.

Some clinicians identify a fourth stage of labor. During this stage, which lasts 1 to 4 hours after expulsion of the placenta, the uterus effectively contracts to control bleeding at the placental site (Cunningham et al., 2005). Nursing care of the laboring woman is discussed in Chapter 24. ∞

The following discussion characterizes the four stages and their accompanying phases.

First Stage

The first stage of labor is divided into the latent, active, and transition phases (Table 22–6). Each phase of labor is characterized by physical and psychologic changes.

LATENT PHASE

The latent phase begins with the onset of regular contractions. As the cervix begins to dilate it also effaces, although little or no fetal descent is evident. For a woman in her first labor (nullipara) the latent phase averages 8.6 hours but should not exceed 20 hours. The latent phase in multiparas averages 5.3 hours but should not exceed 14 hours (Cunningham et al., 2005).

Table 22–6   CHARACTERISTICS OF LABOR

	First Stage			Second Stage
	Latent Phase	**Active Phase**	**Transition Phase**	
Nullipara	8.6 hr	4.6 hr	3.6 hr	Up to 3 hr
Multipara	5.3 hr	2.4 hr	Variable	0–30 min
Cervical dilatation	0–3 cm	4–7 cm	8–10 cm	
Contractions				
Frequency	Every 3–30 min	Every 2–5 min	Every 1½–2 min	Every 1½–2 min
Duration	20–40 sec	40–60 sec	60–90 sec	60–90 sec
Intensity	Begin as mild and progress to moderate; 25–40 mm Hg by intrauterine pressure catheter (IUPC)	Begin as moderate and progress to strong, 50–70 mm Hg by IUPC	Strong by palpation; 70–90 mm Hg by IUPC	Strong by palpation; 70–100 mm Hg by IUPC

RESEARCH IN PRACTICE

THE IMPACT OF PARITY ON COURSE OF LABOR IN A CONTEMPORARY POPULATION

What is this study about? There is considerable evidence that the length of labor for multiparous women is shorter than that of their nulliparous counterparts. However, most studies documenting the length of labor were conducted more than 20 years ago, and so do not reflect contemporary labor management, for example, induction of labor, epidural anesthesia, elective cesarean delivery, and the rarity of forceps use. Additionally, although it is commonly assumed that having more babies leads to even shorter labors, this relationship had not been statistically documented. These researchers sought to determine if the length of labor has changed with contemporary labor management, and if being parous beyond the first birth is related to a continuing shortened length of labor.

How was this study done? A retrospective analysis of data retrieved from the electronic obstetrics record system of a single Delaware hospital was conducted. All mothers who were low risk and delivered a normal, full-term, singleton delivery between January 2002 and March 2004 were included. The researchers computed the median duration of labor for each 1 centimeter of dilation for each of four groups: parity = 0,1,2,3, respectively. The authors used a data analysis technique that is specific for analyzing the time to an event to determine the median length of time for each stage of labor and to test for differences between groups.

What were the results of the study? All groups of multiparous mothers had a faster median length of labor from 4 to 10 centimeters when compared with nulliparous mothers. The median length of active labor was 383 minutes for nulliparas, 293 minutes for parity = 1, 300 minutes for parity = 2, and 313 minutes for mothers whose parity was 3 or greater. All of these median times are longer than those reported in the literature between 1950 and 1990. The researchers suggest that this may be due to the larger number of obese and extremely obese women in the general obstetric population, who have documented longer lengths of labor than women of average weight. Multiparas also had a significantly shorter second stage than nulliparas. There were no significant differences in either active labor or the second stage among the multiparous groups, however. It does not appear that additional childbearing beyond the first baby has an effect on the progression of labor.

What additional questions might I have? These findings were from a tertiary care teaching hospital that serves a large geographic area. Will these findings transfer to a primary care setting? Are these findings different for women undergoing spontaneous versus induced labor?

How can I use this study? Women approaching delivery often want to know what to expect in terms of the length of their impending labor. These findings can help the nurse counsel patients to have realistic expectations about the length of time they will be in active labor, regardless of parity.

Vahrratian, A., Hoffman, M., Troendle, J., & Zhang, J. (2006). The impact of parity on course of labor in a contemporary population. *Birth, 33*(1), 12–17.

Uterine contractions become established during the latent phase and increase in frequency, duration, and intensity. They may start as mild contractions lasting 20 to 40 seconds with a frequency of 3 to 30 minutes. They average 25 to 50 mm Hg by intrauterine pressure catheter (IUPC) at acme (Cunningham et al., 2005).

In the early or latent phase of the first stage of labor, contractions are usually mild. The woman feels able to cope with the discomfort. She may be relieved that labor has finally started. Although she may be anxious, she is able to recognize and express those feelings of anxiety. The woman is often talkative and smiling and is eager to talk about herself and answer questions. Excitement is high, and her partner or other support person is often as elated as she is.

ACTIVE PHASE

When the woman enters the early *active phase*, her anxiety tends to increase as she senses the intensification of contractions and pain. She begins to fear a loss of control and may use a variety of coping mechanisms. Some women exhibit a decreased ability to cope and a sense of helplessness. Women who have support persons and family available may experience greater satisfaction and less anxiety than those without support. During this phase the cervix dilates from about 4 to 7 cm. Fetal descent is progressive. The cervical dilatation should be at least 1.2 cm per hour in nulliparas and 1.5 cm per hour in multiparas (Cunningham et al., 2005).

TRANSITION PHASE

The transition phase is the last part of the first stage. When the woman enters the transition phase, she may demonstrate significant anxiety. She becomes acutely aware of the increasing force and intensity of the contractions. She may become restless, frequently changing position. By the time the woman enters the transition phase, she is often inner directed and tired. She may fear being left alone at the same time the support person may be feeling the need for a break. The nurse should reassure the woman that she will not be left alone. It is crucial that the nurse be available as a relief support at this time and keep the woman informed about where her labor support people are, if they leave the room.

Cervical dilatation slows as it progresses from 8 to 10 cm and the rate of fetal descent increases. The average rate of descent is at least 1 cm per hour in nulliparas and 2 cm per hour in multiparas. The transition phase should not be longer than 3 hours for nulliparas and 1 hour for multiparas (Cunningham et al., 2005). The total duration of the first stage may be increased by approximately 1 hour if epidural anesthesia is used.

During the active and transition phases, contractions become more frequent, are longer in duration, and increase in intensity. At the beginning of the active phase the contractions have a frequency of 2 to 5 minutes, have a duration of 40 to 60 seconds, and are strong in intensity. During transition, contractions have a frequency of 1½ to 2 minutes, have a duration of 60 to 90 seconds, and are strong in intensity (Cunningham et al., 2005).

As dilatation approaches 10 cm, there may be increased rectal pressure and an uncontrollable urge to bear down, an increase in bloody show, and ROM (if this has not already occurred). The woman may also fear that she will be "torn open" or "split apart" by the force of the contractions. The woman may experience a sensation of pressure so great with the peak of a contraction that it seems to her that her abdomen will burst open. The woman should be informed that this is a normal sensation and reassured that such bursting will not happen.

During transition the woman will most likely withdraw into herself. Increasingly she may doubt her ability to cope with labor. The woman may become apprehensive and irritable. Although she may be terrified of being left alone, she may not want anyone to talk to her or touch her. However, with the next contraction she may ask for verbal and physical support. She may need help regaining focus. Other characteristics that may accompany this phase include the following:

- Hyperventilation, as the woman increases her breathing rate
- Restlessness
- Difficulty understanding directions
- A sense of bewilderment and anger at the contractions
- Generalized discomfort, including low back pain, shaking, and cramping in the legs
- Increased sensitivity to touch
- Increased need for partner's and/or nurse's presence or support
- Increased apprehension and irritability
- Statements that she "can't take it anymore"
- Requests for medication
- Hiccupping, belching, nausea, or vomiting
- Beads of perspiration on the upper lip
- Increasing rectal pressure
- Curling of her toes
- Loss of control
- Crying or yelling

The woman in this phase is anxious to "get it over with." She may be amnesic and sleep between her now-frequent contractions. Her support persons may start to feel helpless and may turn to the nurse for increased participation as their efforts to alleviate her discomfort seem less effective.

Second Stage

The second stage of labor begins when the cervix is completely dilated (10 cm) and ends with birth of the infant. The second stage is typically completed within 2 hours after the cervix becomes fully dilated for primigravidas (multiparas average 15

minutes). The use of epidural anesthesia may extend the duration of the second stage an additional hour. Contractions continue with a frequency of 1½ to 2 minutes, a duration of 60 to 90 seconds, and strong intensity. Descent of the fetal presenting part continues until it reaches the perineal floor.

As the fetal head descends, the woman has the urge to push because of pressure of the fetal head on the sacral and obturator nerves. As she pushes, intra-abdominal pressure is exerted from contraction of the maternal abdominal muscles. As the fetal head continues its descent, the perineum begins to bulge, flatten, and move anteriorly. The amount of bloody show may increase. The labia begin to part with each contraction. Between contractions, the fetal head appears to recede. With succeeding contractions and maternal pushing effort, the fetal head descends farther. **Crowning** occurs when the fetal head is encircled by the external opening of the vagina (introitus) and means birth is imminent. Some women feel acute, increasingly severe pain and a burning sensation as the perineum distends. The woman may continue to fear that she will tear apart. The nurse needs to instruct the woman to "push through the pain and burning."

Usually, a childbirth-prepared woman feels relieved that the acute pain she felt during the transition phase is over. She also may be relieved that the birth is near and she can now push. Some women feel a sense of control now that they can be actively involved. Others, particularly those without childbirth preparation, may become frightened. They tend to fight each contraction and any attempt of others to persuade them to push with contractions. The woman may feel she has lost control and become embarrassed and apologetic, or she may demonstrate extreme irritability toward the staff or her supporters in an attempt to regain control over external forces against which she feels helpless. Such behavior may be frightening and disconcerting to her support persons. The nurse needs to provide reassurance to the support person(s) that this is a common reaction.

SPONTANEOUS BIRTH (VERTEX PRESENTATION)

As the head distends the vulva with each contraction, the perineum becomes extremely thin, and the anus stretches and protrudes. As extension occurs under the symphysis pubis, the head is born. When the anterior shoulder meets the underside of the symphysis pubis, a gentle push by the mother aids in birth of the shoulders. The body then follows (Figure 22–11 ◆). Birth of infants in breech presentation is discussed in Chapter 26. ∞

POSITIONAL CHANGES OF THE FETUS

For the fetus to pass through the birth canal, the fetal head and body must adjust to the maternal pelvis by certain positional changes. These changes, called **cardinal movements** or mechanisms of labor, are described in the order in which they occur (Figure 22–12 ◆).

Descent

Descent is thought to occur because of four forces: (1) pressure of the amniotic fluid, (2) direct pressure of the fundus of the uterus on the breech of the fetus, (3) contraction of the abdominal muscles, and (4) extension and straightening of the fetal

EVIDENCE-BASED PRACTICE

PUSHING IN THE SECOND STAGE OF LABOR

Clinical Question

How can the nurse support the mother's pushing in the second stage of labor so that optimal maternal and neonatal outcomes are achieved?

The Evidence

Three sources of evidence were used to review traditional versus naturalistic approaches to second-stage labor coaching. A nurse-midwife undertook a systematic review of the research literature, appraising 47 studies related to effective pushing in the second stage of labor. A multisite clinical trial involving 220 women evaluated the effects of immediate versus delayed pushing during second stage labor, with a specific focus on indicators of fetal well-being. A third trial reported on a multistage trial that tested the effects of coached versus uncoached maternal pushing during the second stage of labor. The studies reviewed the effects of coached closed-glottis pushing immediately at 10-cm cervical dilatation compared with delayed uncoached pushing. In closed-glottis pushing, the mother is directed to bear down at least three to four times with each contraction while holding her breath. With this approach, the Valsalva maneuver is instituted. In the alternative approach, pushing is delayed until the woman feels the urge to push, passive fetal descent is allowed, and open-glottis pushing (vocalizing while pushing) is encouraged when the woman reports the urge to push. The woman bears down as long as she feels the urge. Outcomes that were studied included maternal considerations such as the length of the second stage of labor, method of birth, and perineal lacerations. Fetal indicators included fetal oxygen desaturation, fetal heart rate patterns, Apgar scores, and umbilical cord blood gases.

What Is Effective?

Pushing involves the use of voluntary muscles, but it becomes involuntary when the pressure of the fetal head on the pelvic floor becomes intense. There is no scientific basis that coached closed-glottis pushing has an advantage for the mother or fetus. Although early pushing was associated with a slightly shorter second stage of labor (13 minutes) in one of these studies, no other advantages were discovered (for mother or baby). In one study, delayed pushing was clearly advantageous for the fetus, resulting in less fetal oxygen desaturation. Coached pushing was slightly associated with more variable decelerations of the fetal heart rate, although there was no difference in the number of cesarean births.

What Is Unclear?

Only one of the three reviews found any effect on the length of the second stage of labor. It is not clear from these reviews how many of these women chose epidural anesthesia, in which contractions may be harder to detect and the urge to push may be delayed.

Best Practice

There is insufficient evidence to support the usefulness of coached, closed-glottis pushing for women as soon as 10 cm of cervical dilatation is achieved. Women who are supported in pushing with vocalization (open-glottis) when they feel the urge to push have outcomes that are, in some cases, better than those who are coached for early pushing. Delayed pushing appears to be better for the fetus and is a more naturalistic approach to the second stage of labor. There is no evidence that delayed pushing is harmful to mother or baby. Women should be supported in pushing in a manner that is desirable to them at a time when they feel the strongest urges to push.

Critical Thinking

How can the nurse support the mother in effectively using open-glottis pushing during the second stage of labor?

REFERENCES: Bloom, S., Casey, B., Schaffer, J., McIntire, D., & Leveno, K. (2006). A randomized trial of coached versus uncoached maternal pushing during the second stage of labor. *American Journal of Obstetrics and Gynecology, 194*(1), 10–13.

Chalk, A. (2004). Pushing in the second stage of labour. *British Journal of Midwifery, 12*(8), 502–508.

Simpson, K., & James, D. (2005). Effects of immediate versus delayed pushing during second stage labor on fetal well-being. *Nursing Research, 54*(3), 149–156.

---

body. The head enters the inlet in the occiput transverse or oblique position because the pelvic inlet is widest from side to side. The sagittal suture is an equal distance from the maternal symphysis pubis and sacral promontory.

Flexion

Flexion occurs as the fetal head descends and meets resistance from the soft tissues of the pelvis, the musculature of the pelvic floor, and the cervix. As a result of the resistance, the fetal chin flexes downward onto the chest.

Internal Rotation

The fetal head must rotate to fit the diameter of the pelvic cavity, which is widest in the anteroposterior diameter. As the occiput of the fetal head meets resistance from the levator ani muscles and their fascia, the occiput rotates from left to right, and the sagittal suture aligns in the anteroposterior pelvic diameter.

Extension

The resistance of the pelvic floor and the mechanical movement of the vulva opening anteriorly and forward assist with extension of the fetal head as it passes under the symphysis pubis. With this positional change the occiput, then brow and face, emerge from the vagina.

Restitution

The shoulders of the infant enter the pelvis obliquely and remain oblique when the head rotates to the anteroposterior diameter through internal rotation. Because of this rotation the neck becomes twisted. Once the head emerges and is free of

Figure 22–11 ◆ The birth sequence.
SOURCE: Stella Johnson (www.stellajohnson.com).

pelvic resistance the neck untwists, turning the head to one side (restitution), and aligns with the position of the back in the birth canal.

External Rotation

As the shoulders rotate to the anteroposterior position in the pelvis, the head is turned farther to one side (external rotation).

Expulsion

After the external rotation and through expulsive efforts of the laboring woman, the anterior shoulder meets the undersurface of the symphysis pubis and slips under it. As lateral flexion of the shoulder and head occurs, the anterior shoulder is born before the posterior shoulder. The body follows quickly.

Third Stage

The third stage of labor is defined as the period of time from the birth of the infant until the completed delivery of the placenta.

PLACENTAL SEPARATION

After the infant is born, the uterus contracts firmly, diminishing its capacity and the surface area of placental attachment. The pla-

Figure 22–12 ◆ Mechanisms of labor. *A, B,* Descent. *C,* Internal rotation. *D,* Extension. *E,* External rotation.

centa begins to separate because of this decrease in surface area. This separation is accompanied by bleeding, leading to the formation of a hematoma between the placental tissue and the remaining decidua. This hematoma accelerates the separation process. The membranes are the last to separate. They are peeled off the uterine wall as the placenta descends into the vagina.

Signs of placental separation usually appear around 5 minutes after birth of the infant, but can take up to 30 minutes to manifest. These signs are (1) a globular-shaped uterus, (2) a rise of the fundus in the abdomen, (3) a sudden gush or trickle of blood, and (4) further protrusion of the umbilical cord out of the vagina.

PLACENTAL DELIVERY

When the signs of placental separation appear, the woman may bear down to aid in placental expulsion. If this fails and the certified nurse-midwife or physician has ascertained that the fundus is firm, gentle traction may be applied to the cord while pressure is exerted on the fundus. The weight of the placenta as it is guided into the placental pan (a basin that holds the placenta once it is expelled) aids in the removal of the membranes from the uterine wall. A placenta is considered to be *retained* if more than 30 minutes have elapsed from completion of the second stage of labor.

If the placenta separates from the inside to the outer margins, it is expelled with the fetal (shiny) side presenting (Figure 22–13 ◆). This is known as the *Schultze mechanism* of placental delivery or, more commonly, *shiny Schultze*. If the placenta separates from the outer margins inward, it will roll up and present sideways with the maternal surface delivering first. This is known as the *Duncan mechanism* of placental delivery and is commonly called *dirty Duncan* because the placental surface is rough.

Nursing and medical interventions during the third stage of labor are discussed in Chapter 24. ∞

Fourth Stage

The fourth stage of labor is the time from 1 to 4 hours after birth in which physiologic readjustment of the mother's body begins. With the birth, hemodynamic changes occur. Blood loss at birth ranges from 250 to 500 mL. With this blood loss and the easing of pressure exerted by the pregnant uterus on the surrounding vessels, blood is redistributed into venous beds. This results in a moderate drop in both systolic and diastolic blood pressure, increased pulse pressure, and moderate tachycardia (Cunningham et al., 2005).

The uterus remains contracted and is in the midline of the abdomen. The fundus is usually midway between the symphysis pubis and umbilicus. Its contracted state constricts the vessels at the site of placental implantation. Immediately after birth of the placenta, the cervix is widely spread and thick.

Nausea and vomiting experienced during transition usually cease. The woman may be thirsty and hungry. She may experience a shaking chill, which is thought to be associated with the ending of the physical exertion of labor. The bladder is often hypotonic due to trauma during the second stage and/or the administration of anesthetics that may decrease sensations. Hypotonic bladder leads to urinary retention. Nursing care during this stage is discussed in Chapter 24. ∞

I have had the privilege of practicing nursing in the birthing area for many years. In my head I know all the factors that must work together to bring this new life into the world. But it is in my heart and in working with and watching the laboring woman (and her partner if she has one) that I truly believe each labor and birth is a miracle. I, along with these parents, get to participate in a moment of time that will never occur again for any of us. I will never tire of this, will never get enough.

MEDIALINK

Animation: Placental Delivery

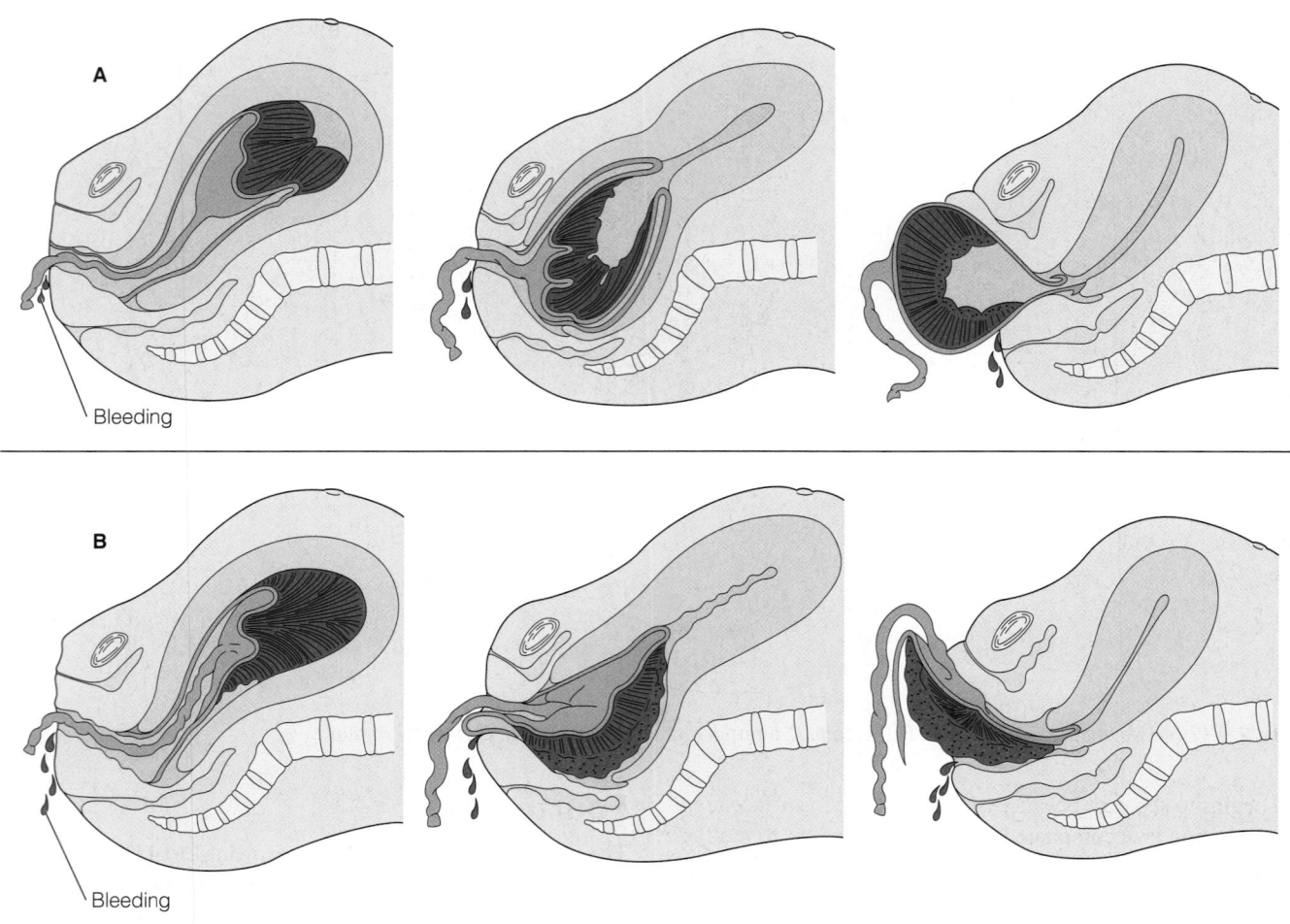

Figure 22–13 ◆ Placental separation and expulsion. *A,* Schultze mechanism. *B,* Duncan mechanism.

MATERNAL SYSTEMIC RESPONSE TO LABOR

The labor process affects nearly every major body system. Each system adapts to these changes through various compensation mechanisms.

Cardiovascular System

The woman's cardiovascular system is stressed both by the uterine contractions and by the pain, anxiety, and apprehension the woman experiences. In pregnancy, the resting pulse rate increases by 10 to 18 beats per minute (Chin, 2006). During labor there is a significant increase in cardiac output. Each strong contraction greatly decreases or completely stops the blood flow in the branches of the uterine artery that supply the intervillous space (in the placenta). This leads to a redistribution of about 300 to 500 mL of blood into the peripheral circulation and an increase in peripheral resistance, resulting in increased systolic and diastolic blood pressure, a slowing of the pulse rate, and an increase of about 30% in cardiac output (Chin, 2006; Cunningham et al., 2005).

Maternal position also affects cardiac output, blood pressure, and pulse. When the laboring woman turns to a side-lying position, cardiac output increases by about 22%, the pulse rate decreases by about 6 beats per minute, and stroke volume increases by 27%. When the woman is supine, cardiac output increases 25%, stroke volume increases 33%, pulse pressure increases more than 26%, blood pressure rises significantly, and pulse rate decreases by 15%.

There is an additional effect on hemodynamics during the bearing-down efforts in the second stage. When the laboring woman holds her breath and pushes against a closed glottis (Valsalva maneuver), intrathoracic pressure rises. As intrathoracic pressure increases, the venous return is interrupted, increasing venous pressure. In addition the blood in the lungs is forced into the left atrium, which leads to a transient increase in cardiac output, blood pressure, and pulse pressure, and causes bradycardia. As venous return to the lungs continues to be diminished while the breath is held, a decrease in blood pressure, pulse pressure, and cardiac output occurs.

When the next breath is taken (Valsalva maneuver is interrupted), the intrathoracic pressure is decreased. Venous return increases, refilling the pulmonary bed and resulting in recovery of the cardiac output and stroke volume. This process is repeated with each pushing effort.

Immediately after birth, cardiac output peaks with an 80% increase over prelabor values. Then in the first 10 minutes it decreases 20% to 25%. Cardiac output further decreases in the first hour after the birth. However, these decreases still leave the woman with an elevated cardiac output for at least 24 hours after the birth (Cunningham et al., 2005).

Blood Pressure

As a result of increased cardiac output, systolic blood pressure rises during uterine contractions. In the first stage, systolic pressure may increase by 35 mm Hg, and there may be further increases in the second stage during pushing efforts. Diastolic pressure also increases by about 25 mm Hg in the first stage and 65 mm Hg in the second stage. These increases begin just before the uterine contraction, with a return to baseline as soon as the contraction ends (Cunningham et al., 2005). Blood pressure may also rise as a result of fear, apprehension, and pain (Varney, Kriebs, & Gegor, 2004).

Blood pressure may drop precipitously when the woman lies in a supine position and experiences aortocaval compression. In addition to hypotension there is an increase in the pulse rate, diaphoresis, nausea, weakness, and air hunger. These changes are attributed to the decreased cardiac output and a subsequent drop in stroke volume.

Women with hydramnios, women with multiple gestation, and obese women have the highest risk of developing aortocaval compression. Other predisposing factors include hypovolemia, dehydration, hemorrhage, metabolic acidosis, administration of narcotics (which results in vasodilation and inhibits compensatory mechanisms), and administration of epidural anesthesia, which results in *sympathetic blockade* (blocking of the sympathetic nervous system, leading to vasodilation and hypotension).

Fluid and Electrolyte Balance

Profuse perspiration (diaphoresis) occurs during labor. Hyperventilation also occurs, altering electrolyte and fluid balance from insensible water loss. The muscle activity elevates the body temperature, which increases sweating and evaporation from the skin. As the woman responds to the work of labor, the rise in the respiratory rate increases the evaporative water volume because each breath of air must be warmed to the body temperature and humidified. With the increased evaporative water volume, maintaining adequate oral fluids/hydration is important. In some instances parenteral intravenous (IV) fluids are administered.

Respiratory System

Oxygen demand and consumption increase at the onset of labor because of the presence of uterine contractions. Approximately 50% of the increased oxygen is used by the placenta, the uterus, and the fetus (Chin, 2006). As anxiety and pain from uterine contractions increase, hyperventilation frequently occurs. With hyperventilation there is a fall in $PaCO_2$, and respiratory alkalosis results (Cunningham et al., 2005).

As labor progresses and contractions become more frequent, stronger, and prolonged, the workload, tension, and anxiety of the woman continue to change. A mild increase in the respiratory rate is normal in labor and is related to the increase in metabolism (Varney et al., 2004).

By the end of the first stage most women have developed a mild metabolic acidosis compensated by respiratory alkalosis. As she pushes in the second stage of labor, the woman's $PaCO_2$ levels may rise along with blood lactate levels (due to muscular activity), and mild respiratory acidosis occurs. By the time the baby is born (end of second stage), there is metabolic acidosis uncompensated by respiratory alkalosis (Cunningham et al., 2005).

The changes in acid-base status that occur in labor are quickly reversed in the fourth stage because of changes in the woman's respiratory rate. Acid-base levels return to pregnancy levels by 24 hours after birth, and nonpregnant values are attained a few weeks after birth.

Renal System

During labor there is an increase in maternal renin, plasma renin activity, and angiotensinogen. This elevation is thought to be important in the control of uteroplacental blood flow during birth and the early postpartal period (Cunningham et al., 2005).

Polyuria is common during labor. This results from the increase in cardiac output, which causes an increase in the glomerular filtration rate and renal plasma flow. Slight proteinuria occurs in one half to one third of women in labor (Varney et al., 2004).

Structurally, the base of the bladder is pushed forward and upward when engagement occurs. The pressure from the presenting part may impair blood and lymph drainage from the base of the bladder, leading to edema of the tissues (Cunningham et al., 2005). Hematuria may be present as a result of trauma to the lower urinary tract.

Gastrointestinal System

During labor, gastric motility and absorption of solid food are reduced. Gastric emptying time is prolonged, and gastric volume (amount of contents that remain in the stomach) remains over 25 mL, regardless of the time the last meal was taken. This is even more marked in women who have received analgesia agents (Cunningham et al., 2005). These women may be at risk for aspiration should general anesthesia need to be used. During labor, anaerobic and aerobic carbohydrate metabolism rise due to an increase in skeletal muscle activity and maternal anxiety (Varney et al., 2004).

The fluid requirements of women in labor have not been clearly established. In some instances oral hydration is the primary goal. In other situations a saline lock may be inserted so that intravenous access is available if needed. If intravenous fluids are used, it is important to remember that when hypertonic glucose infusions are used, there is an increase in maternal blood glucose; this can lead to fetal hyperglycemia and hyperinsulinemia and to hypoglycemia in the newborn.

Immune System and Other Blood Values

The white blood cell (WBC) count increases to 25,000/mm³ to 30,000/mm³ during labor and early postpartum (Chin, 2006). The change in WBC count is due mostly to increased neutrophils resulting from a physiologic response to stress. The increased WBC count makes it difficult to identify the presence of an infectious process.

Maternal blood glucose levels decrease because glucose is used as an energy source during uterine contractions. The decreased blood glucose levels lead to a decrease in insulin requirements (Cunningham et al., 2005). Glucose levels can drop significantly during a prolonged or difficult labor.

Pain

Pain during labor comes from a complexity of physical causes. Each woman will experience and cope with pain differently. Multiple factors affect a woman's reaction to labor pain.

PAIN DURING LABOR

The pain associated with the first stage of labor is unique in that it accompanies a normal physiologic process. Even though perception of the pain is determined to some extent by cultural patterning, there is unquestionably a physiologic basis for pain during labor. Pain during the first stage of labor arises from (1) dilatation of the cervix, (2) hypoxia of the uterine muscle cells during contraction, (3) stretching of the lower uterine segment, and (4) pressure on adjacent structures. The primary source of pain is dilatation or stretching of the cervix. Nerve impulses travel through the uterine plexus, to the pelvis through hypogastric plexes, and then into the lumbar sympathetic chain (Figure 22–14 ◆). They enter the spinal cord through the posterior roots of the 10th through 12th thoracic and 1st lumbar nerves.

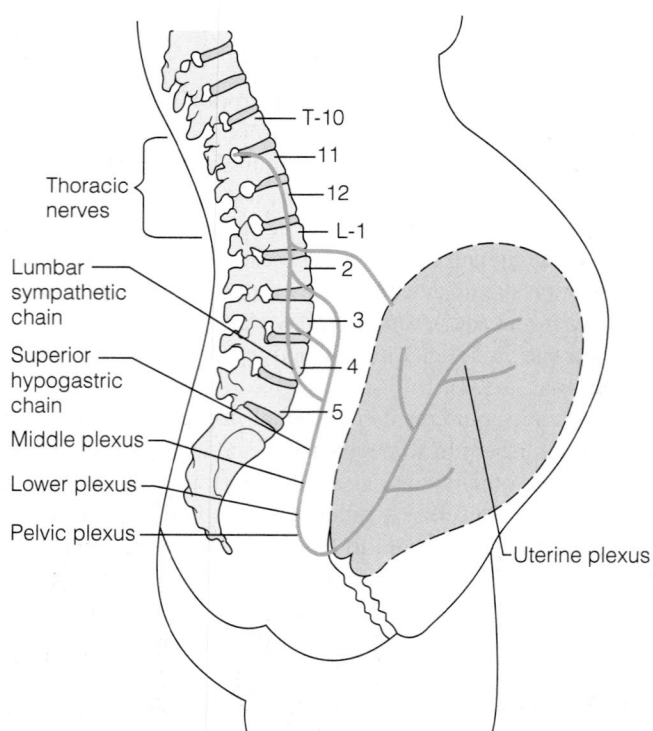

Figure 22–14 ◆ Pain pathway from uterus to spinal cord. Nerve impulses travel through the uterine plexus; pelvic plexus; lower, middle, and superior hypogastric plexus; and lumbar sympathetic chain. They enter the neuroaxis through the 10th, 11th, and 12th thoracic and 1st lumbar spinal segments.
SOURCE: Modified from Bonica, J. J. (1972). *Principles and practice of obstetric analgesia and anesthesia* (p. 492). Philadelphia: Davis.

As with other visceral pain, pain from the uterus is also directly referred to the dermatomes supplied by the 10th through 12th thoracic nerves. The areas of referred pain include the lower abdominal wall and the areas over the lower lumbar region and the upper sacrum (Figure 22–15 ◆).

During the second stage of labor, pain is due to (1) hypoxia of the contracting uterine muscle cells, (2) distention of the vagina and perineum, and (3) pressure on adjacent structures including the lower back, buttocks, and thighs. The nerve impulses from the vagina and perineum are transmitted by way of the pudendal nerve plexus and enter the spinal cord through the posterior roots of the 2nd through 4th sacral nerves. The area of pain increases as shown in Figure 22–16 ◆.

Pain during the third stage results from uterine contractions and cervical dilatation as the placenta is expelled. Sensations of pain are felt above the symphysis pubis bone in the perineal area and in the lower back (Figure 22–17 ◆). The mechanism for the transmission of nerve impulses is the same as for the first stage of labor. The third stage of labor is short, and after this phase anesthesia is needed primarily for episiotomy repair.

FACTORS AFFECTING RESPONSE TO PAIN

Many factors affect the individual's perception of pain impulses. Some psychologic and environmental influences particularly appropriate to labor are discussed here.

Preparation for childbirth has been shown to reduce the need for analgesia during labor. Preparing for labor and birth through reading, talking with others, or attending a childbirth preparation class frequently has positive effects for the laboring woman and her partner. The woman who knows what to expect and what techniques she may use to increase comfort tends to be less anxious during the labor. A tour of the birthing center and an opportunity to see and feel the environment also help reduce anxiety, because during admission (especially with the first child) many new things are happening and they seem to occur all at once. The more the woman and her partner learn during classes and through their own efforts, the more likely they will reduce some anxiety.

Individuals tend to respond to painful stimuli in the way that is acceptable in their culture. In some cultures, it is natural to communicate pain, no matter how mild, whereas members of other cultures stoically accept pain out of fear or because it is expected. Nurses need to be aware of cultural norms and demonstrate culturally sensitive care to women and their families in the intrapartum setting (Atherton, Feeg, & El-Adham, 2004).

Families will react to the healthcare system based on their own cultural beliefs. Nurses need to identify specific cultural norms with each individual family so appropriate care can be provided. Whenever possible, requests that include the family's cultural preferences should be incorporated into the woman's care. Nurses should avoid making generalizations about specific cultures. Instead, individual preferences and beliefs should be explored.

Another factor that may influence response to pain is *fatigue* and *sleep deprivation*. The fatigued woman has less energy and ability to use such strategies as distraction or imagina-

Figure 22–15 ◆ Area of reference of labor pain during the first stage. Pain is most intense in the darker colored areas.
SOURCE: Bonica, J. J. (1972). *Principles and practice of obstetric analgesia and anesthesia* (p. 108). Philadelphia: Davis.

tion to deal with pain. As a result, she may lose her ability to cope with labor and choose analgesics or other medications to relieve the discomfort.

The woman's *previous experience* with pain also affects her ability to manage current and future pain. Those who have had experience with pain seem more sensitive to painful stimuli than those who have not.

Anxiety can affect a woman's response to pain. Unfamiliar surroundings and events can increase anxiety, as does separation from family and loved ones. The woman's anticipation of

Figure 22–16 ◆ Distribution of labor pain during the later phase of the first stage and early phase of the second stage. The darkest colored areas indicate the location of the most intense pain; moderate color, moderate pain; and light color, mild pain. The uterine contractions, which at this stage are very strong, produce intense pain.
SOURCE: Bonica, J. J. (1972). *Principles and practice of obstetric analgesia and anesthesia* (p. 109). Philadelphia: Davis.

Figure 22–17 ◆ Distribution of labor pain during the later phase of the second stage and actual birth. The perineal component is the primary cause of discomfort. Uterine contractions contribute much less.
SOURCE: Bonica, J. J. (1972). *Principles and practice of obstetric analgesia and anesthesia* (p. 109). Philadelphia: Davis.

discomfort and concerns about whether she can cope with the contractions may also increase her anxiety level. It is not uncommon for laboring women to worry about their partner or other family members. Reassurance from family members that things are being "taken care of at home" can help.

Both attention and distraction have an influence on the perception of pain. When pain sensation is the focus of attention, the perceived intensity is greater. A sensory stimulus such as a backrub can be a distraction that focuses the woman's attention on the stimulus rather than the pain. The nurse can offer suggestions to support persons on interventions to initiate physical distractions for the laboring woman.

As part of the culture of health care, nursing and medical professionals have their own (collective and individual) expectations of the woman in labor and those who support her. In one setting, the woman may be expected to use a breathing technique and relaxation methods, whereas in another, most women receive an epidural block. Some nurses may believe that the woman and her support persons should take care of themselves and ask for assistance only if really necessary; other nurses may believe that frequent interaction and support are essential as long as the woman and her support persons are comfortable with the interaction.

The healthcare professional is most likely to interpret pain according to the norms of the healthcare culture, although various other cultures have different ways of responding to pain. The absence of crying and moaning does not necessarily mean that pain is absent, nor does the presence of crying and moaning necessarily mean that pain relief is desired at that moment. It is

very important for the nurse to accept and respect the fact that the pain is whatever the woman says it is and to assist her in coping with it.

FETAL RESPONSE TO LABOR

When the fetus is normal, the mechanical and hemodynamic changes of normal labor have no adverse effects.

Heart Rate Changes

Fetal heart rate decelerations can occur with intracranial pressures of 40 to 55 mm Hg. The currently accepted explanation of this early deceleration is hypoxic depression of the central nervous system, which is under vagal control. The absence of these head compression decelerations (early decelerations) in some fetuses during labor is explained by the existence of a threshold that is reached more gradually in the presence of intact membranes and lack of maternal resistance. Early decelerations are harmless in the normal fetus.

Acid-Base Status in Labor

The blood flow to the fetus is slowed during the acme of the contraction, which leads to a slow decrease in the fetal pH. During the second stage, as uterine contractions become stronger and last longer and the woman pushes with each contraction, there is a more rapid decrease in fetal pH. There is also an increase in fetal base deficit and in $Paco_2$ and a drop in fetal oxygen saturation. Persistent acid-base imbalance can lead to multiorgan dysfunction in the infant, including neurologic impairment.

Hemodynamic Changes

The adequate exchange of nutrients and gases in the fetal capillaries and intervillous spaces depends in part on the fetal blood pressure. Fetal blood pressure is a protective mechanism for the normal fetus during the anoxic periods caused by the contracting uterus during labor. The fetal and placental reserve is enough to see the fetus through these anoxic periods unharmed.

Behavioral States

The human fetus develops behavioral states between 36 and 38 weeks of gestation. The behavioral states seem to continue during labor even in the presence of uterine contractions. Two sleep states (quiet and active) are most prevalent, although quiet and active awake states are occasionally observed. A decrease in fetal heart rate variability accompanies the quiet sleep state, and there is also a decrease in fetal breathing movements and other general body activity. The quiet sleep state generally lasts less than 40 minutes.

Fetal Sensation

Beginning at about 37 or 38 weeks' gestation (full term), the fetus is able to experience sensations of light, sound, and touch. The full-term fetus is able to hear music and the maternal voice. Even in utero, the fetus is sensitive to light and will move away from a bright light source. Additionally, the term baby is aware of pressure sensations during labor such as the touch of the caregiver during a vaginal exam or pressure on the head as a contraction occurs. Although the fetus may not be able to process this input, as the woman labors the fetus is experiencing the labor as well.

CHAPTER REVIEW

FOCUS YOUR STUDY

- Five factors that continually interact during labor and birth are the birth passage, the birth passenger (fetus), the relationship between the birth passage and the fetus, the physiologic forces of labor, and factors associated with the woman's psychosocial status.

- Four types of pelveses have been identified, and each has a different effect on labor. The diameters of gynecoid and anthropoid pelves are usually large enough for labor and birth to progress normally. In the android and platypelloid types, the pelvic diameters are diminished (smaller than in gynecoid and anthropoid). Labor is more likely to be difficult (longer) and a cesarean birth is more likely.

- Important dimensions of the maternal pelvis include the diameters of the pelvic inlet, pelvic cavity, and pelvic outlet.

- The fetal head contains bones in the top portion (cranial vault) that are not fused. This allows them to overlap somewhat in response to the pressures on the fetal head during labor. The pressure and overlapping of the sutures, which are membranous spaces between the cranial bones, result in a change in the shape of the head called molding.

- Fetal attitude refers to the relation of the fetal parts to one another. The head is usually held in midline and not to one side or the other, and the extremities are usually flexed and held close to the body because there is little extra room within the uterine cavity.

- Fetal lie refers to the relationship of the cephalocaudal (head to sacral area) axis of the fetus to the maternal spine. The fetal lie is either longitudinal (both the maternal and fetal spines are vertical) or transverse (the fetal spine is at a right angle to the maternal spine).

- Fetal presentation is determined by the body part lying closest to the inlet of the maternal pelvis. In a longitudinal lie the fetal presentation is usually cephalic (head first) but may also be breech (buttocks or one or both feet first). In a transverse lie the fetal shoulder is usually closest to the pelvic inlet.

- Engagement of the presenting part occurs when the largest diameter of the fetal presenting part reaches or passes through the pelvic inlet.

- Station refers to the relationship of the presenting part to an imaginary line drawn between the maternal ischial spines, which are in the midpoint of the pelvic cavity. The fetal presenting part enters the pelvic inlet at what is termed about a −5 and descends toward the ischial spines, where it is called a 0 (zero) station. Further descent from 0 to +4 occurs as the presenting part descends below the ischial spines toward the vaginal opening.

- Fetal position is the relationship of a specified landmark on the presenting fetal part to the sides, front, or back of the maternal pelvis. Once the position is known, the positions of the fetal head and back can be determined.

- Each uterine contraction has an increment, acme, and decrement.

- Contraction frequency is the time from the beginning of one contraction to the beginning of the next contraction.

- Duration of contractions refers to the period of time from the beginning to the end of one contraction.

- Intensity of contractions refers to the strength of the contraction during acme. Intensity of contractions is termed mild, moderate, or strong.

- Labor stresses the coping skills of women. Women with prenatal education about childbirth usually report more positive responses to labor.

- Women with support persons tend to use their coping skills more effectively than those who lack support.

- Premonitory signs of labor include lightening, Braxton Hicks contractions, cervical softening and effacement, bloody show, sudden burst of energy, weight loss, and, sometimes, rupture of membranes.

- True labor contractions occur regularly with an increase in frequency, duration, and intensity. The contractions usually start in the back and radiate around the abdomen. The discomfort is not relieved by ambulation, rest, or warm tub baths. False labor contractions do not produce progressive cervical effacement and dilatation. They are irregular and do not increase in intensity. The discomfort may be relieved by ambulation, rest, or warm tub baths.

- Possible causes of labor onset include the progesterone withdrawal hypothesis, the prostaglandin hypothesis, and the corticotropin-releasing hormone hypothesis.

- There are four stages of labor and birth. The first stage is from beginning of true labor to complete dilatation of the cervix. The second stage is from complete dilatation of the cervix to birth. The third stage is from birth to expulsion of the placenta. The fourth stage is from expulsion of the placenta to a period of 1 to 4 hours after.

- The fetus accommodates to the maternal pelvis in a series of movements called the cardinal movements of labor, which include descent, flexion, internal rotation, extension, restitution, external rotation, and expulsion.

- Placental separation is indicated by lengthening of the umbilical cord, a small spurt of blood, change in uterine shape, and a rise of the fundus in the abdomen.

- The placenta is expelled by Schultze or Duncan mechanism. This is determined by the way it separates from the uterine wall.

- Maternal systemic responses to labor involve the cardiovascular, respiratory, renal, gastrointestinal, and immune systems. Cardiac output and blood pressure increase, as do oxygen demand and consumption. Polyuria is common, and gastric motility and absorption are reduced. The white blood cell count increases, and blood glucose levels decrease.

- Factors that affect the response to labor pain include education, cultural beliefs, fatigue and sleep deprivation, personal significance of pain, previous experience, anxiety, and the availability of coping techniques.

- The fetus is usually able to tolerate the labor process with no untoward changes.

EXPLORE MediaLink

http://www.prenhall.com/davidson

NCLEX review questions, case studies, and other interactive resources for this chapter can be found on the Web Site at http://www.prenhall.com/davidson. Click on "Chapter 22" to select the activities for this chapter.

For tutorials including animations and videos, more NCLEX review questions, and an audio glossary, access the accompanying Prentice Hall Nursing MediaLink DVD-ROM in this book.

PRENTICE HALL NURSING MEDIALINK DVD-ROM

Audio Glossary

NCLEX Review

Videos: *Fetal Lie; First Stage of Labor; First Stage of Labor—Transition; Second Stage of Labor; Third Stage of Labor—Part 1; Third Stage of Labor—Part 2; Third Stage of Labor—Part 3; Through the Eyes of a Nurse—The Third Trimester*

Animations: *Rupturing Membranes; Placental Delivery*

 COMPANION WEBSITE

Additional NCLEX Review

Case Study: *Client in First Stage of Labor*

Care Plan Activities: *Teenage Client in Uncomplicated Labor; Labor Progress in the First Stage of Labor*

Applications: *Normal Labor and Delivery; Breech Presentation*

Critical Thinking

CRITICAL THINKING IN ACTION

CERVICAL RIPENING USING PROSTAGLANDIN GEL

View the Critical Thinking in Action video in Chapter 22 of the DVD-ROM. Then answer the questions that follow.

 Ann Nelson, a 28-year-old, G2, at 41 weeks' gestation, is admitted to the birthing unit where you are working. She is here for cervical ripening and induction of labor due to postdate pregnancy and decreased amniotic fluid volume. A review of her prenatal chart reveals a pertinent history of infertility (Clomid-induced pregnancy) and asthma (treated with inhalers on a PRN basis). The Doppler picks up a fetal heart rate of 120 bpm. You place Ann on the electronic fetal monitor and obtain the following data: BP 126/76, T 98F, P 82, R 16; vaginal exam reveals a 20% effaced cervix, 1 cm dilatation in the posterior position, and vertex at −2 station. The fetal monitor shows a fetal heart rate baseline of 120 to 128 with occasional mild variable decelerations, accelerations to 140 with fetal activity. No contractions are noted on the monitor or palpated. Ann asks you what to expect with "cervical ripening" using prostaglandin gel.

1. Discuss the action of prostaglandin gel.

2. Ann asks you why cervical ripening and induction of labor are recommended for her and her baby. How would you best respond to her?

3. Ann asks how she will know if she is getting contractions. How would you answer her?

4. Discuss the differences among mild, moderate, and strong contractions.

5. Describe the latent phase of labor.

REFERENCES

Atherton, M. J., Feeg, V., & El-Adham, A. F. (2004). Race, ethnicity, and insurance as determinants of epidural use: Analysis of a national sample survey. *Nursing Economics, 22*(1), 6–13.

Challis, J. R. G. (2004). Characteristics of parturition. In R. Creasy, R. Resnik, & J. Iams (Eds.), *Maternal-fetal medicine* (5th ed., pp. 484–497). Philadelphia: Saunders.

Chin, H. G. (2006). *On call obstetrics and gynecology* (3rd ed.). Philadelphia: W. B. Saunders.

Cunningham, F. G., Leveno, K. J., Bloom, S. L., Hauth, J. C., Gilstrap, L. C., & Wenstrom, K. D. (2005). *Williams obstetrics* (22nd ed.). New York: McGraw-Hill.

Goodman, J. H. (2005). Becoming an involved father of an infant. *Journal of Obstetric, Gynecologic, & Neonatal Nursing, 34*(2), 190–200.

King, T. (2002). Labor pain in the 21st century. *Journal of Midwifery & Women's Health, 47*(2), 67–69.

Mullaly, L. M. (2004). Psychology of pregnancy. In S. Mattson & J. E. Smith (Eds.), *AWHONN: Maternal newborn nursing* (3rd ed.). Philadelphia: Saunders.

Ross, L. E., Murray, B. J., & Steiner, M. (2005). Sleep and prenatal mood disorders: A critical review. *Journal of Psychiatry & Neuroscience, 30*(4), 247–256.

Simkin, P., & Ancheta, R. (2005). *The labor progress handbook* (2nd ed.). Oxford: Blackwell Science.

Varney, H., Kriebs, J. M., & Gegor, C. L. (2004). *Varney's midwifery* (4th ed.). Sudbury, MA: Jones & Bartlett.

Vogel, I., Thorsen, P., Curry, A., Sandager, P., & Uldbjerg, N. (2005). Biomarkers for the prediction of preterm delivery. *Acta Obstetricia et Gynecologica Scandinavica, 84*(6), 516–525.

Wheeler, L. (2002). *A practical guide to prenatal and postpartum care. Nurse-Midwifery Handbook* (2nd ed.). Philadelphia: Lippincott, Williams & Wilkins.

CHAPTER
23 Intrapartal Nursing Assessment

We knew everything was going OK and that I was making progress, but it was so good to hear our nurse check me to see if I was dilating. It was not very uncomfortable, but he was as gentle as he could be, and when he told me I had dilated another 2 centimeters, I felt that I could keep going on. It was nice for us to know that the birth was getting closer with each contraction.

OBJECTIVES

1. Summarize intrapartal physical, psychosocial, and cultural assessments necessary for optimum maternal-fetal outcome.
2. Define the outer limits of normal progress of each of the phases and stages of labor.
3. Compare the various methods of monitoring fetal heart rate and contractions, giving advantages and disadvantages of each.
4. Describe the procedure for performing Leopold's maneuvers and the information that can be obtained.
5. Differentiate between baseline and periodic changes in the fetal heart rate.
6. Identify the differences between fetal tachycardia and fetal bradycardia.
7. Identify fetal heart rates and patterns using National Institute of Child Health and Human Development (NICHD) terminology.
8. Outline the steps to be performed in the systematic evaluation of fetal heart rate tracings.
9. List factors to consider in evaluation of abnormal findings on a fetal heart rate tracing.
10. Identify the interventions that are indicated when a nonreassuring fetal heart rate pattern is identified.
11. Discuss the steps used to perform fetal scalp stimulation.

KEY TERMS

MEDIALINK

Additional resources for this content can be found on the Prentice Hall Nursing MediaLink DVD-ROM and on the Companion Website at http://www.prenhall.com/davidson. Click on "Chapter 23" to select the activities for this chapter.

The labor process is a period of increased physiologic stress for the pregnant woman and her fetus. The physiologic events that occur during the intrapartal period require many changes and rapid adaptations; thus, accurate and frequent assessment is crucial. The primary purpose of the intrapartal assessment is to collect the essential data needed to evaluate the response of the mother and fetus to the changes in labor and the well-being of the "maternal-fetal unit" throughout those changes. The nurse in the birth setting uses a wide variety of assessment skills, including observation, palpation, and auscultation, to provide care for two primary clients, the mother and her child. The expectant mother's partner or support person is also an important member of the birthing team, and assessments of the couple's coping, interactions, and teamwork are integral to the nurse's knowledge base. The nurse's physical presence with the laboring woman provides the best opportunity for ongoing assessment, even as the nurse quietly provides comfort measures and gently assists the "coach" in offering support.

In current practice, "hands-on" techniques can be augmented by the use of technology. For example, the nurse or clinician can use Doppler ultrasound to listen to the fetal heart rate (FHR) or an electronic fetal monitor to assist in recording contractions and the FHR. No matter what technology is used, however, it is important that the nurse remember that "the machine" or "the test" only provides information; it cannot replace the human interaction and support that are provided by the nurse. In the birth setting that provides "high-touch" nursing care, the "high-tech" assessments are easily integrated to provide comprehensive, high-quality care.

This chapter discusses the assessments that are an important part of nursing care in the birth setting.

MATERNAL ASSESSMENT

The goal of a maternal assessment is to create an accurate database of information from which healthcare providers best formulate an optimal plan of care for a patient given her current clinical situation. Assessment of the intrapartal client mother begins with a client history and screening for intrapartal risk factors. Data collection includes a variety of data assessment methods: the prenatal record, admission interviews of the client and family members to obtain historical data, a psychologic assessment, and the initial and ongoing assessments of the mother and fetus throughout labor (Cypher, Adelsperger, & Torgersen, 2003).

Assessment and evaluation of the potential intrapartal client may vary from client to client depending on the client's condition and stage of labor. The professional guidelines for perinatal care state that pregnant women who present to the acute care setting should be evaluated in a timely manner. Clients may often need to be triaged upon presentation to the obstetrical unit; thus, nursing staff may be required to perform intrapartal assessments in various phases to facilitate prompt and efficient care for all clients. For instance, initial evaluation of a pregnant mother who presents for admission may minimally include only the assessment of her vital signs, FHR, status of uterine contractions, and any abnormal symptoms or signs of distress such as vaginal bleeding, acute abdominal pain, temperature above 100.4F, premature labor, premature rupture of membranes, hypertension, or nonreassuring fetal patterns (American Academy of Pediatrics [AAP] & American College of Obstericians and Gynecologists [ACOG], 2002).

If a pregnant client is suspected of being in labor or has ruptured membranes or vaginal bleeding, the nurse should promptly continue to assess and evaluate the mother and initiate appropriate treatment. If a client is in early labor and presents without complications, the nurse may defer the complete physical assessment and admission of the mother once fetal well-being has been determined. With a client who has received prenatal care and has been recently evaluated and had no risk factors found, assessment and evaluation may be limited to the interval between the points of care. On the other hand, a client who has received no prenatal care may require a complete assessment including history and physical, obstetrical evaluation, laboratory tests, ultrasound, and other indicated procedures as her condition warrants (AAP & ACOG, 2002). Regardless of status, the well-being of the mother and fetus are of primary concern, and it is the responsibility of the nursing and medical staff to obtain accurate and appropriate data regarding the client and to provide appropriate services as needed.

Prenatal Record

According to perinatal guidelines, when a pregnant woman approaches approximately 36 weeks' gestation, a copy of the prenatal record should be available at the acute care facility so that the medical record is accessible to members of the healthcare delivery team. If the prenatal record is available, it can provide the foundation for the intrapartum assessment. Health conditions, risk factors, abnormal test results, and ongoing assessments that have been completed during the course of the pregnancy are often useful information in determining client care needs. Information contained in the prenatal record should be verified if possible to avoid the possibility of conflicts during subsequent client interviews.

Historical Data

During assessment interviews, the pregnant client is likely to be the primary source of information. Often her partner or another family member may be present and capable of providing information in the event that the mother cannot concentrate or participate in the interview because of her physical state or stage of labor. The client's privacy must still remain a concern for the nurse in every circumstance, and every measure must be taken to safeguard it and the client's right to confidentiality.

The historical data form the basis for intrapartum assessment. The historical or background data include the client's demographic and socioeconomic information; medical, surgical, family, obstetrical, and gynecological histories; psychosociocultural assessments; and physical examination (Association of Women's Health, Obstetric, and Neonatal Nurses [AWHONN],

THROUGH THE EYES OF A NURSE

Signs and Symptoms of Labor

FAMILY'S EXPERIENCE: At the prenatal visit, the father of the baby expresses concerns about recognizing true labor signs. "She has been having so many of these Braxton Hicks contractions, I am afraid we won't know if it is really labor and she will have the baby at home! Is it that different? I keep having a reoccurring dream that she has the baby at home and we're all alone!"

NURSE'S RESPONSE: "Many couples worry that the baby will come quickly and will be born at home, but this is quite rare. The contractions (Braxton Hicks) that she is having now are for the most part painless tightening although they can be more uncomfortable when you get closer to the due date. They are common and do not have any particular pattern to them.

"True labor is marked by regular contractions that result in cervical change. The only way to know if you are having cervical change is to be examined. Once your contractions become regular and painful, you will come to the hospital where we will monitor your contraction pattern and examine your cervix.

"You will also need to come in to the birth setting if your water breaks or if you have any vaginal bleeding or a decrease in the baby's movement patterns."

NURSE'S ACTIONS AND RATIONALE:

The nurse reassures the couple that labor is usually recognized and that there usually is adequate time to get to the birth setting. The nurse should review the signs of labor and danger signs and advise the couple when they should come to the birth setting. A written information sheet is helpful and allows the couple to review the information at home.

2003). Relevant data include the following (Cypher et al., 2003; Johnston & Herzig, 2006):

- Demographic information
  - Name and age
  - Attending obstetrician or certified nurse-midwife (CNM)
  - Pediatrician/family physician
- Socioeconomic factors
  - Housing, transportation
  - Ability to provide for the new baby
  - Support system
- Medical and surgical histories
  - History of previous illness, such as tuberculosis, heart disease, diabetes, convulsive disorders, immune system abnormalities, hematologic disorders, thyroid disorders, gastrointestinal abnormalities, asthma, sickle cell anemia, Tay-Sachs disease, psychologic disorders, and other inherited disorders
- Family history
  - Genetic disorders, medical conditions, psychiatric conditions
- Obstetrical history
  - Past pregnancies
    - Complications during pregnancy and delivery
    - High-risk factors
    - Previous abortions, term and preterm infants, number of living children, neonatal deaths
    - Mode of birth
  - Current pregnancy
    - Gravidity, parity
    - High-risk factors
    - Blood type; Rh factor; results of serology testing; complete blood count (CBC); quadruple screen results; hepatitis status, rubella status, chlamydia, gonorrhea, and group beta strep culture results, results of any genetic diagnostic testing (nuchal translucency testing, chorionic villus sampling, amniocentesis), and specialized testing (Tay-Sachs, cystic fibrosis, sickle cell)
    - Allergies to medications, foods, or substances
    - Drug and alcohol consumption and smoking during pregnancy
    - Elevated blood pressure, bleeding problems, recurrent urinary tract infection
    - Medications used during the pregnancy, including prescription medication, over-the-counter medications, and herbal supplements
    - Method chosen for infant feeding
    - Type of prenatal education (childbirth preparation classes)

- Woman's preferences regarding labor and birth, such as no episiotomy, no analgesics or anesthetics, or the presence/participation of the father or others at the birth
- Gestational age assessment
- Fetal activity
- Leopold's maneuvers
- Fetal positioning
- Psychosocial assessment
  - Cultural factors
  - Resources and support systems
  - Domestic violence screening
  - Substance abuse/exposure
- Clinical assessment
  - Maternal vital signs
  - Maternal weight, height and weight gain this pregnancy
  - Nutritional status
  - Uterine activity
    - Contraction assessment
      - Onset, duration, frequency of uterine contractions
    - Fetal response to uterine contractions
  - Membrane status
    - Status of membranes, color of amniotic fluid
    - Date and time of rupture
  - Vaginal examination
    - Vaginal bleeding and discharge
    - Cervical exam
- Biochemical examinations during pregnancy
  - Laboratory studies
    - CBC, blood type, and Rh and antibody screen
    - Toxicology screening (if ordered)
    - Blood glucose screening
    - Urine for protein and sugar
  - Infectious disease evaluation
    - Chlamydia, gonorrhea, group beta strep, hepatitis B, rubella, syphilis
    - Optional infectious disease evaluation: cytomegalovirus, tuberculosis, trichomonas, human immunodeficiency virus (HIV), hepatitis A and C, herpes simplex virus
- Fetal assessment
  - Gestational age assessment
    - Last menstrual period (LMP)
    - Fetal movement
    - Ultrasound exams for dating
  - Fetal activity
    - Fetal movement by maternal report
    - Fetal movement by palpation

- Antenatal assessments
  - Nonstress tests (NSTs)
  - Contraction stress tests (CSTs)
  - Biophysical profiles
  - Ultrasounds
  - Amniotic fluid index (AFI)
- Method of monitoring
  - Auscultation
  - External
    - Ultrasound
    - Tocodynamometer
  - Internal
    - Fetal spiral electrode
    - Intrauterine pressure catheter

Intrapartal High-Risk Screening

Screening for intrapartal high-risk factors is an integral part of assessment of the normal laboring woman. While obtaining the history, the nurse notes the presence of any factors that may be associated with a high-risk condition (Joint Commission on Accreditation of Healthcare Organizations [JCAHO], 2004). For example, the woman who reports a physical symptom such as intermittent bleeding needs further assessment to rule out abruptio placentae or placenta previa before the admission process continues. In addition to identifying the presence of a high-risk condition, the nurse must recognize the implications of the condition for the laboring woman and her fetus. For example, in the case of an abnormal fetal presentation, the nurse understands that the labor may be prolonged, prolapse of the umbilical cord may be more likely, and there is a greater possibility of a cesarean birth.

Although physical conditions are frequently listed as the major factors that increase risk in the intrapartal period, sociocultural variables such as poverty, nutrition, the amount of prenatal care, and cultural beliefs regarding pregnancy may also precipitate a high-risk situation in the intrapartal period. Recent research indicates that women who suffer from post-traumatic stress disorder (PTSD) may be at increased risk for some intrapartal complications (Kennedy & MacDonald, 2002). The nurse begins gathering data about sociocultural factors as the woman enters the birthing area.

Communication problems can also affect the course of labor, as well as the nurse's ability to provide support and education. Thus, the nurse observes the communication pattern between the woman and her support person(s) and their responses to admission questions and initial teaching. If the woman and her support persons are not fluent in English or are hearing impaired, the nurse must find some way to provide information in their primary language or an interpreter to sign so that they can make informed decisions. If the nurse or other birthing room staff does not speak the woman's primary language or is hearing impaired, an appropriate interpreter should be obtained. (See further discussion in Appendices C ∞, D ∞, and E ∞). Communica-

tion may also be affected by cultural standards regarding when it is acceptable to speak, who should ask questions, or whether it is acceptable for the woman to let others know if she is experiencing discomfort (Spector, 2004).

A partial list of intrapartal risk factors appears in Table 23–1. The factors precede the Intrapartal Assessment Guide because they must be kept in mind during the assessment.

Intrapartal Physical and Psychosociocultural Assessment

A physical examination is part of the admission procedure and part of the ongoing care of the client. Although the intrapartal physical assessment is not as complete and thorough as the initial prenatal physical examination (see Chapter 15 ∞), it does involve assessment of some body systems and the actual labor process. The Intrapartal Assessment Guide on pages 608–612 provides a framework that the maternity nurse can use when examining the laboring woman.

The physical assessment includes assessments performed immediately on admission as well as ongoing assessments. When labor is progressing very quickly, the nurse may not have time for a complete assessment. In this case, the critical physical assessments would include maternal vital signs, labor status, fetal status, and laboratory findings. Psychologic disorders can also affect the intrapartum course. For example, the woman suffering from clinical depression may exhibit apathy, lack of energy, fear or hopelessness about the outcome of labor, or increased physical symptoms (Beal, Trougakos, Weiss et al., 2006). The woman with a panic disorder may have short-lived, unpredictable episodes of intense anxiety, whereas the woman with a generalized anxiety disorder may experience continual and excessive anxiety or worrying. The woman with obsessive-compulsive disorder may have irrational impulses that are relieved only with performing a ritualistic behavior, such as repetitive handwashing. Psychosis is one of the most disabling psychiatric disorders, and the woman may experience hallucinations and delusions. Women with acute psychosis typically require inpatient hospitalization.

Pregnancy further complicates psychiatric disorders because many of the medications used to treat the symptoms are contraindicated in pregnancy (Timbie, Horvitz-Lennon, Frank et al., 2006). For these reasons, the woman with a psychologic disorder may require additional support from the nurse.

Assessment of psychosocial history is a critical component of intrapartal nursing assessment. Because of the prevalence of physical and sexual assault against women in our society (see Chapter 9 ∞), the nurse needs to consider the possibility that the woman may have experienced such violence at some point in her life. If such is the case, she may be anxious about the labor process, or anxiety may arise during labor. Therefore, it is essential to review the woman's prenatal record and any other available records for information that may indicate abuse.

The cultural assessment provides a starting point for a plan that honors the values and beliefs of the laboring woman (Spector, 2004). Frequently, however, the nurse feels uncertain about what to ask or consider, perhaps because there has

Table 23–1   INTRAPARTAL HIGH-RISK FACTORS

Factor	Maternal Implication	Fetal-Neonatal Implication
Abnormal presentation	↑ Incidence of cesarean birth ↑ Incidence of prolonged labor ↑ Incidence of fibroids	↑ Incidence of placenta previa Prematurity ↑ Risk of congenital abnormality Neonatal physical trauma ↑ Risk of intrauterine growth restriction
Multiple gestation	↑ Uterine distention → ↑ risk of postpartum hemorrhage ↑ Risk of cesarean birth ↑ Risk of preterm labor	Low birth weight Prematurity ↑ Risk of congenital anomalies Feto-fetal transfusion
Hydramnios	↑ Discomfort ↑ Dyspnea ↑ Risk of preterm labor Edema of lower extremities/varicosities	↑ Risk of esophageal or other high alimentary tract atresias ↑ Risk of CNS anomalies (myelocele) ↑ Risk of TORCH infections ↑ Risk of prolapse cord
Oligohydramnios	Maternal fear of "dry birth"	↑ Incidence of congenital anomalies ↑ Incidence of renal lesions ↑ Risk of intrauterine growth restriction ↑ Risk of fetal acidosis ↑ Risk of cord compression Postmaturity
Meconium staining of amniotic fluid	↑ Psychologic stress due to fear for baby	↑ Risk of fetal asphyxia ↑ Risk of meconium aspiration ↑ Risk of pneumonia due to aspiration of meconium
Premature rupture of membranes	↑ Risk of infection (chorioamnionitis) ↑ Risk of preterm labor ↑ Anxiety/fear for the baby Prolonged hospitalization ↑ Incidence of tocolytic therapy	↑ Perinatal morbidity Prematurity ↓ Birth weight ↑ Risk of respiratory distress syndrome Prolonged hospitalization
Induction of labor	↑ Risk of hypercontractility of uterus ↑ Risk of uterine rupture ↑ Length of labor if cervix not ready ↑ Anxiety	Prematurity if gestational age not assessed correctly Hypoxia if hyperstimulation occurs
Abruptio placentae/placenta previa	Hemorrhage Uterine atony ↑ Incidence of cesarean birth ↑ Maternal morbidity	Fetal hypoxia/acidosis Fetal exsanguination ↑ Perinatal mortality
Failure to progress in labor	Maternal exhaustion ↑ Incidence of augmentation of labor ↑ Incidence of cesarean birth	Fetal hypoxia/acidosis Intracranial birth injury
Precipitous labor (less than 3 hours)	Perineal, vaginal, cervical lacerations ↑ Risk of postpartum hemorrhage	Tentorial tears
Prolapse of umbilical cord	↑ Fear for baby Cesarean birth → emergent	Acute fetal hypoxia/acidosis
Fetal heart decelerations	↑ Fear for baby ↑ Risk of cesarean birth, forceps, vacuum Continuous electronic monitoring and intervention in labor	Tachycardia, chronic asphyxic insult, bradycardia Acute asphyxic insult Chronic hypoxia Congenital heart block
Uterine rupture	Hemorrhage Cesarean birth/hysterectomy ↑ Risk of morbidity/mortality	Fetal anoxia Fetal hemorrhage ↑ Neonatal morbidity and mortality
Postdates (greater than 42 weeks)	↑ Anxiety ↑ Incidence of induction of labor ↑ Incidence of cesarean birth ↑ Use of technology to monitor fetus ↑ Risk of shoulder dystocia	Postmaturity syndrome ↑ Risk of fetal-neonatal mortality and morbidity ↑ Risk of antepartum fetal death ↑ Incidence/risk of large baby
Diabetes	↑ Risk of hydramnios ↑ Risk of hypoglycemia or hyperglycemia ↑ Risk of preeclampsia	↑ Risk of malpresentation ↑ Risk of macrosomia ↑ Risk of intrauterine growth restriction ↑ Risk of respiratory distress syndrome ↑ Risk of congenital anomalies
Preeclampsia	↑ Abruptio placentae ↑ Risk of seizures ↑ Risk of stroke ↑ Risk of HELLP	↑ Risk of small-for-gestational-age baby ↑ Risk of preterm birth ↑ Risk of mortality
AIDS/STD	↑ Risk of additional infections	↑ Risk of transplacental transmission

ASSESSMENT GUIDE   Intrapartal—First Stage of Labor

Physical Assessment/ Normal Findings	Alterations and Possible Causes*	Nursing Responses to Data†
VITAL SIGNS		
Blood pressure (BP): less than or equal to 135 systolic and less than or equal to 85 diastolic in adult 18 years of age or older or no more than 15–20 mm Hg rise in systolic pressure over baseline BP during early pregnancy	High blood pressure (essential hypertension, gestational hypertension, preeclampsia, renal disease, apprehension, anxiety or pain) Low blood pressure (supine hypotension) Hemorrhage/hypovolemia Shock Drugs	Evaluate history of preexisting disorders and check for presence of other signs of preeclampsia. Do not assess during contractions; implement measures to decrease anxiety and reassess. Turn woman on her side and recheck BP. Provide quiet environment. Have O₂ available.
Pulse: 60–90 bpm	Increased pulse rate (excitement or anxiety, cardiac disorders, early shock, drug use)	Evaluate cause, reassess to see if rate continues; report to physician/CNM.
Respirations: 12–24/min (or pulse rate divided by 4)	Marked tachypnea (respiratory disease), hyperventilation in transition phase Decreased respirations (Narcotics) Hyperventilation (anxiety/pain)	Assess between contractions; if marked tachypnea continues, assess for signs of respiratory disease or respiratory distress. Encourage slow breaths if woman is hyperventilating.
Pulse ox 95% or greater	Less than 90%: hypoxia, hypotension, hemorrhage	Apply O₂; notify physician/CNM.
Temperature: 36.2–37.6C (98–99.6F)	Elevated temperature (infection, dehydration, prolonged rupture of membranes, epidural regional block)	Assess for other signs of infection or dehydration.
WEIGHT		
25–35 lb greater than prepregnant weight	Weight gain greater than 35 lb (fluid retention, obesity, large infant, diabetes mellitus, preeclampsia), weight gain less than 15 lb (small for gestational age [SGA], substance abuse, psychosocial problems)	Assess for signs of edema. Evaluate dietary patterns. Assess for substance abuse and eating disorders.
LUNGS		
Normal breath sounds, clear and equal	Rales, rhonchi, friction rub (infection), pulmonary edema, asthma	Reassess; refer to physician/CNM
FUNDUS		
At 40 weeks' gestation located just below xiphoid process	Uterine size not compatible with estimated date of birth (SGA, large for gestational age [LGA], hydramnios, multiple pregnancy, placental/fetal anomalies, malpresentation)	Reevaluate history regarding pregnancy dating. Refer to physician for additional assessment.
EDEMA		
Slight amount of dependent edema	Pitting edema of face, hands, legs, abdomen, sacral area (preeclampsia)	Check deep tendon reflexes for hyperactivity; check for clonus; refer to physician.
HYDRATION		
Normal skin turgor, elastic	Poor skin turgor (dehydration)	Assess skin turgor; refer to physician for deviations. Provide fluids per physician/CNM orders.
PERINEUM		
Tissues smooth, pink color (see Prenatal Initial Physical Assessment Guide, Chapter 15 ∞)	Varicose veins of vulva, herpes lesions/genital warts	Note on client record need for follow-up in postpartal period; reassess after birth; refer to physician/CNM.
	*Possible causes of alterations are identified in parentheses.	†This column provides guidelines for further assessment and initial intervention.

ASSESSMENT GUIDE Intrapartal—First Stage of Labor continued

PHYSICAL ASSESSMENT/ NORMAL FINDINGS	ALTERATIONS AND POSSIBLE CAUSES*	NURSING RESPONSES TO DATA†
Clear mucus; may be blood tinged with earthy or human odor.	Profuse, purulent, foul-smelling drainage	Suspected gonorrhea or chorioamnionitis; report to physician; initiate care to newborn's eyes; notify neonatal nursing staff and pediatrician.
Presence of small amount of bloody show that gradually increases with further cervical dilatation	Hemorrhage	Assess BP and pulse, pallor, diaphoresis; report any marked changes. Standard precautions.

LABOR STATUS

Uterine contractions: regular pattern	Failure to establish a regular pattern, prolonged latent phase Hypertonicity Hypotonicity Dehydration	Evaluate whether woman is in true labor; Ambulate if in early labor. Evaluate client status and contractile pattern. Obtain a 20-minute electronic fetal monitoring (EFM) strip. Notify physician or CNM. Provide hydration.
Cervical dilatation: progressive cervical dilatation from size of fingertip to 10 cm (Procedure 23–1)	Rigidity of cervix (frequent cervical infections, scar tissue, failure of presenting part to descend)	Evaluate contractions, fetal engagement, position, and cervical dilatation. Inform client of progress.
Cervical effacement: progressive thinning of cervix (Procedure 23–1)	Failure to efface (rigidity of cervix, failure of presenting part to engage); cervical edema (pushing effort by woman before cervix is fully dilated and effaced, trapped cervix)	Evaluate contractions, fetal engagement and position. Notify physician/CNM if cervix is becoming edematous; work with woman to prevent pushing until cervix is completely dilated. Keep vaginal exams to a minimum.
Fetal descent: progressive descent of fetal presenting part from station −5 to +4 (Figure 23–3 ◆ in Procedure 23–1)	Failure of descent (abnormal fetal position or presentation, macrosomic fetus, inadequate pelvic measurements)	Evaluate fetal position, presentation, and size.
Membranes: may rupture before or during labor	Rupture of membranes more than 12–24 hours before initiation of labor	Assess for ruptured membranes using Nitrazine test tape before doing vaginal exam. Follow standard precautions. Instruct woman with ruptured membranes to remain on bed rest if presenting part is not engaged and firmly down against the cervix. Keep vaginal exams to a minimum to prevent infection. When membranes rupture in the birth setting **immediately assess FHR** to detect changes associated with prolapse of umbilical cord (FHR slows).

Findings on Nitrazine test tape:
Membranes probably intact
  yellow   pH 5.0
  olive   pH 5.5
  olive green pH 6.0
Membranes probably ruptured
  blue-green pH 6.5
  blue-gray pH 7.0
  deep blue pH 7.5
	False-positive results may be obtained if large amount of bloody show is present, previous vaginal examination has been done using lubricant, infection is present, or tape is touched by nurse's fingers.	Assess fluid for consistency, amount, odor; assess FHR frequently. Assess fluid at regular intervals for presence of meconium staining. Follow standard precautions while assessing amniotic fluid.
		Teach woman that amniotic fluid is continually produced (to allay fear of "dry birth").
		Teach woman that she may feel amniotic fluid trickle or gush with contractions.
		Change Chux pads often.

Amniotic fluid clear, with earthy or human odor, no foul-smelling odor	Greenish amniotic fluid (nonreassuring fetal status) Bloody fluid (vasoprevia, abruptio placentae) Strong or foul odor (amnionitis)	Assess FHR; do vaginal exam to evaluate for prolapsed cord; apply fetal monitor for continuous data; report to physician/CNM. Take woman's temperature and report to physician/CNM.
	*Possible causes of alterations are identified in parentheses.	†This column provides guidelines for further assessment and initial intervention.

(Continued on next page)

ASSESSMENT GUIDE   Intrapartal—First Stage of Labor continued

PHYSICAL ASSESSMENT/ NORMAL FINDINGS	ALTERATIONS AND POSSIBLE CAUSES*	NURSING RESPONSES TO DATA†
FETAL STATUS		
FHR: 110–160 bpm	Less than 110 or greater than 160 bpm (nonreassuring fetal status); abnormal patterns on fetal monitor: decreased variability, late decelerations, variable decelerations, absence of accelerations with fetal movement	Initiate interventions based on particular FHR pattern.
Presentation: Cephalic, 97% Breech, 3%	Face, brow, breech, or shoulder presentation	Report to physician; after presentation is confirmed as face, brow, breech, or shoulder, woman may be prepared for cesarean birth.
Position: left-occiput-anterior (LOA) most common	Persistent occipital-posterior (OP) position; transverse arrest	Carefully monitor maternal and fetal status. Reposition mother side-lying or hands/knee to promote rotation of fetal head.
Activity: fetal movement	Hyperactivity (may precede fetal hypoxia)	Carefully evaluate FHR; apply fetal monitor.
	Complete lack of movement (nonreassuring fetal status or fetal demise)	Carefully evaluate FHR; apply fetal monitor. Report to physician/CNM.
LABORATORY EVALUATION		
Hematologic tests **Hemoglobin:** 12–16 g/dL	Less than 11 g/dL. (anemia, hemorrhage, sickle cell disorders, pernicious anemia)	Evaluate woman for problems due to decreased oxygen-carrying capacity caused by lowered hemoglobin.
CBC **Hematocrit:** 38%–47% **RBC:** 4.2–5.4 million/mm³ **WBC:** 4500–11,000/mm³, although leukocytosis to 20,000/mm³ is not unusual **Platelets** 150,000–400,000/mm³	Presence of infection or blood dyscrasias, loss of blood (hemorrhage, disseminated intravascular coagulation [DIC])	Evaluate for other signs of infection or for petechiae, bruising, or unusual bleeding.
Serologic testing Serologic test for syphilis (STS) or Venereal Disease Research Laboratories (VDRL) test: nonreactive Rh	Positive reaction (see Chapter 15, Initial Prenatal Physical Assessment Guide ∞)	For reactive test notify newborn nursery and pediatrician.
	Rh-positive fetus in Rh-negative woman	Assess prenatal record for titer levels during pregnancy. Obtain cord blood for direct Coombs' at birth.
Urinalysis Glucose: negative	Glycosuria (low renal threshold for glucose, diabetes mellitus)	Assess blood glucose; test urine for ketones; ketonuria and glycosuria require further assessment of blood sugars.‡
Ketones: negative	Ketonuria (starvation ketosis)	
Proteins: negative	Proteinuria (urine specimen contaminated with vaginal secretions, fever, infection, kidney disease); proteinuria of 2+ or greater found in uncontaminated urine may be a sign of ensuing preeclampsia	Instruct woman in collection technique; incidence of contamination from vaginal discharge is common. Report any increase in proteinuria to physician/CNM.
Red blood cells: negative	Blood in urine (calculi, cystitis, glomerulonephritis, neoplasm)	Assess collection technique (may be bloody show).
White blood cells: negative	Presence of white blood cells (infection in genitourinary tract)	Assess for signs of urinary tract infection.
Casts: none	Presence of casts (nephrotic syndrome)	

CULTURAL ASSESSMENT§	VARIATIONS TO CONSIDER	NURSING RESPONSES TO DATA†
Cultural influences determine customs and practices regarding intrapartal care.	Individual preferences may vary.	
§These are only a few suggestions. We do not mean to imply that this is a comprehensive cultural assessment; rather, it is a tool to encourage cultural sensitivity.	*Possible causes of alterations are identified in parentheses.	†This column provides guidelines for further assessment and initial intervention. ‡Glycosuria should not be discounted. The presence of glycosuria necessitates follow-up.

ASSESSMENT GUIDE   Intrapartal—First Stage of Labor continued

CULTURAL ASSESSMENT§	VARIATIONS TO CONSIDER	NURSING RESPONSES TO DATA†
Ask the following questions: Who would you like to remain with you during your labor and birth?	She may prefer only her coach to remain or may also want family and/or friends.	Provide support for her wishes by encouraging desired people to stay. Provide information to others (with the woman's permission) who are not in the room.
What would you like to wear during labor?	She may be more comfortable in her own clothes.	Offer supportive materials such as Chux if needed to protect her own clothing. Avoid subtle signals to the woman that she should not have chosen to remain in her own clothes. Have other clothing available if the woman desires. If her clothing becomes contaminated, it will be simple to place it in a plastic bag.
What activity would you like during labor?	She may want to ambulate most of the time, stand in the shower, sit in the jacuzzi, sit on a chair/stool/birthing ball, remain on the bed, and so forth.	Support the woman's wishes; provide encouragement and complete assessments in a manner so her activity and positional wishes are disturbed as little as possible.
What position would you like for the birth?	She may feel more comfortable in lithotomy with stirrups and her upper body elevated, or side-lying or sitting in birthing bed, or standing, or squatting, or on hands and knees.	Collect any supplies and equipment needed to support her in her chosen birthing position. Provide information to the coach regarding any changes that may be needed based on the chosen position.
Is there anything special you would like?	She may want the room darkened or to have curtains and windows open, music playing, a Leboyer birth, her coach to cut the umbilical cord, to save a portion of the umbilical cord, to save the placenta, to videotape the birth, and so forth.	Support requests, and communicate requests to any other nursing or medical personnel (so requests can continue to be supported and not questioned). If another nurse or physician does not honor the request, act as advocate for the woman by continuing to support her unless her desire is truly unsafe.
Ask the woman if she would like fluids, and ask what temperature she prefers.	She may prefer clear fluids other than water (tea, clear juice). She may prefer iced, room-temperature, or warmed fluids.	Provide fluids as desired.
Observe the woman's response when privacy is difficult to maintain and her body is exposed.	Some women do not seem to mind being exposed during an exam or procedure; others feel acute discomfort.	Maintain privacy and respect the woman's sense of privacy. If the woman is unable to provide specific information, the nurse may draw from general information regarding cultural variation: Southeast Asian women may not want any family member in the room during exam or procedures. Her partner may not be involved with coaching activities during labor or birth. Muslim women may need to remain covered during the labor and birth and avoid exposure of any body part. The husband may need to be in the room but remain behind a curtain or screen so he does not view his wife at this time.
If the woman is to breastfeed, ask if she would like to feed her baby immediately after birth.	She may want to feed her baby right away or may want to wait a little while.	

PSYCHOSOCIAL ASSESSMENT	VARIATIONS TO CONSIDER	NURSING RESPONSES TO DATA†
PREPARATION FOR CHILDBIRTH		
Woman has some information regarding process of normal labor and birth.	Some women do not have any information regarding childbirth.	Add to present information base.
Woman has breathing and/or relaxation techniques to use during labor.	Some women do not have any method of relaxation or breathing to use, and some do not desire them.	Support breathing and relaxation techniques that client is using; provide information if needed.
§These are only a few suggestions. We do not mean to imply that this is a comprehensive cultural assessment; rather, it is a tool to encourage cultural sensitivity.		†This column provides guidelines for further assessment and initial intervention.

(Continued on next page)

ASSESSMENT GUIDE   Intrapartal—First Stage of Labor continued

PSYCHOSOCIAL ASSESSMENT	VARIATIONS TO CONSIDER	NURSING RESPONSES TO DATA[†]
PREPARATION FOR CHILDBIRTH (continued)		
Woman and support person have done extensive preparation for childbirth (Bradley Classes, Lamaze).	Some women have strong opinions regarding labor and birth preparation.	Support woman's wishes to participate in her birth experience; support birth plan.
RESPONSE TO LABOR		
Latent phase: relaxed, excited, anxious for labor to be well established	May cope well or feel unable to cope with contractions because of fear, anxiety, or lack of information.	Provide support and encouragement; establish trusting relationship.
Active phase: becomes more intense, begins to tire	May remain quiet and without any sign of discomfort or anxiety, may insist that she is unable to continue with the birthing process.	Provide support and coaching if needed.
Transitional phase: feels tired, may feel unable to cope, needs frequent coaching to maintain breathing patterns		
Coping mechanisms: Ability to cope with labor through use of support system, breathing, relaxation techniques, and comfort measures including frequent position changes in labor, warm water immersion, and massage.	May feel marked anxiety and apprehension, may not have coping mechanisms that can be brought into this experience, or may be unable to use them at this time.	Support coping mechanisms if they are working for the woman; provide information and support if she exhibits anxiety or needs alternative to present coping methods.
	Survivors of sexual abuse may demonstrate fear of IVs or needles, may recoil when touched, may insist on a female caregiver, may be very sensitive to body fluids and cleanliness, and may be unable to labor lying down. May show extreme distress with vaginal examinations.	Encourage participation of coach/significant other if a supportive relationship seems apparent. Establish rapport and a trusting relationship. Provide information that is true and offer your presence.
ANXIETY		
Some anxiety and apprehension is within normal limits	May show anxiety through rapid breathing, nervous tremors, frowning, grimacing, clenching of teeth, thrashing movements, crying, increased pulse and blood pressure.	Provide support, encouragement, and information. Teach relaxation techniques; support controlled breathing efforts. May need to provide a paper bag to breathe into if woman says her lips are tingling. Note FHR.
SOUNDS DURING LABOR		
	Some women are very quiet; others moan or make a variety of noises.	Provide a supportive environment. Encourage woman to do what feels right for her.
SUPPORT SYSTEM		
Physical intimacy between mother and father (or mother and support person/doula) caretaking activities such as soothing conversation, touching	Some women would prefer no contact, others may show clinging behaviors.	Encourage caretaking activities that appear to comfort the woman; encourage support for the woman; if support is limited, the nurse may take a more active role.
Support person stays in close proximity	Limited interaction may come from a desire for quiet.	Encourage support person to stay close (if this seems appropriate).
Relationship between mother and father (or support person): involved interaction	The support person may seem to be detached and maintain little support, attention, or conversation.	Support interactions; if interaction is limited, the nurse may provide more information and support.
		Ensure that coach/significant other has short breaks, especially/prior to transition.
		[†]This column provides guidelines for further assessment and initial nursing intervention.

been no personal opportunity to become aware of varying cultural values and beliefs. It is important to remember that despite one's cultural background, variations in different individuals and families can vary dramatically. Some individuals may not embrace cultural beliefs that are inherent in their cul-

ture. This section of the assessment guide (see pages 610–611) should help.

The final section addresses psychosocial factors. The laboring woman's psychosocial status is an important part of the total assessment. The woman has previous ideas, knowledge, and fears about childbearing. The adequacy of resources, such as housing, transportation, utilities, and access to social services, should also be questioned. By assessing her psychosocial status, the nurse can meet the woman's needs for information and support. The nurse can then support the woman and her partner; in the absence of a partner, the nurse may become the support person.

Evaluating Labor Progress

Intrapartal nursing care requires competent assessment and clinical skills and a comprehensive knowledge of maternal-fetal anatomy and the physiology of the labor process. An ongoing, accurate assessment of both the mother and fetus and their response to labor is necessary to provide the data required to make sound clinical judgments and provide appropriate care. Labor can be monitored in a number of ways, each having its own benefits and limitations. If a "low technology" approach is desired, a nurse can monitor uterine contractions and the FHR intermittently using techniques such as palpation and auscultation. However, if the clinical situation demands, as in the case of a high-risk pregnancy, the laboring client may be monitored electronically. External devices (tocodynanometer and ultrasound) or internal devices (intrauterine pressure catheter and fetal scalp electrode) may be used when a continuous graphic data record is needed to evaluate the mother and fetus during labor.

The method of monitoring during labor may vary, depending on the presence of risk factors at admission, the preferences of the client and healthcare provider, and the institution's policies (AAP & ACOG, 2002; ACOG, 2005). If intermittent monitoring is used, the nurse must perform a "hands-on" assessment, including auscultation of fetal heart tones (FHT) and palpation of uterine contractions (UC). If continuous **electronic fetal monitoring** (EFM) is used, the amount of physical "hands-on" care may vary depending on whether an internal or external mode of monitoring is used. EFM provides a continuous tracing of the FHR.

Professional associations, such as ACOG and AWHONN, and individual healthcare institutions generally set the guidelines for the level of intrapartum monitoring. The frequency of the maternal-fetal assessment and documentation depends on the mother's stage of labor and the presence of risk factors. When EFM is used, ACOG recommends that the nurse or physician review EFM data frequently. For low-risk pregnancies, FHR tracings can be reviewed every 30 minutes in first stage labor and every 15 minutes in second stage labor. The FHR tracings of high-risk pregnancies should be reviewed more frequently—every 15 minutes in first stage labor and every 5 minutes in second stage labor. Periodic documentation should accompany each review of the FHR tracing. See Table 23–2 for the frequency of recommended assessments and documentations.

The recommended frequency of FHR tracing assessment and documentation is only a guideline for practice. At times, the nurse may find it necessary to monitor the FHR more frequently. Certain clinical events such as vaginal exams, rupture of membranes, abnormal uterine activity patterns, administration of medications, or procedures such as epidurals, amniocentesis, external versions, and other events have the potential to adversely affect the FHR tracing. It is beneficial to assess the FHR

Table 23–2   FREQUENCY OF MATERNAL-FETAL ASSESSMENT AND DOCUMENTATION

	First Stage	Second Stage
Low risk	Every 30 minutes	Every 15 minutes
High risk	Every 15 minutes	Every 5 minutes

SOURCES: Data from ACOG, 2005; Cypher, Adelsperger, & Torgersen, 2003.

tracing before and after such events or anytime a nonreassuring FHR tracing is detected (Cypher et al., 2003).

Since its introduction into clinical practice in the late 1960s, EFM has continuously been researched and evaluated in regard to its ability to improve fetal outcomes and reduce morbidity and mortality. In the beginning, EFM was used in high-risk pregnancies, because it was thought that electronic assessment was far more accurate and valuable for diagnosing nonreassuring fetal status in labor. It was believed that continuous fetal monitoring could identify nonreassuring fetal status earlier, facilitate earlier interventions, and prevent fetal morbidity and mortality. Researchers originally thought EFM could prevent cerebral palsy, which was thought to be caused by neurologic damage from nonreassuring fetal status (Cunningham, Leveno, Bloom et al., 2005). Today's research does not support these earlier suppositions.

In 2002, 85% of all labors were monitored electronically, making EFM the most prevalent assessment procedure in maternal-fetal health care (ACOG, 2005). However, despite its widespread use, research has failed to show that it has significantly improved the outcomes at birth. Multiple controlled random trials have failed to show that EFM is beneficial over intermittent auscultation in preventing neonatal morbidity and mortality (ACOG, 2005; AWHONN, 2004; Cunningham et al., 2005). Intermittent assessment of the maternal-fetal couplet labor is generally considered to be as appropriate an assessment technique as electronic monitoring, especially for low-risk pregnancies when proper technique and nurse-to-patient ratio are used (AWHONN, 2003; Will, Hennicke, Jacobs et al., 2006).

UTERINE ACTIVITY ASSESSMENT

Monitoring uterine activity throughout labor is essential and provides data regarding the labor progress and fetal well-being. Numerous internal and external factors affect the maternal and fetal well-being. UCs interrupt the flow of blood to the placenta and reduce the amount of oxygen immediately available to the fetus. Decreased oxygen and blood flow directly affect the FHR. The pattern and intensity of contractions have a direct effect on the duration and progress of labor and the ability of the fetus to adapt to the intrapartal process. It is impossible to interpret the FHR without considering its relationship to the uterine activity (AWHONN, 2003).

UCs occur in wavelike patterns. Beginning at the fundus (top or apex of the uterus), the UC progresses downward through the lower segments of the uterus and is then followed by a similar wave of relaxation. The contraction of the upper uterine segment increases intrauterine pressure and leads to cervical dilatation and effacement and the descent of the fetus. During and between UCs, the fundus changes shape and firmness, reflecting the intensity of the UC. By monitoring the changes in the fundus, the nurse can determine the timing and intensity of the UC and the resting tone of the uterus between contractions (AWHONN, 2004). The intensity and frequency of the UC varies from woman to woman and labor to labor. Three methods of monitoring UCs are currently used: palpation, external electronic monitoring with a tocodynanometer, and internal electronic monitoring with an intrauterine pressure catheter. Each method is discussed.

Palpation

Palpation is the technique of assessing a UC by touch. To assess UCs, the nurse places the fingertips of one hand on the top of the uterus. Hand placement is usually on the fundus, but the location may vary based on maternal or fetal position, uterine size and shape, or maternal body composition. Gentle pressure is applied to the abdomen until the firmness of the underlying uterine wall is felt.

The frequency of the contractions is measured from the beginning of one contraction to the beginning of the next. The length of the contraction, referred to as the *duration,* is measured from the beginning of the contraction, when the muscle begins to tense, to the end of the same contraction, when the muscle is completely relaxed. Uterine resting tone is determined between UCs, when optimum uterine relaxation is achieved.

During the acme (peak) of the contraction, intensity can be evaluated subjectively by estimating the firmness of the fundus. It can be useful to compare the contraction to the firmness of a nose, chin, or forehead. A tense fundus that is easily indented (tip of the nose) is considered mild intensity. When the fundus becomes firm and difficult to indent with the fingertips (chin), the strength of the UC is considered moderate. The fundus that is hard and cannot be indented (forehead) is classified as strong. The nurse should assess successive contractions to provide reliable data. Table 23–3 compares contraction characteristics in different phases of labor. Direct uterine palpation is used with intermittent auscultation of the fetal heart or in conjunction with continuous EFM. The frequency of palpation depends on the risk status of the mother and fetus and the stage of labor.

Palpation has its capabilities, benefits, and limitations. Palpation allows the nurse to assess relative frequency, duration, and subjective strength of the contraction and uterine resting tone. UC assessment by palpation is beneficial over electronic monitoring because it (1) is noninvasive and does not increase the risk for infection or patient injury; (2) is readily accessible, requiring no equipment; (3) increases the "hands-on" care of the client that can be reassuring to the client; and (4) allows the mother freedom from restricting and sometimes uncomfortable abdominal belts, thus permitting her to move freely and ambulate if her condition permits. Palpation is limited because it does not provide actual quantitative measure of uterine pressure; thus subjective differences between nurses and nurse-to-client interpretations may exist. Palpation offers no permanent record, which can hinder interpretation by others. Maternal size and increased adipose tissue from obesity and maternal positioning may prevent direct palpation of the fundus. The limitations of palpation may outweigh the benefits in some clinical situations, and electronic monitoring may be a more appropriate choice for uterine assessment (Will et al., 2006).

Electronic Monitoring with External Tocodynanometer

Electronic monitoring of uterine contractions can be done externally by using a tocodynamometer or tocotransducer (toco). A toco is a pressure monitoring device that is placed on the maternal abdomen at or near the fundus (the area of greatest contractility) and held in place with an elastic belt, belly band, or other adhesive material (Figure 23–1 ◆). By placing the toco over a fetal part in the fundus rather than a pocket of amniotic fluid, a better contraction tracing can be obtained. As the uterus contracts, pressure exerted against the toco is amplified and transmitted to the EFM and recorded on graph paper.

The procedure for applying the tocotransducer begins with palpation of the uterus to locate the fundus. The toco is placed at or near the point of maximum contractility or strength of the uterine muscle. It is then secured with a belt, strap, or other type of adhesive device and plugged into a fetal monitor. The toco monitors uterine activity transabdominally by detecting changes in the abdominal wall and converting the fundal movement into elec-

Table 23–3	CONTRACTION AND LABOR PROGRESS CHARACTERISTICS

Contraction Characteristics

Latent phase:	Every 10–30 min × 20–40 sec; mild, progressing to moderate Every 5–7 min × 30–40 sec; moderate
Active phase:	Every 2–3 min × 40–60 sec; moderate to strong
Transition phase:	Every 1½–2 min × 60–90 sec; strong

Labor Progress Characteristics

Primipara:	1.2 cm/hr dilatation 1 cm/hr descent Less than 2 hr in second stage
Multipara:	1.5 cm/hr dilatation 2 cm/hr descent Less than 1 hr in second stage

Figure 23–1 ◆ Woman in labor with external monitor applied. The tocodynamometer placed on the uterine fundus is recording uterine contractions. The lower belt holds the ultrasonic device that monitors the fetal heart rate. The belts can be adjusted for comfort.
SOURCE: © Stella Johnson (www.stellajohnson.com).

tronic impulses. The toco can be used to assess UCs for *frequency* (timing) and *duration* (length). However, it cannot determine UC intensity (strength). The displayed numbers and graph tracing for UC intensity are arbitrary and are influenced by how tightly the belt is applied around the maternal abdomen and/or the maternal position. Palpation must be used to assess UC intensity when the external toco monitor is used. When the belt is tight enough, the nurse should be able to note the beginning of contractions on the monitor just before or at the same time the woman begins to feel them (Will et al., 2006).

A beltless tocodynamometer system featuring remote telemetry is available. This system consists of an adhesive transducer that is applied to the most prominent part of the woman's abdomen with a double-sided adhesive film. The nonbelted tocodynamometer tends to be preferred by the laboring woman because it allows more freedom of movement, is easily applied, needs readjustment only infrequently, and generally is more convenient (Figure 23–2 ◆). It enables upright positions, which promote fetal descent by gravity, as well as ambulation, which can shorten the labor course and increase comfort for the laboring woman.

The advantages to using a toco for assessing uterine contractions are that it is noninvasive, easy to place, and may be used both before and following rupture of membranes. Because it is noninvasive, it can be used intermittently to allow the woman to ambulate, shower, or use a whirlpool bath. The toco also provides a permanent, continuous recording of the duration and frequency of contractions for future evaluation. Placement of the tocotransducer influences the accuracy of the uterine graphic tracing. As with any type of technology, no toco is flawless, and the monitor cannot fill the role of the nurse. The nurse should routinely palpate the intensity of the contractions and the relaxation of the uterus between contractions and compare the assessment with data recorded by the monitor. Another disadvantage is that sometimes the belt may become uncomfortable because it

Figure 23–2 ◆ The beltless tocodynamometer system features remote telemetry.
SOURCE: Courtesy of Hewlett-Packard Company.

must be worn snugly to monitor UCs accurately. The belt may require frequent readjustment as the mother changes position. The mother may also feel inhibited to move or as though she needs to remain in one position so as not to disturb the belt.

Trying to figure out if I was in labor was quite a task. Here I was, a birthing room nurse, and I couldn't decide if my contractions were the real thing. I timed them, and about the time I decided this was it, they would slow down. How exasperating not to know! It was so hard on me. But now I see that all women are in this spot. They want so much to be right, and we often treat them as if they should be able to sense when it's the real thing. I'd like the birthing room nurses to remember this.

Electronic Monitoring by Internal Pressure Catheter

Electronic monitoring of UCs can be done internally by using an **intrauterine pressure catheter (IUPC).** The IUPC is a catheter that is inserted into the uterine cavity through the cervix os. With correct placement in the uterus, usually in the area of the fetal small parts (arms or legs), the catheter reflects the pressure inside the uterine cavity. As the pressure changes in the uterus, the changes are relayed through a transducer to the fetal monitor, producing a tracing on the graph paper. The IUPC can measure the resting tone of the uterus between contractions and the actual amount of intrauterine pressure during contractions, referred to as UC intensity.

IUPCs can be one of two types: fluid-filled catheters and solid-tipped catheters. Fluid-filled catheters are a single-lumen catheter connected to a pressure-sensitive diaphragm outside the uterus. As intrauterine pressure changes, the column of fluid in the catheter fluctuates and exerts pressure on the diaphragm, sending signals to the transducer and fetal monitor. The solid-tipped catheter uses more recent technology in that the catheter contains a solid-state micropressure transducer (electronic sensor) at its tip, and the catheter that is inserted directly into the uterus. The catheter is then connected by a cable to the EFM. The catheter also incorporates a second lumen, permitting amnioinfusion while simultaneously providing accurate monitoring of intrauterine pressure (Figure 23–3 ◆). Regardless of the type of catheter, fluid filled or solid tipped, the IUPC can be used only after membranes are ruptured and the client has adequate cervical dilation, usually 3 centimeters or more.

The IUPC has several benefits over an external tocotransducer or palpation. Because the IUPC is inserted directly into the uterus, it provides near-exact pressure measurements for contraction intensity and uterine resting tone. The increased sensitivity of the IUPC allows for very accurate timing of UCs, thus making it extremely useful in cases when the provider needs closer uterine monitoring. The IUPC may be the preferred method of monitoring when it is particularly important to avoid hyperstimulation and possible uterine rupture in women with a previous history of cesarean birth who are attempting a vaginal birth after cesarean (VBAC) and are receiving oxytocin. If the woman's labor is prolonged, internal monitoring can be used to accurately assess the frequency and strength of contractions. If a nonreassuring FHR tracing is present, internal monitoring with IUPC and fetal scalp electrode may be essential to correlate UC

Figure 23–3 ◆ INTRAN Plus intrauterine pressure catheter. There is a micropressure transducer (electronic sensor) located at the tip of the catheter and a port for amnioinfusion at the distal end of the catheter.
SOURCE: Photographer, Elena Dorfman.

timing and FHR pattern response. IUPCs are also preferred when amnioinfusion is indicated, such as in cases with meconium-stained amniotic fluid. The IUPC provides a permanent record of the uterine activity for future analysis and documentation, making it useful in client care decision making.

However, with all of its benefits, the IUPC has its limitations and risks. Use of IUPCs is limited by the clinical situation. Membranes must be ruptured and adequate cervical dilation must be achieved for insertion. The procedure is invasive and increases the risk of uterine infection or uterine perforation or trauma. When an intrauterine catheter is used, there is a 1% risk of infection, but this seems to depend on the duration of ruptured membranes and length of labor. Invasive equipment like the IUPC is contraindicated in cases when active infections can be transmitted vertically through the cervix into the uterus to the fetus. Insertion of an IUPC with a low-lying placenta can result in placenta puncture, which can cause hemorrhage and nonreassuring fetal status (Sciscione, Duhl, Pullook et al., 2005). IUPCs also require proper insertion and zeroing procedures; thus competency in insertion technique and equipment maintenance and troubleshooting is essential.

CERVICAL ASSESSMENT

Cervical dilatation and effacement are evaluated directly by vaginal examination (see Procedure 23–1: Performing an Intrapartal Vaginal Examination). The vaginal examination can also provide information regarding fetal position, station of the presenting part, and membrane status (intact or ruptured). To assist in evaluating membrane status, the nurse assesses for the presence of amniotic fluid (Procedure 23–2: Assessing for Amniotic Fluid).

PROCEDURE 23–1 Performing an Intrapartal Vaginal Examination

NURSING ACTION	RATIONALE
Preparation	
• Explain the procedure, the indications for the exam, what the exam may feel like, and that it may cause discomfort.	
• Assess for latex allergies.	
• Position the woman with her thighs flexed and abducted. Instruct her to put the heels of her feet together. Drape the woman with a sheet, leaving a flap to access the perineum.	*This position provides access to the woman's perineum. The drape ensures privacy.*
• Encourage the woman to relax her muscles and legs.	*Relaxation decreases muscle tension and increases comfort.*
• Inform the woman before touching her. Be gentle.	

> **CLINICAL TIP**
> Use nonlatex gloves if the woman has a latex allergy

Equipment and Supplies

Clean disposable gloves if membranes not ruptured
Sterile gloves if membranes ruptured
Lubricant
Nitrazine test tape
Slide
Sterile cotton-tipped swab (Q-tip)

Before the Procedure: Test for Fluid Leakage

If fluid leakage has been reported or noted, use Nitrazine test tape and Q-tip with slide for fern test before performing the exam (see Procedure 23–2).

PROCEDURE 23–1 Performing an Intrapartal Vaginal Examination   continued

NURSING ACTION	RATIONALE

Procedure: Clean Gloves (Sterile if membranes ruptured)

CLINICAL TIP

Digital examination may be deferred if the woman has ruptured membranes but is not in active labor (AAP & ACOG, 2002).

1. Pull glove onto dominant hand.

Single glove is worn when membranes are intact. If a sterile exam is needed, both hands will be gloved with sterile gloves.

2. Using your gloved hand, position the hand with the wrist straight and the elbow tilted downward. Insert your well-lubricated second and index fingers of the gloved hand gently into the vagina until they touch the cervix. Use care when positioning your hand.

This position allows the fingertips to point toward the umbilicus and find the cervix.

3. If the woman verbalizes discomfort, acknowledge it and apologize. Pause for a moment and allow her to relax before progressing.

This validates the woman's discomfort and helps her feel more in control.

4. To determine the status of labor progress, perform the vaginal examination during and between contractions.

Cervical effacement, dilatation, and fetal station are affected by the presence of a contraction.

5. Palpate for the opening, or a depression, in the cervix. Estimate the diameter of the depression to identify the amount of dilatation (Figure 23–4 ◆).

Allows determination of effacement and dilatation.

6. Determine the status of the fetal membranes by observing for leakage of amniotic fluid. If fluid is expressed, test for amniotic fluid.

Determine the presenting part is necessary to assess the position of the fetus and to evaluate fetal descent.

7. Palpate the presenting part (Figure 23–5 ◆.)

8. Assess the fetal descent (Figure 23–6 ◆) and station by identifying the position of the posterior fontanelle.

9. Record findings on woman's chart and on fetal monitor strip if fetal monitor is being used.

Documentation   Document that the procedure was explained to the client, and that the woman verbalized understanding and provided consent before the vaginal examination. The woman's reaction and how the procedure was tolerated should be documented. The findings of the examination should be clearly documented using a facility-appropriate documentation form.

Figure 23–4 ◆ To gauge cervical dilatation, the nurse places the index and middle fingers against the cervix and determines the size of the opening. Before labor begins, the cervix is long (approximately 2.5 cm), the sides feel thick, and the cervical canal is closed, so an examining finger cannot be inserted. During labor, the cervix begins to dilate, and the size of the opening progresses from 1 cm to 10 cm in diameter.

(Continued on next page)

PROCEDURE 23–1 Performing an Intrapartal Vaginal Examination   continued

Figure 23–5 ◆ Palpation of the presenting part (the portion of the fetus that enters the pelvis first). *A,* Left occiput anterior (LOA). The occiput (area over the occipital bone on the posterior part of the fetal head) is in the left anterior quadrant of the woman's pelvis. When the fetus is in LOA, the posterior fontanelles (located just above the occipital bone and triangular in shape) are in the upper left quadrant of the maternal pelvis. *B,* Left occiput posterior (LOP). The posterior fontanelle is in the lower left quadrant of the maternal pelvis. *C,* Right occiput anterior (ROA). The posterior fontanelle is in the upper right quadrant of the maternal pelvis. *D,* Right occiput posterior (ROP). The posterior fontanelle is in the lower right quadrant of the maternal pelvis.
NOTE: The anterior fontanelle is diamond shaped. Because of the roundness of the fetal head, only a portion of the anterior fontanelle can be seen in each of the views, so it appears to be triangular in shape.

FETAL ASSESSMENT

A complete intrapartal fetal assessment requires determination of the fetal position and presentation and evaluation of the fetal status.

Determination of Fetal Position and Presentation

Fetal position is determined in several ways, including the following:

- Inspection of the woman's abdomen
- Palpation of the woman's abdomen (Leopold's maneuvers)
- Vaginal examination to determine the presenting part
- Ultrasound

INSPECTION

The nurse should observe the woman's abdomen for size and shape. The lie of the fetus should be assessed by noting whether

the uterus projects up and down (longitudinal lie) or left to right (transverse lie).

PALPATION: LEOPOLD'S MANEUVERS

Leopold's maneuvers are a systematic way to evaluate the maternal abdomen (Figure 23–7 ◆). Frequent practice increases the examiner's skill in determining fetal position by palpation. Leopold's maneuvers may be difficult to perform on an obese woman or on a woman who has excessive amniotic fluid (hydramnios).

Care should be taken to ensure the woman's comfort during Leopold's maneuvers. The woman should have recently emptied her bladder and should lie on her back with her abdomen uncovered. To aid in relaxation of the abdominal wall, the shoulders should be raised slightly on a pillow and the knees drawn up a little. The procedure should be completed between contractions. The examiner's hands should be warm. The order in which Leopold's maneuvers are performed may vary from one clinician to another.

PROCEDURE 23–1 Performing an Intrapartal Vaginal Examination continued

High head (station −4) Head is ballotable	Flexion and descent (station −2/ −3)	Engaged (at the spines) (zero station)	Deeply engaged (station +2)	On pelvic floor and rotating (station +4)	Rotation into A.P. (station +4/+5)
Membranes intact	Sagittal suture in transverse diameter	Cervix dilating, head descending	→ → →	Occiput rotating forward	Rim of cervix felt

Figure 23–6 ◆ Descent of the fetus through the maternal pelvis can be assessed by determining station (the relationship of the presenting part to an imaginary line between the maternal ischial spines). As the fetus moves downward, cardinal movements occur (see Chapter 22 ∞). The nurse assesses the station and identifies the cardinal movements by determining the position of the posterior fontanelle. The upper panels depict the fetal head progressing downward through the pelvis. From left to right, the first four views depict descent and flexion of the fetal chin onto the fetal chest. In the last two views, internal rotation occurs. Each view also depicts downward movement of the fetal head through the maternal pelvis as measured by the change in station. The lower panels depict the cervix, which is still rather thick (little effacement has occurred). The amniotic membranes are still intact over the fetal head. When the fetus is at −4 station, the fetal head is ballotable (when it is touched by the examining nurse's finger, the head floats upward and resettles downward). In the second view, note the thinner cervix (which indicates that more effacement has occurred). The saggital suture and posterior fontanelle can be palpated. The next two views depict further effacement and descent of the fetal head from 0 station to +2. The last two views depict continuing effacement and position that would be felt on vaginal examination of the presenting part while the fetal head is completing internal rotation.

While inspecting and palpating the maternal abdomen, the nurse should consider the following questions:

- Is the fetal lie longitudinal or transverse?
- What is in the fundus? Am I feeling buttocks or head?
- Where is the fetal back?
- Where are the small parts or extremities?
- What is in the inlet? Does it confirm what I found in the fundus?
- Is the presenting part engaged, floating, or dipping into the inlet?
- Is there fetal movement?
- How large is the fetus (appropriate, large, or small for gestational age)?
- Is there one fetus or more than one?
- Is fundal height proportionate to the estimated gestational age?

First Maneuver

While facing the woman, the nurse palpates the upper abdomen with both hands (see Figure 23–7, *A* ◆). The nurse determines the shape, size, consistency, and mobility of the form that is found. The fetal head is firm, hard, and round and moves independently of the trunk. The breech feels softer and symmetric and has small bony prominences; it moves with the trunk.

Second Maneuver

After ascertaining whether the head or the buttocks occupies the fundus, the nurse tries to determine the location of the fetal back and notes whether it is on the right or left side of the maternal abdomen. Still facing the woman, the nurse palpates the abdomen with deep but gentle pressure, using the palms (see Figure 23–7, *B* ◆). The right hand should be steady while the left hand explores the right side of the uterus. The nurse then repeats the maneuver, probing with the right hand and steadying

PROCEDURE 23–2 Assessing for Amniotic Fluid

NURSING ACTION	RATIONALE

Preparation

- Explain the procedure, indications for the procedure, what the woman will feel, and information that may be obtained.
- Determine whether she has noted the escape of any fluid from her vagina.

Equipment and Supplies

Nitrazine test tape
Sterile speculum
A glass slide and a sterile cotton-tipped swab (Q-tip)
Sterile syringe
Microscope

Procedure: Sterile Gloves

1. Complete this test before doing an examination that requires the use of lubricant.
2. Put on sterile gloves. With one gloved hand, spread the labia, and with the other gloved hand place a small section of Nitrazine tape (approx. 2 in. long) against the vaginal opening. Take care not to touch the tape with bare fingers before the test.

   Contamination of the Nitrazine test tape with lubricant can make the test unreliable. Enough fluid needs to be placed on the test tape to make it wet. Amniotic fluid is alkaline, and an alkaline fluid turns the Nitrazine test tape a dark blue. If the test tape remains a beige color, the test is negative for amniotic fluid.

3. Compare the color on the test tape to the guide on the back of the Nitrazine test tape container to determine test results.

4. Amniotic fluid may also be obtained by speculum exam. This is indicated in preterm premature rupture of membranes. If fluid is present in sufficient amount to draw some into a syringe, a small amount should be collected, or the pool of fluid in the posterior vagina can be obtained with a sterile cotton swab. A small amount of fluid is placed on a glass slide, allowed to dry, and then examined under the microscope. A ferning pattern confirms the presence of amniotic fluid. See Figure 12–4 ∞ for an example of ferning.

   Obtaining a specimen by speculum examination reduces the contamination of the fluid with other substances such as blood and cervical mucus and reduces the chance of infection for the woman who is not actively laboring.

Documentation	Record the findings on the labor record. Documentation of the status of membranes should include whether they are intact or ruptured. Other characteristics, such as color, odor, and amount of fluid present, should also be recorded, along with the time of rupture.

the uterus with the left hand. The fetal back should feel firm and smooth and should connect what was found in the fundus with a mass in the inlet. Once the back is located, the nurse validates the finding by palpating the fetal extremities (small irregularities and protrusions) on the opposite side of the abdomen.

Third Maneuver

Next, the nurse should determine what fetal part is lying above the inlet by gently grasping the lower portion of the abdomen just above the symphysis pubis with the thumb and fingers of the right hand (see Figure 23–7, *C* ◆). This maneuver yields the opposite information from what was found in the fundus and validates the presenting part. If the head is presenting and is not engaged, it may be gently pushed back and forth.

Fourth Maneuver

For this portion of the examination, the nurse faces the woman's feet and attempts to locate the cephalic prominence or brow. Location of this landmark assists in assessing the descent of the presenting part into the pelvis. The fingers of both hands are moved gently down the sides of the uterus toward the pubis (see Figure 23–7, *D* ◆). The cephalic prominence (brow) is located on the side where there is greatest resistance to the descent of the fingers toward the pubis. It is located on the opposite side from the fetal back if the head is well flexed. However, when the fetal head is extended, the occiput is the first cephalic prominence felt, and it is located on the same side as the back. Therefore, when completing the fourth maneuver, if the nurse finds that the first cephalic prominence palpated is on the same side

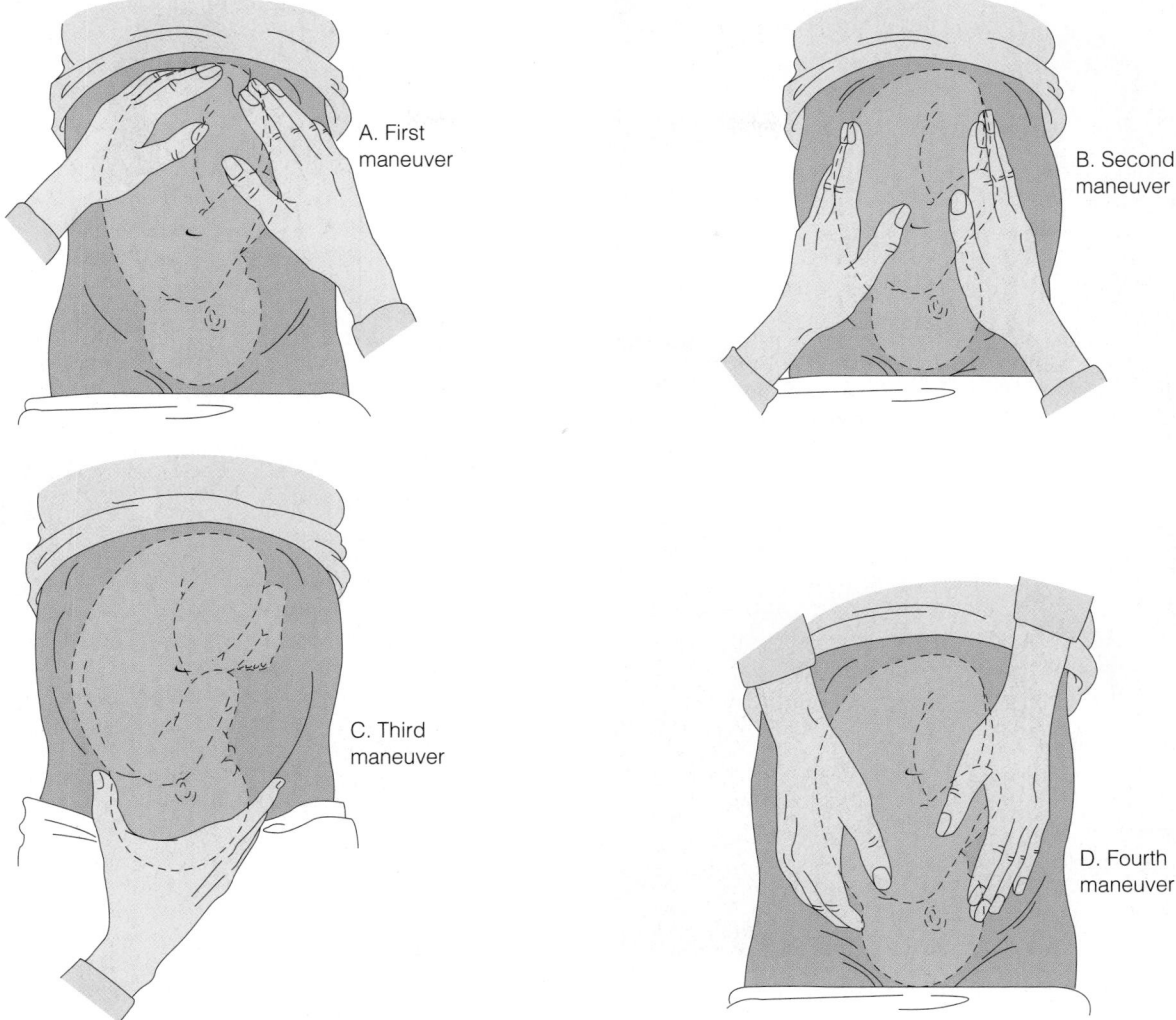

Figure 23–7 ◆ Leopold's maneuvers for determining fetal head position, presentation, and lie.
NOTE: Some practitioners may perform the sequence differently. Many nurses do the fourth maneuver first to identify the part of the fetus in the pelvic inlet.

as the back, the head is not flexed. If the first prominence found is opposite the back, the head is well flexed.

VAGINAL EXAMINATION

The vaginal examination reveals information regarding the fetus such as presentation, position, station, degree of flexion of the fetal head, and any swelling that may be present on the fetal scalp (caput succedaneum).

> **CLINICAL TIP**
>
> If you are having difficulty reaching a posterior cervix, ask the woman to place her fists under her buttocks or use a bedpan to facilitate a pelvic tilt, which will make the cervix more accessible.

ULTRASOUND

Real-time ultrasound is frequently available in the birth setting. It may be used to assess fetal lie, presentation, and position; obtain measurements of biparietal diameter to estimate gestational age; assess for anomalies when a vaginal examination reveals suspicious findings, and assess placement of the placenta. Ultrasound is often helpful to locate the fetal heart location when the nurse is having difficulty locating it, such as in cases where there are multiple fetuses. It can also be used to diagnose a fetal demise. (See Chapter 21 ∞ for further discussion of the use of ultrasound for fetal assessment).

Auscultation of Fetal Heart Rate

Auscultation is the direct auditory monitoring and interpretation of the fetal heart in utero. The number of fetal heart beats per minute (bpm) is referred to as the FHR or FHT. Auscultation uses a handheld instrument, such as a fetoscope or ultrasound Doppler, to listen to and count the FHR (Figure 23–8 ◆). Each instrument uses slightly different technology. Fetoscopes magnify actual fetal heart sounds, whereas Dopplers use ultrasound to convert fetal myocardial movement into sound waves that are then amplified and sent through a speaker from which the heart rate can be counted. Some Dopplers display a digital readout in addition to the audible sound produced.

A

B

Figure 23–8 ◆ *A,* When the fetal heart rate is picked up by the electronic monitor, the sound of the heartbeat can be heard by all persons in the room.
SOURCE: Photographer, Elena Dorfman.
B, The nurse uses a Doppler to assess the fetal heart rate. Doppler monitors can be used for intermittent labor monitoring or in the outpatient or community setting.
SOURCE: Michael Newman/PhotoEdit.

Figure 23–9 ◆ Location of FHR in relation to the more commonly seen fetal positions. The FHR is heard more clearly over the fetal back.

Before listening to the FHR the first time, the nurse may choose to perform Leopold's maneuvers to determine the probable location of the FHR. The FHR is heard most clearly at the fetal back (Figure 23–9 ◆). Thus, in a cephalic presentation, the FHR is best heard in the lower quadrant of the maternal abdomen. In a breech presentation it is heard at or above the level of the maternal umbilicus. In a transverse lie the FHR may be heard best just above or just below the umbilicus. As the presenting part descends and rotates through the maternal pelvis during labor, the FHR tends to descend and move toward the midline. In some instances, the monitor may track the maternal heart rate instead of the FHR. However, the nurse can avoid the error by comparing the maternal pulse with the FHR.

After the FHR is located, it is usually counted for 30 to 60 seconds to obtain the number of beats per minute. The nurse should listen before, during, and just after a contraction to detect

any abnormal heart rate, especially if the FHR is over 160 (tachycardia) or under 110 (bradycardia), or if irregular beats are heard. Listening through a contraction may be difficult because of maternal movement or a muffling of the FHR sounds. It is especially important to listen during and after the contraction to detect any deceleration that might occur. It is also important to listen immediately after each contraction when the woman is pushing during second stage, because fetal bradycardia frequently occurs as pressure is exerted on the fetal head during descent. See Procedure 23–3: Auscultation of Fetal Heart Rate and Table 23–4 for guidelines regarding how often to auscultate FHR.

Auscultation has been used for many years and remains a very valuable assessment technique even though it uses less technology than EFM. Research and standards have shown that intermittent auscultation is equally effective for monitoring the FHR

PROCEDURE 23–3 Auscultation of Fetal Heart Rate

NURSING ACTION	RATIONALE

Preparation

- Explain the procedure, the indications for it, and the information that will be obtained.
- Uncover the woman's abdomen.

Equipment and Supplies

Doppler device
Ultrasonic gel

Procedure

> **CLINICAL TIP**
>
> The fetal heart rate (FHR) is heard most clearly through the fetal back.
> Locate the fetal back using Leopold's maneuvers.

1. To use the Doppler:
   - Place ultrasonic gel on the diaphragm of the Doppler. Gel is used to maintain contact with the maternal abdomen and enhances conduction of sound.
   - Place the Doppler diaphragm on the woman's abdomen halfway between the umbilicus and symphysis and in the midline. You are most likely to hear the FHR in this area. Listen carefully for the sound of the fetal heartbeat.
2. Check the woman's pulse against the fetal sounds you hear. If the rates are the same, reposition the Doppler and try again.
3. If the rates are not similar, count the FHR for 1 full minute. Note that the FHR has a double rhythm and only one sound is counted.
4. If you do not locate the FHR, move the Doppler laterally (see Figure 23–8, *A*).
5. Auscultate the FHR between, during, and for 30 seconds following a uterine contraction (UC).
6. Frequency recommendations:
   - Low-risk women: Every 30 minutes during the first stage, and every 15 minutes in the second stage.
   - High-risk women: Every 15 minutes during the first stage, and every 5 minutes in the second stage.

If the rates are the same, you are probably hearing the maternal pulse and not the FHR.

This evaluation provides the opportunity to assess the fetal status and response to labor.

Documentation	Document that the procedure was explained to the woman and that she verbalized understanding. The location of the FHR, FHR baseline, changes in FHR that occur with contractions, and presence of accelerations or decelerations should be included. Other characteristics should include variability, maternal position, the type of device used, uterine activity, maternal pulse, and nursing interventions that were performed.

The Fetoscope

The fetoscope is an older assessment tool; however, some clinicians prefer it because it is "natural" and does not rely on ultrasound.
To use the fetoscope:

- Place the fetoscope earpieces in your ears and the device support against your forehead; use the handpiece to position the bell of the fetoscope on the mother's abdomen.
- Place the diaphragm halfway between the umbilicus and symphysis and in the midline. *You are most likely to hear the FHR in this area.*
- Without touching the fetoscope, listen carefully for the FHR.

Table 23–4   FREQUENCY OF AUSCULTATION: ASSESSMENT AND DOCUMENTATION

Low-Risk Patients	High-Risk Patients
First stage of labor every 30 min	First stage of labor every 15 min
Second stage of labor every 15 min	Second stage of labor every 5 min

Labor Events

Assess FHR before:
  Initiation of labor-enhancing procedures (e.g., artificial rupture of membranes)
  Periods of ambulation
  Administration of medications
  Administration or initiation of analgesia/anesthesia
Assess FHR following:
  Rupture of membranes
  Recognition of abnormal uterine activity patterns, such as increased basal tone or tachysystole
  Evaluation of oxytocin (maintenance, increase, or decrease of dosage)
  Administration of medications (at time of peak action)
  Expulsion of enema
  Urinary catheterization
  Vaginal examination
  Periods of ambulation
  Evaluation of analgesia and/or anesthesia (maintenance, increase, or decrease of dosage)

as EFM when a 1:1 nurse-to-client ratio is maintained and the pregnant client remains low risk. Low-risk status has been defined as "no pregnancy risk factors, no meconium stained fluid, normal labor patterns, and labor without augmentation or induction" (ACOG, 2005; Will et al., 2006). Outside these parameters, intermittent auscultation may not be appropriate and should not be used to assess high-risk pregnancies (ACOG, 2005).

Auscultation is a learned skill and requires practice and knowledge of its benefits and limitations as an assessment tool. It has many advantages that make it a preferred method of monitoring by both mothers and nurses. Auscultation uses minimum instrumentation, is portable, and allows for maximum maternal movement; thus it is convenient and economical. Its disadvantages include the limited data this technique can provide compared with EFM. Only the baseline FHR (BL FHR), rhythms of the FHR, and obvious increases and decreases can be monitored. Auscultation also does not provide a permanent record, thus making interpretation of the FHR impossible in the future or by another care provider. Identifying patterns and nonreassuring FHR is difficult and requires training. Auscultation must be practiced to ensure accurate interpretation of data.

Identifying UCs and the FHR simultaneously is necessary to determine patterns in the FHR and the relationship between the FHR and the UC. Auscultation does not allow for the detection of small changes in the FHR and cannot determine baseline variability (BL VAR). It may also be limited by maternal obe-

sity and movement by the mother and fetus (AWHONN, 2006). In such instances, it may be essential to monitor using electronic means, regardless of the client's risk status.

ELECTRONIC FETAL MONITORING

Electronic fetal monitoring (EFM) provides a continuous tracing of the FHR, allowing characteristics of the FHR to be observed and evaluated (see Procedure 23–4: Electronic Fetal Monitoring). When the FHR is monitored electronically, the interval between two successive fetal heartbeats is continually measured, and the rate is displayed as if the beats occurred at the same interval for 60 seconds. For example, if the interval between beats is 0.5 seconds, the rate for the full minute would be 120 bpm.

In the late 1990s, standardized definitions for FHR tracings were proposed (NICHD, 1997) in an effort to resolve controversy surrounding the benefits of EFM, the primary interpretation of FHR patterns, and appropriate interventions for nonreassuring tracings (Cunningham et al., 2005). In 2004, JCAHO recommended standardized and consistent use of fetal monitoring terminology among all healthcare professionals and the development of clear guidelines for fetal monitoring of potential high-risk patients (JCAHO, 2004). In response, in May 2005, ACOG issued a bulletin that reviewed FHR assessment terminology and described the management of nonreassuring FHR patterns (ACOG, 2005). At the same time, the AWHONN revised its fetal monitoring courses to incorporate the standardized terminology. In December 2005, ACOG modified its May bulletin to match AWHONN guidelines and the NICHD terminology. This chapter reflects the most recent guidelines instituted by ACOG and AWHONN and the NICHD terminology for FHR tracings.

Indications for Electronic Fetal Monitoring

ACOG states that the frequency of FHR monitoring used during labor should be based on risk factors (ACOG, 2005). Although there is as yet no standardized list, Table 23–5 identifies some common indications for EFM.

External Monitoring

Electronic monitoring of the FHR can be done externally by using an ultrasound (US) transducer. The US transducer is a Doppler device with computerized logic to interpret and count the Doppler signals (Cunningham et al., 2005). The US transducer is placed on the maternal abdomen over the fetal back (as determined by Leopold's maneuvers), where the FHR is usually the loudest, and is held in place with an elastic belt. A water-soluble gel is applied to the underside of the transducer to aid in conduction of the fetal heart sounds. The US transducer then emits ultrasonic beams that reflect off the moving fetal myocardium and return to the transducer. The transducer receives the signal and interprets it before amplifying it in the

PROCEDURE 23–4 Electronic Fetal Monitoring

NURSING ACTION	RATIONALE

Preparation

- Explain the procedure, the indications for it, and the information that will be obtained.

Equipment and Supplies

Monitor
Two elastic monitor belts
Tocodynamometer ("toco")
Ultrasound transducer
Ultrasound gel

Procedure

CLINICAL TIP

Evaluating the FHR tracing provides information about fetal status and response to the stress of labor. The presence of reassuring characteristics is associated with good fetal outcomes. Rapid identification of nonreassuring characteristics allows prompt interventions and the opportunity to determine the fetal response to the interventions.

1. Turn on the monitor.
2. Place the two elastic belts around the woman's abdomen.
3. Place the "toco" over the uterine fundus off the midline on the area palpated to be most firm during contractions. Secure it with one of the elastic belts.
   The uterine fundus is the area of greatest contractility.
4. Note the UC tracing. The resting tone tracing (that is, without a UC) should be recording on the 10 or 15 mm Hg pressure line. Adjust the line to reflect that reading.
   If the resting tone is set on the zero line, there often is a constant grinding noise.
5. Apply the ultrasonic gel to the diaphragm of the ultrasound transducer.
   Ultrasonic gel is used to maintain contact with the maternal abdomen. The ultrasonic beam is directed toward the fetal heart.
6. Place the diaphragm on the maternal abdomen in the midline between the umbilicus and the symphysis pubis.
7. Listen for the FHR, which will have a whiplike or galloping sound. Move the diaphragm laterally if necessary to obtain a stronger sound (see Figure 23–9).
8. When the FHR is located, attach the second elastic belt snugly to the transducer.
   Firm contact is necessary to maintain a steady tracing.
9. Place the following information on the beginning of the fetal monitor paper: date, time, woman's name, gravida, para, membrane status, and name of physician or certified nurse-midwife.

Note: Each birthing unit may have specific guidelines about additional information to include.

Document	Document that the procedure was explained to the woman and that she verbalized understanding. The location of the FHR, FHR baseline, changes in FHR that occur with contractions, and presence of accelerations or decelerations should be included. Other characteristics should include variability, maternal position, the type of device used, and maternal pulse, presence of fetal movement, procedures performed, and contraction characteristics (duration, frequency, strength). Entry documenting FHR, variability, response of FHR to UC, the intervention used, and subsequent positive fetal response to the intervention. 8-3-06 FHR BL 135–140. Minimal variability noted. Late decelerations noted with decrease of FHR to 130 bpm for 20 sec. UC every 3 min × 50–60 sec of moderate intensity by palpation. Client turned to left side. No further deceleration with three subsequent UCs. Two accelerations of 20 bpm × 20 sec noted with fetal movement. Client instructed to remain on left side. B Burch, RNC

Table 23–5   POSSIBLE INDICATIONS FOR ELECTRONIC FETAL MONITORING

Fetal Factors

Decreased fetal movement
Abnormal auscultory FHR
Meconium passage
Abnormal presentations/positions
Intrauterine growth restriction (IUGR) or small-for-gestational-age (SGA) fetus
Postdates (greater than 41 weeks)
Multiple gestation

Maternal Factors

Fever
Infections
Preeclampsia
Disease conditions (e.g., hypertension, diabetes)
Anemia
Rh alloimmunization
Previous perinatal death
Grand multiparity
Previous cesarean birth
Borderline/contracted pelvis

Uterine Factors

Dysfunctional labor
Failure to progress in labor
Oxytocin induction/augmentation
Uterine anomalies

Complications of Pregnancy

Prolonged rupture of membranes
Premature rupture of membranes
Preterm labor
Marginal abruptio placentae
Partial placenta previa
Occult/frank prolapse of cord
Amnionitis

Regional Anesthesia

Elective Monitoring

fetal monitor and recording it on graph paper. The US image can be influenced by other moving structures in the maternal abdomen, such as maternal arterial blood flow and maternal or fetal movement. Interference is generally filtered out; however, on occasion the maternal heart rate is detected by the US transducer and must be distinguished from the FHR by comparing the signal with the maternal pulse.

The external US transducer is beneficial over auscultating the FHR because it produces a continuous graphic recording. The US transducer can show the BL, BL VAR, and changes in the FHR. It is noninvasive and does not require rupture of membranes or minimal cervical dilation. FHR monitoring by US transducer is limited because it is susceptible to interference from maternal and fetal movement, as discussed earlier, and may produce a weak signal. The tracing may become sketchy and difficult to interpret. Repeating the procedure for US placement usually remedies the weak signal and tracing.

Internal Monitoring

Internal fetal monitoring is accomplished with a fetal scalp electrode (FSE), a fine surgical spiral wire, attached to the fetal scalp or other presenting part. The FSE is the most precise method of monitoring because it is a direct ECG of the FHR and produces the most accurate FHR tracing. The FSE is attached to the fetus during a vaginal exam. Once in place, the electrode is connected to the fetal monitor. The monitor determines the time between fetal "R" waves in the "QRS" complex and calculates the findings into a FHR. The FHR is then recorded on graph paper.

For the spiral electrode to be inserted, the cervix must be dilated at least 2 cm, the presenting fetal part must be accessible by vaginal examination, and the membranes must be ruptured. Even though it is not possible to apply the electrode and catheter under strict sterile conditions, the procedure should be performed as aseptically as possible. After determining fetal position by vaginal examination, the examiner (physician or nurse) inserts the electrode, which is encased in a plastic guide, to the level of the internal cervical os and attaches it to the presenting part, being careful not to apply it to the face, suture lines, fontanelles, cervix, or perineum if the fetus is in a breech presentation. The electrode is rotated clockwise until it is attached to the presenting part and is then disengaged from the guide tube. The guide tube is removed, and the end wires are connected to a leg plate that is attached to the woman's thigh. The cable from the leg plate is connected to the monitor. Infections and injuries from internal electrodes and catheters are a small but actual risk. Although nurses in some facilities apply internal monitors, in many settings their application is limited to the physician or CNM.

Because the risk of transmission to the fetus is increased by the small puncture in the fetal scalp, use of internal scalp electrodes should be avoided if at all possible in the presence of known maternal infections such as HIV, hepatitis, or group B streptococcus. Also, women who have had internal monitors and subsequently given birth by cesarean are more likely to have postpartum infections (Chan & Johnson, 2005). Fetal scalp monitors are also avoided in preterm infants because of the increased risk of ventricular hemorrhage.

The FHR tracing at the top of Figure 23–10 ◆ was obtained by internal monitoring, and the uterine contraction tracing at the bottom by external monitoring. A comparison shows that the spiral electrode provides an instantaneous and continuous recording of FHR that is clearer than the data provided by external monitoring. Notice that the FHR is variable (the tracing moves up and down instead of in a straight line), ranging between about 140 and 155 bpm.

Telemetry

As discussed previously, FHR and uterine activity may also be monitored by a telemetry system. Equipment consists of US along with external uterine pressure transducers connected to a small battery-operated transmitter. Signals are transmitted to a receiver connected to a monitor that displays FHR and uterine activity data. A printout provides documentation. This system,

Figure 23–10 ◆ *Top,* An FHR tracing obtained by internal monitoring. Normal FHR range is 110 to 160 bpm. This tracing indicates an FHR range of 140 to 155 bpm. *Bottom,* A uterine contraction tracing obtained by external monitoring. Each dark vertical line marks 1 minute, and each small rectangle represents 10 seconds. The contraction frequency is about every 3 minutes, and the duration of the contractions is 50 to 60 seconds.

which can be worn on a shoulder strap, allows the woman to ambulate, helping her to feel more comfortable and less confined during labor, yet provides for continuous monitoring. Telemetry provides for direct as well as indirect monitoring of FHR, indirect monitoring of uterine pressure, and dual FHR monitoring of twins.

FETAL HEART RATE PATTERNS

FHR is evaluated by assessing the BL rate, the BL VAR, and the periodic and episodic changes that occur in response to the intermittent stress of UCs.

The standardized definitions for FHR tracings developed by NICHD, mentioned previously, have potential benefits. Standardized terminology minimizes variation among care providers and allows for accurate documentation of the fetal status in medical records. If everyone on the perinatal team communicates clearly, treatment can be initiated promptly and there may be a decreased risk of adverse outcomes (AWHONN, 2005). The NICHD definitions were developed for visual interpretation by perinatal care providers, and complete understanding of FHR requires an understanding of the FHR characteristics presented next using these NICHD definitions (ACOG, 2005).

Baseline Rate

The **baseline rate** is the mean (average) FHR during a 10-minute period, rounded to increments of 5 bpm (e.g., 125, 130,

135, 140). The area for selection to determine the BL FHR should be the largest segment of the BL in any given 10-minute segment (Curran & Torgersen, 2006). The average FHR excludes periodic or episodic changes in FHR, periods of marked FHR variability, or segments of BL that differ by more than 25 bpm. The BL must be observed for a minimum of 2 minutes in any 10-minute segment, and it can be determined before, during, or after contractions as long as none of the previous conditions exists (ACOG, 2005). The 2-minute period to determine the BL FHR can be either 2 consecutive minutes or two 1-minute segments that occur within the 10-minute segment (AWHONN, 2006). If a 10-minute window does not contain 2 minutes of readable BL, the BL for that 10-minute period is considered indeterminate and the preceding 10-minute window must be used to determine the BL (Cypher et al., 2003). For example, if FHR over a period of 10 minutes fluctuates between 142 bpm and 156 bpm, the BL FHR would be documented as 150 bpm with moderate variability.

The normal BL rate ranges from 110 to 160 bpm, depending on gestational age. As the gestational age of the fetus increases, the FHR decreases. The FHR decreases an average of 16 bpm between 16 weeks' gestation and term. The slowing of the FHR occurs as the parasympathetic nervous system matures and exerts control over the fetal heart activity (Cunningham et al., 2005).

TACHYCARDIA

Fetal tachycardia is an FHR BL greater than 160 bpm for at least a 10-minute period. The possible causes of tachycardia may be idiopathic, maternal, fetal, or a combination of maternal and fetal. Some of the most common causes are the following:

Maternal

- Fever (Metabolism of the fetus accelerates because of increased maternal temperature.)
- Dehydration
- Anxiety
- Betasympathomimetic drugs, such as ritodrine, terbutaline, atropine, and isoxsuprine (These drugs have a cardiac stimulant effect.)
- Maternal hyperthyroidism (Thyroid-stimulating hormones may cross the placenta and stimulate the FHR.)
- Supraventricular tachycardia

Fetal

- Early fetal hypoxia (This leads to stimulation of the sympathetic nervous system (SNS) as the fetus compensates for reduced blood flow.)
- Asphyxia
- Fetal anemia (The heart rate increases as a compensatory mechanism to improve tissue perfusion.)
- Infection
- Prematurity
- Prolonged fetal stimulation

Tachycardia is considered a nonreassuring sign if it is accompanied by other FHR patterns such as late decelerations, severe variable decelerations, or decreased or absent variability. If tachycardia is associated with maternal fever, treatment may consist of antipyretics, cooling measures, and antibiotics. Fetal arrhythmia or dysrhythmia needs to be ruled out. The pediatrician should be notified, because tachycardia may cause heart failure in the newborn.

Intervention for tachycardia usually requires treatment of the underlying cause. Additional testing and monitoring may be used to further determine fetal well-being.

BRADYCARDIA

Fetal bradycardia is an FHR BL less than 110 bpm for at least a 10-minute period. The lower limits of the FHR have been debated in the past. An FHR as low as 90 bpm with good variability has been classified as benign and reassuring (Freeman, 2003). When bradycardia is accompanied by decreased variability or late decelerations, or both, it is considered ominous and a sign of advanced fetal compromise (Cunningham et al., 2005). The possible causes of bradycardia include the following:

- Stimulation of the vagus nerve (prolonged head compression as in early decelerations, application of the forceps or vacuum extractor, or prolonged scalp stimulation)
- Drugs that stimulate the parasympathetic nervous system or block the sympathetic (anesthesia and regional analgesia)
- Maternal hypotension (Maternal hypotension results in decreased blood flow to the fetus.)

- Prolonged umbilical cord compression (Fetal baroreceptors are activated by cord compression, which produces vagal stimulation, and in turn decreases FHR.)
- Fetal dysrhythmia (This is associated with complete heart block in the fetus.)
- Hypoxemia or late fetal asphyxia (There is depression of myocardial activity.)
- Accidental monitoring of maternal pulse

WANDERING BASELINE

A *wandering baseline* is a smooth, meandering, unsteady BL that fluctuates in the normal BL range without variability (Cunningham et al., 2005). The possible causes of this type of BL may be a congenital defect or metabolic acidosis. Immediate interventions should be taken to enhance fetal oxygenation, and delivery should be anticipated (AWHONN, 2006).

SINUSOIDAL BASELINE

A sinusoidal BL is an FHR pattern consisting of a series of cycles that are extremely smooth and regular (not necessarily identical) in amplitude and duration. The pattern resembles a perfect letter "S" lying on its side. The FHR undulates in a sine pattern between 120 and 160 bpm with variability amplitude of 5 to 15 bpm. Accelerations do not occur spontaneously, nor can they be induced (Figure 23–11 ◆).

Sinusoidal patterns may be benign (pseudosinusoidal) or pathological (true sinusoidal) patterns. Although not recognized by the NICHD, there are additional resources that describe pseudosinusoidal patterns as "sinusoidal patterns falsely induced by medication administration" (Curran & Torgersen, 2006; Cypher et al., 2003). Pseudosinusoidal FHR patterns may be caused by medications, such as meperidine or morphine; rhythmic fetal movement, such as thumb sucking; or infections, such as amnionitis. The wave pattern often lacks the regularity and smoothness of true sinusoidal patterns and is often followed by a normal FHR pattern when the stimulus causing the pattern is removed or corrected. Pathologic sinusoidal patterns are indicative of nonreassuring fetal status and require immediate attention (Cunningham et al., 2005). The possible causes of a true sinusoidal pattern include the following:

- Fetal anemia
- Chronic fetal bleeding
- Fetal isoimmunization
- Twin-to-twin transfusion
- Umbilical cord occlusion
- Central nervous system (CNS) malformations (Cunningham et al., 2005)

If the sinusoidal pattern is uncorrectable and pseudosinusoidal pattern has been ruled out, interventions include immediate notification of the healthcare provider and expeditious delivery.

ARRHYTHMIAS AND DYSRHYTHMIAS

Arrhythmias, a term often used interchangeably with *dysrhythmias,* are disturbances in the FHR pattern that are not

Figure 23–11 ◆ Sinusoidal pattern. Note the undulating waveform evenly distributed between the 120 and 130 bpm baseline. There is minimal variability.

associated with abnormal electrical impulse formation or conduction in the fetal cardiac tissue. An arrhythmic pattern demonstrates a normal P wave and QRS complexes (Curran & Torgersen, 2006; Torgersen, 2003). However, dysrhythmic FHR patterns may exhibit abnormal electrical impulse formation and/or conduction in the fetal cardiac tissues, resulting in abnormal P waves or QRS complexes, or both. Arrhythmic and dysrhythmic patterns get their names from the origin of the pattern, for example, sinus node variants, atrial node patterns, or ventricular patterns (Curran & Torgersen, 2006; Torgersen, 2003).

FHR dysrhythmias are estimated to occur in 2% to 14% of all pregnancies. Whereas 90% of dysrhythmias are benign, 10% can be life threatening and require the consultation of a neona-

tal or pediatric cardiology expert (AWHONN, 2006; Torgersen, 2003). For this reason, it is important to accurately diagnose abnormal FHR patterns and distinguish fetal arrhythmias from artifact and electrical interference. Fetal dysrhythmias can be difficult to diagnose, because detection of the fetal cardiac electrical activity is best accomplished by invasive or advanced monitoring techniques such as fetal scalp electrode, real-time ultrasound, Doppler velocimetry, fetal echocardiogram, and echocardiogram monitoring (e.g., M-Mode EchoCG, and Pulsed Doppler EchoCG) (Torgersen, 2003). With the exception of the fetal scalp electrode, more advanced and expensive diagnostic testing may not be readily available.

The most common causes of FHR dysrhythmias are discussed in Table 23–6.

Table 23–6   COMMON CAUSES OF VARIOUS TYPES OF FETAL DYSRHYTHMIAS

Sinus Node Variants	Atrial Dysrhythmias	Ventricular Dysrhythmias
• Bradycardia • Tachycardia • Marked sinus arrhythmia • Infections • CNS disturbances	• Parasympathetic response to fetal hypoxemia • Maternal ingestion of stimulants (e.g., caffeine, tobacco, alcohol, cocaine) • Abnormal reentry conduction • Cardiomyopathy • Fetal-maternal placental hemorrhage • Nonimmune hydrops fetalis • Wolf-Parkinson White syndrome • Cardiac structural abnormalities (e.g., ASD, VSD, valve malformation)	• Beta-blocker drugs • Complete heart blocks (AV malformation) • Congenital heart disease • Autoimmune disease (AV malformation) • Maternal collagen disorders (AV malformation)

SOURCES: Data from AWHONN, 2004; Cunningham et al., 2005; Torgersen, 2003; Tucker, 2004.

Baseline Variability

Baseline variability (BL VAR) is a reliable indicator of fetal cardiac and neurological function and well-being. The opposing "push-pull" balancing between the sympathetic nervous system and the parasympathetic nervous system directly affects the FHR. The NICHD has defined BL VAR as BL fluctuations of 2 cycles per minute or greater, and it is classified by the visually quantified amplitude of peak-to-trough in beats per minute. Evaluation of BL VAR is based on visual assessment of the amplitude of the BL cycles (AWHONN, 2005). The BL VAR is classified into four categories (ACOG, 2005; Curran & Torgersen, 2006; Cypher et al., 2003):

- Absent—amplitude undetected
- Minimal—amplitude range detectable but 5 bpm
- Moderate—amplitude range of 6 to 25 bpm
- Marked—amplitude greater than 25 bpm

Figures 23–12 ◆ and 23–13 ◆ illustrate examples of each of these categories.

Fetal Heart Rate Changes

In addition to changes in the average FHR BL range, the FHR may also exhibit intermittent or transient deviations or changes from the BL that are commonly referred to as accelerations and decelerations. These transient deviations or changes in BL are classified as episodic or periodic. Episodic changes (formerly referred to as nonperiodic changes) are not associated with UCs. Periodic changes occur with UCs. If a periodic change occurs with 50% or more of UCs in a 20-minute period, it is further classified as a recurrent change or pattern.

The nurse must remember that it is very important to examine all changes in FHR in relation to the surrounding BL and uterine activity. A comprehensive evaluation of the maternal-fetal interaction facilitates effective and efficient treatment and fetal well-being.

ACCELERATIONS

An **acceleration** is described as a visually apparent increase in the BL FHR, with an onset-to-peak of less than 30 seconds beginning at the most recent calculated BL. The duration of the acceleration is defined as the time from the initial change in FHR from the BL to the return of the FHR to the BL. After 32 weeks' gestation, an acceleration must peak 15 beats above the BL and last for a total of 15 seconds from the time it leaves the BL FHR until the time it returns to the FHR BL. At gestations of less than 32 weeks, an acceleration of 10 beats by 10 seconds is acceptable. A *prolonged acceleration* is any acceleration that lasts longer than 2 minutes. Prolonged accelerations that last more than 10 minutes are classified as changes in BL.

Accelerations can be either episodic or periodic. *Episodic,* or *spontaneous, accelerations* are not associated with contractions and tend to be more peaked and abrupt. They are often associated with fetal movement, stimulation, or an environmental stimulus. Episodic accelerations are reassuring FHR patterns, whether or not they are accompanied by fetal movement. *Periodic accelerations* are associated with uterine contractions. When they occur on a repetitive basis, they may be smooth in configuration, multiphasic, and may precede variable decelerations. Various types of accelerations are displayed in Figure 23–14 ◆.

Accelerations are generally associated with the stimulation of the autonomic nervous system (ANS), specifically the SNS, which increases the FHR. If the heart rate increases with CNS stimulation, it usually indicates an intact fetal nervous system and fetal well-being. FHR accelerations can be associ-

Figure 23–12 ◆ *A* and *B,* Moderate variability. *C,* Minimal variability. *D,* Absent variability.

Figure 23–13 ◆ Marked variability. FHR varies markedly between 120 and 190 bpm. With this type of pattern, it is not possible to determine average baseline FHR because of the wide, marked variations.

ated with fetal movement, vaginal exams, application of a fetal scalp electrode, occiput posterior presentation and uterine contractions, fundal pressure, abdominal palpation, vibroacoustic stimulation (VAS), scalp stimulation, and other environmental stimuli (Curran & Torgersen, 2006; Cypher et al., 2003; Tucker

et al., 2003). Infants of extreme prematurity are less likely to accelerate because of their immature parasympathetic nervous system. In fetuses of less than 32 gestational weeks, an acceleration of at least 10 bpm for 10 seconds is reassuring. Fetuses suffering from intrauterine growth restriction (IUGR)

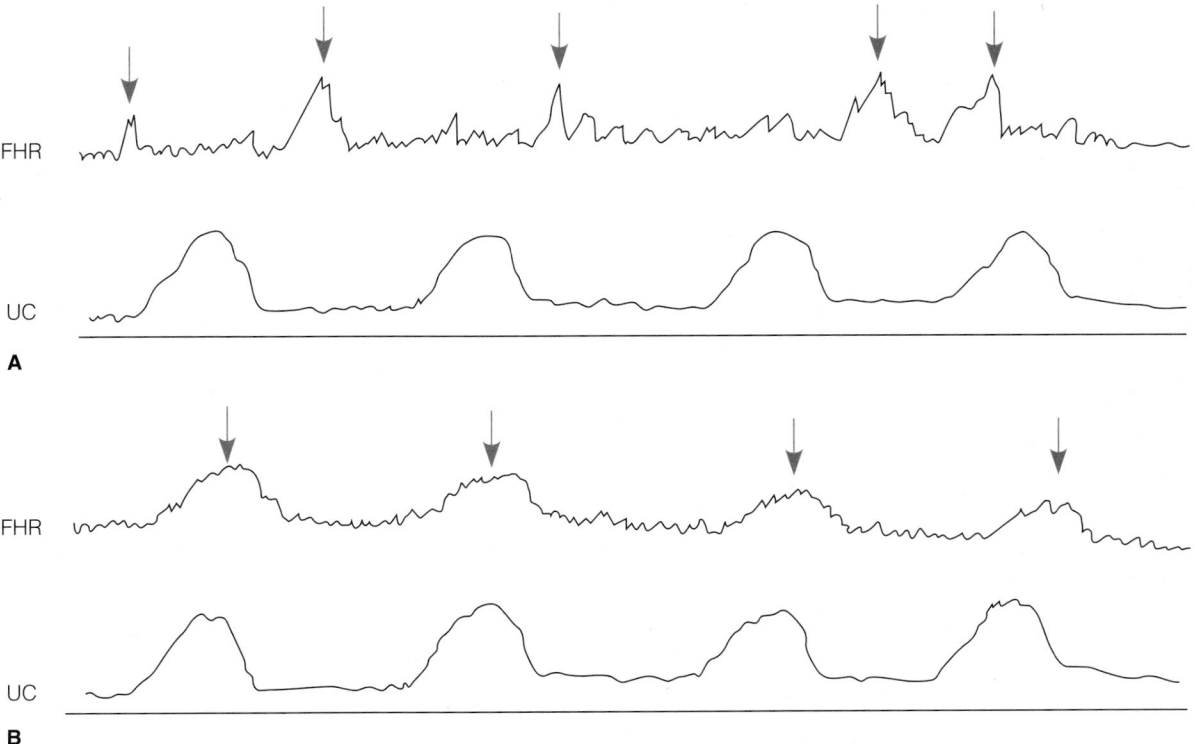

Figure 23–14 ◆ Types of accelerations. *A,* Episodic accelerations. *B,* Periodic accelerations.

experience fewer accelerations than normal, healthy, well-oxygenated fetuses. Medications administered to the mother may inhibit accelerations because of their effect on the SNS. Some of the drugs seen to affect fetuses are beta blockers and CNS depressants. Hypoxia is also a large contributing factor to lack of accelerations and may be the first sign of a nonreassuring FHR tracing.

Accelerations are generally benign because they are associated with an intact fetal nervous system, lack of fetal hypoxia, and acidosis. The patterns are considered reassuring, thus no intervention is required (Cunningham et al., 2005; Curran & Torgersen, 2006; Cypher et al., 2003; Tucker, 2004).

DECELERATIONS

Decelerations, often referred to as *decels,* are generally defined as decreases in the FHR below the BL. Each deceleration has its own unique characteristics, etiology, and significance. Each deceleration consists of several components:

- *Onset:* point at which the deceleration leaves the FHR BL
- *Descent:* time from onset to nadir
- *Nadir:* lowest point of the deceleration
- *Depth:* the level (in beats per minute) a deceleration reaches its nadir
- *Recovery:* time from nadir to return to BL
- *Duration:* the total length of time from onset to return to BL

Decelerations are identified and classified by their shape, appearance, rate of descent, and timing in relationship to uterine contractions (Figure 23–15 ◆).

Abrupt or Gradual

Decelerations are classified into two types based on the rate at which the FHR descends after it leaves the FHR BL. Based on NICHD nomenclature, *abrupt deceleration* of the FHR (onset to nadir) occurs in less than 30 seconds. Variable decelerations de-

	Early deceleration	Late deceleration	Variable deceleration
	Head compression (HC)	Uteroplacental insufficiency (UPI)	Umbilical cord compression (CC)
Shape	Waveform consistently uniform; inversely mirrors contraction	Waveform uniform; shape reflects contraction	Waveform variable, generally sharp drops and returns
Onset	Just prior to or early in contraction	Late in contraction	Abrupt with fetal insult; not related to contraction
Lowest level	Consistently at or before midpoint of contraction	Consistently after the midpoint of the contraction	Variable around midpoint
Range	Usually within normal range of 120–160 bpm	Usually within normal range of 120–130 bpm	Not usually within normal range
Ensemble	Can be single or repetitive	Occasional, consistent, gradually increase—repetitive	Variable—single or repetitive

Figure 23–15 ◆ Types and characteristics of early, late, and variable decelerations.
SOURCE: Hon, E. (1976). *An introduction to fetal heart rate monitoring* (2nd ed., p. 29). Los Angeles: University of Southern California School of Medicine.

scend abruptly. *Gradual deceleration* of the FHR (onset to nadir) requires 30 seconds or longer (ACOG, 2005; AWHONN, 2005). Early and late decelerations both descend gradually but differ in respect to their timing with the UC. Early and late contractions are discussed further later in this section.

Episodic or Periodic

Decelerations can be episodic or periodic. Episodic implies that the decelerations occur without relationship to UCs. They may occur without or between contractions and usually are the result of environmental stimuli, such as vaginal exams, rupture of membranes, the administration of regional anesthesia or medications, or other events. Periodic refers to decelerations that occur in direct association with UCs. Episodic or periodic decelerations are considered *repetitive* if they occur with 50% or more of UCs (ACOG, 2005; AWHONN, 2005).

Early or Late

Periodic decelerations associated with UCs are also classified by their timing in respect to them. There are three types of deceleration patterns: early, late, and variable. **Early decelerations** occur simultaneously with UCs; thus their onset, nadir, and recovery occur at the same time as the onset, acme (peak), and recovery, respectively, of the UC. **Late decelerations** are delayed after the UC in that their onset, nadir, and recovery occur after the beginning, peak, and end of the contraction, respectively (ACOG, 2005). **Variable decelerations** can occur either early or late with respect to a UC.

The etiology and clinical significance of each type of deceleration are unique. Clinical interventions and treatments are based on the systematic assessment of the FHR tracing and the overall evaluation of the mother, the fetus, and labor status. Deceleration characteristics and the discussion of their

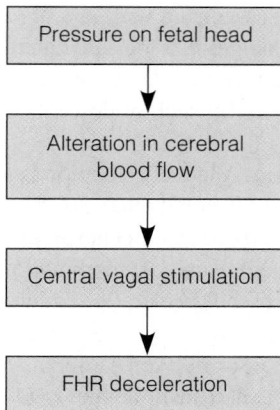

Figure 23–16 ◆ Mechanism of early deceleration (head compression).
SOURCE: Adapted from Freeman, R. K., & Garite, T. J. (1981). The physiologic basis of fetal monitoring. In *Fetal heart rate monitoring* (p. 13). Baltimore, MD: Williams & Wilkins.

clinical significance and interventions are included in the following sections.

Early Decelerations. An early deceleration is a visually apparent, gradual decrease in the FHR with a return to BL. The decrease from the BL is gradual (onset to nadir of 30 seconds or more), and the nadir of the deceleration occurs at the same time as the peak of the contraction. Early decelerations are a result of vagal nerve stimulation caused by fetal head compression that occurs during UCs (Figure 23–16 ◆). Early decelerations are usually uniform in shape and mirror the shape of the UC. The depth of the deceleration is rarely more than 30 to 40 bpm (AWHONN, 2003) (Figure 23–17 ◆). Early decels occur most frequently during the active phase of labor (between 4 and 7 cm dilation) and are considered benign (Cypher et al., 2003; Freeman, 2003).

Figure 23–17 ◆ Early decelerations. Baseline FHR is 150 to 155 bpm. Nadir (lowest point) of decelerations is 130 to 145 bpm.

Early decels are not associated with loss of variability, tachycardia, or other FHR changes that are associated with fetal hypoxia, acidosis, or low Apgar scores. They are viewed as reassuring unless they are seen with the lack of descent of the fetal head into the pelvis.

Late Decelerations. A late deceleration is a visually apparent, gradual (onset to nadir is greater than 30 seconds) decrease in the FHR with a return to BL. The descent (onset to nadir) and the recovery of the FHR are usually smooth and uniform. The onset, nadir, and recovery of the deceleration occur after the beginning, peak, and end of the contraction, respectively.

Late decelerations, often referred to as *lates* or *late decels,* are due to uteroplacental insufficiency and are a result of decreased blood flow and/or oxygen transfer to the fetus through the intervillous space during contractions. Late decels may be one of two types: reflexive or myocardial. The pathophysiology of late decels is complicated and is not always understood (Cunningham et al., 2005; Cypher et al., 2003; Tucker, Parry, Penney et al., 2003).

When uteroplacental reserve is adequate, the fetus normally tolerates the transient stress of repetitive contractions. If a decrease in uteroplacental blood flow (for example, from maternal hypotension or excessive uterine activity) lowers the oxygen level in the intervillous space to a level lower than the oxygen level in the fetus, fetal chemoreceptors are stimulated and FHR decreases. This response to the lowered oxygen level is reflexive, because it is a normal physiological chemical response to low oxygen levels in the blood. The delay in the FHR deceleration is due to the time it takes for the normal physiological response of the neurologic system to respond to the lowered oxygen environment. This type of late decels is generally considered nonacidemic and is associated with moderate BL VAR. The BL VAR is the key to determining an intact fetal CNS and should always be considered when evaluating late decelerations and the level of intervention required.

In some cases, repetitive or chronic episodes of decreased oxygen in the intervillous space exist and the fetus experiences a chronic state of hypoxia that leads to metabolic acidosis. The fetal CNS is affected by the metabolic acidosis and progresses to myocardial depression. Late decelerations are produced by the myocardial depression (Cypher et al., 2003) (Figure 23–18 ◆).

The decrease in heart rate resulting from late decelerations is usually shallow, typically 10 to 20 bpm; however, it may approach 30 to 40 bpm below the BL (Cunningham et al., 2005) (Figure 23–19 ◆). The depth of the late deceleration is usually proportional to the strength of the UC; however, late decels may be of any depth, depending on the preexisting fetal oxygen reserve. Late decelerations are considered a nonreassuring sign. When they are repetitive and uncorrectable and associated with minimal or absent BL VAR and/or BL rate changes, they indicate fetal hypoxia and acidemia and require prompt attention and intervention. The objective of intervention is to improve fetal oxygenation and uteroplacental perfusion while assessing and eliminating the stressor as reflected by the deceleration. If this is not possible, immediate birth may be indicated.

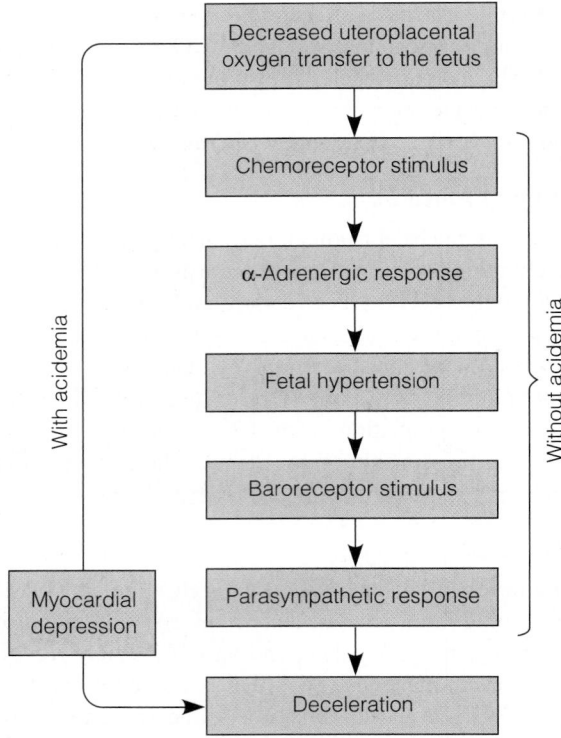

Figure 23–18 ◆ Mechanism of late deceleration.
SOURCE: Freeman, R. K., & Garite, T. J. (1981). The physiologic basis of fetal monitoring. In *Fetal heart rate monitoring* (p. 15). Baltimore, MD: Williams & Wilkins.

Sometimes late or variable decelerations are due to the supine position of the laboring woman. In this case, the decrease in uterine blood flow to the fetus may be alleviated by raising the woman's upper trunk or turning her to the side to displace pressure of the gravid uterus on the inferior vena cava. If the woman remains flat on her back, the fetus will continue to have decelerations because of oxygen compromise. Immediate nursing interventions include changing the maternal position and increasing the administration of intravenous fluids. Oxygen should be provided to the mother via face mask if hypoxia is suspected, such as when there is absent or minimal variability. If oxytocin (Pitocin) is being administered, the infusion should be stopped immediately until the FHR recovers or the physician or CNM has instructed that the infusion be resumed. The physician or CNM should be notified immediately in the event that late decelerations occur.

Late decelerations normally occur within the normal heart range (110 to 160 bpm) and may be quite obvious or very subtle and almost indistinguishable. Some fetuses at highest risk demonstrate a flat FHR BL with late decelerations that are barely noticeable.

Variable Decelerations. A variable deceleration is a visually apparent, abrupt (onset to nadir less than 30 seconds) decrease in the FHR below the BL. The decrease in FHR is 15 bpm or more with a duration of 15 seconds or more but less than 2 minutes (ACOG, 2005). (See Figures 23–20 ◆ through 23–22 ◆).

Prolonged Decelerations. A **prolonged deceleration** is a visually apparent decrease in the FHR below the BL that lasts more than 2 minutes and less than 10 minutes from onset to return to BL (Figure 23–23 ◆).

Figure 23–19 ◆ Late decelerations. Baseline FHR is 130 to 148 bpm. Nadir (lowest point) of decelerations is 110 to 120 bpm. Absent variability.

Figure 23–20 ◆ Variable decelerations with overshoot. The timing of the decelerations is variable, and most have a sharp decline. A rebound acceleration (overshoot) occurs after most of the decelerations. Baseline FHR is 115 to 130 bpm. Nadir of decelerations is 55 to 80 bpm. Variability is minimal.

Evaluation of Tracings

The effective nurse uses a systematic approach in evaluating FHR tracings to avoid interpreting findings on the basis of inadequate or erroneous data. With a systematic approach, the nurse can make a more accurate and rapid assessment; easily communicate data to the woman, physician or CNM, and staff; and have a universal language for documenting the woman's record.

Figure 23–21 ◆ Mechanism of variable deceleration.
SOURCE: Adapted from Freeman, R. K., & Garite, T. J. (1981). The physiologic basis of fetal monitoring. In *Fetal heart rate monitoring* (p. 13). Baltimore, MD: Williams & Wilkins.

Figure 23–22 ◆ Atypical variable decelerations. The presence of any of these types of variable decelerations strongly suggests fetal hypoxia, especially when variability is decreased.
SOURCE: Krebs, H. B., Petrie, R. E., & Dunn, L. J. (1983). Atypical variable decelerations. *American Journal of Obstetrics & Gynecology, 145*(3), 298.

Figure 23–23 ◆ The prolonged deceleration depicted lasts approximately 160 seconds. Note the prolonged contraction of 120 seconds. The deceleration begins after 80 seconds of uterine contraction. Note the beginning return of FHR 30 seconds after uterine tone returns to normal resting tone (contraction ends). Minimal variability is present despite the deceleration.

Evaluation of the electronic monitor tracing begins with a look at the uterine contraction pattern. To evaluate the contraction pattern, the nurse should:

1. Determine the uterine resting tone.

2. Assess the contractions:

   a. What is the frequency?

   b. What is the duration?

   c. What is the intensity (if internal monitoring)?

The next step is to evaluate the FHR tracing.

1. Determine the baseline:

   a. Is the baseline within normal range?

   b. Is there evidence of tachycardia?

   c. Is there evidence of bradycardia?

2. Determine FHR variability:

   a. Is variability absent, minimal, or moderate? Is variability minimal or marked?

3. Determine whether a sinusoidal pattern is present.

4. Determine whether there are periodic changes.

   a. Are accelerations present?

   b. Is there a reassuring tracing or FHR pattern?

   c. Are decelerations present?

   d. Are they uniform in shape? If so, determine if they are early or late decelerations.

   e. Are they nonuniform in shape? If so, determine if they are variable decelerations.

After evaluating the FHR tracing for the factors just listed, the nurse may further classify the tracing as reassuring (normal) or nonreassuring (worrisome). Reassuring patterns contain normal parameters and do not require additional treatment or intervention. Characteristics of reassuring FHR patterns include the following:

- BL rate is 110 to 160 bpm.
- Variability is present and ranges more than 2 cycles per minute.
- Periodic patterns consist of accelerations with fetal movement, and early decelerations may be present.
- No late, variable, or prolonged decelerations.

Nonreassuring patterns indicate that the fetus is becoming stressed and intervention is needed. Characteristics of nonreassuring patterns include the following:

- Variable decelerations (FHR drops below 70 bpm for longer than 30 to 45 seconds and is accompanied by rising BL or decreasing variability.)
- Late decelerations of any magnitude
- Absence of variability
- Prolonged deceleration (Deceleration lasts greater than 2 minutes but less than 10 minutes.)
- Severe (marked) bradycardia (FHR BL is 70 bpm or less.)

Nonreassuring patterns may require continuous monitoring and more involved treatment and intervention.

Table 23-7	GUIDELINES FOR MANAGEMENT OF VARIABLE, LATE, AND PROLONGED DECELERATION PATTERNS
Pattern	**Nursing Interventions**
Variable decelerations Isolated or occasional Moderate	Report findings to physician/CNM and document in chart. Provide explanation to woman and partner. Change maternal position to one in which FHR pattern is most improved. Discontinue oxytocin if it is being administered and other interventions are unsuccessful. Perform vaginal examination to assess for prolapsed cord or change in labor progress. Monitor FHR continuously to assess current status and for further changes in FHR pattern.
Variable decelerations Severe and uncorrectable	Give oxygen if indicated. Report findings to physician/CNM and document in chart. Provide explanation to woman and partner. Prepare for probable cesarean birth. Follow interventions listed above. Prepare for vaginal birth unless baseline variability is decreasing or FHR is progressively rising—then cesarean, forceps, or vaccum birth is indicated. Assist physician with fetal scalp sampling if ordered. Prepare for cesarean birth if scalp pH shows acidosis or downward trend.
Late decelerations	Give oxygen if indicated. Report findings to physician/CNM and document in chart. Provide explanation to woman and partner. Monitor for further FHR changes. Maintain maternal position on left side. Maintain good hydration with IV fluids (normal saline or lactated Ringer's). Discontinue oxytocin if it is being administered and late decelerations persist despite other interventions. Administer oxygen by face mask at 7–10 L/min. Monitor maternal blood pressure and pulse for signs of hypotension; possibly increase flow rate of IV fluids to treat hypotension. Follow physician's orders for treatment for hypotension if present. Increase IV fluids to maintain volume and hydration (normal saline or lactated Ringer's). Assess labor progress (dilatation and station). Assist physician with fetal blood sampling: If pH stays above 7.25, physician will continue monitoring and resample; if pH shows downward trend (between 7.25 and 7.20) or is below 7.20, prepare for birth by most expeditious means.
Late decelerations with tachycardia or decreasing variability	Report findings to physician/CNM and document in chart. Maintain maternal position on left side. Administer oxygen by face mask at 7–10 L/min. Discontinue oxytocin if it is being administered. Assess maternal blood pressure and pulse. Increase IV fluids (normal saline or lactated Ringer's). Assess labor progress (dilatation and station). Prepare for immediate cesarean birth. Explain plan of treatment to woman and partner. Assist physician with fetal blood sampling (if ordered).
Prolonged decelerations	Perform vaginal examination to rule out prolapsed cord or to determine progress in labor status. Change maternal position as needed to try to alleviate decelerations. Discontinue oxytocin if it is being administered. Notify physician/CNM of findings/initial interventions and document in chart. Provide explanation to woman and partner. Increase IV fluids (normal saline or lactated Ringer's). Administer tocolytic if hypertonus noted and ordered by physician/CNM. Anticipate normal FHR recovery following deceleration if FHR previously normal. Anticipate intervention if FHR previously abnormal or deceleration lasts greater than 3 minutes.

It is important to provide information to the laboring woman regarding the FHR pattern and the interventions that will help her fetus. Sharing information with the laboring woman reassures her that a potential or actual problem has been identified and that she is an active participant in the interventions. Occasionally, a problem arises that requires immediate intervention. In that case, the nurse can say something like, "It is important for you to turn on your left side right now because the baby is having a little difficulty. I'll explain what is happening in just a few moments." This type of response lets the woman know that although an action needs to be accomplished rapidly, information will soon be provided. In the haste to act quickly, the nurse must not forget that it is the woman's body and her baby.

Labor and birth nurses must be skilled and competent in evaluating electronic FHR patterns and responding appropriately (Table 23-7). Competence can be maintained through frequent in-services, formal courses, and continuing education programs.

INDIRECT METHODS OF FETAL ASSESSMENT

When there is a question regarding fetal status, indirect methods such as **scalp stimulation** (pressing on the fetal scalp with the examining fingers during a vaginal exam to elicit an acceleration of FHR), *acoustic stimulation* (using a sound device placed against the maternal abdomen to elicit an acceleration in FHR),

RESEARCH IN PRACTICE

USE OF FETAL PULSE OXIMETRY AMONG HIGH RISK WOMEN IN LABOR: A RANDOMIZED CLINICAL TRIAL

What is this study about? Monitoring of fetal status during labor has a twofold purpose: to reassure the practitioner that a healthy birth can be expected and to quickly identify the fetus who is physically compromised. Electronic fetal heart rate (FHR) monitoring has been shown to predict a healthy infant quite well, but it is not as effective in specifically identifying that a fetus is compromised. In fact, an abnormal FHR tracing has only 50% specificity for fetal compromise; this means that about half the time, an abnormal FHR pattern occurs in a healthy baby. Fetal pulse oximetry (FPO) has been proposed as an adjunct fetal assessment, used in concert with FHR monitoring, to improve the accuracy with which fetal compromise is diagnosed. Previous studies showed that FPO reduced the incidence of cesarean birth for a nonreassuring FHR tracing, and FPO was subsequently approved for use in women with singleton pregnancies of at least 36 weeks who were in active labor. The purpose of this study was to determine the effectiveness of FPO in women with high-risk pregnancies.

How was this study done? This prospective randomized trial was conducted over a 3-year period at a single hospital in Mississippi. Three hundred and sixty women met the inclusion criteria and were recruited to participate in the trial. The women were in active or induced labor and were noted by FHR monitoring to have a nonreassuring fetal heart tracing despite maternal/fetal resuscitation. The women were randomly assigned into a study group that received FPO and electronic FHR monitoring or a control group that received FHR monitoring alone. Both groups received standard care under the hospital's protocol. The two groups were similar for maternal age, ethnicity, gestational age at delivery, rate of preterm delivery, and antepartum complications. There were more nulliparous women in the study group when compared to the control group. Outcomes that were measured included the rate of cesarean birth, incidence of dystocia, decision-to-incision time for cesarean births, and indicators of neonatal health.

What were the results of the study? Neonatal outcome was similar in the two groups. The requirement for neonatal resuscitation and admission to the neonatal intensive care unit was both identical in the study and control groups. Contrary to the previous study, the rate of cesarean birth was the same for the two groups, although the decision-to-incision time was considerably shorter in the group that received FPO as an adjunct to FHR monitoring. This measure was used as a surrogate for the sense of urgency for an emergent cesarean delivery and was nearly 10 minutes shorter for those mothers in the experimental group.

What additional questions might I have? Would these results be the same if the proportion of nulliparous women was identical for the two groups? How acceptable was the actual process of fetal pulse oximetry to these mothers, given that it requires the placement of an intrauterine sensor? Is the reduction in decision-to-incision time significant enough to warrant an invasive procedure in high-risk mothers during labor?

How can I use this study? Women in labor need to understand the value of each of the intrapartum monitoring options available to them. Even though physicians may discuss these options, often mothers need additional discussion with the nurse. The nurse can help the laboring mother balance the risks and benefits of each monitoring option, so that an informed decision can be made. The option of fetal pulse oximetry involves the insertion of an invasive sensor but may reduce the time it takes to actually complete a cesarean birth if its necessity becomes evident.

Klauser, C., Christensen, E., Chauham, S., Bufkin, L., Magann, E., Bofill, J., et al. (2005). Use of fetal pulse oximetry among high risk women in labor: A randomized clinical trial. *American Journal of Obstetrics & Gynecology. 192,* 1810–1819.

or stimulation by maternal abdominal palpation (patting or shaking the abdomen) can be used to stimulate the fetus. When one of the indirect methods is used, the fetus who is not in any stress responds with an acceleration of the FHR, described as a reactive response (acceleration of 15 bpm amplitude with a duration of 15 seconds). Whereas reactivity is associated with fetal well-being, the absence of acceleration does not diagnose acidemia or predict fetal compromise. Further observation and assessment measures are indicated.

Scalp Stimulation

Scalp stimulation is the use of direct stimulation to the fetal scalp in utero to elicit an acceleration when auscultating or when interpreting a nonreassuring EFM pattern. Scalp stimulation is accomplished by applying direct digital pressure to the fetal scalp during a vaginal examination. It is considered an indirect method of assessing fetal acid-base balance when the FHR pattern does not show accelerations. Uncompromised fetuses with adequate oxygen reserve will elicit an acceleration of at least 15 bpm for 15 seconds. If the fetus is able to generate an acceleration, it is not acidotic.

Cord Blood Analysis at Birth

In cases in which significant abnormal FHR patterns have been noted before birth, amniotic fluid is meconium stained, or the infant is depressed at birth, umbilical cord blood may be analyzed immediately after birth to assess the infant's respiratory status. The cord is usually clamped before the infant takes his or her first breath to provide an evaluation of blood gas status before the infant interacts with the extrauterine environment, because values can change after only a few seconds of neonatal breathing.

An 8- to 10-inch segment of the umbilical cord is double-clamped and cut, and a small amount of blood is aspirated from one of the umbilical arteries (arterial blood seems to provide the most reliable indication of blood gas status and fetal tissue pH).

Blood is collected in a heparinized syringe unless it is to be analyzed immediately; it should not be allowed to remain in the segment of cord longer than 30 minutes. Some clinicians may collect a segment of cord and send blood samples only if the Apgar score is below 7 at 5 minutes, as recommended by the AAP and ACOG (2002). In this instance, values might be used to clarify the cause of a low Apgar score while minimizing any medical-legal exposure and expense. Determination of pH and base deficit values can differentiate whether fetal acidemia is due to hypoperfusion of the placenta or to cord compression.

CHAPTER REVIEW

FOCUS YOUR STUDY

- Intrapartal assessment includes attention to both physical and psychosociocultural parameters of the laboring woman, assessment of the fetus, and ongoing assessment for conditions that place the woman and her fetus at an increased risk.

- Birthing room nurses have responsibilities for recognizing and interrupting fetal monitoring patterns, notifying the physician or CNM of problems, and initiating corrective and supportive measures when needed.

- Uterine contractions may be assessed externally through palpation or by an electronic monitor. An intrauterine pressure catheter can be placed internally to measure uterine activity more accurately.

- A vaginal examination determines the status of cervical dilatation, effacement, and fetal presentation, position, and station.

- Fetal presentation can also be assessed by inspection, vaginal examination, or ultrasound.

- Leopold's maneuvers provide a systematic evaluation of fetal presentation and position.

- Indications for electronic fetal monitoring include fetal, maternal, and uterine factors; presence of pregnancy complications; regional anesthesia; and elective monitoring.

- The fetal heart rate may be assessed by auscultation or electronic fetal monitoring.

- Electronic fetal monitoring is accomplished by indirect ultrasound or by direct methods that require the placement of a spiral electrode on the fetal presenting part.

- Variability refers to baseline fluctuations of 2 cycles per minute or greater in the FHR and it is classified by the visually quantified amplitude of peak-to-trough in beats per minute.

- The normal range of FHR is 110 to 160 beats per minute.

- Baseline changes in the FHR include tachycardia, bradycardia, and variability.

- Tachycardia is defined as a rate of 160 beats per minute or more for at least a 10-minute segment of time.

- Bradycardia is defined as a rate of 110 beats per minute or less for at least a 10-minute segment of time.

- Baseline variability is an important parameter of fetal well-being.

- Periodic changes in the FHR from baseline include decelerations and accelerations. Accelerations are normally caused by fetal movement.

- Decelerations are categorized as early, late, or variable according to the NICHD categories.

- Early decelerations are due to compression of the fetal head during contractions and are generally considered benign when they occur with ongoing fetal descent. They typically do not require intervention.

- Late decelerations are associated with uteroplacental insufficiency.

- Variable decelerations are associated with compression of the umbilical cord.

- Sinusoidal patterns are characterized by an undulant sine wave.

- Fetal scalp stimulation can be used when there is a question regarding fetal status.

EXPLORE MediaLink

http://www.prenhall.com/davidson

NCLEX review questions, case studies, and other interactive resources for this chapter can be found on the Web Site at http://www.prenhall.com/davidson. Click on "Chapter 23" to select the activities for this chapter.

For tutorials including animations and videos, more NCLEX review questions, and an audio glossary, access the accompanying Prentice Hall Nursing MediaLink DVD-ROM in this book.

PRENTICE HALL NURSING MEDIALINK DVD-ROM

Audio Glossary

NCLEX Review

Videos: *Leopold's Maneuvers; Monitoring a Fetal Heart Rate; Through the Eyes of a Nurse—The Third Trimester*

COMPANION WEBSITE

Additional NCLEX Review

Case Study: *Maternal Assessment During Labor*

Care Plan Activity: *Client with Decelerations*

Applications: *Fetal Monitoring; Fetal Bradycardia*

Critical Thinking

CRITICAL THINKING IN ACTION

BENEFITS OF AMBULATION DURING LABOR

View the Critical Thinking in Action video in Chapter 23 of the DVD-ROM. Then answer the questions that follow.

Cindy Bell, a 20-year-old gravida 2, para 1 at 40 weeks' gestation, presents to you in the birthing unit with contractions every 5 to 7 minutes. She is accompanied by her husband. Spontaneous rupture of membranes occurred 2 hours before admission. Cindy tells you that the fluid was colorless and clear. You orient Cindy and her family to the birthing room and perform a physical assessment, documenting the following data: vital signs are normal, and a vaginal exam demonstrates the cervix is 75% effaced, 4 cm dilated with a vertex at 1 station in the LOP position. You place Cindy on an external fetal monitor. The fetal heart rate baseline is 140 to 147 with accelerations to 156; no decelerations are noted. Contractions are 5 to 6 minutes apart, moderate intensity, and lasting 40 to 50 seconds. Cindy states that she would like to stay out of bed as long as possible because lying down seems to make the contractions more painful, especially in her back.

1. Discuss the benefits of ambulation in labor.

2. Cindy would like her daughter to be present for the baby's birth. What would you discuss with her about the impact of having a young sibling present during labor and birth?

3. What fetal heart rate assessment will best ensure fetal well-being during the period Cindy is ambulating?

4. When a nonreassuring fetal heart pattern is detected, what remedial nursing intervention is carried out?

5. What are indications for continuous fetal monitoring in labor?

REFERENCES

American Academy of Pediatrics (AAP) & American College of Obstetricians and Gynecologists (ACOG). (2002). *Guidelines for perinatal care* (5th ed.). Washington, DC: Author.

American College of Obstetricians and Gynecologists (ACOG). (2005). Intrapartum fetal heart rate monitoring. ACOG Practice Bulletin No. 70. Author: Washington, D.C.

Association of Women's Health, Obstetric, and Neonatal Nurses (AWHONN); E. Breslin & V. Lucas (Eds.). (2003). Women's health nursing: Toward evidence-based practice. Philadelphia: Saunders.

Association of Women's Health, Obstetric, and Neonatal Nurses (AWHONN); S. Mattson & J. Smith (Eds.). (2004). Core curriculum for maternal-newborn nursing, ed. 3. Philadelphia: Saunders.

Association of Women's Health, Obstetric, and Neonatal Nurses (AWHONN). (2005). *Foundations of fetal heart monitoring: An introduction to the AWHONN fetal heart monitoring principles and practices program.* Baltimore: Lippincott, Williams & Wilkins.

Association of Women's Health, Obstetric, and Neonatal Nurses (AWHONN). (2006). In J. Poole (Ed.), *Foundations of fetal heart rate monitoring: An introduction to AWHONN's fetal heart rate monitoring principles and practices program.* Baltimore: Williams & Wilkins.

Beal, D. J., Trougakos, J. P., Weiss, H. M., & Green, S. G. (2006). Episodic processes in emotional labor: Perceptions of affective delivery and regulation strategies. *Journal of Applied Psychology, 91*(5), 1053–1065.

Chan, P. D., & Johnson, S. M. (2005). *Gynecology and obstetrics 2006.* Laguna Hills, CA: Current Clinical Strategies.

Cunningham, G., Leveno, K. J., Bloom, S. L. Hauth, J. C., Gilstrap, L. C., & Wenstrom, K. D. (2005). *Williams obstetrics* (21st ed.). New York: McGraw-Hill.

Curran, C., & Torgersen, K. (2006). *EFM, the textbook: Electronic fetal monitoring.* Virginia Beach, VA: Colley Avenue Copies & Graphics.

Cypher, R., Adelsperger, D., & Torgersen, K. (2003). Interpretation of fetal heart rate patterns. Dubuque, IA: Kendall-Hunt. In N. Feinstein, K. Torgersen, & J. Atterbury, (Eds.), *Fetal heart monitoring principles and practices* (3rd ed., pp. 113–158). Dubuque, IA: Kendall-Hunt.

Freeman, R. K. (2003). The evolution of antepartum fetal testing methods. *American Journal of Obstetrics & Gynecology, 189*(1), 310.

Johnston, M. E., & Herzig, R. M., (2006). The interpretation of "culture": Diverging perspectives on medical provision in rural Montana. *Social Science & Medicine, 63*(9), 2500–2511.

Joint Commission on Accreditation of Healthcare Organizations. (2004, July 21). *Preventing infant death and injury during delivery.* Retrieved September 24, 2006, from http://www.jointcommission.org/SentinelEvents/SentinelEventAlert/sea_30.htm?HTTPJCS ARCH.JCAHO.ORG_CGI_BIN_MSMFIND. EXE?RESMASK5MssResEN.mskhttp%3A//jcserch.jcaho.org/cgibin/MsmFind.exe%3Fhttp%3A//jcsearch.jcaho.org/cgibin/MsmFind.exe%3FRESMASK%3DMssResEN.msk.

Kennedy, H. P., & MacDonald, E. L. (2002). Altered consciousness during childbirth: Potential clues to post traumatic stress disorder? *Journal of Midwifery & Women's Health, 47*(5), 380–382.

National Institute of Child Health and Human Development (NICHD). (1997). *NICHD fetal monitoring workshop.* Bethesda, MD: Author.

Sciscione, A. C, Duhl, A., Pollock, M. A., Hoffman, M. K., Rhee, A., & Colmorgen, G. H. C. (2005). Extramembranous placement of an air-coupled vs. transducer-tipped intrauterine pressure catheter: A randomized comparison. *Journal of Reproductive Medicine, 50*(8), 578–584.

Spector, R. E. (2004). *Cultural diversity in health and illness* (6th ed.). Upper Saddle River, NJ: Pearson-Prentice Hall.

Timbie, J. W., Horvitz-Lennon, M., Frank, R. G., & Normand, S. T. (2006). A meta-analysis of labor supply effects of interventions for major depressive disorder. *Psychiatric Services, 57*(2), 212–218.

Torgersen, K. (2003). Arrhythmias and dysrhythmias. In N. Feinstein, K. Torgersen, & J. Atterbury (Eds.), *Fetal heart monitoring principles and practices* (3rd ed.). Dubuque, IA: Kendall-Hunt.

Tucker, J., Parry, G., Penney, G., Page, M., & Hundley, V. (2003). Is midwife workload associated with quality of process of care (continuous electronic fetal monitoring [CEFM]) and neonatal outcome indicators? A prospective study in consultant-led labour wards in Scotland. *Journal of Paediatric and Perinatal Epidemiology, 17*(4), 369–377.

Will, S. B., Hennicke, K. P., Jacobs, L. S., O'Neill, L. M., & Raab, C. A. (2006). The perinatal patient safety nurse: A new role to promote safe care for mothers and babies. *Journal of Obstetric, Gynecologic, & Neonatal Nursing, 35*(3), 417–423.

CHAPTER
24

The Family in Childbirth: Needs and Care

The moment our daughter was born, time seemed to stand still. We couldn't keep our eyes off of her. I remember vividly the first time I touched her tiny finger and stroked her cheek. Those moments together as a family are forever engraved in my memory.

KEY TERMS

Apgar score   670
Hyperventilation   660
Precipitous birth   680

OBJECTIVES

1. Identify nursing diagnoses specific to the first, second, third, and fourth stages of labor.

2. Describe factors that are assessed in the laboring woman during the admission process.

3. Discuss the components of a social history and its role in caring for the laboring woman.

4. Summarize the importance of incorporating family expectations and cultural beliefs into the nursing care plan.

5. Discuss nursing interventions to meet the care needs of the laboring woman and her partner during each stage of labor.

6. Describe nursing interventions for promoting the woman's comfort during each stage of labor.

7. Summarize immediate nursing care of the newborn following birth.

8. Discuss the components of care for the woman during the third stage of labor.

9. Discuss initial measures to help the woman and family integrate the newborn into family life.

10. Explore the nurse's role in providing sensitive care to adolescent parents.

11. Delineate management of a nurse-managed precipitous birth.

MEDIALINK

Additional resources for this content can be found on the Prentice Hall Nursing MediaLink DVD-ROM and on the Companion Website at http://www.prenhall.com/davidson. Click on "Chapter 24" to select the activities for this chapter.

It is time for a child to be born. The waiting is over; labor has begun. The dreams and wishes of the past months fade as the expectant family faces the reality of the tasks of childbearing and childrearing that are ahead.

The couple is about to undergo one of the most meaningful and stressful events in their life together. Physical and psychologic resources, coping mechanisms, and support systems will all be challenged. Despite months of childbirth education classes, the laboring woman may question her ability to cope with labor and to meet her own expectations of herself. The partner may wonder whether he will be able to provide the support his partner and newborn will need. They may worry about the baby's health. Although they look forward to the birth of their baby, they are entering an unfamiliar landscape where, even with prenatal preparation, unknown possibilities await them.

Many childbearing families look to the nurse for support and guidance. Indeed, for laboring women who are admitted alone, the nurse may be their sole support. It is essential, therefore, to provide holistic care that addresses the client's or couple's physiologic, psychologic, and comfort needs throughout the challenging and emotional process of labor and birth.

The previous two chapters present information that lays the foundation for this chapter. Chapter 22 ∞ presents a database of information regarding physiologic and psychologic changes during labor and birth, and Chapter 23 ∞ discusses intrapartal assessment. This chapter discusses nursing care during labor and birth. The Clinical Pathway on pages 645–647 summarizes nursing care of the childbearing family in the first through fourth stages of labor and birth.

NURSING DIAGNOSIS DURING LABOR AND BIRTH

In devising a plan of care for the intrapartal period, the nurse can develop a general plan that encompasses the whole process, from the beginning of labor through the fourth stage, or the nurse can develop a plan for each stage of labor and birth. The nurse's plan and actions are based on current findngs from nursing and medical research. By providing evidence-based guided care, the nurse ensures that the woman and her family are appropriately cared for during their labor and birth. An overall plan presents an overview of the whole process, but it is usually general in nature. A plan of care that identifies nursing diagnoses for (at least) each stage provides an opportunity to identify more specific nursing interventions.

In the first stage of labor, nursing diagnoses that may apply include the following:

- *Fear/Anxiety* related to discomfort of labor and unknown labor outcome
- *Health-Seeking Behaviors: Information About the Fetal* monitor related to an expressed desire to understand equipment used
- *Compromised Family Coping* related to labor process

- *Acute Pain* related to uterine contractions, cervical dilatation, and fetal descent
- *Deficient Knowledge* related to lack of information about normal labor process and comfort measures
- *Fear/Anxiety* related to unknown birth outcome and anticipated discomfort

Nursing diagnoses for the second and third stages may include the following:

- *Acute Pain* related to uterine contractions, birth process, and/or perineal trauma from birth
- *Deficient Knowledge* related to lack of information about pushing methods
- *Ineffective Coping* related to birth process
- *Fear/Anxiety* related to outcome of birth process

In the fourth stage, possible nursing diagnoses include the following:

- *Acute Pain* related to perineal trauma
- *Deficient Knowledge* related to lack of information about involutional process and self-care needs
- *Readiness for Enhamced Family Processes* related to incorporation of the newborn into the family

NURSING CARE DURING ADMISSION

Many families worry that they will not reach the birthing center in time for the birth or that cues indicating the onset of labor will be missed. Sometimes labor occurs so rapidly that birth is imminent upon admission. Usually, the family is advised to arrive at the birth setting at the beginning of the active phase of labor or when the following occur:

- Rupture of membranes (ROM)
- Decreased fetal movement
- Regular, frequent uterine contractions (nulliparas, about 5 minutes apart for 1 hour; multiparas, 6 to 8 minutes apart for 1 hour)
- Any vaginal bleeding
- Decreased fetal movement

If time permits and the family is not familiar with what will occur during labor, the nurse can provide information on admission. (See Client Teaching: What to Expect During Labor.)

The family may be facing a number of unfamiliar procedures that are routine for healthcare providers. It is important to remember that each woman has the right to determine what happens to her body. Informed consent should be obtained before any procedure that involves touching the body.

Establishing a Positive Relationship

The initial interaction with the nurse and how it is perceived by the woman and her partner greatly influences the course of

CLINICAL PATHWAY For Intrapartal Stages

CATEGORY	FIRST STAGE	SECOND AND THIRD STAGE	FOURTH STAGE BIRTH TO 1 HOUR PAST BIRTH
Referral	Review prenatal record Advise CNM/physician of admission	Labor record for first stage	Report to recovery room nurse ◆ *Expected Outcomes* Appropriate resources identified and utilized
Assessments	Admission assessments: Ask about problems since last prenatal visit; labor status (contraction frequency and duration), membrane status (intact or ruptured); coping level; support; woman's desires during labor and birth; ability to verbalize needs; laboratory testing (blood and UA) Intrapartal assessments: Cervical assessment: from 1 to 10 cm dilatation; nullipara (1.2 cm/h), multipara (1.5 cm/h) Cervical effacement: from 0% to 100% Fetal descent: progressive descent from −4 to +4 Membrane assessment: intact or ruptured; when ruptured, Nitrazine positive, fluid clear, no foul odor Comfort level: woman states is able to cope with contractions Behavioral characteristics: facial expressions, tone of voice, and verbal expressions are consistent with comfort level and ability to cope Latent Phase: • BP, P, R q30min for low-risk women and q15min for high-risk women if in normal range (BP 90–135/60–85 or not greater than 30 mm Hg systolic or 15 mm Hg diastolic over baseline; pulse 60–90; respirations 12–24/min, quiet, easy) • Temp every 4h unless greater than 37.6C (99.6F) or membranes ruptured then q1h • Uterine contractions q30min for low-risk women and q15min for high-risk women (contractions q5–10min, 15–40 sec, mild intensity) • FHR q30min (for low-risk women) and q15min (for high-risk women) if reassuring (reassuring FHR has: baseline 110–160, variability present, average, accelerations with fetal movement, no late decelerations); if nonreassuring, position on side, start O₂, assess for hypotension, monitor continuously, discontinue Pitocin if infusing, notify CNM/physician Active Phase: • BP, P, R, q30min if WNL for low-risk women and q15min for high-risk women. • Temp as above • Uterine contractions q15–30min: contractions q2–3min, 60 sec, moderate to strong • FHR q30min (for low-risk women) and q15min (for high-risk women) if reassuring; if nonreassuring institute interventions Transition: • BP, P, R, q30min • Uterine contractions q30min for low-risk women and q15min for high-risk women; contractions q2min, 60–75 sec, strong • FHR q30min for low-risk women and every 15 minutes for high-risk women if reassuring; if nonreassuring, see above	Second stage assessments: • BP, P, R q5–15min • Uterine contractions palpated continuously • FHR q15min (for low-risk women) and q5min (for high-risk women) if reassuring; if nonreassuring, monitor continuously Fetal descent: descent continues to birth Comfort level: woman states is able to cope with contractions and pushing Behavioral characteristics: response to pushing, facial expressions, verbalization Third stage assessments: • BP, P, R q5min • Uterine contractions, palpate occasionally until placenta is delivered, fundus maintains tone and contraction pattern continues to birth of placenta Newborn assessments: • Assess Apgar score of newborn • Respirations: 30–60, irregular • Apical pulse: 110–160 and somewhat irregular • Temperature: Skin temp above 36.5C (97.8F) • Umbilical cord: two arteries, one vein (if one artery, assess for anomalies and urine output) • Gestational age: 38–42 weeks	Immediate postbirth assessments of mother q15min for 1h: • BP: 90–135/60–85; should return to prelabor level • Pulse: slightly lower than in labor; range is 60–90 • Respirations: 12–24/min; easy; quiet • Temperature: 36.2–37.6C (98–99.6F) • Fundus firm, in midline, at the umbilicus • Lochia rubra; moderate amount; less than 1 pad/h; no free flow or passage of clots with massage • Perineum: sutures intact; no bulging or marked swelling; minimal bruising may be present; no c/o severe pain nor rectal pain • Bladder nondistended; spontaneous void of greater than 100mL clear, straw-colored urine; bladder nondistended following voiding • If hemorrhoids present, no tenseness or marked engorgement; less than 2 cm diameter Comfort level: less than 3 on scale of 1 to 10 Energy level: awake and able to hold newborn Newborn assessments if newborn remains with parents: • Respirations: 30–60; irregular • Apical pulse: 110–160 and somewhat irregular • Temperature: skin temp above 36.5C (97.8F); skin feels warm to touch • Skin color noncyanotic • Mucus: small amount, clear, easily suctioned with bulb syringe without skin color change • Behavioral: newborn opens eyes widely if room is slightly darkened • Movements rhythmic; no hand tremors present ◆ *Expected Outcomes* Findings indicate normal progression with absence of complications

(Continued on next page)

CLINICAL PATHWAY For Intrapartal Stages continued

Category	First Stage	Second and Third Stage	Fourth Stage Birth to 1 Hour Past Birth
Teaching/ psychosocial	Establish rapport Orient to environment, expected assessments, and procedures Answer questions and provide information Orient to EFM if used Teach relaxation, visualization, and breathing pattern if needed Explain comfort measures available Assume advocacy role for woman/family during labor and birth	Orient to expected assessments and procedures Answer questions and provide information Explain comfort measures available Continue advocacy role	Explain immediate assessments and care after this first hour Teach self-massage of fundus and expected findings Instruct to call for assistance if mother desires to get OOB Begin newborn teaching; bulb syringe, positioning; maintaining warmth Assist parents in exploring their newborn Assist with first breastfeeding experience ◆ *Expected Outcomes* Client and partner verbalize/demonstrate understanding of teaching
Nursing care management and report	Straight cath prn if bladder distended If regional block administered monitor BP, FHR, sensation per protocol Provide continuing status reports to CNM/physician Perform sterile vaginal examination as indicated	Indwelling catheter or straight cath prn if bladder distended Continue monitoring VS, FHR, and sensation if regional block has been given	Straight cath if bladder distended Monitor return of motor ability and sensation if regional block has been given Weigh perineal pads if lochia flow greater than 1 saturated pad in 15 min, presence of boggy uterus and close; ↓BP, ↑P ◆ *Expected Outcomes* • Maternal/fetal well-being maintained and supported • Mother and newborn experience safe labor and birth • Family participates in process as desired
Activity	Encourage ambulation unless contraindicated Maintain bed rest immediately after administration of IV pain medication, or following regional block Woman rests comfortably between contractions	Position comfortably for birth Woman rests comfortably between pushing efforts and while awaiting birth of placenta	Position of comfort ◆ *Expected Outcomes* • Activity maintained as desired unless contraindicated • Comfort enhanced by positioning/movement
Comfort	Institute comfort measures: ambulation, frequent position change, effleurage, focal point, patterned paced breathing, visualization, therapeutic touch, backrub, moist cloths to face, holding hand, words of encouragement, changing underpad, shower, whirlpool, staying with the woman/family, warmed blanket at back, sacral pressure Offer pain medication or administer if requested Assist with administration of regional block	Institute comfort measures: • Second stage: cool cloth to forehead, encouragement, coaching, help support legs while pushing, position of comfort for pushing and birth • Third stage: cool cloth to forehead, assist parents to see newborn, position mother to hold newborn, provide encouragement	Institute comfort measures: • Perineal discomfort: gently cleanse and apply ice pack; position to decrease pressure on perineum • Uterine discomfort; palpate fundus gently • Hemorrhoids: ice pack • General fatigue: position of comfort, encourage rest • Administer pain medication PRN ◆ *Expected Outcomes* • Optimal comfort level maintained • Active reduction of pain/discomfort achieved
Nutrition	Ice chips and clear fluids Evaluate for signs of dehydration	Ice chips and clear fluids	Regular diet if assessments are WNL Encourage fluids ◆ *Expected Outcomes* Nutritional needs met
Elimination	Voids at least q2h; urine clear, strawcolored, negative for protein Bladder nondistended May have bowel movement Monitor I & O with IVs	May void spontaneously with pushing May pass stool with pushing	Voids spontaneously ◆ *Expected Outcomes* Urinary bladder and bowel function unimpaired

CLINICAL PATHWAY For Intrapartal Stages continued

CATEGORY	FIRST STAGE	SECOND AND THIRD STAGE	FOURTH STAGE BIRTH TO 1 HOUR PAST BIRTH
Medications	Administer pain medication per woman's request	Local infiltration of anesthetic agent for birth by CNM/physician Pitocin 10–20 units IM, IVP per IV, tubing, or added to IV fluids	Continue Pitocin infusion Administer pain medication PRN ◆ *Expected Outcomes* Comfort enhanced by pain-relieving techniques, administration of analgesia agent or an analgesic or anesthetic block
Discharge planning	Evaluate knowledge of labor and birth process Evaluate support system and need for referral after birth		Provide information if mother to be moved from LDR room Provide opportunity for parents to ask questions regarding newborn Evaluate knowledge of normal postpartum, newborn care ◆ *Expected Outcomes* Mother and newborn transferred to low-risk postpartal and newborn care
Family involvement	Identify available support person(s) Recognize possible impact of culture on responses Observe interaction between woman and partner Create moment alone with woman to identify possible abuse Assess current parenting skills	Provide opportunities for woman and support person(s) to watch newborn assessments Perform newborn assessment on mother's abdomen/chest if possible	Provide opportunity for parents to be with baby Encourage skin-to-skin contact Darken room to encourage eye-to-eye contact Provide quiet time for new family Parenting: demonstrates early culturally expected parenting behaviors ◆ *Expected Outcomes* • Incorporation of newborn into family • Family verbalizes comfort with newborn care
Date			

CNM, certified nurse-midwife; BP, blood pressure; FHR, fetal heart rate; LTV long-term variability; WNL, within normal limits; VS, vital signs; EFM, electronic fetal monitoring; IV, intravenous; I&0, intake and output; IM, intramuscularly; IVP, intravenous push; LDR, labor, delivery, and recovery; OOB, out of bed; UA, urinary analysis; PRN, as needed

her hospital stay. For some women, the hospital environment itself can be perceived as cold, impersonal, and technical and can produce anxiety or emotional stress. If the family is greeted in a brusque, harried manner, they are less likely to look to the nurse for support. A calm, pleasant manner, in contrast, indicates to the family that they are important. It helps instill in the couple a sense of confidence in the staff's ability to provide quality care and ensure safety during this critical time.

It is important to establish rapport and to create an environment in which the family feels free to ask questions. The support and encouragement of the nurse in maintaining a caring environment begins with the initial admission but needs to be attended to with all subsequent actions. Before completing assessments, the nurse may provide the opportunity for questions and may explain the environment and the procedures that will be a part of the labor and birthing care. In many hospitals, the admission process also includes signing an informed consent for treatment, and the client is given information on arranging advance directives or instructions about her wishes if she were to become critically ill. In all cases, an identification bracelet and a bracelet that lists all known drug allergies are attached to her wrist.

Another important aspect of the initial contact is communicating in the woman and family's primary language. In addition to having interpreters available for Hispanic, Korean, Vietnamese, and other clients who do not speak English fluently, the nurse must consider the special needs of the deaf woman or family. There are more than 400,000 Americans who have a bilateral hearing loss, so there is a good chance that the nurse will work with a deaf expectant mother, father, grandparents, or siblings at some point. Table 24–1 provides suggestions for communicating more effectively with a woman or support person who is deaf.

Culture plays a major role in how a woman and her family view the labor and birth process. Trends in American culture are moving toward a shared partnership model between the woman and her partner in which the partner is actively involved in the birth process and often stays with the mother throughout the labor and birth. In contrast, Jordanian women are less likely to have their partner with them in the labor and birth setting. Instead, this is primarily the role of elder women family members and female friends (Safadi, 2005).

CLIENT TEACHING What to Expect During Labor

ASSESSMENT   As the woman is admitted into the birthing area, assess the woman's knowledge regarding the childbirth experience. Her knowledge base will be affected by previous births, attendance at childbirth education classes, and the amount of information she has been able to gather during her pregnancy by asking questions or reading. You may also assess the factors that affect communication and anxiety level. Assess labor progress to determine what to teach and the time available for teaching. If the woman is in early labor and she needs additional information, proceed with teaching.

NURSING DIAGNOSIS   The key nursing diagnosis will probably be *Deficient Knowledge* related to lack of information about nursing care during labor.

NURSING PLAN AND IMPLEMENTATION   The teaching plan will focus on the assessments and support the woman will receive during labor.

CLIENT GOALS   At the completion of teaching, the woman will be able to:

• Verbalize the assessments the nurse will complete during labor

• Discuss the support and comfort measures that are available

TEACHING PLAN

CONTENT	TEACHING METHOD
• Describe aspects of the admission process, including:	Provide information on the basic assessment and care activities.
• Taking an abbreviated history	Allow time for questions and discussion as labor progress permits.
• Physical assessment (maternal vital signs [VS], fetal heart rate [FHR], contraction status, status of membranes)	
• Assessment of uterine contractions (frequency, duration, intensity)	
• Orientation to surroundings	
• Introductions to other support staff	
• Determination of woman's and family support person's expectations of the nurse	
• Present aspects of ongoing physical care, such as when to expect assessment of material VS, FHR, and contractions.	
• If the electronic fetal monitor is used, describe how it works and the information it provides. Orient the woman to the sights and sounds of the monitor. Explain what "normal" data will look like and what characteristics are being watched for.	Demonstrate the fetal monitor.
• Be sure to note that assessments will increase as the labor progresses, especially during the transition phase (usually the time the woman would like to be left alone) to help keep the mother and baby safe by noting deviations from normal course.	
• Describe the vaginal examination and the information it elicits.	Use a cervical dilatation chart to illustrate the amount of dilatation.
• Review comfort techniques that may be used in labor and ascertain what the woman thinks will promote comfort.	Focus on open discussion.
• Review the breathing techniques the woman has learned so that you will be able to support her technique.	Ask the woman to demonstrate the techniques she has learned.
• Review comfort and support measures, such as positioning, backrub, effleurage, touch, distraction techniques, and ambulation.	Focus on open discussion.
• If the woman is in early labor, offer her a tour of the birthing area.	Provide a tour of birthing area, explaining equipment and routines. Include the woman's partner.

EVALUATION

At the end of this teaching session, the woman will be able to describe the assessments that will occur during her labor and to discuss comfort and support measures that may be used.

DOCUMENTATION

Documentation of client teaching should include the teaching information discussed, the client's verbalization of understanding, and specific interventions or warning signs that were given, along with the client's understanding of follow-up, if needed in the future.

Table 24–1   IMPROVING COMMUNICATION WITH A DEAF WOMAN OR SUPPORT PERSON

- Determine how the deaf individual prefers to communicate: speech reading (lip reading), sign language, pantomine, writing, or a combination of methods.
- If speech reading is used, face the person directly, speak with a natural tone and rhythm (exaggerated pronunciation may distort lip movements), and keep your hands away from your face. Do not chew gum.
- Use gestures and pantomime if necessary to enhance your speech.
- Do not assume written communication is the most effective approach. Writing carries a great potential for miscommunication and should not be forced unless the deaf person requests it.
- Most deaf individuals in the United States use American Sign Language (ASL). If the woman signs, call a professional ASL interpreter.
- Only use a family member as an interpreter until the professional interpreter arrives. Family members may not interpret all that is said or may add additional information. Professional ASL interpreters are bound by a code of ethics to maintain strict confidentiality, to transmit accurate messages, and to refrain from editing or adding information.
- Keep the woman's dominant hand and arm free for signing.
- Explain any procedures before they are needed.
- Look at the deaf individual, not the interpreter, when speaking.
- Speak in first person to the client.
- Be alert for signs of "smiling and nodding." Often, when a deaf person does not understand something, the person will simply smile and nod. If that occurs, assess the person's understanding by asking the person to repeat the information to you.

SOURCE: Adapted from Shelp, S. G. (1997). Your patient is deaf, now what? *RN, 60*(2), 37–38, 40. Reprinted by permission of Medical Economics. Montvale, NJ.

Labor Assessment

Following the initial greeting, the woman may either be taken into a labor assessment area (sometimes called a *triage area*) for evaluation or admitted directly into a birthing room. Some couples prefer to remain together during the admission process, and others prefer to have the partner or support person wait outside. The nurse should ask the woman's preference whenever possible. As the nurse helps the woman undress and get into a hospital gown, the nurse can begin to develop rapport and establish the nursing database. The labor and birth nurse can obtain essential information regarding the woman and her pregnancy. By doing an admission history, the nurse can initiate any immediate interventions needed and establish individualized priorities. The nurse is then able to make effective nursing decisions regarding intrapartal care:

- Is the woman in labor or is she a candidate to be sent home with a clear understanding of when to return?
- Are there factors that put the laboring woman or the fetus at risk?
- Should ambulation or bed rest be encouraged?
- Is more frequent monitoring needed?
- What does the woman or couple want during labor and birth?
- Who will be with the laboring woman for social support?

The woman is made comfortable. If she wants to rest in bed, a side-lying or semi-Fowler's position rather than a supine

position is most comfortable and avoids supine hypotensive syndrome (vena caval syndrome).

After obtaining the essential information from the woman and her prenatal records from her certified nurse-midwife (CNM) or physician, the nurse begins the intrapartal assessment. (Chapter 23 ∞ considers intrapartal assessment in depth).

As the assessments begin, the nurse auscultates the fetal heart rate (FHR). (Detailed information on monitoring FHR is presented in Chapter 21 ∞). The woman's blood pressure, pulse, respirations, and oral temperature are assessed. Contraction status (frequency, duration, and intensity), cervical dilatation and effacement, and fetal presentation and station are determined. If the woman is a nullipara in the early latent phase (for example, contractions are 10 to 30 minutes apart, with mild intensity and very little discomfort; cervix is long and thick, with dilatation of 1 to 2 cm; membranes are intact) she may be sent home to ambulate and rest in her own surroundings or directed to remain in a birthing center area and ambulate. When further progress is documented, she is admitted. Women who are admitted in the latent phase are more likely to have a longer duration of labor, increased use of epidural analgesia for pain, and increased use of oxytocin to augment labor than women who are clearly in the active phase at admission.

After the vaginal examination, the nurse shares the findings with the couple. If there are signs of advanced labor (frequent contractions, advanced cervical dilatation, and/or an urge to bear down), the physician or CNM is notified immediately, and actions are taken to prepare for the birth. If there are signs of excessive bleeding upon admission or if the woman reports episodes of painless bleeding in the last trimester, placenta previa may be present; in such cases, vaginal examination is not performed because it may stimulate copious bleeding.

Results of FHR assessment, uterine contraction evaluation, and the vaginal examination help determine whether the rest of the admission process can proceed at a more leisurely pace or whether additional interventions have higher priority. For example, an FHR of 110 beats per minute (bpm) on auscultation indicates that an electronic fetal monitor (EFM) should be applied immediately to obtain additional data. The woman's vital signs will then be assessed immediately (Table 24–2).

Depending on how rapidly labor is progressing, the nurse notifies the CNM or physician before or after completing the admission procedures. If high-risk or emergency data are identified, the nurse immediately reports the findings to the CNM or physician; otherwise all assessment data should be gathered before initiating contact with the healthcare provider (Reece & Hobbins, 2006). The report should include the following information: cervical dilatation and effacement, station, presenting part, status of the membranes, contraction pattern, FHR, vital signs that are not in the normal range, the woman's wishes, and her response to labor.

Collecting Laboratory Data

After admission data are obtained, multiple laboratory tests are performed to provide more extensive physiologic data that are used to determine appropriate care for the woman and her fetus. A clean-voided midstream urine specimen is usually collected.

Table 24–2	INDICATORS OF NORMAL LABOR PROCESS ON ADMISSION
Indicator	**Normal Characteristics**
Uterine contractions	Frequency of not less than 2 minutes Duration of less than 75 seconds Uterine relaxation between contractions Most intense discomfort only with contractions (Some women, especially those with occiput posterior position, complain of less intense lower abdominal and/or back pain between contractions.)
Fetal heart rate	Rate 110–160 with average variability Absence of late decelerations
Maternal vital signs	BP below +140/90 or less than +30/+15 above prepregnancy readings Pulse 60–100 Temperature between 97.8F and 99.6F (36.5C and 37.5C)
If membranes ruptured	Fluid clear without odor

The woman with intact membranes may collect her specimen in the bathroom. The nurse can test the woman's urine for the presence of protein, ketones, glucose, and leukocytes by using a dipstick before sending the sample to the laboratory. This procedure is especially important if nondependent edema or elevated blood pressure is noted on admission. Proteinuria of +1 or more may be a sign of preeclampsia. Glycosuria is found frequently in pregnant women because of the increased glomerular filtration rate in the proximal tubules and the inability of these tubules to increase glucose reabsorption. However, it may also be associated with gestational diabetes and should not be discounted. Leukocytes can be found in the urine when bacteria are present. The presence of a urinary tract infection can contribute to uterine irritability, pelvic pressure, and back pain, all symptoms that can be mistaken for labor.

Laboratory tests can be performed in the outpatient setting before admission but are most commonly done at the time of admission in the birthing center. Hemoglobin and hematocrit values help determine the oxygen-carrying capacity of the circulatory system and the ability of the woman to withstand blood loss at birth. Elevation of the hematocrit indicates hemoconcentration of blood, which occurs with edema or dehydration. A low hemoglobin, in the absence of other evidence of bleeding, suggests anemia. Blood may be typed and cross-matched if the woman is in a high-risk category, has active bleeding, or has a history of blood disorders. A serology test for syphilis is obtained if one has not been done in the last 3 months or if an antepartal serology result was positive. The Centers for Disease Control and Prevention (CDC) recommends that all women undergo voluntary screening for human immunodeficiency virus (HIV) during pregnancy. Women who have not been screened during the pregnancy should be screened for HIV in the intrapartum setting once consent has been obtained (CDC, 2004).

Social Assessment

Once initial physical assessments are performed, the nurse can then take a detailed social history that provides a comprehensive view of both the woman's social habits and psychologic factors that may affect her birth experience. The presence of certain risk factors—including family violence or sexual assault (see Chapter 9 ∞); use of drugs, alcohol, or tobacco; and presence of sexually transmitted infections—can influence a woman's labor, birth, and future childrearing choices. With the prevalence of domestic violence, it is imperative to ask the woman about family violence and sexual assault (Verhey, Levy, & Schmidt, 2004). Because many women find questions about psychosocial risk factors embarrassing, the nurse should always ask such questions when the woman is alone and should use a straightforward, nonjudgmental approach. For example, a question such as "How many times per week do you drink alcohol?" prompts the woman to be specific in her answer. If the woman reports that she does drink alcohol on a daily basis, the nurse then asks about the amount. Drug use can be assessed in a similar manner.

A social assessment should also include data about the woman's current living situation, availability of resources, preparedness for the infant, community resources, and the woman's social support network. This dialog provides an opportunity for the nurse to continue to build support, to provide information when requested, and to be direct yet supportive. Referrals to social services, the Special Supplemental Food Program for Women, Infants, and Children (WIC), and new parent support programs can be initiated. It is important to begin this dialog early in the admission process so that adequate resources can be obtained for the family.

Documentation of Admission

A nursing admission note is entered into the computer or the charting system. The admission note should include the reason for admission; the date, time and method of the woman's arrival; notification of the CNM or physician; the condition of the woman and her baby; labor and membrane status; and pertinent social assessment information (American Academy of Pediatrics [AAP] & American College of Obstetricians and Gynecologists [ACOG], 2002). Her comfort level and support system should also be addressed. For a woman who speaks a different language, an interpreter should be provided, and documentation should include that the interpreter was used and that the woman verbalized understanding.

NURSING CARE DURING THE FIRST STAGE OF LABOR

After completing the nursing assessment and diagnosis steps, the nurse creates a plan of care to achieve nursing goals (Simpson, 2005). During the first stage of labor, the nurse is concerned about the physical safety of the laboring woman and her child, as well as the emotional well-being of the laboring couple and their support system. Therefore, the nurse continually assesses the effects of uterine contractions on the course of labor and the well-being of the fetus, and monitors the woman's vital signs, contraction pattern, cervical changes, and intake and output. Additionally, the nurse monitors the couple's and support system's responses to labor.

Labor support is a primary role for nurses who are caring for couples during the first stage of labor. Couples look to their nurse for information about labor progress, pain management, procedures, and examinations, and for assistance with pain management techniques such as breathing and relaxation. Couples need reassurance that labor is progressing in normal trajectory and explanations when it is not within normal limits. They also need praise for their accomplishments and support during labor. For most couples, the nurse's presence in the room is highly valued as labor advances; however, the nurse should assess the woman's individual preferences, because some women may prefer privacy. Clinical research has established that laboring women have fewer complications and shorter labors when they perceive support from their nurse and/or friends and family members (Hottenstein, 2005).

Integration of Family Expectations

Laboring families have certain expectations of the experience, of themselves, of the nurse, and of the physician or CNM. Some of these expectations may not be realistic. Unrealistic expectations can increase the anxiety level of both the laboring woman and her partner. The labor nurse should assess the family's expectations to integrate them into the labor plan and/or assist the family in reestablishing expectations that are realistic. Some families may present to the facility with a birth plan (discussed in Chapter 13 ∞). The plan should be reviewed and requests should be incorporated into the woman's nursing care plan whenever possible. Requests that cannot be met should be discussed and a clear rationale should be provided.

Laboring families' expectations of the nurse can range from wanting the nurse to be highly involved in the labor, to wanting the nurse to be minimally involved (Hottenstein, 2005). The couple who desires high involvement expects the labor nurse to be in the room continuously and to provide direct labor support. The couple may view the labor nurse as the woman's primary labor coach, providing guidance and emotional support. The couple who desires minimal involvement of the labor nurse prefers that the nurse is present only when assessments and interventions need to be done and when the couple requests the nurse's presence.

With the variety of expectations clients have of nurses, it becomes a challenge to provide individualized care. The nurse needs to assess and respond to the couple's needs and desires. To determine preferences, the nurse can look for cues. When the woman and her coach are admitted, do they seem to take control and know what is going to happen? Do they have a birth plan that they have already worked out, or do they seem hesitant and unsure of the process?

Although these two ends of the spectrum are obvious, they are a starting point. It would be fairly safe to assume that the "situation-is-in-control" couple would want a little less involvement, and the couple who is hesitant and asking questions will want more extensive involvement. The nurse can also gain more information by asking questions such as, "Other than the assessments that I will be making, what kind of involvement would you like from me? Would you like to call me when you need something or have me come in now and then, or would you be more comfortable if I stay in the room most of the time?" This gives the couple an opportunity to make their wishes known. This approach also provides the couple with the opportunity to

ask questions and seek advice as needed. It is also important that the couple knows that the nurse understands that their wishes may change during labor and that the nurse will be available for them throughout the process.

During the labor process, the nurse also serves as an advocate for the woman and her partner. The partner may need support, guidance, or an opportunity for rest periods. The nurse models behavior to family members who may feel uncomfortable or uneasy in the labor and birth setting (Naber, 2005).

Integration of Cultural Beliefs

Values, customs, and practices of different cultures are as important during labor as they are in the prenatal period. Research indicates that an individual's experiences in labor are highly dependent upon social and cultural norms (Cheung, 2002). Without this knowledge, a nurse is less likely to understand a family's behavior and may impose personal values and beliefs upon them. As cultural sensitivity increases, so does the likelihood of providing high-quality care (Spector, 2004).

The following sections briefly present a few possible cultural responses to labor. Additional information on culturally sensitive care is provided in Chapter 2. ∞ It is difficult to present such a limited discussion without appearing to advance stereotypes. No statement of a specific behavior can accurately reflect the preference of all people in a group. Within every culture, each person develops his or her own beliefs and value system. Nurses must regard general information about any culture or belief system as background information to help them determine the person's own needs and desires.

CLINICAL TIP

It is best not to assume that women of any culture have the information they desire regarding birth, self-care, and newborn care, regardless of the number of children they have had. An important aspect of nursing is to teach, so always offer culturally sensitive information. Most nurses are not knowledgeable regarding all cultural practices. So be sensitive, and ask what is important to the mother. For example, is there special clothing she wants the newborn to wear, or does she have any preference about how she wants the umbilical stump cared for? Remain aware that the information you learned in class or a text reflects primarily the nursing culture and the Western, chiefly European, culture. To believe that the healthcare practices of these two cultures are relevant to all people is an example of ethnocentrism. Strive to increase your understanding of other cultures as your clinical practice base grows.

MODESTY

Modesty is an important consideration for women, regardless of the culture to which they belong. However, some women may be more uncomfortable than others with the degree of exposure needed for some procedures during the labor and the birth process. Some women may be particularly uncomfortable when men are present and feel more comfortable with women; others may be uncomfortable with exposure of personal body parts regardless of the gender of the examiner or person who assists them. The nurse needs to be observant of the woman's responses to examinations and procedures and to provide appropriate draping and privacy (Shamshad & Crown, 2005). It is more prudent to assume that embarrassment will occur with exposure and take measures to provide privacy than to assume that it will not matter to the woman.

For example, many Hispanic women may fear loss of privacy, so they labor at home as long as possible. Maintaining dignity for the couple is important (Spector, 2004). Some Asian women are not accustomed to male physicians and attendants, and some Muslims forbid any male (other than the husband) to see a woman who is uncovered. The nurse should be aware that in the Muslim culture, the man is the primary source of information. It may be necessary to speak to the man before interacting with the woman. This communicates respect and shows cultural sensitivity. The nurse should ensure coverage of the woman whenever possible, even during vaginal exams and the second stage (Spector, 2004).

PAIN EXPRESSION

Women's reactions to the discomfort of labor vary greatly. Some turn inward and remain very quiet during the whole process, whereas others may be very vocal, with behaviors such as counting out loud, moaning quietly or loudly, crying, or cursing. They may also turn from side to side or change positions frequently. The nurse supports a woman's individual expression of pain, whatever it may be, to enhance the birthing experience for mother, baby, and family.

In the Korean culture it used to be important for the laboring woman to be silent so she would not bring shame on her family. However, today women are encouraged to be less passive. Vocalization is more common, although older in-laws or other family members may discourage shouting or outcries as aggressive behavior. Hmong women are frequently quiet during labor, although behavior varies from one individual to the next. European Americans demonstrate a wide variety of behaviors in response to pain. Some stay very quiet and seem to turn inward to "keep control"; others move about in bed, change positions frequently, moan, and cry. Especially in the transitional phase, some women want to squeeze their partner's (or the nurse's) hand, and some may be tempted to bite during the most intense part of the contraction. Vietnamese women tend to report more pain, use less pain medication, and regard labor as a negative experience (McLachlan & Waldenstrom, 2005).

EXAMPLES OF CULTURAL BELIEFS

Some differences between cultures are apparent with regard to specific practices related to position and food and drink during labor. In most non-European societies uninfluenced by Westernization, women assume an upright position in childbirth. For example, during birth some Native American women use meditation, self-control, or indigenous plants, and the father may be expected to avoid certain rituals such as eating meat. Some Native Americans may ask to take the placenta home for a ritualistic ceremony that involves returning the placenta to the earth.

For Hmong women from Laos, the beginning of labor signifies the beginning of a transition and entails certain dietary restrictions. The woman usually prefers only "hot" foods, tea made with loose tea leaves, and warm water to drink. The woman usually maintains self-control, and may wish to move about freely during the first stage of labor. She may smile even throughout intense contractions. The husband is frequently present and actively involved in providing comfort. Traditionally, the woman prefers that the amniotic membranes not be ruptured until just before birth. It is thought that the escape of fluid at this time makes the birth easier. She may choose to kneel or squat for the birth of her baby. As soon as the baby is born, a soft-boiled egg must be given to the mother to restore her energy. During the postpartum period, the mother prefers "warm" foods, such as chicken prepared with warm water and warm rice (Her, 2004). The newborn is protected from praise to prevent jealousy.

Latina women often want their partner to stay with them during labor and birth and to reassure them that everything will be all right. The women want the partner to show caring and love as they labor and to speak to them using affectionate words. Standing close to the woman and using touch are important roles for the partner (Spector, 2004).

Muslim women may have their husband, a female friend or relative, or a male relative with them during childbirth. Family support may be particularly important but does not preclude the importance of the nurse's presence. The woman may want to retain her head covering (*khimar*), and two long-sleeved gowns can be offered. Examinations should be done by a female nurse, physician, or CNM whenever possible. Some Muslim women are not comfortable in the presence of a male physician or nurse. If a male physician is involved with their care, they may wish for their husband to remain in the room during all care by the physician. Male providers should only enter the room after receiving permission from the husband. Modesty needs vary, and each individual will need to be assessed. After the birth, Muslim fathers traditionally call praise to Allah (*adhan*) in the newborn's right ear and clean the newborn. It is helpful if the birthing room personnel are aware of these practices so that the family's expectations and wishes can be incorporated into care. Many Middle-Eastern clients also believe that compliments addressed to the parents about their new baby will bring on the evil eye. The "evil eye" is the name given for the passage of sickness from one person to another, either intentionally or unintentionally, as a result of being jealous or envious (Spector, 2004). Thus, the nurse should avoid directly complimenting the couple, but instead direct compliments to God (*Allah*).

> *I am in an area with a very small Muslim population, and one of the nursing students with me had the opportunity to work with a Muslim couple during labor, birth, and then in the postpartum area the following day. During labor, the woman's sister remained at her side, and her husband sat on the other side of a drawn curtain inside the labor room and close to the door. He requested that a sign be placed on the door indicating that no males were to enter the room. We took care to ensure that we asked for a female lab tech for blood drawing, and a female physician attended the birth. The labor and birth went smoothly, and the woman did not utter any sound, even during pushing. After the birth, the father was shown the child before his wife held the newborn boy. The father was very pleased and talked quietly to his son, with his head down beside the newborn's ear. The next day, the student was once again assigned to this family. The sign remained on the*

door, and at all times that day, the sister and father remained in the room, the father always sitting away from the bed, close to the door. This was the woman's fifth child, so at first the student thought that she would not want much self-care, newborn, or breastfeeding information. But she began to talk to the woman, with her husband interpreting all questions and giving answers, and as each topic was brought up, the mother indicated that she wanted more information. Building on the trust that they had established the previous day in labor, the father told the student to "give the instruction," and he left the room. The mother and sister were full of questions about their health and their bodies—questions they had had for years! The student was proud that she did not make assumptions and was able to share so much information with them. It was an experience that the student and I will always remember with great joy.

Sometimes cultural norms are passed down from one generation to the next. African Americans, especially those whose ancestors are from Western Africa, may have beliefs rooted in traditional folk healing. Some African Americans have strong beliefs in healers and faith healers (Quaye, 2005). Some of these beliefs are centered on labor and childrearing. For example, it is widely believed that an infant born with a caul (a piece of the amniotic membrane covering the head at birth) will have the ability to communicate with spirits. This is viewed as a sign of good luck and is widely embraced within this culture.

In working with women from another culture, the nurse needs an awareness of their beliefs, values, and practices to understand their needs. The maternity nurse would do well to make it a priority to become acquainted with the beliefs and practices of the various cultures in the community. In the birthing situation, the nurse supports the family's cultural practices as long as it is safe to do so.

Provision of Care in the First Stage

Throughout the first stage, the nurse needs to evaluate physical parameters of the woman and her fetus. Maternal temperature is monitored every 4 hours unless the temperature is over 37.5C (99.6F); in such cases, it must be taken every hour. Once the amniotic fluid has ruptured, temperature should be monitored every 2 hours.

The nurse monitors blood pressure, pulse, and respirations every hour (Johnson & Taylor, 2005). If the woman's blood pressure is over 140/90 mm Hg or her pulse is more than 100, the CNM or physician must be notified. The blood pressure and pulse are then reevaluated more frequently. The nurse palpates uterine contractions for frequency, intensity, and duration.

Intrapartal vaginal exams are done to assess cervical changes, status of membranes, fetal position, and station. However, frequent vaginal exams increase the risk of infection and should be performed only when needed. Some providers advocate performing vaginal examinations only when a change of management will occur, such as before an epidural or to provide scalp stimulation.

The FHR is auscultated every 30 minutes as long as it remains between 110 and 160 bpm without the presence of decelerations (ACOG, 2005; AWHONN, 2003b). The FHR should be auscultated throughout one contraction and for about 15 seconds after the contraction to ensure that there are no decelerations. If the FHR is not in the 110 to 160 range and/or decelerations are heard, continuous electronic monitoring is recommended. Table 24–3 summarizes nursing assessments in the first stage of labor. The nurse documents labor progress, status of fetus, and interventions in the woman's chart.

CLINICAL TIP

If the monitor is no longer recording the fetal heart tracing, check that there is adequate gel under the transducer and reposition it before you assume there is a problem with the baby.

LATENT PHASE

If the laboring woman has not had childbirth education classes, the latent phase is a time when the nurse can give anticipatory guidance. Most women are not too uncomfortable with contractions at this time and are responsive to teaching about breathing and other techniques for coping with labor contractions. In fact, many women in the latent phase seek information about what to expect. The unprepared woman may hesitate to ask questions and thus can benefit even more from anticipatory guidance by the nurse.

Table 24–3	NURSING ASSESSMENTS IN THE FIRST STAGE	
Phase	**Mother**	**Fetus**
Latent	Blood pressure, respirations each hour if in normal range Temperature every 4 hours unless over 37.5C (99.6F) or membranes ruptured, then every hour Uterine contractions every 15–30 minutes	FHR every 30 minutes for low-risk women and every 15 minutes for high-risk women if normal characteristics present (presence of variability, baseline in the 110–160 bpm range, without late decelerations). Note fetal activity. If electronic fetal monitor in place, assess for reactive NST.
Active	Blood pressure, pulse, respirations every hour if in normal range Uterine contractions palpated every 15–30 minutes	FHR every 30 minutes for low-risk women and every 15 minutes for high-risk women if normal characteristics are present (Reece & Hobbins, 2006).
Transition	Blood pressure, pulse, respirations every 15–30 minutes Contractions palpated at least every 15–30 minutes	FHR every 15–30 minutes if normal characteristics are present.

occurs frequently because of the decreased gastric emptying time. It is not uncommon for women to vomit during the first stage, especially during the transition phase. The nurse should reassure the woman and provide oral care.

ACTIVE PHASE

During the active phase, the contractions have a frequency of 2 to 3 minutes, a duration of 50 to 60 seconds, and moderate intensity. Contractions need to be palpated every 15 to 30 minutes. As the contractions become more frequent and intense, intrapartal vaginal examination may be performed to assess cervical dilatation and effacement and fetal station and position. During the active phase, the cervix dilates from 4 to 7 cm, and vaginal discharge and bloody show increase. The woman should be encouraged to void because a full bladder can interfere with fetal descent. If the woman is unable to void, catheterization may be necessary. Maternal vital signs, including blood pressure, pulse, and respirations, should be assessed every hour for low-risk women (unless previously elevated), and every 30 minutes for high-risk women. The FHR is auscultated every 30 minutes for women without complications and more frequently (every 15 minutes) for women with complications (ACOG, 2005; AWHONN, 2003a).

For the woman experiencing slow progress of labor or the inability to tolerate fluids, an intravenous (IV) electrolyte solution may be started to provide energy and prevent dehydration. If an IV is started, it becomes even more important to encourage voiding every 1 to 2 hours to prevent bladder distention.

CLINICAL TIP

Catheterizing a woman during a contraction is uncomfortable for her and difficult to do because of the increased downward pressure. To avoid these problems, pass the catheter between contractions. If the baby's head is low in the pelvis, you will have to change the direction of the catheter. Visualize passing it up and over the baby's head rather than straight into the urethra.

Women in labor may wish to remain ambulatory to promote comfort and aid in labor progression (Shilling, 2004). Some women who have been ambulatory up to this point may wish to sit in a chair or on a bed. The woman may also need to take periodic rest periods as contractions intensify. If the woman wants to lie in bed, encourage her to assume a side-lying position, help her into a comfortable position, and place support pillows between her knees, under her abdomen, and against the small of the back. To increase comfort, offer a backrub or apply counterpressure to the lower sacral area (Stremler, 2005). Other nursing care measures can include providing effleurage or offering cool washclothes for the forehead or back of the neck. Because vaginal discharge increases, the absorbent pad should be changed frequently. The perineum should be washed with warm soap and water to improve comfort. Standard precautions should be used at all times.

If the amniotic membranes have not ruptured previously, the CNM or physician may do so during this phase. When the membranes rupture, the nurse notes the color and odor of the amniotic fluid and the time of rupture and immediately auscul-

Figure 24–1 ◆ Woman and her partner walking in the hospital during labor.
SOURCE: Photographer, Elena Dorfman.

As long as there are no contraindications (such as vaginal bleeding or ROM with the fetus unengaged), the woman may be encouraged to ambulate, because upright positions shorten labor (Simpson, 2005). A tour of the birthing facility can help decrease anxiety and distract her from her discomfort. Many women feel much more at ease and comfortable if they can move around and do not have to remain in bed. Ambulation also aids in fetal descent, increases the frequency and intensity of contractions, and provides the woman with a sense of control (Figure 24–1 ◆).

The nurse should offer fluids in the form of clear liquids or ice chips at frequent intervals. Because gastric emptying time is prolonged during labor, solid foods are usually avoided. Fasting during labor is the subject of some controversy. Some providers believe that eating and drinking in labor should be an option for women. Research has shown that oral intake during labor does not result in adverse maternal or fetal outcomes (Parsons, 2004; Tramner, 2005). Although women are still advised to avoid solid foods for 6 to 8 hours before elective cesarean birth, modest amounts of clear liquids are recommended for women experiencing a normal labor (ACOG, 2002). Vomiting during labor tates the FHR. The fluid should be clear with no odor. Meconium-stained amniotic fluid may be a sign of a compromised fetus or may be present when the fetus is in a breech presentation. In the case of a breech fetus, meconium staining may not indicate a compromised fetus. In a cephalic presentation, however, meconium staining may indicate a compromised fetal state. When the fetus is compromised, the intestines and anal sphincter relax, leading to the release of meconium into the amniotic fluid. Meconium turns the fluid greenish brown (Bowes, 2005). Whenever the nurse notes meconium-stained fluid, an electronic monitor is applied to continuously assess the FHR (AWHONN, 2003a). The time of rupture is noted because the incidence of amnionitis increases with rupture over 24 hours. An additional concern is prolapse of the umbilical cord, which occurs when membranes rupture and the fetus is not engaged. The concern is that the amniotic fluid coming through the cervix will propel the umbilical cord through the cervix (prolapsed cord). Prolapsed cord is assessed by monitoring for signs of nonreassuring fetal status and performing a vaginal examination with a sterile glove. The FHR is auscultated because a drop in the rate might indicate an undetected prolapsed cord. Immediate intervention is necessary to remove pressure on a prolapsed umbilical cord until a cesarean birth can be performed (see Chapter 27 ∞). (See Table 24–4 for additional deviations from normal.)

TRANSITION PHASE

During transition, the contraction frequency is every 2 to 3 minutes, duration is 60 to 90 seconds, and intensity is strong. Cervical dilatation increases from 8 to 10 cm, effacement is complete (100%), and a heavy amount of bloody show is usually present. Contractions are palpated at least every 15 minutes. Sterile vaginal examination can be done during this stage of labor to assess rapid changes in status. Maternal blood pressure, pulse, and respirations are taken at least every 30 minutes, and FHR is auscultated every 30 minutes for low-risk women and every 15 minutes for high-risk women (ACOG, 2005; AWHONN, 2003a).

Throughout labor the woman's center of focus gradually turns inward. She becomes less aware of what is going on around her and intensely aware of her uterine contractions. She experiences body boundary diffusion, which hampers her ability to know where her body ends and her external environment begins. Women during this time will reach out to others but may be uncomfortable with others touching them.

The woman's ability to speak in coherent sentences can be impaired during the transitional phase. This makes it difficult for the woman to communicate her needs to healthcare providers and her support team. The support person(s) and nurse need to follow the woman's cues and change interventions as needed.

The woman's mouth and lips can become dry because of her breathings being more rapid. The woman can be instructed to breathe in through her nose and out through her mouth. The nurse can also offer small spoons of ice chips to moisten the mouth and apply A and D ointment or a lip emollient to the dry lips. If the woman vomits, the nurse should wipe her mouth and offer water to rinse her mouth.

Table 24–4   DEVIATIONS FROM NORMAL LABOR PROCESS REQUIRING IMMEDIATE INTERVENTION

Problem	Immediate Action
Women admitted with vaginal bleeding or history of painless vaginal bleeding	Do not perform vaginal examination. Assess FHR. Evaluate amount of blood loss. Evaluate labor pattern. Notify physician/CNM immediately.
Presence of greenish or brownish amniotic fluid	Continuously monitor FHR. Evaluate dilatation of cervix and determine if umbilical cord is prolapsed. Evaluate presentation (vertex or breech). Maintain woman on complete bed rest on left side. Notify physician/CNM immediately.
Absence of FHR and fetal movement	Notify physician/CNM. Provide truthful information and emotional support to laboring couple. Remain with the couple.
Prolapse of umbilical cord	Relieve pressure on cord manually. Continuously monitor FHR; watch for changes in FHR pattern. Notify physician/CNM. Assist woman into knee-chest position or place in Trendelenburg position. Administer oxygen.
Woman admitted in advanced labor; birth imminent	Prepare for immediate birth. Obtain critical information: Estimated date of birth (EDB) History of bleeding problems History of medical or obstetric problems Past and/or present use/abuse of prescription/OTC/illicit drugs Problems with this pregnancy FHR and maternal vital signs Whether membranes are ruptured and how long since rupture Blood type and Rh Direct another person to contact physician/CNM. Do not leave woman alone. Provide support to couple. Put on gloves.

The nurse should encourage the woman to rest between contractions by instructing the woman at the end of her contraction to take a deep breath and to let it out slowly while she relaxes her muscles. Helping to maintain a quiet room between contractions can also enhance the woman's ability to rest. The woman during this phase is present focused; thus, providing instruction between contractions should be kept to a minimum.

Some women have difficulty coping with the intensity of labor during this time and need assistance in performing breathing techniques. Either the support person or the nurse can breathe along with the woman during each contraction to help her maintain her pattern. It is helpful to encourage her and assure her that she is doing a good job. The woman will begin to feel increased rectal pressure as the fetal presenting part moves down the birth canal and sometimes a burning sensation as the tissues begin to stretch. The nurse encourages the woman to refrain from pushing until the cervix is completely dilated. For the

MEDIALINK

Video: First Stage of Labor—Transition

woman who is unmedicated, the urge to push may seem unbearable. Specific instructions, such as encouraging the woman to "blow in short breaths like you are blowing out a candle" or "pant like a puppy," can help prevent the woman from involuntarily pushing. This measure also helps prevent cervical edema or lacerations.

The end of transition and beginning of the second stage may be indicated by involuntary passage of flatus or stool and the movement of the fetus from the side of the maternal abdomen to the midline. Other indications include a change in the woman's voice or the sounds she is making. As the fetus moves down and she feels increased pressure and a bearing-down sensation, her voice tends to deepen. A moan during a contraction takes on a more guttural quality. Labor nurses recognize this sound as a sign that the woman may have entered the second stage.

Promotion of Comfort in the First Stage

The first step in planning care for the laboring woman is to talk with the woman and her partner or support person to identify their goals. Usually the couple is concerned with discomfort, so it is important to identify factors that may contribute to discomfort. These factors include uncomfortable positions, diaphoresis, continual leaking of amniotic fluid, a full bladder, dry mouth, anxiety, and fear. Nursing interventions can minimize the effects of these factors. These interventions are discussed later in this section.

There are many responses to pain. As the intensity of the contraction increases with the progression of labor, the woman becomes less aware of the environment and may have difficulty hearing and understanding verbal instructions. The pattern of coping with labor contractions varies from the use of highly structured breathing techniques to turning inward.

In labor, the more common pain reactions, such as increased pulse and respiratory rates, dilated pupils, increased blood pressure, and muscle tension, are transitory because the pain is intermittent. However, increased muscle tension may impede the progress of labor; therefore, the nurse encourages the woman to relax her skeletal muscles and avoid holding her breath.

Sounds are an important part of the labor and birthing process. Some women naturally make sounds such as moans and grunts and feel that it helps them cope and do the work of labor; they are responding to what their body tells them to do. Others begin to make loud sounds (screams) only as they lose their ability to cope and feel they do not have any other options.

Some women may want physical contact during contractions (Figure 24–2 ◆). They may provide verbal and nonverbal signs, such as crying, moaning, and beseeching the coach or nurse to hold their hand or rub their back. They may look at the support person or reach out for help to indicate their anxiety. Touch may be used to convey support and enhance comfort for the woman. She may be soothed by a neck or backrub or by holding the hand of her partner or the nurse. A woman generally wants touching and physical contact during the first part of labor, but when she moves into the transition phase, she may re-

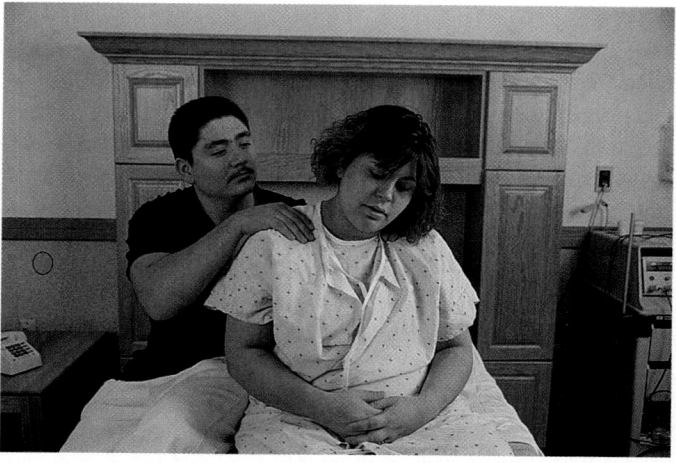

Figure 24–2 ◆ The woman's partner provides support and encouragement during labor.
SOURCE: Photographer, Elena Dorfman.

buff all efforts and pull away. Other women do not want to be touched at all, regardless of the phase of labor.

A decrease in the intensity of discomfort is one of the goals of nursing support during labor. Nursing measures to decrease pain include the following:

- Encouraging position changes
- Assisting with personal comfort measures
- Decreasing anxiety
- Providing information
- Using specific supportive relaxation techniques
- Encouraging paced breathing
- Administering pharmacologic agents as desired by the woman

POSITION CHANGES

As noted earlier, the woman is encouraged to ambulate if the fetal head is engaged and the EFM has shown a reassuring FHR pattern. However, to avoid the risk of umbilical cord prolapse, the woman is generally instructed to remain in bed if membranes are ruptured and the presenting part is not engaged.

If she stays in bed, the woman is encouraged to assume any position that she finds comfortable (Figure 24–3 ◆). A side-lying position is generally the most advantageous for the laboring woman. Care should be taken that all body parts are supported, with the joints slightly flexed. Pillows may be placed against her chest and under the uppermost arm. A pillow or folded bath blanket is placed between her knees to support the uppermost leg and relieve tension or muscle strain. A pillow (or warmed rolled blanket) placed at the woman's midback also helps provide support. If the woman is more comfortable on her back, the head of the bed should be elevated to relieve the pressure of the uterus on the vena cava and the uterus should be tilted by placing a towel or blanket under the woman's back. Pillows may be placed under each arm and under the knees to provide support. Because a pregnant woman is at increased risk for thrombophlebitis, excessive pressure behind the knee and calf should be avoided, and frequent assessment of pressure points needs to be made.

RESEARCH IN PRACTICE

DIMENSIONS OF PROFESSIONAL LABOR SUPPORT FOR INTRAPARTUM PRACTICE

What is this study about? Support for the mother in labor is an important part of intrapartum care. It has been documented that effective labor support is linked to positive outcomes for both the mother and baby. However, although nurses recognize its value, there is no universal definition of exactly what constitutes effective nursing support in labor. When nurses are asked to define and describe labor support, diverse responses are given. This lack of clarity hampers communication between professionals, affects the expectations of nurses and clients, and makes comparisons of data across studies difficult. This latter aspect hinders the creation of evidence-based practice guidelines for labor support. This study sought to define labor support, clarify its meaning, and identify its dimensions in order to promote consistency in research and practice.

How was this study done? The researcher first performed an in-depth literature review to determine if themes or commonalities could be identified. Although many authors defined labor support theoretically, no conclusive definition could be determined. The researcher sent the "Labor Support Questionnaire" to a random sample of Texas nurses registered with the obstetrics and gynecology database. The survey is designed to measure intrapartum nurses' perceptions concerning the importance of professional labor support in their practice. Reliability and validity were well established for the instrument. Of the 541 surveys sent, 223 were returned, for a 41% response rate. Of these, 146 were complete and usable in the study. The data were subjected to factor analysis, a statistical technique that helps the researcher determine if individual items in a dataset have similar characteristics and form into natural groups. The groups of items are then evaluated to determine if an overall descriptor, called a factor, can be identified. The factors represent overall concepts that are reflected by the individual items.

What were the results of the study? Nursing support during labor was clearly a multidimensional concept. Six factors were identified. Of these, three had characteristics in common with emotional support. This finding reinforces that emotional support is intricately interwoven with multiple aspects of labor support. Three factors—reassurance, creating control, and nurse caring behaviors—included elements of emotional support. The remaining factors included tangible support, such as physical assistance and companionship; advocacy, or acting on the client's behalf; and informational support, including instructional advice.

What additional questions might I have? The final sample of responses that were used for analysis was small; are these findings representative of all nurses who support laboring mothers? Would mothers identify the kind of support they need during labor the same as these nurses? What specific interventions represent each of these key dimensions?

How can I use this study? Women in labor have a wide variety of needs for support. Nurses can ensure that they provide comprehensive intrapartal care by specifically designing interventions and care guidelines that incorporate all six of the key dimensions.

Sauls, D. (2006). Dimensions of professional labor support for intrapartum practice. *Journal of Nursing Scholarship, 38*(1), 36–41.

Figure 24–3 ◆ The laboring woman is encouraged to choose a position of comfort. The nurse modifies assessments and interventions as necessary.
SOURCE: Photographer, Elena Dorfman.

Frequent position changes (at least every hour) seem to achieve more efficient contractions, and contribute to comfort and relaxation. It is also helpful for the woman to sit up in a rocking chair or other comfortable chair, or in the shower.

PERSONAL COMFORT MEASURES

The use of hydrotherapy during labor promotes maternal relaxation and pain management and decreases the length of labor. Thus women can be encouraged to use a warm bath, shower, or whirlpool to increase comfort during labor.

Because vaginal discharge increases, the nurse needs to change the underpads frequently. Washing the perineum with warm soap and water removes secretions and increases comfort. The nurse needs to use standard precautions to avoid exposure to vaginal secretions.

Diaphoresis and the constant leaking of amniotic fluid can dampen the woman's gown and bed linen. Fresh, smooth, dry bed linen promotes comfort. To avoid having to change the bottom sheet following ROM, the nurse may replace the underpads at frequent intervals (standard precautions need to be followed). The perineal area should be kept as clean and dry as possible to promote comfort. The woman may also find comfort in applying a cool washcloth to her forehead or behind the back of her neck.

CLINICAL TIP

To promote maternal comfort, dampen a washcloth with cool water and wring it out thoroughly. Hold one corner of the washcloth and swing the cloth in a circular motion for a cooling fanlike effect.

EVIDENCE-BASED PRACTICE

MATERNAL POSITIONS TO SUPPORT LABOR AND BIRTH

Clinical Question

What are the benefits and risks of different maternal positions during the second stage of labor?

The Evidence

Three systematic reviews were conducted for several types of maternal positions in labor and birth. Three researchers independently reviewed 20 trials comparing any upright or lateral position with the supine or lithotomy position. These randomized trials focused on maternal outcomes such as perineal trauma, blood loss, and pain, and involved 6135 participants. Fetal heart rate pattern was assessed. Two other studies focused on the hands and knees posture, both in late pregnancy and in labor. These studies collected data from 2794 women. These studies included evaluation of maternal and fetal outcomes but focused on the effects of maternal position on fetal position, specifically occipitoposterior position. A lateral or posterior fetal position may be associated with a more painful labor, specifically lower back pain.

What Is Effective?

There was a slight reduction in the duration of second stage of labor, assisted births, episiotomies, and perineal tears in those mothers who birthed in any upright or lateral position when compared with the supine or lithotomy position. This was balanced by a slightly increased chance of blood loss greater than 500 mL in the upright group. The hands and knees position was effective in the short term in supporting an optimal fetal position, but the effects were short term. The position does seem to reduce the persistent back pain associated with an occipitoposterior fetal position.

What Is Unclear?

The outcomes that were studied did not include the rate of cesarean birth, so it is not known if any of these maternal positions is associated with an increase in operative births. The differences attributed to the upright positions were quite small and so do not likely make an argument for suggesting the upright position over other positions that may be desirable for the mother.

Best Practice

Women should be encouraged to give birth in the position they find most comfortable. Until the benefits and risks can be weighed with greater certainty, there is no clear advantage for any single position. The supine and lithotomy positions seem the least desirable, but even these positions are not associated with a substantially greater risk of maternal complications. Women should be encouraged to make informed choices about the birth positions they might wish to assume for the birth of their babies.

Critical Thinking

Under what conditions might the nurse suggest a particular position for a mother during labor and birth? What information do mothers need to make informed choices about their position during labor and birth?

REFERENCES: Gupta, J., Hofmeyr, G., & Smyth, R. (2004). Position in the second stage of labour for women without epidural anaesthesia. *The Cochrane Database of Systematic Reviews* (4) (Article No. CD002006.pub2).

Hofmeyr, G., & Kulier, R. (2005). Hands and knees posture in late pregnancy or labour for fetal malposition (lateral or posterior). *The Cochrane Database of Systematic Reviews* (2) (Article No. CD001063.pub2).

Stremler, R., Hodnett, E., Petryshen, P., Steves, B., Weston, J., & Willan, A. (2005) Randomized controlled trial of hands and knees positioning for occipitoposterior position in labor. *Birth, 32*(4), 243–251.

A full bladder adds to the discomfort during a contraction and may prolong labor by interfering with the descent of the fetus. Even though the woman is voiding, urine may be retained because of the pressure of the fetal presenting part. A full bladder can be detected by palpation directly over the symphysis pubis. Some of the procedures for regional analgesia during labor contribute to the inability to void, and catheterization may be necessary. The woman should be encouraged to empty her bladder about every 1 to 2 hours. The nurse should offer the woman a bedpan before catheterization because some women are able to void despite anesthesia, and spontaneous voiding decreases the risk of infection that is associated with repeated catheterizations.

The woman may experience dryness of her mouth. Clear fluids and ice chips are usually offered unless a complication exists that makes cesarean birth a possibility. Some prepared childbirth programs advise the woman to bring lollipops to help combat the dryness that occurs with some of the breathing patterns.

Some women feel discomfort from cold feet. Wearing socks or slippers may increase their comfort. Some women may wish to wear their own nightgown, although they need to know that the gown will most likely be soiled and may be more difficult to move around in.

Birthing balls—large, heavy plastic balls that accommodate an adult's weight—are used by some laboring women to increase comfort (Figure 24–4 ◆). The woman sits on the ball and can roll it back and forth gently. The slow rock is thought to widen the pelvis and enhance fetal descent, while leaning forward on the knees with the head, arms, and chest over the ball simulates a hands-and-knees position and may facilitate rotation of an occiput-posterior. When a birthing ball is used, the nurse should remain close by the woman to help provide balance. Many balls come with aluminum frames to prevent falls.

Some family members or support persons can assist the woman with comfort measures. They may help with position changes, provide ice chips, walk with the laboring woman, and give effleurage or backrubs. If the family is not already involved

Figure 24–4 ◆ A birthing ball is used to promote maternal comfort during labor. The birthing ball facilitates fetal descent and fetal rotation and helps increase the diameter of the pelvis.

in providing comfort measures and seems to want to be, the nurse can act as a role model while providing comfort measures and then invite the support person(s) to join in if they like.

Family members also need to be encouraged to maintain their own comfort. As their attention is directed toward the laboring woman, they may forget their own needs. The nurse may have to encourage them to take breaks, maintain food and fluid intake, and rest.

REDUCING ANXIETY

The anxiety experienced by women entering labor is related to a combination of factors inherent to the process. A moderate amount of anxiety enhances the ability to deal with the pain. But an excessive degree of anxiety decreases the woman's ability to cope with the pain.

To decrease anxiety that is not related to pain, the nurse can give information (which eases fear of the unknown), establish rapport with the couple (which helps them preserve their personal integrity), express confidence in the couple's ability to work with the labor process, and assist with breathing and relaxation techniques. In addition to being a good listener, the nurse needs to demonstrate genuine concern for the laboring woman. Remaining with the woman as much as possible conveys a car-

ing attitude and dispels fear of abandonment. Praise for correct breathing, relaxation efforts, and pushing efforts not only encourages repetition of the behavior but also decreases anxiety about the ability to cope with labor.

The woman's partner and other members of her support team may also experience increasing anxiety as the woman advances through labor. Their anxiety can stem from watching their loved one in pain, feeling helpless about their ability to assist her in reducing the pain, a lack of knowledge or information about the labor experience, and lack of support from the labor nurse. Their anxiety may be reduced or kept at a minimum by keeping them informed about the progress of labor, reassuring them that the sounds and behaviors of the woman in labor are normal, explaining procedures and the use of equipment, and praising them for their assistance in supporting the woman through labor.

PROVIDING INFORMATION

Providing information about the nature of the discomfort that will occur during labor is important and is best achieved in the early portion of labor. Stressing the intermittent nature and maximum duration of the contractions can be most helpful. The woman can cope with pain better when she knows how far she has progressed and that a period of relief will follow. Describing the type of discomfort and specific sensations that will occur as labor progresses helps the woman recognize these sensations as normal and expected when she does experience them.

A thorough explanation of surroundings, procedures, and equipment being used also decreases anxiety, thereby reducing pain. For some clients, attachment to an electronic monitor can produce fear because equipment of this type is associated with critically ill people. For others, hearing their infant's heartbeat is reassuring. The nurse should explain the purpose of the monitor and the monitor strip, and show the woman and her support persons how the monitor can help them use controlled breathing techniques to relieve pain. The monitor may indicate the beginning of a contraction just seconds before the woman feels it. The woman and coach can learn how to read the tracing to identify the beginning of the contraction.

Labor and childbirth may be a time of increased anxiety for the woman with a history of sexual abuse or rape. All women entering the healthcare arena need to be assessed for a history of sexual abuse or rape. It is not uncommon for women to deny sexual abuse or rape, because this information is difficult to share with a stranger. It is important to be alert for nonverbal cues, such as unexplained anxiety, unrelenting pain, or intense fear during vaginal examinations. The nurse should offer support, provide information, and introduce relaxation techniques to aid the woman in coping to offset her anxiety.

SUPPORTIVE RELAXATION TECHNIQUES

Tense muscles increase resistance to the descent of the fetus and contribute to maternal fatigue and anxiety. This fatigue increases pain perception and decreases the woman's ability to cope with the pain. Comfort measures, massage, techniques for decreasing anxiety, and client teaching can conserve energy. The laboring woman needs to be encouraged to use the periods between contractions to rest and relax her muscles.

Distraction is a method of increasing relaxation and coping with discomfort. During early labor, conversation or activities such as light reading, cards, or other games serve as distractions.

Touch is another type of distraction. Although some women regard touching as an invasion of privacy or threat to their independence, others want to touch and be touched during a painful experience. Nurses can make themselves available to the woman who desires touch. The nurse can place a hand on the side of the bed within the woman's reach. The person who needs touch will reach out for contact, and the nurse can pick up and follow through with this behavioral cue.

Mild to moderate abdominal discomfort during contractions may be relieved or lessened by effleurage. Back pain associated with labor may be relieved more effectively by firm pressure on the lower back or sacral area. To apply firm pressure, the nurse or a support person places a hand or a rolled, warmed towel or blanket in the small of the woman's back. Warm compresses can also provide relief.

Visualization techniques also enhance relaxation. For example, the nurse might encourage the woman to imagine herself floating in a warm pool of water, fully supported; to imagine the birth canal slowly opening up as the baby descends; or to visualize a rose opening its petals. Or the woman may simply wish to recall and concentrate on a pleasant experience she has had in the past. Table 24–5 describes a simple visualization method.

In addition to these measures, the nurse can enhance the woman's relaxation by providing encouragement and support for controlled breathing techniques.

BREATHING TECHNIQUES

Breathing techniques may help the laboring woman. Breathing techniques increase the woman's pain threshold, encourage relaxation, provide distraction, enhance the ability to cope with uterine contractions, and allow the uterus to function more efficiently.

Table 24–5   SIMPLE VISUALIZATION METHOD

Direct a visualization by saying something like the following: "Think about a place you have been that has pleasant memories and feelings around it. A place that was relaxing, where all your stress disappeared. As you think about this place, take in a breath and remember the smells around it. If it was outside, feel the warmth of the sun or the way the breeze felt on your face. Sit in the place again in your mind. Let all your tension and tiredness leave your body as you feel the warmth and breezes."

Give the woman a few moments to think about her special place: Ask if she would like to share information about the setting. If the woman chooses to do this, add the information to help her with the visualization (for example, "Think about the mountain cabin and the warmth of the sun on your face as you sit in the rocking chair on the front porch").

After the woman has a visualization set up, suggest thinking about it during contractions as a means of increasing relaxation and focusing concentration. You could say, "As each contraction begins, think about this special place for a moment, and let your body relax. Keep a picture of your place in your mind as you breathe with the contraction. When the contraction is over, let your body stay relaxed. Feel the comfort of this room and support of those around you."

COMPLEMENTARY AND ALTERNATIVE THERAPIES

HYDROTHERAPY

Centuries-old water immersion in hot springs, and more recently in jaccuzis and spas, is used all over the world to promote relaxation and relax muscles. Current evidence supports the use of hydrotherapy in labor as an effective method of pain management in the first stage of labor. Women who use hydrotherapy report less pain and use less analgesia during the first stage of labor (Benfield, 2002; Cluett, Pickering, Getliff et al., 2004). Water immersion has both physical and psychologic benefits, including counterpressure and support of stretching tissues.

Many women learn breathing techniques during prenatal education classes. Patterned-paced breathing, which is commonly used in the Lamaze method, has three levels. The woman tends to begin with the first level and then proceed to the next when she feels the need. Regardless of the level of breathing used, a cleansing breath begins and ends each pattern. A cleansing breath involves only the chest. It consists of inhaling through the nose and exhaling through pursed lips (as if blowing on a spoonful of hot food). See Table 24–6 for information regarding nursing support of patterned-paced breathing.

Other childbirth education models encourage different types of breathing exercises. Abdominal breathing, which is commonly used in the Bradley method, encourages the woman to move the abdominal wall upward as she inhales and downward as she exhales (see Table 24–6). This method tends to lift the abdominal wall off the contracting uterus and thus may provide some pain relief. The breathing is deep and rhythmic. If the woman has not been trained in a particular technique, teaching her the "quick method," which uses a pant-pant-blow breathing pattern, may help her from breathing too rapidly (see Table 24–6).

Hyperventilation may occur when a woman breathes very rapidly over a prolonged period of time. Hyperventilation is the result of an imbalance of oxygen and carbon dioxide (that is, too much carbon dioxide is exhaled, and too much oxygen remains in the body). The signs and symptoms of hyperventilation are tingling or numbness in the tip of nose, lips, fingers, or toes; dizziness; spots before the eyes; or spasms of the hands or feet (carpal-pedal spasms). If hyperventilation occurs, the woman should be encouraged to slow her breathing rate and to take shallow breaths. With instruction and encouragement, many women are able to change their breathing to correct the problem. Encouraging the woman to relax and counting out loud for her so she can pace her breathing during contractions are also helpful. If the signs and symptoms continue or become more severe (that is, if they progress from numbness to spasms), the woman can breathe into a paper surgical mask or into her hands until symptoms abate. Breathing into a mask or her hands causes rebreathing of carbon dioxide. The nurse should remain with the woman to reassure her.

Table 24–6   NURSING SUPPORT OF PATTERNED-PACED BREATHING

Determine which breathing method the woman (couple) has learned. Provide encouragement as needed in maintaining breathing pattern. Provide support to the labor coach and assist as needed.

Lamaze Breathing Pattern Levels

First level (slow paced)
Pattern begins and ends with a cleansing breath (in through the nose and out through pursed lips as if cooling a spoonful of hot food). While inhaling through the nose and exhaling through pursed lips, slow breaths are taken, moving only the chest. The rate should be approximately 6–9 breaths/minute or 2 breaths/15 seconds. The coach or nurse may assist by reminding the woman to take a cleansing breath, and then the breaths could be counted out if needed to maintain pacing. The woman inhales as someone counts "one one thousand, two one thousand, three one thousand, four one thousand." Exhalation begins and continues through the same count.

First level for use during uterine contractions (The level begins and ends with a cleansing breath [CB]).

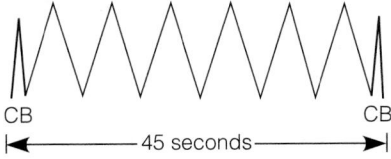

Second level (modified paced)
Pattern begins and ends with a cleansing breath. Breaths are then taken in and out silently through the mouth at approximately 4 breaths/5 seconds. The jaw and entire body need to be relaxed. The rate can be accelerated to 2–2½ breaths/second. The rhythm for the breaths can be counted out as "one and two and one and two and. . ." with the woman exhaling on the numbers and inhaling on "and."

Second level

Third level (pattern paced)
Pattern begins and ends with a cleansing breath. All breaths are rhythmical, in and out through the mouth. Exhalations are accompanied by a "hee" or "hoo" sound in a varying pattern, 2:1, which begins as 3:1 (hee hee hee hoo) and can change to 2:1 (hee hee hoo) or 1:1 (hee hoo) as the intensity of the contraction changes. The rate should not be more rapid than 2–2½ breaths/second. The rhythm of the breaths would match a "one and two and . . ." count.

Third level (Darkened spike represents "hoo.")

Abdominal Breathing Pattern Cues

The abdomen moves outward during inhalation and downward during exhalation. The rate remains slow with approximately 6–9 breaths/minute.

Breathing sequence for abdominal breathing

Quick Method

When the woman has not learned a particular method and is in active phase of labor, the nurse may teach her a combination of two patterns. Abdominal breathing may be used until labor is more advanced. Then a more rapid pattern consisting of two short blows from the mouth followed by a longer blow can be used. (This pattern is called "pant-pant-blow" even though all exhalations are a blowing motion.)

Pant-pant-blow breathing pattern

As the woman uses her breathing technique, the nurse can assess and support the interaction between the woman and her coach or support person. In the absence of a coach, the nurse supports the laboring woman by helping to identify the beginning of each contraction and encouraging her as she breathes through it. Continued encouragement and support with each contraction through labor yield immeasurable benefits.

OTHER COMFORT MEASURES

In some instances, analgesic agents or regional anesthetic blocks may be used to enhance comfort and relaxation during labor. See Chapter 25 ∞ for a discussion of analgesia and anesthesia.

Table 24–7 summarizes labor progress, possible responses of the laboring woman, and nursing care during the first stage of labor.

NURSING CARE DURING THE SECOND STAGE OF LABOR

Nursing care in the second stage entails both physical and psychologic support, continual encouragement, and appropriate client teaching to facilitate birth.

Provision of Care in the Second Stage

The second stage begins when the cervix is completely dilated (10 cm). The uterine contractions continue as in the transition phase. Sterile vaginal examinations are performed to assess fetal descent. Maternal pulse, blood pressure, and FHR are assessed every 5 minutes; some protocols recommend assessment after each contraction (ACOG, 2005). Table 24–8 summarizes nursing assessments in the second stage of labor.

Table 24–7   NORMAL PROGRESS, PSYCHOLOGIC CHARACTERISTICS, AND NURSING SUPPORT DURING FIRST AND SECOND STAGES OF LABOR

Phase	Cervical Dilatation	Uterine Contractions	Woman's Response	Support Measures
Stage 1				
Latent phase	1–4 cm	Every 10–20 minutes, 15–20 seconds' duration Mild intensity *progressing to* Every 5–7 minutes, 30–40 seconds' duration Moderate intensity	Usually happy, talkative, and eager to be in labor Exhibits need for independence by taking care of own bodily needs and seeking information	Establish rapport on admission and continue to build during care. Assess information base and learning needs. Be available to consult regarding breathing technique if needed; teach breathing technique if needed and in early labor. Orient family to room, equipment, monitors, and procedures. Encourage woman and partner to participate in care as desired. Provide needed information. Assist woman into position of comfort; encourage frequent change of position; encourage ambulation during early labor. Offer fluids/ice chips. Keep couple informed of progress. Encourage woman to void every 1 to 2 hours. Assess need for an interest in using visualization to enhance relaxation and teach if appropriate.
Active phase	4–7 cm	Every 2–3 minutes, 50–60 seconds' duration Moderate to strong intensity	May experience feelings of helplessness Exhibits increased fatigue and may begin to feel restless and anxious as contractions become stronger Expresses fear of abandonment Becomes more dependent as she is less able to meet her needs	Encourage woman to maintain breathing patterns. Provide quiet environment to reduce external stimuli. Provide reassurance, encouragement, support; keep couple informed of progress. Promote comfort by giving backrubs, sacral pressure, cool cloth on forehead, assistance with position changes, support with pillows, effleurage. Provide ice chips, ointment for dry mouth and lips. Encourage to void every 1 to 2 hours. Offer shower/whirlpool/warm bath if available.
Transition phase	8–10 cm	Every 2–3 minutes, 60–90 seconds' duration Strong intensity	Tires and may exhibit increased restlessness and irritability May feel she cannot keep up with labor process and is out of control Physical discomforts Fear of being left alone May fear tearing open or splitting apart with contractions	Encourage woman to rest between contractions. If she sleeps between contractions, wake her at beginning of contraction so she can begin breathing pattern (increases feeling of control). Provide support, encouragement, and praise for efforts. Keep couple informed of progress; encourage continued participation of support persons. Promote comfort as listed above but recognize many women do not want to be touched when in transition. Provide privacy. Provide ice chips, ointment for lips. Encourage to void every 1 to 2 hours.
Stage 2	Complete	Every 1½–2 minutes	May feel out of control, helpless, panicky, or may be happy that she can take a more active role in pushing	Assist woman in pushing efforts. Encourage woman to assume position of comfort. Provide encouragement and praise for efforts. Keep couple informed of progress. Provide ice chips. Maintain privacy as woman desires.

As the woman pushes during the second stage, she may make a variety of sounds. At times, these sounds are disturbing for nurses and physicians, and they feel the need to help her or encourage her to be more quiet. Other nurses feel more comfortable with maternal sounds and use them as cues. For example, if the woman begins to feel she is losing control, her sound may change to a high-pitched cry or whimper, or she may even shriek in pain. The nurse stays sensitive to changes in the sounds for clues that the woman needs help coping with her pain. The nurse may encourage her to push harder and not let any breath out, or to put all her effort into the push and not into making noise. But the nurse needs to be aware that maternal sounds may be a coping mechanism for some women and may assist in their pain management.

Several nursing research studies have been conducted focusing on when a woman should push during the second stage of labor. A review article on research focusing on pushing during the second stage recommends that the woman be allowed to rest at the beginning of the second stage and to begin pushing when she feels the natural urge to bear down. There is a decrease in maternal fatigue levels and an increase in fetal oxygenation with fewer decelerations noted when women delay pushing until they feel the urge to push. Furthermore, women who delayed pushing pushed for a shorter period of time (Hansen, Clark, & Foster, 2002).

When the woman reports feeling an uncontrollable urge to push (bear down), the nurse can help her greatly by letting her know that these new sensations are normal. This is because some

Table 24–8 NURSING ASSESSMENTS IN THE SECOND STAGE	
Mother	**Fetus**
Blood pressure, pulse, respiration every 5–15 minutes.	FHR every 5 minutes.
Uterine contraction palpated continuously.	

women interpret the increased rectal pressure as a need to move her bowels. The instinctive response is to tighten muscles rather than bear down. The woman may also report that she fears she is "splitting apart" or that she feels a "ring of fire." The woman who expects these sensations and understands that bearing down contributes to progress at this stage is more likely to do so.

When I tried to push with the contractions, I felt as if I would tear apart. It hurt so badly that I was shaking. I knew it was time to push and my body was telling me, too, but it hurt so much. The nurse kept saying, "Just push and you will feel better." I wanted to scream at her. She had no idea what was happening to me.

When the contraction begins, the nurse tells the woman to take two short breaths, then to take a third breath and hold it while pulling back on her knees and pushing down with her abdominal muscles (Figure 24–5 ◆). Some women prefer to exhale slightly (exhale breathing) while pushing to avoid the physiologic effects of the Valsalva maneuver. With this method the woman takes several deep breaths and then holds her breath for 5 to 6 seconds. Then, through slightly pursed lips, she exhales slowly every 5 to 6 seconds while continuing to hold her breath. The woman takes another breath and continues exhale breathing and pushing during the contraction.

I knew when I was completely dilated. I knew when to push and I did it without tearing. My body told me to listen. I knew what to do.

~HARRIETTE HARTIGAN, *WOMEN IN BIRTH*~

The woman is encouraged to rest between contractions. Although the laboring woman may appear exhausted at this time, most experience relief at being able to push with contractions. Perspiration increases with the pushing efforts, and a cold washcloth for the forehead and face is most soothing. The birthing woman may also appreciate sips of fluid or ice chips at this time.

When I began pushing, I felt in control because I could do something. . . . I could push the baby out. I knew he was ready to be born.

~HARRIETTE HARTIGAN, *WOMEN IN BIRTH*~

The nurse and/or support person can assist the woman into a comfortable position for pushing. Maternal positions, such as standing, squatting while leaning back on a partner or on a birthing bar (Figure 24–6 ◆), lying in a lateral or Sims' position, or crouching on hands and knees, may increase comfort and ef-

Figure 24–5 ◆ The nurse provides encouragement and support during pushing efforts.
SOURCE: Margaret Miller/Photo Researchers, Inc.

Figure 24–6 ◆ Using a birthing bar.
SOURCE: Photographer, Elena Dorfman.

fectiveness of pushing. Some women feel that sitting on a toilet seat is a comfortable position that assists their pushing efforts. This position may cause anxiety in the caregivers, however, for fear that the birth may occur quickly in this most inopportune place. Some women benefit from gripping the hands of the support person or nurse. This technique increases intra-abdominal pressure, which aids in the expulsion effort. Another variation of this technique, which can be quite effective, is to have the woman grip a towel while the support person or nurse pulls the towel in the opposite direction. Care should be taken that the nurse or support person does not suffer a back injury.

Additional comfort measures may be used during this stage. Warm perineal, abdominal, and back compresses may be used to increase muscle relaxation. Perineal massage and stretching with a lubricant (Lubafax) may relieve the tearing and burning sensation as the perineal tissue distends. Providing perineal massage before imminent crowning can result in considerable perineal edema. For this reason, some institutions may limit perineal massage to physicians and CNMs.

Visualization techniques may be helpful. The woman can be encouraged to envision the infant descending the birth canal and the vagina opening up. Phrases such as "Open to your baby" and "Let the baby come; don't try to hold back" can be useful and calming. Many women benefit from visualizing the descent of the fetus in a mirror. The nurse should ask the woman if she would like to watch in the mirror.

If anticipated progress is not made or the laboring woman wants to try other positions for pushing, the nurse should support her. Some nurses have their own preferences and may be more comfortable directing the laboring woman to use these preferred positions; however, it is important to remember that the nurse is there to support the birth, and that frequent changes in position may assist in the descent of the baby.

If the maternal pushing effort diminishes because of frustration or fatigue, many women benefit from short rest periods. Rest periods are appropriate if maternal and fetal assessments are stable. In addition, the physician or CNM should be informed of the actual time that has been spent pushing and not the time that has elapsed since the beginning of the second stage. If the maternal vital signs are stable and the FHR is reassuring, rest peiods can be used to prevent maternal exhaustion (Hansen et al., 2002).

Throughout the second stage, it remains important to provide information regarding progress and what is happening in the labor. It is also imperative to address the woman's questions honestly, to acknowledge her concerns, and to continue to provide support.

A nullipara is usually prepared for birth when the perineum begins to bulge. A multipara usually progresses much more quickly, so she may be prepared for the birth when the cervix is dilated 7 to 8 cm.

The woman's blood pressure and the FHR are monitored between contractions, and the contractions are palpated until the birth. The nurse continues to assist the woman in her pushing efforts. Both the woman and the coach are kept informed of procedures and of progress, and both are supported throughout the birth.

In addition to assisting the woman and her partner, the nurse assists the physician or CNM in preparing for the birth. The physician or CNM usually dons a sterile gown and gloves and may place sterile drapes over the woman's abdomen and legs. Some providers may perform a sterile preparation before birth; others may not do so as part of their normal routine. Although some physicians and CNMs may place the woman in stirrups for birth, others may opt to drop the foot of the bed lower than the upper portion and let the woman rest her feet on the bed to facilitate maternal comfort. An episiotomy may be done just before birth if there is a need for one or if the provider performs them on a routine basis. See the discussion of episiotomy in Chapter 27. ∞

Promotion of Comfort in the Second Stage

Most of the comfort measures that have been used during the first stage remain appropriate at this time. Cool cloths to the face and forehead may help provide cooling as the woman is involved in the intense physical exertion of pushing. If she has been diaphoretic, a dry gown may be comforting. The woman may feel hot and want to remove some of the covering. Care still needs to be taken to provide privacy even though covers are removed. Some women may want to remove all of their clothing. Healthcare providers should allow the woman to give birth in a way that will promote her comfort. The woman can be encouraged to rest and "let all muscles go" during the period between contractions. The nurse and support person(s) can assist the woman into a pushing position with each contraction to further conserve energy. Sips of fluid or ice chips may be used to provide moisture and relieve dryness of the mouth. Constant reassurance is imperative.

Assisting the Couple and Physician or CNM During Birth

Shortly before the birth, the birthing room or delivery room is prepared with equipment and materials that may be needed. Family members do not need to change into other clothing if the birth occurs in a birthing room; they don a disposable scrub suit if the birth is to occur in a delivery room or surgery suite. Meticulous handwashing is required of the nurses and CNM or physician. Nurses who will be in direct contact with the mother at the time of birth need to wear protective clothing, such as an apron or gown with a splash apron, disposable gloves, and eye covering. The CNM or physician will also need to wear a gown with a splash apron or a plastic apron, eye covering, and sterile gloves.

Most facilities now use one room for labor, delivery, and recovery (LDR) rooms. Use of a separate birthing room is rare. If the laboring woman is to give birth in a separate birthing room, she will be moved shortly before birth on her bed or a cart. It is important to preserve her privacy during the transfer, and safety must be provided by raising the side rails into a locked position. In the birthing room, the labor bed or transfer cart must be carefully supported against the delivery table; this ensures the woman's safety during the transfer.

If the woman is to be moved from one bed to another, it should be done between contractions. During the contraction, the woman feels increased discomfort and may be involved in pushing efforts. Perineal bulging may be occurring, which adds to the discomfort and difficulty in moving. All of these factors make moving the woman very uncomfortable. If birth seems imminent (within the next minute), it is safer for the woman to give birth in her labor bed or on the cart. Transfer to the delivery table is then delayed until after the baby is born and the cord has been clamped and cut.

Even though there are differences in the birthing room setting, the family can still be together during the birth. It is important to provide encouragement for family members to participate because the delivery room environment may be unfamiliar and seem less relaxed. The family member may be hesitant to continue to provide support for fear of interfering or being in the way. The nurse can ensure that family members are included throughout the birthing process by giving them simple directions about how they can assist and be involved in the process.

MATERNAL BIRTHING POSITIONS

The woman is usually positioned for birth on a bed, birthing chair, or delivery table. In some instances, she may give birth standing at the side of the bed or on her hands and knees on the floor. The position the woman assumes is determined not only by her individual wishes but also by the CNM or physician.

If stirrups are used, they should be padded to alleviate pressure, and both legs should be lifted simultaneously to avoid strain on abdominal, back, and perineal muscles. The stirrups should be adjusted to fit the woman's legs. The feet are supported in the stirrup holders. The height and angle of the stirrups are adjusted so there is no pressure on the back of the knees or the calf, which might cause discomfort and postpartal vascular problems. This is particularly true of women with epidural anesthesia. The birthing bed is elevated 30 to 60 degrees to help the woman bear down, and handles are provided so she may pull back on them.

The upright posture for birth was considered normal in most societies until modern times. Alternatively, women selected squatting, kneeling, standing, and sitting for birth. Only within the last 200 years has the recumbent position become the norm in the Western world. Its use in this century has been reinforced because of the convenience it offers in applying new technology, and it has thus become the conventional manner in which North American women give birth in hospitals. In searching for alternative positions, consumers and professionals alike continue to refocus on the comfort of the laboring woman and the advantages of alternative positions rather than on the convenience of the CNM or physician (Table 24–9).

Recumbent Position

The recumbent (lithotomy) position for birth is used sometimes to enhance the maintenance of asepsis, assessment of FHR, and performance of episiotomy and repair. In contrast, when the

Table 24–9 COMPARISON OF BIRTHING POSITIONS

Position	Advantages	Disadvantages	Nursing Actions
Recumbent	Enhances ability to maintain sterile field. May be easier to monitor FHR. Easier to perform episiotomy or laceration repair.	May decrease blood pressure. It is difficult for the woman to breathe due to pressure on the diaphragm. There is an increased risk of aspiration. May increase perineal pressure making laceration more likely. May interfere with uterine contractions.	Ensure that stirrups do not cause excess pressure on the legs. Assess legs for adequate circulation and support.
Left lateral Sims'	Does not compromise venous return from lower extremities. Increases perineal relaxation and decreases need for episiotomy. Appears to prevent rapid descent.	It is difficult for the woman to see the birth.	Adjust position so that the upper leg lies on the bed (scissor fashion) or is supported by the partner or on pillows.
Squatting	Size of pelvic outlet is increased. Gravity aids descent and expulsion of newborn. Second stage may be shortened (Roberts, 2003).	It may be difficult to maintain balance while squatting.	Help woman maintain balance. Use a birthing bar if available.
Semi-Fowler's	Does not compromise venous return from lower extremities. Women can view birth process.	If legs are positioned wide apart, relaxation of perineal tissues is decreased.	Assess that upper torso is evenly supported. Increase support of body by changing position of bed or using pillows as props. Ensure that legs and feet have adequate support.
Sitting in birthing bed	Gravity aids descent and expulsion of the fetus. Does not compromise venous return from lower extremities. Woman can view the birth process. Leg position may be changed at will.		
Sitting on birthing stool	Gravity aids descent and expulsion of infant. Does not compromise venous return from lower extremities. Woman can view birth process.	It is difficult to provide support for the woman's back.	Encourage woman to sit in a position that increases her comfort.
Hands and knees	Increases perineal relaxation and decreases need for episiotomy. Increases placental and umbilical blood flow and decreases nonreassuring fetal status. Improves fetal rotation. Better able to assess perineum. Better access to fetal nose and mouth for suctioning at birth. Facilitates birth of infant with shoulder dystocia.	Woman cannot view birth. There is decreased contact with birth attendant. Caregivers cannot use instruments. There may be increased maternal fatigue.	Adjust birthing bed by dropping the foot down. Supply extra pillows for increased support.

comfort and well-being of the woman and fetus are considered, the following disadvantages have been noted (Blackburn, 2003):

- There is a decrease of as much as 30% in the blood pressure of 10% of women.
- Many women experience difficulty breathing because of pressure of the uterus on the diaphragm.
- The uterine axis is directed toward the symphysis pubis instead of the pelvic inlet, thus interfering with fetal alignment.
- Aspiration of vomit is more likely.
- The woman may feel resentment at being forced to assume an "embarrassing" position.
- Supine hypotension syndrome may occur.
- The labor may be prolonged and may lead to the use of medications to augment labor.
- The contractions may seem more uncomfortable, making coping more difficult.
- Tightening of the vagina and perineum as the thighs are flexed may increase the likelihood of an episiotomy or laceration.
- The position may interfere with the frequency and intensity of contractions.
- Stirrups cause excessive pressure on the legs.
- The woman works against gravity.

These disadvantages may be lessened slightly if the woman has her back elevated 30 to 40 degrees.

Left Lateral Sims' Position

A common position favored by some women and birth attendants is the left lateral Sims' or side-lying position (Figure 24–7, A ◆). In assuming this position for birth, the woman lies on her left side with her left leg extended and her right knee drawn against her abdomen or flexed by her side or with both legs bent at the knees. Although the frequency of contractions may decrease in this position, the intensity increases, yielding greater uterine efficiency (Blackburn, 2007). Those who favor this position find that it increases overall comfort, does not compromise venous return from the lower extremities, puts less stress and pressure on the maternal neck, and diminishes the chances of aspiration should vomiting occur. Women also perceive the lateral Sims' as a more natural and comfortable position and less intrusive with no stirrups or overhead lights required. Birth attendants have found that the position has a positive effect on the management of fetal shoulder dystocias. Side-lying positions are also helpful in labors in which the fetus is in a posterior position, because this position allows the uterine weight and the fetus to tip away from the maternal back (Blackburn, 2003). Fewer episiotomies are required in this position because the perineum tends to be more relaxed. The disadvantages cited relate to the difficulty of cutting and repairing large episiotomies and problems with difficult forceps births. These disadvantages, however, can be rectified by repositioning the woman if forceps are needed or if a repair is needed after the birth.

A

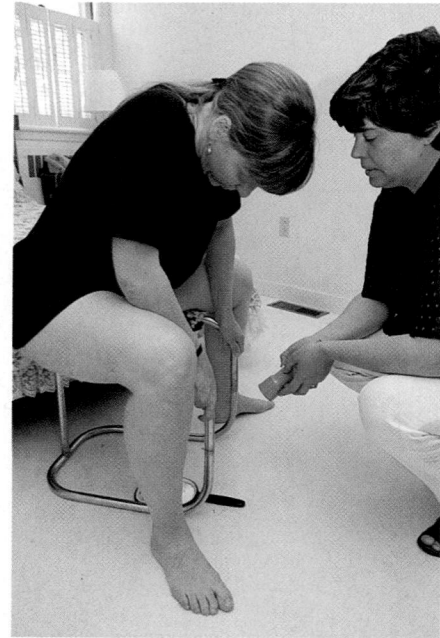

B

Figure 24–7 ◆ Birthing positions. *A,* Side-lying (also known as left lateral Sims') position. SOURCE: Photographer, Elena Dorfman. *B,* Using a birthing stool.
SOURCE: © Stella Johnson (www.stellajohnson.com).

Squatting Position

Squatting is favored by some women primarily for the positive use it makes of gravity that allows the abdominal wall to relax (Blackburn, 2007). Squatting is thought to facilitate the entrance of the presenting part into the pelvic inlet, thus hastening engagement. This engagement facilitates pressure being applied to the cervix, which aids in stretching it. This is turn can stimulate the myometrium to produce more intense uterine contractions and shorten the length of labor. A squatting bar (birthing bar) may be used across a bed or on the floor to increase the woman's balance and provide some support (see Figure 24–6). During the second stage of labor, squatting increases the size of the pelvic outlet by 28% and helps in the woman's pushing efforts. The pressure from the thighs against the uterus can also aid in fetal descent and help facilitate a favorable fetal position (Blackburn, 2007). Some birth attendants object to this position because the perineum is relatively inaccessible, and it is difficult for them to control the birth process. Squatting also increases the difficulty of administering analgesia, using instruments, and monitoring fetal status. Perineal edema can also occur from prolonged squatting. Ice may be applied intermittently to lessen perineal edema. Women with epidural anesthesia may be unable to assume this position because of the heaviness in their lower extremities.

Semi-Fowler's Position

Some care providers advocate a semi-Fowler's position as an appropriate middle ground between the recumbent and upright positions. This position has also been associated with shorter first and second stages of labor than the traditional lithotomy position (Blackburn, 2007). This position enhances the effectiveness of the abdominal muscle efforts while the woman is pushing and thereby shortens the second stage of labor. Raising and supporting the torso helps the woman view the birth process. At the same time the birth attendant has access to the perineum. Supporting a woman in this position is not difficult with most birthing beds.

Sitting Position

The sitting position is becoming an option for more women with the increased availability of birthing chairs. The use of birthing chairs or stools can be traced back to ancient Egypt, and they were broadly used in ancient Greek, Roman, and Incan civilizations. In the wake of the 19th-century battle against puerperal fever, birthing chairs began to vanish on hygienic grounds. Birthing chairs are being used again during the second stage of labor and are perceived by some women as a positive way to participate in the birth process (see Figure 24–7, B ◆). A supported sitting position may also be achieved in a birthing bed.

The upright sitting position offers advantages similar to squatting. It has been associated with stronger, more effective uterine contractions. It has been postulated that the weight of a term fetus is sufficient force in itself to supply much of what is needed to bring the newborn into the world. Proponents of the birthing chair state that it makes possible spontaneous births that would have required operative assistance in the recumbent position. Women experiencing severe back pain have found that use of the chair can diminish or eliminate the pain. The woman can curl forward and grasp her knees and ankles during pushing efforts. She can usually see the birth without aid of mirrors, and following birth she can lift the baby up toward her face.

Duration of the second stage and fetal outcome are not significantly affected by use of the birthing chair. However, it may carry a potential for increased blood loss.

Hands and Knees Position

The hands and knees position is more comfortable for a woman experiencing back labor because there is less pressure on the maternal back from the fetus, and the fetus may be able to rotate more easily from the posterior position. The mother can be well supported by dropping the foot of the birthing bed and supplying extra pillows upon which she can rest her forearms. Because there is less pressure on the perineum, there is less need for an episiotomy, and the incidence of lacerations is less. The birth attendant is better able to assess the perineum for stretching and has good access to the fetal nose and mouth for suctioning at the time of birth. This position may also increase placental and umbilical blood flow during episodes of nonreassuring fetal status. This position also increases the intensity of the uterine contractions. Lastly, the hands and knees position may increase the pelvic diameter and facilitate birth of the infant with shoulder dystocia. Disadvantages of this position include decreased eye contact between the mother and birth attendant, the inability to use instruments, and the potential necessity of repositioning the mother for perineal repair. Women may also become easily fatigued in this position.

CLEANSING THE PERINEUM

If a perineal prep is to be performed, the woman is positioned for the birth, and her vulvar and perineal area is cleansed to increase her comfort and to remove the bloody discharge that is present before the actual birth. An aseptic technique such as the one that follows is recommended.

After thorough handwashing, the nurse opens the sterile prep tray, dons sterile gloves, and cleans the vulva and perineum with the cleansing solution. Beginning with the mons pubis, the area is cleansed up to the lower abdomen. A second sponge is used to clean the inner groin and thigh of one leg, and a third is used to clean the other leg, moving upward to avoid carrying material from surrounding areas to the vaginal outlet. The last three sponges are used to clean the labia and vestibule with one downward sweep each. The used sponges are discarded. Once the cleansing is completed, the woman returns to the desired birthing position. Not all birthing facilities use such formalized cleansing procedures. Some facilities use a spray bottle with povidone-iodine (Betadine) or other cleansing agent and simply spray the perineal area. Because birth is not truly a "sterile procedure" some providers do not perform perineal cleansing techniques.

SUPPORTING THE COUPLE

The nurse assesses the woman's partner or other support person for comfort and knowledge and assists him or her in activities that will support the woman during the second stage. Some support persons will want to take an active role in coaching the woman through the birth process, whereas others will prefer simply to observe the birth process. The nurse assesses the roles the members of the support team desire and provides interventions that enhance these roles. It is important to keep the support team informed of the woman's progress, provide explanations of what is happening, and praise them for their supportive activities. A nurse who provides calm reassurance can help promote a positive experience.

ASSISTING WITH THE BIRTH OF THE INFANT

When the fetal head has distended the perineum, the clinician may perform a hand maneuver, such as supporting the perineum between the thumb and four fingers, which is believed to prevent

Figure 24–8 ◆ A birthing sequence.
SOURCE: © Stella Johnson (www.stellajohnson.com).

undue trauma to the fetal head and maternal soft tissues. The woman may be asked to breathe rapidly, pant, or blow to avoid too rapid birth of the fetal head. The woman may also be instructed to push and take a breath intermittently to avoid rapid expulsion.

After the infant's head is born, the clinician palpates the neck for the presence of a cord, which can be slipped over the fetal head if it is loose. If the cord is tight, it is double-clamped and cut.

Restitution and external rotation occur after the head is born. The only assistance needed during this time is support of the maternal perineum. While awaiting completion of external rotation, the clinician suctions the newborn's nose and mouth to remove mucus. When the newborn's shoulder appears at the symphysis pubis, the clinician may use both hands to grasp the newborn's head gently and pull downward for release of the anterior shoulder. Gentle upward traction facilitates release of the posterior shoulder.

Birth of the newborn's body may be controlled by grasping the posterior shoulder with one hand, palm turned toward the perineum. The left hand may be used for this if the newborn is left occiput anterior (LOA). The right hand then follows along the infant's back, and the feet are grasped as they are expelled. The newborn's head is kept down and to the side as the feet, legs, and body are tucked under the clinician's left arm in a football hold. The clinician's right hand is then free for further care of the newborn, and the newborn is securely held. CNMs often place the newborn directly on the mother's abdomen. The nose and mouth are suctioned with a bulb syringe, and respiratory passages are cleared. Figure 24–8 ◆ depicts an entire birthing experience.

ASSISTING WITH CLAMPING THE CORD

There is controversy about when to clamp and cut the cord. If the newborn is held at or below the vagina as cord clamping is delayed, as much as 50 to 100 mL of blood may be shifted from the placenta to the newborn. If the newborn is held 50 to 60 cm above the vagina, blood may be transferred from the newborn to the placenta. The extra amount of blood added to the newborn's circulation by holding the newborn below the vagina may reduce the frequency of iron deficiency anemia, which can occur later in infancy. However, in some cases the circulatory overload may produce polycythemia and favor hyperbilirubinemia. The newborn is not elevated above the vagina. Some parents may specify a preference in their birth plan regarding exactly when the umbilical cord is to be cut. There is some evidence that suggests that delayed cord clamping in preterm infants results in fewer transfusions and lower rates of intraventricular hemorrhage, although delayed clamping can interfere with immediate resuscitation efforts (Rabe, 2005). Delayed cord clamping may also benefit infants with a nuchal cord. One study that compared cutting the umbilical cord before the birth of the shoulders versus delayed cord cutting by reducing the

cord around the fetal neck showed a reduction in hypovolemia, anemia, shock, hypoxic-ischemic encephalopathy, and cerebral palsy when the delayed approach was used (Mercer, 2005). The pros and cons of early and late cord clamping can be discussed before the birth.

The cord is usually clamped with two Kelly clamps and cut between them. The father, other support person, or the mother may wish to cut the cord after it has been clamped by the physician or CNM.

The physician or CNM may double-clamp the cord so that a section can be made available for the collection of cord blood gases (discussed shortly). After the cord has been cut, cord blood is collected and sent to the lab as needed.

If the physician or CNM has not placed a cord clamp on the newborn's umbilical stump, it is the responsibility of the nurse to do so. Before applying the cord clamp, the nurse examines the cut end for the presence of two arteries and one vein. The umbilical vein is the largest vessel, and the arteries are smaller vessels. The presence of only one artery in the umbilical cord is associated with genitourinary abnormalities. The number of vessels is recorded on the birth and newborn records.

The cord is clamped approximately 1/2 to 1 inch from the abdomen to allow room between the abdomen and clamp as the cord dries (Figure 24–9). Abdominal skin must not be clamped because this will cause necrosis of the tissue. The clamp is removed in the newborn nursery approximately 24 hours after birth if the cord has dried. Some facilities now place an umbilical cord alarm with the cord clamp (Figure 24–10 ◆). This security measure triggers an alarm if the infant comes within a certain distance from the unit's exterior door. The alarm can only be removed with a special removal device.

CORD BLOOD COLLECTION FOR BANKING

Growing numbers of parents are arranging for cord blood banking (see discussion in Chapter 1 ∞). Immediately after the

A   C

B

Figure 24–9 ◆ Hollister cord clamp. *A,* Clamp is positioned 1/2 to 1 inch from the abdomen and then secured. *B,* Cut cord. The one vein and two arteries can be seen. *C,* Plastic device for removing clamp after cord has dried. After the cord is cut, the nurse grasps the Hollister clamp on either side of the cut area and gently separates it.

MEDIALINK Videos: Third Stage of Labor

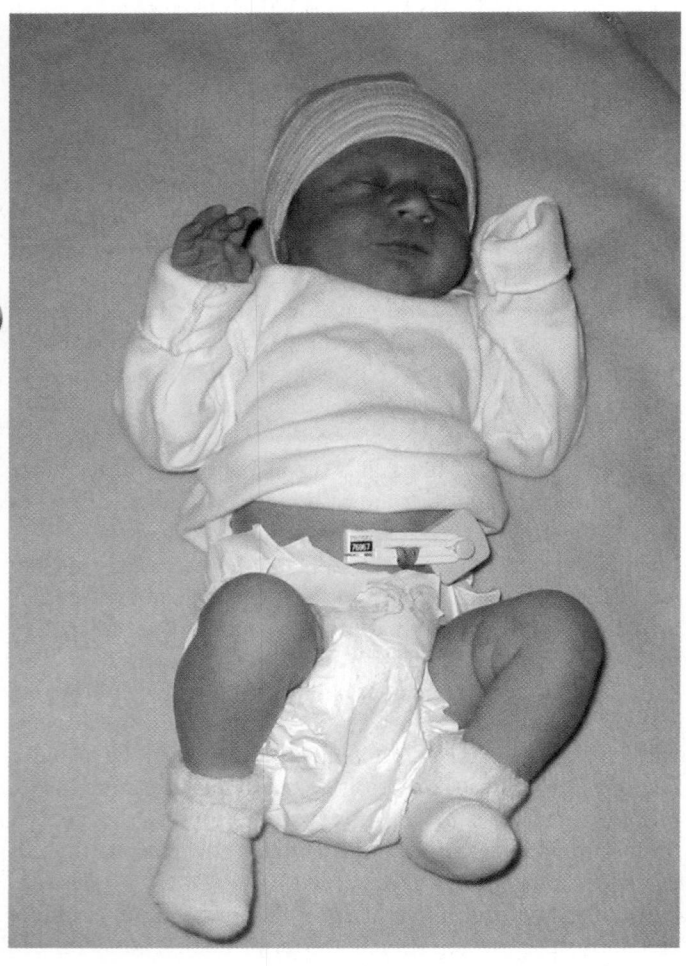

Figure 24–10 ◆ Umbilical alarm in place on a newborn infant.

MEDIALINK Application: Cord Blood Banking

newborn's umbilical cord is clamped and cut and before the placenta is expelled, the physician or CNM withdraws blood from the umbilical cord. The blood is placed in a special container that parents receive from the Cord Blood Registry and bring with them for the birth. The parents will have any special directions that are required for storage and care of the container. Although current recommendations for cord blood banking include a family history of an illness that can be treated with fetal cells and children whose parents are from a nontraditional lineage, such as mixed race backgrounds or other ethnic combinations that are uncommon, many families are now choosing to bank their infants' cord blood. Stem cell transplants are now used to treat many different types of diseases (Table 24–10). The future of stem cell transplantation is promising, with rapid explanation of uses (Moise, 2005).

Table 24–7 on page 662 summarizes labor progress, possible responses of the laboring woman, and nursing care during the second stage of labor.

NURSING CARE DURING THE THIRD STAGE OF LABOR

Nursing care in the third stage focuses on providing initial newborn care and assisting with birth of the placenta.

Provision of Initial Newborn Care

The physician or CNM places the newborn on the mother's abdomen or in the radiant-heated unit to begin the initial care. If the newborn is not placed on the mother's abdomen, the radiant-heated unit is positioned so the parents can see the baby.

Because the first priority is to maintain respirations, the newborn is placed in a modified Trendelenburg position to aid drainage of mucus from the nasopharynx and trachea. The newborn is also suctioned with a bulb syringe or DeLee mucus trap as needed (Procedure 24–1: Performing Nasal Pharyngeal Suctioning).

The second priority is to provide and maintain warmth, so the newborn is dried immediately with warmed, soft infant blankets. Wet blankets should be immediately removed to prevent heat loss. The nurse dries the newborn's head first to minimize heat loss. Warmth can be maintained by putting the newborn in skin-to-skin contact with the mother and placing warmed blankets over both of them. If the newborn is placed in a radiant-heated unit, he or she is dried, laid on a dry blanket, and left uncovered under the radiant heat. Because radiant heat warms the outer surface of objects, a newborn wrapped in blankets will receive no benefit. In many settings a stocking cap is placed on the newborn's head to conserve heat.

APGAR SCORING SYSTEM

The Apgar scoring system (Table 24–11) was designed in 1952 by Dr. Virginia Apgar, an anesthesiologist. The purpose of the **Apgar score** is to evaluate the physical condition of the newborn at birth and the immediate need for resuscitation. The newborn is rated 1 minute after birth and again at 5 minutes and receives a total score ranging from 0 to 10 based on the following criteria:

1. The heart rate is auscultated or palpated at the junction of the umbilical cord and skin. This is the most important assessment. A newborn heart rate of less than 100 bpm indicates the need for immediate resuscitation.

2. The respiratory effort is the second most important Apgar assessment. Complete absence of respirations is termed *apnea.* A vigorous cry indicates good respirations.

3. The muscle tone is determined by evaluating the degree of flexion and resistance to straightening of the extremities. A normal term newborn's elbows and hips are flexed, with the knees positioned up toward the abdomen.

4. The reflex irritability is evaluated as the newborn is dried or by lightly rubbing the soles of the feet. A cry is a score of 2. A grimace is 1 point, and no response is 0.

5. The skin color is inspected for cyanosis and pallor. Newborns generally have blue extremities, and the rest of the body is pink, which merits a score of 1. This condition, termed *acrocyanosis,* is present in 85% of normal newborns at 1 minute after birth. A completely pink newborn scores a 2, and a totally cyanotic, pale infant is scored 0. Newborns with darker skin pigmentation will not be pink. Their skin color is assessed for pallor and acrocyanosis, and a score is selected based on the assessment.

Table 24–10	DISEASES THAT MAY BE TREATED WITH STEM CELL TRANSPLANTS

Arthritis

- Rheumatoid Arthritis
- Osteoarthritis

Blood Disorders and Cancers

- Aplastic Anemia
- Thrombocytopenia
- Leukemias
- Lymphomas
- Immune Deficiencies
- Marrow Failure
- Sickle Cell Disease
- Thalassemia
- Inherited Disorders Caused by Defective Monocytes

Other Cancers

- Brain Tumors
- Ewing Sarcoma
- Neuroblastoma
- Ovarian Cancer
- Renal Cell Carcinoma
- Rhabdomyosarcoma
- Small Cell Lung Cancer
- Testicular Cancer
- Thymoma (Thymic Carcinoma)

Chronic Pain Disorders

Diabetes and Diabetic Complications

- Type 1 Diabetes Mellitus
- Type 2 Diabetes Mellitus
- Diabetic Ulcers

Inflammatory Bowel Disorders

- Crohn's Disease
- Ulcerative Colitis

Diseases and Disorders of the Eye

- Macular Degeneration
- Diabetic Retinopathy

Heart & Circulatory Diseases

- Hypertension
- Coronary Artery Disease
- Congestive Heart Failure

Liver Diseases

- Hepatitis
- Liver cirrhosis

Nervous System Disorders & Spinal Cord Injuries

- Stroke
- Multiple Sclerosis
- Amyotrophic Lateral Sclerosis (Lou Gehrig's disease)
- Parkinson's Disease
- Alzheimer's Disease
- Epileptiform (or trigeminal) neuralgia
- Muscular Dystrophy (Duchenne's Disease)

Myelodysplastic/Myeloproliferative Disorders

Inherited Immune System Disorders

Inherited Metabolic Disorders

A score of 7 to 10 indicates a newborn in good condition and requires only nasopharyngeal suctioning and perhaps some oxygen near the face. An Apgar score between 4 and 7 indicates the need for stimulation; a score under 4 indicates the need for resuscitation (ACOG, 2006). See the discussion in Chapter 33. ∞

NEWBORN PHYSICAL ASSESSMENT BY THE NURSE

An abbreviated systematic physical assessment is performed by the nurse in the birthing area to detect any abnormalities (Table 24–12). First, the nurse notes the size of the newborn and the contour and size of the head in relationship to the rest of the body. The newborn's posture and movements indicate tone and neurologic functioning. The appearance of the head is noted along with palpation of the fontanelles. The face should be inspected along with the ears and neck.

The skin is inspected for discoloration, presence of vernix caseosa and lanugo, and evidence of trauma and desquamation (peeling of skin). *Vernix caseosa* is a white, cheesy substance normally found on newborns. It is absorbed within 24 hours after birth. Vernix is abundant on preterm infants and absent on postterm newborns. A large quantity of fine hair *(lanugo)* is often seen on preterm newborns, especially on their shoulders, foreheads, backs, and cheeks. Desquamation of the skin is seen in postterm newborns.

The nares are observed for flaring. As the newborn cries, the palate can be inspected for cleft palate. Mucus in the nose and mouth can be assessed and removed with the bulb syringe as needed. The chest is inspected for respiratory rate and the presence of retractions. If retractions are present, the newborn is assessed for grunting or stridor. A normal respiratory rate is 30 to 60 per minute. The lungs may be auscultated bilaterally for

PROCEDURE 24–1 Performing Nasal Pharyngeal Suctioning

NURSING ACTION	RATIONALE

Preparation

- Suction equipment is always available in the birthing area to clear secretions from the newborn's nose or oropharnyx if respirations are depressed or if amniotic fluid was meconium stained.
- Tighten the lid on the DeLee mucus trap or other suction device collection bottle.
- Connect one end of the DeLee tubing to low suction.

This avoids spillage of secretions and prevents air from leaking out of the lid.

Equipment and Supplies

DeLee mucus trap or other suction device

Procedure: Clean Gloves

1. Don gloves.
2. Without applying suction, insert the free end of the DeLee tubing 3 to 5 inches into the newborn's nose or mouth (Figure 24–11 ◆).

   Applying suction while passing the tube would interfere with smooth passage of the tube.

3. Place your thumb over the suction control and begin to apply suction. Continue to suction as you slowly remove the tube, rotating it slightly.

   Suctioning during withdrawal removes fluid and avoids redepositing secretions in the newborn's nasopharnyx.

4. Continue to reinsert the tube and provide suction for as long as fluid is aspirated.

Figure 24–11 ◆ A newborn infant being suctioned with a DeLee mucus trap to remove excess secretions from the mouth and nares.
SOURCE: Photographer, Elena Dorfman.

NOTE: Excessive suctioning can cause vagal stimulation, which decreases the heart rate.

5. If it is necessary to pass the tube into the newborn's stomach to remove meconium secretions that the newborn swallowed before birth, insert the tube through the newborn's mouth into the stomach. Apply suction and continue to suction as you withdraw the tube.

   Because the newborn's nares are small and delicate, it is easier and faster to pass the suction tube through the mouth.

6. Document the completion of the procedure and the amount and type of secretions.

   This documentation provides a record of the intervention and the status of the infant at birth.

Documentation   Documentation of client teaching should include the teaching information discussed, the client's verbalization of understanding, and specific interventions or warning signs that were given, along with the client's understanding of follow-up, if needed in the future.

breath sounds. Absence of breath sounds on one side may indicate pneumothorax. Rales may be heard immediately after birth because a small amount of fluid may remain in the lungs; this fluid will be absorbed. Rhonchi indicate aspiration of oral secretions. The abdomen is inspected and palpated for masses. The heart is assessed for heart rate, rhythm, and the presence of any murmurs. The normal newborn heart rate is 110 to 160 bpm. The umbilical cord is inspected, and the number of vessels is recorded.

The genital area, buttocks, and anus are inspected. The elimination of urine or meconium is noted and recorded on the newborn record. The extremities are inspected and compared

Table 24–11   THE APGAR SCORING SYSTEM

Sign	Score 0	1	2
Heart rate	Absent	Slow—below 100	Above 100
Respiratory effort	Absent	Slow—irregular	Good crying
Muscle tone	Flaccid	Some flexion of extremities	Active motion
Reflex irritability	None	Grimace	Vigorous cry
Color	Pale blue	Body pink, blue extremities	Completely pink

SOURCE: Reprinted from *Pediatric Clinics of North America, 13,* V. Apgar, "The Newborn (Apgar) Scoring System, Reflections and Advice, p. 645. Copyright © 1966, with permission from Elsevier.

Table 24–12   INITIAL NEWBORN EVALUATION

Assess	Normal Findings
Respirations	Rate 30–60 irregular
	No retractions, no grunting
Apical pulse	Rate 110–160 and somewhat irregular
Temperature	Skin temp above 36.5C (97.8F)
Skin color	Body pink with bluish extremities
Umbilical cord	Two arteries and one vein
Gestational age	Should be 38–42 weeks to remain with parents for extended time
Sole creases	Sole creases that involve the heel

In general, expect scant amount of vernix on upper back, axilla, groin, lanugo only on upper back; ears with incurving of upper ⅔ of pinnae and thin cartilage that springs back from folding; male genitals—testes palpated in upper or lower scrotum; female genitals—labia majora larger; clitoris nearly covered.

In the following situations, newborns should generally be stabilized rather than remaining with parents in the birth area for an extended period of time.

Apgar less than 8 at 1 minute and less than 9 at 5 minutes or baby requires resuscitation measures (other than whiffs of oxygen)

Respirations below 30 or above 60, with retractions and/or grunting

Apical pulse below 110 or above 160 with marked irregularities

Skin temperature below 36.5C (97.8F)

Skin color pale blue or circumoral pallor

Baby less than 38 or more than 42 weeks' gestation

Baby very small or very large for gestational age

Congenital anomalies involving open areas in the skin (meningomyelocele)

for symmetry. Reflexes are assessed to determine central nervous system maturity. A complete newborn assessment can be found in Chapter 29. ∞

NEWBORN IDENTIFICATION

To ensure correct identification, the nurse gives the mother and the newborn identification bands with identical codes in the birthing or delivery room. One bracelet is placed on the mother's wrist and sometimes on the wrist of her partner or a support person whom she designates. Two bracelets are placed on the newborn—one on the wrist and one on the ankle. The newborn bands must be applied snugly to prevent their loss. Infants should not be removed from the room until these identification bands have been placed. The bands should remain in place until the mother and infant are discharged home.

Some facilities now use security devices that are placed on the umbilical cord clamp or the identification bracelet of the infant. The alarm is left in place until discharge. The alarm sounds if the infant is removed from the hospital unit or if the alarm is cut or disengaged. Some systems activate a "lockdown" of the birthing unit, thus making abduction of an infant more difficult.

Additional security measures are now commonplace in many maternity settings. Staff must wear appropriate identification at all times. Parents are advised not to allow individuals without proper identification to remove their infant under any circumstances. The nurse also advises the parents to keep the infant on the side of the bed furthest from the door. The infant should be returned to the nursery if the mother plans to nap or shower if no other family member is present.

Although infants were once footprinted for security reasons, the practice is now performed to provide a souvenir for parents and is no longer considered a safety measure. To prepare the newborn for footprinting, the nurse wipes the soles of both the newborn's feet to remove any vernix caseosa. The footprint can be placed on a card or in the parents' baby book.

INITIATION OF ATTACHMENT

The birth of the baby is usually an emotionally charged time for all members of the family. The sight of the new baby and the sounds of the first cry may fill the parents with utter amazement. As the baby is placed on the mother's abdomen or chest, she frequently reaches out to touch and stroke her baby. When the newborn is placed in this position, the father also has a very clear, close view and can also reach out to touch his baby.

When the parents feel comfortable in the environment, they may talk to the newborn, and some mothers talk to their babies in a high-pitched voice, which seems to soothe newborns. Some couples verbally express amazement and pride when they see they have produced a beautiful, healthy baby. Their verbalization enhances feelings of accomplishment and ecstasy.

If lights in the birthing area can be dimmed, the newborn will probably open his or her eyes wide and gaze at the surroundings. In this first hour after birth, the newborn is usually quiet and continues to gaze. This is a wonderful opportunity for eye contact with the parents, and many parents are content to gaze quietly at their newborn.

Even though the baby is on the mother's abdomen or chest, the nurse can complete any needed assessments or interventions such as footprinting and applying an identification bracelet to the child. As soon as possible the nurse can assist the mother to a more comfortable position for holding the newborn. Breastfeeding can be encouraged if the mother and baby desire. When the baby is held close to the breast, the baby will seek out the nipple. Even if the newborn does not actively nurse, she or he can lick, taste, and smell the mother's skin.

Videos: Third Stage of Labor   MediaLink

This activity stimulates the maternal release of prolactin, which promotes the onset of lactation.

The initial parental-newborn attachment period can be enhanced if the care providers keep routine investigations to a minimum, delay instillation of ophthalmic antibiotic for the first hour, keep the room slightly darkened, avoid loud noises, talk in quiet tones, and provide privacy. Both parents need to be encouraged to do whatever they feel most comfortable doing. Parents may have differing wishes concerning contact with their newborn. Some want immediate and unlimited time; some prefer to wait until all birth-related activities are completed (the placenta is expelled and episiotomy repair is completed); others prefer limited contact immediately after birth and quiet time later. Although immediate contact may be important for attachment and initiation of breastfeeding, the parents' wishes need to be supported.

Parents can be encouraged to delay phone calls and visits from friends until after the first hour of birth because it is a time when the baby is the most alert. Most facilities have policies in place where the newborn is taken to the nursery for assessment and bathing after an initial visit with the parents. This is an excellent time for phone calls and visits with family and friends. It enables the new family to spend valuable time together and facilitates bonding.

Animation: Placental Delivery   MediaLink

> *I was hungry for the baby as he was born. I wanted to see, hold him. It was hours before I realized or even thought love in relation to him.*
>
> ~HARRIETTE HARTIGAN, *WOMEN IN BIRTH*~

Delivery of the Placenta

After the cord has been clamped and cut, the physician or CNM observes for the following signs of placental separation:

1. The uterus rises upward in the abdomen because the placenta settles downward into the lower uterine segment.
2. As the placenta proceeds downward, the umbilical cord lengthens.
3. A sudden trickle or spurt of blood appears.
4. The uterus changes from a discoid to a globular shape.

Video: Delivery of Placenta   MediaLink

While waiting for these signs, the nurse gently palpates the uterus to check for ballooning caused by uterine relaxation and subsequent bleeding into the uterine cavity.

After the placenta has separated, it may be expelled by various techniques such as maternal bearing-down effort, controlled cord traction, and fundal pressure. Maternal effort allows the placenta to be expelled spontaneously and is best accomplished in an upright position. When the mother is in a dorsal recumbent or lithotomy position, she or the nurse can help the process by splinting or supporting her abdominal muscles. The mother or nurse can place her palms over the lower abdomen, or the mother can flex her thighs over her abdomen. The mother then bears down to expel the placenta.

To help the woman expel her placenta, the physician or CNM first ensures that separation has occurred and then places one hand above the symphysis pubis with the palm against the

DEVELOPING CULTURAL COMPETENCE

MIDWIFE-ATTENDED BIRTHS: MALAYSIA

In Malaysia, 75% of all births are attended by a *dukun* (midwife). In many parts of the country, especially in rural areas, a home setting is preferred over a hospital setting for birth. It is believed that the baby's first cry is symbolic of loyalty to the parents and should be heard at home. The birth itself is a social event in which many women sit with the laboring woman. It is customary for the woman in labor and her female company to chew red-staining betel nuts. At the time of birth, either the mother or a female relative is given the honor of cutting the umbilical cord.

anterior surface of the uterus. The uterus is displaced upward and backward as the mother is asked to relax her abdominal muscles and breathe through an open mouth. The elevation of the uterus straightens out the birth canal and facilitates expulsion of the placenta, as well as protecting the uterus from inversion. Gentle traction is exerted on the umbilical cord. Excessive pulling may increase the risk of uterine involution, snapping off of the cord, and subsequent hemorrhage. During this procedure, the nurse encourages the mother to continue breathing through an open mouth and to relax her abdominal muscles.

Fundal pressure is not a method of choice because it is very uncomfortable for the mother, may damage uterine supports, and may invert the uterus. If this method is needed, the mother is asked to relax her abdominal muscles, and then the hand of the physician or CNM is placed behind the uterus with the fingers directed downward toward the maternal spine. With a quick "scooping" motion, the contracted uterus is pressed downward in an arc. This motion is different from direct downward pressure, which folds the uterus over the lower segment and does not enhance movement of the placenta. During the procedure, the nurse provides continued encouragement to maintain abdominal relaxation. This is very difficult because of the discomfort of the procedure.

After expulsion of the placenta, the physician or CNM inspects the placental membranes to make sure they are intact and that all cotyledons are present. This inspection is especially important with placentas expelled via the Duncan mechanism (the chance of tearing off a portion of a cotyledon is greatest with this mechanism of placental separation). If there is a defect or a part missing from the placenta, a digital uterine examination is done. The time and mechanism (Schultze or Duncan) of expulsion of the placenta are noted on the birth record (see Chapter 22 ∞). The vagina and cervix are inspected for lacerations, and any necessary repairs are made. An episiotomy or laceration may be repaired now if it has not been done previously. (See further discussion of episiotomy in Chapter 27 ∞). The fundus of the uterus is palpated; normal position is at the midline and below the umbilicus. If the fun-

DRUG GUIDE   Carboprost Tromethamine (Hemabate)

Pregnancy Risk Category: D

Overview of Action

Carboprost tromethamine (Hemabate) is used to reduce blood loss secondary to uterine atony. It stimulates myometrial contractions to control postpartum hemorrhaging that is unresponsive to usual techniques. Carboprost tromethamine can also be used to induce labor in women desiring an elective termination of a pregnancy. The drug is also used to induce labor in cases of intrauterine fetal death and hydatidiform mole (Wilson, Shannon, & Stang, 2006).

Route, Dosage, Frequency

In cases of immediate postpartum hemorrhage, the usual intramuscular dose is 250 mcg (1 mL) which can be repeated every 1½ to 3½ hours if uterine atony persists. The dosage can be increased to 500 mcg (2 mL) if uterine contractility is inadequate after several doses of 250 mcg. The total dosage should not exceed 12 mg. The maximum duration of use is 48 hours (Wilson et al., 2006).

Contraindications

The drug is contraindicated in women with active cardiac, pulmonary, or renal disease. It should not be administered during pregnancy or in women with acute pelvic inflammatory disease. It should be used with caution in women with asthma, adrenal disease, hypotension, hypertension, diabetes mellitus, epilepsy, fibroids, cervical stenosis, or previous uterine surgery (Wilson et al., 2006).

Side Effects

The most common side effects are nausea and diarrhea. Fever, chills, and flushing can occur. Headache, muscle, joint, abdominal, or eye pain can also occur (Wilson et al., 2006).

Nursing Considerations

1. The injection should be given in a large muscle. Aspiration should be performed to avoid injection into a blood vessel which can result in bronchospasm, tetanic contractions, and shock.
2. After administration, monitor uterine status and bleeding carefully.
3. Report excess bleeding to the physician/CNM.
4. Check vital signs routinely, observing for an increase in temperature, elevated pulse, and decreased blood pressure.
5. Breastfeeding should be delayed for 24 hours after administration (Wilson et al., 2006).

---

dus is displaced, it may be because of a full bladder or a collection of blood in the uterus.

The medical-nursing culture tends to refer to the placenta as the "afterbirth" and considers that its value is fulfilled once it is expelled and examined. Disposal of the placenta is prescribed by the hospital or birth center, and no more thought is given to it. However, many cultures have other beliefs regarding the placenta. Some clients will have specific beliefs about disposal of the placenta and will ask to take it home with them. Labor nurses will need to review hospital policies for disposal of the placenta before giving the placenta to the woman or family members.

Use of Oxytocics

Some CNMs and physicians advocate the use of an oxytocic drug (Pitocin) to stimulate uterine contractions after birth and to reduce the incidence of third-stage hemorrhage.

The physician or CNM may request that 10 units of oxytocin be given intramuscularly to the woman when the anterior shoulder of the infant appears at the vaginal opening. Some practitioners believe that this procedure facilitates the expulsion of the placenta. Others question whether this method increases the incidence of neonatal hyperviscosity because an additional bolus of blood may be infused into the fetus when the uterus contracts in response to the oxytocin. At other times 10 units of oxytocin may be administered intramuscularly at the time of placental expulsion. Both techniques are thought to prevent uterine atony and excessive bleeding. Some prefer to add 10 to 20 units of oxytocin to IV fluids administered over a period of hours. Additional information and associated nursing implications are presented in the Drug Guide: Oxytocin (Pitocin) in Chapter 27. ∞ Methylergonovine maleate (Methergine), 0.2 mg can be administered intramuscularly. Methergine should not be given if preeclampsia is present. Carboprost tromethamine (Hemabate) 250 mcg/mL can also be administered intramuscularly (See Drug Guide: Carboprost Tromethamine [Hemabate]). Although the use of misoprostol (Cytotec) in treating postpartum hemorrhage is an off-label use, it is used in some settings with favorable results (Moore, 2002).

NURSING CARE DURING THE FOURTH STAGE OF LABOR

The period immediately following expulsion of the placenta is referred to as the fourth stage of labor and birth. Actually, the label is misleading because labor and birth are completed with delivery of the placenta, and the next few hours are actually the immediate recovery phase. The fourth stage is usually defined as lasting from 1 to 4 hours after the birth or until vital signs are stable. Nursing care in this phase involves the basics of postpartum nursing care.

Immediately after the placenta is expelled, the episiotomy or vaginal lacerations are repaired. The uterus is palpated at frequent intervals, usually every 15 minutes for an hour until bleeding is within normal limits, to ensure that it remains firmly contracted. Although labor is completed, the uterus is sensitive to touch. Palpation of the uterine fundus will be uncomfortable for the woman. If the mother has not held her baby, immediate newborn care should be completed at her side and within her reach so that she can touch her baby during this time. As

MEDIALINK Video: Fourth Stage of Labor

soon as immediate care is completed, the new mother is usually eager to cuddle and explore her baby. If she plans to breastfeed and the baby is interested, she should be encouraged and helped to do so right after birth while the baby is awake and alert. Care should be taken not to try to force an uninterested baby to breastfeed because it will just lead to frustration for both mother and baby.

Behavioral characteristics of the mother vary, according to such factors as the length of labor, level of fatigue, extent of interruption in normal sleep patterns, and cultural norms. After the initial excitement of becoming acquainted with their new baby and notifying others of the birth, many new mothers are very tired and want to rest. Others are wide awake, eager to talk about their labor and satisfy basic body needs, such as hunger and thirst.

Provision of Care in the Fourth Stage

As soon as the CNM or physician completes the repair of any perineal lacerations or an episiotomy, drapes (if used) are removed. If the mother is to remain in the birthing bed, the nurse places clean absorbent pads beneath her and applies maternity pads. A cold pack may be placed directly on the perineum if perineal edema is present or an episiotomy has been done. If a mother prefers to shower immediately after birth, the nurse can assist her as needed and change the bed linens while the mother is up.

If stirrups were used, her perineum is cleansed and maternity pads applied before her legs are removed from the stirrups. To avoid muscle strain, both legs are removed from the stirrups at the same time. The legs may be held together and gently pushed toward the woman's abdomen, back to a neutral position and then gently lowered toward her right side and then the left side to promote circulation return. If the woman has given birth on a delivery table she is transferred to a recovery room bed. If the mother has not had a chance to hold her infant, she may do so before she is transferred from the birthing room. The nurse ensures that the mother and father or support person and newborn are given time to begin the attachment process.

In addition to encouraging family celebration of the birth, the immediate recovery period involves assessing both maternal bleeding and newborn stabilization. The most significant source of bleeding is from the site where the placenta was implanted and where uterine vessels previously provided pooling of maternal blood to nourish the fetus. It is therefore critical that the fundus stay well contracted to clamp off these uterine vessels and prevent hemorrhage. It is the nurse's responsibility to assess the mother's blood pressure, pulse, firmness and position of fundus, and amount and character of vaginal blood flow every 15 minutes for the first 1 or 2 hours. Deviations from the normal ranges require more frequent checking. Table 24–13 summarizes maternal changes following birth. Blood pressure should return to the prelabor level, and pulse rate should be slightly lower than it was in labor. The maternal blood pressure should be monitored at 5- to 15-minute intervals. The return of the blood pressure is due to an increased volume of blood returning to the maternal circulation from the uteroplacental shunt. Baroreceptors cause a vagal response, which slows the pulse. The physiologic slowing may be offset by excitement, increased

Table 24–13	MATERNAL ADAPTATIONS FOLLOWING BIRTH
Characteristic	**Normal Finding**
Blood pressure	Returns to prelabor level
Pulse	Slightly lower than in labor
Uterine fundus	In the midline at the umbilicus or 1–2 fingerbreadths below the umbilicus
Lochia	Red (rubra), small to moderate amount (from spotting on pads to ¼–½ of pad covered in 15 minutes)
	Doesn't exceed saturation of one pad in first hour
Bladder	Nonpalpable
Perineum	Smooth, pink, without bruising or edema
Emotional state	Wide variation, including excited, exhilarated, smiling, crying, fatigued, verbal, quiet, pensive, and sleepy

temperature, or dehydration. A rise in the blood pressure may be a response to oxytocic drugs or may be caused by preeclampsia. Blood loss may be reflected by a lowered blood pressure and a rising pulse rate.

The fundus should be firm at the umbilicus or lower and in the midline. The uterus should be palpated but not massaged unless boggy (atonic) (Procedure 24–2). When the uterus becomes boggy, pooling of blood occurs within it, resulting in the formation of clots. Anything left in the uterus prevents it from contracting effectively. Thus if it becomes boggy or appears to rise in the abdomen, the fundus should be massaged until firm. The uterus at this time is very tender, and palpation and massage cause discomfort. All palpation and massage should be done as gently as possible.

A boggy uterus feels very soft instead of firm and hard. The uterus may have relaxed so much that it cannot be found when the nurse attempts to palpate it. In this case the nurse places a hand in the midline of the abdomen at the level of the umbilicus and begins to make kneading motions. This motion stimulates the uterine fundus to contract, and the nurse will feel the fundus tighten to a firm, hard object.

CLINICAL TIP

Teach the woman to gently massage her own uterus by feeling for the uterus at the level of the umbilicus. Describe the uterus as a commonly known identifiable object, such as a grapefruit or a softball, to provide a visual cue for the woman. Once she identifies her uterus, she can gently massage it to increase uterine contractions.

The nurse inspects the bloody vaginal discharge, called *lochia,* for amount and charts it as minimal, moderate, or heavy (see Chapter 34 ∞). It should be bright red. Because different brands of maternity pads absorb varying amounts of blood, it may be necessary to weigh the maternity pad to determine actual blood loss. A gram scale is used, and 1 g is equivalent to approximately 1 mL of blood. If the perineal pad becomes soaked in a 15-minute period or if blood pools under the buttocks, continuous observation is necessary. As long as the woman remains

PROCEDURE 24–2 Assessing the Uterine Fundus following Vaginal Birth

NURSING ACTION	RATIONALE

Preparation

- Explain the procedure, the information it provides, and what it might feel like.
- Ask the woman to void.

- Have the woman lie flat in bed with her head on a pillow. If the procedure is uncomfortable, she may find that it helps to flex her legs.

A full bladder can cause uterine atony.
The supine position prevents falsely high assessment of fundal height. Flexing the legs relaxes the abdominal muscles.

Equipment and Supplies

A clean perineal pad

Procedure Clean Gloves

1. Gently place one hand on the lower segment of the uterus. Using the side of the other hand, palpate the abdomen until you locate the top of the fundus.

One hand stabilizes the uterus while the other hand locates the top of the fundus.

CLINICAL TIP

Gloves may be put on before assessing the abdomen and fundus or when you are ready to assess the perineum and lochia.

2. Determine whether the fundus is firm. If it is, it will feel like a hard round object in the abdomen. If it is not firm, massage the abdomen lightly until the fundus is firm.

A firm fundus indicates that the uterine muscles are contracted and bleeding will not occur.

3. Measure the top of the fundus in fingerbreadths above, below, or at the fundus. See Figure 24–12 ◆.

Fundal height gives information about the progress of involution.

4. Determine the position of the fundus in relation to the midline of the body. If it is not in the midline, locate it and then evaluate the bladder for distention.

The fundus may deviate from the midline when the bladder is full because the enlarged bladder pushes the uterus aside.

5. If the bladder is distended, use nursing measures to help the woman void. If she is not able to void after a specified period of time, catheterization may be necessary.

6. Measure urine output for the next few hours until normal elimination is established.

7. Assess the lochia

Figure 24–12 ◆ Suggested method of palpating the fundus of the uterus during the fourth stage. The left hand is placed just above the symphysis pubis, and gentle downward pressure is exerted. The right hand is cupped around the uterine fundus.

During the postpartum as diuresis occurs, the bladder may fill far more rapidly than normal, putting the woman at risk for uterine atony and hemorrhage.

(Continued on next page)

PROCEDURE 24–2 Assessing the Uterine Fundus following Vaginal Birth   continued

Documentation	The nurse documents the position (midline, deviated to the left or right), fundal height in relation to the umbilicus (F @ U or F @ U ↑ 1 or F @ U ↓ 1), and consistency (firm, boggy). The bladder status should also be recorded (distended, appears empty), along with the time of the last void.

in bed during the first hour, bleeding should not exceed saturation of one pad. Laceration of the vagina, cervix, or an unligated vessel in the episiotomy may be indicated by a continuous trickle of blood even though the fundus remains firm. (See Procedure 34–2: Evaluating Lochia, in Chapter 34 ∞).

If the fundus rises and displaces to the right, the nurse palpates the bladder to determine whether it is distended. All measures should be taken to enable the mother to void. If she is unable to void, catheterization is necessary. Postpartal women have decreased sensations to void as a result of the decreased tone of the bladder caused by the trauma imposed on the bladder and urethra during childbirth. The bladder fills rapidly as the body attempts to rid itself of the extra fluid volume returned from the uteroplacental circulation and of IV fluid that may have been received during labor and birth. If the mother is unable to void, a warm towel placed across the lower abdomen, warm water poured over the perineum, or spirits of peppermint poured into a bedpan may help the urinary sphincter relax and thus facilitate voiding. A distended bladder can cause uterine atony, thus increasing postpartal bleeding.

The perineum is inspected for edema and hematoma formation. With an episiotomy or laceration, an ice pack often reduces swelling and alleviates discomfort. To fully visualize the episiotomy or laceration site, the nurse has the woman lie on her side and lifts her anterior buttock to visualize the suture line. The site should be well approximated and may appear swollen or bruised. No active bleeding at the site should be observed.

The following conditions should be reported to the CNM or physician: hypotension, tachycardia, uterine atony, excessive bleeding, or a temperature over 38C (100F). The nurse should be aware that the blood pressure may not fall rapidly in the presence of dangerous bleeding in postpartal mothers because of the extra systemic volume. However, an increasing pulse rate may be noted before a decrease in blood pressure is detected. A normal blood pressure with the mother in the Fowler's position is a good confirmation of a normotensive woman.

Promotion of Comfort in the Fourth Stage

Women frequently have tremors in the immediate postpartal period. It has been proposed that this shivering response is caused by exhaustion or a difference in internal and external body temperatures (higher temperature inside the body than on the outside). Another theory is that the woman is reacting to the fetal cells that have entered the maternal circulation at the placental site. Shivering is more common in women who have received epidural anesthesia (Blackburn, 2007). A heated bath blanket placed next to the woman and perhaps a warm drink tend to alleviate the problem.

The couple may be tired, hungry, and thirsty. Some hospitals serve the couple a meal. The tired mother may initially have a period of excitement but may then drift off into a welcome sleep because of exhaustion from the energy that was exerted during labor. The partner should also be encouraged to rest because his supporting role is physically and mentally tiring. The mother is usually transferred from the birthing unit to the postpartal unit after 2 hours or more, depending on agency policy and whether the following criteria are met: stable vital signs, stable lochia, nondistended bladder, firm fundus, and sensations fully recovered from any anesthetic agent received during childbirth.

NURSING CARE OF THE ADOLESCENT

Adolescent pregnancy rates have declined by 28% since 1990 (Alan Guttmacher Institute, 2004). Despite these promising statistics, the United States continues to have the highest adolescent pregnancy rate of any Western industrialized nation. Factors associated with teen pregnancy include early puberty, substance abuse, alcohol abuse, childhood sexual abuse, Latino ethnicity, teen girls with live-in boyfriends, lack of community-based contraceptive clinics, and lack of an adult role model with whom a teen can discuss sexuality issues (Chamberlain, 2005; Deardorff, Gonzales, Christopher et al., 2005; Harner, 2005; Kelly, 2005; Talashek, 2006).

Adolescent clients need ongoing support throughout labor and the birth process. Each adolescent in labor is different. The nurse must assess what each client brings to the experience by asking the following questions:

- Has the young woman received prenatal care?

- What are her attitudes and feelings about the pregnancy?

- How does her developmental stage influence her behavior, and how are her specific needs different?

- Who will support her during the birth, and what is the person's relationship to her?

- What preparation has she had for the experience?

- What are her expectations and fears regarding labor and birth?

- How has her culture influenced her?
- What are her usual coping mechanisms?
- Does she have adequate social support?
- Does she plan to keep the newborn? If so, does she need to learn parenting skills?
- Will the father of the baby be involved in the labor and birth experience?

Adolescents are at highest risk for pregnancy and labor complications and must be assessed carefully. Any adolescent who has not had prenatal care requires especially close observation during labor. The status of the fetus is monitored to ensure its well-being. The young woman's prenatal record is carefully reviewed for risks. The adolescent is more likely to have poor nutritional intake, preeclampsia, cephalopelvic disproportion (CPD), anemia, drugs ingested during pregnancy, sexually transmitted infections, fetal death, and size-date discrepancies (gestation appears to be less than dates indicate because of minimal weight gain) (Hill, 2004). Infants born to teenage mothers are more likely to have lower birth weights. They are also more likely to be exposed to alcohol, drugs, and tobacco in utero and in early childhood.

The nurse's support role depends on the young woman's support system during labor. When the client is not accompanied by someone who will stay with her during childbirth, it is even more important for the nurse to establish a trusting relationship with her. In this way, the nurse can help her cope with labor and understand what is happening to her. Establishing rapport without recrimination will provide emotional support and encouragement. The adolescent who is given positive reinforcement for "work well done" will leave the experience with increased self-esteem, despite the emotional stress and difficulty of giving birth at such a young age.

The adolescent who has taken childbirth education classes is generally better prepared than the adolescent who has had no preparation. The nurse must keep in mind, however, that the younger the adolescent, the less she may be able to participate actively in the process.

Age-Related Responses to Labor and Birth

The very young adolescent (under age 14) has fewer coping mechanisms and less experience to draw on than her older counterparts have. Because her cognitive development is incomplete, the younger adolescent may have fewer problem-solving capabilities. Her ego integrity may be more threatened by the experience, and she may be more vulnerable to stress and discomfort.

The very young woman needs someone to rely on at all times during labor. She may be more childlike and dependent than older teens. The nurse must be sure that instructions and explanations are simple and concrete. During the transition phase, the young teenager may become withdrawn and unable to express her need to be nurtured. Touch, soothing encouragement, and measures to promote her comfort help her maintain control and meet her needs for dependence. During the second stage of labor, the young adolescent may feel as if she is losing control and may reach out to those around her. By remaining calm and giving directions, the nurse helps her control feelings of helplessness.

One of the most memorable expectant mothers I cared for during my nursing course was Cara, a 13-year-old. I met her each week as she came into the OB clinic at our hospital and stayed with her as she waited for her appointment and was then seen by the medical student. I noticed that with each passing visit, she became more and more anxious. I did my best to determine the source of her anxiety, provided general teaching, and tried to answer all of her questions. I consulted with my professor, and she sat in with me during some visits. But Cara became more and more anxious. Near term, she began asking if she could just have the baby cut out. Whatever was she afraid of? Finally, in the 38th week, after 2½ months of building trust, she told me she was afraid because her baby had gotten too big, and it would never be able to come out through her belly button. I was speechless for a moment. For 2½ months, I had answered questions and felt so proud of my support and teaching, and for all this time, she had not been able to ask the most important question of all—the question that paralyzed her with fear. I was finally able to provide specific information, made drawings on a paper towel, had the medical student talk with her, and best of all, was able to be on call and be with her in labor and during birth. The beautiful smile on her face as her baby daughter was born was unbelievable. Cara wasn't afraid! It's been 39 years since then, and I still remember her.

The middle adolescent (ages 14 to 16 years) often attempts to remain calm and unflinching during labor. If unable to break through the teenager's stoic barrier, the nurse needs to rise above frustration and realize that a caring attitude will still positively affect the young woman.

Many older adolescents (ages 16 to 19 years) feel that they "know it all," but they may be no more prepared for childbirth than their younger counterparts. The nurse's reinforcement and nonjudgmental manner will help them save face. If the adolescent has not taken classes, she may require preparation and explanations. The older teenager's response to the stresses of labor is similar to that of the adult woman.

The Adolescent Father

Consideration of the adolescent father is a very important aspect of labor and birthing care. Nurses need to be aware that this is a stressful time for the young father. There are some specific interventions that increase comfort, enhance education, and perhaps decrease stress. In the early part of labor, the nurse can talk with the father about his expectations for parenting the newborn and what resources are available in the community. Many adolescents are reluctant to ask questions, but an accepting attitude may help in establishing rapport and gaining trust.

The teen father may need encouragement to provide supportive care and to know what actions are acceptable in the birthing area. He may be encouraged to hold the mother's hand, to sit on the bed beside her, to give a back massage, or to stroke her forehead. He may need assistance in how to give a shoulder rub or backrub; he can watch the nurse first and then perform the action himself with the encouragement of the nurse. He may need more encouragement than the older father to share a Jacuzzi or shower or to support the mother in changing positions and ambulating. It is important for the nurse to speak in lay terms and to anticipate questions, to answer all vocalized questions honestly, and to provide opportunities for the parents to ask for further information.

Other Members of the Support Team

In addition to the adolescent's partner, the mother may want her parents or friends with her as members of her support team. Some teens may want their mother as their primary support person, whereas others may strive to prove their independence and "do this on their own." Still other young women may look to friends for advice and support. The nurse includes parents and friends of the adolescent mother in the client teaching and other aspects of the mother's care. It is important to respect the young woman's privacy and honor her wishes regarding whom she wants in the room for the birth. The nurse may have to advocate for the young woman in certain circumstances.

Teaching the Adolescent Mother

During the latent phase of labor, the nurse can explain to the young woman what changes in body sensations and emotional reactions she might anticipate as labor and birth progress. The adolescent also needs teaching about what possible medical procedures (such as EFM, etc.) might be used, as well as what nursing care measures are available. Some adolescents might not realize that they can request the nurse's presence, touch, or advice, unless the nurse specifically informs them that these options are available.

Adolescents are oriented to the present time and may not adequately predict future needs for themselves or their infant. The nurse should assess to make sure adequate resources are available, including infant and postpartum supplies, transportation to and from follow-up visits, and child care, if the adolescent mother is planning on returning to school or work.

Young mothers may need more information on infant care and feeding choices than older women. Some adolescents may be reluctant to breastfeed because of embarrassment or lack of information. The nurse can assist the young woman to explore her feelings related to breastfeeding and provide information (Figure 24–13 ◆). The nurse should provide encouragement and support the young mother's decision. Sometimes, young women feel "pressured" to breastfeed their infants when they truly do not feel comfortable with this feeding choice. The nurse should give the young mother permission to make her own decision. Young women who choose to use formula should be given clear instructions on the importance of mixing the formula per the manufacturer's directions because overdiluting or underdiluting can cause adverse side effects for the baby.

Although more rare than in previous decades, some adolescents may choose to relinquish their newborns. In these situations, the nurse informs the adolescent that seeing the infant can facilitate the grieving process but lets her know that seeing the newborn is her choice. (See Chapter 35 ∞

Figure 24–13 ◆ An adolescent mother receives breastfeeding assistance in the immediate postpartum period.
SOURCE: Amy Etra/PhotoEdit.

for further discussion of the relinquishing mother and the adolescent parent).

NURSING CARE DURING PRECIPITOUS BIRTH

Occasionally, labor progresses so rapidly that the nurse is faced with the task of managing the birth of the baby. This is called a **precipitous birth.** The attending nurse has the primary responsibility for providing a physically and psychologically safe experience for the woman and her baby.

A woman whose physician or CNM is not present may feel disappointed, frightened, cheated, and abandoned, especially if she is not prepared through childbirth education. The nurse can support the woman by keeping her informed about the labor progress and assuring her that the nurse will stay with her. If birth is imminent, the nurse must not leave the mother alone. Auxiliary personnel can be directed to contact the attending physician or CNM, or other physicians or CNMs who are in the facility. The auxiliary personnel should also retrieve the emergency pack ("precip pack"), which should be readily accessible to the birthing/labor rooms. A typical pack contains the following items: a small drape that can be placed under the woman's buttocks to provide a sterile field, a bulb syringe to clear mucus from the newborn's mouth, two sterile clamps (Kelly or Rochester) to clamp the umbilical cord before applying a cord clamp, sterile scissors to cut the umbilical cord, a sterile umbilical cord clamp, a baby blanket to wrap the newborn in after birth, and a package of sterile gloves.

As the materials are being gathered, the nurse must remain calm. The woman is reassured by the nurse's composure and feels that the nurse is competent. The primary goal of nursing care is the safe birth of the infant.

Birth of Infant

The nurse manages precipitous birth in the hospital by encouraging the woman to assume a comfortable position. If time permits, the nurse scrubs both hands with soap and water and puts on sterile gloves. Sterile drapes are placed under the woman's buttocks.

At all times during the birth, the nurse gives clear instructions to the woman, supports her efforts, and provides reassurance. The nurse needs to remain calm and proceed in a slow, confident manner.

Most infants will be born in vertex presentation. When the infant's head crowns, the nurse instructs the woman to either blow or pant, which decreases her urge to push. The nurse checks whether the amniotic sac is intact. If it is, the nurse tears the sac with a clamp so that the newborn will not breathe in amniotic fluid with the first breath.

The nurse may place an index finger inside the lower portion of the vagina and the thumb on the outer portion of the perineum and gently massage the area to aid in stretching of perineal tissues and to help prevent perineal lacerations. This is called "ironing the perineum."

With one hand, the nurse applies gentle pressure against the fetal head to maintain flexion and prevent it from popping out rapidly. The nurse does not hold the head back forcibly. Rapid birth of the head may tear the woman's perineal tissues. The rapid change in pressure within the fetal head may cause subdural or dural tears. The nurse supports the perineum with the other hand and allows the head to be delivered between contractions.

As the woman continues to blow or pant, the nurse inserts one or two fingers along the back of the fetal head to check for the umbilical cord. If the cord is around the neck, the nurse bends her fingers like a fish hook, grasps the cord, and pulls it over the baby's head, loosens it, or slips it down over the shoulders. It is important to check that the cord is not wrapped around more than one time. If the cord is tightly looped and cannot be slipped over the baby's head, the nurse places two clamps on the cord, cuts it between the clamps, and unwinds the cord. Because this ceases oxygenation to the baby, all efforts should be made to reduce (remove) the cord over the head whenever possible. The head typically rotates (restitutes) to the left or right. The nurse needs to let the head rotate (restitute) to the side before attempting delivery of the head.

Immediately after birth of the head, the nurse suctions first the mouth, throat, and then the nasal passages. The nurse places a hand on each side of the head and instructs the woman to push gently so that the rest of the body can be expelled quickly. The newborn must be supported as it emerges.

Breech vaginal births are quite rare. Because the incidence of breech presentations is only 3%, most breech presentations are scheduled for cesarean births, and women are advised to come to the hospital immediately if labor does begin spontaneously. Because the primary concern in a breech birth is to prevent the entrapment of the head in the cervix, intervention is avoided until the buttocks are born. The nurse then pulls down a loop of cord (to avoid stress on its point of insertion) and supports the breech in both hands. The infant's body is lifted slightly upward for birth of the posterior shoulder and arm. The newborn may then be lowered, and the anterior shoulder and arm will pass under the symphysis pubis. Suprapubic pressure should be applied to maintain the normal flexion of the baby's head and should be continued until the baby is born. The nape of the neck pivots under the symphysis, and the rest of the head is born over the perineum by a movement of flexion.

Regardless of the presentation at birth, the newborn is held at the level of the uterus to facilitate blood flow through the umbilical cord immediately after birth. The combination of amniotic fluid and vernix makes the newborn very slippery, so the nurse must be careful to avoid dropping the baby. Placing the woman in stirrups is not recommended for this reason; instead, the foot of the bed can be lowered. The nurse suctions the nose and mouth of the newborn again, using a bulb syringe. The nurse then dries the newborn quickly to prevent heat loss. Wet blankets should be removed and replaced with warmed, dry blankets.

As soon as the nurse determines that the newborn's respirations are adequate, the infant can be placed on the mother's abdomen. The newborn's head should be slightly lower than the body to aid drainage of fluid and mucus. The weight of the newborn on the mother's abdomen stimulates uterine contractions, which aid in placental separation. The umbilical cord should not be pulled. The Apgar score is assessed at 1 and 5 minutes.

The nurse is alert for signs of placental separation. When these signs are present, the nurse places one hand just above the symphysis pubis to guard the uterus and uses the other hand to maintain gentle downward traction on the cord while instructing the mother to push so that the placenta can be expelled. In some instances the mother can squat, and this usually helps expel the placenta. The nurse inspects the placenta to determine whether it is intact. Because the physician or CNM is usually en route, delivery of the placenta can be delayed until the practitioner arrives. Traction should not be applied because this can result in hemorrhage or detaching the umbilical cord from the placenta.

The nurse checks the firmness of the uterus. Palpation of the uterus should not be performed before separation of the placenta. The fundus may be gently massaged to stimulate contractions and decrease bleeding. Putting the newborn to breast also stimulates uterine contractions through release of oxytocin from the pituitary gland.

The umbilical cord may now be cut. Two sterile clamps are placed approximately 2 to 4 inches from the newborn's abdomen. The cord is cut between them with sterile scissors. A sterile cord clamp (Hollister or Hesseltine) can be placed adjacent to the clamp on the newborn's cord, between the clamp and the newborn's abdomen. The clamp must not be placed snugly against the abdomen because the cord will dry and shrink.

The area under the mother's buttocks is cleaned, and her perineum is inspected for lacerations. Bleeding from lacerations may be controlled by pressing a clean perineal pad against the perineum and instructing the woman to keep her thighs together. Further evaluation by the CNM or physician will be needed to determine if lacerations are present that need to be repaired.

If the arrival of the physician or CNM is delayed or if the newborn is having respiratory distress, the newborn should be transported immediately to the nursery. The newborn must be properly identified before he or she leaves the birthing area.

Record Keeping

The nurse notes and places on the record the following information:

1. Position of fetus at birth
2. Presence of cord around neck or shoulder (nuchal cord)
3. Time of birth
4. Apgar scores at 1 and 5 minutes after birth
5. Gender of newborn
6. Time of expulsion of placenta
7. Method of placental expulsion
8. Appearance and intactness of placenta
9. Mother's condition
10. Any medications that were given to mother or newborn (per agency protocol)

Postbirth Interventions

Postbirth interventions are the same as those listed under Nursing Care During the Third Stage of Labor.

EVALUATION

Evaluation provides an opportunity to determine the effectiveness of nursing care. As a result of comprehensive nursing care during the intrapartal period, the following outcomes may be anticipated:

- The mother's physical needs and the psychologic well-being of the family have been maintained and supported.
- The baby's physical and psychologic well-being has been protected and supported.
- The family has had input into the birth process, and members have participated as much as they desired.
- The birth was safe and promoted family cohesiveness.

CHAPTER REVIEW

FOCUS YOUR STUDY

- Admission to the birth setting involves assessment of many physiologic, psychologic, and social factors. The information gained helps the nurse establish priorities of care.
- Before initiating care, the nurse explains what will be done, the reasons, potential benefits and risks, and possible alternatives if appropriate. This helps the woman determine what happens to her body and is a critical element in the process of obtaining informed consent.
- Behavioral responses to labor vary with the phase of labor, the woman's preparation and previous experience, cultural beliefs, and developmental level.
- Each woman's cultural beliefs affect her need for privacy, her expression of discomfort, her expectations for the birth, and the role she wishes the father to play in the birth event.
- The laboring woman's comfort may be increased by general comfort measures, supportive relaxation techniques, methods of handling anxiety, controlled breathing, and support by a caring person.
- The laboring woman fears being alone during labor. Even though there is a support person available, the woman's anxiety may be decreased when the nurse remains with her.

- Maternal birthing positions include a wide variety of possibilities, such as recumbent, side-lying, sitting, squatting, and crouching on hands and knees.
- Immediate assessments of the newborn include evaluation of the Apgar score and an abbreviated physical assessment. These early assessments help determine whether there is a need for resuscitation and whether the newborn's adaptation to extrauterine life is progressing normally. The newborn who is not experiencing problems may remain with the parents for an extended period of time following birth.
- Immediate care of the newborn following birth also includes maintaining respirations, promoting warmth, preventing infection, and providing accurate identification.
- The new parents and their baby are given time together as soon as possible after birth.
- Nursing assessments continue after the birth and are important to ensure that normal physiologic adaptations are taking place.
- The adolescent has special needs in the birth setting. Her developmental needs require specialized nursing care.
- Nurse-assisted births are sometimes performed in the absence of the CNM or physician when birth is imminent.

EXPLORE MEDIALINK

 http://www.prenhall com/davidson

NCLEX review questions, case studies, and other interactive resources for this chapter can be found on the Web Site at http://www.prenhall.com/davidson. Click on "Chapter 24" to select the activities for this chapter.

For tutorials including animations and videos, more NCLEX review questions, and an audio glossary, access the accompanying Prentice Hall Nursing MediaLink DVD-ROM in this book.

 PRENTICE HALL NURSING MEDIALINK DVD-ROM

Audio Glossary

NCLEX Review

Videos: *First Stage of Labor; First Stage of Labor—Transition; Second Stage of Labor; Third Stage of Labor—Part 1; Third Stage of Labor—Part 2; Third Stage of Labor—Part 3; Newborn Assessment; Delivery of Placenta; Fourth Stage of Labor; Through the Eyes of a Nurse—The Third Trimester*

Animation: *Placental Delivery*

COMPANION WEBSITE

Additional NCLEX Review

Care Plan Activity: *Presence of Extended Family*

Case Study: *Labor and Birth of Client Who Received No Prenatal Care*

Applications: *Developing a Birth Plan; Positioning Options During Labor and Delivery; Cord Blood Banking*

Critical Thinking

CRITICAL THINKING IN ACTION

LABOR STRESS AND ANXIETY REDUCTION

View the Critical Thinking in Action video in Chapter 24 of the DVD-ROM. Then answer the questions that follow.

Anita Grey, a 22-year-old primigravida at 40 weeks' gestation, is admitted to you in the birthing center in labor. Anita was sent from her physician's office after being evaluated at her prenatal visit. While in the office, she was assessed to be 4 cm dilated, 100% effaced, vertex at 0 station with bulging membranes. She tells you that her husband is on his way to the birthing center and she is anxious for him to arrive. A review of her prenatal record shows no complications affecting this pregnancy. Anita's vital signs are within normal limits. You assess the fetal heart rate and contraction pattern with the fetal monitor and observe a fetal heart rate of 140 to 150 bpm with accelerations to 160s. Contractions are every 3 to 4 minutes x 30 seconds of moderate intensity by palpation. Anita seems to be tolerating the contractions well but still seems anxious about her husband's arrival.

1. What steps can you take to reduce the stress and anxiety of the laboring woman and her family?

2. When you notify the physician or midwife, what pertinent information should the report contain?

3. What support measures can you give in the active phase of labor?

4. What measures can be used to decrease discomfort/pain as labor progresses?

5. What observations reflect the physiologic manifestations of pain?

REFERENCES

Alan Guttmacher Institute. (2004). *U.S. pregnancy statistics: Overall trends, trends by race and ethnicity, and state by state information.* New York: Author.

American Academy of Pediatrics (AAP) & American College of Obstetricians and Gynecologists (ACOG). (2002). *Guidelines for perinatal care* (5th ed.). Washington, DC: Author.

American College of Obstetricians and Gynecologists (ACOG). (2002). *Analgesia and cesarean delivery rates* (ACOG Committee Opinion, No. 269). Washington, DC: Author.

American College of Obstericians and Gynecologists (ACOG). (2005). *Intrapartum fetal heart rate monitoring* (ACOG Practice Bulletin, No. 70). Washington, DC: Author.

American College of Obstetricians and Gynecologists (ACOG). (2006). *The Apgar score* (ACOG Committee Opinion No. 333). Washington, DC: Author.

Association of Women's Health, Obstetric, and Neonatal Nurses (AWHONN). (2003a). *Fetal heart rate monitoring: Principles and practice* (3rd ed.). Washington, DC: Author.

Association of Women's Health, Obstetric, and Neonatal Nurses (AWHONN). (2003b). *Standards for professional nursing practice in the care of women and newborns* (6th ed.). Washington, DC: Author.

Benfield, R. D. (2002). Hydrotherapy in labor. *Journal of Nursing Scholarship, 34*(4), 347–352.

Blackburn, S. T. (2007). *Maternal, fetal, and neonatal physiology: A clinical perspective* (3rd ed.). Philadelphia: Saunders.

Bowes, W. A. (2005). Prognostic value of change in amniotic fluid color during labor. *Obstetrical & Gynecological Survey, 60*(7), 425–426.

Chamberlain, L. J. (2005). Child advocacy training: Curriculum outcomes and resident satisfaction. *Archives in Pediatric & Adolescent Medicine, 159*(9), 842–847.

Centers for Disease Control and Prevention (2004). *Routine prenatal testing the opt-out approach.* Atlanta: Author.

Cheung, N. F. (2002). The cultural and social meanings of childbearing for Chinese and Scottish women in Scotland. *Midwifery, 18*(4), 279–295.

Cluett, E. R., Pickering, R. M., Getliffe, K., & St. George-Saunders, N. J. (2004). Randomised controlled trial of labouring in water compared with standard of augmentation for management of dystocia in first stage of labour. *British Medical Journal, 328*(7435), 314.

Deardorff, J., Gonzales, N. A., Christopher, F. S., Roosa, M. W., & Millsap, R. E. (2005). Early puberty and adolescent pregnancy: The influence of alcohol use. *Pediatrics, 116*(6), 1451–1456.

Hansen, S. L., Clark, S. L., & Foster, J. C. (2002). Active pushing versus passive fetal descent in the second stage of labor: A randomized controlled trial. *Obstetrics and Gynecology, 99*, 29–34.

Harner, H. M. (2005). Childhood sexual abuse, teenage pregnancy, and partnering with adult men: Exploring the relationship. *Journal of Psychosocial Nursing and Mental Health Services, 43*(8), 20–28.

Her, C. (2004). Culturally responsive care for Hmong patients. Collaboration is a key treatment component. *Postgraduate Medicine, 116*(6), 39–42, 45–46.

Hill, S. D. (2004). The association between adverse childhood experiences and adolescent pregnancy, long-term psychosocial consequences, and fetal death. *Pediatrics, 113*(2), 320–327.

Hottenstein, S. E. (2005). Continuous labor support: Creating optimal birth experiences through theory-driven nursing care. *AWHONN Lifelines, 9*(3), 242–247.

Johnson, R., & Taylor, W. (2005). *Skills for midwifery practice* (2nd ed.). Oxford: Churchill-Livingstone.

Kelly, L. S. (2005). Why lightning strikes twice: Postpartum resumption of sexual activity during adolescence. *Journal of Pediatrics and Adolescent Gynecology, 18*(5), 327–335.

McLachlan, H., & Waldenstrom, U. (2005). Childbirth experiences in Australia of women born in Turkey, Vietnam, and Australia. *Birth: Issues in Perinatal Care, 32*(4), 272–282.

Mercer, J. S. (2005). Nuchal cord management and nurse-midwifery practice. *Journal of Midwifery & Women's Health, 50*(5), 373–379.

Moise, K. J. (2005). Umbilical cord stem cells. *Obstetrics and Gynecology, 106*, 1393–1407.

Moore, M. L. (2002). Research update: Misoprostol, is more research needed? *Journal of Perinatal Education, 11*(3), 43–47.

Naber, M. (2005). A family affair. *Nursing, 35*(10), 51.

Quaye, R. K. (2005). *African Americans health care practices, perspectives, and needs.* Lanham, MD: University Press of America

Parsons, M. (2004). A midwifery practice dichotomy on oral intake in labour. *Midwifery, 20*(1), 72–81.

Rabe, H. (2005). Early versus delayed umbilical cord clamping in preterm infants. *Cochrane Library* (4).

Reece, A., & Hobbins, J. (2006). *Clinical obstetrics handbook.* Boston: Blackwell Publishing.

Roberts, J. E. (2003). A new understanding of the second stage of labor: Implications for nursing care. *Journal of Obstetric, Gynecologic, & Neonatal Nursing 32*(6), 794–801.

Safadi, R. (2005). Jordanian women: Perceptions and practices in first time pregnancy. *International Journal of Nursing Practice, 11*(6), 269–276.

Shamshad, M., & Crown, L. A. (2005). A Muslim's family experience with acute care. *Family Practice Recertification, 27*(1), 27–30.

Shilling, T. (2004). Care practices that promote normal birth #2: Freedom of movement throughout labor. *Journal of Perinatal Education, 13*(2), 11–15.

Simpson K. R. (2005). The context and clinical evidence for common nursing practices during labor. *American Journal of Maternal/Child Nursing, 30*(6), 356–365.

Spector, R. E. (2004). *Cultural diversity in health and illness* (6th ed.). Upper Saddle River, NJ: Prentice Hall.

Stremler, R. (2005). Randomized controlled trial of hands-and-knees positioning for occipitoposterior position in labor. *Birth: Issues in Perinatal Care, 32*(4), 243–251.

Talashek, M. L. (2006). Untangling the health disparities of teen pregnancy. *Journal of Specialized Pediatric Nursing, 11*(1), 14–27.

Tramner, J. E. (2005, May–June). The effect of unrestricted oral carbohydrate intake on labor progress [includes abstract]. *Journal of Obstetric, Gynecologic, & Neonatal Nursing, 34*(3), 319–328.

Verhey, M. P., Levy, J., & Schmidt, R. (2004, November 16). Abuse in pregnancy. *Cinahl Information Systems* (2).

Wilson, B. A., Shannon, M. T., & Stang, C. L. (2006). *Nurse's drug guide: 2006.* Upper Saddle River, NJ: Prentice Hall.

25 Pain Management During Labor

We had attended childbirth classes and practiced through the last few weeks, and I had hoped to go through all of labor and birth without medication. But when the contractions really came on strong, I just wasn't ready for the amount and the kind of pain that I felt. I've always been able to tolerate pain well, but this was different. My husband and I talked about it and he reassured me that, if I felt I needed something, it was okay with him. My nurse was also very supportive. She helped me feel I was making a good decision and wasn't failing somehow.

OBJECTIVES

1. Discuss the nurse's role in supporting pharmaceutical pain relief measures in labor.
2. Describe the use of systemic analgesics to promote pain relief during labor.
3. Compare the major types of regional analgesia and anesthesia, including area affected, advantages, disadvantages, techniques, and nursing implications.
4. Summarize possible complications of regional anesthesia.
5. Describe the three methods used to provide general anesthesia.
6. Delineate the major complications of general anesthesia.
7. Identify contraindications to specific types of analgesia and anesthesia for high-risk mothers.

KEY TERMS

Epidural block   696
General anesthesia   710
Local anesthesia   709
Pudendal block   708

Regional analgesia   694
Regional anesthesia   693
Spinal block   702

MEDIALINK

Additional resources for this content can be found on the Prentice Hall Nursing MediaLink DVD-ROM and on the Companion Website at http://www.prenhall.com/davidson. Click on "Chapter 25" to select the activities for this chapter.

When a childbearing woman experiences discomfort during labor and birth, the nurse can assist her to have a positive birth experience by providing effective comfort measures. Nursing interventions directed toward pain relief begin with the nonpharmacologic measures described in Chapter 24 ∞ , such as providing information, encouragement, backrubs, and clean linens. Many women need no further interventions.

For other women, the progression of labor brings increasing levels of pain that interfere with their ability to cope effectively. For these women, pharmacologic agents may be used to decrease discomfort, increase relaxation, and reestablish the ability to participate more actively in the labor and birth experience. In addition to systemic analgesics, regional nerve blocks (epidural, spinal, and combined epidural-spinal) and local anesthetic blocks (pudendal and perineal) are available. The methods are not mutually exclusive and may be used in combination with nonpharmacologic comfort measures.

Nurses need to recognize that the decision to have an unmedicated or a medicated birth involves many factors and reflects a great deal of thought and planning for most women and their families. Some of these factors include client and caregiver preferences, availability of anesthesia and analgesia, fear of risks and complications, past life experiences, previous experiences with pain, and cultural influences. Other factors, such as the amount of sleep the woman has had or the length of labor, can also influence the need or desire for pharmacologic pain relief measures. The woman should be supported regardless of her decision even if it changes during the course of labor.

Each year in the United States, over 4 million infants are born. Of these births, 50% of all women will receive epidural anesthesia (Wong, Scavone, Peaceman et al., 2005). Many couples who have had childbirth education approach their birth experience confident that the techniques they have learned will enable them to cope with the pain of labor. Nurses should respect these couples' choices and provide support to help them meet their goals. Analgesics and anesthetics do affect the fetus and can be accompanied by maternal side effects. Following an unmedicated birth, many women report a quicker postpartum recovery. Many are able to ambulate, urinate, shower, and eat within an hour of giving birth. Additionally, many women feel an enormous sense of empowerment after successfully having an unmedicated birth.

For the woman who has advised the nursing staff that she wants no pharmacologic remedies, the nurse should offer alternative comfort measures. All nurses in the intrapartum setting need to be familar with various nonpharmacologic techniques available to help women cope with the pain they may experience. The nurse should avoid offering these women pain medications unless they specifically ask for them or for information about pharmacologic options.

On the other hand, many women are simply unprepared for the intense pain of active labor and may request medication. They may begin labor undecided about whether to use medication, then request pain relief as contractions intensify. Frequently, feelings of inadequacy and guilt accompany such decisions. The nurse plays a special role in assisting the woman and her partner to explore their options for pain relief realistically. The nurse can explain to the couple that, although pharmacologic agents do affect the fetus, so do the pain and stress experienced by the laboring mother. In response to stress, the woman's ventilation and oxygen consumption increase, which decreases the amount of oxygen available to the fetus. In addition, pain and stress can lead to metabolic acidosis and the release of catecholamines, causing the maternal blood vessels to constrict. This in turn decreases oxygen and nutrient supply to the fetus (Florence & Palmer, 2003). Thus, if the woman's pain and anxiety are more than she can cope with, the adverse physiologic effects on the fetus may be as great as would occur with the administration of a small amount of an analgesic agent. The nurse should reassure the woman and her partner that accepting medication for pain is not a failure. The emphasis should be on the goal of a healthy, satisfying outcome for the family.

I felt really prepared for labor! We went through all of the classes and had envisioned the "perfect birth." After 16 hours of labor and no progress, I was exhausted and frustrated; sobbing, I totally broke down. I felt like a failure for getting an epidural. My nurse, Madison, was great! She comforted me and reinforced that I was not a failure. She reassured me that in the end the most important thing would be holding my daughter in my arms. She was right, my despair was forgotten when I was able to enjoy the rest of labor, rest, and get some much needed sleep before Katherine was born. As I gazed at my newborn daughter, I learned what was really important that day, and in my life!

SYSTEMIC ANALGESIA

The goal of systemic analgesia during labor is to provide maximal pain relief with minimal risk for the woman and fetus.

Multiple factors must be considered in the use of analgesic agents:

- Effects on the woman
- Effects on the fetus
- Effects on the labor contractions
- Medical status of the woman
- Progress of labor

The effects on the mother are of primary importance, because the well-being of the fetus depends on adequate functioning of the maternal cardiopulmonary system. Any alteration of function that disturbs the woman's homeostatic mechanism affects the fetal environment. Maintaining the maternal respiratory rate and blood pressure within normal range is thus of prime importance. The use of electronic fetal monitoring (EFM) provides a means of accurately assessing the effects of pharmacologic agents on uterine contractions.

All systemic analgesics can cross the placental barrier by simple diffusion, with some agents crossing more readily than others. Drug action in the body depends on the rate at which the substance is metabolized by liver enzymes and excreted by the kidneys. The fetal liver enzymes and renal systems are inadequate to metabolize analgesic agents, so high doses remain active in fetal circulation for a prolonged period of time. The percentage of blood volume flowing to the fetal brain increases during intrauterine stress, so the hypoxic fetus receives an even larger amount of a depressant drug. The blood-brain barrier is more permeable at the time of birth, a factor that also increases the amount of drug carried to the central nervous system (Kuczkowski, 2004b).

Administration of Analgesic Agents

The optimal time for administering analgesia is determined after a complete assessment of many factors. In the past, an analgesic agent was administered to nulliparas when the active phase of labor was well established (cervix had dilated to 5 or 6 cm) and to multiparas when the cervix had reached 3 or 4 cm dilatation. This practice is now seen as only a generalization, however; the character of each labor must be taken into account. There is debate on the ideal timing of medication administration; however, both the American College of Obstetricians and Gynecologists (ACOG) and the American Society of Anesthesiologists (ASA) agree that a woman's request for pain medications is ample reason to administer them (ACOG, 2002). In general, the woman should receive pain medication when she is uncomfortable and in a well-established labor pattern with contractions occurring regularly and of significant duration with moderate to strong intensity. Analgesia given too early may prolong labor and depress the fetus. Analgesia given too late is of no value to the woman and may cause neonatal respiratory depression. In many institutions, the nurse decides when to give the analgesic agent prescribed by the physician, certified nurse-midwife (CNM), or certified registered nurse-anesthetist (CRNA). The nurse observes the woman for cues that indicate she would benefit from the administration of analgesics. The nurse performs needed assessments (as discussed in the next section) and then notifies the CNM or physician. The decision to administer pain medication is based on a complete assessment of the woman and the progress of labor. The CNM or physician may evaluate the woman at the bedside or may rely on the nurse's assessment and instruct the nurse to administer the medications. In most institutions, the CRNA is available to monitor analgesia-related complications and provide ongoing monitoring for women who later receive an epidural. Some facilities may have anesthesiologists (physicians who specialize in administering anesthesia) provide these services.

MATERNAL ASSESSMENT

The following maternal assessments are critical before administering systemic analgesics:

- The woman is willing to receive medication after being advised about it.
- Vital signs are stable.
- Contraindications (such as drug allergies, respiratory compromise, or current drug dependence) are not present.
- Knowledge of other medications being administered, such as magnesium sulfate or tocolytics.

FETAL ASSESSMENT

The following assessments of the fetus are also required:

The fetal heart rate (FHR) is between 110 and 160 beats per minute, reactive nonstress test (NST) (accelerations of FHR are present with fetal movement), short-term variability is present, long-term variability is average, and periodic late decelerations or nonperiodic (variable) decelerations are absent.

ASSESSMENT OF LABOR

The following assessment parameters must also be evaluated:

- Contraction pattern
- Cervical dilatation
- Fetal presenting part
- Station of the fetal presenting part.

If normal parameters are absent or if nonreassuring maternal or fetal factors are present, the nurse may need to complete further assessments with the physician or CNM. In addition, no complications that would preclude administering an analgesic agent should be present, such as drug allergies or drug-specific contraindications.

Before administering the medication, the nurse once again ascertains whether the woman has a history of any drug reactions or allergies and provides information regarding the medication (Table 25–1). After giving the medication, the nurse records the drug name, dose, route, site, and the woman's blood pressure and pulse (before and after) on the EFM strip and on the woman's record. If the woman is alone, the nurse raises the side rails to provide safety and assesses the FHR for possible side effects of the medication.

Oral analgesics are not used because they are poorly absorbed and gastric emptying time is prolonged during labor. The intramuscular (IM), intravenous (IV), or subcutaneous (SC) routes are used instead. For IM administration, the needle must be of sufficient length to penetrate the muscle and the subcutaneous fat. The IV route is preferred because it results in prompt, smooth, and more predictable action with a smaller total dose required than the IM route. When an agent is given intravenously, it is suggested that the injection be given with the onset of a contraction, when the blood flow to the uterus and the fetus is normally decreased (Wylie, 2005).

When an analgesic medication is administered by IM or SC route, it takes a few minutes for the effect to be felt. The nurse can continue with other supportive measures to enhance

Table 25–1 WHAT WOMEN NEED TO KNOW ABOUT PAIN RELIEF MEDICATIONS

Before receiving medications, the woman should understand the following:
- Type of medication administered
- Route of administration
- Expected effects of medication
- Implications for fetus/newborn
- Safety measures needed (for example, remain in bed with side rails up)
- Side effects/complications

comfort until the effect of the medication is perceived. When the medication begins to take effect, the woman may be able to sleep between contractions. This short period of rest can restore her energy. When an IV route is prescribed, the woman feels the effect of the drug within a minute or two, so if any change of position is necessary or if the woman needs to void, the nurse may suggest that these activities be completed before the drug is administered (Nagoette, 2006). Some women may be so uncomfortable that they do not want anything except the medication. Administering the medication first is more helpful for these women. As in all cases when there is a possibility of coming into contact with body fluids, standard precautions should be used. Consistent handwashing before and after procedures along with wearing disposable gloves can reduce the risk of blood or body fluid exposure. Sometimes analgesics are administered via IV and IM routes simultaneously. The benefit of this technique is that the woman receives a rapid onset from the IV route as well as the longer duration of pain control that is achieved with the IM route (Nagoette, 2006).

Sedatives

In current labor and birth practice, sedatives are used primarily in the early latent phase of labor, when the cervix is long, closed, and thick, and rest is prescribed for the expectant woman. Sedatives promote relaxation and allow the woman to sleep for a few hours. Upon the woman's awakening, contractions have either ceased (i.e., the woman was in false labor) or contractions return and take on a regular pattern that promotes changes in cervical dilatation and effacement. Sedatives should not be given when a woman is in active labor because they can cause respiratory depression in the infant. Sedatives have minimal analgesic properties and can actually increase the reaction to painful stimuli. They should be administered only to decrease anxiety and promote sleep, because they cross the placenta and can cause depression in the newborn (Mattingly, D'Alessio, & Ramanathan, 2003).

BARBITURATES

The most common barbiturates used in labor are secobarbital (Seconal) and zolpidem tartrate (Ambien). Seconal is fast acting, usually providing effects in 10 to 15 minutes with a duration of 3 to 4 hours. It is administered orally and is well tolerated. Its primary role is to treat false labor and produce a sedation effect. Both Seconal and Ambien can be used in latent labor to promote rest and relaxation and thereby prevent maternal exhaustion. Hypnotic effects also occur with many drugs in this category. Seconal has a long half-life and can remain in the maternal and fetal blood for up to 40 hours after administration, whereas Ambien has a half life of 4.5 hours (Florence & Palmer, 2003). For this reason, Ambien may be more desirable for women in early labor. A barbiturate should not be administered to women in active labor because it can cause fetal depression and, in fact, is rarely used at anytime during true labor.

BENZODIAZEPINES

Benzodiazepines, such as diazepam (Valium), are similar to barbiturates in their mechanism of action. They are primarily used to treat anxiety. They can also be used for their anticonvulsant action. They have a rapid onset of action and are absorbed quite easily when ingested orally. Although this class of drugs can be used to decrease anxiety, some have an amnesic effect, which may not be desirable for childbearing women. Fetal side effects have been reported but are usually mild. These include a decrease in variability of the FHR (Braveman, 2006). Midazolam (Versed), which is commonly used during operative procedures, has been associated with low Apgar scores when administered 5 minutes or less before birth. Because of this side effect, it is not advisable to use midazolam for childbearing women (Rayburn & Bogenschutz, 2004). It is primarily used for maternal anxiety during cesarean births and is given after the fetus is born when the surgical procedure is being completed. Flumazenil, the drug used to reverse benzodiazepine sedative effects, should be kept on hand in case of accidental overdose.

H₁-RECEPTOR ANTAGONISTS

H₁-receptor antagonists block the action of histamines at the receptor sites. These drugs cross the blood-brain barrier and inhibit N-methyltransferase, which is a by-product of histamine. It is this mechanism that leads to the sedative effects of this class of drugs. In addition, these drugs also have anti-Parkinson and antiemetic effects. There are seven subtypes of H₁-receptor antagonists. These drugs cause drowsiness and are frequently used in early labor to promote sleep and decrease anxiety. The degree of drowsiness experienced depends on which drug is administered. Common H₁-receptor antagonists used in labor include promethazine (Phenergan), hydroxyzine (Vistaril), and diphenhydramine (Benadryl) (Florence & Palmer, 2003).

Promethazine (Phenergan), which is a phenothiazine, results in marked sedation and is often combined with opiates because it potentiates their effects. It also has strong antiemetic effects and can be combined with opiates to relieve nausea and vomiting, which can be a side effect of certain drugs, like meperidine (Demerol). All phenothiazines cross the placental barrier and can result in decreased beat-to-beat variability. Promethazine has not, however, resulted in lower Apgar scores. Phenothiazines can also bind to bilirubin binding sites in newborns whose mothers are exposed to the drug at term. This can result in an increased incidence of neonatal hyperbilirubinemia and jaundice (Florence & Palmer, 2003).

Hydroxyzine (Vistaril) is a piperazine subtype. It can be given in early or prodromal labor to decrease anxiety and nausea. It also results in sedation so the mother can rest. This drug is administered intramuscularly in a large muscle. Women in false labor are able to rest and frequently will awaken to find that their uterine contractions have dissipated. Commonly, women who receive this drug in early or prodromal labor are able to rest and frequently enter active labor (Braveman, 2006).

Diphenhydramine (Benadryl) is an ethanolamine subtype of the H₁ antagonists. Most commonly, this over-the-counter medication is used to treat allergic rhinitis and urticaria; however, it also possesses sedative and antiemetic properties that can be used to treat women in early labor. The drug has a relatively short half-life (1 to 4 hours) and can last up to 6 to 8 hours (Braveman, 2006). Nurses can advise women to use this drug at home if medically indicated, because it is readily available. It should be noted that this drug causes agitation in some women. If this side effect occurs, women should discontinue the medication (Wilson, Shannon, & Stang, 2006).

NURSING CARE MANAGEMENT

The nurse should carefully assess the woman before administration of analgesic agents. Common indications for various medications are summarized in Table 25–2. Because they are not indicated for women in active labor, the nurse needs to determine the stage of labor. The nurse should evaluate the woman to determine the frequency, duration, and intensity of her contractions (Nagoette, 2006). A vaginal exam is performed to determine if cervical change has occurred. Fetal well-being is established by obtaining electronic fetal monitoring and ensuring a reactive fetal heart tracing. The nurse should explain the desired effects of the medication and possible side effects. If the woman is not in active labor, she can be given the medication and be advised to return home and rest. Since drowsiness can occur, however, the nurse needs to ensure the woman has a safe form of transportation home. Nurses need to review the symptoms of active labor and warning signs and advise the woman to call her healthcare provider should they occur.

Narcotic Analgesics

Narcotic analgesic agents that are injected into the circulation have their primary action at sites in the brain. Specifically, a narcotic that diffuses out of cerebral capillaries and reaches the periventricular/periaqueductal gray matter of the brain activates the neurons that descend to the spinal cord and inhibits the transmission of pain impulses in the substantia gelatinosa. Nausea and vomiting are produced by stimulation of the medullary chemoreceptor trigger zone.

A brief discussion of some selected narcotic analgesic agents follows. The drugs are summarized in Table 25–3.

Table 25–2 COMMON INDICATIONS FOR MEDICATIONS IN LABOR				
Drug	Pain Relief	Anxiety or Apprehension	Sedation	Antiemetic
Demerol (meperidine)	X		X	
Nubain (nalbuphine)	X		X	
Phenergan (promethazine)		X	X	X
Stadol (butorphanol)	X		X	
Vistaril (hydroxyzine)		X	X	
Seconal (secobarbital)		X	X	X
Benadryl (diphenhydramine hydrochloride)		X	X	X

BUTORPHANOL TARTRATE (STADOL)

Butorphanol tartrate (Stadol) is a mixed agonist-antagonist agent. The analgesic potency is 30 to 40 times that of meperidine and 7 times that of morphine (Wilson et al., 2006). Administration of butorphanol reverses the analgesic effect of other opioids or narcotics in the woman's body and precipitates withdrawal in drug-dependent individuals. For this reason, it is important to assess each woman's history of narcotic drug use during the admission assessment; if she has been using drugs, she should not receive butorphanol.

For the woman in labor, butorphanol is most frequently given by the IV route; however, it can also be given by IM injection. When administered intravenously, the recommended dose is 1 to 2 mg (the smaller dose is most frequently used). The onset of action is rapid, peak analgesia occurs in 30 to 60 minutes and duration is 3 to 4 hours (Wilson et al., 2006). If given by IM route, the recommended dose is 1 to 2 mg, although 2 mg is the most usual dose. Onset of action occurs in 10 to 15 minutes, peak analgesia occurs in 30 to 60 minutes, and duration is 3 to 4 hours (Wilson et al., 2006).

Respiratory depression of both the mother and fetus/newborn can occur. The effects of butorphanol (Stadol) can be reversed with naloxone (Narcan). Although not a common side effect, urinary retention can occur. The nurse should frequently assess the woman's bladder for distention. The nurse may need to perform an in-and-out catheterization using sterile technique to alleviate bladder distention. Major side effects include somnolence, dizziness, and feelings of dysphoria (Cunningham, Leveno, Bloom et al., 2005).

NURSING CARE MANAGEMENT

Administering butorphanol with other central nervous system depressants, such as sedatives, phenothiazides, other tranquilizers, hypnotic agents, and general anesthetics, can exacerbate respiratory depression and cause other effects. For this reason, the nurse should evaluate the woman's respiratory and cardiac status by careful observation of vital signs and pulse oximetry. The woman's level of consciousness is also checked frequently. Continuous electronic monitoring of the FHR pattern is recommended. Respiratory depression in the mother or fetus/newborn can be reversed by naloxone (Narcan), which is a specific antagonist for this agent. The nurse ensures that naloxone is readily available should respiratory depression occur. A slightly depressed newborn is not likely to experience prolonged drowsiness or sluggishness, however, because the metabolites of butorphanol are inactive.

NALBUPHINE HYDROCHLORIDE (NUBAIN)

Like butorphanol, nalbuphine hydrochloride (Nubain) is a synthetic agonist-antagonist narcotic analgesic and may precipitate drug withdrawal if the woman is physically dependent on narcotics (Florence & Palmer, 2003). Nalbuphine crosses the

| Table 25–3 | ANALGESICS USED IN LABOR | | | |

Drug/Class	Dosage, Route, Frequency	Common Side Effects	Life-Threatening Reactions	Contraindications
Stadol (butorphanol tartrate): CNS agent, analgesic, narcotic agonist/antagonist	IM 1–4 mg every 3–4 hours IV 0.5–2 mg every 6–8 hours. Intranasal: 1 mg (1 puff) may repeat in 90 seconds (max dose every 3–4 hours)	Sedation	Respiratory depression	Narcotic dependency, breastfeeding
Nubain (nalbuphine hydrochloride): CNS agent, analgesic, narcotic agonist, antagonist	10–20 mg every 3–6 hours prn SC/IM/IV	Sedation; sweaty, clammy skin; nausea and vomiting	Respiratory depression	Hypersensitivity to the drug
Demerol (meperidine hydrochloride): CNS agent, analgesic, narcotic agonist	50–00 mg IM or SC every 3–4 hours 25–50 mg IV every 3–4 hours	Nausea, vomiting, itching, urinary retention, sedation, respiratory depression, dizziness	Respiratory depression in mother and/or newborn, seizures, cardiovascular collapse, cardiac arrest, bronchoconstriction	Narcotic dependency, epilepsy, hypersensitivity to the drug
Morphine (morphine sulfate): CNS agent, analgesic, narcotic, agonist	IV 2.5–15 mg every 4 hours IM/SC 5–20 mg every 4 hours	Pruritus, constipation, nausea	Anaphylactic reaction, respiratory depression; overdose; respiratory arrest, cardiac arrest	Hypersensitivity to opiates, increased intracranial pressure, convulsive disorders, acute alcoholism, acute asthma, chronic pulmonary diseases, decreased respirations, pulmonary edema, biliary tract surgery, anastomosis, pancreatitis, acute ulcerative colitis, liver/renal insufficiency, Addison disease, hypothyroidism
Phenergan (promethazine hydrochloride): GI agent, antiemetic, antivertigo agent, phenothiazine	25–50 mg every 3–4 hours po/pr/IM/IV	Sedation, drowsiness, dry mouth, blurred vision	Respiratory depression, agranulocytosis	Hypersensitivity to phenothiazines, glaucoma, peptic ulcer, pyloroduodenal obstruction, bladder neck obstruction, epilepsy, bone marrow depression, and breastfeeding
Vistaril (hydroxyzine pamoate): antihistamine, antianxiety, sedative, antipruritic, antiemetic	25–100 mg PO/IM every 6 hours	Sedation, dizziness, dry mouth, nausea, headache	Seizures	Hypersensitivity to drug, use with caution in glaucoma, urinary retention
Benadryl (diphenhydramine hydrochloride): antihistamine, antiemetic, antivertigo, antitussive, sedative-hypnotic	25–50 mg every 6 hours PO/IM/IV	Drowsiness, sedation, dry mouth, hypotension, nausea and vomiting, GI symptoms	Anaphylaxis, seizures, coma, respiratory depression	Hypersensitivity to drug, use during an acute asthma attack, use with caution in glaucoma, bladder obstruction, hypertension, hypothyroidism, renal disease

placenta to the fetus and can cause nonreassuring fetal status and neonatal respiratory depression (Florence & Palmer, 2003). Nalbuphine may be given by the IM, SC, or IV route. It is most frequently given by the IV route in the birth setting. The usual dose for adults is 10 mg/70 kg. If given intravenously, onset of action occurs in 2 to 3 minutes, peak of action occurs in 15 to 20 minutes, and duration is 3 to 6 hours. When given by the IM or SC route, the onset of action occurs in less than 15 minutes, peak of action occurs in 30 to 60 minutes, and duration is 3 to 6 hours. When given by the IV route, nalbuphine may be given directly into the tubing of a running IV infusion; 10 mg should be administered over 3 to 5 minutes (Florence & Palmer, 2003). Adverse effects in the woman include respiratory depression, drowsiness, dizziness, crying, blurred vision, nausea, diaphoresis, and urinary urgency (Florence & Palmer, 2003). See Drug Guide: Nalbuphine Hydrochloride (Nubain).

NURSING CARE MANAGEMENT

The nurse assesses the woman's history to identify contraindications to use of nalbuphine, such as the possibility of current narcotic drug dependence, sensitivity to sulfites, and history of asthma (Florence & Palmer, 2003). If no contraindications exist, the IV route is frequently used during labor. The woman's respiratory rate, quality of respirations, and characteristics of the FHR must be carefully assessed. Anticipation of urinary urgency is important. Because the woman may experience dizziness and sedation, use of a bedpan may be necessary.

DRUG GUIDE   Nalbuphine Hydrochloride (Nubain)

Overview of Action

Nubain is a synthetic narcotic analgesic with agonist and weak antagonist properties. Analgesic properties are equal to that produced by morphine. Nubain's potency is 3 to 4 times greater than pentazocine. The incidence of respiratory depression that occurs is equivalent to morphine.

Dosage Route

Nubain is indicated for moderate to severe pain. Adults: 10–20 mg every 3–6 hours prn SC/IM/IV.

Maternal Contraindications

Hypersensitivity or allergy to nalbuphine hydrochloride.

Maternal Side Effects

Sedation; clammy, sweaty skin; dry mouth; bitter taste in mouth; nausea and vomiting; dizziness; vertigo; nervousness; restlessness; depression; crying; euphoria; dysphoria; confusion; hallucinations; unusual dreams; distortion of body image; numbness; tingling sensations; headache; miosis; hypertension; hypotension; bradycardia; tachycardia; flushing; abdominal cramps; dyspnea; asthma; speech difficulty; and urinary urgency.

Nursing Considerations

- Assess client's sensitivity to narcotics on admission.
- Inform woman of potential side effects.
- Monitor and evaluate analgesic effect. Ask client about comfort level and notify anesthesiologist of inadequate pain relief.
- Observe for symptoms of hypersensitivity: pruritus, urticaria, and/or burning sensation.
- May produce an allergic response in clients, with sulfite sensitivity. If allergic reaction (urticaria, edema, or respiratory difficulties) occurs, administer naloxone or diphenhydramine per physician order.
- Assess respiratory rate before administration. Notify healthcare provider if respirations less than 12 per minute.
- Monitor urinary output and assess bladder for distention. Assist client to void.
- Assist client with ambulation after administration.
- Counsel client that use with alcohol or other central nervous system depressants may increase medication effects.
- Counsel client that prolonged use with abrupt discontinuation can result in symptoms consistent with narcotic withdrawal.

MEPERIDINE HYDROCHLORIDE (DEMEROL)

Meperidine hydrochloride is also a synthetic agonist-antagonist narcotic analgesic. Like Nubain, it may also precipitate drug withdrawal if the woman is physically dependent on narcotics (Florence & Palmer, 2003). Meperidine crosses the placenta within 90 seconds of maternal administration, with maternal and fetal concentrations achieving equilibrium at 6 minutes (Braveman, 2006). Meperidine can be administered IM or IV in labor. The subcutaneous and oral routes are not routinely used for laboring women. The typical dose is 50 to 100 milligrams IM or 25 to 50 milligrams IV (Wilson et al., 2006). Whereas IM administration can take up to 40 to 50 minutes to be effective, IV administration can provide pain relief within 5 to 10 minutes after administration (Braveman, 2006). Adverse maternal effects include nausea, vomiting, itching, urinary retention, sedation, respiratory depression, and dizziness (Wilson et al., 2006). Since meperidine can cause convulsions, it should not be given to women with known convulsive disorders, such as epilepsy (Wilson et al., 2006).

Meperidine has multiple fetal side effects, including alteration in fetal electroencephalogram, decreased or absent respiratory movements, a decrease in fetal movements, and decreased variability with the FHR (Braveman, 2006). In addition, newborns who have received meperidine take longer to sustain respirations after birth, have lower Apgar scores, lower oxygen saturation, a higher incidence of respiratory acidosis, and a higher incidence of abnormal neurological examinations at birth (Braveman, 2006). Meperidine has also been associated with delays in initiation of successful breastfeeding. Newborns whose mothers had received meperidine during labor had more

sucking problems, including lack of sucking and incorrect sucking technique (Braveman, 2006).

NURSING CARE MANAGEMENT

The nurse assesses the woman's history to identify if contraindications exist, such as the possibility of current narcotic drug dependence or convulsive disorders (Florence & Palmer, 2003). If no contraindications exist, the IV or IM route is frequently used during labor. Because respiratory depression can occur, the woman's respiratory rate and quality of respirations are routinely assessed. Characteristics of the FHR must be carefully assessed. Although meperidine can cause a decrease in variability, the FHR should be continuously assessed for signs of late decelerations. Anticipation of urinary retention is important. The woman is offered a bedpan and bladder distention is routinely assessed. If her bladder becomes distended and she is unable to void, catherization may be necessary. Because the woman may experience dizziness and sedation, the woman typically remains on bed rest and does not ambulate after the medication is administered. The nurse assesses the woman for side effects and reports undesired side effects to the physician or CNM.

OPIATE ANTAGONIST: NALOXONE (NARCAN)

Because naloxone (Narcan) is an antagonist with little or no agonistic effect, it exhibits little pharmacologic activity in the

THROUGH THE EYES OF A NURSE

Epidural for Pain Management

FAMILY'S EXPERIENCE: "I know I really want to have the option of having something for pain, but I learned in our (childbirth) class that some of the medications can affect the baby's heart rate. I don't want anything that will hurt the baby! What is the safest choice for me and the baby?"

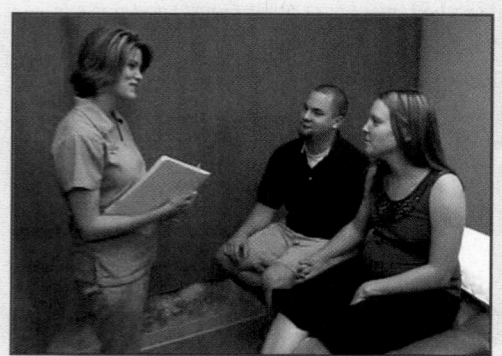

NURSE'S RESPONSE: "Typically, the intravenous medications, such as Demerol or Nubain, can cause some changes in the baby's heartbeat and can cause respiratory problems at birth. For this reason, those medications are not given when birth will occur within a few hours.

"The epidural is another option and gives better pain relief. It can be given throughout labor. It can affect the heartbeat when it is first given if the mother's blood pressure drops immediately after it is administered. This is prevented by giving intravenous fluids to the mother before administering the epidural."

NURSE'S ACTIONS AND RATIONALE:

There are many types of analgesic and anesthesia options to the laboring woman. Analgesics commonly used in labor are summarized in Table 25–2. The nurse reviews the pros and cons of each option. Epidural anesthesia can also have risks and benefits. The medications should be reviewed with the woman before administration. Although complications are rare, the nurse explains possible complications that can occur. The nurse gives clear objective information based on evidence-based practice. All questions should be answered before the onset of labor so the woman can make informed choices when labor occurs.

absence of narcotic agents. Naloxone can be used to reverse the mild respiratory depression, sedation, and hypotension following small doses of opiates (McGuire & Fowlie, 2003). Naloxone exerts its effect by competing for opiate receptors and taking the place of the opiate on the receptor. In this manner, naloxone blocks or reverses the action of the narcotic analgesic (McGuire & Fowlie, 2003). The drug is useful for respiratory depression caused by butorphanol (Stadol) and nalbuphine (Nubain) and meperidine hydrochloride (Demerol) (McGuire & Fowlie, 2003). *Naloxone is the drug of choice when the depressant is unknown because it will cause no further depression.* Naloxone's duration of action is less than that of most narcotic analgesics; however, respiratory depression may return as the antagonistic effect of naloxone wears off. Withdrawal symptoms may occur when Narcan is given to a woman or a newborn who is physically dependent on narcotics. A careful assessment that includes opiate drug use is imperative.

NURSING CARE MANAGEMENT

When naloxone is administered to the laboring mother or to the newborn just after birth, resuscitative measures and trained personnel should be readily available in the event that additional respiratory support is needed. When administered to the laboring mother, naloxone may be injected undiluted at a rate of 0.4 mg over 15 seconds into the tubing of a running IV infusion. Naloxone may also be diluted in an IV infusion of 5% dextrose or normal saline for a titrated dose. Titrated doses of naloxone are more likely to be used in a postoperative setting, when epidural analgesia has been given with a cesarean birth. After the direct IV administration, maternal vital signs should be obtained at 5-minute intervals until the respiratory rate has been stabilized and then every 30 minutes (McGuire & Fowlie, 2003). Neonatal administration can be administered via IV, IM,

or endotracheal (ET) routes. The standard neonatal dosage is 0.01 mg/kg (Wilson et al., 2006).

The duration of the drug is shorter (minutes to hours) than the analgesic drug it is acting as an antagonist for, so the nurse must be alert to the return of respiratory depression and the need for repeated doses. Naloxone should be given with caution in women with known or suspected opiate dependence, because it may precipitate severe withdrawal symptoms in the mother and the newborn.

REGIONAL ANALGESIA AND ANESTHESIA

Regional anesthesia is the temporary and reversible loss of sensation produced by injecting an anesthetic agent (called a local anesthetic) into an area that will bring the agent into direct contact with nervous tissue. Loss of sensation occurs because the local agents stabilize the cell membrane, which prevents initiation and transmission of nerve impulses. The regional anesthetic blocks most commonly used in childbearing include epidural, spinal, or combined epidural-spinal. Epidural blocks may be used for analgesia during labor and vaginal birth and for anesthesia during cesarean birth. A combined epidural-spinal block may also be used. With this approach, the epidural is used to provide analgesia for labor, and the spinal provides anesthesia for birth or analgesia following birth.

An epidural relieves pain associated with the first stage of labor by blocking the sensory nerves supplying the uterus. Pain associated with the second stage of labor and with birth can be alleviated with epidural, combined epidural-spinal, and pudendal blocks (Figure 25–1 ◆ and Table 25–4).

Regional anesthesia carries considerably less risk than general anesthesia. Risk of maternal death with general anesthesia during a cesarean birth is 16.7 times more likely than with regional anesthesia (Tsen, 2005).

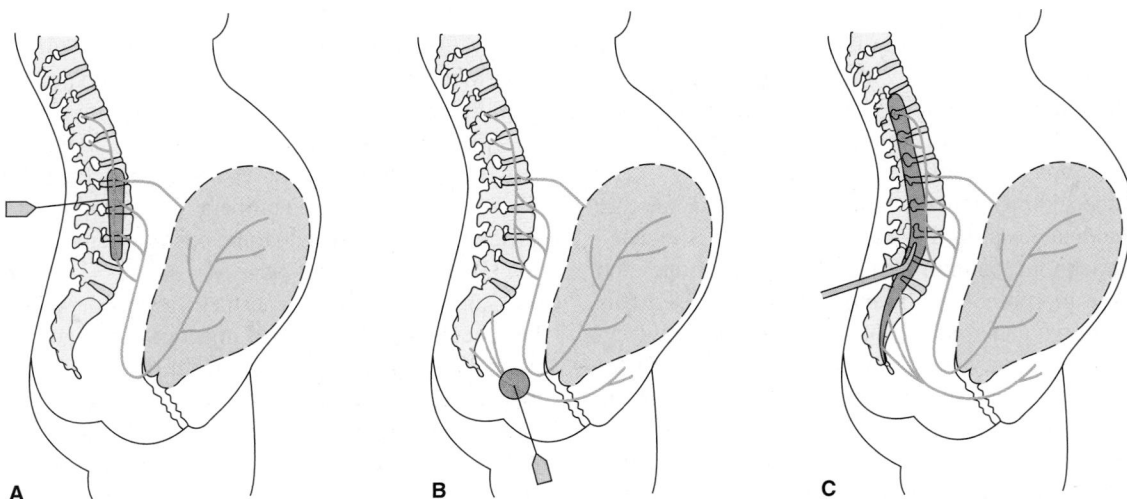

Figure 25–1 ◆ Schematic diagram showing pain pathways and sites of interruption. *A,* Lumbar sympathetic (spinal) block: relief of uterine pain only. *B,* Pudendal block: relief of perineal pain. *C,* Lumbar epidural block: Dark area demonstrates peridural (epidural) space and nerves affected, and the gray tube represents a continuous plastic catheter.
SOURCE: Bonica, J. J. (1972). *Principles and practice of obstetric analgesia and anesthesia* (pp. 492, 512, 521, 614). Philadelphia: Davis.

Table 25–4	**SUMMARY OF COMMONLY USED REGIONAL BLOCKS**		
Type of Block	**Areas Affected**	**Use During Labor and Birth**	**Nursing Actions**
Lumbar epidural	Uterus, cervix, vagina, and perineum	Given in first stage and second stage of labor.	Assess woman's knowledge regarding the block. Act as advocate to help her obtain further information if needed. Monitor maternal blood pressure to detect the major side effect, which is hypotension. Provide support and comfort. See Clinical Pathway for Epidural Anesthesia for further nursing actions.
Combined spinal-epidural	Uterus, cervix, vagina, and perineum	Spinal analgesia may be given in latent phase for pain relief. Epidural is given when active labor begins.	Assess woman's knowledge regarding the block. Monitor maternal vital signs and FHR status. Provide comfort measures.
Pudendal	Perineum and lower vagina	Given in the second stage just before birth to provide anesthesia for episiotomy or for low forceps birth.	Assess woman's knowledge regarding the block. Act as advocate to help her obtain further information if needed.
Local infiltration	Perineum	Administered just before birth to provide anesthesia for episiotomy.	Assess woman's knowledge regarding the block. Provide information as needed. Provide comfort and support. Observe perineum for bruising or other discoloration in the recovery period.
Spinal	Uterus, cervix, vagina, and perineum	Given during first stage for pain relief. Provides immediate onset of anesthesia.	Assess woman's knowledge regarding the block. Monitor maternal vital signs and FHR status.

Until fairly recently, the same anesthetic agents used for regional epidural anesthesia were also used to produce **regional analgesia** (pain relief) during labor. This approach was somewhat problematic because anesthetic agents alter the transmission of impulses to the bladder, making voiding difficult. The agents also interfere with the woman's ability to maintain her blood pressure and move her lower extremities. In addition, the descent of the fetus may be slowed, because the agents also decrease the woman's ability to push effectively during the second stage of labor (Fraser, Cayer, Soeder et al., 2002). To address these problems, regional analgesia is now obtained by injecting a narcotic agent such as fentanyl along with only a small amount of a local anesthetic agent. This approach yields effective pain relief without the troubling side effects of epidural anesthesia. The woman's pain is relieved, her blood pressure remains stable, and, because there is no motor blockage, she may be able to move about freely and ambulate. Urinary retention can still occur, but it can be treated with the placement of an indwelling Foley catheter or an in-and-out catheter (Cunningham et al., 2005). Urinary retention is usually a short-term complication that resolves on its own after the anesthesia has completely worn off.

The intrathecal injection of narcotics results in another type of regional analgesia. In this case, the narcotic is injected into the subarachnoid (spinal) space. Fentanyl citrate and preservative-free morphine are the most frequently used narcotic agents. The woman's pain is usually relieved; however, she may experience urinary retention. Delayed respiratory depression may also occur and seems to be more frequent with the use of morphine (Wilson et al., 2006).

It is important for the laboring woman to have information about the regional analgesia or anesthesia that is to be administered. As with other procedures, the woman needs to know how the block is given, the expected effect on her and the fetus, advantages and disadvantages, and possible risks. Many women discuss possible analgesic and anesthetic blocks with their physician or CNM during the pregnancy. If they have not, they should have an opportunity to ask questions and obtain information before receiving any regional analgesia or anesthesia while in labor. The nurse should answer questions and address concerns in early labor before the onset of acute pain. This ensures that the woman fully understands the information and can make an informed choice. Informed consent is obtained in writing before the administration of the medication.

Action and Absorption of Anesthetic Agents

Local anesthetic agents block nerve conduction by impairing propagation of the action potential in axons along with impairing the transmission of nerve impulses by stabilizing the cell membrane. The agents interact directly with specific receptors on the sodium channel, inhibiting sodium ion influx (Renn & Dorsey, 2005). The types of nerve fibers are differentially sensitive to the various anesthetic agents. In general, the smaller the fiber, the more sensitive it is to local agents. For example, it is possible to block the small C and A delta fibers, which transmit pain, touch, and temperature, without blocking the larger A alpha, A beta, and A gamma fibers, which continue to maintain a sense of pressure, muscle tone, position sense, and motor function (Renn & Dorsey, 2005).

Absorption of local anesthetic agents depends primarily on the vascularity of the area of injection. The agents also increase blood flow by causing vasodilatation (Wylie, 2005). Higher concentrations cause greater vasodilatation. Good maternal physical condition or a high metabolic rate aids absorption. Malnutrition, dehydration, electrolyte imbalance, and cardiovascular and pulmonary problems increase the potential for toxic effects. The pH of tissues affects the rate of absorption, which has implications for fetal complications, such as acidosis (Wylie, 2005). The addition of vasoconstrictors, such as epinephrine, delays absorption and prolongs the anesthetic effect.

Epinephrine decreases uteroplacental blood flow, making it an undesirable additive in many situations. The breakdown of local anesthetics in the body is accomplished by the liver and plasma esterase, and the resulting substance is eliminated by the kidneys. It is important to use the weakest concentration and the smallest amount necessary to produce the desired results (Wylie, 2005).

Types of Local Anesthetic Agents

Three types of local anesthetic agents are currently available—esters, amides, and opiates. The ester type includes procaine hydrochloride (Novocain), chloroprocaine hydrochloride (Nesacaine), and tetracaine hydrochloride (Pontocaine). Esters are rapidly metabolized; therefore, toxic maternal levels are not as likely to be reached, and placental transfer to the fetus is prevented.

Amide types include bupivacaine hydrochloride (Marcaine), mepivacaine hydrochloride (Carbocaine), and lidocaine hydrochloride (Xylocaine). Amide types are more powerful and longer-acting agents. They readily cross the placenta, can be measured in the fetal circulation, and affect the fetus for a prolonged period. Newer amide types of local anesthetic agents, such as rovicaine and levbupivaine, are becoming more commonly used because they have a long action but fewer toxic effects (Buckenmaier & Bleckner, 2005).

Opioids are used with epidural blocks to produce analgesia for labor. Some of the agents used include morphine, fentanyl, butorphanol, and meperidine. When only opioids are used epidurally, the amount of pain relief is not as great. A combination of opioids and a low dose of a local anesthetic agent achieve better pain control with reduced motor impairment (Braveman, 2006). There does appear to be a higher incidence of pruritus (itching) when this combination method is used, however; although the addition of opiates has been associated with undesirable side effects, such as nausea, vomiting, hypotension, respiratory depression, and sedation, the incidence appears to be low. These agents are commonly used, especially in women undergoing a cesarean birth, because of their high effectiveness rates in controlling postpartal pain (Leung, 2005). One study that examined women who had received fentanyl revealed interference with early breastfeeding, with higher dosages having more negative impact than lower dosages (Bowes, 2005). Other evidence supports the use of fentanyl and butorphanol for administration in labor. Bowes (2005) found no differences in cesarean and operative birth rates between women who received epidural opiates and those who had received systemic analgesia. The women who received the epidural opiates had a shorter first stage than those who had received systemic analgesic agents (Bowes, 2005).

A variety of anesthetic agents and a wide range of doses have been used for epidural anesthesia with varying results. The most commonly used agents are lidocaine 2% with epinephrine 1:200,000, bupivacaine 0.25%, and 2-chloroprocaine 3% (Braveman, 2006). Each agent provides adequate anesthesia with 15 to 20 mL of the solution, but each has been associated with side effects. The pharmacology of each drug must be understood before it is used.

Adverse Maternal Reactions to Anesthetic Agents

Reactions to local anesthetic agents range from mild symptoms to cardiovascular collapse. Mild reactions include palpitations, vertigo, tinnitus, apprehension, confusion, headache, and a metallic taste in the mouth. Common side effects include pruritus, vertigo, dizziness, and urinary retention (Foley, Strong, & Garite, 2004). Moderate reactions include more severe degrees of the mild symptoms plus nausea and vomiting, hypotension, and muscle twitching, which may progress to convulsions and loss of consciousness. Severe reactions are sudden loss of consciousness, coma, severe hypotension, bradycardia, respiratory depression, and cardiac arrest (Braveman, 2006). High concentrations of the agents may also cause local toxic effects on tissues. It is important to remember that when the mother experiences an adverse reaction, the fetus is also affected.

Systemic toxic reactions most commonly occur with an excessive dose because of too great a concentration or too large a volume. Pregnant women in labor generally require less medication because of hormonal factors, uterine compression, an increase in cardiac output, and an increased sensitivity of the neural axons (Rosenberg, Veering, & Urmey, 2005). Accidental IV injection that suddenly increases the amount of the drug in maternal circulation results in depression of vasomotor, respiratory, and other medullary centers of the brain (Wylie, 2005). It also depresses the heart and peripheral vascular bed. A massive intravascular dose can result in sudden circulatory collapse within 1 minute. Reactions to subcutaneous and extradural injection occur in 5 to 40 minutes. The short-acting agent procaine can produce toxic reactions in 10 to 15 minutes, and the long-acting agent mepivacaine in 20 to 40 minutes (Wilson et al., 2006). It is imperative that the woman is under close supervision by knowledgeable personnel throughout the time that an agent is being used and that an IV line is in place.

If epinephrine has been added to the anesthetic agent to prolong the anesthesia, it is necessary to differentiate between reaction to the anesthetic agent and to the epinephrine. Reaction to epinephrine is characterized by pallor, perspiration, dyspnea, and a greater increase in blood pressure and pulse than occurs with reactions to anesthetic agents.

Psychogenic reactions such as severe anxiety, hallucinations, inability to move or speak, or catatonic appearance can also occur, with symptoms similar to those occurring with systemic toxic reactions (Braveman, 2006). This phenomenon may occur as the procedure is begun and before the injection of the anesthetic agent. Regardless of the cause, the symptoms must be treated.

Allergic reactions to anesthetic agents may also occur. The manifestations of the antigen-antibody reaction include urticaria, laryngeal edema, joint pain, swelling of the tongue, and bronchospasm.

TREATMENT OF SYSTEMIC TOXICITY

Preferred treatment of mild toxicity involves the administration of oxygen by mask and IV injection of a short-acting barbiturate to decrease anxiety (Braveman, 2006). The clinician should

EVIDENCE-BASED PRACTICE

EFFECTIVENESS OF EPIDURAL ANESTHESIA IN LABOR

Clinical Questions

What is the effectiveness of epidural analgesia for pain control in labor? Are there adverse effects from epidural anesthesia?

The Evidence

Two experts independently reviewed the reports of 21 research studies, appearing in 48 publications and involving 6664 women. All but one of the studies compared epidural anesthesia with opiate pain control, but a variety of other pain control techniques were tested in many of the studies. Some of the other pain control techniques included 1:1 midwife support, transcutaneous electrical stimulation (TENS), and some complementary and alternative techniques. Many of the studies had true control groups that received no external pain control. A range of outcomes were studied relative to the course and length of labor, the nature of the birth, and the safety of mother and baby. Only one study measured the mothers' perceptions of pain using a visual analog scale.

What Is Effective?

The use of epidural anesthesia reduces pain in labor. When epidural anesthesia is used, there is less need for additional pain relief measures, and mothers report a shorter time until relief is felt. The pain relief from epidural anesthesia is better than other methods in both the first and second stages of labor. In these studies, there was no increase in cesarean birth rate or long-term backache among mothers receiving epidural pain relief. The length of the first stage of labor was unaffected by epidural anesthesia. There is apparently no effect on neonatal condition, as 5-minute Apgar scores are the same for mothers receiving epidural anesthesia and mothers using other methods of pain relief. There was, however, an increased rate of instrument-assisted birth, and the second stage of labor was significantly longer for these mothers. The risk of hypotension, urinary

retention, and fever were all higher for mothers receiving epidural anesthesia.

What Is Unclear?

There was significant variability in the results relative to "maternal satisfaction with pain relief." The perception of pain affects satisfaction with the birth experience, and high levels of perceived pain may impact breastfeeding and mother-infant interaction. Pain is a very subjective experience, and only one study captured maternal perceptions; the remaining focused on specific objective outcomes. The specific impact on perceptions, satisfaction, and associated outcomes needs more study. These studies used different measurement scales and statistical techniques, and so comparing results across studies is difficult. Some findings were contradictory across studies (for example, one study showed an increase in cesarean birth rates, whereas several others did not) and so additional study is warranted.

Best Practice

Epidural anesthesia affords mothers superior pain relief, and faster time to relief, and leads to less need for additional pain relief. However, mothers who have epidural anesthesia can expect a longer second stage and a higher possibility of an instrument-assisted birth. The mother should be monitored carefully for hypotension, urinary retention, and fever. Appropriate prevention interventions should be planned for the mother who has an epidural anesthetic.

Critical Thinking

What information about the effectiveness of epidural anesthesia should be incorporated into the prenatal teaching plan? What assessments should be in place to evaluate the mother undergoing epidural anesthesia to prevent complications?

REFERENCE: Anim-Somuah, J., Smyth, R., & Howell, C. (2005). Epidural versus non-epidural or no analgesia in labour. *The Cochrane Database of Systematic Reviews* (4) (Article No. CD000331.Pub2.)

---

anticipate the possibility of convulsions or cardiovascular collapse and make appropriate preparations to treat them. Specific nursing interventions in the treatment of systemic toxicity are included in the Clinical Pathway for Epidural Anesthesia on pages 703–705.

TREATMENT OF CONVULSIONS

The best treatment for convulsions is to establish the airway and administer 100% oxygen. Thiopental or diazepam may be administered to stop convulsions (Braveman, 2006). Small doses are adequate and help avoid cardiorespiratory depression.

TREATMENT OF SUDDEN CARDIOVASCULAR COLLAPSE

In sudden cardiovascular collapse, an airway must be established as cardiopulmonary resuscitation begins. IV fluids are increased, and emergency cesarean birth may be started immediately (Foley et al., 2004).

Lumbar Epidural Block

A lumbar **epidural block** involves injection of a local anesthetic agent into the epidural space. The epidural space is a potential space between the dura mater and the ligamentum flavum, extending from the base of the skull to the end of the sacral canal (Figure 25–2 ◆). It contains areolar tissue, fat, lymphatics, and the internal vertebral venous plexus (Wylie, 2005). This space is accessed through the lumbar area. The technique is most often used as a continuous block to provide analgesia and anesthesia from active labor through the birth and episiotomy repair. Complete pain relief is achieved for 85% of women. Another 12% experience partial relief, whereas only 3% of women report no relief at all (Cunningham et al., 2005).

Lumbar epidural block has become fairly common during labor and birth. In the United States, epidural blocks are used by more than 60% of all women giving birth (Camann, 2005). More-

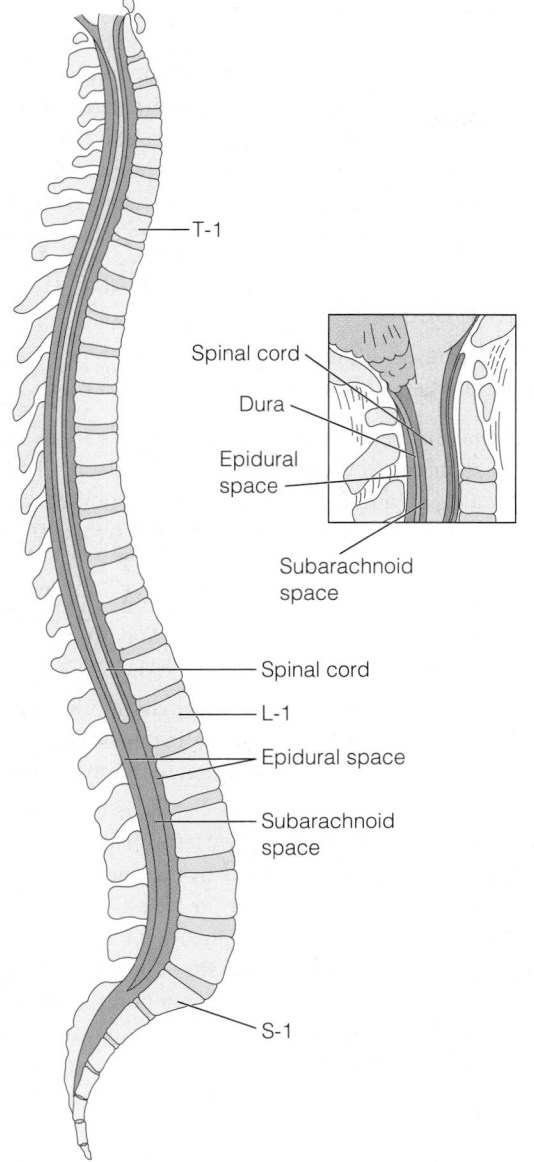

T-1

Spinal cord

Dura

Epidural
space

Subarachnoid
space

Spinal cord

L-1

Epidural space

Subarachnoid
space

S-1

Figure 25–2 ◆ The epidural space lies between the dura mater and the ligamentum flavum, extending from the base of the skull to the end of the sacral canal.

over, recent studies have shown that the use of epidural anesthesia is the preferred method of pain relief for laboring women.

In the United States, epidural rates have continued to rise because of an increase in 24-hour availability of anesthesia services, the rise in cesarean birth rates, and a decline in the number of women who attempt a vaginal birth after a previous cesarean section (VBAC) (Braveman, 2006). However, there are disparities in the use of epidural block that raise questions regarding how and to whom the procedure is offered. In the United States, regrettably, there have been studies that have shown that women with publicly funded insurance, such as Medicaid, are less likely to receive epidurals than women with private insurance. Twice as many privately insured women receive epidural anesthesia compared with those with publicly funded insurance. Although race does not appear to be an issue,

cultural norms significantly affect the request for epidural anesthesia. Hispanic women are twice as likely as non-Hispanic women not to receive an epidural during labor (Atherton, Feeg, & El-Adham, 2004).

Epidural blocks can be administered in a number of ways. To provide analgesia and anesthesia during labor, the block can be administered as a single dose with an epidural needle, as a single dose through an epidural catheter with additional doses (called "top-ups" or "top-offs") given as needed, or as a continuous epidural. Many women equate the quality of their labor experience directly with their satisfaction with the anesthesia they receive while in labor. Although many women desire the pain relief from regional anesthesia, many do not like its side effects, such as inability to void, decreased motor sensation in the lower extremities, and the need to maintain bed rest. Although some procedures require that the woman remain in bed, others—called "walking," "ambulatory," or "mobile" epidurals—are given with analgesic agents or anesthetic agents, or both, that leave the woman with sufficient motor control to be out of bed (Kuczkowski, 2004a).

Although ACOG has recommended postponing epidural administration until active labor is established, the ASA is not in agreement. Although earlier literature indicated there was a slight increased risk of cesarean birth (2%) with early epidural placement, current practice that involves using a low dose of bupivacaine does not increase the risk of cesarean (Bowes, 2005; Santos, 2004).

ADVANTAGES

The lumbar epidural block produces good analgesia that alters maternal physiologic responses to pain. The woman is fully awake during labor and birth. The continuous technique allows different blocking for each stage of labor so that internal rotation of the fetus can be accomplished. In many cases, the dose of anesthetic agent can be adjusted to preserve the woman's reflex urge to bear down.

DISADVANTAGES

The most common complication of an epidural block is maternal hypotension. Hypotension commonly occurs as a result of peripheral vasodilatation (Braveman, 2006). This is increased by the blockade of the sympathetic nerve supply to the adrenal glands, which prevents the release of catecholamines (Braveman, 2006). This is generally prevented by preloading with a rapid infusion of IV fluids, then providing IV fluids continuously. Although hypotension can occur, the incidence of hypotension requiring ephedrine is relatively low, less than 2% (Cunningham et al., 2005). Other serious complications, although rare, have been reported, including postdural puncture seizures, meningitis, cardiorespiratory arrest, and vertigo (vestibulocochlear dysfunction) (Kuczkowski, 2004b). Another disadvantage is that the onset of analgesia may not occur for up to 30 minutes. Epidural block requires skilled personnel for administration and close observation of the woman and her fetus. The anesthesia provider must be careful while administering the block to avoid perforating the dura mater, which would place the needle in the subarachnoid space; if the error is not recognized, the anesthetic agent would be injected into the spinal canal. Skilled nurses are also required to maintain close observation of the laboring woman and her fetus. Variability of the FHR may decrease, and late decelerations may occur if maternal hypotension develops. Finally, epidural anesthesia is more costly than systemic agents. This may be a crucial factor for women and families without insurance who are paying out of pocket for their birthing costs (Atherton et al., 2004).

There are multiple regional anesthesia approaches for women undergoing cesarean birth. When an epidural block is used for cesarean birth, an epidural catheter is inserted and a single dose can be given. This approach allows for a more gradual onset and requires less medication to be administered. This reduces the risk of hypotension (Wickwire & Gross, 2004). The catheter provides access to the epidural space, so that additional anesthetic agents and opioids may be administered if needed and so that opioids may be given to provide pain relief for the 24 hours following birth.

The most commonly used epidural technique for laboring women is the continuous epidural infusion via a pump that allows the woman to get a predetermined amount of medication on a continual basis. If the woman becomes uncomfortable, a bolus of additional medication can be given to achieve comfort.

Some women with epidurals may have decreased sensation and movement, or they may have essentially no control over movement in the anesthetized region. Some studies have demonstrated that epidural use prolonged the first stage of labor and contributed to the need to augment labors with oxytocin (Lieberman, & O'donoghue, 2002). On the other hand, other clinical studies, along with healthcare providers, assert that epidural analgesia may shorten the active and transition phases because of the pain relief (Bowes, 2005). Howell (2002) reviewed 11 research studies that included 3157 women and found that although epidural anesthesia was associated with greater pain relief, it prolonged both the first and second stages of labor. Epidurals also increased the incidence of fetal malposition and the use of oxytocin. In a recent study comparing women who had received epidurals with women who did not receive epidural anesthesia during labor, the women with epidurals had a longer active stage of labor; however, other stages of labor remained the same in the two groups (Vahratian, 2004). In another study, a group who received epidural anesthesia in early labor was compared with a second group who received epidurals later in labor (after being 4 cm or more). The two groups had the same rates of cesarean births (Wong, Scavone et al., 2005). Other studies have shown a relationship between epidural use and the need for instrument-assisted births (Howell, 2002; Lieberman & O'donoghue, 2002), which increases the risk of perineal trauma. The question of epidural use and its effect on labor is an ideal example for the need for evidence-based practice within the nursing and medical professions. Additional research is needed to examine this ongoing issue.

CONTRAINDICATIONS

The absolute contraindications for epidural block are maternal refusal, local or systemic infection, coagulation disorders, actual or anticipated maternal hemorrhage, low platelet counts (below

100,000/mm^3), hypovolemia, allergy to a specific class of local anesthetic agents, suspicion of neurologic disease, long-term use of aspirin or anti-inflammatory agents, abruptio placentae, acute infection at the epidural site, and lack of trained staff (Foley et al., 2004; Schwartz, 2006). Epidurals should not be used in women with heart failure or aortic stenosis because these women cannot compensate for the decrease in vascular resistance that can occur when an epidural is inserted (Schwartz, 2006).

TECHNIQUE FOR CONTINUOUS LUMBAR EPIDURAL BLOCK

In administering a continuous lumbar epidural block the following actions are taken (Schwartz, 2006):

1. Maternal and fetal status and labor progress are assessed. Because maternal blood pressure and pulse will be taken frequently, an automatic blood pressure device may be useful. FHR is continuously monitored by an EFM by the nurse.

2. Oxygen and resuscitative equipment is readied. The nurse ensures all equipment is in the room and properly functioning.

3. An IV infusion is begun, and a preload of 500 to 2000 mL of IV fluid (e.g., 0.45% normal saline or lactated Ringer's) is given over approximately 15 to 30 minutes by the nurse.

4. The woman is positioned on her left or right side, at the edge of the bed (the mattress is firmer and provides more support) with the assistance of the nurse, with her legs slightly flexed, or she is asked to sit on the edge of the bed. She is advised to drop her shoulders, round out the small of her back, and place her chin on her chest. It may be helpful to advise the woman to "arch her back like a cat" to achieve the proper position. This position is especially effective for positioning obese women. The spinal column is not kept convex, as it is for a spinal block, because the convex position reduces the peridural space to a greater degree and stretches the dura mater, making it more susceptible to puncture. The epidural space is decreased during pregnancy because of venous engorgement. It is also smaller in obese and short individuals (Cunningham et al., 2005). A small pillow may be placed under the woman's head and in front of her chest to provide support for her arms (Figure 25–3 ◆). The nurse typically stands beside the woman, offering support and assisting her in maintaining this position. The nurse assists the woman with breathing techniques and alerts the anesthesia provider when a contraction occurs.

5. The skin is prepared with an antiseptic agent by the anesthesia provider.

6. A skin wheal of a small amount of local anesthesia is given intradermally by the anesthesia provider to anesthetize the supraspinous and interspinous ligaments (Wylie, 2005).

7. The anesthesia provider then inserts a short, beveled 16- to 18-gauge needle with stylet that is passed to the

Figure 25–3 ◆ Positioning woman for epidural anesthesia block. *A,* Incorrect maternal positioning for placing subarachnoid or epidural block. The upper shoulder has fallen forward, upper leg has rotated forward, and the client is positioned on the center of the bed so that there is no support from the edge and the back can curve. *B,* Vertebral position with client in incorrect position. The vertebrae rotate forward and, if the needle is inserted in the usual way (needle 1), the apophyseal joints are encountered. Needle 2 shows the proper insertion of the needle entering the epidural space. *C,* Correct maternal positioning. The back is straight and vertical, the shoulders are square, and the upper leg is prevented from rolling forward. *D,* Vertebral position with the woman correctly positioned.
SOURCE: From S. M. Shnider & G. Levinson, *Anesthesia for Obstetrics,* 3rd ed., Copyright © Lippincott, Williams & Wilkins, 1993. Reprinted with permission.

ligamentum flavum in the widest interspace below the second lumbar vertebra (usually in the third or fourth lumbar interspace) (Figure 25–4 ◆). The ligamentum flavum is identified by its resistance to injection of saline or air (called loss of resistance technique). Resistance disappears as the peridural space is entered.

8. The anesthesia provider then injects 5 mL of preservative-free saline in order to pass the catheter into the epidural space more easily.

9. The catheter is inserted approximately 1 to 2 cm into the epidural space by the anesthesia provider. The needle is removed. Aspiration for blood (indicating that a vessel has been inadvertently entered) or cerebrospinal fluid (indicating the dura mater has been punctured) is attempted.

10. If aspiration tests are negative, a test dose of local anesthetic agent containing 1.5% lidocaine with epinephrine 1:200,000 concentration or 3 mL of 0.25% bupivacaine with 1:200,000 concentration of epinephrine is injected. The anesthesiologist usually injects the medication after aspiration and after a uterine contraction to minimize the risk of tachycardia that can occur if the drug is directly injected into a vessel (Cunningham et al., 2005). If the subarachnoid space has been entered, sensory and motor changes occur in the woman's extremities. If there are no untoward effects, additional anesthetic agent is injected. The catheter is securely taped so that its placement will not be disturbed. Pain relief should occur within 15 to 20 minutes after administration (Cunningham et al., 2005).

MEDIALINK

Video: Epidural Placement

Figure 25–4 ◆ Technique for lumbar epidural block. *A,* Proper position of insertion. *B,* Needle in the ligamentum flavum. *C,* Tip of needle in epidural space. *D,* Force of injection pushing dura away from tip of needle.

SOURCE: Bonica, J. J. (1972). *Principles and practice of obstetric analgesia and anesthesia* (p. 631). Philadelphia: Davis.

11. The nurse then assists the woman into a semireclining position with a lateral tilt of her uterus for 10 minutes to allow for distribution of the block. This also prevents aortocaval compression (see Chapter 14 ∞). She is then maintained in a side-lying position to maximize uteroplacental perfusion. If she needs to be turned to a supine position for fetal blood sampling or other procedures, the nurse turns the woman as quickly as possible and repositions her on her side.

12. The anesthesia provider or the nurse then monitors the maternal blood pressure every 1 to 2 minutes for the first 10 minutes past the injection and then every 5 to 15 minutes until the block wears off. Maternal vital signs are evaluated by either the nurse or the anesthesia provider against baseline readings obtained just before the beginning of the procedure. The nurse is responsible for documentation of assessment data that are obtained throughout the procedure.

13. The woman must be attended by a nurse, nurse anesthetist, or an anesthesiologist for the first 20 minutes following the initial dose and after administration of any additional dose.

14. If hypotension (a 20% to 30% fall in systolic pressure or a drop to below 100 mm Hg) occurs, the nurse ensures that

left lateral displacement of the uterus is maintained, and the IV fluids are infused more rapidly. Oxygen is delivered by a face mask to ensure proper oxygenation of the fetus. A 10- to 20-degree Trendelenburg position may be used. If the blood pressure is not restored within 1 to 2 minutes, a vasopressor such as ephedrine, 5 to 15 mg, may be administered IV.

15. The maternal blood pressure and pulse and the FHR continue to be monitored by the nurse.

16. If the epidural is not being administered by continuous pump, the anesthesiologist aspirates the catheter before administering subsequent doses.

TECHNIQUE FOR SINGLE-DOSE LUMBAR EPIDURAL BLOCK

The procedure of a single-dose lumbar epidural block is the same as for the lumbar block just described, except that instead of injecting 5 mL of saline, the anesthesiologist injects a test dose of 2 to 3 mL of anesthetic agent to make sure the dura mater has not been penetrated. After checking again to confirm that the dura mater has not been perforated, the clinician injects a single dose of 10 to 12 mL to provide anesthesia for birth. Subsequent care continues as for the procedure just described, from step 11 (Schwartz, 2006).

PROBLEMS AND ADVERSE EFFECTS

The major adverse effect of epidural anesthesia is maternal hypotension caused by a spinal blockade, which lowers peripheral resistance, decreases venous return to the heart, and subsequently lessens cardiac output and lowers blood pressure. Maternal hypotension results in uteroplacental insufficiency in the fetus, which is manifested as late decelerations on the fetal monitoring strip. The risk of hypotension can be minimized by hydrating the vascular system with 500 to 1000 mL of IV solution (Wickwire & Gross, 2004) before the procedure and changing the woman's position and/or increasing the IV rate afterward.

A potentially distressing maternal problem is an inadequate block, unilateral block, or block failure. Epidural anesthesia has a higher failure rate than spinal anesthesia because the catheter must be properly placed to produce adequate anesthesia (Braveman, 2006). A one-sided block is fairly common and can be overcome by having the woman lie on the unanesthetized side and injecting more of the local anesthetic agent. If the woman has a continuous epidural block, she should turn from side to side every hour to avoid a one-sided block. A block may be effective except for a "spot" ("hot spot") or "window" of pain in the inguinal or suprapubic area. Breakthrough pain may occur at any time during the epidural infusion. It usually occurs when the continuous infusion rate of the anesthetic agent is below the recommended rate for a therapeutic dose. Breakthrough pain can also occur when the woman has a full bladder or when the cervix is completely dilated. The nurse assesses the woman carefully before calling the anesthesia provider for additional medication administration (commonly referred to as a "top-off." It may also occur when the infusion pump rate is altered or the integrity of the epidural line is broken.

Pruritus may occur at any time during the epidural infusion. It usually appears first on the face, neck, or torso and is generally the result of the agent used in the epidural infusion (Braveman, 2006). Frequently Benadryl, an antihistamine, can be administered to manage pruritus.

Maternal temperature may be elevated to 37.8C or higher with the use of epidural anesthesia. Sympathetic blockade may decrease sweat production and, in turn, diminish heat loss. It has also been suggested that heat loss may result from a failure of the central nervous system to regulate temperature. Headaches, migraine headaches, neckaches, and tingling of the hands and fingers have also been reported (Cunningham et al., 2005).

Short-term localized tenderness at the needle puncture site occurs in about 40% of women during the first week after birth. Backache is fairly common and is thought to result from inadvertently maintaining stressed positions during periods of muscle relaxation and pain relief from the epidural block. Long-term back pain is uncommon. Other problems or adverse effects include urinary retention, shivering, nausea, and vomiting.

COMPLICATIONS

One of the most serious complications of regional anesthesia, systemic toxic reaction, has been discussed in "Adverse Maternal Reactions to Anesthetic Agents" on p. 695. Toxic reactions following a lumbar epidural block may be caused by unintentional placement of the drug in the arachnoid or subarachnoid space, excessive amount of the drug in the epidural space (massive epidural), or accidental intravascular injection (Foley et al., 2004). Because large quantities of anesthetic agent are used for epidural block, the likelihood of toxic reactions is higher than with some of the other regional procedures. The incidence of drug reactions is relatively low, but the possibility is always present.

Pain during cesarean birth with epidural anesthesia has been reported by a growing number of women. In light of this, some anesthesiologists use both temperature and pinprick tests to assess sensory loss. Dermatomes from T_4 to S_3 should be tested for sensory loss before beginning a cesarean (Braveman, 2006). The method of assessment and the results should be documented in the anesthesia record.

Spinal headaches can also be a complication that occurs with epidural anesthesia. Spinal headaches occur when the dura is accidently punctured during epidural placement (Braveman, 2006).

NURSING CARE MANAGEMENT

The nurse assesses the maternal vital signs and the FHR for baseline information and to ensure that both maternal and fetal vital signs are within normal limits.

(*Note:* All information regarding assessments, procedures, and other activities is recorded on the fetal electronic monitor strip as well as in the nursing notes. Some facilities may use checklist or computerized charting systems.) Labor progress is also assessed. The procedure and expected results are explained, and the woman's questions are answered. The nurse acts as an advocate and arranges for consultation with the anesthesiologist if questions arise. The family, significant other, or support person should be included to promote a family-centered approach. Informed consent for the epidural should be obtained.

The nurse starts an IV infusion, if one is not already in place. The nurse preloads at a rapid infusion rate to increase both blood volume and cardiac output per physician's order or agency protocol. It is recommended that dextrose-free solutions be used, because dextrose can cause fetal hyperglycemia with rebound hypoglycemia the first few hours after birth (Braveman, 2006). It is helpful to provide an opportunity for the woman to void just before administering the block, because her urge to urinate will be decreased afterward (Schwartz, 2006). The nurse assists the woman with positioning on either side or in a sitting position on the side of the bed or stretcher. The nurse provides physical and emotional support throughout the procedure.

After the epidural block is given, the woman may be positioned in a semireclining position (head at 25 degrees) with lateral uterine tilt to provide equal distribution of the block; then she is turned to a side-lying position (Braveman, 2006). If she is supine for procedures such as sterile vaginal examinations or fetal scalp blood sampling, the nurse places a wedge under her hip to help eliminate aortocaval compression. The nurse takes maternal blood pressure and pulse every 5 minutes for at least 30 minutes and then at least every 30 minutes thereafter while the block is present (Schwartz, 2006). The FHR is monitored and assessed by continuous EFM.

If hypotension (systolic blood pressure below 100 mm Hg) occurs, the nurse assists with corrective measures such as positioning the woman in a left side-lying position, increasing the flow rate of the IV infusion, and placing the bed in a 10- to 20-degree Trendelenburg position (Schwartz, 2006). If maternal blood pressure does not increase within 1 to 2 minutes, 5 to 15 mg of ephedrine may be administered IV per physician or protocol order. These measures are usually sufficient; however, if hypotension persists, oxygen by mask at 7 to 10 L/min and additional vasopressors may be needed (Cunningham et al., 2005). During episodes of maternal hypotension, the nurse observes the FHR for signs of late decelerations related to uteroplacental insufficiency. Nausea and vomiting may be associated with hypotension. An antiemetic may be ordered to increase the woman's comfort. With severe or prolonged hypotension, added treatment includes elevating the woman's legs for 2 or 3 minutes to increase blood return from the extremities (Braveman, 2006).

If additional local anesthetic agents are injected, the regimen of assessing maternal blood pressure and initial surveillance should be repeated each time the epidural catheter is reinjected. If the woman's legs have been in stirrups during a vaginal birth, her blood pressure should be assessed as soon as her legs are taken out of the stirrups. While the legs were elevated, circulating blood volume in the trunk increased. Restoring circulation to the legs decreases the overall blood volume and may precipitate hypotension.

Additional nursing care following the block includes frequent assessment of the bladder to avoid bladder distention. Catheterization may be necessary, because most women are unable to void; however, the nurse should first offer the woman a bedpan, because catheterization increases the risk of urinary tract infections (Wylie, 2005).

Shivering may be caused by heat loss from increased peripheral blood flow or alteration of thermal input to the central nervous system when warm but not cold sensations have been suppressed. Applying warmed blankets and reassuring the woman may make her feel more comfortable (Wylie, 2005).

The nurse assesses the woman's level of pain relief. The nurse can promote equal distribution of the anesthetic agent by assessing the temperature of the woman's feet. If one foot warms more quickly than the other, the woman should be positioned with the cooler side dependent (Wickwire & Gross, 2004). It is important for the woman to turn from side to side every hour to promote equal distribution of the anesthetic agent. Again, the woman should be assessed for advanced cervical dilatation and bladder distention. If positioning changes and emptying the bladder do not help and the woman has inadequate pain relief, the anesthesia provider needs to be notified. During a continuous epidural block, the anesthesiologist should titrate the infusion to maintain a sensory level of T_{10}, and the presence of motor block and height of sensory block should be documented at least hourly (Wickwire & Gross, 2004).

Respiratory rate and quality of the respirations should be assessed at least every 15 to 30 minutes. The nurse should notify the anesthetist of any significant decreases in respiratory rate or respiratory pattern changes. If the respiratory rate falls below 14 respirations per minute, naloxone (Narcan) may be given to remove the effect of the anesthetic agent; respirations will then return to a normal rate (Schwartz, 2006).

The nurse asks the woman if she is experiencing pruritus (itching) and is alert for signs of scratching, especially on the face, neck, and torso. If present, pruritus is usually treated with diphenhydramine (Benadryl), 25 mg administered IV or 50 mg IM per physician's or CNM's order (Schwartz, 2006).

During the second stage of labor, the woman may require assistance with pushing, because she may not feel her contractions or experience the urge to push. If the woman does not feel the urge to push, the nurse may collaborate with the anesthesia provider so that the block can be turned down or temporarily turned off until to urge to push returns. She may also need assistance holding or controlling her legs in order to push. After birth, return of complete sensation and the ability to control the legs are essential before ambulation is attempted. This may take several hours, depending on the agent and the total dose. The woman must also be able to maintain blood pressure in a sitting and then standing position. For further discussion of nursing care, see "Clinical Pathway for Epidural Anesthesia" on pages 703 to 705.

Epidural Analgesia after Birth

To provide analgesia for approximately 24 hours after the birth, the anesthesiologist may inject an opioid, such as morphine (Duramorph) 5 mg or 7.5 mg, into the epidural space immediately following the birth. These agents are typically reserved for women who have had a cesarean birth. The analgesic effect of Duramorph begins approximately 30 to 60 minutes after the injection. The side effects include pruritus, nausea and vomiting, and urinary retention (Wilson et al., 2006). See Drug Guide: Postbirth Epidural Morphine in Chapter 35. ∞

Other agents are being examined that offer equal or better pain control with fewer side effects. Meperidine (Demerol) may be injected during an epidural block for birth, and then continued through use of patient-controlled epidural analgesia (PCEA). Epidural meperidine is associated with fewer side effects than epidural morphine and does not cause hemodynamic changes (Macarthur, 2002). Epidural fentanyl and lidocaine have also been used. The addition of lidocaine has been associated with a more rapid onset of sensory block without the increased side effects (Macarthur, 2002).

Spinal Block

In a **spinal block,** a local anesthetic agent is injected directly into the spinal fluid in the subarachnoid space to provide anesthesia for cesarean birth. The subarachnoid space is the fluid-filled area between the dura mater and the spinal cord. During pregnancy, the space decreases because of the distention of the epidural veins. Thus a specific dose of anesthetic produces a much higher

CLINICAL PATHWAY   For Epidural Anesthesia

Category	First Stage	Second and Third Stage	Fourth Stage Birth to 1 Hour Past Birth
Referral	Review prenatal record Advise CNM/physician of admission	Labor record for first stage	Report to recovery room nurse ◆ *Expected Outcomes* Appropriate resources identified and utilized
Assessments	Admission assessments: Ask about problems since last prenatal visit; labor status (contraction frequency and duration, cervical dilatation, and effacement), membrane status; coping level; support; woman's desires during labor and birth; ability to verbalize needs; laboratory testing (blood and UA) Woman's request for epidural Intrapartal assessment: timing *Latent Phase:* • BP, P, R, q15–30min if in normal range (BP) 90–135/60–85 or no increase greater than 30 mm Hg systolic or 15 mm Hg diastolic over baseline; pulse 60–90; respirations 12–24/min, quiet; easy) • Temp q4h unless greater than 37.6C (99.6F) or membranes ruptured; then q1h. Uterine contractions q15–30min: contractions q5–10min, 15–40 sec, mild intensity) • FHR q30min (for low-risk women) and q15min for high-risk women if reassuring (FHR baseline 110–160, variability present and average, accelerations with fetal movement, no late nor variable decelerations); if nonreassuring, position on side, start O$_2$, assess for hypotension, monitor continuously, notify CNM/physician *Active Phase:* • BP, P, R, every 15–30 min if WNL • Temp as above • Uterine contractions assessed every 15–30 min. Low-risk women may be monitored every 30 min; high-risk women need to be monitored every 15 min. • FHR assessed continuously per EFM • Pulse ox greater than 95% *Transition Phase:* • BP, P, R, q15–30min if in normal range • Uterine contractions q15–30min • FHR q30min (for low-risk women) and q15min (for high-risk women) if reassuring: if nonreassuring, see above • Pulse ox greater than 95% Cervical assessment: from 1–10 cm dilatation; nullipara (1:2 cm/h), multipara (1.5 cm/h) Cervical effacement: from 0% to 100% Fetal descent: progressive descent from −4 to +4 Membrane assessment: when ruptured, Nitrazine positive, fluid clear, no foul odor Behavioral characteristics: response to labor process, facial expressions, verbalizations, tone of voice, changes in behavior during contractions, body movement	Second stage assessments: • BP, P, R, q5–15min • Uterine contractions palpated continuously • FHR q5min if reassuring; if nonreassuring, monitor continuously Fetal descent: descent continues to birth Behavioral characteristics: response to pushing, facial expressions, verbalization Third stage assessments: • BP, P, R q5min • Uterine contractions, palpate occasionally until placenta is delivered, fundus maintains tone and contraction pattern continues to birth of placenta Newborn assessments: • Assess Apgar score of newborn • Respirations: 30–60, irregular • Apical pulse: 110–160 and somewhat irregular • Temperature: skin temp above 36.5C (97.8F) • Umbilical cord: 2 arteries, 1 vein (if 1 artery, assess for anomalies and urine output) • Gestational age: 38 to 42 weeks	Immediate postbirth assessments q15min for one hour • BP; 90–135/60–85; should return to prelabor level • Pulse: slightly lower than in labor; range is 60–90 • Respirations: 12–24/min; easy; quiet • Temperature: 36.2–37.6C (98–99.6F) • Fundus firm, in midline, at the umbilicus or 1–2 fingerbreadths below the umbilicus • Lochia rubra; moderate amount; less than 1 pad/h; no free flow or passage of clots with massage • Perineum: sutures intact; no bulging or marked swelling; minimal bruising may be present; no c/o severe pain nor rectal pain • Bladder nondistended; spontaneous void of greater than 100 mL clear, straw-colored urine; bladder nondistended following voiding (catheterize if necessary) • If hemorrhoids present, no tenseness or marked engorgement: less than 2 cm diameter Comfort level: less than 3 on scale of 1 to 10 Energy level: awake and able to hold newborn Newborn assessments if newborn remains with parents: • Respirations: 30–60; irregular • Apical pulse: 110–160 and somewhat irregular • Temperature: skin temp above 36.5C (97.8F); skin feels warm to touch • Skin color noncyanotic • Mucus: small amount, clear, easily suctioned with bulb syringe without skin color change • Behavioral: newborn opens eyes widely if room is slightly darkened • Movements rhythmic; no hand tremors present ◆ *Expected Outcomes* Assessment findings indicate labor is progressing WNL, maternal vital signs stable and within established parameters, and reassuring fetal heart rate Maternal/fetal well-being unimpaired

(Continued on next page)

CLINICAL PATHWAY For Epidural Anesthesia continued

CATEGORY	FIRST STAGE	SECOND AND THIRD STAGE	FOURTH STAGE BIRTH TO 1 HOUR PAST BIRTH
Teaching/ psychosocial	Establish rapport Orient to environment, expected assessments and procedures Answer questions and provide information/give emotional support Orient to EFM Teach relaxation, visualization, and breathing pattern if needed Explain comfort measures available. Provide information regarding the reason for the block, possible side effects, and nursing care that may be expected Assume advocacy role for woman/family during labor and birth Explain possible delayed effects of anesthetic agents on fetus	Orient to expected assessments and procedures Answer questions and provide information Continue advocacy role Instruct woman to maintain bed rest until full function of lower extremities returns	Explain immediate assessments and care after this first hour Teach self-massage of fundus and expected findings Instruct to call for assistance if mother desires to get OOB Begin newborn teaching; bulb syringe, positioning, maintaining warmth Assist with first breastfeeding experience ◆ *Expected Outcomes* Woman verbalizes/demonstrates understanding of teaching
Nursing care management and reports	Straight cath PRN if bladder distended. If regional block administered monitor BP, FHR, sensation per protocol and obtain consent for procedure Provide continuing status reports Perineal clip per woman's request Small enema per woman's request Perform sterile vaginal examination as indicated Position woman correctly for regional block Assess maternal status: • Obtain baseline vital signs before any anesthetic agent is given • Monitor blood pressure q1–2min for 10 min and then q5–15min following administration of anesthetic agent • Monitor pulse and respiration • Monitor FHR continuously Observe, record, and report complications of anesthesia, including hypotension, fetal stress, respiratory paralysis, changes in uterine contractility, decrease in voluntary muscle effort, trauma to extremities, nausea and vomiting, and loss of bladder tone Observe, record, and report symptoms of hypotension, including systolic pressure less than 100 mm Hg or a 20–30% fall in systolic pressure, apprehension, rest-lessness, dizziness, tinnitus, headache Initiate treatment measures: • Place woman in left lateral position or position as directed with the foot of the bed elevated • Increase IV fluid rate • Administer oxygen by face mask at 7–10 L/min as needed • Administer vasopressors as ordered (usually ephedrine 5–15 mg IV) • Manually displace uterus laterally to left • Keep woman supine (semireclining) for 5–10 min following administration of block to allow drug to diffuse bilaterally. After 5–10 min position woman on side Observe, record, and report fetal bradycardia (FHR less than 110 bpm) and loss of beat-to-beat variability	Indwelling catheter or straight cath PRN if bladder distended Continue monitoring VS, FHR, and sensation Assess for potential problems of epidural infusion: sedation, nausea, vomiting, pruritus, hypotension, and "breakthrough pain"	Straight cath if bladder distended Monitor return of motor ability and sensation if regional block has been given Weigh perineal pads if lochia flow greater than 1 saturated pad in 1 h; presence of boggy uterus and clots; decreased BP, increased P ◆ *Expected Outcomes* Mother and fetus experience safe labor and birth Actual/potential complication identified and minimized Woman and family actively participate in decision making and plan of care

CLINICAL PATHWAY For Epidural Anesthesia continued

CATEGORY	FIRST STAGE	SECOND AND THIRD STAGE	FOURTH STAGE BIRTH TO 1 HOUR PAST BIRTH
Activity	Encourage ambulation unless contraindicated Maintain bed rest immediately after administration of IV pain medication, or following regional block Encourage woman to rest between contractions	Position comfortably for birth Encourage woman to rest between pushing efforts, and while awaiting birth of placenta	Position of comfort ◆ *Expected Outcomes* Activity maintained per protocol. Comfort and uterine perfusion enhanced by position/movement
Comfort	Woman states that she desires regional anesthesia Assist with administration of epidural block	Second stage: assess and inform woman of progress of labor. Provide reassurance throughout labor. Assist with "sitting dose" reinjection for birth. Encouragement, coaching, help support legs while pushing, position of comfort for pushing and birth. Third stage: cool cloth to forehead assist parents to see newborn, position mother to hold newborn, provide encouragement	Institute comfort measures: Perineal discomfort: gently cleanse and apply ice pack; position to decrease pressure on perineum Uterine discomfort: palpate fundus gently Hemorrhoids: ice pack General fatigue: position of comfort, encourage rest Administer pain medication ◆ *Expected Outcomes* Optimal comfort maintained
Nutrition	Ice chips and clear fluids Evaluate for signs of dehydration	Ice chips and clear fluids	Regular diet if assessments are WNL Encourage fluids ◆ *Expected Outcomes* Nutrition and hydration needs met
Elimination	Voids at least q2h; urine clear, straw-colored, negative for protein Bladder nondistended, empty before regional block administered May have bowel movement Monitor I & O with IVs	Monitor bladder at frequent intervals	Monitor bladder status with each assessment ◆ *Expected Outcomes* Intake and output WNL
Medications	Hydrate the woman receiving an epidural block with 500–1000 mL fluid before the procedure (dextrose-free solution is recommended)	Local infiltration of anesthetic agent for birth by CNM/physician Pitocin 10–20 units IM, IVP per IV tubing, or added to IV fluids	Continue Pitocin infusion Administer pain medication ◆ *Expected Outcomes* Perfusion and hydration supported Uterine hemorrhage prevented or successfully treated
Discharge planning/ home care	Evaluate knowledge of labor and birth process Evaluate support system and need for referral after birth		Provide information if mother to be moved from LDR room Provide opportunity for parents to ask questions regarding newborn Evaluate knowledge of normal postpartum, newborn care ◆ *Expected Outcomes* Individualized discharge teaching completed
Family Involvement	Identify available support person(s) Recognize possible impact of culture on responses Observe interaction between woman and partner Create moment alone with woman to identify possible abuse Assess current parenting skills	Provide opportunities for woman and support person(s) to watch newborn assessments Perform newborn assessment on mother's abdomen/chest if possible	Provide opportunity for parents to be with baby Encourage skin-to-skin contact Darken room to encourage eye-to-eye contact Provide quiet time for new family ◆ *Expected Outcomes* Family demonstrates support of family members Parenting: demonstrates early culturally expected parenting behaviors Family able to identify supportive resources in the community
Date			

BP, P, R, blood pressure, pulse, respirations; CNM certified nurse-midwife; EFM, electronic fetal monitor; FHR, fetal heart rate; IV, intravenous; IVP, intravenous push; LDR, labor, delivery, recovery, LTV long-term variability; PRN, as needed or as desired; 0₂, oxygen; OOB, out of bed; temp, temperature; VS, vital signs; WNL, within normal limits; c/o, complaints of.

Figure 25–5 ◆ Levels of anesthesia for vaginal and cesarean births.
SOURCE: Reprinted with permission of Ross Laboratories, Columbus, OH. From Clinical Education Aid No. 17.

level of anesthesia in the pregnant woman than in the nonpregnant woman. When a spinal block is properly administered, failure rate is low. Unlike epidural anesthesia, spinal blocks allow the anesthesia directly to mix with the cerebrospinal fluid, which eliminates "windows" where anesthesia coverage is not obtained (Wickwire & Gross, 2004). Cesarean birth requires anesthetic blockade to the T_4 dermatome (Figure 25–5 ◆).

ADVANTAGES

The advantages of spinal block are immediate onset of anesthesia, relative ease of administration, a smaller drug volume, and maternal compartmentalization of the drug. Spinal anesthesia is frequently the regional block of choice in acute obstetrical emergencies because it is the safest and fastest anesthesia technique (Wickwire & Gross, 2004).

DISADVANTAGES

The primary disadvantage of spinal block is intense blockade of sympathetic fibers, resulting in a high incidence of hypotension. This leads to a greater potential for fetal hypoxia. In addition, uterine tone is maintained, which makes intrauterine manipulation difficult. Spinal anesthesia is traditionally short acting, and it is difficult to maintain adequate anesthesia coverage for prolonged procedures (Schwartz, 2006).

CONTRAINDICATIONS

Spinal anesthesia is contraindicated for women with severe hypovolemia, regardless of cause; central nervous system disease; infection over the site of puncture; maternal coagulation problems; and allergy to local anesthetic agents (Schwartz, 2006). Sepsis and active genital herpes may be considered relative rather than absolute contraindications. Spinal block is also contraindicated for women who do not wish to have spinal procedures or are unable to appropriately consent (Cunningham et al., 2005; Schwartz, 2006).

TECHNIQUE

The following steps are followed in administering a subarachnoid block (Schwartz, 2006):

1. The nurse assists the woman into a sitting or left lateral position.

2. Intravenous infusion is checked for patency.

3. The woman places her arms between her knees, bows her head, and arches her back to widen the intervertebral space.

4. The anesthesiologist or nurse anesthetist prepares the skin carefully, maintaining sterility before initiating the procedure.

5. A skin wheal is made over L3 or L4.

6. An 18- or 19-gauge needle is introduced through the skin and into the interspinous ligament. Then, a 24- to 27-gauge pencil-point needle is introduced inside the larger needle and inserted into the ligamentum flavum, the epidural space through the dura mater, and into the subarachnoid space (Figure 25–6 ◆).

7. The appropriate amount of anesthetic agent is injected slowly, and both needles are removed.

8. Upon removal, a drop of cerebrospinal fluid can be seen in the hub of the needle if the subarachnoid space has been entered.

9. With hyperbaric solutions, the woman remains sitting up for 45 seconds.

10. The nurse assists the woman onto her back with a pillow under her head. Position changes can alter the dermatome level if done within 3 to 5 minutes. After 10 minutes, a position change will not affect the level of anesthesia.

11. The nurse monitors blood pressure, pulse, and respirations every 1 to 2 minutes for the first 10 minutes, then every 5 to 10 minutes.

The nurse provides encouragement and support during the procedure. The nurse informs the physician when a contraction is beginning so the anesthetic agent will not be injected at that time.

In the absence of maternal hypotension or toxic reaction, a spinal block exerts no direct effect on the fetus. The amount of anesthetic used is too small to reach fetal circulation in a quantity that might cause fetal depression. Spinal anesthesia has been shown to be well tolerated by a healthy fetus when a maternal IV fluid preload in excess of 500 to 1000 mL precedes the administration of the spinal.

Figure 25–6 ◆ Double-needle technique for spinal injection. *A,* Large needle in epidural space. *B,* 25-gauge needle in larger needle entering the subarachnoid space.
SOURCE: Bonica, J. J. (1972). *Principles and practice of obstetric analgesia and anesthesia* (p. 563). Philadelphia: Davis.

COMPLICATIONS

The complications of spinal anesthesia include hypotension, drug reaction, total spinal neurologic sequelae, and spinal headache. The side effects include nausea, shivering, and urinary retention.

Hypotension can be minimized by prehydrating with 500 to 2000 mL of non-dextrose-containing fluids and displacing the uterus to a lateral position. The practice of placing an already hypotensive woman in a sitting position following injection to prevent upward spread of hyperbaric solution is dangerous because it will cause venous pooling in the lower extremities, further decreasing the maternal blood pressure (Braveman, 2006). The normal curve of the thoracic spine prevents cranial spread of an intrathecal agent. A pillow is placed under the woman's head to exaggerate the curve (Braveman, 2006).

Treatment of hypotension is the same as with an epidural block: positioning the woman in a lateral position, head-down position and rapidly infusing IV fluids. Preventing cardiovascular collapse requires early detection, supplemental oxygen, assisted ventilation, and measures to maintain the blood pressure. The extent to which the fetus is affected relates to the degree of maternal hypotension. When maternal hypotension has been reversed, it is best to delay the birth for 4 to 5 minutes to allow the fetus to recover. If hypotension does not resolve in a short period of time, ephedrine can be administered IV. Resuscitative equipment and trained personnel must be available to treat the mother and baby.

Complications that involve anesthesia occurring in the phrenic nerve (C3–C5) or higher can occur (Wickwire & Gross, 2004). In a "high-level" block, respiratory function becomes impaired, requiring mechanical ventilation to maintain adequate respiratory functioning until the block recedes. Another extremely rare complication is the "complete spinal" in which respiratory assistance is needed and loss of consciousness also occurs. A "total spinal" block occurs when there is paralysis of the respiratory muscles. It is a relatively rare but critical event. The symptoms include apnea, dilation of pupils, loss of consciousness, and absence of blood pressure. The onset of symptoms usually occurs within minutes of the injection but can occur in a span of time ranging from 30 seconds to 45 minutes. Resuscitative treatment, airway control, and support of blood pressure must begin immediately. If this complication occurs, it is important to remember that this woman is not asleep; although she may be paralyzed, she may be aware of everything going on around her. She requires assurance that her respiratory status will be maintained until she can breathe on her own again (Wickwire & Gross, 2004).

On the other hand, a spinal block can render inadequate anesthesia coverage (in which the anesthesia does not reach the T4 level) and discomfort can occur. During intraoperative procedures, this may warrant the need for a repeat insertion or the need for general anesthesia (Wickwire & Gross, 2004).

Neurologic complications may occur coincidentally with spinal anesthesia, for example, with preexisting disease or faulty positioning of the woman. Hypotension and apnea can occur, requiring prompt treatment to prevent cardiac arrest. The woman should be positioned with a left tilt, and fluids should be administered to treat hypotension (Cunningham et al., 2005). Genuine neurologic sequelae, such as paralysis, are extremely rare.

Although much less serious than other complications, headache may be an unpleasant aftermath of spinal anesthesia. It is the most frequent complication with an incidence of about 1% to 3% (Wickwire & Gross, 2004). Leakage of spinal fluid at the site of dural puncture is thought to be the cause. Several techniques have been suggested to decrease the possibility of headache. The use of a narrow-gauge pencil-point anesthesia needle (24- to 27-gauge) reduces the incidence of spinal headache. Conservative treatment, such as hyperhydration and keeping the woman flat in bed after birth, have been used with minimum success. An abdominal binder may provide some relief. Postdural headaches can last up to 7 days and not only are painful but can also interfere with maternal infant interactions and breastfeeding success (Wickwire & Gross, 2004). In severe cases, a blood patch can be performed. A few milliliters of the woman's blood is drawn and, before coagulation occurs, is injected into the epidural space at the site of the puncture. This technique generally results in immediate pain relief.

NURSING CARE MANAGEMENT

The nurse should assist in positioning the woman, provide oxygen via nasal cannula or mask, assess and record baseline vital signs of the mother and fetus, and start an IV infusion before administration of the block (Schwartz, 2006). A bolus of fluid should be given before initiation of the block whenever possible (Schwartz, 2006). After the block is instilled, the nurse should continue to monitor maternal blood pressure, pulse, and respiration until the anesthesiologist takes over. The nurse monitors the FHR at least every 5 minutes until it is no longer accessible because the abdominal surgical prep is begun. The anesthesiologist is responsible for assessing and recording the level of the spinal block.

The nurse positions the woman as described earlier and supports her in this position. The nurse palpates the woman's uterus to detect the beginning of a contraction. Intrathecal agents are not administered during a contraction because the increased pressure could cause a higher level of anesthesia than desired. After the agent has been administered, the woman is supported upright for the length of time determined by the anesthesiologist and is then assisted to the supine position with a wedge under her right hip to displace the uterus; a pillow is placed under her head. In the surgical setting, a safety belt is placed across the woman's thighs to prevent injury. The nurse regularly monitors blood pressure, pulse, and respirations every 5 minutes until the birth. Some physicians administer oxygen as a prophylactic measure. The woman should be kept informed of everything that is going on in the birthing area, particularly if she is receiving mask oxygen. Raising her legs facilitates venous return from the extremities. If using stirrups, both legs should be raised at the same time to avoid undue tension and possible injury to back muscles.

If hypotension should occur, the IV fluids should be increased and the uterus displaced manually to the left (Braveman, 2006). If the woman reports that she is having difficulty breathing, she needs to be assessed very carefully. Total spinal block rarely occurs, but the possibility must always be kept in mind. The woman should be observed for apnea, unconsciousness, pupil dilation, and unobtainable blood pressure. Prompt treatment, which may include the use of a vasopressor (such as ephedrine), may avert maternal or fetal death. It is essential to establish an airway and give oxygen with positive pressure until the woman can be intubated and other emergency measures instituted.

Following the birth, the woman may be kept flat. Although the effectiveness of the supine position to avoid headache following a spinal is controversial, the physician's orders may include lying flat for 6 to 12 hours.

Combined Spinal-Epidural Block

Spinal anesthesia may be combined with an epidural block. The combined spinal-epidural (CSE) can be used for labor analgesia and for cesarean birth. The anesthetic and analgesic agents used differ according to the purpose of the CSE. A CSE is accomplished by inserting an epidural needle into the epidural space. A narrow-gauge pencil-point anesthesia needle (24- to 27-gauge) is inserted through the epidural needle, through the dura, and into the cerebrospinal fluid. A small amount of local anesthetic agent, opioid, or both, is injected, and the needle is withdrawn. An epidural catheter is then threaded through the epidural needle

into the epidural space. The epidural needle is removed and the epidural catheter is securely placed against the woman with tape.

An advantage of CSE is that the spinal agent will have a faster onset than medications that are injected into the epidural space. A CSE is versatile in that medication can be added to increase the effectiveness. Additional medication can also be added if an instrument-assisted birth or cesarean is needed (Wickwire & Gross, 2004). CSE also preserves motor functioning. Most drugs are used in low dose, so spinal analgesia may be given in early labor to assist with labor pain. The nurse assesses the woman's strength and motor functioning before ambulation occurs. If ambulation is desired, a continuous assessment of the FHR and the maternal blood pressure is needed. Close supervision is needed to prevent falls or other injuries. When CSE is used, there does appear to be a higher incidence of nausea and pruritus. There are no reports of increased risks of fetal or neonatal complications.

Pudendal Block

The **pudendal block** technique provides perineal anesthesia for the second stage of labor, birth, and episiotomy repair. An anesthetic agent is injected below the pudendal plexus, as shown in Figure 25–1. The pudendal plexus arises from the anterior division of the second and third sacral nerves and the entire fourth sacral nerve. Below the plexus, the branches converge into the pudendal nerve, which crosses the sacrosciatic notch and passes the tip of the ischial spine, where it divides into the perineal, dorsal, and inferior hemorrhoidal nerves of the pudendal plexus. The perineal nerve, which is the largest branch of the pudendal plexus, supplies the skin of the vulvar area, the perineal muscles, and the urethral sphincter. The dorsal nerve supplies the clitoris, and the inferior hemorrhoidal nerve supplies the skin and muscles of the perineal region as well as the internal anal sphincter. Pudendal block provides relief of pain from perineal distention but does not relieve pain of uterine contractions (Figure 25–7 ◆).

ADVANTAGES AND DISADVANTAGES

The advantages of pudendal block are ease of administration and absence of maternal hypotension. It also allows the use of low forceps or vacuum extraction for birth.

A moderate dose of anesthetic agent (10 mL per side) has minimal ill effects on the woman and the course of labor. The urge to bear down during the second stage of labor may be decreased, but the woman is able to do so with appropriate coaching. There is usually little effect on the uncompromised fetus unless overly rapid or intravascular injection occurs. The block may be done by a transvaginal or transperineal approach. The woman may experience a burning sensation when the block is administered. Transvaginal injection is simpler, safer, and more direct, making it the procedure of choice.

COMPLICATIONS

A systemic toxic reaction can occur from accidental vascular injection. Other possible maternal complications specific to pudendal block include broad ligament hematoma, perforation of the rectum, and trauma to the sciatic nerve.

Figure 25–7 ◆ *A,* Pudendal block by the transvaginal approach. *B,* Area of perineum affected by pudendal block.

NURSING CARE MANAGEMENT

The nurse explains the procedure and the expected effect and answers any questions. Pudendal block does not alter maternal vital signs or FHR, so assessments in addition to the expected ones are not necessary.

Local Infiltration Anesthesia

Local anesthesia is accomplished by injecting an anesthetic agent into the intracutaneous, subcutaneous, and intramuscular areas of the perineum (Figure 25–8 ◆). It is generally used at the time of birth for episiotomy and repair and is especially useful for women giving birth without previous pharmacologic interventions. The procedure is essentially free from complications. The woman may experience a burning sensation at the time of administration.

ADVANTAGES

The major advantage of the local block is that it involves the use of the least amount of anesthetic agent. It can be done if an episiotomy is needed just before the birth. It can also be used when a laceration has occurred and a repair is needed.

DISADVANTAGES

The major disadvantage is that large amounts of solution must be used. Although any local anesthetic may be used, chloropro-

Figure 25–8 ◆ Local infiltration anesthesia. *A,* Technique of local infiltration for episiotomy and repair. *B,* Technique of local infiltration showing fan pattern for the fascial planes.
SOURCE: Bonica, J. J. (1972). *Principles and practice of obstetric analgesia and anesthesia* (p. 505). Philadelphia: Davis.

caine (Nesacaine), lidocaine (Xylocaine), and mepivacaine (Carbocaine) are the agents of choice in local infiltration because of their capacity for diffusion. A burning sensation at the time of injection is common.

NURSING CARE MANAGEMENT

The nurse explains the procedure and the expected effect and answers any questions. Local anesthetic agents have no effect on maternal vital signs or FHR, so additional assessments are unnecessary.

GENERAL ANESTHESIA

General anesthesia (induced unconsciousness) may be needed for cesarean birth and surgical intervention with some obstetric complications. The method used to achieve general anesthesia may be IV injection, inhalation of anesthetic agents, or a combination of both methods. The use of general anesthesia in the obstetrical setting continues to decline because of adverse fetal effects and the increase in maternal risks. The most common indications for general anesthesia include perceived lack of time for regional anesthesia, contraindications to regional anesthesia, failure to successfully insert regional anesthesia, and client refusal (Tsen, 2005).

Intravenous Anesthetics

Sodium thiopental (Pentothal) is an ultra-short-acting barbiturate, which means that it exerts its effect rapidly and has a brief duration of action. Sodium thiopental produces narcosis within 30 seconds after IV administration. Introduction and emergence from its effects are smooth and pleasant, with little incidence of nausea and vomiting. Sodium thiopental is most frequently used for initiating unconsciousness and as an adjunct to other more potent anesthetics. Ketamine is an intermediate-acting barbiturate that is used for anesthesia induction. The effects typically last 20 to 60 minutes. Hypersalivation can occur but can be treated with an anticholinergic drug to decrease this side effect. The drug is contraindicated in women with preeclampsia or chronic hypertension.

Inhaled Anesthesia Agents

The most commonly used inhaled anesthesia agent is nitrous oxide. Nitrous oxide does not produce significant uterine relaxation. Although it crosses the placenta immediately after administration, fetal tissue uptake occurs 20 minutes after administration, which results in a lower fetal arterial concentration and less neonatal depression. In recent years, the recommended dosage has been decreased to 50% (down from 70%) and the time from administration until birth has been shortened as much as possible. In order to decrease the length of fetal exposure, it is recommended that the woman be fully prepped and the obstetrician be fully prepared to make the initial incision when nitrous oxide is introduced (Braveman, 2006).

The use of other low-dose halogenated agents, such as isoflurane, halothane, sevoflurane, desflurane, and enflurane, are also used, often in combination with nitrous oxide. These agents have been used commonly and have been found to increase maternal inspired oxygen levels and may increase uterine blood flow (Braveman, 2006). One study did find that the use of sevoflurane was associated with uterine relaxation when administered in high dosages, suggesting that the lowest dose possible should be used (Jirasiritham, Tantivitayatan, & Sirivararom, 2005).

Inhaled anesthetic agents have also been used in combination with spinal or epidural techniques when the epidural anesthesia was ineffective or severe maternal anxiety was present (Vallejo, Phelps, Shepherd et al., 2005). Inhaled agents are also an ideal choice for women with aortic stenosis who are not candidates for regional anesthesia. In one study, all women who received inhaled anesthetic agents had cardiovascular stability throughout surgery and no adverse fetal outcomes (Orme, Grange, Ainsworth et al., 2004).

Complications of General Anesthesia

A primary danger of general anesthesia is fetal depression. Most general anesthetic agents reach the fetus in about 2 minutes. The depression of the fetus is directly proportional to the depth and duration of the anesthesia. The long-term significance of fetal depression in a normal birth has not been determined. The poor fetal metabolism of general anesthetic agents is similar to that of analgesic agents administered during labor. General anesthesia is not advocated when the fetus is considered to be at high risk, particularly in preterm birth.

Most general anesthetic agents cause some degree of uterine relaxation although the inhalation agents effect uterine relaxation to a lesser degree than the IV agents. They may also cause vomiting and aspiration.

Pregnancy results in decreased gastric motility, and the onset of labor halts the process almost entirely. Food eaten hours earlier may remain undigested in the stomach. Even when food and fluids have been withheld, the gastric juice produced during fasting is highly acidic and can produce chemical pneumonitis if aspirated. This pneumonitis is known as Mendelson syndrome. The signs and symptoms are chest pain, respiratory distress, cyanosis, fever, and tachycardia. Women undergoing emergency cesarean births appear to be at considerable risk for adverse events. The leading cause of maternal deaths in women who have had general anesthesia is the failure to establish a patent airway (Tsen, 2005).

Care During General Anesthesia

Prophylactic antacid therapy is given to reduce the acidic content of the stomach before general anesthesia. Administration of a nonparticulate antacid (such as Bicitra) may be used. Cimetidine (Tagamet) may also be used (Cunningham et al., 2005).

Before the induction to anesthesia, the woman should have a wedge placed under her hip to displace the uterus and avoid vena caval compression in the supine position. She should also be preoxygenated with 3 to 5 minutes of 100% oxygen. IV fluids should be started so that access to the intravascular space is immediately available.

During the process of rapid induction of anesthesia, the nurse applies cricoid pressure. This is accomplished by depressing the cricoid cartilage 2 to 3 cm posteriorly so that the esophagus is occluded. Cricoid pressure is continued until the anesthesiologist has placed the cuffed endotracheal tube and indicates that the pressure can be released. Figure 25–9 ◆ shows the appropriate technique. The woman's neck should be supported by the nurse's other hand.

Neonatal Neurobehavioral Effects of Anesthesia and Analgesia

Studies have focused on the neurobehavioral effects on the newborn of pharmacologic agents used during labor and birth. Although analgesic and anesthetic agents may alter the behavioral

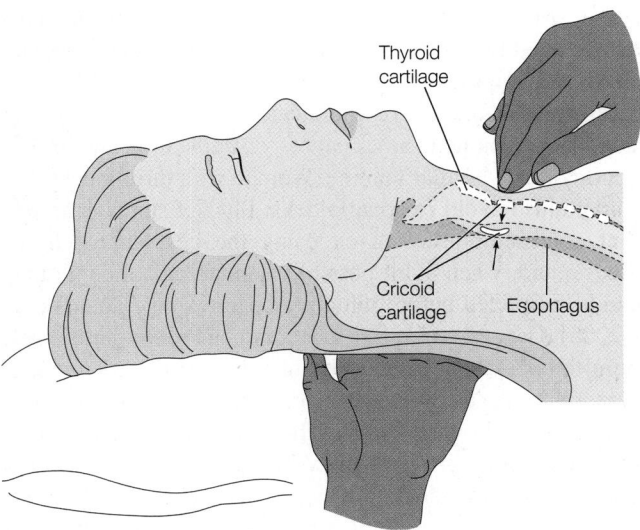

Figure 25–9 ◆ Proper position for fingers in applying cricoid pressure until a cuffed endotracheal tube is placed by the anesthesiologist or certified nurse-anesthetist. The cricoid cartilage is depressed 2 to 3 cm so that the esophagus is occluded.

and adaptive function of the newborn, physiologic factors such as hunger, degree of hydration, and time within the sleep-wake cycle may also exert an influence (Berens, 2004). The long-range importance of these findings has not been well established.

Women who receive general anesthesia are also slower to initiate breastfeeding in the immediate postpartum period, which can have long-term effects on breastfeeding success. Women who receive general anesthesia also have a lower incidence of breastfeeding at 6 months compared with women who have received regional anesthesia (Berens, 2004).

ANALGESIC AND ANESTHETIC CONSIDERATIONS FOR THE HIGH-RISK MOTHER AND FETUS

Up to this point the discussion of obstetric analgesia and anesthesia has dealt with the healthy woman and healthy fetus. Pain relief for high-risk women during labor and birth requires skill in decision making, close observation, and awareness of potential threats to the woman and fetus. Safety for all involved requires the close cooperation of the obstetrician, anesthesiologist, pediatrician, and labor nurse. The pathophysiologic changes that accompany maternal disorders have a direct influence on the choice of agent or technique. It is difficult to separate maternal and fetal complications because whatever alters the woman's response will also affect the fetus. The effects on the woman cannot be considered without the potential effects on the fetus.

Preterm Labor

The preterm fetus has special risks and requirements. An immature fetus is more susceptible to depressant drugs because he or she has less protein available for binding; has a poorly devel-

oped blood-brain barrier, which increases the likelihood that pharmacologic agents will attain a higher concentration in the central nervous system; and has a decreased ability to metabolize and excrete drugs after birth (Wylie, 2005). Analgesia during labor should be avoided whenever possible. If it becomes necessary, the smallest dose that will provide relief should be administered. Emotional support will be very valuable to the woman in this situation (Braveman, 2005).

Preeclampsia

Pregnancies complicated by preeclampsia are high-risk situations, as indicated in Chapter 20. ∞ The potential for chronic placental insufficiency or preterm birth is also present. The woman with mild preeclampsia usually may have the analgesia or anesthesia of choice, although the incidence of hypotension with epidural anesthesia is increased (Wylie, 2005). If hypotension occurs with the epidural block, it provides further stress on an already compromised cardiovascular system. Hypotension can usually be managed with judicious fluid increase and positioning.

The woman with severe preeclampsia poses a real challenge. Regional anesthesia seems to be the preferred method as long as hypotension can be avoided. Raising the central venous pressure by 3 to 4 cm H_2O with IV fluids helps avoid hypotension, but it must be remembered that this woman is already threatened with heart failure (Foley et al., 2004). The effect of fluid intake can be monitored with a pulmonary catheter. Pulmonary artery catheterization is used to correct volume deficits and appears more accurate than central pressure catheters in monitoring left and right side cardiac filling pressures, cardiac output, and systemic vascular resistance (Santos, 2004). It is important to monitor and record the fluid intake and output. Some physicians use vasopressors; others avoid them because of the possible decrease in uterine blood flow to an already compromised fetus and the threat of a maternal cerebral vascular accident (Foley et al., 2004). Spinal anesthesia is rarely used because of the greater potential for hypotension.

The use of general anesthesia poses a risk of aggravating maternal hypertension. In general, the safest method for general anesthesia is intubation, but because it may cause a hypertensive episode, it is avoided if possible. Another important consideration is that women with preeclampsia are more prone to have mucosal edema in the oral cavity and glottis, making intubation more difficult (Santos, 2004).

Diabetes Mellitus

The fetus of a mother with diabetes mellitus may have a reduction in placenta blood flow. Hypotension, which can result during regional anesthesia, can deplete this blood flow even further. If the fetus is tolerating labor well without an indication of nonreassuring fetal status, the continuous epidural technique may be undertaken. If nonreassuring fetal status occurs, cesarean birth may be necessary.

Anesthesia for cesarean birth requires special consideration in this case. The diabetic woman is more likely to experience cardiovascular depression during a regional block because of higher sympathetic blockade (Foley et al., 2004). If a regional block is selected, it is recommended that acute hydration (preload) be provided by administering dextrose-free solution. In addition, left uterine displacement is initiated before the administration of the block and maintained throughout the surgery. Hypotension is treated promptly.

Cardiac Disease

Pregnancy imposes significant risks for the woman with cardiac disease. With mild mitral stenosis, the preferred anesthetic is continual epidural anesthesia with low forceps birth. This method avoids the cardiovascular changes associated with contractions and the Valsalva maneuver during bearing down in the second stage of labor. Hypotension can be avoided with carefully controlled IV fluids and measuring central venous pressure to avoid overload. Epidural block or general anesthesia may be used in cesarean birth. Ketamine should be avoided because it produces tachycardia (Braveman, 2006).

Bleeding Complications

The current trend in treating bleeding complications during labor is to schedule cesarean birth when possible. When the maternal cardiovascular system is stable and there is no evidence of nonreassuring fetal status, an epidural may be given for birth. However, when either of these conditions results in active bleeding, the threat of hypovolemia must be treated immediately. Maternal hypovolemia and shock produce fetal hypoxia, acidosis, and possible fetal death (Foley et al., 2004).

Regional blocks are contraindicated during active bleeding because the sympathetic block causes vasodilatation and further reduction of the vascular volume. Women with thrombocytopenia should also avoid regional blocks. Platelet status is an important consideration when choosing the best approach for anesthesia and, when at all possible, hematological conditions should be corrected before initiating birth (Wong, Chan, & Irwin, 2005). General anesthesia is recommended for these cases. Sodium thiopental may be used, but it is a cardiac depressant and vasodilator, and ketamine may be a more appropriate choice for induction. Following birth of the infant and placenta, oxytocin should not be given as an IV bolus to contract the uterus because it causes vasodilatation, which in turn causes a decrease in blood pressure and in total peripheral resistance. Oxytocin should be given as a dilute infusion to gain an oxytocic effect to treat uterine atony (relaxation) and to control postpartum bleeding. Resources that should be on hand to handle hemorrhagic emergencies include large-bore IV catheters, a fluid warmer, a forced-air body warmer, the woman's specific blood type or O negative blood, and equipment to infuse blood products rapidly (Foley et al., 2004).

CHAPTER REVIEW

FOCUS YOUR STUDY

- Pain relief during labor may be enhanced by nonpharmacologic methods and administration of analgesic agents and regional anesthesia blocks. The nurse can offer alternative comfort measures, avoid offering pain medication to women who do not desire pain medication, provide the woman who does desire pain medication with the opportunity to explore available options, and provide education and reassurance to the expectant woman and her support person.

- The goal of pharmacologic analgesia during labor is to provide maximal pain relief with minimal risk for the woman and fetus.

- The optimal time for administering analgesia is determined after a complete assessment of vital factors, including maternal, fetal, and labor assessments and the woman's perception of her pain level and her need and desire for pain medication.

- Two common analgesic agents are butorphanol (Stadol) and nalbuphine (Nubain).

- Opiate antagonists, such as naloxone (Narcan), counteract the respiratory depressant effect of the opiate narcotics by acting at specific receptor sites in the central nervous system.

- Sedatives, including barbiturates, benzodiazepines, and H_1-receptor antagonists, are primarily used in latent or early labor to promote rest and allow the woman to sleep.

- Regional anesthesia is achieved by injecting local anesthetic agents into an area that will bring the agent into direct contact with nerve tissue. Methods most commonly used in childbearing include lumbar epidural, spinal block, combined spinal-epidural block, pudendal block, and local infiltration.

- Three types of local anesthetic agents used in regional blocks are amides, esters, and opiates. The amides are absorbed quickly and can be found in maternal blood within minutes after administration. The esters are metabolized more rapidly and have only limited placental transfer. Opiates act on specific opiate receptors in the spinal cord and have a greater analgesic effect when combined with a low dose of local anesthetic.

- Possible maternal complications of regional anesthesia, although rare, include systemic toxicity, convulsions, and sudden cardiovascular collapse.

- Agents in use for epidural and spinal routes include the opioids morphine and fentanyl. Adverse reactions of the woman to local anesthetic agents range from mild symptoms, such as palpitations, to cardiovascular collapse. The newer amides, including ropivacaine and levobupivacaine, are longer acting and have fewer side effects.

- Pudendal blocks provide perineal anesthesia during the second stage of labor, birth, episiotomies, or laceration repair.

- General anesthesia can be achieved by intravenous injection, inhalation of anesthetic agents, or a combination of both methods.

- The goal of general anesthesia is to provide maximal pain relief with minimal side effects to the woman and her fetus.

- Complications of general anesthesia include fetal depression, uterine relaxation, vomiting, and aspiration.

- The choice of analgesia and anesthesia for the high-risk woman and fetus requires careful evaluation.

EXPLORE MediaLink

Video: Epidural Placement Video

http://www.prenhall.com/davidson

NCLEX review questions, case studies, and other interactive resources for this chapter can be found on the Web Site at http://www.prenhall.com/davidson. Click on "Chapter 25" to select the activities for this chapter.

For tutorials including animations and videos, more NCLEX review questions, and an audio glossary, access the accompanying Prentice Hall Nursing MediaLink DVD-ROM in this book.

PRENTICE HALL NURSING MEDIALINK DVD-ROM

Audio Glossary

NCLEX Review

Videos: *Epidural Placement; Through the Eyes of a Nurse—The Third Trimester*

COMPANION WEBSITE

Additional NCLEX Review

Case Study: *Client Requesting an Epidural*

Care Plan Activity: *Managing Side Effects of an Epidural*

Applications: *Risks and Benefits of Using IV Medications for Pain Relief During Labor; Epidural Analgesia*

Critical Thinking

CRITICAL THINKING IN ACTION

REGIONAL ANALGESIA DURING LABOR AND BIRTH

View the Critical Thinking in Action video in Chapter 25 of the DVD-ROM. Then answer the questions that follow.

Sandra, a 26-year-old G1, is in active labor when she presents to you at the birthing center. She has been in labor for 5 hours and is clearly tired and seems to be having difficulty coping with the pain. Her contractions are occurring every 2 to 4 minutes, lasting 50 to 60 seconds, and are moderate to strong in intensity. You assess the fetal heart rate of 120 to 130 with early decelerations; moderate variability is present. Sandra's vital signs are stable and her laboratory results are within normal limits. She is requesting an epidural analgesia for pain control. A vaginal exam demonstrates the cervix is 100% effaced, 6 cm dilated with the vertex at 0 station in the LOT position. You notify the physician of Sandra's wish for pain relief and labor progress. You review the client's record for written consent for regional analgesia and assist the anesthesiologist with the procedure.

1. Discuss the advantages of regional analgesia.

2. Describe the nursing responsibility during the administration of regional analgesia.

3. Discuss the side effects of regional analgesia.

4. What are the absolute contraindications for an epidural block?

5. How do you assist Sandra with the second stage of labor when she cannot feel her contractions?

REFERENCES

American College of Obstetricians and Gynecologists (ACOG). (2002). *Obstetric analgesia and anesthesia* (ACOG Practice Bulletin No. 36). Washington, DC: Author.

Atherton, M. J., Feeg, V. D., & El-Adham, A. F. (2004). Race, ethnicity, and insurance as a determinate analysis of a national sample survey. *Nursing Economics, 22*(1), 6–13.

Berens, P. D. (2004). Applied physiology in the peripartum management of lactation. *Obstetrics and Gynecology, 47*(3), 643–655.

Bowes, W. A. (2005). The impact of intrapartum analgesia on infant feeding. *Obstetrical & Gynecological Survey, 60*(12), 790–791.

Braveman, F. R. (2006). *Obstetric and gynecologic anesthesia: The requisites.* St. Louis, MO: Mosby.

Buckenmaier, C. C., & Bleckner, L. (2005). Anesthetic agents for advanced regional anesthesia: A North American perspective. *Drugs, 65*(6), 745–759.

Camann, W. (2005). Pain relief during labor. *Obstetric Anesthesia Digest, 25*(3), 115.

Cunningham, F. G., Leveno, K. J., Bloom, S. L., Hauth, J. C., Gilstrap, L. C., & Wenstrom, K. D. (2005). *Williams obstetrics* (22nd ed.). New York: McGraw-Hill.

Florence, D. J., & Palmer, D. G. (2003). Therapeutic choices for the discomforts of labor. *Journal of Perinatal and Neonatal Nursing, 17*(4), 238–249.

Foley, M. R., Strong, T. H., & Garite, T. J. (2004). Obstetric intensive care manual (2nd ed.). New York: McGraw-Hill.

Fraser, W. D., Cayer, M., Soeder, B. M., Turcot, L., & Marcoux, S. (2002). Risk factors for difficult delivery in nulliparas with epidural analgesia in second stage. *Obstetrics and Gynecology, 99*, 409–418.

Howell, C. J. (2002). Epidural versus non-epidural analgesia for pain relief in labour. *The Cochrane Library* (Oxford) (1) (Article No. CD000331) (1).

Jirasiritham, S., Tantivitayatan, K., & Sirivararom, P. (2005). Over half MAC sevoflurane

in cesarean section. *Journal of the Medical Association of Thailand, 88*(7), 914–920.

Kuczkowski, K. M. (2004a). Ambulatory labor analgesia: What does an obstetrician need to know? *Acta Obstetricia et Gynecologica Scandinavica, 83*(5), 415–424.

Kuczkowski, K. (2004b). Nonobstetric surgery during pregnancy. What are the risks of anesthesia? *Obstetrical & Gynecological Survey, 59*(1), 52–56.

Leung, A. Y. (2005). Postoperative pain management in obstetric anesthesia: New challenges and solutions. *Survey of Anesthesiology, 49*(4), 203–204.

Lieberman, E., & O'donoghue, C. (2002). Unintended effects of epidural analgesia during labor: A systematic review. *American Journal of Obstetrics & Gynecology, 186*(Suppl. 5, Nature), S31–68.

Macarthur, A. (2002). Solving the problem of spinal-induced hypotension in obstetric anesthesia. *Canadian Journal of Anaesthesia, 49*(6), 536–539.

Mattingly, J. E., D'Alessio, J., & Ramanathan, J. (2003). Effects of obstetric analgesics and anesthetics on the neonate: A review. *Pediatric Drugs, 5*(9), 615–627.

McGuire, W., & Fowlie, P. W. (2003). Naloxone for narcotic exposed newborn infants: Systematic review. *Archives of Disease in Childhood; Fetal and Neonatal Edition, 88,* F308.

Nagoette, M. (2006). Timing of conduction analgesia in labor. *American Journal of Obstetrics & Gynecology, 194*(3), 598–599.

Orme, R. M., Grange, C. S., Ainsworth, Q. P., & Grebenik, C. R. (2004). General anaesthesia using remifentanil for caesarean section in parturients with critical aortic stenosis: A series of four cases. *International Journal of Obstetric Anesthesia, 13*(3), 183–187.

Rayburn, W. F., & Bogenschutz, M. P. (2004). Pharmacotherapy for pregnant women with addictions. *American Journal of Obstetrics & Gynecology, 191*(6), 1885–1897.

Renn, C. L., & Dorsey, S. G. (2005). The physiology and processing of pain: A review.

AACN Clinical Issues: Advanced Practice in Acute Care, 16(3), 277–290.

Rosenberg, P. H., Veering, B. T., & Urmey, W. F. (2005). Maximum recommended dosages of local anesthetic agents: A multifactoral concept. *Obstetric Anesthesia Digest, 25*(3), 118–119.

Santos, A. C. (2004). Anesthetic management of the preeclamptic parturient. *ASA Refresher Course in Anesthesia, 32*(1), 197–204.

Schwartz, A. J. (2006). Learning the essentials of epidural anesthesia. *Nursing, 36*(1), 44–50.

Tsen, L. (2005). Anesthesia for cesarean delivery. *ASA Refresher Course in Anesthesia, 33*(1), 235–245.

Vahratian, A. (2004). Maternal prepregnancy overweight and obesity and the pattern of labor progression in term nulliparous women. *Obstetrics and Gynecology, 104*(5, Part 1), 943–951.

Vallejo, M. C., Phelps, A. L., Shepherd, C. J., Kaul, B., Mandell, G. L., & Ramanathan, S. (2005). Nitrous oxide anxiolysis for elective cesarean section. *Journal of Clinical Anesthesia, 17*(7), 543–548.

Wickwire, A. T., & Gross, C. E. (2004). From pre-op to post-op: Cesarean delivery from the anesthesiologist's point of view. *Clinical Obstetrics and Gynecology, 47*(2), 299–316.

Wilson, B. A., Shannon, M. T., & Stang, C. L. (2006). *Prentice Hall nurse's drug guide 2006.* Upper Saddle River, NJ: Pearson Prentice Hall.

Wong, A. Y. C., Chan, R. S. N., & Irwin, M. G. (2005). Anesthetic management of a cesarean delivery with hypoplastic anemia and severe pre-eclampsia. *Obstetric Anesthesia Digest, 25*(2), 103–104.

Wong, C. A., Scavone, B. M., Peaceman, A. M, McCarthy, R. J., & Sullivan, J. T. (2005). The risk of cesarean delivery with neuraxial analgesia given early versus late in labor. *Obstetrical & Gynecological Survey, 60*(7), 424–425.

Wylie, L. (2005). *Essential anatomy and physiology in maternity care.* London: Churchill Livingstone.

CHAPTER
26
Childbirth at Risk: The Intrapartal Period

I couldn't wait to begin labor. I wasn't afraid. We had wonderful plans for our labor and birth. My nurse helped me with my breathing as I entered transition. Everything was going so well. Suddenly, the baby began having decelerations. The nurse assisted me onto my side and called for assistance. Time seemed to stand still as the once rapidly beating heart suddenly sounded so slow. It seemed like it took forever to return to its previous rapid pace. For an instant, I was terrified, but after that one episode, there were no further problems.

OBJECTIVES

1. Describe psychologic disorders that may contribute to difficulty in coping during labor and birth.
2. Discuss dysfunctional labor patterns.
3. Identify the potential maternal risks of precipitous labor and birth.
4. Describe the impact of postterm pregnancy on the childbearing family.
5. Summarize various types of fetal malposition and malpresentation and possible associated problems.
6. Discuss the implications of macrosomia and hydrocephalus on the woman and the fetus.
7. Identify maternal and fetal risks associated with multiple gestations.
8. Compare abruptio placentae and placenta previa.
9. Identify variations that may occur in the umbilical cord and insertion into the placenta.
10. Discuss the identification, management, and nursing care of women with amniotic fluid embolus, hydramnios, and oligohydramnios.
11. Delineate the effects of pelvic contractures on labor and birth.
12. Discuss complications of the third and fourth stages of labor.

KEY TERMS

MEDIALINK

Additional resources for this content can be found on the Prentice Hall Nursing MediaLink DVD-ROM and on the Companion Website at http://www.prenhall.com/davidson. Click on "Chapter 26" to select the activities for this chapter.

The successful completion of the 40-week gestational period requires the harmonious functioning of the five critical factors we discussed in Chapter 22 ∞: the birth passage, the fetus, the relationship between the passage and fetus, forces of labor, and psychosocial considerations. Disruptions in any of these components may result in dystocia (at-risk or difficult labor). Some of the most common at-risk conditions are discussed in this chapter.

CARE OF THE WOMAN AT RISK BECAUSE OF PSYCHOLOGIC DISORDERS

Anxiety and fear are common emotions in many women in labor. The onset of labor is a time of mixed emotions. Joy, happiness, excitement, fear of the unknown, and anxiety related to pain sensations may all occur. Even women who are well prepared can experience anxious feelings. Although these reactions are expected in the woman with normal coping mechanisms and adequate social support, women with psychologic disorders may face additional emotional challenges and need additional nursing care and support in the intrapartum period.

The prevalence of psychologic disorders of adults in the United States is 26.2% (Table 26–1). **Psychologic disorders** are characterized by alterations in thinking, mood, or behavior (Kessler, 2005). Although there are many different types of psychologic disorders, only the most common are presented here. Because an in-depth description is beyond the scope of this text, we focus on the impact of these disorders on labor and birth (Table 26–2). Postpartal psychologic disorders are discussed in Chapter 37. ∞

Depression affects millions of Americans annually. More women are affected than men (National Institute of Mental Health [NIMH], 2006). Depression is believed to be caused by a central nervous system (CNS) imbalance in serotonin and

other neurotransmitters. The hormonal changes associated with pregnancy can directly impact a woman with a previous history of depression. Individuals with depression may have persistent sad mood, anxiety, physical slowing, agitation, energy loss, feelings of worthlessness, difficulty thinking or concentrating, and sleep disturbances (NIMH, 2006).

Depression can affect the labor process in a variety of ways. The woman may be unable to concentrate or process information being provided by healthcare team members. Because depression often causes difficulty sleeping, she may begin labor fatigued or sleep deprived. The labor process may overwhelm her physically and emotionally, because she has no energy "reserves" on which to draw. She may feel unworthy of motherhood or experience hopelessness about the outcome of her labor. However, she may not be able to articulate any of these feelings and may instead appear irritable or withdrawn.

Individuals with *bipolar disorder* can have depressive symptoms that alternate with episodes of mania. Although a complete discussion of bipolar disorder is beyond the scope of this text, students should refer to a psychiatric nursing text for a

Table 26–2   PSYCHOLOGIC DISORDERS THAT CAN AFFECT LABOR AND BIRTH

Anxiety Disorders	Personality Disorders
Generalized anxiety disorder (GAD)	Antisocial personality
Social anxiety disorder	Avoidant personality
Obsessive-compulsive disorder (OCD)	Borderline personality
Post-traumatic stress disorder (PTSD)	Dependent personality
Panic disorder	Narcissistic personality
Specific phobias	Obsessive-compulsive personality
	Schizoid personality
	Schizotypal personality
	Paranoid personality
Depression	**Dissociative Identity Disorder**
Major depression	
Dysthymia	**Schizophrenia**
Bipolar depression	

Table 26–1   PREVALENCE OF PSYCHOLOGIC DISORDERS

Disorder	US Prevalence	Prevalence in Women/Men	Maternal Implication
Generalized anxiety disorder	4 million (2.8%)	Two times higher in women	Anxiety related to the birth process or medical interventions
Bipolar disorder	2.3 million (1.2%)	Women and men equally affected	Depressive or manic symptoms during labor
Depression	19 million (9.5%)	Two times higher in women	Withdrawn behavior, physical fatigue due to insomnia, crying spells, sadness, hopelessness, feelings of guilt, lack of interest in baby, thoughts of suicide, headaches during pregnancy
Obsessive-compulsive disorder	3.3 million (2.3%)	Equal in men and women	Ritualistic behaviors or thoughts, difficulty focusing on directions
Panic disorder	2.4 million (1.7%)	Two times higher in women	Intense fear or sense of panic related to birth process
Phobias	5.3 million (3.6%)	Higher in women	May have specific fear related to an individual(s) or a procedure or place
Post-traumatic stress disorder (PTSD)	5.2 million (3.6%)	Higher in women	Repressed memories may be triggered during labor, causing intense anxiety, fear, and emotional distress
Schizophrenia	2.2 million (1.1%)	Affects men and women equally	Typically starts in the late 20s and early 30s. May have hallucinations or delusions, lack of sense of present events, high risk for suicide

SOURCE: Adapted from National Institute of Mental Health (NIMH). (2006). *Prevalence of psychologic disorders*. Rockville, MD: Author.

more complete discussion. Individuals with bipolar disorder experience the same symptoms as depression (previously discussed) during the depressive phase. Mania is characterized by expansiveness, elation, agitation, hyperactivity, and increased speed of thought and ideas (NIMH, 2006). During manic phases, individuals commonly exhibit poor judgment and hyperexcitability. A pregnant woman experiencing a manic episode may engage in behaviors that are dangerous for herself or her fetus, including alcohol or drug use, fast driving, driving without a seat belt, or engaging in unprotected intercourse with individuals at high risk for sexually transmitted infections (see Chapter 6 ∞). There is also a higher risk of suicide in individuals with mood disorders. Women with a previous diagnosis of bipolar depression are at greater risk for developing a mood disorder in the postpartum period (Freeman & Gelenberg, 2005). Although postpartum psychosis is a rare disorder (see Chapter 38 ∞), it is more common in women with bipolar disorder.

Anxiety disorders include a cluster of diagnoses, such as panic disorder, obsessive-compulsive disorder (OCD), post-traumatic stress disorder (PTSD), generalized anxiety disorder, social phobia, and other specific phobias. These disorders can cause a wide range of symptoms in laboring women. Specifically, women with panic attacks can experience intense feelings of terror without warning that result in physical symptoms (chest pain, shortness of breath, weakness, faintness, or dizziness) and/or psychologic symptoms (fear, terror, or anxiety). Other serious medical conditions need to be excluded (e.g., amniotic fluid embolism, cardiac complications, asthma attack). Women with OCD may need to repeat specific rituals as a means of coping in labor. Ritualistic activities that are safe for the mother and the fetus can be used to reduce anxiety. Women who have a history of rape or sexual abuse may suffer from PTSD. The events of labor may trigger flashbacks, avoidance behaviors, or anxiety symptoms. Generalized anxiety disorder, although not acutely disabling, may make the woman very uncomfortable as she enters labor. She may have a vague sense of something being "wrong" with her labor progress or her fetus and may need repeated reassurances that she and her baby are "doing just fine." A woman with social phobia may feel overwhelmed or embarrassed, especially if excessive numbers of staff are needed to care for her or her newborn. These women may also exhibit symptoms that mimic more serious medical conditions. Women with specific phobias may exhibit fears that seem irrational to healthcare providers, such as fear of needles or of their own contractions. Such phobias may be difficult to manage intrapartally and may require pharmacologic intervention.

Schizophrenia is the most disabling psychologic disorder. It is often difficult to treat schizophrenia in pregnant women because many of the medications are contraindicated because they are teratogenic. Women with uncontrolled schizophrenia may have difficulty managing emotions, interacting with the healthcare team, or thinking clearly. The woman's behavior may be dramatically inappropriate or she may simply be withdrawn.

As a nurse-midwife, all of the women I care for are special, but Karen was one person I will never forget. Karen was diagnosed with bipolar disorder with psychotic episodes that became uncontrolled in pregnancy as a result of discontinuing her medication. In labor, she arrived in a manic state. Her speech was excessively fast-paced and she rocked in her bed violently throughout the labor. We ensured her physical safety throughout the labor, monitored her contractions and the baby as infrequently as possible, and provided continuous encouragement. At one point, Karen was adamant everyone must "get low" and sit on the floor to facilitate fetal descent. Although it did not seem rational to us, we did sit on the floor. Remarkably, her anxiety dramatically decreased and the sense of control she felt enabled her to focus and 15 minutes later, she pushed her baby out. At her 6-week postpartum visit, Karen was back on medication and enjoying her new role as a mother.

In general, women with psychologic disorders tend to exhibit somewhat exaggerated behaviors during labor. They may need absolute control of everything that happens and refuse to participate until they feel secure. Although responses vary with different disorders, the woman may not be able to articulate her fears or needs, may not respond to supportive nursing measures, may be unaware of what will happen in labor and birth, may be unable to understand what is happening, or may be suddenly overwhelmed by terrifying memories.

One young woman I'll call Cheryl Ann was in preterm labor. I was evaluating her, and she was cooperative but anxious. Then the on-call physician began the vaginal exam. Suddenly, Cheryl Ann's face changed, and she began screaming over and over: "Don't hurt me, I'll do anything you want. No, keep the fire away, please, please, please." She was not with us in the room, she was in another event in her life, and she was terrified! I didn't know what to do. I stayed right beside her and kept talking softly. "It's all right, Cheryl Ann, you are here in the birth center. I'm your nurse. I will stay with you, and I won't let anyone hurt you. There is no fire here. Can you look at me? Hold my hand. You are safe here." She held my hand and in a few moments was able to look at me. She became less anxious and finally was able to be present in her experience.

Clinical Therapy

The goal of clinical therapy is to provide support that will help decrease the woman's anxiety, keep her oriented to reality, and promote optimal functioning while in labor. The physician or certified nurse-midwife (CNM) may prescribe a sedative, as needed, to help with symptoms and may seek the assistance of the on-call psychiatrist to assess and talk with the woman. The physician or CNM may also provide written orders for analgesic medications because relieving the pain may decrease the psychologic symptoms.

NURSING CARE MANAGEMENT
Nursing Assessment and Diagnosis

Unless birth is imminent or severe complications exist, the nurse begins the assessment by reviewing the woman's background. Factors such as age, parity, family support, culture, past and present experiences, and knowledge of the labor process affect the woman's psychologic response to labor. Past or current history of psychologic disorders should be evaluated. Current and past treatment can also yield helpful information. A careful history should include documentation of all psychotrophic medications used during pregnancy, because some medications can have adverse effects on pregnancy (Newport, Viguera, Beach et al., 2005).

As labor progresses, the nurse remains alert for the woman's verbal and nonverbal behavioral responses to the pain and anxiety of labor. The woman who is agitated and seems uncooperative or too quiet and compliant may require further appraisal for psychologic symptoms. Questions such as, "Is everything okay?" or "What's going on?" usually indicate some degree of anxiety and concern. Some women may be irritable, require frequent explanations, or repeat the same questions. The nurse further observes for nonverbal cues, including a tense posture, clenched hands, or pain out of context to the stage of labor. Recognizing the impact of fatigue on pain and anxiety is another important nursing responsibility. Women with sudden physical complaints need extensive evaluation to determine if the etiology is physical or psychologic. The nurse should assess what coping mechanisms have been effective for the woman in the past.

Nursing diagnoses that may apply to the woman with a psychologic disorder include the following:

- *Ineffective Coping* related to increased anxiety and stress
- *Compromised Family Coping* related to anxiety associated with labor and birth
- *Fear* related to invasive medical procedures and unknown outcome of birth process
- *Anxiety* related to unfamiliar surroundings and care by unknown medical personnel
- *Disturbed Visual Sensory Perception* related to reactivation of traumatic memories
- *Impaired Adjustment* related to delayed developmental tasks of pregnancy

Nursing Plan and Implementation

Primary nursing interventions center on supporting the laboring woman and her family and support persons. If the woman begins to lose her ability to cope or her orientation to reality, the nurse may be able to help her regain control and orientation by:

- Ensuring that the woman's external environment is free from excessive stimuli.
- Maintaining consistency in care providers to the extent possible.
- Encouraging her to identify and to use coping mechanisms that work well for her.
- Identifying and reducing the source of distress if possible.
- Acknowledging the woman's fears, pain, and other symptoms.
- Repeatedly orienting the woman to person, place, and time by statements such as "Janine, I am Tony Martinez and I am your nurse. It is Tuesday and you are in the birthing center because you are in labor now."

- Offering methods to promote relaxation and comfort (see Chapter 24 ∞).
- Providing clear but succinct information about the labor process, medical procedures, the environment, simple breathing exercises, and relaxation techniques.
- Employing a calm, caring, confident, and nonjudgmental approach.
- Providing frequent attention and therapeutic interaction.

Although providing emotional support and comfort measures is imperative, some women with severe uncontrolled psychologic disorders may continue to have excessive symptoms throughout labor and birth. Care for these women should focus on maintaining a safe environment and ensuring maternal and fetal well-being. Pharmacologic interventions may be needed to control excessive symptoms.

Evaluation

Expected outcomes of nursing care include the following:

- The woman experiences a decrease in physiologic and psychologic stress and an increase in physiologic and psychologic comfort.
- The woman remains oriented to person, place, and time.
- The woman uses effective coping mechanisms to manage her stress and anxiety in labor.
- The woman's and the family's fear is decreased.
- The woman verbalizes feelings about her labor.

CARE OF THE WOMAN EXPERIENCING DYSTOCIA RELATED TO DYSFUNCTIONAL UTERINE CONTRACTIONS

Dystocia is an abnormal labor pattern in which abnormalities occur with the power (uterine contractions or maternal expulsion forces), the passenger (fetal size, position, or presentation), or the passage (soft tissues or pelvis) (American College of Obstetricians and Gynecologists [ACOG], 2003). Dystocia encompasses many problems in labor, the most common of which is dysfunctional (or uncoordinated) uterine contractions that result in a prolongation of labor. This form of dystocia is the most common indication for cesarean birth in nulliparous women, accounting for 60% of cesarean births in this group (ACOG, 2003).

Although there is considerable controversy regarding the definition of a normal labor, there is agreement that women enter the active phase of labor when the cervix is dilated 3 to 4 cm. During this time, contractions occur in a regular pattern and the cervix changes rapidly as plotted against time. As the cervix dilates, the fetal part progressively descends. Alterna-

Figure 26–1 ◆ Comparison of labor patterns. *A,* Normal uterine contraction pattern. Note that the contraction frequency is every 3 minutes; duration is 60 seconds. The baseline resting tone is below 10 mm Hg. *B,* Hypotonic uterine contraction pattern. Note in this example that the contraction frequency is every 7 minutes with some uterine activity between contractions, duration is 50 seconds, and intensity increases approximately 25 mm Hg during contractions.

tively, cervical dilatation may be slower than normal (protraction disorders) or cease altogether (arrest disorders) (ACOG, 2003). Figure 26–1 ◆ depicts normal and hypotonic uterine contraction patterns.

Hypertonic Labor Patterns

In hypertonic labor patterns, ineffectual uterine contractions of poor quality occur in the latent phase of labor, and the resting tone of the myometrium increases. Contractions usually become more frequent. Although the contractions are painful, they are ineffective in dilating and effacing the cervix, and a prolonged latent phase may result.

Maternal risks of hypertonic labor include the following:

- Increased discomfort due to uterine muscle cell anoxia
- Fatigue as the pattern continues and no labor progress results
- Stress on coping abilities
- Dehydration and increased incidence of infection if labor is prolonged

  Fetal-neonatal risks include the following:

- Nonreassuring fetal status because contractions and increased resting tone interfere with the uteroplacental exchange
- Prolonged pressure on the fetal head, which may result in cephalhematoma, caput succedaneum, or excessive molding

CLINICAL THERAPY

Management of hypertonic labor may include bed rest and sedation to promote relaxation and reduce pain. If the hypertonic pattern continues and develops into a prolonged latent phase, oxytocin infusion or amniotomy may be considered (see Chapter 27 ∞). These methods are instituted only after cepha-

lopelvic disproportion (CPD) and fetal malrepresentation have been ruled out. CPD is a disparity between the size of the maternal pelvis and the size of the presenting fetal head due to position, presentation, or increased fetal weight that precludes a vaginal birth. When an oxytocin infusion is used to stimulate uterine contractions, the physician or CNM needs to assess whether vaginal birth is possible (i.e., whether the maternal pelvis is large enough for the fetus to pass through). If the maternal pelvis diameters are less than average, or if the fetus is particularly large or is in a malpresentation or malposition, CPD is said to be present. In the presence of true CPD, labor is not stimulated because vaginal birth is not possible.

NURSING CARE MANAGEMENT
Nursing Assessment and Diagnosis

As part of the labor assessment, the nurse should evaluate the relationship between the intensity of the pain being experienced and the degree to which the cervix is dilating and effacing. The nurse should also note whether anxiety is negatively affecting labor progress. Evidence of increasing frustration and discouragement on the part of the mother and her partner may indicate that the nurse needs to provide some additional information or assurance.

Nursing diagnoses that may apply to the woman in hypertonic labor include the following:

- *Acute Pain* related to the woman's inability to relax secondary to hypertonic uterine contractions
- *Ineffective Coping* related to ineffectiveness of breathing techniques to relieve discomfort
- *Anxiety* related to slow labor progress

Nursing Plan and Implementation

A key nursing responsibility is to provide comfort and support to the laboring woman and her partner. The woman experiencing a hypertonic labor pattern will probably be very uncomfortable because of the increased force of contractions. Her anxiety level and that of her partner may be high. The nurse attempts to reduce the woman's discomfort and promote a more effective labor pattern.

The nurse may suggest supportive measures such as a change of position: left lateral side-lying, high Fowler's, rocking in a rocking chair, sitting up, or walking. Soothing measures include a warm shower, whirlpool, quiet environment, backrub, therapeutic touch, and visualization. Mouth care, change of linens, effleurage, and relaxation exercises may provide comfort. If sedation is ordered, the nurse ensures that the environment is conducive to relaxation. The labor partner may also need assistance in helping the woman cope. A calm, understanding approach by the nurse offers the woman and her partner further support. Providing information about the cause of the hypertonic labor pattern and assuring the woman that she is not overreacting to the situation are important nursing actions.

Client education is key for the woman experiencing hypertonic labor. She needs information about the dysfunctional labor pattern and the possible implications for herself and her baby. Information will help relieve anxiety and thereby increase relaxation and comfort. The nurse needs to explain treatment options and offer opportunities to ask questions.

Evaluation

Anticipated outcomes of nursing care include the following:

- The woman has increased comfort and decreased anxiety.
- The woman and her partner are able to cope with the labor.
- The woman experiences a more effective labor pattern.

Hypotonic Labor Patterns

The specific cause of hypotonic contractions is unknown; however, genetic factors may control the normal physiologic processes of labor. Cesarean birth and operative vaginal birth (use of forceps or vacuum extractor), for example, tend to run in families. Some research suggests there is a relationship between uterine dysfunction and advancing maternal age (ACOG, 2003). The familial tendencies for difficult labor give rise to the theory that genetic processes control normal labor. It is hypothesized that there may be an inheritable tendency toward poor uterine contractions and/or soft-tissue relaxation (Algovik, Nilsson, Cnattingius et al., 2004).

CLINICAL TIP

As you know, normal cervical dilatation in a first-time mother—commonly known as a "primip"—is just over 1 cm per hour, and dilatation in a "multip" is about 1.5 cm per hour. If your assessments reveal that this expected pattern is not occurring, consider that a problem may be developing. The most likely causes of the problem are related to either the contractions or to fetal position or size.

CLINICAL THERAPY

When uterine contractions are irregular and of low amplitude and there is commonly less than 1 cm cervical dilatation per hour (called protracted labor) or there has been no change of cervical dilatation for 2 hours (arrest of progress), the physician or CNM evaluates the woman for the presence of any factor that would preclude the use of oxytocin (Pitocin) augmentation. The physician or CNM evaluates the size of the maternal pelvis, the position and presentation of the fetus, and fetal weight. The physician or CNM carefully considers the possibility of CPD. Station is a key component when evaluating for CPD. If the presenting part is not engaged ("out of the pelvis"), especially in a nulliparous woman, it is possible that CPD is present. The physician or CNM may attempt to push the presenting part into the pelvis with fundal pressure to assess if CPD exists. If CPD exists, oxytocin (Pitocin) augmentation should not be used.

When CPD is ruled out, an amniotomy (artificial rupture of membranes [AROM]) can be performed if membranes are intact. Amniotomy is associated with a reduction of labor duration and a decrease in use of oxytocin (Pitocin) (ACOG, 2003). Amniotomy should not be performed if the presenting part is not well applied to the cervix because this increases the risk of cord prolapse (discussed later in the chapter). However, it is an accepted procedure with the diagnosis of dystocia secondary to uterine hypocontractility. Oxytocin (Pitocin) augmentation can be implemented if adequate contractions do not occur. (See Drug Guide: Oxytocin [pitocin] in Chapter 27 ∞).

ACOG has outlined two regimens of oxytocin administration: a low-dose regimen and a high-dose regimen (see complete discussion in Chapter 27 ∞). Although low-dose regimens are associated with less uterine hyperstimulation, fetal outcomes have not differed between the two groups. High-dose regimens are said to shorten the mean length of labor, decrease the length of second stage, decrease the incidence of chorioamnionitis and neonatal sepsis, and reduce the incidence of cesarean births related to dystocia (ACOG, 2003). The current data do not support the notion that low-dose regimens are safer or superior to high-dose regimens (ACOG, 2003). Continuous electronic fetal monitoring (EFM) is used to provide ongoing information regarding fetal response to the augmentation. With augmentation of labor, the contraction pattern and progressive cervical dilatation pattern should improve, and fetal descent (measured by station) should occur. If there is no improvement in these areas, cesarean birth may be necessary.

Some practitioners support the use of **active management of labor (AMOL).** This method of labor management of nulliparous women has four components: (1) standardized criteria for diagnosis of labor, (2) standardized method of labor management, (3) one-to-one nursing care throughout the course of labor, and (4) prenatal education to teach women about the protocol (ACOG, 2003). In this process labor is managed from the beginning with amniotomy, timed cervical examinations, and augmentation of labor with intravenous oxytocin if adequate progress is not made. AMOL begins with careful assessment of the laboring woman, AROM (if the membranes are still intact) within 1 hour of diagnosis of the presence of actual labor, and hourly cervical examinations for the first 3 hours. Thereafter cervical examinations are performed every 2 hours, and at least an additional 1 cm of dilatation is expected at each examination. If cervical dilatation is less than expected, augmentation with an intravenous oxytocin infusion is begun. AMOL also incorporates a strong one-to-one nursing care program, in which the nurse remains with the woman. This permits ongoing assessment and provides the beneficial aspect of constant nursing support. Recent large-scale studies have shown that AMOL does not increase maternal and infant mortality or morbidity. Proponents have voiced support because it does shorten labor in nulliparous women. Interestingly, the rates of caesarean births are not decreased with AMOL (ACOG, 2003).

Those who oppose AMOL contend that labor needs to be considered a normal process and allowed to progress without automatic intervention. Frequent examinations can increase the risk of maternal fever, intrauterine infection, and fetal compromise. Although some women may not strictly adhere to the expected normal time limits of labor, many will go on to give birth without complications if given an opportunity to progress through labor at their own pace. Just as all women do not have the same emotional reactions to labor, all women do not go through labor at the same pace and speed. Only if problems occur should the labor be augmented.

NURSING CARE MANAGEMENT
Nursing Assessment and Diagnosis

Assessing maternal vital signs, contractions, cervical dilatation, fetal descent, and fetal heart rate characteristics provides the nurse with data to evaluate maternal-fetal status. The nurse also assesses for signs and symptoms of infection and dehydration. During the vaginal examination, the fetal presenting part (usually vertex) is assessed for the development of a caput. If the fetal vertex presses down on the cervix during contractions without further descent, a *caput succedaneum* may occur. As hypotonic labor continues, the caput increases in size; it seems that the head is descending, but it is not (Figure 26–2 ◆).

Because labor progress is slow, the nurse assesses the woman's stress and coping, noting whether anxiety is having a deleterious effect on labor progress. Evidence of increasing frustration and discouragement on the part of the mother and her partner may become apparent as labor continues.

Nursing diagnoses that may apply to the woman experiencing dysfunctional labor include the following:

- *Acute Pain* related to rapid increase in frequency and intensity of uterine contractions
- *Ineffective Coping* related to ineffectiveness of breathing techniques to relieve discomfort
- *Anxiety* related to slow labor progress

Figure 26–2 ◆ Effects of labor on the fetal head. *A,* Caput succedaneum formation. The presenting portion of the scalp area is encircled by the cervix during labor, causing swelling of the soft tissue. *B,* Molding of the fetal head in cephalic presentations: (1) occiput anterior, (2) occiput posterior, (3) brow, (4) face.

Nursing Plan and Implementation

Nursing measures are aimed at promoting maternal and fetal well-being. The nurse frequently monitors maternal vital signs; notes the frequency, duration, and strength of contractions; and assesses the fetal heart rate (FHR). Once the amniotic membranes are ruptured, the nurse assesses the amount of fluid and the presence of blood or meconium (dark green or black stool present in the large intestine of the fetus). Because meconium can be associated with a compromised fetus, ongoing observation of the amniotic fluid is critical. Maternal hydration status can be monitored by recording intake and output. The nurse assesses the bladder every 2 hours for distention; an in-and-out catheterization can be performed for women unable to void on their own. Alternatively, a Foley catheter may be inserted during the first stage of labor to reduce the need for multiple in-and-out catheterizations, which can increase the risk of urinary tract infections. The catheter should be removed before maternal pushing.

Ongoing evaluation for symptoms of infection should be performed, especially for prolonged labors. These symptoms include fever, chills, foul-smelling amniotic fluid, and fetal tachycardia. Vaginal examinations should be kept to a minimum to reduce the incidence of infections.

The laboring woman needs information about the hypotonic labor pattern and the possible implications for herself and her baby. It is particularly important to address the couple's concerns and questions with clear, accurate information. They need to be informed of progress and possible treatment measures. Disadvantages and treatment alternatives also need to be discussed and understood by the woman and her support person.

Evaluation

Expected outcomes of nursing care include the following:

- The woman and her partner understand the labor pattern and its possible implications.
- The woman and her partner are able to cope with the labor.
- The woman's comfort increases and her anxiety decreases.
- The woman experiences a more effective labor pattern.

CARE OF THE WOMAN AND FETUS AT RISK FOR PRECIPITOUS LABOR AND BIRTH

Precipitous labor and birth occurs when the entire process of labor and birth occurs within 3 hours. The most common causes are abnormally low resistance in maternal soft tissues, which allows for rapid cervical dilatation and fetal descent, and abnormally strong uterine contractions (Cunningham, Leveno, Bloom et al., 2005). In precipitous labor, cervical dilatation is 5 cm or more per hour in the primigravida and up to 10 cm per hour for the multipara.

Precipitous labor and birth and precipitous birth are not the same. A precipitous birth is a sudden, and often unattended, birth. See Chapter 24 ∞ for a discussion of precipitous birth and nurse-attended births.

Maternal risks may include abruptio placentae (discussed shortly) because of the abnormally strong contractions. If maternal tissues are not soft, extensive lacerations of the cervix, vagina, and perineum may occur. During the uterine contractions, fetal oxygenation and placenta blood flow may be poor. Fetal risks include meconium-stained fluid that may be aspirated at birth, low Apgar scores, brachial palsy, and intracranial trauma resulting from the rapid birth and resistance of the birth canal to the fetal head (Cunningham et al., 2005). Women who have had a precipitous labor and birth are also at risk for postpartum hemorrhage because the uterus often becomes hypotonic after delivery.

Clinical Therapy

Any woman with a history of precipitous labor requires close medical monitoring and preparation for precipitous birth to facilitate a safe outcome for the mother and fetus. Women with a history of precipitous birth should be closely monitored for cervical effacement and dilatation in the final weeks of pregnancy. An induction can be scheduled to control the birth environment and prevent complications that can occur with an unattended birth. Drugs such as magnesium sulfate or other tocolytic agents have not proven to be effective in these circumstances (Cunningham et al., 2005).

NURSING CARE MANAGEMENT
Nursing Assessment and Diagnosis

During the intrapartal nursing assessment, the nurse can identify a woman at increased risk of precipitous labor (for example, a previous history of precipitate or short labor places a woman at risk). During the labor, accelerated cervical dilatation and fetal descent and intense contractions with little uterine relaxation between contractions are indicative of precipitous labor.

Nursing diagnoses that may apply to the woman with precipitous labor include the following:

- *Risk for Injury* related to rapid labor and birth
- *Acute Pain* related to rapid labor process

Nursing Plan and Implementation

If the woman has a history of precipitous labor, it is imperative that the nurse establish rapport quickly because the nurse and woman may be involved in another precipitous labor and birth, and the situation has the potential to be tense. The physician or CNM should be notified of the woman's status immediately. Rapport and support from the nurse will enhance all other interventions. The nurse closely monitors the woman's contractions and cervical dilatation, and an emergency birth pack is kept near the bed. The nurse stays in constant attendance if at all possible, assists the woman to a comfortable position, and provides a quiet environment. The nurse provides information and support before and after the birth. See Chapter 24 ∞ for a discussion of nurse-managed birth.

The fetus is monitored for signs of hypoxia and other indications of nonreassuring fetal status. If meconium staining of the amniotic fluid is present, the fetal nares and mouth will be suctioned just after the head is born (before the birth of the shoulders) to prevent the baby from drawing more meconium-stained fluid into the lungs with the first breath. After the birth of the baby, the cords will be visualized and additional suctioning carried out as needed. The neonatologist or nursery staff should be present for immediate care of the infant.

Evaluation

Expected outcomes of nursing care include the following:

- The woman and her baby are closely monitored during labor, and a safe birth occurs.
- The couple feels support and enhanced comfort during labor and birth.

CARE OF THE WOMAN WITH POSTTERM PREGNANCY

Postterm pregnancy is one that extends more than 294 days or 42 completed weeks past the first day of the last menstrual period. It is important to understand that 42 completed weeks refers to the completion of 42 weeks, meaning that the 7th day has elapsed. The incidence of postterm pregnancy is approximately 7% of all pregnancies in the United States. Most causes of postterm pregnancies are unknown. Postterm pregnancy has been associated with primiparity, previous postterm pregnancy, placenta sulfatase deficiency, fetal anencephaly, male fetus, and genetic predisposition (ACOG, 2004a).

The most frequent cause of postterm pregnancy is error in determining the time of ovulation and conception according to the first day of the last menstrual period. This error can be corrected by performing an ultrasound scan in early pregnancy. A first-trimester scan is the most accurate ultrasonic gestational age assessment. During the first trimester, the crown-rump length is used. In second-trimester ultrasound, which is less accurate, the biparietal diameter of the fetal head is measured and then compared with conventional dating tables (ACOG, 2004a).

Maternal Risks

Although postterm pregnancy does not pose any significant risk to the woman during the pregnancy, the labor and birth process may be affected. In many instances, labor is induced. Because postterm pregnancy is associated with an increased incidence of large-for-gestational-age (LGA) or macrosomic (weight in excess of 4500 g) fetuses, vaginal birth is frequently associated with the use of forceps or vacuum extractor. Women who deliver postterm fetuses are more likely to encounter perineal damage because of the increased size of the fetus. Maternal hemorrhage may also occur. Cesarean birth rates are doubled in postterm pregnancies. Cesarean births are associated with endometritis, hemorrhage, and thromboembolitic disease (ACOG, 2004a). Many women experience anxiety and are emotionally fatigued as their estimated date of birth (EDB) passes. Normal discomforts associated with late pregnancy persist that can lead to irritability and loss of sleep.

When I went over my due date, I felt so anxious and over-whelmed. I was mentally prepared to carry my baby until a certain date, but once that date was reached, I felt unable to deal with all of the discomforts of pregnancy. I couldn't sleep well. I was uncomfortable eating, walking, even putting on my shoes. Well-wishing friends and family would call and say, "Haven't you had that baby yet?" The calls just made it worse. I can't tell you how relieved I was when labor started and I knew I would soon meet my new baby.

Fetal-Neonatal Risks

True postterm pregnancies are frequently associated with placental changes that cause a decrease in the uterine-placental-fetal circulation. The perinatal mortality rate after 42 weeks is twice that of term infants and increases sixfold during the 43rd gestational week (ACOG, 2004a). This decrease reduces the blood supply, oxygen, and nutrition for the fetus. Oligohydramnios (decreased amount of amniotic fluid) is frequently present and may increase the risk of umbilical cord compression (because the cord does not have as much fluid to float in). In such cases, the fetus is more likely to be small-for-gestational-age (SGA) because of decreased nutrition associated with decreased uteroplacental-fetal circulation. If uteroplacental-fetal circulation is not compromised, the fetus continues to gain weight until the 42nd week; therefore, the fetus is often LGA and macrosomic. The LGA or macrosomic fetus has a higher incidence of birth trauma or shoulder dystocia (difficulty or inability to deliver the baby's shoulders). Macrosomia is also associated with prolonged labor, increased risk of cesarean birth, and CPD (ACOG, 2004a; Cunningham et al., 2005). During labor, the postterm fetus may have meconium staining of the amniotic fluid, which can lead to nonreassuring fetal status and meconium aspiration at birth (Cunningham et al., 2005). Infants born after the 42nd week of pregnancy have low umbilical artery pH and lower 5-minute Apgar scores (ACOG, 2004a).

Approximately 20% of all postterm infants experience *dysmaturity syndrome,* which is associated with uteroplacental insufficiency (resembling intrauterine growth restriction), meconium aspiration, and short-term neonatal complications (ACOG, 2004a). Neonatal complications associated with postterm pregnancies include hypoglycemia seizures and respiratory distress. These fetuses frequently experience nonreassuring fetal heart tracings in the antepartum and intrapartum periods. Infants delivered after the 42nd gestational week are also at an increased risk to die during the first year of life (ACOG, 2004a).

Clinical Therapy

When the 40th week of gestation is completed and birth has not occurred, most practitioners begin using the nonstress test

(NST), biophysical profile (BPP), or a modified BPP (ultrasound measurement of the amniotic fluid volume plus an NST) as assessment tools. According to ACOG, there is no consensus on the frequency of antenatal surveillance; however, many practitioners use twice-weekly testing. Any time that tests indicate fetal problems or there is decreased amniotic fluid volume, induction of labor is recommended (ACOG, 2004a).

NURSING CARE MANAGEMENT
Nursing Assessment and Diagnosis

When the woman is admitted into the birthing area, it is important to establish the EDB and ascertain the type of antenatal testing that has been completed. During labor, ongoing assessments of the FHR by continuous EFM are important to identify reassuring characteristics (lack of decelerations, accelerations with fetal movement) and to determine the presence of variable decelerations so that corrective actions may be taken. When amniotic membranes rupture, the nurse assesses the fluid for the presence of meconium. Ongoing assessments of labor progress (contractions, progressive cervical dilatation and effacement, and fetal descent) may provide clues to the presence of a macrosomic fetus because labor may be lengthened and fetal descent may not occur.

Possible nursing diagnoses for the woman with postterm pregnancy include the following:

- **Fear** related to the unknown outcome for the baby
- **Risk for Ineffective Coping** or **Compromised Family Coping** related to concern regarding the status of the baby

Nursing Plan and Implementation
COMMUNITY-BASED NURSING CARE

If the woman has not been assessing fetal activity every day, the nurse teaches her how to do it so that she can identify inadequate fetal movement and contact her healthcare provider (see Chapter 21 ∞ for further discussion of techniques to detect fetal movement). The nurse encourages the woman to keep all appointments for BPPs and other testing and provides information regarding the postterm pregnancy and the antenatal testing that will be indicated. In addition, the nurse addresses the implications and associated risks for the baby, as well as possible treatment plans, and provides the woman and her partner opportunities to ask questions and clarify information.

HOSPITAL-BASED NURSING CARE

In the birth setting, the response of the fetus during labor is assessed carefully. Continuous electronic monitoring of FHR is important to determine whether reassuring characteristics are present and to detect variable decelerations, especially if oligohydramnios is present. If variable decelerations are present, the laboring woman's position is changed to attempt to take pressure off the umbilical cord, and FHR is reevaluated. When an amnioinfusion is performed to increase the volume of fluid or to

dilute meconium-stained fluid, the nurse assists with the procedure and monitors the infusion and the response of the FHR. (See Chapter 27 ∞ for further discussion).

Evaluation

Expected outcomes of nursing care include the following:

- The woman is able to explain the implications of the postterm pregnancy.
- The woman and her partner and family feel supported and able to cope with the labor and birth.
- Fetal problems are identified quickly.

CARE OF THE WOMAN AND FETUS AT RISK BECAUSE OF FETAL MALPOSITION

Persistent occiput-posterior (OP) position of the fetus is the most common fetal malposition and occurs when the head remains in the direct OP position throughout labor. In early labor approximately 15% of fetuses are in OP position, although only 5% remain in that position at the time of birth (Cunningham et al., 2005). This position may be normal in some races, particularly those whose women tend to have a small pelvis. The position is related to transverse narrowing of the midpelvis. For a fetus in an OP position to rotate to an occiput-anterior (OA) position, it must rotate 135 degrees (ROP to ROT to ROA to OA), and in most cases this rotation is accomplished. In others, however, it is not. Labor progress may cease or the fetus may be born in a posterior position.

Maternal-Fetal-Neonatal Risks

The woman usually experiences intense pain in the small of her back throughout the labor, unless the baby rotates. At birth, if the fetus remains in a posterior position, the woman may suffer a third- or fourth-degree perineal laceration or extension of a midline episiotomy. There is no increased risk of fetal mortality because of the OP position unless labor is protracted or an operative birth is performed. There is a higher incidence of operative vaginal deliveries in fetuses who fail to rotate from the OP position.

Clinical Therapy

Medical treatment focuses on close monitoring of both maternal and fetal status and labor progress to determine whether vaginal or cesarean birth is the safer method. According to Cunningham et al. (2005), vaginal birth is possible via:

1. Spontaneous birth
2. Forceps-assisted birth with the occiput directly posterior
3. Forceps rotation of the occiput to the anterior position and birth (Scanzoni maneuver [Figure 26–3 ◆])
4. Manual rotation to the anterior position followed by spontaneous or forceps-assisted birth (Figure 26–4 ◆)

A   **B**

Figure 26–3 ◆ Scanzoni maneuver, anterior rotation. *A,* Forceps are applied to the fetal head, which is in ROP position. Fetal head is then rotated 45 degrees to ROT, then another 45 degrees to ROA, then a final 45 degrees to OA. *B,* The fetal position has now changed from ROP to OA for a total rotation of 135 degrees. The forceps are now upside down, so they are removed and reapplied to provide the traction necessary for a forceps-assisted birth.

SOURCE: Oxorn, H., and Foote, W. (1986). *Human labor and birth* (5th ed., p. 401). Norwalk, CT: Appleton & Lange. Reproduced with permission of The McGraw-Hill Companies.

A Grasping the head

B ROP to ROT (45°)

C ROT to ROA (45°)

D The manual rotation is completed as the head is rotated another 45° from ROA to OA

Figure 26–4 ◆ Manual rotation of ROP to OA. *A,* The physician's left hand is inserted into the vagina and the back of the fetal head is grasped. *B,* The head is flexed and then rotated 45 degrees to ROT. *C,* The head is rotated another 45 degrees to ROA. *D,* The manual rotation is completed as the head is rotated another 45 degrees from ROA to OA. During the manual rotation, the physician's other hand is placed on the maternal abdomen, and the body is turned in the same direction as the head by applying pressure to the fetal breech or shoulders.

If the pelvis has larger diameters and the perineal muscles are relaxed, as found in grandmultiparity, the fetus may have no particular problem emerging spontaneously in the OP position. If, however, the perineum is rigid, the second stage of labor may be prolonged. A prolonged second stage is one that lasts over an hour in multiparas and 2 hours or more in nulliparas.

In the event of a prolonged second stage with arrest of descent due to the OP position, a forceps or manual rotation may be done if no CPD is present. Forceps rotation has been associated with neonatal high cervical spinal cord injuries in the past. For this reason, obstetricians may choose to perform a cesarean birth (Cunningham et al., 2005). In cases of CPD, cesarean is always the preferred mode of birth. Of women with a persistent OP position,

60% will deliver via cesarean. These account for 12% of all ce-sarean births performed for dystocia (Cunningham et al., 2005).

NURSING CARE MANAGEMENT
Nursing Assessment and Diagnosis

The first sign of OP position is intense back pain in the first stage of labor. The back pain is caused by the fetal occiput compressing the sacral nerves. Other signs and symptoms may include a dysfunctional labor pattern, a prolonged active phase, secondary arrest of dilatation, or arrest of descent. Further assessment may reveal a depression in the maternal abdomen above the symphysis pubis (because the fetal face, rather than the back of its head, is turned up against the symphysis). FHR may be heard far laterally on the maternal abdomen, and on vaginal examination the nurse will find the wide diamond-shaped anterior fontanelle in the anterior portion of the pelvis. This fontanelle may be difficult to feel because of molding of the fetal head.

Nursing diagnoses that may apply to women with persistent OP position include the following:

- *Pain* related to back discomfort secondary to occiput-posterior position
- *Ineffective Coping* related to persistent back pain

Nursing Plan and Implementation

Changing maternal posture has been used for many years to enhance rotation of OP or OT to OA. The woman may be placed on one side and then asked to move to the other side as the fetus begins to rotate. This side-lying position may promote rotation; it also enables the support person to apply counterpressure on the sacral area to decrease discomfort. A knee-chest position provides a downward slant to the vaginal canal, directing the fetal head downward on descent and is often effective in rotating the fetus. In addition to maintaining a hands-and-knees position on the bed, the woman may do pelvic rocking, and the support person may perform firm stroking motions on the abdomen. The stroking begins over the fetal back and swings around to the other side of the abdomen. After the fetus has rotated, the woman lies in Sims' position on the side opposite the fetal back. In addition to assuming these positions, the woman may want to sit on the toilet, walk around the room, stand beside the bed and lean forward with her hands on the bed and do the pelvic rock, rest in a whirlpool, or lie on her side in the bed.

Evaluation

Expected outcomes of nursing care include the following:

- The woman's discomfort is decreased.
- The woman and her partner apply comfort measures and position changes that assist her.
- The woman's coping abilities are strengthened.
- The woman and her partner state that they feel supported and encouraged.

CARE OF THE WOMAN AND FETUS AT RISK BECAUSE OF FETAL MALPRESENTATION

In a normal cephalic presentation, the occiput is the presenting part (Figure 26–5, *A* ◆). Three cephalic presentations are classified as abnormal presentations: military (sinciput), brow, and face (Figure 26–5, *B –D*). The fetal body straightens out in these malpresentations from the classic fetal position to an S-shaped position. Of these, the military presentation is probably the least difficult for the woman and fetus. In most cases, as soon as the head reaches the pelvic floor, flexion occurs and a vaginal birth results. Thus, of the cephalic malpresentations, only brow and face are discussed here.

In addition to the cephalic malpresentations, the breech, shoulder (transverse lie), and compound presentations can cause significant difficulty during labor. These malpresentations are also discussed in this chapter.

Brow Presentation

Brow presentations are the least common of all presentations, with an incidence of 1 in 500 births to 1 in 3543 births (Parker & Napolitano, 2005). In a brow presentation, the forehead of the fetus becomes the presenting part. The fetal head is slightly extended instead of flexed, with the result that the fetal head enters the birth canal with the widest diameter of the head (occipitomental) foremost (Figure 26–5, *C*). Although no specific cause can be identified, proposed causes include high parity, placenta previa, uterine anomaly, hydramnios, fetal anomaly, low birth weight, and large fetus (Simonsen, Lyon, Adler et al., 2005).

In labors in which a brow presentation exists, 33% to 50% will result in a prolonged labor or a secondary arrest of labor (Parker & Napolitano, 2005). Cesarean birth is preferred in the presence of CPD or failure of a brow presentation to convert to a normal vertex or face presentation. If a vaginal birth is attempted, the woman will probably have an episiotomy and may require extension of the episiotomy at the moment of birth.

Fetal mortality is increased because of injuries received during the birth. Trauma during the birth process can include cerebral and neck compression and damage to the trachea and larynx.

Clinical Therapy

Active medical intervention is not necessary as long as cervical dilatation and fetal descent are occurring. If labor progress is slow, clinical pelvimetry findings and ultrasound to determine the presence of fetal anomalies are important. Brow presentations should be managed expectedly because a cesarean birth may be warranted (Stitley & Gherman, 2005). Oxytocin may be used with caution to correct an inadequate labor pattern. Use of forceps or manual conversion is contraindicated (Parker & Napolitano, 2005). If problems occur, cesarean birth is indicated.

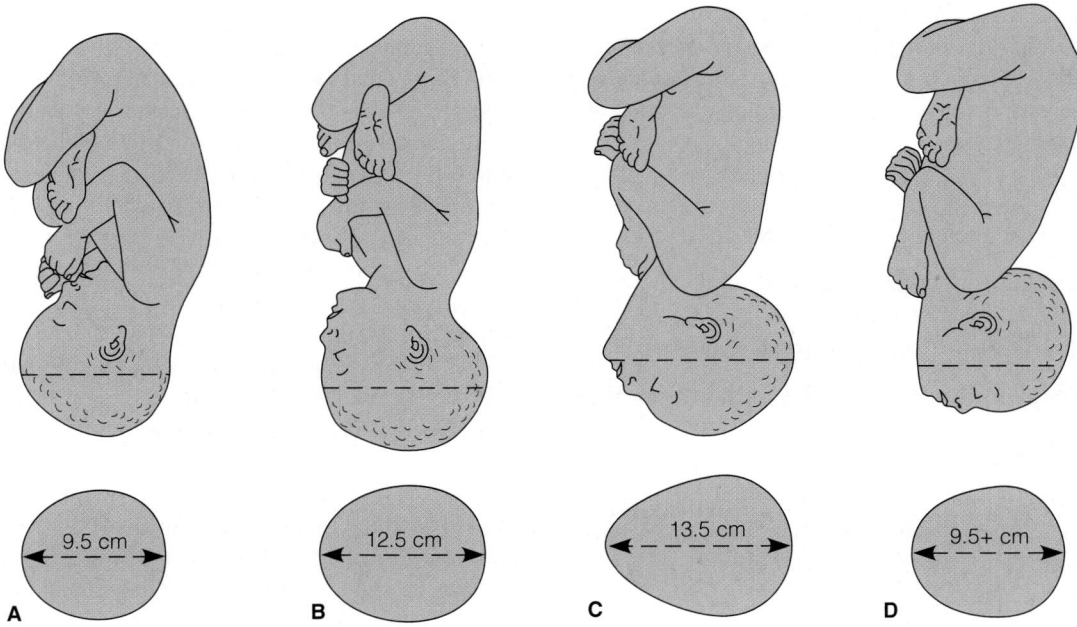

Figure 26–5 ◆ Types of cephalic presentations. *A,* The occiput is the presenting part because the head is flexed and the fetal chin is against the chest. The largest anteroposterior (AP) diameter that presents and passes through the pelvis is approximately 9.5 cm. *B,* Military (sinciput) presentation. The head is neither flexed nor extended. The presenting AP diameter is approximately 12.5 cm. *C,* Brow presentation. The largest diameter of the fetal head (approximately 13.5 cm) presents in this situation. *D,* Face presentation. The AP diameter is 9.5 cm.
SOURCE: Danforth, D. N., & Scott, J. R. (Eds.). (1990). *Obstetrics and gynecology* (5th ed., p. 170, fig. 8–9). New York: Lippincottt. Copyright Lippincott, Williams & Wilkins. Reprinted with permission.

NURSING CARE MANAGEMENT
Nursing Assessment and Diagnosis

Leopold's maneuvers suggest a brow presentation when both the chin and occiput are palpable. A brow presentation may be detected on vaginal examination by palpation of the diamond-shaped anterior fontanelle and orbital ridges (Figure 26–6 ◆).

Nursing diagnoses that may apply to brow presentation include the following:

* *Anxiety* or *Fear* related to outcome for fetus
* *Deficient Knowledge* related to lack of information about possible maternal-fetal effects of brow presentation
* *Risk for Injury to the fetus* related to pressure on fetal structures secondary to brow presentation

Nursing Plan and Implementation

Nursing management of the brow presentation includes close observation of the woman for labor aberrations and of the fetus for signs of nonreassuring fetal status. The fetus should be observed closely during labor for signs of hypoxia as evidenced by late decelerations.

The nurse may need to explain the position of the fetus to the laboring couple or to interpret what the physician or CNM has told them. The nurse should stay close at hand to reassure the couple, inform them of any changes, and assist them with labor-coping techniques.

In both brow and face presentations, the appearance of the newborn may be affected. The couple may need help in

Figure 26–6 ◆ Brow presentation. *A,* Descent. *B,* Internal rotation in the pelvic cavity.
SOURCE: Oxorn, H., & Foote, W. (1986). *Human labor and birth* (5th ed., p. 211). Norwalk, CT: Appleton & Lange. Reproduced with permission of The McGraw-Hill Companies.

beginning the attachment process because of the newborn's facial appearance. After the infant is inspected for gross abnormalities, the pediatrician and nurse can assure the couple that the facial edema and excessive molding are only temporary and will subside in a few days.

Evaluation

Expected outcomes of nursing care include the following:

- The woman and her partner understand the implications and associated problems of brow presentation.
- The mother and her baby have a safe labor and birth.

Face Presentation

In a face presentation, the face of the fetus is the presenting part. The fetal head is hyperextended even more than in the brow presentation. Face presentation occurs frequently in multi-parous women or women with a pendulous abdomen. Women with a contracted pelvis account for 10% to 40% of all face presentations. Fetal factors include macrosomia or a nuchal cord around the neck. The presence of anencephaly accounts for 30% and fetal malformations occur in up to 60% of all face presentations (Napolitano & Parker, 2005). The incidence of face presentation is about 1 in 500 births overall or 0.2% of all births (Napolitano & Parker, 2005).

The risks of CPD and prolonged labor are increased with face presentation. As with any prolonged labor, the chance of infection is increased.

The fetus may develop edema, making vaginal examination for placement of heart rate electrodes difficult. If a fetal scalp electrode is applied, it should be placed on the mentum (Napolitano & Parker, 2005). After birth the edema gives the newborn an unusual appearance. As with the brow presentation, the neck and internal structures may swell as a result of trauma received during descent. Petechiae and ecchymoses are often seen in the superficial layers of the facial skin because of the birth trauma.

CLINICAL THERAPY

If no CPD is present, the mentum (chin) is anterior, and the labor pattern is effective, the objective of medical treatment is a vaginal birth (Figure 26–7 ◆). The success rate of vaginal delivery is 60% to 70%. Oxytocin may be administered as needed for hypotonic labor patterns. Attempts at manual rotation should not be made, because this increases perinatal mortality and maternal morbidity (Napolitano & Parker, 2005). Mentum posteriors can become wedged on the anterior surface of the sacrum (Figure 26–8 ◆). In this case as well as in the presence of CPD, cesarean is the preferred method of birth.

Figure 26–7 ◆ Face presentation. Mechanism of birth in mentoanterior position. *A,* The submentobregmatic diameter at the outlet. *B,* The fetal head is born by movement of flexion.

Figure 26–8 ◆ Face presentation. Mechanism of birth in mentoposterior position. Fetal head is unable to extend farther. The face becomes impacted.

NURSING CARE MANAGEMENT
Nursing Assessment and Diagnosis

When performing Leopold's maneuvers, the nurse finds that the back of the fetus is difficult to outline, and a deep furrow can be palpated between the hard occiput and the fetal back (Figure 26–9 ◆). Fetal heart tones can be heard on the side where the fetal feet are palpated. It may be difficult to determine by vaginal examination whether a breech or a face is presenting, especially if facial edema is already present. During the vaginal examination, palpation of the saddle of the nose and the gums should be attempted. When assessing engagement, the nurse needs to remember that the face has to be deep within the pelvis before the biparietal diameter has entered the inlet.

Nursing diagnoses that may apply to the woman with a fetus in face presentation include the following:

- *Fear* related to unknown outcome of the labor and appearance of the baby
- *Risk for Injury* to the newborn's face related to edema secondary to the birth process

Nursing Plan and Implementation

Nursing interventions are the same as for the brow presentation.

Evaluation

Expected outcomes of nursing care include the following:

- The woman and her partner understand the implications and problems of face presentation.
- The mother and her baby have a safe labor and birth.

Breech Presentation

Breech presentation is the most common malpresentation, with an overall incidence of approximately 4% of births. The incidence of breech presentation is directly related to gestational age: at 25 to 26 weeks' gestation, the incidence is about 25%, but by 32 weeks, the incidence has decreased to 7% (Fischer, 2005).

Frank breech is the most common type of breech (especially at term) and is characterized by flexed hips and extended knees. It occurs in about 50% to 70% of breech births (Figure 26–10, A ◆). Single or double footling breech (incomplete breech), characterized by one or both hips extended and a foot presenting, accounts for about 10% to 30% of breech births (Figure 26–10, B) and occurs more frequently in preterm fetuses. The remaining 5% to 10% of breech presentations are complete breech presentations (Fischer, 2005) (Figure 26–10, C).

Breech presentation is most frequently associated with placenta previa, implantation of the placenta in either cornual area, hydramnios, high parity, oligohydramnios, hydrocephaly, anencephaly, previous breech presentation, uterine anomalies, pelvic tumors, multiple gestation, and fetal anomalies (Cunningham et al., 2005). Because the presenting part does not completely fill the space in the lower uterine segment, once membranes rupture, cord prolapse is more likely. The incidence of cord prolapse is more likely in a breech presentation. Infants born after breech presentation have higher infant mortality and neonatal complications. These birth defects can be associated with factors that caused the breech presentation (birth defects or intrauterine growth restriction) or with damage that occurred during birth (Eide, Oyen, Skjaerven et al., 2005).

Head trauma during vaginal birth is more likely in breech presentation because it does not allow for the slow molding that occurs in a cephalic presentation as the fetal head moves through the birth canal. The head is the largest and least resilient part of the fetal body. It is the last to come through the maternal pelvis in breech presentations; thus molding does not occur. In the case of a preterm breech, a single or double footling and the torso may emerge through a cervix that is not completely dilated, leaving the larger head entrapped by the cervix. Entrapment may also occur with cesarean birth if the incision is

Figure 26–9 ◆ Face presentation. *A,* Palpation of the maternal abdomen with the fetus in right mentum posterior (RMP). *B,* Vaginal examination may permit palpation of facial features of the fetus.

Figure 26–10 ◆ Breech presentation. *A*, Frank breech. *B*, Incomplete (footling) breech. *C*, Complete breech in left sacral anterior (LSA) position. *D*, On vaginal examination, the nurse may feel the anal sphincter. The tissue of the fetal buttocks feels soft.

inadequate or uterine relaxation is less than optimum. Vaginal breech birth also carries higher risks of meconium aspiration and fetal asphyxia (Eide et al., 2005).

A recent multicenter trial demonstrated that planned cesarean births of breech fetuses had a lower risk of perinatal morbidity and mortality than planned vaginal births (Molkenboer, Reijners, Nijhuis et al., 2004).

CLINICAL THERAPY

An external cephalic version (ECV) is usually attempted at 37 to 38 weeks' gestation. The ECV can reduce breech presentation by 50% (Fischer, 2005). Complementary/alternative therapies have also been used with some success. *Moxibustion* is a technique in which certain herbs are burned to stimulate an acupressure point at the outside of the fifth toenail (see Complementary and Alternative Therapies: Moxibustion to Promote Version in Breech Presentation). This technique stimulates the pressure point, much like acupressure or acupuncture. Moxibustion has been shown to decrease the need for ECV and reduce the use of oxytocin before and during labor (Coyle, Smith, & Peat, 2005). If the version is unsuccessful or the fetus spontaneously turns back into a breech presentation, the physician will evaluate the possibility of a vaginal birth or plan a cesarean birth. Many physicians recommend a cesarean birth when a breech presentation is detected, especially if the woman is nulliparous because breech births

COMPLEMENTARY AND ALTERNATIVE THERAPIES

MOXIBUSTION TO PROMOTE VERSION IN BREECH PRESENTATION

Traditional Chinese medicine (TCM) uses the herb mugwort in the form of moxa to promote version in a breech presentation. *Moxa* is a system of treatment, often combined with acupuncture, in which an herb is dried, rolled into cones (like incense cones), and placed on certain meridian parts of the body. The moxa is then lit and allowed to burn close to the skin, hence the *-bustion* component of the name. The heat and pungency of mugwort stimulates the point, and energy moves through. It is believed that the effect of moxibustion increases fetal activity.

The meridian point used in moxibustion to promote version in breech presentations is acupoint BL67, located beside the outer corner of the fifth toenail (Coyle, Smith, & Peat, 2005). Treatment may take from 7 days to 2 weeks. In two recent clinical trials, moxibustion was found to be an effective modality in the management of breech presentations (Coyle, Smith, & Peat, 2005).

have higher mortality and morbidity rates as well as an increased incidence of cord prolapse, birth trauma, and fetal cervical spinal cord injuries due to hyperextension of the head (Kayem, Goffinet, Thomas et al., 2002). Contraindications for labor and vaginal birth include the following:

- Fetal weight less than 1500 g or more than 3800 g
- Hyperextension of the fetal neck of more than 90 degrees
- Extension of the fetal arms over the head
- Anomalies, such as hydrocephalus
- Diminished maternal pelvic measurements

If a vaginal birth is being attempted, narcotic agents or an epidural block may be used for pain relief. Epidural anesthesia may be advantageous during the latter portion of labor because it will help prevent the pushing sensation the woman may feel before complete dilatation. If the woman pushes before cervical dilatation is complete, the fetal body may be expelled and the head entrapped. At the time of birth the physician may have an assistant available in case forceps are needed. Once the fetal body is born, an assistant supports the fetal body as the physician applies Piper forceps to assist in birth of the fetal head (called the *aftercoming head*) (Cunningham et al., 2005).

NURSING CARE MANAGEMENT
Nursing Assessment and Diagnosis

At times, the nurse is the first person to recognize a breech presentation. On palpation using Leopold's maneuvers, the nurse feels the hard vertex in the fundus and can perform ballottement of the head independently of the fetal body. The wider sacrum is palpated in the lower part of the abdomen. If the sacrum has not descended, on ballottement the entire fetal body will move. Furthermore, fetal heart tones (FHTs) are usually auscultated above the umbilicus. Passage of meconium from compression of the infant's intestinal tract during descent may occur.

The nurse is particularly alert for a prolapsed umbilical cord, especially in single or double footling breeches, because there is space between the cervix and presenting part through which the cord can slip. If the infant is small and the membranes rupture, the danger is even greater. This is one reason why any woman admitted to the birthing area with a history of ruptured membranes should not ambulate until a full assessment, including vaginal examination, is performed.

Nursing diagnoses that may apply to breech presentation include the following:

- *Risk for Impaired Gas Exchange in the fetus* related to interruption in umbilical blood flow secondary to compression of the cord

- *Health-Seeking Behavior: Information about Breech Presentation* related to an expressed desire to understand the implications of the procedure

Nursing Plan and Implementation

During labor, the fetus is at increased risk for prolapse of the cord. Some agency protocols may therefore call for continuous fetal monitoring even though there are no current research studies to support the use of an EFM. Ongoing assessments of contractions, cervical dilatation, effacement, and fetal descent are also important to monitor labor progress. Emotional support and sharing of information are critical to the childbearing woman and her support person. They need to be kept apprised of the labor's current status as well as the possible treatment plans so they can continue to make informed choices.

During a vaginal birth, the nurse continues to assess the FHR and to provide encouragement and support for the couple. Piper forceps need to be readily available to the physician; the nurse may assist the physician if the forceps are needed for the birth.

Evaluation

Expected outcomes of nursing care include the following:

- The woman and her partner can describe the implications and associated problems with breech presentation.

- The mother and baby have a safe labor and birth.

- Major complications are recognized early, and corrective measures are instituted.

Shoulder Presentation (Transverse Lie) of a Single Fetus

It is not uncommon in multiple gestations for one or more of the fetuses to be in a transverse lie. An incidence of transverse lie of a single fetus is approximately 1 in 300 term births (Cunningham et al., 2005). The infant's long axis lies across the woman's abdomen, and on inspection the contour of the maternal abdomen appears widest from side to side (Figure 26–11 ◆).

Figure 26–11 ◆ Transverse lie. *A,* Shoulder presentation. *B,* On vaginal examination, the nurse may feel the acromion process as the fetal presenting part.

Maternal conditions associated with a transverse lie are grandmultiparity with lax uterine musculature (the most common cause); obstructions such as bony dystocia, placenta previa, neoplasms, and fetal anomalies; hydramnios; and preterm fetus.

Vaginal birth is impossible with a transverse lie. Labor should not be allowed to continue, and a cesarean birth is done quickly. Frequently a vertical incision is made in the uterus because the fetal head and fetal feet lie in the upper portion of the uterus; a low transverse incision may lead to difficulties in extracting the fetus (Cunningham et al., 2005).

If labor is allowed to continue, the fetal shoulder will be forced down into the pelvis and the fetus will become impacted. With no relief, uterine rupture may occur (Cunningham et al., 2005).

CLINICAL THERAPY

Transverse lie may be diagnosed using Leopold's maneuvers and can then be confirmed by ultrasound. At the time of the ultrasound examination, it is important to confirm fetal position, fetal biparietal diameters (to confirm gestational age), and location of the placenta and to carry out an examination for the presence of fetal anomalies and structural abnormalities of the uterus such as leiomyoma (fibroid tumor) or adnexal tumors.

Management varies, depending on the length of gestation, because many transverse lies convert to either cephalic or breech presentation by term (38 weeks). If the fetus is still in a transverse lie at term, an ECV may be done if (1) there is no contraindication to vaginal birth (for example, a fetal anomaly, complete placenta previa, or a structural problem in the uterus); and (2) fetal pulmonary lung maturity is confirmed either by ultrasound measurements or by amniocentesis for assessment of phospholipids (2:1 lecithin/sphingomyelin [L/S] ratio and the presence of phosphatidylglycerol). An ECV is most likely to be successful close to term. Spontaneous version will likely occur if performed before 37 weeks. The use of tocolytics for the procedure may be helpful for nulliparas. The fetus is assessed with an NST or BPP before the procedure. If the version is successful, the woman may be induced if she is at term and her cervix is favorable. However, scientific studies do not support immediate induction as a routine to minimize the chance the fetus will return to the original position (Hofmeyr, 2004).

NURSING CARE MANAGEMENT
Nursing Assessment and Diagnosis

The nurse can identify a transverse lie by inspection and palpation of the abdomen, by auscultation of FHTs in the midline of the abdomen (not conclusive), and by vaginal examination.

On palpation, no fetal part is felt in the fundal portion of the uterus or above the symphysis pubis. The head may be palpated on one side and the breech on the other. FHTs are usually auscultated just below the midline of the umbilicus. On vaginal examination, if a presenting part is palpated, it is the ridged thorax or possibly an arm that is compressed against the chest. Women with a transverse lie may report less shortness of breath, pelvic pressure, and urinary frequency than other women because pressure is not exerted on the diaphragm and the bladder.

Nursing diagnoses that may apply when transverse lie is present include the following:

- **Risk for Impaired Gas Exchange in the fetus** related to decrease in blood flow secondary to cord compression associated with prolapsed cord
- **Risk for Ineffective Coping** related to unknown outcome
- **Fear** related to unknown outcome of birth

Nursing Plan and Implementation

The primary nursing actions are to help evaluate the fetal presentation and to provide information and support to the couple. If an ECV has been accomplished and an induction is started, the nurse completes all interventions related to the induction (see the discussion in Chapter 27 ∞). If transverse lie is discovered when the woman is admitted to the birthing unit in labor, the nurse provides information regarding the need for either an ECV or a cesarean birth and assists with preparation for the birth. If an ECV is not performed or is unsuccessful, a cesarean birth will be performed. Before the cesarean, the nurse watches for rupture of membranes and the possibility of prolapse of the umbilical cord. (See Chapter 27 ∞ for further information regarding teaching with cesarean birth).

Evaluation

Expected outcomes of nursing care include the following:

- The transverse lie is recognized promptly, and crucial assessments are completed.

- Measures to perform an ECV or a cesarean birth are completed.
- The mother and baby have a safe birth.
- The couple can describe the implications and associated problems of transverse lie.

Compound Presentation

A compound presentation is one in which there are two presenting parts. It can occur when the pelvic inlet is not totally occluded by the primary presenting part. If the prolapsed part is a hand, the birth is generally not difficult. Sometimes the hand slips back, and occasionally it is born alongside the head. This may increase the chance of laceration. Cesarean birth is indicated in the presence of uterine dysfunction or nonreassuring fetal status (Cunningham et al., 2005).

CARE OF THE WOMAN AND FETUS AT RISK BECAUSE OF MACROSOMIA

Fetal **macrosomia** is defined as weight of more than 4500 g. It is important to remember that the mean birth weight varies throughout the world. For instance, mean birth weight in Sweden is 3490 g, whereas in Pakistan the mean birth weight is 2770 g. In Latino cultures, "fat" babies are more desirable and are viewed as more healthy. Nurses working with Latino women may encounter resistance if counseling is focused on preventing a large baby. Instead, nurses should stress the importance of the baby's health status (Leininger & McFarland, 2005). The definition of macrosomia will thus differ according to the ethnic group being discussed.

A woman who is obese is 3 to 4 times more likely to have a macrosomic fetus (4500 g) (Ramos & Caughey, 2005). Obesity has been defined a number of ways. For a complete discussion on maternal obesity, see Chapter 18. ∞ There is also an association between macrosomia and both pregestational and gestational diabetes. Increased maternal glucose levels have also been shown to increase fetal weight to more than 4500 g (Ramos & Caughey, 2005). Other risk factors include postterm pregnancy, multiparity, previous macrosomic infant, previous shoulder dystocia, male sex, excessive weight gain, and maternal birth weight.

A woman's pelvis that is adequate for an average-sized fetus may be disproportionately small for an oversized fetus. Distention of the uterus causes overstretching of the myometrial fibers, which may lead to dysfunctional labor and an increased incidence of postpartal hemorrhage. If the oversized fetus is not able to descend, the chance of uterine rupture during labor increases. Vaginal birth poses an increased risk of perineal lacerations and extensions of an episiotomy. The mother is also at risk for postpartum hemorrhage and puerperal infection. The incidence of vacuum and forceps birth increases with fetal size.

The most significant complication in macrosomia is *shoulder dystocia,* which is an obstetric emergency. However, shoulder dystocia may occur with fetuses weighing less than 4000 g, and risk factors are not reliable predictors. Following birth of the head, the anterior shoulder of the macrosomic fetus may not emerge either spontaneously or with gentle traction (Cunningham et al., 2005). If shoulder dystocia is not managed correctly, permanent injury to the baby may result. Brachial plexus injury (due to improper or excessive traction applied to the fetal head) and fractured clavicles may occur. Asphyxia and neurologic damage can also occur.

CLINICAL THERAPY

The occurrence of the maternal and fetal problems associated with macrosomic infants may be somewhat lessened by identifying macrosomia before the onset of labor. The diagnosis is not precise. There is good evidence to show that estimating fetal size with ultrasound is no more accurate than a clinical estimate from Leopold's maneuvers (ACOG, 2000). Additional studies show that ultrasound estimation of fetal weight can be in error of 300 to 550 g (Mongelli & Tambyraja, 2003). If a large fetus is suspected, the maternal pelvis should be evaluated carefully. An estimation of fetal size can be made by palpating the crown-rump length of the fetus in utero, but the greatest errors in estimation occur on both ends of the spectrum—the macrosomic fetus and the very small fetus. Whenever the uterus appears excessively large, hydramnios, an oversized fetus, or a multiple pregnancy must be considered.

Labor and vaginal birth for a fetus greater than 5000 g may warrant a cesarean birth to reduce the risks associated with vaginal births (ACOG, 2000). If a vaginal birth is attempted and difficulty extracting the shoulders occurs during the birth, the obstetrician or CNM may direct the woman to sharply flex her thighs up against her abdomen (McRoberts maneuver). This position is thought to change the maternal pelvic angle and therefore reduce the force needed to extract the shoulders, thereby decreasing the incidence of brachial plexus stretching and clavicular fracture (Figure 26–12 ◆) (Varney, Krebs, & Gegor, 2004). McRoberts maneuver has a high success rate. The maternal head should be lowered and the nurse applies suprapubic pressure directly over the symphysis pubis to aid release of the anterior shoulder. Fundal pressure (pressure exerted at the top of the maternal fundus) should not be performed, because this can further wedge the shoulder against the suprapubic bone.

In addition, the obstetrician or CNM may incorporate other interventions, such as checking the placement of the shoulder, performing an episiotomy, and using the Woods Screw maneuver (which consists of rotating the anterior shoulder 180 degrees to the posterior position). In cases where these interventions fail, the obstetrician or CNM may electively break the clavicle to facilitate extraction of the shoulders.

NURSING CARE MANAGEMENT
Nursing Assessment and Diagnosis

The nurse assists in identifying factors associated with macrosomic infants. During the intrapartum period, the risk factors in-

Figure 26–12 ◆ McRoberts maneuver. *A,* The woman flexes her thighs up onto her abdomen. *B,* The angle of the maternal pelvis before McRoberts maneuver. *C,* The angle of the pelvis with McRoberts maneuver.

clude slow descent of the fetus and prolonged second stage. Because women with these risk factors are prime candidates for dystocia and its complications, the nurse frequently assesses the FHR for nonreassuring heart rate patterns, which may indicate fetal stress; evaluates the rate of cervical dilatation; and assesses fetal descent.

Nursing diagnoses that may apply to the woman with a macrosomic fetus include the following:

- *Risk for Injury to the fetus* related to trauma during the birth process
- *Risk for Infection* related to traumatized tissue secondary to maternal tissue damage during birth

Nursing Plan and Implementation

The nurse monitors labor closely for a dysfunctional pattern, assessing FHR and reporting any sign of labor dysfunction or nonreassuring heart rate patterns to the physician or CNM. The nurse notes any arrest of descent, excessive molding of the fetal head, or the presence of caput succedaneum, which can also indicate a large fetus or CPD.

The nurse provides support for the laboring woman and her partner and information regarding the implications and possible associated problems. The nurse can provide the couple with directions for proper positioning at the time of birth to facilitate extraction of the shoulders. If the nurse anticipates a possible shoulder dystocia, additional staff should be notified and appropriate support personnel for the newborn should be informed. During the birth, the nurse continues to provide support and encouragement to the couple. Informing the woman that possible suprapubic pressure may be needed can help reduce anxiety for the couple.

After the birth, the nurse inspects the newborn for cephalhematoma, Erb palsy (caused by overstretching of the brachial plexus and damage to C5, C6, C7), and fractured clavicles (exhibited by nonmovement of one arm) and informs the admission nursery of any problems. The newborn will need to be observed closely for cerebral and neurologic damage.

Postpartally, the nurse checks the uterus for potential atony and the maternal vital signs for deviations suggesting hypovolemic shock. Frequent fundal checks should be performed to evaluate the woman for postpartum bleeding.

Evaluation

Expected outcomes of nursing care include the following:

* The woman and her partner can describe the implications of macrosomia and possible associated problems.
* The mother and baby have a safe labor and birth.

CARE OF THE WOMAN WITH A MULTIPLE GESTATION

The incidence of twins in the United States accounts for 3.2% of all pregnancies; however, with advances in reproductive technologies, the incidence is increasing (Martin, Hamilton, Sutton et al., 2005). It is estimated that triplets and higher order multiples account for 1.8% of all births. In 2002, 130,000 infants were born as a result of a multifetal gestation (ACOG, 2004b). The incidence of these higher order births is declining because of recent recommendations from the ACOG (Martin et al., 2005) to reduce the number of fetuses transferred during in vitro fertilization procedures. Because twin birth is by far the most common multiple birth, the discussion focuses on this type. The chapter also identifies specific variations for triplets and higher order multiple gestations as appropriate.

Embryology of Multiple Gestation

Terminology related to various types of twins is presented in Table 26–3. Twins can develop from either the fertilization of two separate ova or from the division of one fertilized ovum. Twins that occur from two separate ova are called *dizygotic* (two zygotes, also referred to as fraternal twins). In this type, the fe-

tuses may be the same sex or different sexes and there are two complete amnions and two chorions. The fetuses are no more closely related genetically than any other siblings.

In contrast, 33% of twins are *monozygotic* (also referred to as identical twins); that is, they develop from one fertilized ovum (Blackburn, 2007). These twins are genetically identical, and thus always of the same sex (see Table 26–3). If the zygote divides within the first 72 hours past fertilization, the twins will be diamniotic and dichorionic. If the division occurs from the fourth to the eighth day past fertilization, the embryos will develop with two separate amnions and one chorion. If the division happens after the eighth day, the two fetuses will share both a common amniotic sac and chorion. The terminology is important because the perinatal morbidity and mortality rates differ greatly among different types of twins (Blackburn, 2007). For example, monozygotic twins have a high incidence of cord entrapment, twin-to-twin transfusion, and fetal demise (Blackburn, 2003).

Pregnancy Loss in Multiple Gestation

The development of sensitive human chorionic gonadotropin (hCG) assays and increasingly sensitive ultrasound techniques has made it possible to determine more accurately the early pregnancy loss rate of twins, including both complete pregnancy loss and spontaneous resorption of one twin (called the "vanishing twin" phenomenon). Of all twin pregnancies, approximately 25% are lost before the end of the first trimester (Malinowski, Koktysz, & Stawerski, 2005). Causative factors in the loss of both twins in the first trimester include environmental factors, infectious organisms, trophoblast dysfunction, poor embryo quality, or a lower concentration of placentally produced substances. Although loss of one twin can occur at any time during the pregnancy, it more commonly occurs in the first trimester. Marginal and velamentous cord insertions (to be discussed shortly) are more likely to be present when there is a vanishing twin, and the presence of a monochorionic placenta is more likely to result in either a singleton gestation (because of a vanishing twin) or complete pregnancy loss (Malinowski et al., 2005).

Pregnancy loss of twins in the second trimester is associated with congenital anomalies, growth restriction, chromosomal abnormalities, and cervical incompetence. In a monochorionic placenta, there may be a vascular anastomosis that leads to twin-to-twin transfusion syndrome. When this syndrome is present, blood is chronically drained from one fetus to the other. The donor fetus becomes growth restricted, and oligohydramnios develops. The recipient fetus becomes polycythemic and hydropic, and hydramnios develops. If the fetuses become severely affected during the second trimester, untreated mortality may be 100% (ACOG, 2004b).

The incidence of preterm birth is also higher in multiple gestations. Preterm birth occurs in 55% to 57% of all multiple gestations. Preterm births before 32 gestational weeks, when the risk of mortality and morbidity are greatest, occur in 12% of twin pregnancies, 36% of triplet pregnancies, and 60% of quadruple pregnancies (ACOG, 2004b). In singletons, the perinatal mortality is at the lowest point at 40 weeks' gestation; for twins, the

Table 26–3	CHARACTERISTICS OF TWIN PREGNANCY			
Type	**Time of Division**	**Characteristics**	**Frequency**	**Mortality Rate**
Dizygotic				
(Two separate ova) Fraternal twins Dichorionic-diamniotic twins	Develop from two ova released at the same time.	Each twin has own placenta, chorion, amnion. Dizygotic twins are called fraternal twins. They may be the same or different sex.	67% of all twins	11.5%
Monozygotic				
(Single ovum) Identical twins Dichorionic-diamniotic twins	Division occurs within 72 hours past fertilization.* Inner cell mass not yet developed.	Each twin has own chorion, amnion, placenta.	33% of all twins 30% of monozygotic twins	9%
Monochorionic-diamniotic twins	Division occurs at blastocyst stage, 4 to 8 days after fertilization.* Inner cell mass divides in two.	Placenta has one chorion and two amnions. Each twin lies in own sac.	68% of monozygotic twins	25%
Monochorionic-monoamniotic twins	Division occurs in primitive germ disk, 9 to 13 days past fertilization.*	Twins lie in the same amniotic sac. Increased risk of umbilical cords becoming tangled or knotted.	2% of monozygotic twins	Less than 50%

*Chasen, S. T., & Chervanak, F. A. (1998). What is the relationship between the universal use of ultrasound, the rate of detection of twins, and outcome differences? *Clinical Obstetrics and Gynecology, 41*, 67–77.

perinatal mortality rate decreases until 37 weeks and then increases steadily from 38 to 42 weeks. The optimal delivery time for triplet pregnancies is 35 weeks (ACOG, 2004b). A woman pregnant with twins who has not spontaneously begun labor by 40 gestational weeks is typically induced at her due date.

IMPLICATIONS

Women with a multiple gestation are more likely to develop complications, which include the following (ACOG, 2004b):

- Spontaneous abortions are more common, as previously discussed.

- Gestational diabetes occurs more often in multiple gestations. Three percent to 6% of twin pregnancies and 22% to 39% of triplet pregnancies are complicated by gestational diabetes.

- Hypertension is the major maternal complication. The risk of developing severe hypertension or preeclampsia is 2.6 times higher in twins and significantly higher in triplets.

- Multiple gestations are more likely to acquire HELLP syndrome, a complication resulting from eclampsia or preeclampsia.

- Women with multiple gestations are more likely to develop acute fatty liver, which is manifested by severe coagulopathy, hypoglycemia, and hyperammonemia, which can lead to maternal and fetal death.

- Pulmonary embolism is 6 times more likely to develop during pregnancy with multiple gestations.

- Maternal anemia occurs because of demands of the multiple gestation. The hemoglobin averages 10 g/dL from the 20th week on. Anemia is indicated by hemoglobin levels below 11 g/dL in the first or third trimester or below 10.5 g/dL in

the second trimester. When decreased hemoglobin is accompanied by serum ferritin concentration of less than 12 mg/dL, iron deficiency anemia is diagnosed.

- Hydramnios may be due to increased renal perfusion from cross-vessel anastomosis of monozygotic twins.

- Premature rupture of membranes, incompetent cervix, and intrauterine growth restriction occur more commonly.

- Rare complications associated with twins include twin-to-twin transfusion (previously discussed), conjoined (Siamese) twins, and *acardia* (twin reversed arterial perfusion sequence).

- Complications during labor include preterm labor, uterine dysfunction due to an overstretched myometrium, abnormal fetal presentations, instrumental or cesarean birth, and postpartum hemorrhage.

The woman with a multiple gestation may experience more physical discomfort during her pregnancy, such as shortness of breath, dyspnea on exertion, backaches, round ligament pain, heartburn, pelvic or suprapubic pressure, and pedal edema because of the oversized uterus.

CLINICAL THERAPY

The goals of medical care are to promote normal fetal development to prevent maternal complications, to prevent preterm birth, and to diminish fetal trauma during labor.

Ultrasound examinations play a crucial role in the care and treatment of multiple gestations. Ultrasound assists with identifying the presence of more than one fetus early in the pregnancy, providing accurate dating of the pregnancy, and detecting fetal anomalies. Because the incidence of perinatal mortality and morbidity is increased in twins, use of ultrasound in the first and second trimesters can be particularly helpful. Evidence supports the use of ultrasound for accurately determining chorionicity and amnionicity in multiple pregnancies (ACOG, 2004b). Knowledge of chorionicity is essential in differentiating twin-to-twin transfusion from fetal growth restriction secondary to abnormal placental blood flow. Knowledge of chorionicity is also important in determining the management of a multiple pregnancy in which one twin is sonographically abnormal. If the twins are dichorionic/diamniotic (DC/DA), then selective termination could be considered. Determination of amnionicity is based on ultrasound visualization or the lack of visualization of an intertwin membrane. Visualization of this membrane becomes more difficult as the gestation advances because of progressive thinning of the intertwin membrane, fetal crowding, and an increasing incidence of oligohydramnios. Knowledge regarding the presence of one amnion is crucial, because management of monochorionic/monoamniotic (MC/MA) twins requires more intensive surveillance and earlier birth, usually by cesarean (ACOG, 2004b). Women with (MC/MA) twins are frequently cared for by perinatologists in a facility that has high-risk services available.

Preventing preterm labor is a major goal. Prenatal care should begin early, and more frequent visits are usually scheduled. Many practitioners perform vaginal examinations at each visit after 28 weeks to identify cervical changes, such as cervical shortening, effacement, or dilatation, or the beginning of bulging membranes. Although digital vaginal examinations are somewhat objective, they have positive predictive values of predicting preterm labor in 60% to 70% of twin and triplet gestations (ACOG, 2004b). Although the use of fetal fibronectin (ffN) as a predictor of preterm labor has been well established in singleton pregnancies, the results have been conflicting in multiple gestations (ACOG, 2004b). Further research is needed to determine if this test has a place in determining preterm labor in pregnancies resulting in more than one fetus.

There is evidence to support routine cervical measurements for preterm prevention. Women having cervical measurements less than 25 mm at 24 weeks' gestation were the best predictor of a preterm birth (ACOG, 2004b). There is insufficient evidence, however, to support policies for routine cervical cerclage, reduced activity and work, and prophylactic bed rest (ACOG, 2004b). A systematic review of studies of hospitaliza-

---

EVIDENCE-BASED PRACTICE

HOSPITALIZATION AND BED REST FOR MULTIPLE PREGNANCY

Clinical Question

Is hospitalization and/or bed rest effective for women with a multiple pregnancy, for prevention of preterm birth and other adverse fetal, neonatal, and maternal outcomes?

The Evidence

Six randomized trials were appraised for evidence of effectiveness of bed rest in preventing various maternal and fetal outcomes. The trials involved more than 600 women and 1400 babies. The trials all included subjects who had multiple pregnancies. The studies were variously representative of women with uncomplicated twin pregnancy, women with a triplet pregnancy, and women with a twin pregnancy complicated by preterm labor.

What Is Effective?

The evidence in the case of bed rest and/or hospitalization for multiple pregnancies does not support the effectiveness of this intervention. No differences were found for mothers with preterm labor in terms of preterm birth, perinatal mortality, fetal growth, or in other neonatal outcomes. Likewise, although mothers who were on bed rest for triplet pregnancy had slightly beneficial effects, the differences were not statistically significant. For women with uncomplicated twin pregnancy, the risk of preterm birth was not reduced; indeed, the risk of very preterm birth was higher for this group. No differences were seen in perinatal mortality or in other neonatal outcomes. There was a trend for a smaller number of low-birth-weight infants when all of the trials were considered, but these differences were slight. No differences were seen in the number of

very low-birth-weight infants, and no support for the policy was found in other neonatal outcomes.

What Is Unclear?

No benefits were measured or described for ongoing development of the infants after birth. Acceptability of the treatment is often difficult for mothers—particularly if they have young children in the home—and so its benefits should be distinct and of a sufficient magnitude to warrant such a serious disruption for the family's life. However, some positive effects were suggested, and so this intervention warrants further study for some groups, specifically for women with triplet pregnancy.

Best Practice

There is currently not enough evidence to support a policy of routine hospitalization and/or bed rest for mothers with multiple pregnancy. No reduction in the risk of preterm birth or perinatal death was clear. There is a suggestion that fetal growth is improved, but only if the mother is at risk of preterm birth. For women with an uncomplicated twin pregnancy, this review suggests that bed rest may actually be harmful in that the risk of very preterm birth appears to be increased. Until further substantive evidence is produced, the policy of hospital admission and bed rest cannot be recommended as a routine clinical practice in uncomplicated multiple pregnancies.

Critical Thinking

Are there any conditions under which it might be beneficial to recommend bed rest for a mother with a multiple pregnancy?

REFERENCE: Crowther, C. (2006). Hospitalization and bed rest for multiple pregnancy. *The Cochrane Database of Systematic Reviews* (1) (Article No.: Cd000110).

Figure 26–13 ◆ Twins may be in any of these presentations while in utero.

tion and bed rest for multiple pregnancy showed insufficient evidence to support routine bed rest (ACOG, 2004b). Although home monitoring was commonly used in the 1990s, the effectiveness of this intervention has been disputed by large randomized studies and is no longer endorsed for preterm labor monitoring (ACOG, 2004b).

Some areas offer twin clinics, which provide many advantages for the woman with multiple gestation. These advantages include consistent evaluation, intensive prenatal education, counseling, and support from the same healthcare providers.

Intrapartal management and assessment require careful attention to maternal and fetal status. The mother should have an intravenous infusion in place with a large-bore needle. Anesthesia and cross-matched blood should be readily available. The twins are monitored by dual EFM. The labor may progress very slowly or very quickly.

The decision about method of birth may not be made until labor occurs, and the method depends on a variety of factors. The presence of maternal complications such as placenta previa, abruptio placentae, or severe preeclampsia usually indicates the need for cesarean birth. Fetal factors such as severe intrauterine growth restriction (IUGR), preterm birth, fetal anomalies, nonreassuring fetal status, or unfavorable fetal position or presentation also require cesarean birth. Typically, a cesarean birth is performed if the presenting twin is in a presenting position other than vertex and cannot be turned to a vertex presentation.

Birth of three or more fetuses is best accomplished by cesarean because of the risk of fetal insult due to decreased placental perfusion and hemorrhage from the separating placenta during the intrapartal period (Cunningham et al., 2005). Complicated obstetric maneuvers such as breech extraction and podalic version, the risk of prolapse of the cord, and an increase in fetal collision provide additional reasons for cesarean birth.

Any combination of presentations and positions can occur with twins (Figure 26–13 ◆). Approximately 50% of twins are born by cesarean, which is chosen in the hope of reducing complications for the twins, especially birth asphyxia (Cunningham et al., 2005).

The placentas are examined after the birth. If the twins are of the same sex, the placentas are sent to the pathology laboratory for examination to determine whether they are monozygotic or dizygotic twins.

NURSING CARE MANAGEMENT
Nursing Assessment and Diagnosis

When obtaining a maternal history at the beginning of antenatal care, the nurse should identify any family history of twinning. Equally important is a history of medication taken to enhance fertility. These facts should be noted on the antepartal record.

At each antepartal clinic visit, the nurse should measure the fundal height. During the prenatal period, a fundal height greater than expected for the weeks of gestation and auscultation of two heartbeats that differ by at least 10 beats per minute are the most likely clues of twin pregnancy. Some women experience severe nausea and vomiting and develop severe anemia despite the intake of multiple-vitamin therapy. The α-fetoprotein level may be elevated (ACOG, 2004b).

Any growth, fetal movement, or heart tone auscultation out of proportion to gestational age by dates is indicative of twins. During palpation, the nurse may feel many small parts on all sides of the abdomen (Figure 26–14 ◆). If twins are suspected, the nurse should attempt to auscultate two separate heartbeats in different quadrants of the maternal abdomen. Use of the Doppler device may be helpful. Conclusive evidence of twins is found on sonography.

During the prenatal visits the nurse should determine the family's level of preparation for integrating more than one new member. Although the thought of having twins can be very exciting, the reality of attaching to two infants and adapting to the parental role may be trying.

During labor it is important to monitor each fetus. In the case of twins, an external electronic monitor can be applied to both, or if conditions permit, the internal monitor can be applied to twin A and the external monitor to twin B. The heart rates may be auscultated on different quadrants of the maternal abdomen, but continuous monitoring is more beneficial. Signs of nonreassuring heart rate patterns should be reported to the CNM or obstetrician.

After a multiple birth, the mother is closely monitored for postpartal hemorrhage. Nursing diagnoses that may apply to a woman with a multiple gestation include the following:

- *Fear* related to unknown outcome of the birth process
- *Ineffective Coping* related to uncertainty about the labor and birth plan
- *Deficient Knowledge* related to lack of information about the problems associated with multiple gestation
- *Risk for Impaired Gas Exchange in the fetuses* related to decreased oxygenation secondary to cord compression

Nursing Plan and Implementation
COMMUNITY-BASED NURSING CARE

Antepartally, the woman may need counseling about diet and daily activities. The nurse can help her plan meals to meet her increased needs. A daily intake of 4000 kcal (minimum) and 135 g of protein is recommended for optimal weight gain and fetal growth. A prenatal vitamin and 1 mg of folic acid and iron should also be taken daily. A weight gain of 35 to 45 lb is recommended.

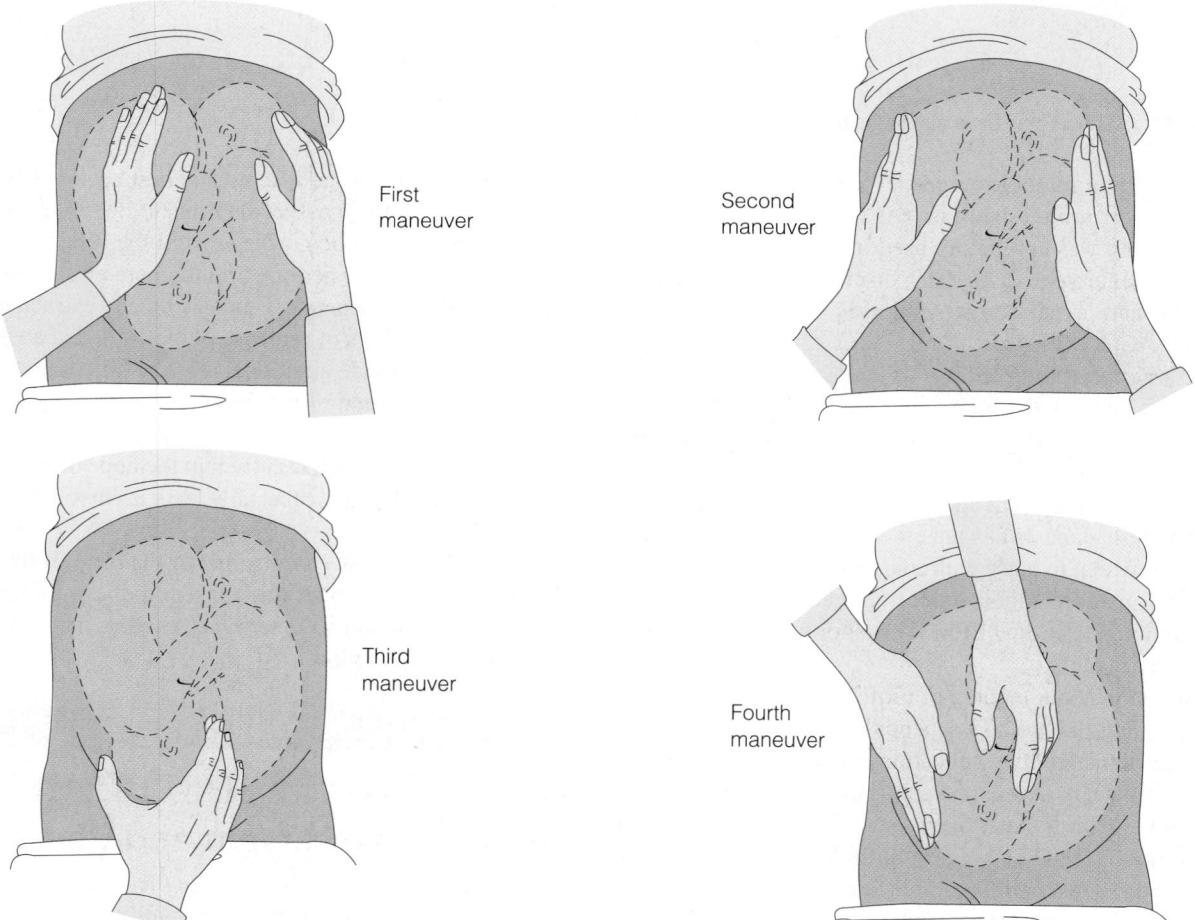

First maneuver

Second maneuver

Third maneuver

Fourth maneuver

Figure 26–14 ◆ Leopold's maneuvers in twin pregnancy. The fetus on the mother's right side is in cephalic presentation, and the fetus on the left is in breech presentation. Leopold's maneuvers may be done in a different sequence.

Maternal hypertension is treated with bed rest in the lateral position to increase uterine and kidney perfusion. Back discomfort can be alleviated by pelvic rocking, good posture, and good body mechanics. The nurse can help the woman schedule frequent periods of rest during the day. Family members or friends may be willing to care for the woman's other children periodically to allow her time to get rest. Community support systems, such as neighbors or church members, may be available to assist the family with meals, grocery shopping, and household chores. Many communities now have support groups specifically designed for mothers of multiples. Members provide invaluable peer support throughout pregnancy and the postpartum period. Teaching regarding prevention and recognition of preterm labor is very important. For further discussion see Chapter 20. ∞

HOSPITAL-BASED NURSING CARE

The nurse needs to prepare to receive multiple newborns. This means a multiplication of resuscitation equipment and newborn identification papers and bracelets. The newborns may be placed in individual radiant warmers or in the same one once identification bands have been applied. Additional staff members should be available for newborn resuscitation, monitoring, and newborn care. Special precautions should be observed to ensure correct identification of the newborns. The first born is usually tagged Baby A; the second, Baby B; and so on.

Evaluation

Expected outcomes of nursing care include the following:

- The woman is able to discuss the implications and problems associated with multiple gestation.
- The woman feels she is able to cope with the pregnancy and birth.
- The woman understands the treatment plan and how to gain further information.
- The mother, father, and babies have a safe prenatal course, labor, and birth and a safe postpartal and newborn course.

CARE OF THE WOMAN AND FETUS IN THE PRESENCE OF NONREASSURING FETAL STATUS

When the oxygen supply is insufficient to meet the physiologic demands of the fetus, a nonreassuring fetal status may result. *Nonreassuring fetal status* is the term used to identify data describing the fetal status. Previously, the term *nonreassuring*

RESEARCH IN PRACTICE

EFFICACY OF INTRAUTERINE RESUSCITATION TECHNIQUES IN IMPROVING FETAL OXYGEN STATUS DURING LABOR

What is this study about? There are several standard procedures for treating suspected fetal hypoxemia when it is exhibited in a nonreassuring fetal heart rate (FHR) pattern. It is common practice to administer a bolus of either 500 or 1000 mL of fluid; to position the mother in the left lateral position; and to administer oxygen by mask at 10 L/min. However, little data exist supporting the efficacy of these procedures in relieving nonreassuring fetal status. This study undertook a randomized trial to document the efficacy of these intrauterine resuscitation techniques.

How was this study done? The researchers recruited healthy, nulliparous women admitted at term for elective induction of a birth. Routine FHR monitoring was applied. Women who subsequently met the standard criteria for fetal oxygen saturation monitoring (FSpO$_2$) were admitted to the study. This resulted in a sample of 56 mothers. The mothers were assigned to an intravenous bolus group intervention first; mothers were randomized to either 500 mL or 1000 mL fluid bolus. Subsequently, maternal positioning was tested. One hour before the epidural anesthesia, mothers were randomized to one of six positions. All of the positions were sequentially applied for 15 minutes at a time. One hour after the position sequence, mothers were administered oxygen with a nonrebreather face mask at 10 L/min. After 15 minutes, the oxygen was discontinued. FHR patterns and FSpO$_2$ were monitored per standard protocol throughout the experiment.

What were the results of the study? Both the 500 and 1000 mL intravenous boluses of fluid were effective in improving FSpO$_2$ and FHR. The 1000 mL had greater effects that were longer lasting than the smaller volume. Either lateral position was superior to the supine position in improving indicators of fetal oxygenation; the differences between the left and right lateral positions were not statistically significant. Oxygen administration improved fetal oxygenation. The effect persisted for 30 minutes even after the oxygen was removed. The effect was greater and longer lasting for fetuses that started out in the low normal range, and appeared to have more benefit than those that started in the normal range.

What additional questions might I have? Does the sequence with which these interventions are applied make a difference? In this case, the fluid bolus was first, followed by positioning and finally oxygen application. Are the effects cumulative? Can simultaneous application of all three interventions improve fetal oxygenation status and outcomes even better?

How can I use this study? Nonreassuring FHR patterns should be assessed by the nurse and immediate actions taken. Increasing the rate of administration of fluids, putting the mother into the lateral position, and administering oxygen should be part of the standard care plans for laboring mothers. These interventions can improve fetal oxygenation status and FHR patterns, and the effects of the interventions may persist even after the interventions are discontinued.

Simpson, K., & James, D. (2005). Efficacy of intrauterine resuscitation techniques in improving fetal oxygen status during labor. *Obstetrics and Gynecology, 105*(6), 1362–1368.

Figure 26–15 ◆ Intrapartal management of nonreassuring fetal status.
Note: bl = baseline; FAST = fetal acoustic stimulation test; SST = scalp stimulation test.
SOURCE: From Zuspan, F. P., & Quilligan, E. J. *Handbook of obstetrics, gynecology, and primary care.* Copyright 1998, Mosby; reprinted with permission from Elsevier Science.

fetal status was used; however, its use implied an ill fetus despite the fact that the condition is often transient, not chronic.

A variety of factors may contribute to a nonreassuring fetal status. The most common are related to cord compression and uteroplacental insufficiency associated with placental abnormalities and preexisting maternal or fetal disease. If the resultant hypoxia persists and metabolic acidosis follows, the situation can be life threatening to the fetus.

The most common initial signs of nonreassuring fetal status are meconium-stained amniotic fluid (in a vertex presentation) and changes in the FHR. The presence of ominous FHR patterns, such as late or severe variable decelerations, decrease in or lack of variability, and progressive acceleration in the FHR baseline, are indicative of hypoxia. Fetal scalp blood samples demonstrating a pH value of 7.2 or less provide a more sophisticated indication of fetal problems and are generally obtained when questions about fetal status arise. (See also Chapter 23 ∞).

Clinical Therapy

When there is evidence of possible nonreassuring fetal status, treatment centers on relieving the hypoxia and minimizing the effects of anoxia on the fetus. Initial interventions include changing the mother's position, increasing infusion rates of intravenous fluids, and administering oxygen by mask at 6 to 10 L per minute. If EFM has not yet been used, it is usually instituted at this time. If oxytocin is in use, it should be discontinued. Fetal scalp stimulation can be performed. Fetal scalp blood samples can be taken. If EFM is ineffective, the CNM or physician may utilize internal monitoring devices to more accurately assess FHR changes. Figure 26–15 ◆ depicts intrapartal management of nonreassuring fetal status heart rate patterns.

NURSING CARE MANAGEMENT
Nursing Assessment and Diagnosis

The nurse reviews the woman's prenatal history to anticipate the possibility of nonreassuring fetal status. When the membranes rupture, it is important to assess FHR and to observe for meconium staining. As labor progresses, the nurse is particularly alert for even subtle changes in the FHR pattern and the fetal scalp pH, if available. Reports by the mother of increased or greatly decreased fetal activity may also be associated with nonreassuring fetal status. For further discussion of FHR patterns and characteristics, see evaluation of fetal status during labor in Chapter 23. ∞

Nursing diagnoses that may apply in the presence of non-reassuring fetal status include the following:

- *Decreased Cardiac Output in fetus* related to decreased uteroplacental perfusion secondary to maternal hypotension, decreased blood volume, or vasoconstriction with preeclampsia
- *Anxiety* related to knowledge of nonreassuring fetal status

Nursing Plan and Implementation

Staff members may become so involved in assessing fetal status and initiating corrective measures that they fail to give explanations and emotional support to the woman, her partner, and other family members. It is imperative that the nurse provide both full explanations of the problem and comfort to the couple. In many instances, if birth is not imminent, the woman must undergo cesarean birth. Anticipation of this surgery may cause fear and frustration for the couple, especially if they were committed to a shared, prepared birth experience.

Evaluation

Expected outcomes of nursing care include the following:

- The woman and her family become less anxious and more able to cope with their situation.
- The FHR remains in normal range, or, alternatively, supportive measures maintain the FHR as normal as possible.

CARE OF THE WOMAN AND FETUS AT RISK BECAUSE OF PLACENTAL PROBLEMS

Maintaining placental function is paramount to ensuring fetal well-being and continuation of the pregnancy. Because the placenta is highly vascular, problems that develop are usually associated with maternal and possibly fetal hemorrhage. Causes and sources of hemorrhage are reviewed in Table 26–4.

Abruptio Placentae

Abruptio placentae is the premature separation of a normally implanted placenta from the uterine wall. The incidence of abruptio placentae is 0.5% to 2% of all pregnancies but it accounts for 15% of perinatal mortality (Perinatal Institute, 2006). It is more frequent in pregnancies complicated by smoking, premature rupture of membranes, and hypertension (Perinatal Institute, 2006). The risk of recurrence is 10 times higher if a previous abruption has occurred (Perinatal Institute, 2006).

The cause of abruptio placentae is largely unknown. Theories have been proposed relating its occurrence to decreased blood flow to the placenta through the sinuses during the last trimester. It is estimated that maternal hypertension is the most common cause (44%) with maternal trauma accounting for 2%

Table 26–4   CAUSES AND SOURCES OF HEMORRHAGE

Causes and Sources	Signs and Symptoms
Antepartal Period	
Abortion	Vaginal bleeding Intermittent uterine contractions Rupture of membranes
Placenta previa	Painless vaginal bleeding after seventh month
Abruptio placentae	
Partial	Vaginal bleeding: no increase in uterine pain
Severe	Vaginal bleeding may or may not be present Extreme tenderness of abdominal area Rigid, boardlike abdomen Increase in size of abdomen
Intrapartal Period	
Placenta previa	Bright red vaginal bleeding
Abruptio placentae	Same signs and symptoms listed above
Uterine atony in stage III	Bright red vaginal bleeding Ineffectual contractility
Postpartal Period	
Uterine atony	Boggy uterus Dark vaginal bleeding Presence of clots
Retained placental fragments	Boggy uterus Dark vaginal bleeding Presence of clots
Lacerations of cervix or vagina	Firm uterus Bright red blood

Table 26–5   CLASSIFICATION OF ABRUPTION

Class 0	Asymptomatic; diagnosed after birth
Class I	Mild; most common, occurring in 48% of cases
Class II	Moderate; both mother and fetus show signs of distress; 27% of cases
Class III	Severe; maternal shock and fetal death likely; 24% of cases

SOURCE: Used with permission from Gaufberg, S. A. "Abrupto Placenta" *eMedicine Journal* (series online). Available at: http:www.emedicine.com/emerg/topic12.htm

to 10% of the cases. Domestic violence, abdominal trauma, presence of fibroids, uterine overdistention, fetal growth restriction, advanced maternal age, alcohol consumption, cocaine use, a short umbilical cord, and high parity also contribute (Perinatal Institute, 2006). Abruptions also appear to be more common in certain ethnic groups. Caucasian and African American women have higher incidences of abruptions than Asian and Latin American women (Cunningham et al., 2005). Classification of abruption is based on the extent of separation (Table 26–5).

PATHOPHYSIOLOGY

Premature separation of the placenta may be divided into three types (Figure 26–16 ◆):

1. *Marginal.* The blood passes between the fetal membranes and the uterine wall and escapes vaginally. Separation

Figure 26–16 ◆ Abruptio placentae. *A,* Marginal abruption with external hemorrhage. *B,* Central abruption with concealed hemorrhage. *C,* Complete separation.

begins at the periphery of the placenta; this marginal sinus rupture may or may not become more severe.

2. *Central.* The placenta separates centrally, and the blood is trapped between the placenta and the uterine wall. Entrapment of the blood results in concealed bleeding.

3. *Complete.* Massive vaginal bleeding is seen in the presence of almost total separation.

In severe cases of central abruptio placentae, a blood clot forms behind the placenta. With no place to escape, the blood invades the myometrial tissues between the muscle fibers. This occurrence accounts for the uterine irritability that is a significant sign of premature separation of the placenta. If hemorrhage continues, eventually the uterus turns entirely blue in color. After the baby is born, the uterus contracts only with difficulty. This syndrome is known as a *Couvelaire uterus* and frequently necessitates hysterectomy.

As a result of the damage to the uterine wall and the retroplacental clotting with covert abruption, large amounts of thromboplastin are released into the maternal blood supply, which in turn triggers the development of disseminated intravascular coagulation (DIC) and the resultant hypofibrinogenemia. Fibrinogen levels, which are ordinarily elevated in pregnancy, may drop to incoagulable amounts within a matter of minutes as a result of rapidly developing premature separation of the placenta. Additional information on DIC may be found in a medical-surgical nursing textbook.

MATERNAL RISKS

Maternal mortality is now uncommon, although maternal morbidity is still common (Cunningham et al., 2005). Problems following the birth depend in large part on the severity of the intrapartal bleeding, coagulation defects (DIC), hypofibrinogenemia, and length of time between separation and the birth. Moderate to severe hemorrhage results in hemorrhagic shock, which ultimately may prove fatal to the mother if not reversed. In the postpartal period, women who have suffered this disorder are at risk for hemorrhage and renal failure due to shock, vascular spasm, intravascular clotting, or a combination of the three. Another cause of renal failure is incompatible emergency blood transfusion. Failure is directly proportional to the number of units transfused. In some cases, hysterectomy is performed if bleeding cannot be controlled.

FETAL-NEONATAL RISKS

Perinatal mortality associated with abruptio placentae is approximately 25% (Cunningham et al., 2005). In severe cases in which separation occurs to approximately 50% of the placenta, infant mortality is 100%. In less severe separation, fetal outcome depends on the level of maturity. The most serious complications in the newborn arise from preterm labor, anemia, and hypoxia. If fetal hypoxia progresses unchecked, irreversible brain damage or fetal demise may result. Neurologic defects within the first year of life occur in approximately 14% of infants who survive (Cunningham et al., 2005). With thorough assessment and prompt action on the part of the healthcare team, fetal and maternal outcome can be optimized.

CLINICAL THERAPY

Because of the risk of DIC, evaluating the results of coagulation tests is imperative. In DIC, fibrinogen levels and platelet counts are usually decreased; prothrombin times (PT) and partial thromboplastin times (PTT) are normal to prolonged. If the values are not markedly abnormal, serial testing may be helpful in establishing an abnormal trend that is indicative of coagulopathy. Another very sensitive test determines fibrin degradation products; these levels rise with DIC.

After the diagnosis is established, emphasis is placed on maintaining the cardiovascular status of the mother and developing a plan for effecting the birth of the fetus. Intravenous access with a large-gauge cannula is warranted along with continuous EFM. Which birth method is selected depends on the condition of the woman and fetus; in many circumstances cesarean birth may be the safest option.

If the separation is mild and gestation is near term, labor may be induced, and the fetus may be born vaginally with as little trauma as possible. If rupture of membranes and oxytocin infusion by pump do not initiate labor within a short time, a cesarean birth is usually done. A longer delay would increase the risk of hemorrhage, with resulting hypofibrinogenemia. Supportive treatment to decrease risk of DIC includes typing and cross-matching for blood transfusions (at least three units), clotting mechanism evaluation, and intravenous fluids.

In cases of moderate to severe placental separation, a cesarean birth is done after hypofibrinogenemia has been treated by intravenous infusion of cryoprecipitate or fresh frozen plasma (FFP). Vaginal birth is impossible in the event of a Couvelaire uterus because it could not contract properly in labor. Cesarean birth is necessary in the face of severe hemorrhage to allow an immediate hysterectomy to save both woman and fetus.

The hypovolemia that accompanies severe abruptio placentae is life threatening and must be combated with whole blood. If the fetus is alive but experiencing stress, emergency cesarean birth is the method of choice. With a stillborn fetus, vaginal birth is preferable unless shock from hemorrhage is uncontrollable. Intravenous fluids of a balanced salt solution such as lactated Ringer's solution are given through a 16- or 18-gauge cannula (Cunningham et al., 2005). Central venous pressure (CVP) monitoring may be needed to evaluate intravenous fluid replacement. Hemodynamic monitoring is an essential aspect of nursing care for the woman with abruption. If there is any evidence of hypovolemia, two venous lines should be started. Urine output should be monitored with an indwelling catheter. If the output drops below 30 mL per hour with adequate fluid replacement, CVP should be used to assess for hypovolemia. CVP will be the guide to fluid replacement. An absolute level is not as significant as the response to fluid replacement. Pulmonary artery catheter measurement, such as with a Swan-Ganz catheter, may be necessary to manage the hemodynamic changes. However, a significant abruption may preclude placing a catheter in the jugular or subclavian vein because the DIC is causing bleeding from multiple sites. The CVP is evaluated hourly, and results are communicated to the physician. Elevations of CVP may indicate fluid overload and pulmonary edema. The hematocrit is maintained at 30% through the administration of packed red cells or whole blood, or both (Cunningham et al., 2005).

Laboratory testing is ordered to provide ongoing data regarding hemoglobin, hematocrit, and coagulation status. A clot observation test may be done at the bedside to evaluate coagulation status. A red top glass tube containing 5 mL of maternal blood is inverted four to five times. If a clot fails to form in 6 minutes, a fibrinogen level of less than 150 mg/dL is suspected. If a clot is not formed in 30 minutes, the fibrinogen level may well be less than 100 mg/dL. A clot observation test may be completed by a physician or a nurse.

Measures are taken to stimulate labor to effect vaginal birth as indicated by the condition of the mother and fetus. The birth may be hastened by performing an amniotomy and by oxytocin stimulation. Previously, birth within 6 hours of the diagnosis of severe placental abruption was recommended to reduce maternal mortality and morbidity. Currently, changing medical practice directed to ensuring adequate fluid replacement, especially blood, appears to accomplish the same outcome (Cunningham et al., 2005).

NURSING CARE MANAGEMENT
Nursing Assessment and Diagnosis

Electronic monitoring of the uterine contractions and resting tone between contractions provides information regarding the labor pattern and effectiveness of the oxytocin induction. Because uterine resting tone is frequently increased with abruptio placentae, it must be evaluated frequently for further increase. Abdominal girth measurements may be ordered hourly and are obtained by placing a tape measure around the maternal abdomen at the level of the umbilicus. Another method of evaluating uterine size, which increases as more bleeding occurs at the site of abruption, is to place a mark at the top of the uterine fundus. The distance from the symphysis pubis to the mark may be evaluated hourly.

Nursing diagnoses that may apply to the woman with abruptio placentae include the following:

- **Fluid Volume Deficit** related to hypovolemia secondary to excessive blood loss
- **Risk for Ineffective Tissue Perfusion** related to blood loss secondary to uterine atony following birth
- **Anxiety** related to concern for personal status and the baby's safety
- **Risk for Impaired Gas Exchange** in the fetus related to decreased blood volume and hypotension

Nursing Plan and Implementation

The psychologic aspects of nursing care are very important. Maternal apprehension increases as the clinical picture changes. Factual reassurance and an explanation of the procedures and what is happening are essential for the emotional well-being of the expectant couple. The nurse can reinforce positive aspects of the woman's condition, such as normal FHR, normal vital signs, and decreased evidence of bleeding.

Other nursing care measures are addressed in the Clinical Pathway for Hemorrhage in Third Trimester and at Birth on pages 744–745.

CLINICAL PATHWAY For Hemorrhage in Third Trimester and at Birth

CATEGORY	IMMEDIATE CARE	OUTCOMES
Referral	Perinatologist Neonatologist	◆ *Expected Outcomes* Appropriate resources identified and utilized
Assessments	Obtain history to identify if any factors are present predisposing to hemorrhage: • Presence of preeclampsia-eclampsia • Overdistention of the uterus; multiple pregnancy; hydramnios • Grandmultiparity • Advanced maternal age • Uterine contractile problems: hypotonicity; hypertonicity • Painless vaginal bleeding after seventh month • Presence of hypertension • Presence of diabetes • History of previous hemorrhage or bleeding problems, blood coagulation defects, abortion • Retention of placental fragments • Cervical and/or vaginal lacerations Determine religious preference to establish whether client will permit a blood transfusion	◆ *Expected Outcomes* • Potential/actual hemorrhage identified • Related complications minimized
Teaching/ psychosocial	Keep woman informed of present status Provide accurate information Provide opportunities for questions Establish a trusting relationship with client Encourage the woman to participate in decision making if at all possible Instruct client to keep bladder empty Notify RN if vag bleeding or leaking noted, decreased fetal movement, abdominal pain/discomfort or uterine contractions Report saturation greater than 1 pad within 1 h or less	◆ *Expected Outcomes* Woman verbalizes/demonstrates understanding of teaching
Nursing care management and reports	Observe, record, and report blood loss Evaluate using the following parameters: • Monitor rate and quality of respirations frequently • Measure pulse rate • Assess pulse quality by direct palpation • Determine pulse deficit by comparing apical-radial rates • Compare present BP with woman's baseline BP; note pulse pressure • Inspect skin for presence of pallor and cyanosis, coldness, and clamminess • Evaluate state of consciousness frequently • Measure CVP: normal CVP is 5–10 cm H_2O • Assess amount of blood loss: • Count pads • Weigh pads and Chux (1 g = approximately 1 mL blood) • Record amount in a specific amount of time (e.g., 50 mL bright red blood on pad in 20 min) Relieve decreased blood pressure by administering whole blood per physician order While waiting for whole blood to be available, infuse isotonic fluids, plasma, plasma expanders, or serum albumin, per physician order If marginal abruptio placentae is present: • Evaluate blood loss • Assess uterine contractile pattern, tenderness, and height • Start continuous monitoring of uterine contractions by EFM • Monitor maternal vital signs • Assess fetal status per continuous EFM • Assess cervical dilatation and effacement to determine labor progress if uterine contractions are present • Rule out placenta previa • Assist with amniotomy, and begin oxytocin infusion per physician order if labor does not start immediately or is ineffective • Review and evaluate diagnostic lab tests (hemoglobin, hematocrit, PT, PTT, fibrin split products, fibrinogen, platelets)	◆ *Expected Outcomes* • Blood loss reduced, controlled, or halted • Perfusion and oxygenation supported

CLINICAL PATHWAY For Hemorrhage in Third Trimester and at Birth continued

CATEGORY	IMMEDIATE CARE	OUTCOMES
Nursing care management and reports continued	If central abruptio placentae with severe blood loss is present: • Perform same assessments as for marginal abruptio placentae • Monitor CVP • Replace blood loss • Observe for signs and symptoms of disseminated intravascular coagulation (DIC) Woman is at risk for uterine atony following birth: • Assess contractility of uterus and amount of vaginal bleeding • Assess uterus every 15 min × 4, every 30 min × 2, every 60 min × 2–4. Evaluate more frequently if uterus is boggy or not in the midline. Administer oxytocin per protocol or physician order.	
Activity	Complete bed rest Diversional activity	◆ *Expected Outcomes* No exacerbation of hemorrhage occurs
Comfort	Assess comfort of woman	◆ *Expected Outcomes* Woman's comfort maintained
Nutrition	IV fluids infusing NPO	◆ *Expected Outcomes* Optimal hydration and blood volume maintained
Elimination	Monitor urine output (decrease to less than 30 mL/h is sign of shock): • Insert Foley catheter • Measure output hourly • Measure specific gravity to determine concentration of urine	◆ *Expected Outcomes* Urinary output maintained
Medications	IV—lactated Ringer's at 150 mL/h If premature—Betamethasone O₂ as indicated	◆ *Expected Outcomes* Circulation and perfusion maintained
Discharge planning/ home care	Determine need for assistance in the home Provide information regarding community resources	◆ *Expected Outcomes* Woman is discharged with plan for follow-up care related to fatigue and blood loss
Family involvement	Establish a trusting relationship with family	◆ *Expected Outcomes* Family development and newborn attachment unimpaired
Date		

BP, blood pressure; CVP, central venous pressure; EFM, electronic fetal monitor; NPO, nothing by mouth

Evaluation

Expected outcomes of nursing care include the following:

• The woman and her baby have a safe labor and birth without further complications for the mother or child.

• The woman and family verbalize understanding of reasons for medical therapy and risks.

Placenta Previa

In **placenta previa,** the placenta is improperly implanted in the lower uterine segment. This implantation may be on a portion of the lower segment or over the internal os (Figure 26–17 ◆). As the lower uterine segment contracts and dilates in the later weeks of pregnancy, the placental villi are torn from the uterine wall, thus exposing the uterine sinuses at the placental site. Bleeding begins, but because the amount depends on the number of sinuses exposed, it may initially be either scanty or profuse.

The cause of placenta previa is unknown. Statistically, it occurs in about 1 in 200 pregnancies (Cunningham et al., 2005). Factors associated with placenta previa are multiparity, increasing age, placenta accreta (discussed shortly), defective development of blood vessels in the decidua, prior cesarean birth, smoking, a recent spontaneous or induced abortion, and a large placenta (Cunningham et al., 2005).

Placenta previa is classified in four degrees:

1. *Total placenta previa.* Internal os is covered completely by the placenta.

MEDIALINK   Application: Placenta Previa

A   B   C

Figure 26–17 ◆ Placenta previa. *A,* Low placental implantation. *B,* Partial placenta previa. *C,* Total placenta previa.

2. *Partial placenta previa.* Internal os is partially covered by the placenta.

3. *Marginal placenta previa.* Edge of the placenta is at the margin of the internal os.

4. *Low-lying placenta.* Placenta is implanted in the lower segment but does not reach the os although it is in close proximity of it (Cunningham et al., 2005).

Another condition, **vasa previa,** occurs when the fetal vessels course through the amniotic membranes and are present at the cervical os. Although this is a rare cause of antepartum bleeding, it is associated with a high rate of fetal death (Cunningham et al., 2005).

CLINICAL THERAPY

Women who present with vaginal bleeding should be questioned regarding any history of abnormal placenta placement that was diagnosed during the pregnancy. When possible, prenatal records should be reviewed. Women who have not had a routine ultrasound examination and have no history of bleeding during the pregnancy may have an undiagnosed placenta previa. The goal of medical care is to identify the cause of bleeding and to provide treatment that will ensure birth of a mature newborn. It must be determined whether the cause of the bleeding is placenta previa or advanced labor with copious bloody show (which is normal). Indirect diagnosis is made by localizing the placenta via tests that require no vaginal examination. The most commonly employed diagnostic test is the transabdominal ultrasound scan. Abdominal or transvaginal sonography is used to identify the presence of placenta previa. If placenta previa is ruled out, a vaginal examination can be performed with a speculum to determine the cause of bleeding (such as cervical lesions or polyps).

Direct diagnosis of placenta previa can be made only by feeling the placenta inside the cervical os. However, such an examination may cause profuse bleeding because of tearing of tissue in the cotyledons of the placenta. Because of the danger of bleeding, a vaginal examination is generally contraindicated

and is performed only if ultrasound is not available, the pregnancy is near term, and there is already profuse vaginal bleeding. The examination is done by a physician using a double setup procedure; that is, the delivery room is set up for the vaginal examination and normal vaginal birth and for a cesarean birth should placenta previa be present and the examination precipitate brisk bleeding. Adequate personnel must be present to respond to treatment decisions.

The differential diagnosis of placental or cervical bleeding takes careful consideration. Table 26–6 provides a comparison of the signs and symptoms of placenta previa and abruptio placentae. Partial separation of the placenta may also present with painless bleeding, and a true placenta previa may not demonstrate overt bleeding until labor begins, thus confusing the di-

Table 26–6   DIFFERENTIAL SIGNS AND SYMPTOMS OF PLACENTA PREVIA AND ABRUPTIO PLACENTAE

	Placenta Previa	Abruptio Placentae
Onset	Quiet and sneaky	Sudden and stormy
Bleeding	External	External or concealed
Color of blood	Bright red	Dark venous
Anemia	= Blood loss	greater than apparent blood loss
Shock	= Blood loss	greater than apparent blood loss
Toxemia	Absent	May be present
Pain	Only labor	Severe and steady
Uterine tenderness	Absent	Present
Uterine tone	Soft and relaxed	Firm to stony hard
Uterine contour	Normal	May enlarge and change shape
Fetal heart tones	Usually present	Present or absent
Engagement	Absent	May be present
Presentation	May be abnormal	No relationship

SOURCE: Oxorn, H., and Foote, W. (1986). *Human labor and birth* (5th ed., p. 507). Norwalk, CT: Appleton & Lange. Reproduced with permission of The McGraw-Hill Companies.

Figure 26–18 ◆ Management of placenta previa.
SOURCE: Reprinted from Zuspan, F. P., & Quilligan, E. J. *Handbook of obstetrics, gynecology, and primary care.* Copyright 1998, with permission from Elsevier Science.

agnosis. In fact, the causes of slight to moderate antepartal bleeding episodes in 20% to 25% of women are never accurately diagnosed.

Care of the woman with painless late gestational bleeding depends on (1) the week of gestation during which the first bleeding episode occurs and (2) the amount of bleeding (Figure 26–18 ◆). If the pregnancy is less than 37 weeks' gestation, expectant management is employed to delay birth until about 37 weeks' gestation to allow the fetus to mature. Expectant management involves stringent compliance with the following:

1. Bed rest with bathroom privileges only as long as the woman is not bleeding

2. No vaginal examinations

3. Monitoring of blood loss, pain, and uterine contractility

4. Evaluation of FHRs with external monitor

5. Monitoring of maternal vital signs

6. Complete laboratory evaluation: hemoglobin, hematocrit, Rh factor, and urinalysis

7. Administration of intravenous fluid (lactated Ringer's solution) with drip rate monitored

8. Availability of two units of cross-matched blood for possible transfusion

9. Administration of betamethasone to facilitate fetal lung maturity

If frequent, recurrent, or profuse bleeding persists or if fetal well-being appears threatened, a cesarean birth needs to be performed.

NURSING CARE MANAGEMENT
Nursing Assessment and Diagnosis

Assessment of the woman with placenta previa must be ongoing to prevent or treat complications that are potentially lethal to the mother and fetus. Painless, bright red vaginal bleeding is the best diagnostic sign of placenta previa. If this sign should develop during the last 3 months of a pregnancy, placenta previa should always be considered until ruled out by ultrasound examination. The first bleeding episode is generally scanty. If no vaginal examinations are performed, it often subsides spontaneously. However, each subsequent hemorrhage is more profuse.

The uterus remains soft, and if labor begins, it relaxes fully between contractions. The FHR usually remains stable unless profuse hemorrhage and maternal shock occur. As a result of the placement of the placenta, the fetal presenting part is often unengaged, and transverse lie is common.

The nurse appraises blood loss, pain, and uterine contractility from both subjective and objective perspectives. Maternal vital signs and the results of blood and urine tests provide the nurse with additional data about the woman's condition. FHR is evaluated with an external fetal monitor. Another nursing responsibility is observing and verifying the family's ability to cope with the anxiety associated with an unknown outcome.

Nursing diagnoses that may apply to the woman experiencing placenta previa are as follows:

• *Fluid Volume Deficient* related to hypovolemia secondary to excessive blood loss

- *Risk for Ineffective Tissue Perfusion* related to blood loss secondary to uterine atony following birth
- *Anxiety* related to concern for own personal status and the baby's safety
- *Risk for Impaired Gas Exchange* related to decreased blood volume and hypotension

Nursing Plan and Implementation

The nurse continues to monitor the woman and her fetus to determine the status of the bleeding and to determine the mother's and baby's responses. Vital signs, intake and output, and other pertinent assessments must be made frequently. The nurse evaluates the electronic monitor tracing to evaluate the fetal status.

Emotional support for the family is an important nursing care goal. When active bleeding is occurring, the assessments and management must be directed toward physical support. However, emotional aspects need to be addressed simultaneously. The nurse can explain the assessments being completed and the treatment measures that need to be done. Time can be provided for questions, and the nurse can act as an advocate in obtaining information for the family. The nurse can also offer emotional support by staying with the family and by the use of touch.

The newborn's hemoglobin, cell volume, and erythrocyte count should be checked immediately after birth and then monitored closely. The newborn may require oxygen and administration of blood and admission into a neonatal intensive care unit.

Additional information regarding nursing care is addressed in the Clinical Pathway for Hemorrhage in Third Trimester and at Birth.

Evaluation

Expected outcomes of nursing care include the following:

- The cause of hemorrhage is recognized promptly, and corrective measures are taken.
- The woman's vital signs remain in the normal range.
- The woman and her baby have a safe labor and birth.
- The family understands what has happened and the implications and associated problems of placenta previa.

Other Placental Problems

Other problems of the placenta can be divided into those that are developmental and those that are degenerative. Developmental problems of the placenta include placental lesions, succenturiate placenta, circumvallate placenta, and battledore placenta (Table 26–7). Degenerative changes include infarcts and placental calcification.

SUCCENTURIATE PLACENTA

In *succenturiate placenta,* one or more accessory lobes of fetal villi have developed on the placenta, with vascular connections of fetal origin (see Table 26–7). Vessels from the major to the minor lobe(s) are supported only by the membranes, thus increasing the risk of the minor lobe's being retained during the third stage of labor.

The gravest maternal danger is postpartal hemorrhage if this minor lobe is severed from the placenta and remains in the uterus. All placentas should be examined closely for intactness. If vessels appear to be severed at the margin of the placenta, the uterus should be explored for retained placental tissue. This condition is not usually diagnosed until after the birth of the placenta.

Fetal/newborn implications can be life threatening if the vascular connections rupture between the placenta lobes because a fatal fetal hemorrhage can result. Examination of the fetal membrane following birth may reveal a small hole with vessels running toward it. This is another indication of a retained lobe (Cunningham et al., 2005). At birth, the infant should be inspected for pallor, cyanosis, retractions, tachypnea, tachycardia, and feeble pulse. The infant's cry will be weak and the muscle tone flaccid.

CIRCUMVALLATE PLACENTA

In *circumvallate placenta,* the fetal surface of the placenta is exposed through a ring opening around the umbilical cord (see Table 26–7). The vessels descend from the cord and end at the margin of the ring instead of coursing through the entire surface area of the placenta. The ring is composed of a double fold of amnion and chorion with some degenerative decidua and fibrin between. The cause of this condition is unknown. Maternal-fetal problems include an increased incidence of late abortion or fetal death, antepartal hemorrhage, prematurity, and abnormal maternal bleeding during or following the third stage of labor, resulting from improper placental separation or shearing of membranes from the placenta.

BATTLEDORE PLACENTA

In *battledore placenta,* the umbilical cord is inserted at or near the placental margin (see Table 26–7). As a result, all fetal vessels transverse the placental surface in the same direction. The chances of preterm labor are high because of interference with fetal circulation and nutrition. Nonreassuring fetal status or bleeding during labor is also likely because of cord compression or vessel rupture.

PLACENTAL INFARCTS AND CALCIFICATIONS

As the placenta grade matures (previously discussed in Chapter 21 ∞), the placenta may develop infarcts and calcifications. They become significant if they cover a large enough area to interfere with the uterine-placental-fetal exchange. Altered exchange can also occur with certain maternal disease processes, such as hypertension. Infarcts are most often seen in cases of severe preeclampsia and in women who smoke.

CARE OF THE WOMAN AND FETUS AT RISK BECAUSE OF PROBLEMS ASSOCIATED WITH THE UMBILICAL CORD

Prolapsed Umbilical Cord

An umbilical cord that precedes the fetal presenting part is known as a **prolapsed umbilical cord.** It occurs when the cord

Table 26–7	**PLACENTAL AND UMBILICAL CORD VARIATIONS**	
Placental Variation	**Maternal Implications**	**Fetal-Neonatal Implications**

Succenturiate placenta

| One or more accessory lobes of fetal villi will develop on the placenta. | Postpartal hemorrhage from retained lobe | None, as long as all parts of the placenta remain attached until after birth of the fetus | |

Circumvallate placenta

| A double fold of chorion and amnion form a ring around the umbilical cord, on the fetal side of the placenta. | Increased incidence of late abortion, antepartal hemorrhage, and preterm labor | Intrauterine growth restriction, prematurity, fetal death | |

Battledore placenta

| The umbilical cord is inserted at or near the placental margin. | Increased incidence of preterm labor and bleeding | Prematurity, fetal stress | |

Velamentous insertion of the umbilical cord

| The vessels of the umbilical cord divide some distance from the placenta in the placental membranes. | Hemorrhage if one of the vessels is torn | Fetal stress, hemorrhage | |

falls or is washed down through the cervix into the vagina and becomes trapped between the presenting part and the maternal pelvis. The incidence of cord prolapse is 3% of vertex presentations and 3.7% of all breech presentations (Morgan & Ross, 2005). Because of this entrapment, the vessels carrying blood to and from the fetus are compressed. In rare circumstances a prolapsed cord may be visible at the lower edge of the vagina. In other cases, the umbilical cord lies beside or just ahead of the fetal head; this is called *occult cord prolapse.*

Any time that the pelvic inlet is not completely filled by the fetus or the presenting part is not firmly against the cervix, and the membranes rupture, the umbilical cord can be washed down into the birth canal in front of the presenting part (Figure 26–19 ◆). The incidence of prolapse of the cord is 20 times greater with abnormal axis lie (Cunningham et al., 2005)—especially footling breech and shoulder presentations—low birth weight, a multipara with more than five previous births, multiple gestation, obstetric manipulation (amniotomy), and

Figure 26–19 ◆ Prolapse of the umbilical cord.

the presence of a long cord (longer than 80 cm). Approximately 50% of cord prolapses occur in the second stage of labor. An additional 47% of cord prolapses occur as a result of some obstetric intervention, such as amniotomy, application of fetal scalp electrode, intrapressure catheter, or external cephalic version (Nasser, Roberts, Barratt et al., 2006).

MATERNAL-FETAL-NEONATAL RISKS

Although a prolapsed cord does not directly precipitate physical alterations in the woman, her immediate concern for the baby creates enormous stress. The woman may need to deal with some unusual interventions, a cesarean birth, and, in some circumstances, death of the fetus.

The fetus is affected because compression of the umbilical cord occludes blood flow through the umbilical vessels. Bradycardia (FHR baseline below 110 beats per minute) and persistent variable decelerations may develop. If labor is occurring, the cord is compressed further with each contraction. If the pressure on the cord is not relieved, the fetus will die.

CLINICAL THERAPY

Preventing the occurrence of cord prolapse is the preferred medical approach. For all laboring women with a history of ruptured membranes, bed rest is usually indicated until engagement with no cord prolapse has been documented. When prolapse does occur, it is usually discovered by the nurse, and relieving the compression of the cord by pushing back the presenting part (discussed shortly) is critical for the fetus. The method of birth will most likely be cesarean.

NURSING CARE MANAGEMENT
Nursing Assessment and Diagnosis

In the intrapartal area, the nurse reviews the nursing history and ascertains whether the woman is likely to be at risk for prolapse of the cord. Particularly when the presenting part is not engaged and spontaneous or artificial rupture of the membranes occurs, the nurse observes the perineum and assesses the FHR for bradycardia and severe, recurrent, variable decelerations.

Nursing diagnoses that may apply to the woman with a prolapsed cord include the following:

- **Risk for Impaired Gas Exchange** in the fetus related to decreased blood flow secondary to compression of the umbilical cord
- **Fear** related to unknown outcome

Nursing Plan and Implementation

Because there are few outward signs of cord prolapse, each pregnant woman is advised to call her physician or CNM when the membranes rupture and to go immediately to the office, clinic, or birthing facility. A sterile vaginal examination determines whether there is danger of cord prolapse. If the presenting part is well engaged, the risk is minimal and ambulation may be encouraged. If the presenting part is not well engaged, bed rest is recommended to prevent cord prolapse. Maintaining bed rest after rupture of membranes can lead to conflict if the laboring woman and her partner do not hold the same beliefs. The nurse can ease this situation by helping communication between the physician or CNM and the couple.

If membranes have not yet ruptured when the woman arrives at the facility, at the time of spontaneous rupture or amniotomy the FHR should be monitored by EFM or auscultated for at least a full minute and again at the end of a contraction and after a few contractions. In the presence of cord prolapse, EFM tracings show baseline bradycardia or severe, moderate, or prolonged nonperiodic decelerations. If these patterns are found, the nurse performs a vaginal examination.

If a loop of cord is discovered, the nurse's gloved fingers are left in the vagina, and the presenting part is pushed upward to lift the fetal part off the cord and relieve cord compression until the physician or CNM arrives. This is a lifesaving measure. Oxygen is administered, and FHR is monitored by EFM to see if the cord compression is adequately relieved (baseline will rise above 110 beats per minute, and variable decelerations are lessened or relieved). The nurse may also feel pulsation in the cord; however, in some instances a pulsation cannot be felt, and FHR can be detected only by EFM. A large-gauge intravenous cannula is inserted and intravenous fluids should be initiated. Anesthesia and neonatology services should be notified of impending birth.

In some cases, another nurse may insert an indwelling bladder catheter and, using a sterile asepto syringe or infusion device, fill the bladder with approximately 500 mL of warmed, sterile normal saline. The filled bladder lifts the fetal head upward and relieves pressure on the umbilical cord (Varney et al., 2004). Filling her bladder and maintaining the woman in a side-lying position may be all that is needed to relieve the pressure on the cord. If the bladder is not filled, the force of gravity can be incorporated. In this instance, the nurse maintains pressure on the presenting part and instructs the woman to bring her knees to her chest or adjusts the bed to the Trendelenburg position. The nurse maintains pressure on the presenting part while the woman is transported to the birthing or operating room in this position. The nurse maintains this position until the fetus is born via cesarean birth.

Evaluation

Expected outcomes of nursing care include the following:

- The FHR remains in normal range with supportive measures.
- The fetus is born safely.
- The woman and her partner feel supported.
- The woman and her partner understand the problem and the corrective measures that are undertaken.

Umbilical Cord Abnormalities

Umbilical cord abnormalities include congenital absence of an umbilical artery, insertion variations, cord length variations, and knots and loops of the cord. Insertion variations include velamentous insertion and vasa previa, and cord length problems include long and short cords.

CONGENITAL ABSENCE OF UMBILICAL ARTERY

Absence of an umbilical artery may have serious fetal implications. The incidence of all types of fetal anomalies is 15.4% in infants born with two-vessel cords (Cristina, Ana, Ines et al., 2005).

Immediately after the umbilical cord is cut, it should be inspected to determine whether the correct number of vessels is present. If an artery is absent, the nurse should examine the newborn closely for anomalies and gestational age problems and alert the attending pediatrician.

INSERTION VARIATIONS

In a *velamentous insertion,* the vessels of the umbilical cord divide some distance from the placenta in the placental membranes (see Table 26–7). Velamentous insertions occur more frequently in multiple gestations than in singletons. Other placental anomalies, such as succenturiate placenta, often accompany this condition. The velamentous insertion is more easily compressed or kinked during pregnancy or labor because of the lack of Wharton's jelly to protect it. If the vessels become torn during labor, fetal hemorrhage can occur, and the blood can escape from the vagina. When fetal hemorrhage occurs, it results in FHR abnormalities.

When the vessels of a velamentous insertion transverse the internal os and appear in front of the fetus, a vasa previa has occurred. Fetal hemorrhage with asphyxia is likely to result because as the fetal blood escapes out of the vagina the hemorrhage will probably be diagnosed as maternal.

CORD LENGTH VARIATIONS

The average length of the umbilical cord is 55 cm. Although short cords rarely cause complications directly, they have been associated with umbilical hernias in the fetus, abruptio placentae, and cord rupture. Long cords tend to twist and tangle around the fetus, causing transient variable decelerations. A long cord rarely causes fetal death, however, because it is generally not pulled tight until descent at the time of birth. With a long cord and an active fetus, one or more true knots can result. Again, these knots usually are not pulled tight enough to cause fetal

stress until the infant has been born, and the cord can then be clamped and cut.

CLINICAL THERAPY

The goals of medical treatment are to prevent serious fetal complications and to examine the newborn for anomalies that coexist with umbilical cord abnormalities.

Any vaginal bleeding during labor warrants continuous monitoring of the fetus, preferably with an external electronic monitor. Any signs of nonreassuring heart rate patterns should be reported immediately. In the presence of bleeding, laboratory tests may be used to differentiate fetal from maternal red blood cells. Fetal hemorrhage is resolved by terminating the pregnancy vaginally or through cesarean birth and by correcting neonatal anemia. Expediting the birth, whether vaginally or surgically, is paramount when a severe nonreassuring heart rate pattern is apparent. Following the birth, the pediatric team identifies and treats any neonatal complications or anomalies.

NURSING CARE MANAGEMENT
Nursing Assessment and Diagnosis

Umbilical abnormalities may not become evident until the birth of the fetus. During labor the nurse should observe for signs of nonreassuring fetal status and excessive bleeding (with velamentous insertion and vasa previa).

Nursing diagnoses that may apply include the following:

- ***Risk for Impaired Gas Exchange in the fetus*** related to decreased blood flow secondary to placental abnormalities
- ***Health-Seeking Behavior: Information about Placental Abnormalities*** related to an expressed desire to understand the implications of the finding

Nursing Plan and Implementation

The nurse is alert for an unusual amount of bleeding during the labor and birth. Following the birth, the placenta is inspected for abnormalities. Examination of the placenta by a pathologist may be indicated.

Often any mild or moderate variable deceleration can be successfully managed by the nurse. Repositioning of the woman often alleviates pressure on the cord if this is the reason for the deceleration.

Evaluation

Expected outcomes of nursing care include the following:

- The mother and baby have a safe labor and birth.
- The woman's bleeding is assessed quickly, and corrective measures are taken.
- The family is able to cope successfully with fetal or neonatal anomalies, if they exist.

CARE OF THE WOMAN AND FETUS AT RISK BECAUSE OF AMNIOTIC FLUID-RELATED COMPLICATIONS

Complications related to amniotic fluid include amniotic fluid embolism, hydramnios, and oligohydramnios.

Amniotic Fluid Embolism

Amniotic fluid embolism occurs when a bolus of amniotic fluid enters the maternal circulation and then the maternal lungs. The cause of this obstetric emergency is unknown but has a 60% to 80% mortality rate (Demianczuk & Corbett, 2005). It is the second leading cause of maternal deaths, resulting in 10% of all maternal deaths per year in the United States (Demianczuk & Corbett, 2005). Because amniotic fluid embolism is a rare complication, a national registry was initiated in 1988 to collect retrospective data for analysis.

Hydramnios

Hydramnios (also called *polyhydramnios*) occurs when there is over 2000 mL of amniotic fluid. It typically occurs in 1% of all pregnancies (Cunningham et al., 2005). The exact cause of hydramnios is unknown; however, it often occurs in cases of major congenital anomalies. It is postulated that a major source of amniotic fluid is found in special amnion cells that lie over the placenta (Cunningham et al., 2005). In cases of hydramnios, no pathology has been found in this amniotic epithelium. However, during the second half of the pregnancy, the fetus normally begins to swallow and inspire amniotic fluid and to urinate, which contributes to the amount present. Fetal malformations that affect this swallowing mechanism—as well as neurologic disorders in which the fetal meninges are exposed in the amniotic cavity—can result in hydramnios.

This condition is also found in cases of anencephaly, in which the fetus is thought to urinate excessively because of overstimulation of the cerebrospinal centers. When a monozygotic twin manifests hydramnios, it is possible that the twin with the increased blood volume urinates excessively. The weight of the placenta has been found to be increased in some cases of hydramnios, indicating that increased functioning of the placental tissue may contribute to the problem.

There are two types of hydramnios: chronic and acute. The chronic type, in which the fluid volume gradually increases, is a problem of the third trimester. Most cases are of this variety. In acute cases, the volume increases rapidly over a period of a few days. The acute type is usually diagnosed between 20 and 24 weeks' gestation.

When the amount of amniotic fluid is over 3000 mL, the woman experiences shortness of breath and edema in the lower extremities from compression of the vena cava. If hydramnios is severe enough, she can experience intense pain. The acute form of hydramnios tends to be more severe. Milder forms of hydramnios occur more frequently and are associated with minimal symptoms. Hydramnios is associated with such maternal disorders as diabetes and Rh sensitization. It can also occur as a result of infections such as syphilis, toxoplasmosis, cytomegalovirus, herpes, and rubella.

Fetal malformations and preterm birth are common with hydramnios; thus there is a fairly high rate of perinatal mortality. Prolapsed umbilical cord can occur when the membranes rupture, which adds a further complication for the fetus. The incidence of malpresentations is also increased.

CLINICAL THERAPY

Hydramnios is managed with supportive treatment unless the intensity of the woman's distress and symptoms dictate otherwise.

If the accumulation of amniotic fluid is severe enough to cause maternal dyspnea and pain, hospitalization and removal of the excessive fluid are required. This can be done vaginally by AROM or by amniocentesis. The dangers of performing AROM vaginally are prolapsed cord and the inability to remove the fluid slowly. A *needle amniotomy* may be preferred because this releases the fluid at a slower rate and allows the presenting part to descend gradually. A needle amniotomy is performed by the CNM or physician. A needle or a fetal scalp electrode is used to make a small puncture in the amniotic sac. There is a risk that the force of the fluid could make a larger hole in the amniotic sac, thus increasing the risk of a prolapsed cord. If amniocentesis is performed, it should be done with the aid of sonography to prevent inadvertent damage to the fetus and placenta.

A prostaglandin synthesis inhibitor (indomethacin) is often used to treat hydramnios. Indomethacin has been shown to decrease amniotic fluid volume by decreasing fetal urine output (Cunningham et al., 2005).

NURSING CARE MANAGEMENT

Nursing Assessment and Diagnosis

Hydramnios should be suspected when the fundal height increases out of proportion to the gestational age.

With increased fluid, the nurse may have difficulty palpating the fetus and auscultating the FHR. In more severe cases the maternal abdomen appears extremely tense and tight on inspection. On sonography large spaces can be identified between the fetus and the uterine wall.

Nursing diagnoses that may apply for a woman with hydramnios include the following:

- *Risk for Impaired Gas Exchange* related to pressure on the diaphragm secondary to hydramnios
- *Fear* related to unknown outcome of the pregnancy

Nursing Plan and Implementation

When amniocentesis is performed, sterile technique is used to prevent infection. The nurse can offer support to the couple by explaining the procedure to them.

If the fetus has been diagnosed with a congenital defect in utero or is born with the defect, psychologic support is needed to assist the family. Often the nurse collaborates with social services to offer the family this additional help. The nurse can also offer to contact chaplain services at the family's request.

Evaluation

Expected outcomes of nursing care include the following:

*   The woman and her partner can discuss the procedure, implications, risks, and characteristics that need to be reported to the caregiver.

Oligohydramnios

Oligohydramnios is defined as a less than normal amount of amniotic fluid (approximately 500 mL is considered normal). Although no exact amount of fluid has been definitively identified as diagnostic of this condition, oligohydramnios is diagnosed when the largest vertical pocket of amniotic fluid visible on ultrasound examination is 5 cm or less (Cunningham et al., 2005). The exact cause of oligohydramnios is unknown. It is found in cases of postmaturity, with IUGR secondary to placental insufficiency, and in fetal conditions associated with major renal malformations, including renal aplasia with dysplastic kidneys and obstructive lesions of the lower urinary tract. If oligohydramnios occurs in the first part of pregnancy, there is a danger of fetal adhesions (one part of the fetus may adhere to another part).

During the gestational period, fetal skin and skeletal abnormalities may occur because fetal movement is impaired as a result of inadequate amniotic fluid volume. Because there is less fluid available for the fetus to use during fetal breathing movements, pulmonary hypoplasia may develop. During the labor and birth, the lessened amounts of fluid reduce the cushioning effect for the umbilical cord, and cord compression is more likely to occur.

CLINICAL THERAPY

During the antepartum period, oligohydramnios may be suspected when the uterus does not increase in size in accordance with established gestational dating, the fetus is easily palpated and outlined by the examiner, and the fetus is not ballottable. The fetus can be assessed by BPP, NSTs, and serial ultrasounds. During labor the fetus will be monitored by continuous EFM to detect cord compression, which will be indicated by nonperiodic decelerations. Amnioinfusion can replace some fluid volume and remove pressure on the umbilical cord (see Chapter 27 ∞).

NURSING CARE MANAGEMENT

Continuous EFM is an important part of assessment during the labor and birth. The nurse evaluates the EFM tracing for the presence of nonperiodic decelerations or other nonreassuring signs (such as increasing or decreasing baseline, decreased variability, or presence of periodic decelerations). If nonperiodic decelerations are noted, the nurse can change the woman's position (to relieve pressure on the umbilical cord) and must then notify the physician or CNM. If position changes are insufficient to relieve the pattern, an amnioinfusion may be performed.

After the birth, the newborn is evaluated for signs of congenital anomalies, pulmonary hypoplasia, or postmaturity.

CARE OF THE WOMAN WITH CEPHALOPELVIC DISPROPORTION

The birth passage includes the maternal bony pelvis, beginning at the pelvic inlet and ending at the pelvic outlet, and the maternal soft tissues within these anatomic areas. A contracture (narrowing) in any of the described areas can result in **cephalopelvic disproportion (CPD).** Abnormal fetal presentations and positions occur in CPD as the fetus moves to accommodate passage through the maternal pelvis.

The gynecoid and anthropoid pelvic types are usually adequate for vertex birth, but the android and platypelloid types predispose to CPD. Certain combinations of types also can result in pelvic diameters inadequate for vertex birth. (See Chapter 10 ∞ for a description of the types of pelves and their implications for childbirth). Clues that may lead to suspicion of contractures of the maternal pelvis are presented in Table 26–8. Women with a history of pelvic fractures may also be at risk for CPD.

TYPES OF CONTRACTURES

Contractures of the Inlet

The pelvic inlet is contracted if the shortest anterior-posterior diameter is less than 10 cm or the greatest transverse diameter is less than 12 cm. The anterior-posterior diameter may be approximated by measuring the diagonal conjugate, which in the contracted inlet is less than 11.5 cm. Clinical and x-ray pelvimetry are used to determine the smallest anterior-posterior diameter through which the fetal head must pass.

The treatment goal is to allow the natural forces of labor to push the biparietal diameter of the fetal head beyond the potential interspinous obstruction. Although forceps may be used, they cause difficulty because pulling on the head destroys flexion and because they further diminish the available space. A bulging perineum and crowning indicate that the obstruction has been passed.

Table 26–8	**CLUES TO CONTRACTURES OF MATERNAL PELVIS**

Diagonal conjugate less than 11.5 cm (contracture of inlet), outlet less than 8 cm (contracture of outlet)

Unengaged fetal head in early labor in primigravidas (consider contracture of inlet, malpresentation, or malposition)

Hypotonic uterine contraction pattern (consider contracted pelvis)

Deflexion of fetal head (fetal head not flexed on fetal chest; may be associated with occiput posterior)

Uncontrollable pushing before complete dilatation of cervix (may be associated with occiput posterior)

Failure of fetal descent (consider contracture of inlet, midpelvis, or outlet)

Edema of anterior portion (lip) of cervix (consider obstructed labor at the inlet)

Contractures of the Outlet

An interischial tuberous diameter of less than 8 cm constitutes an outlet contracture. Outlet and midpelvic contractures frequently occur simultaneously. Whether vaginal birth can occur depends on the woman's interischial tuberous diameters and the fetal posterosagittal diameter.

IMPLICATIONS OF PELVIC CONTRACTURES

Labor is prolonged and protracted in the presence of CPD, and premature rupture of the membranes (PROM) can result from the force of the unequally distributed contractions being exerted on the fetal membranes. In obstructed labor (the fetus is not able to pass through the birth canal) uterine rupture can also occur. With delayed descent, necrosis of maternal soft tissues can result from pressure exerted by the fetal head. Eventually, necrosis can cause fistulas from the vagina to other nearby structures. Difficult forceps-assisted births can also result in damage to maternal soft tissue.

If the membranes rupture and the fetal head has not entered the inlet, there is a danger of cord prolapse. Extreme molding of the fetal head can result. Traumatic forceps-assisted births can damage the fetal skull and CNS.

CLINICAL THERAPY

Fetopelvic relationships can be assessed by comparing the estimated weight of the fetus as obtained by ultrasound measurements to pelvic measurements obtained by a manual examination before labor and by computed tomography (CT). Occasionally, in high-risk centers magnetic resonance imaging (MRI) is used to identify adequacy of pelvic diameters.

When the pelvic diameters are borderline or questionable, a trial of labor (TOL) may be advised. In this process the woman continues to labor, and careful assessments of uterine contractions, cervical dilatation, and fetal descent are made by the CNM or physician and nurse. As long as there is continued progress, the TOL continues. If progress ceases, the decision for a cesarean birth is made.

NURSING CARE MANAGEMENT
Nursing Assessment and Diagnosis

The adequacy of the maternal pelvis for a vaginal birth should be assessed intrapartally as well as antepartally. During the intrapartal assessment, the size of the fetus and its presentation, position, and lie must also be considered. (See Chapter 23 ∞ for intrapartal assessment techniques).

The nurse should suspect CPD when labor is prolonged, cervical dilatation and effacement are slow, and engagement of the presenting part is delayed or lack of fetal descent occurs.

Nursing diagnoses that may apply include the following:

- *Deficient Knowledge* related to lack of information about implications of CPD
- *Fear* related to unknown outcome of labor

Nursing Plan and Implementation

Nursing actions during the TOL are similar to care during any labor, with the exception that the assessments of cervical dilatation and fetal descent are done more frequently. Contractions should be monitored and the labor progress charted. The fetus should also be monitored frequently. Any signs of fetal stress are reported to the physician or CNM immediately.

The woman may be positioned in a variety of ways to increase the pelvic diameters. Sitting or squatting increases the outer diameters and may be effective in instances where there is failure of or slow fetal descent. Changing from one side to the other or maintaining a hands-and-knees position may assist the fetus in OP position to change to an OA position. The woman may instinctively want to assume one of these positions. If not, the nurse may encourage a change of position. Women with an epidural may use position changes with adequate support.

A couple may need help in coping with the stresses of complicated labor. The nurse should keep the couple informed of what is happening and explain the procedures that are being used. This should reassure the couple that measures are being taken to resolve the problem.

Evaluation

Expected outcomes of nursing care include the following:

- The woman's fear is lessened.
- The woman has additional knowledge regarding the problems, implications, and treatment plans.

CARE OF THE WOMAN AT RISK BECAUSE OF COMPLICATIONS OF THIRD AND FOURTH STAGES OF LABOR

Common complications of the third and fourth stages of labor include retained placenta, lacerations, and placenta accreta.

Retained Placenta

Retention of the placenta beyond 30 minutes after birth is termed **retained placenta.** It occurs in 2% to 3% of all vaginal births. Bleeding as a result of a retained placenta can be excessive. If placenta expulsion does not occur, a manual removal of the placenta by the physician or CNM is attempted. In women who do not have an epidural in place, intravenous sedation may be required because of the discomfort caused by the procedure. Retained placenta may be a symptom of an accreta, increta, or percreta. Failure to retrieve the placenta via manual removal usually necessitates surgical removal by curettage. If the woman does not have an epidural in place, the procedure can be performed under general anesthesia.

Lacerations

Lacerations of the cervix or vagina may be present when bright red vaginal bleeding persists in the presence of a well-contracted uterus. The incidence of lacerations is higher among childbearing women who are young, are nulliparous, have an epidural block, undergo forceps-assisted or vacuum-assisted birth, or undergo an episiotomy. Vaginal and perineal lacerations are often categorized in terms of degree:

- First-degree laceration is limited to the fourchette, perineal skin, and vaginal mucous membrane.

- Second-degree laceration involves the perineal skin, vaginal mucous membrane, underlying fascia, and muscles of the perineal body; it may extend upward on one or both sides of the vagina.

- Third-degree laceration extends through the perineal skin, vaginal mucous membranes, and perineal body and involves the anal sphincter; it may extend up the anterior wall of the rectum.

- Fourth-degree laceration is the same as the third degree but extends through the rectal mucosa to the lumen of the rectum; it may be called a third-degree laceration with a rectal wall extension.

Placenta Accreta

In **placenta accreta,** the chorionic villi attach directly to the myometrium of the uterus. Two other types of placental adherence are **placenta increta,** in which the myometrium is invaded, and **placenta percreta,** in which the myometrium is penetrated. These placenta adherent disorders can be life threatening. The adherence itself may be total, partial, or focal, depending on the amount of placental involvement. The incidence of placenta accreta is 1 in 2500 births (Cunningham et al., 2005). Placenta accreta is the most common type of adherent placenta.

The primary complication of placenta accreta is maternal hemorrhage and failure of the placenta to separate following birth of the infant. An abdominal hysterectomy may be the necessary treatment, depending on the amount and depth of involvement. Chapter 38 ∞ discusses hemorrhage following birth.

CHAPTER REVIEW

FOCUS YOUR STUDY

- Intense anxiety; fear; loss of orientation to person, place, or time; or other inappropriate behaviors may be associated with an underlying psychologic disorder that results in difficulties with coping.

- Hypotonic labor patterns begin normally and then progress to infrequent, less intense contractions. If there are no contraindications, oxytocin is administered intravenously as treatment.

- Precipitous labor and birth is extremely rapid labor and birth that lasts less than 3 hours. It is associated with an increased risk to the mother and newborn infant.

- Postterm pregnancy is one that extends more than 294 days, or 42 weeks, past the first day of the last menstrual period.

- The occiput-posterior position of the fetus prolongs the labor process, causes severe back discomfort in the laboring woman, and predisposes her to vaginal and perineal trauma and lacerations during birth.

- The types of fetal malpresentations include face, brow, breech, and shoulder.

- A fetus or newborn weighing more than 4500 g is termed *macrosomic*. Macrosomia may lead to problems during labor and birth and in the early neonatal period.

- In multiple gestation, preventing and treating problems that infringe on the development and birth of normal fetuses are significant medical-nursing activities.

- Major bleeding problems in the intrapartal period are abruptio placentae and placenta previa.

- Abruptio placentae is the separation of the placenta from the side of the uterus before birth of the infant. Abruptio placentae may be central, marginal, or complete.

- Placenta previa occurs when the placenta implants low in the uterus near or over the cervix. A low-lying or marginal placenta is one that lies near the cervix. In partial placenta previa, part of the placenta lies over the cervix. In complete placenta previa, the cervix is completely covered.

- Prolapsed umbilical cord results when the umbilical cord precedes the fetal presenting part. When this occurs, pressure is placed on the umbilical cord, and blood flow to the fetus is diminished.

- Amniotic fluid embolism occurs when a bolus of amniotic fluid enters the maternal circulation and then enters the maternal lungs. Maternal mortality is very high with this complication.

- Hydramnios (also called polyhydramnios) is the presence of over 2000 mL of amniotic fluid contained within the amniotic membranes. Hydramnios can be associated with fetal malformations that affect fetal swallowing and with maternal diabetes mellitus, Rh sensitization, and multiple gestations.

- Oligohydramnios is a severely reduced volume of amniotic fluid. Oligohydramnios is associated with intrauterine growth restriction, postterm pregnancy, and fetal renal or urinary malfunctions. The fetus is more likely to experience variable decelerations because the amniotic fluid is insufficient to keep pressure off the umbilical cord.

- Cephalopelvic disproportion occurs when there is a narrowed diameter in the maternal pelvis. The narrowed

diameter is called a contracture, and it may occur in the pelvic inlet, midpelvis, or outlet. If pelvic measurements are borderline, a trial of labor may be attempted. Failure of cervical dilatation or fetal descent would then necessitate a cesarean birth.

- Third- and fourth-stage complications usually involve a hemorrhage. Causes of hemorrhage include lacerations of the birth canal or cervix, retained placenta, and placenta accreta.

- Nonreassuring fetal status is indicated by persistent late decelerations, persistent severe variable decelerations, and prolonged decelerations. If fetal stress is recognized and treated appropriately, the fetus may be spared any permanent damage.

EXPLORE MediaLink

http://www.prenhall.com/davidson

NCLEX review questions, case studies, and other interactive resources for this chapter can be found on the Web Site at http://www.prenhall.com/davidson. Click on "Chapter 26" to select the activities for this chapter.

For tutorials including animations and videos, more NCLEX review questions, and an audio glossary, access the accompanying Prentice Hall Nursing MediaLink DVD-ROM in this book.

PRENTICE HALL NURSING MEDIALINK DVD-ROM
Audio Glossary
NCLEX Review

COMPANION WEBSITE
Additional NCLEX Review
Case Study: *Client with Placental Problems*
Care Plan Activity: *Prevention of Cord Prolapse*
Applications: *Placenta Previa; Umbilical Cord Prolapse*
Critical Thinking

CRITICAL THINKING IN ACTION

OXYTOCIN LABOR INDUCTION OR AUGMENTATION

View the Critical Thinking in Action video in Chapter 26 of the DVD-ROM. Then answer the questions that follow.

June Dice, a 25-year-old G3, P1011, is admitted to you in labor and delivery at 38 weeks with a moderate amount of dark red vaginal bleeding. June's prenatal history is significant for late prenatal care (20 weeks' gestation by ultrasound) and cocaine abuse. An ultrasound is done upon admission that demonstrates a marginal placenta abruption. You place June on the fetal monitor and observe a fetal heart rate baseline of 146 to 155 with accelerations to 166 with fetal movement. There are occasional mild variable decelerations with a quick return to baseline. Contraction pattern is interpreted as an irritable uterus. An intravenous infusion with Ringer's lactate is started with a #18 intracath. June's vital signs are within normal limits. Her hematocrit is 29%. You assist the physician with a vaginal exam to rupture membranes and insert a fetal scalp electrode and intrauterine pressure catheter. A small amount of light yellow-green amniotic fluid is observed. The exam shows June is 4 cm dilated, 50% effaced, vertex at 21 station. You follow protocol and start an oxytocin induction/augmentation. June is asking why oxytocin is needed.

1. Explain the goal of labor induction/augmentation in response to June's question.

2. Explain potential risk factors associated with oxytocin induction of labor.

3. You observe a nonreassuring fetal heart rate of 144 to 150 with decreased variability and persistent late decelerations

with each contraction. What interventions would you immediately take?

4. What supportive actions are taken to decrease the risk of hypofibrinogenemia?

5. What complications might be present in the newborn at birth?

REFERENCES

Algovik, M., Nilsson, E., Cnattingius, S., Lichtenstein, P., Nordenskjöld, A., & Westgren, M. (2004). Genetic influence on dystocia. *Acta Obstetricia et Gynecologica Scandinavica, 83*(9), 832–837.

American College of Obstetricians and Gynecologists (ACOG). (2000). *Fetal macrosomia* (ACOG Practice Bulletin No. 22). Washington, DC: Author.

American College of Obstetricians and Gynecologists (ACOG). (2003). *Dystocia and augmentation of labor* (ACOG Practice Bulletin No. 49). Washington, DC: Author.

American College of Obstetricians and Gynecologists (ACOG). (2004a). *Management of postterm pregnancy* (ACOG Practice Bulletin No. 55). Washington, DC: Author.

American College of Obstetricians and Gynecologists (ACOG). (2004b). *Multiple gestation: Complicated twin, triplet and high-order multifetal births* (ACOG Practice Bulletin No. 56). Washington, DC: Author.

Blackburn, S. (2007). *Maternal, fetal, and neonatal physiology: A clinical perspective.* (3rd ed.). Philadelphia: Saunders.

Coyle, M. E., Smith, C. A., & Peat, B. (2005). Cephalic version by moxibustion for breech presentation. *The Cochrane Database of Systematic Reviews* (2) (Article No.: CD003928.pub2. DOI: 10.1002/14651858.CD003928.pub2).

Cristina, M. P., Ana, G., Ines, T., Manuel, G. E., & Enrique, I. G. (2005). Perinatal results following the prenatal ultrasound diagnosis of single umbilical artery. *Acta Obstetricia et Gynecologica Scandinavica, 84*(11), 1068–1074.

Cunningham, F. G., Leveno, K. J., Bloom, S. L., Hauth, J. C., Gilstrap, L. C., & Wenstrom, K. D. (2005). *Williams obstetrics* (22nd ed.). New York: McGraw-Hill.

Demianczuk, C. E., & Corbett, T. F. (2005). Successful pregnancy after amniotic fluid embolism: A case report. *Journal Obstetrics & Gynaecology Canada, 27*(7), 699–701.

Eide, M. G., Oyen, N., Skjaerven, R., Irgens, L. M., Bjerkedel, T., & Nielson, S. T. (2005). Breech delivery and intelligence: A population-based study of 8,738 breech infants. *Obstetrics and Gynecology, 105*(1), 4–11.

Fischer, R. (2005). Breech presentation. *E-Medicine.* Retrieved February 3, 2006, from http://www.emedicine.com/med/topic3272.htm

Freeman, M. P., & Gelenberg, A. J. (2005). Bipolar disorder in women: Reproductive events and treatment considerations. *Acta Psychiatrica Scandinavica, 112*(2), 88–96.

Hofmeyr, G. J. (2004). Obstructed labor: Using better technologies to reduce mortality. *International Journal of Gynaecology and Obstetrics, 85* (Suppl. 1), S62–72.

Kayem, C. F., Goffinet, D. F., Thomas, C., & Clement, D. (2002). Conservative versus extirpative management in cases of placenta accreta. *Obstetrics and Gynecology, 104*(3), 531–536.

Kessler, R. C. (2005). Prevalence and severity of mental illness in the United States. *Archives of General Psychiatry, 62,* 617–627.

Leininger, M. M., & McFarland, M. (2005). *Cultural care diversity and universality: A worldwide nursing theory.* London: Jones & Bartlett.

Malinowski, W., Koktysz, R., & Stawerski, P. (2005). Intrauterine death of one fetus during the first trimester of monochorionic diamniotic twin gestation. *Ginekologia Polska, 76*(1), 54–60.

Martin, J. A., Hamilton, B. E., Sutton, P. D., Ventura, S. J., Menacker, F., & Munson, M. L. (2005). Births: Final data for 2003. *National Vital Statistics Reports, 54*(2), 1–116.

Molkenboer, J. F., Reijners, E. P., Nijhuis, J. G., & Roumen, F. J. (2004). Moderate neonatal morbidity after vaginal term breech delivery. *Journal of Maternal-Fetal and Neonatal Medicine, 16*(6), 357–361.

Mongelli, M., & Tambyraja, R. (2003). Ultrasonic fetal weight estimation and tolerance to measurement error: A comparative analysis. *Australasian Radiology, 47*(4), 389–392.

Morgan, B. L. G., & Ross, M. G. (2005). Umbilical cord complications. *E-Medicine.* Retrieved February 14, 2006, from http://www.emedicine.com/med/topic3276.htm

Napolitano, P. G., & Parker, J. (2005). Face presentation. *E-Medicine.* Retrieved February 3, 2006, from http://www.emedicine.com/med/topic3273.htm

Nasser, N., Roberts, C. L., Barratt, A., Bell, J. C., Olive, E. C., & Peat, B. (2006). Systematic review of adverse outcomes of external cephalic version and persisting breech presentation at term. *Paediatric Perinatal Epidemiology, 20*(2), 163–171.

National Institute of Mental Health (NIMH). (2006). *Depression.* Retrieved February 2, 2006, from http://www.nimh.nih.gov/healthinformation/depressionmenu.cfm

Newport, D. J., Viguera, A. C., Beach, A. J., Ritchie, J. C., Cohen, L. S., & Stowe, Z. N. (2005). Lithium placental passage and obstetrical outcome: Implications for clinical management during late pregnancy. *American Journal of Psychiatry, 162*(11), 2162–2170.

Parker, J., & Napolitano, P. G. (2005). Brow presentation. *E-Medicine.* Retrieved February 15, 2006, from http://www.emedicine.com/med/topic3274.htm

Perinatal Institute. (2006). Perinatal review: Obstetric emergencies, placenta abruption. Retrieved October 21, 2006. http://www.perinatal.nhs.uk/reviews/oe/oe_placental_abruption.htm

Ramos, G. A., & Caughey, A. B. (2005). The interrelationship between ethnicity and obesity on obstetric outcomes. *American Journal of Obstetrics & Gynecology, 193*(3, Pt. 2), 1089–1093.

Simonsen, S. M., Lyon, J. L., Adler, S. C., & Varner, M. W. (2005). Effect of grandmultiparity on intrapartum and newborn complications in young women. *Obstetrics and Gynecology, 106*(3), 454–460.

Stitley, M. L., & Gherman, R. B. (2005). Labor with abnormal presentation and position. *Obstetrics and Gynecology Clinics of North America, 32*(2), 165–179.

Varney, H., Krebs, J. M., & Gegor, C. E. (2004). *Varney's midwifery* (4th ed.). London: Jones & Bartlett.

CHAPTER 27

Birth-Related Procedures

With our first baby I suddenly had to have a cesarean. Everything happened so fast, but our son was OK, and that's all that mattered. With our second baby I wanted to try for a vaginal birth but nevertheless I was afraid. I don't know what I would have done without my nurse. She stayed with me the whole time I labored and kept giving me support. She explained everything, so I knew what was happening. I felt safe. I had a beautiful baby girl after 8 hours of labor. Everything went well postpartally, and I am so glad I was able to avoid another cesarean. We don't plan to have another baby, but if we did, I wouldn't be so afraid.

OBJECTIVES

1. Describe the impact of selected procedures on the childbearing woman and her family or support system.

2. Contrast the methods of external cephalic version and internal version and the related nursing management.

3. Discuss the use of amniotomy in current maternal-newborn care.

4. Compare methods for inducing labor, explaining their advantages and disadvantages.

5. Discuss the use of transcervical intrapartum amnioinfusion.

6. Describe the types of episiotomies performed, the rationale for each, and the associated nursing interventions.

7. Summarize the indications for forceps-assisted birth, types of forceps that may be used, complications, and related interventions.

8. Discuss the use of vacuum extraction, including indications, procedure, complications, and related nursing management.

9. Explain the indications for cesarean birth, impact on the family unit, preparation and teaching needs, and associated nursing management.

10. Discuss vaginal birth following cesarean birth.

KEY TERMS

Amnioinfusion 773
Amniotomy 771
Cervical ripening 762
Cesarean birth 782
Episiotomy 774
External cephalic version (ECV) 759
Forceps-assisted birth 777
Labor augmentation 765
Labor induction 765
Podalic version 759
Vacuum extraction 779
Vaginal birth after cesarean (VBAC) 786

MEDIALINK

Additional resources for this content can be found on the Prentice Hall Nursing MediaLink DVD-ROM and on the Companion Website at http://www.prenhall.com/davidson. Click on "Chapter 27" to select the activities for this chapter.

Most births occur without the need for operative obstetric intervention. In some instances, however, obstetric procedures are necessary to maintain the safety of the woman and the fetus. The most common obstetric procedures are version, amniotomy, induction of labor, episiotomy, cesarean birth, and vaginal birth following a previous cesarean birth.

Generally, women are aware of the possible need for an obstetric procedure during their labor and birth, and many women accept whatever procedure is recommended based on the belief that the caregiver knows what is needed and that it is in the baby's best interest. However, some women expect to have a "natural" birth experience and do not desire or anticipate any medical intervention. These women may feel disappointed or even guilty when an unanticipated obstetric procedure is needed. This conflict between expectation and the need for intervention presents a challenge to maternity nurses. The nurse can provide information regarding any procedure to enhance the woman's and her partner's understanding of what is proposed, the anticipated benefits and possible risks, and any possible alternative treatments.

The nurse must provide emotional support to the woman and her family to assist them in accepting the unanticipated procedure. Although the physical responses to interventions are constantly monitored and documented, it is especially important for nurses to continually assess and document the family's emotional responses to interventions. Many times it is the nurse who plays a key role in emotional support and teaching. The importance of this role is just as imperative to any physical care that the nurse performs for the laboring woman and her family.

CARE OF THE WOMAN DURING VERSION

Version, or turning the fetus, is a procedure used to change the fetal presentation by abdominal or intrauterine manipulation. The most common type of version is **external cephalic version (ECV)** in which the fetus is changed from a breech, transverse, or oblique lie to a cephalic presentation by external manipulation of the maternal abdomen (Figure 27–1 ◆). The success rates for version are the highest for transverse presentations. Overall, success rates for version average 60% (Cunningham, Leveno, Bloom et al., 2005). Successful ECVs decrease the chances of nonvertex and cesarean births (Hofmeyr & Kulier, 2002).

The other type of version, called a **podalic version,** is used only with the second twin during a vaginal birth. In an internal version, the obstetrician places a hand inside the uterus, grabs the fetus's feet, and then turns the fetus from a transverse or noncephalic presentation to a breech presentation (Figure 27–2 ◆). The fetus is then born in a breech presentation. This maneuver is used only when the second twin is not in a cephalic position. It is considered superior to an external cephalic version because it causes fewer decelerations (Cunningham et al., 2005). Some obstetricians may elect to have the second twin be born by cesarean if the twin is not in a cephalic presentation.

Figure 27–1 ◆ External (or cephalic) version of the fetus. A new technique involves applying pressure to the fetal head and buttocks so that the fetus completes a "backward flip" or "forward roll."

External Cephalic Version

If breech or shoulder presentation (transverse lie) is detected in the later weeks of pregnancy, an ECV may be attempted. The version is usually done after 36 to 37 weeks' gestation because most fetuses still in breech presentation at this time will not spontaneously change back to a vertex presentation. In addition, if complications arise from the procedure, the risk of prematurity is eliminated. Even when ECV is successful, there is some evidence that the stress of the procedure may increase the rate of intrapartum cesarean births. Breech fetuses have some variances from fetuses that present in a cephalic presentation. Breech fetuses have been shown to have smaller head circumferences, lower birth weight, and lower fetoplacental ratios. Fetuses that were previously breech tend to have higher rates of nonreassuring fetal status and dystocia. These mothers may also have a smaller pelvis, which may be the cause of the breech presentation in the first place (Chan, Tang, Tsoi et al., 2004). Factors associated with higher success rates include higher parity, adequate amniotic fluid, lack of fetal engagement, and transverse lie. Factors associated with higher failure rates include nulliparity, advanced dilatation, fetal weight less than 2500 g, anterior placenta, a low station, maternal obesity, and anterior or posterior positioning of the fetal spine (Cunningham et al., 2005).

A

B

C

D

Figure 27–2 ◆ Use of podalic version and extraction of the fetus to assist in the vaginal birth of the second twin. *A,* The physician reaches into the uterus and grasps a foot. Although a vertex birth is always preferred in a singleton birth, in this instance of assisting in the birth of a second twin it is not possible to grasp any other fetal part. The fetal head would be too large to grasp and pull downward, and grasping the fetal arm would result in a transverse lie and make vaginal birth impossible. *B,* While applying pressure on the outside of the abdomen to push the baby's head up toward the top of the uterus with one hand, the physician pulls the baby's foot down toward the cervix. *C,* Both feet have been pulled through the cervix and vagina. *D,* The physician now grasps the baby's trunk and continues to pull downward on the baby to assist the birth.

Criteria for External Version

The following criteria should be met before performing ECV (Hofmeyr & Kulier, 2002):

- A single fetus (also called a singleton) must be present. If a multiple gestation exists, a variety of concerns preclude an external version. For example, a cesarean rather than vaginal birth may need to be considered, and the fetuses might become entangled during a version.

- The fetal breech is not engaged. Once the presenting part is engaged, it is difficult, if not impossible, to do a version.
- An adequate amount of amniotic fluid must exist. The amniotic fluid helps ease movement of the fetus and provides adequate room for the umbilical cord to float without being compressed.
- A reactive nonstress test (NST) should be obtained immediately before performing the version. A reactive NST indicates fetal well-being.

- The fetus must be 36 to 37 or more weeks' gestation. A version may be accompanied by complications that require immediate birth by cesarean. If gestation is less than 37 weeks, a preterm birth would result.

- (*Note:* Occasionally, a physician may do an external version while the woman is in labor.)

Contraindications for External Version

Absolute contraindications to ECV include the following (Cunningham et al., 2005):

- *Suspected intrauterine growth restriction.* The fetus has been stressed and amniotic fluid may be decreased.

- *Fetal anomalies.* This category includes major abnormalities.

- *Presence of an abnormal fetal heart rate (FHR) tracing.* A nonreassuring FHR pattern might indicate that the fetus is already stressed and other action needs to be taken.

- *Rupture of the membranes.* Rupture of the membranes would result in an inadequate amount of amniotic fluid.

- *Cesarean birth indicated anyway.* For example, if a complete previa is present, birth will be by cesarean. If a placenta previa, marginal previa, or low-lying placenta is present, the manipulation during the version may precipitate bleeding.

- *Maternal problems.* Maternal problems such as gestational diabetes that has required insulin, uncontrolled chronic hypertension, preeclampsia, or maternal cardiac disease.

- *Amniotic fluid abnormalities.* Oligohydramnios (amniotic fluid index less than 5 cm) makes the fetus difficult to maneuver and increases risk of umbilical cord compression. Hydramnios (amniotic fluid index greater than 25 cm) stretches the uterine walls, increasing pressure and decreasing the chance the fetus will remain in a cephalic presentation.

Relative contraindications to ECV include the following:

- Previous lower uterine segment cesarean birth. Prior scarring of the uterus may increase the risk of uterine tearing or uterine rupture.

- Nuchal cord. A nuchal cord may tighten around the fetal neck and decrease circulation to the fetus.

- Multiple gestation

- Evidence of uteroplacental insufficiency

- Significant third trimester bleeding

- Uterine malformation

External Version Procedure

The external version is accomplished in a birthing unit, rather than an outpatient setting, in case further intervention (such as emergency cesarean birth) is necessary. There have been no reported fetal deaths from the procedure since 1980. The risk of

major complications resulting from an ECV has been reported as 1% to 2%. These risks include "abnormal cardiotocography (CTG) patterns (5.7%), persisting pathological CTG readings (0.37%), and vaginal bleeding (0.47%). The incidence of placental abruption was even lower, at 0.12%. Fetomaternal transfusion was absent in five out of seven studies, with a mean incidence of 3.7%. Emergency cesareans were performed in 0.43% of all versions. Perinatal mortality was 0.16%" (Collaris & Oei, 2004).

The woman is instructed to fast for 8 hours preceding the version in case a cesarean birth needs to be performed because of complications. The physician uses ultrasound to confirm the presence of a single fetus, the amount of amniotic fluid, the location of the placenta, the position of the umbilical cord, and that a breech presentation still exists. Maternal vital signs are assessed, and continuous electronic fetal monitoring (EFM) is done to evaluate the FHR, to obtain a reactive NST, and to evaluate the presence of uterine contractions or uterine wall tenseness. Blood work is drawn, including a complete blood count (CBC) and a blood type and antibody screen. The physician explains the procedure and the client signs a consent form.

An intravenous line is established for medication administration and in case of difficulties. A beta-mimetic agent (a subcutaneous dose of terbutaline) or intravenous infusion of magnesium sulfate (if a beta-mimetic agent is contraindicated because of a medical condition) is administered to achieve uterine relaxation. Occasionally, some physicians do not use a beta-mimetic agent during the version. However, it greatly enhances the comfort of the woman (Theron & Theron, 2002). The use of epidural analgesia has been found to increase success rates, although further research is needed (Cunningham et al., 2005).

The woman is placed in a supine or slight Trendelenburg position. Once uterine relaxation is achieved, the maternal abdomen is copiously covered with warmed ultrasound gel to decrease excessive manipulation and friction, and the physician grasps the fetal breech between the index finger and the thumb. First the presenting part is gently pushed upward or lifted out of the maternal pelvis by exerting pressure over the skin on the maternal abdomen. If the fetal breech can be lifted out, then the breech and head are rotated or moved out in opposite directions. In most cases, a direction similar to a forward roll is attempted initially. If that is not successful, a roll in the opposite direction is attempted. The procedure should be concluded when any of the following occur: the fetal head is moved to a head-down position; repeated failures have occurred; the woman has indicated that the procedure has become too painful or stressful; or signs of maternal or fetal problems occur, including a nonreassuring FHR pattern (Cunningham et al., 2005). The intravenous tocolytic agent is discontinued, and frequently the fetus is held in the new presentation by either the physician or the nurse until the uterus regains tone. In the event of a failed version, a repeat attempt can be made within a week if the procedure was well tolerated by the woman and her fetus. If the woman is Rh negative, an adequate amount of Rh immune globulin must always be administered after the version because there is a 4% risk of maternal-fetal hemorrhage (Cunningham et al., 2005) (see

Chapter 20). A vaginal examination and ultrasound are done to evaluate cervical dilatation and to confirm position and fetal descent. Spontaneous reversion can also occur.

NURSING CARE MANAGEMENT

The nurse begins by ensuring that the expectant woman understands the procedure, knows that the procedure may be uncomfortable or very painful, and realizes that she can tell the physician to stop if the pain is too great.

The possibility of failure of the ECV and the slight risk of a cesarean birth if the fetus exhibits a nonreassuring fetal status should also be discussed. Explaining what will occur in either of these circumstances better prepares the woman and partner if intervention becomes necessary. Before the version, the nurse completes initial maternal and fetal assessments, provides ongoing evaluation of FHR, performs the NST, and obtains blood work. The nurse provides psychologic support throughout the procedure through reassurance. The nurse also provides continuous explanations about the procedure while the version is being performed and answers any questions. The nurse continues to monitor maternal blood pressure and pulse about every 2 minutes throughout the period of time the beta-mimetic agent is used and for about 30 minutes after. The FHR is monitored for approximately 1 to 2 hours following the ECV. The nurse also assesses the maternal-fetal response to the to-colytic agent. The nurse continues to provide information by reiterating aftercare instructions, such as monitoring for uterine contractions, being aware of fetal movement (fetal kick counts), and recognizing signs of reversion (excessive movement or a sensation described as the fetus "turning around"). RhoGAM should be administered to all Rh negative women (Cunningham et al., 2005).

CARE OF THE WOMAN DURING CERVICAL RIPENING

Prostaglandin E_2 (PGE_2) gel for **cervical ripening** (softening and effacing the cervix) may be used for the pregnant woman at or near term when there is a medical or obstetric indication for induction of labor. The two most commonly used types of gel are Prepidil and Cervidil. Prepidil gel contains 0.5 mg dinoprostone (a form of prostaglandin E_2 for intracervical application) and is placed intracervically. Cervidil is packaged in an intravaginal insert that resembles a 2-cm-square piece of cardboard-like material. It is placed in the posterior vagina and is left in place to provide a slow release of 10 mg dinoprostone at a rate of 0.3 mg/hr over 12 hours (Thornton & Whaites, 2004).

 DRUG GUIDE   Dinoprostone (Cervidil) Vaginal Insert

Pregnancy Risk Category: C

Overview of Maternal-Fetal Action
Dinoprostone is a naturally occurring form of prostaglandin E_2. Dinoprostone can be used at term to ripen the cervix and can stimulate the smooth muscle of the uterus to enhance uterine contractions. A single vaginal insert may be used to ripen the cervix and then oxytocin can be administered 30 minutes later (Forrest Pharmaceuticals, 1995).

Route, Dosage, Frequency
The vaginal insert contains 10 mg of dinoprostone. The insert is placed transversely in the posterior fornix of the vagina, and the client is kept supine for 2 hours but then may ambulate. The dinoprostone is released at approximately 0.3 mg/hr over a 12-hour period. The vaginal insert should be removed by pulling on the retrieval string upon onset of uterine contractions or after 12 hours (Forrest Pharmaceuticals, 1995).

Contraindications
• Client with known sensitivity to prostaglandins
• Presence of nonreassuring fetal status
• Unexplained bleeding during pregnancy
• Strong suspicion of cephalopelvic disproportion
• Client already receiving oxytocin
• Client with six or more previous term pregnancies
• Client who is not anticipated to be able to give birth vaginally

Dinoprostone vaginal insert should be used with CAUTION in clients with ruptured membranes, a fetus in breech presentation, presence of glaucoma, or history of asthma (Forrest Pharmaceuticals, 1995).

Maternal Side Effects
Uterine hyperstimulation with or without nonreassuring fetal status has occurred in a very small number (2.8%–4.7%) of clients. Fewer than 1% of clients have experienced fever, nausea, vomiting, diarrhea, or abdominal pain (Forrest Pharmaceuticals, 1995).

Effects on Fetus/Newborn
Nonreassuring fetal heart rate patterns

Nursing Considerations
• Assess for presence of contraindications.
• Monitor maternal vital signs, cervical dilatation, and effacement carefully.
• Monitor fetal status for presence of reassuring fetal heart rate pattern (baseline 110–160 bpm, presence of short-term variability, average variability presence of accelerations with fetal movement, absence of late or variable decelerations).
• Remove vaginal insert if uterine hyperstimulation, sustained uterine contractions, nonreassuring fetal status, or any other maternal adverse actions occur.

SOURCE: Forrest Pharmaceuticals. (1995). *Cervidil manufacturer's fact sheet.* St. Louis: Forrest Pharmaceuticals.

DRUG GUIDE   Dinoprostone (Prepidil)

Pregnancy Risk Catergory: C

Overview of Maternal-Fetal Action

Dinoprostone is a synthetically prepared form of prostoglandin E_2. Dinoprostone can be given at term and acts directly on the myometrial fibers to stimulate uterine contractility. Dinoprostone directly softens the cervix, relaxing smooth muscle in the cervix itself, and assists the uterus in producing coordinated contractions with lower doses of pitocin (Sciarra, 2004).

Route, Dosage, and Frequency

Prepidil is packaged as a single-dose syringe that contains 0.5 mg of dinoprostone in a 2.5 mL viscous gel. The package contains two soft plastic catheters that are used for intracervical administration. The plastic catheter is introduced into the external cervical os for placement. The catheters come in two different lengths and have a shield to prevent instillation of the medication into the internal os. The medication can be placed directly during a digital examination, or a speculum can be used to visualize the cervix. The woman is placed in a reclining position and bed rest is maintained to prevent the medication from leaking from the vagina. The woman should be monitored using electronic fetal monitoring for at least 30 minutes and up to 2 hours after placement to assess the contraction pattern and the fetal status. Prepidil may be repeated every 6 hours up to 3 doses. Pitocin should not be administered for at least 6 to 12 hours because the effects of dinoprostone can be heightened when oxytocin is administered (Sciarra, 2004).

Contraindications

- Known sensitivity to prostaglandins
- Presence of nonreassuring fetal status
- Unexplained vaginal bleeding during pregnancy

- Current use of oxytocin
- Grandmultiparous women with more than six previous term vaginal births
- Known contraindications for vaginal birth
- Suspected cephalopelvic disproportion
- Previous surgical scar on uterus

Dinoprostone should be used with caution in women with a history of asthma; ruptured membranes; or renal, hepatic, or cardiovascular disease (Wilson, Shannon, Strang, 2006).

Maternal Side Effects

Uterine hyperstimulation can occur, resulting in a nonreassuring fetal heart rate pattern. Rarely, fever, nausea, vomiting, and diarhea have also been noted to occur. In the past, women who have had a previous cesarean birth and have been given dinoprostone have had a uterine rupture as a result.

Effects on Fetus/Newborn

Nonreassuring fetal heart rate patterns.

Nursing Considerations

- Assess fetal status before administration.
- Assess for contractions.
- Monitor vital signs, cervical changes, and potential side effects.
- Monitor for reassuring fetal status (fetal heart rate of 110–160, presence of variability, accelerations with fetal movement, absence of late or variable decelerations).
- Report uterine hyperstimulation, sustained uterine contractions, nonreassuring fetal status, or adverse maternal reactions to physician or CNM immediately.

Advantages and Disadvantages of Prostaglandin Administration

The advantage of Cervidil is that it can be removed easily if uterine hyperstimulation occurs (Deglin & Vallerand, 2005). Both preparations have been demonstrated to cause cervical ripening, shorter labor, and lower requirements for oxytocin during labor induction. Vaginal birth is achieved within 24 hours for most women. The incidence of cesarean birth is reduced when prostaglandin agents are used before labor induction (Mahlmeister, 2005).

Risks of prostaglandin administration include uterine hyperstimulation, nonreassuring fetal status, a higher incidence of postpartum hemorrhage, and uterine rupture that can occur even in the absence of a previous uterine incision (Mahlmeister, 2005). Contraindications to labor induction are found in Table 27–1. Women with a previous uterine incision should not receive prostaglandin agents, as the risk of uterine rupture is greatly increased (Mahlmeister, 2005). Prostaglandin should be used with caution in women with compromised cardiovascular, hepatic, or renal function and in women with asthma or glaucoma (Thornton & Whaites, 2004).

Table 27–1   ABSOLUTE CONTRAINDICATIONS TO LABOR INDUCTION OR AUGMENTATION

- Complete placenta previa
- Vasa previa
- Abruptio placentae
- Prolapsed umbilical cord
- Fetal bradycardia
- Acute nonreassuring fetal status (persistent nonreassuring fetal status)
- Previous classic uterine incision or transfundal uterine surgery
- Previous myomectomy
- Vaginal bleeding with unknown cause
- Pelvic structure abnormality
- Active genital herpes (HSV) infection
- Invasive cervical cancer
- Cephalopelvic disproportion

SOURCE: Adapted from American College of Obstetricians and Gynecologists. *Induction of Labor.* (Practice Bulletin No. 10). Washington, DC: © ACOG, November 1999.

Prostaglandin Agent Insertion Procedure

It is recommended that prostaglandin gel be used only in a hospital birthing unit and that an obstetrician be readily available in case an emergency cesarean birth is needed. The use of PGE in outpatient settings and birth centers is currently under study. When Prepidil is used, it is introduced by means of a prefilled syringe with a catheter attached to the hub. The catheter is inserted through the vagina and into the endocervix, where the gel is injected. The catheter has a small shield at the top so that the gel cannot be deposited above the internal os. Dinoprostone is available as a gel that may be placed in a diaphragm and applied to the cervix and as a suppository that is placed in the posterior fornix of the vagina.

When Cervidil is used, the vaginal insert is placed in the posterior vagina. The woman should be instructed to call the nurse if it becomes dislodged so it can be reinserted. The woman is then monitored so her contractions and the fetus can be assessed. If hyperstimulation does occur, the insert can be removed. If active labor is established, the insert should also be removed. Women who receive Cytotec typically remain in the acute care setting and oxytocin is started to facilitate birth.

Use of Misoprostol (Cytotec)

Misoprostol (Cytotec) is a synthetic PGE_1 analogue that can be used to soften and ripen the cervix and to induce labor. It is available as a tablet that is inserted into the vagina, or it can be taken orally. When Cytotec was widely used in the 1990s for cervical ripening and induction of labor, several reports showed an increase in the rates of uterine rupture. The drug manufacturer subsequently issued a statement that the drug should not be used for labor induction (Tenore, 2003). Many hospitals responded by discontinuing use of the drug; however, it is still used in some agencies.

Research since that time has shown that Cytotec used in ripening the cervix and inducing labor is more effective than oxytocin or prostaglandin agents. Women who receive Cytotec to induce labor typically deliver within 24 hours of administration. The use of Cytotec is also associated with lower cesarean birth rates. When compared with women who have been induced using prostaglandin agents or oxytocin, the adverse outcomes do not differ among the three methods (Goldberg & Wing, 2003). The use of Cytotec for cervical ripening or induction of labor should be carefully considered. The American College of Obstetricians and Gynecologists ([ACOG] 2004a) issued the following recommended guidelines for administration:

- Use only in the third trimester for cervical ripening or induction of labor.
- One fourth of a tablet or 25 mcg should be the initial dose.
- Recurrent administration should not exceed dosing intervals of more than 3 to 6 hours.
- Pitocin should not be administered less than 4 hours after the last Cytotec dose.

Absolute contraindications for Cytotec include the following (ACOG, 2004a):

- Presence of uterine contractions three times in 10 minutes
- Significant maternal asthma
- Previous cesarean birth or other uterine scar
- Bleeding during the pregnancy
- Presence of placenta previa
- Nonreassuring fetal status

Use of Transcervical Catheter

Balloon catheters have been used for cervical ripening for many years to promote mechanical dilatation. A Foley catheter with a 25-mL to 80-mL balloon is passed through the undilated cervix and then inflated. The weighted balloon applies pressure on the internal os of the cervix and acts to ripen the cervix. This technique can be used alone or in conjunction with other induction methods, such as vaginal misoprostol, intravenous Pitocin, or extra-amniotic saline infusion where additional saline is inserted into the Foley bulb, which is pulled snugly against the cervial os (Cunningham et al., 2005).

One study examined cervical ripening after Foley catheter insertion with either 30 mL or 80 mL of sterile saline contained in a Foley catheter that was inserted and left in place in the cervical canal. The group with 80 mL had higher Bishop scores (3 cm or more). Of the primiparous women in the group, the women with the 80-mL balloon catheters had a higher rate of vaginal deliveries that occurred within 24 hours and had less need for intravenous oxytocin (Levy, Kanengiser, Furman et al., 2004).

NURSING CARE MANAGEMENT

Physicians, certified nurse-midwives (CNMs), and labor and delivery nurses who have had special education and training may administer agents for cervical ripening (Thornton & Whaites, 2004). Maternal vital signs are assessed for a baseline, and an electronic fetal monitor is applied for at least 30 minutes to obtain an external tracing of uterine activity, fetal heart rate (FHR) pattern, and a reactive NST. If a nonreactive test is obtained, consultation with the physician or CNM is required. After the gel, intravaginal insert, or tablet is inserted, the woman is instructed to remain lying down with a rolled blanket or hip wedge under her right hip to tip the uterus slightly to the left for the first 30 to 60 minutes to maintain the cervical ripening agent in place. Gel may leak from the endocervix. The nurse monitors the woman for uterine hyperstimulation and FHR abnormalities (changes in baseline rate, variability, and presence of decelerations) for 30 minutes to 2 hours if a prostaglandin gel agent is used (Deglin & Vallerand, 2005). If tachysystole (hyperstimulation) of the uterus greater than five contractions in 10 minutes occurs, the woman is positioned on her left side and oxygen is administered if fetal stress is noted. The administration of a tocolytic agent (such as a subcutaneous injection of 0.25 mg terbutaline) should be considered if the uterine hyperstimulation pattern continues. The gel may be removed if hyperstimulation, severe nausea, vomiting, or tachysystole develops (Wilson et al., 2006). Treatment with antiemetics, antipyretics, and antidiarrheal agents usually is not indicated. Women who receive Cervidil or Cytotec tend to remain in the acute care setting so the contraction pattern and fetal status can be continually monitored.

Women undergoing induction via balloon catheters do not need continous fetal monitoring. The nurse can perform intermittent monitoring along with the maternal vital signs. The nurse should also assess the location of the catheter to ensure the catheter has not become displaced. This can be achieved by marking the catheter tubing at the introitus and noting whether movement has occurred. After the catheter is inserted, the woman should remain in a recumbent position. Vaginal examinations should not be performed. A bedpan should be used as ambulation should be avoided.

CARE OF THE WOMAN DURING INDUCTION OR AUGMENTATION OF LABOR

The ACOG defines **labor induction** as the stimulation of uterine contractions before the spontaneous onset of labor, with or without ruptured fetal membranes, for the purpose of accomplishing birth (ACOG, 2003). **Labor augmentation** refers to the "stimulation of uterine contractions when spontaneous contractions have failed to result in progressive cervical dilation or the descent of the fetus" (ACOG, 2003, p. 416).

Induction or augmentation may be indicated in the presence of the following:

- Diabetes mellitus
- Renal disease
- Preeclampsia
- Hypertensive disorders
- Premature rupture of membranes (PROM)
- Chorioamnionitis
- Fetal demise
- Postterm gestation
- Intrauterine growth restriction (IUGR)
- Isoimmunization
- History of rapid labor (precipitous labor and birth) to prevent an unattended birth
- Mild abruptio placentae, no fetal stress or unreassuring FHR
- Nonreassuring antepartal testing (poor biophysical profile score)
- Severe oligohydramnios
- Macrosomia

Contraindications to Labor Induction or Augmentation

All contraindications to spontaneous labor and vaginal birth are contraindications to the induction or augmentation of labor (see Table 27–1). Relative maternal contraindications to induction are included in Table 27–2.

Before induction is attempted, appropriate assessment must indicate that both the woman and fetus are ready for the onset of labor. This includes evaluation of fetal maturity and cervical readiness.

The gestational age of the fetus is best evaluated by accurate menstrual dating, ultrasound visualization of the gestational sac between 5 and 6 weeks' gestation, and quickening at 18 to 20 weeks. Serial ultrasounds are helpful in validating gestational age. When needed, amniotic fluid studies for lecithin/sphingomyelin (L/S) ratio and phosphatidylglycerol are also beneficial in assessing fetal lung maturity (see Chapter 21 ∞).

The findings on vaginal examination will help determine whether cervical changes favorable for induction have occurred. Bishop (1964) developed a prelabor scoring system that is still helpful in predicting the inducibility of women (Table 27–3). Components evaluated are cervical dilatation, effacement,

Table 27–2   RELATIVE CONTRAINDICATIONS TO LABOR INDUCTION

- Abnormal fetal heart rate patterns
- Breech presentation
- Unknown fetal presentation
- Multiple gestation
- Polyhydramnios
- Presenting fetal part above the maternal pelvic inlet
- Severe hypertension
- Maternal heart disease

SOURCE: Adapted from American College of Obstetricians and Gynecologists. *Induction of Labor* (Practice Bulletin No. 10). Washington, DC: © ACOG, November 1999.

Table 27–3   PRELABOR STATUS EVALUATION SCORING SYSTEM

Factor	Assigned Value			
	0	1	2	3
Cervical dilatation	Closed	1–2 cm	3–4 cm	5 cm or more
Cervical effacement	0% to 30%	40% to 50%	60% to 70%	80% or more
Fetal station	−3	−2	−1, 0	+1, or lower
Cervical consistency	Firm	Moderate	Soft	
Cervical position	Posterior	Midposition	Anterior	

SOURCE: Bishop, E. H. (1964). Pelvic scoring for elective inductions. *Obstetrics and Gynecology, 24,* 266.

consistency, and position, as well as the station of the fetal presenting part. A score of 0, 1, 2, or 3 is given to each assessed characteristic. The higher the total score for all the criteria, the more likely that labor will occur. The lower the total score, the higher the failure rate. A favorable cervix is the most important criterion for a successful induction (Cunningham et al., 2005). The presence of a cervix that is anterior, soft, 50% effaced, and dilated at least 2 cm, with the fetal head at +1 station or lower (Bishop score of 9), is favorable for successful induction (Bishop, 1964). Low Bishop scores have been correlated with prolonged labors and a higher incidence of cesarean births (Cunningham et al., 2005).

Fetal fibronectin assay (fFN) has been suggested as a biochemical marker for predicting impending term labor and successful labor induction (Tekesin, Wallwiener, & Schmidt, 2005). The presence of fetal fibronectin in the cervicovaginal secretions has been associated with successful induction of labor. Currently, the high cost of fFN testing has limited its use to the detection of preterm births (see Chapter 21 ∞).

Methods of Inducing or Augmenting Labor

When the cervix is favorable, the most frequently used methods of induction or augmentation are stripping the amniotic membranes, amniotomy, intravenous oxytocin (Pitocin) infusion, and complementary methods. Amniotomy is discussed later in this section.

STRIPPING THE MEMBRANES

A nonpharmacologic method of induction or augmentation frequently used by physicians and CNMs is called *stripping* (or *sweeping*) *the amniotic membranes.* The CNM or physician inserts a gloved finger as far as possible into the internal cervical os and rotates the finger 360 degrees, twice. This motion separates the amniotic membranes that are lying against the lower uterine segment and internal os from the distal part of the lower uterine segment. The stripping or sweeping is thought to release $PGF_{2\alpha}$ from the amniotic membranes or PGE_2 from the cervix. Women who undergo sweeping of the membranes tend to have a reduction in pregnancy length and tend to give birth before 41 gestational weeks (Boulvain & Irion, 2005). Women should be advised that this procedure can cause discomfort. In addition, uterine contractions, cramping, and a bloody discharge can occur after the procedure is performed. Although the procedure is not 100% effective as a labor induction method, if labor is initiated, it typically begins within 24 to 48 hours. As an augmentation method, stripping of the membranes can be performed in the birthing room in an attempt to strengthen contractions without the need for oxytocin administration. If contractions fail to become adequate, however, oxytocin may need to be considered.

OXYTOCIN INFUSION

Intravenous administration of oxytocin is an effective method of initiating uterine contractions to induce labor. The goal is to achieve three uterine contractions with a duration of 40 to 60 seconds in 10 minutes with good uterine relaxation and return to the baseline tone between contractions (Medifocus, 2002). When augmentation is needed because of an arrest of labor or failure to descend, oxytocin is given intravenously to achieve a desirable labor pattern with strong contractions that will achieve cervical dilatation and fetal descent.

Typically, augmentation is warranted if there are fewer than three contractions in a 10-minute period or if the intensity is less than 25 mm Hg as indicated by an internal uterine pressure catheter. An assessment of the maternal pelvis, fetal station, and fetal position is performed before starting the oxytocin infusion. In addition, cephalopelvic disproportion should be ruled out because it is a contraindication. The other contraindications for labor augmentation are the same as for labor induction (see Table 27–1).

A primary bottle of intravenous fluid is prepared and used to start and maintain the infusion. This avoids the risk of infusing a large dose of oxytocin as the line is begun and provides additional fluids while the oxytocin solution is being kept at a low infusion rate. After the infusion is started, the oxytocin solution is piggybacked into the primary tubing port closest to the catheter insertion. This allows only a small amount of oxytocin to back flow into the tubing and ensures greater dosage accuracy. The oxytocin should be administered with a device that permits precise control of the flow rate. Oxytocin should not be administered intramuscularly or without the aid of an intravenous electric pump. Over the past few years, differences in opinion regarding oxytocin dosage have surfaced.

Ten to 20 units of oxytocin (Pitocin) are added to 1 L of a secondary line of intravenous fluid (usually 5% dextrose in balanced saline solution—for example, 5% dextrose in lactated Ringer's solution). The resulting mixture will contain 10 or 20 milliunits of oxytocin per milliliter (1 milliunit/min/6 milliunit/hr or 2 milliunit/min/12 milliliters/hr), and the prescribed dose can be calculated easily. Some facilities are now using 30 units of oxytocin (Pitocin) per 500 mL of intravenous fluid to reduce the risk of pulmonary edema in the postpartum period. Other dilutions can also be used. Other dosage concentrations are presented in the Drug Guide: Oxytocin (Pitocin) on pages 767–768. It is imperative that the nurse be familiar with the specific dosage used within the institution to avoid medication errors.

ACOG (2003) cites the use of both a low-dose and a high-dose regimen. The low-dose regimen uses a starting dose of 0.5 to 2 milliunits/min with increases of 1 to 2 milliunits/min every 15 to 40 minutes until an adequate labor pattern is established. The high-dose regimen has a starting dose of up to 6 milliunits/min with incremental increases of 1 to 6 milliunits/min every 20 to 40 minutes. Higher dose regimens have been associated with a shorter labor, less incidence of dystocia, lower cesarean birth rates, and a lower incidence of chorioamniotis (ACOG, 2003).

Oxytocin induction is not without some associated risks: hyperstimulation of the uterus, resulting in uterine contractions that are too frequent (more often than every 2 minutes), uterine contractions that are too intense, or an increased uterine resting tone. Other risks include uterine rupture and water intoxication.

DRUG GUIDE   Oxytocin (Pitocin)

Overview of Obstetric Action

Oxytocin (Pitocin) exerts a selective stimulatory effect on the smooth muscle of the uterus and blood vessels. Oxytocin affects the myometrial cells of the uterus by increasing the excitability of the muscle cell, increasing the strength of the muscle contraction, and supporting propagation of the contraction (movement of the contraction from one myometrial cell to the next). Its effect on the uterine contraction depends on the dosage used and on the excitability of the myometrial cells. During the first half of gestation, there is little excitability of the myometrium, and the uterus is fairly resistant to the effects of oxytocin. However, from midgestation on, the uterus responds increasingly to exogenous intravenous oxytocin. Cautious use of diluted oxytocin administered intravenously at term results in a slow rise of uterine activity.

The circulatory half-life of oxytocin is 3 to 5 minutes. It takes approximately 40 minutes for a particular dose of oxytocin to reach a steady-state plasma concentration (Wilson et al., 2006).

The effects of oxytocin on the cardiovascular system can be pronounced. Blood pressure initially may decrease but after prolonged administration increase by 30% above the baseline. Cardiac output and stroke volume increase. With doses of 20 milliunits/min or above, oxytocin exerts an antidiuretic effect decreasing free water exchange in the kidney and markedly decreasing urine output.

Oxytocin is used to induce labor at term and to augment uterine contractions in the first and second stages of labor. Oxytocin may also be used immediately after birth to stimulate uterine contraction and thereby control uterine atony.

Route, Dosage, Frequency

For induction of labor: Add 10 units of Pitocin (1 mL) to 1000 mL of intravenous solution. (The resulting concentration is 10 mU oxytocin per 1 mL of intravenous fluid.) Using an infusion pump, administer IV, starting at 0.5–1 milliunit/min and increase by 1–2 milliunits/min every 40–60 minutes. Alternatively, start at 1–2 milliunits/min and increase by 1 milliunit/min every 15 minutes until a good contraction pattern (every 2–3 minutes and lasting 40–60 seconds) is achieved.

Maternal Contraindications

- Severe preeclampsia-eclampsia
- Predisposition to uterine rupture (in nullipara over 35 years of age, multigravida 4 or more, overdistention of the uterus, previous major surgery of the cervix or uterus)
- Cephalopelvic disproportion
- Malpresentation or malposition of the fetus, cord prolapse
- Preterm infant
- Rigid, unripe cervix; total placenta previa
- Presence of nonreassuring fetal status

Maternal Side Effects

Hyperstimulation of the uterus results in hypercontractility, which in turn may cause the following:

- Abruptio placentae
- Impaired uterine blood flow, leading to fetal hypoxia

- Rapid labor, leading to cervical lacerations
- Rapid labor and birth, leading to lacerations of cervix, vagina, or perineum, uterine atony; fetal trauma
- Uterine rupture
- Water intoxication (nausea, vomiting, hypotension, tachycardia, cardiac arrhythmia) if oxytocin is given in electrolyte-free solution or at a rate exceeding 20 milliunits/min; hypotension with rapid IV bolus administration postpartum

Effect on Fetus-Newborn

- Fetal effects are primarily associated with the presence of hypercontractility of the maternal uterus. Hypercontractility decreases the oxygen supply to the fetus, which is reflected by irregularities or decrease in fetal heart rate (FHR).
- Hyperbilirubinemia (Wilson et al., 2006)
- Trauma from rapid birth

Nursing Considerations

- Explain induction or augmentation procedure to client.
- Apply fetal monitor, and obtain 15- to 20-minute tracing and nonstress test (NST) to assess FHR before starting IV oxytocin.
- For induction or augmentation of labor, start with primary IV, and piggyback secondary IV with oxytocin and infusion pump.
- Ensure continuous monitoring of the fetus and uterine contractions.
- The maximum rate is 40 milliunits/min (Blackburn, 2007). Not all protocols recommend a maximum dose. When indicated, the maximum dose is generally between 16 and 40 milliunits/min. Decrease oxytocin by similar increments once labor has progressed to 5–6 cm dilatation. Protocols may vary from one agency to another.

0.5 milliunit/min = 3 mL/hr

1.0 milliunit/min = 6 mL/hr

1.5 milliunit/min = 9 mL/hr

2 milliunit/min = 12 mL/hr

4 milliunit/min = 24 mL/hr

6 milliunit/min = 36 mL/hr

8 milliunit/min = 48 mL/hr

10 milliunit/min = 60 mL/hr

12 milliunit/min = 72 mL/hr

15 milliunit/min = 90 mL/hr

18 milliunit/min = 108 mL/hr

20 milliunit/min = 120 mL/hr

- Assess FHR, maternal blood pressure, pulse, frequency and duration of uterine contractions, and uterine resting tone before each increase in the oxytocin infusion rate.
- Record all assessments and IV rate on monitor strip and on client's chart.
- Record oxytocin infusion rate in milliunits/min and mL/hr (e.g., 0.5 milliunits/min [3 mL/hr]).

(Continued on next page)

DRUG GUIDE Oxytocin (Pitocin) continued

- Record on monitor strip all client activities (such as change of position, vomiting), procedures done (amniotomy, sterile vaginal examination), and administration of analgesic agents to allow for interpretation and evaluation of tracing.
- Assess cervical dilatation as needed.
- Apply nursing comfort measures.
- Discontinue IV oxytocin infusion and infuse primary solution when (1) nonreassuring fetal status is noted (bradycardia, late or variable decelerations; (2) uterine contractions are more frequent than every 2 minutes; (3) duration of contractions exceeds more than 60 seconds; or (4) insufficient relaxation of the uterus between contractions or a steady increase in resting tone are noted (Blackburn, 2007). In addition to discontinuing IV oxytocin infusion, turn client to side, and if nonreassuring fetal status is present, administer oxygen by tight face mask at 7–10 L/min; notify physician.
- Maintain intake and output record.

For augmentation of labor:

Prepare and administer IV Pitocin as for labor induction. Increase rate until labor contractions are of good quality. The flow rate is gradually increased at no less than every 30 minutes to a maximum of 10 milliunits/min (Blackburn, 2007). In some settings or in a situation when limited fluids may be administered, a more concentrated solution may be used. When 10 units Pitocin are added to 500 mL IV solution, the resulting concentration is 1 milliunit/min = 3 mL/hr. If 10 units Pitocin are added to 250 mL IV solution, the concentration is 1 milliunit/min = 1.5 mL/hr.

For administration after expulsion of placenta:

- One dose of 10 units of Pitocin (1 mL) is given intramuscularly or added to IV fluids for continuous infusion.
- Assess FHR, maternal blood pressure, pulse, frequency and duration of uterine contractions, and uterine resting tone before each increase in oxytocin infusion rate.
- Record all assessments and IV rate on monitor strip and on client's chart. Record oxytocin infusion rate in milliunits/min and mL/hr (e.g., 0.5 milliunits/min [3 mL/hr]).
- Record on monitor strip all client activities (such as change of position, vomiting), procedures done (amniotomy, sterile vaginal examination), and administration of analgesic agents to allow for interpretation and evaluation of tracing.
- Assess cervical dilatation as needed.
- Apply nursing comfort measures.
- Discontinue IV oxytocin infusion and infuse primary solution when (1) nonreassuring fetal status is noted (tachycardia or bradycardia, late or variable decelerations), (2) uterine contractions are more frequent than every 2 minutes, (3) duration of contractions exceeds 60 seconds, or (4) insufficient relaxation of the uterus between contractions or a steady increase in resting tone are noted (Blackburn, 2007). In addition to discontinuing IV oxytocin infusion, turn client to side, and if nonreassuring fetal status is present, administer oxygen by tight face mask at 7–10 L/min; notify physician.
- Maintain intake and output record. Assess intake and output every hour.

Nonreassuring FHR patterns have also been observed (Deglin & Vallerand, 2005).

Researchers continue to investigate a new method of labor induction with pulsatile oxytocin administration by a computer-controlled pump.

COMPLEMENTARY METHODS

In addition to the allopathic cervical ripening and induction methods previously discussed, there are a variety of more "natural" and noninvasive methods that CNMs tend to suggest or administer either in the home setting or in tertiary care centers. These methods include the following: sexual intercourse/lovemaking; self or partner stimulation of the woman's nipples and breasts; the use of herbs, such as blue/black cohosh, evening primrose oil, and red raspberry leaves; the use of homeopathic solutions, such as caulophyllum or pulsatilla; castor oil; enemas; and acupressure/acupuncture. Mechanical dilation of the cervix with balloon catheters is another technique used.

Although not widely described in nursing and medical textbooks, the use of complementary and alternative medicine (CAM) has risen dramatically. It is estimated that 40% of American adults use some type of CAM therapy (Sierpina & Frenkel, 2005). Natural methods are very effective and are frequently the preferred choice of many CNMs and their clients. It is important for nursing students, nurses, and consumers to be aware of all aspects of pregnancy care.

Sexual intercourse is a logical method of stimulating cervical ripening and uterine contractions; female orgasm stimulates uterine contractions, and the male ejaculate contains a rich source of natural prostaglandins. Breast and nipple stimulation are also a frequent part of lovemaking, and this stimulates the release of endogenous oxytocin, which in turn stimulates the uterus to contract. Until recently, most literature about sexual intercourse and lovemaking during pregnancy has focused on the possible harmful effects that may arise; however, more research is needed to determine if sexual intercourse will initiate labor (Tillett, 2005). Sexual intercourse is not used to augment labor.

Nipple stimulation for cervical ripening may be done at term or to augment labor. Nipple stimulation is found to increase endogenous oxytocin and stimulate uterine contractions. It also has been found to intitiate spontaneous labor (Schaffir, 2002). There are multiple suggested methods, including manual manipulation and use of the electric breast pump. In one study, women who used a breast pump were found to have shorter labors than those receiving intravenous Pitocin. Care should be taken to monitor uterine contractility because hyperstimulation can occur (Schaffir, 2002).

Herbal preparations such as blue and black cohosh, evening primrose oil, and red raspberry leaf teas are used for both cervical ripening and induction of labor. Although extensive scientific data are not available, they have been widely used to promote uterine contractions and stimulate and augment labor (Born & Barron, 2005).

Homeopathic solutions, such as caulophyllum, cimicifuga, pulsatilla, and others, are used for cervical ripening and induction of labor. There are no current guidelines for their use in augmenting labor. The midwife or physician needs thorough personal knowledge of homeopathic remedies or ongoing consultation with a homeopathic physician.

Castor oil has been used for many years but has not been studied frequently as a method of labor induction and augmentation. The method by which castor oil stimulates uterine contractions is not understood. Although some studies have examined the effectiveness of castor oil, further research is needed to determine the effectiveness of this method (Schaffir, 2002).

Acupressure and acupuncture are not as accepted in the United States as in other countries. However, the rising interest in and use of holistic practices and alternative medicine is prompting a closer look at acupuncture as a method of inducing and augmenting labor and relieving labor pain. In acupuncture, sterile needles are inserted into the body at specific predetermined sites to elicit a desired response, such as initiation of contractions or relief of pain (Sierpina & Frenkel, 2005). Although acupuncture requires extensive education and training, some CNMs can work with an acupressurist/acupuncturist to learn manual massage of acupuncture and acupressure points, shiatsu, and other touch techniques.

NURSING CARE MANAGEMENT

No matter which induction or augmentation method is used, close observation and accurate assessments are mandatory to provide safe, optimal care for both woman and fetus. The nurse obtains maternal vital signs (temperature, pulse, respirations, and blood pressure) before beginning an oxytocin infusion. Induction protocols also recommend obtaining a 20- to 30-minute electronic fetal monitor recording demonstrating a reassuring FHR and a reactive NST and contraction status before the infusion is started. Client teaching includes the purpose and procedure for the induction, as well as a review of the care that will be provided, including assessments and comfort measures. A Clinical Pathway for Induction of Labor appears on pp. 770 to 771.

During the oxytocin infusion, an obstetrician should be readily accessible to manage any complication that occurs. A fetal monitor is used to provide continuous data. Women may ambulate if a portable or walking monitor is available.

Women who are undergoing alternative methods of induction also need continuous assessment and nursing support. For women who have entered labor after stripping of the amniotic membranes, a normal labor pattern should ensue. Intermittent external fetal monitoring can be used if the fetus is reactive and

COMPLEMENTARY AND ALTERNATIVE THERAPIES

EVENING PRIMROSE OIL

Evening primrose oil is a natural substance that is extracted from the plant's seeds. It has been widely used for centuries by midwives as a means of softening the cervix, vagina, and perineum to facilitate the onset of labor. Evening primrose oil contains a fatty acid called gamma linolenic acid, which is converted into a prostaglandin compound. Prostaglandins play a key role in ripening the cervix so labor can begin. Women can be advised to begin evening primrose oil supplementation during the 36th week of pregnancy. The recommended dose is 2500 mg per day taken either orally or vaginally until birth. Side effects are rare but can include headaches, nausea, or skin rashes. Women who experience side effects should be counseled to discontinue the supplement unless advised otherwise by their CNM or physician (Midwifery Today E-News, 2002).

the maternal vital signs are within normal parameters. Women should be advised that they may continue to have a blood-tinged discharge from the procedure. Women who have their membranes stripped are less likely to go past their due dates (Rayburn, 2002). The nurse continues to assess the contraction pattern, including the frequency, intensity, and duration of the contractions.

Women who choose to use nipple stimulation as a means of inducing labor should be continuously monitored with the external fetal monitor while the electric breast pump is in use. Release of oxytocin stimulated by breast pumping can result in surges of oxytocin release, which can lead to nonreassuring fetal status. Some fetuses who are unable to tolerate the release of oxytocin from breast pumping may react without stress to intravenous oxytocin administration, as this results in a small amount of oxytocin being released in a controlled manner.

In cases where homeopathic or herbal remedies have been used to induce labor, normal intermittent monitoring and assessment of maternal vital signs can be performed. If oxytocin is to be administered, the nurse should inform the physician or CNM of what has been given, the dose, the last time administered, and the immediate effects that were achieved. An assessment is performed before administration of pharmacologic substances.

Expected outcomes of nursing care include the following:

• The woman and family understand the induction process and are able to relate the advantages, disadvantages, risks, and possible outcomes.

• The woman's labor is successfully induced.

• The labor progresses at a normal rate and maternal vital signs remain in normal range.

• The fetal status remains reassuring throughout the labor period.

MEDIALINK   Care Plan Activity: Client with Pitocin for Labor Augmentation

MEDIALINK   Case Study: Client Undergoing Labor Induction

CLINICAL PATHWAY For Induction of Labor

Category	Immediate Care	Outcomes
Referral	Review prenatal record Advise CNM or physician of admission Anesthesia	◆ *Expected Outcomes* Appropriate resources identified and utilized
Assessments	Previous pregnancies, present pregnancy, and childbirth preparation Estimated gestational age of the fetus Assess woman's feelings regarding induction as well as knowledge base regarding the induction process Assess knowledge of breathing techniques. If woman does not have a method to use, teach breathing techniques before starting oxytocin infusion.	◆ *Expected Outcomes* Potential/actual complications identified
Teaching/ psychosocial	Provide emotional support through teaching and answering all questions	◆ *Expected Outcomes* Woman verbalizes/demonstrates understanding of information given
Nursing care management and reports	Examination of pregnant uterus (Leopold's maneuvers to determine fetal size and position) Vaginal examination to evaluate cervical readiness: • Ripe cervix feels soft to the examining finger, is located in a medial to anterior position, is more than 50% effaced, and is 2–3 cm dilated • Unripe cervix feels firm to the examining finger, is long and thick, is perhaps in a posterior position, and is dilated little or not at all Presence of contractions Membranes intact or ruptured Maternal vital signs and a 20 min baseline fetal monitoring strip prior to induction to determine fetal well-being Diagnostic studies: • Fetal maturity tests (L/S ratio, creatinine concentrations, ultrasonography), NST, CST, BPP • Maternal blood studies (CBC, hemoglobin, hematocrit, blood type, Rh factor) • Urinalysis Monitor for nausea, vomiting, hypotension, tachycardia, cardiac arrhythmias, headache, mental confusion, decreased urinary output Monitor FHR by continuous electronic fetal monitoring. Do not start infusion or advance rate (if induction has already begun) if FHR is not in range of 110–160 bpm, if decelerations are present, or if variability decreases. Evaluate and document maternal BP and pulse before beginning induction and then before each increase in infusion rate. Do not advance infusion rate in presence of maternal hypertension or hypotension or radical changes in pulse rate. If the woman becomes hypotensive: • Keep her on her side. May change to other side. • Discontinue oxytocin infusion • Increase rate of primary IV • Monitor FHR • Notify physician • Assess for cause of hypotension Evaluate and document contraction frequency, duration, and intensity prior to each increase in infusion rate Discontinue oxytocin infusion if: • Contractions are more frequent than every 2 min • Contraction duration exceeds 90 sec • Uterus does not relax between contractions Increase oxytocin IV infusion rate every 20 min until adequate contractions are achieved. Do not exceed an infusion rate of 20–40 mL/min. (Note: Protocols directing how often oxytocin is increased may vary from 15–60 min. See institutional protocol.) Check infusion pump to assure oxytocin is infusing. Check whether pump is on, chamber refills and empties, level of fluid in IV bottle becomes lower. If problem is found, correct and restart infusion at beginning dose. Check main IV site frequently. Check piggyback connection to primary tubing to assure solution is not leaking. Evaluate cervical dilatation by vaginal examination as indicated. Monitor FHR continuously (normal range is 110–160 bpm). In episodes of bradycardia (less than 110 bpm) lasting for more than 30 sec, administer oxygen by face mask at 7–10 L/min. Stop oxytocin infusion. Position woman on left side if quick recovery of FHR does not occur. Carefully evaluate fetal tachycardia (greater than 160 bpm). Sustained tachycardia may necessitate discontinuation of oxytocin infusion. Assess for presence of meconium staining. Notify physician.	◆ *Expected Outcomes* • Progression of labor and birth without difficulty • Potential/actual complications minimized

CLINICAL PATHWAY   For Induction of Labor continued

CATEGORY	IMMEDIATE CARE	OUTCOMES
Activity	Ambulate until 5–10 cm then bed rest Position woman in left lateral or semi-Fowler's position Encourage her to avoid supine position	◆ *Expected Outcomes* Activity individualized for woman
Comfort	Provide support to woman as she uses breathing techniques Encourage use of effluerage, backrub, and other supportive measures Assess need for analgesia or anesthesia	◆ *Expected Outcomes* Optimal comfort level maintained
Nutrition	IV/lactated Ringer's Ice chips, clear fluids	◆ *Expected Outcomes* Nutritional and hydration needs met
Elimination	Encourage voiding every 2 h. Monitor and record I&O.	◆ *Expected Outcomes* Intake and output WNL
Medications	Start primary IV as ordered Administer oxytocin in electrolyte solution (Piggyback oxytocin onto primary IV at closest site to IV needle insertion.) Pain meds PRN	◆ *Expected Outcomes* Induction/augmentation of labor occurs within expected parameters
Discharge planning/ home care	Photo packet Birth certificate worksheet Sibling visitation Car seat	◆ *Expected Outcomes* Individualized discharge teaching completed
Family involvement	Family visitation policy per institutional protocol Encourage significant other to stay close and assist with breathing of woman	◆ *Expected Outcomes* Family/support person involvement maximized
Date		

BP, blood presure; bpm, beats per minute; BPP, biophysical profile; CBC, complete blood count; CST, contraction stress test; FHR, fetal heart rate; I&O, intake and output; IV, intravenous; NST, nonstress test; PRN, as needed; WNL, within normal limits

CARE OF THE WOMAN DURING AN AMNIOTOMY

Amniotomy is the artificial rupture of the amniotic membranes (AROM). It is probably the most common procedure performed in obstetrics. Because the amniotomy requires that an instrument be inserted through the cervix, at least 2 cm of cervical dilatation must be present. The amniotomy may be performed as a method of induction of labor (to stimulate the beginning of labor), or it may be done to augment labor. If an amniotomy is done, the labor will probably be shortened by 1 to 2 hours (Simpson & Thorman, 2005). The use of amniotomy in early labor is associated with a higher incidence of cesarean birth (Simpson & Thorman, 2005). Amniotomy may also be performed during labor to allow access to the fetus in order to apply an internal fetal heart monitoring electrode to the scalp, to insert an intrauterine pressure catheter, or to obtain a fetal scalp blood sample for acid-base determination.

Advantages and Disadvantages of Amniotomy

Amniotomy as a method of labor induction has the following advantages:

1. The contractions elicited are similar to those of spontaneous labor.

2. There is usually no risk of hypertonus or rupture of the uterus, as with intravenous oxytocin induction.

3. The woman does not require the same intensive monitoring as with intravenous oxytocin induction.

4. EFM is facilitated because, once the membranes are ruptured, a fetal scalp electrode may be applied, an intrauterine catheter may be inserted, and scalp blood sampling for pH determinations may be done to assist in evaluating an FHR pattern.

5. The color and composition of amniotic fluid can be evaluated.

The disadvantages of amniotomy are as follows (Simpson & Thorman, 2005):

1. Once an amniotomy is done, birth should occur within 24 hours, because microorganisms can now invade the intrauterine cavity and cause amnionitis.

2. The danger of a prolapsed cord is increased once the membranes have ruptured, especially if the fetal presenting part is not firmly pressed down against the cervix.

3. Compression and molding of the fetal head are increased because of loss of the cushioning effect of the amniotic fluid for the fetal head during uterine contractions.

THROUGH THE EYES OF A NURSE

Labor Induction

FAMILY'S EXPERIENCE: "I can't take it anymore! I can't sleep; I can't bend over; I am exhausted! I have contractions all of the time. We sit and time them, and just when we think it is time to call and come to the hospital, they space out and go away! I am miserable; I just want to get this over. I really want to be induced at this point. I can't take it, I really can't!"

Her husband is concerned as well. "We have been to the hospital twice. She is having contractions on the (electronic fetal) monitor but they keep sending us home. She is crying and miserable. She is up all night and can't rest. What are the dangers of inducing her?"

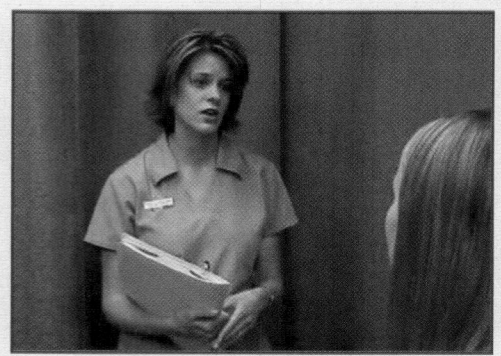

NURSE'S RESPONSE: "What you are feeling is very typical at this stage of pregnancy. It is often uncomfortable at the end stages of pregnancy. We can certainly let the nurse-midwife know that you would like to consider an induction.

"There are a variety of factors to consider. It is important to determine if there are any contraindications to induction and to review the risks with you. You are overdue, which is one of the indications for induction. The midwife will need to examine your cervix to determine if your cervix is ripe or favorable for induction. You can also explore whether you would like to try complementary methods first or if you would like to schedule a medical induction where oxytocin is administered."

NURSE'S ACTIONS AND RATIONALE:

The nurse provides reassurance that her feelings and the physical discomforts that she is experiencing are normal at this stage in pregnancy. The nurse explains that there are some contraindications to induction and these need to be reviewed with the healthcare provider. Tables 27–1 and 27–2 list absolute and relative contraindications to induction. The midwife will perform a vaginal examination to determine if the woman's cervix is favorable for induction. The Bishop score (see Table 27–3) is a measure of prelabor status criteria that is commonly used to determine if induction is likely to be successful. A score of 9 indicates that labor will most likely occur if induction is attempted.

4. Fetal injury can occur if the amniohook causes a laceration on the presenting part.

5. Bleeding can occur if an undiagnosed vasa previa is present.

6. Severe variable decelerations can occur, which increases the likelihood of a cesarean birth.

Amniotomy Procedure

Before an amniotomy is performed, the fetus is assessed for presentation, position, station, and FHR. Unless the fetal head is well engaged in the pelvis, some practitioners do not advocate an amniotomy because of the danger of prolapsed cord (refer to Chapter 26 ∞ for discussion of prolapsed cord). Other risks are abruptio placentae (because of rapid decompression of the uterus with the rapid loss of amniotic fluid), infection (because of the introduction of organisms into the cervix and intrauterine cavity), and amniotic fluid embolus (because of rapid decompression of the uterus and small amounts of fluid entering the maternal vascular system from under the edge of the placenta). These complications may also be associated with spontaneous rupture of membranes.

While performing a sterile vaginal examination, the physician or CNM introduces an amnihook (or other rupturing device) into the vagina, through the cervix, and against the amniotic membrane, which is in front of the fetal presenting part. A small tear is made in the amniotic membrane. Following rupture of the membrane, amniotic fluid is allowed to escape slowly.

NURSING CARE MANAGEMENT

The nurse explains the procedure to the woman. The fetal presentation, position, and station are assessed because amniotomy is usually delayed until engagement has occurred (to decrease the risk of a prolapsed cord when the fluid is expelled). The woman is positioned in a semireclining position and draped to provide privacy. Disposable underpads and/or towels are placed under the woman's buttocks to absorb the amniotic fluid. The FHR is assessed just before and immediately after the amniotomy, and the two FHR assessments are compared. If there are marked changes, the nurse should check for prolapse of the cord. The amniotic fluid is inspected for amount, color, odor, and the presence of meconium or blood. While wearing disposable gloves, the nurse cleanses and dries the perineal area and changes the disposable underpads. The nurse advises the woman that fluid will continue to be expelled from her vagina. Frequent pericare and pad changes should be done to increase client comfort. Because there is now an open pathway for organisms to ascend into the uterus, strict sterile technique must be observed during vaginal examinations. In addition, the number of vaginal examinations must be kept to a minimum to reduce the chance of introducing an infection, and the woman's temperature should be monitored every 2 hours. Bed rest is maintained unless the presenting part is engaged and is firmly against the cervix (to decrease the risk of prolapsed cord). The nurse needs to provide information about the amniotomy and the expected effects. Some

couples may worry that all the amniotic fluid will be gone and that they will experience a "dry birth." It is important for them to know that amniotic fluid is constantly produced.

CARE OF THE WOMAN DURING AMNIOINFUSION

Amnioinfusion (AI) is a technique by which a volume of warmed, sterile, normal saline or Ringer's lactate solution is introduced into the uterus through the use of an intrauterine pressure catheter (IUPC). AI can be used intrapartally to increase the volume of fluid when oligohydramnios is present and the physician wants either to prevent the possibility of variable decelerations by increasing the volume of amniotic fluid or to treat nonperiodic decelerations that are already occurring. The AI increases the volume of fluid, relieving pressure on the umbilical cord and promoting increased perfusion to the fetus. When AI is used for this indication or for prolonged decelerations in FHR patterns, the abnormal FHR pattern is usually relieved in 20 to 30 minutes (Ross, 2005).

AI has also been used for meconium dilution in the presence of medium to heavy meconium staining. Debate has ensued regarding the effectiveness of this regimen. A recent study revealed that 2000 women who had received AI for thick, meconium-stained amniotic fluid that was identified during labor did not show a decrease in the incidence of meconium aspiration syndrome, perinatal death, or major maternal or fetal disorders following AI (Fraser, Hofmeyr, Lede et al., 2005). The possibility that the meconium had already entered the fetal tracheobronchial tree before the onset of labor or that affected fetuses have been exposed to prolonged periods of nonreassuring fetal status are other factors that may contribute to the study's findings (Ross, 2005). Even with these findings, many practitioners continue to administer AIs in the presence of moderate to severe meconium staining. Further research is needed to examine these factors.

Contraindications to AI include amnionitis, hydramnios, uterine hypertonus, multiple gestation, known fetal anomaly, uterine anomaly, nonreassuring fetal status requiring immediate birth, nonvertex presentation, scalp pH below 7.2, placenta previa, vasa previa, or abruptio placentae (Hofmeyr, 2002). AI can also be associated with rare serious risk factors, including umbilical cord prolapse, amniotic fluid embolism, and uterine rupture (Fraser et al., 2005).

There is no one accepted protocol for AI. However, most procedures involve infusing a bolus of from 250 to 500 mL of warmed normal saline through an intrauterine catheter using an infusion pump over 20 to 30 minutes and then a constant administration of warmed saline until birth occurs.

NURSING CARE MANAGEMENT

The nurse is frequently the first person to detect changes in FHR associated with cord compression or to observe thick,

EVIDENCE-BASED PRACTICE

VAGINAL DISINFECTION FOR PREVENTING MOTHER-TO-CHILD TRANSMISSION OF INFECTION

Clinical Question

Is vaginal disinfection an effective procedure for preventing mother-to-child transmission of harmful pathogens, including human immunodeficiency virus (HIV) and group B streptococcus (GBS)?

The Evidence

Two systematic reviews focused on the effectiveness of vaginal disinfection. One review selected studies related to the prevention of mother-to-child transmission of HIV infection. Three reviewers independently appraised randomized trials comparing vaginal disinfection during labor with placebo or no treatment in known HIV-infected pregnant women. Outcome measures focused on infant and maternal mortality and morbidity. Only two studies met these criteria, but these studies were multisite and involved 708 women. A second review focused on GBS infections. Three authors assessed five randomized trials comparing vaginal disinfection, specifically with chlorhexidine, to placebo or no treatment. The studies that met the criteria included 2190 term and preterm infants. Outcomes included both colonization of GBS from newborn and the development of neonatal GBS infections, including skin infections, pneumonia, and meningitis.

What Is Effective?

A woman's vagina normally contains numerous bacteria that, in general, pose no danger to the newborn during passage through the birth canal. A notable exception is mother-to-child transmission of HIV infection, which is the primary mechanism through which children are infected. There is no evidence of an effect of vaginal disinfection on the transmission of HIV from mother to baby. Vaginal disinfection with chlorhexidine was effective in reducing the colo-

nization of GBS on neonatal skin, but had no effect on the actual development of GBS-related disease in these babies.

What Is Unclear?

Larger studies are needed to determine if vaginal disinfection might have an additive effect in protecting babies of HIV-infected mothers who are being treated with antiretroviral drugs. Given the low cost and ease of administration of this intervention, there continues to be a need for large-scale study of the effectiveness of this procedure in reducing neonatal infections. The authors of these reviews admit that the number of studies is too small to reach a definitive conclusion about the effectiveness (or lack of effectiveness) of vaginal disinfection in reducing both the colonization of pathogens and the subsequent development of disease.

Best Practice

There is insufficient evidence to support the usefulness of vaginal disinfection in the prevention of transmission of HIV infection from mother to the newborn. Although the procedure may reduce the actual pathogens that are colonized from the newborn's skin, it does not appear that this is protective against subsequent morbidity. Further study is needed before this procedure should be adopted as a routine nursing intervention.

Critical Thinking

Are there any conditions under which prevention of skin colonization of GBS is desirable and for whom vaginal disinfection is recommended?

REFERENCES: Stade, B., Shah, V., & Ohlsson, A. (2004). Vaginal chlorhexidine during labour to prevent early-onset neonatal group B streptococcal infection. *The Cochrane Database of Systematic Reviews* (3) (Article No.: CD003520.pub2).

Wiysonge, C., Shey, M., Shang, J., Sterne, J., & Brocklehurst, P. (2005). Vaginal disinfection for preventing mother-to-child transmission of HIV infection. *The Cochrane Database of Systematic Reviews* (4) (Article No.: CD003651.pub2).

---

meconium-stained amniotic fluid. When cord compression is suspected, the immediate intervention is to assist the laboring woman to another position in an effort to relieve the compression and to apply O₂ via face mask (see Chapter 26 ∞ for further discussion). If this intervention is not successful, an AI will be considered. The nurse helps with the AI and monitors the woman's vital signs (blood pressure, pulse, and respiration) and contraction status (frequency, duration, intensity, resting tone, and associated maternal discomfort). FHR is monitored by continuous EFM. The nurse should provide ongoing information to the laboring woman and her partner and answer questions as they arise. Comfort measures and positioning are very important because AI requires the woman to be on bed rest.

The AI should not cause pain or discomfort for the laboring woman other than the need for bed rest. The nurse needs to ensure that the fluid infused is being expelled from the woman's vagina. This is achieved with frequent examination of the woman's sanitary pad or an absorbent pad that is placed beneath

her buttocks. The woman should be advised that fluid will leak from her vagina. The nurse should change absorbent pads and provide pericare on a regular basis.

CARE OF THE WOMAN DURING AN EPISIOTOMY

An **episiotomy** is a surgical incision of the perineal body. Traditionally some physicians and CNMs performed episiotomies to prevent damage to the periurethra, perineum, anal sphincter, and rectum from lacerations during the birth; to prevent damage to the posterior wall of the vagina; to prevent jagged tears from lacerations; to reduce mechanical and metabolic risk to the fetus/newborn; to protect the maternal bladder; and to prevent future perineal relaxation. However, new research indicates that routine episiotomy is now typically performed because of time pressures, conventional education practices, birth setting, malpractice concerns, lack of experience with perineal stretching techniques, and interventionist practice patterns (Webb & Culhane, 2002).

Although the incidence of episiotomies in the United States has declined, it is still performed in one third of all vaginal births. Typically, nurse-midwives tend to perform fewer episiotomies than physicians (Davidson, 2002). Residents and hospital-based physicians tend to perform fewer routine episiotomies than physicians in private practice (Howden, Weber, & Meyn, 2004).

Even though the procedure is very common, its routine use has been questioned. The most current research indicates that there are no maternal advantages in performing routine episiotomies (Agency for Healthcare Research & Quality, 2005). Research suggests that, rather than protecting the perineum from lacerations, the presence of an episiotomy makes it more likely that the woman will have deep perineal tears. It has also been suggested that perineal lacerations heal more quickly in the absence of episiotomy (Agency for Healthcare Research & Quality, 2005). Major perineal trauma (extension to or through the anal sphincter) is *more* likely to occur if a midline episiotomy is performed. It is estimated that one in five women will experience an anal sphincter injury as a result of a vaginal delivery (Goetz & Lowry, 2005). Women who are allowed to tear spontaneously have less sexual dysfunction than women who have undergone episiotomies (Simpson & Thorman, 2005).

Additional complications associated with an episiotomy are blood loss, infection, pain, and perineal discomfort that may continue for days or weeks past birth, including dyspareunia (painful intercourse). Flatal incontinence (uncontrollable passage of gas) has also been reported (Eason, Labrecque, Marcoux et al., 2002). There are no scientific data to support the beliefs that episiotomies yield a shorter second stage, improved Apgar scores, or a decrease in perinatal asphyxia (Youssef, Ramalingam, MacLeod et al., 2005). In light of the debate over the value of episiotomy, it is now suggested that the procedure be used selectively to facilitate birth in the presence of maternal or fetal stress or when a shoulder dystocia is anticipated. There is debate on whether episiotomies should be performed to create more room in the presence of a breech presentation, multiple gestation, or a large-for-gestational-age infant (greater than 4000 g), or for the use of an instrument (forceps or vacuum extractor) to assist birth. Some researchers argue that midline episiotomy and vacuum-assisted birth should be avoided when a large baby is anticipated. Although many practitioners perform episiotomies when an instrument is being used to assist birth, new research suggests this may result in more third- and fourth-degree extensions (Youssef et al., 2005).

Risk Factors That Predispose Women to Episiotomy

Overall factors that place a woman at increased risk for an episiotomy are primigravid status, large or macrosomic fetus, occiput-posterior position, use of forceps or vacuum extractor, shoulder dystocia, and white race (Fitzpatrick & O'Herlihy, 2005). Other factors that predispose a woman to episiotomy

may be mitigated by nurses and physicians or CNMs. These include the following:

- Use of lithotomy position or other recumbent position (causes excessive perineal stretching)
- Encouraging or requiring sustained breath holding during second-stage pushing (causes excessive perineal stretching, can adversely affect blood flow in the mother and fetus, and encourages the woman to be responsive to caregiver directions rather than to her own urges to push spontaneously)
- Arbitrary time limit placed by the physician or CNM on the length of the second stage

Nursing advocacy is needed to promote selective rather than routine episiotomies. The nurse can begin by encouraging pregnant women to read about prenatal perineal preparation and to talk with the physician or CNM about their personal beliefs and the incidence of episiotomy in their practice. Nurses can share current research with nursing colleagues through staff meetings and explore and strongly encourage nursing care interventions that avoid the lithotomy position. The woman should be encouraged to respond to her body's urges to push during the second stage. Just as clients ask physicians and CNMs about their episiotomy philosophy and incidence, clients may at some time in the future ask labor and birthing nurses to provide information about their actions to help decrease episiotomy rates. It is imperative that each nurse continue to stay current about new information and research in order to maintain current practice standards.

Episiotomy Procedure

The episiotomy is performed with a sharp scissors that has rounded points, just before birth, when approximately 3 to 4 cm of the fetal head is visible during a contraction (Cunningham et al., 2005). There are two types of episiotomy: midline and mediolateral (Figure 27–3 ◆). A midline episiotomy is performed along the median raphe of the perineum. It extends down from the vaginal orifice to the fibers of the rectal sphincter. This type of episiotomy avoids muscle fibers and major blood vessels because it divides the insertions of the superficial perineal muscles (Blackburn, 2007). A midline episiotomy is preferred if the perineum is of adequate length and no difficulty is anticipated during the birth, because it entails less blood loss, is easy to repair, and heals with less discomfort for the mother. The major disadvantage is that a tear of the midline incision may extend through the anal sphincter and rectum (Myers & Goldberg, 2006).

In the presence of a short perineum, macrosomia, and instrument-assisted birth (use of forceps or vacuum extractor), a mediolateral episiotomy provides more room and decreases the possibility of a traumatic extension into the rectum. The mediolateral episiotomy begins in the midline of the posterior fourchette (to avoid incision into the Bartholin's gland) and extends at a 45-degree angle downward to the right or left (the direction depending on the handedness of the clinician). The mediolateral episiotomy may be complicated by greater blood loss, a longer healing period, and more postpartal discomfort (Myers & Goldberg, 2006).

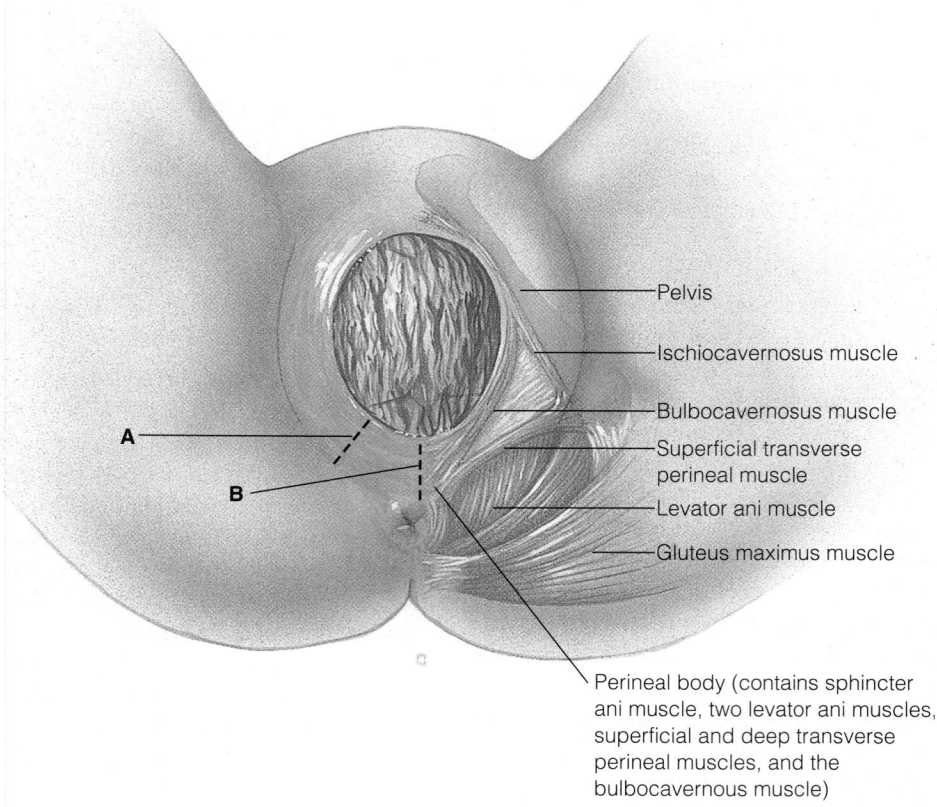

Pelvis

Ischiocavernosus muscle

Bulbocavernosus muscle

Superficial transverse perineal muscle

Levator ani muscle

Gluteus maximus muscle

Perineal body (contains sphincter ani muscle, two levator ani muscles, superficial and deep transverse perineal muscles, and the bulbocavernous muscle)

Figure 27–3 ◆ The two most common types of episiotomies are midline and mediolateral. *A,* Right mediolateral. *B,* Midline.

The episiotomy is usually performed with regional or local anesthesia but may be performed without anesthesia in emergency situations. It is generally suggested that as crowning occurs, the distention of the tissues causes numbing. Adequate anesthesia must be given for the repair.

Repair of the episiotomy (episiorrhaphy) and any lacerations is performed either during the period between birth of the baby and before expulsion of the placenta or after expulsion of the placenta. Many providers wait until after expulsion of the placenta in case a manual removal of the placenta or a uterine exploration is indicated (Myers & Goldberg, 2006).

NURSING CARE MANAGEMENT

The woman needs to be supported during the episiotomy and the repair because she may feel some pressure sensations. It is not uncommon for the woman to feel a "pulling" or "tugging" sensation. In the absence of adequate anesthesia, she may feel pain. Placing a hand on her shoulder and talking with her can provide comfort and distraction from the repair process. If the woman is having more discomfort than she can comfortably handle, the nurse needs to act as an advocate in communicating the woman's needs to the physician or CNM. At all times, the woman needs to be the one who decides whether the amount of discomfort is tolerable, and she should never be told, "This

doesn't hurt." She is the person experiencing the discomfort, and her evaluation needs to be respected. If there are just a few (three to five) stitches left, she may choose to forgo more local anesthesia, but she should be given the choice. For women with severe pain or anxiety, intravenous medication such as Demerol or Nubain can be administered for both pain and anxiety control.

The nurse notes the type of episiotomy on the birth record. This information should also be included in a report to the postpartum nurse so that adequate assessments can be made and relief measures can be instituted if necessary.

Pain relief measures may begin immediately after birth with application of an ice pack to the perineum. For optimal effect, the ice pack should be applied for 20 to 30 minutes and removed for at least 20 minutes before being reapplied. This is advisable because the ice causes vasoconstriction; however, if the ice pack is left in place more than 30 minutes, vasodilation and subsequent edema may occur. The perineal tissues should be assessed frequently to prevent injury from the ice pack. The episiotomy site is inspected every 15 minutes during the first hour after the birth for redness, swelling, tenderness, and hematomas. As a part of postpartal care, the mother will need instruction in perineal hygiene care and comfort measures. (See Chapter 35 ∞ for additional discussion of relief measures for the immediate postpartum period).

It is important for nurses to recognize that perineal pain continues for a period of time. Women who experience prolonged pain tend to have other problems, such as breastfeeding

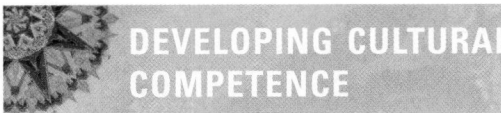

CANADIAN ORTHODOX JEWISH WOMEN

Although many North American women have specific beliefs and expectations for childbirth, other cultural or religious groups may not verbalize specific requests or ideas for their labor experience. Canadian Orthodox Jewish women typically do not express their preferences but instead depend on their healthcare practitioner to make decisions regarding procedures that may be indicated. They typically view healthcare providers as authority figures and participate less in their own healthcare decision making.

difficulties and depression, and are more reluctant to reestablish sexual activity. Risk factors for subsequent lacerations include use of repeat episiotomy and instrument-assisted births (Youssef et al., 2005).

CARE OF THE WOMAN DURING FORCEPS-ASSISTED BIRTH

Forceps are designed to assist the birth of a fetus by providing traction or by providing the means to rotate the fetal head to an occiput-anterior position. In medical literature and practice, **forceps-assisted birth** is also known as *instrumental delivery, operative delivery,* or *operative vaginal delivery.* There are many different types of forceps, each with special functions. For example, Piper forceps are designed to be used with a breech presentation (buttocks as presenting part); they are applied after the birth of the body, when the fetal head is still in the birth canal and assistance is needed. In conversational language, Piper forceps are said to be applied to the aftercoming head. All other forceps are used in situations when the fetus is in a cephalic (head down) presentation. In such situations, the forceps are applied to the sides of the head. The type of forceps used is determined by the physician assisting with the birth.

Criteria for Forceps Application

ACOG has classified the definitions of forceps applications into three categories: outlet, low, and midforceps. Criteria for *outlet forceps* application are as follows (Cunningham et al., 2005):

1. Forceps are applied when the fetal skull has reached the pelvic floor and is at or on the perineum. (There is bulging of the perineum.)

2. The scalp is visible between contractions without separating the labia. (Earlier in labor, as the woman pushes during the contraction, the fetal scalp may be visible, but when the pushing effort ceases, the scalp recedes and is no longer visible. This criterion indicates that the scalp remains visible even when the woman is not pushing.)

3. The sagittal suture is not more than 45 degrees from the midline. The sagittal suture is the anterior-posterior suture on the top of the fetal head. At this point in a spontaneous birth, extension has almost been completed, external rotation is beginning, and the sagittal suture is between the midline and 45 degrees from the midline. (For example, think of a clock face. If 12:00 is the maternal symphysis pubis and the fetus is in left occiput anterior (LOA), the sagittal suture and the occiput are between 12:00 and 1:30.) (See Chapter 22 ∞). The important aspect of this criterion is that with outlet forceps, the fetal head is moving naturally from extension to external rotation, and the forceps are being used to guide or lift the head out.

The criterion for *low forceps* application is that the leading edge (presenting part) of the fetal skull must be at a station of plus 2 (+ 2) or below (for example, + 3) but not on the pelvic floor. The rotation (internal rotation, which is part of the cardinal movements) of the fetal head is less than 45 degrees (right or left occiput anterior to occiput anterior, or right or left occiput posterior to occiput posterior) (Cunningham et al., 2005).

The criterion for *midforceps* application is that the fetal head must be engaged (largest diameter of the head reaches or passes through the pelvic inlet), but the leading edge (presenting part) of the fetal skull is above a plus 2 (+ 2) station (for example + 1, 0, − 1, − 2). When midforceps are used, the goal is to apply traction, and, frequently, to rotate the head and facilitate the vaginal birth.

High forceps are not indicated in current obstetric practice. A woman whose fetus is at a station of −3 or is above the pelvic inlet should give birth by cesarean. Types of forceps are depicted in Figure 27–4 ◆.

Indications for Use of Forceps

Indications for the use of forceps include the presence of any condition that threatens the mother or fetus and that can be relieved by birth. Conditions that put the woman at risk include heart disease, acute pulmonary edema or pulmonary compromise, certain neurological conditions, intrapartal infection, prolonged second stage, or exhaustion. Fetal conditions include premature placental separation, prolapsed umbilical cord, and nonreassuring fetal status. Forceps may be used electively to shorten the second stage of labor and spare the woman's pushing effort (when exhaustion or heart disease is present) or when regional anesthesia has affected the woman's motor innervation and she cannot push effectively. In the past, outlet forceps have been used to protect the head of a preterm infant during birth; however, the advantages of this practice are now being questioned (Cunningham et al., 2005).

Risk factors for a forceps- or vacuum-assisted birth (discussion to follow) are as follows (Cunningham et al., 2005):

- Nulliparity
- Maternal age (35 and over)
- Maternal height of less than 150 cm (4 ft 11 in)
- Pregnancy weight gain of more than 15 kg (33 lb)
- Postdate gestation (41 weeks or more)

MEDIALINK

Forceps Delivery

Figure 27–4 ◆ Forceps are composed of a blade, shank, and handle and may have a cephalic and pelvic curve. (Note labels on Piper and Tucker-McLean forceps.) The blades may be fenestrated (open) or solid. The front and lateral views of these forceps illustrate differences in blades, open and closed shanks, and cephalic and pelvic curves. Elliot, Simpson, and Tucker-McLean forceps are used as outlet forceps. Kielland and Barton forceps are used for midforceps rotations. Piper forceps are used to provide traction and flexion of the aftercoming head (the head comes after the body) of a fetus in breech presentation.

- Epidural anesthesia
- Infant presentation other than occipitoanterior
- Presence of dystocia
- Presence of a midline episiotomy
- Abnormal FHR tracing

Neonatal and Maternal Risks

Some newborns may develop a small area of ecchymosis or edema, or both, along the sides of the face as a result of forceps application. Caput succedaneum or cephalhematoma (and subsequent hyperbilirubinemia) may occur as well as transient facial paralysis. Other reported complications include low Apgar scores, retinal hemorrhage, corneal abrasions, ocular trauma, other trauma (Erb's palsy, fractured clavicle), elevated neonatal bilirubin levels, and prolonged infant hospital stay (Cunningham et al., 2005).

Maternal risks may include trauma such as lacerations of the birth canal, periurethral lacerations, and extensions of a median episiotomy into the anus, resulting in increased bleeding, bruising, hematomas, and pelvic floor injuries (Caughey, Sandberg, Zlatnik et al., 2005). Women who give birth with the assistance of forceps are more likely to have a third- or fourth-degree laceration and report more perineal pain and sexual problems in the postpartum period (Caughey et al., 2005; Thompson, Roberts, Currie et al., 2002). In addition, an increase in postpartum infections, cervical lacerations, and prolonged hospital stays has been reported (Caughey et al., 2005). Women who have given birth with forceps may also experience urinary and rectal incontinence, anal sphincter injury, and postpartum metritis (Cunningham et al., 2005).

Prerequisites for Forceps Application and Birth

It is very important that all of the prerequisites be met before the forceps procedure is attempted. The prerequisites are as follows (Cunningham et al., 2005):

- The physician must be knowledgeable about the advantages and disadvantages of different types of forceps and their use.
- The cervix must be completely dilated.
- The fetal head must be engaged and the station, presentation, and exact position of the head must be known. The fetus should be in a vertex or a face presentation with the chin anterior.
- Amniotic membranes must be ruptured to allow a firm grasp on the fetal head.
- The type of pelvis should be identified, because certain pelvic types do not permit rotation. In addition, there must be no disproportion between the fetal head and the maternal pelvis.
- Maternal bladder should be empty.
- There must be no obstructions to the birth below the fetal head, such as an incurving coccyx that will not allow the fetus to pass or a disproportion between the size of the head and the outlet or the midpelvis.
- Adequate anesthesia must be given for the type of forceps procedure that is anticipated. For instance, low forceps may be done with a pudendal block; however, midforceps or a rotation of more than 45 degrees requires an epidural, spinal-epidural, or general anesthesia.

Trial or Failed Forceps Procedure

The use of forceps or vacuum may be considered when the clinician believes a successful outcome can occur. In a trial forceps procedure, the physician attempts to use forceps with the knowledge that there could be a degree of cephalopelvic disproportion. A complete setup for immediate cesarean birth needs to be available before the forceps are applied. If a good application cannot be obtained or if no descent occurs with the application, a vacuum technique can be attempted. If this yields no descent, then a cesarean birth is the method of choice.

NURSING CARE MANAGEMENT

The nurse directs nursing care measures toward the variable(s) that may be positively affected by specific nursing interventions. For instance, dystocia may be corrected by changing maternal position, ambulation, rocking, frequent bladder emptying, and so on. FHR abnormalities may be af-

fected by utero-placental-fetal circulation, so the nurse could support ambulation (if not contraindicated), frequent position changes, intake of adequate fluids, and monitoring to detect early FHR changes.

If a forceps-assisted birth is required, the nurse explains the procedure briefly to the woman. With adequate regional anesthesia, the woman should feel some pressure but no pain. The nurse encourages her to avoid pushing during application of the forceps (Figure 27–5 ◆ depicts the application). The nurse monitors contractions and advises the physician when one is present because traction is applied only with a contraction. During the contraction, as the forceps are applied, the nurse again advises the woman to avoid pushing. With each contraction, *after the forceps are in place,* the physician provides traction on the forceps as the woman pushes. It is not uncommon to observe mild bradycardia as traction is applied to the forceps. This bradycardia results from head compression and is transient.

Following birth, the newborn is assessed for facial edema, bruising, caput succedaneum, cephalhematoma, and any sign of cerebral edema. In the fourth stage, the nurse assesses the woman for perineal swelling, bruising, hematoma, excessive bleeding, and hemorrhage. In the postpartum period it is important to assess for signs of infection if lacerations occurred during the procedure (Mazouni, Bretelle, Collette et al., 2005).

The nurse answers questions and reiterates explanations provided, reviews nursing assessments of the woman and her newborn, and provides opportunities for the woman and family to ask further questions. Some women may feel a sense of loss or failure as a result of needing forceps for birth. The nurse provides reassurance to the woman and her family.

CARE OF THE WOMAN DURING VACUUM EXTRACTION

Vacuum extraction is an obstetric procedure used to assist the birth of a fetus by applying suction to the fetal head. The vacuum extractor accounts for 68% of all operative vaginal births. Its use has increased by 41% since 1990 and continues to rise (Demissie, Rhoads, Smulian et al., 2004). The vacuum extractor is composed of a soft suction cup attached to a suction bottle (pump) by tubing. The suction cup, which comes in various sizes, is placed against the occiput of the fetal head. Care must be taken to ensure that no cervical or vaginal tissue is trapped under the cup. The pump is used to create negative pressure (suction) of approximately 50 to 60 mm Hg. An artificial caput ("chignon") is formed as the fetal scalp is pulled into the cup. The physician or CNM then applies traction in coordination with uterine contractions. The fetal head should descend with each contraction until it emerges from the vagina (Figure 27–6 ◆).

Research indicates that negative suction applied for more than 10 minutes is associated with a greater incidence of scalp injury. The longer the duration of suction, the more likely the newborn will have scalp injury. Although there are no data on

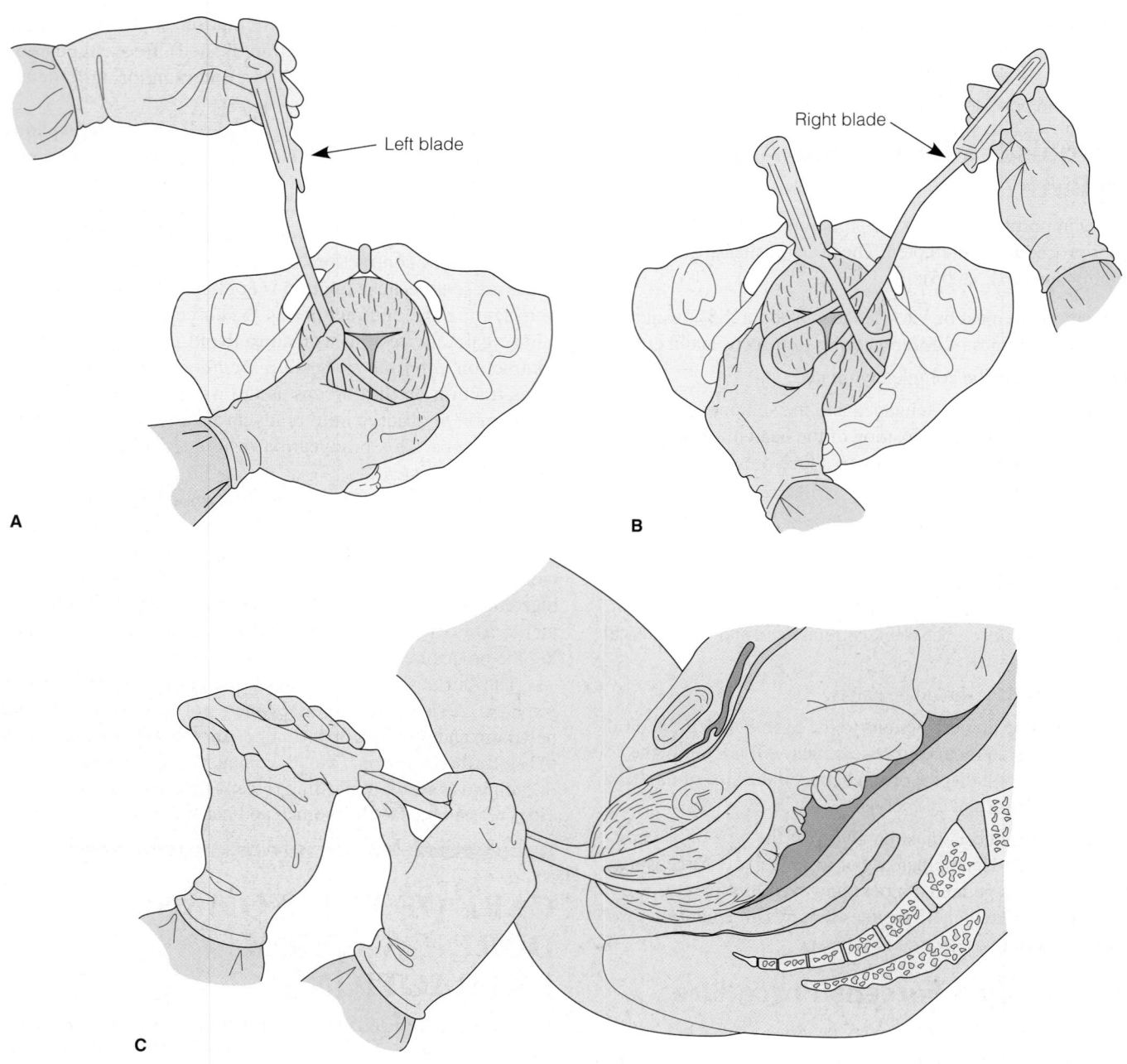

Figure 27–5 ◆ Application of forceps in occiput-anterior (OA) position. *A,* The left blade is inserted along the left side wall of the pelvis over the parietal bone. *B,* The right blade is inserted along the right side wall of the pelvis over the parietal bone. *C,* With correct placement of the blades, the handles lock easily. During uterine contractions, traction is applied to the forceps in a downward and outward direction to follow the birth canal.

the duration of use, ACOG advises a 30-minute time limit (Liu, Heaman, Joseph et al., 2005). Many practitioners limit the time to 20 minutes. Although there are no specifications on the number of attempts, failure to descend with multiple attempts is an indicator that a cesarean birth may be needed. In addition, if more than three "pop-offs" occur (the suction cup pops off the fetal head), the procedure should be discontinued.

The most common indication for the use of the vacuum extractor is a prolonged second stage of labor or nonreassuring heart rate pattern. Vacuum extraction is also used to relieve the woman of pushing effort, or when analgesia or fatigue interferes

with her ability to push effectively, or in cases of nonreassuring fetal status when prompt birth is indicated. The vacuum extractor is preferred to forceps in cases of borderline cephalopelvic disproportion (CPD), when successful passage of the fetal head requires all potential space inside the vaginal canal. True CPD is an absolute contraindication to vacuum extraction. Other contraindications include nonvertex presentations, maternal or suspected fetal coagulation defects, known or suspected hydrocephalus, and fetal scalp trauma (Cunningham et al., 2005). Relative contraindications include suspected fetal macrosomia, high fetal station, face or breech presentation, gestation less

RESEARCH IN PRACTICE

FACTORS PREDICTING SEVERE PERINEAL TRAUMA DURING CHILDBIRTH: ROLE OF FORCEPS DELIVERY ROUTINELY COMBINED WITH MEDIOLATERAL EPISIOTOMY

What is this study about? Severe trauma to the perineal region during birth is associated with a number of postpartum complications. In the immediate postpartum period, mothers with third- and fourth-degree tears are at higher risk of infection and rectovaginal fistulae. Although primary surgical repair is generally associated with good outcomes, long-term consequences may include perineal pain, fecal incontinence, or sexual dysfunction for years after birth. Although fourth-degree tears to the anal sphincter are relatively rare, these injuries are a severe complication of birth. The objective of this study was to determine the variables that may influence the occurrence of perineal lacerations that involve the external sphincter. The researchers sought to identify those women with a higher risk for severe perineal trauma.

How was this study done? Data were collected from chart review of 5377 women who experienced vaginal birth over a 5-year period in two European hospitals. Of the 5044 spontaneous vaginal births and 233 instrument-assisted births, 4.8% experienced third- or fourth-degree perineal trauma. One hundred fifty-five comparison subjects were randomly selected from mothers who did not have severe perineal trauma. Variables collected from the records included maternal age, parity, gestational age, tobacco use, gestational diabetes or hypertension, use of peridural anesthesia, duration of the first and second stages of labor, birth weight, use of mediolateral episiotomy with and without forceps, induction of la-

bor, and infant head diameter and shoulder circumference. Data were analyzed using a statistical technique that determines if the individual variables are associated with the traumatic outcome, but which can also determine if interactions between variables may be responsible for the injury.

What were the results of the study? Severe perineal tears were not associated with maternal age, gestational age, gestational diabetes, hypertension, or tobacco use. The use of peridural anesthesia, labor induction, and head or shoulder circumference of the infant were unrelated to perineal trauma. Women with greater than third-degree tearing were more likely to be nulliparous, have longer first and second stages of labor, have an episiotomy and/or forceps delivery, and have babies higher in birth weight. These variables were inter-related; the only independent factors that had a clear effect were higher birth weight and forceps birth.

What additional questions might I have? Is it possible that some of these risk factors would be more significant if larger samples were studied? Which risk factors are associated with less severe perineal injury?

How can I use this study? If a mother has a number of risk factors identified in this study, then the nurse can include assessments for perineal trauma in the postpartum nursing care plan. First-time mothers with prolonged labor, high birth weight, and assisted birth should be carefully evaluated for signs of perineal trauma so that infection and fistulae can be avoided in the postpartum period.

Hudelist, G., Gell'n, J., Singer, C., Ruecklinger, E., Czerwenka, K., Kandolf, O., et al. (2005). Factors predicting severe perineal trauma during childbirth: Role of forceps delivery routinely combined with mediolateral episiotomy. *American Journal of Obstetrics & Gynecology, 192,* 875–881.

than 34 weeks, incompletely dilated cervix, and previous fetal scalp blood sampling (Cunningham et al., 2005).

Neonatal complications include scalp lacerations, bruising, subgaleal hematomas, cephalhematomas, intracranial hemorrhages, subconjunctival hemorrhages, neonatal jaundice, fractured clavicle, Erb's palsy, damage to the sixth and seventh cranial nerves, retinal hemorrhage, and fetal death. In addition, there is an increased incidence of shoulder dystocia (Cunningham et al., 2005). There appear to be more neonatal complications and injuries with use of a metal suction cup device than with soft cup devices. In the presence of a preterm gestation, risk of periventricular-intraventricular hemorrhage (PV-IVH) has been a concern, and some studies provide conflicting recommendations. Maternal complications include perineal trauma, edema, third- and fourth-degree lacerations, postpartum pain, and infection (Demissie et al., 2004). Women who give birth with the aid of a vacuum extractor report more sexual difficulties in the postpartum period. Maternal genital tract and anal sphincter injuries occur less frequently with the vacuum extractor than with forceps.

In 1998, the US Food and Drug Administration (FDA) released a health advisory statement that vacuum extraction can

cause serious or fatal complications. Twelve deaths and nine serious injuries occurred between 1994 and 1998. The FDA recommended caution in using rocking movements when using the device. They also recommended that pediatricians be alerted when a vacuum-assisted birth occurred so the infant can be closely monitored for related injuries. In addition, the following guidelines are recommended when a birth is facilitated by a vacuum extractor (Cunningham et al., 2005):

1. The criteria used to evaluate the appropriateness of a forceps birth should also be used to determine the appropriateness of a vacuum birth (station).

2. The same indications and contraindications should be used for both forceps and vacuum births.

3. The presenting part must be vertex and must be at 0 station or below.

4. Vacuum-assisted births should be performed only by an experienced practitioner.

5. The procedure should be terminated immediately if descent does not occur or if the vacuum device pops off more than three times.

MEDIALINK

Application: Vacuum Extraction Delivery

Figure 27–6 ◆ Vacuum extractor traction. *A,* The cup is placed on the fetal occiput, creating suction. Traction is applied in a downward and outward direction. *B,* Traction continues in a downward direction as the fetal head begins to emerge from the vagina. *C,* Traction is maintained to lift the fetal head out of the vagina.

NURSING CARE MANAGEMENT

There are different types of vacuum extractors. The nurse must be familiar with the types used within the birthing setting and learn the pressure limits of each type.

The nurse should inform the woman about what is happening during the procedure. If adequate regional anesthesia has been administered, the woman feels only pressure during the procedure. The nurse pumps the vacuum to the appropriate level to provide suction by the physician or CNM. The FHR is auscultated at least every 5 minutes or assessed by continuous EFM. The parents need to be informed that the caput (chignon) on the baby's head will disappear within 2 to 3 days.

The nurse continues to assess the newborn for complications such as bruising, newborn jaundice, cephalhematomas, intracranial hemorrhage, and retinal hemorrhages.

CARE OF THE FAMILY DURING CESAREAN BIRTH

Cesarean birth is the birth of the infant through an abdominal and uterine incision. Cesarean birth is one of the oldest surgical procedures known. Until the 20th century, cesareans were primarily equated with an attempt to save the fetus of a dying woman. As the maternal and perinatal morbidity and mortality rates associated with cesarean birth steadily decreased throughout the 20th century, the rate of cesarean births increased. In 1965, cesarean births constituted 4.5% of all births and progressed to a high of 29.1% in 2004 (Cunningham et al., 2005; Martin, Hamilton, Menacker et al., 2005). The cesarean birth rate has risen by 40% since 1996 (Martin et al., 2005). In some countries, the incidence has been much lower throughout the 20th century. Boliva has one of the lowest cesarean birth rates in the world, accounting for only 5% of all births. Sweden and the Netherlands have maintained cesarean birth rates of 10% for decades. Many Latin American countries also have low rates, including Peru with a cesarean birth rate below 10%, and Honduras with a rate of 12%. England and Canada have rates below 20%. However, some countries, such as Chile, have rates as high as 40% (Walker, Turnbull, & Wilkinson, 2002).

The rising cesarean birth rate has created marked concern among various practitioner groups. ACOG created a task force in 2000 to address concerns regarding the rise in cesarean birth rates. The committee recommended two benchmarks be achieved by 2010. They recommended a primary cesarean rate of 15.5% for women who were greater than 37 gestational weeks with a cephalic singleton presentation and a vaginal birth rate of 37% in women who have had one previous cesarean birth after 37 gestational weeks (Cunningham et al., 2005).

Many factors affect the cesarean birth rate, and they need to be considered in discussions about decreasing the current rate in the United States. These factors include a rising number of nulliparous women, who are at an increased risk for cesareans, giving birth; a rise in the maternal age, which is associated with a higher incidence of cesarean birth; changing philosophies regarding the best method of birth with a breech presentation; interpretations of EFM tracings; a decrease in the use of forceps and vacuum extractors to facilitate a vaginal birth; and a dramatic rise in obesity, another risk factor for cesarean birth. Other risks include changing practice related to vaginal birth after cesarean birth, increased use of epidural anesthesia, physician convenience, and type of provider (Cunningham et al., 2005). Interestingly, some women are now requesting a primary cesarean birth because of fear of labor, convenience, and concern about pelvic floor damage that could result in long-term medical complications (Nygaard & Cruikshank, 2003).

One of the most significant factors that has dominated the 21st century is the concern related to medical malpractice litigation. Failure to perform a cesarean birth is one of the most common malpractice claims in obstetrical practice. Although there is no association between performing a cesarean birth and a reduction in childhood neurological problems, including a decline in neonatal seizures or cerebral palsy, fear of litigation remains a driving force in obstetrical practice (Physicians Insurance Association of America, 2002). The malpractice crisis has become so grave that some CNMs and physicians are abandoning obstetrical practice because of fear of litigation and high malpractice premiums.

Indications

Cesarean births are performed in the presence of a variety of maternal and fetal conditions. Commonly accepted indications include complete placenta previa, CPD, placental abruption, active genital herpes, umbilical cord prolapse, failure to progress in labor, proven nonreassuring fetal status, and benign and malignant tumors that obstruct the birth canal. Indications that are more controversial include breech presentation, previous cesarean birth, major congenital anomalies, cervical cerclage, severe Rh isoimmunization, and maternal preference for cesarean birth. The majority of cesarean births performed in the United States are done because of a previous cesarean birth and dystocia (Cunningham et al., 2005).

Maternal Mortality and Morbidity

Cesarean births have a higher maternal mortality rate than vaginal births. In the United States, women undergoing a cesarean birth have a fourfold risk of death when compared with women who give birth vaginally (Harper, Byington, & Espeland, 2003). In England, emergency cesarean birth has a ninefold risk of death when compared with vaginal delivery, and elective cesarean births have a threefold risk (Cunningham et al., 2005). Perinatal morbidity is also considerably higher in women who have had a cesarean. Common postoperative complications include infection, reactions to anesthesia agents, blood clots, and bleeding. Women who have had a cesarean birth are twice as likely to be rehospitalized within 60 days of birth when compared with women who have had a vaginal birth. Other sources of maternal morbidity that are directly associated with cesarean birth include ureteral injury, bladder laceration, and wound infection (Cunningham et al., 2005).

Surgical Techniques

Cesarean birth requires both a skin and a uterine incision, which are not necessarily the same type of incision.

SKIN INCISIONS

The skin incision for a cesarean birth is either transverse (Pfannenstiel) or vertical and is not indicative of the type of incision made into the uterus. The type of skin incision is determined by time factor, client preference, cosmetic reasons, or physician preference.

The transverse incision is made across the lowest and narrowest part of the abdomen. Because the incision is made just below the pubic hair line, it is almost invisible after healing. Other advantages of this type of incision include less bleeding and better healing. The limitations of this type of skin incision are that it does not allow for extension of the incision if needed. Because it usually requires more time, this incision is used when time is not of the essence (e.g., with failure to progress and no fetal or maternal stress). This type of incision may result in suboptimal visualization, especially in obese women. This type of incision may also develop more scar tissue if subsequent surgeries, such as repeat cesarean, are performed (Kadir, Khan, Wilcock et al., 2006).

The vertical (infraumbilical midline) incision is made between the navel and the symphysis pubis. This incision is quicker and is therefore preferred in cases of nonreassuring fetal status when rapid birth is indicated, with preterm or macrosomic infants, or when the woman is obese (Kadir et al., 2006).

UTERINE INCISIONS

The type of uterine incision depends on the need for the cesarean. The choice of incision affects the woman's opportunity for a subsequent vaginal birth and her risks of a ruptured uterine scar with a subsequent pregnancy.

The two major locations of uterine incisions are the lower uterine segment and the upper segment of the uterine corpus (Figure 27–7 ◆).

The most common lower uterine segment incision is a transverse incision (Figure 27–7, A), which is preferred for the following reasons (Cunningham et al., 2005):

1. The lower segment is the thinnest portion of the uterus and involves less blood loss.
2. It requires only moderate dissection of the bladder from underlying myometrium.
3. It is easier to repair, although repair takes longer.
4. The site is less likely to rupture during subsequent pregnancies.
5. There is a decreased chance of adherence of bowel or omentum to the incision line.

The disadvantages include the following:

1. It takes longer to make a transverse incision.
2. It is limited in size because of the presence of major blood vessels on either side of the uterus.
3. It has a greater tendency to extend laterally into the uterine vessels.

Figure 27–7 ◆ Uterine incisions for a cesarean birth. *A*, This transverse incision in the lower uterine segment is called a Kerr incision. *B*, The Sellheim incision is a vertical incision in the lower uterine segment. *C*, This view illustrates the classic uterine incision that is done in the body (corpus) of the uterus. The classic incision was commonly done in the past and is associated with increased risk of uterine rupture in subsequent pregnancies and labor.

4. The incision may stretch and become a thin window, but it usually does not create problems clinically until subsequent labor ensues.

The lower uterine segment vertical incision is preferred for multiple gestation, abnormal presentation, if the woman has had no labor, and for preterm and macrosomic fetuses (Figure 27–7, *B* ◆).

Disadvantages of this incision are as follows:

1. The incision may extend downward into the cervix.
2. More extensive dissection of the bladder is needed to keep the incision in the lower uterine segment.
3. If the incision extends upward into the upper segment, hemostasis and closure are more difficult.
4. The vertical incision carries a higher risk of rupture with subsequent labor. Consequently, once a vertical incision is performed, future births need to be via cesarean.

One other incision, the classic incision, was the method of choice for many years but it is used infrequently now (Figure 27–7, *C* ◆). This vertical incision was made into the upper uterine segment. More blood loss resulted, and it was more difficult to repair. Most important, it carried an increased risk of uterine rupture with subsequent pregnancy, labor, and birth, because the upper uterine segment is the most contractile portion of the uterus.

The primary indications for a classical incision include a very small fetus in breech presentation when the lower uterine segment is not thinned out, morbid maternal obesity that precludes safe access to the lower uterine segment, a macrosomic fetus in transverse position with the shoulder impacted in the birth canal, inability to expose the lower uterine segment because of scarring of the maternal bladder associated with previous surgery, myoma in the lower uterine segment, cervical cancer, and placenta percreta (Cunningham et al., 2005). Students should recognize that these situations are very rare and that classical uterine incisions are rarely performed.

Analgesia and Anesthesia

There is no perfect anesthesia for cesarean birth. Each has its advantages, disadvantages, possible risks, and side effects. Goals for analgesia and anesthesia administration include safety, comfort, and emotional satisfaction for the client. See Chapter 25. ∞

NURSING CARE MANAGEMENT
Preparation for Cesarean Birth

Because one out of every four births is a cesarean, preparing the woman and family for this possibility is an integral part of prenatal education (Martin et al., 2005). Nurses should encourage all pregnant women and their partners to discuss with their obstetrician or CNM what approach would be taken in the event of a cesarean. They can also discuss their needs and desires as a couple under those circumstances. Their preferences may include the following:

- Participating in the choice of anesthetic
- Presence of the father (or significant other) during the procedures in the recovery or postpartum room
- Audio or video recording and/or photographing of the birth
- Delayed instillation of eye drops to promote eye contact between parent and infant in the first hour after birth
- Physical contact or holding the newborn while on the operating room table or in the recovery room (If the mother cannot hold the newborn, the father can hold the baby for her.)
- Breastfeeding immediately after the surgery has been completed
- Preparation that may be done, such as abdominal prep, insertion of an indwelling bladder catheter, and starting an intravenous infusion and epidural placement
- Description or viewing of the operating room
- Types of anesthesia for birth and analgesia available postpartum
- Sensations that may be experienced
- Roles of significant others
- Interaction with the newborn
- Immediate recovery phase
- Postpartal phase

Preparing the woman for surgery involves more than the procedures of establishing intravenous lines and a urinary indwelling catheter or doing an abdominal prep. As discussed previously, good communication skills are essential in assisting the couple. Therapeutic use of touch and eye contact (if culturally acceptable and possible) do much to maintain reality orientation and control. These measures reduce anxiety for the woman during the stressful preparatory period.

If the cesarean birth is scheduled and not an emergency, the nurse has ample time for preoperative teaching. The woman needs to practice her turning, coughing, and deep breathing. It is helpful if she is taught to splint her abdominal muscles when she coughs. An informed consent for surgery needs to be signed.

To prepare the woman for the surgery, she is given nothing by mouth. To reduce the likelihood of serious pulmonary damage should aspiration of gastric contents occur, antacids may be administered within 30 minutes of surgery. If epidural anesthesia is used, the nurse may assist with the procedure, monitor the woman's blood pressure and response, and continue EFM. An abdominal and perineal prep is done, and an indwelling catheter is inserted to prevent bladder distention. For women receiving epidural anesthesia, it may be more comfortable to place the Foley catheter after the epidural has been placed. An intravenous line is started with a needle of adequate size to permit blood administration, and preoperative medication may be ordered. The pediatrician, neonatologist, or neonatal intensive care unit should be notified and adequate preparation made to receive the infant. The nurse should make sure that the infant warmer is functional and that appropriate resuscitation equipment is available.

The nurse assists in positioning the woman on the operating table. FHR should be ascertained before surgery and during preparation because fetal hypoxia can result from aortocaval compression. The operating table may be adjusted so it slants slightly to one side, or a wedge (folded blanket or towels) may be placed under the right hip. The uterus should be displaced about 15 degrees from the midline. This helps relieve the pressure of the heavy uterus on the vena cava and lessens the incidence of vena caval compression and supine maternal hypotension. The woman is strapped onto the table to prevent falls or injuries from occurring during the surgery. If a cauterization device is being used, the grounding source is secured on the woman's leg after the device has been checked to make sure it is in working order. The suction should be in working order, and the urine collection bag should be positioned under the operating table to ensure proper urinary drainage. Auscultation or electronic monitoring of the FHR needs to continue until immediately before the surgery. A last-minute check is done to ensure that the fetal scalp electrode has been removed if the fetus was internally monitored. The nurse should continue to provide reassurance and describe the various procedures being performed, along with a rationale, to ease anxiety and give the woman a sense of control.

Before beginning the procedure, a count of all instruments that will be used during the operative procedure is performed and recorded. Typically, this count is repeated three times throughout the operation to ensure that no instruments are left in the woman's abdomen. The nurse is responsible for ensuring that the instrument count is correct. In the event the count is not correct or if a count was not done initially because of emergency circumstances, a portable x-ray screening is performed to ensure no instruments remain in the maternal abdomen.

Preparation for Repeat Cesarean Birth

When a couple is anticipating a repeat cesarean birth, they have time to reflect on their past experiences, analyze and synthesize the new information they are given, and prepare for the experience. Couples who have had previous negative experiences need an opportunity to describe what they felt contributed to these events. They should be encouraged to identify what they would like to have altered and to list interventions that would make the experience more positive. Those who have had positive experiences need reassurance that their needs and desires will be met in the same manner. In addition, the nurse should provide an opportunity for the couple to discuss any fears or anxieties. Some women undergoing an elective repeat cesarean birth may continue to grieve the loss of the ideal birth experience or continue to exhibit mixed emotions regarding their choices for the birth. These women need reassurance and support throughout the birth process.

Preparation for Emergency Cesarean Birth

The period preceding surgery must be used to its greatest advantage. If possible, the couple needs some time for privacy to assimilate the information given to them and to ask for additional information. It is imperative that caregivers use their most effective communication skills. The nurse must address what the couple may anticipate during the next few hours. Asking the couple, "What questions do you have about the decision?" gives the couple an opportunity for further clarification. The nurse can prepare the woman in stages, giving her information and the rationale for each procedure before commencing. Before carrying out a procedure, it is essential to tell the woman (1) what is going to happen, (2) why it is being done, and (3) what sensations she may experience. This allows the woman to be informed and to consent to the procedure. The woman experiences a sense of control and therefore less helplessness and powerlessness.

Supporting the Father/Partner

Every effort should be made to include the father/partner or support person in the cesarean birth experience. When the father or support person attends the cesarean birth, he or she must wear a surgical gown and mask as do others in the operating suite. The father or support person can sit on a stool placed beside the woman's head to provide physical touch, visual contact, and verbal reassurance to his partner.

Many support persons worry about their own reactions to the operative procedure. A sterile drape is placed between the woman's head and the sterile field. The nurse can advise the support person that this can be used as a partition if he or she does not wish to view the procedure itself. The nurse should encourage support persons to eat if possible before the surgery. Most fathers or support persons who fear "fainting" or "feeling queasy" do not have difficulties in the operating room and frequently forget these fears as they are swept away in the excitement of the birth.

Other measures, such as the following, can be taken to promote the participation of the father or partner who chooses not to be present in the delivery room:

• Allowing the father or partner to be near the operating room, where he can hear the newborn's first cry

• Encouraging the father/partner to carry or accompany the infant to the nursery for the initial assessment

• Involving the father/partner in postpartal care in the recovery room

In the event that a support person cannot be with the woman during the cesarean birth, such as in situations involving emergencies, the nurse may obtain consent from the woman before the surgery and then provide updates to the support person to alleviate undue fear and anxiety.

Immediate Postpartal Recovery Period

After birth, the nurse assesses the Apgar score and completes the initial assessment and identification procedures as after a vaginal birth. Every effort must be made to assist the parents in bonding with the infant. If the mother is awake, one of her arms should be freed to enable her to touch and stroke the infant. The baby can be given to the father to hold until she or he must be taken to the nursery.

The nurse caring for the postpartal woman should check her vital signs every 5 minutes until they are stable, then every 15 minutes for an hour, then every 30 minutes until she is discharged to the postpartal unit. The nurse should remain with the woman until she is stable.

The dressing and perineal pad must be checked every 15 minutes for at least an hour, and the fundus should be gently palpated to determine whether it is remaining firm. The fundus may be palpated by placing a hand to support the incision. Intravenous oxytocin is usually administered to promote the contractility of the uterine musculature. If the woman has had general anesthesia, she should be positioned on her side to facilitate drainage of secretions, turned, and assisted with coughing and deep breathing every 2 hours for at least 24 hours. If she has received a spinal or epidural anesthetic, the level of anesthesia should be checked every 15 minutes. It is important to monitor intake and output and to observe the urine for bloody tinge, which could mean surgical trauma to the bladder. The physician prescribes medication to relieve the mother's pain and nausea, and this should be administered as needed. Some physicians use a single dose of epidural morphine (5 to 7.5 mg) for postsurgical pain relief. Facilitation of parent-infant interaction following birth and postpartal care is discussed in Chapter 35. ∞ Pertinent areas of nursing care are addressed in the Cesarean Birth Clinical Pathway in Chapter 35. ∞

CARE OF THE WOMAN UNDERGOING VAGINAL BIRTH AFTER CESAREAN

In the late 1980s there was an increasing trend to have a trial of labor and **vaginal birth after cesarean (VBAC)** birth in cases of nonrecurring indications for a cesarean (for example, twins, umbilical cord prolapse, placenta previa, nonreassuring fetal status). This trend was influenced by consumer demand and studies that support VBAC as a viable and safe alternative. Recent media reports have reintroduced the debate regarding the safety of VBACs.

The 2004 ACOG guidelines state that the following aspects should be met when identifying candidates for a trial of labor:

• One previous cesarean birth and a low transverse uterine incision.

• An adequate pelvis.

• No other uterine scars or previous uterine rupture.

• A physician who is able to do a cesarean needs to be available throughout active labor.

• In-house anesthesia personnel are available for emergency cesarean births if warranted.

Recent debate and research have led to a considerable rise in cesarean births and a significant reduction in women attempting VBACs. In the late 1980s, a movement to increase vaginal births after a previous cesarean birth was advocated because of the increases in morbidity, mortality, and costs associated with cesarean births. This resulted in a decline in the cesarean birth rate and a rise in the VBAC rates. Research in the 1990s, however, changed this trend when reports of rising numbers of uterine ruptures were reported in women attempting VBACs.

Table 27–4	COMPLICATIONS ASSOCIATED WITH VBAC

Uterine rupture
Uterine dehiscence
Hysterectomy
Uterine infection
Maternal death
Neonatal death
Antepartum stillbirth
Intrapartum stillbirth
Transfusion
Hypoxic ischemic encephalopathy

Although the absolute risks of VBAC are small, there is a 0.1% to 0.7% risk of uterine rupture when women attempt a trial of labor after previously undergoing a cesarean birth. The significance is that, in the studies, there were no uterine ruptures in the group of women who had undergone an elective repeat cesarean birth. There were, however, higher rates of stillbirths and hypoxia in infants born to mothers who underwent a trial of labor (Chauhan, Martin, & Hendrichs, 2003; National Institutes of Child Health & Human Development, 2004). These findings are primarily responsible in the decline of VBACs in the United States since the 1990s. Other risks associated with VBAC are included in Table 27–4.

Although VBACs remain controversial, success rates for VBAC have been encouraging. Women whose previous cesarean was performed because of nonrecurring indications have been reported to have approximately a 60% to 80% chance of success with VBAC (ACOG, 2004b). Women whose previous cesarean was performed for breech presentation had the highest success rates for VBAC (91%). Women who had a previous cesarean birth for nonreassurring fetal status had an 84% success rate, whereas a woman diagnosed with previous dystocia had a 67% success rate. Women who were previously diagnosed with dystocia before 5-cm dilatation had a 67% success rate, whereas women who had previously progressed to 6 to 9 cm had a 73% success rate. Women who had been labeled as having dystocia in the second stage had a 75% success rate (Cunningham et al., 2005).

NURSING CARE MANAGEMENT

The nursing care of a woman undergoing VBAC varies according to institutional protocols. Generally, if the woman is at very low risk (has had one previous cesarean with a lower uterine segment incision), her blood count, type, and screen are obtained on admission; a heparin lock is inserted for intravenous access if needed; continuous EFM is used; and clear fluids may be taken. If the woman is at higher risk, NPO status should be maintained, and, in addition to the care listed, an intrauterine catheter may be inserted to monitor intrauterine pressures during labor.

Supportive and comfort measures are very important. The woman may be excited about this opportunity to experience labor and vaginal birth, or she may be hesitant and frightened about the possibility of complications. The nurse provides information and encouragement for the laboring woman and her partner.

CHAPTER REVIEW

FOCUS YOUR STUDY

- An external (or cephalic) version may be done after 37 weeks' gestation to change a breech presentation to a cephalic presentation, thereby making a lower risk vaginal birth more possible.

- The version is accomplished with the use of tocolytic agents to relax the uterus. An internal (podalic) version is used only when needed during the vaginal birth of a second twin.

- Amniotomy (AROM) is performed to hasten labor. The risks are prolapse of the umbilical cord and infection.

- Prostaglandin E$_2$ may be used before an induction of labor to soften the cervix (called cervical ripening). Prepidil and Cervidil are inserted into the vagina to make the cervix more favorable for induction.

- Labor is induced for many reasons. The methods include amniotomy, stripping of the membranes, intravenous oxytocin infusion, and alternative and complementary methods. Nursing responsibilities are heightened during an induced labor.

- Amnioinfusions are used in cases of oligohydramnios or nonperiodic decelerations to increase the volume of amniotic fluid, which relieves cord compression and promotes perfusion to the fetus.

- An episiotomy may be performed just before birth of the fetus. Although it is still prevalent in the United States, it is becoming somewhat controversial.

- Forceps-assisted birth can be accomplished using outlet forceps, low forceps, or midforceps. Outlet forceps are the most common and are associated with few maternal-fetal complications. Midforceps are associated with more complications but, when needed, are an important aid to birth.

- A vacuum extractor is a soft, pliable cup attached to suction that can be applied to the fetal head and used in much the same way as forceps.

- At least one in four births is accomplished by cesarean. The nurse has a vital role in providing information, support, and encouragement to the couple participating in a cesarean birth.

- Vaginal birth after cesarean (VBAC) carries a low risk of uterine rupture; however, many physicians perform repeat cesarean births out of fear of malpractice issues. Overcoming the old fears of uterine rupture is a high priority for both the parents and the medical and nursing community.

EXPLORE MediaLink

 http://www.prenhall.com/davidson

NCLEX review questions, case studies, and other interactive resources for this chapter can be found on the Web Site at http://www.prenhall.com/davidson. Click on "Chapter 27" to select the activities for this chapter.

For tutorials including animations and videos, more NCLEX review questions, and an audio glossary, access the accompanying Prentice Hall Nursing MediaLink DVD-ROM in this book.

 PRENTICE HALL NURSING MEDIALINK DVD-ROM

Audio Glossary

NCLEX Review

Videos:
  Vacuum Extraction
  Types of Incisions
  Cesarean Birth
    Epidural Placement
    Delivery of Infant
    Assessment of Infant
    Bonding
    Suturing of Uterus
    Scrub Nurse Roles
  Through the Eyes of a Nurse—The Third Trimester

 COMPANION WEBSITE

Additional NCLEX Review

Case Study: *Client Undergoing Labor Induction*

Care Plan Activity: *Client with Pitocin for Labor Augmentation*

Applications: *Vacuum Extraction Delivery; Cesarean Birth*

Critical Thinking

CRITICAL THINKING IN ACTION

CEPHALIC VERSION PROCEDURE (EXTERNAL)

View the Critical Thinking in Action video in Chapter 27 of the DVD-ROM. Then answer the questions that follow.

Betsy Jones, a 28-year-old G1 P0 at 39 weeks' gestation, and her husband present to you in the labor suite for an external cephalic version procedure by her obstetrician. You introduce yourself and review her record for any significant risk factors or contraindications to the version procedure. Her prenatal chart is significant in that the fetus has been in a persistent frank breech position. You encourage Betsy and her husband to express their understanding and ex-

pectations of the procedure. You discuss certain criteria to be met before the procedure and obtain vital signs as follows: T 98.8F, P 88, R 14, BP 110/80, urine screening negative for sugar, albumin, and ketones. You place Betsy on the external electronic fetal monitor, which demonstrates a fetal heart rate baseline of 140 to 152 with moderate variability. There are no contractions observed by the monitor or Betsy. After explaining how to record fetal movement on the monitor, you proceed with an NST.

1. Explain the contraindications to the version procedure.

2. Discuss the criteria that should be met before performing external version.

3. How would you explain to Betsy and her husband what to expect during the version procedure?

4. What support would you give Betsy during the procedure?

5. Explain postversion discharge teaching.

REFERENCES

Agency for Healthcare Research & Quality. (2005, May 3). Routine use of episiotomy in uncomplicated births offers no benefits to women [Press release]. Agency for Healthcare Research and Quality, Rockville, MD. Retrieved December 8, 2005, from http://www.ahrq.gov/news/press/pr2005/episobpr.htm

American College of Obstetricians and Gynecologists (ACOG). (2003). Dystocia and augmentation of labor (ACOG Practice Bulletin No. 49). Washington, DC: Author.

American College of Obstetricians and Gynecologists (ACOG). (2004a). Response to Searle's drug warning on misoprostol (ACOG Committee Opinion No. 248). Washington, DC: Author.

American College of Obstetricians and Gynecologists (ACOG). (2004b). Vaginal birth after previous cesarean delivery (ACOG Practice Bulletin No. 54). Washington, DC: Author.

Bishop, E. H. (1964). Pelvic scoring for elective induction. Obstetrics and Gynecology, 24, 266.

Blackburn, S. (2007). Maternal, fetal, and neonatal physiology: A clinical perspective. Philadelphia: Saunders.

Born, D., & Barron, M. L. (2005). Herb use in pregnancy: What nurses should know. American Journal of Maternal/Child Nursing, 30(3), 201–206.

Boulvain, M. S., & Irion, O. (2005). Membrane sweeping for induction of labour. Birth, 32(2), 152.

Caughey, A. B., Sandberg, P. L., Zlatnik, M. G., Thiet, M. P., Parer, J. T., & Laros, R. K. (2005). Forceps compared with vacuum: Rates of neonatal and maternal morbidity. Obstetrics and Gynecology, 106(5, Pt. 1), 908–912.

Chan, L. Y., Tang, J. L., Tsoi, K. F., Fok, W. Y., Chan, L. W., & Lau, T. K. (2004, July). Intrapartum cesarean delivery after successful external cephalic version: A meta-analysis [Review]. Obstetrics and Gynecology, 104(1), 155–160.

Chauhan, S. P., Martin, J. N., & Hendrichs, C. E. (2003). Maternal and perinatal complications with uterine rupture in 142,075 patients who attempted vaginal birth after cesarean delivery: A review of the literature. Obstetrics & Gynecology, 189, 408.

Collaris, R. J., & Oei, S. G. (2004). External cephalic version: A safe procedure? A systematic review of version-related risks. Acta Obstetricia et Gynecologica Scandinavica, 83(6), 511–518.

Cunningham, F. G., Leveno, L. J., Bloom, S. L., Hauth, J. C., Gilstrap, L. C., & Wenstrom, K. D. (2005). Williams obstetrics (22nd ed.). New York: McGraw-Hill.

Davidson, M. R. (2002). Outcomes of high-risk women cared for by certified nurse-midwives. Journal of Midwifery & Women's Health, 47(1), 46–49.

Deglin, J. H., & Vallerand, A. H. (2005). Davis's drug guide for nurses (9th ed.). Philadelphia: Davis.

Demissie, K., Rhoads, G. G., Smulian, J. C., Balasubramanian, B. C., Gandhi, K., Joseph, K. S., et al. (2004). Operative vaginal delivery and neonatal and infant adverse outcomes: Population based retrospective analysis. British Medical Journal, 329(7456), 24–29.

Eason, E., Labrecque, M., Marcoux, S., & Mondour, M. (2002). Anal incontinence after childbirth. Canadian Medical Association Journal, 166(3), 326–330.

Fitzpatrick, M., & O'Herlihy, C. (2005). Short-term and long-term effects of obstetric anal sphincter injury and their management. Current Opinions in Obstetrics & Gynecology, 17(6), 605–610.

Forrest Pharmaceuticals. (1995). Cervidil manufacturer's fact sheet. St. Louis: Forrest Pharmaceuticals.

Fraser, W. D., Hofmeyr, J., Lede, R., Faron, G., Alexander, S., Goffinet, F., et al. (Amnioinfusion trial group). (2005). New England Journal of Medicine, 353, 909–917.

Goetz, L. H., & Lowry, A. C. (2005). Fetal incontinence: Overlapping sphincteroplasty: Is it the standard of care? Clinics in Colon & Rectal Surgery, 18(1), 22–31.

Goldberg, A. B., & Wing, D. A. (2003). Induction of labor: The misoprostol controversy. Journal of Midwifery & Women's Health, 48(4), 244–248.

Harper, M. A., Byington, R. P., & Espeland, M. A. (2003). Pregnancy-related death and health care services. Obstetrics and Gynecology, 101, 80.

Hofmeyr, G. J. (2002). Amnioinfusion for meconium-stained liquor in labour [Update]. Cochrane Database Systematic Review, 2000(2) (CD000014;10796085).

Hofmeyr, G. J., & Kulier, R. (2002). External cephalic version for breech presentation at term. Cochrane Library (Oxford) 1 (CD000083) (1).

Howden, N. L. S., Weber, A. M., & Meyn, L. A. (2004). Episiotomy use among residents and faculty compared with private practitioners. Obstetrics and Gynecology, 103, 114–118.

Kadir, R. A., Khan, A., Wilcock, F., & Chapman, L. (2006, April 16). Is inferior dissection of the rectus sheath necessary during Pfannenstiel incision for lower segment Caesarean section? A randomised controlled trial. *European Journal of Obstetrics, Gynecology, & Reproductive Biology, 42*(6), 94–99.

Levy, R., Kanengiser, B., Furman, B., Arie, A., Brown, D., & Hagay, Z. J. (2004). A randomized trial comparing a 30-mL and an 80-mL Foley catheter balloon for preinduction cervical ripening. *American Journal of Obstetrics & Gynecology, 191*(5), 1632–1636.

Liu, S., Heaman, M., Joseph, K. S., Liston, R. M., Huang, L., Sauve, R., et al. (Maternal Health Study Group of the Canadian Perinatal Surveillance System). (2005). Risk of maternal postpartum readmission associated with mode of delivery. *Obsterics & Gynecology, 105,* 836–842.

Mahlmeister, L. (2005). Best practices in perinatal and neonatal nursing: Cervical ripeners and the induction of labor. *Journal of Perinatal and Neonatal Nursing, 19*(2), 97–99.

Martin, J. A., Hamilton, B. E., Menacker, F., Sutton, P. D., & Mathews, T. J. (2005). *Preliminary births for 2004: Infant and maternal health.* Health E-stats. Retrieved November 29, 2005, from http://www.cdc.gov/nchs/products/pubs/pubd/hestats/prelimbirths04/prelimbirths04health.htm

Mazouni, C., Bretelle, F., Collette, E., Heckenroth, H., Bonnier, P., & Gamerre, M. (2005). Maternal and neonatal morbidity after first vaginal delivery using Thierry's spatulas. *Australian & New Zealand Journal of Obstetrics & Gynaecology, 45*(5), 405–409.

Medifocus. (2002). *Electronic fetal monitoring.* Silver Spring, MD: Author.

Midwifery Today E-News. (2002). Herbs. *Midwifery Today Forums, 1,* 44. Retrieved December 20, 2002, from http://www.midwiferytoday.com/enews

Myers, V., & Goldberg, J. (2006). Episiotomy: An evidence-based approach. *Obstetric Gynecology Survey, 61*(8), 491–492.

National Institutes of Child Health & Human Development. (2004, December 14). Risk from labor after prior cesarean delivery low [Press release]. Retrieved December 9, 2005, from http://www.nih.gov/news/pr/dec2004/nichd-14.htm

Nygaard, I., & Cruikshank, D. P. (2003). Should all women be offered elective cesarean delivery? *Obstetrics and Gynecology, 102,* 217.

Physicians Insurance Association of America. (2002). *Risk management review: 2002, Obstetrics 2002.* Rockville, MD. Retrieved June 19, 2006, from http://www.thepiaa.org

Rayburn, W. F. (2002). Preinduction cervical ripening: Basis and methods of current practice. *Obstetrical & Gynecological Survey, 57*(10), 683–692.

Ross, M. G. (2005). Meconium aspiration syndrome: More than intrapartum meconium. *New England Journal of Medicine, 353*(9), 946–948.

Schaffir, J. (2002). Survey of folk beliefs about induction of labor. *Birth, 29*(1), 47–51.

Sciarra, J. J. (2004). *Obstetrics and gynecology.* Philadelphia: Lippincott Williams & Wilkins.

Sierpina, V., & Frenkel, M. A. (2005). Acupuncture: A clinical review. *Southern Medical Journal, 98*(3), 330–337.

Simpson, K. R., & Thorman, K. E. (2005). Obstetric "conveniences": Elective induction of labor, cesarean birth on demand, and other potentially unnecessary interventions. *Journal of Perinatal and Neonatal Nursing, 19*(2), 134–144.

Tekesin, I., Wallwiener, D., & Schmidt, S. (2005). The value of quantitative ultrasound tissue characterization of the cervix and rapid fetal fibronectin in predicting preterm delivery. *Journal of Perinatal Medicine, 33*(5), 383–391.

Tenore, J. L. (2003). Methods for cervical ripening and induction of labor. *American Family Physician, 67,* 2123–2128.

Theron, G. B., & Theron, A. M. (2002). Routine external version by physicians in training for abnormal presentation. *International Journal of Gynaecology & Obstetrics, 76*(2), 173–174.

Thompson, J. F., Roberts, C. L., Currie, M., & Ellwood, D. A. (2002). Prevalence and persistence of health problems after childbirth: Associations with parity and method of birth. *Birth, 29*(2), 83–94.

Thornton, C., & Whaites, M. (2004). Protocol audit of dinoprostone gel induction of labour. *Australian Journal of Midwifery, 17*(4), 22–25.

Tillett, J. (2005). Obstetric rituals: Is practice supported by evidence? *Journal of Perinatal and Neonatal Nursing, 19*(2), 91–93.

Tzeng, Y. L., Shih, Y. J., Chiu, C. Y., & Huang, M. Y. (2005). Enema prior to labor: A controversial routine in Taiwan. *Journal of Nursing Research, 13*(4), 263–270.

Walker, R., Turnbull, D., & Wilkinson, C. (2002). Strategies to address global cesarean section rates: A review of the evidence. *Birth, 29*(1), 28–39.

Webb, D. A., & Culhane, J. (2002). Hospital variation in episiotomy use and the risk of perineal trauma during childbirth. *Birth, 29*(2), 132–136.

Wilson, B. A., Shannon, M. T., & Stang, C. L. (2006). *Prentice Hall nurse's drug guide: 2006.* Upper Saddle River, NJ: Prentice Hall Health.

Youssef, R., Ramalingam, U., MacLeod, M., & Murphy, D. J. (2005). Cohort study of maternal and neonatal morbidity in relation to use of episiotomy at instrumental vaginal delivery. *Obstetrical & Gynecological Survey, 60*(12), 787–788.

UNIT
6

The Newborn

28 Physiologic Responses of the Newborn to Birth

The incredible attributes of the newborn have a major purpose. They prepare the baby for interaction with the family and for life in the world.

~Marshall H. Klaus & Phyllis H. Klaus,
The Amazing Newborn~

KEY TERMS

Active acquired immunity   812
Brown adipose tissue (BAT)   805
Cardiopulmonary adaptation   796
Conduction   805
Convection   804
Evaporation   804
Habituation   814
Meconium   810
Neonatal transition   793
Neutral thermal environment (NTE)   803

Orientation   814
Passive acquired immunity   812
Periodic breathing   798
Periods of reactivity   813
Physiologic anemia of infancy   801
Physiologic jaundice   807
Radiation   804
Self-quieting ability   814
Surfactant   793
Total serum bilirubin   806

OBJECTIVES

1. Summarize the respiratory and cardiovascular changes that occur during the transition to extrauterine life and during stabilization.

2. Describe how various factors affect the newborn's blood values.

3. Correlate the major mechanisms of heat loss in the newborn to the process of thermogenesis in the newborn.

4. Explain the steps involved in conjugation and excretion of bilirubin in the newborn.

5. Discuss the reasons why the newborn may develop jaundice.

6. Delineate the functional abilities of the newborn's gastrointestinal tract and liver.

7. Identify the reasons the newborn's kidneys have difficulty maintaining fluid and electrolyte balance.

8. List the immunologic responses available to the newborn.

9. Explain the physiologic and behavioral responses of newborns during the periods of reactivity, and identify possible interventions.

10. Describe the normal sensory/perceptual abilities and behavioral states present in the newborn period.

MEDIALINK

Additional resources for this content can be found on the Prentice Hall Nursing MediaLink DVD-ROM and on the Companion Website at http://www.prenhall.com/davidson. Click on "Chapter 28" to select the activities for this chapter.

The newborn period is the time from birth through the first 28 days of life. During this period, the newborn adjusts from intrauterine to extrauterine life. The nurse needs to be knowledgeable about a newborn's normal physiologic and behavioral adaptations and be able to recognize alterations from normal.

The first few hours of life, in which the newborn stabilizes respiratory and circulatory functions, are called **neonatal transition.** All other newborn body systems change their level of functioning or become established over a longer period of time during the neonatal period.

RESPIRATORY ADAPTATIONS

To begin life as a separate being, the baby must immediately establish respiratory gas exchange, which occurs in conjunction with marked circulatory changes. These radical and rapid changes are crucial to the maintenance of extrauterine life.

Intrauterine Factors Supporting Respiratory Function

Even before the significant respiratory events occur at birth, certain intrauterine factors also enhance the newborn's ability to breathe. Adequate fetal lung development allows the newborn to expand his or her lungs and exchange oxygen and carbon dioxide gases. Even before birth the fetus practices breathing movements, which allow him or her to breathe immediately after birth.

FETAL LUNG DEVELOPMENT

The respiratory system is in a continuous state of development during fetal life, and lung development continues into early childhood. During the first 20 weeks of gestation, lung development is limited to the differentiation of pulmonary, vascular, and lymphatic structures. At 20 to 24 weeks, alveolar ducts begin to appear, followed by primitive alveoli at 24 to 28 weeks. During this time, the alveolar epithelial cells begin to differentiate into type I cells (structures necessary for respiratory gas exchange) and type II cells (structures that provide for the synthesis and storage of surfactant). **Surfactant** is composed of a group of surface-active phospholipids (lecithin and sphingomyelin), which are critical for alveolar stability.

At 28 to 32 weeks of gestation, the number of type II cells increases further, and surfactant is produced by a choline pathway within them. Surfactant production by this pathway peaks at about 35 weeks of gestation and remains high until term, paralleling late fetal lung development. At this time, the lungs are structurally developed enough to maintain good lung expansion and adequate exchange of gases.

Clinically, the peak production of lecithin—one component of surfactant—corresponds closely to the marked decrease in incidence of idiopathic respiratory distress syndrome for babies born after 35 weeks' gestation. Production of sphingomyelin—the other component—remains constant during gestation. The newborn born before the lecithin/sphingomyelin (L/S) ratio is 2:1 will have varying degrees of respiratory distress. (See discussion of L/S ratio in Chapters 21 ∞ and 33 ∞).

FETAL BREATHING MOVEMENTS

The newborn's ability to breathe air immediately after his or her birth appears to result from weeks of intrauterine practice. In this respect, breathing can be seen as a continuation of an intrauterine process; the lungs convert from a fluid-filled organ to an air-filled organ capable of gas exchange.

Fetal breathing movements (FBM) occur as early as 11 weeks' gestation (see Biophysical Profile in Chapter 21 ∞ for discussion). These breathing movements are essential for developing the chest wall muscles and the diaphragm and, to a lesser extent, for regulating lung fluid volume and resultant lung growth.

Initiation of Breathing

To maintain life the lungs must function immediately after birth. Two radical changes must take place for the lungs to function:

1. Pulmonary ventilation must be established through lung expansion following birth.

2. A marked increase in the pulmonary circulation must occur.

The first breath of life—the gasp in response to mechanical and reabsorptive, chemical, thermal, and sensory changes associated with birth—starts the serial opening of the alveoli. So begins the transition from a fluid-filled environment to an air-breathing, independent, extrauterine life. Figure 28–1 ◆ summarizes the initiation of respiration.

MECHANICAL EVENTS

During the latter half of gestation, the fetal lungs continuously produce fluid. This fluid production expands the lungs almost completely, filling the air spaces. Some of the lung fluid moves up into the trachea and out into the amniotic fluid. The amniotic fluid is then swallowed by the fetus.

Production of lung fluid diminishes 2 to 4 days before onset of labor, and fetal breathing movements decrease 24 to 36 hours before the onset of labor (Laughlin & Knuppel, 2003). However, approximately 80 to 110 mL of fluid remains in the respiratory passages of a normal term fetus at the time of birth. This fluid must be removed from the lungs to permit adequate movement of air (Polin, Fox, & Abman, 2004).

As the fetus experiences labor, there is a fetal gasp and active exhalation that initiates the removal of fluid from the lungs (Polin et al., 2004). During the birth process the fetal chest is compressed, increasing intrathoracic pressure and squeezing a small amount of fluid out of the lungs. After the birth of the newborn's trunk, the chest wall recoils. This chest recoil creates negative intrathoracic pressure, which is thought to produce a small, passive inspiration of air that replaces the fluid that was squeezed out. The significance of the "thoracic squeeze" is controversial, and it is now thought that the process of labor is primarily responsible for the initial movement of lung fluid out of the lungs (Polin et al., 2004).

After this first inspiration, the newborn exhales, with crying, against a partially closed glottis, creating a positive intrathoracic pressure. The high positive intrathoracic pressure distributes the inspired air throughout the alveoli and begins the establishment of *functional residual capacity (FRC)*, the air left

Figure 28–1 ◆ Initiation of respiration in the newborn.

in the lungs at the end of a normal expiration. The higher intrathoracic pressure also increases absorption of lung fluid via the capillaries and lymphatic system. The negative intrathoracic pressure created when the diaphragm moves down with inspiration causes lung fluid to flow from the alveoli across the alveolar membranes into the pulmonary interstitial tissue.

At birth the alveolar epithelium is temporarily more permeable. This, combined with decreased cellular resistance at the onset of breathing, may facilitate passive liquid absorption. With each succeeding breath, the lungs continue to expand, stretching the alveolar walls and increasing the alveolar volume. Protein molecules are too large to pass through capillary walls. The presence of more protein molecules in the pulmonary capillaries than in the interstitial tissue creates oncotic pressure. This pressure draws the interstitial fluid into the capillaries and lymphatic tissue to balance the concentration of protein. The expansion of the lung facilitates movement of the remaining lung fluid into the interstitial tissue. As pulmonary vascular resistance decreases, pulmonary blood flow increases, and more interstitial fluid is absorbed into the bloodstream. In the healthy term newborn, lung fluid moves rapidly into the interstitial tissue but may take several hours to move into the lymph and blood vessels. Figure 28–2 ◆ depicts the changes in fetal lung fluid with the first and subsequent breaths. Most of the lung fluid

is reabsorbed within 2 hours after birth, and it is completely absorbed within 12 to 24 hours after birth (Polin et al., 2004).

Although the initial chest compression and recoil should clear the airways of accumulated fluid and permit further inspiration, most clinicians feel it is wise to suction mucus and fluid from the newborn's mouth, nose, and throat. They use a bulb syringe or mucus trap attached to suction as soon as the newborn's head and shoulders are born and again as the newborn adapts to extrauterine life and stabilizes (see Procedure 24–1 and Chapter 24 ∞).

Newborns may have problems clearing the fluid in the lungs and beginning respiration for a variety of reasons:

- The lymphatic system may be underdeveloped, thus decreasing the rate at which the fluid is absorbed from the lungs.

- Complications that occur before or during labor and birth can interfere with adequate lung expansion, causing failure to decrease pulmonary vascular resistance, resulting in decreased pulmonary blood flow. These complications include inadequate compression of the chest wall in a very small newborn, the absence of the chest wall compression in the newborn born by cesarean birth, respiratory depression secondary to maternal anesthesia, or aspiration of amniotic fluid or meconium.

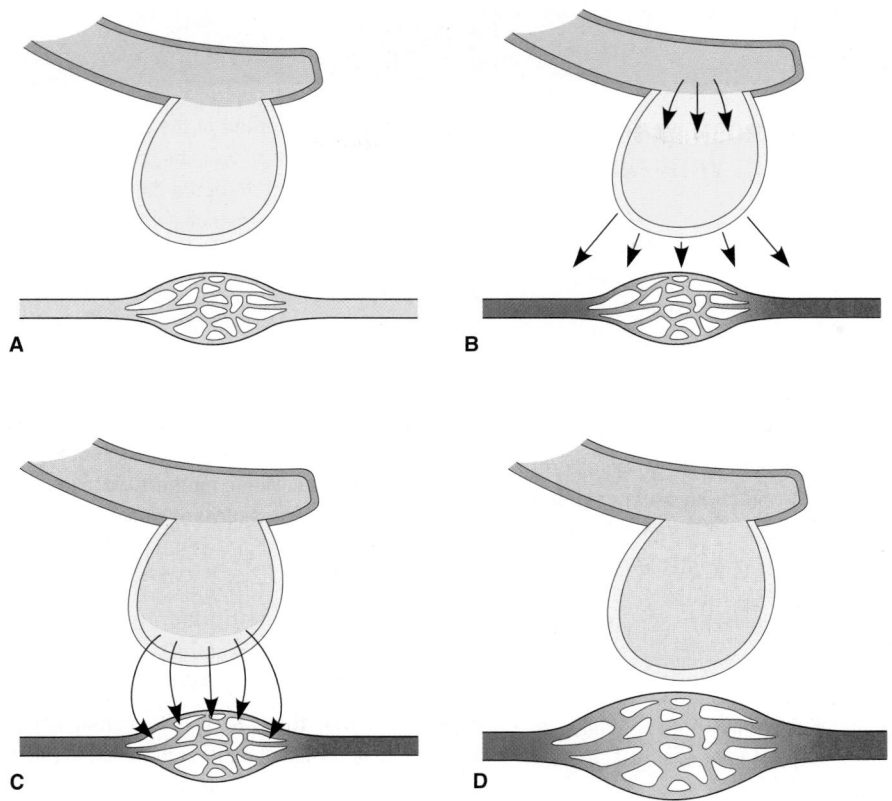

Figure 28–2 ◆ Process of absorption of fetal lung fluid during breathing after birth. *A,* Fetal alveoli filled to functional residual capacity with fetal lung fluid. Fetal lung fluid is produced by the alveoli, fills the airways, and eventually enters the amniotic fluid. *B,* After fetal chest compression, one third of the fetal lung fluid is squeezed out, allowing air to enter passively as the chest recoils. *C,* With each subsequent breath, the lungs expand, facilitating the movement of the remaining fetal lung fluid into the capillaries and lymphatic system. Pulmonary blood flow is increasing. *D,* Normal alveoli after removal of fetal lung fluid and dilatation of pulmonary arteries. Surfactant has lined the inside of the alveoli to prevent collapse.

CHEMICAL STIMULI

An important chemical stimulator that contributes to the onset of breathing is transitory asphyxia of the fetus and newborn. The first breath is really an inspiratory gasp triggered by the elevation in P_{CO_2} and decrease in pH and P_{O_2}, which are the natural result of normal vaginal birth with cessation of placental gas exchange when the cord is clamped. These changes, present in all newborns to some degree, stimulate the aortic and carotid chemoreceptors, initiating impulses that trigger the brain's respiratory center. Although this brief period of asphyxia is a significant stimulator, prolonged asphyxia is abnormal and depresses respiration.

THERMAL STIMULI

A significant decrease in ambient temperature after birth—from 37C to 21 to 23.9C (98.6F to 70 to 75F) results in sudden chilling of the moist newborn (Cheffer, 2004). The cold stimulates skin nerve endings and the newborn responds with rhythmic respirations. Normal temperature changes that occur at birth are apparently within acceptable physiologic limits. Excessive cooling, however, may result in profound respiratory depression and evidence of cold stress (see Chapter 33 ∞ for discussion of cold stress).

SENSORY STIMULI

During intrauterine life, the fetus is in a dark, sound-dampened, fluid-filled environment and is nearly weightless. After birth the newborn experiences light, sounds, and the effects of gravity for the first time. As the fetus moves from a familiar, comfortable, quiet environment to one of sensory abundance, a number of physical and sensory influences help respiration begin. They include the numerous tactile, auditory, and visual stimuli of birth. Joint movement results in enhanced proprioreceptor stimulation to the respiratory center to sustain respirations. Thoroughly drying the newborn and placing him or her in skin-to-skin contact with the mother's chest and abdomen provides stimulation in a far more comforting way and also decreases heat loss.

CLINICAL TIP

Historically, slapping the buttocks or heels of the newborn was a common way to stimulate breathing, but today the emphasis is on gentle physical contact. Thoroughly dry the newborn and place the baby in skin-to-skin contact with the mother's chest and abdomen. This will provide ample stimulation in a far more comforting way and also decrease heat loss.

RESEARCH IN PRACTICE

TEMPERATURE VARIATION IN NEWBORN BABIES: IMPORTANCE OF PHYSICAL CONTACT WITH THE MOTHER

What is this study about? After birth, the newborn must physiologically control his or her temperature. Hypothermia is one of the most common causes of death during the first weeks of life. A primary focus for care of the newborn is preservation of body temperature. Thermoregulation in newborns has been studied by evaluation of surface and core temperature, but this assessment is generally under standardized conditions in a controlled environment. Research that focuses on the newborn when physically removed from his or her mother does not reflect the usual care of a newborn in the hospital setting. In a natural setting, the newborn would have considerable physical contact with his or her mother. This study sought to determine natural patterns of temperature variation in newborn babies related to the influence of external factors, including physical contact with the mother.

How was this study done? Abdominal and peripheral skin temperatures of 27 healthy newborns were measured continuously during the first 2 days of life. Measurements started 4 to 8 hours after birth. The newborns wore diapers and were dressed similarly. When in their cribs, the babies were covered with a cotton blanket. Central skin temperature was measured below the umbilicus under the diaper. Peripheral skin temperature was measured on the sole of the foot. Newborn skin temperatures were recorded once a minute and were transmitted wirelessly to a receiver located under the infant's crib. The transmitter range was about 30 feet, allowing unrestricted access to the newborn and the provision of normal care within the mother's room or in the hospital. Environmental air temperature was recorded at the same time as the skin temperature. Rectal temperature was measured twice a day. The mothers were given a log sheet to record the times of specific activities, including feeding, diaper changes, whether the child was in the crib or in contact with the mother, and clothing changes.

What were the results of the study? Mean rectal and skin temperatures were all lower on day 1 than on day 2. The foot skin temperature was directly related to the care that was reported and was significantly higher when the baby was in physical contact with the mother. The abdominal skin temperature was less influenced by external factors than the foot temperature, but it did affect heat balance. When mothers were in physical contact with the newborns, the measures indicated a positive heat balance. This balance indicated more heat loss when the newborn was lying in the crib.

What additional questions might I have? Do these findings also apply to newborns who have more difficulty regulating their temperature, for example, preterm newborns?

How can I use this study? This study emphasizes the importance of close physical contact between the newborn and mother during the first few postnatal days. Periods of time in the crib result in heat loss, whereas physical contact results in a positive heat balance. Mothers in the immediate postnatal period should be encouraged to have frequent, extended physical contact with their newborn. This contact may be most important in influencing neonatal body temperature during the first day of life.

Fransson, A., Karlsson, H., & Nilsson, K. (2005). Temperature variation in newborn babies: Importance of physical contact with the mother. *Archives of Disease in Childhood: Fetal and Neonatal Edition, 90,* F500–F504.

Factors Opposing the First Breath

Three major factors may oppose the initiation of respiratory activity: (1) the contracting force between alveoli—called *alveolar surface tension;* (2) viscosity of lung fluid within the respiratory tract, which is influenced by surfactant levels; and (3) the ease with which the lung is able to fill with air—called *lung compliance.*

Alveolar surface tension is the contracting force between the moist surfaces of the alveoli. This tension is necessary for healthy respiratory function but would cause the small airways and alveoli to collapse after each inspiration if surfactant were not present. Surfactant is important because it reduces the attracting force between alveoli. This prevents the alveoli from completely collapsing with each expiration and thus promotes lung expansion. Similarly, surfactant promotes lung compliance, the ability of the lung to fill with air easily. When surfactant is decreased, compliance is also decreased, and the pressure needed to expand the alveoli with air increases.

Resistive forces of the fluid-filled lung, combined with the small radii of the airways, necessitates pressures of 30 to 40 cm of water pressure, which are needed to open the lung initially (Thureen, Deacon, Hernandez et al., 2005).

The first breath usually establishes FRC that is 30% to 40% of the fully expanded lung volume. This FRC allows alveolar sacs to remain partially expanded on expiration, decreasing the need for continuous high pressures for each of the following breaths. Subsequent breaths require only 6 to 8 cm H_2O pressure to open alveoli during inspiration. Thus, the first breath of life is usually the most difficult.

Cardiopulmonary Physiology

The onset of respiration stimulates cardiovascular system changes necessary for successful transition to extrauterine life, hence the term **cardiopulmonary adaptation.** As air enters the lungs, Po_2 rises in the alveoli, relaxing the pulmonary arteries and triggering a decrease in the pulmonary vascular resistance. As pulmonary vascular resistance decreases, the vascular flow in the lung increases very rapidly and achieves 100% normal flow volume at 24 hours of life. This delivery of greater blood volume to the lungs contributes to the conversion from fetal circulation to newborn circulation.

After pulmonary circulation is established, blood is distributed throughout the lung, although the alveoli may or may not be fully open. For adequate oxygenation to occur, the heart must deliver sufficient blood to functional open alveoli. Shunting of blood is common in the early newborn period. Bidirectional blood flow, or right-to-left shunting through the ductus arteriosus, may divert a significant amount of blood away from the lungs, depending on the pressure changes of respiration, crying, and the cardiac cycle. This shunting in the newborn period is also responsible for the unstable transitional period in cardiopulmonary function.

Oxygen Transport

The transportation of oxygen to the peripheral tissues depends on the type of hemoglobin in the red blood cell (RBC). In the fetus and newborn, a variety of hemoglobins exists, the most significant being fetal hemoglobin (HbF) and adult hemoglobin (HbA). Approximately 70% to 90% of hemoglobin in the fetus and newborn is HbF. The greatest difference between HbF and HbA is related to the transport of oxygen.

The oxygen-carrying capacity of fetal hemoglobin is lower than that of adult hemoglobin. Although each gram of HbF carries less oxygen, it has a greater affinity for the oxygen molecules it carries. At any given arterial oxygen level, HbF has a greater oxygen saturation than HbA. Thus the oxygen-hemoglobin dissociation curve for HbF lies to the left of that for HbA (Figure 28–3 ◆). HbF's greater affinity for oxygen benefits the fetus and newborn because it facilitates oxygen transfer across the placenta and into the newborn's tissues. In utero, the fetus has an arterial oxygen tension (Pao$_2$) between 30 and 40 mm Hg. Because of the nature of the HbF as depicted in the curve, small changes in fetal Pao$_2$ result in a great amount of oxygen loading in the placenta or unloading to the tissues as compared with the adult. HbF's greater affinity for oxygen also requires that a lower tissue oxygen level exist before oxygen unloading than is required by HbA. Because of this phenomenon, the newborn will have both a lower arterial oxygen level and lower oxygen saturation than the adult before cyanosis becomes clinically apparent.

In addition to the specific characteristics of HbF, other conditions affect the transport of oxygen. Alkalosis (increased pH) and hypothermia can result in less oxygen being available to the body tissues, whereas acidosis, hypercarbia, and hyperthermia can result in less oxygen being bound to hemoglobin and more oxygen being released to the body tissues. Therefore, as blood is perfusing active tissues that are producing acids and carbon dioxide, hemoglobin's affinity for oxygen decreases, allowing oxygen unloading and carbon dioxide and acid uptake. This blood is then transferred to the placenta or the lungs, where its lower carbon dioxide and acid content results in uploading of these waste products from hemoglobin and the uptake of oxygen to be transferred to the tissues.

Other factors that regulate oxygen delivery to the tissues are oxygen-carrying capacity and cardiac output. The oxygen-carrying capacity of blood is defined as the product of the hemoglobin concentration and the maximum amount of oxygen that 1 g of hemoglobin can hold when it is fully saturated. The amount of oxygen bound to hemoglobin divided by the oxygen-carrying capacity yields a percentage that signifies oxygen saturation. Oxygen saturation usually reaches a value between 96% and 98% after several hours of life. Although HbF can hold only 1.26 mL of oxygen per gram of hemoglobin, compared with 1.34 mL of oxygen per gram of HbA, the newborn's hemoglobin level at birth (17 g/dL) is substantially greater than in adults (13 g/dL). Therefore, the absolute oxygen-carrying capacity of fetal blood (21.42 vol %) is greater than in adult blood (17.42 vol %) and allows the fetus to tolerate the relatively hypoxic intrauterine environment.

A significant reduction in the oxygen-carrying capacity results in an increased cardiac output to compensate for hemoglobin's decreased oxygen concentration. Lastly, cardiac output of the fetus and newborn is relatively greater per body weight than in the adult, which contributes to the rapid delivery of oxygenated blood to tissues with high metabolic demands.

Maintaining Respiratory Function

The lungs' ability to maintain oxygen and carbon dioxide exchange (ventilation) is influenced by such factors as lung compliance and airway resistance. Lung compliance is influenced by the elastic recoil of the lung tissue and by anatomic differences in the newborn. The newborn has a relatively large heart as well as mediastinal structures that reduce available lung space. Also, the newborn chest is equipped with weak intercostal muscles, a rib cage with horizontal ribs, and a high diaphragm that restricts the space available for lung expansion. The large abdomen further encroaches on the high diaphragm to decrease lung space. Another factor that limits ventilation is airway resistance, which depends on the radii, length, and number of airways. Airway resistance is increased in the newborn when compared with adults.

Figure 28–3 ◆ Fetal oxygen-hemoglobin dissociation curve.
SOURCE: Reprinted from Klaus, M., & Fanaroff, A. A. *Care of the high risk infant* (3rd ed., p. 234). Copyright 1986, with permission from Elsevier Science.

Characteristics of Newborn Respiration

The normal newborn respiratory rate is 30 to 60 breaths per minute. Initial respirations may be largely diaphragmatic, shallow, and irregular in depth and rhythm. The abdomen's movements are synchronous with chest movements. When the breathing pattern is characterized by pauses lasting 5 to 15 seconds, **periodic breathing** is occurring. Periodic breathing is rarely associated with differences in skin color or heart rate changes, and it has no prognostic significance. Tactile or other sensory stimulation stimulates the respiratory center and converts periodic breathing patterns to normal breathing patterns during neonatal transition. With deep sleep, the pattern is reasonably regular. Periodic breathing occurs with rapid eye movement (REM) sleep, and grossly irregular breathing is evident with motor activity, sucking, and crying. Cessation of breathing lasting more than 20 seconds is defined as *apnea* and is abnormal in term newborns. Apnea may or may not be associated with changes in skin color or heart rate (drop below 100 beats per minute [bpm]). Apnea always needs to be further evaluated.

The newborn must breathe through the nose. Any obstruction will cause respiratory distress, so it is important to keep the throat and nose clear. Immediately after birth and for about the next 2 hours, respiratory rates of 60 to 70 breaths per minute are normal. Some cyanosis and acrocyanosis are normal for several hours; thereafter, a steady improvement in color occurs. If respirations drop below 30 or exceed 60 per minute when the baby is at rest, or if dyspnea, cyanosis, or nasal flaring and expiratory grunting occur, the clinician should be notified. Any increased use of the intercostal muscle (retractions) may indicate respiratory distress. (See Respiratory Distress Syndrome in Chapter 33 ∞ and Table 33–1 ∞ for signs of respiratory distress).

CARDIOVASCULAR ADAPTATIONS

As described earlier, the onset of respiration triggers increased pulmonary blood flow after birth. This greater blood volume contributes to the conversion from fetal circulation to neonatal circulation.

Fetal-Newborn Transitional Physiology

During fetal life, blood with the highest oxygen content is directed to the heart and brain. Blood in the descending aorta is less oxygenated and supplies the kidneys and intestinal tract before it is returned to the placenta. Limited amounts of blood, pumped from the right ventricle toward the lungs, enter the pulmonary vessels. In the fetus, increased pulmonary resistance forces most of the blood through the ductus arteriosus into the descending aorta (Table 28–1). See the fetal heart animation on the CD-ROM.

Marked changes occur in the cardiovascular system at birth. Expansion of the lungs with the first breath decreases the pulmonary vascular resistance and increases pulmonary blood

Table 28–1 FETAL AND NEONATAL CIRCULATION		
System	**Fetal**	**Neonatal**
Pulmonary blood vessels	Constricted with very little blood flow; lungs not expanded.	Vasodilation and increased blood flow; lungs expanded; increased oxygen stimulates vasodilation.
Systemic blood vessels	Dilated with low resistance; blood mostly in placenta.	Arterial pressure rises due loss of placenta; increased systemic blood volume and resistance.
Ductus arteriosus	Large with no tone; blood flow from pulmonary artery to aorta.	Reversal of blood flow. Now from aorta to pulmonary artery because of increased left atrial pressure. Ductus is sensitive to increased oxygen and body chemicals and begins to constrict.
Foramen ovale	Patent with large blood flow from right atrium to left atrium.	Increased pressure in left atrium attempts to reverse blood flow and shuts one-way valve.

flow. Pressure in the left atrium increases as blood returns from the pulmonary veins. Pressure in the right atrium drops, and systemic vascular resistance increases as umbilical venous flow is halted when the cord is clamped. These physiologic mechanisms mark the beginning of transition from fetal to neonatal circulation and show the interplay of the cardiovascular and respiratory systems (Figure 28–4 ◆).

Five major areas of change in cardiopulmonary adaptation (Figure 28–5 ◆) are:

1. *Increased aortic pressure and decreased venous pressure.* Clamping of the umbilical cord eliminates the placental vascular bed and reduces the intravascular space. Consequently, aortic (systemic) blood pressure increases. At the same time, blood return via the inferior vena cava decreases, resulting in decreased right atrial pressure and a small decrease in pressure within the venous circulation.

2. *Increased systemic pressure and decreased pulmonary artery pressure.* With the loss of the low-resistance placenta, systemic resistance increases, resulting in greater systemic pressure. At the same time, lung expansion increases pulmonary blood flow, and the increased blood PO_2 associated with initiation of respirations dilates pulmonary blood vessels. The combination of vasodilation and increased pulmonary blood flow decreases pulmonary artery resistance. As the pulmonary vascular beds open, the systemic vascular pressure increases, enhancing perfusion of the other body systems.

3. *Closure of the foramen ovale.* Closure of the foramen ovale is a function of changing atrial pressures. In utero, pressure is greater in the right atrium, and the

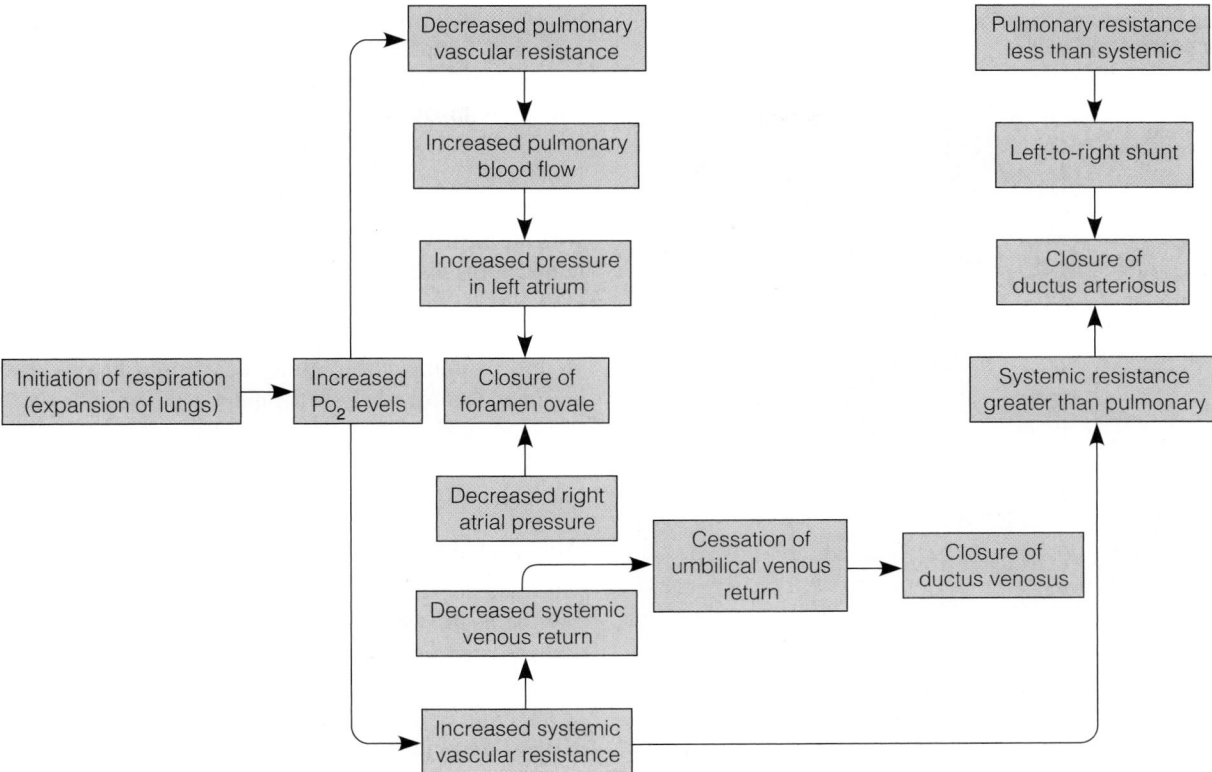

Figure 28–4 ◆ Transitional circulation: conversion from fetal to neonatal circulation.

foramen ovale is open after birth. Decreased pulmonary resistance and increased pulmonary blood flow increase pulmonary venous return into the left atrium, thereby increasing left atrial pressure slightly. The decreased pulmonary vascular resistance and the decreased umbilical venous return to the right atrium also cause a decrease in right atrial pressure. The pressure gradients across the atria are now reversed, with left atrial pressure greater, and the foramen ovale is functionally closed 1 to 2 hours after birth. However, a slight right-to-left shunting may occur in the early neonatal period. Any increase in pulmonary resistance or right atrial pressure, such as occurs in crying, acidosis, cold stress, or induced hypoxia, may cause the foramen ovale to reopen, causing a right-to-left shunt. Permanent closure of the foramen ovale occurs within 6 months.

4. *Closure of the ductus arteriosus.* Initial elevation of the systemic vascular pressure above the pulmonary vascular pressure increases pulmonary blood flow by reversing the flow through the ductus arteriosus. Blood now flows from the aorta into the pulmonary artery. Furthermore, although the presence of oxygen causes the pulmonary arterioles to dilate, an increase in blood Po_2 triggers the opposite response in the ductus arteriosus—it constricts.

In utero the placenta produces prostaglandin E_2 (PGE_2), which causes ductus vasodilation. With the loss of the placenta and increased pulmonary blood flow, PGE_2

levels drop, leaving the active constriction by Po_2 unopposed. If the lungs fail to expand or if Po_2 levels drop, the ductus remains patent. Functional closure is accomplished within 15 hours of birth, and fibrosis of the ductus occurs within 3 weeks after birth (Blackburn, 2003).

5. *Closure of the ductus venosus.* Although the mechanism of initiating closure of the ductus venosus is not known, it appears to be related to mechanical pressure changes that result from severing of the cord, redistribution of blood, and cardiac output. Closure of the ductus venosus forces perfusion of the liver. Fibrosis of the ductus venosus occurs within 2 months. Figure 28–6 ◆ depicts the changes in blood flow and oxygenation as the fetal cardiopulmonary circulation adapts to extrauterine life.

Characteristics of Cardiac Function

Evaluation of the newborn's heart rate, blood pressure, heart sounds, and cardiac workload provides data for evaluating cardiac function.

HEART RATE

Shortly after the first cry and the start of changes in cardiopulmonary circulation, the newborn heart rate accelerates to 180 bpm. The average resting heart rate in the first week of life is 120 to 160 bpm in a healthy full-term newborn but may vary significantly during deep sleep or active awake states. In full-term newborns, the heart rate may drop to a low of 80 bpm during sleep (Thureen et al., 2005).

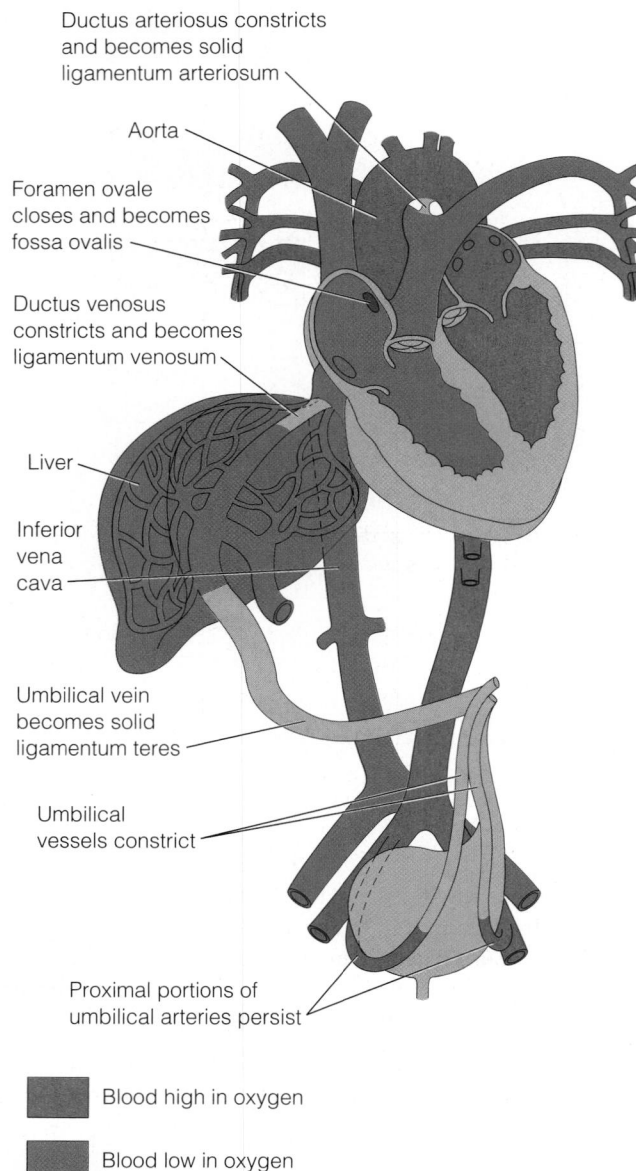

Ductus arteriosus constricts
and becomes solid
ligamentum arteriosum

Aorta

Foramen ovale
closes and becomes
fossa ovalis

Ductus venosus
constricts and becomes
ligamentum venosum

Liver

Inferior
vena
cava

Umbilical vein
becomes solid
ligamentum teres

Umbilical
vessels constrict

Proximal portions of
umbilical arteries persist

Blood high in oxygen

Blood low in oxygen

Figure 28–5 ◆ Major changes that occur in the newborn's circulatory system.
SOURCE: Hole, J. W. (1990). *Human anatomy and physiology* (5th ed.). Dubuque, IA: William C. Brown. All rights reserved.

Apical pulse rates should be obtained by auscultation for a full minute, preferably when the newborn is asleep. The heart rate should be evaluated for abnormal rhythms or beats. Peripheral pulses of all extremities should also be evaluated to detect any lags or unusual characteristics. Peripheral radial pulses are difficult to palpate in the newborn. They can be assessed when blood pressure is measured if blood pressure readings are taken on all four extremities.

BLOOD PRESSURE

The blood pressure tends to be highest immediately after birth, and then it descends to its lowest level at about 3 hours of age. By 4 to 6 days of life, the blood pressure rises and plateaus at a level approximately the same as the initial level. Blood pressure is sensitive to the changes in blood volume that occur in the transition to newborn circulation. Figure 28–7 ◆ diagrams this response. Peripheral perfusion pressure is a particularly sensitive indicator of the newborn's ability to compensate for alterations in blood volume before changes in blood pressure. Capillary refill should be less than 2 to 3 seconds when the skin is blanched.

Blood pressure values during the first 12 hours of life vary with the birth weight. The mean blood pressure is 5 to 55 mm Hg in newborns over 3 kg during the first 12 hours of life (Thureen et al., 2005). In the preterm newborn, the mean blood pressure varies according to weight. Crying may cause an elevation of 20 mm Hg in both the systolic and diastolic blood pressure; thus accuracy is more likely in the quiet newborn. The measurement of blood pressure is best accomplished by using the Doppler technique or a 1- to 2-inch cuff and a stethoscope over the brachial artery.

HEART MURMURS

Murmurs are usually produced by turbulent blood flow. They may be heard when blood flows across an abnormal valve or across a stenosed valve, when there is an atrial septal or ventricular septal defect, or when there is increased flow across a normal valve. In newborns, 90% of all murmurs are transient and *not associated with anomalies*. They usually involve incomplete closure of the ductus arteriosus or foramen ovale. Soft murmurs may be heard as the pulmonary branch arteries increase their blood flow from 7% to 50% of the combined ventricular output during transition, causing a physiologic peripheral pulmonary stenosis. Clicks may normally be heard at the lower left sternal border as the great vessels dilate to accommodate systolic blood flow in the first few hours of life. Because of the current practice of early discharge, murmurs associated with ventricular septal defect and patent ductus arteriosus are often not detected until the first well-baby checkup at 4 to 6 weeks of age. Murmurs are sometimes absent in seriously malformed hearts.

CARDIAC WORKLOAD

In the first 2 hours after birth, when the ductus arteriosus remains mostly patent, about one third of the left ventricular output is returned to the pulmonary circulation. As a result, the left ventricle has a significantly greater volume load than the right ventricle after birth. In the adult, right and left ventricular outputs are equal; in the newborn, right ventricular output reflects systemic venous return, and left ventricular output reflects pulmonary venous return. Systemic blood volume and pulmonary blood volume are not equal in the newborn. The newborn's combined cardiac output (left and right ventricular) is greater per unit of body weight than it will be in later childhood.

Before birth, the right ventricle does approximately two thirds of the cardiac work, resulting in increased size and thickness of the right ventricle at birth. After birth, the left ventricle must assume a larger share of the cardiac workload, and it progressively increases in size and thickness. This may explain why right-sided heart defects are better tolerated than left-sided lesions and why left-sided heart defects rapidly become symptomatic after birth.

Figure 28–6 ◆ Fetal-neonatal circulation. *A,* Pattern of blood flow and oxygenation in fetal circulation. *B,* Pattern of blood flow and oxygenation in transitional circulation of the newborn. *C,* Pattern of blood flow and oxygenation in neonatal circulation.

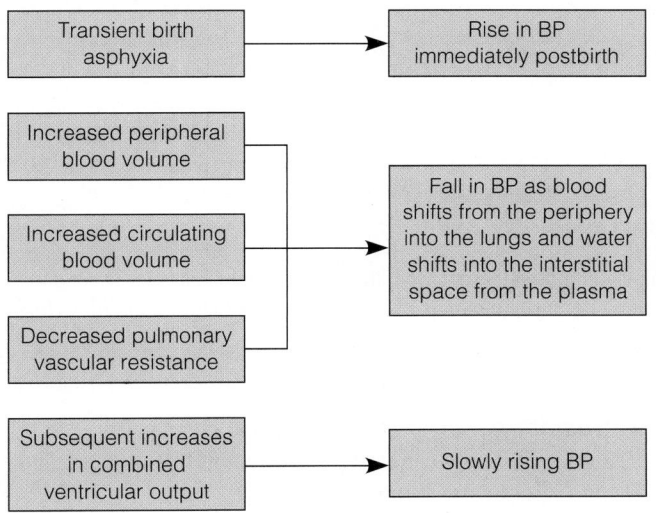

Figure 28–7 ◆ Response of blood pressure (BP) to changes in neonatal blood volume.

HEMATOPOIETIC ADAPTATIONS

Fetal blood flowing through the umbilical vein in utero is 50% oxygen saturated; this relative hypoxia causes increased amounts of erythropoietin to be secreted, resulting in active erythropoiesis (an increase in nucleated red blood cells and reticulocytes). After birth, the increases in oxygen saturation and arterial oxygen levels shut off the production of erythropoietin. In the first days of life, hemoglobin concentration may rise 1 to 2 g/dL above fetal levels as a result of placental transfusion, low oral fluid intake, and diminished extracellular fluid volume. By 1 week postnatally, peripheral hemoglobin is comparable to fetal blood counts. The hemoglobin level declines progressively thereafter during the first 2 months after birth (Polin et al., 2004). This initial decline in hemoglobin creates a phenomenon known as **physiologic anemia of infancy.** A factor that influ-

ences the degree of physiologic anemia is the nutritional status of the newborn. Supplies of vitamin E, folic acid, and iron may be inadequate given the amount of growth in the later part of the first year of life. Hemoglobin values fall, mainly from a decrease in red cell mass rather than from the dilutional effect of increasing plasma volume.

The fact that red cell survival is lower in newborns than in adults, and that red cell production is less, also contributes to this anemia. Neonatal RBCs have a lifespan of 80 to 100 days, approximately two thirds of an adult's RBC lifespan.

Leukocytosis is a normal finding because the stress of birth stimulates increased production of neutrophils during the first few days of life. Neutrophils then decrease to 35% of the total leukocyte count by 2 weeks of age. Lymphocytes play a role in antibody formation and eventually become the predominant type of leukocyte, and the total white blood count falls. Also, megakaryocytes appear in the liver and spleen as platelets at about 11 weeks' gestation and approach adult values by 30 weeks' gestation.

Blood volume of the term infant is estimated to be 80 mL/kg of body weight. For example, a 3.6 kg (8 lb) newborn has a blood volume of 290 to 309 mL. Blood volume varies according to the amount of placental transfusion received during the expulsion of the placenta as well as other factors, including the following:

1. *Delayed cord clamping and the normal shift of plasma to the extravascular spaces.* Newborn hemoglobin and hematocrit values are higher when a placental transfusion occurs at birth. Placental vessels contain about 75 to 125 mL of blood at term, most of which can be transfused into the newborn through the umbilical vein by holding the newborn below the level of the placenta and by delaying clamping of the cord (Figure 28–8 ◆). Blood volume increases by 50% with delayed cord clamping (Polin et al., 2004). The increase is reflected by a rise in hemoglobin level and an increase in the hematocrit. Cord blood provides the most accurate assessment of the newborn's initial hemoglobin and hematocrit.

Figure 28–8 ◆ Schematic illustration of the mechanisms in placental transfusion (normal term births) through the umbilical vein. The mean neonatal blood volume at 30 minutes is plotted against the time of cord clamping after birth (mean + 1 SE, data from 114 full-term infants). Note episodic, stepwise increments in blood volume at 10, 60, and 180 seconds.
SOURCE: Yao, A. C., & Lind, J. (1982). *Placental transfusion: A clinical and physiological study.* Springfield, IL: Charles C. Thomas.

Table 28–2   NORMAL TERM NEWBORN CORD BLOOD VALUES

Laboratory Data	Normal Range
Hemoglobin	14–20 g/dL
Hematocrit	43%–63%
WBC	10,000–30,000/mm³
Neutrophils	40%–80%
Platelets	150,000–350,000/mm³
Reticulocytes	3%–7%
Blood volume	82.3 mL/kg (third day after early cord clamping), 92.6 mL/kg (third day after delayed cord clamping)
Sodium	129–144 mEq/L
Potassium	3.4–9.9 mEq/L
Chloride	103–111 mEq/L
Calcium	8.2–111 mg/dL
Glucose	45–94 mg/dL

SOURCE: Adapted from Fanaroff, A. A., & Martin, R. J. (Eds.). (2006). *Neonatal-perinatal medicine* (8th ed., pp. 1801, 1810). St. Louis: Mosby.

2. *Gestational age.* There appears to be a positive association between gestational age, RBC numbers, and hemoglobin concentration.

3. *Prenatal or perinatal hemorrhage.* Significant prenatal or perinatal bleeding decreases the hematocrit level and causes hypovolemia.

4. *Site of the blood sample.* Hemoglobin and hematocrit levels taken simultaneously are significantly higher in capillary blood than in venous blood. Sluggish peripheral blood flow creates red blood cells stasis, increasing RBC concentration in the capillaries. Consequently, blood samples taken from venous blood sites are more accurate than those from capillary sites.

The concentration of serum electrolytes in the blood indicates the fluid and electrolyte status of the newborn. See Table 28–2 for normal electrolyte and blood values of the normal term newborn.

TEMPERATURE REGULATION

Temperature regulation is the maintenance of thermal balance by losing heat to the environment at a rate equal to heat production. Newborns are *homeothermic;* they attempt to stabilize their internal (core) body temperatures within a narrow range in spite of significant temperature variations in their environment. At birth, the fetus moves from a warm intrauterine environment to the relatively colder extrauterine environment. The newborn's temperature may fall 2C to 3C after birth mainly because of evaporative losses; this triggers cold-induced metabolic responses and heat production. Term newborns can increase their metabolic rate by 100% by 15 to 30 minutes after birth.

Thermoregulation in the newborn is closely related to the rate of metabolism and oxygen consumption. Within a specific environmental range called the **neutral thermal environment (NTE),** the rates of oxygen consumption and metabolism are minimal, and internal body temperature is maintained because of thermal balance (Table 28–3) (Thureen et al., 2005). For an unclothed full-term newborn, the NTE range is an ambient environmental temperature of 32C to 34C (89.6F to 93.2F)

within 50% relative humidity. The limits for an adult are 26C to 28C (78.8F to 82.4F) (Polin et al., 2004). Thus the normal newborn requires higher environmental temperatures to maintain a neutral thermal environment.

Several newborn characteristics affect establishment of thermal stability.

- The newborn has less subcutaneous fat than an adult and a thin epidermis.
- Blood vessels of the newborn are closer to the skin than those of an adult. Therefore, the circulating blood is influenced by changes in environmental temperature and in turn influences the hypothalamic temperature-regulating center.
- The flexed posture of the term infant decreases the surface area exposed to the environment, thereby reducing heat loss.

Table 28–3   NEUTRAL THERMAL ENVIRONMENTAL TEMPERATURES

Age and Weight*	Range of Temperature (C)	Age and Weight*	Range of Temperature (C)
0–6 Hours		**72–96 Hours**	
Under 1200 g	34–35.4	Under 1200 g	34–35
1200–1500 g	33.9–34.4	1200–1500 g	33–34
1501–2500 g	32.8–33.8	1501–2500 g	31.1–33.2
Over 2500 (and greater than 36 weeks)	32–33.8	Over 2500 (and greater than 36 weeks)	29.8–32.8
6–12 Hours		**4–12 Days**	
Under 1200 g	34–35.4	Under 1500 g	33–34
1200–1500 g	33.5–34.4	1501–2500 g	31–33.2
1501–2500 g	32.2–33.8	Over 2500 (and greater than 36 weeks)	
Over 2500 (and greater than 36 weeks)	31.4–33.8	4–5 days	29.5–32.6
		5–6 days	29.4–32.3
		6–8 days	29–32.2
12–24 Hours		8–10 days	29–31.8
Under 1200 g	34–35	10–12 days	29–31.4
1200–1500 g	33.3–34.3		
1501–2500 g	31.8–33.8	**12–24 Days**	
Over 2500 (and greater than 36 weeks)	31–33.7	Under 1500 g	32.6–34
		1500–2500 g	31–33.2
24–36 Hours		Over 2500 (and greater than 36 weeks)	29–30.8
Under 1200 g	34–35		
1200–1500 g	33.1–34.1	**2–3 Weeks**	
1501–2500 g	31.6–33.6		
Over 2500 (and greater than 36 weeks)	30.7–33.5	Under 1500 g	32.2–34
		1500–2500 g	30.5–33
36–48 Hours		**3–4 Weeks**	
Under 1200 g	34–35	Under 1500 g	31.6–33.6
1200–1500 g	33–34.1	1500–2500 g	30–32.7
1501–2500 g	31.4–33.5		
Over 2500 (and greater than 36 weeks)	30.5–33.3	**4–5 Weeks**	
		Under 1500 g	31.2–33
		1500–2500 g	29.5–32.2
48–72 Hours			
Under 1200 g	34–35	**5–6 Weeks**	
1200–1500 g	33–34		
1501–2500 g	31.2–33.4	Under 1500 g	30.6–32.3
Over 2500 (and greater than 36 weeks)	30.1–33.2	1500–2500 g	29–31.8

*Generally speaking, the smaller infants in each weight group will require a temperature in the higher portion of the temperature range. Within each time range, the younger the infant, the higher the temperature required.

SOURCE: Adapted from Scopes and Ahmed (1966) (For his table Scopes had the walls of the incubator 1 to 2 degrees warmer than the ambient air temperatures.) Reproduced with permission, from Klaus, M. H., & Fanaroff, A. A. (1986). *Care of the high-risk neonate* (3rd ed. p. 103). Philadelphia: Saunders.

Size and age may also affect the establishment of an NTE. For example, the preterm or small-for-gestational-age (SGA) newborn has less adipose tissue and is hypoflexed, and therefore requires higher environmental temperatures to achieve a thermal neutral environment. A larger, well-insulated newborn may be able to cope with lower environmental temperatures. If the environmental temperature falls below the lower limits of the NTE, the newborn responds with increased oxygen consumption and raised metabolism, which results in greater heat production. Prolonged exposure to the cold may result in depleted glycogen stores and acidosis. Oxygen consumption also increases if the environmental temperature is above the NTE.

Heat Loss

A newborn is at a distinct disadvantage in maintaining a normal temperature. With a large body surface in relation to mass and a limited amount of insulating subcutaneous fat, the full-term newborn loses about four times as much heat as an adult does. The newborn's poor thermal stability is due primarily to excessive heat loss rather than to impaired heat production. Because of the risk of hypothermia and possible cold stress, minimizing heat loss in the newborn after birth is essential. (See Provision of Initial Newborn Care in Chapter 24 ∞ and Chapter 30 ∞ for nursing measures).

Two major routes of heat loss are from the internal core of the body to the body surface and from the external body surface to the environment. Usually the core temperature is higher than the skin temperature, resulting in continuous transfer or conduction of heat to the surface. The greater the difference in temperatures between core and skin, the more rapidly heat transfer occurs. The transfer is accomplished through an increase in oxygen consumption, depletion of glycogen stores, and metabolizing of brown fat. Heat loss from the body surface to the environment takes place by four avenues—convection, radiation, evaporation, and conduction (Figure 28–9 ◆).

- **Convection** is the loss of heat from the warm body surface to the cooler air currents. Air-conditioned rooms, air currents with a temperature below the infant's skin temperature, oxygen by mask, and removal of the infant from an incubator for procedures increase convective heat loss of the newborn.

- **Radiation** losses occur when body heat rises to cooler surfaces and objects not in direct contact with the body. The walls of a room or of an incubator are potential causes of heat loss by radiation, even if the ambient temperature of the incubator is within the neutral thermal range for the infant. Placing cold objects (such as ice for blood gases) onto the incubator or near the infant in the radiant warmer will increase radiant heat losses.

- **Evaporation** is the loss of heat incurred when water is converted to a vapor. The newborn is particularly prone to heat loss by evaporation immediately after birth (when the baby is wet with amniotic fluid) and during baths; thus drying the newborn is critical.

A

B

C

D

Figure 28–9 ◆ Methods of heat loss. *A,* Convection. *B,* Radiation. *C,* Evaporation. *D,* Conduction.

- **Conduction** is the loss of heat to a cooler surface by direct skin contact. Chilled hands, cool scales, cold examination tables, and cold stethoscopes can cause heat loss by conduction. Even if objects are warmed to the incubator temperature, there still may be a significant temperature difference between the infant's core temperature and the ambient temperature. This difference results in heat transfer.

Once the infant has been dried after birth, the highest losses of heat generally result from radiation and convection because of the newborn's large ratio of body surface to weight, and from thermal conduction because of the marked difference between core temperature and skin temperature. The newborn can respond to the cooler environmental temperature with adequate peripheral vasoconstriction, but this mechanism is less effective because of the minimal amount of fat insulation present, the large body surface, and ongoing thermal conduction. Because of these factors, minimizing the baby's heat loss and preventing hypothermia are imperative. Nursing measures for preventing hypothermia are described in Chapter 30. ∞

Heat Production (Thermogenesis)

When exposed to a cool environment, the newborn requires additional heat. The newborn has several physiologic mechanisms that increase heat production, or *thermogenesis*. These include increased basal metabolic rate, muscular activity, and chemical thermogenesis (also called *nonshivering thermogenesis [NST]*) (Polin et al., 2004).

Nonshivering thermogenesis, an important mechanism of heat production, is unique to the newborn. It occurs when skin receptors perceive a drop in environmental temperature and, in response, transmit sensations to stimulate the sympathetic nervous system. NST uses the newborn's stores of **brown adipose tissue (BAT)** (also called *brown fat*) to provide heat. Brown fat receives its name from the dark color caused by its enriched blood supply, dense cellular content, and abundant nerve endings. These characteristics promote rapid metabolism, heat generation, and heat transfer to the peripheral circulation. The large numbers of brown fat cells increase the speed with which triglycerides are metabolized to produce heat.

Thus, NST from BAT is the primary source of heat in the hypothermic newborn. It first appears in the fetus at 26 to 30 weeks' gestation and continues to increase until 2 to 5 weeks after the birth of a term infant, unless it is depleted by cold stress. Brown fat is deposited in the midscapular area, around the neck, and in the axillas, with deeper placement around the trachea, esophagus, abdominal aorta, kidneys, and adrenal glands (Figure 28–10 ◆). BAT constitutes 2% to 6% of the newborn's total body weight.

Shivering, a form of muscular activity common in the cold adult, is rarely seen in the newborn, although it has been observed at ambient temperatures of 15C (59F) or less (Polin et al., 2004). If the newborn does shiver, it means the newborn's metabolic rate has already doubled. The extra muscular activity does little to produce needed heat.

Thermographic studies of newborns exposed to cold show an increase in the skin heat over the brown fat deposits in the

Figure 28–10 ◆ The distribution of brown adipose tissue (brown fat) in the newborn.
SOURCE: Adapted from Davis, V. (1980). Structure and function of brown adipose tissue in the neonate. *Journal of Obstetric, Gynecologic, & Neonatal Nursing, 9,* 364.

newborn between 1 and 14 days of age (Polin et al., 2004). However, if the brown fat supply has been depleted, the metabolic response to cold will be limited or lacking. An increase in basal metabolism as a result of hypothermia results in an increase in oxygen consumption. A decrease in the environmental temperature of 2C, from 33C to 31C, is a drop sufficient to double the oxygen consumption of a term newborn. Keeping the normal newborn warm promotes normal oxygen requirements, whereas chilling can cause the newborn to show signs of respiratory distress.

When exposed to cold, the normal term newborn is usually able to cope with the increase in oxygen requirements, but the preterm newborn may be unable to increase ventilation to the necessary level of oxygen consumption. (See Chapter 33 ∞ for discussion of cold stress.) Because oxidation of fatty acids depends on the availability of oxygen, glucose, and adenosine triphosphate (ATP), the newborn's ability to generate heat can be altered by pathologic events such as hypoxia, acidosis, and hypoglycemia or by medications that block the release of norepinephrine. The effect of certain drugs such as meperidine

NEWBORN BATHS IN JORDAN

In Jordan, the birth of a male infant is a much celebrated event. The newborn is bathed daily during the first week of life. During the final bath, salt is added to the water to help the newborn's skin adjust to the external environment and protect it from changes in the weather.

(Demerol) may also prevent metabolism of brown fat. Meperidine given to the laboring woman leads to a greater fall in the newborn's body temperature during the neonatal period. Neonatal hypothermia prolongs as well as potentiates the effects of many analgesic and anesthetic drugs in the newborn.

Response to Heat

Sweating is the usual initial response of the term newborn to hyperthermia. The newborn sweat glands have limited function until after the fourth week of extrauterine life; heat is lost through peripheral vasodilation and evaporation of insensible water loss. In term SGA infants, the onset of sweating is delayed; it is virtually nonexistent in preterm infants of less than 30 weeks' gestation because of the underdevelopment of the sweat glands. The term infant will be flaccid and assume a position of extension to facilitate heat loss (Kenner, 2003). Oxygen consumption and metabolic rate also increase in response to hyperthermia. Severe hyperthermia can lead to death or to gross brain damage if the baby survives.

HEPATIC ADAPTATIONS

The newborn's liver is frequently palpable 2 to 3 cm below the right costal margin. It is relatively large and occupies about 40% of the abdominal cavity. The newborn's liver plays a significant role in iron storage, carbohydrate metabolism, conjugation of bilirubin, and coagulation.

Iron Storage and Red Blood Cell Production

As RBCs are destroyed after birth, their iron content is stored in the liver until needed for new RBC production. Newborn iron stores are determined by total body hemoglobin content and length of gestation. The term newborn has about 270 mg of iron at birth, and about 140 to 170 mg of this amount is in the hemoglobin. If the mother's iron intake has been adequate, enough iron will be stored to last until 5 months of age. After about 6 months of age, foods containing iron or iron supplements must be given to prevent anemia.

Carbohydrate Metabolism

At term the newborn's cord blood glucose is 70% to 80% of the maternal blood glucose level (Kalhan & Parimi, 2006). Neonatal carbohydrate reserves are relatively low. One third of this reserve is in the form of liver glycogen. Neonatal glycogen stores are twice that of the adult. The newborn enters an energy crunch at the time of birth with the removal of the maternal glucose supply and the increased energy expenditure associated with the birth process and extrauterine life. Fuel sources are consumed at a faster rate because of the work of breathing, loss of heat when exposed to cold, activity, and activation of muscle tone.

Glucose is the main source of energy in the first 4 to 6 hours after birth. During the first 2 hours of life, the serum blood glucose level declines, then rises, and finally reaches a steady state 2 to 3 hours after birth (Kalhan & Parimi, 2006)

The nurse may assess the glucose level on admission to the newborn nursery if risk factors are present or per agency protocol. As stores of liver and muscle glycogen and blood glucose decrease, the newborn compensates by changing from a predominantly carbohydrate metabolism to fat metabolism. Energy is derived from fat and protein as well as from carbohydrates. The amount and availability of each of these "fuel substrates" depends on the ability of immature metabolic pathways (i.e., lacking specific enzymes or hormones) to function in the first few days of life.

Conjugation of Bilirubin

Conjugation of bilirubin is the conversion of yellow lipid-soluble pigment into water-soluble pigment. Unconjugated (indirect) bilirubin is a breakdown product derived from hemoglobin that is released primarily from destroyed RBCs. Unconjugated bilirubin is not in an excretable form and is a potential toxin. **Total serum bilirubin** is the sum of conjugated (direct) and unconjugated (indirect) bilirubin.

Fetal unconjugated bilirubin crosses the placenta to be excreted, so the fetus does not need to conjugate bilirubin. Total bilirubin at birth is less than 3 mg/dL unless an abnormal hemolytic process has been present. After birth, the newborn's liver must begin to conjugate bilirubin. This produces a rise in serum bilirubin in the first few days of life. The bilirubin formed, after RBCs are destroyed, is transported in the blood bound to albumin. The bilirubin is transferred into the hepatocytes and bound to intracellular proteins. These proteins determine the amount of bilirubin that is held in the liver cells for processing and consequently determine the amount of bilirubin uptake into the liver. The activity of uridine diphosphoglucuronosyl transferase (UDPGT) enzyme results in the attachment of unconjugated bilirubin to glucuronic acid (a product of liver glycogen), producing bilirubin glucuronides (conjugated, direct bilirubin). Direct bilirubin is excreted into the tiny bile ducts, then into the common duct and duodenum. The (direct) conjugated bilirubin then progresses down the intestines, where bacteria transform it into urobilinogen (urine bilirubin) and stercobilinogen. Stercobilinogen is not reabsorbed but is excreted as a yellow-brown pigment in the stools.

Even after the bilirubin has been conjugated and bound, it can be changed back to unconjugated bilirubin via the enterohepatic circulation. In the intestines, β-glucuronidase enzyme acts to split off (deconjugate) the bilirubin from bilirubin glucuronides if it is not first acted upon by gut bacteria to produce urobilinogen; the free bilirubin is reabsorbed through the intestinal wall and brought back to the liver via portal vein circulation. This recycling of the bilirubin and decreased ability to clear bilirubin from the system are prevalent in babies who have very high β-D-glucuronidase activity levels as well as delayed bacterial colonization of the gut (such as with the use of antibiotics) and further increases the newborn's susceptibility to jaundice. Conjugation of bilirubin in newborns is depicted in Figure 28–11 ◆.

The newborn liver has relatively less metabolic and enzymatic activity at birth and in the first few weeks of life than an adult liver. This reduction in hepatic activity, along with a rela-

Figure 28–11 ◆ Conjugation of bilirubin in newborns.

SOURCE: Adapted from Avery, G. B., Fletcher, M. A., & MacDonald, M. G. *Neonatology: Pathophysiology and management of the newborn* (5th ed., p. 767, fig. 38–5). Copyright © 1999 Lippincott, Williams & Wilkins. Reprinted with permission.

tively large bilirubin load, decreases the liver's ability to conjugate bilirubin and increases susceptibility to jaundice.

Physiologic Jaundice

Physiologic jaundice is caused by accelerated destruction of fetal RBCs, impaired conjugation of bilirubin, and increased bilirubin reabsorption from the intestinal tract. This condition does not have a pathologic basis, but rather is a normal biologic response of the newborn.

Maisels (2005) describes six factors—several of which can also be related to pathologic events—whose interactions may give rise to physiologic jaundice:

1. *Increased amounts of bilirubin delivered to the liver.* The increased blood volume due to delayed cord clamping combined with faster RBC destruction in the newborn leads to an increased bilirubin level in the blood. A proportionately larger amount of nonerythrocyte bilirubin is formed in the newborn. Therefore, newborns

have two to three times greater production or breakdown of bilirubin. The use of forceps or vacuum extraction that sometimes causes facial bruising or cephalhematoma (entrapped hemorrhage) can increase the amount of bilirubin to be handled by the liver.

2. *Defective uptake of bilirubin from the plasma.* If the newborn does not ingest adequate calories, the formation of hepatic intracellular binding proteins diminishes, resulting in higher levels of bilirubin.

3. *Defective conjugation of the bilirubin.* Decreased uridine diphosphoglucuronosyl activity, as in hypothyroidism, or inadequate caloric intake causes the intracellular binding proteins to remain saturated and results in greater unconjugated bilirubin levels in the blood. The fatty acids in maternal breast milk compete with bilirubin for albumin binding sites; this process is thought to impede bilirubin processing.

4. *Defect in bilirubin excretion.* Delay in introduction of bacterial flora and decreased intestinal motility can also delay excretion and increase enterohepatic circulation of bilirubin.

5. *Inadequate hepatic circulation.* Decreased oxygen supplies to the liver associated with neonatal hypoxia or congenital heart disease lead to a rise in the bilirubin level.

6. *Increased reabsorption of bilirubin from the intestine.* Reduced bowel motility, intestinal obstruction, or delayed passage of meconium increases the circulation of bilirubin in the enterohepatic pathway, resulting in higher bilirubin values.

About 50% of full-term and 80% of preterm newborns exhibit physiologic jaundice on about the second or third day after birth. The characteristic yellow color results from increased levels of unconjugated bilirubin, which are a normal product of RBC breakdown and reflect a temporary inability of the body to eliminate bilirubin. Serum levels of bilirubin are about 4 to 6 mg/dL before yellow coloration of the skin and sclera appears. The signs of physiologic jaundice appear *after* the first 24 hours postnatally. This differentiates physiologic jaundice from pathologic jaundice (see Chapter 33 ∞), which is clinically seen at birth or within the first 24 hours of postnatal life.

Peak bilirubin levels are reached between days 3 and 5 in the full-term infant and between days 5 and 7 in the preterm infant. But these values are established for European and American Caucasian newborns. Chinese, Japanese, Korean, and Native American newborns have considerably higher bilirubin levels that are not as apparent and that persist for longer periods with no apparent ill effects (Maisels, 2005).

The nursery or postpartum room environment, including lighting, can hinder the early detection of the degree and type of jaundice. Pink walls and artificial lights mask the beginning of jaundice in newborns. Daylight assists the observer in early recognition by eliminating distortions caused by artificial light.

If jaundice is suspected, the nurse can quickly assess the newborn's coloring by pressing the skin, generally on the fore-

head or nose, with a finger. As blanching occurs, the nurse can observe the icterus (yellow coloring).

Several newborn care procedures will decrease the probability of high bilirubin levels:

- Maintain the newborn's skin temperature at 36.5C (97.8F) or above, because cold stress results in acidosis. Acidosis decreases available serum albumin-binding sites, weakens albumin-binding powers, and causes elevated unconjugated bilirubin levels.

- Monitor stool for amount and characteristics. Bilirubin is eliminated in the feces; inadequate stooling may result in reabsorption and recycling of bilirubin. Encourage early breastfeeding because the laxative effect of colostrum increases excretion of meconium and transitional stool.

- Encourage early feedings to promote intestinal elimination and bacterial colonization and to provide caloric and protein intake necessary for the formation of hepatic binding proteins.

If jaundice becomes apparent, nursing care is directed toward keeping the newborn well hydrated and promoting intestinal elimination. For specific nursing management and therapies, see Nursing Care Plan: Newborn with Hyperbilirubinemia in Chapter 33. ∞

Physiologic jaundice may be very upsetting to parents; they require emotional support and thorough explanation of the condition. If the baby is placed under phototherapy, a few additional days of hospitalization may be required, which may also be disturbing to parents. They can be encouraged to provide for the emotional needs of their newborn by continuing to feed, hold, and caress the infant. If the mother is discharged, the parents should be encouraged to return for feedings and telephone or visit whenever they wish. In many instances the mother, especially if she is breastfeeding, may elect to remain hospitalized with her newborn; the nurse should support this decision. If insurance limitations make this unrealistic, it may be possible to find an empty room for the discharged mother and her family to use while visiting the newborn. As an alternative to continued hospitalization, some newborns are treated with home phototherapy. (See Phototherapy in Chapter 33 ∞ for more information).

Breastfeeding Jaundice and Breast Milk Jaundice

Breastfeeding is implicated in jaundice in some newborns. *Breastfeeding jaundice* occurs in the first days of life in breast-fed newborns. It appears to be associated with poor feeding practices and not with any abnormality in milk composition. Prevention of early breastfeeding jaundice includes encouraging frequent (every 2 to 3 hours) breastfeeding, avoiding supplementation, and accessing maternal lactation counseling.

In *breast milk jaundice,* the bilirubin begins to rise after the first week of life, when physiologic jaundice is waning after the mother's milk has come in. The level peaks at 5 to 10 mg/dL at 2 to 3 weeks of age and declines over the first several months of life (Maisels, 2005).

In contrast to breastfeeding jaundice, breast milk jaundice is related to milk composition. Some women's breast milk may contain several times the normal concentration of certain free fatty acids. These free fatty acids may compete with bilirubin for binding sites on albumin and inhibit the conjugation of bilirubin or increase lipase activity, which disrupts the RBC membrane. Increased lipase activity enhances absorption of bile across the gastrointestinal tract membrane, thereby increasing the entero-hepatic circulation of bilirubin. In the past it was thought that the breast milk of women whose newborns have breast milk jaundice contained an enzyme that inhibited glucuronyl transferase, but this hypothesis has not been proven (Thureen et al., 2005).

Newborns with breast milk jaundice appear well, and at present an absence of documented kernicterus (toxic levels of bilirubin in the brain) with this type of jaundice has not been documented. Temporary cessation of breastfeeding may be advised if bilirubin reaches presumed toxic levels of approximately 20 mg/dL or if the interruption is necessary to establish the cause of the hyperbilirubinemia. Most physicians believe that breastfeeding may be resumed once other causes of jaundice have been ruled out and as long as serum bilirubin levels remain below 20 mg/dL. In cases of breast milk jaundice, within 24 to 36 hours after breastfeeding is discontinued, the newborn's serum bilirubin levels begin to fall dramatically. With resumption of breastfeeding, the bilirubin concentration may show a slight rise of 2 to 3 mg/dL with a subsequent decline. Breastfeeding mothers need encouragement and support in their desire to breastfeed their infants, assistance and instruction regarding pumping and expressing milk during the interrupted breastfeeding period, and reassurance that nothing is wrong with their milk or their mothering abilities. Table 28–4 summarizes key factors in physiologic and breast milk jaundice.

> **CLINICAL TIP**
>
> Breastfeeding mothers need encouragement and support in their desire to breastfeed their infants, assistance and instruction about pumping and expressing milk during the interrupted breastfeeding period, and reassurance that nothing is wrong with their milk or mothering abilities.

Coagulation

The liver plays an important part in blood coagulation during fetal life and continues this function following birth. Coagulation factors II, VII, IX, and X (synthesized in the liver) are activated under the influence of vitamin K and therefore are considered vitamin K dependent. The absence of normal intestinal flora needed to synthesize vitamin K in the newborn gut results in low levels of vitamin K and creates a transient blood coagulation alteration between the second and fifth day of life. From a low point at about 2 to 3 days after birth, these coagulation factors rise slowly but do not approach adult levels until 9 months of age or later. Other coagulation factors with low cord blood levels are XI, XII, and XIII. Fibrinogen and factors V and VII are near adult ranges.

Although newborn bleeding problems are rare, an injection of vitamin K (AquaMEPHYTON) is given prophylactically on the day of birth to combat potential clinical bleeding problems.

DEVELOPING CULTURAL COMPETENCE

INTERPRETING ILLNESS THROUGH CULTURAL BELIEFS

Cultural beliefs lead mothers to interpret illness within their cultural framework, especially when left without clear and understood explanations (Hannon, Willis, & Scrimshaw, 2001). For example, some Latina women believe that showing strong maternal emotions during pregnancy and during breastfeeding can be detrimental. They may blame jaundice in their newborn on "bili" associated with anger. Such maternal reactions can be lessened by careful explanations to the mothers about the diagnosis, prognosis, duration, and management options for jaundice, and possibility for recurrence.

Table 28–4   JAUNDICE

Physiologic Jaundice

Physiologic jaundice occurs after the first 24 hours of life.

During the first week of life, bilirubin should not exceed 13 mg/dL. Some pediatricians allow levels up to 15 mg/dL.

Bilirubin levels peak at 3 to 5 days in term infants.

Breast Milk Jaundice

Bilirubin levels begin to rise about the fourth day after mature breast milk comes in.

Peak of 5–10 mg/dL is reached at 2 to 3 weeks of age.

It may be necessary to interrupt breastfeeding for a short period when bilirubin reaches 20 mg/dL.

(Hemorrhagic disease of the newborn is discussed in more depth in Chapter 33 ∞).

Platelet counts at birth are in the same range as for older children, but newborns may manifest mild transient difficulty in platelet aggregation functioning. Phototherapy accentuates this platelet problem. Prenatal maternal therapy with phenytoin sodium (Dilantin) or phenobarbital also causes abnormal clotting studies and newborn bleeding in the first 24 hours after birth. Infants born to mothers receiving warfarin (Coumadin) compounds may bleed because these agents cross the placenta and accentuate existing vitamin K-dependent factor deficiencies. Transient neonatal thrombocytopenia may occur in infants born to mothers with severe hypertension or HELLP syndrome (hemolysis, elevated liver enzymes, and low platelet count) and in infants born to mothers who have idiopathic isoimmune thrombocytopenic purpura.

GASTROINTESTINAL ADAPTATIONS

By 36 to 38 weeks of fetal life, the gastrointestinal tract is adequately mature, with the presence of enzymatic activity and the ability to transport nutrients.

Digestion and Absorption

The full-term newborn has adequate intestinal and pancreatic enzymes to digest most simple carbohydrates, fat, and proteins. The carbohydrates requiring digestion in the newborn are usually disaccharides (lactose, maltose, sucrose), which are split into monosaccharides (galactose, fructose, and glucose) by the enzymes of the intestinal mucosa. Lactose is the primary carbohydrate in the breastfeeding newborn and is generally easily digested and well absorbed. The only enzyme lacking at birth is pancreatic amylase, which remains relatively deficient during the first few months of life. Newborns have trouble digesting starches (changing more complex carbohydrates into maltose), so they should not eat them until after the first few months of life.

Although proteins require more digestion than carbohydrates, they are well digested and absorbed from the newborn intestine. The newborn digests and absorbs fats less efficiently because of the minimal activity of pancreatic lipase. The newborn excretes 10% to 20% of the dietary fat intake, compared with 10% for the adult. The fat in breast milk is absorbed more completely by the newborn than is the fat in cow's milk because it consists of more medium-chain triglycerides and contains lipase. (See Chapter 31 ∞ for a more detailed discussion of infant nutrition).

By birth the newborn has experienced swallowing, gastric emptying, and intestinal propulsion. In utero, fetal swallowing is accompanied by gastric emptying and peristalsis of the fetal intestinal tract. By the end of gestation, peristalsis becomes much more active in preparation for extrauterine life. Fetal peristalsis is also stimulated by anoxia, causing the expulsion of meconium into the amniotic fluid in more mature fetuses.

Air enters the stomach immediately after birth. The small intestine is air filled within 2 to 12 hours, and the large bowel within 24 hours. The salivary glands are immature at birth, and little saliva is manufactured until the infant is about 3 months old. The newborn's stomach has a capacity of 50 to 60 mL. It empties intermittently, starting within a few minutes of the beginning of a feeding and ending between 2 and 4 hours after feeding. Bowel sounds are present within the first 30 to 60 minutes of birth and the newborn can successfully feed during this time. The newborn's gastric pH becomes less acidic about a week after birth and remains less acidic than that of adults for the next 2 to 3 months.

The cardiac sphincter is immature, as is neural control of the stomach, so some regurgitation may be noted in the neonatal period. Regurgitation of the first few feedings during the first day or two of life can usually be lessened by avoiding overfeeding and by burping the newborn well during and after the feeding.

When no other signs and symptoms are evident, vomiting is limited and ceases within the first few days of life. Continuous vomiting or regurgitation should be monitored closely. If the newborn has swallowed bloody or purulent amniotic fluid, lavage of the stomach may be indicated in the term newborn to relieve the problem. Bilious vomiting is abnormal and must be evaluated thoroughly because it might represent a condition that warrants prompt surgical intervention.

Adequate digestion and absorption are essential for newborn growth and development. If optimal nutritional support is available, postnatal growth ideally should parallel intrauterine growth. After 30 weeks of gestation the fetus gains 30 g per day and adds 1.2 cm to body length daily. To gain weight at the intrauterine rate, the term newborn requires 120 kcal/kg/day. Following birth, caloric intake is often insufficient for weight gain until the newborn is 5 to 10 days old. During this time there may be a weight loss of 5% to 10% in term newborns. A shift of intracellular water to extracellular space and insensible water loss account for the 5% to 10% weight loss. Thus failure to lose weight when caloric intake is limited may indicate fluid retention.

Term newborns normally pass meconium within 8 to 24 hours of life—and almost always within 48 hours. **Meconium** is formed in utero from the amniotic fluid and its constituents, with intestinal secretions and shed mucosal cells. It is recognized by its thick, tarry, black (or dark green) appearance. Transitional (thinner brown to green) stools consisting of part meconium and part fecal material are passed for the next day or two, after which the stools become entirely fecal. Generally, the stools of a breast-fed newborn are pale yellow (but may be pasty green); they are more liquid and more frequent than those of formula-fed newborns, whose stools are paler (Figure 28–12 ◆). Frequency of

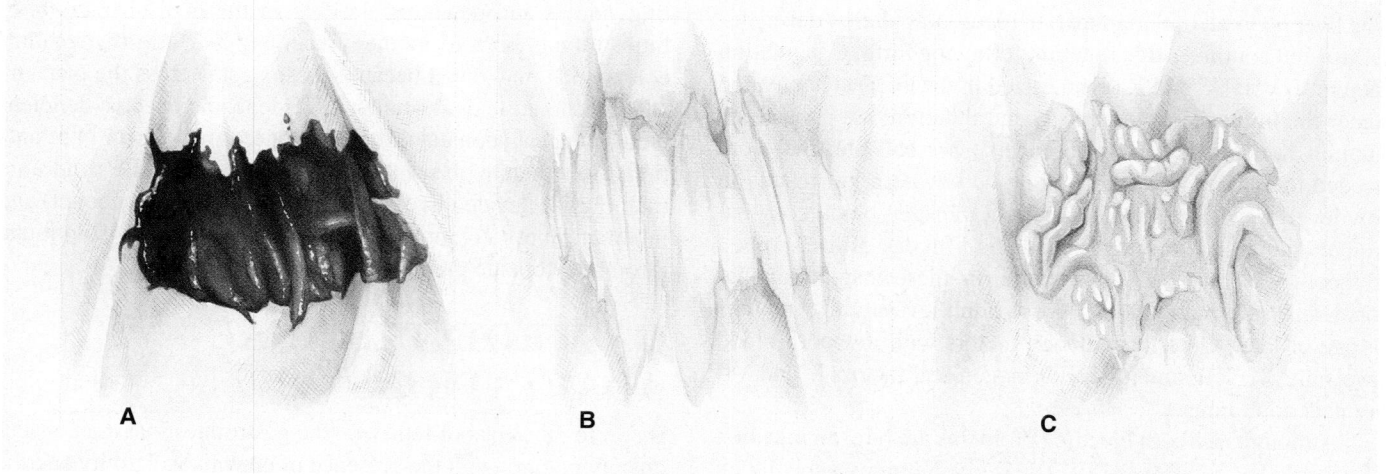

A   B   C

Figure 28–12 ◆ Newborn stool samples. *A,* Meconium stool. *B,* Breast milk stool. *C,* Cow's milk stool.

Table 28–5	PHYSIOLOGIC ADAPTATIONS TO EXTRAUTERINE LIFE
Periodic breathing may be present.	
Desired skin temperature 36C–36.5C (96.8F–97.7F), stabilizes 4 to 6 hours after birth.	
Desired blood glucose level reaches 60–70 mg/dL by third postnatal day.	
Stools (progress from):	
Meconium (thick, tarry, black)	
Transitional stools (thin, brown to green)	
Breastfed infants (yellow gold, soft, or mushy)	
Formula-fed infants (pale yellow, formed, and pasty)	

Table 28–6	NEWBORN URINALYSIS VALUES
Protein less than 5–10 mg/dL	
WBC less than 2–3/hpf	
RBC 0	
Casts 0	
Baleria 0	
Color pale yellow	

bowel movement varies but initially ranges from one every 2 to 3 days to as many as 10 daily. Totally breastfed infants often progress to stools that occur every 5 to 7 days. Mothers should be counseled that this is not constipation as long as the bowel movement remains soft. Table 28–5 describes the progression of stools and other physiologic adaptations to extrauterine life.

When the nurse took my first child and put him to my breast his tiny mouth opened and reached for me as if he had known forever what to do.

~LESLIE KENTON, *ALL I EVER WANTED WAS A BABY* ~

URINARY ADAPTATIONS
Kidney Development and Function

Certain physiologic features of the newborn's kidneys may affect the newborn's ability to handle body fluids and excrete urine:

1. The term newborn's kidneys have a full complement of functioning nephrons by 34 to 36 weeks of gestation.

2. The glomerular filtration rate of the newborn's kidneys is low in comparison with the adult rate. Because of this physiologic decrease in kidney glomerular filtration, the newborn's kidneys are unable to dispose of water rapidly when necessary.

3. The juxtamedullary portion of the nephron has limited capacity to reabsorb HCO_3 and H and concentrate urine. The limitation of tubular reabsorption can lead to inappropriate loss of substances present in the glomerular filtrate, such as amino acids, bicarbonate, glucose, and sodium.

Full-term newborns are less able than adults to concentrate urine (reabsorb water back into the blood) because the tubules are short and narrow. Also, the reduced ability to concentrate urine is caused by the limited tubular reabsorption of water and limited excretion of solutes (principally sodium, potassium, chloride, bicarbonate, urea, and phosphate) in the growing newborn. The ability to concentrate urine fully is attained by 3 months of age. Feeding practices may affect the osmolarity of the urine but have limited effect on concentration of the urine.

Because the newborn has difficulty concentrating urine, the effect of excessive insensible water loss or restricted fluid intake

is unpredictable. The newborn kidney is also limited in its dilutional capabilities. Concentrating and dilutional limitations of renal function are important considerations in monitoring fluid therapy to avoid dehydration and overhydration.

Characteristics of Newborn Urinary Function

Many newborns void immediately after birth, and the voiding frequently goes unnoticed. Among normal newborns, 93% void by 24 hours after birth, and 100% void by 48 hours after birth (Thureen et al., 2005). A newborn who has not voided by 48 hours should be assessed for adequacy of fluid intake, bladder distention, restlessness, and symptoms of pain. The appropriate clinical personnel should be notified if indicated.

The initial bladder volume is 6 to 44 mL of urine. Unless edema is present, normal urinary output is often limited, and the voidings are scanty until fluid intake increases. (The fluid of edema is eliminated by the kidneys, so infants with edema have a much higher urinary output.) The first 2 days postnatally, the newborn may void two to six times daily, with a urine output of 15 mL/kg/day. The newborn subsequently voids 5 to 25 times every 24 hours, with a volume of 25 mL/kg/day.

Following the first voiding, the newborn's urine frequently appears cloudy (because of mucus content) and has a high specific gravity, which decreases as fluid intake increases. Occasionally, pink stains ("brick dust spots") appear on the diaper. These are caused by urates and are innocuous. Blood may occasionally be observed on the diapers of female infants. This *pseudomenstruation* is related to the withdrawal of maternal hormones. Males may have bloody spotting from a circumcision. In the absence of apparent causes for bleeding, the clinician should be notified. During early infancy, normal urine is straw colored and almost odorless, although odor occurs when there is a metabolic disorder or when infection is present. Table 28–6 summarizes urinalysis values of the normal newborn.

IMMUNOLOGIC ADAPTATIONS

The newborn's immune system is not fully activated until sometime after birth. The limitations in the newborn's inflammatory response result in failure to recognize, localize, and destroy invasive bacteria. Thus the signs and symptoms of infection are often subtle and nonspecific in the newborn. The newborn also has a poor hypothalamic response to pyrogens; therefore, fever is not a reliable indicator of infection. In the neonatal period, hypothermia is a more reliable sign of infection.

Of the three major types of immunoglobulins primarily involved in immunity—IgG, IgA, and IgM—only IgG crosses the placenta. The pregnant woman forms antibodies in response to illness or immunization. This process is called **active acquired immunity.** When IgG antibodies are transferred to the fetus in utero, **passive acquired immunity** results because the fetus does not produce the antibodies himself or herself. IgG is very active against bacterial toxins.

Because the maternal immunoglobin is transferred primarily during the third trimester, preterm newborns (especially those born before 34 weeks) may be more susceptible to infection. In general, newborns have maternally induced immunity to tetanus, diphtheria, smallpox, measles, mumps, poliomyelitis, and a variety of other bacterial and viral diseases. The period of resistance varies: Immunity against common viral infections such as measles may last 4 to 8 months, whereas immunity to certain bacteria may disappear within 4 to 8 weeks.

The normal newborn does produce antibodies in response to an antigen but not as effectively as an older child does. It is customary to begin immunization at 2 months of age so the infant can develop active acquired immunity.

IgM immunoglobulins are produced in response to blood group antigens, gram-negative enteric organisms, and some viruses in the expectant mother. Because IgM does not normally cross the placenta, most or all is produced by the fetus beginning at 10 to 15 weeks' gestation. Elevated levels of IgM at birth may indicate placental leaks or, more commonly, fetal antigenic stimulation in utero. Consequently, elevations suggest that the infant was exposed to an intrauterine infection such as syphilis or TORCH syndrome (toxoplasmosis, rubella, cytomegalovirus, or herpes virus hominis type 2 infection). (For in-depth discussion, see Chapter 20 ∞ and Table 33–5 ∞). The lack of available maternal IgM in the newborn also accounts for the infant's susceptibility to gram-negative enteric organisms such as *Escherichia coli.*

The functions of IgA immunoglobins are not fully understood. IgA appears to provide protection mainly on secreting surfaces such as the respiratory tract, gastrointestinal tract, and eyes. Serum IgA does not cross the placenta and is not normally produced by the fetus in utero. Unlike the other immunoglobins, IgA is not affected by gastric action. Colostrum, the forerunner of breast milk, is very high in the secretory form of IgA. It may provide some passive immunity to the infant of a breastfeeding mother. Newborns begin to produce secretory IgA in their intestinal mucosa at about 4 weeks after birth.

NEUROLOGIC AND SENSORY/PERCEPTUAL FUNCTIONING

The newborn's brain is about one quarter the size of an adult's, and myelination of nerve fibers is incomplete. Unlike the cardiovascular or respiratory systems, which undergo tremendous changes at birth, the nervous system is minimally influenced by the actual birth process. Because many biochemical and histologic changes have yet to occur in the newborn's brain, the post-

natal period is considered a time of risk in regard to the development of the brain and nervous system. For neurologic development—including development of intellect—to proceed, the brain and other nervous system structures must mature in an orderly, unhampered fashion. For discussion of cranial nerves, see Chapter 29. ∞

Intrauterine Factors Influencing Newborn Behavior

Newborns respond to and interact with the environment in a predictable pattern of behavior that is shaped somewhat by their intrauterine experience. This intrauterine experience is affected by intrinsic factors such as maternal nutrition and external factors such as the mother's physical environment. Depending on the newborn's intrauterine experience and individual temperament, newborn behavioral responses to different stresses vary. Some newborns react quietly to stimulation, others become overreactive and tense, and some may exhibit a combination of the two.

Factors such as exposure to intense auditory stimuli in utero can eventually be manifested in the behavior of the newborn. For example, the fetal heart rate (FHR) initially increases when the pregnant woman is exposed to an auditory stimuli, but repetition of the stimuli leads to decreased FHR. Thus the newborn who was exposed to intense noise during fetal life is significantly less reactive to loud sounds postnatally.

Characteristics of Newborn Neurologic Function

- Partially flexed extremities with the legs near the abdomen is the usual position of the normal newborn. When awake, the newborn may exhibit purposeless, uncoordinated bilateral movements of the extremities. The organization and intensity of the newborn's motor activity are influenced by a number of factors, including the following (Brazelton, 1984):
  - Sleep-wake states
  - Presence of environmental stimuli, such as heat, light, cold, and noise
  - Conditions causing a chemical imbalance, such as hypoglycemia
  - Hydration status
  - State of health
- Recovery from the stress of labor and birth

Eye movements are observable during the first few days of life. An alert newborn is able to fixate on faces and geometric objects or patterns such as black and white stripes. A bright light shining in the newborn's eyes elicits the blinking reflex.

The cry of the newborn should be lusty and vigorous. High-pitched cries, weak cries, or no cries are all causes for concern.

The newborn's body grows in a cephalocaudal (head-to-toe), proximal-distal fashion. The newborn is somewhat hypertonic; that is, there is resistance to extending the elbow and knee joints. Muscle tone should be symmetric. Diminished muscle tone and flaccidity may indicate neurologic dysfunction.

Specific symmetric deep tendon reflexes can be elicited in the newborn. The knee jerk is brisk; a normal ankle clonus may involve three or four beats. Plantar flexion is present. Other reflexes, including the Moro, grasping, rooting, Babinski, and sucking reflexes, are characteristics of neurologic integrity. (For further discussion, see Chapter 29 ∞).

Complex behavioral patterns reflect the newborn's neurologic maturation and integration. Newborns who can bring a hand to the mouth are demonstrating motor coordination as well as a self-quieting technique, thus increasing the complexity of the behavioral response. Newborns also possess complex organized defensive motor patterns as exhibited by the ability to remove an obstruction such as a cloth across the face.

Periods of Reactivity

The baby usually shows a predictable pattern of behavior during the first several hours after birth, characterized by two **periods of reactivity** separated by a sleep phase.

FIRST PERIOD OF REACTIVITY

The first period of reactivity lasts approximately 30 minutes after birth. During this period the newborn is awake and active and may appear hungry and have a strong sucking reflex. This is a natural opportunity to initiate breastfeeding if the mother has chosen it (Figure 28–13 ◆). Bursts of random, diffuse movements alternating with relative immobility may occur. Respirations are rapid, as high as 80 breaths per minute, and there may be retraction of the chest, transient flaring of the nares, and grunting. The heart rate is rapid, and rhythm may be irregular. Bowel sounds are usually absent.

PERIOD OF INACTIVITY TO SLEEP PHASE

After approximately half an hour, the newborn's activity gradually diminishes. The heart rate and respirations decrease as the newborn enters the sleep phase. The sleep phase may last from a few minutes to 2 to 4 hours. During this period the newborn will be difficult to awaken and will show no interest in sucking. Bowel sounds become audible, and cardiac and respiratory rates return to baseline values.

Figure 28–13 ◆ Mother and baby gaze at each other. This quiet alert state is the optimal state for interaction.

SECOND PERIOD OF REACTIVITY

During the second period of reactivity, the newborn is again awake and alert. This period lasts 4 to 6 hours in the normal newborn. Physiologic responses are variable during this stage. The heart and respiratory rates increase; however, the nurse must be alert for apneic periods, which may cause a drop in the heart rate. The newborn is stimulated to continue breathing during such times. The newborn may develop rapid color changes and become mildly cyanotic or mottled during these fluctuations. Production of respiratory and gastric mucus increases, and the newborn responds by gagging, choking, and regurgitating.

Continued close observation and intervention may be required to maintain a clear airway during this period of reactivity. The gastrointestinal tract becomes more active. The newborn often passes the first meconium stool and may also have an initial voiding. The newborn shows he or she is ready to be fed by such behaviors as sucking, rooting, and swallowing. If feeding was not initiated in the first period of reactivity, it is done at this time. See Initial Feeding in Chapter 31 ∞ for further discussion of this first feeding.

Behavioral States of the Newborn

The behavior of the newborn can be divided into two categories: the sleep state and the alert state (Brazelton, 1999). These postnatal behavioral states are similar to those that have been identified during pregnancy. Subcategories are identified under each major category.

SLEEP STATES

The sleep states are as follows:

1. *Deep or quiet sleep.* The baby has closed eyes with no eye movements, regular even breathing, and jerky motion or startles at regular intervals. Behavioral responses to external stimuli are likely to be delayed. Startles are rapidly suppressed, and changes in state are not likely to occur. Heart rate may range from 100 to 120 bpm.

2. *Active rapid eye movement (REM).* The baby has irregular respirations, eyes closed with REM, irregular sucking motions, minimal activity, and irregular but smooth movement of the extremities. Environmental and internal stimuli initiate a startle reaction and a change of state.

Newborn sleep cycles have been recognized and defined according to duration. The length of the cycle depends on the age of the newborn. At term, REM active sleep and quiet sleep occur in intervals of 50 to 60 minutes (Gardner & Goldson, 2002). About 45% to 50% of the total sleep of the newborn is active sleep, 35% to 45% is quiet (deep) sleep, and 10% of sleep is transitional between these two periods. Growth hormone secretion depends on regular sleep patterns. Any disturbance of the sleep-wake cycle can result in irregular spikes of growth hormone. REM sleep stimulates the highest peaks of growth hormone and the growth of the neural system. Over time, the newborn's sleep-wake patterns become diurnal; that is, the newborn sleeps at night and stays awake during the day. (See "Newborn Behavioral Assessment" in Chapter 29 ∞ for in-depth discussion of Brazelton's assessment of newborn states).

MediaLink   Care Plan Activity: Physiologic Responses of the Newborn

MediaLink   Newborn Sleep

ALERT STATES

In the first 30 to 60 minutes after birth, many newborns display a quiet alert state, characteristic of the first period of reactivity. Nurses should use these alert states to encourage bonding and breastfeeding. These periods of alertness tend to be short the first 2 days after birth to allow the baby to recover from the birth process. Subsequently, alert states are of choice or of necessity (Brazelton, 1999). The newborn's increasing choice of wakefulness by the newborn indicates a maturing capacity to achieve and maintain consciousness. Heat, cold, and hunger are but a few of the stimuli that can cause wakefulness by necessity. Once the disturbing stimuli are removed, the baby tends to fall back asleep.

The following are subcategories of the alert state (Brazelton, 1999):

1. *Drowsy or semidozing.* The behaviors common to the drowsy state are open or closed eyes; fluttering eyelids; semidozing appearance; and slow, regular movements of the extremities. Mild startles may be noted from time to time. Although the reaction to a sensory stimulus is delayed, it often causes a change of state.

2. *Wide awake.* In the wide awake state, the newborn is alert and follows and fixates on attractive objects, faces, or auditory stimuli. Motor activity is minimal, and the response to external stimuli is delayed.

3. *Active awake.* The eyes are open, and motor activity is quite intense, with thrusting movements of the extremities in the active awake state. Environmental stimuli increase startles or motor activity, but individual reactions are difficult to distinguish because of generalized high activity level.

4. *Crying.* Intense crying is accompanied by jerky motor movements. Crying serves several purposes for the newborn. It may be used as a distraction from disturbing stimuli such as hunger and pain. Fussiness often allows the newborn to discharge energy and reorganize behavior. Most important, crying elicits an appropriate response of help from the parents.

Behavioral and Sensory Capacities of the Newborn

Newborns have several behavioral capacities that assist in their adaptation to extrauterine life. For example, **self-quieting ability** is the ability of newborns to use their own resources to quiet and comfort themselves. Their repertoire includes hand-to-mouth movements, sucking on a fist or tongue, and attending to external stimuli.

Neurologically impaired newborns are unable to use self-quieting activities and require more frequent comforting from caregivers when stimulated. For example, drug-positive newborns often exhibit abnormal sleep and feeding patterns and irritability.

Habituation is the newborn's ability to process and respond to complex stimulation. For example, when a bright light is flashed into the newborn's eyes, the initial response is blinking, constriction of the pupil, and perhaps a slight startle reaction. However, with repeated stimulation the newborn's response repertoire gradually diminishes and disappears. The capacity to ignore repetitious disturbing stimuli is a neonatal defense mechanism readily apparent in the noisy, well-lighted nursery.

Sensory abilities include visual, auditory, olfactory, taste, and tactile capacities.

VISUAL CAPACITY

Orientation is the newborn's ability to be alert to, to follow, and to fixate on complex visual stimuli that have a particular appeal and attraction. The newborn prefers the human face and eyes and bright, shiny objects. As the face or object is brought into the line of vision, the newborn responds with bright, wide eyes; still limbs; and fixed staring. This intense visual involvement may last several minutes, during which time the newborn is able to follow the stimulus from side to side. Figure 28–14 ◆ illustrates this response. The newborn uses this sensory capacity to become familiar with family, friends, and surroundings.

AUDITORY CAPACITY

The newborn responds to auditory stimulation with a definite, organized behavior repertoire. The stimulus used to assess auditory response should be selected to match the state of the newborn. A rattle is appropriate for light sleep, a voice for an awake state, and a clap for deep sleep. As the newborn hears the sound, the cardiac rate rises, and a minimal startle reflex may be seen. If the sound is appealing, the newborn will become alert and search for the site of the auditory stimulus.

OLFACTORY CAPACITY

Newborns can select their mother by smell (Klaus, Kennell, & De Pompei, 2006). Newborns were able to distinguish their mothers' breast pads from those of other mothers' at just 1 week postnatally.

TASTE AND SUCKING

The newborn responds differently to varying tastes. Sugar, for example, increases sucking. Newborns fed with a rubber nipple versus the breast also show sucking pattern variations. When breastfeeding, the newborn sucks in bursts with frequent regu-

Figure 28–14 ◆ Head turning to follow an object.
SOURCE: Photographer, Elena Dorfman.

lar pauses. The bottle-fed newborn tends to suck at a regular rate with infrequent pauses.

When awake and hungry, the newborn displays rapid searching motions in response to the rooting reflex. Once feeding begins, the newborn establishes a sucking pattern according to the method of feeding. Finger sucking happens not only postnatally, but also in utero. The newborn frequently uses nonnutritive sucking as a self-quieting activity, which assists in the development of self-regulation. For bottle-fed infants, there is no reason to discourage nonnutritive sucking with a pacifier. Pacifiers should be offered to breastfed infants only after breastfeeding is well established. If the pacifier is offered too soon, a phenomenon called "nipple confusion" may occur in which the breastfed infant has difficulty learning to suck from the breast and nurse less. (See Supplementary Bottle Feeding in Chapter 31 ∞ for a more in-depth discussion).

TACTILE CAPACITY

The newborn is very sensitive to being touched, cuddled, and held. Often a mother's first response to an upset or crying newborn is touching or holding. Swaddling, placing a hand on the abdomen, or holding the arms to prevent a startle reflex are other ways to soothe the newborn. The settled newborn is then able to attend to and interact with the environment.

CHAPTER REVIEW

FOCUS YOUR STUDY

- Newborn respiration is initiated primarily by chemical and mechanical events in association with thermal and sensory stimulation.

- The production of surfactant is crucial to keeping the lungs expanded during expiration by reducing alveolar surface tension.

- The newborn is an obligatory nose breather. Respirations move from being primarily shallow, irregular, and diaphragmatic to synchronous abdominal and chest breathing.

- Normal respiratory rate is 30 to 60 breaths per minute.

- Periodic breathing is normal, and newborn sleep states affect breathing patterns.

- The status of the cardiopulmonary system may be measured by evaluating the heart rate, blood pressure, and presence or absence of murmurs. The normal heart rate is 120 to 160 bpm.

- Oxygen transport in the newborn is significantly affected by the presence of greater amounts of HbF (fetal hemoglobin) than HbA (adult hemoglobin). HbF holds oxygen more efficiently but releases it to the body tissues only at low PO_2 levels.

- Blood values in the newborn are modified by several factors, such as site of the blood sample, gestational age, prenatal or perinatal hemorrhage, and the timing of the clamping of the umbilical cord.

- The newborn is considered to have established thermoregulation when oxygen consumption and metabolic activity are minimal.

- Evaporation is the primary heat loss mechanism in newborns who are wet from amniotic fluid or a bath. In addition, excessive heat loss occurs from radiation and convection because of the newborn's larger surface area compared with weight and from thermal conduction because of the marked difference between core temperature and skin temperature.

- The primary source of heat in the cold-stressed newborn is brown adipose tissue.

- Blood glucose levels should reach a steady state by 3 hours of age.

- The newborn's liver plays a crucial role in iron storage, carbohydrate metabolism, conjugation of bilirubin, and coagulation.

- Controversy continues about the relationship of breastfeeding and the development of prolonged jaundice.

- The normal newborn possesses the ability to digest and absorb nutrients necessary for newborn growth and development.

- The newborn's stools change from meconium (thick, tarry, black) to transitional stools (thinner, brown to green) and then to the distinct forms for either breastfed newborns (yellow-gold, soft, or mushy) or formula-fed newborns (pale yellow, formed, and pasty). Most newborns pass their first stool within 48 hours of birth.

- The newborn's kidneys are characterized by a decreased rate of glomerular flow, limited tubular reabsorption, limited excretion of solutes, and limited ability to concentrate urine. Most newborns void within 48 hours of birth.

- The immune system in the newborn is not fully activated until sometime after birth, but the newborn does possess some immunologic abilities.

- Neurologic and sensory perceptual functioning in the newborn is evident from the newborn's interaction with the environment, presence of synchronized motor activity, and well-developed sensory capacities.

- The first period of reactivity lasts for 30 minutes after birth. The newborn is alert and hungry at this time, making this a natural opportunity to promote attachment.

- The second period of reactivity requires close monitoring by the nurse because apnea, decreased heart rate, gagging, choking, and regurgitation are likely to occur and require nursing intervention.

- Behavioral states in the newborn can be divided into sleep states and alert states.

- Sensory development proceeds in a specific order: tactile/vestibular, olfactory/gustatory, and auditory/visual.

EXPLORE MEDIALINK

http://www.prenhall.com/davidson

NCLEX review questions, case studies, and other interactive resources for this chapter can be found on the Web Site at http://www.prenhall.com/davidson. Click on "Chapter 28" to select the activities for this chapter.

For tutorials including animations and videos, more NCLEX review questions, and an audio glossary, access the accompanying Prentice Hall Nursing MediaLink DVD-ROM in this book.

PRENTICE HALL NURSING MEDIALINK DVD-ROM

Audio Glossary

NCLEX Review

COMPANION WEBSITE

Additional NCLEX Review

Case Study: *Normal Range of Newborn's Vital Signs*

Care Plan Activity: *Physiologic Responses of the Newborn*

Applications: *Newborn Thermoregulation; Physiologic Jaundice*

Critical Thinking

CRITICAL THINKING IN ACTION

NEWBORN ASSESSMENT

View the Critical Thinking in Action video in Chapter 28 of the DVD-ROM. Then answer the questions that follow.

Sandra Dee, a 21-year-old, G1, P0000, at 38 weeks' gestation, has been in labor for the last 12 hours and is fully dilated with caput visible on the perineum. The fetal heart rate is 148 to 152 with early deceleration down to 142 with contraction and pushing.

Sandra's mother and sister are present for the birth. Her prenatal record shows no significant pregnancy problems or complications, and her vital signs have been stable within normal limits. Sandra has received two doses of Stadol for a total of 2 mg IV for pain relief during her labor. The last dose was given 2 hours ago. You assist with the vaginal birth of a live baby without an episiotomy. You observe the sex and time as the midwife places the infant girl on the mother's abdomen, suctions out the baby's mouth and nose, and proceeds to clamp the cord. You dry and stimulate the infant to breathe, remove the wet blanket and replace it with a dry one, and place the infant skin to skin on the mother's chest. You assess the need for infant resuscitation. The baby has a lusty cry spontaneously less than 30 seconds after birth. You palpate the cord, obtaining a heart rate of 120, and observe that the baby's chest and face are pink, and the legs and arms are flexed with open fist.

1. Explain the changes that must occur in the infant's cardiopulmonary system at birth.

2. What criteria do you look for when you assess the newborn for adequate cardiopulmonary adaptation at birth?

3. What steps do you take to maintain a neutral thermal environment at birth?

4. Sandra plans to breastfeed. When would you initiate the first feeding?

5. Discuss nursing actions that can decrease the probability of high bilirubin levels in the newborn.

REFERENCES

Blackburn, S. T. (2003). *Maternal, fetal, & neonatal physiology: A clinical perspective* (2nd ed.). St. Louis, MO: Saunders.

Brazelton, T. B. (1984). *Neonatal behavioral assessment scale* (2nd ed.). London: Heineman.

Brazelton, T. B. (1999). Behavioral competence. In G. B. Avery, M. A. Fletcher, & M. G. MacDonald (Eds.), *Neonatology: Pathophysiology and management of the newborn* (5th ed., pp. 321–332). Philadelphia: Lippincott.

Cheffer, N. D. (2004). Adaptation to extrauterine life and immediate nursing care. In S. Mattson & J. E. Smith (Eds.), *Core curriculum for maternal-newborn nursing* (3rd ed., pp. 421–436). St. Louis, MO: Saunders.

Gardner, S. L., & Goldson, E. (2002). The neonate and the environment: Impact on development. In G. B. Merenstein & S. L. Gardner (Eds.), *Handbook of neonatal intensive care* (5th ed., pp. 219–282). St. Louis, MO: Mosby.

Hannon, P. R., Willis, S. K., & Scrimshaw, S. C. (2001). Persistence of maternal concerns surrounding neonatal jaundice. An exploratory study. *Archives of Pediatrics & Adolescent Medicine, 155,* 1357–1363.

Kalhan, S. C., & Parimi, P. (2006). Disorders of carbohydrate metabolism. In A. A. Fanaroff, R. J. Martin, & M. C. Walsh (Eds.), *Fanaroff and Martin's neonatal-perinatal medicine* (8th ed., pp. 1467–1596). St. Louis, MO: Mosby.

Kenner, C. (2003). Resuscitation and stabilization of the newborn. In C. Kenner & J. W. Lott (Eds.), *Comprehensive neonatal nursing: A physiologic perspective* (3rd ed., pp. 210–228). Philadelphia: Saunders.

Klaus, M. H., Kennell, J. H., & De Pompei, P. M. (2006). Care of the mother, father, and infant. In A. A. Fanaroff, R. J. Martin, & M. C. Walsh (Eds.), *Fanaroff and Martin's neonatal-perinatal medicine* (8th ed., pp. 645–659). St. Louis, MO: Mosby.

Laughlin, D., & Knuppel, R. A. (2003). Maternal-placental-fetal unit: Fetal and early neonatal physiology. In A. H. DeCherney & L. Nathan (Eds.), *Current obstetric & gynecologic diagnosis & treatment* (9th ed., pp. 163–191). New York: Lang Medical Books /McGraw-Hill.

Maisels, M. J. (2005). Jaundice. In M. G. MacDonald, M. D. Mullett, & M. Seshia (Eds.), *Avery's neonatology: Pathophysiology & management of the newborn* (6th ed., pp. 768–846). Philadelphia: Lippincott Williams & Wilkins.

Polin, R. A., Fox, W. W., & Abman, S. H. (2004). *Fetal and neonatal physiology* (3rd ed.). Philadelphia: Saunders.

Thureen, P. J., Deacon, J., Hernandez, J., & Hall, D. M. (2005). *Assessment and care of the well newborn* (2nd ed.). Philadelphia: Saunders.

CHAPTER 29

Nursing Assessment of the Newborn

Something very special occurs within the first hour after birth. If the environment is quiet, the birthing without complications, the lights lowered, the handling diminished, newborn infants—aside from all the physiological adaptations they must make—begin in a uniquely human way to adapt to the new experience of being in the world.

~Marshall H. Klaus & Phyllis H. Klaus,
The Amazing Newborn~

OBJECTIVES

1. Explain the various components of the gestational age assessment.

2. Describe the normal physical and behavioral characteristics of the newborn.

3. Summarize the components of a complete newborn assessment and the significance of normal variations and abnormal findings.

4. Discuss the neurologic and neuromuscular characteristics of the newborn and the reflexes that may be present at birth.

5. Describe the categories of the newborn behavioral assessment.

KEY TERMS

Acrocyanosis   831
Apgar score   819
Babinski reflex response   845
Barlow maneuver   843
Brazelton's Neonatal Behavioral Assessment Scale   847
Caput succedaneum   834
Cephalhematoma   834
Chemical conjunctivitis   836
Dubowitz tool   820
Epstein's pearls   837
Erb-Duchenne paralysis (Erb's palsy)   842
Erythema toxicum   832
Forceps marks   832
Gestational age assessment tools   820
Grasping reflex   844
Harlequin sign   832
Jaundice   832
Lanugo   820
Milia   832
Molding   833

Mongolian blue spots   832
Moro reflex   844
Mottling   832
Nevus flammeus (port wine stain)   833
Nevus vasculosus (strawberry mark)   833
New Ballard score   820
Ortolani's maneuver   843
Pseudomenstruation   841
Rooting reflex   844
Skin turgor   822
Subconjunctival hemorrhage   836
Sucking reflex   845
Telangiectatic nevi (stork bites)   832
Thrush   837
Tonic neck reflex   844
Trunk incurvation (Galant reflex)   845
Vernix caseosa   832

MEDIALINK

Additional resources for this content can be found on the Prentice Hall Nursing MediaLink DVD-ROM and on the Companion Website at http://www.prenhall.com/davidson. Click on "Chapter 29" to select the activities for this chapter.

Unlike adults, newborns communicate their needs primarily by their behavior. Because nurses are the most consistent professional observer of the newborn, they can translate this behavior into information about the newborn's condition and to respond with appropriate nursing interventions. This chapter focuses on the assessment of the newborn and interpretation of findings. Assessment of the newborn is a continuous process used to evaluate development and adjustments to extrauterine life. In the birthing area, Apgar scoring (see Chapter 24 ∞ for discussion) and careful observation of the newborn form the basis of the assessment and are correlated with information such as the following:

- Maternal prenatal care history

- Birthing history

- Maternal analgesia and anesthesia

- Complications of labor or birth

- Treatment instituted immediately after birth, in conjunction with determination of clinical gestational age

- Consideration of the newborn's classification by weight and gestational age and by neonatal mortality risk

- Physical examination of the newborn

The nurse incorporates data from these sources with the assessment findings during the first 1 to 4 hours after birth to formulate a plan for nursing intervention.

The various newborn assessments and the data obtained from them are only valuable to the degree to which they are shared with the parents. The parents must be included in the assessment process from the moment of their child's birth. The **Apgar score** and its meaning should be explained immediately to the family. As soon as possible, the parents should take part in the physical and behavioral assessments as well.

The nurse encourages the parents to identify the unique behavioral characteristics of their newborn and to learn nurturing activities. Attachment is promoted when parents have the opportunity to explore their newborn in private, identifying individual physical and behavioral characteristics. The nurse's supportive responses to the parents' questions and observations are essential throughout the assessment process. The newborn physical examination is the beginning of newborn health surveillance and health education for the newborn's family that continues into the community setting.

TIMING OF NEWBORN ASSESSMENTS

During the first 24 hours of life, the newborn makes the critical transition from intrauterine to extrauterine life. The risk of mortality and morbidity is statistically high during this period. Assessment of the newborn is essential to ensure that the transition is proceeding successfully

There are three major time frames for assessing newborns while they are in the birth facility.

Table 29–1	TIMING AND TYPES OF NEWBORN ASSESSMENTS

Assess immediately after birth:

Need for resuscitation

If newborn is stable and can be placed with parents to initiate early attachment/bonding

Assessments within 1 to 4 hours after birth:

Progress of newborn's adaptation to extrauterine life

Determination of gestational age

Ongoing assessment for high-risk problems

Assessment procedures within first 24 hours or before discharge:

Complete physical examination (Depending on agency protocol, the nurse may complete some components independently with the certified nurse-midwife/physician/nurse practitioner completing the exam before discharge.)

Nutritional status and ability to formula-feed or breastfeed satisfactorily

Behavioral state organization abilities

- The first assessment is done in the birthing area immediately after birth to determine the need for resuscitation or other interventions. The stable newborn can stay with the family after birth to initiate early attachment. The newborn with complications is usually taken to the nursery for further evaluation and intervention.

- A second assessment is done by the nursery nurse as part of the routine admission procedure. During this assessment, the nurse carries out a brief physical examination to estimate gestational age and evaluate the newborn's adaptation to extrauterine life. The accuracy of gestational age assessment decreases when performed more than 24 hours after birth. No later than 2 hours after birth, the admitting nursery nurse should evaluate the newborn's status and any problems that place the newborn at risk (American Academy of Pediatrics [AAP] & the American College of Obstetricians and Gynecologists [ACOG], 2002).

- Before discharge a certified nurse-midwife, physician, or nurse practitioner will carry out a behavioral assessment and a complete physical examination to detect any emerging or potential problems.

This chapter presents the procedures for estimating gestational age and performing the complete physical examination and behavioral assessment (Table 29–1). Chapter 24 ∞ discusses the immediate postbirth assessment. Chapter 30 ∞ describes the brief assessment performed during the first 4 hours of life.

ESTIMATION OF GESTATIONAL AGE

It is essential to establish the newborn's gestational age in the first 4 hours after birth so that careful attention can be given to age-related problems. Traditionally, a newborn's gestational age was determined from the date of the pregnant woman's last menstrual period. This method was accurate only 75% to 85% of the time. Because of the problems that develop with the newborn who is preterm or whose weight is inappropriate for gestational age, a more accurate system was developed to evaluate the newborn. Once learned, the procedure can be done in a few minutes. *It is essential that the nurse wear gloves when assessing the newborn in these early hours after birth and before the first bath until amniotic fluid, vaginal, and bloody secretions on the skin are removed.*

Clinical **gestational age assessment tools** have two components: external physical characteristics and neurologic or neuromuscular development evaluations. Physical characteristics generally include sole creases, amount of breast tissue, amount of lanugo, cartilaginous development of the ear, testicular descent, and scrotal rugae or labial development. These objective clinical criteria are not influenced by labor and birth and do not change significantly within the first 12 hours after birth.

Neurologic examination facilitates assessment of functional or physiologic maturation in addition to physical development. However, the newborn's nervous system is unstable during the first 24 hours of life; neurologic evaluation findings based on reflexes or assessments dependent on the higher brain centers may not be reliable. If the neurologic findings drastically deviate from the gestational age derived by evaluation of the external characteristics, a second assessment is done in 24 hours.

The neurologic assessment components (excluding reflexes) are especially helpful in assessing the gestational age of newborns less than 34 weeks' gestation. Between 26 and 34 weeks, neurologic changes are significant, whereas significant physical changes are less evident. One significant neuromuscular change is that muscular tone develops from extension to having the ability to flex the extremity as neurologic maturity develops in a caudocephalad (tail-to-head) progression.

Ballard et al. (1991) developed the estimation of gestational age by maturity rating, a simplified version of the well-researched **Dubowitz tool.** The Ballard tool omits some of the neuromuscular tone assessments, such as head lag, ventral suspension (which is difficult to assess in very ill newborns or those on respirators), and leg recoil. In Ballard's tool, each physical and neuromuscular finding is given a point value, and the total score is matched to a gestational age (Figure 29–1 ◆). The maximum score on the Ballard tool is 50, which corresponds to a gestational age of 44 weeks.

For example, on completing a gestational assessment of a 1-hour-old newborn, the nurse gives a score of 3 to all the physical characteristics, for a total of 18, and gives a score of 3 to all the neuromuscular assessments, for a total neurologic score of 18. The physical characteristics score of 18 is added to the neurologic score of 18 for a total score of 36, which correlates with 38 or more weeks' gestation. Because all newborns vary slightly in the development of physical characteristics and maturation of neurologic function, scores will usually vary instead of all being 3, as in this example.

Postnatal gestational age assessment tools can overestimate preterm gestational age and underestimate postterm gestational

age. The tools have been shown to lose accuracy when newborns of less than 28 weeks' or more than 43 weeks' gestation are assessed. Ballard et al. (1991) in the **New Ballard score** (NBS) added criteria for more accurate assessment of the gestational age of newborns between 20 and 28 weeks' gestation and less than 1500 g. They suggest that the assessment be made within 12 hours of birth to optimize accuracy, especially in infants of less than 26 weeks' gestational age. Also the Ballard assessment may be overstimulating to infants of less than 27 weeks' gestation.

Some maternal conditions such as preeclampsia, diabetes, and maternal analgesia and anesthesia, may affect certain gestational assessment components and warrant further study. Maternal diabetes, although it appears to accelerate fetal physical growth, seems to retard maturation. Maternal hypertension states, which retard fetal physical growth, seem to speed maturation.

Newborns of women with preeclampsia have a poor correlation with the criteria involving active muscle tone and edema. Maternal analgesia and anesthesia may cause the baby to have respiratory depression. Babies with respiratory distress syndrome (RDS) tend to be flaccid and edematous and to assume a "froglike" posture. These characteristics affect the scoring of the neuromuscular components of the assessment tool used. The NBS gestational age assessment tool is used throughout this chapter to demonstrate the assessment of the physical and neuromuscular criteria associated with gestational age.

Assessment of Physical Maturity Characteristics

The nurse first evaluates observable characteristics without disturbing the baby. Selected physical characteristics common to the Dubowitz and Ballard gestational assessment tools are presented here in the order in which they might be most effectively evaluated:

1. *Resting posture,* although a neuromuscular component, should be assessed as the baby lies undisturbed on a flat surface (Figure 29–2 ◆).

2. *Skin* in the preterm newborn appears thin and transparent, with veins prominent over the abdomen early in gestation. As the newborn approaches term, the skin appears opaque because of increased subcutaneous tissue. Disappearance of the protective vernix caseosa promotes skin desquamation and this is commonly seen in postmature infants (infants greater than 42 weeks' gestational age and those showing signs of placental insufficiency; see Chapter 32 ∞).

3. *Lanugo,* a fine hair covering, decreases as gestational age increases. The amount of **lanugo** is greatest at 28 to 30 weeks and then disappears, first from the face, then from the trunk and extremities.

4. *Sole (plantar) creases* are reliable indicators of gestational age in the first 12 hours of life. Later, the skin of the foot begins drying, and superficial creases appear. Development of sole creases begins at the top (anterior)

NEWBORN MATURITY RATING & CLASSIFICATION

ESTIMATION OF GESTATIONAL AGE BY MATURITY RATING
Symbols: X - 1st Exam O - 2nd Exam

NEUROMUSCULAR MATURITY

	−1	0	1	2	3	4	5
Posture							
Square Window (wrist)	>90°	90°	60°	45°	30°	0°	
Arm Recoil		180°	140°−180°	110°−140°	90°−110°	<90°	
Popliteal Angle	180°	160°	140°	120°	100°	90°	<90°
Scarf Sign							
Heel to Ear							

Gestation by Dates _____ wks

Birth Date _____ Hour _____ am pm

APGAR _____ 1 min _____ 5 min

MATURITY RATING

score	weeks
−10	20
−5	22
0	24
5	26
10	28
15	30
20	32
25	34
30	36
35	38
40	40
45	42
50	44

PHYSICAL MATURITY

Skin	sticky friable transparent	gelatinous red, translucent	smooth pink, visible veins	superficial peeling &/or rash, few veins	cracking pale areas rare veins	parchment deep cracking no vessels	leathery cracked wrinkled
Lanugo	none	sparse	abundant	thinning	bald areas	mostly bald	
Plantar Surface	heel-toe 40–50 mm:−1 <40 mm:−2	>50 mm no crease	faint red marks	anterior transverse crease only	creases ant. 2/3	creases over entire sole	
Breast	imperceptible	barely perceptible	flat areola no bud	stippled areola 1–2 mm bud	raised areola 3–4 mm bud	full areola 5–10 mm bud	
Eye/Ear	lids fused loosely:−1 tightly:−2	lids open pinna flat stays folded	sl. curved pinna; soft; slow recoil	well curved pinna; soft but ready recoil	formed & firm instant recoil	thick cartilage ear stiff	
Genitals male	scrotum flat, smooth	scrotum empty faint rugae	testes in upper canal rare rugae	testes descending few rugae	testes down good rugae	testes pendulous deep rugae	
Genitals female	clitoris prominent labia flat	prominent clitoris small labia minora	prominent clitoris enlarging minora	majora & minora equally prominent	majora large minora small	majora cover clitoris & minora	

SCORING SECTION

	1st Exam = X	2nd Exam = 0
Estimating Gest Age by Maturity Rating	_____Weeks	_____Weeks
Time of Exam	Date _____ Hour_____ am pm	Date _____ Hour_____ am pm
Age at Exam	_____ Hours	_____ Hours
Signature of Examiner	_____ M.D.	_____ M.D.

Figure 29–1 ◆ Newborn maturity rating and classification. If a 1-hour-old newborn is given a score of 3 for each of the physical characteristics and neuromuscular assessments, the newborn's total score would be 36. A total score of 36 correlates with 38 or more weeks' gestation.
SOURCE: Ballard, J. L., et al. (1991). New Ballard score, expanded to include extremely premature infants. *Journal of Pediatrics, 119,* 417.

A   **B**   **C**

Figure 29–2 ◆ Resting posture. *A,* Infant exhibits beginning of flexion of the thigh. The gestational age is approximately 31 weeks. Note the extension of the upper extremities. Score 1 or 2. *B,* Infant exhibits stronger flexion of the arms, hips, and thighs. The gestational age is approximately 35 weeks. Score 3. *C,* The full-term infant exhibits hypertonic flexion of all extremities. Score 4.

portion of the sole and, as gestation progresses, proceeds to the heel (Figure 29–3 ◆). Peeling may also occur. Plantar creases vary with race. In newborns of African descent, sole creases may be less developed at term.

5. The nurse inspects the *areola* and gently palpates the breast bud tissue by applying the forefinger and middle finger to the breast area and measuring the tissue between them in centimeters or millimeters (Figure 29–4 ◆). At term gestation, the tissue will measure between 0.5 and

1 cm (5 to 10 mm). During the assessment, the nipple should not be grasped firmly because skin and subcutaneous tissue will prevent accurate estimation of size. The nurse must perform this procedure gently to avoid causing trauma to the breast tissue.

As gestation progresses, the breast tissue mass and areola enlarge. However, a large breast tissue mass can occur as a result of conditions other than advanced gestational age or the effects of maternal hormones on the baby. In the

A   **B**   **C**

Figure 29–3 ◆ Sole creases. *A,* Infant has a few sole creases on the anterior portion of the foot. Note the slick heel. Score 2. The gestational age is approximately 35 weeks. *B,* Infant has a deeper network of sole creases on the anterior two thirds of the sole. Note the slick heel. Score 3. The gestational age is approximately 37 weeks. *C,* The full-term infant has deep sole creases down to and including the heel as the skin loses fluid and dries after birth. Score 4. Sole (plantar) creases can be seen even in preterm newborns.

A   B   C

Figure 29–4 ◆ Breast tissue. *A,* Newborn has a visible raised area greater than 0.75 cm diameter. Score 3. The gestational age is 38 weeks. *B,* Newborn has a breast tissue area of 10 mm. Score 4. The gestational age is 40 to 44 weeks. *C,* Gently compress the tissue between the middle and index fingers, and measure the tissue in centimeters or millimeters. Absence of or decreased breast tissue often indicates premature or SGA newborn.
SOURCE: *B,* Used with permission from V. Dubowitz, MD, Hammersmith Hospital, London, England.

large-for-gestational-age infant of a diabetic mother, accelerated development of breast tissue is a reflection of subcutaneous fat deposits. Small-for-gestational-age term or postterm newborns may have used subcutaneous fat (which would have been deposited as breast tissue) to survive in utero; as a result their lack of breast tissue may indicate a gestational age of 34 to 35 weeks, even though other factors indicate a term or postterm newborn.

6. *Ear form and cartilage distribution* develop with gestational age. The cartilage gives the ear its shape and substance (Figure 29–5 ◆). In a newborn of less than 34 weeks' gestation, the ear is relatively shapeless and flat; it has little cartilage, so the ear folds over on itself and remains folded. By approximately 36 weeks' gestation, some cartilage and slight incurving of the upper pinna are present, and the pinna springs back slowly when folded.

A   B   C

Figure 29–5 ◆ Ear form and cartilage. *A,* The ear of the infant at approximately 36 weeks' gestation shows incurving of the upper two thirds of the pinna. Score 2. *B,* Infant at term shows well-defined incurving of the entire pinna. Score 3. *C,* If the auricle stays in the position in which it is pressed or returns slowly to its original position, it usually means that the gestational age is less than 38 weeks.

A

B

Figure 29–6 ◆ Male genitals. *A,* Preterm infant's testes are not within the scrotum. The scrotal surface has few rugae. Score 2. *B,* Term infant's testes are generally fully descended. The entire surface of the scrotum is covered by rugae. Score 3.

(The nurse tests this response by holding the top and bottom of the pinna together with the forefinger and thumb and then releasing it, or by folding the pinna of the ear forward against the side of the head and releasing it, and observing the response.) By term, the newborn's pinna is firm, stands away from the head, and springs back quickly from the folding.

7. *Male genitals* are evaluated for size of the scrotal sac, the presence of rugae (wrinkles and ridges in the scrotum), and descent of the testes (Figure 29–6 ◆). Before 36 weeks, the small scrotum has few rugae, and the testes are palpable in the inguinal canal. By 36 to 38 weeks, the testes are in the upper scrotum, and rugae have developed over the anterior portion of the scrotum. By term, the testes are generally in the lower scrotum, which is pendulous and covered with rugae.

8. The appearance of the *female genitals* depends in part on subcutaneous fat deposition and therefore relates to fetal nutritional status (Figure 29–7 ◆). The clitoris varies in size and occasionally is so large that it is difficult to

identify the sex of the newborn. This swelling may be caused by adrenogenital syndrome, which causes the adrenals to secrete excessive amounts of androgen and other hormones. At 30 to 32 weeks' gestation, the clitoris is prominent, and the labia majora are small and widely separated. As gestational age increases, the labia majora increase in size. At 36 to 40 weeks, they nearly cover the clitoris. At 40 weeks and beyond, the labia majora cover the labia minora and clitoris.

Other physical characteristics assessed by some gestational age scoring tools include the following:

1. *Vernix* covers the preterm newborn. The postterm newborn has no vernix. After noting vernix distribution, the birthing area nurse (wearing gloves) dries the newborn to prevent evaporative heat loss, thus disturbing the vernix and potentially altering this gestational age criterion. The birthing area nurse must communicate to the neonatal nurse the amount of vernix and the areas of vernix coverage.

A

B

C

Figure 29–7 ◆ Female genitals. *A,* Infant has a prominent clitoris. The labia majora are widely separated, and the labia minora, viewed laterally, would protrude beyond the labia majora. Score 1. The gestational age is 30 to 36 weeks. *B,* The clitoris is still visible. The labia minora are now covered by the larger labia majora. Score 2. The gestational age is 36 to 40 weeks. *C,* The term infant has well-developed, large labia majora that cover both clitoris and labia minora. Score 3.

2. *Hair* of the preterm newborn has the consistency of matted wool or fur and lies in bunches rather than in the silky, single strands of the term newborn's hair.

3. *Skull firmness* increases as the fetus matures. In a term newborn, the bones are hard, and the sutures are not easily displaced. The nurse should not attempt to displace the sutures forcibly.

4. *Nails* appear and cover the nail bed at about 20 weeks' gestation. Nails extending beyond the fingertips may indicate a postterm newborn.

Assessment of Neuromuscular Maturity Characteristics

The central nervous system of the human fetus matures at a fairly constant rate. Tests have been designed to evaluate neurologic status as manifested by development of neuromuscular tone. As noted earlier, neuromuscular tone in the fetus develops in a caudocephalic direction, from the lower to the upper extremities.

The neuromuscular evaluation requires more manipulation and disturbances than the physical evaluation of the newborn. The neuromuscular evaluation (see Figure 29–1) is best performed when the infant has stabilized. The following characteristics are evaluated:

1. The *square window sign* is elicited by flexing the baby's hand toward the ventral forearm until resistance is felt. The angle formed at the wrist is measured (Figure 29–8 ◆).

2. *Recoil* is a test of flexion development. Because flexion first develops in the lower extremities, recoil is first tested in the legs. The nurse places the newborn on his or her back on a flat surface. With a hand on the newborn's knees and while manipulating the hip joint, the nurse

places the baby's legs in flexion, and then extends them parallel to each other and flat on the surface. The response to this maneuver is recoil of the newborn's legs. According to gestational age, they may not move, or they may return slowly or quickly to the flexed position. Preterm infants have less muscle tone than term infants so preterm infants have less recoil.

Arm recoil is tested by flexion at the elbow and extension of the arms at the newborn's side. While the baby is in the supine position, the nurse completely flexes both elbows, holds them in this position for 5 seconds, extends the arms at the baby's side, and releases them. Upon release, the elbows of a full-term newborn form an angle of less than 90 degrees and rapidly recoil back to a flexed position. The elbows of preterm newborns have slower recoil time and form a greater than 90-degree angle. Arm recoil is also slower in healthy but fatigued newborns after birth; therefore, arm recoil is best elicited after the first hour of birth, when the baby has had time to recover from the stress of birth. The deep sleep state also decreases the arm recoil response. Assessment of arm recoil should be bilateral to rule out brachial palsy.

3. The *popliteal angle* (degree of knee flexion) is determined with the newborn flat on his or her back. The thigh is flexed on the abdomen and chest, and the nurse places the index finger of the other hand behind the newborn's ankle to extend the lower leg until resistance is met. The angle formed is then measured. Results vary from no resistance in the very immature newborn to an 80-degree angle in the term newborn.

4. The *scarf sign* is elicited by placing the newborn supine and drawing an arm across the chest toward the newborn's opposite shoulder until resistance is met. The location of the elbow is then noted in relation to the

A   B   C

Figure 29–8 ◆ Square window sign. *A,* This angle is 90 degrees and suggests an immature newborn of 28 to 32 weeks' gestation. Score 0. *B,* A 30–40-degree angle is commonly found in newborns from 38 to 40 weeks' gestation. Score 2–3. *C,* A 0-degree angle occurs in newborns from 40 to 42 weeks' gestation. Score 4.
SOURCE: *C,* Used with permission from V. Dubowitz, MD, Hammersmith Hospital, London, England.

A

B

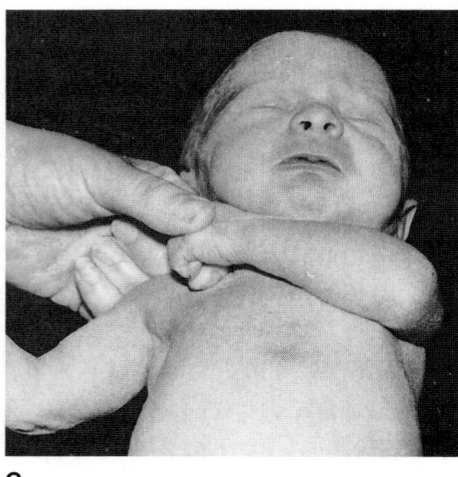
C

Figure 29–9 ◆ Scarf sign. *A,* No resistance is noted until after 30 weeks' gestation. The elbow can be readily moved past the midline. Score 1. *B,* The elbow is at midline at 36 to 40 weeks' gestation. Score 2. *C,* Beyond 40 weeks' gestation, the elbow will not reach the midline. Score 4.
SOURCE: *C,* Used with permission from V. Dubowitz, MD, Hammersmith Hospital, London, England.

midline of the chest (Figure 29–9 ◆). A preterm infant's elbow will cross the midline of the chest, whereas a full term infant's elbow will not cross midline.

5. The *heel-to-ear extension* is performed by placing the newborn in a supine position and then gently drawing the foot toward the ear on the same side until resistance is felt. The nurse should allow the knee to bend during the test. It is important to hold the buttocks down to keep from rolling the baby. Both the proximity of foot to ear and degree of knee extension are assessed. The leg of a preterm, immature newborn remains straight and the foot goes to the ear or beyond. With advancing gestational age, the newborn demonstrates increasing resistance to this maneuver. Maneuvers involving the lower extremities of newborns who had frank breech presentation should be delayed to allow for resolution of leg positioning (Figure 29–10 ◆).

6. *Ankle dorsiflexion* is determined by flexing the ankle on the shin. The nurse uses a thumb to push on the sole of the newborn's foot while the fingers support the back of the

leg. Then the angle formed by the foot and the interior leg is measured (Figure 29–11 ◆). This sign can be influenced by intrauterine position and congenital deformities.

7. *Head lag* (neck flexors) is measured by pulling the baby to a sitting position and noting the degree of head lag. Total lag is common in infants up to 34 weeks' gestation, whereas the postmature newborn (42 or more weeks) will hold the head in front of the body line. Full-term newborns are able to support their heads momentarily.

8. *Ventral suspension* (horizontal position) is evaluated by holding the newborn prone on the examiner's hand. The position of head and back and degree of flexion in the arms and legs are then noted. Some flexion of arms and legs indicates 36 to 38 weeks' gestation; fully flexed extremities, with head and back even, are characteristic of a term newborn.

9. Major reflexes such as sucking, rooting, grasping, Moro, tonic neck, Babinski, and others are also evaluated during the newborn exam. These reflexes are discussed later in the chapter.

A supplementary method for estimating gestational age (done by the physician or nurse practitioner) is to view the vascular network of the cornea with an ophthalmoscope. The nurse should delay administration of prophylactic eye ointment until after the eye exam. The amount of vascularity present over the surface of the lens has excellent correlation with infants of 27 through 34 weeks' gestational age. In babies less than 27 weeks' gestation, the cornea is cloudy, and the vascular network is not visible; after 34 weeks' gestation the vascular network has generally disappeared completely.

When the gestational age determination and birth weight are considered together, the newborn can be identified as one whose *growth is below the 10th percentile,* or *small for gestational age (SGA); appropriate for gestational age (AGA);* or *above the 90th percentile,* or *large for gestational age (LGA)* (Figure 29–12 ◆). This determination enables the nurse to

Figure 29–10 ◆ Heel-to-ear. No resistance. Leg fully extended. Score 0.

A   **B**

Figure 29–11 ◆ Ankle dorsiflexion. *A,* A 45-degree angle indicates 32 to 36 weeks' gestation. A 20-degree angle indicates 36 to 40 weeks' gestation. Score 2–3. *B,* A 15 to 0-degree angle is common at 40 weeks' or more gestational age. Score 4.

Figure 29–12 ◆ Classification of newborns by birth weight and gestational age. The newborn's birth weight and gestational age are placed on the graph. The newborn is then classified as large for gestational age (LGA), appropriate for gestational age (AGA), or small for gestational age (SGA).

SOURCE: Battaglia, F. C., & Lubchenco, L. O. (1967). A practical classification of newborn infants by weight and gestational age. *Journal of Pediatrics, 71,* 161.

Symbols: X-1st Exam O-2nd Exam

	1st Exam (X)	2nd Exam (O)
LARGE FOR GESTATIONAL AGE (LGA)		
APPROPRIATE FOR GESTATIONAL AGE (AGA)		
SMALL FOR GESTATIONAL AGE (SGA)		
Age at Exam	hrs	hrs
Signature of Examiner	M.D.	M.D.

Figure 29–13 ◆ Classification of newborns based on maturity and intrauterine growth.

SOURCE: Adapted from Lubchenco, L. O., Hansman, C., & Boyd, E. (1966). *Pediatrics, 37,* 404, Figure 1. Reprinted with permission from the American Academy of Pediatrics. Battaglia, F. C., & Lubchenco, L. O. (1967). A practical classification of newborn infants by weight and gestational age. *Journal of Pediatrics, 71,* 161.

anticipate possible physiologic problems. This information is used in conjunction with a complete physical examination to establish a plan of care appropriate for the individual newborn. For example, an SGA newborn often requires frequent glucose monitoring and early feedings. See Chapter 32 ∞ for discussion of these categories and their potential problems.

The nurse also plots the gestational age against the newborn's length, head circumference, and weight on the appropriate growth chart to determine whether these measurements fall within the average range—the 10th to 90th percentile for the corresponding gestational age (Figure 29–13 ◆). These correlations further document the level of maturity and appropriate category for the newborn. The comparison of the newborn's ratio of weight to length further facilitates identification of SGA newborns as being symmetrically or asymmetrically growth restricted. See Chapter 32 ∞ for more detail.

CLINICAL TIP

Measuring weight and height often aggravate newborns and may alter their vital signs. For better accuracy, take the newborn's vital signs before weighing and measuring.

PHYSICAL ASSESSMENT

After the initial determination of gestational age and related potential problems, the nurse carries out a more extensive physical assessment in a warm, well-lighted area that is free of drafts. Completing the physical assessment in the presence of the parents provides an opportunity to acquaint them with their unique newborn. The examination is performed in a systematic, head-to-toe manner, and all findings are recorded. When assessing the physical and neurologic status of the newborn, the nurse should first consider general appearance and then proceed to specific areas.

The Assessment Guide: Newborn Physical Assessment on pages 848–858 outlines how to systematically assess the newborn. Normal findings, alterations, and related causes are presented and correlated with suggested nursing responses. The findings are typical for a full-term newborn.

General Appearance

The newborn's head is disproportionately large for the body. The neck looks short because the chin rests on the chest. Newborns have a prominent abdomen, sloping shoulders, narrow hips, and a rounded chest. The center of the baby's body is the umbilicus rather than the symphysis pubis, as in the adult. The body appears long and the extremities short.

Newborns tend to stay in a flexed position similar to the one maintained in utero and will offer resistance when the extremities are straightened. The flexed position that the newborn maintains contributes to the short appearance of the extremities. The hands are tightly clenched. After a breech birth, the feet are usually dorsiflexed, and it may take several weeks for the newborn to assume typical newborn posture.

Weight and Measurements

The normal full-term Caucasian newborn has an average birth weight of 3405 g (7 lb, 8 oz). Newborns of African, Asian, or Mexican descent are usually somewhat smaller at term, whereas Native American infants are often heavier at term (Mandleco, 2004; Wu & Daniel, 2001). Other factors that influence weight are age and size of parents, health of mother (smoking and malnutrition decrease birth weight), and the interval between pregnancies (short intervals, such as every year, result in lower birth weight). After the first week and for the first 6 months, the newborn's weight will increase about 198 g (7 oz) weekly.

Approximately 70% to 75% of the newborn's body weight is water. During the initial newborn period (the first 3 or 4 days), term newborns have a physiologic weight loss of about 5% to 10% because fluid shifts. This weight loss may reach 15% for preterm newborns. Large babies tend to lose more weight because of greater fluid loss in proportion to birth weight. If weight loss is greater than 10%, clinical reappraisal is necessary. Factors contributing to weight loss include small fluid intake resulting from delayed breastfeeding or a slow adjustment to formula, increased volume of meconium excreted, and urination. Weight loss may be marked in the presence of temperature elevation (because of associated dehydration) or consistent chilling (because of nonshivering thermogenesis).

The length of the normal newborn is difficult to measure because the legs are flexed and tensed. To measure length, the nurse should place newborns flat on their backs with legs extended as much as possible (Figure 29–14 ◆). The average length is 50 cm (20 in.), with the range being 48 to 52 cm (18 to 22 in). The newborn will grow approximately 1 inch a month for the next 6 months. This is the period of most rapid growth.

At birth the newborn's head is one third the size of an adult's head. The circumference of the newborn's head is 32 to 37 cm (12.5 to 14.5 in). For accurate measurement, the nurse places the tape over the most prominent part of the occiput and

Figure 29–14 ◆ Measuring the length of the newborn.
SOURCE: Courtesy of Vanessa Howell, RNC, BSN.

A

B

Figure 29–15 ◆ *A,* Measuring the head circumference of the newborn. *B,* Measuring the chest circumference of the newborn.
SOURCE: Courtesy of Vanessa Howell, RNC, BSN.

brought to just above the eyebrows (Figure 29–15, *A* ◆). The circumference of the newborn's head is approximately 2 cm greater than the circumference of the newborn's chest at birth and will remain in this proportion for the next few months. (Factors that alter this measurement are discussed under the "Head" section.) It is best to take another head circumference on the second day if the newborn experienced significant head molding or caput from the birth process.

The average circumference of the chest at birth is 32 cm (12.5 in.) and ranges from 30 to 35 cm (12 to 14 in.). Chest measurements should be taken with the tape measure at the lower edge of the scapulas and brought around anteriorly directly over the nipple line (Figure 29–15, *B* and Table 29–2). The abdominal circumference or girth may also be measured at this time by placing the tape around the newborn's abdomen at the level of the umbilicus, with the bottom edge of the tape at the top edge of the umbilicus.

Temperature

Initial assessment of the newborn's temperature is critical. In utero the temperature of the fetus is about the same as, or slightly higher than, the expectant mother's. When babies enter the outside world, their temperatures can suddenly drop as a result of exposure to cold drafts and the skin's heat loss mechanisms.

If no heat conservation measures are initiated, the normal term newborn's core temperature falls 0.1C (0.2F) per minute; skin temperature decreases 0.3C (0.5F) per minute. Skin temperature markedly decreases within 10 minutes after exposure to room air. The temperature should stabilize within 8 to 12 hours. Temperature should be monitored when the newborn is admitted to the nursery and at least every 30 minutes until the newborn's status has remained stable for 2 hours. Thereafter the nurse should assess temperature at least once every 8 hours or according to institutional policy (AAP & ACOG, 2002). (See Chapter 28 ∞ for a discussion of the physiology of temperature regulation).

Table 29–2   NEWBORN MEASUREMENTS
Weight
Average: 3405 g (7 lb, 8 oz)
Range: 2500–4000 g (5 lb, 8 oz–8 lb, 13 oz)
Weight is influenced by racial origin and maternal age and size.
Physiologic weight loss: 5%–10% for term newborns, up to 15% for preterm newborns
Growth: 198 g (7 oz) per week for first 6 months
Length
Average: 50 cm (20 in.)
Range: 48–52 cm (18–22 in.)
Growth: 2.5 cm (1 in.) per month for first 6 months
Head Circumference
32–37 cm (12.5–14.5 in.)
Approximately 2 cm larger than chest circumference
Chest Circumference
Average: 32 cm (12.5 in.)
Range: 30–35 cm (12–14 in.)

Temperature can be assessed by the axillary skin method, a continuous skin probe, the rectal route, or a tympanic thermometer. Axillary temperature reflects body (core) temperature and the body's compensatory response to the thermal environment. Axillary temperatures are the preferred method and are considered to be a close estimation of the rectal temperature. In preterm and term newborns there is less than 0.1C (0.2F) difference between the two sites and the axillary method is preferred. If the axillary method is used, the thermometer must remain in place at least 3 minutes, unless an electronic thermometer is used (Figure 29–16 ◆). Axillary temperature ranges from 36.5C to 37C (97.7F to 98.6F). Keep in mind that axillary tempera-

Figure 29–16 ◆ Axillary temperature measurement. The axillary temperature should be taken for 3 minutes. The newborn's arm should be tightly but gently pressed against the thermometer and the newborn's side, as illustrated.

tures can be misleading because the friction caused by apposition of the inner arm skin and upper chest wall and the nearness of brown fat to the probe may elevate the temperature.

Skin temperature is measured most accurately by continuous skin probe, especially for small newborns or newborns maintained in incubators or under radiant warmers. Normal skin temperature is 36C to 36.5C (96.8F to 97.7F). Assessing skin temperature allows time for interventions to be initiated before a more serious fall in core temperature occurs (Figure 29–17 ◆).

Rectal temperature is assumed to be the closest approximation to core temperature, but the accuracy of this method depends on the depth to which the thermometer is inserted. Normal rectal temperature is 36.6C to 37.2C (97.8F to 99F). The rectal route is **not** recommended as a routine method because it may predispose to rectal mucosal irritation and increase chances of perforation.

Many institutions use tympanic thermometers. These are portable sensor probes with disposable covers that are placed in the auditory canal. The probe uses infrared technology to measure the temperature of the internal carotid artery blood flow within several seconds. Research suggests that tympanic and digital thermometer axillary temperatures provide accurate estimations of body temperature in *healthy* newborns (Blackburn, 2003). Current research still questions the accuracy of tympanic

thermometer readings from sick or potentially ill newborns (Blackburn, 2003).

Temperature instability, a deviation of more than 1C (2F) from one reading to the next, or a subnormal temperature may indicate an infection. In contrast with an elevated temperature in older children, an increased temperature in a newborn may indicate a reaction to too many coverings, too hot a room, or dehydration. Dehydration, which tends to increase body temperature, occurs in newborns whose feedings have been delayed for any reason. Newborns respond to overheating (temperature greater than 37.5C or 99.5F) by increased restlessness and eventually by perspiration. The perspiration is initially seen on the head and face, then on the chest. Many newborns initially cannot perspire, so they increase their respiratory and heart rates, which increases oxygen consumption.

Skin Characteristics

Although the newborn's skin color varies with genetic background, all healthy newborns have a pink tinge to their skin. The ruddy hue results from increased red blood cell concentration in the blood vessels and from limited subcutaneous fat deposits.

Skin pigmentation is slight in the newborn period, so color changes may be seen even in darker skinned babies. A newborn who is cyanotic at rest and pink only with crying may have choanal atresia (congenital blockage of the passageway between the nose and pharynx). If crying increases the cyanosis, heart or lung problems should be suspected. Very pale newborns may be anemic or have hypovolemia (low blood volume) and should be evaluated for these problems.

Acrocyanosis (bluish discoloration of the hands and feet) may be present in the first 2 to 6 hours after birth (Figure 29–18 ◆). This condition is due to poor peripheral circulation, which results in vasomotor instability and capillary stasis, especially when the baby is exposed to cold. If the central circulation is adequate, the blood supply should return quickly (2 to 3 seconds) to the extremity after the skin is blanched with a finger. Blue hands and nails are a poor indicator of oxygenation in a newborn. The face and mucous membranes should be assessed for pinkness reflecting adequate oxygenation.

Figure 29–17 ◆ Temperature monitoring for the newborn. A skin thermal sensor is placed on the newborn's abdomen, upper thigh, or arm and secured with porous tape or a foil-covered foam pad.
SOURCE: Photographer, Elena Dorfman.

Figure 29–18 ◆ Acrocyanosis.

Mottling (lacy pattern of dilated blood vessels under the skin) occurs as a result of general circulation fluctuations. It may last several hours to several weeks or may come and go periodically. Mottling may be related to chilling, prolonged apnea, sepsis, or hypothyroidism.

Harlequin sign (clown) color change is occasionally noted. A deep color develops over one side of the newborn's body while the other side remains pale, so that the skin resembles a clown's suit. This color change results from a vasomotor disturbance in which blood vessels on one side dilate while the vessels on the other side constrict. It usually lasts from 1 to 20 minutes. Affected newborns may have single or multiple episodes, but they are transient and clinically insignificant. The nurse should document its occurrence.

Jaundice is first detectable on the face (where skin overlies cartilage) and the mucous membranes of the mouth (Varney, Kriebs, & Gegor, 2004). Jaundice advances from head to toe and regresses in the opposite direction. It is evaluated by blanching the tip of the nose, the forehead, the sternum, or the gum line. This procedure must be carried out in appropriate lighting. If jaundice is present, the area will appear yellowish immediately after blanching. Another area to assess for jaundice is the sclera. Jaundice must be evaluated and its cause determined immediately to prevent possible serious sequelae. Jaundice may be related to breastfeeding (in some cases), hematomas, immature liver function, or bruises from forceps, or it may be caused by blood incompatibility, oxytocin (Pitocin) augmentation or induction, or a severe hemolytic process. Any jaundice noted before 24 hours of age should be reported to the physician or nurse practitioner. For a detailed discussion of the causes and assessment of jaundice, see Chapter 33. ∞

Erythema toxicum is an eruption of lesions in the area surrounding a hair follicle that are firm, vary in size from 1 to 3 mm, and consist of a white or pale yellow papule or pustule with an erythematous base. It is often called "newborn rash" or "flea bite" dermatitis. The rash may appear suddenly, usually over the trunk and diaper area, and is frequently widespread (Figure 29–19 ◆). The lesions do not appear on the palms of the hands or the soles of the feet. The peak incidence is at 24 to 48 hours of life. The condition rarely presents at birth or after 5 days of life. The cause is unknown and no treatment is neces-

sary. Some clinicians feel it may be caused by irritation from clothing. The lesions disappear in a few hours or days. If a maculopapular rash (eruption consisting of both macules and papules) appears, a smear of the aspirated papule will show numerous eosinophils on staining; no bacteria will be cultured.

Milia, which are exposed sebaceous glands, appear as raised white spots on the face, especially across the nose (Figure 29–20 ◆). No treatment is necessary, because they will clear up spontaneously within the first month. Infants of African heritage have a similar condition called transient neonatal pustular melanosis.

Skin turgor is assessed to determine hydration status, the need to initiate early feedings, and the presence of any infectious processes. The usual place to assess skin turgor is over the abdomen, forearm, or thigh. Skin should be elastic and should return rapidly to its original shape.

Vernix caseosa, a whitish cheeselike substance, covers the fetus while in utero and lubricates the skin of the newborn. The skin of the term or postterm newborn has less vernix and is frequently dry; peeling is common, especially on the hands and feet.

Forceps marks may be present after a difficult forceps birth. The newborn may have reddened areas over the cheeks and jaws. It is important to reassure the parents that these will disappear, usually within 1 or 2 days. Transient facial paralysis resulting from the forceps pressure is a rare complication. Vacuum extractor suction marks on the vertex of the scalp are often seen when vacuum extractors are used to assist with the birth. These are benign and do not indicate any underlying brain lesions.

Birthmarks

Telangiectatic nevi (stork bites) appear as pale pink or red spots and are frequently found on the eyelids, nose, lower occipital bone, and nape of the neck (Figure 29–21 ◆). These lesions are common in light-complexioned newborns and are more noticeable during periods of crying. These areas have no clinical significance and usually fade by the second birthday.

Mongolian blue spots are macular areas of bluish black or gray-blue pigmentation found on the dorsal area and the but-

Figure 29–19 ◆ Erythema toxicum.

Figure 29–20 ◆ Facial milia.

Figure 29–21 ◆ Stork bites.

Figure 29–22 ◆ Mongolian spots.

Figure 29–23 ◆ Port wine stain.

tocks (Figure 29–22 ◆)(Johnston, Flood, & Spinks, 2003). They are common in newborns of Asian, Hispanic, and African descent and other dark-skinned races and can be seen in 1% to 9% of Caucasians. They gradually fade during the first or second year of life. They may be mistaken for bruises and should be documented in the newborn's chart.

Nevus flammeus (port wine stain) is a capillary angioma directly below the epidermis. It is a nonelevated, sharply demarcated, red to purple area of dense capillaries (Figure 29–23 ◆). In infants of African descent it may appear as a purple-black stain. The size and shape varies, but it commonly appears on the face. It does not grow in size, does not fade with time, and does not blanch as a rule. The birthmark may be concealed by using an opaque cosmetic cream. If convulsions and other neurologic problems accompany the nevus flammeus, the clinical picture is suggestive of Sturge-Weber syndrome with involvement of the fifth cranial nerve (the ophthalmic branch of the trigeminal nerve).

Nevus vasculosus (strawberry mark) is a capillary hemangioma. It consists of newly formed and enlarged capillaries in the dermal and subdermal layers. It is a raised, clearly delineated, dark red, rough-surfaced birthmark commonly found in the head region. Such marks usually begin to grow (often rapidly) during the second or third week of life and may not reach their full size for 1 to 3 months (Thureen, Deacon, Hernandez et al., 2005). They begin to shrink and start to resolve spontaneously several weeks to months after they reach peak growth. A pale purple or gray spot on the surface of the hemangioma sig-

nals the start of resolution. The best cosmetic effect is achieved when the lesions are allowed to resolve spontaneously.

Birthmarks are frequently a cause of concern for the parents. The mother may be especially anxious, fearing that she is to blame ("Is my baby marked because of something I did?"). Guilt feelings are common in the presence of misconceptions about the cause. Birthmarks should be identified and explained to the parents. By providing appropriate information about the cause and course of birthmarks, the nurse frequently relieves the fears and anxieties of the family. The nurse should note any bruises, abrasions, or birthmarks seen on the newborn's admission to the nursery.

Head

GENERAL APPEARANCE

The newborn's head is large (approximately one fourth of the body size), with soft, pliable skull bones. For most term infants, the occipital-frontal circumference (OFC) is 32 to 37 cm. The head may appear asymmetric in the newborn of a vertex presentation. This asymmetry, called **molding,** is caused by the overriding of the cranial bones during labor and birth (Figure 29–24 ◆). The degree of molding varies with the amount and length of pressure exerted on the head. Within a few days after birth, the overriding usually diminishes, and the suture lines become palpable. Because head measurements are affected by molding, a second measurement is indicated a few days after birth. The heads of breech-born newborns and those born by elective cesarean birth are characteristically round and well shaped because pressure was not exerted on them during birth. Any extreme differences in head size may indicate microcephaly (an abnormally small head) or hydrocephalus (an abnormal buildup of fluid in the brain). Variations in the shape, size, or appearance of the head may be due to *craniosynostosis* (premature closure of the cranial sutures), which needs to be corrected through surgery to allow brain growth, or *plagiocephaly* (asymmetry caused by pressure on the fetal head during gestation) (Thureen et al., 2005).

Two *fontanelles* ("soft spots") may be palpated on the newborn's head. Fontanelles, which are openings at the juncture of the cranial bones, can be measured with the fingers. Accurate measurement necessitates that the examiner's finger be measured

Figure 29–24 ◆ Overlapped cranial bones produce a visible ridge in a small premature infant. Easily visible overlapping does not occur often in term infants.
SOURCE: Korones, S. B. *High-risk newborn infants* (4th ed.). Copyright © 1986, with permission from Elsevier.

Figure 29–25 ◆ Cephalhematoma is a collection of blood between the surface of a cranial bone and the periosteal membrane. This is a cephalhematoma over the left parietal bone.
SOURCE: Photo reprinted from Potter, E. L., & Craig, J. M. *Pathology of the fetus and infant* (3rd ed.). Copyright © 1975, with permission from Elsevier.

in centimeters. The assessment should be carried out with the newborn in sitting position and not crying. The diamond-shaped *anterior fontanelle* is 3 to 4 cm long by 2 to 3 cm wide. It is located at the juncture of the frontal and parietal bones. The *posterior fontanelle,* smaller and triangular, is formed by the parietal bones and the occipital bone and is 0.5 cm by 1 cm. Because of molding, the fontanelles tend to be smaller immediately after birth than several days later. The anterior fontanelle closes within 18 months, whereas the posterior fontanelle closes within 8 to 12 weeks.

The fontanelles are a useful indicator of the newborn's condition. The anterior fontanelle may swell when the newborn cries or passes a stool or may pulsate with the heartbeat, which is normal. A bulging fontanelle usually signifies increased intracranial pressure, and a depressed fontanelle indicates dehydration (Kiesler & Ricer, 2003). The sutures between the cranial bones should be palpated for amount of overlap. In newborns whose growth has been restricted, the sutures may be wider than normal, and the fontanelle may also be larger because of impaired fetal growth of the cranial bones. In addition to being inspected for degree of molding and size, the head should be evaluated for soft-tissue edema and bruising.

CEPHALHEMATOMA

Cephalhematoma is a collection of blood resulting from ruptured blood vessels between the surface of a cranial bone (usually parietal) and the periosteal membrane (Figure 29–25 ◆).

The scalp in these areas feels loose and slightly edematous. These areas emerge as defined hematomas between the first and second days. Although external pressure may cause the mass to fluctuate, it does not increase in size when the newborn cries. Cephalhematomas may be unilateral or bilateral and do not cross suture lines. They are relatively common in vertex births and disappear within 2 weeks to 3 months. They may be associated with physiologic jaundice, because there are extra red blood cells being destroyed within the cephalhematoma. A large cephalhematoma can lead to anemia and hypotension.

CAPUT SUCCEDANEUM

Caput succedaneum is a localized, easily identifiable soft area of the scalp, generally resulting from a long and difficult labor or vacuum extraction. The sustained pressure of the presenting part against the cervix results in compression of local blood vessels, and venous return is slowed. Slowed venous return causes an increase in tissue fluids, an edematous swelling, and occasional bleeding under the periosteum. The caput may vary from a small area to a large area covering a severely elongated head. The fluid in the caput is reabsorbed within 12 hours to a few days after birth. Caputs resulting from vacuum extractors are sharply outlined, circular areas up to 2 cm thick. They disappear more slowly than naturally occurring edema. It is possible to distinguish between a cephalhematoma and a caput because the caput overrides suture lines (Figure 29–26 ◆), whereas the cephalhematoma, because of its location, never crosses a suture line (Table 29–3). Caput succedaneum is present at birth, whereas cephalhematoma generally is not.

Hair

The term newborn's hair is smooth with texture variations depending on ethnic background. Scalp hair is usually high over the eyebrows. Assessment of the newborn's hair characteristics such as color, quantity, hairlines, direction of growth, and hair whorls can identify genetic, metabolic, and neurologic disorders (Furdon & Clark, 2003). For example, coarse, brittle, and dry hair may indicate hypothyroidism.

Figure 29–26 ◆ Caput succedaneum is a collection of fluid (serum) under the scalp.
SOURCE: Photo courtesy of Mead Johnson Nutritionals, Evansville, IN.

 Table 29–3   COMPARISON OF CEPHALHEMATOMA AND CAPUT SUCCEDANEUM

Cephalhematoma

Collection of blood between cranial (usually parietal) bone and periosteal membrane

Does not cross suture lines

Does not increase in size with crying

Appears on first and second days

Disappears after 2 to 3 weeks or may take months

Caput Succedaneum

Collection of fluid, edematous swelling of the scalp

Crosses suture lines

Present at birth or shortly thereafter

Reabsorbed within 12 hours or a few days after birth

Face

The newborn's face is well designed to help the newborn suckle. Sucking (fat) pads are located in the cheeks, and a labial tubercle (sucking callus) is frequently found in the center of the upper lip. The chin is recessed, and the nose is flattened. The lips are sensitive to touch, and the sucking reflex is easily initiated.

Symmetry of the eyes, nose, and ears is evaluated. See Assessment Guide: Newborn Physical Assessment for deviations in symmetry and variations in size, shape, and spacing of facial features. Facial movement symmetry should be assessed to determine the presence of facial palsy. Facial paralysis appears when the newborn cries; the affected side is immobile, and the palpebral (eyelid) fissure widens (Figure 29–27 ◆). Paralysis may result from forceps-assisted birth or pressure on

Figure 29–27 ◆ Facial paralysis. Paralysis of the right side of the face from an injury to the right facial nerve.
SOURCE: Photo reprinted from Potter, E. L., & Craig, J. M. *Pathology of the fetus and infant* (3rd ed.). Copyright © 1975, with permission from Elsevier.

the facial nerve from the maternal pelvis during birth. Facial paralysis usually disappears within a few days to 3 weeks, although in some cases it may be permanent.

Eyes

The eyes of newborns of northern European descent are a blue or slate blue-gray. Dark-skinned newborns tend to have dark eyes at birth. The scleral color tends to be white to bluish white because of its relative thinness. A blue sclera is associated with osteogenesis imperfecta. The infant's eye color is usually established at approximately 3 months, but it may change any time up to 1 year.

The eyes should be checked for size, equality of pupil size, reaction of pupils to light, blink reflex to light, and edema and inflammation of the eyelids. The eyelids can be edematous during the first few days of life because of the pressure associated with birth.

Erythromycin and tetracycline are frequently used prophylactically instead of silver nitrate and usually do not cause chemical irritation of the eye. The instillation of silver nitrate drops in the newborn's eyes may cause edema and **chemical conjunctivitis,** which may appear a few hours after instillation and disappear in 1 to 2 days. If infectious conjunctivitis exists, the newborn has the same purulent (greenish yellow) discharge as in chemical conjunctivitis, but it is caused by gonococcus, *Chlamydia,* staphylococci, or a variety of gram-negative bacteria and requires treatment with ophthalmic antibiotics. Onset is usually after the second day. Edema of the orbits or eyelids may persist for several days until the newborn's kidneys can evacuate the fluid.

Small **subconjunctival hemorrhages** appear in about 10% of newborns and are commonly found on the sclera. These hemorrhages are caused by the changes in vascular tension or ocular pressure during birth. They will remain for a few weeks and are of no pathologic significance. Parents need reassurance that the infant is not bleeding from within the eye and that vision will not be impaired.

The newborn may demonstrate transient strabismus (pseudostrabismus) or squinting caused by neuromuscular control of eye muscles (Figure 29–28 ◆). It gradually regresses in 3 to 4 months. The "doll's eye" phenomenon is also present for about 10 days after birth. As the newborn's head position is changed to the left and then to the right, the eyes move to the opposite direction. "Doll's eye" results from underdeveloped integration of head-eye coordination.

The nurse should observe the newborn's pupils for opacities or whiteness and for the absence of a normal red retinal reflex. Red retinal reflex is a red-orange flash of color observed when an ophthalmoscope light reflects off the retina. In a newborn with dark skin color, the retina may appear paler or more grayish. Absence of red reflex occurs with cataracts. Congenital cataracts should be suspected in infants of mothers with a prenatal history of rubella, cytomegalic inclusion disease, or syphilis.

The cry of the newborn is commonly tearless because the lacrimal structures are immature at birth and are not usually fully functional until the second month of life. However, some babies may produce tears during the newborn period.

Figure 29–28 ◆ Transient strabismus in the newborn may be due to poor neuromuscular control.
SOURCE: Courtesy of Mead Johnson Nutritionals, Evansville, IN.

Poor oculomotor coordination and absence of accommodation limit visual abilities, but newborns do have peripheral vision and can fixate on near objects (8 to 10 in.) in front of their faces for short periods, can accommodate to large objects (3 in. tall by 3 in. wide), and can seek out high-contrast geometric shapes. Newborns can perceive faces, shapes, and colors and begin to show visual preferences early. Newborns generally blink in response to bright lights, to a tap on the bridge of the nose (glabellar reflex), or to a light touch on the eyelids. Pupillary light reflex is also present. The eye is best examined by rocking the newborn from an upright position to the horizontal a few times or by other methods, such as diminishing overhead lights, which will elicit an opened-eye response.

Nose

The newborn's nose is small and narrow. Infants are characteristically nose breathers for the first few months of life. The newborn generally removes obstructions by sneezing. The nose is patent if the newborn breathes easily with the mouth closed. If respiratory difficulty occurs, the nurse checks for choanal atresia (congenital blockage of the passageway between the nose and pharynx). Historically, choanal atresia can be checked by attempting to gently pass a soft #5 French catheter into both nostrils. Because of possible trauma, a cold, flat metal object may also be held under the nose to observe for fogging (Thureen et al., 2005).

The newborn has the ability to smell after the nasal passages are cleared of amniotic fluid and mucus. Newborns demonstrate this ability by the search for milk. They will turn their heads toward the milk source, whether bottle or breast. Newborns react to strong odors, such as alcohol, by turning their heads away or blinking.

Mouth

The lips of the newborn should be pink, and a touch on the lips should produce sucking motions. Saliva is normally scant. The taste buds are developed before birth, and the newborn can easily discriminate between sweet and bitter flavors.

Figure 29–29 ◆ The nurse inserts the index finger (or "pinky") into the newborn's mouth and feels for any openings along the hard and soft palates.
Note: Gloves or a finger cot are always worn to examine the palate.
SOURCE: Courtesy of Vanessa Howell, RNC, BSN.

The easiest way to examine the mouth completely is to stimulate infants to cry by gently depressing their tongue, thereby causing them to open the mouth fully. It is extremely important to observe the entire mouth to look for a cleft palate, which can be present even in the absence of a cleft lip. The examiner moves a gloved index finger along the hard and soft palate to feel for any openings (Figure 29–29 ◆). Glove powder should always be removed before examining the newborn's mouth.

Occasionally, an examination of the gums will reveal precocious teeth over the area where the lower central incisor will erupt. If they appear loose, they should be removed to prevent aspiration. Gray-white lesions (inclusion cysts) on the gums may be confused with teeth. On the hard palate and gum margins, **Epstein's pearls,** small glistening white specks (keratin-containing cysts) that feel hard to the touch, are often present. They usually disappear in a few weeks and are of no significance. **Thrush** may appear as white patches that look like milk curds adhering to the mucous membranes, and bleeding may occur when patches are removed. Thrush is caused by *Candida albicans,* often acquired from an infected vaginal tract during birth, antibiotic use, or poor handwashing when handling the newborn. Thrush is treated with a preparation of nystatin (Mycostatin).

A newborn who is tongue-tied has a ridge of frenulum tissue attached to the underside of the tongue at varying lengths from its base, causing a heart shape at the tip of the tongue. "Clipping the tongue," or cutting the ridge of tissue, is not recommended. This ridge does not affect speech or eating, but cutting does create an entry for infection.

Transient nerve paralysis resulting from birth trauma may be manifested by asymmetric mouth movements when the newborn cries or by difficulty with sucking and feeding.

Ears

The ears of the newborn are soft and pliable and should recoil readily when folded and released. In the normal newborn, the top

of the ear (pinna) should be parallel to the outer and inner canthus of the eye. The ears should be inspected for shape, size, position, and firmness of ear cartilage. *Low-set ears* are characteristic of many syndromes and may indicate chromosomal abnormalities (especially trisomies 13 and 18), mental retardation, or internal organ abnormalities, especially bilateral renal agenesis as a result of embryologic developmental deviations (Figure 29–30 ◆). A preauricular skin tag may be present just in front of the ear. Visualization of the tympanic membranes is not usually done soon after birth because blood and vernix block the ear canal.

Following the first cry, the newborn's hearing becomes acute as mucus from the middle ear is absorbed, the eustachian tube is aerated, and the tympanic membrane becomes visible. The newborn's hearing initially can be evaluated by response to loud or moderately loud noises unaccompanied by vibrations. The sleeping newborn should stir or awaken in response to the nearby sounds. (This is not a very accurate test, but it may help to alert the examiner to possible problems.) The newborn can discriminate the individual characteristics of the human voice and is especially sensitive to sound levels within the normal conversation range. The newborn in a noisy nursery may be able to habituate to the sounds and not stir unless the sound is sudden or much louder.

The AAP has endorsed universal newborn hearing screening (UNHS) in birthing units as the standard of care (Thureen et al., 2005). The current goal is to screen all infants by 1 month of age, confirm hearing loss with audiologic examination by 3 months of age, and treat with comprehensive early intervention services before 6 months of age (AAP & ACOG, 2002). Families need to be educated about appropriate interpretation of screening test results and the appropriate steps for follow-up.

Risk factors (AAP & ACOG, 2002) associated with potential hearing loss include the following:

- The presence of familial hearing loss
- Serum bilirubin level greater than 20 mg/dL for the full-term newborn or hyperbilirubinemia with a level exceeding indications for exchange transfusion because of toxic drugs
- Prolonged mechanical ventilation of more than 5 days
- Congenital infection with rubella, herpes, cytomegalovirus, toxoplasmosis, or syphilis

A   B

Figure 29–30 ◆ The position of the external ear may be assessed by drawing a line across the inner and outer canthus of the eye to the insertion of the ear. *A,* Normal position. *B,* True low-set position.
SOURCE: Courtesy of Mead Johnson Nutritionals, Evansville, IN.

- Bacterial meningitis or sepsis
- Congenital defects of the ear, nose, or throat
- Small preterm newborns, particularly less than 1500 g at birth
- Perinatal asphyxia
- Ototoxic medications

If congenital hearing loss risk factors exist, two types of tests are commonly used: otoacoustic emissions (OAEs) and auditory brainstem response (ABR). Typically, screening programs use a two-stage screening approach (OAE repeated twice, OAE followed by ABR, or automated ABR repeated twice). Families need to be educated about appropriate interpretation of screening test results and appropriate steps for follow-up.

> **CLINICAL TIP**
>
> Vital sign assessments are most accurate if the newborn is at rest, so measure pulse and respirations first if the baby is quiet. To soothe a crying baby, try placing your moistened gloved finger in the baby's mouth, and then complete your assessment while the baby suckles.

Neck

A short neck, creased with skin folds, is characteristic of the normal newborn. Because muscle tone is not well developed, the neck cannot support the full weight of the head, which rotates freely. The head lags considerably when the newborn is pulled up from a supine to a sitting position, but the prone newborn is able to raise the head slightly. The neck is palpated for masses and presence of lymph nodes and is inspected for webbing. Adequate range of motion and neck muscle function is determined by fully extending the head in all directions. Injury to the sternocleidomastoid muscle (congenital torticollis) must be considered in the presence of neck rigidity.

The clavicles are evaluated for evidence of fractures, which occasionally occur during difficult births or in newborns with broad shoulders. The normal clavicle is straight. If fractured, a lump and a grating sensation (crepitus) during movements may be palpated along the course of the side of the break. The Moro reflex (see pages 844 and 846) is also elicited to evaluate bilateral equal movement of the arms. If the clavicle is fractured, this response will be demonstrated only on the unaffected side.

Chest

The thorax is cylindric and symmetric at birth, and the ribs are flexible. The general appearance of the chest should be assessed. A protrusion at the lower end of the sternum, called the xiphoid cartilage, is frequently seen. It is under the skin and will become less apparent after several weeks as the infant accumulates adipose tissue.

Engorged breasts occur frequently in both male and female newborns. This condition, which appears by the third day, is a result of maternal hormonal influences and may last up to 2 weeks (Figure 29–31 ◆). A whitish secretion from the nipples may also be noted. The infant's breast should not be massaged or squeezed because this practice may cause a breast abscess. Extra nipples or supernumerary nipples are occasionally noted

Figure 29–31 ◆ Breast hypertrophy.
SOURCE: Korones, S. B. *High-risk newborn infants* (4th ed.). Copyright © 1986, with permission from Elsevier.

below and medial to the true nipples. These harmless pink or brown (in darker skinned newborns) spots vary in size and do not contain glandular tissue. Accessory nipples can be differentiated from a pigmented nevus (mole) by placing the fingertips alongside the accessory nipple and pulling the adjacent tissue laterally. The accessory nipple will appear dimpled. At puberty the accessory nipple may darken.

Cry

The newborn's cry should be strong, lusty, and of medium pitch. A high-pitched, shrill cry is abnormal and may indicate neurologic disorders or hypoglycemia. Periods of crying vary in length after consoling measures are used. A baby's cries are an important method of communication and alert caregivers to changes in the baby's condition and needs.

Respiration

Normal breathing for a term newborn is 30 to 60 respirations per minute and predominantly diaphragmatic, with associated rising and falling of the abdomen during inspiration and expiration. Any signs of respiratory distress, nasal flaring, intercostal or xiphoid retractions, expiratory grunting or sighing, seesaw respirations, or tachypnea (sustained or greater than 60 respirations per minute) should be noted. Hyperexpansion (chest appears high) or hypoexpansion (chest appears low) of the anteroposterior diameter of the chest should also be noted. Both the anterior and posterior chest are auscultated. Some breath sounds are heard best when the newborn is crying, but it is difficult to localize and identify breath sounds in the newborn. Upper airway noises and bowel sounds can be heard over the chest wall, making auscultation difficult. Because sounds may be transmitted from the unaffected lung to the affected lung, the absence of breath sounds may not be diagnosed. Air entry may be noisy in the first couple of hours until lung fluid resolves, especially in cesarean births. Brief periods of apnea (episodic breathing) may occur, but no color or heart rate changes occur in healthy, term newborns. Sepsis should be suspected in full-term infants experiencing apneic episodes.

Heart

Heart rates can be as rapid as 180 beats per minute in newborns and fluctuate a great deal, especially if the baby moves or is startled. Normal range is 120 to 160 beats per minute. Auscultation provides the nurse with valuable assessment data. The heart is examined for rate and rhythm, position of the apical impulse, and heart sound intensity. Dysrhythmias should be evaluated by a physician.

The pulse rate is variable and is influenced by physical activity, crying, state of wakefulness, and body temperature. Auscultation is performed over the entire heart region (precordium), below the left axilla, and below the scapula. Apical pulse rates are obtained by auscultation for a full minute, preferably when the newborn is asleep.

The placement of the heart in the chest should be determined when the newborn is in a quiet state. The heart is relatively large at birth and is located high in the chest, with its apex somewhere between the fourth and fifth intercostal space.

A shift of heart tones in the mediastinal area to either side may indicate pneumothorax, dextrocardia (heart placement on the right side of the chest), or a diaphragmatic hernia. The experienced nurse can diagnose these and many other problems early with a stethoscope. Normally, the heartbeat has a "toc tic" sound. A slur or slushing sound (usually after the first sound) may indicate a murmur. Although 90% of all murmurs are transient and are considered normal, they should be monitored closely by a physician. Many murmurs are related to a patent ductus arteriosus, which should close 1 to 2 days after birth.

In newborns, a low-pitched, musical murmur heard just to the right of the apex of the heart is fairly common. Occasionally, significant murmurs will be heard, such as the murmur of a patent ductus arteriosus, aortic or pulmonary stenosis, or small

RESEARCH IN PRACTICE

CAPILLARY REFILL TIME IS AN UNRELIABLE INDICATOR OF CARDIOVASCULAR STATUS IN TERM NEONATES

What is this study about? It is commonly believed that circulatory status can be evaluated by blanching an area of skin and measuring the time elapsed until baseline color returns. This procedure, which is referred to as capillary refill time (CRT), has been widely used as a clinical tool in the assessment of circulatory status. It is so well accepted that it has been incorporated into well-recognized clinical scoring systems such as the Trauma Score. The results of the CRT may be used by clinicians to guide clinical decisions, and so it is imperative that it accurately represents underlying cardiovascular status. However, recent research shows that CRT varies considerably with age, temperature, site of measurement, and duration of pressure. The purpose of this study was to examine the relationship between CRT and indicators of cardiovascular status in normal newborns.

How was this study done? This study was conducted in the newborn nursery of a single, tertiary medical center in Texas. A sample of 42 healthy, term babies were in the study. CRT was measured within 4 hours of birth. Three anatomical sites for determining CRT were studied: the finger, heel, and lower sternum. CRT was measured with a stopwatch after brief pressure (1 to 2 seconds) and extended pressure (3 to 4 seconds) at each of the six sites. All assessments were collected by one investigator so that the measurement procedure was consistent. The outcomes investigated were heart rate (as detected by auscultation) and blood pressure, as measured by oscillometry using the appropriate size cuff on the arm and leg. The relationship between CRT and the outcomes was analyzed using correlation statistics.

What were the results of the study? Regardless of site, CRT was greater when extended versus brief pressure was used. There was no significant variation in these results by site. There was a moderate, direct relationship between blood pressure and CRT over the sternum. This is a significant finding, as a direct correlation indicates that increased capillary refill time was associated with *increased* blood pressure. The authors hypothesize that this result was due to an increase in circulating vasoactive substances in the immediate newborn period. This paradoxical result is not definitive in this small sample, but does raise the question of the reliability of CRT in detecting deteriorating cardiovascular status in the first 4 hours of life. CRT in the finger reflected only systolic blood pressure, and that relationship was a weak one. There was no association between CRT on the heel and any cardiovascular indicator.

What additional questions might I have? At what age does the infant's capillary refill time reflect circulatory status as reliably as it does in an older child? Would a larger sample have detected a more significant effect between CRT and these indicators?

How can I use this study? Capillary refill time may be a reliable indicator of blood pressure in the newborn if extended pressure (3 to 4 seconds) is applied to the skin over the sternum. However, it does not appear that CRT is a reliable indicator of cardiovascular status in the first 4 hours after birth. The finger and heel are not better sites to assess capillary refill. Consistent assessment by the same nurse is desirable, as results were affected by variations in procedure.

LeFlore, J., & Engle, W. (2005). Capillary refill time is an unreliable indicator of cardiovascular status in term neonates. *Advances in Neonatal Care, 5*(3), 147–154.

A

B

Figure 29–32 ◆ *A*, Bilaterally palpate the femoral arteries for rate and intensity of the pulses. Press fingertip gently at the groin as shown. *B*, Compare the femoral pulses to the brachial pulses by palpating the pulses simultaneously for comparison of rate and intensity.
SOURCE: Photographer, Elena Dorfman.

Figure 29–33 ◆ Blood pressure measurement using the Dinemapp and Doppler devices. The cuff can be applied to either the newborn's upper arm or the thigh.
SOURCE: Courtesy of Vanessa Howell, RNC, BSN.

CLINICAL TIP:

If possible, obtain blood pressure (BP) measurement during quiet sleep or sleep state. Place cuff on arm or leg and give infant time to quiet. Obtain average of 2 to 3 measurements when making clinical decisions. Follow mean BP to monitor changes, as it is less likely to be erroneous. Noninvasive BP may overestimate BP in very low-birth-weight infants.

Blood pressure may not be measured routinely on healthy newborns but is an essential measurement in newborns who are having distress, are premature, or are suspected of having a cardiac anomaly (Thureen et al., 2005). Infants who have birth asphyxia and are on ventilators have significantly lower systolic and diastolic blood pressures than healthy infants. If a cardiac anomaly is suspected, blood pressure is palpated in all four extremities (Table 29–4). At birth, systolic values usually range from 70 to 50 mm Hg and diastolic values from 45 to 30 mm Hg. By the 10th day of life, blood pressure may rise to 90/50 mm Hg.

Abdomen

The nurse can learn a great deal about the newborn's abdomen without disturbing the infant. The abdomen should be cylindrical, protrude slightly, and move with respiration. A certain amount of laxness of the abdominal muscles is normal. A scaphoid (hollow-shaped) appearance suggests the absence of abdominal contents, seen in diaphragmatic hernia. No cyanosis should be present, and few if any blood vessels should be apparent to the eye. There should be no gross distention or bulging. The more distended the abdomen, the tighter the skin becomes, and engorged vessels appear. Distention is the first sign of many of the abnormalities found in the gastrointestinal tract.

Before palpation of the abdomen, the nurse should auscultate the presence or absence of bowel sounds in all four quadrants. Bowel sounds should be present by 1 hour after birth. Palpation can cause a transient decrease in bowel sound intensity.

Abdominal palpation should be carried out systematically. The nurse palpates each of the four abdominal quadrants, mov-

ventricular septal defect. See Chapter 32 ∞ for a discussion of congenital heart defects.

Peripheral pulses (brachial, femoral, pedal) are also evaluated to detect any lags or unusual characteristics. Brachial pulses are palpated bilaterally for equality and compared with the femoral pulses. Femoral pulses are palpated by applying gentle pressure with the middle finger over the femoral canal (Figure 29–32 ◆). Decreased or absent femoral pulses may indicate coarctation of the aorta or hypovolemia and require additional investigation. A wide difference in blood pressure between the upper and lower extremities also indicates coarctation.

The measurement of blood pressure is best accomplished by using a noninvasive blood pressure device (Figure 29–33 ◆). If a blood pressure cuff is used, the newborn's extremities must be immobilized during the assessment, and the cuff should cover two thirds of the upper arm or upper leg. Movement, crying, and inappropriate cuff size can give inaccurate measurements of the blood pressure.

Table 29–4	NEWBORN VITAL SIGNS
Pulse	**Blood Pressure**
120–160 bpm	70–50/45–30 mm Hg at birth
During sleep as low as 100 bpm; if crying, up to 180 bpm	90/60 mm Hg at day 10
Apical pulse counted for 1 full minute	**Temperature**
Respirations	Normal range: 36.5C–37.5C (97.7F–99.4F)
30–60 respirations/minute	Axillary: 36.4C–37.2C (97.5F–99F)
Predominantly diaphragmatic but synchronous with abdominal movements	Skin: 36C–36.5C (96.8F–97.7F)
Respirations are counted for 1 full minute	Rectal: 36.6C–37.2C (97.8F–99F)

DEVELOPING CULTURAL COMPETENCE

NATIVE AMERICANS AND UMBILICAL CORD CARE

In the Woodland Indian tribe, upon birth, the umbilical cord is tied and a small piece is saved. This section of the umbilical cord is sewn into a deerskin diamond-shaped pocket. The pocket is hung over the infant's crib to provide protection for the infant.

Figure 29–34 ◆ Umbilical hernia.

ing in a clockwise direction, checking for softness, tenderness, and the presence of masses. The nurse should place one hand under the back for support during palpation. When palpating the abdomen, the nurse may feel for the liver. The newborn's liver is large in proportion to the rest of the body and can usually be felt between 1 and 2 cm below the right costal margin. Depending on institutional protocol, palpation of the kidney may be performed by the staff nurse. Kidneys are more difficult to feel but can be more easily examined within 4 to 6 hours after birth, before the intestines become distended with air and feedings are initiated. By placing a finger at the posterior flank and pushing upward while pressing downward with the opposite hand, each kidney may be palpated as a firm oval mass between the examiner's finger and hand. The lower pole of the kidney is usually found 1 to 2 cm above the umbilicus. The spleen tip may be palpated in the lateral aspect of the left upper quadrant in the normal newborn.

Umbilical Cord

Initially, the umbilical cord is white and gelatinous in appearance, with the two umbilical arteries and one umbilical vein readily apparent. Because a single umbilical artery is frequently associated with congenital anomalies, the vessels should be counted as part of the newborn assessment. The cord begins drying within 1 or 2 hours after birth and is shriveled and blackened by the second or third day. Within 7 to 10 days it sloughs off, although a granulated area may remain for a few days longer.

Cord bleeding is abnormal and may result because the cord was inadvertently pulled or because the cord clamp was loosened. Foul-smelling drainage is also abnormal and is generally caused by infection, which requires immediate treatment to prevent septicemia. If the newborn has a patent urachus (abnormal connection between the umbilicus and bladder), moistness or draining urine may be apparent at the base of the cord. Another umbilical cord anomaly that can occur is umbilical cord hernia and associated patent omphalomesenteric duct (Figure 29–34 ◆). Umbilical hernias are more common in infants of African descent than in Caucasian infants (Thureen et al., 2005).

Serous or serosanguineous drainage that continues after the cord falls off may indicate a granuloma. It appears as a small, red button deep in the umbilicus. Treatment involves cauterization by a physician with a silver nitrate stick (Thureen et al., 2005).

Genitals

FEMALE INFANTS

The nurse examines the labia majora, labia minora, and clitoris, noting the size of each as appropriate for gestational age. A vaginal tag or hymenal tag is often evident and will usually disappear in a few weeks. During the first week of life, the female newborn may have a vaginal discharge composed of thick whitish mucus. This discharge, which can become tinged with blood, is referred to as **pseudomenstruation** and is caused by the withdrawal of maternal hormones. *Smegma*, a white cheese-like substance, is often present between the labia. Removing it may traumatize tender tissue.

MALE INFANTS

The penis is inspected to determine whether the urinary orifice is correctly positioned. *Hypospadias* occurs when the urinary meatus is located on the ventral surface of the penis. It occurs most commonly among people of Western European descent. *Phimosis* is a condition occurring in newborn males in which the opening of the foreskin (prepuce) is small, and the foreskin cannot be pulled back over the glans at all. This condition may interfere with urination, so the adequacy of the urinary stream should be evaluated.

The scrotum is inspected for size and symmetry and should be palpated to verify the presence of both testes and to rule out *cryptorchidism* (failure of testes to descend). The testes are palpated separately between the thumb and forefinger, with the thumb and forefinger of the other hand placed together over the inguinal canal. Scrotal edema and discoloration are common in breech births. *Hydrocele* (a collection of fluid surrounding the testes in the scrotum) is common in newborns and should be identified. It usually resolves without intervention. The presence of a discolored or dusky scrotum and solid testis should raise the suspicion of testicular torsion, which should be reported immediately.

Anus

The anal area is inspected to verify that it is patent and has no fissure. Imperforate anus and rectal atresia may be ruled out by observation. A digital examination, if necessary, is done by a physician or nurse practitioner. The passage of the first meconium stool is also noted. Atresia of the gastrointestinal tract or meconium ileus with resultant obstruction must be considered if the newborn does not pass meconium in the first 24 hours of life.

> **CLINICAL TIP**
> Always examine more closely any infant who is reluctant to move an extremity. Fractures are often asymptomatic in the newborn; paralytic injuries are characterized by immobility of an extremity.

Extremities

Extremities are examined for gross deformities, extra digits or webbing, clubfoot, and range of motion. Normal newborn extremities appear short, are generally flexible, and move symmetrically.

ARMS AND HANDS

Nails extend beyond the fingertips in term newborns. Fingers and toes should be counted. *Polydactyly* is the presence of extra digits on either the hands or the feet. *Syndactyly* refers to fusion (webbing) of fingers or toes. Hands should be inspected for normal palmar creases. A single palmar crease, called a simian line (see also Figure 12–21 ∞), is frequently present in children with Down syndrome.

Brachial palsy, which is partial or complete paralysis of portions of the arm, results from trauma to the brachial plexus during a difficult birth. It occurs most commonly when strong traction is exerted on the head of the newborn in an attempt to deliver a shoulder lodged behind the symphysis pubis in the presence of shoulder dystocia. Brachial palsy may also occur during a breech birth if an arm becomes trapped over the head and traction is exerted.

The portion of the arm affected is determined by the nerves damaged. **Erb-Duchenne paralysis (Erb's palsy)** involves damage to the upper arm (fifth and sixth cervical nerves) and is the most common type. Injury to the eighth cervical and first thoracic nerve roots and the lower portion of the plexus produces the relatively rare *lower arm injury*. The *whole arm type* results from damage to the entire plexus.

With Erb-Duchenne paralysis, the newborn's arm lies limply at the side (Figure 29–35 ◆). The elbow is held in extension, with the forearm pronated. The newborn is unable to ele-

Figure 29–35 ◆ Right Erb's palsy resulting from injury to the fifth and sixth cervical roots of brachial plexus.
SOURCE: Photo reprinted from Potter, E. L., & Craig, J. M. *Pathology of the fetus and infant* (3rd ed.). Copyright © 1975, with permission from Elsevier.

vate the arm, and therefore the Moro reflex cannot be elicited on the affected side (see Figure 29–35). When a lower arm injury occurs, paralysis of the hand and wrist results; complete paralysis of the limb occurs with the whole arm type.

The nurse carefully instructs the parents in the correct method of performing passive range-of-motion exercises (to prevent muscle contractures and restore function) and arranges supervised practice sessions. In more severe cases, splinting of the arm is indicated until the edema decreases. The arm is held in a position of abduction and external rotation with the elbow flexed 90 degrees, often called the "Statue of Liberty" position. The "Statue of Liberty" splint is commonly used, although similar results are obtained by attaching a strip of muslin to the head of the crib and tying the other end around the wrist, thereby holding the arm up.

Prognosis is related to the degree of nerve damage resulting from trauma and hemorrhage within the nerve sheath. Complete recovery occurs within a few months with minimal trauma. Moderate trauma may result in some partial paralysis. Recovery is unlikely with severe trauma, and muscle wasting may develop.

LEGS AND FEET

The legs of the newborn should be of equal length, with symmetric skin folds. However, they may assume a "fetal posture" secondary to position in utero, and it may take several days for the legs to relax into normal position.

To evaluate for hip dislocation or hip instability, the Ortolani and Barlow maneuvers are performed (Figure 29–36 ◆). The nurse (or, more commonly, the physician or nurse practi-

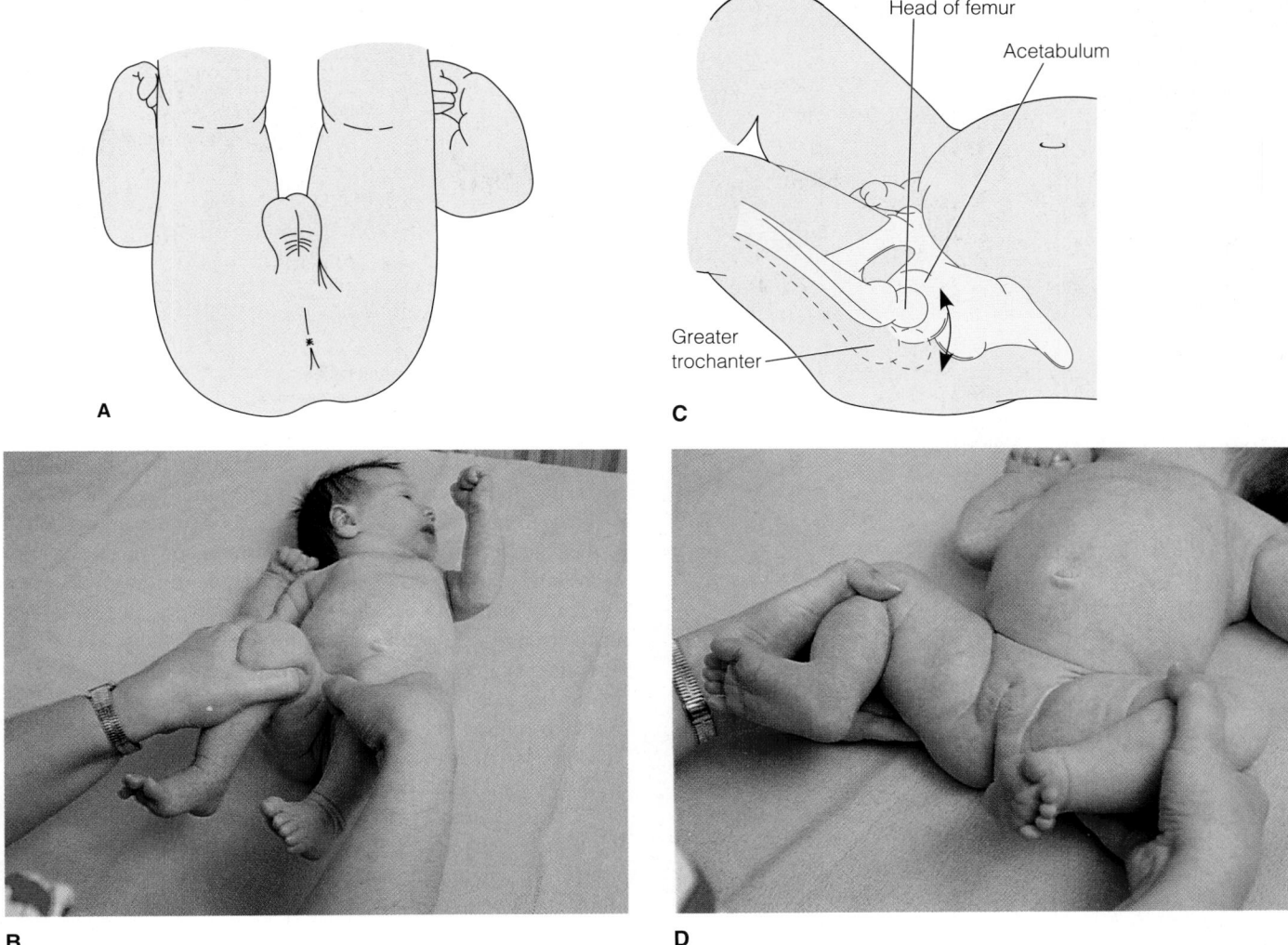

Figure 29–36 ◆ *A,* The asymmetry of gluteal and thigh fat folds seen in infant with left developmental dysplasia of the hip. *B,* Barlow (dislocation) maneuver. Baby's thigh is grasped and adducted (placed together) with gentle downward pressure. *C,* Dislocation is palpable as femoral head slips out of acetabulum. *D,* Ortolani's maneuver puts downward pressure on the hip and then inward rotation. If the hip is dislocated, this maneuver will force the femoral head back into the acetabular rim with a noticeable "clunk."

tioner) performs the **Ortolani's maneuver** to rule out the possibility of congenital hip dysplasia (hip dislocatability). With the newborn relaxed and quiet on a firm surface, the hips and knees flexed at a 90-degree angle, the examiner grasps the infant's thigh with the middle finger over the greater trochanter and lifts the thigh to bring the femoral head from its posterior position toward the acetabulum. With gentle abduction of the thigh, the femoral head is returned to the acetabulum and the examiner feels a sense of reduction or a "clunk." This reduction is palpable and may be heard. With the **Barlow maneuver,** the examiner grasps and adducts the infant's thigh and applies gentle downward pressure. Dislocation is felt as the femoral head slips out of the acetabulum. The femoral head is then returned to the acetabulum using the Ortolani maneuver, confirming the diagnosis of an unstable or dislocatable hip.

The feet are then examined for evidence of a talipes deformity (clubfoot). Intrauterine position frequently causes the feet to appear to turn inward (Figure 29–37 ◆); this is termed a "positional" clubfoot. If the feet can easily be returned to midline

by manipulation, no treatment is indicated. Range-of-motion exercises can be taught to the family. Further investigation is indicated when the foot will not turn to the midline position or align readily. This is considered the most severe type of "true clubfoot," or talipes equinovarus.

Back

With the baby prone, the nurse examines the back. The spine should appear straight and flat because the lumbar and sacral curves do not develop until the infant begins to sit. The base of the spine is examined for a dermal sinus. The nevus pilosus ("hairy nevus") is occasionally found at the base of the spine in newborns. It is significant because it is frequently associated with spina bifida. A pilonidal dimple should be examined to ascertain that there is no connection to the spinal canal.

Assessment of Neurologic Status

The nurse should begin the neurologic examination with a period of observation, noting the general physical characteristics

A

B

Figure 29–37 ◆ *A*, Unilateral talipes equinovarus (clubfoot). *B*, To determine the presence of clubfoot, the nurse moves the foot to the midline. Resistance indicates true clubfoot.
SOURCE: *A*, Courtesy of Mead Johnson Nutritionals, Evansville, IN.

and behavior of the newborn. Important behaviors to assess are the *state of alertness, resting posture, cry,* and *quality of muscle tone* and *motor activity.*

The usual position of the newborn is partially flexed extremities with the legs abducted to the abdomen. When awake, the newborn may exhibit purposeless, uncoordinated bilateral movements of the extremities. If these movements are absent, minimal, or obviously asymmetric, neurologic dysfunction should be suspected. Eye movements are observable during the first few days of life. An alert newborn is able to fixate on faces and brightly colored objects. Shining a bright light in the newborn's eyes elicits the blinking response.

The nurse evaluates muscle tone by moving various parts of the newborn's body while the newborn's head remains in a neutral position. The newborn is somewhat hypertonic; that is, the newborn resists the examiner's attempts to extend the elbow and knee joints. Muscle tone should be symmetric. Diminished muscle tone and flaccidity require further evaluation.

Tremors or jitteriness (tremorlike movements) in the full-term newborn must be evaluated to differentiate the tremors from convulsions. Tremors may be related to hypoglycemia, hypocalcemia, or substance withdrawal. Environmental stimuli may initiate tremors. Jitteriness may be distinguished from tonic-clonic seizure activity because it usually can be stopped

Figure 29–38 ◆ Tonic neck reflex.
SOURCE: © Stella Johnson (www.stellajohnson.com).

by the infant's sucking on the extremity or by the nurse holding or flexing the involved extremity. A fine jumping of the muscle is likely to be a central nervous system disorder and requires further evaluation. Neonatal seizures may consist of no more than chewing or swallowing movements, deviations of the eyes, rigidity, or flaccidity because of central nervous system immaturity. In contrast to tremors, seizures are not usually initiated by stimuli and cannot be stopped by holding.

Specific deep tendon reflexes can be elicited in the newborn but have limited value unless they are obviously asymmetric. The knee jerk is brisk; a normal ankle clonus may involve three or four beats. Plantar flexion is present.

The immature central nervous system of the newborn is characterized by a variety of reflexes. Because the newborn's movements are uncoordinated, methods of communication are limited, and control of body functions is restricted, the reflexes serve a variety of purposes. Some are protective (blink, gag, sneeze); some aid in feeding (rooting, sucking) and may not be very active if the infant has eaten recently; and some stimulate human interaction (grasping).

The most common reflexes found in the normal newborn are the following:

- The **tonic neck reflex** (fencer position) is elicited when the newborn is supine and the head is turned to one side. In response, the extremities on the same side straighten, whereas on the opposite side they flex (Figure 29–38 ◆). This reflex may not be seen during the early newborn period, but once it appears, it persists until about the third month.

- The **grasping reflex** is elicited by stimulating the newborn's palm with a finger or object. The newborn will grasp and hold the object or finger firmly enough to be lifted momentarily from the crib (Figure 29–39 ◆).

- The **Moro reflex** is elicited when the newborn is startled by a loud noise or is lifted slightly above the crib and then suddenly lowered. In response the newborn straightens arms and hands outward while the knees flex. Slowly, the arms return to the chest, as in an embrace. The fingers spread, forming a C, and the newborn may cry (Figure 29–40 ◆). This reflex may persist until about 6 months of age.

- The **rooting reflex** is elicited when the side of the newborn's mouth or cheek is touched. In response the

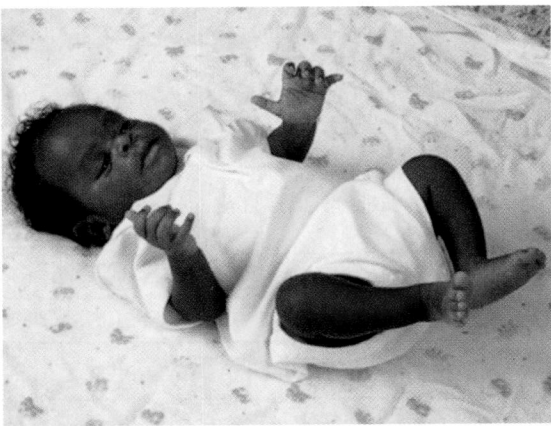

Figure 29–39 ◆ Palmar grasping reflex.

Figure 29–41 ◆ Rooting reflex.

Figure 29–40 ◆ Moro reflex.

newborn turns toward that side and opens the lips to suck (if not fed recently) (Figure 29–41 ◆).

- The **sucking reflex** is elicited when an object is placed in the newborn's mouth or anything touches the lips. Newborns suck even while sleeping; this is called nonnutritive sucking, and it can have a quieting effect on the baby.

- The **Babinski reflex response,** or fanning and hyperextension of all toes and dorsiflexion of the big toe, occurs when the lateral aspect of the sole is stroked from the heel upward across the ball of the foot (Mandleco, 2004). In children older than 24 months, it is considered an abnormal response if there is extension or fanning of all the toes; this Babinski response indicates upper motor neuron abnormalities (Figure 29–42 ◆).

- **Trunk incurvation (Galant reflex)** is seen when the newborn is prone. Stroking the spine causes the pelvis to turn to the stimulated side.

In addition to these reflexes, newborns can *blink, yawn, cough, sneeze,* and draw back from pain (protective reflexes). They can even move a little on their own. When placed on their stomachs, they push up and try to crawl (prone crawl). When held upright with one foot touching a flat surface, the newborn puts one foot in front of the other and "walks" (stepping reflex) (Figure 29–43 ◆). This reflex is more pronounced at birth and is lost in 4 to 8 weeks. Table 29–5 summarizes the stimulus for and response of the common newborn reflexes.

Figure 29–42 ◆ The Babinski reflex (response).

Figure 29–43 ◆ The stepping reflex disappears between 4 and 8 weeks of age.

MEDIALINK

Application: Newborn Reflexes

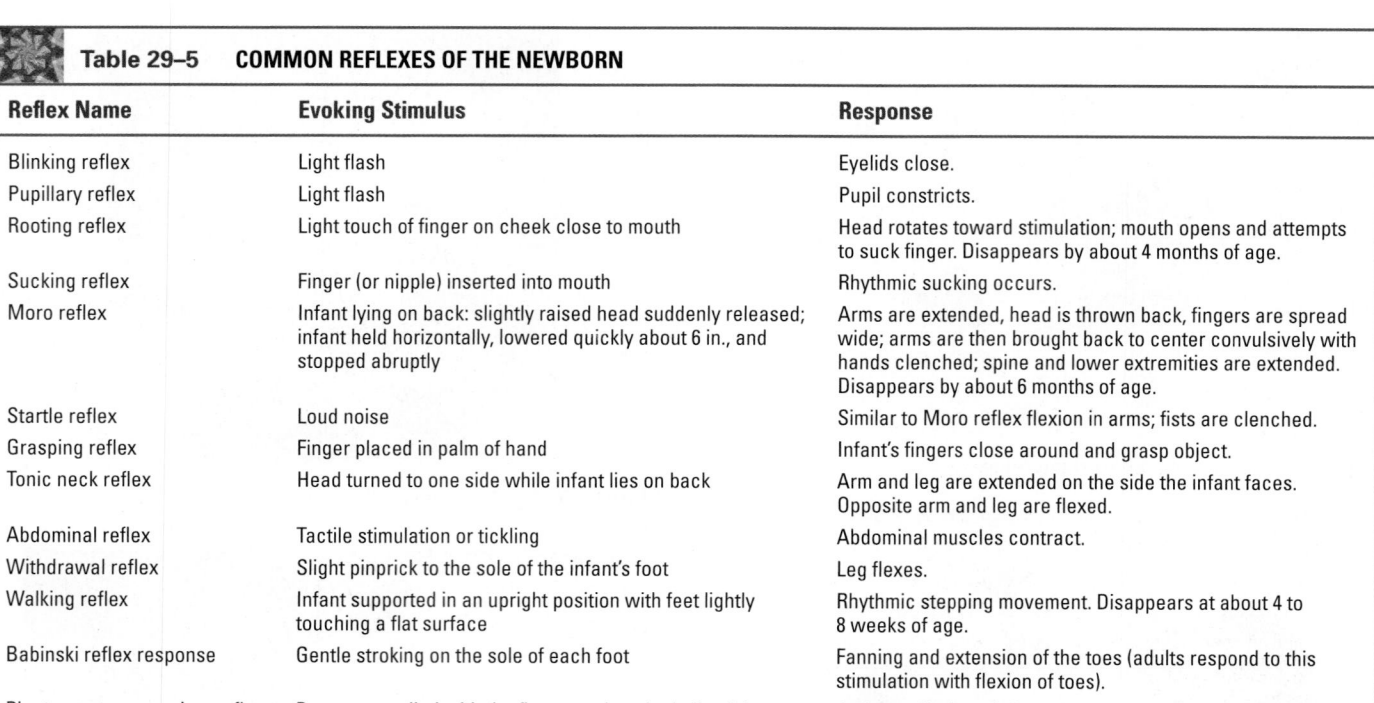

Table 29–5   COMMON REFLEXES OF THE NEWBORN

Reflex Name	Evoking Stimulus	Response
Blinking reflex	Light flash	Eyelids close.
Pupillary reflex	Light flash	Pupil constricts.
Rooting reflex	Light touch of finger on cheek close to mouth	Head rotates toward stimulation; mouth opens and attempts to suck finger. Disappears by about 4 months of age.
Sucking reflex	Finger (or nipple) inserted into mouth	Rhythmic sucking occurs.
Moro reflex	Infant lying on back: slightly raised head suddenly released; infant held horizontally, lowered quickly about 6 in., and stopped abruptly	Arms are extended, head is thrown back, fingers are spread wide; arms are then brought back to center convulsively with hands clenched; spine and lower extremities are extended. Disappears by about 6 months of age.
Startle reflex	Loud noise	Similar to Moro reflex flexion in arms; fists are clenched.
Grasping reflex	Finger placed in palm of hand	Infant's fingers close around and grasp object.
Tonic neck reflex	Head turned to one side while infant lies on back	Arm and leg are extended on the side the infant faces. Opposite arm and leg are flexed.
Abdominal reflex	Tactile stimulation or tickling	Abdominal muscles contract.
Withdrawal reflex	Slight pinprick to the sole of the infant's foot	Leg flexes.
Walking reflex	Infant supported in an upright position with feet lightly touching a flat surface	Rhythmic stepping movement. Disappears at about 4 to 8 weeks of age.
Babinski reflex response	Gentle stroking on the sole of each foot	Fanning and extension of the toes (adults respond to this stimulation with flexion of toes).
Plantar, or toe-grasping, reflex	Pressure applied with the finger against the balls of the infant's feet	A plantar flexion of all toes. Disappears by the end of the first year of life.

SOURCE: Adapted from Mott, S. R., James, S. R., & Sperhac, A. M. (1990). *Nursing care of children and families: A holistic approach* (2nd ed.). Menlo Park, CA: Addison-Wesley Nursing.

The nurse uses the following steps to assess CNS integration:

1. Insert a gloved finger into the newborn's mouth to elicit a sucking reflex.
2. As soon as the newborn is sucking vigorously, assess hearing and vision responses by noting sucking changes in the presence of a light, a rattle, and a voice.
3. The newborn should respond with a brief cessation of sucking followed by continuous sucking with repeated stimulation.

This examination demonstrates auditory and visual integrity as well as complex behavioral interactions. Refer to the Newborn Physical Assessment Guide in this chapter for a summary of stimulus for, and response of, the common newborn reflexes.

As healthcare providers carry out the newborn physical and neurologic assessment, they are always on the alert to recognize possible alterations and possible injuries related to the birth process that require further investigation and intervention. (See Table 29–6 for potential birth injuries.)

Newborn Physical Assessment Guide

Following is a guide for systematically assessing the newborn (pages 848–858). Normal findings, alterations, and related causes are presented in correlation with suggested nursing responses. The findings are typical for a full-term newborn.

Newborn Behavioral Assessment

Two conflicting forces influence parents' perceptions of their newborn. One is the parents' preconceptions, based on hopes

Table 29–6   POTENTIAL BIRTH INJURIES

Classification	Examples*
Soft-tissue injuries	Lacerations, abrasions, bruising, fat necrosis
Skull injuries	Cephalhematoma,* fractures
Scalp laceration	Fetal scalp electrode
Scalp abscess	Fetal scalp electrode
Intracranial hemorrhage	Subdural, subarachnoid
Eye injuries	Subconjunctival* and retinal hemorrhages
Fractures	Clavicle,* facial bones, humerus, femur
Dislocations	
Torticollis	Sternocleidomastoid muscle
Nerve injuries	Facial nerve,* brachial plexus,* phrenic nerve, recurrent laryngeal nerve (vocal cord paralysis), Horner syndrome
Spinal cord injuries	
Visceral rupture	Liver, spleen

*Most common birth injuries seen in newborns.

and fears, of what their newborn will be like. The other is their initial reaction to their baby's temperament, behaviors, and physical appearance. Nurses can assist parents in identifying their baby's specific behaviors.

> *One of the newborn's first responses is to move into a quiet but alert state of consciousness. The baby is still; his body molds to yours; his hands touch your skin; his eyes open wide and are bright and shiny. He looks directly at you.*

EVIDENCE-BASED PRACTICE

NEONATAL PAIN ASSESSMENT

Clinical Question

What is the most reliable, accurate, and clinically useful method to assess pain in newborns?

The Evidence

Two systematic reviews were conducted appraising instruments that help nurses determine the presence and severity of pain in newborns. In one study, two independent reviewers used a structured approach to evaluate the quality of 35 published and unpublished neonatal pain assessment tools. The raters used predetermined criteria to evaluate the reliability, validity, and clinical utility of the instruments. Of the instruments reviewed, 18 were one dimensional (measuring pain by focusing on primarily physical manifestations) and 17 were multidimensional (combines behavioral, contextual, and physiological information). A second group of reviewers specifically evaluated the Neonatal Infant Pain Scale (NIPS), the CRIES tool, and the Pain Assessment in Neonates (PAIN) tool. All three of these instruments are multidimensional.

What Is Effective?

Measuring newborns' level of pain is challenging because they are unable to verbalize the presence and intensity of their pain. Minimizing neonatal pain is required to promote normal growth and development, and to reduce the potential long-term sequelae of unmanaged pain. The first step in managing neonatal pain is assessment. An assessment tool must be both reliable and valid to be clinically useful. A reliable instrument is one that yields a consistent result when applied consistently. Validity indicates that a tool is accurate, meaning it measures what it purports to measure. None of the existing instruments fulfilled all the criteria for an ideal measure. However, given that the use of any pain tool is only one factor in the context of an infant's overall condition, there are several available tools that were judged as clinically useful. The Comfort Scale, the CRIES instrument, the Modified Infant Pain Scale, and the PAIN tool are all effective for normal newborns. The NIPS and the Premature Infant Pain Profile are both useful for preterm infants. Mechanically ventilated infants demonstrate pain behaviors that are reliably observed with the Modified Postoperative Comfort Scale and the Behavioral Pain Score. Postoperative pain can be evaluated with the Riley Infant Pain Scale or the Childrens' and Infants' Postoperative Pain Scale.

What Is Unclear?

Intuitively, it is expected that a multidimensional tool would demonstrate superior performance in evaluating pain. However, these reviewers were able to find adequate documentation of reliability and validity for only 6 of the 17 multidimensional tools. These tools are more complex to administer and so the simpler one-dimensional instruments may perform as well. Untested instruments are not recommended, as it is difficult to evaluate changes in the infant's pain level over time. Only a small minority of the tools had been tested for ease and efficiency of use. The subjectivity of the rater affects virtually all of these tools, and so instruments with the best inter-rater reliability are recommended. All of the assessments are affected by environmental stimuli, which may inflate pain scores. Very ill newborns may not be able to generate a pain score because they are incapable of an observable pain response, and so it is not clear if any of these tools are effective for evaluation of the sickest babies.

Best Practice

The application of established neonatal pain assessment tools supports clinical judgment that is evidence based. When using any pain assessment tool, first consider the infant population, the setting, and the type of pain experience. The nurse should have several tools available because different pain assessment tools work well in different circumstances and for different reasons. These neonatal assessment instruments could be classified into four broad uses: for normal, term infants; for preterm neonates; for mechanically ventilated babies; and for postoperative pain evaluation. Each baby should have an assessment tool applied and a baseline pain measure recorded within the first few hours of birth. This baseline gives the clinician an opportunity to assess the presence and severity of pain over time.

Critical Thinking

What factors should the nurse consider in selecting a pain assessment tool for use with newborns? Why is reliability of measurement of pain important in the neonatal care setting?

REFERENCES: Clifford, P., Stringer, M., Christensen, H., & Mountain, D. (2004). Pain assessment and intervention for term newborns. *Journal of Midwifery & Women's Health, 49*(6), 514–519.

Duhn, L., & Medves, J. (2004). A systematic integrative review of infant pain assessment tools. *Advances in Neonatal Care, 4*(3), 126–140.

This special alert state, this innate ability to communicate, may be the initial preparation for becoming attached to other human beings. One feels awed by the intensity and appealing power of this little bud of humanity meeting the world for the first time.

~ THE AMAZING NEWBORN ~

Brazelton's Neonatal Behavioral Assessment Scale provides valuable guidelines for assessing the newborn's state changes, temperament, and individual behavior patterns. It provides a way for the healthcare provider, in conjunction with the parents (primary caregivers), to identify and understand the individual newborn's states and capabilities. Families learn which responses, interventions, or activities best meet the special needs of their newborn, and this understanding fosters positive attachment experiences.

The assessment tool attempts to identify the newborn's repertoire of behavioral responses to the environment and also documents the newborn's neurologic adequacy and capabilities.

ASSESSMENT GUIDE   Newborn Physical Assessment

PHYSICAL ASSESSMENT/ NORMAL FINDINGS	ALTERATIONS AND POSSIBLE CAUSES*	NURSING RESPONSES TO DATA†
VITAL SIGNS		
Blood pressure (BP): At birth: 70–50/45–30 mm Hg	Low BP (hypovolemia, shock)	Monitor BP in all cases of distress, prematurity, or suspected anomaly.
Day 10: 90–60/50–40 mm Hg (may be unable to measure diastolic pressure with standard sphygmomanometer)		Low BP: Refer to physician immediately so measures to improve circulation are begun.
Pulse: 120–160 bpm (if asleep, as low as 80 bpm; if crying, up to 180 bpm)	Weak pulse (decreased cardiac output) Bradycardia (severe asphyxia, arrhythmia) Tachycardia (over 160 bpm at rest) (infection, CNS problems, arrhythmia, stress, hypovolemia)	Assess skin perfusion by blanching (capillary refill test–normal: 2–3 sec.) Correlate finding with BP assessments; refer to physician. Carry out neurologic and thermoregulation assessments. Check blood pressure and Hct.
Respirations: 30–60 breaths/min		
Synchronization of chest and abdominal movements	Tachypnea (pneumonia, respiratory distress syndrome [RDS])	Identify sleep-wake state; correlate with respiratory pattern.
Diaphragmatic and abdominal breathing	Rapid, shallow breathing (hypermagnesemia due to large doses given to mothers with preeclampsia) Respirations below 30 breaths/min (maternal anesthesia or analgesia)	Evaluate for all signs of respiratory distress; report findings to physician.
Transient tachypnea	Expiratory grunting; subcostal and substernal retractions; flaring of nares (respiratory distress); apnea (cold stress, respiratory disorder)	Evaluate for cold stress. Report findings to physician or neonatal nurse practitioner.
Crying: Strong and lusty Moderate tone and pitch	High pitched, shrill (neurologic disorder, hypoglycemia)	Discuss newborn's use of cry for communication. Assess and record abnormal cries.
Cries vary in length from 3 to 7 min after consoling measures are used	Weak or absent (CNS disorder, laryngeal problem)	Reduce environmental noises.
Temperature: Axilla 36.4–37.2C (97.5–99F)	Elevated temperature (room too warm, too much clothing or covers, dehydration, sepsis, brain damage)	Notify physician of elevation or drop.
Rectal 36.6–37.2C (97.8–99F); 36.8C (98.8F) desired	Subnormal temperature (brainstem involvement, cold, sepsis)	Counsel parents on possible causes of elevated or low temperatures, appropriate home care measures, when to call physician.
Heavier newborns tend to have higher body temperatures	Swings of more than 2°F from one reading to next or subnormal temperature (infection)	Teach parents how to take an axillary temperature; assess parents' knowledge regarding use of thermometer; provide teaching as needed.
Weight: 2500–4000 g (5 lb, 8 oz-8 lb, 13 oz)	Less than 2748 g (less than 6 lb) = SGA or preterm infant Greater than 4050 g (greater than 9 lb) = LGA or infants of diabetic mothers	Plot weight and gestational age on growth chart to identify high-risk infants. Ascertain body build of parents. Counsel parents regarding appropriate caloric intake. Feed the infant early post birth. Check blood glucose according to hospital policy.
Within first 3 to 4 days, normal weight loss of 5%–10% Large babies tend to lose more due to greater fluid loss in proportion to birth weight except infants of diabetic mothers	Loss greater than 15% (low fluid intake, loss of meconium and urine, feeding difficulties, diabetes insipidus)	Notify physician of net losses or gains. Calculate fluid intake and losses from all sources (insensible water loss, radiant warmers, phototherapy lights). Daily weights and before discharge.
Length: 48–52 cm (18–22 in.)	Less than 45 cm (congenital dwarf)	Assess for other signs of dwarfism.
Grows 10 cm (3 in.) during first 3 months	Short/long bones proximally (achondroplasia) Short/long bones distally (Ellis-van Creveld syndrome)	Determine other signs of skeletal system adequacy. Plot progress at subsequent well-baby visits.
	*Possible causes of alterations are identified in parentheses.	†This column provides guidelines for further assessment and initial nursing intervention.

ASSESSMENT GUIDE   Newborn Physical Assessment continued

PHYSICAL ASSESSMENT/ NORMAL FINDINGS	ALTERATIONS AND POSSIBLE CAUSES*	NURSING RESPONSES TO DATA†
POSTURE		
Body usually flexed, hands may be tightly clenched, neck appears short because chin rests on chest	Only extension noted, inability to move from midline (trauma, hypoxia, immaturity)	Record spontaneity of motor activity and symmetry of movements.
In breech births, feet are usually dorsiflexed	Constant motion (maternal caffeine intake or drug withdrawal)	If parents express concern about newborn's movement patterns, reassure and further evaluate if appropriate.
SKIN		
Color: Color consistent with ethnic background	Pallor of face conjunctiva (anemia, hypothermia, anoxia)	Discuss with parents common skin color variations to allay fears. Skin color can vary widely within African-American infants.
Newborns of European descent: pink-tinged or ruddy color over face, trunk, extremities Newborns of African or Native American descent: pale pink with yellow or red tinge Newborns of Asian descent: pink or rosy red to yellow tinge	Beefy red (hypoglycemia, immature vasomotor reflexes, polycythemia)	Document extent and time of occurrence of color change.
Common variations: acrocyanosis, circumoral cyanosis, harlequin color change, or mongolian spots	Meconium staining (nonreassuring fetal status) Jaundice (hemolytic reaction from blood incompatibility within first 24 hours, sepsis)	Obtain Hgb and hematocrit values; obtain bilirubin levels. Assess for respiratory difficulty and temperature instability. Differentiate between physiologic and pathologic jaundice.
Mottled when undressed	Cyanosis (choanal atresia, CNS damage or trauma, respiratory or cardiac problem, cold stress)	Assess degree of (central or peripheral) cyanosis and possible causes; refer to physician.
Minor bruising over buttocks in breech presentation and over eyes and forehead in facial presentations		Discuss with parents cause and course of minor bruising related to labor and birth.
Texture: Smooth, soft, flexible; may have dry, peeling hands and feet	Generalized cracked or peeling skin (SGA or postterm; blood incompatibility; metabolic, kidney dysfunction) Seborrheic-dermatitis (cradle cap) Absence of vernix (postmature) Yellow vernix (bilirubin staining)	Report to physician. Instruct parents to shampoo the scalp and anterior fontanelle areas daily with mild soap or baby shampoo; rinse well; avoid use of oil.
Turgor: Elastic, returns to normal shape after pinching	Maintains tent shape (dehydration)	Assess for other signs and symptoms of dehydration.
Pigmentation: Clear; milia across bridge of nose, forehead; or chin will disappear within a few weeks		Advise parents not to pinch or prick these pimplelike areas.
Café-au-lait spots (one or two)	Six or more (neurologic disorder such as von Recklinghausen disease, cutaneous neurofibromatosis)	If there are six or more café-au-lait spots, refer for genetic and neurologic consult.
Mongolian blue spots common over dorsal area and buttocks in dark-skinned infants		Assure parents of normality of this pigmentation; it will fade in first year or two.
Erythema toxicum	Impetigo (group A β-hemolytic streptococcus or *Staphylococcus aureus* infection)	If impetigo occurs, instruct parents about handwashing and linen precautions during home care.
Telangiectatic nevi	Hemangiomas: Nevus flammeus (port-wine stain) Nevus vasculosus (strawberry hemangioma) Cavernous hemangiomas	Collaborate with physician. Counsel parents about birthmark's progression to allay misconceptions. Record size and shape of hemangiomas. Refer for follow-up at well-baby clinic.
	*Possible causes of alterations are identified in parentheses.	†This column provides guidelines for further assessment and initial nursing intervention.

(Continued on next page)

ASSESSMENT GUIDE   Newborn Physical Assessment continued

PHYSICAL ASSESSMENT/ NORMAL FINDINGS	ALTERATIONS AND POSSIBLE CAUSES*	NURSING RESPONSES TO DATA†
SKIN (continued)		
Rashes	Rashes (infection)	Assess location and type of rash (macular, papular, vesicular). Obtain history of onset, prenatal history, and related signs and symptoms.
Petechiae of head or neck (breech presentation, cord around neck)	Generalized petechiae (clotting abnormalities)	Determine cause; advise parents if further health care is needed.
HEAD		
General appearance, size, movement Round, symmetric, and moves easily from left to right and up and down; soft and pliable	Asymmetric, flattened occiput on either side of the head (plagiocephaly) Head held at angle (torticollis) Unable to move head side to side (neurologic trauma)	Instruct parents to change infant's positions frequently when awake. When awake, needs to spend "tummy time." Infants should be placed supine for sleep per "Back to sleep" guidelines. Determine adequacy of all neurologic signs.
Circumference: 32–37 cm (12.5–14.5 in.); 2 cm greater than chest circumference Head one fourth of body size	Extreme differences in size may be due to microencephaly (Cornelia de Lange syndrome, cytomegalic inclusion disease [CID]), rubella, toxoplasmosis, chromosome abnormalities, hydrocephalus (meningomyelocele, achondroplasia), anencephaly (neural tube defect) Head is 3 cm or more larger than chest circumference (preterm, hydrocephalus)	Measure circumference from occiput to frontal area using metal or paper tape. Measure chest circumference using metal or paper tape and compare to head circumference. Record measurements on growth chart. Reevaluate at well-baby visits.
Common variations: Molding	Cephalhematoma (trauma during birth, may persist up to 3 months)	Evaluate neurologic response.
Breech and cesarean newborns' heads are round and well shaped	Caput succedaneum (long labor and birth; disappears in 1 week)	Observe for hyperbilirubinemia. Check Hct. Reassure parents regarding common manifestations due to birth process and when they should disappear.
Fontanelles: Palpation of juncture of cranial bones	Overlapping of anterior fontanelle (malnourished or preterm newborn)	Discuss normal closure times with parents and care of "soft spots" to allay misconceptions.
Anterior fontanelle; 3–4 cm long by 2–3 cm wide, diamond shaped	Premature closure of sutures (craniosynostosis)	Refer to physician. Assess fontanelles and sutures daily.
Posterior fontanelle: 1–2 cm at birth, triangle shaped	Late closure (hydrocephalus)	Observe for signs and symptoms of hydrocephalus.
Slight pulsation	Moderate to severe pulsation (vascular problems)	Refer to physician.
Moderate bulging noted with crying, stooling; pulsations with heartbeat	Bulging (increased intracranial pressure, meningitis) Sunken (dehydration)	Report to physician. Evaluate neurologic status. Evaluate hydration status.
HAIR		
Texture: Smooth with fine texture variations (*Note:* Variations depend on ethnic background.)	Coarse, brittle, dry hair (hypothyroidism) White forelock (Waardenburg syndrome)	Instruct parents regarding routine care of hair and scalp.
Distribution: Scalp hair high over eyebrows (Spanish-Mexican hairline begins midforehead and extends down back of neck)	Low forehead and posterior hairlines may indicate chromosomal disorders	Assess for other signs of chromosomal aberrations. Refer to physician.
	*Possible causes of alterations are identified in parentheses.	†This column provides guidelines for further assessment and initial nursing intervention.

ASSESSMENT GUIDE   Newborn Physical Assessment continued

PHYSICAL ASSESSMENT/ NORMAL FINDINGS	ALTERATIONS AND POSSIBLE CAUSES*	NURSING RESPONSES TO DATA†
FACE Symmetric movement of all facial features, normal hairline, eyebrows and eyelashes present		Assess and record symmetry of all parts, shape, regularity of features, sameness or differences in features.
Spacing of features: Eyes-ears at same level, nostrils equal size, cheeks full, and sucking pads present	Eyes wide apart—ocular hypertelorism (Apert syndrome, Cri-du-chat, Turner syndrome)	Observe for other signs and symptoms indicative of disease states or chromosomal aberrations.
Lips equal on both sides of midline	Atypical face (Down syndrome, cretinism, gargoylism)	
Chin recedes when compared with other bones of face	Atypical small jaw—micrognathia (Pierre Robin syndrome, Treacher Collins syndrome)	Maintain airway; do not position supine. Initiate surgical consultation and referral.
Movement: Makes facial grimaces	Inability to suck, grimace, and close eyelids (cranial nerve injury)	Initiate neurologic assessment and consultation.
Symmetric when resting and crying	Asymmetry (paralysis of facial cranial nerve)	Assess and record symmetry of all parts, shape, regularity of features, and sameness or differences in features.
EYES *General placement and appearance:* Bright and clear; even placement; slight nystagmus (involuntary cyclic eye movements)	Gross nystagmus (damage to third, fourth, and sixth cranial nerves)	
Concomitant strabismus	Constant and fixed strabismus	Reassure parents that strabismus is considered normal up to 6 months.
Move in all directions Blue-gray or slate–blue-gray	Lack of pigmentation (albinism) Brushfield spots may indicate Down syndrome (a light or white speckling of the outer two thirds of the iris)	Discuss with parents any necessary eye precautions. Assess for other signs of Down syndrome.
Brown color at birth in dark-skinned infants		Discuss with parents that permanent eye color is usually established by 3 months of age.
Eyelids: Position: above pupils but within iris, no drooping	Elevation or retraction of upper lid (hyperthyroidism). "Sunset sign" lid retraction and downward gaze (hydrocephalus), ptosis (congenital or paralysis of oculomotor muscle)	Assess for signs of hydrocephalus and hyperthyroidism. Evaluate interference with vision in subsequent well-baby visits.
Eyes on parallel plane	Upward slant in non-Asians (Down syndrome)	Assess for other signs of Down syndrome.
Epicanthal folds in Asian and 20% of newborns of northern European descent	Epicanthal folds (Down syndrome, Cri-du-chat syndrome)	
Movement: Blink reflex in response to light stimulus. Eyes open wide in dimly lighted room	Blink absent (CNS injury)	Evaluate neurologic status. Refer to physician.
Inspection: Edematous for first few days of life, resulting from birth; no lumps or redness	Purulent drainage (infection); infectious conjunctivitis (gonococcus, chlamydia, staphylococcus, or gram-negative organisms) Marginal blepharitis (lid edges red, crusted, scaly)	Initiate good handwashing. Refer to physician. Evaluate infant for seborrheic dermatitis; scales can be removed easily.
Cornea: Clear	Ulceration (herpes infection); large cornea or corneas of unequal size (congenital glaucoma)	Refer to ophthalmologist.
Corneal reflex present	Clouding, opacity of lens (cataract)	Assess for other manifestations of congenital herpes; institute nursing care measures.
Sclera: May appear bluish in newborn, then white; slightly brownish color frequent in newborns of African descent	True blue sclera (osteogenesis imperfecta)	Refer to physician.
	*Possible causes of alterations are identified in parentheses.	†This column provides guidelines for further assessment and initial nursing intervention.

(Continued on next page)

ASSESSMENT GUIDE   Newborn Physical Assessment continued

PHYSICAL ASSESSMENT/ NORMAL FINDINGS	ALTERATIONS AND POSSIBLE CAUSES*	NURSING RESPONSES TO DATA†
EYES (continued)		
Pupils: Pupils equal in size, round, and react to light by accommodation	Anisocoria—unequal pupils (CNS damage) Dilation or constriction (intracranial damage, retinoblastoma, glaucoma) Pupils nonreactive to light or accommodation (brain injury)	Refer for neurologic examination.
Slight nystagmus in newborn who has not learned to focus Pupil light reflex demonstrated at birth or by 3 weeks of age	Nystagmus (labyrinthine disturbance, CNS disorder)	
Conjunctiva: Chemical conjunctivitis Subconjunctival hemorrhage	Pale color (anemia)	Obtain hematocrit and hemoglobin. Reassure parents that chemical conjunctivitis will subside in 1 to 2 days and subconjunctival hemorrhage disappears in a few weeks.
Palpebral conjunctival (red but not hyperemic)	Inflammation or edema (infection, blocked tear duct)	
Vision: 20/200 Tracks moving object to midline Fixed focus on objects at a distance of about 10–20 inches; may be difficult to evaluate in newborn Prefers faces, geometric designs, and black and white to colors	Cataracts (congenital infection)	Record any questions about visual acuity and initiate follow-up evaluation at first well-baby checkup. May suggest toys for parents to purchase— see Chapter 33. ∞
Lashes and lacrimal glands: Presence of lashes (lashes may be absent in preterm newborns)	No lashes on inner two thirds of lid (Treacher Collins syndrome), bushy lashes (Hurler syndrome), long lashes (Cornelia de Lange syndrome)	
Cry commonly tearless	Excessive tearing (plugged lacrimal duct, natal narcotic withdrawal), glaucoma	Demonstrate to parents how to milk blocked tear duct. Refer to ophthalmologist if tearing is excessive before third month of life.
NOSE		
Appearance of external nasal aspects: May appear flattened as a result of birth process	Continued flat or broad bridge of nose (Down syndrome)	Arrange consultation with specialist. May be normal racial variation—Asian or African ancestry.
Small and narrow in midline, even placement in relationship to eyes and mouth	Low bridge of nose, beaklike nose (Apert syndrome, Treacher Collins syndrome) Upturned (Cornelia de Lange syndrome)	Initiate evaluation of chromosomal abnormalities.
Patent nares bilaterally (nose breathers)	Blockage of nares (mucus or secretions), choanal atresia	Inspect for obstruction of nares.
Sneezing common to clear nasal passages	Flaring nares (respiratory distress)	Maintain oral airway until surgical correction is made.
Responds to odors, may smell breast milk	No response to stimulating odors	Inspect for obstruction of nares.
MOUTH		
Function of facial, hypoglossal, glossopharyngeal, and vagus nerves: Symmetry of movement and strength	Mouth draws to one side (transient seventh cranial nerve paralysis due to pressure in utero or trauma during birth, congenital paralysis)	Initiate neurologic consultation.
	Fishlike shape (Treacher Collins syndrome)	Administer artificial tears if eye on affected side of face is unable to close.
Presence of gag, swallowing, coordinated with sucking reflexes	Suppressed or absent reflexes	Evaluate other neurologic functions of these nerves.
Adequate salivation		
	*Possible causes of alterations are identified in parentheses.	†This column provides guidelines for further assessment and initial nursing intervention.

ASSESSMENT GUIDE   Newborn Physical Assessment continued

PHYSICAL ASSESSMENT/ NORMAL FINDINGS	ALTERATIONS AND POSSIBLE CAUSES*	NURSING RESPONSES TO DATA†
MOUTH (continued)		
Palate (soft and hard): Hard palate dome shaped. Uvula midline with symmetric movement of soft palate	High-steepled palate (Treacher Collins syndrome), bifid uvula (congenital anomaly)	Assess for other congenital anomalies.
Palate intact, sucks well when stimulated	Clefts in either hard or soft palate (polygenic disorder)	Initiate a surgical consultation referral. Use special feeding devices.
Epithelial (Epstein's) pearls appear on mucosa		Assure parents that these are normal and will disappear at 2 or 3 months of age.
Esophagus patent, some drooling common in newborn	Excessive drooling or bubbling (esophageal atresia)	Test for patency of esophagus.
Tongue: Free moving in all directions, midline	Lack of movement or asymmetric movement (neurologic damage) Tongue-tied Fasiculations (fine tremors), Spinal muscular atrophy	Further assess neurologic functions. Test reflex elevation of tongue when depressed with tongue blade.
Pink color, smooth to rough texture, noncoated	Deviations from midline (cranial nerve damage) White cheesy coating (thrush) Tongue has deep ridges	Check for signs of weakness or deviation. Differentiate between thrush and milk curds by wiping: if white patches don't come off easily, it is thrush. Reassure parents that tongue pattern may change from day to day.
Tongue proportional to mouth	Large tongue with short frenulum (cretinism, Down syndrome, other syndromes)	Evaluate in well-baby clinic to assess development delays. Initiate referrals.
EARS		
External ear: Without lesions, cysts, or nodules	Nodules, cysts, or sinus tracts in front of ear Adherent earlobes Low set (Genetic abnormality or syndrome) Preauricular skin tags	Evaluate characteristics of lesions. Counsel parents to clean external ear with washcloth only; discourage use of cotton-tip applicators. Refer to physician for ligation.
Hearing: Eustachian tubes are cleared with first cry		
Absence of all risk factors	Presence of one or more risk factors	Assess history of risk factors for hearing loss.
Attends to sounds; sudden or loud noise elicits Moro reflex	No response to sound stimuli (deafness)	Test for Moro reflex.
NECK		
Appearance: Short, straight, creased with skin folds	Abnormally short neck (Turner syndrome) Arching or inability to flex neck (meningitis, congenital anomaly)	Report findings to physician.
Posterior neck lacks loose extra folds of skin	Webbing of neck (Turner syndrome, Down syndrome, trisomy 18)	Assess for other signs of the syndromes.
Clavicles: Straight and intact	Knot or lump on clavicle (fracture during difficult birth)	Obtain detailed labor and birth history; apply figure-eight bandage. Consider oral analgesic.
Moro reflex elicitable	Unilateral Moro reflex response on unaffected side (fracture of clavicle, brachial palsy, Erb-Duchenne paralysis)	
Symmetric shoulders	Hypoplasia	
	*Possible causes of alterations are identified in parentheses.	†This column provides guidelines for further assessment and initial nursing intervention.

(Continued on next page)

ASSESSMENT GUIDE   Newborn Physical Assessment continued

PHYSICAL ASSESSMENT/ NORMAL FINDINGS	ALTERATIONS AND POSSIBLE CAUSES*	NURSING RESPONSES TO DATA†
CHEST		
Appearance and size: Circumference: 32.5 cm, 1–2 cm less than head Wider than it is long		Collaborate with physician. Measure at level of nipples after exhalation.
Normal shape without depressed or prominent sternum	Funnel chest (congenital or associated with Marfan syndrome)	Determine adequacy of other respiratory and circulatory signs.
Lower end of sternum (xiphoid cartilage) may be protruding; less apparent after several weeks	Continued protrusion of xiphoid cartilage (Marfan syndrome, "pigeon chest")	Assess for other signs and symptoms of various syndromes.
Sternum 8 cm long	Barrel chest	
Expansion and retraction: Bilateral expansion	Unequal chest expansion (pneumonia, pneumothorax, respiratory distress)	Assess respiratory effort regularity, flaring of nares, difficulty on both inspiration and expiration.
No intercostal, subcostal, or supraclavicular retractions	Retractions (respiratory distress) Seesaw respirations (respiratory distress)	
Auscultation: Breath sounds are louder in infants	Decreased breath sounds (decreased respiratory activity, atelectasis, pneumothorax)	Obtain transilluminator. Record findings and consult physician.
Chest and axilla clear on crying	Increased breath sounds (resolving pneumonia or in cesarean births)	Perform assessment and report to physician any positive findings.

Bronchial breath sounds (heard where trachea and bronchi closest to chest wall, above sternum and between scapulae):
 	
  Bronchial sounds bilaterally
  Air entry clear
  Rales may indicate normal newborn atelectasis
  Cough reflex absent at birth, appears in 2 or more days
	Adventitious or abnormal sounds (respiratory disease or distress)	Evaluate color for pallor or cyanosis. Monitor every shift or more frequently. Report to physician.

Breasts: Flat with symmetric nipples	Lack of breast tissue (preterm or SGA)	
Breast tissue diameter 5 cm or more at term	Discharge	Evaluate for infection.
Average distance between nipples 8 cm	Breast abscesses	
Breast engorgement occurs on third day of life; liquid discharge may be expressed in term newborns	Enlargement	Reassure parents of normality of breast engorgement.
Nipples	Supernumerary nipples Dark-colored nipples	No intervention is necessary.
HEART		
Auscultation: Location: lies horizontally, with left border extending to left of midclavicle		
Regular rhythm and rate	Arrhythmia (anoxia), tachycardia, bradycardia	Refer all arrhythmia and gallop rhythms. Initiate cardiac evaluation.
Determination of point of maximal impulse (PMI)	Malpositioning (enlargement, abnormal	
Usually lateral to midclavicular line at third or fourth intercostal space	placement, pneumothorax, dextrocardia, diaphragmatic hernia)	
Functional murmurs	Location of murmurs (possible congenital cardiac anomaly)	Evaluate murmur: location, timing, and duration; observe for accompanying cardiac pathology symptoms; ascertain family history.
No thrills		
Horizontal groove at diaphragm shows flaring of rib cage to mild degree	Marked rib flaring (vitamin D deficiency) Inadequacy of respiratory movement	Initiate cardiopulmonary evaluation; assess pulses and blood pressures in all four extremities for equality and quality.
	*Possible causes of alterations are identified in parentheses.	†This column provides guidelines for further assessment and initial nursing intervention.

ASSESSMENT GUIDE   Newborn Physical Assessment continued

Physical Assessment/ Normal Findings	Alterations and Possible Causes*	Nursing Responses to Data†
ABDOMEN		
Appearance: Cylindric, with some protrusion; appears large in relation to pelvis; some laxness of abdominal muscles	Distention, shiny abdomen with engorged vessels (gastrointestinal abnormalities, infection, congenital megacolon)	Examine abdomen thoroughly for mass or organomegaly. Measure abdominal girth.
No cyanosis, few vessels seen Diastasis recti–common in infants of African descent	Scaphoid abdominal appearance (diaphragmatic hernia)	Report deviations of abdominal size.
	Increased or decreased peristalsis (duodenal stenosis, small bowel obstruction)	Assess other signs and symptoms of obstruction.
	Localized flank bulging (enlarged kidneys, ascites, absent abdominal muscles)	Refer to physician.
Umbilicus: No protrusion of umbilicus (protrusion of umbilicus common in infants of African descent)	Umbilical hernia Patent urachus (congenital malformation)	Measure umbilical hernia by palpating the opening and record; it should close by 1–2 years of age; if not, refer to physician. Be aware of cultural practices. Taping or belly bands do not enhance closure.
Bluish white color	Omphalocele (covered defect) Gastroschisis (uncovered defect)	Cover omphalocele and gastroschisis with sterile, moist dressing or plastic sterile bag.
Cutis navel (umbilical cord projects), granulation tissue present in navel	Redness or exudate around cord (infection) Yellow discoloration (hemolytic disease, meconium staining)	Instruct parents on cord care and hygiene.
Two arteries and one vein apparent	Single umbilical artery (congenital anomalies)	Refer anomalies to physician.
Begins drying 1 to 2 hours after birth	Discharge or oozing of blood from the cord	
No bleeding		
Auscultation and percussion: Soft bowel sounds heard shortly after birth every 10–30 seconds	Bowel sounds in chest (diaphragmatic hernia) Absence of bowel sounds Hyperperistalsis (intestinal obstruction)	Collaborate with physician. Assess for other signs of dehydration or infection.
Femoral pulses: Palpable, equal, bilateral	Absent or diminished femoral pulses (coarctation of aorta)	Monitor blood pressure in upper and lower extremities.
Inguinal area: No bulges along inguinal area	Inguinal hernia	Initiate referral.
No inguinal lymph nodes felt		Continue follow-up in well-baby clinic.
Bladder: Percusses 1–4 cm above symphysis	Failure to void within 24–48 hours after birth	Determine whether baby voided at birth.
Emptied about 3 hours after birth; if not, at time of birth	Exposure of bladder mucosa (exstrophy of bladder)	Consult with clinician. Cover exstrophy with sterile moist gauze.
Urine–inoffensive, mild odor	Foul odor (infection)	Obtain urine specimen if infection is suspected.
GENITALS		
Gender clearly delineated	Ambiguous genitals	Refer for genetic consultation.
MALE		
Penis: Slender in appearance, about 2.5 cm long, 1 cm wide at birth	Micropenis (congenital anomaly) Meatal atresia	Observe and record first volding.
Normal urinary orifice, urethral meatus at tip of penis	Hypospadias, epispadias	Collaborate with physician in presence of abnormality, Delay circumcision.
	*Possible causes of alterations are identified in parentheses.	†This column provides guidelines for further assessment and initial nursing intervention.

(Continued on next page)

ASSESSMENT GUIDE   Newborn Physical Assessment continued

PHYSICAL ASSESSMENT/ NORMAL FINDINGS	ALTERATIONS AND POSSIBLE CAUSES*	NURSING RESPONSES TO DATA†
MALE (continued)		
Noninflamed urethral opening	Urethritis (infection)	Palpate for enlarged inguinal lymph nodes and record painful urination.
Foreskin adheres to glans	Ulceration of meatal opening (infection, inflammation)	Evaluate whether ulcer is due to diaper rash; counsel regarding care.
Uncircumcised foreskin tight for 2 to 3 months	Phimosis–if still tight after 3 months	Instruct parents on how to care for uncircumcised penis.
Circumcised		Teach parents how to care for circumcision. Check for voiding after procedure and evaluate for excessive bleeding.
Erectile tissue present		
Scrotum: Skin loose and hanging or tight and small; extensive rugae and normal size	Large scrotum containing fluid (hydrocele) Red, shiny scrotal skin (orchitis)	Shine a light through scrotum (transilluminate) to verify diagnosis.
Normal skin color Scrotal discoloration common in breech	Minimal rugae, small scrotum	Assess for prematurity.
Testes: Descended by birth; not consistently found in scrotum	Undescended testes (cryptorchidism)	If testes cannot be felt in scrotum, gently palpate femoral, inguinal, perineal, and abdominal areas for presence.
Testes size 1.5–2 cm at birth	Enlarged testes (tumor) Small testes (Klinefelter syndrome or adrenal hyperplasia)	Refer to and collaborate with physician for further diagnostic studies.
FEMALE		
Mons: Normal skin color, area pigmented in dark-skinned infants		
Labia majora cover labia minora in term and postterm newborns; symmetric size appropriate for gestational age	Hematoma, lesions (trauma) Labia minora prominent	Evaluate for recent trauma. Assess for prematurity.
Clitoris: Normally large in newborn Edema and bruising in breech birth	Hypertrophy (hermaphroditism)	Refer for genetic workup.
Vagina: Urinary meatus and vaginal orifice visible (0.5 cm circumference)	Inflammation; erythema and discharge (urethritis) Congenital absence of vagina	Collect urine specimen for laboratory examination. Refer to physician.
Vaginal tag or hymenal tag disappears in a few weeks		
Discharge; smegma under labia	Foul-smelling discharge (infection)	Collect data and further evaluate reason for discharge.
Bloody or mucoid discharge	Excessive vaginal bleeding (blood coagulation defect)	
BUTTOCKS AND ANUS		
Buttocks symmetric	Pilonidal dimple	Examine for possible sinus. Instruct parents about cleansing this area.
Anus patent and passage of meconium within 24–48 hours after birth	Imperforate anus, rectal atresia (congenital gastrointestinal defect)	Evaluate extent of problems. Initiate surgical consultation.
No fissures, tears, or skin tags	Fissures	Perform digital examination to ascertain patency if patency uncertain.
	*Possible causes of alterations are identified in parentheses.	†This column provides guidelines for further assessment and initial nursing intervention.

ASSESSMENT GUIDE   Newborn Physical Assessment continued

PHYSICAL ASSESSMENT/ NORMAL FINDINGS	ALTERATIONS AND POSSIBLE CAUSES*	NURSING RESPONSES TO DATA†
EXTREMITIES AND TRUNK		
Short and generally flexed; extremities move symmetrically through range of motion but lack full extension	Unilateral or absence of movement (spinal cord involvement) Fetal position continued or limp (anoxia, CNS problems, hypoglycemia)	Review birth record to assess possible cause.
All joints move spontaneously; good muscle tone, of flexor type, birth to 2 months	Spasticity when infant begins using extensors (cerebral palsy, lack of muscle tone, "floppy baby" syndrome) Hypotonia (Down syndrome)	Collaborate with physician.
Arms: Equal in length	Brachial palsy (difficult birth)	Report to clinician.
Bilateral movement	Erb-Duchenne paralysis	
Flexed when quiet	Muscle weakness, fractured clavicle Absence of limb or change of size (phocomelia, amelia)	
Hands: Normal number of fingers	Polydactyly (Ellis-van Creveld syndrome) Syndactyly—one limb (developmental anomaly) Syndactyly—both limbs (genetic component)	Report to clinician.
Normal palmar crease	Simlan line on palm (Down syndrome)	Refer for genetic workup.
Normal-sized hands	Short fingers and broad hand (Hurler syndrome)	Evaluate for history of distress in utero.
Nails present and extend beyond fingertips in term newborn.	Cyanosis and clubbing (cardiac anomalies) Nails long or yellow stained (postterm)	Carry out cardiac and respiratory assessments. Check pulse oximetry.
Spine: C-shaped spine	Spina bifida occulta (nevus pilosus)	Evaluate extent of neurologic damage; initiate care of spinal opening.
Flat and straight when prone	Dermal sinus	
Slight lumbar lordosis	Myelomeningocele	
Easily flexed and intact when palpated	Head lag, limp, floppy trunk (neurologic problems)	
At least half of back devoid of lanugo		
Full-term infant in ventral suspension should hold head at 45-degree angle, back straight		Elicit reflex to assess degree of involvement.
Hips: No sign of instability	Sensation of abnormal movement; jerk, or snap of hip dislocation	Physician or nurse practitioner examines all newborn infants for dislocated hip prior to discharge from birthing center.
Hips abduct to more than 60 degrees		If this is suspected, refer to orthopedist for further evaluation. Reassess at well-baby visits.
Inguinal and buttock skin creases: Symmetric inguinal and buttock creases	Asymmetry (dislocated hips)	Refer to orthopedist for evaluation. Counsel parents regarding symptoms of concern and discuss therapy.
Legs: Legs equal in length	Shortened leg (dislocated hips)	Refer to orthopedist for evaluation.
Legs shorter than arms at birth	Lack of leg movement (fractures, spinal defects)	Counsel parents regarding symptoms of concern and discuss therapy.
Feet: Foot is in straight line	Talipes equinovarus (true clubfoot)	Discuss differences between positional and true clubfoot with parents.
Positional clubfoot—based on position in utero		Teach parents passive manipulation of foot. Refer to orthopedist if not corrected by 3 months of age.
Fat pads and creases on soles of feet	Incomplete sole creases in first 24 hours of life (premature)	
Talipes planus (flat feet) normal under 3 years of age		Reassure parents that flat feet are normal in infants.
	*Possible causes of alterations are identified in parentheses.	†This column provides guidelines for further assessment and initial nursing intervention.

(Continued on next page)

ASSESSMENT GUIDE   Newborn Physical Assessment continued

PHYSICAL ASSESSMENT/ NORMAL FINDINGS	ALTERATIONS AND POSSIBLE CAUSES*	NURSING RESPONSES TO DATA†
NEUROMUSCULAR		
Motor function: Symmetric movement and strength in all extremities	Limp, flaccid, or hypertonic (CNS disorders, infection, dehydration, fracture)	Appraise newborn's posture and motor functions by observing activities and motor characteristics.
May be jerky or have brief twitchings	Tremors (hypoglycemia, hypocalcemia, infection, neurologic damage)	Evaluate for electrolyte imbalance, hypoglycemia, and neurologic functioning.
Head lag not over 45 degrees	Delayed or abnormal development (preterm, neurologic involvement)	
Neck control adequate to maintain head erect briefly	Asymmetry of tone or strength (neurologic damage)	Refer for genetic evaluation.
REFLEXES		
Blink: Stimulated by flash of light; response is closure of eyelids	Lack of blink response (damage to cranial nerve, CNS injury)	Assess neurologic status.
Pupillary reflex: Stimulated by flash of light; response is constriction of pupil	Lack of reflex (damage to cranial nerve, CNS injury)	
Moro: Response to sudden movement or loud noise should be one of symmetric extension and abduction of arms with fingers extended; then return to normal relaxed flexion	Asymmetry of body response (fractured clavicle, injury to brachial plexus)	Discuss normality of this reflex in response to loud noises or sudden movements.
Infant lying on back: slightly raised head suddenly released; infant held horizontally, lowered quickly about 6 inches, and stopped abruptly	Consistent absence (brain damage)	Absence of reflex requires neurologic evaluation.
Fingers form a C		
Present at birth; disappears by 6 months of age		
Rooting and sucking: Turns in direction of stimulus to cheek or mouth; opens mouth and begins to suck rhythmically when finger or nipple is inserted into mouth; difficult to elicit after feeding; disappears by 4 to 7 months of age	Poor sucking or easily fatigable (preterm, breastfed infants of drug-addicted mothers, possible cardiac problem) Absence of response (preterm, neurologic involvement, depressed newborns)	Evaluate strength and coordination of sucking. Observe newborn during feeding, and counsel parents about mutuality of feeding experience and newborn's responses.
Sucking is adequate for nutritional intake and meeting oral stimulation needs; disappears by 12 months		
Palmar grasp: Fingers grasp adult finger when palm is stimulated and held momentarily; lessens at 3 to 4 months of age	Asymmetry of response (neurologic problems)	Evaluate other reflexes and general neurologic functioning.
Plantar grasp: Toes curl downward when sole of foot is stimulated; lessens by 8 months	Absent (defects of lower spinal column)	Assess for other lower extremity neurologic problems.
Stepping: When held upright and one foot touching a flat surface, will step alternately; disappears at 4 to 8 weeks of age	Asymmetry of stepping (neurologic abnormality)	Evaluate muscle tone and function on each side of body. Refer to specialist.
Babinski: Fanning and extension of all toes when one side of sole is stroked from heel upward across ball of foot; disappears at about 12 months	Absence of response (low spinal cord defects)	Refer for further neurologic evaluation.
Tonic neck: Fencer position—when head is turned to one side, extremities on same side extend and on opposite side flex; this reflex may not be evident during early neonatal period; disappears at 3 to 4 months of age	Absent after 1 month of age or persistent asymmetry (cerebral lesion)	Assess neurologic functioning.
Response often more dominant in leg than in arm		
Prone crawl: While on abdomen, newborn pushes up and tries to crawl	Absence or variance of response (preterm, weak, or depressed newborns)	Evaluate motor functioning. Refer to specialist.
Trunk Incurvation (Galant): In prone position, stroking of spine causes pelvis to turn to stimulated side	Failure to rotate to stimulated side (neurologic damage)	
	*Possible causes of alterations are placed in parentheses.	†This column provides guidelines for further assessment and initial nursing interventions.

The examination usually takes 20 to 30 minutes and involves about 30 tests. Some items are scored according to the newborn's response to specific stimuli. Others, such as consolability and alertness, are scored as a result of continuous behavioral observations throughout the assessment. (For a complete discussion of all test items and maneuvers, see Brazelton & Nugent, 1995.)

Because the first few days after birth are a period of behavioral disorganization, the complete assessment should be done on the third day after birth. The nurse should make every effort to elicit the best response. This may be accomplished by repeating tests at different times or by testing during situations that facilitate the best possible response, such as when parents are holding, cuddling, rocking, or singing to their baby.

The assessment of the newborn should be carried out initially in a quiet, dimly lighted room, if possible. The nurse should first determine the newborn's state of consciousness, because scoring and introduction of the test items correlate with the sleep or awake state. The newborn's state depends on physiologic variables, such as the amount of time from the last feeding, positioning, environmental temperature, and health status; presence of such external stimuli as noises and bright lights; and the sleep-wake cycle of the infant. An important characteristic of the neonatal period is the pattern of states, as well as the transitions from one state to another. The pattern of states is a predictor of the newborn's receptivity and ability to respond to stimuli in a cognitive manner. Babies learn best in a quiet, alert state and in an environment that is supportive and protective and that provides appropriate stimuli.

The nurse should observe the newborn's sleep-wake patterns (as discussed in Chapter 28 ∞) and the rapidity with which the newborn moves from one state to another, the newborn's ability to be consoled, and the newborn's ability to diminish the impact of disturbing stimuli. The following questions may provide the nurse with a framework for assessment:

- Does the newborn's response style and ability to adapt to stimuli indicate a need for parental interventions that will alert the newborn to the environment so that the baby can grow socially and cognitively?

- Are parental interventions necessary to lessen the outside stimuli, as in the case of the baby who responds to sensory input with intensity?

- Can the baby control the amount of sensory input to be dealt with?

The behaviors and the sleep-wake states in which they are assessed are categorized as follows:

- *Habituation.* The newborn's ability to diminish or shut down innate responses to specific repeated stimuli, such as a rattle, bell, light, or pinprick to heel.

- *Orientation to inanimate and animate visual and auditory assessment stimuli.* How often and where the newborn attends to auditory and visual stimuli are observed. Orientation to the environment is determined by an ability to respond to cues given by others and by a natural ability to fix on and to follow a visual object horizontally and vertically. This capacity and parental appreciation of it are important for positive communication between infant and parents; the parents' visual (*en face*) and auditory (soft, continuous voice) presence stimulates their infant to orient to them. Inability or lack of response may indicate visual or auditory problems. It is important for parents to know that their newborn can turn to voices usually soon after birth or by 3 days of age and can become alert at different times with a varying degree of intensity in response to sounds.

- *Motor activity.* Several components are evaluated. Motor tone of the newborn is assessed in the most characteristic state of responsiveness. This summary assessment includes overall use of tone as the newborn responds to being handled—whether during spontaneous activity, prone placement, or horizontal holding—and overall assessment of body tone as the newborn reacts to all stimuli.

- *Variations.* Frequency of alert states, state changes, color changes (throughout all states as examination progresses), activity, and peaks of excitement are assessed.

- *Self-quieting activity.* Assessment is based on how often, how quickly, and how effectively newborns can use their resources to quiet and console themselves when upset or distressed. Considered in this assessment are such self-consolatory activities as putting hand to mouth, sucking on a fist or the tongue, and attuning to an object or sound (Figure 29–44 ◆). The newborn's need for outside consolation must also be considered—for example, seeing a face; being rocked, held, or dressed; using a pacifier; and being swaddled.

- *Cuddliness or social behaviors.* This area encompasses the infant's need for and response to being held. Also considered is how often the newborn smiles. These behaviors influence the parents' self-esteem and feelings of acceptance

Figure 29–44 ◆ The newborn can bring hand to mouth as a self-soothing activity.

or rejection. Cuddling also appears to be an indicator of personality. Cuddlers appear to enjoy, accept, and seek physical contact; are easier to placate; sleep more; and form earlier and more intense attachments. Noncuddlers are active, are restless, have accelerated motor development, and are intolerant of physical restraint. Smiling, even as a grimace reflex, greatly influences parent-infant feedback. Parents identify this response as positive.

CHAPTER REVIEW

FOCUS YOUR STUDY

- A perinatal history, determination of gestational age, physical examination, and behavioral assessment form the basis for complete newborn assessment.

- The common physical characteristics included in the gestational age assessment are skin, lanugo, sole (plantar) creases, breast tissue and size, ear form and cartilage, and genitals.

- The neuromuscular components of gestational age scoring tools are usually posture, square window sign, popliteal angle, arm recoil, heel-to-ear extension, and scarf sign.

- By assessing the physical and neuromuscular components specified in a gestational age tool, the nurse can determine the gestational age of the newborn.

- After determining the gestational age of the baby, the nurse can assess how the newborn will make the transition to extrauterine life and can anticipate potential physiologic problems.

- The nurse identifies the newborn as small for gestational age (SGA), appropriate for gestational age (AGA), or large for gestational age (LGA), and prioritizes individual needs.

- Normal ranges for vital signs assessed in newborns are heart rate of 120 to 160 beats per minute; respiratory rate of 30 to 60 respirations per minute; axillary temperature of 36.4C to 37.2C (97.5F to 99F); skin temperature of 36C to 36.5C (96.8F to 97.7F); rectal temperature of 36.6C to 37.2C (97.8F to 99F); and blood pressure of 70/45 to 50/30 mm Hg (at birth).

- Normal newborn measurements include weight from 2500 to 4000 g (5 lb, 8 oz to 8 lb, 13 oz), with weight dependent on maternal size and age; length from 48 to 52 cm (18 to 22 in.); and head circumference from 32 to 37 cm (12.5 to 14.5 in.). Head circumference is approximately 2 cm larger than the chest circumference.

- Commonly elicited newborn reflexes are tonic neck, Moro, grasping, rooting, sucking, and blink.

- Newborn behavioral abilities include habituation, orientation to visual and auditory stimuli, motor activity, cuddliness, and self-quieting activity.

- An important role of the nurse during the physical and behavioral assessments of the newborn is to teach parents about their newborn and involve them in their baby's care. This facilitates the parents' identification of their newborn's uniqueness and allays their concerns.

EXPLORE MediaLink

Video: Palmar grasp

http://www.prenhall.com/davidson

NCLEX review questions, case studies, and other interactive resources for this chapter can be found on the Web Site at http://www.prenhall.com/davidson. Click on "Chapter 29" to select the activities for this chapter.

For tutorials including animations and videos, more NCLEX review questions, and an audio glossary, access the accompanying Prentice Hall Nursing MediaLink DVD-ROM in this book.

PRENTICE HALL NURSING MEDIALINK DVD-ROM

Audio Glossary

NCLEX Review

Videos:

Assessment of an Infant

Newborn Reflexes

Gross and Fine Motor Activity

Maternal-Newborn Reflexes

Moro Reflex

Palmar Grasp

Rooting

Sucking

Babinski

Trunk Incurvation (Galant Reflex)

COMPANION WEBSITE

Additional NCLEX Review

Case Study: *Newborn Maturity Assessment*

Care Plan Activity: *Assessment of the Uncomplicated Newborn*

Applications: *Newborn Gestational Assessment; Newborn Reflexes; Newborn Assessment*

Critical Thinking

CRITICAL THINKING IN ACTION

MOTHER LEARNS ABOUT HER NEWBORN

View the Critical Thinking in Action video in Chapter 29 of the DVD-ROM. Then answer the questions that follow.

Susan Pine, a 21-year-old G2, now P1011, delivers a 39-weeks'-gestation female newborn. The vaginal birth is assisted with a vacuum extractor. The prenatal record is significant for an increase of maternal blood pressure to 140/90 on the day of birth. Susan is treated with magnesium sulfate during her labor and has an epidural analgesia for the pain of labor. The baby's Apgar is 8 and 9 at 1 and 5 minutes,

and she has been admitted to the newborn nursery. The newborn's admission exam is normal except for a 2-cm round caput succedaneum. Now, 8 hours later, the baby's condition is stable and she needs to be bottle-fed. You take her to her mother's room where you observe that Susan does not reach out to take her from you. She seems unsure when handling her baby. Susan asks you about the swelling on her baby's head and wonders if it will ever go away.

1. How would you explain the cause of Susan's baby's caput succedaneum?

2. Compare the difference between a cephalhematoma and caput succedaneum.

3. Explore with Susan her baby's reflexes and state of alertness.

4. Susan asks you how she will know what her baby needs. How would you respond?

REFERENCES

American Academy of Pediatrics (AAP) Committee on Fetus and Newborn & American College of Obstetricians and Gynecologists (ACOG) Committee on Obstetrics. (2002). *Guidelines for perinatal care* (5th ed.). Evanston, IL: Author.

Ballard, J. L., Khoury, J. C., Wedig, K., Wang, L., Eilers-Walsman, B. L., & Lipp, R. (1991). New Ballard score, expanded to include extremely premature infants. *Journal of Pediatrics, 119*(3), 417–423.

Blackburn, S. T. (2003). *Maternal, fetal, and neonatal physiology: A clinical perspective.* St. Louis, MO: Saunders.

Brazelton, T. B., & Nugent, J. K. (1995). *The neonatal behavioral assessment scale* (3rd ed.). London: MacKeith.

Furdon, S. A., & Clark, D. A. (2003). Scalp hair characteristics in the newborn infant. *Advances in Neonatal Care, 3*(6), 286–296.

Johnston, P., Flood, K., & Spinks, K. (2003). *The newborn child* (9th ed.). Edinburgh: Churchill Livingstone.

Kiesler, J., & Ricer, R. (2003). The abnormal fontanel. *American Family Physician, 67*(12), 2547–2552.

Mandleco, B. L. (2004). *Growth and development handbook: Newborn through*

adolescence. Clifton Park, NY: Thomson Delmar Learning.

Thureen, P. J., Deacon, J., Hernandez, J. A., & Hall, D. M. (2005). *Assessment and care of the well newborn* (2nd ed.). St. Louis, MO: Elsevier.

Varney, H., Kriebs, J. M., & Gegor, C. L. (2004). *Varney's midwifery* (4th ed.). Sudbury, MA: Jones and Bartlett.

Wu, T. Y., & Daniel, L. (2001). Growth of immigrant Chinese infants in the first year of life. *American Journal of Maternal Child Nursing, 26*(4), 202–207.

CHAPTER
30

The Normal Newborn: Needs and Care

This moment of meeting seemed to be a birth time for both of us; her first and my second life. Nothing, I knew, could ever be the same again.

~Laurie Lee, Two Women~

KEY TERMS

Circumcision   874
Newborn screening tests   883
Parent-newborn attachment   872

OBJECTIVES

1. Summarize the essential areas of information to be obtained about a newborn's birth experience and immediate postnatal period.

2. Relate the physiologic and behavioral responses of newborns to possible interventions needed.

3. Discuss the major nursing considerations and activities to be carried out during the first 4 hours after birth (admission and transitional period) and subsequent daily care.

4. Identify activities that should be included in a daily care plan for a normal newborn.

5. Determine the common concerns of families regarding their newborns.

6. Describe topics and related content to be included in parent teaching on newborn and infant care.

7. Identify opportunities to individualize parent teaching and enhance each parent's abilities and confidence while providing infant care in the birthing unit.

8. Delineate the information to be included in discharge planning with the newborn's family.

MEDIALINK

Additional resources for this content can be found on the Prentice Hall Nursing MediaLink DVD-ROM and on the Companion Website at http://www.prenhall.com/davidson. Click on "Chapter 30" to select the activities for this chapter.

At the moment of birth, numerous physiologic adaptations begin to take place in the newborn's body. Because of these dramatic changes, newborns require close observation to determine how smoothly they are making the transition to extrauterine life. Newborns also require special care that enhances their chances of making the transition successfully.

The two broad goals of nursing care during this period are (1) to promote the physical well-being of the newborn, and (2) to support the establishment of a well-functioning family unit. The nurse meets the first goal by providing comprehensive care to newborns while in the mother-baby unit. The nurse meets the second goal by teaching family members how to care for their new baby and by supporting their efforts so that they feel confident and competent. Thus, the nurse must be knowledgeable about family adjustments that need to be made as well as the healthcare needs of the newborn. It is important that the family return home with the positive feeling that they have the support, information, and skills to care for their newborn. Equally important is the need for each member of the family to begin a unique relationship with the newborn. The cultural and social expectations of individual families and communities affect the way normal newborn care is carried out.

The previous two chapters present an informational database of the physiologic and behavioral changes occurring in the newborn and the pertinent nursing assessments that are needed. This chapter discusses nursing care management while the newborn is in the birthing unit. The Clinical Pathway for Newborn Care starts on page 865.

NURSING CARE DURING ADMISSION AND THE FIRST FOUR HOURS OF LIFE

Immediately after birth, the baby is formally admitted to the healthcare facility.

Nursing Assessment and Diagnosis

Before the birth of an infant, the nurse reviews the prenatal record of the mother for information concerning possible risk factors for the infant. These include infectious disease screening results, drug or alcohol use by the mother, gestational diabetes, and any other data determined to be of use in anticipating the needs of the newborn. In addition, the nurse reviews the delivery record for prolonged rupture of membranes, instrument or vacuum delivery, use of narcotic analgesia, presence of meconium, and any other data that may impact the infant's ability to successfully transition to the extrauterine environment.

During the first 4 hours after birth, the nurse carries out a preliminary physical examination, including an assessment of the newborn's physiologic adaptations. In many birthing units, the nurse performs and documents the initial head-to-toe physical assessment during the first hour of transition. The nurse is responsible for notifying the physician or nurse practitioner of any deviations from normal. A complete physical examination is also performed later by the physician or nurse practitioner,

within the first 24 hours after birth and within 24 hours before discharge. This can be accomplished with one physical examination (American Academy of Pediatrics [AAP] & American College of Obstetricians and Gynecologists [ACOG], 2002). (See Chapter 29 ∞ and Table 29–1 ∞).

Nursing diagnoses are based on an analysis of the assessment findings. Physiologic alterations of the newborn form the basis of many nursing diagnoses, as does the family's incorporation of them in caring for their new baby. Nursing diagnoses that may apply to the newborn include the following:

* ***Ineffective Airway Clearance*** related to presence of mucus and retained lung fluid
* ***Risk for Altered Body Temperature*** related to evaporative, radiant, conductive, and convective heat losses
* ***Altered Peripheral Tissue Perfusion*** related to ineffective thermoregulation
* ***Acute Pain*** related to heel sticks for glucose or hematocrit tests or vitamin K injection

As discussed in Chapter 28 ∞, the newborn's physiologic adaptation to extrauterine life occurs rapidly. All body systems are affected. Therefore, many of these nursing diagnoses and associated interventions must be identified and implemented in a very short period (Table 30–1).

Nursing Plan and Implementation

The nurse initiates newborn admission procedures and evaluates the newborn's need to remain under observation. This evaluation may take place in a special transition area or at the mother's bedside. It includes the following:

* Maternal and birth history
* Airway clearance
* Vital signs
* Body temperature

 Table 30–1 SIGNS OF NEWBORN TRANSITION

Normal findings for the newborn during the first few days of life include the following:

Pulse: 120–160 beats/minute

   During sleep as low as 100 beats/minute

   If crying, up to 180 beats/minute

   Apical pulse is counted for 1 full minute because rate may fluctuate

Respirations: 30–60 respirations/minute

   Predominantly diaphragmatic but synchronous with abdominal movements

   Brief periods of apnea (less than 15 seconds) with no color or heart rate changes

Temperature:

   Axillary: 36.5C–37C (97.5F–98.6F)

   Skin: 36C–36.5C (96.8F–97.7F)

Blood pressure: 90–60/50–40 mm Hg at birth; 100/50 mm Hg at day 10

Blood glucose: greater than or equal to 40 mg%

Hematocrit: less than 65% to 70% central venous sample

- Neurologic status
- Ability to feed
- Evidence of complications

If the evaluation is normal, the baby is successfully making the transition to extrauterine life and may need less frequent observations. In some settings, this may also be a time for moving the mother and baby to another care unit.

INITIATION OF ADMISSION PROCEDURES

After birth the baby is formally admitted to the healthcare facility. The admission procedures include a review of prenatal and birth information for possible risk factors, a gestational age assessment, and an assessment to ensure that the newborn's adaptation to extrauterine life is proceeding normally. This evaluation for risk factors and the status of the newborn must be done no later than 2 hours after birth (AAP & ACOG, 2002).

If the initial assessment indicates that the newborn is not at risk physiologically, the nurse performs many of the routine admission procedures in the presence of the parents and others in the birthing area. Some care measures indicated by the assessment findings may be performed by the nurse or by family members under the guidance of the nurse in an effort to educate and support the family. Other interventions might best be delayed if the newborn must be transferred to an observational nursery.

The nurse responsible for the newborn first checks and confirms the newborn's identification with the mother's identification and then obtains and records all significant information. The essential data to be recorded as part of the newborn's chart include the following:

1. *Condition of the newborn.* Pertinent information includes the newborn's Apgar scores at 1 and 5 minutes, resuscitative measures required in the birthing area, physical examination, vital signs, voidings, and passing of meconium. Complications to be noted include excessive mucus, delayed spontaneous respirations or responsiveness, abnormal number of cord vessels, and obvious physical abnormalities.

2. *Labor and birth record.* A copy of the labor and birth record should be placed in the newborn's chart or be accessible on computer. The record contains all the significant data about the birth, for example, duration, course, and status of mother and fetus throughout labor and birth and any analgesia or anesthesia administered to the mother. Particular care is taken to note any variation or difficulties such as prolonged rupture of membranes, abnormal fetal position, meconium-stained amniotic fluid, signs of nonreassuring fetal status during labor, nuchal cord (cord around the newborn's neck at birth), precipitous birth, use of forceps or vacuum extraction assisted device, maternal analgesia and anesthesia received within 1 hour of birth, and administration of antibiotics during labor.

3. *Antepartal history.* Any maternal problems that may have compromised the fetus in utero—such as preeclampsia, spotting, illness, recent infections, rubella status, serology results, hepatitis B screen results, exposure to group B streptococci, or a history of maternal substance abuse—are of immediate concern in newborn assessment. The chart should also include information about maternal age, estimated date of birth (EDB), previous pregnancies, and presence of any congenital anomalies. A human immunodeficiency virus (HIV) test result, if obtained, is also relevant. State statutes vary as to who may have access to this information (AAP & ACOG, 2002).

4. *Parent-newborn interaction information.* The nurse notes parents' interactions with their newborn and their desires regarding care, such as rooming-in, circumcision, and type of feeding. Information about other children in the home, available support systems, and patterns of interaction within each family unit assists the nurse in providing comprehensive care.

As part of the admission procedure, the nurse weighs the newborn in both grams and pounds. In the United States, parents understand weights best when stated in pounds and ounces (Figure 30–1 ◆). The nurse cleans and covers the scales each time a newborn is weighed to prevent cross-infection and heat loss from conduction.

The nurse then measures the newborn, recording the measurements in both centimeters and inches. Three routine measurements are length, circumference of the head, and circumference of the chest. In some facilities, abdominal girth may also be measured. The nurse rapidly assesses the baby's color, muscle tone, alertness, and general state. Remember that the first period of reactivity may have concluded, and the baby may be in the sleep-inactive phase, which makes the infant hard to arouse. The nurse does basic assessments for estimating gestational age and completes the physical assessment. (For more discussion of the process of newborn assessment, see Chapter 29 ∞).

In addition to obtaining vital signs, the nurse performs hematocrit and blood glucose evaluations on at-risk newborns or as clinically indicated (such as for small-for-gestational-age [SGA] or large-for-gestational-age [LGA] infants or if the new-

Figure 30–1 ◆ Weighing a newborn. The scale is balanced before each weighing, with the protective pad in place.

CLINICAL PATHWAY For Newborn Care

CATEGORY	FIRST 4 HOURS	4–8 HOURS PAST BIRTH	8–24 HOURS PAST BIRTH
Referral	Review labor/birth record Review transitional nursing record Check ID bands Consult prn: orthopedics, genetics, infectious disease	Check ID bands Transfer to mother-baby care at 4–6 hours of age if stable As parents desire, obtain circumcision permit after their discussion with physician Check ID bands and crib cards to ensure they are in the correct crib Lactation consult prn	Check ID bands q shift ◆ *Expected Outcomes* Mother/baby ID bands correlate at time of discharge; consults completed prn
Assessments	Continue assessments begun first hour after birth Vital signs: TPR, BP prn, q1h 4 times (skin temp 97.7–98.6F (36.5C–37C), resp may be irregular but within 30–60 per min) ◆ *Newborn Assessments* • Respiratory status with resp distress scale × 1 then prn. If resp distress, assess every 5–15 min • Cord: bluish white color, clamp in place and free of skin • Color: skin, mucous membranes, extremities, trunk pink with slight acrocyanosis of hands and feet • Wt (5 lb, 8 oz–8 lb, 13 oz) 2500–4000 g, length (18–22 in.) 46–56 cm, HC (12.5–14.5 in.) 32–37 cm, CC (32.5 cm, 1–2 cm less than head) • Extremity movement—may be jerky or brief twitches • Gestational age classification—term AGA • Anomalies (cong. anomalies can interfere with normal extrauterine adaptation)	Assess newborn's progress through periods of reactivity Vital signs: TPR q8h; and prn or per agency protocol, BP prn ◆ *Newborn Assessments* • Skin color q4h prn (circulatory system stabilizing, acrocyanosis decreased) • Eyes for drainage, redness, hemorrhage • Auscultate lungs q4h (noisy, wet breath sounds clear and equal) • Increased mucus production (normal in 2nd period of reactivity) • Check apical pulse q4h • Umbilical cord base for redness, drainage, foul odor, drying, damp in place • Extremity movements q4h • Check for expected reflexes (suck, rooting, Moro, grasp, blink, yawn, sneeze, tonic neck, Babinski) • Note common normal variations • Assess suck and swallow during feeding • Note behavioral characteristics • Temp before and after admission bath	VS q8h; normal ranges: T, 97.5–99F (36.3C–37.2C); P, 120–160; R, 30–60; BP, 90–60/50–40 mm Hg ◆ *Continue Newborn Assessments* • Skin color q4h prn • Signs of drying or infection in cord area • Check out clamp in place until removed before discharge • Check circ for bleeding after procedure, then q30 min 2 times, then q4h and prn • Observe for jaundice, obtain total serum bili (TsB) if infant visibly jaundiced before 24 hours of age. Obtain transcutaneous bili on all infants not previously tested before discharge ◆ *Expected Outcomes* Vital signs medically acceptable, color pink, assessments WNL, circ site without s/s infection, cord site without s/s of infection and clamp removed; newborn behavior WNL
Teaching/ psychosocial	Admission activities performed at mother's bedside if possible, orient to nursery prn, handwashing, assess teaching needs Teach parents use of bulb syringe, signs of choking, positioning, and when to call for assistance Teach reasons for use of radiant warmer, infant hat, and warmed blankets when out of warmer Discuss/teach infant security, identification	Reinforce teaching about choking, bulb syringe use, positioning, temperature maintenance with clothing and blankets Teach infant positioning to facilitate breathing and digestion Teach new parents holding and feeding skills Teach parents soothing and calming techniques Teach parents about introducing newborn to sibling	Final discharge teaching: diapering, normal void and stool patterns, bathing, nail and cord care, circumcision/uncircumcised penis/genital care and normal characteristics, rashes, jaundice, sleep-wake cycles, soothing activities, taking temperatures, thermometer reading Explain s/s of illness and when to call healthcare provider Infant safety: car seats, immunizations, metabolic screening ◆ *Expected Outcomes* Mother/family verbalize comprehension of teaching; demonstrate care capabilities
Nursing care management and reports	Place under radiant warmer Place hat on newborn (decreases convection heat loss) Suction nares/mouth with bulb syringe prn Keep bulb syringe with infant Attach security sensor Obtain lab tests: blood glucose, as needed Obtain blood type, Rh, Coombs on cord blood, HSV culture if parental hx	Wean from radiant warmer (T 98.6F [37C] axillary) Chemstrips prn; BP prn Oxygen saturation prn Bathe infant if temp greater than 97.7F (36.5C) Position on side Suction nares prn (esp during 2nd period of reactivity) Obtain peripheral Hct per protocol	Check for hearing test results Weigh before discharge Cord assessment every shift DC cord clamp before discharge[1] Perform newborn metabolic screening blood tests before discharge Circumcision if indicated; circumcision care: change diaper prn, noting ability to void; follow policy for circumcision clamp or Plastibell care

1. In the case of very early discharge, the cord may still be moist enough that the decision may be made to leave it in place until the follow-up visit with the physician.

(Continued on next page)

CLINICAL PATHWAY For Newborn Care continued

CATEGORY	FIRST 4 HOURS	4–8 HOURS PAST BIRTH	8–24 HOURS PAST BIRTH
Nursing care management and reports (continued)	Notify physician's office of infant's birth and any change in status Maintain standard precautions	Cord care per protocol Fold diaper below cord (for plastic diapers, turn plastic layer away from skin)	◆ *Expected Outcomes* Newborn maintains temp, lab test WNL, cord dry without s/s infection and clamp removed, screening tests accomplished, circ site without s/s infection or bleeding
Activity and comfort	Place under radiant warmer or wrap in prewarmed blankets until stable Soothe baby as needed with voice, touch, cuddling, nesting in warmer	Leave in warmer until stable, then swaddle Position on back after each feeding	Place in open crib Swaddle to allow movement of extremities in blanket, including hands to face ◆ *Expected Outcomes* Infant maintains temp WNL in open crib; infant attempts self-calming
Nutrition	Assist newborn to breastfeed as soon as mother/baby condition allows Supplement breast only when medically indicated or per agency policy Initiate formula-feeding within first hour Gavage feed if necessary to prevent hypoglycemia	Breastfeed on demand, at least q3-4h Teach positions, observe/assist with feeding, breast/nipple care, establishing milk supply, breaking suction, feeding cues, latching-on techniques, nutritive suck, burping Formula-feed on demand, at least q3-4h Determine readiness to feed and feeding tolerance	Continue breastfeeding or formula-feeding pattern Assess feeding tolerance q4h Discuss normal feeding requirements, signs of hunger and satiation, handling feeding problems, and when to seek help ◆ *Expected Outcomes* Mother verbalizes knowledge of feeding information; breastfeeds on demand without supplement; bottle—tolerates formula feeding, nipples without problems
Elimination	Note first void and stool if not noted at birth	Note all voids, amount and color of stools q4h	Evaluate all voids and stool color q8h ◆ *Expected Outcomes* Voids qs; stools qs without difficulty; stool character WNL, diaper area without s/s of skin breakdown or rashes
Medication	Prophylactic ophthalmic ointment both eyes after baby makes eye contact with parents within 1 hr after birth Administer AquaMEPHYTON IM, dosage according to infant weight per MD/NP order and within 1 hr of birth	Hepatitis B injection as ordered by physician after consent signed by parents	Hepatitis B vaccine within 2 hr of birth or before discharge ◆ *Expected Outcomes* Baby has received ophthalmic ointment and vitamin K injection; baby has received first Hep B vaccine if ordered and parental permission received
Discharge planning/ home care	Hepatitis B consent signed Hearing screen consent signed Plan discharge call with parent or guardian in 24 hr to 2 days Assess parents' discharge plans, needs, and support systems	Review/reinforce teaching with mother and significant other Review home preparedness Present birth certificate instructions	Initial newborn screening tests (hearing, blood tests, metabolic screen; i.e., PKU) before discharge Bath and feeding classes, videos, or written information given Give written copy of discharge instructions Newborn photographs Set up appointment for follow-up PKU test Have car seat available before discharge. All discharge referrals made, follow-up appt. scheduled ◆ *Expected Outcomes* Infant discharged home with family; mother verbalizes follow-up appt. time/date

CLINICAL PATHWAY   For Newborn Care continued

CATEGORY	FIRST 4 HOURS	4–8 HOURS PAST BIRTH	8–24 HOURS PAST BIRTH
Family involvement	Facilitate early investigation of baby's physical characteristics (maintain temp during unwrapping), hold infant *en face* Dim lights to help infant keep eyes open	Assess parents' knowledge of newborn behaviors, such as alertness, suck and rooting, attention to human voice, response to calming techniques Facilitate parent interaction with infant by performing care in presence of parents and encouraging parents to participate in care	Assess mother-baby bonding/interaction Incorporate father and siblings in care Enhance parent-infant interaction by sharing characteristics and behavioral assessment Support positive parenting behaviors Identify community referral needs and refer to community agencies ◆ *Expected Outcome* Demonstrates caring and family incorporation of infant
Date			

AGA, average for gestational age; Appt, appointment; CC, chest circumference; cong, congenital; esp, especially; HC, head circumference; Hct, hematocrit; Hx, history; ID, identification; PKU, phenylketonuria; qs, quantity sufficient; s/s, signs and symptoms; temp, temperature; TPR, temperature, pulse, respirations; VS, vital signs; WNL, within normal limits.

born is jittery). These procedures may be done on admission or within the first 2 hours after birth (AAP & ACOG, 2002). (See Procedure 33–1.)

MAINTENANCE OF A CLEAR AIRWAY AND STABLE VITAL SIGNS

Free-flow oxygen should be readily available. The nurse positions the newborn on his or her back (or side, if the infant has copious secretions). If necessary, a bulb syringe or DeLee wall suction (see Procedure 24–1) is used to remove mucus from the nasal passages and oral cavity. A DeLee catheter attached to suction may be used to remove mucus from the stomach to help prevent possible aspiration. When possible, this procedure should be delayed for 10 to 15 minutes after birth, reducing the potential for severe vasovagal reflex apnea.

In the absence of any newborn distress, the nurse continues with the admission by taking the newborn's vital signs. The initial temperature is taken by the axillary method. A wider range of normal exists for axillary temperature, specifically 36.5C to 37C (97.7F to 98.6F).

Once the initial temperature is taken, the nurse monitors the core temperature either by obtaining axillary temperatures at intervals or by placing a skin sensor on the newborn for continuous reading. The usual skin sensor placement site is on the newborn's abdomen, but placement on the upper thigh or arm can give a reading closely correlated with the mean body temperature. The vital signs for a healthy term newborn should be monitored at least every 30 minutes until the newborn's condition has remained stable for 2 hours (AAP & ACOG, 2002). The newborn's respirations may be irregular yet still be normal. Brief periods of apnea, lasting only 5 to 10 seconds with no color or heart rate changes, are considered normal. The normal pulse range is 120 to 160 beats per minute (bpm), and the normal respiratory range is 30 to 60 respirations per minute.

MAINTENANCE OF A NEUTRAL THERMAL ENVIRONMENT

A neutral thermal environment is essential to minimize the newborn's need for increased oxygen consumption and use of calories to maintain body heat in the optimal range of 36.5C to 37C (97.7F to 98.6F). If the newborn becomes hypothermic, the body's response can lead to metabolic acidosis, hypoxia, and shock.

The nurse can best achieve a neutral thermal environment by performing the assessment and interventions with a newborn unclothed and under a radiant warmer. The radiant warmer's thermostat is controlled by the thermal skin sensor taped to the newborn's abdomen, upper thigh, or arm (Figure 30–2 ◆). The sensor indicates when the newborn's temperature exceeds or falls below the acceptable temperature range. The nurse should be aware that leaning over the newborn may block the radiant heat waves from reaching the newborn.

It is common practice in some institutions to cover the newborn's head with a cap made of wool lined with gauze and cotton, Thinsulate, or cotton and polyester terry cloth to prevent further heat loss in addition to placing the baby under a radiant warmer (Blackburn, 2003).

CLINICAL TIP
A cap can be fashioned from a piece of stockinette to help reduce heat loss from the head.

When the newborn's temperature is normal and vital signs are stable (about 2 to 4 hours after birth), the baby may be given a sponge bath. However, this admission bath may be postponed for some hours if the newborn's condition dictates or the parents wish to give the first bath. In light of early discharge practices (12 to 48 hours), healthy term infants can be safely bathed immediately after the admission assessment is completed (Behring, Vezeau, & Fink, 2003). The baby is bathed while still

PROCEDURE 30–1 Thermoregulation of the Newborn

NURSING ACTION	RATIONALE

Preparation

- Prewarm the incubator or radiant warmer. Make sure warm towels and/or lightweight blankets are available.
- Maintain the temperature of the birthing room at 22C (71F), with a relative humidity of 60% to 65%.

The change from a warm, moist intrauterine environment to a cool, dry, drafty environment stresses the newborn's immature thermoregulation system.

Equipment and Supplies

Prewarmed towels or blankets
Infant stocking cap
Servocontrol probe
Infant T-shirt and diaper
Open crib

Procedure: Clean Gloves

1. Don gloves.

   Gloves are worn whenever there is the possibility of contact with body fluids—in this case, a newborn wet with amniotic fluid, vernix, and maternal blood.

2. Place the newborn under the radiant warmer. Wipe the newborn free of blood, fluid, and excess vernix, especially from the head, using prewarmed towels.

   The radiant warmer creates a heat-gaining environment. Drying is important to prevent the loss of body heat through evaporation.

3. If the newborn is stable, wrap him or her in a prewarmed blanket, apply a stocking cap, and carry the newborn to the mother. The mother and her support person can hold and enjoy the newborn together. Alternatively, carry the newborn wrapped to the mother, loosen the blanket, and place the infant skin to skin on the mother's chest under a warmed blanket.

   Use of a prewarmed blanket reduces convection heat loss and facilitates maternal-newborn contact without compromising the newborn's thermoregulation. Skin-to-skin contact with the mother or father helps maintain the newborn's temperature.

4. After the newborn has spent time with the parents, return him or her to the radiant warmer and apply a diaper. Leave the newborn uncovered (except for the cap and diaper) under the radiant warmer.

   Radiant heat warms the outer skin surface, so the skin needs to be exposed.

5. Tape a servocontrol probe on the newborn's anterior abdominal wall, with the metal side next to the skin. Do not place it over the ribs. Secure the probe with porous tape or a foil-covered aluminum heat deflector patch. Figure 30–2 shows a newborn with a skin probe. Note that in this picture the newborn is no longer wearing a stocking cap.

6. Turn the heater to servocontrol mode so that the abdominal skin is maintained at 36.5C to 37C (97.7F to 98.6F).

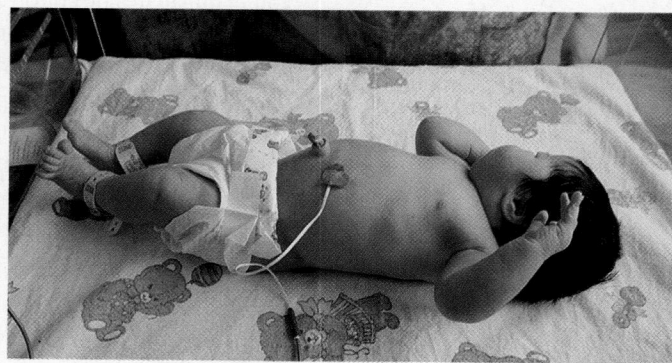

Figure 30–2 ◆ Temperature monitoring for the newborn. A skin thermal sensor is placed on the newborn's abdomen, upper thigh, or arm and secured with porous tape or a foil-covered foam pad.
SOURCE: Photographer, Elena Dorfman.

PROCEDURE 30–1   Thermoregulation of the Newborn   continued

NURSING ACTION	RATIONALE
7. Monitor the newborn's axillary and skin probe temperatures per agency protocol.	The temperature indicator on the radiant warmer continually displays the newborn's probe temperature. The axillary temperature is checked to ensure that the machine is accurately recording the newborn's temperature.
8. When the newborn's temperature reaches 37C (98.6F), add a T-shirt, double-wrap the infant (two blankets), and place the newborn in an open crib.	
9. Recheck the newborn's temperature in 1 hour and regularly thereafter according to agency policy.	It is important to monitor the newborn's ability to maintain his or her own thermoregulation.
10. If the newborn's temperature drops below 36.1C (97F), rewarm the infant gradually. Place the infant (unclothed except for a diaper) under the radiant warmer with a servocontrol probe on the anterior abdominal wall.	Rapid heating can lead to hyperthermia, which is associated with apnea, insensible water loss, and increased metabolic rate.
11. Recheck the newborn's temperature in 30 minutes, then hourly.	
12. When the temperature reaches 37C (98.6F), dress the newborn, remove him or her from the radiant warmer, double-wrap, and place in an open crib. Check the temperature hourly until stable, then regularly according to agency policy.	

Note: An infant who repeatedly requires rewarming should be observed for other signs and symptoms of illness and a physician notified, because it may warrant screening for infection.

under the radiant warmer; the bathing may be done in the parents' room and by the parents (Medves & O'Brien, 2004). Bathing the newborn offers an excellent opportunity for teaching and welcoming parent involvement in the care of their baby.

The nurse rechecks the temperature after the bath and, if it is stable, dresses the newborn in a shirt, diaper, and cap; wraps the baby; and places the baby in an open crib at room temperature. If the baby's axillary temperature is below 36.5C (97.7F), the nurse returns the baby to the radiant warmer. The rewarming process should be gradual to prevent the possibility of hyperthermia. Once the newborn is rewarmed, the nurse implements measures to prevent further neonatal heat loss, such as keeping the newborn dry, swaddled in one or two blankets with hat on, and away from cool surfaces or instruments. The nurse also protects the newborn from drafts, open windows or doors, and air conditioners. Blankets and clothing are stored in a warm place. See "Temperature Regulation" in Chapter 29 ∞ and Procedure 30–1. Newborns are often "double-wrapped" in two or more blankets for temperature maintenance.

CLINICAL TIP

Take action to help the newborn maintain a stable temperature:
- Keep the newborn's clothing and bedding dry.
- Double-wrap the newborn and put a stocking cap on him or her.
- Use the radiant warmer during procedures.
- Reduce the newborn's exposure to drafts.
- Warm objects that will be in contact with the newborn (e.g., stethoscopes).
- Encourage the mother to snuggle with the newborn under blankets or to breastfeed the newborn with hat and light cover.

PREVENTION OF VITAMIN K DEFICIENCY BLEEDING

A prophylactic injection of vitamin K_1 (AquaMEPHYTON) is given to prevent hemorrhage, which can occur because of low prothrombin levels in the first few days of life (see the Drug Guide: Vitamin K_1 Phytonadione [AquaMEPHYTON]). The potential for hemorrhage results from the absence of gut bacterial flora, which influences the production of vitamin K in the newborn. (See Chapter 33 ∞ for further discussion.) Newborns receive a single parenteral dose of 0.5 to 1 mg of natural vitamin K_1 oxide (phytonadione) within 1 hour of birth (AAP & ACOG, 2002; Wilson, Shannon, Shields, & Stang, 2007). Current recommendations underscore the need for treatment in infants who are exclusively breastfed (AAP, 2003).

Vitamin K injection is given intramuscularly in the middle third of the vastus lateralis muscle located in the lateral aspect of the thigh (Figure 30–3 ◆). Before injecting, the nurse must clean the newborn's skin site for the injection thoroughly with a small alcohol swab. The nurse uses a 25-gauge, 5/8-inch needle for the injection. An alternative site is the rectus femoris muscle in the anterior aspect of the thigh. However, this site is near the sciatic nerve and femoral artery and should be used with caution (Figure 30–4 ◆).

PREVENTION OF EYE INFECTION

The nurse is also responsible for giving the legally required prophylactic eye treatment for *Neisseria gonorrhoeae*, which may have infected the newborn of an infected mother during the birth process. A variety of topical agents appear to be equally effective. Ophthalmic ointments that are used include 0.5% erythromycin

DRUG GUIDE   Vitamin K₁ Phytonadione (AquaMEPHYTON)

Overview of Neonatal Action

Phytonadione is used in prophylaxis and treatment of vitamin K deficiency bleeding (VKDB), formerly known as hemorrhagic disease of the newborn. It promotes liver formation of the clotting factors II, VII, IX, and X. At birth, the newborn does not have the bacteria in the colon that are necessary for synthesizing fat-soluble vitamin K₁. Therefore, the newborn may have decreased levels of prothrombin during the first 5 to 8 days of life, reflected by a prolongation of prothrombin time.

Pregnancy Risk Category: C

Route, Dosage, Frequency

Intramuscular injection is given in the vastus lateralis thigh muscle. A one-time-only prophylactic dose of 0.5 to 1 mg is given intramuscularly in the birthing area or within 1 hour of birth (Wilson et al., 2007).

 If the mother received anticoagulants during pregnancy, an additional dose may be ordered by the physician and is given 6 to 8 hours after the first injection. IM concentration: 1 mg/0.5 mL (neonatal strength); can use 10 mg/mL concentration to minimize volume injected.

Neonatal Side Effects

Pain and edema may occur at the injection site. Allergic reactions, such as rash and urticaria, may also occur.

Nursing Considerations

• Protect the drug from light.
• Observe for signs of local inflammation.
• Observe for jaundice and kernicterus, especially in preterm infants.
• Give vitamin K₁ before circumcision procedure.
• Observe for bleeding (usually occurs on second or third day). Bleeding may be seen as generalized ecchymoses or bleeding from the umbilical cord, circumcision site, nose, or gastrointestinal tract. Results of serial prothrombin time (PT) and international normalized ratio (INR) should be assessed.

Figure 30–3 ◆ Procedure for vitamin K injection. Cleanse area thoroughly with alcohol swab, and allow skin to dry. Bunch the tissue of the upper thigh (vastus lateralis muscle) and quickly insert a 25-gauge 5/8-inch needle at a 90-degree angle to the thigh. Aspirate, then slowly inject the solution to distribute the medication evenly and minimize the baby's discomfort. Remove the needle and massage the site with an alcohol swab.
SOURCE: Photographer, Elena Dorfman.

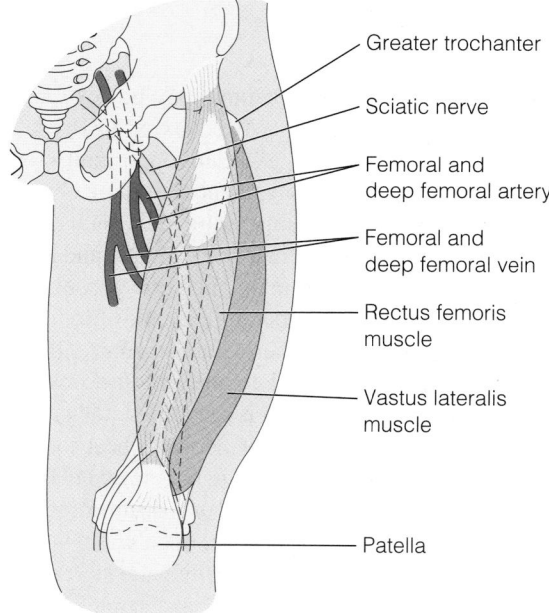

Figure 30–4 ◆ Injection sites. The middle third of the vastus lateralis muscle is the preferred site for intramuscular injection in the newborn. The middle third of the rectus femoris is an alternative site, but its proximity to major vessels and the sciatic nerve necessitates caution in using this site for injection.

(Ilotycin Ophthalmic) (see the Drug Guide: Erythromycin Ophthalmic Ointment [Ilotycin Ophthalmic], 1% silver nitrate, 1% tetracycline, and opthalmic solution of povidone-iodine (2.5%). All are also effective against chlamydia, which has a higher incidence rate than gonorrhea.

 Successful eye prophylaxis requires that the medication be instilled into the lower conjunctival sac of each eye (Figure 30–5 ◆). The nurse massages the eyelid gently to distribute the ointment. Instillation may be delayed up to 1 hour after birth to allow eye contact during parent-newborn bonding.

Eye prophylaxis medication can cause chemical conjunctivitis, which gives the newborn some discomfort and may interfere with the baby's ability to focus on the parents' faces. The resulting edema, inflammation, and discharge may cause concern if the parents have not been informed that the side effects will clear in 24 to 48 hours and that this prophylactic eye treatment is necessary for the newborn's well-being.

DRUG GUIDE   Erythromycin Ophthalmic Ointment (Ilotycin Ophthalmic)

Overview of Neonatal Action

Erythromycin (Ilotycin Ophthalmic) is used as prophylactic treatment of ophthalmia neonatorum, which is caused by the bacteria *Neisseria gonorrhoeae*. Preventive treatment of gonorrhea in the newborn is required by law. Erythromycin is also effective against ophthalmic chlamydial infections. It is either bacteriostatic or bactericidal, depending on the organisms involved and the concentration of the drug.

Pregnancy Risk Category: B

Route, Dosage, Frequency

Ophthalmic ointment (0.5%) is instilled as a narrow ribbon or strand, 0.5 to 1 cm long, along the lower conjunctival surface of each eye, starting at the inner canthus. It is instilled only once in each eye. The ointment may be administered in the birthing area or, alternatively, later in the nursery so that eye contact between infant and parent is facilitated and the bonding process immediately after birth is not in-

terrupted. After administration, gently close the eye and manipulate to ensure spread of ointment (Wilson et al., 2007).

Neonatal Side Effects

Sensitivity reaction; may interfere with ability to focus and may cause edema and inflammation. Side effects usually disappear in 24 to 48 hours.

Nursing Considerations

- Wash hands immediately before instillation to prevent introduction of bacteria.
- Do not irrigate the eyes after instillation. Use new tube or single-use container for ophthalmic ointment administration shortly after birth. May wipe away excess after 1 minute.
- Observe for hypersensitivity.
- Teach parents about need for eye prophylaxis. Educate them regarding side effects and signs that need to be reported to the healthcare provider.

Figure 30–5 ◆ Ophthalmic ointment. Retract lower eyelid outward to instill a 1/4-inch strand of ointment from a single-dose ampule along the lower conjunctival surface.

EARLY ASSESSMENT OF NEONATAL DISTRESS

During the first 24 hours of life, nurses are constantly alert for signs of distress. If the newborn is with the parents during this period, the nurse must take extra care to teach them how to maintain their newborn's temperature, recognize the hallmarks of newborn distress, and respond immediately to signs of respiratory problems. The parents should learn to observe the newborn for changes in skin color or activity, rapid breathing with chest retractions, nasal flaring, or facial grimacing. Their interventions should include nasal and oral suctioning with bulb syringe, positioning, and vigorous fingertip stroking of the newborn's spine to stimulate respiratory activity if necessary. The

Table 30–2   SIGNS OF NEONATAL DISTRESS

Increased respiratory rate (more than 60/minute) or difficult respirations

Sternal, substernal, intercostal retractions

Nasal flaring

Grunting

Excessive mucus

Facial grimacing

Cyanosis (central: skin, lips, tongue)

Abdominal distention or mass

Vomiting of bile-stained material

Absence of meconium elimination within 24 hours of birth

Absence of urine elimination within 24 hours of birth

Jaundice of the skin within 24 hours of birth or because of hemolytic process

Temperature instability (hypothermia or hyperthermia)

Jitteriness or glucose less than 40 mg%

SOURCE: Adapted from Tappero, E. P., & Honeyfield, M. E. (1996). *Physical assessment of the newborn* (2nd ed.). Petaluma, CA: NICU Inc.

nurse must be immediately available to provide appropriate interventions should the newborn develop distress (Table 30–2).

A common cause of neonatal distress is early-onset group B streptococcal (GBS) disease. Infected mothers transmit GBS infection to their infants during labor and birth; thus it is recommended that at-risk mothers receive intrapartum antimicrobial prophylaxis (IAP) for GBS disease. All infants of mothers identified as at risk should be assessed and observed for signs and symptoms of sepsis.

INITIATION OF FIRST FEEDING

The timing of the first feeding varies, depending on whether the newborn is to be breastfed or formula-fed and whether there were any complications during pregnancy or birth, such as maternal diabetes or intrauterine growth restriction (IUGR).

Mothers who choose to breastfeed their newborns should be encouraged to put their baby to breast during the first period of reactivity. This practice should be encouraged because successful, long-term breastfeeding during infancy appears to be related to beginning breastfeedings in the first few hours of life. Sleep-wake states affect feeding behavior and need to be considered when evaluating the newborn's sucking ability (Karl, 2004).

Formula-fed newborns usually begin the first feedings by 5 hours of age, during the second period of reactivity, when they awaken and appear hungry. Signs indicating newborn readiness for the first feeding are licking of the lips, placing a hand in or near the mouth, mouthing the blanket, active bowel sounds, absence of abdominal distention, and a lusty cry that quiets with rooting and sucking behaviors when a stimulus is placed near the lips. Observing the earlier, more subtle cues that baby is ready to nurse provides an opportunity for the nurse to teach the parents to recognize these cues and respond before the baby is frustrated and crying.

FACILITATION OF PARENT-NEWBORN ATTACHMENT

To facilitate **parent-newborn attachment,** eye-to-eye contact between parents and their newborn is extremely important during the early hours after birth, when the newborn is in the first period of reactivity. The newborn is alert during this time, the eyes are wide open, and direct eye contact is made with human faces within optimal range for visual acuity (7 to 8 inches). It is theorized that this eye contact is an important foundation in establishing attachment in human relationships (Klaus & Klaus, 1985). Consequently, the prophylactic eye medication is often delayed, but no more than 1 hour, to provide an opportunity for this period of eye contact between parents and their newborn, thus facilitating the attachment process (AAP & ACOG, 2002). Parents who cannot be with their newborns in this first period because of maternal or infant distress may need reassurance that the bonding process can proceed normally as soon as both mother and baby are stable.

Another situation that can facilitate attachment is the interactive bath. While bathing their newborn for the first time, parents attend closely to their baby's behavior. In this way the newborn becomes an active participant and parents are drawn into an interaction with their newborn. The nurse can interpret the infant's behavior, model ways to respond to the behavior, and support parental strategies for doing so (Karl, 2004).

Now I believe in love at first sight!

~A NEW MOTHER HOLDING HER INFANT FOR THE FIRST TIME~

Evaluation

When evaluating the nursing care provided during the period immediately after birth, the nurse may anticipate the following outcomes:

- The newborn baby's adaptation to extrauterine life is supported and complete.
- The baby's physiologic and psychologic integrity is supported.
- Positive interactions between parent and infant will be supported.

NURSING MANAGEMENT OF THE NEWBORN FOLLOWING TRANSITION

Once healthy newborns have demonstrated successful adaptation to extrauterine life, they need appropriate observations for the first 6 to 12 hours after birth and the remainder of their stay in the birthing facility.

Nursing Diagnosis

Examples of nursing diagnoses that may apply during daily care of the newborn include the following:

- *Risk for Ineffective Breathing Pattern* related to periodic breathing
- *Altered Nutrition: Less than Body Requirements* related to limited nutritional or fluid intake and increased caloric expenditure
- *Altered Urinary Elimination* related to meatal edema secondary to circumcision
- *Risk for Infection* related to umbilical cord healing, circumcision site, immature immune system, or potential birth trauma (forceps or vacuum extraction birth)
- *Health-Seeking Behaviors* related to lack of information about basic baby care, male circumcision, and breast-and/or formula-feeding
- *Altered Family Processes* related to integration of newborn into family unit or demands of newborn care and feeding
- *Risk for Neurologic Impairment* related to hyperbilirubinemia

Nursing Plan and Implementation
MAINTENANCE OF CARDIOPULMONARY FUNCTION

The nurse assesses vital signs every 6 to 8 hours or more, depending on the newborn's status. The newborn should be placed on his or her back (supine) for sleeping. A bulb syringe is kept within easy reach should the baby need oral-nasal suctioning. If the newborn has respiratory difficulty, the airway is cleared. Vigorous fingertip stroking of the baby's spine will frequently stimulate respiratory activity. A cardiorespiratory monitor can be used on newborns who are not being observed at all times and are at risk for decreased respiratory or cardiac function. Indicators of risk are pallor, cyanosis, ruddy color, apnea, or other signs of instability. Changes in skin color may indicate the need for closer assessment of temperature, cardiopulmonary status, hematocrit, glucose, and bilirubin levels.

MAINTENANCE OF A NEUTRAL THERMAL ENVIRONMENT

The nurse makes every effort to maintain the newborn's temperature within the normal range. The nurse must make certain the newborn is dried completely after the bath, dressed, and exposed to the air as little as possible. A head covering should be used initially, and continued with the small newborn, who has less subcutaneous fat to act as insulation in maintaining body heat. Ambient temperature of the room where the newborn is kept should be monitored to prevent excessive cooling. Parents may be advised to dress the newborn in one more layer of clothing than is necessary for an adult to maintain thermal comfort. The use of clothes layering allows for flexibility as the infant is moved from one area to another.

A newborn whose temperature falls below optimal levels will use calories to maintain body heat rather than for growth. Chilling also decreases the affinity of serum albumin for bilirubin, thereby increasing the likelihood of newborn jaundice. It also increases oxygen use and may cause respiratory distress.

An overheated newborn will increase activity and respiratory rate in an attempt to cool the body. Both measures deplete caloric reserves. In addition, the increased respiratory rate leads to increased insensible fluid loss (Blackburn, 2003).

PROMOTION OF ADEQUATE HYDRATION AND NUTRITION

Newborn nutrition is addressed in depth in Chapter 31. ∞ The nurse records the newborn's caloric and fluid intake and enhances adequate hydration by maintaining a neutral thermal environment and offering early and frequent feedings. Early feedings promote gastric emptying and increase peristalsis, thereby decreasing the degree of hyperbilirubinemia by limiting the amount of time fecal material is in contact with the enzyme β-glucuronidase in the small intestine. This enzyme acts to free the bilirubin from the stool, allowing bilirubin to be reabsorbed into the vascular system. The nurse records voiding and stooling patterns. The first voiding should occur within 24 hours and passage of stool within 48 hours. When they do not occur, the nurse continues the normal observation routine while assessing for abdominal distention, bowel sounds, hydration, fluid intake, voiding pattern, and temperature stability.

The newborn should be weighed at the same time each day for accurate comparisons and must be kept warm during the weighing. A weight loss of up to 10% for term newborns is considered within normal limits during the first week of life. This weight loss is the result of limited intake, loss of excess extracellular fluid, and passage of meconium. Parents should be told about the expected weight loss, the reason for it, and the expectations for regaining the birth weight. Birth weight should be regained by 2 weeks if feedings are adequate.

Excessive handling can cause an increase in the newborn's metabolic rate and calorie use and cause fatigue. The nurse should be alert to the baby's subtle cues of fatigue, including a decrease in muscle tension and activity in the extremities and neck, as well as loss of eye contact, which may be manifested by fluttering or closing the eyelids. The nurse quickly ceases stimulation when signs of fatigue appear and demonstrates to the parents the need to be aware of newborn cues of fatigue and to wait for periods of alertness for contact and stimulation. The nurse is also responsible for assessing the woman's comfort and latching-on techniques, if breastfeeding, or bottle-feeding techniques.

PROMOTION OF SKIN INTEGRITY

Newborn skin care, including bathing, is important for the health and appearance of the individual newborn and for infection con-

Figure 30–6 ◆ The umbilical cord base is carefully cleaned.

trol within the nursery. Ongoing skin care involves cleansing the buttock and perianal areas with fresh water and cotton, or with a mild soap and water, with diaper changes. If commercial baby wipes are used, those without alcohol should be selected. Wipes that are perfume- and latex-free are also available.

The umbilical cord is assessed for signs of bleeding or infection. Removal of the cord clamp within 24 to 48 hours of birth reduces the chance of tension injury to the area. Keeping the umbilical stump clean and dry can reduce the chance for infection (Figure 30–6 ◆). Many types of routine cord care are practiced, including the use of triple-dye or an antimicrobial agent such as bacitracin or application of 70% alcohol to the cord stump. These practices are largely based on tradition rather than current research findings. The skin absorption and toxicity of triple-dye agents in newborns have not been carefully studied (AAP & ACOG, 2002). Recent studies have shown that alcohol may not be helpful in promoting drying or preventing infection. Folding the diaper down to prevent coverage of the cord stump can prevent contamination of the area and promote drying. The nurse is responsible for cord care per agency policy. It is also the nurse's responsibility to instruct parents in caring for the cord and observing for signs and symptoms of infection after discharge, such as foul smell, redness and drainage, localized heat and tenderness, or bleeding.

PROMOTION OF SAFETY

Safety of the newborn is paramount. It is essential that the nurse and other caregivers verify the identity of the newborn by comparing the numbers and names on the identification bracelets of mother and newborn before giving a baby to a parent. Another form of identification band or sensor attached to the umbilical cord has a built-in sensor unit that sounds an alarm if the baby is transported beyond set birthing unit boundaries. Individual birthing units should practice safety measures to prevent infant abduction and provide information to parents regarding their role in this area. Parental measures to prevent abduction include the following:

- Checking that identification bands are in place as they care for their infant and, if missing, asking that they be replaced immediately

MediaLink   Care Plan Activity: Infant Care During Transition

- Allowing only people with proper birthing unit identification to remove their baby from their room
- Returning baby to nursery or having baby accompany the parent when leaving the room
- Reporting the presence of any suspicious people on the birthing unit

PREVENTION OF COMPLICATIONS

Newborns are at continued risk for the complications of hemorrhage, late-onset cardiac symptoms, jaundice, and infection. Pallor may be an early sign of hemorrhage and must be reported to the physician. The newborn is placed on a cardiorespiratory monitor to permit continuous assessment. Several newborn conditions or procedures such as circumcision put the newborn at risk for bleeding. Cyanosis that is not relieved by oxygen administration requires emergency intervention, may indicate a congenital cardiac condition or shock, and requires immediate and ongoing assessment.

Infection in the nursery is best prevented by requiring that all personnel having direct contact with newborns scrub for 2 to 3 minutes from fingertips to and including elbows at the beginning of each shift. The hands must be washed with soap and rubbed vigorously for 15 seconds before and after contact with every newborn or after touching any soiled surface, such as the floor or one's hair or face. Parents are instructed to practice good handwashing and/or use of an antiseptic hand cleaner before touching the baby. They are also instructed that anyone holding the baby should wash hands as well, even after the family returns home. In some clinical settings family members are requested to wear a gown (preferably disposable) over their street clothes during contact with infants. These are good opportunities for the nurse to reinforce the efficacy of handwashing in preventing the spread of infection.

Jaundice in newborns is caused by the accumulation of the pigment *bilirubin* in the skin. Jaundice occurs in most newborn infants. Most jaundice is benign, but because of the potential toxicity of bilirubin, newborn infants must be monitored to identify those who might develop severe hyperbilirubinemia and, in rare cases, acute bilirubin encephalopathy or kernicterus (AAP, 2004). Current recommendations include obtaining a total serum bilirubin level in any infant who is visibly jaundiced in the first 24 hours of life, and obtaining either a serum or transcutaneous bilirubin level before discharge. Nomograms for evaluating risk factors based on bilirubin levels and age of infant are available.

CIRCUMCISION

Circumcision is a surgical procedure in which the prepuce, an epithelial layer covering the tip of the penis, is separated from the glans penis and excised. This permits exposure of the glans for easier cleaning.

Circumcision was originally a religious rite practiced by Jews and Muslims. The practice gained widespread cultural acceptance in the United States but is much less common in Europe. Many parents choose circumcision because they want the male child to have a physical appearance similar to that of the father or the majority of other children, or they may feel that it

is expected by society. Another commonly cited reason for circumcising newborn males is to prevent the need for anesthesia, hospitalization, pain, and trauma should the procedure be needed later in life (AAP & ACOG, 2002). During the prenatal period, the nurse ensures that parents have clear and current information regarding the risks and benefits of circumcision.

The parents make the decision about circumcision for their newborn male child. In most cases, the choice is based on cultural, social, and family tradition. To ensure informed consent, parents should be informed about possible long-term medical effects of circumcision and noncircumcision.

Current Recommendations

As in the past, recommendations regarding circumcision have varied. The 1999 AAP policy statement does not recommend routine circumcision but acknowledges that medical indications for circumcision still exist (AAP Task Force on Circumcision, 1999). The policy recommends that analgesia (e.g., EMLA cream, dorsal penile nerve block [DPNB], or subcutaneous ring block) be used during circumcision to decrease procedural pain (AAP & ACOG, 2002). The DPNB and subcutaneous ring block are the most effective options. If a circumcision is to be performed it should be done using the least painful method. Recent studies show that using oral sucrose for painful procedures can be effective in managing pain for newborns. "The unique response of the neonate to an oral sucrose solution allows for a very safe and effective measure in minimizing procedural pain" (Thompson, 2004).

Circumcision *should not be performed* if the newborn is premature or compromised, has a known bleeding problem, or is born with a genitourinary defect, such as hypospadias or epispadias, that may necessitate the use of the foreskin in future surgical repairs.

Nurse's Role

The nurse plays an essential role in providing parents with current information regarding the medical, social, and psychologic aspects of newborn circumcision. A well-informed nurse can allay parents' anxiety, answer questions, and provide an opportunity for parents to express their concerns. In order for parents to make a truly informed decision, they must be knowledgeable about the potential risks and outcomes of circumcision. Hemorrhage, infection, difficulty in voiding, separation of the edges of the circumcision, pain, and restlessness are early potential problems. Later there is the risk that the glans and urethral meatus can become irritated and inflamed from contact with ammonia from urine. Ulcerations and progressive stenosis may develop. Adhesions, progressive stenosis, entrapment of the penis, and damage to the urethra are all potential complications that could require surgical correction (AAP & ACOG, 2002).

The parents of an uncircumcised male infant require information from the nurse about good hygiene practices. They should be told that the foreskin and glans are two similar layers of cells that separate from each other. The separation process begins prenatally and is normally completed at between 3 and 5 years of age. In the process of separation, sterile sloughed cells build up between the layers. This buildup looks similar to the

RESEARCH IN PRACTICE

THE USE OF NON-NUTRITIVE SUCKING TO DECREASE THE PHYSIOLOGIC PAIN RESPONSE DURING NEONATAL CIRCUMCISION: A RANDOMIZED CONTROLLED TRIAL

What is this study about? The majority of male babies are circumcised in the United States. As would be expected, this procedure constitutes a stressful event for the newborn. While routine analgesia and local anesthesia are used for circumcision, a single form of pain control is unlikely to completely manage the pain associated with the procedure. This study sought to evaluate the pain-control effect of offering the baby a gloved finger to suck on while the procedure was underway. Described as non-nutritive sucking (NNS), the researchers sought to determine the effect of this simple intervention on neonatal pain, as reflected by several indicators.

How was this study done? Forty-four infants met the inclusion criteria, in that they were healthy term newborns. The babies were randomized into two groups. All the infants received oral Tylenol and a dorsal penile nerve block before the circumcision. The experimental group also received a gloved finger for the baby to suck on during the procedure. The primary physiologic outcomes that were measured were heart rate, pulse oximetry, crying time, and salivary cortisol levels. These measures were recorded every 4 minutes. In addition to the physical measures, a pain profile score was calculated, using the Premature Infant Pain Profile (PIPP). The circumcision procedure was filmed, and the PIPP score was calculated by a blinded rater after reviewing the film.

What were the results of the study? There was no difference in mean heart rate or pulse oximetry scores between the babies who were allowed to suck on a gloved finger during the procedure and those who were not. There was, however, a statistically significant decrease in salivary cortisol levels and crying time for those in the intervention group. The control group cried for longer periods of time and showed physiologic signs of stress when compared with those allowed to suck. Review of the actual size of the effect indicated that non-nutritive sucking took the children from a mild pain status to a minimum or no pain state.

What additional questions might I have? Would these results be similar in small or preterm babies, who may have a weaker suck reflex? Would NNS help neonates deal with pain from other types of procedures? Does a pacifier work as well as a gloved finger?

How can I use this study? Allowing an infant to suck on a gloved finger during stressful or potentially painful procedures is an efficient and inexpensive method of soothing the baby. This study demonstrated the value of this simple act in comforting the baby during a stressful time.

South, M., Strauss, R., South, A., Boggess, J., & Thorp, J. (2005). The use of non-nutritive sucking to decrease the physiologic pain response during neonatal circumcision: A randomized controlled trial. *American Journal of Obstetrics & Gynecology, 193,* 537–543.

smegma secreted after puberty, and it is harmless. Occasionally during the daily bath, the parents can gently test for retraction. If retraction has occurred, daily gentle washing of the glans with soap and water is sufficient to maintain adequate cleanliness. The parents should teach the child to incorporate this practice into his daily self-care activities. Most uncircumcised males have no difficulty doing so.

If circumcision is desired, the procedure should be performed after the newborn is well stabilized and has received his initial physical examination by a healthcare provider. The parents may also choose to have the circumcision done after discharge. However, they need to be advised that if the baby is older than 1 month, the current practice is to hospitalize him for the procedure.

Before a circumcision, the nurse ascertains that the physician has explained the procedure, determines whether the parents have any further questions about the procedure, and checks that the circumcision permit is signed. As with any surgical procedure, the identification band of the infant should be checked to verify his identity before the procedure begins. The nurse gathers the equipment and prepares the newborn by removing the diaper and placing him on a circumcision board or some other type of restraint, but restraining only the legs. In Jewish circumcision ceremonies, the infant is held by the father or grandfather and given wine before the procedure.

There are a variety of devices (Gumco clamp, Plastibel, Mogen clamp) used for circumcision (Figures 30–7 ◆ and 30–8 ◆), and all produce minimal bleeding. Therefore the nurse should make special note of infants with a family history of bleeding disorders or with mothers who took anticoagulants, including aspirin, prenatally. During the procedure, the nurse assesses the newborn's response. One important consideration is pain experienced by the newborn. A DPNB or ring block using 1% lidocaine without epinephrine or similar anesthetic significantly minimizes the pain and the shifts in behavioral patterns, such as crying, irritability, and erratic sleep cycles associated with circumcision. Other studies of pain control measures involve the use of topical anesthetic applied 60 to 90 minutes before prepuce removal and the use of sucrose pacifiers before and during the procedure, acetaminophen, and cryoanalgesia. Studies indicate that a combination of methods is most effective in reducing pain during circumcision (Razmus, Dalton, Wilson et al., 2004).

During the procedure, the nurse can provide comfort measures such as lightly stroking the baby's head, providing a pacifier, and talking to him. Following the circumcision, the infant should be held and comforted by a family member or the nurse. The nurse must be alert to any cues that these measures are overstimulating the newborn instead of comforting him. Such cues include turning away of the head, increased generalized body movement, skin color changes, hyperalertness, and hiccuping.

MEDIALINK Circumcision Resources

Figure 30–7 ◆ Circumcision using the Yellen or Gomco clamp. *A,* The prepuce is drawn over the cone. *B,* The clamp is applied. Pressure is maintained for 3 to 4 minutes, and then excess prepuce is cut away.

Figure 30–8 ◆ Circumcision using the Plastibel. The bell is fitted over the glans. A suture is tied around the bell's rim, and the excess prepuce is cut away. The plastic rim remains in place for 3 to 4 days until healing occurs. The bell may be allowed to fall off; it is removed if still in place after 8 days.

Ideally, the circumcision should be assessed for signs of hemorrhage and infection every 30 minutes for at least 2 hours following the procedure. It is important to observe for the first voiding after a circumcision to evaluate for urinary obstruction related to penile injury and/or edema. Petroleum and gauze are applied to the site immediately following the procedure to help prevent bleeding and can be used to protect the healing tissue afterward.

The nurse must also teach family members how to assess for unusual bleeding, how to respond if it is present, and how to care for the newly circumcised penis. Parents of babies circumcised with a method other than Plastibel should receive the following information:

Figure 30–9 ◆ Following circumcision, petroleum ointment may be applied to the site for the next few diaper changes.

- Apply petroleum ointment for the next few diaper changes to help prevent further bleeding (Figure 30–9 ◆).
- If bleeding does occur, apply light pressure with a sterile gauze pad to stop the bleeding within a short time. If this is not effective, contact the physician immediately, or take the baby to the healthcare provider's office.
- The glans normally has granulation tissue (a yellowish film) on it during healing. Continued application of a petroleum ointment (or ointment suggested by the healthcare provider) can help protect the granulation tissue that forms as the glans heals.
- Report to the care provider any signs or symptoms of infection, such as increasing swelling, pus drainage, and cessation of urination.
- When diapering, ensure that the diaper is not loose enough to cause rubbing with movement, or tight enough to cause pain.
- If the infant's care provider recommends oral analgesics, follow instructions for proper measuring and administration.

If the Plastibel is used, parents should receive information about normal appearance and how to observe for infection. The parents are informed that the Plastibel should fall off within 8 days. If it still remains after 8 days, they should consult with their physician. Though no ointments or creams should be used while the bell remains, use of petroleum ointment to protect granulation tissue may be useful afterward.

ENHANCEMENT OF PARENT-NEWBORN ATTACHMENT

Parent-newborn attachment is promoted by encouraging all family members to be involved with the new member of the family. Some specific interventions are examined in Chapters 24 ∞ and 35 ∞ and the accompanying Client Teaching: Enhancing Attachment. Infant massage is a common childcare practice in many parts of the world, especially Africa and Asia,

CLIENT TEACHING Enhancing Attachment

CLIENT GOALS   At the completion of teaching, the parents will be able to:

1. Demonstrate appropriate nurturing behaviors such as touching, bonding, talking to, kissing, and holding their baby.

2. Discuss the normal characteristics and emotional needs of the newborn.

3. List at least three comforting techniques.

TEACHING PLAN

CONTENT	TEACHING METHOD
• Present information on periods of reactivity and expected newborn responses.	Focus on open discussion.
• Describe normal physical characteristics of the newborn.	Present slides showing newborn characteristics.
• Explain the bonding process, its gradual development, and the reciprocal interactive nature of the process.	
• Discuss the infant's capabilities for interaction, such as nonverbal communication abilities. The nonverbal communications include movement, gaze, touch, facial expressions, and vocalizations—including crying. Emphasize that eye contact is considered one of the cardinal factors in developing infant-parent attachment and will be integrated with touching and vocal behaviors.	Show a video on the interactive capabilities of newborns.
• Explain that touching, including stroking, patting, massaging, and kissing, will progress to interactive touch between the parents and their infant; discuss their need to assimilate these behaviors into their daily routine with the baby.	Provide handouts, and use a doll to demonstrate behaviors.
• Describe and demonstrate comforting techniques, including the use of sound, swaddling, rocking, massage, and stroking.	Demonstrate the techniques and ask for a return demonstration.
• Describe the progression of the infant's behaviors as the infant matures, and the importance of the parents' consistent response to their infant's cues and needs.	Allow time for questions and discussion.
• Provide information about available pamphlets, videos, and support groups in the community.	

DOCUMENTATION	EVALUATION
The nurse should document the information that was given, the type of teaching method used, indicate if the parent performed nurturing behaviors such as touching and comfort techniques, and if verbal or written directions were given. Verbalization of understanding and clarification of any information should be documented. Safety issues and instructions on newborn physical characteristics and normal progression of infant behaviors were given.	Evaluate the learning by providing time for discussion, questions, and return demonstrations in the birthing unit, and during the postpartal return visit or home visit. Continue to observe the parents' positive interaction with their baby during the remainder of their stay in the birthing unit.

and has recently gained attention in the United States. Parents can be taught to use infant massage as a method to facilitate the bonding process and to reduce the stress and pain associated with teething, inoculations, constipation, and colic. Infant massage not only induces relaxation for the infant, but also provides a calming and "feel good" interaction for the parents that fosters the development of warm, positive relationships.

The nurse can discuss waking activities such as talking with the baby while making eye contact, holding the baby in an upright position (sitting or standing), gently bending the baby back and forth while grasping under the knees and supporting the head and back with the other hand, and gently rubbing the baby's hands and feet. Quieting activities may include swaddling the baby to increase a sense of security; using slow,

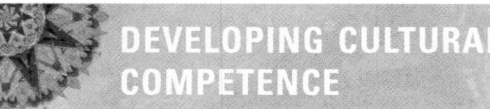

DEVELOPING CULTURAL COMPETENCE

INFANT NAMING IN KENYA

In Kenya, the naming of the child is an important event. Names are commonly selected to mirror important or current events. For example, an infant who is born while traveling may be given a name that means "wanderer" or "traveler." Other names may be chosen after a relative who is among the "living-dead" (deceased). It is believed that this results in a partial reincarnation of that relative, especially if the child has characteristics in common with that individual. It is also believed there is a connection between newborns and the spirit world. In some parts of the country, the name is chosen when the child is crying. Different names of the living-dead are called, and when the child quits crying when a particular name is called, that is the given name. In some areas, the name is given on the third day and is marked by a celebration with feasting and rejoicing. On the fourth day, the father of the child commonly hangs an iron necklace on the child's neck. It is at this time that the infant is considered a full human being and the connection with the spirit world is lost.

calming movements; and talking softly, singing, or humming to the baby (Figure 30–10 ◆). The nurse must also be aware of cultural variations in newborn care such as timing of naming of the newborn, giving compliments about the baby, and using good luck charms (see Developing Cultural Competence: Infant Naming in Kenya). The nurse plays a vital role in fostering parent-infant attachment. It is important to be sensitive to the cultural beliefs and values of the family.

Evaluation

When evaluating the nursing care provided during the newborn period, the nurse may anticipate the following outcomes:

- The baby's physiologic and psychologic integrity is supported.
- The newborn feeding pattern will be satisfactorily established.
- The parents express understanding of the bonding process and display attachment behaviors.

NURSING MANAGEMENT IN PREPARATION FOR DISCHARGE

Although the adjustment to parenting is a normal process, going home presents a critical transition for the family. The parents become the primary caregivers for the newborn and must provide a nurturing environment in which the emotional and physical needs of the newborn can be met. Nursing interventions focus on promoting health and preventing possible problems.

A Letter From Your Baby

Dear Parents:

I come to you a small, immature being with my own style and personality. I am yours for only a short time; enjoy me.

1. Please take time to find out who I am, how I differ from you, and how much I can bring you joy.

2. Please feed me when I am hungry. I never knew hunger in the womb, and clocks and time mean little to me.

3. Please hold, cuddle, kiss, touch, stroke, and croon to me. I was always held closely in the womb and was never alone before.

4. Please don't be disappointed when I am not the perfect baby that you expected, nor disappointed with yourselves that you are not the perfect parents.

5. Please don't expect too much from me as your newborn baby, or too much from yourself as a parent. Give us both six weeks as a birthday present—six weeks for me to grow, develop, mature, and become more stable and predictable, and six weeks for you to rest and relax and allow your body to get back to normal.

6. Please forgive me if I cry a lot. Bear with me and in a short time, as I mature, I will spend less and less time crying and more time socializing.

7. Please watch me carefully and I can tell you the things that soothe, console, and please me. I am not a tyrant who was sent to make your life miserable, but the only way I can tell you that I am not happy is with my cry.

8. Please remember that I am resilient and can withstand the many natural mistakes you will make with me. As long as you make them with love, you cannot ruin me.

9. Please take care of yourself and eat a balanced diet, rest, and exercise so that when we are together, you have the health and strength to take care of me.

10. Please take care of your relationship with others. Relationships that are good for you, support both you and me.

Although I may have turned your life upside down, please realize that things will be back to normal before long.

Thank you,

Your Loving Child

Figure 30–10 ◆ A letter from your baby.

Nursing Assessment and Diagnosis

When preparing for discharge, assess whether parents have realistic expectations of the newborn's behavior and the depth of their knowledge in caring for their newborn.

Nursing diagnoses that may apply to the newborn's family include the following:

- *Readiness for Enhanced Parenting* related to appropriate behavioral expectations for the newborn
- *Readiness for Enhanced Family Processes* related to integration of newborn into family unit or demands of newborn care and feeding

Planning and Implementation

PARENT TEACHING

To meet parent needs for information, the nurse who is responsible for the daily care of the mother and newborn should assume the primary responsibility for parent education. Nearly every contact with the parents presents an opportunity for sharing information that can facilitate their sense of competence in newborn care. The nurse also needs to recognize and respect the fact that there are many good ways to provide safe care. Unless their care methods are harmful to the newborn, the parents' methods of giving care should be reinforced rather than contradicted.

Caring for newborns in the hospital setting means that the nurse will have contact with patients from a wide variety of racial, religious, and cultural backgrounds. Though it may not be possible to be conversant with all cultures, the nurse can demonstrate cultural competence with both colleagues and patients when she or he:

- Shows respect for the inherent dignity of every human being, whatever their age, gender, religion
- Accepts the rights of individuals to choose their care provider, participate in care, and refuse care
- Acknowledges personal biases and prevents them from interfering with the delivery of quality care to persons of other cultures
- Recognizes cultural issues and interacts with clients from other cultures in culturally sensitive ways
- Incorporates cultural preferences, health beliefs and behaviors, and traditional practices into the management plan
- Develops client-appropriate educational materials that address the language and cultural beliefs of the client
- Accesses culturally appropriate resources to deliver care to clients from other cultures
- Assists clients to access quality care within a dominant culture
   (Green-Hernandez, Quinne, Falkenstern et al., 2004)

The nurse must be sensitive to the cultural beliefs and values of the family. (See Developing Cultural Competence: Examples of Cultural Beliefs and Practices Regarding Baby Care.)

The information that follows is provided to increase the nurse's knowledge of newborn care and is used to meet parents' needs for information. Parents may be familiar with handling and caring for infants, or this may be their first time to interact with a newborn. If they are new parents, the sensitive nurse gently teaches them by example and provides instructions geared to their needs and previous knowledge about the various aspects of newborn care.

The length of stay in the birthing unit for mother and baby after birth is often 48 hours or less. The challenge for the nurse is to use every opportunity to teach, guide, and support parents, fostering the parents' capabilities and confidence in caring for their newborn. Including mother-baby care and home care instruction on the night shift can help meet the teaching needs of early discharge parents.

The nurse observes how parents interact with their infant during feeding and caregiving activities. Even during a short stay, there will be opportunities for the nurse to provide information and evaluate whether the parents are comfortable with changing diapers and wrapping, handling, and feeding their newborn (Figure 30–11 ◆). Do both parents get involved in the infant's care? Is the mother depending on someone else to help her at home? Does the mother give excuses ("I am too tired," "My stitches hurt," or "I will learn later") for not wanting to be involved in her baby's care? As the family provides care, the nurse can enhance parental confidence by giving them positive feedback. If the family encounters problems, the nurse can express confidence in the family's abilities to master the new skill or information, suggest alternatives, and serve as a role model. All these considerations need to be taken into account when evaluating the educational needs of the parents.

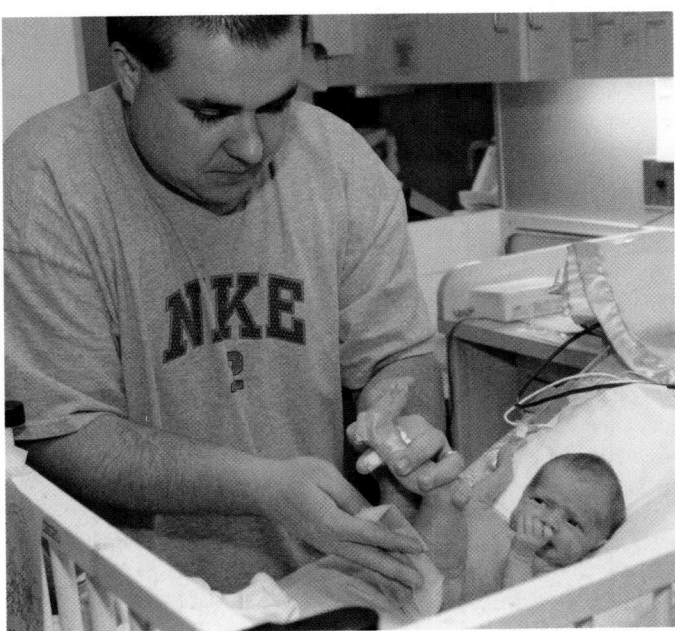

Figure 30–11 ◆ A father demonstrates competence and confidence in diapering his newborn daughter.

DEVELOPING CULTURAL COMPETENCE

EXAMPLES OF CULTURAL BELIEFS AND PRACTICES REGARDING BABY CARE*

Umbilical Cord

People of Latin American or Filipino cultural background may use an abdominal binder or bellyband to protect against dirt, injury, and umbilical hernia. They may also apply oils to the stump of the cord or tape metal to the umbilicus to ward off evil spirits.

People of northern European ancestry may expect a sterile cutting of the cord at birth. They may allow the stump to air-dry and discard the cord once it falls off.

Some Latin American cultures cauterize the stump with a hot flame, hot coal, or the like (World Health Organization [WHO], 1999).

In Kenya, women may express colostrum to the cord stump (WHO, 1999).

In Ecuador, the cord is left long in girls to prevent a small uterus and problems with childbirth (WHO, 1999).

Parent-Infant Contact

People of Asian ancestry may pick up the baby as soon as he or she cries, or they may carry the baby at all times.

Some Native Americans, notably the Navajos, may use cradle boards so the infant can be with the family even during work (Andrews, 2003).

Korean mothers may be reluctant to pick up or touch their infant, deferring infant care to the paternal grandmother (Schneiderman, 1996).

The Muslim father traditionally calls praise to Allah in the newborn's right ear and cleans the infant after birth (Hedayat, 2001).

Feeding

Some women of Asian heritage may breastfeed their babies for the first 1 to 2 years of life. Many Cambodian refugees practice breast-feeding on demand without restriction, or, if formula-feeding, provide a "comfort bottle" in between feedings (Rasbridge & Kulig, 1995).

People of Iranian heritage may breastfeed female babies longer than male babies. Some people of African ancestry may wean their babies after they begin to walk.

Most Korean mothers resist breastfeeding in the hospital, contending that they do not have "milk," and state that they will begin breastfeeding at home (Schneiderman, 1996).

Some Asians, Hispanics, Eastern Europeans, and Native Americans may delay breastfeeding because they believe colostrum is "bad" (D'Avanzo & Geissler, 2003).

Circumcision

People of Muslim and Jewish ancestry practice circumcision as a religious ritual (Ott, Al-Khashuri, & Al-Junaibi, 2003).

Many natives of Africa and Australia practice circumcision as a puberty rite.

Native Americans and people of Asian and Latin American cultures rarely perform circumcision.

Only 15% of the world's male population is circumcised.

Health and Illness

Some people from Latin American cultural backgrounds may believe that touching the face or head of an infant when admiring it will ward off the "evil eye." They may also neglect to cut the baby's nails to avoid nearsightedness and instead put mittens on the baby's hands to prevent scratching. They also may believe that fat babies are healthy (Andrews, 2003).

Some people of Asian heritage may not allow anyone to touch the baby's head without asking permission.

Some Orthodox Jews believe that saying the baby's name before the formal naming ceremony will harm the baby.

Some Asians and Haitians delay naming their infants (D'Avanzo & Geissler, 2003).

Some people of Vietnamese ancestry believe that cutting a baby's hair or nails will cause illness.

*NOTE: The information is meant only to provide examples of some of the behaviors that may be found within certain cultures. Not all members of a culture practice the behaviors described.

Several methods may be used to teach parents about newborn care. Daily newborn care videos or classes are a nonthreatening way to convey general information. Individual instruction is helpful to answer specific questions or to clarify an item that may have been confusing in class. Currently many birthing centers have 24-hour educational video channels or videos to be viewed in the mother's room on a variety of postpartum and newborn care issues.

CLINICAL TIP

For clients who are hearing-impaired, videotapes with information in both spoken and signed formats are most helpful. Also, birthing centers should have handouts available for families who do not speak English as well as either birthing center interpreters (not family members) or language interpreter phones.

One-to-one teaching while the nurse is in the mother's room is shown to be the most effective educational model. Both first-time and experienced postpartum mothers rate individual teaching as the most effective method of instruction. Individual instruction is helpful both to answer specific questions and to clarify something that the parents may have found confusing in the educational video. With shorter stays, most teaching unfortunately tends to focus on infant feeding and immediate physical needs of the mothers, with limited anticipatory guidance provided in other areas. (Table 30–3, "What Parents Need to Know about Newborn Care," illustrates a broad range of information important to share with new parents. These topics are discussed in more detail next.)

With the new life come new rhythms. Or perhaps I should say no rhythms. The day is divided into phone calls, meals eaten on the run,

Table 30–3   WHAT PARENTS NEED TO KNOW ABOUT NEWBORN CARE

Immediate Safety Measures for the Newborn

Watch for excessive mucus: use bulb syringe to remove mucus.

Have baby sleep on his or her back in crib or in someone's arms.

Voiding and Stool Characteristics and Patterns

Urine is straw to amber color without foul smell. Small amounts of uric acid crystals are normal in first days of life (may be mistaken by parents as blood in diaper because of reddish "brick dust" appearance).

At least 6 to 10 wet diapers a day after the first few days of life.

Normal progression of stool changes: (1) meconium (thick, tarry, dark green); (2) transitional stools (thin, brown to green); (3a) breastfed infant: yellow gold, soft or mushy stools; (3b) formula-fed infant: pale yellow, formed and pasty stools.

Only 1 to 2 stools a day for formula-fed baby.

Six to 10 small, loose yellow stools per day or only one stool every few days after breastfeeding is well established (after about 1 month).

Cord Care

Wash hands with clean water and soap before and after care. Keep the cord dry and exposed to air or loosely covered with clean clothes. (If cultural custom demands binding of the abdomen, a sanitary method such as the use of a clean piece of gauze can be recommended.)

Clean cord and skin around base with a cotton swab or cotton ball. Clean 2 to 3 times a day or with each diaper change. Touching the cord, applying unclean substances to it, and applying bandages should be avoided. Do not give tub baths until cord falls off in 7 to 14 days.

Fold diapers below umbilical cord to air-dry the cord (contact with wet or soiled diapers slows the drying process and increases the possibility of infection).

Check cord each day for any odor, oozing of greenish yellow material, or reddened areas around the cord. Expect tenderness around the cord and darkening and shriveling of cord. Report to healthcare provider any signs of infection.

Normal changes in cord: Cord should look dark and dry up before falling off. A small drop of blood may present when cord falls off.

Never pull the cord or attempt to loosen it.

Care Required for Circumcision and Uncircumcised Infants

Circumcision Care
Squeeze soapy water over circumcision site once a day.

Rinse area off with warm water and pat dry.

Apply small amount of petroleum jelly (unless a Plastibel is in place) with each diaper change.

Fasten diaper over penis snugly enough so that it does not move and rub the tender glans.

Because the glans is sensitive, avoid placing baby on his stomach for the first day after the procedure.

Check for any foul-smelling drainage or bleeding at least once a day.

Let Plastibel fall off by itself (about 8 days after circumcision).

Plastibel should not be pulled off.

Light, sticky, yellow drainage (part of healing process) may form over head of penis.

Uncircumcised Care
Clean uncircumcised penis with water during diaper changes and with bath.

Do not force foreskin back over the penis; foreskin will retract normally over time (may take 3 to 5 years).

Techniques for Waking and Quieting Newborns

Techniques for Waking Baby
Loosen clothing, change diaper.

Hand-express milk onto baby's lips.

Talk with baby while making eye contact.

Hold baby in upright position (sitting or standing).

Have baby do sit-ups (gently and rhythmically bend baby back and forth while grasping the baby under his or her knees and supporting baby's head and back with your other hand).

Play patty-cake with baby.

Stimulate rooting reflex (brush one cheek with hand or nipple).

Increase skin contact (gently rub hands and feet).

Techniques for Quieting Baby

Check for soiled diaper.

Swaddle or bundle baby (bring arms and legs into midline, which increases sense of security).

Hold swaddled baby upright against mid-chest, supporting bottom and back of head. Baby can hear heartbeat, feel warmth, and hear your softly spoken words or calming sounds.

Use slow, calming movements with baby.

Softly talk, sing, or hum to baby.

Signs of Illness and Use of Thermometer

See Table 30–4: When Parents Should Call Their Healthcare Provider.

---

visitors who've come to see the baby, trips from hospital to home to walk the dog.

The new life brings new thoughts, new perceptions of the world.

Why don't men take paternity leave? Why is time off, if any, basically reserved for women? Why don't we take a month off? In those first few chaotic days, filled with ecstasy and fear, the family needs to be together. Being together in times of joy and sadness is what a family is. A month's distance from the office grind, from the bottom line, could not help but create a healthier world.

~DENNIS DONZIGER, *DADDY*~

GENERAL INSTRUCTIONS FOR NEWBORN CARE

How to pick up a newborn is one of the first concerns of anyone who has not had experience. The newborn is easily picked up by sliding one hand under the neck and shoulders and the other hand under the buttocks or between the legs, then gently lifting the newborn. This technique provides security and support for the head (which the baby is unable to consistently support until 3 or 4 months of age).

The nurse can be an excellent role model for families in the area of safety. Safety topics include proper positioning of the newborn on the back to sleep and correct use of the bulb syringe (discussed shortly). The baby should never be left alone anywhere but in the crib. The mother is reminded that while she and the newborn are together in the birthing unit, she should never leave the baby alone for security reasons and because newborns spit up frequently the first day or two after birth.

Demonstrating a bath (see Chapter 36 ∞), cord care, and temperature assessment is the best way for the nurse to provide information on these topics to parents. Parents should be told to

MEDIALINK
Case Study: Newborn Care

call their healthcare provider if redness, foul odor, bright red bleeding, or greenish yellow drainage occurs at the cord site or if the area remains unhealed 2 to 3 days after the cord stump has sloughed off. Current evidence does not support the routine application of topical antimicrobials to the drying cord (WHO, 1999). See Table 30–3: What Parents Need to Know about Newborn Care.

The nurse demonstrates and reviews the taking of an axillary or tympanic temperature with the family and discourages the use of mercury thermometers. It is important that families understand the differences and know how to select a thermometer. The newborn's temperature needs to be taken only when signs of illness are present. Parents are advised to call their physician or pediatric nurse practitioner immediately if they observe any signs of illness.

NASAL AND ORAL SUCTIONING

Most newborns are obligatory nose breathers for the first months of life. They generally maintain air passage patency by coughing or sneezing. During the first few days of life, however, the newborn has increased mucus, and gentle suctioning with a bulb syringe may be indicated. The nurse can demonstrate the use of the bulb syringe in the nose and mouth and have the parents do a return demonstration. The parents should repeat this demonstration before discharge so they will feel more confident and comfortable with the procedure. Care should be taken to apply only gentle suction to prevent nasal bleeding.

To suction the newborn, the bulb syringe is compressed and the tip is placed in the nostril. The nurse or parent must take care not to occlude the passageway. The bulb is permitted to reexpand slowly by releasing the compression on the bulb (Figure 30–12 ◆). The bulb syringe is removed from the nostril, and drainage is then compressed out of the bulb onto a tissue. The bulb syringe may also be used in the mouth if the newborn is spitting up and unable to handle the excess secretions. The bulb is compressed, the tip of the bulb syringe is placed about 1 inch to one side of the newborn's mouth, and compression is re-

leased. This draws up the excess secretions. The procedure is repeated on the other side of the mouth. The roof of the mouth and back of the throat are avoided because suction in these areas might stimulate the gag reflex. The bulb syringe should be washed in warm, soapy water and rinsed in warm water daily and as needed after use. Rinsing with a half-strength white vinegar solution followed by clear water may help to extend the useful life of the bulb syringe by inhibiting bacterial growth. A bulb syringe should always be kept near the newborn. New parents and nurses who are inexperienced with babies may fear that the baby will choke and may be relieved if they know how to take action if such an event occurs. They should be advised to turn the newborn's head to the side or hold the newborn with his or her head down as soon as there is any indication of gagging or vomiting and to use the bulb syringe as needed.

Some infants may have transient edema of the nasal mucosa following suctioning of the airway after birth. The nurse can demonstrate the use of normal saline to loosen secretions, and instruct parents in the gentle and moderate use of the bulb syringe to avoid further irritation of the mucous membranes. If parents will be using humidifiers at home, they should be instructed to follow the manufacturer's cleaning instructions carefully so that molds, spores, and bacteria from a dirty humidifier do not enter the baby's environment.

CLINICAL TIP

You'll find that left-handed people tend to hold the baby over their right shoulder, and right-handed people do the opposite. This keeps the dominant hand free. However, most health personnel wear their name tags on the left side. To avoid scratching the baby's face, wear your name tag on the same side as your dominant hand.

SWADDLING THE NEWBORN

Swaddling (wrapping) helps the newborn maintain body temperature, provides a feeling of closeness and security, and may be effective in quieting a crying baby by having the newborn's hands near the mouth to allow for sucking (Roach, 2004). A blanket is placed on the crib (or secure surface) in the shape of a diamond. The top corner of the blanket is folded down slightly, and the newborn's body is placed with the head at the upper edge of the blanket. The right corner of the blanket is wrapped around the infant and tucked under the left side (not too tightly—newborns need a little room to move and to allow for hands to get to the mouth). The bottom corner is then pulled up to the chest, and the left corner is wrapped around the baby's right side (Figure 30–13 ◆). The nurse can show this wrapping technique to a new mother so she will feel more skilled in handling her baby.

SLEEP AND ACTIVITY

The National Institute of Child Health and Human Development and the American Academy of Pediatrics recommend that healthy term infants be placed on their back to sleep. Parents are taught the importance of following "Back to Sleep Guidelines" to reduce the incidence of sudden infant death syndrome (SIDS). Though infants may need to be placed on their sides initially because of copious or thick secretions, placing them on their backs in the newborn period serves to educate parents re-

Figure 30–12 ◆ Nasal and oral suctioning. The bulb is compressed, the tip is placed in either the mouth or the nose, and the bulb is released.
SOURCE: © Stella Johnson (www.stellajohnson.com)

Figure 30–13 ◆ Steps in wrapping a baby.

Figure 30–14 ◆ Infant car restraint for use from birth to about 12 months of age.

garding infant positioning. Studies indicate that parents position their babies in the same positions they observe in the hospital setting, so nurses must demonstrate this behavior to reduce the risk of SIDS. If exceptions are warranted, these should be explained to families so they do not misinterpret what they observe. The placement of babies in a prone position during wakeful play sessions should be encouraged as well (National Institute of Child Health and Human Development, 2002).

Perhaps nothing is more individual to each baby than the sleep-activity cycle. It is important for the nurse to recognize the individual variations of each newborn and to assist parents as they develop sensitivity to their infant's communication signals and rhythms of activity and sleep (Roach, 2004). See Chapter 29 ∞ for more detailed discussion of the sleep-activity cycle.

CAR SAFETY CONSIDERATIONS

Half the children killed or injured in automobile accidents could have been protected by the use of a federally approved car seat. Newborns should go home from the birthing unit in a car seat adapted to fit newborns (Figure 30–14 ◆). Babies should never be in the front seat of a car equipped with a passenger-side air bag. The safest spot in any car is the middle of the back seat. The car seat should be positioned to face the rear of the car until the baby is a year old or weighs 20 pounds (9.09 kg) (AAP Committee on Injury and Poison Prevention, 2002). Nurses need to ensure that all parents are knowledgeable about the benefits of child safety seat use and proper installation. Nurses can encourage parents to have their infant safety seats checked by local groups trained specifically for that purpose. The Seat Check Initiative provides locations and information about child safety seats.

NEWBORN SCREENING AND IMMUNIZATION PROGRAM

Before the newborn and mother are discharged from the birthing unit, the nurse informs the parents about **newborn screening tests** and tells them when to return to the birthing center or clinic

if further tests are needed. Some of the disorders that can be identified from a few drops of blood obtained by a heel stick are cystic fibrosis, galactosemia, congenital adrenal hyperplasia, hypothyroidism, maple syrup urine disease (MSUD), sickle cell trait, biotinidase deficiency, phenylketonuria (PKU), and hemoglobinopathies.

The Expanded Newborn Screening Program allows parents to have their babies screened for more than 20 disorders. Early newborn discharge puts infants at risk for delayed or even missed diagnosis of PKU and congenital hypothyroidism because of decreased sensitivity of screening before 24 hours of age. Newborns should be retested by 2 weeks of age if the first test was done before 24 hours of age. New technology is quickly increasing the number of metabolic and other disorders that can be detected in the newborn period. Although controversy exists over the need for such comprehensive testing, many states already have programs in place or will soon have programs that test for more than 20 additional disorders through a process known as Tandem Mass Spectrometry (Banta-Wright & Steiner, 2004).

Hearing loss is found in 1 to 3 per 1000 infants in the normal newborn population (Thureen, Deacon, Hernandez et al., 2005). The AAP Task Force on Newborn and Infant Hearing endorses the Joint Committee on Infant Hearing recommendations of implementing universal newborn screening before discharge in all hospitals providing obstetric services (AAP, 1999).

Immunization programs against the hepatitis B virus during the newborn period and infancy are in place in many states, at least 20 countries, and high-incidence areas such as American Samoa. Universal vaccination of infants is recommended. Infants should receive the first dose of hepatitis B (Hep B) vaccine at birth to 2 months of age. The second dose should be at least 1 month after the first dose. The third dose should be

EVIDENCE-BASED PRACTICE

REDUCING THE RISK OF SUDDEN INFANT DEATH SYNDROME

Clinical Question

What actions are recommended to reduce the risk of sudden infant death syndrome (SIDS) in infants?

The Evidence

The American Academy of Pediatrics appointed five MDs and a PhD to a task force to study SIDS prevention methods and make evidence-based revisions to the 2000 recommendations. The 2000 recommendations are widely believed to be responsible for a dramatic decrease in SIDS in the past decade. The task force was asked to determine if the evidence continues to support the effectiveness of the original recommendations. The members reviewed 122 research articles that met strict criteria for methodological quality and relevance.

What Is Effective?

The supine position continues to be the optimal position for reducing the risk of SIDS in infants younger than 6 months. However, while the original recommendations identified any nonprone position as optimal, current evidence reveals that the supine position confers the lowest risk. The side-lying position, while associated with lower SIDS rates than the prone position, has higher risk than the supine position. If the side-lying position must be used, then it is recommended that the arm be brought forward to prevent the infant from rolling to prone. A firm sleep mattress covered only with a sheet is best; the baby should be dressed so that he or she is warm but not overheated. Soft pillows, toys, and bedding should be kept out of the crib. The highest risk was among babies placed in the prone position on soft bedding. Although *room* sharing with the parents is associated with a lower risk of SIDS, *bed* sharing is associated with a higher risk. Although the infant can be brought into the bed for breastfeeding or comforting, the infant should be returned to the crib as soon as possible. The baby should not be brought into the bed at all if the parents are overly tired, and sleeping with the infant on a couch is risky and never recommended. The task force recommends that the infant sleep in a crib in the parents' room for the first 6 months. A new—and controversial—recommendation is the use of a pacifier. Although the exact mechanism of action is unknown, it is thought that a pacifier lowers the infant's arousal threshold. The evidence that pacifier use is associated with a lower SIDS rate is compelling, and the evidence that a pacifier causes harm in the first 6 months is not. The task force recommends that the pacifier be initiated at 1 month, after breastfeeding is firmly established, at the point when the risk of SIDS begins to rise. The original recommendations against maternal smoking, smoking in the infant's environment, and overheating the infant were reiterated in these recommendations.

What Is Unclear?

There are commercial devices available that claim to alert the parents if a child stops breathing. These devices have not been adequately tested for effectiveness, and the task force could find no evidence that use of these devices is associated with a lower SIDS rate. Breastfeeding as a strategy to reduce SIDS was also not supported. Although SIDS is lower in infants who are breastfed, the effect appears to be due to factors associated with breastfeeding (e.g., maternal nonsmoking), not the breastfeeding itself. There does appear to be an overall increase in the incidence of plagiocephaly, and although many have attributed this change to the use of the prone sleeping position, there was no evidence of a causal effect. Whether the increase is due to an actual increase in incidence or an increase in reporting plagiocephaly was unclear. Many newborn nurseries continue to place newborns on their side, under the assumption that this practice helps the newborn clear the lungs of amniotic fluid more quickly. There is no evidence that this is the case.

Best Practice

Newborns and infants should be placed in the supine position any time they are in a crib. Mothers tend to copy the practices at home that they observe from healthcare practitioners, particularly if the contact is extensive (such as with preterm infants) so this practice should be conscientiously observed. Advise new parents to keep their infant in a crib with a firm mattress in their bedroom until the infant is 6 months old, and to keep soft bedding, pillows, and stuffed animals out of the crib. Suggest the use of a pacifier when the infant is put to bed, but advise the parents to clean the pacifier frequently and replace it often. Wean the infant from the pacifier after 6 months of age, when the risk of SIDS declines dramatically. As with the existing recommendations, counsel the parents to keep the infant in a smoke-free environment that is not overly warm. Inform the parents that there continues to be no evidence suggesting a causal relationship between immunizations and SIDS.

Critical Thinking

How can you devise a teaching plan that will ensure that all new parents are aware of the recommendations for prevention of SIDS? How can you model these behaviors consistently in the newborn nursery and the neonatal intensive care unit?

REFERENCES: American Academy of Pediatrics Task Force on Sudden Infant Death Syndrome. (2005). The changing concept of sudden infant death syndrome: Diagnostic coding shifts, controversies regarding the sleeping environment, and new variables to consider in reducing risk. *Pediatrics, 116,* 1245–1255.

Haupt, F., Omojokum, O., & Siadaty, M. (2005). Do pacifiers reduce the risk of sudden infant death syndrome? A meta-analysis. *Pediatrics, 116,* E716.

McCartney, P. (2006). New recommendations to reduce the risk of sudden infant death syndrome. *American Journal of Maternal/Child Nursing, 31*(2), 128.

DRUG GUIDE   Hepatitis B Vaccine (Engerix-B, Recombivax HB)

Overview of Neonatal Action

Recombinant hepatitis B vaccine is used as a prophylactic treatment against all subtypes of the hepatitis B virus. It provides passive immunization for newborns of HBsAg-negative and HBsAg-positive mothers. Hepatitis B can be transmitted across the placenta, but most newborns are infected during birth.

The vaccine is produced from baker's yeast and plasmid containing the HBsAg gene.

Hepatitis B (thimerosal free) vaccine contains more than 95% HBsAg protein and is an inactivated (noninfective) product. Universal immunization is recommended.

Infants of HBsAg-positive mothers should concurrently receive 0.5 mL of hepatitis B immunoglobulin (HBIG) prophylaxis at separate injection sites (CDC, 2004).

Pregnancy Risk Category: C

Route, Dosage, Frequency

The first dose of 0.5 mL (10 mcg) is given intramuscularly into the anterolateral thigh within 12 hours of birth for infants born to HBsAg-positive mothers. The second dose of vaccine is given at 1 month of age and followed by a final dose at 6 months of age.

Infants born to HBsAg-negative mothers receive their first dose of vaccine at birth, the second dose at 1 to 2 months, and the third dose at 6 to 18 months (Thureen et al., 2005).

Infants whose mother's HBsAg status is unknown should receive the same doses of vaccine as infants born to HBsAg-positive mothers.

Neonatal Side Effects

The only common side effect is soreness at the injection site. Occasionally, there is erythema, swelling, warmth, and induration at the injection site; irritability; or a low-grade fever (37.7C [99.8F]).

Nursing Considerations

Delay administration during active infection; the vaccine will not prevent infection during its incubation period.
- The vaccine should be used as supplied. Do not dilute. Shake well.
- Do not inject intravenously or interdermally.
- Monitor for adverse reactions. Monitor temperature closely.
- Have epinephrine available to treat possible allergic reactions.
- Responsiveness to the vaccine is age dependent. Preterm infants weighing less than 1000 g have lower seroconversion rates. Consider delaying the first dose until the infant is term postconceptual age (PCA) or use a 4-dose schedule.

administered at least 4 months after the first dose and at least 2 months after the second dose, but not before 6 months of age (Centers for Disease Control and Prevention [CDC], 2004). See the Drug Guide: Hepatitis B Vaccine (Engerix-B, Recombivax HB). Parents need to be advised whether their birthing center provides newborn hepatitis vaccination so that an adequate follow-up program can be set in motion.

Early discharge has affected both the timing of newborn metabolic screening tests and the acquisition of subsequent immunization. For example, the accuracy of the test for PKU is directly related to the newborn's age. The likelihood of detecting PKU increases as the infant grows older, and the infant must be at least 24 hours old for a valid test. A second test is required in most states, usually between 1 week and 1 month of age, to minimize the chance of a positive child going undetected.

The nurse should teach the family all necessary caregiving methods before discharge. A checklist may be helpful to determine whether the teaching has been completed and to verify the parents' knowledge on leaving the birthing unit (Figure 30–15 ◆). The nurse needs to review all areas for understanding or any outstanding questions with the mother and father, without rushing, taking time to answer all queries. Any concerns of the parents or nurse are noted.

COMMUNITY-BASED NURSING CARE

The nurse discusses with parents ways to meet their newborn's needs, ensure safety, and appreciate the newborn's unique characteristics and behaviors. By assisting parents in establishing links with their community-based healthcare provider, the nurse can get the new family off to a good start. Parents also need to know the signs of illness, how to reach the pediatrician or after-

Table 30–4   WHEN PARENTS SHOULD CALL THEIR HEALTHCARE PROVIDER

Temperature above 38C (100.4F) axillary or below 36.6C (97.8F) axillary

Continual rise in temperature

More than one episode of forceful vomiting or frequent vomiting over a 6-hour period

Refusal of two feedings in a row

Lethargy (listlessness), difficulty in awakening baby

Cyanosis (bluish discoloration of skin) with or without a feeding

Absence of breathing longer than 20 seconds

Inconsolable infant (quieting techniques are not effective) or continuous high-pitched cry

Discharge or bleeding from umbilical cord, circumcision, or any opening (except vaginal mucus or pseudomenstruation)

Two consecutive green watery or black stools or increased frequency of stools

No wet diapers for 18 to 24 hours or fewer than six to eight wet diapers per day after 4 days of age

Development of eye drainage

hours clinic, and the importance of follow-up after discharge. See Table 30–4. Parents should also check with their clinician for advice about over-the-counter medications to be kept in the medicine cabinet.

The family should have the care provider's phone number, address, and any specific instructions. Having the birthing unit or nursery phone number is also reassuring to a newborn's family. They are encouraged to call with questions. Follow-up calls lend added support by providing another opportunity for parents to have their questions answered.

MEDIALINK   Application: Newborn Screening Tests

FOR NURSES
ONLY

NURSERY TEACHING CHECKLIST

Please read the *Mother/Baby* information booklet given to you after birth. After reading it, please go through the following list and check whether you understand each topic or need to know more.

		I know this already	Doesn't apply to me	I need to know more	Taught/ reviewed/ demonstrated
Baby Care	What to do if baby is choking or gagging				
	Safety				
	How to do skin care/cord care				
	How to take care of the circumcision or genital area				
	How to know if my baby is sick and what to do				
	What is jaundice and how to detect it				
	Use of thermometer				
	Use of bulb syringe				
	How and when to burp baby				
	Newborn behavior: crying/comforting				
	How to position baby after feeding				
	What does demand scheduling mean?				
Breastfeeding	I attended breastfeeding class/watched breastfeeding video	YES ☐ NO ☐			
	How to position baby for feeding				
	How to get baby to latch on to my nipple properly				
	When and how long to breastfeed				
	Removal of baby from my nipple				
	What is the supply and demand concept?				
	What is the let-down reflex?				
	When does breast milk come in?				
	Supplementing				
	Proper diet for breastfeeding mothers				
	Prevention and comfort measures for sore nipples				
	Prevention and comfort measures for engorgement				
	When and how to use a breast pump				
	How to express milk by hand				
	How to go back to work and continue to breastfeed				
Bottle-Feeding	How to feed my baby a bottle				
	Reasons for NOT propping bottles				
	How to clean nipple/bottle				
	How to prepare formula				
	What formula should my baby drink				
Safety	**Use of infant car seat**				
	Back to Sleep				
	Shaken Baby Syndrome				

Other information:

_____

_____

_____

_____

_____

I have received and understand the instructions given on the above topics.

_____   _____
MOTHER'S SIGNATURE   DATE

Videos viewed/ Literature given:

_____

Language Spoken by Mother:

☐ English ☐ Spanish ☐ Other _____

Interpreter Used? ☐ Yes ☐ No ☐ Family Interprets

Nurse's Signature(s):

_____

_____

_____

Figure 30–15 ◆ An infant teaching checklist is completed by the time of discharge.

SOURCE: Adapted from Presbyterian/St. Luke's Medical Center, Denver, CO.

Some institutions have initiated postpartum and/or newborn follow-up visits 48 to 72 hours after birth when the family is unable to visit their primary care physician within that time period (Lieu, Braverman, Escobar et al., 2000). The newborn visit focuses on normal newborn care, assessment for hyperbilirubinemia (jaundice), extreme weight loss, feeding problems, and knowledge deficits related to newborn care and feeding within the family unit.

Routine well-baby visits should be scheduled with the clinic, pediatric nurse practitioner, or physician. Regardless of the type of follow-up services available in the community, the nurse contributes to the newborn's health by stressing the importance of routine care and by helping families who have no follow-up plans to connect to local resources for care.

Evaluation

When evaluating the nursing care provided during the newborn period, the nurse may anticipate the following outcomes:

- The parents demonstrate safe techniques for caring for their newborn.
- The parents verbalize developmentally appropriate behavioral expectations of their newborn and knowledge of community-based newborn follow-up care.

CHAPTER REVIEW

FOCUS YOUR STUDY

- The overall goal of newborn nursing care is to provide comprehensive care while promoting the establishment of a well-functioning family unit.
- The period immediately following birth, during which adaptation to extrauterine life occurs, requires close monitoring to identify any deviations from normal.
- Nursing goals during the first 4 hours after birth (admission and transitional period) are to maintain a clear airway, maintain a neutral thermal environment, prevent hemorrhage and infection, initiate oral feedings, and facilitate attachment.
- The newborn is routinely given prophylactic vitamin K to prevent possible hemorrhagic disease of the newborn.
- Prophylactic eye treatment for *Neisseria gonorrhoeae* is legally required on all newborns.
- Nursing goals in daily newborn care include maintaining cardiopulmonary function, maintaining a neutral thermal environment, promoting adequate hydration and nutrition, preventing complications, promoting safety, and enhancing attachment and family knowledge of child care.
- Essential daily care includes assessing vital signs, weight, overall color, intake, output, umbilical cord and circumcision, newborn nutrition, parent education, and attachment.
- Following a circumcision, the newborn must be observed closely for signs of bleeding, inability to void, and signs of infection.
- Signs of illness in newborns include temperature above 38C (100.4F) axillary or below 36.6C (97.8F) axillary, more than one episode of forceful vomiting, refusal of two feedings in a row, lethargy, cyanosis with or without a feeding, and absence of breathing for longer than 20 seconds.
- Newborn screening for congenital hypothyroidism and phenylketonuria may be done on all newborns in the first 1 to 3 days.

EXPLORE MediaLink

http://www.prenhall.com/davidson

NCLEX review questions, case studies, and other interactive resources for this chapter can be found on the Web Site at http://www.prenhall.com/davidson. Click on "Chapter 30" to select the activities for this chapter.

For tutorials including animations and videos, more NCLEX review questions, and an audio glossary, access the accompanying Prentice Hall Nursing MediaLink DVD-ROM in this book.

PRENTICE HALL NURSING MEDIALINK DVD-ROM

Audio Glossary

NCLEX Review

Videos: *Newborn Care; Through the Eyes of a Nurse—Welcoming the New Arrival at the Postpartal Visit*

COMPANION WEBSITE

Additional NCLEX Review

Case Study: *Newborn Care*

Care Plan Activity: *Infant Care During Transition*

Applications: *Circumcision; Newborn Screening Tests*

Critical Thinking

CRITICAL THINKING IN ACTION

INSTRUCTING THE MOTHER IN CARE OF HER NEWBORN

View the Critical Thinking in Action video in Chapter 30 of the DVD-ROM. Then answer the questions that follow.

Alice Fine, age 32, G1, spontaneously delivers a 7.25-pound baby girl over a median episiotomy. The baby's Apgars are 7 and 9 at 1 and 5 minutes. The baby is suctioned, stimulated, and given free-flow oxygen at birth. As the nurse on duty, you admit baby Fine to the newborn nursery, place her under a radiant heater, and perform a newborn assessment. You obtain the vital signs of temperature 97F, heart rate 128, respiration 55. A physical exam demonstrates no abnormalities, and you note that there were no significant problems with the pregnancy, the mother's blood type is A positive, and she plans to bottle-feed. You monitor the baby until her vital signs are stable and then take her to the mother's room for her first bottle-feeding at 60 minutes old.

1. How would you review measures to promote the safety of the newborn from abduction?

2. How would you explain the technique to suction the newborn with a bulb syringe?

3. Describe the care of the newborn's cord.

4. How would you review bottle-feeding with the mother?

REFERENCES

American Academy of Pediatrics (AAP). (1999). Newborn and infant hearing loss: Detection and intervention. *Pediatrics, 103,* 527–530.

American Academy of Pediatrics (AAP) Clinical Practice Guideline. (2004). Management of hyperbilirubinemia in the newborn infant 35 or more weeks of gestation. *Pediatrics, 114*(1), 297–316.

American Academy of Pediatrics (AAP) Committee on Fetus and Newborn & American College of Obstetricians and Gynecologists (ACOG) Committee on Obstetrics. (2002). *Guidelines for perinatal care* (5th ed.). Evanston, IL: Author.

American Academy of Pediatrics (AAP) Committee on Fetus and Newborn. (2003). Controversies concerning vitamin K and the newborn. *Pediatrics, 112*(1), 191–192.

American Academy of Pediatrics (AAP) Committee on Injury and Poison Prevention. (2002). Selecting and using the most appropriate car safety seats for growing children: Guidelines for counseling parents. *Pediatrics, 109*(3), 550–553.

American Academy of Pediatrics (AAP) Task Force on Circumcision. (1999). Circumcision policy statement. *Pediatrics, 103*(3), 686–693.

Andrews, M. M. (2003). Transcultural perspectives in the nursing care of children and adolescents. In M. M. Andrews & J. S. Boyle (Eds.), *Transcultural concepts in nursing care* (4th ed., pp. 132–180). Philadelphia: Lippincott.

Banta-Wright, S., & Steiner, R. (2004). Tandem mass spectrometry in newborn screening: A primer for neonatal and perinatal nurses. *Journal of Perinatal and Neonatal Nursing, 18*(1), 41–58. Retrieved October 21, 2005, from http://web33.epnet.com/

Behring, A., Vezeau, T. M., & Fink, R. (2003). Timing of the newborn first bath: A replication. *Neonatal Network, 22*(1), 39–46.

Blackburn, S. T. (2003). *Maternal, fetal, & neonatal physiology: A clinical perspective.* St. Louis, MO: Saunders.

Centers for Disease Control and Prevention (CDC) Advisory Committee on Immunization Practices. (2004). *Recommended childhood and adolescent immunization schedule, United States 2004.* Retrieved September 20, 2004, from http://www.cdc.gov/NLP/acip

D'Avanzo, C. E., & Geissler, E. M. (2003). *Pocket guide to cultural assessment* (3rd ed.). St. Louis, MO: Mosby.

Green-Hernandez, G., Quinne, A., Falkenstern, S., Denman-Vitale, S., & Judge-Ellis, T. (2004, July/August). Making nursing care culturally competent. *Holistic Nursing Practice,* 215–218.

Hedayat, K. M. (2001). Issues in Islamic biomedical ethics: A primer for the pediatrician. *Pediatrics, 108*(4), 965–971.

Karl, D. J. (2004). Using principles of newborn behavioral state organization to facilitate breastfeeding. *American Journal of Maternal/Child Nursing, 29*(5), 292–298.

Klaus, M., & Klaus, P. (1985). *The amazing newborn.* Menlo Park, CA: Addison-Wesley.

Lieu, T. A., Braverman, P. A., Escobar, G. J., Fischer, A. F., Jensvold, N. G., & Capra, A. M. (2000). A randomized comparison of home and clinic follow-up visits after early postpartum hospital discharge. *Pediatrics, 105*(5), 1058–1065.

Medves, J. M., & O'Brien, B. (2004). The effect of bather and location of first bath on maintaining thermal stability in newborns. *Journal of Obstetric, Gynecologic, & Neonatal Nursing, 33*(2), 175–182.

National Institute of Child Health and Human Development. (2002). *Babies sleep best on their backs: Reduce the risk of sudden infant death syndrome.* Retrieved January 10, 2003, from http://www.NIH.gov

Ott, B., Al-Khashuri, J., & Al-Junaibi, S. (2003). Preventing ethical dilemmas: Understanding Islamic health care practice. *Pediatrics, 29*(3), 227–230.

Rasbridge, L. A., & Kulig, J. C. (1995). Infant feeding among Cambodian refugees. *American Journal of Maternal/Child Nursing, 20*(4), 213–218.

Razmus, I., Dalton, M., Wilson, D., & Hayes, J. (Eds.). (2004). Pain management for newborn circumcision. *Pediatric Nursing, 30*(5), 414–417, 427.

Roach, J. A. (2004). Newborn stimulation: Preventing over-stimulation is key for optimal growth and well-being. *AWHONN Lifelines, 7*(6), 531–535.

Schneiderman, J. U. (1996). Postpartum nursing for Korean mothers. *American Journal of Maternal/Child Nursing, 21*(3), 155–158.

Thompson, D. G. (2004). Utilizing an oral sucrose solution to minimize neonatal pain. *Journal for Specialists in Pediatric Nursing, 10,* 1, 3–10.

Thureen, P. J., Deacon, J., Hernandez, J. A., & Hall, D. M. (2005). *Assessment and care of the well newborn* (2nd ed.). St. Louis, MO: Elsevier Saunders.

Wilson, B. A., Shannon, M. T., Shields, K. M., & Stang, C. L. (2007). *Prentice Hall nurse's drug guide 2007.* Upper Saddle River, NJ: Pearson Education.

World Health Organization (WHO). (1999). *Care of the umbilical cord: A review of the evidence.* Retrieved February 2000, from http://www.whoint/rht/documents/MSM98-4

CHAPTER
31 Newborn Nutrition

I had been told that most babies ate every three or four hours and slept the rest of the time. Not mine! She wanted to nurse every two hours, and sometimes more often than that. Sometimes she would sleep for an hour, sometimes for fifteen minutes. I loved her, but I also felt consumed by her needs. It was hard to adjust to the fact that I couldn't get anything finished, whether it was an article I was reading or folding the laundry. At the end of the day I would realize I hadn't accomplished anything. Once I accepted the fact that I was not going to function at my old efficient rate (at least for a while) and stopped feeling guilty about what I wasn't getting done, I felt free to enjoy the time I was spending with my baby.

~ The Boston Women's Health Collective,
The New Our Bodies, Ourselves ~

OBJECTIVES

1. Compare the nutritional value and composition of breast milk and formula preparations.
2. Discuss the advantages and disadvantages of breastfeeding and formula-feeding for both mother and newborn.
3. Develop guidelines for helping both breastfeeding and formula-feeding mothers to feed their infants successfully.
4. Delineate nursing responsibilities for client teaching regarding infant feeding issues.
5. Incorporate knowledge of newborn nutrition and normal growth patterns into parent education and infant assessment.
6. Recognize the influence of cultural values on infant care, especially feeding practices.

KEY TERMS

Colostrum 904
Foremilk 904
Hindmilk 904
La Leche League
   International 919
Let-down reflex 904

Mature milk 904
Milk/plasma ratio 902
Oxytocin 904
Prolactin 903
Transitional milk 904

 MEDIALINK

Additional resources for this content can be found on the Prentice Hall Nursing MediaLink DVD-ROM and on the Companion Website at http://www.prenhall.com/davidson. Click on "Chapter 31" to select the activities for this chapter.

Early nutrition has a significant impact on the present and future health and well-being of the infant because this is a period of rapid growth and brain development. Good nutrition fosters physical growth and helps maintain a healthy immune system. In addition, infant feeding itself is an important component of newborn socialization that promotes cognitive and emotional development.

Whether choosing to breastfeed or use infant formula, parents find feeding their newborn an exciting, satisfying, but often worrisome task. Meeting this essential need of their new child helps parents strengthen their attachment to their baby and fosters their self-images as nurturers and providers. It is important that the nurse is well informed about infant nutrition and feeding methods, because the parents look to the nurse for this guidance. Parents need accurate and consistent information from the nursing staff. They need to learn the skills to feed their infant successfully. Through each interaction with the parents, there is an opportunity for the nurse to support the parents and promote the family's sense of confidence.

In this chapter an emphasis is placed on feeding the full-term healthy infant of normal birth weight during the neonatal period. We will look at the nutritional needs of the newborn in the context of both breast milk and formula composition, discuss feeding methods, explore community-based nursing care, and finally look at a nutritional assessment of the newborn.

NUTRITIONAL NEEDS AND MILK COMPOSITION

The newborn's diet must supply all the nutrients required by the body in the proper quantities to meet the rapid rate of physical and neurologic growth and development. A neonatal diet should provide adequate hydration and sufficient calories and include protein, carbohydrates, fat, vitamins, and minerals. Exclusive breast milk and/or iron-fortified 20-calorie/ounce formula are sufficient as sole sources of nutrition to meet the dietary needs of the newborn from birth up to 6 months of age. Complementary solid foods are introduced in the second half of the first year, and the infant continues to receive breast milk and/or formula until at least 12 months of age (American Academy of Pediatrics [AAP] Section on Breastfeeding, 2005).

This next section discusses the nutritional requirements of the newborn and how these are met by breast milk and cow's milk-based formula. There are three categories of commercial infant formulas: (1) standard cow's milk-based formulas, (2) soy protein-based formulas, and (3) specialized or therapeutic formulas. Further information on the latter two may be found in the section "Specialty Formula."

Dietary Reference Intakes

Before discussing the nutritional needs of the infant, the nurse should note that the new title *dietary reference intake (DRI)* is an updated generic term that replaces the well-known nutritional reference term *recommended dietary allowances (RDAs)*. The term *RDA* previously served as a benchmark for nutritional adequacy in the United States, but it reflected primarily disease prevention from nutrient deficiency. The term *DRI* encompasses four aspects of nutrient-based reference values: (1) estimated average requirement (EAR), (2) RDA, (3) adequate intake (AI), and (4) tolerable upper intake level (UL). The DRIs represent a framework that links nutrition and health across the lifespan (Gregory, 2005).

Growth

It is normal for both breastfed and formula-fed infants to lose weight in the first 3 to 4 days of life. Formula-feeding infants generally lose up to 3.5% of their birth weight; breastfeeding infants should not exceed a weight loss greater than 7% of their birth weight (Association of Women's Health, Obstetric and Neonatal Nurses (AWHONN), 2000; International Lactation Consultant Association, 2005, MacDonald, Ross, Grant, et al., 2003). Infants lose weight with the passage of meconium and because their fluid intake is normally low in the first few days while transitioning to enteral feedings. This loss is normal and does not result in dehydration, as infants draw on their extracellular water reserves (Biancuzzo, 2003). Infants should begin gaining weight by day of life 5 or sooner and should be at or above birth weight by 10 to 14 days of age. Weight gain during the first 4 weeks should be about 10 g/kg/day or 5 to 7 oz/week (Riordan, 2005).

Breastfed and formula-fed babies have different growth rates. This is understandable because the compositions of breast milk and formula are different. See Table 31–1 to compare breast milk and formula compositions. Most physicians (as well as formula companies) consider breastfeeding as the "gold standard" from which to compare nutritional outcomes (AAP, 2005; Lawrence & Lawrence, 2005).

Formula-fed infants tend to regain their birth weight earlier than breastfed infants because the formula-fed infant has a greater fluid intake early on. The breastfeeding infant's fluid intake depends on mother's milk supply and breastfeeding efficiency. It is noteworthy that breastfeeding infants born to multiparous mothers often do not lose as much weight as infants born to primiparous mothers, because the multiparous mother's milk typically "comes in" quicker (Lawrence & Lawrence, 2005). If a healthy full-term infant with normal birth weight has a weight loss exceeding 7%, then a feeding evaluation is indicated. If an infant has a weight loss of 10% or greater, then an evaluation, an intervention, and a follow-up is indicated to make certain that the infant receives sufficient fluid and calories. In this case, a follow-up weight check is recommended to ascertain if the feeding problem is resolved.

Growth rates for breastfed and formula-fed infants are somewhat different once feedings are established. Exclusively breastfed infants have the same or slightly higher weight gain than their formula-fed and mixed-fed peers in the first 3 to 4 months. Thereafter, formula-fed and mixed-fed infants have a greater weight gain pattern compared with breastfed infants. This characteristic weight gain pattern results in a leaner body build in the breastfed group by the latter half of the first year of life (Riordan, 2005). Measurements of length and head circumference are the same for both groups. An infant typically grows

Table 31–1   COMPARISON OF SELECTED NUTRIENTS IN MILK

Nutrients per 30 mL	Human Milk	Similac Advance®	Enfamil Lipil®	Whole Milk
Calories	20	20	20	19
Protein, grams	0.31	0.41	0.42	1.1
% of cal	6%	8%	8%	22%
Source	Human milk	Nonfat milk, Whey protein	Nonfat milk, Whey protein	Cow's milk
Whey: casein	90:10 greater than 50:50*	52:48	60:40	20:80
Fat, grams	1.15	1.1	1.1	1.1
% of cal	52%	49%	48%	49%
Source	Human milk (contains DHA, ARA**, etc.)	Safflower, soy, coconut DHA, ARA**	Palm, soy, coconut, sunflower, DHA, ARA**	Butterfat
Carbohydrate, grams	2.1	2.2	2.2	1.5
% of cal	42%	43%	43%	31%
Source	Lactose (human milk)	Lactose (nonfat milk)	Lactose (nonfat milk)	Lactose (whole milk)
Linoleic acid, mg	110	200	172	26
Calcium, mg	8.2	15.6	15.6	39
Phosphorus, mg	4.2	8.4	10.6	30.4
Iron, mcg	8	360	360	16
Copper, mcg	7.4	18	15	4.2
Selenium, mcg	0.4	0.4	0.6	0
Sodium, mg	5.2	4.8	5.4	16
Potassium, mg	15.6	21	21.6	49.8
Chloride, mg	12.4	13	12.6	32.8
Solute load, mOsm	2.9	3.7	3.8	10
Osmolality, mOsm/l	286	300	300	285
Vitamin A, international unit	66	60	60	41
Vitamin D, international unit	0.6	12	12	13.4
Vitamin E, international unit	0.12	0.3	0.4	0.02
Vitamin K, mcg	0.06	1.6	1.6	1.2
Folate, mcg	1.4	3	3.2	1.6

*Whey:casein ratio in human milk changes after birth.

**Docosahexaenoic acid (DHA), arachidonic acid (ARA) additives derived from algae, mycotic sources.

Data from Mead-Johnson Nutritionals. (2004). *Pediatric Products Handbook.* New York: Bristol-Myers Squibb Company (http://www.meadjohnson.com) and Ross Products Division. (2004). *Pediatric Nutritionals Product Guide.* Columbus, OH: Abbott Laboratories. (http://www.ROSS.com)

1 inch per month in the first 6 months, and then 0.5 inch for the next 6 months. Length is a greater indicator of growth than is weight. Infants generally double their birth weight by 5 months, triple their birth weight by 1 year of age, and quadruple their birth weight by 2 years (Riordan, 2005). Growth charts for tracking an infant's weight, length, and head circumference can be downloaded from the Centers for Disease Control and Prevention (CDC) Web site.

CLINICAL TIP

Following are newborn caloric and fluid needs:
- Caloric intake: 45.5 to 52.5 kcal/lb/day or 100 to 115 kcal/kg/day
- Fluid requirements: 64 to 73 mL/lb/day or 140 to 160 mL/kg/day
- First 6 months weight gain: Formula fed—1 oz/day;
  Breastfed— 0.5 oz/day

Fluid

Requirements. Fluid requirements during the neonatal period are high (140 to 160 mL/kg/day) because of the newborn's decreased ability to concentrate urine and increased overall metabolic rate. Although the infant's total body water content is high (75% to 80%) compared with an adult's (60%), the infant has an increased surface area to mass ratio and decreased renal absorptive capacity that makes the infant more susceptible to dehydration from insufficient fluid intake or increased fluid loss due to diarrhea, vomiting, or other source of fluid loss. Parents and caretakers should be aware of the signs of dehydration. Dry or chapped lips, dry oral cavity, decreased urine output, concentrated urine, general weakness, lethargy, poor skin turgor, sunken eyes, and sunken fontanelle are some of the signs of dehydration. The infant's fluid intake will need to be increased above the baseline fluid needs when the infant has a fever or is in a warm environment for an extended period of time. For infants under 6 months of age, increased fluid requirements should be met with additional breast milk or formula, rather than water.

Milk Composition. Breast milk and formula contain almost 90% water, which meets the infant's water needs. Feeding supplemental water is not recommended routinely for infants under 6 months of age who are still on an exclusively milk diet (breast milk or formula), because the increased water can cause hyponatremia and may result in seizures if water consumption is excessive. In some cases in which the infant has become more severely dehydrated or will not tolerate increased breast milk or formula, a physician may recommend use of a water/electrolyte solution for initial rehydration.

Energy

Requirements. The basal metabolic rate (BMR) refers to the energy needed for thermoregulation, cardiorespiratory function, cellular activity, and growth. The healthy full-term infant's BMR is about twice that of an adult's, based on body weight (Rolfes, Pinna, & Whitney, 2006). A newborn requires 100 to 115 kcal/kg/day at 1 month and 85 to 95 kcal/kg/day from 6 to 12 months of age. When infants do not receive sufficient calories, they risk losing weight, may experience tissue breakdown, and are at risk for delayed growth and development (Gregory, 2005).

Milk Composition. Healthy full-term newborns derive about half of their required calories from fat (breast milk 52%, formula 49%). The remaining calories are derived from carbohydrates (breast milk 42%, formula 43%) and to a lesser extent from protein (breast milk 6%, formula 8%) (Mead-Johnson Nutritionals, 2004; Ross Products Division, 2004). Often, calories derived from protein are not counted in the total daily caloric intake as there is a metabolic cost to breaking down protein that at least partially negates the caloric benefits.

Fats

Requirements. As noted, infants receive approximately 50% of their calories from fat. Fats also help the body absorb the fat-soluble vitamins A, D, E, and K. Fats are a precursor of prostaglandins and other hormones. Essential fatty acids and their derivatives docosahexaenoic acid (DHA) and arachidonic acid (ARA) are associated with improved visual acuity and cognitive ability (Riordan, 2005).

Milk Composition. Triglycerides make up 98% to 99% of milk fat. Triglycerides break down to free fatty acids and glycerol. The lipid fraction of breast milk provides essential fatty acids, including linoleic acid and linolenic

acid, as well as their longer chain derivatives DHA and ARA. In 2001 the Food and Drug Administration (FDA) approved the addition of DHA and ARA to infant formula. Fat content is the most variable component in breast milk, ranging from 30 to 50 grams/liter. It is influenced by maternal parity, duration of pregnancy, the stage of lactation, diurnally, and even during a single feeding. Multiparous mothers produce milk with a lower content of fatty acids. Mothers of preterm infants have a greater concentration of long-chain polyunsaturated fatty acids (LCPUFAs) in their milk compared with mothers of term infants. Phospholipids and cholesterol levels are higher in colostrum compared with mature milk, although overall fat content is higher in mature breast milk compared with colostrum. Fat content is generally higher in the evening and lower in the early morning. Within a single feeding session an infant initially receives the low-fat foremilk before receiving the higher calorie, high-fat hindmilk. Finally, the fat content of breast milk is also affected by maternal diet and maternal fat stores. Mothers on low-fat diets have increased production of medium chain fatty acids (C6-C10), and mothers with high levels of body fat produce breast milk with a higher fat content (Lawrence & Lawrence, 2005).

The fats in the milk-based formulas are modified to parallel the fat profile of breast milk by removing the butterfat from cow's milk and adding vegetable oils. There are quite a few differences in the fat sources and amounts used among the major formula brands (see Table 31–1). The different blends of fats all provide a fatty acid profile in the end that is similar to breast milk in terms of amount of saturated, monounsaturated, and polyunsaturated fats present. In 2002, the formula companies in the United States added long-chain polyunsaturated fatty acids (LCPUFAs), namely, DHA for brain development and ARA for visual acuity (AAP, 2002).

Carbohydrates

Requirements. Carbohydrates (sugars) serve as the other main source of energy for the infant, providing about 40% of the calories in the infant's diet. By weight, both breast milk and formula contain more carbohydrates than fat, but the caloric value of carbohydrates is 4 calories/gram, whereas fat provides 9 calories/gram.

Milk Composition. In breast milk, the primary carbohydrate is lactose. In addition to providing energy, lactose also functions to enhance the absorption of calcium, magnesium, and zinc (Lawrence & Lawrence, 2005). Breast milk also contains trace amounts of other carbohydrates such as glucosamines and nitrogen-containing oligosaccharides (Biancuzzo, 2003). Glucosamines are one of the building blocks for connective tissues and help strengthen and hold together ligaments and tendons. Oligosaccharides promote the growth of *Lactobacillus bifidus,* which promotes an intestinal acidic environment, creating a hostile environment for bacteria to thrive (Riordan, 2005).

In comparing carbohydrates among the milk-based formulas, both Enfamil® and Similac® provide all of their carbohydrate calories from lactose. Carnation Good Start® uses a blend of 70% lactose and 30% maltodextrin (a table sugarlike carbohydrate) (Sears, n.d.).

Protein

Requirements. Proteins are the building blocks for muscle and organ structure. They are key to just about every metabolic process in the body, including energy metabolism, cell-signaling, growth, and immune function. Some dietary proteins are absorbed intact, although the majority are broken down into component amino acids and utilized by the infant to build new proteins to support rapid growth and repair of body cells. The protein requirement for an infant is about 0.8 to 0.9 gram per deciliter (Riordan, 2005).

Milk Composition. Milk proteins are often grouped into whey proteins and casein. Casein is the major phosphoprotein found in milk. It is not easily denatured and is relatively insoluble in water. It is the predominant protein that forms the curds seen when milk interacts with acid or the enzyme renin in the stomach. Whey proteins are the remaining proteins suspended in the liquid portion of milk after curds are formed. Cow's milk contains a high amount of casein (a low ratio of whey to casein—approximately 20:80) compared with human milk (60:40 whey:casein). Because of its tendency to form curds, milk with high amounts of casein is less easily digested. Cow's milk-based formulas are usually modified to get closer to the whey:casein ratio of human milk. For example, the whey:casein ratio in Enfamil® is 60:40. Although Similac® has a ratio of 48:52, the company claims this produces an amino acid profile in the blood that is closer to that found in the breastfeeding infant. Carnation Good Start® contains hydrolyzed whey protein, which the company states decreases the incidence of constipation, but which makes comparison difficult (Sears, n.d.). It should also be noted that the whey and casein components in breast milk are not static and change over time to meet the needs of the growing infant. In early lactation, the whey:casein ratio is 90:10. As lactation progresses, the whey:casein ratio in mature breast milk is 60:40. Finally, during late lactation, the whey:casein ratio is 50:50 (Riordan, 2005).

Whey protein in breast milk is composed of five major components: (1) alpha-lactalbumin, (2) serum albumin, (3) lactoferrin, (4) immunoglobulins, and (5) lysozyme. The latter three components are involved in immunologic activities. Breast milk contains many other kinds of proteins as well. These include enzymes, growth modulator, and hormones (Riordan, 2005). The major whey components in cow's milk-based formula are beta-lactoglobulin and alpha-lactalbumin. The former can trigger allergic reactions in some infants (Groenewald, 1996; Vonlanthen, 1998).

Vitamins, Minerals, and Trace Elements

VITAMINS

Requirements. Vitamins can be grouped into fat-soluble and water-soluble vitamins. The fat-soluble vitamins are vitamins A, D, E, and K and are found in both cow's milk-based formula and breast milk. Vitamin K is also synthesized in the infant's intestinal tract by bacteria that are colonized there. After absorption via the lymphatic system, vitamins enter the blood and are transported to the various tissues where they are needed. Excess fat-soluble vitamins are stored in adipose tissue and the liver (Rolfes et al., 2006). Excessive amounts of fat-soluble vitamins may result in toxicity, and there is general agreement that no routine fat-soluble vitamin supplementation is needed with the exception of vitamin D. To prevent rickets the AAP recommends that all infants receive 200 international units of oral vitamin D drops daily during the first 2 months of life, and the infants should continue to take the vitamin supplement until feeding at least 500 mL per day (about 16.6 oz/day) of vitamin D-fortified formula or milk. Most healthy, full-term formula-feeding infants of average birth weight will receive sufficient vitamin D intake before they are 2 months old and, therefore, may not require vitamin D supplementation. However, the breastfeeding infant should continue to take vitamin D until weaned to the recommended minimum 500 mL per day of vitamin D-fortified formula or milk (AAP, 2003).

Milk Composition. Breast milk is naturally low in vitamin D (25 international units per liter or less) and may be of concern particularly among breastfeeding infants who have limited sunlight exposure. Factors that place an infant at high risk for vitamin D deficiency include: having increased skin pigmentation, living in a geographic location where there is little sunlight, having one's skin consistently covered with clothing or sunscreen, not spending much time outdoors, living in an area that consistently has heavy pollution that blocks sunlight, and having a mother who is vitamin D deficient. Some breastfeeding advocates argue that infants require only a few minutes of sunlight exposure per day to stimulate vitamin D production in their skin to protect them from vitamin D deficiency (Mohrbacher & Stock, 2003). The AAP contends that it is difficult to know what is adequate sunlight exposure for an individual, and it also recommends against direct sunlight exposure of infants (AAP, 2003).

The vitamin B complex and vitamin C are water-soluble vitamins that pass readily from serum to breast milk. However, mothers who follow a strict vegetarian diet or macrobiotic diet may have insufficient vitamin B_{12} in their milk. In that case the exclusively breastfed infant should receive vitamin B_{12} supplementation. Formula is fortified with adequate amounts of the water-soluble vitamins to meet the DRI. Unlike fat-soluble vitamins, any excess water-soluble vitamins ingested are simply excreted and the threat of toxicity is low (Lawrence & Lawrence, 2005).

MINERALS

Requirements. Minerals have diverse regulatory functions throughout the body. For example, calcium is important in the clotting mechanisms; phosphorus is a component in adenosine triphosphate (ATP), deoxyribonucleic acid (DNA), ribonucleic acid (RNA), and phospholipids; calcium and phosphorus are necessary for bone formation; sodium is involved in fluid balance; calcium, sodium, and potassium are needed for nerve and muscle function; chlorine is involved in acid-base balance; cobalt works with vitamin B_{12} to form blood cells; copper and iron aid in extracting energy from the citric acid cycle and are also involved in blood production; iodine is needed for thyroid hormone synthesis; and magnesium, manganese, and zinc are needed to help with many enzymatic processes (Thibodeau & Patton, 2002).

Iron is an important mineral required by the body to make hemoglobin and is needed for neurologic function. Neurotransmitters require adequate iron levels to function properly, and, therefore, infants with chronic anemia are at risk for cognitive and developmental delays. Infants deficient in iron may look pale, appear sleepy or tire easily while feeding, and be tachycardic or tachypneic at rest. The infant's iron status is affected by the amount of iron accumulated in utero, the infant's diet after birth, and the general health of the infant. The amount of iron transferred to the fetus during the third trimester of pregnancy is influenced by maternal iron status (O'Brien, Zavaleta, Abrams et al., 2003).

Milk Composition. Both breast milk and infant formulas contain several major and trace minerals to satisfy the needs of the growing infant. The mineral content of breast milk does not appear to be influenced by maternal diet. The vitamins and minerals among the three formulas being compared are essentially the same, although all generally contain higher levels of minerals than breast milk to compensate for their lower bioavailability.

Much has been written about iron content of breast milk and formula and its bioavailability to the infant. The AAP does not advocate the use of low-iron fortified formulas because of the increased risk for anemia associated with their use (AAP, 1999). Low-iron formula is fortified with only 2 mg of iron per liter compared with "iron-fortified" formula, which is fortified with 12 mg of iron per liter. It should be noted that the iron concentration in breast milk is 0.5 to 1 mg per liter, which is considerably lower than in iron-fortified formulas. However, the iron in breast milk is much more completely absorbed—the infant receiving breast milk absorbs 50% to 80% of the iron in breast milk compared with less than 12% of the iron in formula. Researchers continue to study iron nutrition to determine the best level of iron fortification in infant formula. Healthy term infants with normal birth weights receiving breast milk or an iron-fortified infant formula during the first 5 to 6 months of life are unlikely to develop iron-deficiency anemia because these infants have sufficient iron stores to sustain them until they start solid feedings in the second half of the first year of life (Riordan, 2005).

Nurses have a responsibility to educate parents who have a misconception that infants fed iron-fortified formula are likely to have constipation. The iron added to formula is in an ionic form and does not cause constipation (Katz, Levin, Cotton et al., n.d.). The casein in formula (which is different from the casein in breast milk) creates large, rubbery curds that are slow to metabolize and have been associated with constipation in formula-fed infants. In addition, there is evidence that palm olein oil (an additive to some formulas) also may contribute to constipation. Palm olein oil is added to some formulas to provide palmitic acid in an attempt to match the natural palmitic acid profile in breast milk. However, the chemical arrangements are different. Palmitic acid derived from olein oil is poorly absorbed. The unabsorbed palmitic acid in formula reacts with calcium to create insoluble soaps during digestion. Research reveals that there is a correlation between the amount of insoluble soap present and the hardness of the stools (Lloyd, Halter, Kuchan et al., 1999).

TRACE ELEMENTS

New additives to formulas not yet mentioned include nucleotides (building blocks for DNA and RNA that appear to enhance the immune system, among other things), carnitine (derived from the amino acid lysine and functioning in part to transport fatty acids to the mitochondria for oxidation), and taurine (a conditionally essential nonprotein sulfur amino acid with a number of functions, including a role in growth, and in central nervous system (CNS) and auditory function development). There are many other breast milk components not yet duplicated in formula (and many will never be because of the cost). Also, not all components in breast milk have been identified. In general, though, formula companies are always striving to improve their products to develop the best "humanized" milk possible. There is no question that formulas today are far superior to formulas from the past.

Specialty Formula

If an infant has medical problems related to inability to metabolize components of breast milk or standard formula, or if the parents are vegans, the family should consult with the baby's healthcare provider to discuss the issue of supplements or switching their infant to another infant formula.

Soy protein-based formulas (e.g., Enfamil Prosobee LIPIL®, Isomil®, Isomil Advance®, Isomil DF®, and Good

Start Supreme Soy®) do not contain any bovine protein or lactose. Soy protein-based formulas use a soy protein harvested from soybeans and supplemented with methionine (an essential amino acid), carnitine, and taurine. Because soy protein-based formulas do not contain lactose, the formula is usually sweetened with corn syrup or sucrose. The latter may cause dental decay after teeth have erupted. Phytates present in soy formulas decrease the absorption of iron, calcium, and zinc, so greater concentrations of minerals and vitamins are added to soy formulas.

Soy protein-based formula is not intended as a first-choice formula except for infants with primary lactase deficiency or galactosemia and for term infants of formula-feeding vegan parents. The AAP Committee on Nutrition (1998) recommends against the use of soy protein-based formula for preterm infants who weigh less than 1800 grams or infants with renal failure because of the high aluminum level in soy formulas. Breast milk contains 4 to 65 ng/mL of aluminum; soy protein-based formulas contain 600 to 1300 ng/mL.

The AAP states that the "isolated soy protein-based formulas are safe and effective alternatives to provide appropriate nutrition for normal growth and development" for term infants whose nutritional needs are not being met from breast milk or cow's milk-based formulas. However, there is no advantage to using soy protein-based formula over cow's milk-based formula as a supplement for breastfeeding babies. According to the AAP (1998), there is no proof that soy protein-based formula will prevent or lessen the symptoms of colic or prevent atopic disease, and infants who have a sensitivity to cow's milk protein may have a sensitivity to soy protein as well. Therefore, the AAP does not recommend routinely switching an infant from cow's milk-based formula to soy-based formula (AAP, 1998).

Infants with an allergic response to standard formulas may require a hypoallergenic "hydrolysate" formula. Hydrolyzed formulas (i.e., Nutramigen®, Alimentum®, and Pregestimil®) are sometimes referred to as "predigested" formulas because the dietary proteins have been broken down in a process that mimics digestion (hydrolysis). The simple protein compounds are usually too small to be recognized by the infant's immune system as an antigen, thereby decreasing the infant's allergic response. These formulas are also used in infants who have difficulties with normal digestion or absorption.

The other group of hypoallergenic formulas is the elemental amino acid-based formulas, such as Neocate® and Elecare®. The proteins in these formulas have been completely broken down to their amino acid constituents. These formulas are the most hypoallergenic formulas available and virtually eliminate the possibility of allergic reaction. They are intended for severely allergenic infants with multiple dietary protein intolerances or infants with severe absorption disorders.

Other specialized formulas are intended for infants with particular medical conditions and should be fed to infants only under a physician's supervision. There are specific specialized formulas intended for infants born prematurely to promote rapid growth. There are other specialized formulas for infants with heart disease, kidney disease, malabsorption syndromes, metabolic diseases, and allergies. These formulas vary in caloric content, nutrient composition and ingredients, digestibility, taste/odor, and cost.

After the First Year

Parents frequently ask when their child can begin feeding cow's milk or soy milk (whole milk, low-fat, or skim). Parents need to be informed that it is recommended that the infant receive breast milk or formula for 12 months, before weaning to whole milk. The protein content in cow's milk is markedly higher than both breast milk or modified cow's milk used for formulas and is much less easily digested. The high alpha-casein content in cow's milk also decreases iron absorption. Therefore, cow's milk is a poor source for iron. Some infants experience microscopic gastrointestinal bleeding while on cow's milk and this can further lead to anemia. Cow's milk, compared with breast milk or formula, has higher levels of calcium, phosphorus, sodium, and potassium, which increase the renal solute load and result in greater obligatory water loss. It also is deficient in vitamin C, zinc, and essential fatty acids. When switching to cow's milk at 12 months the infant should start off on whole milk. Low-fat milk and skim milk lack adequate calories, fat content, and essential fatty acids necessary for proper neurologic development. Nutritionists advise waiting until a toddler is 2 years of age to give low-fat milk (2% or 1% milk) or skim milk, and then only provided the child is growing well.

CHOICE OF FEEDING: BREAST VERSUS BOTTLE

The Evolution of Formula

Finding an acceptable breast milk substitute following maternal death, infant abandonment, low milk supply, and other situations has been a challenge for centuries. Although there are no written records describing infant feedings from ancient times to the Renaissance period, there is physical evidence of societies using alternative feedings dating back to 2000 BC. Throughout Europe spouted feeding cups and other feeding receptacles have been found in the graves of infants. Records from written works show that from 1500 to 1700, "wet nurses" (a lactating woman whose purpose of employment was to nurse another woman's infant, sometimes abandoning her own infant to gain employment) were hired at foundling homes (orphanages) and by wealthy European women, because it was customary for noblewomen to delegate all physical work, including infant care (Lawrence & Lawrence, 2005).

By the 19th century wet-nursing was falling out of favor, and "dry-nursing" was attempted. Dry-nursing is the practice of feeding an infant milk obtained from another mammal (goats, cows, mares, donkeys, etc.) (Schuman, 2003). Cow's milk was most commonly used because of its availability, not because it was closer in composition to human milk. This practice was used in foundling homes and was associated with very high infant mortality (Lawrence & Lawrence, 2005).

Recognizing the need for an improved alternative breast milk substitute, a few physicians continued attempts to develop a "humanized" animal milk substitute. In the late 1830s, a German scientist published a report of the content of human milk and cow's milk. This served as the basis for a number of "formulas" for modifying cow's milk to make it more like human milk. Around the 1860s, the first commercially available baby food and infant formula was developed in Europe and became available in the United States by the 1870s. The first formula was comprised of only malt, cow's milk, and wheat flour and required reconstitution with water (Schuman, 2003). Between 1860 and 1920 there were additional scientific discoveries that contributed to overall infant survival among nonbreastfeeding infants. These included the discovery of the germ theory and subsequent development of pasteurization of milk, the invention of the bottle and rubber nipple to replace feeding devices that required skill to use and were difficult to clean, and the invention of the "ice box" to refrigerate the baby milk (Baumslag & Michels, 1995).

Two of the biggest commercial advances in milk science were the invention of sweeetened condensed milk in the 1830s and evaporated milk in 1883. Condensed milk was made by boiling milk and permitting it to evaporate to one-fourth its original volume, and then adding 6 ounces of sugar per pint to the milk as a preservative (Baumslag & Michels, 1995). The invention of sweetened condensed milk and evaporated milk meant that for the first time in history, a family did not have to have access to a cow in order to feed their infant milk (if not breastfeeding). From evaporated milk, a home-made evaporated milk formula recipe was created and made available to the public. The evaporated milk formula was a simple mixture of evaporated milk, water, and sugar or corn syrup. The evaporated milk formula gained acceptance because it was affordable, widely available, and appeared to support growth equal to that of breastfed infants. It is estimated that by 1960 about 80% of bottle-fed infants were being fed with evaporated milk formula and given supplements of vitamins and iron. However, poor infant outcomes were still being observed.

In the 1960s proprietary commercial formulas began to gain acceptance because parents were impressed with the advances in science and wanted to raise their children scientifically "by the book." Using formula seemed to be a progressive idea to embrace. By this time more and more women were working outside the home than ever before. "Modern women" saw formula use as more convenient than breastfeeding. Formula companies appealed to these women. In addition to a changing social climate in America, advances in agriculture created a surplus of cow's milk and offered a new marketing opportunity for global commercialization of formula (Baumslag & Michels, 1995).

Artificial baby milk that was originally intended as a lifesaving product for extreme situations was now being aggressively marketed as a food for all infants. To this end formula companies began an aggressive marketing campaign. One of their marketing tactics was to provide free formula to hospitals, enabling hospitals to phase out their formula preparation rooms. Mothers viewed commercial formula as an acceptable breast milk substitute that appeared to have medical endorsement, it was easy to use and affordable, and it freed her up to do other things such as work outside the home. By 1972, formula use

peaked and breastfeeding rates in the United States plummeted (only 25% of women were breastfeeding at hospital discharge) (Schuman, 2003). Again, the public was led to believe that commercial formula was as good as, if not better than, breast milk.

Research efforts beginning in the 1970s showed that breast milk was unquestionably superior to evaporated milk and proprietary infant formulas as evidenced by a significant rise in infant morbidity and mortality, especially in developing countries (Baumslag & Michels, 1995). The revelation of the research findings from the 1970s up to the present has led to a resurgence in breastfeeding. By 2003, 66% of mothers in the United States were breastfeeding at hospital discharge. However, only 33% of infants were still receiving some breast milk at 6 months of age (Ross Products Division, 2004).

Over the last 50 years or so, considerable time, effort, and money have been allocated to the development of commercial infant formulas in an attempt to better imitate the content and performance of human milk. In 1954, the executive board of the AAP established a Committee on Nutrition to set the standards for nutritional requirements and feeding practices for infants, children, and adolescents. This committee makes recommendations for nutritional requirements in infant formulas to the federal FDA. In 1971 the FDA created the first regulation for commercial formula, which established minimum requirements for fat, protein, linoleic acid, and vitamins and minerals (Schuman, 2003). In 1980 Congress passed the Infant Formula Act, which was later amended in 1986. The safety and nutritional quality of formula are now significantly regulated.

Although breastfeeding is increasing in popularity, formula-feeding continues to be a viable and nurturing choice, particularly in developed countries, and meets the goal of successful growth of the baby. The closeness and warmth that can occur during breastfeeding is also an integral part of formula-feeding. An advantage of formula-feeding is that parents can share equally in this nurturing, caring experience with their baby.

Advantages of Breast Milk

In its breastfeeding policy statement, the AAP recommends exclusive breastfeeding as the preferred feeding for all infants, with a few exceptions, for the first 6 months and continued breastfeeding during the introduction of solids until the infant is 12 months old or older, as desired. There is overwhelming scientific evidence that shows that breastfeeding provides newborns and infants with specific nutritional, immunologic, and psychosocial advantages over formula-feedings (AAP, 2005).

NUTRITIONAL ADVANTAGES

Human milk provides optimum nutrition for the human infant because it is species specific. The macronutrients such as protein, fat, and carbohydrates (lactose) are synthesized by the mother in the alveoli of the breasts by specialized secretory cells. Micronutrient elements such as vitamins and minerals derive from the circulating maternal plasma. There are more than 200 distinct components in breast milk, with more remaining to be identified (Lawrence & Lawrence, 2005).

As noted earlier, lactose is the primary carbohydrate in mammalian milk and plays a crucial role in the nourishment of

EVIDENCE-BASED PRACTICE

GUIDELINES FOR THE ESTABLISHMENT OF EXCLUSIVE BREASTFEEDING

Clinical Question

How can the nurse support the new mother in establishing exclusive breastfeeding for her infant?

The Evidence

The International Lactation Consultant Association convened a task force of four lactation consultant experts to perform a systematic review of the literature and develop a practice guideline. The task force members devised a search strategy and independently appraised 258 studies, concluding with the development of standards for supporting exclusive breastfeeding after birth.

What Is Effective?

Breastfeeding should be established within the first hour after birth. Continuous skin-to-skin contact between mother and infant should take place until the first feeding, and procedures for both should be avoided until breastfeeding has been attempted. Keeping the mother and infant together for the entire postpartum stay encourages exclusive breastfeeding. The new mother should be taught to recognize and respond to early infant feeding cues, and to recognize that crying is a late cue that may interfere with effective feeding. The nurse should assess both mother and baby for signs of effective breastfeeding, such as weight changes, quality and frequency of neonatal bowel movements, signs of dehydration, and the appearance that the newborn is satisfied. If supplemental nutrition is medically indicated, the method that is least likely to compromise the transition to exclusive breastfeeding should be used. The mother's own stored milk should be used first, followed by pasteurized donor milk. Mothers should be given access to community resources and appropriate breastfeeding materials, as both are likely to support the mother in continuing exclusive breastfeeding.

What Is Unclear?

Pacifiers, artificial nipples, and supplements do not appear to be productive in helping the baby learn to latch on the nipple. Although the mother should eat a variety of foods and drink to satisfy thirst, there is little evidence to determine if common dietary restrictions are necessary. It appears that few infants are affected by foods eaten by the mother, but the evidence is not from randomized trials.

Best Practice

The nurse should plan strategies that help the mother be successful in early breastfeeding attempts. Mothers who have access to supportive resources and educational materials are more likely to establish and maintain exclusive breastfeeding.

Critical Thinking

What should be included in the postpartum breastfeeding teaching plan? What strategies can the nurse employ to support the mother in her choice to exclusively breastfeed?

REFERENCE: International Lactation Consultant Association. (2005, June 28). *Clinical guidelines for the establishment of exclusive breastfeeding.* Raleigh, NC: Author.

---

our offspring. Human milk has a very high lactose content compared with the milk of other mammal species (Biancuzzo, 2003). After lactose is hydrolyzed into galactose and glucose, the galactose is used in the formation of cerebral galactolipids and contributes to brain and CNS development. Glucose is used by many tissues, but especially by the brain, which consumes 20% of the body's energy requirements and derives this almost exclusively from glucose. In addition to providing a cellular energy source, lactose enhances the absorption of calcium, magnesium, and zinc (Lawrence & Lawrence, 2005).

As noted previously, the sole or primary carbohydrate in milk-based formulas is lactose. However, some of the specialty formulas use other carbohydrates such as corn syrup solids, sucrose, tapioca starch, and dextrose. This raises concerns about the long-term use of lactose-free formulas when an infant's sole source of food is formula. All too often, fussy breastfeeding or cow's milk-based formula-fed infants are switched to a lactose-free formula because of concerns about lactose intolerance. It is important to distinguish true lactose intolerance from cow's milk protein allergy or other source of feeding intolerance.

Lactose intolerance is defined as a "deficiency of the intestinal enzyme lactase that splits lactose into two smaller sugars, glucose and galactose, and allows lactose to be absorbed from the intestine" (Marks, 2003). This condition causes diarrhea, flatulence, abdominal pain, and, sometimes, abdominal bloating, abdominal distension, and nausea. There are three causes of lactose intolerance: (1) congenital lact*ase* deficiency, (2) secondary lact*ose* intolerance, and (3) developmental or acquired lact*ose* intolerance (Marks, 2003).

Congenital lactase deficiency is common in premature infants because of inability to produce the enzyme lactase until they have matured, but it is exceedingly rare in term infants, with fewer than 50 cases known (Jarvela, Sabri, Kokkonen et al., 1998). Secondary lactose intolerance occurs as a result of damage to the mucosal lining of the small intestine, where the lactase enzyme is produced. Any condition that causes gastroenteritis, especially if prolonged, can create this condition. Following a severe bout of diarrhea, transient lactose intolerance may persist for a brief time until the brush border of the intestinal mucosa heals.

The most common cause of lactose intolerance is developmental or acquired. Many parents will assume that their infant has lactose intolerance because they or the child's older sibling has lactose intolerance. However, this is an age-related condition that develops after 2 to 5 years of age and therefore not a common condition affecting newborns. Its prevalence and onset varies by ethnicity. Nearly 100% of Asians, 80% to 100% of Native Americans, up to 80% of African Americans and Latinos, and up to 20% of American Caucasians acquire lactose intolerance during their lifetime (Marks, 2003; Swagerty, Walling, & Klein, 2002).

Infants with symptoms similar to those of lactose intolerance are more likely to be reacting to cow's milk protein (mostly because of the beta-lactoglobulin component in cow's milk) or to some other antigen. This can occur even with exclusively breastfed infants who are allergic to bovine protein, as some of the cow's milk protein antigens consumed by the mother can pass into her breast milk. Elimination of the antigen from the mother's diet may resolve the problem.

Approximately 98% of the human milk fat is in the form of triglycerides, and a very small but clinically significant amount is from cholesterol. Some researchers believe that the cholesterol in breast milk may play a role in myelination and neurologic development. Cholesterol levels in breast milk may also stimulate the production of enzymes that lead to more efficient metabolism of cholesterol, thereby reducing its harmful long-term effects on the cardiovascular system (Biancuzzo, 2003).

Fatty acids are another key component to brain development. Prenatally, fatty acids transfer across the placenta. Postnatally, they are obtained from the diet. Omega-3 and omega-6 fatty acids are two classes of essential fatty acids found in breast milk, although the level can vary with maternal diet. Fish is a rich source of these kinds of fatty acids.

DHA and ARA are LCPUFAs derived from linoleic acid and α-linolenic acid. They are major components of the cell membranes of the retina, brain, and other neural tissues. Along with oleic acid, these LCPUFAs are needed for myelination of the spinal cord and other nerves, and they have an impact on visual acuity and cognitive and behavioral functions. Since 2002 some infant formulas have been supplemented with DHA and ARA. However, breast milk still contains 167 other fatty acids of uncertain function and that are absent from formula (Lawrence & Lawrence, 2005). It seems reasonable that many of these will turn out to be important as well.

Another advantage of breast milk is that its composition varies according to gestational age and stage of lactation. For example, the milk of a mother who delivers a preterm infant has a greater concentration of DHA and ARA than does the milk of a mother who gives birth to a full-term infant. Babies born prematurely miss receiving the continuous placental transfer of DHA and ARA while developing during the third trimester. By receiving breast milk, these preterm infants receive the increased concentrations of DHA and ARA intended for the premature infant (Lawrence & Lawrence, 2005).

Breast milk provides newborns with minerals in more appropriate doses than do formulas (Blackburn, 2003). As mentioned earlier in this chapter, the iron found in breast milk, even though much lower in concentration than that of prepared formulas, is much more readily and fully absorbed and appears sufficient to meet the infant's iron needs for the first 6 months. Additional iron that is not absorbed may increase the growth of pathogenic bacteria as well as cause cellular oxidative injury. In addition, formula does not contain lactoferrin, an iron-binding protein that scavenges iron in the gut and enhances its absorption (Lawrence & Lawrence, 2005).

There is research supporting additional health advantages for the breastfed infant. Breastfed infants have a reduced risk of developing type 1 or type 2 diabetes mellitus, lymphoma, leukemia, Hodgkin's disease, obesity, hypercholesterolemia, and asthma. Finally, the mother who breastfeeds has health advantages as well. After delivery there is decreased postpartum bleeding and more rapid uterine involution. The breastfeeding mother also burns additional calories making milk (quicker return to prepregnancy weight), has a decreased risk of developing breast cancer and ovarian cancer, and may have a decreased risk of developing postmenopausal osteoporosis (AAP, 2005).

IMMUNOLOGIC ADVANTAGES

The immunologic advantages of breast milk include varying degrees of protection from respiratory tract and gastrointestinal tract infections, necrotizing enterocolitis, urinary tract infections, otitis media, bacterial meningitis, bacteremia, and allergies (AAP, 2005). Transplacental passage of maternal immunoglobulin gradually diminishes over the first 6 months of life until the infant can begin to produce his or her own immunoglobulins. Breast milk-derived immunologic protection helps supplement this protection.

Secretory IgA, an immunoglobulin present in colostrum and breast milk, has antiviral, antibacterial, and antigenic-inhibiting properties, specifically across mucosal surfaces such as the intestinal tract. Secretory IgA plays a role in decreasing the permeability of the small intestine to help prevent large protein molecules from triggering an allergic response. Other constituents of colostrum and breast milk that act to inhibit the growth of bacteria or viruses are *Lactobacillus bifidus,* lysozymes, lactoperoxidase, lactoferrin, transferrin, and various immunoglobulins (Biancuzzo, 2003).

Some mothers wonder if there are special considerations for breastfed infants regarding immunizations, in particular the oral polio virus (OPV) vaccination because it is a live virus vaccine. These mothers worry that their antibodies will inactivate the live polio virus. The CDC recommends that all babies be on the same schedule; there is no indication for withholding breastfeeding in relationship to OPV administration, and no extra doses of the vaccine are indicated. Furthermore, breastfed babies actually have better antibody responses to parenteral and oral vaccines than formula-fed infants (Lawrence & Lawrence, 2005).

PSYCHOSOCIAL BENEFITS OF BREASTFEEDING

The psychosocial advantages of breastfeeding are primarily those associated with maternal-infant attachment. For some mothers the attachment process begins when the decision to become pregnant is made. The hormonal changes associated with pregnancy strengthen that bond. Events that occur during pregnancy, such as hearing the fetal heart beat, feeling the fetus move within her, and watching her abdomen grow bigger, further promote the bonding. At delivery there may be intense bonding. For other mothers bonding develops over the next few days (Lawrence & Lawrence, 2005). Some hospital practices inadvertently interfere with the attachment process. Rooming-in and breastfeeding have been shown to increase maternal-infant attachment.

When a mother chooses to breastfeed, she often has more frequent direct skin-to-skin contact with her infant than if she were bottle feeding (bottle-feeding parents should be encouraged to have frequent skin-to-skin contact too, however). Infants with skin-to-skin contact have greater physiologic stability, cry less, sleep longer, and tend to breastfeed better. The newborn's sense of touch is highly developed at birth and is a primary means of communication. The tactile stimulation associated with breastfeeding can communicate warmth, closeness, and comfort. The increased closeness provides both newborn and mother with the opportunity to learn each other's behavioral cues and needs. Mothers may feel more affectionate toward their newborns, have improved let-down response while pumping, and breastfeed more frequently and for longer periods of time (Klaus, 1998; Mohrbacher & Stock, 2003).

The mother who breastfeeds has a different hormonal state compared with the mother who does not breastfeed. Prolactin levels double each time the infant suckles at the breast, regardless of the age of the infant or duration of lactation (Biancuzzo, 2003). If a mother does not stimulate her breasts by breastfeeding or pumping, her prolactin levels return to prepregancy levels by 14 days postpartum (Lawrence & Lawrence, 2005). Prolactin increases feelings of relaxation and euphoria (Biancuzzo, 2003). Oxytocin levels also increase with breastfeeding. Oxytocin produces feelings of relaxation and sleepiness, heightens responsiveness and receptivity toward the infant, and increases the frequency of nurturing behaviors (Lawrence & Lawrence, 2005).

Another psychologic advantage to the breastfeeding mother is satisfaction derived from the knowledge that she is providing her infant with the optimal nutritional start in life. For many mothers breastfeeding takes effort, understanding, and an emotional commitment to endure the demands of this lifestyle choice. The mother's sense of accomplishment in being able to satisfy her baby's needs for nourishment and comfort can be a tremendous source of personal satisfaction.

There are significant cost savings for the family who chooses breastfeeding. The cost of standard formula is approximately $1,200 annually per infant. There are also healthcare cost savings for families resulting from the decreased incidence of illness in the infant. Because breastfed babies access healthcare resources less often, the family saves money on medical visits and prescription medications and loses less time from work.

Potential societal benefits to breastfeeding include decreased spending on public assistance programs (e.g., Women Infant Children Supplemental Nutrition Program [WIC]), and environmental benefits in terms of use of natural resources and solid waste disposal. Breastfeeding is not dependent on modern technology and can provide the infant with a fresh, clean, naturally warm source of nutrition independent of transportation, supply, electricity, refrigeration, clean water, bottles, nipples, and so on. There are also substantial medical cost savings to society, estimated to be approximately $400 in excess medical costs per never-breastfed infant (Ball & Wright, 1999). With current breastfeeding initiation rates of approximately 66%, this amounts to an additional $544 million per year in potential healthcare costs that could be saved by breastfeeding.

Potential Disadvantages and Contraindications to Breastfeeding

DISADVANTAGES

Following is a list of sometimes cited potential disadvantages to breastfeeding:

1. *Pain with breastfeeding.* Breastfeeding is a natural process but requires a certain knowledge base that formerly was passed on from generation to generation. With the decline in the extended family structure, this source of knowledge and assistance is often missing for the new mother. Nipple tenderness is the most common source of discomfort and is usually related to improper positioning and/or not obtaining a proper attachment of the infant on the breast. Pain can also be related to engorgement or infection. Breastfeeding with proper technique should not hurt and these mothers should be encouraged to seek assistance from a knowledgeable person skilled in lactation.

2. *Leaking milk.* Some women will leak milk when their breasts are full and it is nearly time to breastfeed again or whenever they experience "let-down," which can be triggered by hearing, seeing, or even thinking of their babies. If this causes concern to the mother, she can be instructed on how to apply gentle pressure directly over her nipple for a minute or so to stop the leaking momentarily. The use of nursing pads (with instructions to change wet pads frequently), wearing printed tops that camouflage small leaks, and reassurance that the problem lessens with time may help alleviate this problem.

3. *Embarrassment.* Some mothers feel uncomfortable about breastfeeding because the mother is modest, or the mother may feel embarrassed because our society views breasts as sexual objects, and/or an unfriendly social environment makes it difficult to breastfeed in public. This is not an easy issue to overcome. Some mothers will feel some reassurance after learning how to breastfeed discreetly while in public.

4. *Stress.* Finding time and feeling tied down to the demands of breastfeeding can be stressful, expecially for the mother attending school or working outside of the home. This is a common reason mothers cite for weaning their infant prematurely. Mothers can be offered the option to decrease the frequency of pumping rather than quitting altogether. Of course this will decrease the mother's milk supply, but there are numerous studies showing that babies who receive some breast milk are still healthier than babies who do not receive any breast milk at all.

5. *Unequal feeding responsibilities/fathers left out.* Some parents want feedings to be a shared responsibility. The parents should be informed that it is advisable for the father to wait to bottle feed the baby with expressed breast milk until after breastfeeding is established. In the meantime, encourage the father to be supportive of the

breastfeeding mother, to have a lot of skin-to-skin contact with his infant, and to share the responsibilities of all other aspects of infant care (bathing, dressing, diapering, burping, rocking, etc.).

6. *Diet restriction.* Some mothers think that they have to give up eating certain foods when they breastfeed. This is, for the most part, a myth. Generally, mothers can still eat all the foods they are accustomed to eating. There are rare instances in which some infants are intolerant to something in the mother's milk. The most common problem comes from dairy products. In this case switching to cow's milk-based formula will not help as the infant will react to the cow's milk proteins in the formula. Often these infants will have cross-reaction to other types of proteins and will not tolerate soy-based formulas either. These babies may need to be on an expensive specialty formula such as a "predigested" hydrolysate formula if the mother quits breastfeeding. Again, this is not a common problem, but when it comes up, it is advisable to refer the mother to a lactation consultant for its management.

7. *Limited hormonal birth control options.* Some mothers think that they cannot use a hormonal method of birth control while breastfeeding. Mothers should be informed that using birth control pills containing progesterone and estrogen can cause a decrease in milk volume and may affect the quality of breast milk. It is preferred that the mother who wants to use a hormonal birth control method consider using the progestin-only minipill (i.e., Micronor®, Nor-QD®, Aygestin®, or Norlutate®); receive Depo-Provera®, a progestin-only injection administered every 90 days; or have a progestin-only implant. Although progestin-only hormonal birth control is compatible with lactation, they should not be started at the time of discharge. It is recommended that the mother wait 6 to 8 weeks before taking the hormonal medication to ensure a good milk supply (ACOG, 2000). Mothers can be reassured that barrier methods of birth control and natural family planning do not interfere with lactation at all and are good options to consider as well.

8. *Vaginal dryness associated with breastfeeding.* Some mothers experience vaginal dryness related to a low level of estrogen while lactating. Mothers can be given reassurance that this is only a temporary side effect while breastfeeding. A water-based lubricant such as K-Y® jelly or Astroglide® can be used during intercourse until she weans and estrogen levels increase again.

9. *Medications and breastfeeding.* Some mothers are concerned about the safety of breastfeeding while they are taking medications. Mothers can be reassured that most prescription and over-the-counter medications are safe for the breastfeeding infant. However, the mother needs to inform her healthcare provider and her infant's healthcare provider that she needs to take a medication for a period of time. The healthcare provider has a responsibility to research the medication, look at alternatives if indicated, and inform the mother whether the medication is compatible with breastfeeding. If the medication is not compatible with breastfeeding but is needed for only a short time, the mother can use a breast pump to maintain lactation and discard the milk. For additional information on medications and their compatibility with breastfeeding, see the list of resources at the end of the chapter.

POTENTIAL CONTRAINDICATIONS

There are some instances when breastfeeding is or may be contraindicated:

- Mother who is positive for the human immunodeficiency virus (HIV) or has acquired immunodeficiency virus syndrome (AIDS) is counseled against breastfeeding except in countries where the risk of neonatal death from diarrhea and other disease (excluding AIDS) is high (Jackson, Chopra, Witten et al., 2003).
- Mother uses illicit drugs (e.g., cocaine, heroin).
- Mother is an alcoholic.
- Maternal smoking can result in breastmilk concentrations of nicotine of 1.5 to 3 times the maternal plasma concentration. Although there is no documented infant health risk related to breastfeeding and smoking, smoking cessation is urged for maternal health reasons (Thureen, Deacon, Hernandez et al., 2005).
- Specific medications (e.g., radioactive isotopes, antimetabolites, chemotherapy drugs, and a few others). A mother with a diagnosis of breast cancer should not breastfeed so that she can begin treatment immediately.
- Mother has active, untreated tuberculosis.
- Infant has galactosemia.
- Mother has active herpes on her breast—the infant may still feed on the unaffected side only until the lesion has healed.
- Mother has varicella.
- Mother is human T-cell leukemia virus type 1–positive (HTLV1).
- Mother has another illness, on a case-by-case basis.

In addition concern is expressed about whether women with breast implants should breastfeed or are able to breastfeed. Some research on breast augmentation using the periareolar approach suggests increased incidence of lactation insufficiency (inadequate expressed milk volume and/or infant growth). Factors that may influence the ability of a mother with breast augmentation to breastfeed include: the surgical approach used, alterations in nipple sensation, amount of breast tissue present, and lack or little breast changes during pregnancy with little or no postpartum engorgement (Hill, Wilhelm, Aldag et al., 2004).

Another concern is related to the possible toxicity of the silicone in some breast implants. The silicone concentrations in formula and cow milk is higher than that found in the milk of mothers with implants; therefore, silicone breast implants are not a contraindication to breastfeeding (Thureen et al., 2005).

MEDICATIONS

It has long been recognized that medications taken by the breastfeeding mother may penetrate breast milk to some degree. Over the past 20 years, numerous studies have been published providing a better understanding of the kinetics of drug entry into breast milk, as well as factors influencing its bioavailability to the nursing infant. Understanding medications in breast milk and the implications to the infant is important, because use of medication has been identified as a barrier to breastfeeding and a major reason women cite for discontinuing it (Hale, 2004).

It should be noted that although most drugs penetrate into breast milk to some degree (usually less than 1% of the maternal dosage), very few drugs are contraindicated for breastfeeding women. (See the reference list at the end of the chapter for resources on medications in breast milk) (AAP Committee on Drugs, 2001; Briggs, Freeman, & Yaffe, 2005; Hale, 2004; and Lawrence & Lawrence, 2005).

Characteristics of a drug that influences its passage into breast milk include the following:

1. *Degree of protein binding.* Unbound drugs are more likely to enter the breast milk.
2. *Degree of ionization.* Drugs tend to cross into breast milk in un-ionized form.
3. *Molecular weight.* Drugs with lower molecular weight are more likely to cross.
4. *Degree of solubility in fat and water.* Lipid-soluble drugs pass more easily into breast milk across the alveolar epithelium, although all drugs pass more easily during the initial days postpartum when there are larger gaps between the alveolar epithelial cells.
5. *Mechanism of transport.* Most drugs enter breast milk by simple diffusion, but occasionally active transport or carrier-mediated diffusion may be involved.
6. *The pH.* Breast milk, which is acidic, attracts drugs that are weak bases.
7. *Half-life.* Rates of absorption, metabolism, and excretion determine a drug's half-life, or how fast it leaves the body. The longer the half-life, the greater the risk of accumulation in breast milk.

The net measurement of these effects determines the **milk/plasma ratio,** which relates the concentration of the drug in the breast milk to the concentration in the maternal plasma. For drugs that have equivalent dosing levels for the mother *and* equivalent safety profiles in the infant, it is preferable to use the drug with a lower milk/plasma ratio. Also, for any particular drug, it is preferable to use the lowest effective dose in the mother. Finally, the route and timing of the maternal dosing affects the maternal plasma level and therefore also the amount of drug seen by the baby.

The mother should be advised to inform her healthcare provider that she is breastfeeding when a drug is prescribed for her. In counseling the breastfeeding mother, the healthcare provider should weigh the benefits of the medication against the possible risk to the infant and its possible effects on the breast-feeding process. The potential risk to the infant must also be weighed against the effect of interrupting breastfeeding. Table 31–2 compares several factors for parents to consider when choosing between breastfeeding and formula-feeding.

THE FEEDING PROCESS
Breast Milk Production
BREAST ANATOMY

The female breast is divided into 15 to 20 lobes, separated from one another by fat and connective tissue, and interspersed with blood vessels, lymphatic vessels, and nerves. These lobes are subdivided into lobules composed of small units called alveoli where milk is synthesized by the alveolar secretory epithelium. The lobules have a system of lactiferous ductules that join larger ducts and eventually open onto the nipple surface. Mothers are often surprised to see milk coming out of multiple nipple pores when they express their milk. See Figure 31–1 ◆ to view the anatomy of the breast.

LACTOGENESIS

During pregnancy, increased levels of estrogen stimulate breast duct proliferation and development, and elevated progesterone levels promote the development of lobules and alveoli in preparation for lactation. Prolactin levels rise from approximately 10 ng/mL prepregnancy to 200 ng/mL at term. However, lactation is suppressed during pregnancy by elevated progesterone levels secreted by the placenta. Once the placenta is expelled at delivery, progesterone levels fall and

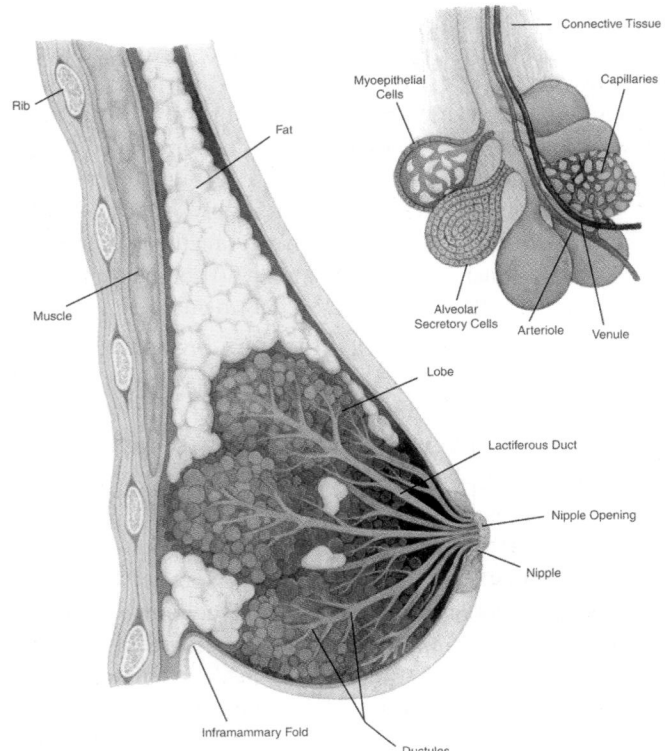

Figure 31–1 ◆ Anatomy of the breast.
SOURCE: From Riordan, J. (2005). *Breastfeeding and human lactation* (3rd ed., pp. 118–119). Boston: Jones & Bartlett. Copyright © 2005 Jones and Bartlett Publishers, Sudbury, MA. www.jbpub.com. Reprinted with permission.

Table 31–2 COMPARISON OF BREASTFEEDING AND FORMULA-FEEDING	
Breastfeeding	**Formula (Iron-Enriched)**
Infant Nutrition	
Species specific. An ideal balance of nutrients, efficiently absorbed. High bioavailability of iron leaves lower iron for bacterial growth, cell injury.	Derived from bovine milk and/or plant sources. Lower bioavailability of nutrients requires higher concentrations in milk. Additives may cause intolerance.
Higher levels of essential fatty acids, lactose, cystine, and cholesterol, necessary for brain and nerve growth.	Still missing numerous ingredients. Formulas do not contain cholesterol. Soy and hydrolysate formulas do not contain lactose. DHA and ARA now added.
Composition varies according to gestational age and stage of lactation, meeting changing nutritional needs.	Nutritional value not varied. Nutritional adequacy depends on proper preparation/dilution.
Long-term decreased incidence of diabetes, cancer, obesity, asthma.	
Contains unsaturated fats.	Contains saturated fats.
Infants determine the volume of milk consumed.	Parents or healthcare provider determine the volume consumed. Overfeeding may occur if caregiver is determined that baby empty bottle.
Frequency of feeding is determined by infant cues. May feed more frequently as milk digestion is faster.	Frequency of feeding is determined by infant's cues. May feed less frequently as milk digestion is slower.
Immunologic Properties	
Contains immunoglobulins, enzymes, and leukocytes that protect against pathogens. Nutrients promote growth of *Lactobacillus,* protective bacteria. Lower rates of urinary tract infections, otitis media, and other infectious diseases.	No anti-infective properties. Formula is linked to an increased incidence of gastrointestinal and respiratory tract infections.
Anti-infective properties present in the milk permit longer storage duration.	Potential for bacterial contamination exists during preparation and storage.
Breast milk is hypoallergenic, with minimal risk of protein allergy/intolerance.	Cow's milk protein allergy relatively common.
Maternal Health	
Faster return to prepregnancy weight.	Provides infant nutrition when breast milk not available because of maternal illness, medication/drug use, or lactation failure (breast surgery, endocrine disease).
Breastfeeding associated with lower risk of breast, ovarian cancer.	
Psychosocial Aspects	
Skin-to-skin contact enhances bonding.	Both parents can participate in positive parent-infant interaction during feeding.
Hormones of lactation promote maternal feelings and sense of well-being.	Father can assume feeding responsibilities.
The value system of modern society can create barriers to successful breastfeeding.	
Some mothers may feel ashamed or embarrassed.	
Breastfeeding after returning to work may be difficult.	
Cost	
Healthy diet for mother.	Formula cost per year: $1200 for standard formula, $2500/year for hypoallergenic formulas.
Savings for infant medical costs: approximately $400 average in first year of life.	Ancillary costs: bottles or bottle liners, nipples, cleaning costs.
Ancillary costs: nursing pads, nursing bras.	
A breast pump may be needed.	
Refrigeration is necessary for storing expressed milk.	Refrigeration is needed if preparing more than one bottle at a time.
Convenience	
Milk is always the perfect temperature. No preparation time is needed.	Formula must be purchased commercially. Preparation is time consuming. Less convenient for traveling or for night feedings.
The mother must be available to feed or will need to provide expressed milk to be given in her absence.	Mother need not be present—anyone can feed the infant.
If she misses a feeding, the mother must express milk to maintain lactation.	
The mother may experience slight discomfort in the early days of lactation.	

the inhibition is removed, triggering milk production. This occurs whether the mother has breast stimulation or not. However, if by the third or fourth day breast stimulation is not occurring, prolactin levels begin to drop. By 2 weeks postpartum, prolactin levels will be back to prepregnancy levels and milk production will cease.

PHYSIOLOGIC CONTROL OF BREASTFEEDING

Initially, lactation is under endocrine control. The hormone **prolactin** is released from the anterior pituitary in response to breast stimulation from suckling or the use of a breast pump. Prolactin stimulates the milk-secreting cells in the alveoli to produce milk, then rapidly drops back to baseline. If more than approximately 3 hours occurs between stimulation, prolactin levels begin to drop below baseline. To reverse the overall decline in prolactin level, the mother can be encouraged to stimulate her breasts more frequently (e.g., every 1.5 to 2 hours). Mothers should be strongly encouraged to stimulate their breasts frequently if their infants are not effective feeders or if they are separated from their infants. Prolactin receptors are established during the first 2 weeks postpartum in response to frequency of breast stimulation (Human Milk Banking Association of North America [HMBANA], 2005). Inadequate development of prolactin receptors during this time is likely to negatively impact the mother's long-term milk volume.

The milk that flows from the breast at the start of a feeding or pumping session is called **foremilk.** The foremilk is watery milk high in protein and low in fat (1% to 2%). This is milk that has trickled down from the alveoli between feedings to fill the lactiferous ducts. It is low-fat milk because the fat globules made in the alveoli stick to each other and to the walls of the alveoli and do not trickle down. In addition to prolactin release, stretching of the nipple and compression of the areola signal the hypothalamus to trigger the posterior pituitary gland to release oxytocin. **Oxytocin** acts on the myoepithelial cells surrounding the alveoli in the breast tissue to contract, ejecting milk, including the fat globules present, into the ducts. This process is called the milk-ejection reflex, better known in lay terms as the **"let-down" reflex.** The average initial let-down response occurs about 2 minutes after an infant begins to suckle, and there will be 4 to 10 let-down responses during a feeding session. The milk that flows during let-down is called hindmilk. As noted, **hindmilk** is rich in fat (can exceed 10%) and therefore high in calories. In a sample of expressed breast milk, the average total fat concentration is about 4% and the total caloric content is about 20 calories/ounce.

By 6 months of breastfeeding prolactin levels are only 5 to 10 ng/mL (Neville, 1999) yet milk production continues. A whey protein called feedback inhibitor of lactation (FIL) has been identified as influencing milk production through a negative feedback loop. FIL is present in breast milk and functions to decrease milk production. The more milk that remains in the breast for a longer period of time, the more milk production is decreased. On the other hand, the more often the breasts are emptied, the lower the level of FIL and the faster milk is produced. This mechanism of regulating milk at the local level is called autocrine control. This process is key to understanding how a mother maintains or loses her milk supply (Edgar, 2005).

There are a number of factors that can delay or impair lactogenesis. Maternal factors include cesarean birth, postpartum hemorrhage, diabetes type 1, untreated hypothyroidism, obesity, polycystic ovary syndrome, retained placenta fragments, vitamin B$_6$ deficiency, history of previous breast surgery, insufficient glandular breast tissue, and significant stress (Mohrbacher & Stock, 2003; Riordan, 2005). Other factors that can interfere with breastfeeding include smoking and use of alcohol and some prescription and over-the-counter medications (e.g., antihistamines, combined birth control pills).

STAGES OF HUMAN MILK

During the establishment of lactation there are three stages of human milk: colostrum, transitional milk, and mature milk.

Colostrum is the initial milk that begins to be secreted during midpregnancy and is immediately available to the baby at delivery. It provides the infant with all the nutrition required until the mother's milk becomes more abundant in a few days. No routine supplementation of other fluids is necessary unless there is a medical indication. Colostrum is a thick, creamy yellowish fluid with concentrated amounts of protein, fat-soluble vitamins, and minerals, and it has lower amounts of fat and lactose compared with mature milk. It also contains antioxidants and high levels of lactoferrin and secretory IgA. It promotes the establishment of *Lactobacillus bifidus* flora in the digestive tract, which helps to protect the infant from disease and illness. Colostrum also has a laxative effect on the infant, which helps the baby pass meconium stools, which in turn helps decrease hyperbilirubinemia.

Between day 2 and day 5, maternal milk production normally becomes noticeably more abundant. The milk "coming in" is called transitional milk. **Transitional milk** has qualities intermediate to colostrum and mature milk. It is still light yellow in color but is more copious than colostrum and contains more fat, lactose, water-soluble vitamins, and calories. By day 5, most mothers are producing about 500 mL/day.

Mature milk is white or slightly blue-tinged in color. It is present by 2 weeks postpartum and continues thereafter until lactation ceases. Mature milk contains about 13% solids (carbohydrates, proteins, and fats) and 87% water. Although mature human milk appears similar to skim cow's milk and may cause mothers to question whether their milk is "rich enough," mothers should be reassured that this is the normal appearance of mature human milk and that it provides the infant with all the necessary nutrients. Although gradual changes in composition do occur continuously over periods of weeks to accommodate the needs of the growing newborn over time, in general the composition of mature milk is fairly consistent with the exception of the fat content as noted previously. Milk production continues to increase slowly over the first month. By 6 months postpartum a mother produces about 800 mL/day (Hartmann, 1987; Hartmann & Prosser, 1984).

Timing of Newborn Feedings

The timing of newborn feedings is ideally determined by physiologic and behavioral cues rather than a set schedule.

INITIAL FEEDING

The nurse should assess for active bowel sounds, absence of abdominal distention, and a lusty cry that quiets and is replaced with rooting and sucking behaviors when a stimulus is placed near the lips. These signs indicate that the newborn is hungry and physically ready to tolerate the initial feeding.

If there are no complications at the birth and the mother is not overly sedated, the infant may be placed on the mother's chest after birth. Throughout the first 2 hours after birth, but especially during the first hour of life, the infant is usually alert and ready to breastfeed. Because colostrum is not irritating if aspirated (which may occur because of the newborn's initial uncoordinated sucking and swallowing abilities) and is readily absorbed by the respiratory system, breastfeeding can usually begin immediately after birth. The mother benefits psychologically from early breastfeeding through enhancement of maternal-infant bonding and physiologically by the release of oxytocin, which helps contract the uterus, expelling the placenta and decreasing the risk of postpartum hemorrhage. Early feedings benefit the newborn because they help prevent hypoglycemia, promote the passage of meconium, provide the newborn receives the immunologic protection of colostrum, and begin to stimulate further maternal milk production, helping prevent later feeding difficulties.

If the mother plans to bottle-feed, she and her newborn can still enjoy skin-to-skin contact initially. Formula-feedings are not typically initiated in the birthing room. Formula-feeding newborns are offered formula as soon as they show interest/feeding cues or per hospital policy. For both breastfed and formula-fed infants, early feeding stimulates peristalsis, helping to eliminate the by-products of bilirubin conjugation (which decreases the risk of jaundice), and enhances maternal-infant attachment.

Assessment of the newborn's physiologic status is a primary and ongoing concern to the nurse throughout the first feeding. Extreme fatigue coupled with rapid respiration, circumoral cyanosis, and diaphoresis of the head and face may indicate cardiovascular complications and should be assessed further.

The first feeding also provides an opportunity for the nurse to assess the effectiveness of the newborn's suck, swallow, and gag reflexes. The nurse should also remain alert to the possibility of medical problems during this time, including respiratory disorders, congenital cardiovascular problems, or more rare disorders such as tracheoesophageal fistula and esophageal atresia (see Chapter 32 ∞). Findings associated with esophageal anomalies include maternal polyhydramnios and increased oral mucus in the infant. In cases of esophageal atresia, the feeding is taken well initially, but as the esophageal pouch fills, the feeding is quickly regurgitated unchanged by stomach contents. If a fistula is present, the infant gags, chokes, regurgitates mucus, and may become cyanotic as fluid passes through the fistula into the lungs.

It is not unusual for the newborn to regurgitate some mucus and water following a feeding, even if it was taken without difficulty, because of initial uncoordinated suck and swallow abilities. It is important to observe the newborn closely and position the baby on the side after the feeding to aid drainage and facilitate gastric emptying. Once the infant is tolerating feeding, the normal position after feeding is on his or her back.

ESTABLISHING A FEEDING PATTERN

An "on-demand" feeding program facilitates each baby's own rhythm and helps a new mother establish lactation. The newborn rapidly digests breast milk and may want to nurse 8 to 10 times in a 24-hour period. After the initial period of alertness and eagerness to suckle, the infant progresses to light sleep, then deep sleep, followed by increased wakefulness and interest in breastfeeding. As wakefulness and interest in nursing increase, the infant will often cluster 5 to 10 feeding episodes over 2 to 3 hours, followed by a 4- to 5-hour deep sleep. After this cluster of minifeeds and deep sleep, the infant will feed frequently but at more regular intervals. Crying is considered a late feeding cue. Often newborn arousal from sleep is the first sign of hunger.

Early feeding cues include rooting, smacking, or attempting to suck on anything near his or her mouth (especially the hand). Although people often accept crying as normal and healthy behavior for newborns, it may actually delay the transition to extrauterine life. Crying involves a Valsalva maneuver that increases pulmonary vascular pressure, which may cause unoxygenated blood to be shunted into systemic circulation through the foramen ovale and ductus arteriosus. If no one has responded to the newborn by this time, then the infant may begin to fuss and eventually work up to a full cry. A newborn who is left to cry and not given the opportunity to feed at this point may subsequently become very disorganized and have a difficult time latching on to the breast or coordinating his or her suck correctly.

Certain hospital practices/policies may contribute to delays in feeding by prolonging the feeding intervals and even decreasing the number of feedings in a 24-hour period. *Couplet care* or rooming-in practices promote cue-based feedings. Therefore, it may be advantageous for the baby to be in the room with the mother; she will respond to the baby's needs more quickly than the nursery staff may be able to, resulting in less infant crying.

Couplet care permits the mother to learn about and respond to her infant's early feeding cues. Early cues that indicate a newborn is interested in feeding include hand-to-mouth or hand-passing-mouth motion, whimpering, sucking, and rooting (Mulford, 1992). Satiety behaviors can include withdrawal of head from the nipple, falling asleep, relaxation of hands, and relief of body tension. When couplet care is not available, a supportive nursing staff and flexible nursery policies allow the mother to feed her infant on cue. It is very frustrating to a new mother to attempt to feed a newborn who is sound asleep because he or she is either not hungry or exhausted from crying.

Feeding intervals are counted from the time of the start of one feeding to the start of the next feeding. Breastfeeding babies typically feed every 1.5 to 3 hours (8 to 12 times in a 24-hour period), but often in an irregular pattern known as "cluster feeding," in which the infant feeds as frequently as every hour for a few feedings followed by a longer sleep period. The normal newborn sleeps a total of 16 to 18 hours per day, but generally with no more than one sleep stretch of up to 5 hours in length. It is more important to focus on the number of feedings in 24 hours than the exact feeding interval time. Formula-fed infants generally eat every 3 to 4 hours and typically 6 to 8 times per day. It is important that families are taught about the normal feeding/sleeping pattern of a newborn. Many parents are distressed by their infant's early erratic feeding pattern. Parents need to be informed that their infant will have a more predictable sleep and feeding pattern when he or she is 2 to 4 months of age.

Maternal medications received during labor may affect newborn feeding behavior by delaying these early cluster feedings. Delays in normal feeding patterns depend on the specific drug and its half-life. Newborns whose mothers received epidural analgesia have been noted to be irritable and demonstrate reduced motor organization, poor self-quieting skills, and decreased visual skills and alertness (Biancuzzo, 2003). Because breastfeeding infants generally have only one long sleep stretch in a 24-hour period, parents can help their infant to take the long sleep stretch at night if they attempt to awaken their infant during the day when the infant is in a light state of sleep and has already slept longer than 3 hours. Parents can attempt to encourage cluster feedings during the day, and, after awhile, the infant may sleep a 5-hour sleep stretch at night. In the meantime, the mother can be encouraged to take "cat naps" during the day while her infant is sleeping. At night the mother can keep stimulation down (lights low, noise low, and diaper change only when necessary).

Both breastfeeding and formula-feeding infants have the same fluid requirements, but because they have different diets, their rates of digestion are different. Digestion of formula produces large, rubbery curds that take about 4 hours to digest compared with the softer, smaller curds produced by breast milk. For this reason formula-fed newborns generally sleep longer at a stretch and awaken to feed every 3 to 4 hours, It is not uncommon that formula-fed newborns may take one or two 5-hour sleep stretches in a 24-hour period. As a result they will often take a larger volume at each feed. Babies may begin skipping the night feeding about 8 to 12 weeks after birth. The need for a night feeding is individual and depends on the size and development of the infant.

Satiety behaviors are the same for formula-fed babies as for breastfed babies. These behaviors include longer pauses toward the end of the feeding, noticeable total body relaxation (the baby lies limp with hands down at his side and unclenched), the infant may release his mother's nipple or the bottle nipple, and many fall asleep. If a baby is satiated and content following feedings, is meeting daily output expectations, and is gaining weight as expected, then feedings are going well.

Both breastfed and formula-fed infants experience growth spurts at certain times and require increased feeding. The breastfeeding mother may meet these increased demands by nursing more frequently to increase her milk supply. It takes about 72 hours for the milk supply to increase adequately to meet the new demand (Biancuzzo, 2003). A slight increase in feedings meets the formula-fed infant's needs.

Some mothers may find fixed feeding schedules attractive. These mothers should be informed that although strict feeding schedules may work for some babies, they often do not work for all babies because they do not take into account differences among breastfeeding women and differences among infants. There are documented cases of infants diagnosed with failure to thrive, poor weight gain, dehydration, breast milk supply failure, and involuntary early weaning associated with this feeding method (Aney, 1998). The AAP released a media alert in April 1998 reaffirming its position that "the best feeding schedules are ones babies design themselves. Scheduled feedings designed by parents may put babies at risk for poor weight gain and dehydration."

Nourishing her newborn is a major concern of the new mother. Her feelings of success or failure may influence her self-concept as she assumes her maternal role. With proper instruction, support, and encouragement from professionals, feeding becomes a source of pleasure and satisfaction to both the parents and infant.

Client Education: Feeding Technique
BREASTFEEDING POSITION AND LATCHING

Breastfeeding is not instinctive, it is learned. It is a natural process, but it takes "know-how." Ideally, each breastfeeding mother should have a breastfeeding evaluation to determine any knowledge deficits, acknowledge any concerns, provide instructions, and assist with breastfeeding.

Positioning. There are many breastfeeding positions, but only the four classic breastfeeding positions are discussed here. In addition, there are minor variations of hand placement and body position even among the four classic positions. The four positions discussed here include (1) modified cradle position, (2) cradle position, (3) football (or clutch) hold position, and (4) side-lying position (Figures 31–2 ◆ through 31–5 ◆). After a mother has fed using one position, encourage her to try a different position when she offers her second breast. Alternating positions facilitates drainage of the breasts and changes the pressure points on the breast. This will provide some relief to the mother with sore nipples.

- Have mother sit comfortably in upright position using good body alignment. Use pillows for support (may use Boppy, body pillow, or standard bed pillows). Lap pillow should help bring baby up to breast level so mother does not lean over baby.
- Place baby on mother's lap and turn baby's entire body toward mother (baby is in side-lying position). Position baby's body so that the baby's nose lines up to the nipple. Maintain baby's body in a horizontal alignment.
- To feed at left breast, mother supports baby's head with her right hand at nape of baby's neck (allow head to slightly lag back), mother's right thumb by baby's left ear, and right forefinger near baby's right ear.
- With mother's free left hand, she can offer her left breast.

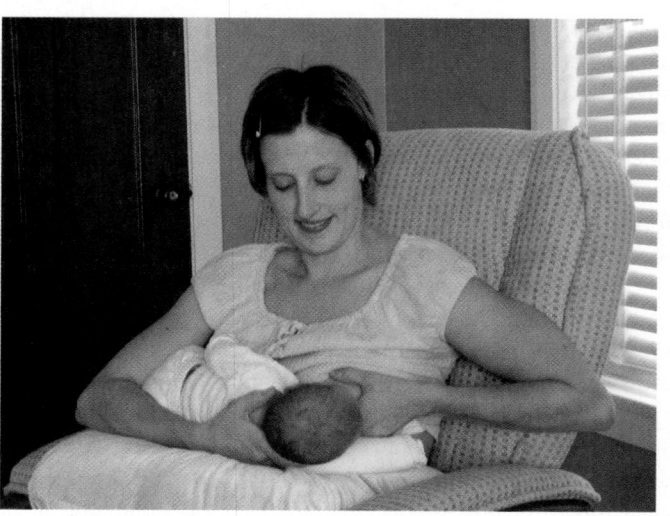

Figure 31–2 ◆ Modified cradle position.
SOURCE: Courtesy of Brigette Hall, MSN, IBCLC.

Figure 31–3 ◆ Cradle position.
SOURCE: Courtesy of Brigette Hall, MSN, IBCLC.

- Have mother sit comfortably in upright position using good body alignment. Use pillows for support (may use Boppy, body pillow, or standard bed pillows). Lap pillow should help bring baby up to breast level so mother does not lean over baby.
- Place baby on mother's lap and turn baby's entire body toward mother (baby is in side-lying position). Position baby's body so that the baby's nose lines up to the nipple. Maintain baby's body in a horizontal alignment.
- If feeding from the left breast, have mother cradle baby's head near the crook of her left arm while supporting her baby's body with her left forearm.
- With mother's free right hand, she can offer her left breast.

Figure 31–4 ◆ Football hold position.
SOURCE: Courtesy of Brigette Hall, MSN, IBCLC.

- Have mother sit comfortably and use pillows to raise baby's body to breast level. If using a Boppy and the Boppy is in "normal" position on mother's lap, turn it counterclockwise slightly (if feeding at left breast) to provide extended support for baby's body resting along mother's left side and near the back of mother's chair.
- If feeding at left breast, place baby on the left side of mother's body, heading baby into position feet first. Baby's bottom should rest on the pillow near mother's left elbow.
- Turn baby slightly on her side so that she faces the breast.
- Mother's left arm clutches baby's body close to mother's body. Baby's body should feel securely tucked in under mother's left arm.
- Have mother support baby's head with her left hand. With mother's free right hand, she can offer her breast. (Good position for mother with c-section).

Figure 31–5 ◆ Side-lying position.
SOURCE: Courtesy of Brigette Hall, MSN, IBCLC.

- Have mother rest comfortably lying on her side (left side for this demonstration). Use pillows to support mother's head and back, and provide support for mother's hips by placing a pillow between her bent knees.
- Place baby in side-lying position next to mother's body. Baby's body should face mother's body. Baby's nose should line up to mother's nipple. Place a roll behind baby's back, if desired.
- With mother's free right hand, she can offer her left breast. After baby is securely attached, mom can rest her right hand anywhere that is comfortable for her.

CLINICAL TIP

The cradle position is challenging, especially when attempted during early lactation by inexperienced mothers because the mother is attempting to support her baby's head near the crook of her arm. This makes it difficult to control the head position and may allow the baby's head to bend forward (chin toward chest), making attachment difficult. It is better to have the infant's head lag slightly backward (chin tilted slightly upward) so that the infant leads into the breast chin first. Some mothers find it easier to start in the modified cradle position and then switch into the cradle position.

Latching On. It is important to have the mother and baby positioned properly in order to achieve an optimal attachment. If, for example, the infant is lying flat on his or her back (supine position) to feed in the modified cradle position, cradle position, or side-lying position, the infant can obtain only a shallow latch (not attached far back onto the areola). The infant's shoulder becomes an obstacle putting distance between the infant's mouth and the mother's breast. Anything that contributes to a shallow latch is going to cause sore nipples and other complications. Nipple trauma, although relatively common, is not normal. See Chapter 36 ∞ for discussion of breastfeeding with inverted or flat nipples.

The infant needs to attach his or her lips onto the breast, or rather more accurately, far back onto the areola, not on the nipple. If the infant attaches just to the nipple, the mother will have sore nipples and pain may inhibit the let-down reflex. To obtain a deep latch, the mother needs to be taught how to elicit the infant's rooting reflex, stimulating the infant to open his or her mouth as widely as possible (like a big yawn). Once the infant does this, the mother should quickly but gently draw her baby in toward her. During the first few days of life, the newborn typically only opens his or her mouth widely for a second or so, and then begins to close the mouth again. If the mother misses her chance to get her baby latched on, she needs to simply start over again.

Figures 31–6 ◆ through 31–11 ◆ demonstrate various positions and techniques used in latching on.

Figure 31–6 ◆ C-hold hand position.
SOURCE: Courtesy of Brigette Hall, MSN, IBCLC.

To be ready to draw baby's mouth onto mother's breast, as soon as the baby opens her or his mouth widely enough, the mother needs to have her hand supporting her breast in ready position. She can use various hand holds, but she needs to keep her fingers well behind the areola. One such hand position is called the "C-hold." In this hold, the thumb is placed on top of the breast near 12 o'clock position and the other four fingers are placed on the underside of the breast near at the 6 o'clock position (depends on mother's hand size and length of fingers). The key point is in keeping the fingers at least 1½ inches back from the base of the nipple as the fingers support the breast. Mothers are not often aware of where they place their fingers, especially on the underside of the breast. If the fingers are too far forward (too close to the nipple), then the infant cannot grasp a large amount of areola in her or his mouth and this results in a "shallow" latch. A shallow latch is associated with nipple pain and ineffective drainage of the breast.

An alternate hand hold not shown is a "U-hold" hand position. The thumb and forefinger are near the 3 o'clock and 9 o'clock positions on the breast again with fingers at least 1½ inches back from the base of the nipple; the body of the hand rests on the lower portion of the breast. Using this hand hold, the mother's arm position is down at her side rather than sticking outward as it is when supporting the breast using in the C-hold position.

The scissor hold is often discouraged because mothers (especially mothers with small hands) have a difficult time keeping their fingers off the areola or at least 1½ inches back from the base of the areola. Here, the mother is able to support her breast well without letting her fingers encroach onto the areola.

The mother should be instructed to gently support the breast and not press too deeply, which can obstruct the flow of milk through the ducts.

Figure 31–7 ◆ Scissor hold hand position.
SOURCE: Courtesy of Brigette Hall, MSN, IBCLC.

Figure 31–8 ◆ Nose to nipple.
SOURCE: Courtesy of Brigette Hall, MSN, IBCLC.

Before eliciting the rooting reflex, it is important to have the baby in good alignment. When the infant opens her or his mouth to latch on, the goal is to achieve a deep, asymmetric latch attachment. The goal is *not* to center the nipple in the baby's mouth. The rationale for this is to optimize oral-motor function. The jaw is a hinge joint. The upper jaw is immobile; the lower jaw compresses the breast. The breast is efficiently drained if more areola is drawn into the baby's mouth from the inferior aspect of the breast and a smaller amount drawn in from the superior aspect of the areola. Aligning the infant to the mother with baby's nose facing mother's nipple permits the jaw to be in a lower position. The next step is to let the infant drop his or her head back (head in "sniff position"), so that the infant leads into the breast with the chin.

Figure 31–9 ◆ Initial attempt to elicit the rooting reflex.
SOURCE: Courtesy of Brigette Hall, MSN, IBCLC.

To trigger the rooting reflex, teach the mother to use her nipple to stroke downward in a vertical motion across the middle of baby's lower lip. Initially, the infant may respond by licking or smacking. This is a normal response to the stimulus. Encourage the mother to keep stimulating the infant's lower lip until the infant finally opens her or his mouth widely. If the infant is not responding at all, then the infant is probably too sleepy and may need help waking up. After trying wake up techniques, the infant may be ready to try breastfeeding again.

Figure 31–10 ◆ Continued attempt to elicit rooting reflex.
SOURCE: Courtesy of Brigette Hall, MSN, IBCLC.

Teach the mother to be patient and wait for the infant's mouth to gape open as widely as possible. Here the infant needs to open the mouth even wider before the mother draws her baby toward the breast. The mother should be encouraged to continue stroking the infant's lip until the infant opens the mouth wider.

Figure 31–11 ◆ Baby is latched-on.
SOURCE: Courtesy of Brigette Hall, MSN, IBCLC.

Once baby has latched onto the breast, the mother should check that baby is latched on properly. The infant's chin should be embedded into the mother's breast. The infant's nose should be very close but not actually touching the breast. The nose should be centered. If the mother feels a little pinch on her areola, she can slowly release the hand supporting her breast so she can have a free hand to attempt to move her baby's jaw gently downward. To do this maneuver, the mother needs to place her thumb or forefinger of her free hand (the hand that just released the breast) on baby's lower jaw (there is a horizontal groove to use as leverage—the groove on baby's chin is parallel with the baby's lips). With gentle downward pressure the mother should feel relief of any persistent tenderness. This procedure opens the jaw wider and it also helps to roll out the infant's lower lip that may have been inadvertently drawn into the baby's mouth. As the baby begins to suckle, there should be no dimpling of the infant's cheeks and no smacking or clicking noises.

CLINICAL TIP

As you assist new mothers with breastfeeding, it is important to create a relaxed environment and approach to breastfeeding. Encourage the mother to get into a comfortable position, well supported with pillows. Remind her to bring the baby to her breast rather than leaning forward to the baby.

BREASTFEEDING ASSESSMENT

During the birthing unit stay, the nurse must carefully monitor the progress of the breastfeeding pair. A systematic assessment of several breastfeeding episodes provides the opportunity to teach the new mother about lactation and the breastfeeding process, provide anticipatory guidance, and evaluate the need for follow-up care after discharge. Criteria for evaluating a breastfeeding session include maternal and infant cues, latch-on, position, let-down, nipple condition, infant response, and maternal response. The literature provides various tools to guide the assessment and documentation of the breast-feeding efforts. The LATCH Scoring Table is one example (Figure 31–12 ◆). Table 31–3 identifies signs of successful breastfeeding.

CLINICAL TIP

With a sleepy baby, unwrap the baby, encourage lots of skin-to-skin contact between mother and baby, have the mother rest with baby near her breast so that the baby can feel and smell the breast. Encourage the mother to watch for feeding cues, such as hand-to-mouth activity, fluttering eyelids, vocalization but not necessarily crying, and mouthing activities.

BOTTLE-FEEDING BREAST MILK (EXPRESSION, PUMPS, STORAGE)

There are a number of different reasons for bottle-feeding breast milk. The nurse should evaluate the indications in order to recommend the best technique for the mother and her particular need. Some mothers prefer to hand express their milk rather than use a breast pump, and many find that in the immediate

---

 Table 31–3   SUCCESSFUL BREASTFEEDING EVALUATION

Babies are probably getting enough milk if:

- They are nursing at least eight times in 24 hours.
- In a quiet room, their mothers can hear them swallow while nursing.
- Their mother's breasts appear to soften after breastfeeding.
- The number of wet diapers increases daily until the fourth or fifth day after birth, and there are at least six to eight wet diapers every 24 hours after day 5.
- Their stools are beginning to lighten in color by the third day after birth, or have changed to yellow no later than day 5.
- Offering a supplemental bottle is not a reliable indicator because most babies will take a few ounces even if they are getting enough breast milk.

---

postpartum period hand expression of milk may be a more effective method of removing drops of colostrum than using an electric breast pump. Nurses should teach all mothers the skill of hand expressing breast milk as it is possible the mother will find herself in a situation without a breast pump but needing to relieve herself from engorgement.

To hand express breast milk, have the mother follow steps 1 through 4 of the pumping instructions provided in Table 31–4. Next the mother should use the Marmet technique of hand expression described next. It is important that the mother take care to place her hands exactly as directed. The steps are as follows:

1. The mother will position her thumb at the 12 o'clock position on the top edge of the areola (about 1 to 1½ inches back from the tip of her nipple) and her forefinger and middle finger pads at the 6 o'clock position on the bottom edge of the areola (about 1 to 1½ inches from the tip of her nipple). If positioned correctly, a line between the thumb and fingers will cross the nipple. See Figure 31–13 ◆.

2. Next the mother will stretch her areola back toward her chest wall without lifting her fingers off her breast.

	0	1	2
L Latch	Too sleepy or reluctant No latch achieved	Repeated attempts Hold nipple in mouth Stimulate to suck	Grasps breast Tongue down Lips flanged Rhythmic sucking
A Audible swallowing	None	A few with stimulation	Spontaneous and intermittent > 24 hours old Spontaneous and frequent < 24 hours old
T Type of nipple	Inverted	Flat	Everted (after stimulation)
C Comfort (breast/nipple)	Engorged Cracked, bleeding, large blisters or bruises Severe discomfort	Filling Reddened/small blisters or bruises Mild/moderate discomfort	Soft Nontender
H Hold (positioning)	Full assist (staff holds infant at breast)	Minimal assist (e.g., elevate head of bed, place pillows for support) Teach one side; mother does other Staff holds and then mother takes over	No assist from staff Mother able to position and hold infant

Figure 31–12 ◆ LATCH: A breastfeeding charting and documentation tool. LATCH was created to provide a systematic method for breastfeeding assessment and charting. It can be used to assist the new mother in establishing breastfeeding and to define areas of needed intervention.
SOURCE: *Used with permission from AWHONN.* (1994). Jensen, D., Wallace, S., & Kelsay, P. Breastfeeding charting system and documentation tool. *Journal of Obstetric, Gynecologic, & Neonatal Nursing, 23*(1), 27–32. (Table 1 Latch Scoring Table, p. 29.) Washington, DC: Author. © 1994 by the Association of Women's Health, Obstetric, and Neonatal Nurses. All rights reserved.

Table 31–4   PUMPING INSTRUCTIONS

1. Once a day rinse your breasts with water during your bath or shower. Avoid using soap on your nipples.
2. Wash your hands well with soap and water before preparing to pump.
3. Take a few minutes to massage your breasts and relax (e.g., do some deep breathing, think about your baby, look at a picture of your baby). Being relaxed is very important for letting down your milk. (Stress causes the release of adrenalin, which blocks receptors for let-down.)
4. You should sit up straight or lean slightly forward (perhaps even place a pillow behind your back so that your posture is tilted slightly forward), as gravity aids in the flow of your milk.
5. For single-sided pumping, pump each breast for 10–15 minutes. Some mothers find that they empty their breasts more efficiently if they switch back and forth from one side to the other as the milk flow diminishes until they have stimulated each breast for 15 minutes.
6. Pump your milk into glass or plastic bottle containers. Mothers of healthy infants may also use bottle bags/liners intended for breast milk storage to collect and store their milk. *[Because of the loss of antibodies that can occur with bottle bags/liners, mothers of preemies and fragile infants should probably avoid using these.]* Do not fill containers more than ¾ full, because milk expands during freezing.
7. Feed freshly expressed breast milk when breastfeeding is not an option/choice. If the expressed breast milk is not needed immediately, store the expressed breast milk in the refrigerator if it is likely to be used within 5–8 days. (The sooner it is used, the greater the quality of the milk.) Otherwise, freeze the expressed breast milk. Avoid placing breast milk in the freezer door or on the bottom of a self-defrosting freezer because the temperature fluctuates more in those areas.
8. Store expressed breast milk in volumes your infant is likely to consume at a single feeding or in a volume your infant will consume in a day.
9. Frozen breast milk can be thawed safely using one of two methods. To quickly thaw breast milk, remove the frozen bottle of breast milk from the freezer, place the bottle in a bowl in the sink, and run warm water over it. To thaw out more slowly, take the frozen bottle of breast milk, place it in the refrigerator and let it thaw out over several hours. The time it takes to do this depends on the volume in the bottle. Note that breast milk that has been sitting will normally separate. To remix it, simply swirl the bottle until the milk is evenly mixed. If the amount in the bottle is more than you will use in one feeding, pour the amount you want into a clean bottle, and put the rest back in the refrigerator. Take the bottle for feeding, place it in a bowl in the sink, and run warm water over it before feeding. The bottle should remain upright and not float in the bowl. The water level in the bowl should remain below the lid of the bottle/milk container. *Note: never use a microwave oven to thaw or warm breast milk.*
10. Thawed breast milk is good in the refrigerator for 24 hours.

---

3. Now she should roll her thumb and fingers simultaneously forward. This action compresses the ducts beneath the areola and stimulates the breast to empty the breast both manually and by triggering the let-down reflex.

4. The mother should repeat the sequence multiple times to completely drain her breasts. She should try to maintain a steady rhythm, cycling 45 to 60 times/minute. It is also more effective if the mother repositions her fingers to other positions on the same breast (3 and 9 o'clock, 1 and 7 o'clock, etc.) when the milk flow slows.

The mother should take care not to traumatize her breasts or nipples. Hand expression should not be painful. Most mothers

Figure 31–13 ◆ Hand expression.
SOURCE: Courtesy of Brigette Hall, MSN, IBCLC.

Figure 31–14 ◆ Manual breast pump.
SOURCE: Courtesy of Brigette Hall, MSN, IBCLC.

will need assistance in learning this technique initially. Reassure the mother that it is a skill that is learned, and with practice, she can become an expert at hand expression.

Although hand expression can be efficient, many mothers will choose to use a mechanical breast pump to express their milk. Not all breast pumps are of the same quality, even within the same category (see Table 31–5, Figure 31–14 ◆, Figure 31–15 ◆). Pumps generally cycle from low to high suction at a frequency similar to that of a breastfeeding infant (about 45 to 60 cycles per minute). However, differences in the quality of the pump motor or the presence or absence of controls over suction pressure mean that some pumps will generate inadequate pressure or cycle too slowly to be effective, whereas others may exert too high a suction that can cause injury. Flange size, proper fit, and comfort are other variables to consider. The nurse should refer the mother to a lactation consultant or other person knowledgeable regarding different breast pumps.

Figure 31–15 ◆ Hospital-grade, double electric breast pump.

Table 31–5	**TYPES OF BREAST PUMPS AND INDICATIONS FOR USE**			
Indication	**Manual Breast Pump (Figure 31–14)**	**Small Battery/Electric Breast Pump**	**Individual Double Electric Breast Pump**	**Hospital-Grade Multiuser Double Electric Breast Pump (Figure 31–15)**
A missed feeding	■	▲		
An evening out	■	▲		
Working part-time	■	▲		
Convenience—occasional use	■	▲		
Working full-time			*	*
Premature/hospitalized infant				*
Low milk supply				*
Sore nipples/engorgement			*	*
Latch-on problems/infection			■	*
Drawing out flattish nipples	■	▲	*	*

■ Good   ▲ Better   * Best

SOURCE: Modified from the Medela Breastfeeding Information Guide Tips and Products. (2002). *Table: Which Breast pump Is Best for You?* (p. 3). McHenry, IL: Medela, Inc. Copyright © Medela, Inc. All rights reserved.

Table 31–6	STORAGE GUIDELINES FOR BREAST MILK AND FORMULA	

Milk	Environment	Time Until Discard
Breast milk or formula, opened/reconstituted	Being fed	Finish feed within 1 hour
Breast milk or formula, opened/reconstituted	Environment greater than 79°F	1 hour
Breast milk or formula, opened/reconstituted	Room temperature	4 hours
Breast milk or formula, opened/reconstituted	Cooler pack less than 59°F	24 hours
Thawed breast milk	Refrigerator	24 hours
Formula, opened/reconstituted	Refrigerator	24–48 hours (see label)
Fresh breast milk	Refrigerator	8 days
Formula powder, opened can	Room temperature	1 month
Fresh breast milk	Freezer	3 month
Formula/powder in sealed container	Avoid excessive heat	Printed expiration date
Thawed breast milk	Freezer	Do not refreeze
Formula	Freezer	Do not freeze

SOURCE: Data from Human Milk Banking Association of North America (HMBANA). (2005). *Best practice for expressing, storing and handling human milk in hospitals, homes and child care settings.* Raleigh, NC: Author; Mead-Johnson Nutritionals. (2004). *Pediatric products handbook.* New York: Bristol-Myers Squibb Company (http://www.meadjohnson.com); and Ross Products Division. (2004). *Pediatric nutritionals product guide.* Columbus, OH: Abbott Laboratories (http://www.ROSS.com).

There are different guidelines for storage of expressed breast milk (EBM) depending on whether the infant is a healthy full-term infant or a premature or sick infant in the hospital. The guidelines in Table 31–6 are intended as a resource for the mother of a healthy, full-term infant.

SUPPLEMENTARY BOTTLE-FEEDING

Supplementary bottle-feedings for the breastfeeding infant after birth are not recommended routinely. Routine supplementation has been strongly implicated in early breastfeeding termination (Hall, Mercer, Teaslet et al., 2002). Routine supplements are not only unnecessary, they can also contribute to maternal and infant health problems, including delayed early maternal milk production, maternal engorgement after her milk production has increased, infant milk-protein intolerance, and difficulties with learning to breastfeed.

"Nipple confusion" or "nipple preference" can occur in some babies, causing them to develop an incorrect sucking technique, or to simply refuse to breastfeed again. This potential problem occurs because the techniques for breastfeeding and bottle-feeding are different. In breastfeeding, the infant has to open his or her mouth very wide in order to latch on. To transfer milk the baby has to extend the tongue forward, cupping the nipple and drawing it from back to front in a milking motion. With bottle-feeding, the infant keeps the tongue retracted and uses the tip of the tongue to block the flow of milk, which otherwise drips rapidly. Some babies can switch back and forth between breast and bottle without obvious difficulty, but for other infants, it is a

problem. To reduce this possibility, experts in the field of lactation recommend introducing the bottle when the infant is between 3 and 6 weeks of age and breastfeeding is well established.

Parents are often concerned because they have no visual assurance of the amount of breast milk consumed. The mother should be taught to observe the infant for effective breastfeeding. The infant should have a rhythmic suckling pattern (the slight pause between jaw compressions on the breast permits the mouth to fill with milk before swallowing). To note if the jaw compressions are strong enough, the mother should observe or feel if there is movement at the bilateral temporomandibular joints located in front of the infant's ears. The infant should maintain a rhythmic feeding pattern with only brief pauses (lasting only seconds, not minutes) between spurts of active feeding, with the feeding session typically lasting for 10 to 20 minutes on the first breast: the infant may feed only a few minutes on the second breast or not at all. The mother should visually observe for swallowing, and, later, as her milk is abundant, she will hear the infant's swallows. Discourage the mother from watching the clock to determine when the infant needs to switch breast sides but rather encourage her to watch the newborn's feeding pattern to note when active feeding ceases. When satiated, the infant will either pull away from the breast or fall asleep. The infant will be extremely relaxed at the end of the feeding and will sleep until the next feeding is due (at least an hour). As the infant matures, the feeding intervals will lengthen. Another indicator of breastfeeding efficiency is softening of mother's breasts, although this is not a reliable indicator in the first few days postpartum while breast milk volume is low. Within a week, however, this is a good indicator of milk transfer.

The infant who feeds well will have a characteristic output. See Figure 31–16 ◆ for breastfeeding intake and output expectations. The infant should also have the characteristic weight loss followed by weight gain pattern discussed earlier in this chapter.

Finally, the most reliable measurement of effective breastfeeding is measuring the breast milk that actually transfers. This is done by obtaining pre- and postbreastfeeding weight checks using an accurate infant scale. The difference in prefeed and postfeed weights is the amount of milk transferred to the infant and may be useful with assessing weight gain in near-term infants.

At times there are valid medical indications for supplementation of the breastfeeding infant. These include delayed lactogenesis, unavailability of the mother because of severe illness or separation, primary lactation failure, hypoglycemia, significant dehydration, weight loss of 8% to 10% with exclusive breastfeeding, delayed passage of stool (presence of meconium on day 5), hyperbilirubinemia related to poor intake, prematurity, or low birth weight, and refusal of or ineffective breastfeeding.

For those times when supplementation is indicated, the first choice is to use the mother's own milk (fresh, previously expressed, or frozen/thawed). If maternal breast milk is not available, pasteurized donor milk is the next choice, and then formula. Supplementation can be admininistered using a bottle or one of the following alternative feeding methods: cup-feeding, spoon-feeding, eyedropper- or syringe-feeding, or a nursing supplementer. The method chosen is based on the particular situation and parental preference.

Breastfeeding Intake and Output Expectations

- Baby should breastfeed 8 to 12 times/day and appear satisfied after feeding.
- Colostrum is all that the newborn needs in the first few days of life in most cases.
- It is normal for the infant to lose up to 7% (or between 5% and 10%) of birth weight in the first few days of life.
- Baby should gain 10 grams/kg/day after the milk is abundant (about day 4 of life).
- Baby should be back to birth weight by 2 weeks of age.
- Baby's stool should change in color, consistency, and frequency during the first few days of life. The color of stools changes from tarry black to dark greenish-black to greenish-brown, to brownish-yellow, to light greenish-yellow, to bright yellow or yellowish-orange. The consistency of stools changes from tarry-sticky to thinner consistencies to curdy or seedy and "explosive." Volume of stool increases as volume of intake increases.

Day 1 and Day 2

Minimum Output:

On day 1, the infant should produce at least one wet diaper and one meconium stool by 24 hours of age.

On day two, the infant should produce at least two wet diapers and 2 meconium stools. The stools may be thinning but remain dark (tarry black to greenish-brown).

Day 3 and Day 4

On day 3, the infant should produce at least three wet diapers and three transitional stools.

On day 4, the infant should produce at least four wet diapers and three to four transitional stools. The transitional stools are greenish-brown to greenish-yellow. Some infants will have transitioned to bright yellow milk stools by now.

Day 5

On day 5, the infant should produce at least five wet diapers and three to four yellow milk stools.

Hereafter, breastfeeding babies will always produce at least six well-saturated wet diapers per day. They typically produce at least 3 to 4 stools per day (not uncommon to have up to 10 stools per day) for the first month of life. After a month of age, breastfeeding infants may drastically reduce the number of stools per day, even skipping several days.

Because stools are an indicator of caloric intake, low stool output (especially in the first couple of weeks of life) warrants a weight check and evaluation.

Figure 31–16 ◆ Breastfeeding intake and output expectations.
SOURCE: Courtesy of Brigette Hall, MSN, IBCLC.

BOTTLE-FEEDING TECHNIQUE

With more attention placed on promoting and assisting breast-feeding mothers, the teaching needs of the mother who is formula-feeding may inadvertently get overlooked. Nurses may assume that families can simply follow the formula preparation instructions on the side of the formula containers. However, research shows that these parents also need teaching, counseling, and support. In one study the authors found that "33% of mothers mixed formula with warm tap water and up to 48% heated bottles in a microwave [oven]," both of which are not recommended (Fein & Falci, 1999). In a systematic review of five studies from developed countries looking at how parents prepare formula, all the studies revealed "errors in reconstitution with a tendency to over-concentrate feeds, although under-concentrating also occurred" (Renfrew, Ansell, & Macleod, 2003). Parents need to learn about the feeding pattern for a formula-feeding infant. They need to know intake and output expectations, the recommended type of formula for their infant, how to prepare and store formula, what equipment they will need, the feeding technique, and safety precautions.

Commercial formulas are available in three forms: powder, concentrate, and ready-to-feed. There are situations in which one formula may be better to use than another, but, in general, convenience and cost usually influence the parents' decision.

- *Powdered formula* is the least expensive type of formula. This formula can be made up one bottle at a time, or multiple bottles can be prepared, but they must be used within 24 to 48 hours. Standard powdered formula is made by adding one level scoop of powdered formula to 60 mL of water (the powder is added to the water). Powdered formulas are not sterile. Powdered formula is made from pasteurized liquid that is then freeze-spray dried into a powder; contamination with microorganisms can occur in the final stages of production. Preparation of any infant formula, but especially powdered formulas, requires careful handling to avoid contamination with microorganisms.

- *Formula concentrate* is more expensive than powder but is not as expensive as ready-to-feed formula. Formula concentrate is commercially sterile. This formula requires being diluted with an equal part of water. By adding boiled water that has been cooled, sterility can be maintained.

- *Ready-to-feed* formula is the easiest to use because it is does not require any mixing; however, this convenience comes at a cost—it is the most expensive formula. It is indicated for use when adequate water is not available, when the infant is immunocompromised and requires commercially sterile (pasteurized) formula, when an inexperienced babysitter will be feeding the infant, and for convenience.

Whatever the type of formula chosen, the nurse should underscore the importance of proper preparation and prompt refrigeration. Parents will need to be briefed on safety precautions during formula preparation. A primary concern is proper mixing to reconstitute formula. Parents need clear instructions to avoid unintentional harm to their infant. Parents should be instructed to follow the directions on the formula can label precisely as written. They should know that adding too much water during preparation dilutes the nutrients and caloric density. This contributes to undernourishment, insufficient weight gain, and, possibly, water intoxication, which can cause hyponatremia and seizures. Not adding enough water concentrates nutrients and calories and can tax an infant's immature kidneys and digestive system as well as cause dehydration (Morin, 2005). See Table 31–6 for storage guidelines for breast milk and formula.

Some recommended sanitary precautions and additional safety precautions are listed here:

- Check the expiration date on the formula container.
- Ensure good handwashing before preparing formula; never dip into the can without clean hands.
- Clean bottles, nipples, rings, disks, and bottle caps.
    a. Washing in a dishwasher when available (small items and heat-sensitive items on top rack secured in a basket), or
    b. Boiling briefly (1 to 2 minutes) in a pot of water, or
    c. Cleaning using a microwave sterilization kit, or
    d. Cleaning using very warm soapy water and a nipple and bottle brush
- Wash the top of the formula container before piercing the lid.
- Shake the liquid formulas well before pouring off desired amount.
- Shake prepared milk that has been sitting in the refrigerator before feeding.
- Allow tap water to run for 1 minute before obtaining water to use for mixing—this helps clear any lead standing in the pipes. Also, always use cold tap water as warm water tends to contain higher levels of lead as well. Water should be warmed (or cooled after boiling) before being added to the formula.
- Use only the scoop supplied in the can of formula when formula preparation instructions call for a "scoop" of powdered formula.
    a. A scoop should not be "packed" and should be leveled off (e.g., with the back of a knife).
- Do not add anything else to the bottle, except under direction of baby's healthcare provider.
- Warm up milk in a bottle by placing the bottle in a bowl of warm tap water. Do not fill the bowl with water higher than the rim of the bottle. (Babies can take cold formula but most young infants will prefer it warm.)
- Do not freeze formula.
- Allow freshly prepared (unused) formula to sit out at room temperature for no longer than 2 hours; use an insulated pack to transport formula. Milk left over in the bottle after a feeding should be discarded.
- In warm weather, transport reconstituted or formula concentrate from an open can in an insulated pack with frozen gel packs.
- Travel with water and formula separated—carry premeasured water bottles and carry bottles with premeasured amounts of powdered formula, or carry

premeasured commercially prepared formula packets, or have the can of formula available.

- Inspect and replace bottle nipples as soon as they show wear—worn nipples can break apart and can become a choking hazard.

- Holding the infant during feeding (even when the infant can hold the bottle for himself or herself) promotes bonding and prevents supine feedings.

- Do not allow the infant to bottle-feed in a supine position because this increases the risk of otitis media and dental caries in the older infant.

- Never prop a bottle—this is a choking hazard.

- Allow infants to take what they want *and* to stop when they want. Overfeeding can lead to obesity.

Parents also need guidance about what kind of water to use to reconstitute formula (see Table 31–7 to review types of water sources) and should discuss with their infant's healthcare provider whether to boil the water before use. If boiling is used, parents need to be instructed to heat the water until it reaches a rolling boil, continue to let the water boil for 1 to 2 minutes, and, most importantly, to allow the water to cool before using it to reconstitute the formula. Parents should also be instructed not to let the water boil down to a low level in the pan because this can cause minerals in the water to become concentrated.

Use of distilled bottle water and filtered tap water raises concerns with regard to fluoride. The AAP recommends that no fluoride supplements should be given to an infant before 6 months of age, but does recommend supplementary flouride for infants and children aged 6 months to 3 years of age if the water source contains less than 0.3 ppm (AAP, 2005). Parents should

be encouraged to read the labels on bottled water to see if fluoride has been added and to determine if the water source is suitable for their infant depending on his or her age (Table 31–7).

Parents often have questions about the kind of bottles and nipples to purchase. Plastic, glass, or disposable bottle bags may all be used based on preference. Mothers who bottle-feed expressed breast milk may want to avoid the use of bottle liners/bottle bags, especially if they have a fragile infant. Research shows that up to 60% of secretory immunoglobulin A (SIgA) found in breast milk binds to the polyethylene material used in these and is therefore lost to the infant (Lawrence & Lawrence, 2005). There are no human antibodies in formula so this is not a concern for bottle-feeding formula.

There are many different bottle nipples on the market. Parents will want to consider a slow-flow nipple for all newborns and for older breastfeeding babies learning to bottle-feed—over time the infant will graduate to medium-flow and high-flow nipples. Nipples come in different shapes. Generally, nipple shape plays a greater importance for breastfeeding babies receiving expressed breast milk or supplemental formula in a bottle. Breastfed babies transition best going from breast to bottle and back to breast again when using a bottle nipple that has a relatively wide base (to help maintain a wide-open latch) and a medium to long nipple length. Another variable to consider is nipple construction. Nipples are generally made from either rubber or silicone. Families with a sensitivity to latex are advised to use silicone nipples. Silicone nipples also have less of an odor, which may be an issue for some infants who are breastfed.

Many newly designed bottles are marketed to lessen air intake while an infant feeds. There is not a particular bottle design that is best for all babies. Different families find different bottles and nipple assembly products better than others. A key point to emphasize to the families is feeding technique. Parents should try to avoid situations in which an infant is crying for a prolonged time. Crying results in increased ingestion of air even before the infant has started feeding. Infants who are very hungry also gulp more air. For these situations, instruct the parents to burp their infant frequently to prevent the infant from having a large emesis (Figure 31–17 ◆). The parent may even want to attempt to pat the baby's back briefly before starting the feeding to calm the infant and and possibly burp as well. Another tip to avoid excessive ingestion of air is to have the parent hold his or her infant cradled in the arms while bottle-feeding and have the parent tilt the baby's bottle at a 45-degree angle (at least) in order for fluid to cover the nipple. This prevents the infant from sucking in air and swallowing it. See Figure 31–18 ◆ to view this technique.

To know if an infant is bottle-feeding well, the nurse needs to observe a bottle-feeding session. Parents should be informed that if the infant is sucking effectively, the parents should observe bubbles rising in the fluid (except if they are using plastic-lined bottles which contract as they empty). If the parent unintentionally placed the bottle nipple under the infant's tongue, preventing him or her from sucking, the infant may make sucking efforts but will not receive any fluid and no bubbles will be visualized. Infants who persistently leak milk from the side of the mouth may be getting fluid too quickly. The nurse could suggest using a slower flowing nipple. If symptoms persist, the in-

MediaLink
Application: Formula Feeding

Table 31–7	WATER SOURCES
Type	**Description**
Distilled water	Minerals and most other impurities have been removed. It will not contain any flouride. An acceptable water source for reconstituting formula.
Filtered tap water	Some minerals and impurities removed during filtration, including fluoride. This is an acceptable water source for reconstituting formula.
Natural mineral water	Comes from protected ground water and by law cannot be treated. Naturally contains high levels of minerals and sodium and so is not suitable for infants or for reconstituting formula.
Spring water	Comes from a single nonpolluted ground water, but unlike natural mineral water, it can be further treated. Because there is no regulation requiring the mineral content to be printed on the bottle label, it is best to avoid this water source for reconstituting formula.
Tap water	Water from the municipal water supply and regulated by drinking water regulations. It is treated and considered safe for use in reconstituting formula.
Well water	Needs to be tested before use. Higher risk of nitrate poisoning. Untested water is not recommended for use in reconstituting formula.

fant should have an oral evaluation. The infant could have a short lingual frenulum (tongue-tie) and not be able to properly cup his tongue under the nipple and channel fluid to the back of the throat, or the infant may have an oral-motor dysfunction and need speech therapy or occupational therapy evaluation.

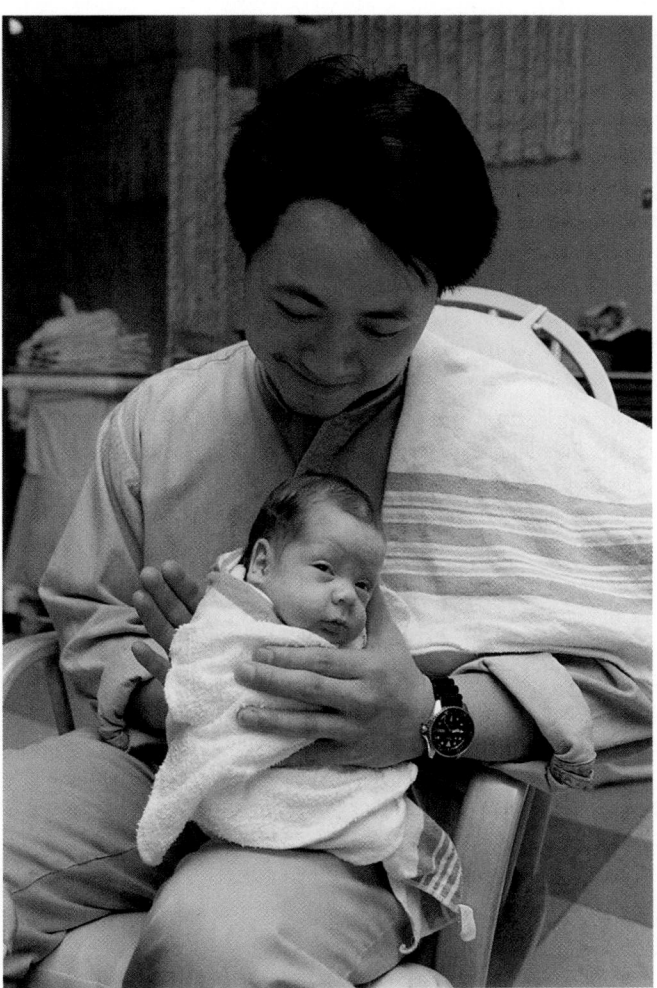

Figure 31–17 ◆ Burping.
SOURCE: © Stella Johnson (www.stellajohnson.com).

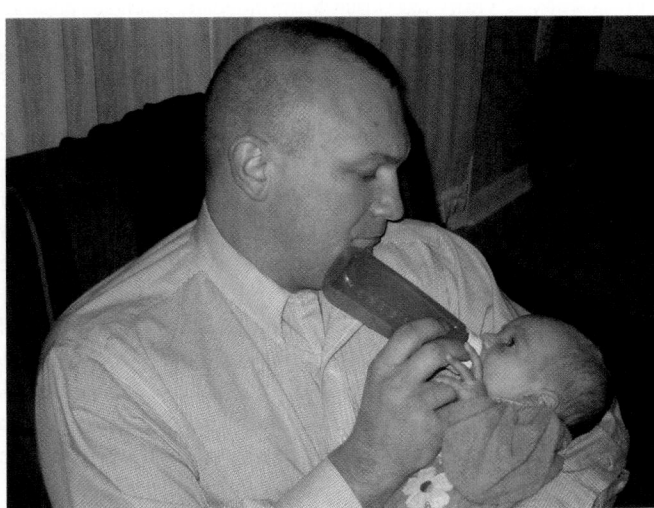

Figure 31–18 ◆ Bottle feeding.

CLINICAL TIP

Parents should be instructed not to put honey or corn syrup on their infant's pacifier to encourage an infant to accept it. Honey and possibly corn syrup may be contaminated with Clostridium botulinum, *a bacterium that causes infantile botulism. This is not a risk for the older child. Botulism is rare, but when it occurs it causes serious illness.*

COMMUNITY-BASED NURSING CARE
Promotion of Successful Infant Feeding

To promote a supportive hospital environment for breastfeeding, some hospitals have applied for Certificates of Intent to become "Baby Friendly." The World Health Organization (WHO) and the United Nations Children's Emergency Fund (UNICEF) have collaborated to create a global program, the Baby-Friendly Hospital Initiative (BFHI), to recognize hospitals and birthing centers that offer optimal lactation services (WHO/UNICEF, 1994). Only hospitals that have been certified as complying with the 10 steps outlined in Table 31–8 have been awarded the designation as "Baby Friendly." Baby-friendly status is not easy to achieve. One obstacle, among many, is having to agree not to accept free or low-cost formula. There are approximately 53 hospitals in the United States with Baby-Friendly designation as of May 2006, according to an update on the Baby-Friendly Hospital Initiative USA Web site (BFHI USA, 2006).

Childbirth and the beginning of motherhood are critical times in a woman's life, so physical, psychologic, and social supports are of paramount importance. The nurse needs to explore the family's social support base. The father or other partner is the

Table 31–8   BABY-FRIENDLY REQUIREMENTS
Baby Friendly 10 Steps to Successful Breastfeeding
• Have a written breastfeeding policy that is routinely communicated to all healthcare staff.
• Train all healthcare staff in skills necessary to implement this policy.
• Inform all pregnant women about the benefits and management of breastfeeding.
• Help mothers initiate breastfeeding within one half-hour of birth.
• Show mothers how to breastfeed and maintain lactation, even if they should be separated from their infants.
• Give newborn infants no food or drink other than breast milk, unless medically indicated.
• Practice rooming in - that is, allow mothers and infants to remain together 24 hours a day.
• Encourage breastfeeding on demand.
• Give no artificial teats or pacifiers (also called dummies or soothers) to breastfeeding infants.
• Foster the establishment of breastfeeding support groups and refer mothers to them on discharge from the hospital or clinic.

SOURCE: World Health Organization/United Nations Children's Emergency Fund (WHO/UNICEF). (1994). *U.S. committee for UNICEF interim program in the United States to promote the baby friendly ten steps to successful breastfeeding.* Washington, DC: Government Printing Office.

MEDIALINK

Breastfeeding Resources

RESEARCH IN PRACTICE

TEMPORAL CHANGES IN THE DETERMINANTS OF BREASTFEEDING INITIATION

What is this study about? Breastfeeding is universally considered the optimal way to feed an infant for the first 6 months of life. It is encouraging that the rate of breastfeeding has increased in most countries. However, the prevalence of breastfeeding is variable across the international community, and so identification of the factors that predict a woman's infant feeding choice is important. Determining which women are unlikely to pursue breastfeeding can help the nurse plan interventions to encourage breastfeeding. These determinants, though, are likely not static over time. This study had as its purpose the comparison of determinants of breastfeeding at discharge from the hospital in 2002/2003 with those reported for 1992/1993.

How was this study done? Both studies were conducted at two regional hospitals in Australia. The studies were conducted 10 years apart, and the same methodology was employed in both studies. Women were considered eligible if they delivered a live infant with no serious health conditions. The women agreed to complete a baseline questionnaire while in the hospital or shortly after discharge. The instruments used in the two studies were the same and included questions about the mother's body mass index, smoking history, and attitude about infant feeding. These variables were then used to identify the determinants of *any* breastfeeding and *exclusive* breastfeeding at discharge from the hospital. In the earlier study, 556 women participated, and 587 participated in the most recent study.

What were the results of the study? There was a significant increase in the proportion of women breastfeeding at discharge from the hospital. In 1992/1993, 83.8% of the women left the hospital breastfeeding, and this increased to 93.8% by 2002/2003. In both

studies, psychosocial factors, such as the mother's perception of her partner's and her own mother's attitude toward breastfeeding, were strong predictors of breastfeeding at discharge. These factors were stronger than any of the sociodemographic and biomedical factors considered. The factors were studied as a group and for any individual effects. The strongest independent predictor of breastfeeding at discharge was the father's infant feeding attitude, as reported by the mother. Women who perceived their partners to prefer breastfeeding were more likely to be breastfeeding at discharge than women who perceived their husbands preferred formula-feeding or were ambivalent about feeding methods. However, although these factors were the strongest predictors of making the decision to breastfeed, biomedical conditions—such as delivery method and infant health problems—were stronger predictors of exclusive breastfeeding at the time of discharge.

What additional questions might I have? What were the primary influences for single mothers or for mothers with no significant male partner? What interventions might be effective to influence the paternal attitude about breastfeeding as well as the mother's?

How can I use this study? The decision to initiate breastfeeding appears to be influenced by family considerations, particularly the attitude of the infant's father. Future interventions should aim to influence these modifiable factors. In particular, fathers play an important role in the infant feeding decision-making process. The nurse should seek ways to include the father in breastfeeding discussions. Fathers should be encouraged to attend antenatal classes that allow time for explanation of the supportive role fathers play in feeding decisions.

Scott, J., Binns, C., Graham, K., & Oddy, W. (2006). Temporal changes in the determinants of breastfeeding initiation. *Birth, 33*(1), 37–45.

---

most important support person for her, although the baby can also provide some support in the form of positive feedback. However, extensive family support systems may not be available. The mother, mother-in-law, sisters, and other females who could mentor and care for the new mother may live at a distance or work full-time.

Many families will have adequate income, a good knowledge base, and good coping skills to handle problems. Some families will have support from a large extended family group, friends, church, or other organization. However, that is not the case for everyone; as evidenced by the frequent discontinuing of breastfeeding in the early postpartum weeks, there is a need for assistance and follow-up in this area. When inadequate support is identified, it may be beneficial to request a referral for the family to have an outpatient case manager involved to make sure the mother knows how to access the community resources and is making a good adjustment. Nurses, dietitians, childbirth educators, certified nurse-midwives, lactation consultants, mother-to-mother support groups, and physicians must collaborate to provide consistent, timely information and support and to attend to the new mother's special needs.

Breastfeeding mothers who work outside the home and are supported in their decision tend to breastfeed their infants for longer periods than mothers who work but do not receive support. A baby-friendly workplace needs to be seen as another item in a benefit package offered by a company. Families and nurses who believe in breastfeeding need to be part of the solution to breastfeeding and workplace issues by educating employers in their communities (Rojjanasrirat, 2004).

With a national nursing shortage and the trend toward earlier discharge from the birthing center, there is limited time for inpatient education. Teaching moments, when they occur, may not be optimal because of the distraction of visitors and the mother's being sleep deprived, uncomfortable, or feeling the effects of an analgesic. It is important that parents receive verbal and written instructions and community resource information to which they can later refer. See also Chapter 36 ∞ for a complete discussion of self-care measures the nurse can suggest to a woman with a breastfeeding problem after discharge from the birthing center.

When parents leave the birthing center, the center staff need to have the name and phone number for both mother and baby's healthcare providers and know the indications to contact them. The breastfeeding mother needs a list of lactation resources available in the community. If no resource handout is available, the mother should be given the phone number to **La Leche League International** or the International Lactation Consultant Association (see MediaLink), which can provide assistance with finding the closest lactation support. Many hospitals around the country have a lactation program and may provide lactation services for a fee to anyone seeking services. Some cities have outpatient lactation centers that provide comprehensive lactation services, including consultation services, breastfeeding classes, and an infant scale for assessing baby's weight, as well as telephone-based lactation advice. Some cities have lactation consultants in private practice who have an outpatient office or may do home visits. The WIC may have a lactation consultant on staff or may have a contract with a lactation consultant in private practice in the community. Another potential resource is a home health agency. Some home health agencies provide outpatient lactation services in the patient's home. Some military facilities provide lactation services to their service members and dependents. The local library is also an excellent resource, and there are many books available commercially. Finally, the Internet can be a tremendous resource, although the quality of information cannot always be ensured. It is very helpful to have a handout listing some good sites that have been reviewed for accuracy.

Both breastfeeding and formula-feeding mothers who may be eligible for WIC should be encouraged to enroll themselves and their infants in the WIC nutrition program. WIC provides a specific number of cans of powdered formula to eligible mothers free of charge. The number of cans the mother receives is based on an agreement in the current government contract that WIC has with one of the two major formula companies (Mead Johnson, the maker of Enfamil®, or Ross, the maker of Similac®) and whether a mother is partially breastfeeding (in this case she usually receives 4 cans per month) or entirely formula-feeding (usually receives 9 to 10 cans per month, depending on the formula ordered and how many ounces of formula the can provides). The breastfeeding mother can also receive additional food vouchers for herself. The amount of formula the mother receives *does not* increase as the infant grows and the parents need to understand that 10 cans will not be sufficient over time and that they will need to purchase the difference when the infant's needs exceed the amount supplied. Mothers with an extremely low income and who lack family support may need the numbers for emergency food assistance programs in the area. These might include local food banks, local churches (including the Salvation Army), and United Way programs. Low-income mothers also need to be reminded to enroll their infant in the Food Stamp Program so they can receive additional food vouchers each month.

Cultural Considerations in Infant Feeding

All groups of people are influenced by their cultural background. Every culture shares a set of values, beliefs, behaviors, and a language unique for that group. These are learned characteristics shared among their members. A person's culture influences every aspect of their life. By learning about other cultures, the nurse will gain an understanding of the "context," or unstated assumptions that influence behavior, thus avoiding misunderstanding and improving the nurse's ability to communicate with the person. Of course, it is also true that not all individuals within a particular cultural group subscribe to each of the values, beliefs, and behaviors characteristic of that group. People need to be seen as individuals within the context of their culture.

Within the United States, many people agree that breastfeeding is the optimum infant feeding method. However, breast exposure is often viewed in a sexual context, leading to disapproval of the mother attempting to breastfeed in public. Although this norm may be changing, it is important for the nurse to recognize that not only do "others" often hold these views, but the mother herself may feel this way. It is therefore important to determine the attitudes of the mother—based on her feelings, it may be very important or not important at all to spend time discussing methods of breastfeeding discreetly.

With regard to the feeding of colostrum, although many recognize that it has properties uniquely suited to the newborn, there are people who consider colostrum "unclean" and do not offer it to their newborns. This belief is found among some groups of Hispanics, Navajo Indians, Filipinos, and Vietnamese (Galanti, 2004). In a situation like this, in which a cultural custom is harmful or denies the infant benefits, it is the nurse's responsibility to try to educate the family about the value of colostrum. A possible approach to this situation is as follows. First, reinforce the parents' desire to protect their baby from infection. Next, validate the assumption that because colostrum looks similar to pus from a wound, it makes sense that one might think it is also unclean. Next, point out that the reason pus looks the way it does is because of the white cells that the body sends to fight infection. Last, explain that as in the case of a wound, colostrum *is* one of the body's ways of helping fight infection—only in this case it is sending the white cells to the baby even before there is an infection. This last point again reinforces the initial validation of the parents' concern for infection but now uses that concern as motivation to feed the colostrum, rather than to avoid it.

In these cultures and in some countries (Guinea, Pakistan, Bangladesh), breastfeeding begins only after milk flow is established (Riordan, 2005). In many Asian cultures, the newborn is given boiled water until the mother's milk flows. The newborn is fed on demand, and cries are responded to immediately. If the crying continues, evil spirits may be blamed and a priest's blessing may be sought. Although many of the Hmong women of Laos combine breastfeeding with some formula-feeding, they usually find expressing their milk or pumping their breasts unacceptable. Thus other methods of providing relief should be suggested if breast engorgement develops. Most Muslim mothers breastfeed because the Qur'an (Koran) encourages it until the child is 2 years old (Ott, Al-Khadhuri, & Al-Junaibi, 2003). Japanese women are returning to breastfeeding as the method of feeding for the baby's first year.

Language is one of the most culturally sensitive behaviors and the source of much confusion. African Americans may refer to their infant as "greedy," which may be interpreted as a concern that the infant is taking too much. However, rather than an expression of concern, this term is often used as an expression of approval of the infant's vigorous feeding. African American culture tends to emphasize plentiful feeding, and solid foods are introduced early—possibly even added to the infant's formula. If the nurse misinterprets the expression, he or she may think that the mother is limiting the baby's feeding and may attempt to convince the mother that she should be encouraging higher intake, which could lead to overfeeding. African American mothers view frequent feeding as an expression of hardiness and a positive behavioral characteristic for their children for the future (Biancuzzo, 2003). For traditional Mexicans, a fat baby is considered healthy and infants are fed on demand. "Soiling" is encouraged.

These are but a few of the multitude of cultural influences related to feeding. (See Developing Cultural Competency: Breastfeeding in Other Cultures.) When faced with an infant care practice different from the ones to which they are accustomed, nurses need to evaluate the effect of the practice. Different practices are not necessarily inferior. The nurse should intervene only if the practice is actually harmful to the mother or baby.

Complementary and Alternative Practices

HERBS

Herbs have been used since antiquity and are still commonly used worldwide. However, during the 20th century as the medical model was embraced in this country, herb use fell out of favor in the United States. Recently there has been a growing interest in herb use among women of childbearing age. Nurses working with this population should become familiar with common herbal preparations used by these women. It is also important to remember that most herbs are classified as dietary supplements and therefore are not bound by the same regulations as medications (Born & Barron, 2005).

Herbs of interest to lactating women include a group of herbs called galactagogues. Galactogogues are commonly used to increase a mother's milk production when her supply is decreased, to assist in reestablishing a milk supply after weaning, and to assist in initiating lactation such as when an adoptive mother desires to nurse her infant. Herbal galactogogues include fenugreek, goat's rue, milk thistle, anise, basil, blessed thistle, fennel seeds, and marshmallow, to name a few (Academy of Breastfeeding Medicine [ABM], 2004). Before taking a galactogogue, women are advised to consult with a knowledgeable healthcare provider first. The healthcare provider will want to obtain a thorough lactation assessment so that the cause of an underlying problem can be determined (e.g., the reason for the low milk supply), guidance and support (including follow-up) can be offered for the management of the problem, and contraindications to any galactogogue can be considered. Most of the herbal galactogogues are taken as a tea, although capsules are also available. Fenugreek is probably the most commonly used herbal galactagogue because it seems to have the fewest adverse side effects. Women who drink it as a tea generally drink 2 to 3 cups per day. The tea is made by adding ¼ teaspoon of fenugreek seeds steeped in 8 ounces of water for 10 minutes. Women who take the capsules generally take one to four capsules (580 to 610 mg capsules) three to four times per day (ABM, 2004). Mothers usually notice an increase in their milk production in 2 to 3 days. Goat's rue, fennel seed, or milk thistle (not blessed thistle) tea is made with 1 teaspoon of dried leaves steeped in 8 ounces of water for 10 minutes; women usually have two to three cups of tea per day (ABM, 2004; Wagner, Graham, & Hope, 2004).

There are also antigalactogogues (e.g., sage, parsley, and peppermint) that may or may not be used in combination with cabbage leaves and ice to decrease severe engorgement, to diminish an oversupply, and to "dry up" when weaning an infant from the breast (Humphrey, 2003). The type of herb, the dosage, and the method of administration are variable depending on the problem to resolve and personal preference.

CLINICAL TIP

To treat severe engorgement that may occur on days 3 and 4, some mothers find relief applying chilled, green cabbage leaves. The mother applies cleaned cabbage leaves (rinsed and dried) after first "crunching" the "veins" in the leaves to help release a chemical to aid in decreasing the swelling. The prepared cabbage leaves are applied topically to the swollen breasts. The cabbage leaves are spread over the breasts (excluding the nipples) and secured in place with a bra. The leaves are changed out every couple of hours when they have become wilted or when the mother awakens during the night. This remedy is discontinued as soon as the mother notices the breast swelling has decreased.

DIETARY SUPPLEMENTS

To treat recurrent breast plugs or mastitis, it is suggested that mothers replace saturated fats with polyunsaturated fats in their diet and consider taking a dietary supplement of lecithin. Lecithin is a natural nutrient present in dairy products, meat, egg yolks, fish, and soybeans. (However, note that meat and dairy products contain saturated fats.) Lecithin is also a liquid constituent of breast milk (Lawrence & Lawrence, 2005).

Lecithin is commonly used as an additive in foods as an emulsifier—for example, it is used in chocolate to make it smooth and is used as an ingredient in no-stick cooking spray to prevent food from sticking on baking cookware. Lecithin is available at health food stores and can be purchased in the form of granules, liquids, or capsules. In the liquid form, lecithin can be used as an oil on salads (Lawrence & Lawrence, 2005).

Women with current breast plugs sometimes take lecithin daily to prevent future bouts with this problem. "Suggested dosages are one tablespoon per day" (Lawrence & Lawrence, 2005) and "one tablespoon three to four times a day or one to two capsules (1200 mg each) three or four times per day" (Mohrbacher & Stock, 2003; Newman & Pitman, 2000).

HOMEOPATHY

This type of alternative therapy utilizes minute doses of a drug to treat a particular disease or problem; the particular drug chosen is the same drug that, if administered in massive amounts, would actually produce symptoms of the disease or problem for which it is being used to treat. Therefore, homeopathic remedies are used with the smallest dose required to relieve symptoms and for the shortest duration possible. Homeopathic remedies come in a variety of forms, such as mother tincture (strongest form), ointments, suppositories, and pills or tablets (also called pellets). Pellets are not handled with fingers because the remedy is on the outside of the pellet. Pellets are administered by being placed on or under a person's tongue to dissolve. The strength of a remedy is designated (noted weakest to strongest) as follows: 6x, 30x, 6c, 30c, 200c, L, and M. An example of a homeopathic remedy is Lac Caninum; it is used to treat engorgement (Humphrey, 2003).

ESSENTIAL OILS

Essential oils are derived from aromatic plants through a distillation process. Water, alcohol, and other plant parts are separated during this process and what is left behind is the fragrant essence of the plant. The oils that are derived are highly concen-

COMPLEMENTARY AND ALTERNATIVE THERAPIES

HERBS, HOMEOPATHY, AND ESSENTIAL OILS FOR BREASTFEEDING

Herbs: Herbs thought to increase milk supply include alfalfa, dandelion, fennel, horsetail, red raspberry, caraway, and anise. The mother may drink caraway tea to reduce colic in the breastfeeding infant. Caraway tea also may be given directly to infants to treat colic (Skidmore-Roth, 2004). The following herbs may decrease milk supply, so they should be avoided until a woman is no longer breastfeeding: black walnut, sage, parsley, and yarrow (Balch & Balch, 2001). Black cohosh, blessed thistle, cascara sagrada, horseradish, garlic, cinnamon bark, kava kava, and senna are also contraindicated during lactation (Blumenthal, 2000).

Homeopathy: Pulsatilla, a homeopathic remedy, is used to improve a deficient flow of milk or dry up the milk if the mother is weaning the child.

Essential Oils: Cracked nipples often respond to calendula cream or ointment, found in health food stores. The nursing mother should wash her nipples off very well before feeding her child. Oil of peppermint, as a cold compress, may relieve breast engorgement or assist in the process of weaning. Place 4 to 5 drops of peppermint oil in ice cold water. Although essential oils feel like water, chemically they are oils and as such do not mix with the water. Dip a piece of clean fabric into the water so that the cloth picks up the essential oil on the surface. Wring out the fabric and place it on the breasts. Again, the breast should be washed completely before feeding. Women who are allergic to ragweed may find that they are also allergic to calendula.

trated and require being diluted with a base oil (e.g., a vegetable oil) before being applied to the skin, ingested, or used in aromatherapy (Humphrey, 2003).

Essential oils are used for their antiseptic, calming, stimulating, and soothing properties, but care must be taken when using them. Because essential oils are potent and can be toxic, mothers are advised to consult with a knowledgeable aromatherapist who will inform her as to which essential oils to avoid and how to safely use them. It is suggested that breastfeeding mothers avoid using essential oils on or near her breasts because even if wiped away, the oil may leave a residue on her skin. Essential oils are potentially allergenic, irritating, and hazardous depending on the type of oil, how it is diluted, and how it is applied (Humphrey, 2003).

NUTRITIONAL ASSESSMENT

A nutritional assessment is an integral part of a thorough health appraisal and is commonly performed by the infant's primary care provider, a nurse, a lactation consultant, a registered dietitian, or a speech therapist. The nutritional assessment will include all or some of the following parameters to measure wellness:

- Nutritional intake (i.e., breast milk, type of formula, other foods)
- Anthropometric measurements (i.e., measurements of weight, length, and head circumference)
- Biochemical status (i.e., the newborn metabolic screening, iron level, etc.)
- Physical examination (i.e., vital signs, total body examination, developmental milestones)
- Sociodemographic data (i.e., parity, maternal age, impact of cultural practices on feeding)

Parents will be asked to present a feeding diary for the provider to review, or the parents will need to recall the infant's feeding pattern over the last 24 to 48 hours. The parents will also be asked to describe the infant's urine and stool output, including quantity and quality. The healthcare professional is interested in the infant's behavior pattern, especially during and immediately after feeding. If the newborn is not gaining sufficient weight, the infant's feeding history must be examined more closely. If the infant is breastfeeding, a relevant maternal history is needed to determine if the mother is having breastfeeding difficulties and to help determine the root cause of the problem. If the infant is formula-feeding, the healthcare professional will first want to investigate the family's formula-feeding practices (including formula preparation technique). While gathering these data, the healthcare professional should be sensitive to the family's cultural practices. However, if a cultural practice has harmful effects, then the provider needs to tactfully educate the family to that fact.

The provider should plot the infant's measurements for length, head circumference, and weight on a growth chart, denoting the infant's individual percentile measurement compared with the general population. Because there are variations among infants at the same age, it is important to monitor the infant's individual growth pattern over time. Ideally, the provider wants to see an infant track along the same growth curve. A drop of 20% or more on the growth curve is cause for concern.

As the healthcare provider begins the infant's physical exam, the provider first obtains a subjective impression of the infant's overall appearance. The provider performs a head-to-toe physical examination, carefully noting any deviations from normal. The physical exam helps identify any nutritional disorders. If the infant's primary healthcare provider has any concerns about the infant's nutritional status, the provider may order relevant laboratory studies (i.e., hemoglobin, hematocrit, transferrin, albumin, creatinine, nitrogen, and others), may evaluate the infant for malabsorption disorders, and may see a need to refer the infant to a pediatric gastroenterologist for further evaluation.

With all the infant data available, it is now possible to determine an infant's nutritional status and potential risks.

The following example shows the effectiveness of these assessments and interventions:

Scenario: *Baby girl Torres was born at 37 weeks' gestation to an 18-year-old, G1P0 via cesarean section. Baby*

Torres is now 76 hours postpartum and she and her mother are expected to go home today. While weighing the infant for a discharge weight, the mother mentions that she does not think her daughter is getting much breast milk when she feeds because her infant keeps falling asleep during the feeding. Baby Torres weighed 3542 grams at birth and her present weight is 3173 grams. (The difference is 369 grams. 369/3542 = 0.104 X 100 = 10.4% weight loss.) A quick assessment of the mother's breasts reveal soft breasts and normal-shaped nipples, with nipples intact. After contacting the infant's healthcare provider to report the significant weight loss, the nurse is now ready to formulate a plan of care.

The nurse makes the following nursing diagnoses:

Ineffective Breastfeeding related to:

- Mother's lack of knowledge about breastfeeding
- Mother's not responding to infant's feeding cues
- Mother's inability to facilitate effective breastfeeding

As evidenced by a weight loss of 10.4% in baby.

Risk for Ineffective Breastfeeding related to:

- Insufficient knowledge regarding newborn's reflexes and breastfeeding techniques
- Lack of support by father of baby or other support persons
- Lack of maternal self-confidence
- Maternal fatigue
- Maternal ambivalence
- Poor infant sucking reflex
- Difficulty waking the sleepy baby

Risk for Imbalanced Nutrition: Less than Body Requirements related to:

- Mother's increased caloric and nutrient needs status postcesarean section
- Infant's inability to correctly latch on and transfer milk

Expected Outcomes of Care

The expected outcomes for the infant include:

- Infant will arouse to feed at least every 3 hours and will stay awake until the end of each feeding.
- The infant will correctly latch on to the breasts and effectively breastfeed 8 to 12 times/day.
- The infant will maintain weight and will gain at least 10 g/kg/day.
- The infant will have four wet diapers, three-four bowel movements on day 4; five wet diapers, three-four bowel movements on day 5; and six-eight wet diapers, three-four bowel movements every day thereafter during the first month of life.

- Infant's stools will transition from black to yellow by day 5 and will change in consistency from thick and sticky to loose and explosive with small curds or seedy appearance.
- Infant will not have any uric acid crystals in her diaper after day 4.
- Infant will be satiated after feeding, as evidenced by relaxed muscle tone and sleepiness.

The expected outcomes for the mother include:

- Mother will verbalize/demonstrate an understanding of breastfeeding technique, including positioning and latch-on, signs of adequate feeding, self-care.
- Mother will breastfeed pain-free.
- Mother will express satisfaction with the breastfeeding experience.
- Mother will consume a nutritionally balanced diet with appropriate caloric and fluid intake to support breastfeeding.

Plan of Care and Interventions

1. Review the mother's history.
   - Maternal demographics—for example, mother's date of birth, parity, marital status
   - Pregnancy history—for example, complications during pregnancy, gestation at delivery
   - Complications of delivery—for example, cesarean section, excessive blood loss
   - Current medical issues—for example, hypothyroidism? diabetes?
   - History of breast surgery or radiation—for example, breast reduction, radiation to treat previous breast cancer
   - Use of medications, herbs, alcohol, cigarettes
   - Psychosocial history—maternal support system, hx depression, and so on
   - History of previous breastfeeding experience
2. Maternal assessment.
   - Assess the breasts and nipples.
   - Obtain a description of lochia drainage.
3. Infant assessment.
   - Obtain the infant's weight and compare with previous weight measurements. *If this were an older infant, then it would be appropriate to obtain head circumference, length, and weight measurements and track the infant's trend on the growth chart; however, because this infant is only 3 days old, daily tracking of the other growth parameters is not applicable for this situation.*
   - Examine the infant, with emphasis on oral anatomy and oral-motor function, infant reflexes, overall behavior, skin color (jaundice).
   - Assess the infant for signs of dehydration.

4. Infant feeding history.
   - Diet
   - Feeding frequency and duration
   - History of supplementation
   - Review elimination pattern
     - Number of wet diapers, quality of urine
     - Number of bowel movements, quality of stool
5. Pre- and postbreastfeeding weight check.
   - Calculate milk transfer during breastfeeding. *Postfeed weight minus prefeed weight equals net breast milk transfer. Note: the nurse must use a digital electronic scale accurate within 2 grams. The infant does not have to be naked but the clothing and diaper the infant is wearing cannot be changed during this test measurement.*
6. Observation of breastfeeding technique.
   - Positioning and latch-on technique, infant responses, suckling pattern, satiated after feeding
7. Review feeding requirement/caloric requirement based on the infant's birth weight (3.542 kg).
   - Fluid requirement: 140 to 160 mL/kg/day
     - Should be up to full volume by day 6; should then receive 496 to 567 mL/day. To calculate mL to oz: take 496 mL, divide by 30 mL/oz, this equals to 16.5. The infant should receive 16.5 to 18.9 oz/day.
     - The infant should feed 8 to 12 times/day. If the infant feeds 10 times/day, then the infant should feed 496/10 = 49.6 mL/feeding.
     - On day 3, the infant will not be expected to feed approximately 50 mL/feeding (minimum full volume); the infant may only feed 30 mL/feeding but will be increasing volume daily as tolerated until up to full volume in the next couple of days.
   - Caloric requirement 100 to 115 kcal/kg/day
     - Should be up to full caloric requirement by day 6; should receive 354 to 407 kcal/day. Breast milk has 20 kcal/oz; standard infant formula has 20 kcal/oz. To determine how many ounces the infant will require per day, take 354 kcal/day divided by 20 equals 17.7 oz/day. *Note: The infant should be gradually increasing her volume of milk each day and will soon be up to full volume.*
8. Assess teaching needs.
   - Review benefits of breastfeeding.
   - Review the process of breastfeeding (principle of supply and demand).
   - Review breastfeeding technique (reading infant cues, positioning, and latch-on).

- Review infant intake and output expectations.
- Review infant weight gain expectations.
- Provide breast pump instructions and review collection and storage.
- Provide information on maternal nutrition and fluid requirements.

9. Provide written instructions.

- *Provide frequent skin-to-skin contact.*
- *Watch the infant for early feeding cues.* If the infant is too dehydrated and weak to exhibit these feeding behaviors, then help the infant to wake up at least every 3 hours.
- *Start pumping each time the infant feeds (8 to 12 times/day),* if the mother's breasts are still very soft and light (delay in milk coming in). All expressed breast milk should be fed to the infant. If the mother is not able to express enough milk, then the infant should be supplemented with iron-fortified cow's milk-based formula unless specified otherwise.

- *Practice proper breastfeeding technique.* Encourage the mother to breastfeed as often as possible and observe for signs of effective breastfeeding.
- *Maintain a feeding diary to monitor the infant's intake and output; call a lactation consultant if the infant is not meeting expectations.*
- *Rest as much as possible and be concerned only about self-care needs (prevention of engorgement, etc.), and caring for the infant right now.*
- *Eat healthy foods and drink plenty of fluids to quench thirst.*
- *Follow-up weight check on infant in 1 to 2 days and assess nutritional status.*

Follow-up lactation consultation visit in 2 days to determine milk transfer efficiency and evaluate maternal milk production.

CHAPTER REVIEW

FOCUS YOUR STUDY

- The American Academy of Pediatrics (AAP) recommends exclusive breastfeeding for the first 6 months and continued breastfeeding until the infant is 1 year old or older.
- During the first few days after birth, the minimum output expectations for an exclusively breastfeeding infant will be: one wet/one stool on day 1; two wets/two stools on day 2; three wets/three to four stools on day 3; four wets/three to four stools on day 4; five wets/three to four stools on day 5. Thereafter, an exclusively breastfeeding infant has six to eight wet diapers and three to four yellow milk stools each day, generally during the first month of life.
- Infants' stools start as black and sticky at birth and transition to yellow, curdy, and seedy by day 5 or sooner.
- Formula-feeding infants lose about 3.5% of their birth weight. Breastfeeding infants lose up to 7% of their birth weight. A weight loss of more than 7% is excessive and requires an evaluation and follow-up. Infants should be back to their birth weight by 10 to 14 days of age.
- Growth rate over the lifespan is greatest during infancy. The healthy full-term infant gains approximately 10 g/kg/day for

the first month of life. Exclusively breastfed infants have the same or slightly greater weight gain in the first 3 to 4 months of life than mixed-fed and formula-fed infants. Thereafter, formula-fed and mixed-fed infants are heavier than breastfed infants.

- Increases in body length and head circumference between breastfed and formula-fed infants is the same. An infant gains 1 inch per month in the first 6 months, and then 0.5 inch for the following 6 months. Length is a better indicator of growth than is weight.
- Generally, infants double their birth weight by 5 months, triple their birth weight by 1 year of age, and quadruple their birth weight by 2 years.
- The dietary reference intake (DRI) for calories for the newborn is 100 to 115 kcal/kg/day.
- The dietary reference intake (DRI) for fluid intake for the newborn is 140 to 160 mL/kg/day.
- Breast milk has immunologic and nutritional properties that make it the optimal food for the first year of life.

- Mature breast milk and standard commercially prepared formulas provide 20 kcal/oz.

- The breastfed infant's iron stores in full-term infants are usually depleted by the time the infant is 6 months old. Breastfeeding infants over 6 months of age who are eating supplementary foods rich in iron and infants consuming iron-enriched formula need no other vitamin or mineral supplements.

- There are three types of commercial infant formulas: cow's milk-based formula, soy milk-based formulas, and specialized formulas including hydrolysated formulas.

- Neither cow's milk nor soy milk should be given to infants before 1 year of age. The use of skim milk or low-fat cow's milk is not recommended for children under 2 years old.

- Signs indicating a newborn's readiness to feed include hand-to-mouth movements, rooting, smacking, fussing, and crying (a late-feeding cue).

- By learning about cultural variations, the nurse will gain an understanding of the "context" or unstated assumptions that influence behavior, thus avoiding misunderstanding and improving the ability of the nurse to communicate with clients.

- Infants should not receive water supplements until they start solid foods.

- Although most maternal medications are transmitted through breast milk, few are actually contraindicated. The bioavailability of transmitted drugs to the infant depends on a variety of factors, including route of administration, protein binding, degree of ionization, molecular weight, timing of the dose with respect to feeding time, and absorption across the infant's intestinal tract. Mothers should consult with a healthcare provider knowledgeable about medications and lactation.

- Breastfeeding mothers should be taught to use proper positioning and latch-on technique. The mother should be advised to alternate feeding positions periodically to promote efficient drainage of all the ducts in the breast.

- The formula-feeding mother may need help learning about the types of formulas and how to prepare and store formula. Like the breastfeeding mother, she will benefit from understanding feeding cues and proper technique for feeding her infant.

- Nutritional assessment of the infant includes the infant's dietary history, anthropometric measurements, physical examination, and laboratory tests, if indicated.

EXPLORE MediaLink

Video: Breastfeeding

http://www.prenhall.com/davidson

NCLEX review questions, case studies, and other interactive resources for this chapter can be found on the Web Site at http://www.prenhall.com/davidson. Click on "Chapter 31" to select the activities for this chapter.

For tutorials including animations and videos, more NCLEX review questions, and an audio glossary, access the accompanying Prentice Hall Nursing MediaLink DVD-ROM in this book.

PRENTICE HALL NURSING MEDIALINK DVD-ROM

Audio Glossary

NCLEX Review

Videos: *Breastfeeding; Through the Eyes of a Nurse—Welcoming the New Arrival at the Postpartal Visit*

COMPANION WEBSITE

Additional NCLEX Review

Case Study: *Client Undecided on Formula Feeding or Breastfeeding*

Care Plan Activity: *Breastfeeding Concerns*

Applications: *Breastfeeding; Formula Feeding*

Critical Thinking

CRITICAL THINKING IN ACTION

BREASTFEEDING TECHNIQUES

View the Critical Thinking in Action video in Chapter 31 of the DVD-ROM. Then answer the questions that follow.

Patty Kline, age 28, G1, now P1, delivers a 7.3-pound baby girl by spontaneous vaginal birth over a median episiotomy. The newborn's Apgar scores are 8 and 9 at 1 and 5 minutes. The infant is suctioned in the nose and mouth and given free-flow oxygen on the mother's abdomen. Patty received an epidural during her labor and birth. Patty initiated breastfeeding within the first hour after the birth, but at that time the newborn did not latch on. The infant was held to the mother's breast, rooted, and licked the nipple. You are the nurse caring for the infant at 2 hours of age. The admission assessment is significant for asymmetric head with a 3-cm caput succedaneum. The infant's temperature is stable. You bring the infant to the mother's room to assist her with breastfeeding.

1. Describe clues that indicate the infant is ready to breastfeed with the mother.
2. How would you explain how to position the infant at the breast?
3. Explain what to observe for the infant's proper latch-on.
4. Explain the basics of milk production.
5. Explore helpful measures the mother can attempt in support of breastfeeding.

REFERENCES

Academy of Breastfeeding Medicine (ABM). (2004). Protocol #9: Use of galactogogues initiating or augmenting maternal milk supply. *ABM News and Views, 10*(3), 20–22. http://www.bfmed.org/

American Academy of Pediatrics (AAP) Committee on Drugs. (2001). Transfer of drugs and other chemicals into human milk. *Pediatrics, 108*(3), 776–789. Retrieved November 22, 2006, from http://www.aap.org/healthtopics/breastfeeding.cfm

American Academy of Pediatrics (AAP) Committee on Nutrition. (1998). Policy statement: Soy protein-based formulas: Recommendations for use in infant feeding. *Pediatrics, 101*(1), 148–153.

American Academy of Pediatrics (AAP) Committee on Nutrition. (1999). Iron fortification of infant formulas. *Pediatrics, 104*(1), 119–123.

American Academy of Pediatrics (AAP) Committee on Nutrition. (2002). New infant formula additives approved by FDA. *AAP News and Feature, 20*(5), 209–211.

American Academy of Pediatrics (AAP) Media Alert. (1998, April 20). *AAP addresses scheduled feedings vs. demand feedings.* Retrieved October 9, 2005, from http://www.ezzo.info/Aney/aapmediaalert.pdf

American Academy of Pediatrics (AAP) Section on Breastfeeding. (2005). Policy statement: Breastfeeding and the use of human milk. *Pediatrics, 115*(2), 496–506.

American Academy of Pediatrics (AAP) Section on Breastfeeding and Committee on Nutrition. (2003). Prevention of rickets and vitamin deficiency: New guidelines for vitamin D intake. *Pediatrics, 111*(4), 908–910.

American College of Obstetricians and Gynecologists (ACOG). (2000). *Breastfeeding:*

Maternal and infant aspects (Educational Bulletin No. 258). Washington, DC: Author.

Aney, M. (1998). Commentary: "Babywise" advice linked to dehydration, failure to thrive. *AAP News, 14*(4), 21.

Association of Women's Health, Obstetric, and Neonatal Nurses (AWHONN). (2000, January). *Breastfeeding support: Prenatal care through the first year. Evidence-based clinical practice guideline* (pp. 1–33). Washington, DC: Author.

Baby-Friendly Hospital Initiative USA (BFHI USA). (2006). *Implementing the UNICEF/WHO baby-friendly hospital initiative in the U.S.* Retrieved May 22, 2006, from http://www.babyfriendlyusa.org/eng/03.html

Balch, J. F., & Balch, P. A. (2001). *Prescription for nutritional healing* (3rd ed.). Garden City, NY: Avery.

Ball, T. M., & Wright, A. L. (1999). Health costs of formula-feeding in the first year of life. *Pediatrics, 103*(4), 870–876.

Baumslag, N., & Michels, D. L. (1995). *Milk, money, and madness: The culture and politics of breastfeeding.* Westport, CT: Bergin & Garvey.

Biancuzzo, M. (2003). *Breastfeeding the newborn: Clinical strategies for nurses* (2nd ed.). St. Louis, MO: Mosby.

Blackburn, S. T. (2003). *Maternal, fetal, & neonatal physiology: A clinical perspective* (2nd ed.). St. Louis, MO: Saunders.

Blumenthal, M. (2000). *Herbal medicine: Expanded commission E monographs.* Austin, TX: American Botanical Council.

Born, D., & Barron, M. (2005). Herb use in pregnancy: What nurses should know. *American Journal of Maternal/Child Nursing, 30*(3), 201–208.

Briggs, G. G., Freeman, R. K., & Yaffe, S. J. (2005). *Drugs in pregnancy and lactation: A reference guide to fetal and neonatal risk* (7th ed.). Baltimore: Lippincott Williams & Wilkins.

Edgar, A. (2005, March–April). Anatomy of a working breast. *New Beginnings, 22*(2), 44–50. Retrieved November 22, 2006, from http://www.lalecheleague.org

Fein, S. B., & Falci, C. (1999). Infant formula preparation, handling, and related practices in the United States. *Journal of the American Dietetic Association, 99,* 1234–1240.

Galanti, G. A. (2004). *Caring for patients from different cultures* (3rd ed.). Philadelphia: University of Pennsylvania Press.

Gregory, K. (2005). Update on nutrition for preterm and full-term infants. *Journal of Obstetric, Gynecologic, & Neonatal Nursing, 34*(1), 98–108.

Groenewald, M. (1996). Milk allergy & intolerance. *Allergy Society of South Africa.* Retrieved September 22, 2005, from http://www.allergysa.org/milk.htm

Hale, T. W. (2004). *Medications and mothers' milk.* Amarillo, TX: Pharmasoft.

Hall, R. T., Mercer, A. M, Teaslet, S. L., McPherson, D. M., Simon, S. D., Santos, S. R., et al. (2002). A breastfeeding assessment score to evaluate the risk for cessation of breast-feeding by 7–10 days of age. *Journal of Pediatrics, 141,* 659–664.

Hartmann, P. E. (1987). Lactation and reproduction in western Australian women. *Journal of Reproductive Medicine, 32,* 543–557.

Hartmann, P. E., & Prosser, C. E. (1984). Physiologic basis of longitudinal changes in human milk yield and composition. *Federation Proceedings, 43,* 2448–2453.

Hedayat, K. M. (2001). Issues in Islamic biomedical ethics: A primer for the pediatrician. *Pediatrics, 108*(4), 965–991.

Hill, P. D., Wilhelm, P. A., Aldag, J. C., & Chatterton, R. T. (2004). Breast augmentation & lactation outcome: A case report. *American Journal of Maternal Child Nursing, 29*(4), 238–242.

Human Milk Banking Association of North America (HMBANA). (2005). *Best practice for expressing, storing and handling human milk in hospitals, homes and child care settings.* Raleigh, NC: Author.

Humphrey, S. (2003). *The nursing mother's herbal.* Minneapolis, MN: Fairview Press.

International Lactation Consultant Association (ILCA). (2005). *Clinical guidelines for the establishment of exclusive breastfeeding* (2nd ed.). Raleigh, NC: Author.

Jackson, D. J., Chopra, M., Witten, C., & Sengwana, M. J. (2003). HIV and infant feeding: Issues in developed and developing countries. *Journal of Obstetric, Gynecologic, & Neonatal Nursing, 32*(1), 117–127.

Jarvela, I., Sabri, E. N., Kokkonen, J., Varilo, T., Savilahti, E., & Peltonen, L. (1998). Assignment of the locus for congenital lactase deficiency to 2q21, in the vicinity of but separate from the lactase-phlorizin hydrolase gene. *American Journal of Human Genetics, 63*(4), 1078–1085.

Katz, N., Levin, M. B., Cotton, J. M., Patrick-Miller, T. J., & Tesoro, L. J. (n.d.). The pediatric group brochure on formula feeding: Formula feeding information. Retrieved October 7, 2005, from http://www.pedgroup.com/frmlabrc.htm

Klaus, M. (1998). Mother and infant: Early emotional ties. *Pediatrics, 102*(5), 1244–1246.

Lawrence, R. A., & Lawrence, R. M. (2005). *Breastfeeding: A guide for the medical profession* (6th ed.). Philadelphia: Mosby.

Lloyd, B., Halter, R. J., Kuchan, M. J., Baggs, G. E., Ryan, A. S., & Masor, M. L. (1999). Formula tolerance in postbreastfed and exclusively formula-fed infants [Electronic version]. *Pediatrics, 103*(1), e7.

Macdonald, P. D., Ross, S. R. M., Grant, L., & Young, D. (2003). Neonatal weight loss in breast and formula fed infants. *Archives of Disease in Childhood: Fetal and Neonatal Edition, 88,* F472–F476.

Marks, J. W. (2003). *Lactose intolerance (lactase deficiency)* (D. Lee, Ed.). Retrieved September 18, 2005, from http://www.medicinenet.com/lactose_intolerance/article.htm

Mead-Johnson Nutritionals. (2004). *Pediatric products handbook.* New York: Bristol-Myers Squibb Company.

Mohrbacher, N., & Stock, J. (2003). *La Leche League International: The breastfeeding answer book* (3rd ed.). Schaumburg, IL: La Leche League International.

Morin, K. (2005). Information parents need about preparing formula. *American Journal of Maternal/Child Nursing, 30*(5), 334.

Mulford, C. (1992). The mother-baby assessment (MBA): An "Apgar score" for breastfeeding. *Journal of Human Lactation, 8*(2), 79–82.

Neville, M. (1999). Physiology of lactation. In C. L. Wagner & D. M. Purohit (Eds.), *Clinics in perinatology: Clinical aspects of human milk and lactation* (pp. 251–279). Philadelphia: W. B. Saunders.

Newman, J., & Pitman, T. (2000). *The ultimate breastfeeding book of answers.* Roseville, CA: Prima.

O'Brien, K. O., Zavaleta, N., Abrams, S. A., & Caulfield, L. E. (2003). Maternal iron status influences iron transfer to the fetus during the third trimester of pregnancy. *American Journal of Clinical Nutrition, 77*(4), 924–930.

Ott, B. B., Al-Khadhuri, J., & Al-Junaibi, S. (2003). Preventing ethical dilemmas: Understanding Islamic health care practices. *Pediatric Nursing, 29*(3), 227–230.

Rasbridge, L. A., & Kulig, J. C. (1995). Infant feeding among Cambodian refugees. *American Journal of Maternal/Child Nursing, 20*(4), 213–218.

Renfrew, M. J., Ansell, P. L., & Macleod, K. L. (2003). Formula feed preparation: Helping reduce risks; a systematic review. *Archives of Diseases of Children, 88,* 855–858.

Riordan, J. (2005). *Breastfeeding and human lactation* (3rd ed.). Boston: Jones & Bartlett.

Rolfes, S. R., Pinna, K., & Whitney, E. (2006). *Understanding normal and clinical nutrition* (7th ed.). Belmont, CA: Thomson Wadsworth, a part of the Thomson Corporation.

Rojjanasrirat, W. (2004). Working women's breastfeeding experience. *American Journal of Maternal/Child Nursing, 29*(4), 222–228.

Ross Products Division. (2004). *Pediatric nutritionals product guide.* Columbus, OH: Abbott Laboratories.

Schneiderman, J. U. (1996). Postpartum nursing for Korean mothers. *American Journal of Maternal/Child Nursing, 21*(3), 155–158.

Schuman, J. (2003, February 1). A concise history of infant formula (twists and turns included). *Contemporary Pediatrics.* Retrieved October 4, 2005, from http://www.contemporarypediatrics.com/contpeds/article/articleDetail.jsp?id=111702

Sears, W. (n.d.). *A word about bottle-feeding.* Retrieved October 21, 2005, from http://www.askdrsears.com/html/0/T000100.asp#T031010

Skidmore-Roth, L. (2004). *Mosby's handbook of herbs and natural supplements.* St. Louis, MO: Mosby.

Swagerty, D. L., Walling, A. D., & Klein, R. M. (2002). Lactose intolerance. *American Family Physician, 65*(9), 1845–1850, 1855–1856.

Thibodeau, G., & Patton, K. T. (2002). *The human body in health & disease* (3rd ed.). St. Louis, MO: Mosby.

Thureen, P. J., Deacon, J., Hernandez, J. A., & Hall, D. M. (2005). *Assessment and care of the well newborn* (2nd ed.). St. Louis, MO: Elsevier Saunders.

Vonlanthen, M. (1998). Lactose intolerance, diarrhea, and allergy. *Breastfeeding Abstracts, 18*(2), 11–12.

Wagner, C. L., Graham, E. M., & Hope, W. W. (2004). *Counseling the breastfeeding mother.* e-Medicine.com., Inc. Retrieved October 11, 2005, from http://www.emedicine.com/ped/topic2774.htm

World Health Organization/United Nations Children's Emergency Fund (WHO/UNICEF). (1994). *U.S. committee for UNICEF interim program in the United States to promote the baby friendly ten steps to successful breastfeeding.* Washington, DC: Government Printing Office.

CHAPTER 32

The Newborn at Risk: Conditions Present at Birth

The rhythmic tides of her sleeping and feeding spaciously measured her days and nights. Her frail absorption was a commanding presence, her helplessness strong as a rock.

~ *Laurie Lee,* Two Women ~

KEY TERMS

Alcohol-related birth defect (ARBD) 964

Fetal alcohol effects (FAE) 964

Fetal alcohol syndrome (FAS) 964

Inborn errors of metabolism 977

Infant of diabetic mother (IDM) 939

Infant of substance-abusing mother (ISAM) 964

Intrauterine drug-exposed infants 965

Intrauterine growth restriction (IUGR) 930

Large for gestational age (LGA) 938

Neonatal morbidity 929

Neonatal mortality risk 929

Phenylketonuria (PKU) 977

Postmaturity 941

Postterm newborn 941

Preterm infant 942

Small for gestational age (SGA) 930

OBJECTIVES

1. Identify factors present at birth that help identify an at-risk newborn.

2. Compare the underlying etiologies of the physiologic complications of small-for-gestational-age (SGA) newborns and preterm appropriate-for-gestational-age (Pr AGA) newborns.

3. Describe the impact of maternal diabetes mellitus on the newborn.

4. Compare the characteristics and underlying etiologies of potential complications of the postterm newborn and the newborn with postmaturity syndrome.

5. Discuss the physiologic characteristics of the preterm newborn that predispose each body system to various complications and are used in development of a plan of care.

6. Identify the information used in developing the nursing diagnoses required to plan interventions for the care of the Pr AGA newborn.

7. Summarize the nursing assessments of and initial interventions for a newborn born with selected congenital anomalies.

8. Explain the special care needed by a drug-exposed newborn.

9. Relate the consequences of maternal human immunodeficiency virus/acquired immunodeficiency syndrome (HIV/AIDS) to the management of the infant in the neonatal period.

10. Identify physical examination findings suggestive of a congenital cardiac defect.

11. Explain the special care needed by a newborn with an inborn error of metabolism.

MEDIALINK

Additional resources for this content can be found on the Prentice Hall Nursing MediaLink DVD-ROM and on the Companion Website at http://www.prenhall.com/davidson. Click on "Chapter 32" to select the activities for this chapter.

The field of neonatology has expanded greatly. Many levels of nursery care have evolved in response to increasing knowledge about the newborn: special care, intensive care, and convalescent or transitional care. Along with the newborn's parents, the nurse is an important caregiver in all these settings. As a professional member of the multidisciplinary healthcare team, the nurse provides the holistic care necessary in the often high-tech perinatal environment.

In addition to the availability of excellent intensive care services, a variety of other factors influences the outcomes of at-risk infants, including the following:

- Birth weight
- Gestational age
- Type and length of newborn illness
- Environmental factors
- Maternal factors
- Maternal-infant separation

IDENTIFICATION OF AT-RISK NEWBORNS

An at-risk newborn is one who is susceptible to illness (morbidity) or even death (mortality) because of dysmaturity, immaturity, physical disorders, or complications during or after birth. In most cases, the infant is the product of pregnancy involving one or more predictable risk factors, including the following:

- Low socioeconomic level of the mother
- Limited or no prenatal care
- Exposure to environmental dangers, such as toxic chemicals and illicit drugs
- Preexisting maternal conditions, such as heart disease, diabetes, hypertension, hyperthyroidism, and renal disease
- Maternal factors such as age or parity
- Medical conditions related to pregnancy and their associated complications
- Pregnancy complications such as abruptio placentae, oligohydramnios, preterm labor, premature rupture of membranes, preeclampsia

Various risk factors and their specific effects on the pregnancy outcome are identified in Table 15–2. ∞ Because these factors and the perinatal risks associated with them are known, the birth of at-risk newborns can often be anticipated. The pregnancy can be closely monitored, treatment can be started as necessary, and arrangements can be made for birth to occur at a facility with appropriate resources to care for both mother and baby.

Whether or not prenatal assessment indicates that the fetus is at risk, the course of labor and birth and the infant's ability to withstand the stress of labor cannot be predicted. The nurse's use of electronic fetal heart monitoring or fetal heart auscultation by Doppler plays a significant role in detecting stress or distress in the fetus. Immediately after birth, the Apgar score is a helpful tool in identifying the at-risk newborn, but it is not the only indicator of possible long-term outcome.

The newborn classification and neonatal mortality risk chart is another useful tool in identifying newborns at risk. Before this classification tool was developed, birth weight of less than 2500 g was the sole criterion for determination of immaturity. Clinicians then recognized that newborns could weigh more than 2500 g but still be immature. Conversely, an infant weighing less than 2500 g might be functionally mature at term or beyond. Birth weight and gestational age together became the criteria used to assess neonatal maturity and mortality risk.

According to the newborn classification and neonatal mortality risk chart, gestation is divided as follows:

- Preterm: less than 37 (completed) weeks
- Term: 38 to 41 (completed) weeks
- Postterm: greater than 42 weeks

As shown in Figure 32–1 ◆, large-for-gestational-age (LGA) infants are those who plot above the 90th percentile growth curve. Appropriate-for-gestational-age (AGA) infants are those between the 10th percentile and 90th percentile growth curve. Small-for-gestational-age (SGA) infants are those below the 10th percentile growth curve. A newborn is assigned to a category depending on birth weight, length, occipital-frontal circumference, and gestational age. For example, a newborn classified as Pr SGA is preterm and small for gestational age. The full-term newborn whose weight is appropriate for gestational age is classified F AGA. It is important to remember that the intrauterine growth curve charts are influenced by altitude and the ethnicity of the newborn population used to create the chart. Also the assigned newborn classification may vary according to the intrauterine growth curve chart used; therefore, the chart used should correlate with the characteristics of the client populations.

Neonatal mortality risk is the chance of death within the neonatal period, that is, within the first 28 days of life. Seventy-five percent of all neonatal deaths occur within the first week, with the highest rates occurring during the first day of life. As indicated in Figure 32–1, the neonatal mortality risk decreases as both gestational age and birth weight increase. Infants who are Pr SGA have the highest neonatal mortality risk. The previously high mortality rates for LGA infants have decreased at most perinatal centers because of improved management of diabetes in pregnancy and recognition of potential complications of LGA newborns.

Neonatal morbidity can also be anticipated based on birth weight and gestational age. In Figure 32–2 ◆, the infant's birth weight is located on the vertical axis, and the gestational age in weeks is found along the horizontal axis. The area where the two meet on the graph identifies common problems. This tool assists in determining the needs of particular infants for special observation and care. For example, an infant of 2000 g at 40 weeks' gestation should be carefully assessed for evidence

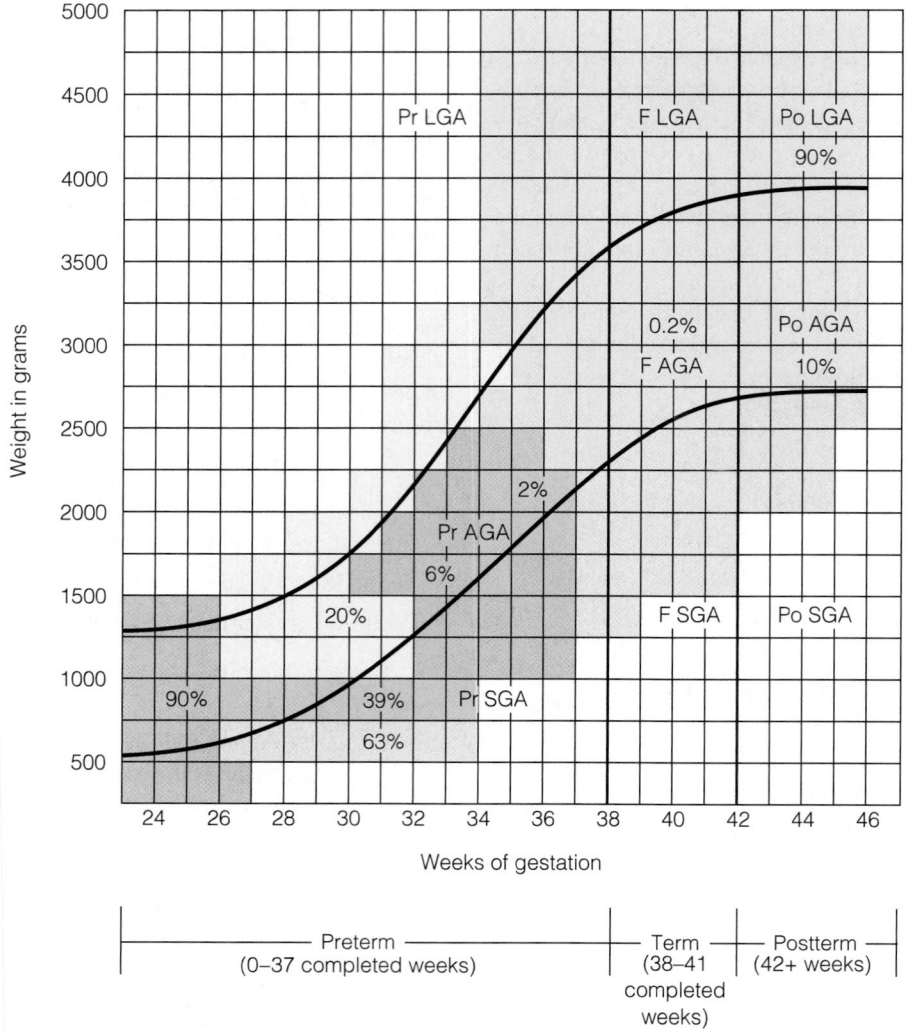

Figure 32–1 ◆ Newborn classification and neonatal mortality risk chart. Infants are classified according to weight as small for gestational age (SGA), appropriate for gestational age (AGA), or large for gestational age (LGA) and by weeks of newborn as preterm (Pr), term (F), or postterm (Po). Corresponding neonatal mortality risks are indicated by the percentages in the various colored regions.
SOURCE: Reprinted from *Journal of Pediatrics, 101*(6), Koops, B. L., Morgan, L. P., & Battaglia, F. C., "Neonatal Mortality Risk in Relationship to Birth Weight and Gestational Age," p. 969. Copyright 1982 with permission from Elsevier.

of nonreassuring fetal status, hypoglycemia, congenital anomalies, congenital infection, and polycythemia.

Identifying the nursing care needs of the at-risk newborn depends on minute-to-minute observations of the changes in the newborn's physiologic status. The nursing care management should be directed toward the following:

- Decreasing physiologically stressful situations
- Constantly observing for subtle signs of change in clinical condition
- Interpreting laboratory data and coordinating interventions
- Conserving the infant's energy for healing and growth
- Providing for developmental stimulation and maintenance of sleep cycles
- Assisting the family in developing attachment behaviors
- Involving the family in planning and providing care

CARE OF THE SMALL-FOR-GESTATIONAL-AGE/INTRAUTERINE GROWTH RESTRICTION NEWBORN

Infants are considered **small for gestational age (SGA)** when they are less than two standard deviations below the population norm or at less than the third percentile (10th percentile for Denver curves because of the lower birth weight at higher altitudes) (see Figure 32–1). When possible, the birth weight charts used to assign the SGA classification to a newborn should be based on the local population into which the newborn is born (Martinez & Simmons, 2005). A SGA newborn may be preterm, term, or postterm. An undergrown newborn may be also said to have **intrauterine growth restriction (IUGR)**, which describes the pregnancy circumstance of advanced gestation and

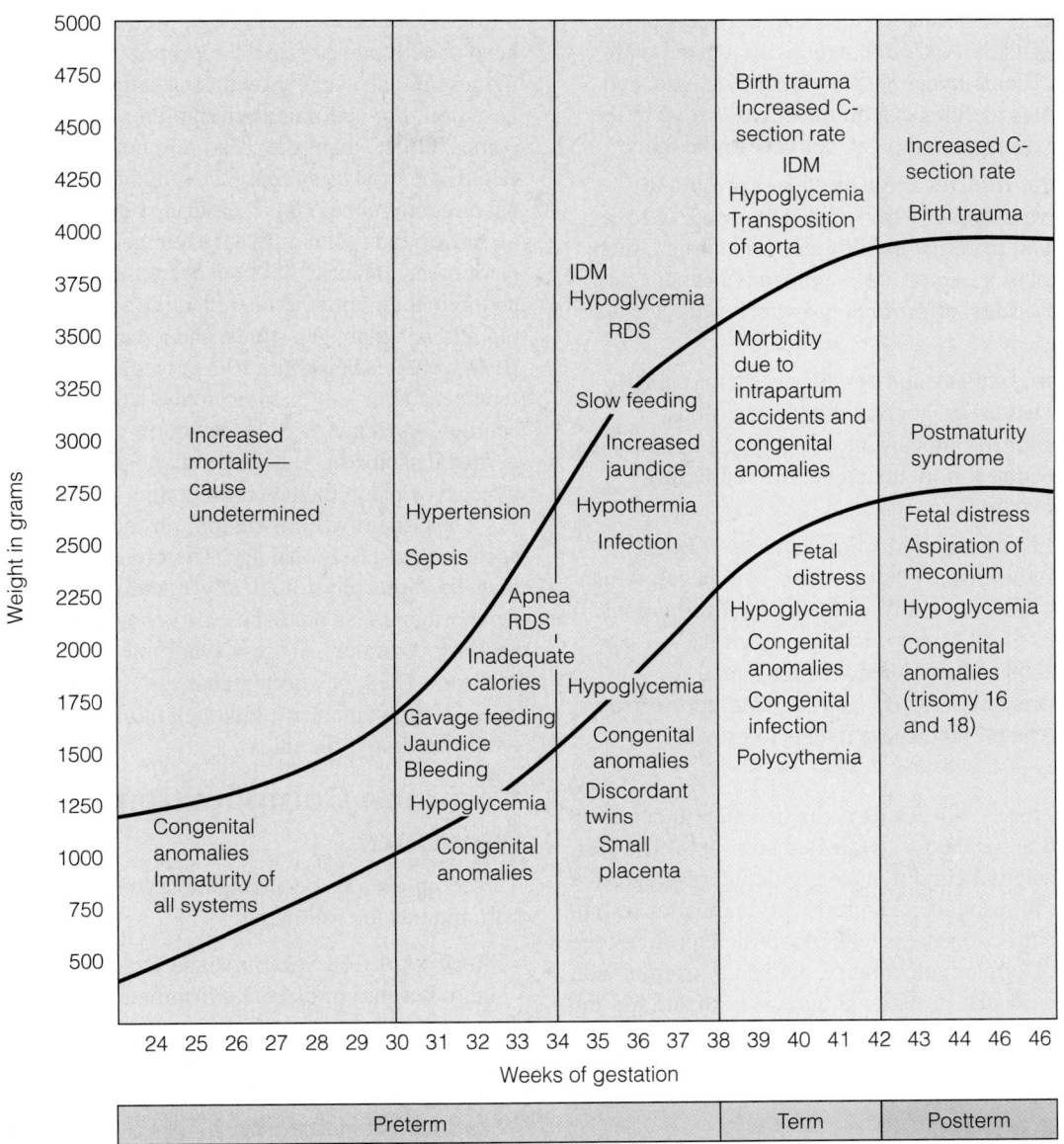

Figure 32–2 ◆ Neonatal morbidity by birth weight and gestational age.
SOURCE: Reprinted from *The High-Risk Infant,* by L. O. Lubchenco, p. 122. Copyright 1976 with permission from Elsevier.

limited fetal growth. The terms SGA and IUGR are not necessarily interchangeable.

SGA infants are commonly seen with mothers who smoke or have high blood pressure, causing these infants to have an increased incidence of perinatal asphyxia and perinatal mortality when compared with AGA infants (Resnik & Creasy, 2004). Intrauterine exposure to certain viruses is often associated with SGA infants. The incidence of polycythemia and hypoglycemia are also higher in this group of infants.

Factors Contributing to Intrauterine Growth Restriction

IUGR may be caused by maternal, placental, or fetal factors and may not be apparent antenatally. In the normal pregnancy, intrauterine growth is linear from approximately 28 to 38 weeks'

gestation. After 38 weeks, growth is variable, depending on the genetic growth potential of the fetus and placental function. The most common causes of growth restriction are the following:

• *Maternal factors.* Primiparity, grand multiparity, multiple-gestation pregnancy (twins and higher order multiples), lack of prenatal care, age extremes (under 16 or over 40), and low socioeconomic status (which can result in inadequate health care, inadequate education, inadequate living conditions, and malnutrition) affect IUGR (Martinez & Simmons, 2005). Before the third trimester, the nutritional supply to the fetus far exceeds his or her needs. Only in the third trimester is maternal malnutrition a limiting factor in fetal growth.

• *Maternal disease.* Maternal heart disease, substance abuse (drugs, tobacco, alcohol), sickle cell anemia, phenylketonuria (PKU), and asymptomatic pyelonephritis are associated with SGA. Complications associated with preeclampsia, chronic hypertensive vascular disease, and advanced diabetes mellitus can diminish blood flow to the uterus, thereby decreasing oxygen delivery to the fetus.

- *Environmental factors.* High altitude, exposure to x-rays, excessive exercise, work-related exposure to toxins, hyperthermia, and maternal use of teratogenic drugs, such as tobacco, alcohol, antimetabolics, anticonvulsants, narcotics, and cocaine, affect fetal growth (Resnik & Creasy, 2004).

- *Placental factors.* Placental conditions such as small placenta, infarcted areas, abnormal cord insertions, placenta previa, or thrombosis may affect circulation to the fetus, which becomes more deficient with increasing gestational age.

- *Fetal factors.* Congenital infections such as TORCH infections (*t*oxoplasmosis, *o*ther, *r*ubella, *c*ytomegalovirus, *h*erpes simplex virus), syphilis, congenital malformations, discordant twins (see Chapter 11 ∞), sex of the fetus (females tend to be smaller), chromosomal abnormalities (trisomies 13, 18, and 21), and inborn errors of metabolism can all predispose a fetus to growth disturbances.

Identifying fetuses with IUGR is the first step in detecting common disorders associated with affected newborns. The perinatal history of maternal conditions, early dating of pregnancy by first trimester ultrasound measurements, antepartal testing (nonstress test, contraction stress test, biophysical profile—see Chapter 21 ∞), Doppler velocimetry, pathology examination of the placenta, cord pH, gestational age assessment, and the physical and neurologic assessment of the newborn are also important (Resnik & Creasy, 2004).

Patterns of IUGR

Intrauterine growth occurs by an increase in cell number and cell size. If insult occurs early during the critical period of organ development in the fetus, fewer new cells are formed, organs are small, and organ weight is subnormal. In contrast, growth failure that begins later in pregnancy does not affect the total number of cells, only their size. The organs are normal, but their size is diminished. There are two clinical pictures of IUGR newborns.

Symmetric (proportional) IUGR is caused by long-term maternal conditions (such as chronic hypertension, severe malnutrition, chronic intrauterine infection, substance abuse, and anemia) or fetal genetic abnormalities (Martinez & Simmons, 2005). Symmetric IUGR can be noted by ultrasound in the first half of the second trimester. In symmetric IUGR there is chronic, prolonged restriction of growth in size of organs, body weight, body length, and, especially, head circumference.

Asymmetric (disproportional) IUGR is associated with an acute compromise of uteroplacental blood flow. Some causes are placental infarcts, preeclampsia, and poor weight gain in pregnancy. The growth restriction may not be evident before the third trimester because although weight is decreased, length and head circumference remain appropriate for that gestational age. In these infants, head growth is usually spared. After 36 weeks' gestation, the abdominal circumference of a normal fetus becomes larger than the head circumference. In asymmetric IUGR, the head circumference remains larger than the abdominal circumference. Thus measuring only the biparietal diameter on ultrasound will not reveal asymmetric IUGR. An early indicator of asymmetric SGA is a decrease in the growth rate of the abdominal circumference, reflecting subnormal liver growth, a reduction in glycogen stores, and a scarcity of subcutaneous fat. Birth weight is below the 10th percentile, whereas head circumference, and/or length, may plot between the 10th and 90th percentiles. Asymmetric SGA newborns are particularly at risk for perinatal asphyxia, pulmonary hemorrhage, hypocalcemia, and hypoglycemia in the newborn period.

Despite growth restriction, physiologic maturity develops according to gestational age. Therefore, the term SGA newborn may be more physiologically mature than the preterm AGA newborn and less predisposed to complications of prematurity such as respiratory distress syndrome and hyperbilirubinemia. The term SGA newborn's chances for survival are better because of organ maturity, although this newborn still faces many other potential difficulties.

Common Complications of the SGA Newborn

The complications occurring most frequently in the SGA newborn include the following:

- *Asphyxia.* The SGA infant suffers chronic hypoxia in utero because of placental insufficiency, which leaves little reserve to withstand the demands of labor and birth. Thus intrauterine asphyxia occurs with its potential systemic problems. Cesarean birth may be necessary.

- *Aspiration syndrome.* In utero, hypoxia can cause the fetus to gasp during birth, resulting in aspiration of amniotic fluid into the lower airways. It can also lead to relaxation of the anal sphincter and passage of meconium. This may result in aspiration of the meconium in utero or with the first breaths after birth.

- *Hypothermia.* Diminished subcutaneous fat (used for survival in utero), depletion of brown fat in utero, and a large surface area decrease the IUGR newborn's ability to conserve heat. The flexed position assumed by the term SGA newborn diminishes the effect of surface area.

- *Hypoglycemia.* An increase in metabolic rate in response to heat loss and poor hepatic glycogen stores cause hypoglycemia. In addition, the infant is compromised by inadequate supplies of enzymes to activate gluconeogenesis (conversion of nonglucogen sources, such as fatty acids and proteins, to glucose).

- *Polycythemia.* The number of red blood cells is increased in the SGA newborn. This finding is considered a physiologic response to in utero chronic hypoxic stress. Polycythemia may contribute to hypoglycemia.

Newborns with significant IUGR tend to have a poor prognosis, especially when born before 37 weeks' gestation. Factors contributing to poor outcome include:

- *Congenital malformations.* Congenital malformations occur in 8% of SGA infants (Martinez & Simmons, 2005); the more severe the IUGR, the greater the chance for malformation as a result of impaired mitotic activity and cellular hypoplasia.
- *Intrauterine infection.* Fetuses exposed to intrauterine infections such as rubella and cytomegalovirus are profoundly affected by direct invasion of the brain and other vital organs by the offending virus, resulting in IUGR.
- *Continued growth difficulties.* SGA newborns tend to be shorter than newborns of the same gestational age. Asymmetric IUGR infants can be expected to catch up in weight and approach their inherited growth potential when given an optimal environment. Symmetric IUGR infants reportedly have varied growth potential but tend not to catch up to their peers (Martinez & Simmons, 2005).
- *Cognitive difficulties.* Often SGA newborns can exhibit subsequent learning disabilities. The disabilities are characterized by hyperactivity, short attention span, and poor fine motor coordination (writing and drawing). Some hearing loss and speech defects also occur.

CLINICAL TIP

In assessing a growth-restricted infant resulting from unexplained maternal etiology (e.g., hypertension, placental insufficiency), an in utero viral infection may be the answer.

Clinical Therapy

The goal of medical therapy for SGA infants is early recognition and implementation of medical management of the potential problems.

NURSING CARE MANAGEMENT
Nursing Assessment and Diagnosis

The nurse is responsible for assessing gestational age and identifying signs of potential complications associated with SGA infants. All body parts of the symmetric IUGR infant are in proportion, but they are below normal size for the baby's gestational age. Therefore, the head does not appear overly large or the length excessive in relation to the other body parts. These newborns are generally vigorous.

The asymmetric IUGR infant appears long, thin, and emaciated, with loss of subcutaneous fat tissue and muscle mass (Figure 32–3 ◆). The baby may have loose skin folds; dry, desquamating skin; and a thin and often meconium-stained cord. The head appears relatively large (although it approaches normal size) because the chest size and abdominal girth are de-

Figure 32–3 ◆ Thirty-five-week gestational age twins. Twin B is SGA and weighs 1260 g. Twin A is AGA and weighs 2605 g.
SOURCE: Courtesy of Carol Harrigan, RNC, MSN, NNP.

creased. The baby may have a vigorous cry and appear alert and wide eyed.

Nursing diagnoses that may apply to the SGA newborn include the following:

- *Impaired Gas Exchange* related to aspiration of meconium
- *Hypothermia* related to decreased subcutaneous fat
- *Risk for Injury to Tissues* related to decreased glycogen stores and impaired gluconeogenesis
- *Altered Nutrition: Less than Body Requirements* related to SGA's increased metabolic rate
- *Risk for Altered Tissue Perfusion* related to polycythemia and increased blood viscosity
- *Risk for Altered Parenting* related to prolonged separation of newborn from parents secondary to illness

Nursing Plan and Implementation
HOSPITAL-BASED NURSING CARE

Hypoglycemia, the most common metabolic complication of IUGR, produces such sequelae as central nervous system abnormalities and mental retardation. Conditions such as asphyxia, hyperviscosity, and cold stress may also affect the baby's outcome. Paying meticulous attention to physiologic parameters is essential for immediate nursing management and reduction of long-term disorders (see Nursing Care Plan: For the Small-for-Gestational-Age Newborn on pages 934–938).

COMMUNITY-BASED NURSING CARE

The long-term needs of the SGA newborn include careful follow-up evaluation of patterns of growth and possible disabilities that may later interfere with learning or motor functioning. Long-term follow-up care is especially necessary for those infants with congenital malformations, congenital infections, and

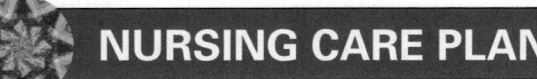

NURSING CARE PLAN

For the Small-for-Gestational-Age Newborn

INTERVENTION	RATIONALE	EXPECTED OUTCOMES
1. Nursing Diagnosis: Risk for Impaired Gas Exchange related to meconium aspiration		
Goal: The infant's respirations will be within normal limits, no periods of apnea or evidence of worsening distress.		
		• The infant will maintain adequate respiratory gas exchange as evidenced by: respirations of 30–60/min and pulse oximetry and arterial blood gases within normal limits.
• Obtain maternal prenatal, labor, and birth records.	• Provides information of fetal stress that may have occurred during the prenatal or intrapartal period. In addition, the birth record will provide information concerning infant's respiratory status at birth; for example, the Apgar score.	
• Maintain airway patency through judicious suctioning.	• Respiratory distress in SGA newborns is due to in utero hypoxia and aspiration of meconium.	
• Observe for worsening signs of respiratory distress such as generalized cyanosis; worsening retractions, grunting, and nasal flaring, as evidenced by Silverman respiratory index; sustained tachypnea; apnea episodes; inequality of breath sounds; presence of rales and rhonchi, decreased oxygenation saturation (less than 86%).		
• Monitor and maintain adequate body temperature (36C±0.2C [97.7F±0.5F]) to avoid increased oxygen consumption.	• Temperature elevation may cause metabolic rate and oxygen needs to increase when associated with meconium aspiration.	
• Administer oxygen or other interventions (e.g., nasal continuous positive airway pressure [CPAP], intubations) per order for relief of respiratory distress signs. (See Chapter 31 ∞ for nursing care and treatment of meconium aspiration, infant resuscitation).	• Provides healthcare personnel with differential information on cardiac and pulmonary status.	
• Implement treatment plan for respiratory distress.		
• Monitor glucose levels.	• Respiratory distress increases consumption of glucose.	
• **Collaborative:** Obtain arterial blood gases (ABGs) per physician/neonatal nurse practitioner (NNP) orders.		

NURSING CARE PLAN

For the Small-for-Gestational-Age Newborn continued

INTERVENTION	RATIONALE	EXPECTED OUTCOMES
• Monitor infant's cardiac status and pulmonary status pulse oximetry and ABGs.	• Oxygen demands increase with meconium aspiration. Obtaining ABGs will provide medical personnel baseline information of infant's respiratory status, and effective medical interventions can be initiated.	

2. Nursing Diagnosis: Risk for Ineffective Thermoregulation and Cold Stress secondary to decreased subcutaneous fat

Goal: The infant's temperature will be stable and maintained within normal limits.

INTERVENTION	RATIONALE	EXPECTED OUTCOMES
• Provide neutral thermal zone (NTZ) range for infant based on postnatal weight.	• Neutral thermal environment charts used for preterm infant are not reliable for weight of SGA infant.	*The infant will not exhibit signs and symptoms of hypothermia as evidenced by temperature maintenance of 36.5–37.3C (97.7–99.1F) and no signs and symptoms of respiratory distress.*
• Place incubator/overhead warmer on servocontrol mode. Use a skin probe to maintain infant's skin temperature at 36C–36.5C (96.8–97.7F).	• A neutral thermal environment requires minimal oxygen consumption to maintain a normal core temperature.	
• Obtain axillary temperatures and compare with registered skin probe temperature. If discrepancy exists, evaluate potential cause.	• Discrepancies between axillary and skin probe monitor temperatures may be due to mechanical causes or the burning of brown fat.	
• Adjust and monitor incubator or radiant warmer to maintain skin tempertature.		
• Minimize heat losses and prevent cold stress by: 1. Warming and humidifying oxygen without blowing over face to avoid increasing oxygen consumption 2. Keeping skin dry 3. Keeping incubators, radiant warmers, and cribs away from windows and cold external walls and out of drafts 4. Avoiding placing infant on cold surfaces such as metal treatment tables, cold x-ray plates 5. Padding cold surfaces with diapers and using radiant warmers during procedures 6. Warming blood for exchange transfusions	• Physical principles of heat loss effects include: 1. Evaporation—lungs and skin when cooling occurs as a result of water evaporation 2. Convection—air currents 3. Conduction—skin contact with cooler object 4. Radiation—loss of warmth to cooler surrounding objects	
• Observe for signs and symptoms of cold stress: decreased temperature, lethargy, pallor (for further discussion see Chapter 33)	• Hypothermia is a potential problem for an SGA infant because: 1. SGA infant has decreased stores of brown fat available for thermogenesis, because SGA infant has used these stores in utero for survival.	

(Continued on next page)

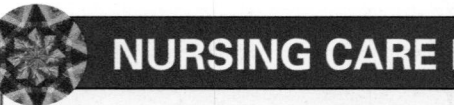

NURSING CARE PLAN

For the Small-for-Gestational-Age Newborn continued

INTERVENTION	RATIONALE	EXPECTED OUTCOMES
	2. SGA infant has poor insulation due to use of subcutaneous tissues in utero for survival.	

3. Nursing Diagnosis: Risk for Injury related to decreased glycogen stores and impaired gluconeogenesis

Goal: Newborn will have a normal blood glucose level.

• Monitor blood glucose levels per SGA protocol and report values less than 45 mg/dL. • Observe, record, and report signs of hypoglycemia: cyanosis, lethargy, jitteriness, seizure activity, and apnea. • Initiate feeding schedule for SGA newborns per agency protocol. • Provide glucose intake either through early enteral feeding (before 4 hr) or by intravenous (IV) per physician/NNP order. See further discussion of hypoglycemia in Chapter 33. ∞	• Combined with depletion of glycogen stores, impaired gluconeogenesis predisposes SGA infants to profound hypoglycemia within first 2 days of life. • Hypoglycemia in SGA infant is indicated by whole blood sugar less than 20 mg/dL. • Frequent monitoring of Dextrostix assists in identifying decreasing glucose levels. • Provision of glucose through early feedings (begin before 4 hr of age) assists in maintaining glucose levels.	• *The infant will not exhibit signs and symptoms of hypoglycemia as evidenced by an euglycemic state and blood glucose greater than 45 mg/dL.*

4. Nursing Diagnosis: Altered Nutrition: Less than Body Requirements related to increased metabolic needs in the infant

Goal: Newborn will gain weight and tolerate nipple feedings without tiring.

• Assess suck, swallow, gag, and cough reflexes. • Initiate test water or per protocol formula-feeding at 1 hour of age, then proceed to 5% glucose/water. Move early to formula-feeding every 2–3 hr. • Use concentrated formulas that supply more calories in less volume, such as 24 cal/oz.	• Prevents feeding problems and assists in determining the best method of feeding for infant. • Sterile water may be used for first feedings because it causes fewer pulmonary complications in the presence of gastrointestinal tract abnormalities and/or aspiration of feeding. • SGA newborns require more calories/kg for growth than AGA newborns because of increased metabolic activity and oxygen consumption secondary to increased percentage of body weight made up by visceral organs. • Small, frequent feedings of high caloric formula are used because of limited gastric capacity and decreased gastric emptying.	• *The infant will maintain steady weight gain as evidenced by less than 2%/day weight loss, tolerates oral feedings, and urine output is 1–3 mL/kg/hour.*

NURSING CARE PLAN

For the Small-for-Gestational-Age Newborn continued

INTERVENTION	RATIONALE	EXPECTED OUTCOMES
• Supplement oral feedings with IV intake per orders. • Promote growth by providing caloric intake of 120–150 cal/kg/day in small amounts. • Observe, record, and report signs of respiratory distress or fatigue occurring during feedings. • Supplement gavage or nipple feedings with IV therapy per physician order until oral intake is sufficient to support growth. • Establish a nipple feeding program that is begun slowly and progresses slowly, such as nipple feed once per day, nipple feed once per shift, and then nipple feed every other feeding. • Monitor daily weight with anticipation of small amount of weight loss when nipple feedings start.	• Growth is evaluated by increase in weight (about 20 g/day), length, and body measurements. • Decrease in exhaustion is an important consideration in feeding SGA infant. • Adequate nutritional intake promotes growth and prevents such complications as metabolic catabolism and hypoglycemia. • Gavage feedings require less energy expenditure on the part of the newborn. • Nipple feeding, an active rather than passive intake of nutrition, requires energy expenditure and burning of calories by infant.	

5. Nursing Diagnosis: Risk for Altered Parenting related to lack of knowledge of infant care and prolonged separation of infant and her or his parents secondary to illness

Goal: Parents will bond with their infant and have realistic expectations about their infant. Parents are comfortable taking infant home. They are able to demonstrate normal infant care and assessments of possible complications, and know when to return for follow-up.

• Support emotionally the psychologic well-being of family, including positive parent-infant attachment and sensory stimulation of infant. • Include parents in determining infant's plan of care and encourage their participation. Encourage parents to visit frequently. Provide opportunities for parents to touch, hold, talk to, and care for infant. Determine the type and amount of appropriate sensory stimulation and implement sensory stimulation program.	• Parent-infant attachment begins in first few hours or days following birth. SGA infants may experience prolonged periods of separation from their parents, which necessitates intervention to ensure parent-infant attachment.	• *The parent will demonstrate ability to perform basic infant care tasks as evidenced by exhibiting appropriate attachment behaviors (i.e., talking and holding infant), feeding infant, and bathing infant.*

(Continued on next page)

NURSING CARE PLAN

For the Small-for-Gestational-Age Newborn continued

INTERVENTION	RATIONALE	EXPECTED OUTCOMES
• Prepare for discharge by instructing parents in such areas as feeding techniques, formula preparation, and breastfeeding; bathing, diapering, and hygiene; temperature monitoring; administration of vitamins, care of complications and preventing exposure to infections; normal elimination patterns, normal reflexes and activity, and how to promote normal growth and development without being overprotective; returning for continued medical care; and availability of community resources if indicated.	• Parents should receive the same postpartum teaching as any parent taking a new infant home. • Parents need to understand the changes to expect in color of the infant's stool and number of bowel movements plus odor from formula- or breastfeeding to avoid unnecessary concern. SGA infants usually do not require referral to community agencies such as visiting nurse associations unless there is a specific problem requiring assistance.	

obvious sequelae from physiologic problems. Parents of the IUGR newborn need support, because a positive atmosphere can enhance the baby's growth potential and the child's ultimate outcome.

Evaluation

Expected outcomes of nursing care include the following:

- The SGA newborn is free from respiratory compromise.
- The SGA newborn maintains a stable temperature.
- The SGA infant is free from hypoglycemic episodes and maintains glucose hemostasis.
- The SGA newborn gains weight and takes breast- or formula-feedings without physiologic distress or fatigue.
- The parents verbalize their concerns surrounding their baby's health problems and understand the rationale behind management of their newborn.

CARE OF THE LARGE-FOR-GESTATIONAL-AGE NEWBORN

A newborn whose birth weight is at or above the 90th percentile on the intrauterine growth curve (at any week of gestation) is considered **large for gestational age (LGA)**. Some AGA newborns have been incorrectly categorized as LGA because of miscalculation of the date of conception due to postconceptional bleeding. Careful gestational age assessment is essential to identify the potential needs and problems of such infants.

The best known condition associated with excessive fetal growth is maternal diabetes (White's classes A, B, C, D; see Table 19–4 ∞); however, only a small fraction of LGA newborns are born to mothers with diabetes. The cause of the ma-

jority of cases of LGA infants is unclear, but certain factors or situations have been found to correlate with their births (Martinez & Simmons, 2005):

- Genetic predisposition is correlated proportionally to the mother's prepregnancy weight and to weight gain during pregnancy. Large parents tend to have large infants.
- Multiparous women have two to three times the number of LGA infants as primigravidas.
- Male infants are typically larger than female infants.
- Infants with erythroblastosis fetalis, Beckwith-Wiedemann syndrome (a genetic condition associated with macroglossia, omphalocele, and newborn hypoglycemia and hyperinsulinemia), or transposition of the great vessels are usually large.

The increase in the LGA infant's body size is characteristically proportional, although head circumference and body length are in the upper limits of intrauterine growth. The exception to this rule is the infant of the diabetic mother, whose body weight is higher but whose length and head circumference may be in the normal range. Macrosomic infants have poor motor skills and have more difficulty in regulating behavioral states. LGA infants tend to be more difficult to arouse and may have problems maintaining a quiet alert state. They may also have feeding difficulties.

Common Complications of the LGA Newborn

Complications of the LGA infant can include the following:

- *Birth trauma due to cephalopelvic disproportion (CPD).* Often LGA newborns have a biparietal diameter greater than 10 cm (4 in.) or are associated with a maternal fundal height measurement greater than 42 cm (16 in.) without the presence of polyhydramnios. Because of their excessive size or macrosomia, there are more breech presentations and shoulder dystocia. These complications may result in asphyxia, fractured clavicles, fractured humerus, brachial plexus palsy, facial paralysis, phrenic nerve palsy, depressed skull fractures, cephalhematoma, and intracranial hemorrhage, all due to birth trauma.

- *Increased incidence of cesarean births and oxytocin-induced births due to fetal size.* Mothers and infants have all the risk factors associated with cesarean births (Martinez & Simmons, 2005).

- *Hypoglycemia, polycythemia, and hyperviscosity.* These disorders are most often seen in infants of diabetic mothers and infants with erythroblastosis fetalis or Beckwith-Wiedemann syndrome.

NURSING CARE MANAGEMENT

The perinatal history, in conjunction with ultrasonic measurement of fetal skull (biparietal diameter) and gestational age testing, is important in identifying an at-risk LGA newborn. Nursing care is directed toward early identification and immediate treatment of the common disorders. Essential components of the nursing assessment are monitoring vital signs, screening for hypoglycemia and polycythemia, and observing for signs and symptoms related to birth trauma. The nurse should address parental concerns about the visual signs of birth trauma and the potential for continuation of the excess weight pattern. The nurse should help parents learn to arouse and console their newborn and facilitate nutritional intake and attachment behaviors. Mothers of LGA infants with bruising of the face or head may be reluctant to interact with their infants because they fear hurting their infants. The nursing care for complications associated with LGA newborns is similar to the care needed by the infant of a diabetic mother and is discussed in the next section.

CARE OF THE INFANT OF A DIABETIC MOTHER

Infants of diabetic mothers (IDMs) are considered at risk and require close observation the first few hours to the first few days of life. Mothers with severe diabetes or diabetes of long duration associated with vascular complications may give birth to SGA infants. The infant of the typical IDM, when the diabetes is poorly controlled or gestational, is LGA. The infant is macrosomic, ruddy in color, and has excess adipose fat tissue (Figure 32–4 ◆). The umbilical cord is thick and the placenta is large. There is a higher incidence of macrosomic infants born to certain ethnic groups (Native Americans, Mexican Americans, African Americans, and Pacific Islanders) (Chmait & Moore, 2005).

IDMs have decreased total body water, particularly in the extracellular spaces, and are therefore not edematous. Their ex-

Figure 32–4 ◆ Macrosomic infant of a Class B insulin-dependent diabetic mother born at 38 weeks' gestation weighing 3402 grams.
SOURCE: Courtesy of Carol Harrigan, RNC, MSN, NNP.

cessive weight is due to increased weight of the visceral organs, cardiomegaly (hypertrophy), and increased body fat. The only organ not affected is the brain.

The excessive fetal growth of the IDM is caused by exposure to high levels of maternal glucose, which readily crosses the placenta. The fetus responds to these high glucose levels with increased insulin production and hyperplasia of the pancreatic beta cells. The main action of insulin is to facilitate the entry of glucose into muscle and fat cells. Once in the cells, glucose is converted to glycogen and stored. Insulin also inhibits the breakdown of fat to free fatty acids, thereby maintaining lipid synthesis; increases the uptake of amino acids; and promotes protein synthesis. Insulin is an important regulator of fetal metabolism and has a "growth hormone" effect that results in increased linear growth. IDMs may be obese as children.

Common Complications of the IDM

Although IDMs are usually large, they are immature in physiologic functions and exhibit many of the problems of the preterm (premature) infant. The complications most often seen in an IDM are as follows:

- *Hypoglycemia.* Hypoglycemia is defined as a blood sugar less than 40 mg/dL. Even though the high maternal blood sugar supply is lost, the IDM continues to produce high levels of insulin, which deplete the infant's blood glucose within hours after birth. IDMs also have less ability to release glucagon and catecholamines, which normally stimulate glucagon breakdown and glucose release. The incidence of hypoglycemia in IDMs varies from 30% to 50% according to the degree of success in controlling the maternal diabetes, the maternal blood sugar level at the time of birth, the length of labor, the class of maternal diabetes, and early versus late feedings of the newborn (Moore, 2004). Signs and symptoms of hypoglycemia include tremors, cyanosis, apnea, temperature instability, poor feeding, and hypotonia. Seizures may occur in severe cases.

CLINICAL TIP

When beginning fluids on an IDM, it is sometimes best to start at a higher concentration of dextrose to avoid hypoglycemic episodes. Usual glucose infusion rates are 6 to 8 mg/kg/minute.

- *Hypocalcemia.* Tremors are the obvious clinical sign of hypocalcemia. They may be due to the IDM's prematurity and to the stresses of difficult pregnancy, labor, and birth, which predispose any infant to hypocalcemia. Women who have diabetes tend to have decreased serum magnesium levels at term secondary to increased urinary calcium excretion, which causes secondary hypoparathyroidism in their infants. Other factors may include vitamin D antagonism, which results from elevated cortisol levels, hypophosphatemia from tissue catabolism, and decreased serum magnesium levels.

- *Hyperbilirubinemia.* This condition may be seen at 48 to 72 hours after birth. It may be caused by slightly decreased extracellular fluid volume, which increases the hematocrit level. This elevation facilitates an increase in red blood cell breakdown, thereby increasing bilirubin levels. The presence of hepatic immaturity may impair bilirubin conjugation. Enclosed cranial hemorrhages resulting from a complicated vaginal birth may also contribute to hyperbilirubinemia.

- *Birth trauma.* Because most IDMs are macrosomic, trauma may occur during labor and birth from shoulder dystocia.

- *Polycythemia.* Fetal hyperglycemia and hyperinsulinism result in increased oxygen consumption, which can lead to fetal hypoxia (Moore, 2004). Hemoglobin A_{1c} binds to oxygen, decreasing the oxygen available to the fetal tissues. This tissue hypoxia stimulates increased erythropoietin production, which increases both the hematocrit level and the potential for hyperbilirubinemia. See Chapter 19 ∞ for discussion of hemoglobin A_{1c}.

- *Respiratory distress syndrome (RDS).* This complication occurs more frequently in newborns of White's classes A through C diabetic mothers who are not well controlled. Insulin antagonizes the cortisol-induced stimulation of lecithin synthesis that is necessary for lung maturation. Therefore, IDMs may have lungs that are less mature than expected for their gestational age. There is also a decrease in the phospholipid phosphatidylglycerol (PG), which stabilizes surfactant. The insufficiency of PG increases the incidence of RDS. Therefore, it is important to test for fetal lung maturity, or the presence of PG, in the amniotic fluid before birth.

  RDS does not appear to be problematic for infants born to diabetic mothers in White's classes D through F; instead,

the stresses of poor uterine blood supply may lead to increased production of steroids, which accelerates lung maturation. IDMs may also have a delay in closure of the ductus arteriosus and decreases in postnatal pulmonary artery pressure (Moore, 2004).

- *Congenital malformations.* These may include transposition of the great vessels, ventricular septal defect, left or right ventricular wall hypertrophy, small left colon syndrome, and sacral agenesis (caudal regression) (Moore, 2004). Early careful regulation of maternal glucose before and during pregnancy, especially during the first trimester, decreases the risk of birth defects. See Chapter 19. ∞

Clinical Therapy

Prenatal management is directed toward controlling maternal glucose levels, which minimizes the common complications of IDMs. Because the onset of hypoglycemia occurs within 1 and 3 hours following delivery in IDMs (with a spontaneous rise to normal levels by 4 to 6 hours), blood glucose determinations should be performed on capillary or venous blood samples hourly during the first 4 hours after birth and at 4-hour intervals until the risk period (about 48 hours) has passed or per nursery protocol.

IDMs whose serum glucose falls below 40 mg/dL should have early feedings with formula or breast milk (colostrum). If normal glucose levels cannot be maintained with oral feeding, an intravenous (IV) infusion of glucose will be necessary. An infusion of D10W at a rate of 6 to 8 mg/kg/min usually maintains normoglycemia in the IDM. If higher glucose concentrations (greater than 12.5%) are needed to maintain normal serum glucose levels, a central line will need to be placed to minimize tissue extravasation. Newborns with refractory hypoglycemia may benefit by the administration of IV corticosteroids. Once the blood glucose has been stable for 24 hours, the infusion rate can be decreased as oral feedings are increased. The newborn's blood glucose levels must be carefully monitored. Repeated dextrose as a bolus infusion is contraindicated because it may lead to severe rebound hypoglycemia following an initial brief increase in glucose level.

NURSING CARE MANAGEMENT
Nursing Assessment and Diagnosis

The nurse should not be lulled into thinking that a big baby is a mature baby. In almost every case, because of the infant's large size, the IDM will appear older than gestational age scoring indicates. The nurse must consider both the gestational age and whether the baby is AGA or LGA in planning and providing safe care. In caring for the IDM, the nurse assesses for signs of respiratory distress, hyperbilirubinemia, birth trauma, and congenital anomalies.

Nursing diagnoses that may apply to IDMs include the following:

- *Altered Nutrition: Less than Body Requirements* related to increased glucose metabolism secondary to hyperinsulinemia

- *Impaired Gas Exchange* related to respiratory distress secondary to impaired production of surfactant
- *Alteration in Calcium Homeostasis* related to inappropriate parathyroid response
- *Increased Incidence of Congenital Anomalies* related to poor maternal glucose control
- *Alteration in Hematologic Status: Polycythemia* related to increased synthesis of erythropoietin secondary to hypoxia due to increased metabolic rate
- *Ineffective Family Coping: Compromised* related to the illness of the baby

Nursing Plan and Implementation

Nursing care of the IDM is directed toward early detection and ongoing monitoring of hypoglycemia (by performing glucose tests) and polycythemia (by obtaining central hematocrits), respiratory distress, and hyperbilirubinemia. For specific nursing interventions for RDS, hypoglycemia, hyperbilirubinemia, and polycythemia, see Chapter 33. ∞ Also assess for signs of birth trauma and congenital anomalies.

Parent teaching is directed toward preventing macrosomia and the resulting fetal-newborn problems and instituting early and ongoing diabetic control. Parents are advised that with early identification and care, most IDMs' complications have no significant sequelae.

Evaluation

Expected outcomes of nursing care include the following:

- The IDM's respiratory and metabolic alteration problems are minimized.
- The parents understand the etiology of the baby's health problems and preventive steps they can initiate to decrease the impact of maternal diabetes on subsequent pregnancies.
- The parents verbalize their concerns surrounding their baby's health problems and understand the rationale behind management of their newborn.

CARE OF THE POSTTERM NEWBORN

The **postterm newborn** is any newborn born after 42 weeks' gestation. Postterm or prolonged pregnancy occurs in approximately 4% to 14% of all pregnancies (Resnik & Resnik, 2004). The cause of most postterm pregnancies is not completely understood, but several factors are known to be associated factors (see Chapter 26 ∞). Many pregnancies classified as prolonged are thought to be a result of inaccurate determination of the estimated date of confinement (EDC). Postterm pregnancy is more common in Australian, Greek, and Italian ethnic groups.

Most babies born as a result of prolonged pregnancy are of normal size and health; some keep on growing and are over 4000 g at birth, which supports the contention that the postterm fetus can remain well nourished. Potential intrapartum problems for these healthy but large fetuses include CPD and shoulder dystocia. See Chapter 26 ∞ for discussion of the necessary assessments and interventions for CPD and shoulder dystocia.

Common Complications of the Newborn with Postmaturity Syndrome

The term **postmaturity** applies only to the infant who is born after 42 completed weeks of gestation and also demonstrates characteristics of *postmaturity syndrome*. Only about 5% of postterm newborns are also postmature.

The truly postmature newborn is at high risk for morbidity and has a mortality rate two to three times higher than that of term infants. Although today the percentages are extremely low, the majority of postmature fetal deaths occur during labor, because by that time the fetus has used up necessary body reserves.

Postmaturity syndrome is characterized by decreased placental function, which impairs nutrition transport and oxygenation, leaving the fetus prone to hypoglycemia and hypoxemia when the stresses of labor begin. The following are common disorders of the postmature newborn:

- Hypoglycemia from nutritional deprivation resulting in depleted glycogen stores.
- Meconium aspiration in response to in utero hypoxia. Oligohydramnios increases the danger of aspirating thick meconium. Severe meconium aspiration syndrome increases the baby's chance of developing persistent pulmonary hypertension, pneumothorax, and pneumonia.
- Polycythemia due to increased production of red blood cells (RBCs) in response to hypoxia.
- Congenital anomalies of unknown cause.
- Seizures due to hypoxic insult.
- Cold stress due to loss or poor development of subcutaneous fat.

The long-term effects of postmaturity syndrome are unclear. At present, studies do not agree on the effect of postmaturity syndrome on weight gain and IQ scores (Resnik & Resnik, 2004).

Prolonged pregnancy by itself is not responsible for the postmaturity syndrome. The characteristics of the postmature newborn are caused primarily by a combination of placental aging and subsequent insufficiency and continued exposure to amniotic fluid.

Clinical Therapy

The aim of antenatal management is to differentiate the fetus who has postmaturity syndrome from the fetus who is large, well nourished, and active and who is tolerating the prolonged (postterm) pregnancy. Antenatal tests that can be done to evaluate fetal status and determine obstetric management are discussed in more depth in Chapters 21 ∞ and 26. ∞ If the amniotic fluid is meconium stained, an amnioinfusion may be done during labor. This procedure dilutes the meconium by directly infusing either normal saline or Ringer's lactate into the uterus, decreasing the risk of meconium aspiration syndrome.

(For detailed discussion of clinical management and care of the newborn at risk for meconium aspiration, see Chapter 33 ∞).

Hypoglycemia is monitored by serial glucose determinations as per agency protocols. If not in respiratory distress, the baby may be placed on glucose infusions or given early feedings if respiratory distress is not present, but these measures must be instituted with caution because of the frequency of asphyxia in the first 24 hours. Postmature newborns are often voracious eaters.

For the SGA infant who is postmature, peripheral and central hematocrits are tested to determine the presence of polycythemia. Fluid resuscitation can be initiated. In extreme cases a partial exchange transfusion may be necessary to manage polycythemia and adverse sequelae such as hyperviscosity. Oxygen is provided for respiratory distress. In addition, decreased liver glycogen stores can cause temperature instability and excessive loss of body heat. See Chapter 30 ∞ for thermoregulation techniques.

NURSING CARE MANAGEMENT
Nursing Assessment and Diagnosis

The newborn with postmaturity syndrome appears alert. This wide-eyed, alert appearance is not necessarily a positive sign because it may indicate chronic intrauterine hypoxia. The infant has dry, cracking, parchmentlike skin without vernix or lanugo (Figure 32–5 ◆). Fingernails are long, and scalp hair is profuse. The infant's body appears long and thin. The wasting involves depletion of previously stored subcutaneous tissue, causing the skin to be loose. Fat layers are almost nonexistent.

Postmature newborns frequently have meconium staining, which colors the nails, skin, and umbilical cord. The varying shades (yellow to green) of meconium staining can give some clue about whether the expulsion of meconium was a recent or a chronic problem. Green coloring indicates a more recent event.

Figure 32–5 ◆ The skin of the postterm infant exhibits deep cracking and peeling.
SOURCE: Dubowitz, L., & Dubowitz, V. (1977). *The gestational age of the newborn.* Menlo Park, CA: Addison-Wesley. Reprinted by permission of V. Dubowitz, MD, Hammersmith Hospital, London, England.

Nursing diagnoses that may apply to the postmature newborn include the following:

* ***Hypothermia*** related to decreased liver glycogen and brown fat stores
* ***Altered Nutrition: Less than Body Requirements*** related to increased use of glucose secondary to stress in utero and decreased placental perfusion
* ***Impaired Gas Exchange in the Lungs and at the Cellular Level*** related to airway obstruction from meconium aspiration
* ***Risk for Altered Tissue Perfusion*** related to increased blood viscosity due to polycythemia

Nursing Plan and Implementation
HOSPITAL-BASED NURSING CARE

Nursing interventions are primarily supportive measures. They include the following:

* Monitor cardiopulmonary status because the stresses of labor are poorly tolerated and can result in hypoxemia in utero and possible asphyxia at birth.
* Provide warmth via an external heat source to counterbalance the infant's poor response to cold stress and decreased liver glycogen and brown fat stores.
* Frequently monitor blood glucose and initiate early feeding (at 1 or 2 hours of age) or IV glucose per physician order.
* Obtain a central hematocrit to determine accurately the presence of polycythemia.

The nurse encourages parents to express their feelings and fears regarding the newborn's condition and potential long-term problems. The nurse also gives careful explanations of procedures, includes the parents in developing care plans for their baby, and encourages follow-up care as needed.

Evaluation

Expected outcomes of nursing care include the following:

* The postterm newborn establishes effective respiratory function.
* The postmature baby is free of metabolic alterations (hypoglycemia) and maintains a stable temperature.

CARE OF THE PRETERM (PREMATURE) NEWBORN

A **preterm infant** is an infant born before the completion of 37 weeks' gestation (Figure 32–6 ◆). With the help of modern technology, infants are surviving at younger gestational ages but not without significant morbidity. The incidence of all preterm births in the United States is approximately 12%; and 18% of African American newborns are preterm (Als & Lawhon, 2004). The rise in multiple birth rates has markedly influenced overall rates of low-birth-weight (LBW) infants. Prematurity and LBW are common in single women and adolescents. (See Chapter 20 ∞ for a discussion of preterm labor).

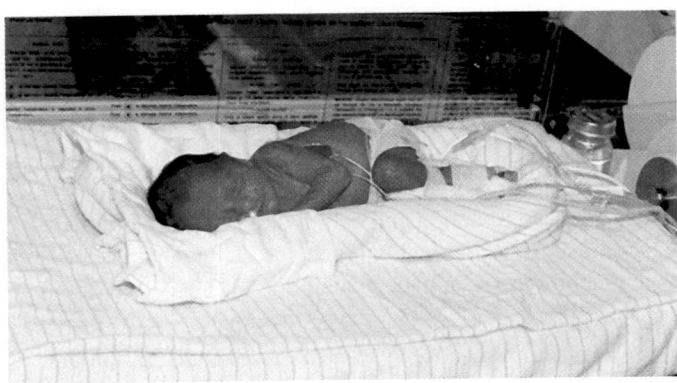

Figure 32–6 ◆ A 6-day-old, 28 weeks' gestational age, 960-g preterm infant.
SOURCE: Courtesy of Carol Harrigan, RNC, MSN, NNP.

The major problem of the preterm newborn is variable immaturity of all systems, the degree of which depends on the length of gestation. The preterm newborn must traverse the same complex, interconnected pathways from intrauterine to extrauterine life as the term newborn. Immaturity means the premature newborn is ill equipped to make this transition smoothly. Maintenance of the preterm newborn falls within narrow physiologic parameters.

Alteration in Respiratory and Cardiovascular Physiology

The preterm newborn is at risk for respiratory problems because the lungs are not fully mature and not fully ready to take over the process of oxygen and carbon dioxide exchange until 37 to 38 weeks' gestation. Critical factors in the development of respiratory distress include the following:

1. The preterm infant is unable to produce adequate amounts of surfactant. (See Chapter 28 ∞ for discussion of respiratory adaptation and development). Inadequate surfactant lessens compliance (ability of the lungs to fill with air easily), thereby increasing the inspiratory pressure needed to expand the lungs with air. The collapsed (or atelectatic) alveoli will not facilitate an exchange of oxygen and carbon dioxide. As a result, the infant becomes hypoxic, pulmonary blood flow is inefficient, and the preterm newborn's available energy is depleted.

2. The muscular coat of the pulmonary blood vessels is incompletely developed. Consequently the pulmonary arterioles do not constrict as well in response to decreased oxygen levels. This lowered pulmonary vascular resistance leads to increased left-to-right shunting through the ductus arteriosus, which increases the blood flow back into the lungs.

3. Normally the ductus arteriosus responds to increasing oxygen and prostaglandin E levels by vasoconstriction; in the preterm infant, who has higher susceptibility to hypoxia, the ductus may remain open. A patent ductus increases the blood volume to the lungs, causing pulmonary congestion, increased respiratory effort, carbon dioxide retention, and bounding femoral pulses.

The common complications of the cardiopulmonary system in preterm infants are discussed later in the chapter and in Chapter 33. ∞

Alteration in Thermoregulation

Heat loss is a major problem in preterm newborns, but the nurse can do much to prevent it. Two limiting factors in heat production, however, are the availability of glycogen in the liver and the amount of brown fat available for heat production. Both glycogen and brown fat appear in the third trimester. In the cold-stressed newborn, norepinephrine is released, which in turn stimulates the metabolism of brown fat for heat production. As a complicating factor, the hypoxic newborn cannot increase oxygen consumption in response to cold stress because of the already limited reserves and thereby becomes progressively colder. Because the muscle mass is small in preterm infants and voluntary muscular activity is diminished (they are unable to shiver), heat production is further limited.

Five physiologic and anatomic factors increase heat loss in the preterm infant:

1. The preterm baby has a high ratio of body surface to body weight. This means that the baby's ability to produce heat (based on body weight) is much less than the potential for losing heat (based on surface area). The loss of heat in a preterm infant weighing 1500 g is five times greater per unit of body weight than in an adult.

2. The preterm baby has very little subcutaneous fat, which is the human body's insulation. Without adequate insulation, heat is easily conducted from the core of the body (warmer temperature) to the surface of the body (cooler temperature). Heat is lost from the body as the blood vessels, which lie close to the skin surface in the preterm infant, transport blood from the body core to the subcutaneous tissues.

3. The preterm baby has thinner, more permeable skin than the term infant. This increased permeability contributes to a greater insensible water loss as well as heat loss.

4. The posture of the preterm baby influences heat loss. Flexion of the extremities decreases the amount of surface area exposed to the environment. Extension increases the surface area exposed to the environment and thus increases heat loss. The gestational age of the infant influences the amount of flexion, from completely hypotonic and extended at 28 weeks to strong flexion displayed by 36 weeks.

5. The preterm baby has a decreased ability to vasoconstrict superficial blood vessels and conserve heat in the body core.

In summary, gestational age is directly proportional to the ability to maintain thermoregulation; thus the more preterm the newborn, the less the infant is able to maintain heat balance. Preventing heat loss by providing a neutral thermal environment using a servocontrol skin probe is one of the most important considerations in nursing management of the preterm infant. Cold stress, with its accompanying severe complications, can be prevented (see Chapter 33 ∞).

Alteration in Gastrointestinal Physiology

The basic structure of the gastrointestinal (GI) tract is formed early in gestation. Maturation of the digestive and absorptive processes is more variable, however, and occurs later in gestation. As a result of GI immaturity, the preterm newborn has the following ingestion, digestion, and absorption problems:

- A marked danger of aspiration and its associated complications due to the infant's poorly developed gag reflex, incompetent esophageal cardiac sphincter, and poor sucking and swallowing reflexes.

- Difficulty in meeting high caloric and fluid needs for growth due to small stomach capacity.

- Limited ability to convert certain essential amino acids to nonessential amino acids. Certain amino acids, such as histidine, taurine, and cysteine, are essential to the preterm infant but not to the term infant.

- Inability to handle the increased osmolarity of formula protein due to kidney immaturity. The preterm infant requires a higher concentration of whey protein than casein.

- Difficulty absorbing saturated fats due to decreased bile salts and pancreatic lipase. Severe illness of the newborn may also prevent intake of adequate nutrients.

- Difficulty with lactose digestion initially because processes may not be fully functional during the first few days of a preterm infant's life. The preterm newborn can digest and absorb most simple sugars.

- Deficiency of calcium and phosphorus may exist because two thirds of these minerals are deposited in the last trimester. Rickets and significant bone demineralization due to deficiency of calcium and phosphorus, which are deposited primarily in the last trimester, are also problems.

- Increased basal metabolic rate and increased oxygen requirements due to fatigue associated with sucking.

- Feeding intolerance and necrotizing enterocolitis (NEC) due to diminished blood flow and tissue perfusion to the intestinal tract due to prolonged hypoxia and hypoxemia at birth.

Alteration in Renal Physiology

The kidneys of the preterm infant are immature in comparison with those of the full-term infant, which poses clinical problems in the management of fluid and electrolyte balance. Specific characteristics of the preterm infant include the following:

- The glomerular filtration rate (GFR) is lower because of decreased renal blood flow. The GFR is directly related to lower gestational age, so the more preterm the newborn, the lower the GFR. The GFR is also decreased in the presence of diseases or conditions that decrease renal blood flow and perfusion, such as severe respiratory distress, hypotension, and asphyxia. Anuria or oliguria may also be observed.

- The preterm infant's kidneys are limited in their ability to concentrate urine or to excrete excess amounts of fluid. This means that if excess fluid is administered, the infant is at risk for fluid retention and overhydration. If too little is administered, the infant will become dehydrated because of the inability to retain adequate fluid.

- The kidneys of the preterm infant begin excreting glucose at a lower serum glucose level than those of the term infant. Therefore, glycosuria with hyperglycemia can lead to osmotic diuresis and polyuria.

- The kidney's buffering capacity is reduced, predisposing the infant to metabolic acidosis. Bicarbonate is excreted at a lower serum level, and acid is excreted more slowly. Therefore, after periods of hypoxia or insult, the preterm infant's kidneys require a longer time to excrete the lactic acid that accumulates. Sodium bicarbonate is frequently required to treat the metabolic acidosis.

- The immaturity of the renal system affects the preterm infant's ability to excrete drugs. Because excretion time is longer, many drugs are given over longer intervals (for example, every 24 hours instead of every 12 hours). Urine output must be carefully monitored when the infant is receiving nephrotoxic drugs, such as gentamicin and vancomycin. In the event of oliguria, drugs can become toxic in the infant much more quickly than in the adult.

Alteration in Hepatic and Hematologic Physiology

Immaturity of the preterm newborn's liver predisposes the infant to several problems. After birth, the glycogen stores in the liver are rapidly used for energy. Glycogen deposits are affected by asphyxia in utero and after birth by both asphyxia and cold stress. The baby born preterm has decreased glycogen stores at birth and frequently experiences stress, which rapidly uses up these limited stores. Therefore, the preterm newborn is at high risk for hypoglycemia and its complications.

Iron is also stored in the liver, especially during the last trimester of pregnancy. Therefore, the preterm newborn is born with low iron stores. If subject to hemorrhage, rapid growth, and excess blood sampling, the preterm infant is likely to become iron depleted more quickly than the term infant. Many preterm babies require transfusions of packed cells to treat symptomatic anemia as a consequence of frequent blood sampling. As the premature infant grows and convalesces, oral iron supplementation may be started, as well as doses of erythropoietin, to enhance RBC production.

Conjugation of bilirubin in the liver is impaired in the preterm infant. Thus bilirubin levels increase more rapidly and to a higher level than in the full-term infant. Early clinical assessment of jaundice associated with indirect hyperbilirubinemia is more difficult in preterm newborns because they lack subcutaneous fat.

The normal cord hemoglobin in an infant of 34 weeks' gestation is approximately 16.8 g/dL, and total blood volume ranges from 80 mL/kg to 100 mL/kg (Blackburn, 2003). Because of the small total blood volume, any blood loss is highly significant to the preterm infant. Therefore, periodic assessments of hemoglobin values are performed during the first weeks of life.

Alteration in Immunologic Physiology

The preterm infant is at a much greater risk for infection than the term infant. This increased susceptibility may be the result of an infection acquired in utero that may have precipitated preterm labor and birth. However, all preterm infants have immature specific and nonspecific immunity.

In utero the fetus receives passive immunity against a variety of infections from maternal IgG immunoglobulins, which cross the placenta (see Chapter 28 ∞). Because most of this immunity is acquired in the last trimester of pregnancy, the preterm infant has few antibodies at birth. These provide less protection and become depleted earlier than in a full-term infant. This may be a contributing factor in the higher incidence of recurrent bacterial infection during the first year of life as well as in the immediate neonatal period.

The other immunoglobulin significant for the preterm infant is secretory IgA, which does not cross the placenta but is found in breast milk in significant concentrations. Breast milk's secretory IgA provides immunity to the mucosal surfaces of the GI tract, protecting the newborn from enteric infections such as those caused by *Escherichia coli* and *Shigella*.

Another altered defense against infection in the preterm infant is the skin surface. In very small infants the skin is easily excoriated, and this factor, coupled with many invasive procedures, places the infant at great risk for nosocomial infections. It is vital to use good handwashing techniques in the care of these infants to prevent unnecessary infection.

> **CLINICAL TIP**
> The sudden onset of apnea and bradycardia, coupled with metabolic acidosis in an otherwise healthy, growing premature infant, may by suggestive of bacterial sepsis, especially if there is a central line present.

Alteration in Neurologic Physiology

The general shape of the brain is formed during the first 6 weeks of gestation. Between the second and fourth months of gestation the brain's total complement of neurons proliferate; these neurons migrate to specific sites throughout the central nervous system (CNS), and nerve impulse pathways organize. The final step in neurologic development is the covering of these nerves with myelin, which begins in the second trimester of gestation and continues into adult life (Volpe, 2001).

Because the period of most rapid brain growth and development occurs during the third trimester of pregnancy, the closer to term an infant is born, the better the neurologic prognosis. A common interruption of neurologic development in the preterm infant is caused by intraventricular hemorrhage (IVH) and intracranial hemorrhage (ICH). Hydrocephalus may develop as a consequence of an IVH due to the obstruction at the cerebral aqueduct.

Alteration in Reactivity Periods and Behavioral States

The newborn infant's response to extrauterine life is characterized by two periods of reactivity, as discussed in Chapter 31. ∞ The preterm infant's periods of reactivity are delayed. In the very ill infant, these periods of reactivity may not be observed at all because the infant may be hypotonic and unreactive for several days after birth.

As the preterm newborn grows and the condition stabilizes, identifying behavioral states and traits unique to each infant becomes increasingly possible. In general, stable preterm infants do not demonstrate the same behavioral states as term infants. Preterm infants are more disorganized in their sleep-wake cycles and are unable to attend as well to the human face and objects in the environment. Neurologically, their responses (sucking, muscle tone, states of arousal) are weaker than full-term infants' responses.

By observing each infant's patterns of behavior and responses, especially the sleep-wake states, the parent and nurse can plan nursing care around the times when the infant is alert and best able to attend. The more knowledge parents have about the meaning of their infant's responses and behaviors, the better prepared they will be to meet their newborn's needs and to form a positive attachment with their child. See discussion of developmental care for the preterm newborn later in this section.

> **CLINICAL TIP**
> After observing an infant's pattern of behavior and responses, especially the sleep-wake states, use the time when the infant is alert and best able to attend to help parents learn about and provide newborn care.

Management of Nutrition and Fluid Requirements

Early feedings are extremely valuable in maintaining normal metabolism and lowering the possibility of such complications as hypoglycemia, hyperbilirubinemia, hyperkalemia, and azotemia. However, the preterm newborn is at risk for complications that may develop because of the immaturity of the digestive system.

NUTRITIONAL REQUIREMENTS

Oral (enteral) caloric intake necessary for growth in an uncompromised healthy preterm infant is 95 to 130 kcal/kg/day (Blackburn, 2003). In addition to these relatively high caloric needs, the preterm infant requires more protein than full-term infants. To meet these needs, many institutions use fortified breast milk or special preterm formulas.

Whether breast milk or formula is used, feeding regimens are established based on the infant's weight and estimated stomach capacity (Table 32–1). Initial formula-feedings are gradually increased as the infant tolerates them. It may be necessary to supplement the oral feedings with parenteral fluids to maintain adequate hydration and caloric intake until the baby is on

Table 32–1   SUGGESTED FEEDING GUIDELINES FOR THE PRETERM INFANT

Weight (g)	Feeding Interval	Beginning Volume (mL/kg/d)	Feeding Increments (mL/kg/d)	Days to Full Feedings†
Less than 1000	Every 3 hours	10–20	10–20	16–13
1000–1500	Every 3 hours	10–20	15–20	10–7
1501–1800 sick‡	Every 3 hours	10–20	20–30	7–5
1501–1800 healthy‡	Every 3 hours	20–40	30–50	5–3
Greater than 1800 sick‡	Every 3 hours	20–40	30–75	5–2

†Full feedings are defined as 120 kcal/kg/day of a 24 kcal/oz formula or human milk.

‡Sick refers to infants who have had symptoms of any medical or surgical condition, other than uncomplicated prematurity.

Healthy refers to term or preterm infants who have had no symptomatic medical or surgical conditions.

Advancement of feedings should occur only as the infant demonstrates tolerance of enteral feedings. Clinical signs of feeding intolerance or illness dictate discontinuing or holding the advancement of feedings.

Infants are started on either full-strength human milk or 24 kcal/oz premature infant formula.

At 100–120 mL/kg, fortifier is added to human milk.

Iron supplements are added at 2–4 mg/kg/day for the human milk fed infant at full feeds.

SOURCE: Courtesy of Lisa Vanatta.

full oral feedings. Those preterm infants who cannot tolerate any oral (enteral) feedings are given nutrition by total parenteral nutrition (TPN).

In addition to a higher calorie and higher protein formula, preterm infants should receive supplemental multivitamins, which include vitamins A, D, and E, iron, and trace minerals. A diet high in polyunsaturated fats (which preterm infants tolerate best) increases the requirement for vitamin E. Preterm infants fed iron-fortified formulas have higher red cell hemolysis and lower vitamin E concentrations and thus require additional vitamin E. Preterm formulas also need to contain medium-chain triglycerides (MCT) and additional amino acids such as cysteine, as well as calcium, phosphorus, and vitamin D supplements to increase mineralization of bones. Rickets and significant bone demineralization have been documented in very-low-birth-weight infants and otherwise healthy preterm infants.

Nutritional intake is considered adequate when there is consistent weight gain of 20 to 30 g per day. Initially, no weight gain may be noted for several days, but total weight loss should not exceed 15% of the total birth weight or more than 1% to 2% per day. Some institutions add the criteria of head circumference growth and increase in body length of 1 cm per week once the newborn is stable.

METHODS OF FEEDING

The preterm infant is fed by various methods, depending on the infant's gestational age, health and physical condition, and neurologic status. The three most common oral feeding methods are bottle, breast, and gavage.

Bottle-Feeding

Preterm infants who have a coordinated as well as rhythmic suck-swallow-breathing pattern are usually between 35 and 36 weeks' postconceptual age and may be fed by bottle. Oral readiness to feed is best described by the following behaviors: remaining engaged in the feeding, to organize oral-motor func-

tioning, to coordinate the suck-swallow-breath skill, and to maintain physiological stable (Thoyre, Shaker, & Pridham, 2005). Those premature infants who root when their cheek is stroked and actively search for the nipple are neurodevelopmentally ready to initiate oral feeding. To avoid excessive expenditure of energy, a soft, yellow, single-hole nipple is usually used (milk flow is less rapid). The infant is fed in a semisitting position and burped gently after each half ounce or ounce. The feeding should take no longer than 15 to 20 minutes (nippling requires more energy than other methods). Preterm infants who are progressing from gavage feedings to bottle-feeding should be assessed for feeding readiness (see Table 32–2) and started with one session of bottle-feeding a day. The number of times a day a bottle is offered should be increased slowly until the baby tolerates all feedings from a bottle.

The nurse also assesses the infant's ability to suck. Sucking may be affected by postconceptional age, asphyxia, chronic lung disease, intraventricular hemorrhage, or other neurologic insult. Before initiating nipple feeding, the nurse observes the infant for any signs of stress, such as tachypnea (more than 60 respirations per minute), respiratory distress, or hypothermia, which may increase the risk of aspiration. During the feeding, the infant should be observed for signs of difficulty with feeding (tachypnea, a decrease in oxygen saturation levels, bradycardia, lethargy, and uncoordinated suck and swallow). Difficulty in bottle-feeding is often associated with a milk bolus that is too large for the infant's oral cavity that can lead to aspiration. Demand feeding protocols, based on the infant's hunger cues, should be considered for a growing premature infant only when there is sufficient caloric intake to promote consistent weight gain (Crosson & Pickler, 2004).

Breastfeeding

Mothers who wish to breastfeed their preterm infants should be given the opportunity to put the infant to breast as soon as the infant has demonstrated a coordinated suck and swallow reflex,

Table 32–2   EXAMPLES OF EARLY FEEDING SKILLS (EFS) ITEMS WITHIN EACH SECTION

Oral Feeding Readiness

Able to hold body in a flexed position with arms/hands toward midline	Yes	No
Demonstrates energy for feeding—maintains muscle tone and body flexion through assessment period	Yes	No

Oral Feeding Skill

Ability to Remain Engaged in Feeding				
Predominant muscle tone (energy infant demonstrates for feeding)	Maintains flexed body position with arms toward midline	Inconsistent tone, variable muscle tone	Some tone consistently felt, but somewhat hypotonic	Little or no tone felt; flaccid, limp most of the time
Ability to Organize Oral-Motor Functioning				
Opens mouth promptly when lips are stroked at feeding onsets	All	Most	Some	None
Once feeding is under way, maintains a smooth, rhythmic pattern of sucking				
Ability to Coordinate Swallowing and Breathing				
Able to engage in long sucking bursts (7–10 sucks) without behavioral stress signs or an adverse or negative cardiorespiratory response				
Ability to Maintain Physiologic Stability				
In the first 30 seconds after each feeding onset, oxygen saturation is stable, and behavioral stress cues absent				
Stops to breathe before behavioral stress cues appear				
Clear breath sounds—no grunting breath sounds (prolonging the exhale, partially closing glottis on exhale)				

Oral Feeding Recovery (During the First Five Minutes Postfeeding)

Predominant state	Quiet alert	Drowsy	Sleep	Fuss/Cry
Range of oxygen saturation (%):				

SOURCE: From Thoyre, S. M., Shaker, C. S., & Pridham, K. F. The early feeding skills assessment for preterm infants. *Neonatal Network*, vol. 25, no. 3, p. 9, May/June 2005. Reprinted with permission.

is showing consistent weight gain, and can control body temperature outside of the incubator, regardless of weight. Preterm infants tolerate breastfeeding with higher transcutaneous oxygen pressures and better maintenance of body temperature than during bottle-feeding. Besides breast milk's many benefits for the infant, it allows the mother to contribute actively to the infant's well-being (Figure 32–7 ◆). Mothers should be encouraged to breastfeed if they choose to do so. It is important for the nurse to be aware of the advantages of breastfeeding as well as the possible disadvantages if breast milk is the sole source of food for the preterm infant. See Chapter 31 ∞ for a detailed discussion of the advantages and disadvantages of breastfeeding. Even if the infant cannot be put to the breast, mothers can pump their breasts, and the breast milk can be given via gavage. A double-pumping system produces higher levels of prolactin than sequential pumping of the breasts (see Figure 31–15 ∞).

By initiating skin-to-skin holding of LBW infants in the early intensive care phase, mothers can significantly increase milk volume, thereby overcoming lactation problems (Turnage-Carrier, 2004). Preterm infants tolerate breastfeeding with higher transcutaneous oxygen pressure and better maintenance of body temperature than during bottle-feeding.

It has been suggested that the football hold is a convenient position for breastfeeding preterm babies. Feeding time may

Figure 32–7 ◆ Mother breastfeeding her premature infant.

take up to 45 minutes, and babies should be burped as they alternate breasts. Length of feeding time must be monitored so that the preterm infant does not expend too many calories.

The nurse should coordinate a flexible feeding schedule so babies can breastfeed during alert times and be allowed to set their own pace. Feedings should be on demand, but a maximum number of hours between feedings should be set. A similar regimen should be used for the baby who is progressing from gavage feeding to breastfeeding. The mother begins with one feeding at the breast and then gradually increases the number of times during the day that the baby breastfeeds. When breastfeeding is not possible because the infant is too small or too weak to suck at the breast, an option for the mother may be to express her breast milk into a cup. The milk touches the infant's lips and is lapped by the protruding motions of the tongue.

Gavage Feeding

The tube or gavage feeding method is used with preterm infants (less than 34 weeks' gestation) who lack or have a poorly coordinated suck-swallow-breathing pattern or are ill and ventilator dependent. Gavage feeding may be used as an adjunct to nipple feeding if the infant tires easily or as an alternative if an infant is losing weight because of the energy expenditure required for nippling, which increases the chance of aspiration. See Procedure 32–1: Performing Gavage Feeding. Gavage feedings are administered by either the nasogastric or orogastric route and by intermittent bolus or continuous drip method. Bolus feedings may be preferred because it is thought to be more like normal feedings than the continuous feeding method and enhances the release of certain GI hormones that are necessary for gut development (Smith, 2005). Currently, there are no conclusive studies supporting one method over the other. In common practice, bolus feedings are usually initiated, but if intolerance occurs, then the feedings are changed to continuous.

Early initiation of minimal enteral nutrition (MEN) via gavage is now advocated in the preterm newborn as a supplement to parenteral nutrition. MEN refers to small-volume feedings of formula or human milk (usually less than 24 mL/kg/day) which are designed to "prime" the intestinal tract, thereby stimulating many of its hormonal and enzymatic functions (Smith, 2005). Benefits of early feedings (as early as 24 to 72 hours of life) include the following: no increase in the incidence of NEC; fewer days on TPN, thereby decreasing the incidence of cholestatic jaundice; increased weight gain; increased muscle maturation of the gut as well as muscle growth; increase in gut peristalsis; increased gut hormone levels, which can lead to improved feeding tolerance; lower risk of osteopenia; and a possible decrease in the total number of hospital days in the neonatal intensive care unit (NICU) (Smith, 2005).

CLINICAL TIP

For an otherwise healthy, growing premature infant who is receiving total enteral intake and has started to experience apnea and bradycardia, one differential diagnosis to think about is reflux rather than sepsis, although sepsis may need to be ruled out.

Transpyloric Feeding

An alternative method of feeding in which the stomach is bypassed is known as transpyloric feeding. This particular feeding method is thought to minimize gastroesophageal reflux. However, transpyloric feedings are associated with adverse effects including the bypassing of gastric digestion, abdominal distension, and intestinal perforation (McGuire & McEwan, 2004). The Cochrane database has concluded that those preterm infants receiving transpyloric feedings had more adverse effects and did not support its use over gastric tube feedings. If deemed medically necessary, this feeding method should be used only in specially equipped and staffed high-risk nurseries.

Total Parenteral Nutrition (TPN)

TPN is used in situations when feeding is contraindicated through the GI tract. Contraindications include GI anomalies requiring surgical intervention, NEC, intolerance of feedings, sepsis, and birth depression. TPN may also be used in adjunct with enteral feedings during the early stages of feeding advancement.

The TPN method provides complete nutrition to the infant intravenously. TPN includes use of hyperalimentation and intralipids. Hyperalimentation provides vitamins, minerals, protein (in the form of amino acids), and glucose. Appropriate amino acid intake (1 to 3.5 g/kg/day) is necessary to avoid catabolism and maintain the newborn in a positive-nitrogen balance, and it can be initiated on the first day of life. A percutaneous central venous catheter (PCVC/PICC) is often used with the LBW infant to deliver higher concentrations of glucose (greater than D12.5) as well as to provide an energy substrate. Intralipids (1 to 3 g/kg/day) are also administered to provide essential fatty acids.

The nurse needs to monitor serum glucose levels and serum chemistries carefully during TPN. The IV rate is monitored hourly to maintain accurate intake. The rate should not be increased to "catch up" if administration lags behind. The IV site should be observed hourly for signs of infiltration—hyperalimentation is extremely caustic and causes severe tissue destruction if it infiltrates. Intake and output are carefully monitored (hyperglycemia causing an osmotic diuresis can lead to dehydration). If hyperglycemia occurs, continuous insulin infusions may be initiated to enhance glucose uptake and utilization. Prolonged administration of TPN combined with little to no enteral intake can result in cholestatic jaundice. Monitoring liver enzymes as well as fractionated bilirubin levels is essential in long-term TPN use. The nurse needs to be aware of the potential complications associated with intralipid infusions, including increased free bilirubin concentrations, impaired pulmonary functions, and interference with platelet function. Therefore, serum triglyceride levels need to be followed. Daily lipid infusion should be spread out over a 24-hour period.

FLUID REQUIREMENTS

The calculation of fluid requirements takes into account the infant's weight and postnatal age. Recommendations for fluid therapy in the preterm infant are approximately 80 to 100 mL/kg/day for day 1, 100 to 120 mL/kg/day for day 2, and 120 to

PROCEDURE 32–1 Performing Gavage Feeding

NURSING ACTION	RATIONALE

Preparation

- When choosing the catheter size, consider the size of the infant, the area of insertion (oral or nasal), and the desired rate of flow.
- Explain the procedure to the parents.
- Elevate the head of the bed and position the infant on the back or side to allow easy passage of the tube.
- Measure the distance from the tip of the ear to the nose to the xiphoid process, and mark the point with a small piece of paper tape (Figure 32–8 ◆) to ensure enough tubing to enter the stomach.

Figure 32–8 ◆ Measuring gavage tube length.

The size of the catheter will influence the rate of flow.

Equipment and Supplies

No. 5 or no. 8 Fr. feeding tube. See the Clinical Tip below for guidelines for choosing tube size.
3- to 5-mL syringe, for aspirating stomach contents
1/4-inch paper tape, to mark the tube for insertion depth and to secure the catheter during feeding
Stethoscope, for auscultating the rush of air into the stomach when testing the tube placement
Appropriate formula
Small cup of sterile water to act as lubricant

CLINICAL TIP

The very small infant (less than 1600 g) requires a 5 Fr. feeding tube; an infant greater than 1600 g may tolerate a larger tube. Long-term indwelling enteral feeding tubes may be used as an alternative to the standard "in and out" gavage tubes, and they come in sizes 5 Fr. and 8 Fr.

Orogastric insertion is preferable to nasogastric because most infants are obligatory nose breathers. If nasogastric is used, a 5 Fr. catheter should be used to minimize airway obstruction.

Procedure: Clean Gloves

Inserting and Checking Placement of Tube

1. If inserting the tube nasally, lubricate the tip in a cup of sterile water. Use water instead of an oil-based lubricant, in case the tube is inadvertently passed into a lung. Shake any excess drops to prevent aspiration.
2. If inserting the tube orally, the oral secretions are enough to lubricate the tube adequately.
3. Stabilize the infant's head with one hand and pass the tube via the mouth (or nose) into the stomach to the point previously marked. If the infant begins coughing or choking or becomes cyanotic or phonic, remove the tube immediately as the tube has probably entered the trachea.

(Continued on next page)

PROCEDURE 32–1 Performing Gavage Feeding   continued

NURSING ACTION	RATIONALE

4. If respiratory distress is not apparent, lightly tape the tube in position, draw up 0.5 to 1.0 mL of air in the syringe, and connect the syringe to the tubing. Place the stethoscope over the epigastrium and briskly inject the air (Figure 32–9 ◆). You will hear a sudden rush as the air enters the stomach.

5. Aspirate the stomach contents with the syringe, and note the amount, color, and consistency to evaluate the infant's feeding tolerance. Return the residual to the stomach unless you are requested to discard it. It is usually not discarded because of the potential for electrolyte imbalance.

Figure 32–9 ◆ Auscultation for placement of gavage tube.

Administering the Feeding

1. Hold the infant for feeding, or position the infant on the right side.

2. Separate the syringe from the tube, remove the plunger from the barrel, reconnect the barrel to the tube, and pour the formula into the syringe.

3. Elevate the syringe 6 to 8 inches over the infant's head, and allow the formula to flow by gravity at a slow, even rate. You may need to initiate the flow of formula by inserting the plunger of the syringe into the barrel just until you see formula enter the feeding tube. Do not use pressure.

4. Regulate the rate to prevent sudden stomach distention leading to vomiting and aspiration. Continue adding formula to the syringe until the infant has absorbed the desired volume.

This position decreases the risk of aspiration in case of emesis during feeding.

Clearing and Removing the Tube

1. Clear the tubing with 2 to 3 mL of air.

2. To remove the tube, loosen the tape, fold the tube over on itself, and quickly withdraw the tube in one smooth motion to minimize the potential for fluid aspiration as the tube passes the epiglottis. If the tube is to be left in, position it so that the infant is unable to remove it. Replace the tube per hospital policy.

This ensures that the infant has received all of the formula. If the tube is going to be left in place, clearing it will decrease the risk of occlusion and bacterial growth in the tube.

Maximize the Feeding Pleasure of the Infant

1. Whenever possible, hold the infant during gavage feeding. If it is too awkward to hold the infant during feeding, be sure to take time for holding after the feeding.

2. Offer a pacifier to the infant during the feeding.

Feeding time is important to the infant's tactile sensory input.

Sucking during feeding comforts and relaxes the infant, making the formula flow more easily. Infants can lose their sucking reflexes when fed by gavage for long periods.

150 mL/kg/day by day 3 of life. These amounts may be increased up to 200 mL/kg/day if the infant is extremely premature, receiving phototherapy, or under a radiant warmer because of increased insensible water losses. If the infant is not hydrated properly, excessive insensible water loss can lead to hypernatremia, hyperkalemia, hypovolemia, hypotension, and oliguria. Fluid losses can be minimized through the use of heat shields and added humidification in the incubator. Daily weights, and sometimes twice-a-day weights, are the best indicator of fluid status in the preterm infant. The expected weight loss during the first 3 to 5 days of life in a preterm infant is 15% to 20% of birth weight.

Common Complications of Preterm Newborns and Their Clinical Management

The goals of medical and nursing care are to meet the growth and development needs of the preterm newborn and to anticipate and manage the complications associated with prematurity. Complications associated with prematurity that require clinical intervention are RDS, patent ductus arteriosus (PDA), apnea, intraventricular hemorrhage, and sepsis. Long-term problems include retinopathy of prematurity, bronchopulmonary dysplasia (BPD) that can lead to chronic lung disease (CLD), pulmonary interstitial emphysema (PIE), and posthemorrhagic hydrocephalus.

An in-depth discussion of RDS, BPD/CLD, and sepsis, including pathophysiology, clinical management, and nursing care, is contained in Chapter 33. ∞ PDA, apnea, IVH, retinopathy of prematurity, and other complications are discussed as follows.

PATENT DUCTUS ARTERIOSUS (PDA)

By definition, the ductus arteriosus is the large vessel that is a conduit between the left pulmonary artery and the descending aorta. In the fetus, the ductus arteriosus shunts blood away from the fluid-filled lungs, which are nonfunctional during gestation, toward the placenta for gas exchange. The functional closure of the ductus arteriosus is related to birth weight; the incidence of a symptomatic PDA increases with a decrease in birth weight. For example, in infants 30 weeks and less, functional closure may take several days to weeks to occur.

The incidence of a PDA in an infant weighing less than 1000 g is approximately 80%. Initially, as the pulmonary vascular resistance (PVR) falls and the systemic vascular resistance (SVR) rises, a left-to-right shunt via the PDA results. Blood flows from the aorta into the pulmonary artery, thereby increasing pulmonary blood flow. This leads to left ventricular volume overload, pulmonary edema, and congestive failure. Oxygenation is compromised, and ventilator requirements will increase, leading to the possible difficulty in weaning from the ventilator and long-term pulmonary sequelae. Clinical findings include tachypnea, hyperactive precordium, bounding peripheral pulses, hypotension, widened pulse pressure, tachycardia, and hepatomegaly.

Early identification of symptomatic infants and prompt clinical intervention will minimize long-term complications. There are a multitude of medical management regimens of the PDA. Initial medical management consists of providing adequate respiratory support, restricting fluids, and using diuretics (to decrease pulmonary edema) and perhaps digoxin (to treat congestive heart failure) while waiting for spontaneous closure of the ductus to occur. The administration of prostaglandin synthetase inhibitors, such as indomethacin (Indocin), impairs synthesis of the E series prostaglandins responsible for dilatation of the ductus and can cause ductal closure. Courses of indomethacin therapy vary; the standard, short course consists of three doses of indomethacin, 0.2 mg/kg IV every 12 hours. As an alternative, a long course of indomethacin may be chosen in-

volving dosing over approximately 7 days. A decrease in renal side effects is thought to be the advantage of the longer dosing schedule. Indomethacin is effective, but it is not without side effects and must be used cautiously. Adverse side effects include transient renal dysfunction, oliguria, platelet dysfunction, and GI bleeding.

If medical management is unsuccessful or contraindicated, then the ductus may be surgically ligated. PDA will often prolong the course of illness in a preterm newborn and may lead to chronic pulmonary dysfunction.

> **CLINICAL TIP**
>
> A growing premature infant showing clinical signs of worsening respiratory status (i.e., increased oxygen needs, increased ventilatory settings), acidosis, and hypotension may be exhibiting signs and symptoms of a PDA.

APNEA

Apnea of prematurity refers to cessation of breathing for 20 seconds or longer or for less than 20 seconds when associated with cyanosis, pallor, and bradycardia. Apnea is the most common problem in the preterm infant presenting between day 2 and day 7 of life. The etiology of apnea is multifactorial but is thought to be primarily a result of neuronal immaturity, a factor that contributes to the preterm infant's irregular breathing patterns (central apnea). Obstructive apnea can occur in the premature infant when there is a cessation of airflow associated with blockage of the upper airway (small airway diameter, increased pharyngeal secretions, improper body alignment and positioning).

Differential diagnoses with regard to apnea include sepsis, electrolyte disturbances, hypoglycemia, lung disease (atelectasis, pneumonia), cardiovascular changes (PDA, hypotension), CNS disturbances (seizures, intraventricular hemorrhage, meningitis), medication use (narcotics, opioids), thermoregulation problems (hypo- and hyperthermia), and GI disturbances (NEC, distention, obstruction, gastroesophageal reflux). Gastroesophageal reflux is defined as a movement of gastric contents into the lower esophagus due to poor lower esophageal sphincter tone, activating the laryngeal chemoreflex causing apnea. Apnea of prematurity is then a diagnosis of exclusion.

Apneic onset is often insidious; cardiorespiratory monitoring allows for early recognition and intervention, thus decreasing the need for resuscitative efforts. Apnea may occur during feeding, suctioning, or stooling. However, there may be no observable activity related to apnea. All episodes of apnea are documented. The documentation includes activity at the time of apnea, length of episode (along with any bradycardia, color change, or desaturation on pulse-oximeter associated with the apneic episode), and treatment required to bring the baby out of the apneic spell. These data are useful in determining etiology and possible treatment.

The nurse makes careful observations, quickly assessing the need for intervention or ascertaining that the infant is having periodic breathing. The intervention required depends on the severity of the apneic episode and the baby's response. Gentle stimulation of the infant may be sufficient. Respiratory support is provided if needed, and pharmacologic intervention using caffeine citrate (a methylxanthine) is often used to treat apnea of prematurity. Conservative management of apnea associated with gastroesophageal reflux would include dietary modification by adding rice cereal to thicken feedings. Feedings may also be small and frequent to decrease gastric distention. Following feedings, the infant should be placed in a side-lying or prone position with the head of the bed elevated 30 degrees for 20 to 30 minutes to facilitate gastric emptying. Often, metoclopramide (Reglan) is begun to increase the resting tone of the esophageal sphincter, to facilitate gastric emptying, and to improve GI motility.

INTRAVENTRICULAR HEMORRHAGE

Intraventricular hemorrhage (IVH) is the most common type of intracranial hemorrhage in the small preterm infant, especially those weighing less than 1500 g or of less than 34 weeks' gestation.

The most common site of hemorrhage is the periventricular subependymal germinal matrix in the lateral ventricles of the brain, where there is a rich blood supply and the capillary walls are thin and fragile. The matrix provides little supportive tissue for the fragile blood vessels. Before 32 weeks' gestation, an infant is much more susceptible to hemorrhage of these tiny vessels because they are vulnerable to wide fluctuations in blood pressure and to hypoxic events (such as respiratory distress, birth trauma, birth depression) that damage and rupture vessel walls.

Prenatal interventions include preventing premature birth, administering antenatal steroids, and transporting the pregnant mother to a tertiary care center. Administration of phenobarbital and vitamin K to the mother is being studied for their preventive effect. Postnatal preventive interventions include careful resuscitation, correction or prevention of major hemodynamic disturbances, and correction of coagulation abnormalities. Potential postnatal preventive pharmacologic interventions include phenobarbital to control seizures, narcotics for sedation, and vitamin E for its antioxidant abilities (Volpe, 2001).

The outcome for the infant depends on the size of the intracerebral bleed and the gestational age of the infant. The most severe hemorrhages may cause motor deficits, posthemorrhagic hydrocephalus, hearing loss, and blindness. Less severe bleeds may have no observable effects. In caring for the infant with an IVH, the nurse provides continuing support for the parents, identifying their level of understanding and facilitating interdisciplinary communication with them.

CLINICAL TIP

An extreme premature, low-birth-weight infant who presents with a sudden drop in hemoglobin along with the onset of severe metabolic acidosis, a "waxy" color, and hypotension may have experienced an intracranial hemorrhage.

ANEMIA OF PREMATURITY

The preterm infant is at risk for anemia because of the rapid rate of growth required, shorter RBC life, excessive blood sampling,

decreased iron stores, and deficiency of vitamin E. The hemoglobin usually reaches its lowest level by 3 to 12 weeks and remains low for 3 to 6 months. Interventions include iron supplementation and administration of recombinant human erythropoietin (r-HuEPO). Iron supplementation ensures adequate stores for RBC production once erythropoiesis starts. The use of r-HuEPO is reported to increase neonatal erythropoiesis, thereby increasing the hematocrit and reticulocyte count. In addition, it has been shown to reduce the need for late blood transfusions (those beyond 2 to 3 weeks of age) in preterm infants (Blackburn, 2003).

LONG-TERM COMPLICATIONS

The care of the preterm infant and the family does not stop on discharge from the nursery. Follow-up care is extremely important because many developmental problems are not noted until the infant is older and begins to demonstrate motor delays or sensory disability.

Within the first year of life, LBW preterm infants face higher mortality than term infants. Causes of death include sudden infant death syndrome (SIDS)—which occurs about five times more frequently in the preterm infant—respiratory infections, and neurologic defects. Morbidity is also much higher among preterm infants, with those weighing less than 1500 g at highest risk for long-term complications.

The most common long-term problems observed in preterm infants include retinopathy of prematurity, speech defects, neurologic defects, and auditory defects.

Retinopathy of Prematurity

Premature newborns are particularly susceptible to injury of the delicate capillaries of the retina causing characteristic retinal changes known as retinopathy of prematurity (ROP). It is this injury to the developing vascular system of the retina that leads to ischemia resulting in hemorrhage, scarring, and, in extreme cases, retinal detachment and impaired vision. The disease is now viewed as multifactorial in origin with hyperoxemia (increased oxygen levels) as one factor. Other risk factors include IVH, CLD, apnea, hypoxia, sepsis, acidosis, multiple gestation, exposure to bright lights, and blood transfusions. Increased survival of very-low-birth-weight infants may be the most important factor in the increased incidence of ROP.

Treatment of the acute stages of ROP with laser photocoagulation and cryotherapy is an option. Because most acute cases of ROP regress spontaneously with no long-term visual impairment, the possibility of regression must be weighed against the risk of an unfavorable outcome from treatment. For infants with bilateral traction and retinal detachment, surgical vitrectomy and scleral buckling are performed. Nursing care for the visually impaired infant must concentrate on parental support and education. When the crisis of premature birth is quickly followed by the devastating news of suspected visual impairment (poor visual acuity, myopia, strabismus, amblyopia, and glaucoma) or blindness, the parents will need extensive support by all members of the interdisciplinary health team. The parents again experience overwhelming anxiety and uncertainty about their infant's future abilities. Premature infants with blindness due to ROP may be at increased risk of cognitive and emotional problems. The evidence suggests that this increased risk may be due to environmental factors rather than to inherent intellectual or neurologic factors.

Speech Defects

The most frequently observed speech defects involve delayed development of receptive and expressive ability that may persist into the school-age years.

Neurologic Defects

The most common neurologic defects include cerebral palsy, hydrocephalus, seizure disorders, lower IQ scores, and learning disabilities. However, the socioeconomic climate and family support systems have been shown to be important factors influencing the child's ultimate school performance in the absence of major neurologic defects. Families can be reminded that risk does not equal injury, injury does not equal damage, and description of damage does not allow a precise prediction about recovery or outcome.

Auditory Defects

Preterm infants have a 1% to 4% incidence of moderate to profound hearing loss and should have a formal audiologic examination before discharge and at 3 to 6 months (corrected age). One test currently used to measure hearing functions of the newborn is the evoked otoacoustic emissions (EOAE) test. Earphones are used on each ear and independently measure sounds produced in the inner ear in response to acoustic stimuli. Another test, the automated auditory brain response (AABR), measures electroencephalogram (EEG) waves in response to sound waves generated by the test. The AABR provides information about the auditory pathway to the brainstem. Any infant with repeated abnormal results should be referred to speech-and-language specialists. Infants at increased risk include those with congenital viral infections, hyperbilirubinemia, severe perinatal asphyxia, meningitis, and birth trauma. Damage from ototoxic drugs such as gentamicin and furosemide (Lasix) is variable and related to multiple factors, including renal function, age, duration of treatment, and concomitant administration of other ototoxic agents.

When evaluating an infant's abilities and disabilities, parents must understand that the developmental progress must be evaluated based on chronologic age from the expected date of birth, not from the actual date of birth (corrected age). In addition, the parents need the consistent support of healthcare professionals in the long-term management of their infant. Many new and ongoing concerns arise as the high-risk infant grows and develops; the goal is to promote the highest quality of life possible.

NURSING CARE MANAGEMENT
Nursing Assessment and Diagnosis

Accurate assessment of the physical characteristics and gestational age of the preterm newborn is imperative to anticipate the special needs and problems of this baby. Physical characteris-

tics vary greatly, depending on the gestational age, but the following characteristics are frequently present:

- *Color.* Usually pink or ruddy but may be acrocyanotic (Cyanosis, jaundice, or pallor are abnormal and should be noted.)
- *Skin.* Reddened, translucent, blood vessels readily apparent, lack of subcutaneous fat
- *Lanugo.* Plentiful, widely distributed
- *Head size.* Appears large in relation to body
- *Skull.* Bones pliable, fontanelle smooth and flat
- *Ears.* Minimal cartilage, pliable, folded over
- *Nails.* Soft, short
- *Genitals.* Male: nonrugated, small scrotum; testes may or may not be descended. Female: prominent clitoris and labia minora
- *Resting position.* Flaccid, froglike
- *Cry.* Weak, feeble
- *Reflexes.* Poor suck, swallow, and gag
- *Activity.* Jerky, generalized movements (Seizure activity is abnormal.)

Determining gestational age in preterm newborns requires knowledge and experience in administering gestational assessment tools. The tool used should be specific, reliable, and valid. For a discussion of gestational age assessment tools, see Chapter 29. ∞

Nursing diagnoses that may apply to the preterm newborn include:

- *Impaired Gas Exchange* related to immature pulmonary vasculature and inadequate surfactant production
- *Ineffective Breathing Pattern* related to immature central nervous system
- *Alteration in Cardiovascular Status* related to hypotension related to decreased tissue perfusion secondary to PDA
- *Ineffective Thermoregulation* related to hypothermia secondary to decreased glycogen and brown fat stores
- *Altered Nutrition: Less than Body Requirements* related to weak suck and swallow reflexes and decreased ability to absorb nutrients
- *Alteration in Tissue Perfusion* related to anemia of prematurity
- *Fluid Volume Deficit* related to high insensible water losses and inability of kidneys to concentrate urine
- *High Risk for Intraventricular Hemorrhage* related to fragile capillary network in the germinal matrix
- *Ineffective Family Coping* related to anger or guilt at having given birth to a premature baby

Nursing Plan and Implementation
MAINTENANCE OF RESPIRATORY FUNCTION

Preterm newborns have increased danger of respiratory obstruction. Their bronchi and trachea are so narrow that mucus can obstruct the airway. The nurse must maintain patency through judiciously suctioning, but only on an as-needed basis.

Positioning of the newborn can also affect respiratory function, especially in the preterm newborn. If the baby is in the supine position, the nurse should slightly elevate the infant's head to maintain the airway, being careful not to hyperextend the neck because the trachea will collapse. Also, because the newborn has weak neck muscles and cannot control head movement, the nurse should ensure that this head position is maintained by using a small roll under the shoulders. The prone position splints the chest wall and decreases the amount of respiratory effort used to move the chest wall. The prone position therefore facilitates chest expansion and improves air entry and oxygenation. Weak or absent cough or gag reflexes increase the chance of aspiration in the premature newborn. The nurse should ensure that the infant's position facilitates drainage of mucus or regurgitated formula.

The nurse monitors heart and respiratory rates with cardiorespiratory monitors as well as through physical assessments to identify alterations in the newborn's cardiopulmonary status. Signs of respiratory distress include the following:

- Cyanosis (serious sign when generalized)
- Tachypnea (sustained respiratory rate greater than 60/minute after first 4 hours of life)
- Retractions
- Expiratory grunting
- Nasal flaring
- Apneic episodes
- Presence of crackles or rhonchi on auscultation
- Diminished air entry

If respiratory distress occurs, the nurse administers oxygen per physician or nurse practitioner order to relieve hypoxemia. If hypoxemia is not treated immediately, it may result in PDA or metabolic acidosis. If oxygen is administered to the newborn, the nurse monitors the oxygen concentration with devices such as the transcutaneous oxygen monitor ($tcPo_2$) or the pulse oximeter. Periodic arterial blood gas sampling to monitor oxygen concentration in the baby's blood is essential because hyperoxemia may lead to ROP.

The nurse also needs to consider respiratory function before initiation of feedings as well as during feeding. To prevent aspiration, increased energy expenditure, and increased oxygen consumption, the nurse needs to ensure that the infant's gag and suck reflexes are intact before starting oral feedings.

MAINTENANCE OF NEUTRAL THERMAL ENVIRONMENT

Providing a neutral thermal environment minimizes the oxygen consumption required to maintain a normal core temperature; it also prevents cold stress and facilitates growth by minimizing caloric expenditure to maintain body temperature. The preterm infant's immature CNS, as well as small brown fat stores, provides poor temperature control. A small infant (less than 1200 g) can lose 80 kcal/kg/day through radiation of body heat.

The nurse should implement all the usual thermoregulation measures discussed in Chapter 30. ∞

In addition, to minimize heat loss and the effects of temperature instability for preterm and LBW newborns, the nurse should do the following:

1. Allow skin-to-skin contact between mother and newborn to maintain warmth and foster security (see "Kangaroo care" discussion later in this chapter).
2. Warm and humidify oxygen to minimize evaporative heat loss and decrease oxygen consumption.
3. Place the baby in a double-walled incubator, or use a Plexiglas heat shield over small preterm infants in single-walled incubators to avoid radiative heat losses. Some institutions use radiant warmers over the baby and pipe in humidity (swamping). Do not use Plexiglas shields on radiant warmer beds because it blocks the infrared heat.
4. Avoid placing the baby on cold surfaces, such as metal treatment tables and cold x-ray plates (conductive heat loss). Pad cold surfaces with diapers and use radiant warmers during procedures; place the preterm infant on prewarmed mattresses; and warm hands as well as the stethoscope before examining the baby to prevent heat transfer via conduction.
5. Use warmed ambient humidity. The use of humidity and its role in decreasing insensible water loss remains controversial (Blackburn, 2003).
6. Keep the skin dry (evaporative heat loss), and place a cap on the baby's head. The head makes up 25% of the total body size.
7. Keep radiant warmers, incubators, and cribs away from windows and cold external walls (radiative heat loss) and out of drafts (conductive heat loss).
8. Open incubator portholes and doors only when necessary, and use plastic sleeves on portholes to decrease convective heat loss.
9. Use a skin probe to monitor the baby's skin temperature. Correlate ambient temperatures with the skin probe in the incubator using the servocontrol rather than the manual mode. The temperature should be 36C to 37C (96.8F to 98.6F). Temperature fluctuations indicate hypothermia or hyperthermia. Be careful not to place skin temperature probes over bony prominences; areas of brown fat; poorly vasoreactive areas, such as extremities; or excoriated areas.
10. Warm formula or stored breast milk before feeding.
11. Use reflector patch over the skin temperature probe when using a radiant warmer bed so that the probe does not sense the higher infrared temperature as the baby's skin temperature and therefore decrease the heater output.

Once preterm infants are medically stable, they should be clothed with a double-thickness cap, cotton shirt, and diaper. If possible, they should be swaddled in a blanket. The nurse begins the process of weaning to a crib when the premature infant is medically stable, does not require assisted ventilation, weighs approximately 1500 g, has 5 days of consistent weight gain, and is taking oral feedings, and when apnea and bradycardia episodes have stabilized. The nurse should be familiar with the individual institution's protocol for weaning to crib for preterm infants.

MAINTENANCE OF FLUID AND ELECTROLYTE STATUS

Hydration is maintained by providing adequate intake based on the newborn's weight, gestational age, chronologic age, and volume of sensible and insensible water losses. Adequate fluid intake should provide sufficient water to compensate for increased insensible losses and to provide the amount needed for renal excretion of metabolic products. Insensible water losses can be minimized by providing a high-ambient humidity, humidifying oxygen, using heat shields, and placing the infant in a double-walled incubator.

The nurse evaluates the baby's hydration status by assessing and recording signs of dehydration. Signs of dehydration include the following:

- Sunken fontanelles
- Loss of weight
- Poor skin turgor (skin returns to position slowly when squeezed gently)
- Dry oral mucous membranes
- Decreased urine output
- Increased urine specific gravity (greater than 1.013)

The nurse must also identify signs of overhydration by observing the newborn for edema or excessive weight gain and by comparing urine output with fluid intake.

The preterm infant should be weighed at least once daily at the same time each day. *Weight change is the most sensitive indicator of fluid balance.* Weighing diapers is also important for accurate input and output measurement (1 mL equals 1 g). A comparison of intake and output measurements over an 8-hour or 24-hour period provides important information about renal function and fluid balance. Assessment of patterns—in particular, whether they show a net gain or loss over several days—is also essential to fluid management. Monitor blood serum levels and pH to evaluate for electrolyte imbalances.

Accurate hourly intake calculations should be maintained when administering IV fluids. Because the preterm infant is unable to excrete excess fluid, it is important that the nurse maintain the correct amount of IV fluid to prevent fluid overload. This can be accomplished by using neonatal or pediatric infusion pumps. To prevent electrolyte imbalance, overhydration, and dehydration, the nurse must take care to give the correct IV solutions and volumes and concentrations of formulas. Urine specific gravity and pH are obtained periodically. Urine osmolality provides an indication of hydration, although this factor must be correlated with other assessments (e.g., serum sodium). Hydration is considered adequate when the urine output is 1 to 3 mL/kg/hr.

PROVISION OF ADEQUATE NUTRITION AND PREVENTION OF FATIGUE DURING FEEDING

The feeding method depends on the preterm newborn's feeding abilities and health status. Both nipple and gavage methods are initially supplemented with IV therapy until oral intake is sufficient to support growth (110 to 130 kcal/kg/day). Early, small-volume enteral feedings called *minimal enteral nutrition via gavage* have proved to be of benefit to the very-low-birth-weight infant. (See "Methods of Feeding," earlier in this chapter.) GI priming with these small-volume feedings is not intended to contribute to the total nutritional intake but rather to enhance gut metabolism. Trophic feedings may also help encourage earlier advancement to full feedings, thereby decreasing the development of NEC and the complications of parenteral nutrition. Formula or breast milk (with or without fortifiers to increase caloric content) is incorporated into the feedings slowly. This is done to avoid overtaxing the digestive capacity of the preterm newborn. The nurse should carefully watch for any signs of feeding intolerance, including:

- Increasing gastric residuals
- Abdominal distention (measured routinely before feedings) with visible bowel loops
- Guaiac-positive stools (occult blood in stools)
- Lactose in stools (reducing substance in the stools)
- Vomiting
- Diarrhea
- Water-loss stools

Before each feeding, the nurse measures abdominal girth and auscultates the abdomen to determine the presence and quality of bowel sounds. Such assessments permit early detection of abdominal distention and decreased peristaltic activity, which may indicate NEC or paralytic ileus. The nurse also checks for residual formula in the stomach before each feeding. This is done when the newborn is fed by gavage method. This procedure also can be performed when the nipple-fed newborn presents with abdominal distention. The presence of residual formula may indicate intolerance to the type or amount of feeding. Carefully watch for other signs of feeding intolerance including guaiac-positive stools (occult blood in stools), lactose in stools (reducing substance in the stools), vomiting, and diarrhea. Preterm newborns who are ill or fatigue easily with nipple feedings are usually fed by gavage. The infant is essentially passive with these methods, thus conserving energy and calories. As the baby matures, gavage feedings are replaced with nipple (breast or formula) feedings to assist in strengthening the sucking reflex and meeting oral and emotional needs. Signs that indicate readiness are a strong gag reflex, presence of nonnutritive sucking, and rooting behavior. Both LBW and preterm infants nipple-feed more effectively in a quiet state. The nurse establishes a gradual nipple-feeding program, such as one nipple feeding per day, then one nipple feeding per shift, and then a nipple feeding every other feeding. Daily weights are monitored because often there is a small weight loss when nipple feedings are started. After feedings, the baby is placed on the left side (with support to maintain this position) or on the abdomen to enhance gastric emptying and decrease the chance of aspiration if regurgitation occurs. Gastroesophageal reflux is not uncommon in preterm newborns. Long-term gavage feeding may create nipple aversion that will require developmental occupational therapy interventions.

The nurse involves the parents in feeding their preterm baby (Figure 32–10 ◆). This is essential to the development of attachment between parents and infant. In addition, such involvement increases parental knowledge about the care of their infant and helps them cope with the situation.

> **CLINICAL TIP**
>
> Residual feeding may indicate early NEC and should be called to the attention of the clinician.

PREVENTION OF INFECTION

The nurse is responsible for minimizing the preterm newborn's exposure to pathogenic organisms. The preterm newborn is susceptible to infection because of an immature immune system and thin, permeable skin. Invasive procedures, techniques such as umbilical catheterization, peripheral venipunctures, and mechanical ventilation, and prolonged hospitalization place the infant at greater risk for infection.

Strict handwashing and the use of separate equipment for each infant help minimize exposure of the preterm newborn to infectious agents. Most nurseries have adopted the standard

Figure 32–10 ◆ Father participates in feeding experience with his premature infant.

precautions recommended by the Centers for Disease Control and Prevention (CDC) of isolating every baby and the Joint Commission on Accreditation of Healthcare Organizations (JCAHO) requirement that staff members have short-trimmed nails and no artificial nails. Staff members are required to scrub

---

RESEARCH IN PRACTICE

EFFECT OF BATHING ON SKIN FLORA OF PRETERM NEWBORNS

What is this study about? Routine bathing may harm the fragile skin of the preterm infant. There is some evidence that routine bathing may actually result in increased colonization of bacteria. Soaps in general are irritating, and they may be harmful for newborn skin in that they disturb the protective lipid layer. Bathing the infant's skin with soap changes its pH so that bacterial colonization and drying of the skin are more likely to happen. This study sought to determine if bathing with water alone was as effective in reducing skin bacteria as soap and water. This study compares the type of microorganisms and quantity of colonies present on the skin of preterm newborns both before and after bathing and between soap and no-soap groups.

How was this study done? Preterm newborns with gestational age between 28 and 35 weeks were eligible for this randomized controlled trial. The babies were from a single tertiary medical center. Babies were excluded if they had skin breakdown or other serious health problems. Seventy-three preterm newborns met the criteria and were randomly assigned to a group that was given daily baths either with water only, or with soap and water for 7 or more days. The groups were similar in age, birth weight, and gestational

age. Skin cultures in both groups were obtained at an average of 19 days of age. On the final day of bathing, bacterial cultures were obtained from the axillary area both before and after bathing. The persons obtaining and reading the cultures were blinded as to group assignment.

What were the results of the study? Coagulase-negative *Staphylococcus* was the most prevalent microorganism in both groups, although there was little systemic disease. No difference was found in the count of microorganism colonies between the groups. Both groups had significantly fewer bacteria on the skin after bathing than before, whether soap was used or not.

What additional questions might I have? Do these findings apply to babies who are healthy and born at term? If soap is only as effective as water—and perhaps harmful to the preterm's skin—are there any situations in which soap baths are recommended?

How can I use this study? The skin of the preterm infant is fragile and prone to breakdown. The bath is an opportunity to maintain the integrity of the skin by bathing with water only. The nurse should incorporate these recommendations into teaching plans for the parents of preterm infants.

Chollopetz da Cunha, M., & Procianoy, R. (2005). Effect of bathing on skin flora of preterm newborns. *Journal of Perinatology, 25,* 375–379.

2 to 3 minutes using antibacterial solutions, which inhibit the growth of gram-positive cocci and gram-negative rod organisms. Other nursing interventions include limiting visitors; requiring visitors to wash their hands; and maintaining strict aseptic practices when changing IV tubing and solutions (IV solutions should be changed every 24 hours or per agency protocols), administering parenteral fluids, and assisting with sterile procedures. Incubators and radiant warmers should be changed weekly. Pressure-area breakdown is prevented by changing the baby's position, doing range-of-motion exercises, and using water-bed pillows or an air mattress. To avoid skin tears, a protective transparent covering can be applied over vulnerable joints, but use it very sparingly (Association of Women's Health, Obstetric, and Neonatal Nurses [AWHONN], 2001). Chemical skin preps and tape may cause skin trauma and should be avoided as much as possible.

If infection (sepsis) occurs in the preterm newborn, the nurse may be the first to identify the associated subtle clinical signs, such as lethargy and increased episodes of apnea and bradycardia. The nurse informs the clinician of the findings immediately and implements the treatment plan per clinician orders in the presence of infection. For specific nursing care required for the newborn with an infection, see Chapter 33. ∞

PROMOTION OF PARENT-INFANT ATTACHMENT

Preterm newborns can be separated from their parents for prolonged periods after illness or complications that are detected in the first few hours or days following birth. The resultant interruption in parent-newborn bonding necessitates intervention to ensure successful attachment.

Nurses should take measures to promote positive parental feelings toward the newborn. Photographs of the baby are given to parents to have at home or to the mother if she is in a different hospital or too ill to come to the nursery and visit. The infant's first name is placed on the incubator as soon as it is known to help the parents feel that their infant is a unique and special person. A weekly card with the baby's footprint, weight, and length is also sent to promote attachment. The nurse provides the parents with the telephone number of the nursery or intensive care unit and names of staff members so that they have access to information about their baby at any time of the day or night. The nurse encourages visits from siblings and grandparents to foster attachment.

Early involvement in the care and decisions regarding their baby provides parents with realistic expectations for their baby. The unique personality characteristics of the infant and the parents influence bonding and contribute to the interactive process for the family. By observing each infant's patterns of behavior and responses, especially sleep-wake states, the nurse can teach parents optimal times for interacting with their infant. Parents need education to develop caregiving skills and to understand the premature infant's behavioral characteristics. Their daily participation (if possible) is encouraged, as are early and frequent visits. The nurse provides opportunities for the parents to touch, hold, talk to, and care for their baby. Skin-to-skin holding *(kangaroo care)* helps parents feel close to their small in-

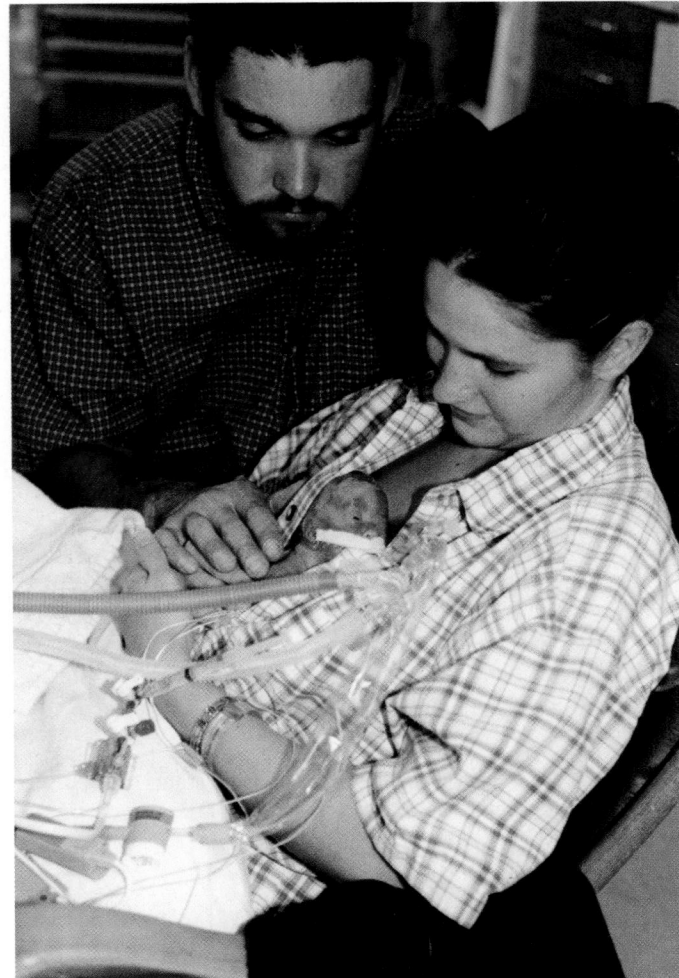

Figure 32–11 ◆ Kangaroo (skin-to-skin) care facilitates a closeness and attachment between parents and their premature infant.
SOURCE: Courtesy of Carol Harrigan, RNC, MSN, NNP.

fants. Kangaroo care has been shown to improve sleep periods and parents' perception of their caregiving ability (Turnage-Carrier, 2004) (Figure 32–11 ◆).

The parents and nurse can plan nursing care around the times when the infant is alert and best able to attend. The more knowledge parents have about the meaning of their infant's responses, behaviors, and cues for interaction, the better prepared they will be to meet their newborn's needs and form a positive attachment with their child. Parental involvement in difficult care decisions is essential and discussed in greater detail in Chapter 33. ∞

Some parents may progress easily to touching and cuddling their infant; others will not (Figure 32–12 ◆). Parents need to know that their apprehension is normal and the progression of acquaintanceship is slow. Rooming-in or "nesting" can provide another opportunity for the stable preterm infant and family to get acquainted. This becomes most beneficial for both the infant and family before discharge, as it offers a quiet, private environment where help is readily available.

Figure 32–12 ◆ Family bonding occurs when parents have opportunities to spend time with their infant.
SOURCE: Courtesy of Carol Harrigan, RNC, MSN, NNP.

Figure 32–13 ◆ An 8-day-old, 30 weeks' gestational age, 860-gram IUGR infant is "nested." Hand-to-face behavior facilitates self-consoling and soothing activities.
SOURCE: Courtesy of Carol Harrigan, RNC, MSN, NNP.

PROMOTION OF DEVELOPMENTALLY SUPPORTIVE CARE

Prolonged separation and the NICU environment necessitate individualized baby sensory stimulation programs. The nurse plays a key role in determining the appropriate type and amount of visual, tactile, and auditory stimulation.

Some preterm infants are not developmentally able to deal with more than one sensory input at a time. The assessment of preterm infant behavior (APIB) scale identifies the individual preterm newborn behaviors according to five areas of development (Als, Lester, Tronick et al., 1982). The preterm infant's physiologic and behavioral subsystems are autonomic, motor control, state differentiation, attention maintenance and social interaction, and, finally, overall system regulation or self-regulation. Integration of these subsystems improves with increasing gestational and postconceptual age. If the premature infant's self-regulatory capacity is exceeded and the infant is not able to return to previously integrated subsystem functioning, maladaptive behaviors may result when the infant is confronted with environmental demands. The nurse observes the baby's behavioral reactions to stimulation and then bases developmental interventions on reducing detrimental environmental stimuli to the lowest possible level and providing appropriate opportunities for development (Blackburn, 2003). Providing developmentally supportive, as well as family-centered, care has been proven to improve the outcomes of the critically ill neonate (Bowie, Hall, Faulkner et al., 2003). With

this in mind, specially designed NICUs with the single-room care concept are being developed to minimize lighting and noise exposure as well as to provide privacy for the parents of the convalescing neonate.

The NICU environment contains many detrimental stimuli that the nurse can help reduce. Noise levels can be lowered by replacing alarms with lights or silencing alarms quickly and keeping conversations away from the baby's bedside. Dimmer switches should be used to shield the baby's eyes from bright lights with blankets over the top portion of the incubator. Dimming the lights may encourage infants to open their eyes and be more responsive to their parents. Nursing care should be planned to decrease the number of times the baby is disturbed. Signs (e.g., "Quiet Please") can be placed near the bedside to allow the baby some periods of uninterrupted sleep (Blackburn, 2003). Some other suggested developmentally supportive interventions include:

- Facilitate handling by using containment measures when turning or moving the infant or doing procedures such as suctioning. Use the hands to hold the infant's arms and legs, flexed, close to the midline of the body. This helps stabilize the infant's motor and physiologic subsystems during stressful activities.

- Touch the infant gently, and avoid sudden postural changes.

- Promote self-consoling or soothing activities, such as placing blanket rolls or approved manufactured devices next to the infant's sides and against the feet, to provide "nesting." Swaddle the infant to maintain extremities in a flexed position while ensuring that the hands can reach the face. This permits the infant to do hand-to-mouth activities, which can be consoling (Figure 32–13 ◆).

- Stimulate the kinesthetic advantages of the intrauterine environment by using sheepskin and approved water beds.

COMPLEMENTARY AND ALTERNATIVE THERAPIES

COMPLEMENTARY AND ALTERNATIVE MEDICINE (CAM) IN THE NICU

As NICUs are becoming more and more "developmentally" friendly, complementary and alternative medicine (CAM) has now become an adjunct to that nurturing environment. This holistic approach in caring for the LBW infant attempts not only to mimic the intrauterine environment, but also to foster parent-infant bonding by simultaneously caring for the body, spirit, and mind.

Aromatherapy is the use of scent to alter mood or behavior to produce a calming and sedating effect. There is an enhanced bonding process between mothers and newborns associated with the natural body odor emitted from the mother (Jones, Kassity, & Duncan, 2001). Aromatherapy is utilized in the NICU by placing an article of clothing belonging to the mother next to the infant to produce a soothing and consoling effect on the infant in her absence. Researchers are also investigating other aromatherapies, including peppermint as a respiratory stimulant, chamomile as a method to regulate sleep-wake cycles, Brazilian guava for its analgesic effects, and lavendar sitz baths for management of diaper rash.

Skin-to-skin (kangaroo) care is becoming more prevalent in NICUs across the United States. It was first practiced in Bogota, Colombia, in the early 1980s because of the fear of the spread of infection from sharing incubators (Eichel, 2001). Skin-to-skin care is defined as the practice of holding infants skin to skin next to their parents. The infant is usually naked, except for a diaper, and placed on his or her parent's bare chest. They are then both covered with a blanket. Benefits of skin-to-skin care as a developmental intervention include the following: improved oxygenation as evidenced by an increase in transcutaneous oxygen levels, enhanced temperature regulation, a decline in the episodes of apnea and bradycardia, increased periods of quiet sleep, stabilization of vital signs, positive interaction between parent and infant which enhances attachment and bonding, increased growth parameters, and early discharge (Kledzik, 2005). Limitations to skin-to-skin care may be due to staff uneasiness when moving the infant while attached to multiple IV lines, monitor leads, and a ventilator, including high-frequency oscillatory ventilation. The restricted confines of the nursery may be another limiting factor as well as the lack of protocols or guidelines to safely maneuver, position, and hold the infant. *Music therapy* as a noninvasive auditory stimulus has been shown to be advantageous for the premature infant (Standley, 2001). The music used in NICUs includes primarily lullabies and soft acoustical pieces which are pleasant, soothing, and calming. Such music has been shown to effect newborn physiologic responses, improving oxygenation and increasing weight gain. It also has behavioral effects, leading to enhanced parental bonding and increased intervals of nonnutritive sucking periods. Language development is also enhanced if the music is live and sung by the mother or another female, which is preferential to the infant (Standley, 2001). The overall noise level in the NICU needs to be considered before including any extra auditory stimulation, including music therapy.

Infant massage and gentle touch have been practiced for many centuries. The types of stimulation include massage with stroking, gentle touch without stroking, and therapeutic touch or "hands on" containment. When infant massage therapy is applied to preterm infants, physiologic benefits such as stimulating blood and lymphatic flow, promoting weight gain, improving developmental scores, and regulating sleep patterns may be seen (Beachy, 2003). Many emotional and behavioral benefits are also cited by practitioners. Classes are available to teach parents how to perform massage on their infants. Massage demonstrates compassion while increasing the parent's empathy and understanding of the baby. It helps parents learn to interpret their baby's behavioral cues such as facial expression, various crying patterns, and other body language. At the same time it helps infants learn about their various body parts and boundaries and feel how they integrate into the whole. Therapeutic touch reduces motor activity and energy expenditure by the infant and promotes comfort (Harrison, 2001). Infant massage therapy should be incorporated into the daily developmental care regimen of the stable preterm infant.

Water bed and pillow use has been reported to improve sleep and decrease motor activity as well as lead to more mature motor behavior, fewer state changes, and a decreased heart rate.

- Provide opportunities for nonnutritive sucking with a pacifier. This improves transcutaneous oxygen saturation; decreases body movement; improves sleep, especially after feedings; and increases weight gain.
- Provide objects for the infant to grasp (e.g., a piece of blanket, oxygen tubing, or a finger) during caregiving. Grasping may comfort the baby.

Teaching the parents to read behavioral cues will help them move at their infant's pace when providing stimulation. Parents are ideally equipped to meet the baby's need for stimulation. Stroking, rocking, cuddling, quiet singing, and talking to the baby can all be an integral part of the baby's care. Visual stimulation in the form of *en face* interaction with the caregivers and mobiles is also important.

PREPARATION FOR HOME CARE

Parents are often anxious when their premature infant is transferred out of the NICU or is discharged home. Parents of preterm babies should receive the same postpartum teaching as any parent taking a new infant home. In preparing for discharge, the nurse encourages the parents to spend time caring directly for their baby. This familiarizes them with their baby's behavior patterns and helps them establish realistic expectations about the infant. Some hospitals have a special room near the nursery where a mother can spend the night with her baby before discharge.

Discharge instruction includes breastfeeding and formula-feeding techniques, formula preparation, and vitamin administration. If the mother wishes to breastfeed, the nurse teaches her to pump her breasts to keep the milk flowing and provide milk even before discharge. The nurse gives information on bathing, diapering, hygiene, and normal elimination patterns and prepares the parents to expect changes in the color of the baby's stool, number of bowel movements, and timing of elimination when the infant is switched from formula-feeding to breastfeeding. This information can prevent unnecessary concern by the parents. The nurse also discusses normal growth and development patterns, reflexes, and activity for preterm infants. In these discussions, the nurse should emphasize ways to promote bonding behaviors and deal with newborn crying. Care of the preterm infant with complications, preventing infections, recognizing signs of a sick baby, and the need for continued medical follow-up are other key issues.

Families with preterm infants usually do not need to be referred to community agencies, such as visiting nurse assistance. Referral may be necessary if the infant has severe congenital abnormalities, feeding problems, or complications with infections or respiratory problems or if the parents seem unable to cope with an at-risk baby. Parents of preterm infants can benefit from meeting with others in a similar situation to share common experiences and concerns. Nurses should refer parents to support groups sponsored by the hospital or by others in the community and make connections for parents with early education intervention centers.

Preterm and LBW infants are at greater risk of increased morbidity from vaccine-preventable diseases (Saari & Committee on Infectious Diseases, 2003). The medically stable preterm infant and LBW infant should receive full doses of diphtheria, tetanus, acellular pertussis, *Haemophilus influenzae* type b, hepatitis B, poliovirus, and pneumococcal conjugate vaccines at a chronologic age consistent with the schedule recommended for full-term infants (Saari & Committee on Infectious Diseases, 2003). The influenza vaccine should be administered at 6 months of age before the beginning of and during the influenza season.

Parents of preterm infants can benefit from meeting with others in a similar situation to share common experiences and concerns. Refer parents to support groups and make connections for parents with early education intervention centers.

Evaluation

Expected outcomes of nursing care include the following:

- The preterm newborn is free of respiratory distress and establishes effective respiratory function.
- The preterm newborn gains weight and shows no signs of fatigue or aspiration during feedings.
- The preterm newborn demonstrates a serial head circumference growth rate of 1 cm per week.
- The parents are able to verbalize their anger, anxieties, and guilt feelings about the birth of a preterm baby and show attachment behavior such as frequent visits and growing confidence in their participatory care activities.

CARE OF THE NEWBORN WITH CONGENITAL ANOMALIES

The birth of a baby with a congenital defect places both newborn and family at risk. Many congenital anomalies can be life threatening if not corrected within hours after birth; others are very visible and cause the families emotional distress. When one congenital anomaly is found, healthcare providers should look for other ones, particularly in body systems that develop at the same time during gestation. Table 32–3 identifies some of the more common anomalies and their early management and nursing care in the newborn period.

Table 32–3   CONGENITAL ANOMALIES: IDENTIFICATION AND CARE IN NEWBORN PERIOD

Congenital Anomaly	Nursing Assessments	Nursing Goals and Interventions
Congenital hydrocephalus (Enlarged head)	Enlarged or full fontanelles Split or widened sutures "Setting sun" eyes Head circumference greater than 90% on growth chart	Assess presence of hydrocephalus; Measure and plot occipital-frontal baseline measurements; then measure head circumference once a day. Check fontanelle for bulging and sutures for widening. Assist with head ultrasound and transillumination. Maintain skin integrity: Change position frequently. Clean skin creases after feeding or vomiting. Use sheepskin pillow under head. Postoperatively, position head off operative site. Watch for signs of infection.
Choanal atresia (Occlusion of posterior nares)	Cyanosis and retractions at rest Noisy respirations Difficulty breathing during feeding Obstruction by thick mucus	Assess patency of nares: Listen for breath sounds while holding baby's mouth closed and alternately compressing each nostril. Assist with passing feeding tube to confirm diagnosis. Maintain respiratory function: Assist with taping airway in mouth to prevent respiratory distress. Position with head elevated to improve air exchange.

Table 32–3   CONGENITAL ANOMALIES: IDENTIFICATION AND CARE IN NEWBORN PERIOD   continued

Congenital Anomaly	Nursing Assessments	Nursing Goals and Interventions
Cleft lip (Unilateral or bilateral visible defect)	May involve external nares, nasal cartilage, nasal septum, and alveolar process Flattening or depression of midfacial contour 	Provide nutrition: Feed with special nipple. Burp frequently (increased tendency to swallow air and reflex vomiting). Clean cleft with sterile water (to prevent crusting on cleft before repair). Support parental coping: Assist parents with grief over loss of idealized baby. Encourage verbalization of their feelings about visible defect. Provide role model in interacting with infant: Parents internalize others' responses to their newborn. (At left) Bilateral cleft lip with cleft abnormality involving both hard and soft palates. Courtesy of Carol Harrigan, RNC, MSN, NNP.
Cleft palate (Fissure connecting oral and nasal cavity)	May involve uvula and soft palate May extend forward to nostril involving hard palate and maxillary alveolar ridge Difficulty in sucking Expulsion of formula through nose	Prevent aspiration/infection: Place prone or in side-lying position to facilitate drainage. Suction nasopharyngeal cavity (to prevent aspiration or airway obstruction). During newborn period feed in upright position with head and chest tilted slightly backward (to aid swallowing and discourage aspiration). Provide nutrition: Feed with special nipple that fills cleft and allows sucking. Also decreases chance of aspiration through nasal cavity. Clean mouth with water after feedings. Burp after each ounce (tend to swallow large amounts of air). Thicken formula to provide extra calories. Plot weight gain patterns to assess adequacy of diet. Provide parental support: Refer parents to community agencies and support groups. Encourage verbalization of frustrations because feeding process is long and frustrating. Praise all parental efforts. Encourage parents to seek prompt treatment for upper respiratory infection (URI) and teach them ways to decrease URI.
Tracheoesophageal fistula (type 3) (Connection between trachea and esophagus)	History of maternal polyhydramnios Excessive oral secretions Constant drooling Abdominal distention beginning soon after birth Periodic choking and cyanotic episodes Immediate regurgitation of feeding Clinical symptoms of aspiration pneumonia (tachypnea, retractions, rhonchi, decreased breath sounds, cyanotic spells) Inability to pass nasogastric tube 	Maintain respiratory status and prevent aspiration: Withhold feeding until esophageal patency is determined. Quickly assess patency before putting to breast in birth area. Place on low intermittent suction to control saliva and mucus (to prevent aspiration pneumonia). Place in warmed, humidified incubator (liquefies secretions, facilitating removal). Elevate head of bed 20–40 degrees (to prevent reflux of gastric juices). Keep quiet (crying causes air to pass through fistula and to distend intestines, causing respiratory embarrassment). Maintain fluid and electrolyte balance. Give fluids to replace esophageal drainage and maintain hydration. Provide parent education: Explain staged repair—provision of gastrostomy and ligation of fistula, then repair of atresia. Keep parents informed; clarify and reinforce physician's explanations regarding malformation, surgical repair, pre- and postoperative care, and prognosis (knowledge is ego strengthening). Involve parents in care of infant and in planning for future; facilitate touch and eye contact (to dispel feelings of inadequacy, increase self-esteem and self-worth, and promote incorporation of infant into family). *(at left)* The most frequently seen type of congenital tracheoesophageal fistula with esophageal atresia. Courtesy of Nancy Houck, RNC, BSN, NNP.

Labels on image 2: Trachea, Lung, Esophagus with atresia, Distal esophageal fistula to the trachea, Stomach

(Continued on next page)

Table 32–3   CONGENITAL ANOMALIES: IDENTIFICATION AND CARE IN NEWBORN PERIOD   continued

Congenital Anomaly	Nursing Assessments	Nursing Goals and Interventions
Diaphragmatic hernia (Portion of intestines in the thoracic cavity through abnormal opening in diaphragm).	Difficulty initiating respirations Gasping respirations with nasal flaring and chest retraction Barrel chest and scaphoid abdomen Asymmetric chest expansion Breath sounds may be absent, usually on left side Heart sounds displaced to right Spasmodic attacks of cyanosis and difficulty in feeding Bowel sounds may be heard in thoracic cavity	Nurse should never ventilate with bag and mask O_2 because the stomach will inflate, further compressing the lungs. Maintain respiratory status: Immediately administer oxygen. Initiate gastric decompression. Place in high semi-Fowler's position (to use gravity to keep abdominal organs' pressure off diaphragm). Turn to affected side to allow unaffected lung expansion. Carry out interventions to alleviate respiratory and metabolic acidosis. Assess for increased secretions around suction tube (denotes possible obstruction). Aspirate and irrigate tube with air or sterile water.

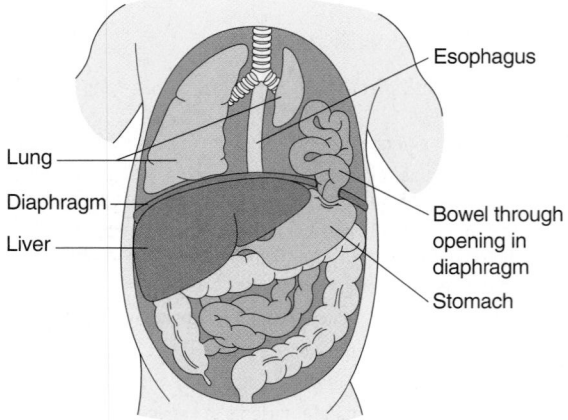

(At left) Diaphragmatic hernia. Note compression of the lung by the intestine on the affected side.
Courtesy of Nancy Houck, RNC, BSN, NNP.

| **Omphalocele** (Herniation of abdominal contents into base of umbilical cord) | May have an enclosed transparent sac covering | Maintain hydration and temperature.
Provide D_5LR and albumin for hypovolemia.
Place infant in sterile bag up to and covering defect.
Initiate gastric decompression by insertion of nasogastric tube attached to low suction (to prevent distention of lower bowel and impairment of blood flow).
Prevent infection and trauma to defect.
Position to prevent trauma to defect.
Administer broad-spectrum antibiotics. |

Newborn with omphalocele
Courtesy of Carol Harrigan, RNC, MSN, NNP.

Table 32–3   CONGENITAL ANOMALIES: IDENTIFICATION AND CARE IN NEWBORN PERIOD   continued

Congenital Anomaly	Nursing Assessments	Nursing Goals and Interventions
Gastroschisis (Full-thickness defect in abdominal wall allowing viscera outside the body to the right of an intact umbilical cord.)	No sac covering. Intestines exposed to the caustic amniotic fluid. Associated with intestinal atresia, malrotation	Maintain hydration and temperature. Prevent trauma and infection to defect. Provide D_5LR normal saline, and/or albumin for hypovolemia Place infant in sterile bag up to axilla Initiate gastric decompression by insertion of nasogastric tube attached to low suction. Administer broad-spectrum antibiotics.

Term newborn with gastroschisis. Note the externalized loops of bowel visible through the bag.
Courtesy of Carol Harrigan, RNC, MSN, NNP.

Congenital Anomaly	Nursing Assessments	Nursing Goals and Interventions
Prune belly syndrome (congenital absence of one or more layers of abdominal muscles)	Oligohydramnious leading to pulmonary hypoplasia common Deficiency of the abdominal wall musculature causing the abdomen to be shapeless Skin hangs loosely and is wrinkled in appearance Associated with urinary abnormalities (urethral obstruction) In males, cryptorchidism is common; rarely occurs in females	Maintain respiratory status: May need to be immediately intubated and ventilated. Prevent trauma and infection. Administer broad-spectrum antibiotics. Place a urinary catheter and monitor urinary output. Carry out interventions to alleviate respiratory and metabolic acidosis. Keep parents updated and informed about prognosis.

Prune belly syndrome.
Courtesy of Carol Harrigan, RNC, MSN, NNP.

(Continued on next page)

Table 32–3	CONGENITAL ANOMALIES: IDENTIFICATION AND CARE IN NEWBORN PERIOD continued	
Congenital Anomaly	**Nursing Assessments**	**Nursing Goals and Interventions**
Myelomeningocele (Saclike cyst containing meninges, spinal cord, and nerve roots in thoracic and/or lumbar area)	Myelomeningocele directly connects to subarachnoid space so hydrocephalus often associated No response or varying response to sensation below level of sac May have constant dribbling of urine Incontinence or retention of stool Anal wink may or may not be present Newborn with lumbar myelomeningocele. Courtesy of Carol Harrigan, RNC, MSN, NNP.	Prevent trauma and infection. Position on abdomen or on side and restrain (to prevent pressure and trauma to sac). Meticulously clean buttocks and genitals after each voiding and defecation (to prevent contamination of sac and decrease possibility of infection). May put protective covering over sac (to prevent rupture and drying). Observe sac for oozing of fluid. Credé bladder (apply downward pressure on bladder with thumbs, moving urine toward the urethra) as ordered to prevent urinary stasis. Assess amount of sensation and movement below defect. Observe for complications. Obtain occipital-frontal circumference baseline measurements; then measure head circumference once a day (to detect hydrocephalus). Check fontanelle for fullness and bulging.
Imperforate anus, congenital dislocated hip, and clubfoot	See discussion in Chapter 29 ∞, Anus and Extremities	Identify defect and initiate appropriate referral early.

CARE OF THE INFANT OF A SUBSTANCE-ABUSING MOTHER

An **infant of a substance-abusing mother (ISAM)** may also be alcohol or drug dependent. After birth, when an infant's connection with the maternal blood supply is severed, the baby may suffer withdrawal. In addition the drugs the mother ingested may be teratogenic, resulting in congenital anomalies or developmental problems.

Alcohol Dependence

The **fetal alcohol syndrome (FAS)**, a leading cause of mental retardation that is potentially preventable, includes a series of malformations (identified shortly) frequently found in infants exposed to alcohol in utero. It has been estimated that complete FAS occurs in up to 5 live births per 1000 (Martinez, Partridge, & Taeusch, 2005). FAS rates are increased among Native Americans and Alaska natives and those of low economic status. **Fetal alcohol effects (FAE)**, or **alcohol-related birth defects (ARBD)**, are usually determined only by a positive maternal drinking history and cognitive difficulties, specifically a reduction in the size of the cerebral cortex, and usually do not exhibit the classic facial dysmorphology (Jones, 2003; Moran, 2004). Another term applied to these children is *alcohol-related neurodevelopmental disorder* (ARND). These children have CNS abnormalities, behavior, and cognitive abnormalities (Moran, 2004). The new diagnostic categories for FAS take into consideration the various clinical manifestations of FAS, the social and family environment, and, if available, the maternal alcohol history.

Although it is known that ethanol freely crosses the placenta to the fetus, it is still not known whether the alcohol alone or the breakdown products of alcohol cause the damage. For in-depth discussion of alcohol abuse in pregnancy, see Chapter 19. ∞ The effects of other substances that are often combined with alcohol, such as nicotine, diazepam (Valium), marijuana, and caffeine, as well as poor diet, enhance the likelihood of FAS.

LONG-TERM COMPLICATIONS FOR THE INFANT WITH FAS

The long-term prognosis for the FAS newborn is less than favorable. Because of the failure-to-thrive appearance, many FAS infants are often evaluated for deficiencies in organic and inorganic amino acids. These infants have a delay in oral feeding development but have a normal progression of oral motor function. Many FAS infants feed poorly and have persistent vomiting until 6 to 7 months of age. They have difficulty adjusting to solid foods and show little spontaneous interest in food.

CNS dysfunctions are the most common and serious problems associated with FAS. Hypotonicity and increased placidity are seen in these infants. They also have a decreased ability to habituate repetitive stimuli. Children exhibiting FAS can be severely mentally retarded or have normal intelligence. The degree of mental retardation is directly proportional to the severity of the dysmorphic findings, meaning the more abnormal the facial features, the lower the IQ will be (Jones, 2003). Often there is little improvement in intelligence (as measured by IQ) despite positive environmental and educational factors (Moran, 2004). These children show impulsivity, cognitive impairment, speech and language abnormalities, and learning disabilities indicative of CNS involvement (Moran, 2004). As they progress through the adolescent years, they change from a very thin and underweight child to one who is overweight and often obese. Short stature and microcephaly persists.

NURSING CARE MANAGEMENT
Nursing Assessment and Diagnosis

The nurse assesses the newborn for the following characteristics typical of FAS:

- *Abnormal structural development and CNS dysfunction.* These include mental retardation, microcephaly, and hyperactivity.

- *Growth deficiencies.* Infants with FAS are often growth retarded with weight, length, and head circumference being affected. These infants continue to show a persistent postnatal growth deficiency with head circumference and linear growth most affected.

- *Distinctive facial abnormalities.* These include short palpebral fissures, epicanthal folds, broad nasal bridge, flattened midfacies, short upturned or beaklike nose, micrognathia (abnormally small lower jaw), hypoplastic maxilla, thin upper lip or vermilion border, and smooth philtrum (groove on upper lip) (Martinez et al., 2005).

- *Associated anomalies.* Abnormalities affecting the heart (primarily septal and valvular defects), eyes (optic nerve hypoplasia), ears (conductive and sensorineural hearing loss), kidneys, and skeletal system (especially those involving joints, such as congenital dislocated hips) are often noted.

Alcohol-exposed newborns in the first week of life may show symptoms that include sleeplessness, excessive arousal states, inconsolable crying, abnormal reflexes, hyperactivity with little ability to maintain alertness and attentiveness to environment, jitteriness, abdominal distention, and exaggerated mouthing behaviors such as hyperactive rooting and increased nonnutritive sucking. Seizures may be common. These symptoms commonly persist throughout the first month of life but may continue longer. Alcohol dependence in the infant is physiologic, not psychologic. Signs and symptoms of withdrawal often appear within 6 to 12 hours and at least within the first 3 days of life. Seizures after the neonatal period are rare.

Nursing diagnoses that may apply to the FAS newborn include the following:

- *Altered Nutrition: Less than Body Requirements* related to decreased oral intake and hyperirritability

- *Alteration in Neurodevelopmental Status* related to central nervous system involvement secondary to maternal alcohol use

- *Ineffective Coping* related to dysfunctional family dynamics and substance-dependent mother

- *Altered Physical Appearance* related to facial dysmorphology secondary to FAS

Nursing Plan and Implementation
HOSPITAL-BASED NURSING CARE

Nursing care of the FAS newborn is aimed at avoiding heat loss, providing adequate nutrition, and reducing environmental stimuli. The FAS baby is most comfortable in a quiet, dimly lighted environment. Because of feeding problems, these infants require extra time and patience during feedings. It is important to provide consistency in the staff working with the baby and parents and to keep personnel and visitors to a minimum at any one time.

The nurse should inform the alcohol-dependent mother that breastfeeding is not contraindicated but that excessive alcohol consumption may intoxicate the newborn and inhibit the letdown reflex. The nurse should monitor the newborn's vital signs closely and observe for evidence of seizure activity and respiratory distress.

COMMUNITY-BASED NURSING CARE

Infants affected by maternal alcohol abuse are also at risk psychologically. Restlessness, sleeplessness, agitation, resistance to cuddling or holding, and frequent crying can be frustrating to parents as their efforts to relieve the distress are unrewarded. Feeding dysfunction can also result in frustrations for the caregiver and digestive upsets for the infant. Frustration may cause the parents to punish the baby or result in the unconscious desire to stay away from the infant. Either outcome may create an unstable family environment and result in the infant's failure to thrive.

The nurse should focus on providing support for the parents and reinforcing positive parenting activity. Before discharge, parents should be given opportunities to provide baby care so that they can feel confident in their interpretations of their baby's cues and their ability to meet the baby's needs. Referring the family to social services and visiting nurse or public health nurse associations is essential for the well-being of the infant. Follow-up care and teaching can strengthen the parents' skills and coping abilities and help them create a stable, healthy environment for their family. The infant with FAS/ARBD should be involved in intervention programs that monitor the child's developmental progress, health, and home environment.

Evaluation

Expected outcomes of nursing care include the following:

- The FAS newborn is able to tolerate feedings and gain weight.

- The FAS infant's hyperirritability is controlled, and the baby has suffered no physical injuries.

- The parents are able to identify and meet the special needs of their newborn and accept outside assistance as needed.

Drug Dependence

Drugs of abuse by the pregnant woman can include the following singularly or in combination: tobacco, cocaine, phencyclidine (PCP), methamphetamines, inhalants, marijuana, heroin,

966 Unit Six The Newborn

antidepressants, and methadone. Patterns of abuse of alcohol, marijuana, and heroin in childbearing women have changed very little in the past few years. The incidence of cocaine (especially "crack") use may have stabilized but oxycodone (oxycontin) use has risen dramatically (see "Substances Commonly Abused During Pregnancy" in Chapter 19 ∞ for more discussion of maternal substance abuse). Marijuana, alcohol, and nicotine are sometimes used in conjunction with cocaine.

Intrauterine drug-exposed infants are predisposed to a number of problems. Almost all narcotic drugs cross the placenta and enter the fetal circulation, so the fetus can develop problems in utero or soon after birth. The effects of polydrug use on the newborn must always be taken into consideration.

The greatest risks to the fetus of the drug-dependent mother include the following:

- *Intrauterine asphyxia.* Asphyxia is often a direct result of fetal withdrawal secondary to maternal withdrawal. Fetal withdrawal is accompanied by hyperactivity with increased oxygen consumption. Insufficiency of oxygen can lead to fetal asphyxia. Moreover, narcotic-addicted women tend to have a higher incidence of preeclampsia, abruptio placentae, and placenta previa, resulting in placental insufficiency and fetal asphyxia.

- *Intrauterine infection.* Sexually transmitted infections, HIV infection, and hepatitis are often connected with the pregnant addict's lifestyle. Such infections can involve the fetus.

- *Alterations in birth weight.* These may depend on the type of drug the mother uses. Women using predominantly heroin or cocaine have infants of lower birth weight who are SGA. Women maintained on methadone have higher-birth-weight infants, some of whom are LGA.

- *Low Apgar scores.* These may be related to the intrauterine asphyxia or the medication the woman received during labor. The use of a narcotic antagonist (nalorphine or naloxone) to reverse respiratory depression is contraindicated because it may precipitate acute withdrawal in the infant.

Common Complications of the Drug-Exposed Newborn

The newborn of a woman who abused drugs during her pregnancy is predisposed to the following problems:

- *Respiratory distress.* The heroin-addicted newborn frequently suffers respiratory stress, mainly meconium-aspiration pneumonia and transient tachypnea. Meconium aspiration is usually secondary to increased oxygen consumption and activity experienced by the fetus during intrauterine withdrawal. Transient tachypnea may develop secondary to the inhibitory effects of narcotics on the reflex responsible for clearing the lungs. RDS, however, occurs less often in heroin-addicted newborns, even in those who are premature, because they have tissue-oxygen unloading capabilities comparable to those of a 6-week-old term infant. In addition, heroin stimulates

production of glucocorticoids via the anterior pituitary gland.

- *Jaundice.* Newborns of methadone-addicted women may develop jaundice due to prematurity. By contrast, infants of mothers addicted to heroin or cocaine have a lower incidence of hyperbilirubinemia because these substances contribute to early maturity of the liver.

- *Congenital anomalies and growth restriction.* The incidence of anomalies of the genitourinary and cardiovascular systems is slightly increased in infants of heroin- and cocaine-addicted mothers. Infants of cocaine-addicted mothers exhibit congenital malformations involving bony skull defects, such as microencephaly, and symmetric IUGR, cardiac defects, and genitourinary defects. In addition, there is a higher incidence of SIDS. Congenital anomalies, however, are rare. Infants exposed to methamphetamines during gestation may show a higher incidence of cleft lip and palate, cardiac anomalies, microcephaly, and LBW (Beauman, 2005).

- *Behavioral abnormalities.* Babies exposed to cocaine have poor state organization. They exhibit decreased interactive behaviors when tested with the Brazelton Neonatal Behavioral Assessment Scale. These infants also have difficulty moving through the various sleep and awake states and have problems attending to and actively engaging in auditory and visual stimuli.

- *Withdrawal.* The most significant postnatal problem of the drug-addicted newborn is narcotic withdrawal (usually from heroin or methadone). Withdrawal manifestations often begin after discharge, especially with short birthing unit stays. See Table 32–4 for a discussion of withdrawal symptoms.

LONG-TERM EFFECTS

During the first 2 years of life, many cocaine-exposed infants demonstrate susceptibility to behavior lability and are unable to express strong feelings such as pleasure, anger, or distress, or even a strong reaction to being separated from their parents. Cocaine-exposed infants may be at higher risk for motor development problems, delays in expressive language skills, and feeding difficulties due to swallowing problems (Martinez et al., 2005). State control is poorly developed in drug-exposed infants, who tend to rapidly progress from sleep to a wakeful state of crying without smooth transition from one state to the next (Greene & Goodman, 2003). As a result, these infants have poor social interaction skills; cannot habituate to external stimuli; and become easily overstimulated, having difficulty sleeping.

Infants of drug-addicted mothers often demonstrate a higher incidence of GI and respiratory illnesses. These illnesses can be related not to drug exposure but to the mothers' lack of education regarding proper infant care, feeding, and hygiene. After birth the infant born to a drug-dependent mother may also be subject to neglect or abuse, or both.

CLINICAL THERAPY

For optimal fetal and newborn outcome, the heroin-addicted woman should receive complete prenatal care as early as possi-

Table 32–4	**CLINICAL MANIFESTATIONS OF NEWBORN WITHDRAWAL**	

Central nervous system signs	**Gastrointestinal signs**	**Vasomotor signs**
• Hyperactivity	• Disorganized, vigorous suck	• Stuffy nose, yawning, sneezing
• Hyperirritability (persistent shrill cry)	• Vomiting	• Flushing
• Increased muscle tone	• Drooling	• Sweating
• Exaggerated reflexes	• Sensitive gag reflex	• Sudden, circumoral pallor
• Tremors and myoclonic jerks	• Hyperphagia	**Cutaneous signs**
• Sneezing, hiccups, yawning	• Diarrhea	• Excoriated buttocks, knees, elbows
• Short, unquiet sleep	• Poor feeding (less than 15 mL on first day of life; takes longer than 30 minutes per feeding)	• Facial scratches
• Fever (accompanies the increased neuromuscular activities)		• Pressure-point abrasions
Respiratory signs		
• Tachypnea (greater than 60 breaths per minute when quiet)		
• Excessive secretions		

ble to reduce maternal morbidity and mortality rates and to promote fetal stability and growth (McCarthy, Leamon, Parr et al., 2005). For those women dependent on narcotics, it is not recommended that the woman be withdrawn completely while pregnant because this induces fetal withdrawal with poor newborn outcomes. Unfortunately, however, pregnant women may be denied access to programs for substance abusers.

Newborn treatment may include management of complications; serologic tests for syphilis, HIV, and hepatitis B; urine drug screen and meconium analysis; and social service referral (Beauman, 2005). Drugs used to control withdrawal symptoms vary and may be regionally based. They include phenobarbital, tincture of opium, oral morphine sulfate, oral methadone, and diazepam (Blackburn, 2003; Beauman, 2005). Nutritional support is important in light of the increase in energy expenditure that withdrawal may entail.

NURSING CARE MANAGEMENT
Nursing Assessment and Diagnosis

Early identification of the newborn needing clinical or pharmacologic interventions decreases the incidence of mortality and morbidity. During the newborn period, nursing assessment focuses on the following:

- Discovering the mother's last drug intake and dosage level through the prenatal history and laboratory tests. Women may be reluctant to disclose this information; therefore, a nonjudgmental interview technique is essential (Andres, 2004).

- Assessing for congenital malformations and the complications related to intrauterine withdrawal, such as SGA, asphyxia, meconium aspiration, and prematurity.

- Identifying the signs and symptoms of newborn withdrawal or neonatal abstinence syndrome (see Table 32–4).

Although many of the signs and symptoms of narcotic withdrawal are similar to those seen with hypoglycemia and hypocalcemia, drug-addicted babies have glucose and calcium values within normal limits.

Neonatal abstinence syndrome includes both physiologic and behavioral responses. The severity of withdrawal can be assessed by a scoring system based on observations and measurement of the responses to neonatal abstinence such as the Finnegan scale. It evaluates the infant on potentially life-threatening signs, such as vomiting, diarrhea, weight loss, irritability, tremors, and tachypnea (Table 32–5).

Nursing diagnoses that may apply to drug-dependent newborns include the following:

- **High Risk for Infant CNS Injury** related to perinatal substance abuse

- **Risk for Ineffective Airway Clearance** related to suppression of respiratory system

- **Altered Nutrition: Less than Body Requirements** related to vomiting and diarrhea, uncoordinated suck and swallow reflex, hypertonia secondary to withdrawal

- **Impaired Skin Integrity** related to constant activity, diarrhea

- **Altered Parenting** related to hyperirritable behavior of the infant and lack of knowledge of infant care

- **Ineffective Family Coping: Disabling** related to drug-dependent parent

- **Sleep Pattern Disturbance** related to CNS excitation secondary to drug withdrawal

Nursing Plan and Implementation
HOSPITAL-BASED NURSING CARE

Care of the drug-exposed newborn is based on reducing withdrawal symptoms and promoting adequate respiration, temperature, and nutrition. See the Nursing Care Plan: The Newborn of a Substance-Abusing Mother for specific nursing care measures. Some general nursing care measures include the following:

- Performing neonatal abstinence scoring per hospital protocol

- Monitoring temperature for hyperthermia

- Carefully monitoring pulse and respirations every 15 minutes and pulse oximetry until stable; stimulation if apnea occurs

- Providing small, frequent feedings, especially in the presence of vomiting, regurgitation, and diarrhea

Table 32–5	**NEONATAL ABSTINENCE SCORE SHEET**

Neonatal Abstinence Scoring System

System	Signs and Symptoms	Score	AM	PM	Comments
Central Nervous System Disturbances	Excessive high-pitched (or other) cry Continuous high-pitched (or other) cry	2 3			Daily weights
	Sleeps < 1 hour after feeding Sleeps < 2 hours after feeding Sleeps < 3 hours after feeding	3 2 1			
	Hyperactive Moro reflex Markedly hyperactive Moro reflex	2 3			
	Mild tremors disturbed Moderate-severe tremors disturbed	1 2			
	Mild tremors undisturbed Moderate-severe tremors undisturbed	3 4			
	Increased muscle tone	2			
	Excoriation (specific area)	1			
	Myoclonic jerks	3			
	Generalized convulsions	5			
Metabolic/Vasomotor/ Respiratory Disturbances	Sweating	1			
	Fever < 101 (99–100.8F/37.2–38.2C) Fever > 101 (38.4C and higher)	1 2			
	Frequent yawning (> 3–4 times/interval)	1			
	Mottling	1			
	Nasal stuffiness	1			
	Sneezing (> 3–4 times/interval)	1			
	Nasal flaring	2			
	Respiratory rate > 60/min Respiratory rate > 60/min with retractions	1 2			
Gastrointestinal Disturbances	Excessive sucking	1			
	Poor feeding	2			
	Regurgitation Projectile vomiting	2 3			
	Loose stools Watery stools	2 3			
	Total Score				
	Initials of Scorer				

SOURCE: Reproduced from "Neonatal Abstinence Syndrome," by L. P. Finnegan, in *Current Therapy in Neonatal-Perinatal Medicine,* 2e, N. Nelson (ed.), 1990, by permission of the publisher, BC Decker In.

- Administering IV therapy as needed
- Administering medications as ordered, such as oral morphine, phenobarbital, and tincture of opium
- Properly positioning on the right side-lying or semi-Fowler's to avoid possible aspirations of vomitus or secretions
- Monitoring frequency of diarrhea and vomiting, and weighing infant every 8 hours during withdrawal
- Observing for problems of SGA or LGA newborns
- Swaddling with hands near mouth to minimize injury and achieve more organized behavioral state. (Offer a pacifier for nonnutritive, excessive sucking. Gentle, vertical rocking can be successful in calming an infant who is out of control [Figure 32–14 ◆].)
- Protecting face and extremities from excoriation by using mittens and soft sheets or sheepskin
- Applying protective skin emollient to the groin area with each diaper change
- Placing newborn in quiet, dimly lighted area of nursery

COMMUNITY-BASED NURSING CARE

Parents need assistance to prepare for what they can expect for the first few months at home. At the time of discharge, the mother should be instructed to anticipate mild jitteriness and irritability in the newborn, which may persist from 6 days to 8 weeks, depending on the initial severity of the withdrawal (Blackburn, 2003). Because infants with neonatal abstinence syndrome are at a significantly higher risk for SIDS when the mother used heroin or cocaine, the infant should be put to sleep in a supine position. The nurse should demonstrate and help the mother learn feeding techniques, comforting measures, how to recognize newborn cues, and appropriate parenting responses.

Figure 32–14 ◆ Nonnutritive suckling on a pacifier has a calming effect on newborn.

Parents are to be counseled regarding available resources, such as support groups, and signs and symptoms that indicate the need for further care. Ongoing evaluation is necessary because of the potential for long-term problems. Follow-up on missed appointments can bring parents back into the healthcare system, thereby improving parent and infant outcomes and promoting a positive, interactive environment after birth.

Evaluation

Expected outcomes of nursing care include the following:

- The newborn tolerates feedings, gains weight, and has a decreased number of stools.
- The parents learn innovative ways to comfort their newborn.
- The parents are able to cope with their frustrations and begin to use outside resources as needed.

Infants of Mothers Who Are Tobacco Dependent

Despite increased knowledge about the dangers of smoking to the fetus and newborn, 15% to 20% of women continue to smoke during pregnancy (Martinez et al., 2005). The common consequence of tobacco use is addiction to nicotine. Most smokers report true enjoyment, associated with a sense of relaxation during stress, especially with the first cigarette of the day (CDC, 2005). The tobacco-induced hazards on the pregnant woman and her developing fetus may be one of the most underrated health issues, at least in public opinion.

Preconceptual cigarette smoking has been found to increase infertility. Fortunately, the reduction in fertility is reversible if the woman stops smoking. Smoking during pregnancy has been associated with spontaneous abortion, placenta previa, and abruptio placentae. See "Tobacco" in Chapter 16 ∞ for discussion of maternal care.

RISKS OF TOBACCO TO THE FETUS AND NEWBORN

The most studied compound found in cigarette smoke that can adversely affect the intrauterine environment is carbon monoxide. Carbon monoxide binds hemoglobin to form carboxyhemoglobin, which reduces the oxygen-carrying capacity of the blood. It also increases the binding of hemoglobin to oxygen, which impairs the release of oxygen to the tissues. Therefore, the fetus can experience intrauterine hypoxia (Martinez et al., 2005). Mothers who smoke during pregnancy are nearly twice as likely to have an LBW infant, and smoking during pregnancy is responsible for 20% to 30% of all LBW infants (Law et al., 2003). The nicotine in cigarettes acts as a neuroteratogen that interferes with fetal development, specifically the developing nervous system. The greatest risks to the fetus and newborn of the mother who smokes include the following (Law et al., 2003):

- *Intrauterine growth restriction and/or prematurity* secondary to cigarette metabolites crossing the placenta, causing vasoconstriction and decreased uterine blood flow
- *Intrauterine distress* presenting as meconium staining and low Apgar scores
- *Neonatal neurobehavioral abnormalities* such as impaired habituation, orientation, consolability, orientation to sound
- *Hypertonia or hypotonia, tremors, increased Moro reflex*
- *Signs of nicotine toxicity* (tachycardia, irritability, poor feeding)

CLINICAL THERAPY

Prevention is always the best intervention. Inquiry into tobacco and smoke exposure should be a routine part of the prenatal history. Preconception and prenatal counseling about the effects of cigarette smoking on pregnancy and the fetus should occur. It is estimated that there would be a 10% reduction in perinatal mortality and an 11% reduction in the incidence of LBW if smoking during pregnancy were eliminated (American Academy of Pediatrics [AAP] & American College of Obstetricians and Gynecologists [ACOG], 2002).

Cotinine, a metabolite of nicotine, has been found in fetal body fluids. There is also a positive correlation between the number of cigarettes smoked per day and concentration of cotinine in maternal urine. Other factors that influence fetal and maternal serum cotinine concentrations are nicotine content of the cigarette and the time elapsed between the last cigarette smoked and the sampling. These findings indicate that cotinine may be used as a marker of maternal-fetal tobacco exposure during pregnancy (Martinez et al., 2005).

NURSING CARE MANAGEMENT

Mothers should be counseled that eliminating or reducing smoking even late in pregnancy can improve fetal growth. The use of nicotine patches (instead of smoking) reduces the absorption of nicotine and thereby may result in increased birth weight of the fetus. See "Tobacco" in Chapter 16 ∞ for further

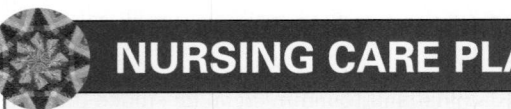

NURSING CARE PLAN

The Newborn of a Substance-Abusing Mother

INTERVENTION	RATIONALE	EXPECTED OUTCOMES
1. Nursing Diagnosis: High Risk for Infant CNS Injury related to perinatal substance abuse		
Goal: The newborn will be free of signs and symptoms of CNS injury.		
• Obtain prenatal records and question the mother about history of drug use. Include duration, type of drug or drugs used, time and amount of last dose taken before delivery.	• Noting the mother's last drug ingestion will provide the medical staff with an approximate time frame to expect the infant to exhibit withdrawal symptoms.	*Infant will have no signs and symptoms of CNS injury as evidenced by reduced hyperactivity, irritability, normal sleep-wake pattern, no jitteriness, and no seizure activity.*
• Record newborn for signs and symptoms of withdrawal (e.g., high-pitched shrill cry, sneezing, vomiting, diarrhea, hypertonicity, restlessness, and wakefulness) using neonatal abstinence scoring tool every 3 hours.	• The average symptoms of withdrawal occur 72 hours after birth; however, symptoms may appear as early as 6–24 hours after birth.	
• Provide a quiet, calm, darkened environment. Swaddle infant tightly and place in a side-lying or prone position.	• Providing a quiet environment decreases stimuli, therefore reducing CNS symptoms.	
• Carefully plan tests and/or treatments to avoid excessive stimuli.	• Planning care promotes rest and reduces external stimuli.	
• Use soothing techniques such as rocking, cuddling, soft music, and soft tones when speaking.	• These activities promote comfort, security, and infant bonding.	
• Administer appropriate medications (e.g., oral morphine, oral methadone, phenobarbital) as ordered by physician. Monitor efficacy and side effects of these medications.	• These medications aid the infant in alleviating symptoms related to withdrawal.	
2. Nursing Diagnosis: Risk for Ineffective Airway Clearance related to suppression of respiratory system		
Goal: Infant will be free of signs and symptoms of respiratory distress after birth.		
• Obtain maternal prenatal, labor, and delivery records.	• Provides information about fetal stress that may have occurred during the prenatal or intrapartal period. In addition, the delivery record will provide information concerning the infant's respiratory status at birth; for example, the Apgar score.	*The newborn will maintain adequate respiratory effort as evidenced by respirations of 30–60/min; no signs of retractions, grunting, or cyanosis; and arterial blood gases are within normal range.*
• Assess infant's respiratory rate and effort, skin color, heart rate, presence or absence of cough reflex, and symptoms of respiratory distress.	• Maternal narcotic consumption may depress the cough reflex and respiratory center of the newborn after birth. Symptoms such as cyanosis, tachycardia, grunting, retractions, and nasal flaring may indicate hypoxia.	
• Position infant in a side-lying or semi-Fowler's position.	• Prevents aspiration.	

NURSING CARE PLAN

The Newborn of a Substance-Abusing Mother continued

INTERVENTION	RATIONALE	EXPECTED OUTCOMES
• Monitor infant for temperature elevation.	• Temperature elevation may cause metabolic rate and oxygen needs to increase when associated with CNS stimulation.	
Collaborative: Obtain arterial blood gases (ABGS) as ordered by physician. • Monitor infant's cardiac status and pulmonary status using electrocardiogram (ECG) and pulse oximetry.	• Oxygen demands increase with drug withdrawal. Obtaining ABGs will provide medical personnel baseline information on infant's respiratory status, and effective medical interventions can be initiated. • Provides medical personnel with cardiac and pulmonary status.	

3. Nursing Diagnosis: Altered Nutrition: Less than Body Requirements related to vomiting and diarrhea, uncoordinated suck and swallow reflex, and hypertonia secondary to withdrawal

Goal: The infant will gain or maintain weight.

• Review gestational age assessment.	• Oral feeding may be difficult because of CNS hyperactivity and GI hypermobility.	• *The infant will tolerate feedings, maintain weight, or gain weight as evidenced by no regurgitation or aspiration of feedings, adequate weight gain according to weight graph.*
• Assess infant's sucking and swallowing reflexes.	• GI hypermobility, irritation, and CNS stimulation can increase nutritional needs.	
• Monitor regurgitation, vomiting, diarrhea. • Use bulb syringe before feedings if newborn is having problems with nasal stuffiness and congestion.	• Allows infant to breathe easier by ridding the nasal passages of excessive mucus.	
• Initiate appropriate feedings per physician's orders (e.g., oral, gavage, or IV feedings). • Provide small frequent feedings of a high-calorie formula.	• Facilitates nutritional intake because SGA infants require 120–150 kcal/kg/day for adequate nutrition.	
• Position infant on right side after feedings. • Monitor infant's weight and document on graph.	• Prevents regurgitation and promotes gastric emptying. • Identifies abnormalities in weight gain/loss and allows for early intervention when necessary.	
• Offer pacifier between feedings for nonnutritive sucking.	• Nonnutritive sucking allows for sucking practice.	

(Continued on next page)

NURSING CARE PLAN

The Newborn of a Substance-Abusing Mother continued

INTERVENTION	RATIONALE	EXPECTED OUTCOMES
4 Nursing Diagnosis: Risk for Altered Parenting related to lack of knowledge of infant care		
Goal: The parent will demonstrate ability to independently provide infant care.		
• Assess mother's desire to learn infant care tasks as well as evaluate her present physical and emotional stability.	• Provides knowledge of mother's ability to care for infant.	• *The parent will demonstrate ability to perform basic infant care tasks as evidenced by exhibiting appropriate attachment behaviors (i.e., talking to and holding infant), feeding infant, and bathing infant.*
• Instruct mother on coping strategies (e.g., exercise, listening to music, and discussing concerns openly) to manage stressful situations.	• Gives mother the tools to handle stress, thereby decreasing the chances of exhibiting abusive behavior.	
• Assess mother's insight into her own chemical dependency.	• Assistance in enrollment into a chemical dependency program may be necessary before mother can independently care for infant.	
• Instruct mother on signs and symptoms of withdrawal and treatment interventions.	• Assists the mother in understanding infant's behaviors and gives her the tools to intervene without feeling anxious.	
• Encourage mother and family members to perform basic infant care tasks. Offer a night of "nesting in" with infant before discharge.	• Facilitates attachment and increases parenting competence.	
• Initiate social service consult.	• Assists parents to care for infant by themselves, but with nursing support nearby.	

discussion of prenatal smoking cessation and other intervention programs. Newborns of mothers who are tobacco dependent may be screened with the NICU Network Neurobehavioral Scale (NNNS) to assess their neurologic, behavioral, and stress/abstinence neurobehavioral function (Law et al., 2003). The potential for long-term respiratory problems such as asthma, as well as cognitive and receptive language delays that may persist into school age, should be evaluated.

CARE OF THE NEWBORN EXPOSED TO HIV/AIDS

Increasing numbers of newborns are born infected with HIV or at risk for acquiring it in the newborn period or early infancy. Transmission during the perinatal and newborn periods can occur across the placenta or through breast milk or contaminated blood. Maternal-to-newborn vertical transmission rates are about 13% to 40% in the United States (Thureen, Deacon, Hernandez et al.,

2005). The risk of vertical transmission can be decreased in mothers taking zidovudine during gestation. For further discussion of maternal and fetal HIV/AIDS, see Chapter 19. ∞ Opportunistic diseases such as gram-negative sepsis and problems associated with prematurity are the primary causes of mortality in HIV-infected babies. Some infants infected by maternal-fetal transmission suffer from severe immunodeficiency, with HIV disease progressing more rapidly during the first year of life.

Early identification of babies with or at risk for HIV/AIDS is essential during the newborn period. However, the currently available HIV serologic tests (enzyme-linked immunosorbent assay [ELISA] and Western blot test) cannot distinguish between maternal and infant antibodies; therefore, they are inappropriate for infants up to 15 months of age. It may take up to 15 months for infected infants to form their own antibodies to HIV (Venkatesh, Merestein, Adams et al., 2006). Testing by HIV deoxyriboneucleic acid (DNA) polymerase chain reaction (PCR) is the preferred test. Results can be made available within 24 hours (Venkatesh et al., 2006). A viral culture may also be performed at birth but it is more expensive. The first DNA PCR test should be performed on the newborn before 48 hours of age. The test is repeated when the infant is 1 month of age. Umbilical cord blood should not be used for HIV testing. If PCR and viral culture are unavailable, the p24 antigen may be used to assess HIV infection status in infants older than 1 month, but the sensitivity of p24 antigen testing is substantially less than that of the other tests. For infants who have three negative (at birth and at 1 and 4 months of age) HIV virologic antibody tests, a negative HIV-specific IgG assay (ELISA) at 18 months of age definitively rules out HIV in exposed infants. AZT (zidovudine [ZDV]) is started prophylactically 2 mg/kg/dose PO every 6 hours. If the infant is confirmed to be HIV positive, ZDV is changed to a multidrug antiretroviral regimen.

NURSING CARE MANAGEMENT
Nursing Assessment and Diagnosis

Many newborns exposed to HIV/AIDS are premature or SGA, or both, and show failure to thrive during the newborn and infant periods. They can show signs and symptoms of disease within days of birth. Signs that may be seen in the early infancy period include enlarged spleen and liver, swollen glands, recurrent respiratory infections, rhinorrhea, interstitial pneumonia (rarely seen in adults), recurrent GI problems (diarrhea and weight loss), organic failure to thrive, urinary system infections, persistent or recurrent oral and genital candidiasis infections, and loss of developmental milestones (Venkatesh et al., 2006). There is also a high risk of acquiring *Pneumocystis carinii* pneumonia. Nursing diagnoses that may apply to the infant exposed to HIV/AIDS include the following:

- *Altered Nutrition: Less than Body Requirements* related to formula intolerance and inadequate intake
- *Risk for Impaired Skin Integrity* related to chronic diarrhea
- *Risk for Infection* related to perinatal exposure and immunoregulation suppression secondary to HIV/AIDS
- *Impaired Physical Mobility* related to decreased neuromuscular development
- *Altered Growth and Development* related to lack of attachment and stimulation
- *Altered Parenting* related to diagnosis of HIV/AIDS and fear of future outcome

Nursing Plan and Implementation
HOSPITAL-BASED NURSING CARE

Nursing care of the newborn exposed to HIV/AIDS includes all the normal care required for any newborn in a nursery. In addition, the nurse must include care for a newborn suspected of having a blood-borne infection, as with hepatitis B. Standard precautions should be used when caring for the newborn immediately after birth until all maternal blood is removed and when obtaining blood samples via vein puncture or heel stick. (The blood of all newborns must be considered potentially infectious because the status of the infant's blood is often not known until after the infant is discharged. There is also a window of time be-

fore seroconversion occurs, during which the baby is still considered infectious.)

Nursing care involves providing for comfort; keeping the newborn well nourished and protected from opportunistic infections; and facilitating growth, development, and attachment. Most institutions recommend that their caregivers wear gloves during all diaper changes and examination of babies. Disposable gloves are worn when changing diapers or cleaning the diaper area, especially in the presence of diarrhea, because blood may be in the stool (AAP Committee on Pediatric AIDS and Committee on Infectious Diseases, 1999). Good skin care is essential to prevent skin rashes. See Table 32–6.

COMMUNITY-BASED NURSING CARE

Handwashing is crucial when caring for newborns at risk for AIDS; thus, parents must be taught proper handwashing technique. Nutrition is essential because failure to thrive and weight loss are common. Small, frequent feedings and food supplementation are helpful. The nurse should discuss with the parents sanitary techniques for preparing formula. The nurse should also inform parents that the baby should not be put to bed with juice or formula because of potential bacteria growth. Parents need to be alert to the signs of feeding intolerance, such as increasing regurgitation, abdominal distention, and loose stools. The newborn should be weighed three times a week.

The baby should have his or her own skin care items, towels, and washcloths. Most clothing and linens can be washed with other household laundry. Linen that is visibly soiled with blood or body fluids should be kept separate and washed separately in hot, sudsy water with household bleach. Prompt diaper changing and perineal care can prevent or minimize diaper rash and promote comfort. The diaper-changing area in the home should be separate from the food preparation and serving areas. The diapers are to be placed in plastic bags, sealed, and disposed of daily. Diaper-changing areas should be cleaned with a 1:10 dilution of household bleach after each diaper change. Toys should be kept as clean as possible, and they should not be shared with other children. Toys should be checked for sharp edges to prevent scratches.

The nurse should instruct parents in what signs of infection to be alert for and when to call their healthcare provider. The inability to feed without pain may indicate esophageal yeast infection and may require administration of nystatin (Mycostatin) for oral thrush. Topical Mycostatin or Desitin ointment is used for diaper rashes and oral Mycostatin for oral thrush. If diarrhea occurs, the baby requires frequent perineal care and fluid replacements. Antidiarrheal medications are often ineffective. Taking rectal temperatures should be avoided, as it may stimulate diarrhea. Fluids, antipyretics, and sponging with tepid water are of use in managing fever. Irritability may be the first sign of fever. Preventive care for exposed infants is the same as for other infants and includes routine immunizations, except that the live polio vaccine should be avoided. If the infant is exposed to varicella, the parents should notify their healthcare professional because the baby may need varicella zoster immune globulin [VZIG] within 96 hours of exposure or if exposed to measles (may need vaccination within 72 hours of exposure).

Parents and family members need to be reassured that there are no documented cases of people contracting HIV/AIDS from

Table 32–6   ISSUES FOR CAREGIVERS OF INFANTS AT RISK FOR HIV/AIDS

Resuscitation	For suctioning use a bulb syringe, mucus extractor, or meconium aspirator with wall suction on low setting. Use masks, goggles, and gloves.	Specimens	Blood and other specimens should be double bagged and/or sealed in an impervious container and labeled according to agency protocol.
Admission care	To remove blood from baby's skin, give warm water-mild soap bath using gloves as soon as possible after admission.	Equipment and linen	Articles contaminated with blood or body fluids should be discarded or bagged according to isolation or institution protocol.
Handwashing	Thorough handwashing is indicated before and after caring for infant. Hands must be washed immediately if contaminated with blood or body fluids. Wash hands after removal of gloves.	Body fluid spills	Blood and body fluids should be cleaned promptly with a solution of 5.25% sodium hypochlorite (household bleach) diluted 1:10 with water. Apply for at least 30 seconds then wipe after the minimum contact time.
Gloves	Gloves are indicated with touching blood or other high-risk fluids. Gloves should also be worn when handling newborns before and during their initial baths, cord care, eye prophylactics, and vitamin K administration.	Education and support	Provide education and psychologic support family and staff. Caregivers who avoid contact with baby at risk or who overdress in unnecessary isolation garb subtly exacerbate an already difficult family situation.
Mask, goggle, and gown	Not routinely needed unless coming in contact with placenta or the blood and amniotic fluid on the skin of the newborn.		Information resources include the National AIDS Hotline (1–800–342–2437) and HIV/AIDS. Treatment Enforcement Service Web http://www.hevatis.org
Needles and syringes	Used needles should not be recapped or bent; they should be disposed of in a puncture-resistant plastic container belonging specifically to that baby. After the newborn is discharged the container is discarded.	Exempted personnel	Immunologically compromised staff (pregnant women may be included in this group) and possibly infectious staff members should not care for these infants.

SOURCE: Adapted from American Academy of Pediatrics, Committee on Pediatric AIDS and Committee on Infectious Diseases. (1999). Issues related to human immunodeficiency transmission in schools child care, medical settings, the home, and community. *Pediatrics, 104*(2), 318–324; Mendez, H., & Jule, J. E. (1990). Care of the infant born exposed to AIDS. *Obstetric and Gynecologic Clinics of North America, 17*(3), 637; Krist, A. H., & Crawford-Faucher, A. (2002). Management of newborns exposed to maternal HIV infection. *American Family Physician, 65*(10), 2049–2056.

routine care of infected babies. Emotional support for the family is essential because of the stress and social isolation they may face. Because of these stresses, parents may not bond with the baby or may fail to provide the baby with enough sensory and tactile stimulation. The nurse should instruct the parents to hold the baby during feedings because the infant will benefit from frequent, gentle touch. Auditory stimulation may also be provided using music or tapes of parents' voices. The nurse should offer information to families about support groups, available counseling, and information resources. Current therapeutic information regarding HIV disease is available to both healthcare providers and families through the AIDS Clinical Trials Information Service (1-800-TRIALS-A). The CDC recommends that HIV-infected women in developed countries not breastfeed because HIV can be transmitted via breast milk. Therefore, if there is a viable alternative feeding method, it should be used (Vankatesh et al., 2006).

Infants of infected mothers should be given antiretroviral drug therapy such as zidovudine (AZT) beginning at 8 to 12 hours of life and continuing for 6 weeks. All infants born to HIV-positive mothers require regular clinical, immunologic, and virologic monitoring. At 1 month of age, the baby's physical examination should include a developmental assessment and a complete blood count, including differential blood count, CD4+ count, and platelet count. Prophylaxis for *Pneumocystis carinii* pneumonia for all infants born to HIV-infected women should be initiated at 4 to 6 weeks of age, regardless of the infant's CD4+ lymphocyte count. Pediatric HIV disease raises many healthcare issues for the family. The parents, depending on their health status, may or may not be able to care for their infant, and they must deal with many psychosocial and economic issues.

Evaluation

Expected outcomes of nursing care include the following:

- The parents are able to bond with their infant and have realistic expectations about the baby.
- Potential opportunistic infections are identified early and treated promptly.
- The parents verbalize their concerns surrounding their baby's existing and potential health problems and accept outside assistance as needed.

CARE OF THE NEWBORN WITH CONGENITAL HEART DEFECT

Congenital heart defects occur in 1% of live births. Because accurate diagnosis and surgical treatment are now available, many deaths can be prevented (American Heart Association, 2005). Corrective cardiac surgery is being done at earlier ages; for example, more than one half of children undergoing surgery are less than 1 year of age, and one fourth are less than 1 month old. It is crucial for the nurse to have comprehensive knowledge of congenital heart disease to detect deviations from normal and to initiate interventions.

Overview of Congenital Heart Defects

In the majority of the cases of congenital heart malformations, the cause is multifactorial with no specific trigger. Other factors that might influence development of congenital heart malformations can be classified as environmental or genetic. Infections of the pregnant woman, such as rubella, cytomegalovirus, coxsackie B, and influenza, have been implicated. Thalidomide, steroids, alcohol, lithium, and some anticonvulsants have been shown to cause malformations of the heart. Seasonal spraying of pesticides has also been linked to an increase in congenital heart defects.

Clinicians are also beginning to see cardiac defects in infants of mothers with phenylketonuria who do not follow their diets. Infants with Down syndrome, Turner's syndrome, Holt-Oram syndrome, trisomy 13, and trisomy 18 frequently have heart lesions. Increased incidence and risk of recurrence of specific defects occur in families.

The common cardiac defects seen in the first 6 days of life are left ventricular outflow obstructions (mitral stenosis, aortic stenosis, or atresia), hypoplastic left heart, coarctation of the aorta, PDA (the most common defect), transposition of the great vessels, tetralogy of Fallot, and large ventricular septal defect or atrial septal defects. Many cardiac defects may not clearly manifest themselves until after discharge from the birthing unit.

CLINICAL TIP

When cyanosis occurs in an otherwise healthy 12- to 24-hour-old newborn displaying no respiratory distress and is unresolved with oxygen, think about a cardiac, especially a ductal-dependent, lesion.

NURSING CARE MANAGEMENT

The primary goals of the neonatal nurse are early identification of cardiac defects and initiation of referral to the physician. The three most common manifestations of cardiac defect are cyanosis, detectable heart murmur, and signs of congestive heart failure (tachycardia, tachypnea, diaphoresis, hepatomegaly, and cardiomegaly). Table 32–7 presents the clinical manifestations and medical/surgical management of these cardiac defects.

Initial repair of heart defects in the newborn period is becoming more commonplace. The NICU staff is now more involved in both the preoperative and postoperative care of cardiac newborns. The benefits for the cardiac infant of being cared for by NICU staff include the staff's knowledge of neonatal anatomy and physiology, experience in supporting the family, and an awareness of the developmental needs of the newborn.

After the baby is stabilized, decisions are made about the special ongoing care needs. The parents need careful and complete explanations and the opportunity to take part in decision making. They also require ongoing emotional support. Families of any baby born with a congenital abnormality need genetic counseling regarding future conception. Parents need to verbalize their concern about their baby's health maintenance and to understand the rationale for follow-up care.

CARE OF THE NEWBORN WITH INBORN ERRORS OF METABOLISM

Inborn errors of metabolism are a group of hereditary disorders that are transmitted by mutant genes. Each causes an enzyme defect that blocks a metabolic pathway and leads to an accumulation of toxic metabolites. Most of the disorders are transmitted by an autosomal recessive gene, requiring two heterozygous parents to produce a homozygous infant with the disorder. Heterozygous parents carrying some inborn errors of metabolism disorders can be identified by special tests, and some inborn errors of metabolism can be detected and treated in utero. Some of the inborn errors of metabolism (especially those associated with mental retardation) are now detected neonatally through newborn screening programs.

Types of Inborn Errors of Metabolism

Phenylketonuria (PKU) is the most common of the group of metabolic errors known as amino acid disorders. Newborn screenings have set its incidence at about 1 in 11,000 live births in the United States; however, the incidence varies considerably among ethnic groups (Kenner & Dreyer, 2000). The highest incidence worldwide is noted in white populations from northern Europe and the United States. It is rarely observed in people of African, Jewish, or Japanese descent.

Phenylalanine is an essential amino acid (found in dietary protein) used by the body for growth, and in the normal individual any excess is converted to tyrosine. The newborn with PKU lacks this converting ability, which results in an accumulation of phenylalanine in the blood. Phenylalanine produces two abnormal metabolites, phenylpyruvic acid and phenylacetic acid, which are eliminated in the urine, producing a musty odor. Excessive accumulation of phenylalanine and its abnormal metabolites in the brain tissue leads to progressive mental retardation.

Maple syrup urine disease (MSUD) is an inborn error of metabolism that, when untreated, is a rapidly progressing and often fatal disease caused by an enzymatic defect in the metabolism of the branched chain amino acids leucine, isoleucine, and valine. Diagnosis of MSUD is made by analyzing blood levels of leucine, isoleucine, and valine. Confirmation of the diagnosis depends on blood assay for the enzyme oxidative decarboxylase.

Homocystinuria is a disorder caused by a deficiency of the enzyme cystathionine β-synthase, which causes an elevated excretion of homocystine and methionine. No symptoms are usually seen in the newborn period. Treatment consists of high doses of vitamin B_6.

Galactosemia is an inborn error of carbohydrate metabolism in which the body is unable to use the sugars galactose and lactose. Enzyme pathways in liver cells normally convert galactose and lactose to glucose. In galactosemia, one step in that conversion pathway is absent, either because of the lack of the enzyme galactose 1-phosphate uridyltransferase or because of the lack of the enzyme galactokinase. High levels of unusable galactose circulate in the blood, causing cataracts, brain damage, and liver damage. There appear to be ethnic differences in age of

Table 32–7	**CARDIAC DEFECTS OF THE EARLY NEWBORN PERIOD**	
Congenital Heart Defect	**Clinical Findings**	**Medical/Surgical Management**

Increased Pulmonary Blood Flow

Patent ductus arteriosus (PDA) ↑ in females, maternal rubella, RDS, less than 1500 g preterm newborns, high-altitude births 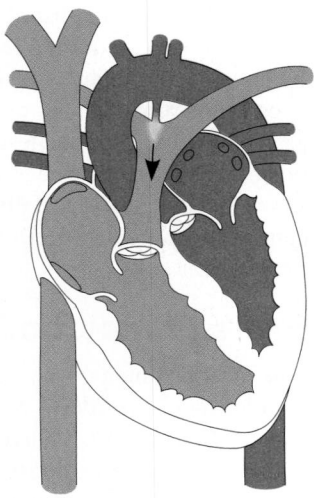	Harsh grade 2–3 machinery murmur upper left sternal border (LSB) just beneath clavicle ↑ difference between systolic and diastolic pulse pressure Can lead to right heart failure and pulmonary congestion ↑ left atrial (LA) and left ventricular (LV) enlargement, dilated ascending aorta ↑ pulmonary vascularity	Indomethacin—0.2 mg/kg IV (prostaglandin inhibitor) 3 doses; one every 12 hours Surgical ligation, occlusion coil Use of O₂ therapy and blood transfusion to improve tissue oxygenation and perfusion Fluid restriction and diuretics

The patent ductus arteriosus is a vascular connection that, during fetal life, short-circuits the pulmonary vasuclar bed and directs blood from the pulmonary artery to the aorta. Postnatally, blood shunts through the ductus from the aorta to the pulmonary artery.

SOURCE: Used with permission: Clinical Education Series No. 7: Columbus, Ohio: Ross Product Division, Abbott Laboratories.

Atrial septal defect (ASD) ↑ in females and Down syndrome	Initially frequently asymptomatic Systolic murmur second left intercostal space (LICS) With large ASD, diastolic rumbling murmur lower left sternal (LLS) border Failure to thrive, upper respiratory infection (URI), poor exercise tolerance	Surgical closure with patch or suture Umbrella occluder
Ventricular septal defect (VSD) ↑ in males	Initially asymptomatic until end of first month or large enough to cause pulmonary edema Loud, blowing systolic murmur between the third and fourth intercostal space (ICS) pulmonary blood flow Right ventricular hypertrophy Rapid respirations, growth failure, feeding difficulties Congestive right heart failure at 6 weeks–2 months of age	Follow medically—some spontaneously close Use of Lanoxin and diuretics in congestive heart failure (CHF) Surgical closure with Dacron patch or umbrella occluder

Obstruction to Systemic Blood Flow

Coarctation of aorta Can be preductal or postductal 	Absent or diminished femoral pulses Increased brachial pulses Late systolic murmur left intrascapular area Systolic BP in lower extremities Enlarged left ventricle Can present in CHF at 7–21 days of life	Surgical resection of narrowed portion of aorta Prostaglandin E₁ to maintain peripheral perfusion No afterload reducer drugs

Coarctation of the aorta is characterized by a narrowed aortic lumen. The lesion produces an obstruction to the flow of blood through the aorta, causing an increased left ventricular pressure and workload.

SOURCE: Used with permission: Clinical Education Series No. 7: Columbus, Ohio: Ross Product Division, Abbott Laboratories.

Table 32–7   CARDIAC DEFECTS OF THE EARLY NEWBORN PERIOD   continued

Congenital Heart Defect	Clinical Findings	Medical/Surgical Management
Hypoplastic left heart syndrome	Normal at birth—cyanosis and shocklike congestive heart failure develop within a few hours to days Soft systolic murmur just left of the sternum Diminished pulses Aortic and/or mitral atresia Tiny, thick-walled left ventricle Large, dilated, hypertrophied right ventricle X-ray examination: cardiac enlargement and pulmonary venous congestion	PGE₁ until decision made Norwood procedure Transplant

Decreased Pulmonary Blood Flow

Congenital Heart Defect	Clinical Findings	Medical/Surgical Management
Tetralogy of Fallot (Most common cyanotic heart defect) Pulmonary stenosis Ventricular septal defect (VSD) Overriding aorta Right ventricular hypertrophy 	May be cyanotic at birth or within first few months of life Harsh systolic murmur LSB Crying or feeding increases cyanosis and respiratory distress X-ray: boot-shaped appearance secondary to small pulmonary artery Right ventricular enlargement	Prevention of dehydration, intercurrent infections Alleviation of paroxysmal dyspneic attacks Palliative surgery to increase blood flow to the lungs Corrective surgery—resection of pulmonic stenosis, closure of VSD with Dacron patch

In tetralogy of Fallot, the severity of symptoms depends on the degree of pulmonary stenosis, the size of the ventricular septal defect, and the degree to which the aorta overrides the septal defect.

SOURCE: Used with permission: Clinical Education Series No. 7: Columbus, Ohio: Ross Products Division, Abbott Laboratories.

Mixed Defects*

Congenital Heart Defect	Clinical Findings	Medical/Surgical Management
Transposition of great vessels (TGA) (↑ females, IDMs, LGAs) 	Cyanosis at birth or within 3 days Possible pulmonic stenosis murmur Right ventricular hypertrophy Polycythemia "Egg on its side" x-ray finding	Prostaglandin E to vasodilate ductus to keep it open Initial surgery to create opening between right and left side of heart if none exists Total surgical repair—usually the arterial switch procedure—done within first few days of life

Complete transposition of great vessels is an embryologic defect caused by a straight division of the bulbar trunk without normal spiraling. As a result, the aorta originates from the right ventricle, and the pulmonary artery from the left ventricle. An abnormal communication between the two circulations must be present to sustain life.

SOURCE: Used with permission: Clinical Education Series No. 7: Columbus, Ohio: Ross Products Division, Abbott Laboratories.

SOURCE: Illustrations from *Congenital Heart Abnormalities*. Clinical Education Aid No. 7, Ross Laboratories, Columbus, OH.
*NOTE: Mixed defects-postnatal survival is dependent upon mixing of systemic and pulmonary blood flow.

onset of symptoms and in severity of course. Caucasians have more severe symptoms and earlier onset (3 to 14 days) than people of African descent (14 to 28 days).

Another disorder frequently included in mandatory newborn blood screening tests is *congenital hypothyroidism (CH)*. An inborn enzymatic defect, lack of maternal dietary iodine, or maternal ingestion of drugs that depress or destroy thyroid tissue can cause CH.

The incidence of metabolic errors is relatively low, but for affected infants and their families these disorders pose a threat to survival and frequently require lifelong treatment.

Clinical Therapy

All states have universal screening of newborns for PKU and CH (Matthews & Robin, 2002). Mandatory newborn screening for other inborn errors of metabolism, including homocystinuria, MSUD, galactosemia, sickle cell anemia, and congentital adrenal hypoplasia, varies among states. In several states newborn screening includes an enzyme assay for galactose 1-phosphate uridyltransferase; however, this test does not detect galactosemia if it is caused by a deficiency of the enzyme galactokinase.

Identification via newborn screening and early clinical intervention for inborn errors of metabolism becomes more difficult with the advent of early discharge of newborns. If the initial specimen is obtained before 24 hours of age, then a second specimen should be obtained before 5 days of age (Zinn, 2002). Early collection of specimens may yield false-positive results for certain metabolic disorders. Conversely, certain metabolic disorders may go undetected. Newborns in the NICU who require interhospital transfers and early-discharged healthy newborns are at risk for nonscreening. Newborn screen specimens are always collected before a blood transfusion.

NURSING CARE MANAGEMENT

The nurse assesses the newborn for signs of inborn errors of metabolism and carries out state-mandated newborn testing. Parents of affected newborns should be referred to support groups. The nurse should also ensure that parents are informed about centers that can provide them with information about biochemical genetics and dietary management.

Infant with PKU

The clinical picture of a PKU baby involves a normal-appearing newborn, most often with blond hair, blue eyes, and fair complexion. Decreased pigmentation may be related to the competition between phenylalanine and tyrosine for the available enzyme tyrosinase. Tyrosine is needed for the formation of melanin pigment and the hormones epinephrine and thyroxine. Without treatment, the infant fails to thrive and develops vomiting and eczematous rashes. By about 6 months of age, the infant exhibits behavior indicative of mental retardation and other CNS involvement, including seizures and abnormal electroencephalogram (EEG) patterns.

The Guthrie blood test for PKU is required for all newborns before discharge. The Guthrie test uses a drop of blood collected from a heel stick and placed on filter paper. It should be done at least 24 hours after the initiation of feedings containing the usual amounts of breast milk or formula so its metabolites begin to build up in the baby with PKU once milk feedings are initiated. High-risk newborns should be receiving a 60% milk intake, with no more than 40% of their total intake coming from nonprotein IV fluids. The PKU testing of high-risk newborns should be deferred for at least 48 hours after hyperalimentation is initiated. It is vital that the parents understand the need for the screening procedure, and a follow-up check is necessary to confirm that the test was done.

The nurse advises parents that once identified, an afflicted PKU infant can be treated by a special diet that limits ingestion of phenylalanine. Special formulas low in phenylalanine, such as Lofenalac, Minafen, and Albumaid XP, are available. Special food lists are helpful for parents of a PKU child (Blackburn, 2003). If treatment is begun before 1 month of age, CNS damage can be minimized. There is an increased risk of producing a child with mental retardation if the mother with PKU is not on a low-phenylalanine diet during pregnancy. It is recommended that the woman reinstate her low-phenylalanine diet a few months before becoming pregnant (Blackburn, 2003).

Infant with MSUD

Newborns with MSUD have feeding problems and neurologic signs (seizures, spasticity, opisthotonos) during the first week of life. A maple syrup odor of the urine is noted, and when ferric chloride is added to the urine, its color changes to gray-green. An ear swab within 6 to 12 hours after birth has a similar smell (Robinson & Drumm, 2001). Diagnosis is confirmed with plasma amino acid analysis.

Newborns with MSUD must be given a formula that is low in the branched-chain amino acids leucine, isoleucine, and valine. This diet must be continued indefinitely. Dietary treatment before 12 days of life has been reported to result in normal intelligence.

Infant with Homocystinuria

Homocystinuria varies in its presentation, but the more common characteristics are skeletal abnormalities, dislocation of ocular lenses, intravascular thromboses, and mental retardation. Abnormalities occur because of the toxic effects of the accumulation of methionine and the metabolite homocystine in the blood.

Infants with homocystinuria are managed on a diet that is low in methionine but supplemented with cystine and pyridoxine (vitamin B_6). Early diagnosis and careful management may prevent mental retardation.

Infant with Galactosemia

Clinical manifestations of galactosemia include vomiting soon after ingestion of milk-based formula or breast milk, diarrhea, poor weight gain, hepatosplenomegaly, jaundice, and mental retardation. The condition is frequently associated with anemia, sepsis, and cataracts in the newborn period (Zinn, 2002). Except for cataracts and mental retardation, those findings are reversible when galactose is excluded from the diet. Mental retardation can be prevented by early diagnosis and careful dietary management.

A baby with galactosemia is placed on a galactose-free diet. Galactose-free formulas include Nutramigen (a protein hydrolysate process formula), meat-based formulas, or soybean formulas. As the infant grows, parents must be educated not only to avoid giving their child milk and milk products but also to read all labels carefully and avoid any foods containing dry milk products. Even with early treatment, children may have learning disabilities, speech problems, and female ovarian failure (Zinn, 2002).

Infant with Congenital Hypothyroidism (CH)

A large tongue, umbilical hernia, cool and mottled skin, low hairline, hypotonia, and large fontanelles (especially the posterior fontanelle in term infants) are frequently associated with congenital hypothyroidism. Early symptoms include prolonged newborn jaundice, poor feeding, constipation, low-pitched cry, poor weight gain, inactivity, and delayed motor development. In addition, premature infants of less than 30 weeks' gestation frequently have lower T4 and thyroid-stimulating hormone (TSH) values than those of term infants. This difference may reflect the premature infant's inability to bind thyroid hormone and a risk for hypothyroidism.

Babies with CH need frequent laboratory monitoring and adjustment of thyroid medication to accommodate their growth and development. With adequate treatment, children remain free of symptoms, but if the condition is untreated, stunted growth and mental retardation occur.

Evaluation

Expected outcomes of nursing care include the following:

- The risk of inborn errors of metabolism is promptly identified, and early intervention is initiated.

- The parents verbalize their concerns about their baby's nutritional status, health problems, long-term care needs, and potential outcomes.

- The parents are aware of available community health resources and use them as indicated.

CHAPTER REVIEW

FOCUS YOUR STUDY

- Early identification of potential high-risk fetuses through assessment of preconception, prenatal, and intrapartal factors facilitates strategically timed nursing observations and interventions.

- High-risk newborns, whether they are premature, SGA, LGA, postterm, or infants of a diabetic or substance-abusing mother, have many similar problems, although their problems are based on different physiologic processes.

- SGA newborns are associated with perinatal asphyxia and resulting aspiration syndrome, hypothermia, hypoglycemia, hypocalcemia, polycythemia, congenital anomalies, and intrauterine infections. Long-term problems include continued growth and learning difficulties.

- LGA newborns are at risk for birth trauma as a result of cephalopelvic disproportion, hypoglycemia, polycythemia, and hyperviscosity.

- Infants of diabetic mothers are at risk for hypoglycemia, hypocalcemia, hyperbilirubinemia, polycythemia, and respiratory distress due to delayed maturation of their lungs.

- Postterm newborns often encounter intrapartal problems such as CPD, shoulder dystocia, and birth traumas, hypoglycemia, polycythemia, meconium aspiration, cold stress, and possible seizure activity. Long-term complications may involve poor weight gain and low IQ scores.

- The common problems of the preterm newborn are results of the baby's immature body systems. Potential problem areas include respiratory distress (RDS), PDA, hypothermia and cold stress, feeding difficulties and NEC, marked insensible water loss and loss of buffering agents through the kidneys, infection, anemia of prematurity, apnea and IVH, retinopathy of prematurity, and behavioral state disorganization. Long-term needs and problems include bronchopulmonary dysplasia, speech defects, sensorineural hearing loss, and neurologic defects.

- Newborns of alcohol-dependent mothers are at risk for alterations in physical characteristics and the long-term complications of feeding problems; CNS dysfunction, including lower IQ, hyperactivity, and language abnormalities; and congenital anomalies.

- Newborns of drug-dependent mothers experience drug withdrawal as well as respiratory distress, jaundice, congenital anomalies, and behavioral abnormalities. With early recognition and intervention, the potential long-term physiologic and emotional consequences of these difficulties can be avoided or at least lessened in severity.

- Newborns of mothers with AIDS require early recognition and treatment so that the physiologic and emotional consequences may be lessened in severity and CDC guidelines implemented.

- Cardiac defects are a significant cause of morbidity and mortality in the newborn period. Early identification and nursing and medical care of newborns with cardiac defects are essential to the improved outcome of these infants. Care is directed toward lessening the workload of the heart and decreasing oxygen and energy consumption.

- Inborn errors of metabolism such as galactosemia, PKU, homocystinuria, and MSUD are usually included in a newborn screening program designed to prevent mental retardation through dietary management and medication.

- The nursing care of the newborn with special problems involves understanding normal physiology, the pathophysiology of the disease process, clinical manifestations, and supportive or corrective therapies. Only with this theoretical background can the nurse make appropriate observations concerning responses to therapy and development of complications.

- The nurse facilitates interdisciplinary communication with the parents. Parents of at-risk newborns need support from nurses and healthcare providers to understand the special needs of their baby and feel confident in their ability to care for their baby at home.

EXPLORE MediaLink

http://www.prenhall.com/davidson

NCLEX review questions, case studies, and other interactive resources for this chapter can be found on the Web Site at http://www.prenhall.com/davidson. Click on "Chapter 32" to select the activities for this chapter.

For tutorials including animations and videos, more NCLEX review questions, and an audio glossary, access the accompanying Prentice Hall Nursing MediaLink DVD-ROM in this book.

PRENTICE HALL NURSING MEDIALINK DVD-ROM

Audio Glossary

NCLEX Review

Video: *Through the Eyes of a Nurse—Welcoming the New Arrival at the Postpartal Visit*

COMPANION WEBSITE

Additional NCLEX Review

Case Study: *Infant with Postmaturity Syndrome*

Care Plan Activity: *Infant of a Diabetic Mother*

Applications: *Care of the Preterm Infant; Congenital Defects*

Critical Thinking

CRITICAL THINKING IN ACTION

BIRTH OF AN ILL OR AT-RISK INFANT

View the Critical Thinking in Action video in Chapter 32 of the DVD-ROM. Then answer the questions that follow.

As the nurse on duty, you are caring for baby Erin, a 38-week IDM female born by repeat cesarean birth to a 32-year-old G3 now P3 mother. Erin's Apgar scores are 7 and 9 at 1 and 5 minutes. At 2 hours of age, the baby has an elevated respiratory rate of 100 to 110, heart rate of 165 with Grade II/VI intermittent machinery murmur, and mild cyanosis. She is now receiving 30% oxygen and has a respiratory rate of 70 to 80. The baby's clinical course, chest

x-ray, and lab results are all consistent with transient tachypnea of the newborn and patent ductus arteriosus. The mother calls you to ask about how her baby is doing. She tells you that her last child was born at 30 weeks and had to be hospitalized for 6 weeks. She says, "I really tried to do it right this time," and asks you if this baby will have the same respiratory problem.

1. What should you tell the mother?

2. What can you do to facilitate mother–infant attachment?

3. Discuss the emotional response of parents to the birth of an ill or at-risk infant. (See Chapter 33 ∞ for additional information).

4. Discuss the four psychologic tasks essential for coping with the stress of an at-risk newborn and providing a basis for the maternal-infant relationship. (See Chapter 33 ∞).

5. Baby Erin is being discharged tomorrow. Review the elements of discharge and home care instructions.

REFERENCES

Als, H., & Lawhon, G. (2004). Theoretic perspective for developmentally supportive care. In C. Kenner & J. M. McGrath (Eds.), *Developmental care of newborns & infants: A guide for health professionals*. St. Louis: Elsevier Mosby.

Als, H., Lester, B. M., Tronick, E., & Brazelton, T. B. (1982). Assessment of preterm infant behavior (APIB). In B. M. Fitzgerald Lester & M. W. Yogman (Eds.), *Theory and research in behavioral pediatrics* (Vol. 1). New York: Plenum.

American Academy of Pediatrics (AAP) Committee on Pediatric AIDS and Committee on Infectious Diseases. (1999). Issues related to human immunodeficiency virus transmission in schools, child care, medical settings, the home, and community. *Pediatrics, 104*(2), 318–324.

American Academy of Pediatrics (AAP) & American College of Obstetricians and Gynecologists (ACOG). (2002). *Guidelines for perinatal care* (5th ed.). Elk Grove Village, IL: Author.

American Heart Association. (2005). *Congenital cardiovascular disease statistics*. Retrieved October 21, 2005, from http://www.americanheart.org/children

Andres, R. L. (2004). Effects of therapeutic, diagnostics and environmental agents and exposure to social and illicit drugs. In R. K. Creasy & R. Resnik (Eds.), *Maternal-fetal medicine: Principles and practice* (5th ed., pp. 281–305). Philadelphia: Saunders.

Association of Women's Health, Obstetric, and Neonatal Nurses (AWHONN). (2001). *Evidence-based clinical practice guidelines. Neonatal skin care*. Washington, DC: Author.

Beachy, J. M. (2003). Premature infant massage in the NICU. *Neonatal Network, 22*(3), 39–45.

Beauman, S. (2005). Identification and management of neonatal abstinence syndrome. *Journal of Infusion Nursing, 28*(3), 159–167.

Blackburn, S. (2003). *Maternal-fetal-neonatal physiology: A clinical perspective* (2nd ed.). Philadelphia: Saunders.

Bowie, B., Hall, R., Faulkner, J., & Anderson, B. (2003). Single-room infant care: Future trends in special care nursery planning and design. *Neonatal Network, 22*(3), 27–34.

Centers for Disease Control and Prevention (CDC), National Center for Chronic Disease Prevention and Health Promotion. (2005). *Pattern of tobacco use among women and girls: Fact sheet*. Retrieved January 31, 2005, from http://www.cdc.gov/tobacco/sgr_forwomen/factsheet_tabaccouse.htm

Chmait, R., & Moore, T. R. (2005). Endrocrine disorders in pregnancy. In H. W. Taeusch, R. A. Ballard, & C. A. Gleason (Eds.), *Avery's disease of the newborn* (8th ed., pp. 71–86). Philadelphia: Saunders.

Crosson, D., & Pickler, R. (2004). An integrated review of the literature on demand feedings for the preterm infant. *Advances in Neonatal Care, 4*(4), 216–225.

Eichel, P. (2001). Kangaroo care: Expanding our practice to critically ill neonates. *Newborn and Infant Nursing Reviews, 1*(4), 224–228.

Greene, C., & Goodman, M. (2003). Neonatal abstinence syndrome: Strategies for care of the drug-exposed infant. *Neonatal Network, 22*(4), 15–24.

Harrison, L. (2001). The use of comforting touch and massage to reduce stress for preterm infants in the neonatal intensive care unit. *Newborn and Infant Nursing Reviews, 1*(4), 235–241.

Jones, M. (2003). Fetal alcohol syndrome. *Neonatal Network, 22*(3), 63–69.

Jones, J., Kassity, N., & Duncan, K. (2001). Complementary care: Alternatives for the neonatal intensive care unit. *Newborn and Infant Nursing Reviews, 1*(4), 207–210.

Kenner, C., & Dreyer, L. A. (2000). Prenatal and neonatal testing and screening: A double-edged sword. *Nursing Clinics of North America, 35*(3), 627–641.

Kledzik, T. (2005). Holding the very low birth weight infant: Skin-to-skin techniques. *Neonatal Network, 24*(1), 7–14.

Law, K. L., Stroud, L. R., LaGasse, L. L., Niaura, R., Liu, J., & Lester, B. M. (2003). Smoking during pregnancy and newborn neurobehavior. *Pediatrics, 111*(6), 1318–1332.

Martinez, A., Partridge, J. C., & Taeusch, H. W. (2005). Perinatal substance abuse. In H. W. Taeusch, R. A. Ballard, & C. A. Gleason (Eds.), *Avery's disease of the newborn* (8th ed., pp. 106–126). Philadelphia: Saunders.

Martinez, A., & Simmons, R. (2005). Abnormalities of fetal growth. In H. W. Taeusch, R. A. Ballard, & C. A. Gleason (Eds.), *Avery's disease of the newborn* (8th ed., pp. 32–45). Philadelphia: Saunders.

Matthews, A. L., & Robin, N. H. (2002). Genetic disorders, malformations, and inborn errors of metabolism. In G. B. Merenstein & S. L. Gardner (Eds.), *Handbook of neonatal intensive care* (5th ed., pp. 679–701). St. Louis, MO: Mosby.

McCarthy, J., Leamon, M., Parr, M., & Anamia, B. (2005). High-dose methadone maintenance in pregnancy: Maternal and neonatal outcomes. *American Journal of Obstetrics & Gynecology, 193*, 606–610.

McGuire, W., & McEwan, P. (2004). Systematic review of transpyloric versus gastric tube feeding

for preterm infants. *Archives of Disease in Childhood Fetal Neonatal Edition, 89*(3), 245–248.

Moore, T. R. (2004). Diabetes in pregnancy. In R. K. Creasy & R. Resnik (Eds.), *Maternal-fetal medicine: Principles and practice* (5th ed., pp. 1023–1061). Philadelphia: Saunders.

Moran, B. A. (2004). Substance abuse in pregnancy. In S. Mattson & J. E. Smith (Eds.), *Core curriculum for maternal-newborn nursing* (3rd ed., pp. 750–770). St. Louis, MO: Elsevier Saunders.

Resnik, J. L., & Resnik, R. (2004). Post-term pregnancy. In R. K. Creasy & R. Resnik (Eds.), *Maternal-fetal medicine: Principles and practice* (5th ed., pp. 663–669). Philadelphia: Saunders.

Resnik, R., & Creasy, R. K. (2004). Intrauterine growth restriction. In R. K. Creasy & R. Resnik (Eds.), *Maternal-fetal medicine: Principles and practice* (5th ed., pp. 495–512). Philadelphia: Saunders.

Robinson, D., & Drumm, L. (2001). Maple syrup disease: A standard of nursing care. *Pediatric Nursing, 27*(3), 255–264, 270.

Saari, T. N., & Committee on Infectious Diseases. (2003). Immunization of preterm and low birth weight infants. *Pediatrics, 112*(1), 193–198.

Smith, J. R. (2005). Early enteral feeding for the very low birth weight infant: The development and impact of a research-based guideline. *Neonatal Network, 24*(4), 9–17.

Standley, J. M. (2001). Music therapy for the neonate. *Newborn and Infant Nursing Reviews, 1*(4), 211–216.

Thoyre, S. M., Shaker, C. S., & Pridham, K. F. (2005). The early feeding skills assessment for preterm infants. *Neonatal Network, 24*(3), 7–14.

Thureen, P. J., Deacon, J., Hernandez, J., & Hall, D. M. (2005). *Assessment and care of the well newborn*. St. Louis, MO: Elsevier Saunders.

Turnage-Carrier, C. S. (2004). Caregiving and the environment. In C. Kenner & J. M. McGrath (Eds.), *Developmental care of newborns & infants: A guide for health professionals*. St. Louis, MO: Elsevier Mosby.

Venkatesh, M., Merestein, G. B., Adams, K. M., & Weisman, L. E. (2006). Infection in the neonate. In G. B. Merenstein & S. L. Gardner (Eds.), *Handbook of neonatal intensive care* (6th ed., pp. 569–593). St. Louis, MO: Mosby.

Volpe, J. J. (2001). *Neurology of the newborn*. Philadelphia: Saunders.

Zinn, A. B. (2002). Inborn errors of metabolism. In A. A. Fanaroff & R. J. Martin (Eds.), *Neonatal-perinatal medicine: Diseases of the fetus and infant* (7th ed., pp. 1468–1516). St. Louis, MO: Mosby.

CHAPTER
33
The Newborn at Risk: Birth-Related Stressors

I watched her breathe every precious breath on the respirator. I saw her covered with wires and tubes. I kept watch. She was special to me and I would tell her over and over, "Daddy is here. Daddy loves you." The three days she lived were hell—not knowing if she would make it, uncertain about what plans we should make. Somehow I thought she would live; I was hopeful. When she died, at least I was there with her. The grief was unbearable. But there was also a sense of relief. The uncertainty, the waiting were finally over.

~ Susan Borg, When Pregnancy Fails *~*

KEY TERMS

Bilirubin encephalopathy   1009
Bronchopulmonary dysplasia (BPD)/chronic lung disease of prematurity (CLD)   1002
Cold stress   1004
Erythroblastosis fetalis   1009
Hemolytic disease of the newborn   1009
Hyperbilirubinemia   1009
Hypoglycemia   1005
Jaundice   1008
Kernicterus   1009

Meconium aspiration syndrome (MAS)   998
Persistent pulmonary hypertension of the newborn (PPHN)   1000
Phototherapy   1011
Physiologic anemia of infancy   1021
Polycythemia   1021
Respiratory distress syndrome (RDS)   988
Sepsis neonatorum   1022

OBJECTIVES

1. Discuss how to identify infants in need of resuscitation and the appropriate method of resuscitation based on the antepartal/labor record and physiologic indicators apparent at birth.

2. Based on clinical manifestations, differentiate among the various types of respiratory distress (respiratory distress syndrome, transient tachypnea of the newborn, meconium aspiration syndrome, and persistent pulmonary hypertension) in the newborn and the nursing care related to each type.

3. Discuss selected metabolic abnormalities (including cold stress and hypoglycemia), their effects on the newborn, and their nursing implications.

4. Differentiate between physiologic and pathologic jaundice according to timing of onset (in hours), cause, possible sequelae, and specific management.

5. Explain how Rh incompatibility or ABO incompatibility can lead to the development of hyperbilirubinemia.

6. Identify the nursing responsibilities in caring for the newborn receiving phototherapy.

7. Discuss selected hematologic problems such as anemia and polycythemia and the nursing implications associated with each.

8. Describe the nursing assessment that would lead the nurse to suspect newborn sepsis.

9. Relate the consequences of selected maternally transmitted infections, such as maternal syphilis, gonorrhea, herpesviridae family (HSV or CMV), and chlamydia, to the management of the infant in the neonatal period.

10. Describe interventions to facilitate parental attachment with the at-risk newborn.

11. Identify the special initial and long-term needs of parents of at-risk infants.

 MEDIALINK

Additional resources for this content can be found on the Prentice Hall Nursing MediaLink DVD-ROM and on the Companion Website at http://www.prenhall.com/davidson. Click on "Chapter 33" to select the activities for this chapter.

Marked homeostatic changes occur during the transition from fetal to newborn life. The most rapid anatomic and physiologic changes of this period occur in the cardiopulmonary system. Thus the major problems of the newborn are usually related to this system. These problems include asphyxia, respiratory distress syndrome (RDS), cold stress, jaundice, hemolytic disease, and anemia. Ideally, problems are anticipated and identified prenatally, some treatment may be initiated in the prenatal period, and appropriate intervention measures are begun at or immediately after birth.

CARE OF THE NEWBORN AT RISK DUE TO ASPHYXIA

Neonatal asphyxia occurs in 1% to 1.5% of live births, and the incidence increases as the gestational age decreases (Cloherty, Eichenwald, & Stark, 2004). Newborn asphyxia results from circulatory, respiratory, and biochemical factors. Circulatory patterns that accompany asphyxia indicate an inability to make the transition to extrauterine circulation—in effect, a return to fetal circulatory patterns. Failure of lung expansion and establishment of respiration rapidly produces serious biochemical changes, including hypoxemia (decreased oxygen in blood), metabolic acidosis (increased acidity of blood reflected by low pH), and hypercapnia (excess levels of carbon dioxide in the blood) (Leuthner & Das, 2004).

These biochemical changes result in pulmonary vasoconstriction and high pulmonary vascular resistance in relation to the lower systemic vascular resistance (following birth the pulmonary vascular resistance should be markedly lower than the systemic vascular resistance), hypoperfusion of the lungs, and a large right-to-left shunt through the ductus arteriosus, bypassing the lungs and impeding oxygenation of the blood. As right atrial pressure exceeds left atrial pressure, the foramen ovale reopens, and blood flows from right to left. See Chapter 28 ∞ for review of normal newborn cardiopulmonary adaptation.

However, the most serious biochemical abnormality caused by hypoxia is a change from aerobic to anaerobic metabolism. This change results in the buildup of lactate, combining with hydrogen to form lactic acid, and subsequently developing metabolic acidosis. Lactic acidosis can develop after prolonged tissue hypoxia (oxygen starvation) as active cells rely on anaerobic metabolism.

Simultaneously, respiratory acidosis may also occur in response to a rapid increase in carbon dioxide (PCO_2) during asphyxia. In response to hypoxia and anaerobic metabolism, the amounts of free fatty acids (FFA) and glycerol in the blood increase. Glycogen stores are mobilized to provide a continuous glucose source for the brain. Hepatic and cardiac stores of glycogen may be used up rapidly during an asphyxial attack.

The newborn has several protective mechanisms against hypoxic insults. These include a relatively immature brain and a resting metabolic rate lower than that observed in the adult, an ability to mobilize substances within the body for anaerobic metabolism and to use the energy more efficiently, and an intact circulatory system able to redistribute lactate and hydrogen ions in tissues still being perfused. Unfortunately, the body's stores of glycogen may be used up rapidly during an asphyxia attack. Severe prolonged hypoxia will overcome these protective mechanisms, resulting in brain damage or death of the newborn. The newborn suffering apnea requires immediate resuscitative efforts. The need for resuscitation can be anticipated if specific risk factors are present during the pregnancy or labor and birth period.

Risk Factors Predisposing to Asphyxia

The need for resuscitation may be anticipated if the mother demonstrates the antepartal and intrapartal risk factors described in Tables 15–1 ∞ and 23–1. ∞ Fetal/neonatal risk factors are as follows (Cloherty et al., 2004; Dildy, 2005; Gomella, Cunningham, Eyal et al., 2004; Thureen, Deacon, Hernandez et al., 2005):

- Nonreassuring fetal heart rate (FHR) pattern/sustained bradycardia
- Difficult birth, prolonged labor
- Fetal scalp/capillary blood sample-acidosis pH less than 7.2
- History of meconium in amniotic fluid
- Prematurity
- Macrosomia
- Male infant
- Small for gestational age
- Multiple births
- Significant intrapartum bleeding
- Structural lung abnormality/oligohydramnios (congenital diaphragmatic hernia, lung hypoplasia)
- Gastrointestinal obstruction/polyhydramnios
- Congenital heart disease
- Maternal infection/sepsis with cardiovascular collapse
- Narcotic use in labor
- Infant of a diabetic mother
- Arrhythmias
- Cardiomyopathy
- Anemia: isoimmunization, fetal-maternal hemorrhage, parvovirus

Risk factors are not always apparent prenatally. Particular attention must be paid to all at-risk pregnancies during the intrapartal period. Certain aspects of labor and birth challenge the oxygen supply to the fetus, and often the at-risk fetus has less tolerance to the stress of labor (indicated by decelerations or lack of variability of the FHR) and birth.

Clinical Therapy

The initial goal of clinical management is to identify the fetus at risk for asphyxia so that resuscitative efforts can begin at birth.

Fetal biophysical assessment (see Chapter 21 ∞) combined with monitoring of fetal pH, FHRs, and fetal oximetry if available during the intrapartal period may help identify the presence of nonreassuring fetal status. If nonreassuring fetal status is present, appropriate measures can be taken to deliver the fetus immediately, before major damage occurs, and to treat the asphyxiated newborn.

The fetal biophysical profile enhances the ability to predict an abnormal perinatal outcome. In addition, fetal scalp blood sampling may indicate asphyxic insult and the degree of fetal acidosis, when considered in relation to the stage of labor, uterine contractions, and nonreassuring FHR patterns. The stress of labor causes an intermittent decrease in exchange of gases in the placental intervillous space, which causes the fall in pH and fetal acidosis. The acidosis is primarily metabolic.

During labor a fetal pH of 7.25 or higher is considered normal (nonacidemia). A pH value of 7.2 or less is considered an ominous sign of intrauterine asphyxia (acidemia), and a pH of less than 7 is considered pathologic acidemia (Dildy, 2005). However, low fetal pH without associated hypoxia can be caused by maternal acidosis resulting from prolonged labor, dehydration, and maternal lactate production.

Assessment of the newborn's need for resuscitation begins at the time of birth. The nurse should note the time of the first gasp, first cry, and onset of sustained respirations in order of occurrence. The Apgar score (see information in Chapter 24 ∞) may be helpful in determining the severity of the neonatal depression and may be predictive of neonatal survival (de Ungria & Steinhorn, 2003; Fanaroff, Martin, & Rodriguez, 2004; Leuthner & Das, 2004). Initial well-being of the fetus/newborn is best analyzed using the umbilical arterial blood sample (Dildy, 2005).

The treatment of fetal or newborn asphyxia is resuscitation. Resuscitative efforts are required by 10% of all newborns (Hermansen & Hermansen, 2005). The goals of resuscitation are to provide an adequate airway with expansion of the lungs, to decrease the PCO_2 and increase the PO_2, to support adequate cardiac output, and to minimize oxygen consumption by reducing heat loss.

RESUSCITATION MANAGEMENT

Initial resuscitative management of the newborn is extremely important. Suctioning is always performed before resuscitation so that the mucus, blood, or meconium is not aspirated into the lungs. Caregivers should keep the newborn in a head-down position before the first gasp to avoid aspiration of the oropharynx secretions and must suction the oropharynx and nasopharynx immediately. Clearing the nasal and oral passages of obstructive fluids, with a bulb syringe or suction catheter attached to low continuous suction, establishes a patent airway.

After the first few breaths, the nurse places the newborn in a level position under a radiant heat source and dries the baby quickly with warm blankets to maintain skin temperature at about 36.5C (97.7F). The stable newborn may be placed on the mother's chest or abdomen "skin to skin" as another heat source (American Academy of Pediatrics [AAP] & American College of Obstetricians and Gynecologists [ACOG], 2002). The extremely preterm newborn may be covered with a plastic wrap or placed in a plastic bag up to the neck to attempt to prevent evaporative heat loss under the radiant warmer (Gomella et al., 2004). Drying is also a good stimulus for breathing. Heat loss through evaporation is tremendous during the first few minutes of life. The temperature of a wet 1500-g baby in a cold room (16C [62F]) drops 1C every 3 minutes. Hypothermia increases oxygen consumption. In an asphyxiated infant, it increases the hypoxic insult and may lead to severe acidosis and development of respiratory distress.

Breathing is established by employing the simplest form of resuscitative measures initially, with progression to more complicated methods, as required, for example:

1. Position and clear airway as necessary. Simple stimulation is provided by rubbing the back with a blanket or towel, while simultaneously drying the baby.

2. If respirations have not been initiated or are inadequate (gasping or occasional respirations), the lungs must be inflated with positive pressure. The proper sized mask is positioned securely on the face (over the nose and mouth, avoiding the eyes) with the head in the "sniffing" or neutral position (Figure 33–1 ◆). Hyperextension of the infant's neck will obstruct the trachea and must be avoided. An airtight connection is made between the baby's face and the mask (thus allowing the bag to inflate). The lungs are inflated rhythmically by squeezing the bag. Oxygen can be delivered at 100% with an anesthesia bag with manometer or modified self-inflating bag and adequate liter flow of at least 8 L/min. The self-inflating (Ambu or Hope) bag delivers only 40% oxygen unless it has been adapted with an attached oxygen reservoir (Cloherty et al., 2004). It may not be possible to maintain adequate inspiratory pressure with Ambu or

Figure 33–1 ◆ Demonstration of resuscitation of an infant with bag and mask. Note that the mask covers the nose and mouth and that the head is in a neutral position. The resuscitation bag is placed to the side of the baby so that chest movement can be seen.

Hope bags. In a crisis situation, it is crucial that 100% O_2 be delivered with adequate pressure.

3. Chest movement is observed for proper ventilation. Air entry and heart rate (HR) are checked by auscultation; HR may be quickly checked by palpating the base of the umbilical cord stump and counting the pulsations for 6 seconds and then multiplying by 10. Manual resuscitation is coordinated with any voluntary efforts. During positive pressure ventilation, squeeze the resuscitation bag just enough to improve HR, color, and muscle tone. Pressure should be adequate to move the chest wall. The pressure gauge (manometer) must be in place to avoid overdistention of the newborn's lungs and other problems such as pneumothorax or abdominal distention. Increasing the positive to 30 cm H_2O or greater is occasionally necessary if there is no improvement in these parameters (HR, color, muscle tone) (American Academy of Pediatrics [AAP] & American Heart Association [AHA], 2006). If ventilation is adequate, the chest moves symmetrically with each inspiration, there is rapid rise in HR, bilateral breath sounds are audible, the lips and mucous membranes become pink, and muscle tone improves. Distention of the stomach is controlled by inserting a nasogastric tube for decompression.

4. Endotracheal intubation (Figure 33–2 ◆) may be needed. However, most newborns, except for very-low-birth-weight (VLBW) (less than 1500 g) infants, can be effectively resuscitated by bag-and-mask ventilation. With preterm newborns, positive end-expiratory pressure (PEEP) is required to help prevent alveolar collapse during exhalation. If the baby is intubated and the color and HR fail to respond to ventilatory efforts, poor or improper placement of an endotracheal tube may be the cause. If the baby is intubated properly, pneumothorax, diaphragmatic hernia, or hypoplastic lungs (Potter's association) may exist. An increasing HR and CO_2 detection are the primary methods for confirming endotracheal tube placement.

Once breathing has been established, the HR should increase to over 100 beats per minute. If the HR is absent or the HR remains less than 60 beats per minute after 30 seconds of effective positive pressure with 100% oxygen, external cardiac massage (chest compression) is begun. Chest compressions are started immediately if there is no detectable heartbeat. The procedure for performing chest compression is as follows:

1. The infant is positioned properly on a firm surface.

2. The resuscitator stands at the foot or head of the infant and the examiner places both thumbs over the lower third of the sternum (just below an imaginary line drawn between the nipples) with the fingers wrapped around and supporting the back (Figure 33–3, A ◆). Alternatively, the examiner can use two fingers instead of the thumbs (Figure 33–3, B). The two-thumb method is preferred because it may provide better coronary perfusion pressure; however, it makes access to the umbilical cord for medication administration more difficult (Cloherty et al., 2004; Gomella et al., 2004).

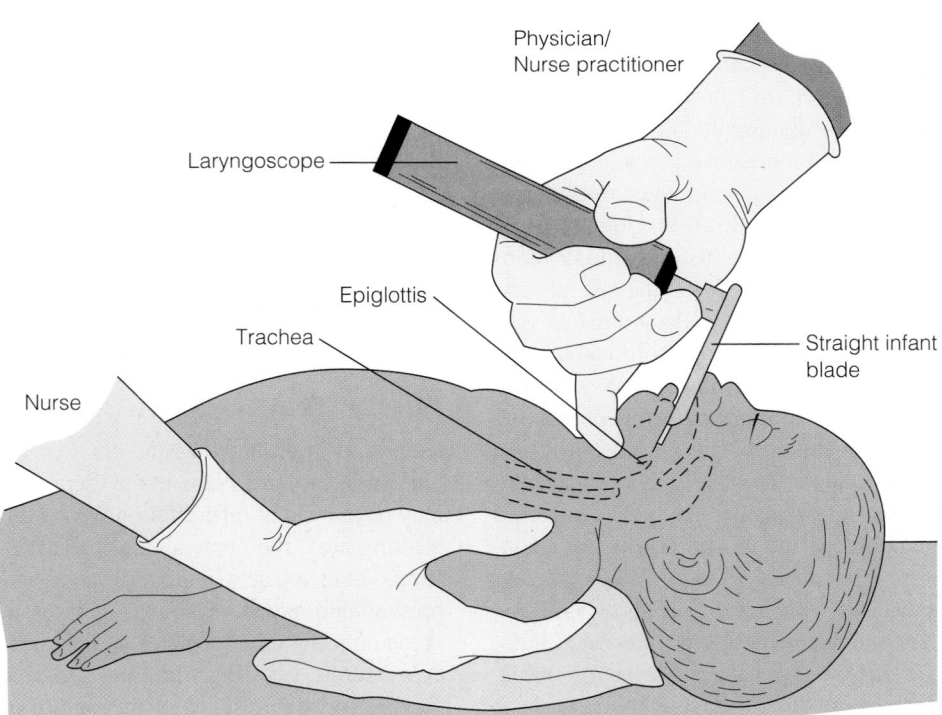

Figure 33–2 ◆ Endotracheal intubation is accomplished with the infant's head in the "sniffing" position. The clinician places the fifth finger under the chin to hold the tongue forward and inserts the laryngoscope blade. Once the blade is in position as shown, an endotracheal tube is inserted through the groove in the laryngoscope blade. The endotracheal tube is not seen in this illustration.

A

B

Figure 33–3 ◆ External cardiac massage. The lower third of the sternum is compressed with two fingertips or thumbs at a rate of 90 beats per minute. *A,* In the thumb method, the fingers support the infant's back, and both thumbs compress the sternum. *B,* In the two-finger method, the tips of two fingers of one hand compress the sternum, and the other hand or a firm surface supports the infant's back.

3. The sternum is depressed to sufficient depth to generate a palpable pulse or approximately one third of the anterior-posterior depth of the chest at a rate of 90 beats per minute (AAP & AHA, 2006; Cloherty et al., 2004; Gomella et al., 2004). Use a 3:1 ratio of heartbeat to assisted ventilation.

Drugs that should be available in the birthing area include those needed in the treatment of shock, cardiac arrest, and narcosis. Oxygen is the drug used most often because of its effectiveness in ventilation. After 30 seconds of ventilation and coordinated cardiac compression, the newborn's cardiopulmonary status is reassessed by palpating the umbilical cord for a pulse. If the newborn has not responded with spontaneous respirations and an HR above 60 beats per minute, resuscitative medications are necessary (Cloherty et al., 2004; Gomella et al., 2004). The most accessible route for administering medications is the umbilical vein (intravenous [IV]). When the HR remains below 60 beats per minute, despite 30 seconds of assisted ventilation followed by another 30 seconds of coordinated chest compression, epinephrine, a cardiac stimulant, is indicated (AAP & AHA, 2006). If bradycardia is present, epinephrine (0.1 to 0.3 mL/kg of a 1:10,000 solution (0.1 mg/mL) is given through the umbilical vein catheter as rapidly as possible. Endotracheal administration may be considered while IV access is being established. When epinephrine is administered by endotracheal tube, consider a higher dose (0.3 to 1 mL/kg). The endotracheal route is associated with unreliable absorption and may not be effective at the lower dose (AAP & AHA, 2006). *Sodium bicarbonate is rarely given in the birthing room.* Sodium bicarbonate is given only to correct metabolic acidosis that results from lactic acid buildup due to insufficient tissue oxygenation and after effective ventilation is established. Dextrose (2 mL/kg) is given to prevent progression of hypoglycemia. A 10% dextrose in water IV solution (D10W) is

usually sufficient to prevent or treat hypoglycemia in the birthing area. Naloxone hydrochloride (0.1 mg/kg), a narcotic antagonist, is used to reverse known iatrogenic narcotic depression (AAP & AHA, 2006). See Drug Guide: Naloxone Hydrochloride (Narcan).

If shock develops (e.g., low BP, pallor, or poor peripheral perfusion), the baby may be given a volume expander such as normal saline or Ringer's lactate in a dose of 10 mL/kg via umbilical vein route. If there is a known fetal hemorrhage or fetal anemia, whole blood (O Rh-negative cross-matched against the mother's blood) and packed red blood cells (RBCs) given over a 5- to 10-minute period can be used for volume expansion and treatment of hypovolemic shock. In some instances of prolonged resuscitation associated with shock and poor response to resuscitation, dopamine (starting at 5 mcg/kg/min) may be necessary.

NURSING CARE MANAGEMENT
Nursing Assessment and Diagnosis

Communication between the obstetric office or clinic and the birthing area nurse helps in the identification of newborns who may be in need of resuscitation. When the woman arrives in the birthing area, the nurse should have the antepartal record and should note any contributory prenatal history factors and assess present fetal status. As labor progresses, nursing assessments include ongoing monitoring of fetal heartbeat and its response to contractions, assisting with fetal scalp blood sampling, and observing for the presence of meconium in the amniotic fluid to help identify possible fetal asphyxia. In addition, the nurse should alert the resuscitation team and the practitioner responsible for the care of the newborn of any potential high-risk laboring women.

DRUG GUIDE   Naloxone Hydrochloride (Narcan)

Overview of Neonatal Action

Naloxone hydrochloride (Narcan) is used to reverse respiratory depression due to acute narcotic toxicity when the mother received a narcotic within 4 hours of delivery. It displaces morphine-like drugs from receptor sites on the neurons; therefore, the narcotics can no longer exert their depressive effects. It is essentially a pure opioid antagonist. Naloxone reverses iatrogenic narcotic-induced respiratory depression, analgesia, sedation, hypotension, and pupillary constriction.

Route, Dosage, Frequency

The dose is 0.1 mg/kg (0.25 mL/kg of 0.4 mg/mL preparation or 0.1 mL/kg of 1 mg/mL) concentration at birth, including premature infants. This drug is usually given through the umbilical vein or endotracheal tube (ET), although naloxone can be given intramuscularly (delays onset of action) if adequate perfusion exists. For IV push, infuse over at least 1 minute; for ET administration, dilute in 1 to 2 millimeters of normal saline (NS).

Reversal of drug depression occurs within 1 to 2 minutes after IV administration and within 15 minutes of intramuscular (IM) administration. The duration of action is variable (minutes to hours) and depends on the amount of the drug present and the rate of excretion. Duration of narcotic often exceeds that of the naloxone. Dose may be repeated in 3 to 5 minutes. If initial reversal occurs, repeat dose as needed (Young & Mangum, 2006).

Neonatal Contraindications

Naloxone should not be administered to infants of narcotic-addicted mothers or those on methadone maintenance because it may precipitate acute withdrawal syndromes (increased HR and blood pressure (BP), vomiting, seizures, and tremors).

Respiratory depression may result from nonmorphine drugs, such as sedatives, hypnotics, anesthetics, or other nonnarcotic central nervous system (CNS) depressants.

Neonatal Side Effects

Excessive doses may result in irritability, increased crying, and possible prolongation of partial thromboplastin time (PTT).

Tachycardia may occur.

Nursing Considerations

- Monitor respirations—rate and depth—closely for improved respiratory effort.
- Assess for return of respiratory depression when naloxone effects wear off and effects of longer-acting narcotics reappear.
- Assess continued respiratory depression after positive-pressure ventilation has restored normal HR and color.
- Have resuscitative equipment, O_2, and ventilatory equipment available.
- Note that naloxone is incompatible with alkaline solutions such as sodium bicarbonate.
- Store at room temperature and protect from light.
- Naloxone is compatible with heparin.

Nursing diagnoses that may apply to the newborn with asphyxia and the newborn's parents include the following:

- **Ineffective Breathing Pattern** related to lack of spontaneous respirations at birth secondary to in utero asphyxia
- **Decreased Cardiac Output** related to impaired oxygenation
- **Ineffective Family Coping: Compromised** related to baby's lack of spontaneous respirations at birth and fear of losing their newborn

Nursing Plan and Implementation

HOSPITAL-BASED NURSING CARE

Following identification of possible high-risk situations, the next step in effective resuscitation is assembling the necessary equipment and ensuring proper functioning.

In the high-risk nursery, the need for resuscitation may occur at any time. The reliability of the equipment must be maintained before an emergency arises, and the equipment must be restocked immediately after use. The nurse inspects all equipment—bag and mask, pressure manometer, oxygen and flow meter, laryngoscope bulb/battery, and suction machine—for damaged or nonfunctioning parts before a birth or when setting up an admission bed. A systematic check of the emergency cart and equipment is a routine responsibility of each shift. It is a good idea to be prepared by assembling equipment for pH and blood gas determination.

During resuscitation it is essential that the nurse keep the infant warm. The nurse dries the newborn quickly with warmed towels or blankets and places a hat to prevent evaporative heat loss, then places the baby under a prewarmed radiant warmer with servocontrol set at 36.5C (97.7F). The radiant warmer provides an overhead radiant heat source (a thermostatic mechanism that is secured to the infant's abdomen, over a solid organ like the liver, triggers the radiant warmer to turn on or off to maintain a constant temperature). An open bed is necessary for easy access to the newborn.

Training and knowledge about resuscitation are vital to personnel in the birth setting for both normal and high-risk births. Resuscitation is at least a two-person effort, and the nurse should call for additional support as needed. One member must have the skill to perform airway management and ventilation. The resuscitative efforts are recorded on the newborn's chart so that all members of the healthcare team will have access to this information.

PARENT TEACHING

The new cardiopulmonary resuscitation (CPR) guidelines favor family members being present during resuscitation in the birthing room and in the neonatal intensive care unit (NICU), but the procedure is particularly distressing for the parents. If the need for resuscitation is anticipated, advise the parents that a support person will be available for them also. As soon as the infant's condition has been stabilized, a member of the interdisciplinary team needs to discuss the baby's condition with the parents. The parents may have many fears about the reasons for resuscitation and the condition of their baby following the resuscitation.

Evaluation

Expected outcomes of nursing care include the following:

- The newborn requiring resuscitation is promptly identified, and intervention is started early.
- The newborn's metabolic and physiologic processes are stabilized, and recovery proceeds without complications.
- The parents can verbalize the reason for resuscitation and what was done to resuscitate their newborn.
- The parents can verbalize their fears about the resuscitation process and potential implications for their baby's future.

CARE OF THE NEWBORN WITH RESPIRATORY DISTRESS

One of the severest conditions to which the newborn may fall victim is respiratory distress—an inappropriate respiratory adaptation to extrauterine life. Respiratory distress affects from 2.9% to 7.6% of neonates, with 4.3% requiring oxygen therapy (Sasidharan, 2004). The nurse caring for a baby with respiratory distress needs to understand the normal pulmonary and circulatory physiology (see "Respiratory Adaptations" in Chapter 28 ∞), the pathophysiology of the disease process, clinical manifestations, and supportive and corrective therapies. Only with this knowledge can the nurse make appropriate observations concerning responses to therapy and development of complications. Unlike the verbalizing adult client, the newborn communicates needs only by exhibiting behaviors or physiologic parameters that must be interpreted by the NICU nurse. The neonatal nurse interprets this behavior as clues about the individual baby's condition. In this section, we discuss (RDS), transient tachypnea of the newborn, meconium aspiration syndrome, and persistent pulmonary hypertension.

Respiratory Distress Syndrome

Respiratory distress syndrome (RDS), also referred to as *hyaline membrane disease (HMD)*, is the result of a primary absence, deficiency, or alteration in the production of pulmonary surfactant. It is a complex disease that affects approximately 20,000 to 30,000 infants a year in the United States, most of whom are preterm. RDS is a complication of about 1% of pregnancies. The syndrome occurs more frequently in premature Caucasian infants than in infants of African or Hispanic descent and almost twice as often in males as in females.

Not all the factors precipitating the pathologic changes of RDS have been determined, but the two main factors associated with its development are as follows:

1. *Prematurity.* All preterm newborns—whether appropriate for gestational age (AGA), small for

gestational age (SGA), or large for gestational age (LGA)—and especially infants of diabetic mothers are at risk for RDS. The incidence of RDS increases with the degree of prematurity, with most deaths occurring in newborns weighing less than 1500 g. The maternal and fetal factors resulting in preterm labor and birth, complications of pregnancy, indications for cesarean birth, and familial tendency are all associated with RDS.

2. *Surfactant deficiency disease.* Normal pulmonary adaptation requires adequate surfactant, a lipoprotein that coats the inner surface of the alveoli. Surfactant provides alveolar stability by decreasing the alveoli's surface tension and tendency for collapse. Surfactant is produced by type II alveolar cells starting at about 24 weeks' gestation. In the normal or mature newborn lung, it is continuously synthesized, oxidized during breathing, and replenished. Adequate surfactant levels lead to better lung compliance and permit breathing with less work. RDS is due to alterations in surfactant quantity, composition, function, or production.

> **CLINICAL TIP**
>
> An alveolus can be thought of as a small balloon filled with water and no air. When the balloon is emptied, the water droplets that remain inside the balloon increase the surface tension. As a result, the sides of the balloon stick together. The increased surface tension makes reinflation very difficult and requires an increased amount of energy.

Development of RDS indicates a failure to synthesize surfactant, which is required to maintain alveolar stability (see "Factors Opposing the First Breath" in Chapter 28 ∞). Upon expiration, the instability increases atelectasis, which causes hypoxia and acidosis because of the lack of gas exchange. These conditions further inhibit surfactant production and cause pulmonary vasoconstriction. The resulting lung instability causes the biochemical problems of hypoxemia (decreased PO_2), hypercarbia (increased PCO_2), and acidemia (decreased pH), which further increases pulmonary vasoconstriction and hypoperfusion. The cycle of events of RDS leading to eventual respiratory failure is diagrammed in Figure 33–4 ◆.

Because of these pathophysiologic conditions, the newborn must expend increasing amounts of energy to reopen the collapsed alveoli with every breath, so that each breath becomes more difficult than the last. The progressive expiratory atelectasis upsets the physiologic homeostasis of the pulmonary and cardiovascular systems and prevents adequate gas exchange. Breathing becomes progressively harder as lung compliance decreases, which makes it more difficult for the newborn to inflate the lungs and breathe.

The physiologic alterations of RDS produce the following complications:

1. *Hypoxia.* As a result of hypoxia, the pulmonary vasculature constricts, pulmonary vascular resistance increases, and pulmonary blood flow is reduced. Increased pulmonary vascular resistance may precipitate a return to fetal circulation as the ductus arteriosus opens

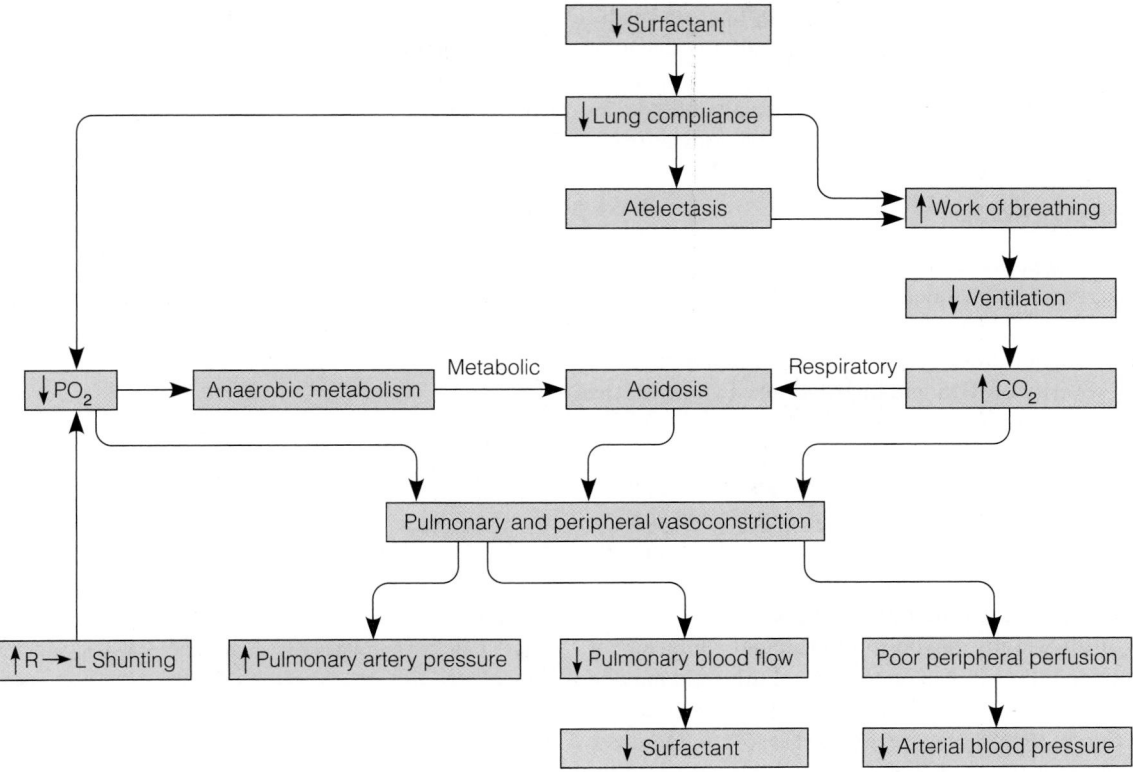

Figure 33–4 ◆ Cycle of events of RDS leading to eventual respiratory failure.
SOURCE: Reprinted from *Pediatric Clinics of North America,* vol. 20, L. Gluck & M. V. Kulovich, "Fetal Lung Development," p. 375, Copyright © 1973, with permission from Elsevier.

and blood flow is shunted around the lungs in a right-to-left blood flow. This shunting increases the hypoxia and further decreases pulmonary perfusion. Hypoxia also causes impairment or absence of metabolic response to cold; reversion to anaerobic metabolism, resulting in lactate accumulation (acidosis); and impaired cardiac output, which decreases perfusion to vital organs.

2. *Respiratory acidosis.* Increased PCO_2 and decreased pH are results of alveolar hypoventilation. A persistent rise in PCO_2 is a poor prognostic sign of pulmonary function and adequacy because increased PCO_2 and decreased pH are results of alveolar hypoventilation

3. *Metabolic acidosis.* Because cells lack oxygen, the newborn begins an anaerobic pathway of metabolism, with an increase in lactate levels and a resulting base deficit (loss of bicarbonate). As the lactate levels increase, the pH decreases in an attempt to maintain acid-base homeostasis.

The classic radiologic picture of RDS is diffuse bilateral reticulogranular (ground glass appearance) density, with portions of the air-filled tracheobronchial tree (air bronchogram) outlined by the opaque ("white-out") lungs with widespread atelectasis, potentially obliterating the heart borders (Cloherty et al., 2004; Thureen et al., 2005) (Figure 33–5 ◆). Opacification of the lungs on x-ray image may be due to massive atelectasis, diffuse alveolar infiltrate, or pulmonary edema. The progression of x-ray findings parallels the pattern of resolution,

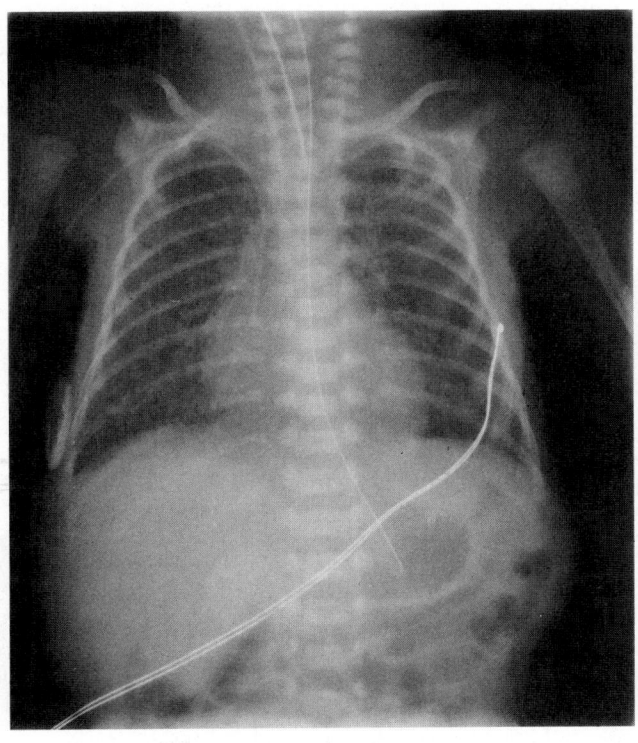

Figure 33–5 ◆ RDS chest x-ray. Chest radiograph of respiratory distress syndrome characterized by a reticulogranular pattern with areas of microatelectasis of uniform opacity and air bronchograms.
SOURCE: Courtesy of Carol Harrigan, RNC, MSN, NNP.

which usually occurs in 7 to 10 days, and the time of surfactant reappearance, unless surfactant replacement therapy and mechanical ventilation have been used (Cloherty et al., 2004; Gomella et al., 2004). Echocardiography is a valuable tool in diagnosing vascular shunts that shunt blood either away from, right to left, or toward the lungs.

CLINICAL THERAPY

The primary goal of prenatal management is to prevent preterm birth through aggressive treatment of preterm labor and administration of steroids to enhance fetal lung development if birth is imminent (see Chapter 20 ∞). Antenatal steroids reduce the incidence and severity of RDS and improve survivability of the extremely low-birth-weight newborn (less than 1250 grams) (Vohr, Wright, Poole et al., 2005); however, there is a decrease in development and maturation of the brain. The goals of postnatal therapy are to maintain adequate oxygenation and ventilation, to correct acid-base abnormalities, and to provide the supportive care required to maintain homeostasis.

Surfactant replacement therapy decreases the severity of RDS in low-birth-weight newborns. Surfactant replacement therapy is delivered through an endotracheal tube and may be given either in the birthing room or the nursery, as indicated by the severity of RDS. Repeat doses are often required. The most frequently reported response to treatment is rapidly improved oxygenation and decreased need for ventilatory support.

Supportive medical management consists of ventilatory therapy, transcutaneous oxygen and carbon dioxide monitoring, blood gas monitoring, correction of acid-base imbalance, environmental temperature regulation, adequate nutrition, and protection from infection. Ventilatory therapy is directed toward preventing hypoventilation and hypoxia. Mild cases of RDS may require only increased humidified oxygen concentrations. Use of continuous positive airway pressure (CPAP) may be required in moderately afflicted infants. Babies with severe cases of RDS require mechanical ventilatory assistance from a respirator (Figure 33–6 ◆). High-frequency ventilation (HFV)

Figure 33–6 ◆ One-day-old, 29 weeks' gestational age, 1450-g baby on respirator and in isolette.
SOURCE: Courtesy of Carol Harrigan, RNC, MSN, NNP.

can be tried when conventional ventilator therapy is not successful, and it sometimes can be the primary mode of ventilation (Cloherty et al., 2004; Gomella et al., 2004). With this type of ventilation the rate is 300 to 1500 breaths per minute. This type of machine applies continuous pressure, preventing collapse of the alveoli. Nitric oxide inhalation therapy may also be useful adjunctive therapy for infants with RDS (Gomella et al., 2004). In some institutions, morphine or fentanyl is used for its analgesic and sedative effects. Sedation may be indicated for infants most likely to have air leak respiratory problems. Use of pancuronium for muscle relaxation in infants with RDS is controversial.

> **CLINICAL TIP**
>
> In babies with RDS who are on ventilators, increased urination/diuresis (determined by weighing diapers) may be an early clue that the baby's condition is improving. As fluid moves out of the lungs into the bloodstream, alveoli open, and kidney perfusion increases; this results in increased voiding. At this point, the nurse must monitor chest expansion closely. If chest expansion is increasing, pulmonary compliance is improving and ventilator settings may have to be decreased, sometimes quite soon after surfactant dosing. Too high a ventilator setting may "blow the lungs," resulting in pneumothorax.

NURSING CARE MANAGEMENT
Nursing Assessment and Diagnosis

Characteristics of RDS the nurse should look for are increasing cyanosis, tachypnea (greater than 60 respirations per minute), grunting respirations, nasal flaring, significant retractions, and apnea. Table 33–1 reviews clinical findings associated with respiratory distress in general. The Silverman-Andersen index (Figure 33–7 ◆) may be helpful in evaluating the signs of respiratory distress and can be done in the birthing area.

Nursing diagnoses that may apply to the newborn with RDS include the following:

- *Impaired Gas Exchange* related to inadequate lung surfactant
- *Ineffective Thermoregulation* related to increased respiratory effort
- *Altered Nutrition: Less than Body Requirements* related to increased metabolic needs of stressed infants
- *Risk for Fluid Volume Deficit* related to increased insensible water losses
- *Risk for Infection* related to invasive procedures

Nursing Plan and Implementation
HOSPITAL-BASED NURSING CARE

Based on clinical parameters, the neonatal nurse implements therapeutic approaches to maintain physiologic homeostasis and provides supportive care to the newborn with RDS. See Nursing Care Plan: For the Newborn with Respiratory Distress Syndrome on pages 992 to 995.

Table 33–1	CLINICAL ASSESSMENTS ASSOCIATED WITH RESPIRATORY DISTRESS
Clinical Picture	**Significance**
Skin Color	
Pallor or mottling	These represent poor peripheral circulation due to systemic hypotension and vasoconstriction and pooling of independent areas (usually in conjunction with severe hypoxia).
Cyanosis (bluish tint)	Depending on hemoglobin concentration, peripheral circulation, intensity and quality of viewing light, and acuity of observer's color vision, this is frankly visible in advanced hypoxia. Central cyanosis is most easily detected by examination of mucous membranes and tongue.
Jaundice (yellow discoloration of skin and mucous membranes due to presence of unconjugated [indirect] bilirubin)	Metabolic alterations (acidosis, hypercarbia, asphyxia) of respiratory distress mean the newborn is predisposed to having bilirubin dissociate from albumin-binding sites and be deposited in the skin and central nervous system.
Edema (presents as slick, shiny taut skin)	This is characteristic of preterm infants because their total protein concentration is low, with a decrease in colloidal osmotic pressure and transudation of fluid. Edema of hands and feet is frequently seen within first 24 hours and resolved by fifth day in infants with severe RDS.
Respiratory System	
Tachypnea (normal respiratory rate 30–60/minute, elevated respiratory rate 60+ minute)	Increased respiratory rate is the most frequent and easily detectable sign of respiratory distress after birth. This compensatory mechanism attempts to increase respiratory dead space to maintain alveolar ventilation and gas exchange in the face of an increase in mechanical resistance. As a decompensatory mechanism, it increases workload and energy output by increasing respiratory rate, which causes increased metabolic demand for oxygen and thus increases alveolar ventilation on an already overstressed system. Shallow, rapid respirations increase dead space ventilation, thus decreasing alveolar ventilation.
Apnea (episode of nonbreathing for more than 20 seconds; periodic breathing, a common "normal" occurrence in preterm infants, is defined as apnea of 5–10 seconds alternating with 10–15 seconds of ventilation that is sometimes quite rapid.	This poor prognostic sign indicates cardiorespiratory disease, CNS disease, metabolic alterations, intracranial hemorrhage, sepsis, or immaturity. Physiologic alterations include decreased oxygen saturation, respiratory acidosis, and bradycardia.
Chest	Inspection of the thoracic cage includes shape, size, and symmetry of movement. Respiratory movements should be symmetric and diaphragmatic; asymmetry reflects pathology (pneumothorax, diaphragmatic hernia). Increased anteroposterior diameter indicates air trapping (meconium aspiration syndrome).
Labored respirations (Silverman-Andersen index in Figure 33–7 indicates severity of retractions, grunting, and nasal flaring, which are signs of labored respirations)	Indicates marked increase in the work of breathing.
Retractions (inward pulling of soft parts of the chest cage—suprasternal, substernal, intercostal, subcostal—at inspiration)	These reflect the significant increase in negative intrathoracic pressure necessary to inflate stiff, noncompliant lungs. Infants try to increase lung compliance by using accessory muscles. Lung expansion markedly decreases. Seesaw respirations are seen when the chest flattens with inspiration and the abdomen bulges. Retractions increase the work of breathing and oxygen need so that assisted ventilation may be necessary due to exhaustion.
Flaring nares (inspiratory dilation of nostrils)	This compensatory mechanism attempts to lessen the resistance of the narrow nasal passage.
Expiratory grunt (Valsalva maneuver in which the infant exhales against a closed glottis, thus producing an audible moan)	This increases transpulmonary pressure, which decreases or prevents atelectasis, thus improving oxygenation and alveolar ventilation. Intubation should not be tried unless the infant's condition is rapidly deteriorating, because it prevents this maneuver and allows the alveoli to collapse.
Rhythmic body movement with labored respirations (chin tug, head bobbing, retractions of anal area)	This is a result of using abdominal and other respiratory accessory muscles during prolonged forced respirations.
Auscultation of chest reveals decreased air exchange, with harsh breath sounds or fine inspiratory rales; rhonchi may be present	Decrease in breath sounds and distant quality may indicate interstitial or intrapleural air or fluid.
Cardiovascular System	
Continuous systolic murmur may be audible	Patent ductus arteriosus is common with hypoxia, pulmonary vasoconstriction, right-to-left shunting, and congestive heart failure.
Heart rate usually within normal limits (fixed heart rate may occur with a rate of 110–120/minute)	A fixed heart rate indicates a decrease in vagal control.
Point of maximal impulse usually located at fourth to fifth intercostal space, left sternal border	Displacement may reflect dextrocardia, pneumothorax, or diaphragmatic hernia.
Hypothermia	This is inadequate functioning of metabolic processes that require oxygen to produce necessary body heat.
Muscle Tone	
Flaccid, hypotonic, unresponsive to stimuli	These may indicate deterioration in the newborn's condition and possible CNS damage due to hypoxia, acidemia, or hemorrhage.
Hypertonia and/or seizure activity	

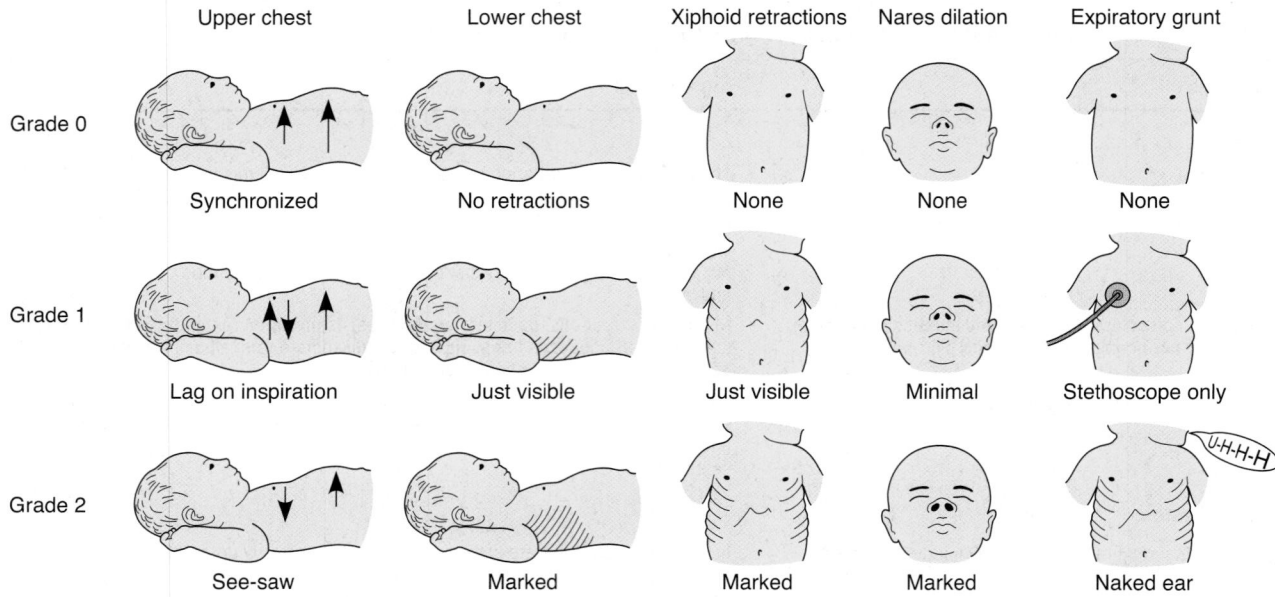

Figure 33–7 ◆ Evaluating respiratory status using the Silverman-Andersen index. The baby's respiratory status is assessed. A grade of 0, 1, or 2 is determined for each area, and a total score is charted in the baby's record or on a copy of this tool and placed in the chart.
SOURCE: Used with permission: Clinical Education Series No. 2: Columbus, Ohio: Ross Products Division, Abbott Laboratories.

NURSING CARE PLAN

For the Newborn with Respiratory Distress Syndrome

INTERVENTION	RATIONALE	EXPECTED OUTCOMES
1. Nursing Diagnosis: Risk for Ineffective Breathing Pattern related to immature lung development		
Goal: The infant will maintain an effective breathing pattern.		
• Review maternal birth records, noting medications given to mother before birth and the infant's condition at birth such as Apgar scores and resuscitative measures.	• Several drugs suppress respiratory function in the newborn.	• *The infant will maintain an effective breathing pattern as evidenced by respirations of 30–60 breaths/min., arterial blood gases are within normal range, infant is free of signs of retractions or nasal flaring, and blood pH is 7.35–7.45.*
• Initiate cardiac and respiratory monitoring and calibrate these monitors every 8 hours. • Monitor infant's respiratory rate and rhythm, pulse, blood pressure, and activity.	• Close monitoring detects periodic apneic spells and allows for medical intervention if necessary. • Increases in respiratory rate and pulse and alteration in rhythm and blood pressure may indicate respiratory distress.	
• Assess skin color; note signs of cyanosis, duskiness, and pallor.	• Any changes in the normal skin color may indicate a physiologic change occurring.	
• Clear infant's airway by suctioning PRN with bulb syringe. • Administer warmed, humidified oxygen by oxygen hood and monitor the oxygen concentrations every 30 minutes.	• Opens airway by clearing mucus and allows maximum respiratory effort. • Prevents mucosal dryness and maintains an even level of oxygen administration.	

NURSING CARE PLAN

For the Newborn with Respiratory Distress Syndrome continued

INTERVENTION	RATIONALE	EXPECTED OUTCOMES
• Do not allow oxyhood to touch infant's face; maintain a stable oxygen concentration by increasing and decreasing oxygen by 5%–10% increments. **Collaborative:** Obtain arterial blood gases (ABGs) per physician orders. a. Maintain constant O_2 concentration for 15–30 minutes before sample is obtained. b. Avoid stimulating infant for 15 minutes before obtaining sample. c. Avoid suctioning infant before obtaining sample. d. Obtain sample in heparinized tuberculin syringe and maintain the temperature of the sample. e. Assess the patency of the IV line to prevent clot formation, then replace blood used to clear line. f. Flush line with 2 mL heparinized solution before restarting flow of IV fluids. g. Monitor transcutaneous pulse oximeter continuously or hourly and record. Rotate sensor site every 3–4 hours. • Assess infant's need for mechanical ventilation: apnea present, hypoxia (PaO_2 less than 50 mm Hg), hypercapnia ($PaCO_2$ greater than 60 mm Hg), respiratory acidosis (pH less than 7.2). • Administer mechanical ventilation per hospital protocol.	• Allowing oxyhood to touch infant's face may cause apnea by stimulating the facial nerve. • Obtaining ABGs is essential in managing an infant receiving oxygen. Suctioning may cause a discrepancy in ABG readings and should be avoided. • Mechanical ventilation improves oxygenation and ventilation, resulting in rise in PaO_2 and decrease in $PaCO_2$. • CPAP or PEEP can be administered by nasal prongs, nasopharyngeal or oral intubation.	

2. Nursing Diagnosis: Ineffective Thermoregulation related to increased respiratory effort

Goal: The infant will exhibit no signs of hypothermia.

INTERVENTION	RATIONALE	EXPECTED OUTCOMES
• Review maternal prenatal and intrapartum records. Note any medications mother received during these times. • Assess infant's temperature frequently. Place servoprobe on infant's skin over a solid organ.	• Medications such as Demerol and magnesium sulfate used by the mother during the prenatal or intrapartum periods significantly interfere with the infant's ability to retain heat. • Hypothermia leads to pulmonary vasoconstriction because of the increase in oxygen consumption. Cold stress leads to increased oxygen needs; thereby, brown fat is used to maintain body temperature.	*The infant will not exhibit signs and symptoms of hypothermia as evidenced by temperature maintenance of 97.7–99.1F and no signs and symptoms of respiratory distress.*

(Continued on next page)

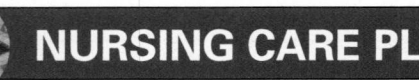

NURSING CARE PLAN

For the Newborn with Respiratory Distress Syndrome continued

INTERVENTION	RATIONALE	EXPECTED OUTCOMES
• Observe for signs of increased oxygen consumption and metabolic acidosis. • Warm all inspired gases and record temperature of delivered gases. • Use radiant warmers or incubators with servocontrols, and open cribs with appropriate clothing. • Note signs and symptoms of respiratory distress, including tachypnea, apnea, cyanosis, acrocyanosis, bradycardia, lethargy, weak cry, and hypotonia.	• Hypoxia and acidosis further depresses surfactant production. • Cold air/oxygen blown in face of newborn is stimulus for consumption of oxygen and glucose and increased metabolic rate. • Maintains neutral thermal environment. • These signs can predispose the infant to metabolic acidosis.	

3. Nursing Diagnosis: Altered Nutrition: Less than Body Requirements related to increased metabolic needs in the infant

Goal: Infant will gain weight in a normal curve.

• Assess suck, swallow, gag, and cough reflexes. • Assess respiratory status of infant. If problems are noted, notify physician. • Monitor IV rates per infusion pump (starting at 80 mL/kg/day) as ordered by physician. • Record hourly intake and output (I&O) and daily weights. • Provide total parenteral nutrition (TPN) when indicated. • Advance, based on tolerance, from IV to gastrointestinal (GI) feedings. Gavage or nipple feedings are used, and IV is used as supplement (discontinued when oral intake is sufficient).	• Prevents feeding problems and assists in determining the best method of feeding for infant. • In the presence of respiratory distress, avoid oral fluids and initiate parenteral nutrition per physician's orders. • Allows for close monitoring of fluid intake. • IV fluids are administered to replace sensible and insensible water loss, as well as evaporative water loss secondary to respiratory distress. Monitoring I&O will prevent circulatory system overload that can lead to pulmonary edema and cardiac problems. • TPN is used as nutritional alternative if bowel sounds are not present and/or infant remains in acute distress. • If IV is discontinued before oral intake is established, baby will not receive adequate calories. • Formula or breast milk stimulate GI hormones necessary for a functional absorptive GI tract. • Avoid complications associated with nutrition by IV route only.	*The infant will maintain steady weight gain as evidenced by less than 2%/day weight loss, tolerates oral feedings, and urine output of 1–3 mL/kg/hour.*

NURSING CARE PLAN

For the Newborn with Respiratory Distress Syndrome continued

INTERVENTION	RATIONALE	EXPECTED OUTCOMES
• Provide adequate caloric intake: consider amount of intake, type of formula, route of administration, and need for supplementation of intake by other routes. • Assess infusion site for signs and symptoms of infection including: erythema, edema, and drainage with a foul odor.	• Calories are essential to prevent catabolism of body proteins and metabolic acidosis due to starvation or inadequate caloric intake. • Appropriate intervention can be initiated when signs and symptoms of infection are detected early. Treatment may avoid infection and sepsis in the infant.	

4. Nursing Diagnosis: Risk for Fluid Volume Deficit related to increased insensible water losses

Goal: The infant will not exhibit signs of dehydration and will display appropriate weight gain.

• Observe for weight fluctuations by obtaining daily weights.	• Fluctuations in weight may indicate water imbalance or inadequate caloric intake.	*The infant will be free of signs and symptoms of dehydration as evidenced by intake equaling output, urine specific gravity in normal range, and a weight gain of at least 20–30 grams/day.*
• Document cumulative balances of intake (IV fluid administration and feedings) and output (urine collection bags, weighing or counting diapers) hourly. • Obtain urinalysis, monitor closely specific gravity and nitrites.	• Balanced fluid intake and output suggest homeostasis. • Specific gravity greater than 1.013 and nitrites present in the urine are indicative of not enough fluid intake.	
• Monitor vital signs including blood pressure, pulse, temperature, and mean arterial pressure (MAP). • Assess client for signs of dehydration (i.e., poor skin turgor, pale mucous membranes, and sunken anterior fontanelle). • Assess IV site for signs of infection (erythema and edema) and infiltration.	• A MAP of less than 20 mm Hg may indicate hypotension. • Detecting signs and symptoms of dehydration early in the infant are important because early interventions are vital to prevent further damage. • If signs and symptoms of infection are noted, intervention is necessary and IV site should be changed.	
Collaborative: Obtain labs for hematocrit (Hct), serum calcium, serum magnesium, serum potassium, blood urea nitrogen (BUN), creatinine, and uric acid levels. • Administer fluids, blood products, and electrolytes as ordered by physician.	• Determines necessity for TPN administration. • Replaces low nutrient stores and treats anemia if present.	

Nursing interventions and criteria for instituting mechanical ventilatory assistance are done per institutional protocol. Methods of noninvasive oxygen monitoring and nursing interventions are described in Table 33–2. The nursing care of infants on ventilators or with umbilical artery catheters is not discussed here.

These infants have severe respiratory distress and are cared for in NICUs by nurses with advanced knowledge and training. Ventilator assistance with high-frequency ventilators has shown positive results. The parents of a baby born having respiratory distress will need a very supportive environment (Figure 33–8 ◆).

Table 33–2 OXYGEN MONITORS		
Type	**Function and Rationale**	**Nursing Interventions**
Pulse Oximetry–SpO$_2$		
Estimates beat-to-beat arterial oxygen saturation.	Calibration is automatic.	Understand and use oxyhemoglobin dissociation curve.
Microprocessor measures saturation by the absorption of red and infrared light as it passes through tissue.	Less dependent on perfusion than TcPO$_2$ and TcPCO$_2$; however, functions poorly if peripheral perfusion is decreased due to low cardiac output.	Monitor trends over time and correlate with arterial blood gases.
Changes in absorption related to blood pulsation through vessel determine saturation and pulse rate.	Much more rapid response time than TcPO$_2$–offers real-time readings.	Check disposable sensor at least every 8 hr.
	Can be located on extremity, digit, or palm of hand, leaving chest free; not affected by skin characteristics.	Use disposable cuffs (reusable cuffs allow too much ambient light to enter, and readings may be inaccurate).
	Requires understanding of oxyhemoglobin dissociation curve.	
	Pulse oximeter reading of 87% to 95% reflects clinically safe range of saturation.	
	Extreme sensitivity to movement; decreases if average of 7th or 14th beat is selected rather than beat to beat.	
	Poor correlation with extreme hyperoxia.	
Transcutaneous Oxygen Monitor–TcPO$_2$		
Measures oxygen diffusion across the skin.	When transcutaneous monitors are properly calibrated and electrodes are appropriately positioned, they provide reliable, continuous, noninvasive measurements of PO$_2$, PCO$_2$, and oxygen saturation.	Use TcPO$_2$ to monitor trends of oxygenation with routine nursing care procedures.
Clark electrode is heated to 43C (preterm) or 44C (term) to warm the skin beneath the electrode and promote diffusion of oxygen across the skin surface. PO$_2$ is measured when oxygen diffuses across the capillary membrane, skin, and electrode membrane (Askin & Diehl-Jones, 2004).	Readings vary when skin perfusion is decreased.	Clean electrode surface to remove electrolyte deposits; change solution and membrane once a week.
	Reliable as trend monitor.	Allow machine to stabilize before drawing arterial gases; note reading when gases are drawn and use values to correlate.
	Frequent calibration necessary to overcome mechanical drift.	Ensure airtight seal between skin surface and electrode; place electrodes on clean, dry skin on upper chest, abdomen, or inner aspect of thigh; avoid bony prominences.
	Following membrane change, machine must "warm up" 1 hour before initial calibration; otherwise, after turning it on, it must equilibrate for 30 minutes before calibration.	Change skin site and recalibrate at least every 4 hours; inspect skin for burns; if burns occur, use lowest temperature setting and change position of electrode more frequently.
	When placed on infant, values will be low until skin is heated; approximately 15 minutes required to stabilize.	Adhesive disks may be cut to a smaller size, or skin prep may be used under the adhesive circle only; allow membrane to touch skin surface at center.
	Second-degree burns are rare but possible if electrodes remain in place too long.	
	Decreased correlations noted with older infants (related to skin thickness), with infants with low cardiac output (decreased skin perfusion), and with hyperoxic infants.	
	The adhesive that attaches the electrode may abrade the fragile skin of the preterm infant.	
	May be used for both preductal and postductal monitoring of oxygenation for observations of shunting.	

Evaluation

Expected outcomes of nursing care include the following:

- The newborn at risk of RDS is promptly identified, and early intervention is initiated.

- The newborn is free of respiratory distress and metabolic alterations.

- The parents verbalize their concerns about their baby's health problem and survival and understand the rationale behind management of their newborn.

Transient Tachypnea of the Newborn

Some newborns, primarily LGA and late preterm infants, may develop progressive respiratory distress that can resemble classic RDS. They may have had intrauterine or intrapartal asphyxia due to maternal oversedation or poor uterine perfusion, maternal bleeding, prolapsed cord, breech birth, or maternal diabetes. The newborn then fails to clear the airway of lung fluid, mucus, and other debris, or an excess of fluid in the lungs due to aspiration of amniotic or tracheal fluid. Transient tachypnea of the newborn (TTN) occurs in 11 per 1000 live births. It is more prevalent in cesarean-born newborns who have not had the tho-

Figure 33–8 ◆ This baby born at 36 weeks' gestational age had severe RDS. He has ongoing oxygen needs provided by a nasal cannula but still can be held by his proud big brother.
SOURCE: Courtesy of Lisa Smith-Pedersen, RNC, MSN, NNP.

racic squeeze that occurs during vaginal birth and removes some of the lung fluid (Cloherty et al., 2004; Gomella et al., 2004).

Usually the newborn experiences little or no difficulty at the onset of breathing. However, shortly after birth, expiratory grunting, flaring of the nares, subcostal retractions, and mild cyanosis may be noted in the newborn breathing room air. Air will become trapped and an increase in the anterior/posterior diameter of the chest will be observed. Tachypnea is usually present by 6 hours of age, with respiratory rates consistently greater than 60 breaths per minute. Mild respiratory and metabolic acidosis may be present within the first 6 hours. These clinical signs usually improve within 24 hours with mild TTN but may continue for up to 72 hours when more severe.

CLINICAL THERAPY

Initial x-ray findings may be identical to those showing RDS within the first 3 hours. However, radiographs of infants with transient tachypnea usually reveal a generalized overexpansion of the lungs (hyperaeration of alveoli), which is identifiable principally by flattened contours of the diaphragm. Dense streaks

Figure 33–9 ◆ Premature infant under oxygen hood. Infant is nested and has a nonnutritive sucking pacifier.
SOURCE: Courtesy of Lisa Smith-Pedersen, RNC, MSN, NNP.

(increased vascularity) radiate from the hilar region and represent engorgement of the lymphatic vessels, which clear alveolar fluid on initiation of air breathing. Within 48 to 72 hours the chest x-ray examination is normal (Cloherty et al., 2004; Gomella et al., 2004).

Ambient oxygen concentrations of 30% to 50%, usually under an oxyhood, may be required to correct the hypoxemia (Figure 33–9 ◆). Fluid and electrolyte requirements should be met with IV fluids during the acute phase of the disease. Oral feedings are contraindicated because of rapid respiratory rates and the subsequent risk of aspiration. The infant should be improving by 8 to 24 hours. The duration of the clinical course of transient tachypnea is approximately 72 hours (Cloherty et al., 2004; Gomella et al., 2004).

When hypoxemia is severe and tachypnea continues, persistent pulmonary hypertension must be considered and treatment measures initiated. If pneumonia is suspected initially, antibiotics may be administered prophylactically.

NURSING CARE MANAGEMENT

For nursing actions, see the Nursing Care Plan: For the Newborn with Respiratory Distress Syndrome on pages 992 to 995.

Care of the Newborn with Meconium Aspiration Syndrome

Because the body's physiologic response to asphyxia is increased intestinal peristalsis and relaxation of the anal sphincter, the presence of meconium in the amniotic fluid indicates that the fetus may be suffering asphyxia. However, if the fetus is in a breech position, the presence of meconium in the amniotic fluid does not necessarily indicate asphyxia.

RESEARCH IN PRACTICE

EFFECTS OF FETAL HEMOGLOBIN ON ACCURATE MEASUREMENTS OF OXYGEN SATURATION IN NEONATES

What is this study about? Fetal hemoglobin (HbF) is different from adult hemoglobin (HbA) in that it has a high affinity for oxygen and so does not release its oxygen molecules to the tissues easily. With a high HbF content, newborns have low oxygen flow to the tissues, resulting in low oxygen content. If other stresses are placed on the newborn as well, such as bradycardia or desaturation, the newborn's tissue oxygenation status may be further compromised. It is necessary, then, to know how oxygen saturation measures may be affected by the amount of circulating HbF, in order to appropriately evaluate the newborn's physiological condition. This researcher sought to determine the association between various measures of neonatal oxygenation and measures of HbF.

How was this study done? Twenty preterm newborns with gestational ages ranging from 25 to 34 weeks were recruited to the study from a single, tertiary care medical center. Babies were excluded from the study if drawing repeated blood samples would compromise their care or physical status. HbF and all oxygen saturation parameters were measured from the blood samples by using a hemoximeter. The instrument allowed in vitro measurements of SO_2, hemoglobin, and HbF. Blood samples of 0.2 mL were collected every 6 hours from the umbilical artery catheter or umbilical venous catheter lines that were already established per the routine care in the NICU. Clinical monitors were used to detect HR, skin temperature, and respiratory rate. SpO_2 readings were recorded using a pulse oximeter. Statistical tests were used to determine the association between these indicators of oxygenation status and the amount of circulating HbF. The variables were then compared with a standard sample of HbA to determine if differences existed when compared with this usual standard.

What were the results of the study? The differences between measurements of these substances showed that circulating HbF does affect readings of oxygen saturation. The blood-based measures were more reactive to circulating HbF than were the pulse oxymetry measures. The venous and arterial SO_2 values were 4% to 7% higher using HbA comparison values than using HbF mode analysis for these preterm newborns.

What additional questions might I have? Can a standard interpretive curve be calculated that would reflect oxygen saturation of tissues accurately? Does this association also present itself with term newborns who are healthy?

How can I use this study? Very young preterm infants may have circulating HbF that reduces the capacity of the tissue to extract its oxygen. This may result in lower oxygen saturation, a condition that can be exacerbated by other morbidities. The nurse should consider that indicators of circulatory oxygenation may be inaccurate by as much as 4% to 7% and so should use multiple indicators of neonatal oxygenation status to evaluate the baby's status.

Shiao, S. (2005). Effects of fetal hemoglobin on accurate measurements of oxygen saturation in neonates. *Journal of Perinatology and Neonatal Nursing, 19*(4), 348–361.

Approximately 13% of live born, close-to-term or term infants are born through meconium-stained amniotic fluid (MSAF). Of the newborns born through MSAF, an average of 5% develop **meconium aspiration syndrome (MAS)** (Gelfand, Fanaroff, & Walsh, 2004a). This fluid may be aspirated into the tracheobronchial tree by the fetus in utero or during the first few breaths taken by the newborn. This syndrome primarily affects term, SGA, and postterm newborns and those who have experienced a long labor.

Presence of meconium in the lungs produces:

- Mechanical obstruction of airways: ball-valve action (air is allowed in but not exhaled), so that alveoli overdistend.

- Chemical pneumonitis; with oxygen and carbon dioxide trapping and hyperinflation, air leaks such as pneumothorax are common, occurring in 15% to 33% of babies with MAS; secondary bacterial pneumonias can occur.

- Vasoconstriction of pulmonary vessels; allowing development of persistent pulmonary hypertension (PPHN).

- Inactivation of natural surfactant (Gelfand et al., 2004a).

CLINICAL MANIFESTATIONS OF MAS

Clinical manifestations of MAS include (1) fetal hypoxia in utero a few days or a few minutes before birth, indicated by a sudden increase in fetal activity followed by diminished activity, slowing of FHR or weak and irregular heartbeat, loss of beat-to-beat variability, and meconium staining of amniotic fluid or particulate meconium; and (2) presence of signs of distress at birth, such as pallor, cyanosis, apnea, slow heartbeat, and low Apgar scores (below 6) at 1 and 5 minutes. Newborns with intrauterine asphyxia, meconium-stained newborns, or newborns who have aspirated particulate meconium often have respiratory depression at birth and require resuscitation to establish adequate respiratory effort.

After the initial resuscitation, the severity of clinical symptoms correlates with the extent of aspiration. Many infants require mechanical ventilation at birth because of immediate signs of distress (generalized cyanosis, tachypnea, and severe retractions). An overdistended, barrel-shaped chest with increased anteroposterior diameter is common. Auscultation reveals diminished air movement with prominent rales and rhonchi. Abdominal palpation may reveal a displaced liver caused by diaphragmatic depression resulting from the overexpansion of the lungs. Yellowish/pale green staining of the skin, nails, and umbilical cord is usually present, especially if the incident occurred some time before birth.

The chest x-ray film for newborns with MAS reveals asymmetric, coarse, patchy, diffuse densities, with possible hyperinflation (9- to 11-rib expansion), which may predispose the newborn to air leak syndromes such as pneumothorax or pneumomediastinum (Gelfand, Fanaroff, & Walsh, 2004b). Evidence of pulmonary air leak is frequently present. These infants have serious biochemical alterations, which include (1) extreme metabolic acidosis resulting from the cardiopulmonary shunting and hypoperfusion; (2) extreme respiratory acidosis due to shunting and alveolar hypoventilation; and (3) extreme hypoxia, even in 100% O_2 concentrations and with ventilatory assistance. The extreme hypoxia is also caused by the cardiopulmonary shunting and resultant failure to oxygenate and can lead to PPHN, discussed shortly.

CLINICAL THERAPY

The maternity and pediatric teams must work together to prevent MAS. The most effective form of preventive management is outlined as follows:

1. After the head of the newborn is delivered and the shoulders and chest are still in the birth canal, the baby's oropharynx and then the nasopharynx are suctioned by the birth attendant with use of a bulb syringe or DeLee attached to wall suction. (This is also done with a cesarean birth.) To decrease the possibility of human immunodeficiency virus (HIV) transmission, low-pressure wall suction is used.

2. If the infant is vigorous even if there is thick or thin meconium in the amniotic fluid, no subsequent special resuscitation is indicated (de Ungria & Steinhorn, 2003).

3. If the infant has absent or depressed respirations, HR less than 100 beats per minute, or poor muscle tone, direct tracheal suctioning by specially trained personnel such as a neonatal nurse practitioner, an experienced NICU nurse trained in those skills, a respiratory therapist, or a nurse anesthetist is recommended. The glottis is visualized with a laryngoscope and the trachea suctioned (Gelfand et al., 2004b).

If the newborn's head is not adequately suctioned on the perineum at the time the head is delivered but the shoulder and chest are still in the vagina, respiratory or resuscitative efforts will push meconium into the airway and into the lungs. Stimulation of the newborn should be avoided to minimize respiratory movements. Further resuscitative efforts are undertaken as indicated, following the same principles of clinical therapy as for asphyxia (discussed earlier in this chapter). Resuscitated newborns should be immediately transferred to the nursery for closer observation. An umbilical arterial line may be used for direct monitoring of arterial blood pressures and blood sampling for pH and blood gases. An umbilical venous catheter may be placed for infusion of IV fluids, blood, or medications.

Treatment usually involves delivery of high oxygen concentrations and high-pressure ventilation. Low PEEPs are preferred to avoid air leaks such as pneumothorax. Unfortunately, high pressures may be needed to cause sufficient expiratory expansion of the obstructed terminal airways or to stabilize airways that are weakened by inflammation so that the most distal atelectatic alveoli are ventilated.

Naturally occurring surfactant may be inactivated by the presence of meconium and the subsequent inflammatory response that occurs. Surfactant replacement therapy is most effective when given as a prophylactic measure. Providing exogenous surfactant possibly decreases the incidence of air leaks (Gelfand et al., 2004b). Systemic blood pressure and pulmonary blood flow must be maintained. Dopamine or dobutamine or volume expanders, or both, may be used to maintain systemic blood pressure.

Newborns with respiratory failure who are not responding to conventional ventilator therapy may require treatment with high-frequency ventilation and/or nitric oxide therapy or extracorporeal membrane oxygenation (ECMO) if baby is greater than 2 kg (Gelfand et al., 2004b). Inhaled nitric oxide has proven successful for newborns with meconium aspiration, pneumonia, and PPHN who are not responding to traditional treatment modalities, and it avoids the need for ECMO (Gelfand et al., 2004b).

Treatment also includes chest physiotherapy (chest percussion, vibration, and drainage) to remove the debris. Prophylactic antibiotics are frequently given. Continuous infusion of bicarbonate to correct metabolic acidosis may be necessary for several days for severely ill newborns. Mortality in term or postterm infants is very high because the cycle of hypoxemia and acidemia is difficult to break.

NURSING CARE MANAGEMENT
Nursing Assessment and Diagnosis

During the intrapartal period, the nurse should observe for signs of fetal hypoxia and meconium staining of amniotic fluid. At birth the nurse assesses the newborn for signs of distress. During the ongoing assessment of the newborn, the nurse carefully observes for complications such as pulmonary air leaks; anoxic cerebral injury manifested by seizures/convulsions; myocardial injury evidenced by congestive heart failure or cardiomegaly; disseminated intravascular coagulation (DIC) resulting from hypoxic hepatic damage with depression of liver-dependent clotting factors; anoxic renal damage demonstrated by hematuria, oliguria, or anuria; fluid overload; sepsis secondary to bacterial pneumonia; and any signs of intestinal necrosis from ischemia, including GI obstruction or hemorrhage.

Nursing diagnoses that may apply to the newborn with MAS and the infant's parents include the following:

- *Ineffective Gas Exchange* related to aspiration of meconium and amniotic fluid during birth
- *Altered Nutrition: Less than Body Requirements* related to respiratory distress and increased energy requirements
- *Ineffective Family Coping: Compromised* related to life-threatening illness in a term newborn

Nursing Plan and Implementation
HOSPITAL-BASED NURSING CARE

Initial interventions are aimed primarily at preventing the aspiration by assisting with the removal of the meconium from the

MediaLink   Application: Meconium Aspiration Syndrome

infant's oropharynx and nasopharynx before the first extrauterine breath.

When significant aspiration occurs, therapy is supportive with the primary goals of maintaining appropriate gas exchange and minimizing complications. Nursing interventions after resuscitation should include maintaining adequate oxygenation and ventilation, regulating temperature, performing glucose testing by glucometer to check for hypoglycemia, observing IV fluids, calculating necessary fluids (which may be restricted in the first 48 to 72 hours because of cerebral edema), providing caloric requirements possibly with TPN, and monitoring IV antibiotic therapy.

Evaluation

Expected outcomes of nursing care include the following:

- The newborn at risk of MAS is promptly identified, and early intervention is initiated.
- The newborn is free of respiratory distress and metabolic alterations.
- The parents verbalize their concerns about their baby's health problem and survival and understand the rationale behind management of their newborn.

Persistent Pulmonary Hypertension of the Newborn

Persistent pulmonary hypertension of the newborn (PPHN) is a serious disorder that may affect on average 0.2% of live-born term newborns annually (Farrow, Fliman, & Steinhorn, 2005). PPHN has also been called *persistent fetal circulation (PFC)* because the problems that occur are a result of right-to-left (R-L) shunting of blood away from the lungs and through the fetal ductus arteriosus and patent foramen ovale, consequently bypassing the lungs and the ability to be oxygenated, causing worsening hypoxemia and acidosis (Farrow et al., 2005).

Depending on the cause, PPHN is classified as primary or secondary. Primary disease results from pulmonary vascular changes before birth, which cause abnormally high pulmonary vascular resistance (PVR). Secondary PPHN occurs when the initial sequences of respiration and change in circulation after birth are interrupted by events that increase the PVR. Hypoxemia and acidosis are the most potent stimulants of pulmonary vasoconstriction. The increased vascular resistance increases pulmonary artery pressure, hypoxemia, and R-L shunting of pulmonary blood across fetal shunts. Once this process has begun, it is self-perpetuating and difficult to interrupt. Clinical deterioration is rapid.

CLINICAL THERAPY

The first goal of medical management is early diagnosis of this disorder to halt the progressive worsening of the R-L shunt. Certain diagnostic tests are often used to evaluate the increased PVR and shunting. Simultaneous preductal and postductal blood gases or pulse oximetry and/or transcutaneous monitoring can be used to demonstrate ductal shunting. A difference greater than 10% to 15% between preductal and postductal oxygen saturation is indicative of a right-to-left ductal shunt. The hyperoxia-hyperventilation test is the most definitive test for PPHN. A positive indication of PPHN is when the prehypertension PaO_2 is less than 50 mm Hg and rises to greater than 100 mm Hg with hyperoxia and hyperventilation. The improved oxygenation can be noted clinically if the infant's mucous membranes turn pink. Echocardiography can demonstrate R-L shunting and a prolonged ratio of right ventricular ejection period to right ventricular ejection time in infants with PPHN. The goal of therapeutic intervention is to lower the PVR and reverse the process of shunting. This can be accomplished with the use of nitric oxide, which is a selective pulmonary vasodilator, when other methods fail (Farrow et al., 2005). Inhaled nitric oxide (INO) improves oxygenation in many infants with PPHN by selectively decreasing PVR. The INO is inhaled by the newborn at a dose of 20 parts per million (Farrow et al., 2005). Maintaining tissue oxygenation in the presence of R-L shunting presents the greatest therapeutic challenge but is essential to minimize complications. With PPHN, oxygen acts as a potent vasodilator and these babies are very labile so it is important to be careful in weaning them from oxygen. Ventilatory management is undertaken to decrease the PVR and increase oxygenation. Hyperventilation to achieve respiratory alkalosis will cause pulmonary vasodilatation, which increases oxygenation; however, it may have detrimental CNS effects, specifically sensorineural hearing loss. Sodium bicarbonate infusions (0.5 to 1 mEq/kg/h) may be required to induce alkalosis (pH greater than 7.45). To prevent respiratory interference and achieve hypocarbia, most infants require paralysis with a neuromuscular blocking agent such as pancuronium (Pavulon) and use of a sedative like Versed in conjunction with an analgesic like morphine sulfate. Either respiratory or metabolic alkalosis may decrease PVR.

If alkalosis alone does not lead to a decrease in the PVR, pharmacologic vasodilators may be given to decrease PVR. In the presence of systemic hypotension, volume expanders such as isotonic crystalloids (normal saline) should be administered; colloids, albumin, or plasma protein fraction (Plasmanate) should be used with caution. Packed RBCs should be used if there is anemia. Infusion of vasopressors (such as dopamine, dobutamine, or isoproterenol) and/or afterload reducers (nitroprusside) are also advocated. Vasopressors increase the systemic vascular resistance, thereby decreasing the amount of R-L shunting, which increases cardiac output. Oxygenation, ventilation, and drug therapy efforts continue until the PaO_2 can be consistently maintained greater than 100 mm Hg. Alkalosis and hyperoxia may have to be maintained for several days to avoid a sudden return of hypoxemia and increased PVR.

NURSING CARE MANAGEMENT

The nurse assesses for the onset of symptoms, which usually occur in the first 12 to 24 hours of life. Affected newborns exhibit signs of respiratory distress (grunting, nasal flaring, tachypnea), with increased anteroposterior diameter and cyanosis. They typically fail to respond to conventional methods of oxygenation and ventilation. Significant unexplained hypoxemia exists in the absence of congenital heart disease. The chest radiograph might show no evidence of pulmonary parenchymal disease (depending on the underlying disease). The hypoxemia and cyanosis associated with PPHN are characteristic of extreme changeability. Marked, rapid changes in PaO_2 and color are seen with agitation, stimulation, therapeutic intervention (suctioning), or rapid changes in ambient oxygen.

Infants with PPHN are critically ill and require experienced, highly skilled nurses to provide optimal care with minimal manipulation/stimulation. Any disturbance may cause agitation, which leads to hypoxemia. If a paralyzing agent is used, nursing care includes monitoring the newborn's response to artificial oxygenation and mechanical ventilation. The nurse ensures that the oxygen is delivered in correct amounts and route and records the percentage of oxygen flow. The ventilator settings are checked frequently and recorded per unit policy. The nurse carefully suctions the endotracheal tube only as necessary while assessing the effect of the procedure on the baby's oxygenation and perfusion. The amount and type of secretions are noted. The nurse carefully assesses arterial blood gases and notifies the clinician if the results are out of the acceptable range. Oxygen monitoring is essential for identifying activities that may compromise the infant's status. (Nursing interventions required for noninvasive oxygen monitoring are discussed in Table 33–2.) Continuous monitoring of vital signs and blood pressure is required, and careful inspection of the skin during positioning is necessary to avoid pressure necrosis.

Pharmacologic vasodilation may lead to precipitous central hypotension, which must be quickly identified and corrected. Tolazoline therapy, previously commonly used, has not been found to be beneficial long term and actually causes profound systemic vasodilation after the initial beneficial pulmonary vasodilation.

Aggressive ventilation poses a potential risk for pneumothorax. The nurse can best prevent complications by advanced preparation and close monitoring for signs of compromise. (See "Pneumothorax" later in this chapter for appropriate nursing interventions.)

Many infants suffering PPHN are born at or near term at a time when parents least expect problems—especially life-threatening problems—to occur. The magnitude of the infant's illness and the rapid deterioration may be overwhelming to parents. The nurse should assess their level of understanding and assist them by providing information about their baby's condition and therapies in easily understandable terms.

Attachment becomes difficult when the infant responds poorly to touching (as seen by decreased PaO_2). Instead, the nurse can encourage parents to talk very softly to their infant because this will usually not compromise the baby's condition. Continuity of nursing care is helpful because it will be less threatening for the parents to relate to a smaller group of nurses.

Evaluation

Expected outcomes of nursing care include the following:

- The risks for development of PPHN are identified early, and immediate action is taken to minimize the development of sudden, severe illness.
- The newborn is free of respiratory distress and establishes effective respiratory function.
- The parents verbalize their concerns about their baby's illness and understand the rationale behind the management of their newborn.

CARE OF THE NEWBORN WITH COMPLICATIONS DUE TO RESPIRATORY THERAPY

Oxygen and mechanical ventilation, although required as therapeutic interventions to reduce hypoxia, hypercarbia, ischemia, and infarction to vital organs, may also have harmful effects. The concentrations of ambient oxygen administered to the newborn must be titrated according to oxygen tension within arterial blood to avoid development of retinopathy of prematurity or bronchopulmonary dysplasia/chronic lung disease. In addition, pulmonary air leaks occur in up to 15% of mechanically ventilated newborns; however, air leaks can be a consequence of injury due to the disease rather than the mechanical ventilation.

Pulmonary Interstitial Emphysema

Pulmonary interstitial emphysema (PIE) is the accumulation of air in lung tissues. It may be unilateral or bilateral. Extra-alveolar air collections are most common with use of positive pressure ventilation. Air collections outside the lung are a function of lung compliance and use of increased pressures to ventilate. Overdistention of alveoli may progress to PIE when rupture occurs and air escapes into the interstitial spaces. Air moves along perivascular spaces but not into the pleural space or mediastinum. As the air collections increase, blood vessels are constricted, and blood gas exchange is impaired. The air does not decrease on expiration. This condition is highly associated with subsequent bronchopulmonary dysplasia (BPD). It may also precede pneumothorax or pneumomediastinum.

Pneumothorax

Pneumothorax, a common complication of respiratory therapy, is an accumulation of air in the thoracic cavity between the parietal and visceral pleura. Pneumothorax occurs when alveoli are overdistended, usually by excessive intra-alveolar pressure and rupture; air then leaks into the thoracic cavity. It may occur spontaneously or as a complication of assisted ventilation.

Pneumothorax in the newborn causes several physiologic changes: collapse of the lung, compression of the heart and lungs, compromise of venous return to the right heart with mediastinal air, and development of tension in the pleural space. Symptoms of pneumothorax include a sudden, unexplained deterioration in the newborn's condition; decreased breath sounds;

apnea; bradycardia; cyanosis; increased oxygen requirements; higher PCO_2; decrease in pH; mottled, asymmetric chest expansion; decreased arterial blood pressure; shock-like appearance; and a shift in the apical cardiac impulses to the side opposite the pneumothorax, often with muffled heart sounds.

Transillumination of the chest is used for rapid evaluation of pneumothorax. Transillumination is the visualization of light through the air in the affected side (or sides, for bilateral pneumothorax) of the baby's chest. However, x-ray examination is the main method of diagnosing this complication (Figure 33–10 ◆).

Pneumothorax is a potentially life-threatening situation for the newborn and may demand immediate removal of the accumulated air. The thoracentesis procedure is done only as an emergency measure and carries a risk of damaging the lung pleura with needle tracks as the air is evacuated and the collapsed lung reexpands. Only skilled and specifically trained personnel should perform this procedure. For complete resolution of the pneumothorax, a chest tube may be inserted.

Figure 33–10 ◆ Chest x-ray of a left-sided pneumothorax. A rupture of the alveoli sacs allows air to leak through the pleura, forming collections of air outside the lung (air shows on x-ray as dark area over lung).
SOURCE: Courtesy of Carol Harrigan, RNC, MSN, NNP.

Bronchopulmonary Dysplasia/Chronic Lung Disease

Bronchopulmonary dysplasia (BPD), also known as **chronic lung disease of prematurity (CLD),** most commonly occurs in very compromised low-birth-weight (LBW) infants who require oxygen therapy and assisted mechanical ventilation for the treatment of RDS. It has also been associated with neonatal pneumonia, MAS, PPHN, congenital heart disease (patent ductus arteriosus), other congenital anomalies requiring high levels of ventilatory support, and low-grade or asymptomatic pulmonary infection with *Ureaplasma urealyticum.* The cause is multifactorial. The process of BPD is one of continuous lung tissue injury and repair, delaying both lung and body growth. The definition of BPD uses dependence on oxygen at 36 weeks' gestational age: Mild BPD requires oxygen greater than or equal to 28 days but not at 36 weeks' gestational age; moderate BPD requires the use of oxygen greater than or equal to 28 days at 36 weeks' gestational age with less than 30% oxygen required; severe BPD requires supplemental oxygen greater than or equal to 30% at greater than or equal to 28 days and/or positive pressure support at 36 weeks' gestational age (Sahni, Ammari, Suri et al., 2005).

CLINICAL THERAPY

The goals of therapeutic intervention for the newborn with BPD are to provide adequate oxygenation and ventilation, prevent further lung damage, promote optimal nutrition, and give supportive care to ensure adequate rates of growth and development. New therapies, such as exogenous surfactant administration, high-frequency ventilation, and steroids (prenatal and postnatal) have altered the severity of BPD, but chronic lung disease remains a major clinical problem. A low vitamin A level in LBW infants less than 1250 grams during the first month of life increases the risk for development of chronic lung disease (Spears, Cheney, & Zerzan, 2004). Because of the chronic nature of BPD, therapeutic intervention must be individualized to meet the specific needs of the infant. Diuretics and fluid restriction (130 mL/kg/day) are frequently used to control pulmonary fluid retention and to improve lung function; electrolyte supplements are necessary to offset the results of chronic diuretic therapy (Cloherty et al., 2004; Gomella et al., 2004). In addition, bronchodilators are indicated to decrease airway resistance and to control bronchospasm. The infant with chronic lung disease is often on long-term steroids. Serial echocardiography is used to monitor cardiac response to the chronic pulmonary disease.

NURSING CARE MANAGEMENT

HOSPITAL-BASED NURSING CARE

The nurse observes carefully any changes in the newborn's oxygenation, giving special attention to maintaining the prescribed oxygen concentration during all activities, especially during periods of stress, such as when the infant is crying; when blood is drawn; while starting an IV infusion; and during a lumbar puncture (LP), suctioning, chest physiotherapy (CPT), and feeding (Figure 33–11 ◆).

The current goal is to adjust the level of supplemental oxygen to consistently keep O_2 saturations between 90% and 94%, depending on the presence of associated clinical problems such as poor growth, recurrent bradycardia, and pulmonary hypertension. PaO_2 should be kept greater than 55 mm Hg. The nurse obtains blood gases based on the institution's chronic blood gas protocol—for example, every 3 days, 20 minutes after a permanent change in ambient oxygen concentration (FiO_2), or more frequently if the infant experiences increasing respiratory distress or increasing lethargy.

Postural drainage, CPT, and vibration followed by suctioning are carried out with close attention to the baby's tolerance. It is essential to time the care activities with rest periods to avoid fatiguing the infant. The nurse maintains the infant's body temperature because hypothermia or hyperthermia will increase oxygen consumption and may increase oxygen requirements. Positioning on the abdomen helps the baby maintain higher transcutaneous oxygen saturation ($TcPO_2$) and improved ventilation.

Bronchodilators such as theophylline, albuterol, and terbutaline; diuretics; steroids; and electrolyte supplements may be used in the clinical management of the BPD infant (Cloherty et al., 2004; Gomella et al., 2004). Appropriate timing of administration is essential to maintain adequate blood levels. Many of the side effects of these drugs, such as hypokalemia and mineral losses (fractures), can be avoided by giving the diuretics every other day.

Providing for adequate nutrition enhances formation of new alveoli and enlargement of the airway diameter. The nurse helps provide adequate nutrition and monitors the newborn's caloric intake and the energy expended during the feeding process. The more severely ill the baby, the higher the caloric need to meet the greater expenditure of energy for survival and healing. As soon as tolerated, a 24 kcal/oz formula for preterm infants is started, especially if the baby is on fluid restriction (Figure 33–12 ◆). More oxygen may be required during feeding, and the least energy-consuming feeding method should be used. If the feeding schedule is too stressful, smaller, more frequent feedings may be initiated (Cloherty et al., 2004; Gomella et al., 2004).

Infants with BPD frequently experience negative oral sensations due to suctioning and intubation. These can adversely affect their transition to nipple or spoon feeding. Positioning is often the key to adequate intake and decreasing gastroesophageal reflux (GER). In addition, most infants receive numerous, possibly unpalatable, medications with meals. Attempts must be made to include pleasurable activities such as cuddling at mealtime to develop positive associations with appropriate feeding behaviors. Premature infants with BPD frequently require some type of feeding therapy to help them eat successfully.

Infants with BPD are very susceptible to infection, especially if they are on long-term steroids; therefore, it is important to discourage anyone with early signs of infectious disease from having contact with them. The infant's behavior and vital signs should be monitored for changes that might indicate early developing infection. Changes in color, quantity, or quality of pulmonary secretions are noted and reported. The frequency of CPT and suctioning may need to be increased.

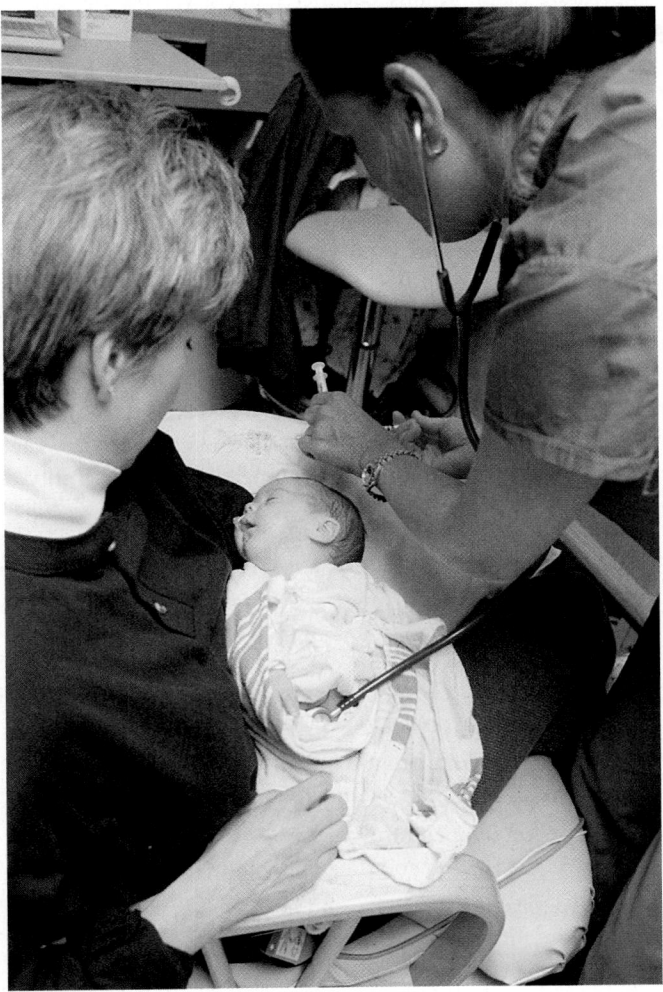

Figure 33–11 ◆ The baby with BPD has ongoing oxygen and nutritional needs as well as the need for gentle individualized care.
SOURCE: © Stella Johnson (www.stellajohnson.com).

Figure 33–12 ◆ A baby requiring oxygen at greater than 36 weeks' gestational age. She still needs to be fed through a NG tube, because she tires with nipple feeds.
SOURCE: Courtesy of Lisa Smith-Pedersen, RNC, MSN, NNP.

Because BPD infants require prolonged hospitalization and/or home care, the nurse should give special attention to formulating a program of early stimulation activities. Psychomotor delays are seen frequently in these infants and are most likely due in part to prolonged exposure to the hospital environment. Because the illness limits these infants' tolerance level for activity, the nurse must individualize activities for each baby. Families need to be included in the plans for their baby.

COMMUNITY-BASED NURSING CARE

When the infant develops BPD and the family becomes aware of the implications of chronic illness and prolonged hospitalization, they may experience despair and find it difficult to cope with this added burden. The nurse can help the family cope by encouraging them to take an active role in their infant's daily activities. Their involvement will help dispel feelings of inadequacy and prepare them to perform the unique tasks necessary to meet their infant's needs.

Parents need to demonstrate their ability to provide all the care their child will require at home before leaving the hospital. This may include feeding, adjusting O_2 support, O_2 saturation monitoring, suctioning and airway management, CPT, bathing, and giving medications. They also need to know when to call the home health nurse who is providing care. Parents should be taught how to assess the infant's respiratory condition and understand the BPD baseline respiratory pattern (frequency of respiration, rhythm, degree of retractions, and color of skin and mucous membranes). Finally, parents must be taught to evaluate their infant's tolerance of activities and to recognize signs of distress due to poor oxygenation, inadequate ventilation, infection, fluid retention, and bronchospasm.

CARE OF THE NEWBORN WITH COLD STRESS

Cold stress is excessive heat loss resulting in the use of compensatory mechanisms (such as increased respirations and nonshivering thermogenesis/use of brown fat stores) to maintain core body temperature. Heat loss that results in cold stress occurs in the newborn through the mechanisms of evaporation, convection, conduction, and radiation. (See Chapter 28 ∞ for a detailed discussion of thermoregulation).

Heat loss at birth that leads to cold stress can play a significant role in the severity of RDS and the ultimate outcome for the infant. Both preterm and SGA newborns are at increased risk for cold stress because they have decreased adipose tissue, brown fat stores, and glycogen available for metabolism.

As discussed in Chapter 28 ∞, the newborn's major source of heat production in nonshivering thermogenesis (NST) is brown fat metabolism. The ability of an infant to respond to cold stress by NST is impaired in the presence of several conditions:

- Hypoxemia (PO_2 less than 50 torr)
- Intracranial hemorrhage or any CNS abnormality
- Hypoglycemia (blood glucose less than 40 mg/dL)

When these conditions occur, the infant's temperature should be monitored more closely and the neutral thermal environment conscientiously maintained. The nurse must recognize these conditions and treat them as soon as possible. The metabolic consequences of cold stress can be devastating and potentially fatal to an infant. Oxygen requirements increase; even before noting a change in temperature, glucose use increases; acids are released into the bloodstream; and surfactant production decreases. The effects are graphically depicted in Figure 33–13 ◆.

NURSING CARE MANAGEMENT

The amount of heat lost by an infant depends to a large extent on the actions of the nurse or caregiver. Following the transfer of an NICU newborn from one bed to another, a transient, although not significant, decrease in temperature for up to 1 hour may be noted. Prevention is especially critical in the VLBW infant. Placing the VLBW newborn in a polyethylene wrapping immediately following birth can decrease the postnatal fall in temperature that normally occurs. Both convective and evaporative heat loss can be reduced (Sedin, 2004).

The nurse observes the baby for signs of cold stress. These include increased movements and respirations, decreased skin temperature and peripheral perfusion, development of hypoglycemia, and, possibly, development of metabolic acidosis.

Vasoconstriction is the initial response to cold stress; because it initially decreases skin temperature, monitor and assess skin temperature instead of rectal temperature. A decrease in rectal temperature means that the infant has long-standing cold stress. By monitoring skin temperature, possible decrease will become apparent before the infant's core temperature is affected.

If a decrease in skin temperature is noted, the nurse determines whether hypoglycemia is present. Hypoglycemia is a result of the metabolic effects of cold stress and is suggested by glucometer values below 40 mg/mL, tremors, irritability or lethargy, apnea, or seizure activity.

If hypothermia occurs, the following nursing interventions should be initiated (Gomella et al., 2004):

- Maintain a neutral thermal environment (NTE); adjust based on the gestational age and postnatal age.
- Warm the newborn slowly, because rapid temperature elevation may cause hypotension and apnea.
- Increase the air temperature in hourly increments of 1C (33.8F) until the infant's temperature is stable.
- Monitor skin temperature every 15 to 30 minutes to determine whether the newborn's temperature is increasing.
- Remove plastic wrap, caps, and heat shields while rewarming the infant so that cool air as well as warm air is not trapped.
- Warm IV fluids before infusion.
- Initiate efforts to block heat loss by evaporation, radiation, convection, and conduction. Maintain the newborn in NTE.

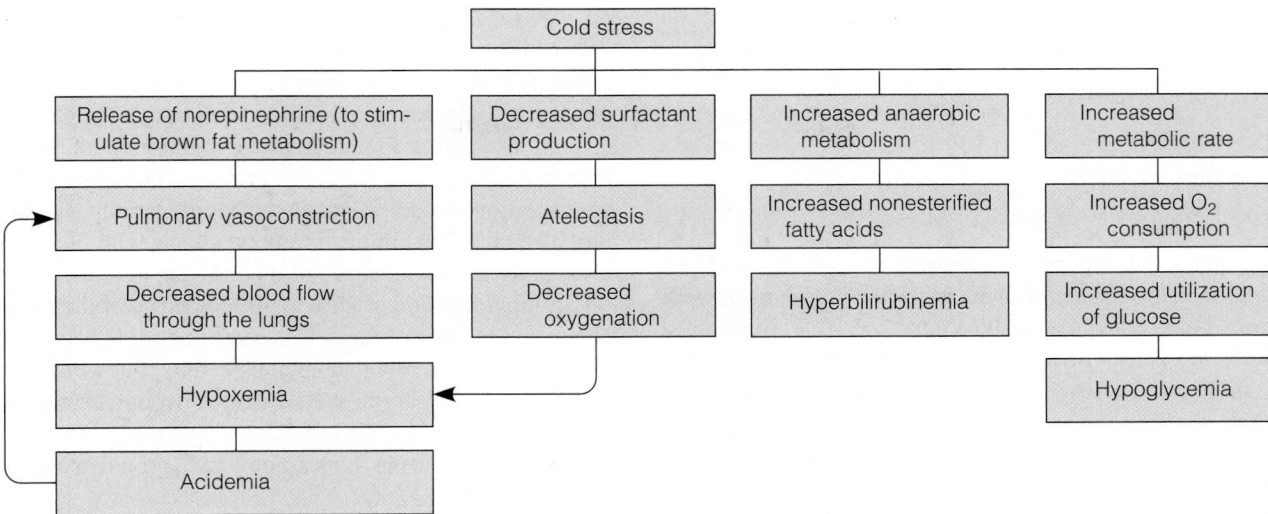

Figure 33–13 ◆ Cold stress chain of events. The hypothermic, or cold-stressed, newborn attempts to compensate by conserving heat and increasing heat production. These physiologic compensatory mechanisms initiate a series of metabolic events that result in hypoxemia and altered surfactant production, metabolic acidosis, hypoglycemia, and hyperbilirubinemia.

The nurse assesses the presence of anaerobic metabolism and initiates interventions for the resulting metabolic acidosis. Attempts to burn brown fat increase oxygen consumption, lactic acid levels, and metabolic acidosis. Hypoglycemia may be reversed by adequate glucose intake, as described in the following section.

CARE OF THE NEWBORN WITH HYPOGLYCEMIA

A widely used cutoff point or threshold for intervention in newborn hypoglycemia is a plasma blood glucose concentration of 40 to 50 mg/dL (Sperling & Menon, 2004). Plasma glucose values less than 20 to 25 mg/dL should be treated with parenteral glucose D10W, regardless of the age or gestation. **Hypoglycemia** is the most common metabolic disorder occurring in infants of diabetic mothers (IDM), SGA infants, the smaller of twins, infants born to mothers with preeclampsia, male infants, and preterm AGA infants. The pathophysiology of hypoglycemia differs for each classification.

AGA preterm infants have not been in utero a sufficient time to store glycogen and fat. As a result, they have a decreased ability to carry out gluconeogenesis. This situation is further aggravated by increased use of glucose by the tissues (especially the brain and heart) during stress and illness (chilling, asphyxia, sepsis, and RDS).

Infants of White's classes A through C or type 1 diabetic mothers (women with diagnosed or gestational diabetes) have increased stores of glycogen and fat (see Chapters 19 ∞ and 32 ∞). Circulating insulin and insulin responsiveness are also higher when compared with other newborns. Because the high glucose loads present in utero stop at birth, the newborn experiences rapid and profound hypoglycemia (Sperling & Menon, 2004).

The SGA infant has used up glycogen and fat stores because of intrauterine malnutrition and has a blunted hepatic en-

zymatic response with which to produce and use glucose. Any newborn stressed at birth from asphyxia or cold also quickly uses up available glucose stores and becomes hypoglycemic. Also epidural anesthesia may alter maternal-fetal glucose homeostasis, resulting in hypoglycemia.

Clinical Therapy

The goal of medical management includes early identification of hypoglycemia through observation and screening of newborns at risk (Sperling & Menon, 2004). The baby may be asymptomatic, or any of the following may occur:

- Lethargy, jitteriness
- Poor feeding, poor sucking
- Vomiting
- Hypothermia
- Pallor
- Apnea, irregular respirations, respiratory distress, cyanosis
- Hypotonia, possible loss of swallowing reflex
- Tremors, jerkiness, seizure activity
- High-pitched cry
- Exaggerated Moro reflex, coma

Aggressive treatment is recommended after a single low blood glucose value if the infant shows any of these symptoms. In at-risk infants, routine screening should be done frequently during the first 4 hours of life and then whenever any of the noted clinical manifestations appears or at 4-hour intervals until the risk period has passed.

Differential diagnosis of a newborn with nonspecific hypoglycemic symptoms includes determining whether the newborn has any of the following:

- CNS disease
- Sepsis

- Metabolic aberrations
- Polycythemia
- Congenital heart disease
- Drug withdrawal
- Temperature instability
- Hypocalcemia

Hypoglycemia may also be defined as a *glucose oxidase reagent strip* below 40 mg/dL, but only when corroborated with laboratory blood glucose (see Procedure 33–1: Performing a Heel Stick on a Newborn). Common bedside methods use whole blood, an enzymatic reagent strip, and a reflectance meter or color chart. Bedside glucose oxidase strip tests can screen for hypoglycemia, but laboratory determinations must confirm the results before a diagnosis of hypoglycemia can be made. Glucose reagent strips should not be used by themselves to screen and diagnose hypoglycemia because their results depend on the baby's hematocrit (they react to the glucose in the plasma, not the RBCs), and there is a wide variance (5 to 15 mg/dL) when compared with laboratory determinations.

CLINICAL TIP

Wrapping the foot in a warm washcloth or disposable diaper is a simple way to create adequate vasodilation for taking a blood specimen.

Blood glucose sampling techniques can significantly affect the accuracy of the blood glucose value. It is important to note that whole blood glucose concentrations are 10% to 15% lower than plasma glucose concentration. The higher the hematocrit, the greater the difference between whole blood and plasma values. Also, venous blood glucose concentrations are approximately 15% to 19% lower than arterial blood glucose concentrations because the tissues extract some glucose before the blood enters the venous system. Newer techniques, such as using a glucose oxidase analyzer or an optical bedside glucose analyzer, are more reliable for bedside screening but must also be validated with laboratory chemical analysis.

CLINICAL TIP

Blood samples for the laboratory should be placed on ice and analyzed within 30 minutes of drawing to prevent the RBCs from continuing to metabolize glucose and giving a falsely low reading.

Adequate caloric intake is important. Early breastfeeding or formula-feeding is one of the major preventive approaches. If early feeding or IV glucose is started to meet the recommended fluid and caloric needs, the blood glucose is likely to remain above the hypoglycemic level. During the first hours after birth, asymptomatic newborns may be given oral glucose contained in formula or breast milk (glucose water should not be used because it causes a rapid increase in glucose followed by an abrupt decrease), and then another plasma glucose measurement is obtained within 30 to 60 minutes after feeding.

IV infusions of a dextrose solution D5W to D10W (5% to 10%) begun immediately after birth should prevent hypo-

glycemia. Plasma glucose levels are obtained when the parenteral infusion is started. However, in the very small AGA infant, infusions of 10% dextrose solution may cause hyperglycemia to develop, requiring an alteration in the glucose concentration. Infants require 6 to 8 mg/kg/min of glucose to maintain normal glucose concentrations. Therefore an IV glucose solution should be calculated based on body weight of the infant and fluid requirements and correlated with blood glucose tests to determine adequacy of the infusion treatment.

A rapid infusion of 25% to 50% dextrose or the use of glucose water in place of formula is contraindicated because it may lead to profound rebound hypoglycemia following an initial brief increase. In more severe cases of hypoglycemia, corticosteroids may be administered. It is thought that steroids enhance gluconeogenesis from noncarbohydrate protein sources (Armentrout, 2004).

NURSING CARE MANAGEMENT
Nursing Assessment and Diagnosis

The objective of nursing assessment is to identify newborns at risk and to screen symptomatic infants. For newborns who are diagnosed with hypoglycemia, assessment is ongoing with careful monitoring of glucose values. Glucose strips, urine dipsticks, and urine volume (monitor only if above 1 to 3 mL/kg/hr) are evaluated frequently for osmotic diuresis and glycosuria.

Nursing diagnoses that may apply to the newborn with hypoglycemia include the following:

- *Altered Nutrition: Less than Body Requirements* related to increased glucose use secondary to physiologic stress
- *Ineffective Breathing Pattern* related to tachypnea and apnea
- *Acute Pain* related to frequent heel sticks for glucose monitoring

Nursing Plan and Implementation

The nurse should monitor blood glucose levels in at-risk groups no later than 2 hours after birth and before feedings or whenever there are abnormal signs (Armentrout, 2004). Monitor the IDM within 30 minutes of birth. Once an at-risk infant's blood sugar level is stable, glucose testing every 2 to 4 hours (or per agency protocol), or before feedings, adequately monitors glucose levels. See Procedure 33–1: Performing a Heel Stick on a Newborn. The infant's lateral heel is the preferred site for the glucose sample, so that the posterior tibial nerve and artery and the important longitudinally oriented fat pad of the heel will not be damaged.

Calculating glucose requirements and maintaining IV glucose will be necessary for any symptomatic infant with low serum glucose levels. The method of feeding greatly influences glucose and energy requirements; thus pay careful attention to glucose monitoring during the transition from IV to oral feedings. Titration of IV glucose may be required until the infant is able to take adequate amounts of formula or breast milk to

PROCEDURE 33–1 Performing a Heel Stick on a Newborn

NURSING ACTION	RATIONALE

Preparation

- Explain to parents what will be done.
- Select a clear, previously unpunctured site.

- The infant's lateral heel is the site of choice because it precludes damaging the posterior tibial nerve and artery, plantar artery, and the important longitudinally oriented fat pad of the heel, which in later years could impede walking (Figure 33–14 ◆). This is especially important for infants undergoing multiple heel stick procedures. Toes are acceptable sites if necessary.

The selection of a previously unpunctured site minimizes the risk of infection and excessive scar formation.

Equipment and Supplies

Microlancet (do not use a needle)
Alcohol swabs
2 × 2 sterile gauze squares
Small bandage
Transfer pipette or capillary tubes
Glucose reagent strips or reflectance meters
Gloves

Puncture sites

Figure 33–14 ◆ Potential sites for heel sticks. Avoid shaded areas to prevent injury to arteries and nerves in the foot and the important longitudinally oriented fat pad of the heel, which in later years could impede walking.

A needle may nick the periosteum. Gloves are used to implement standard precautions and prevent nosocomial infections.

Procedure: Clean Gloves

1. Apply gloves.
2. Use a warm wet wrap or specially designed chemical heat pad to warm the infant's heel for 5 to 10 seconds to facilitate blood flow.

Performing the Heel Stick

1. Grasp the infant's lower leg and foot so as to impede venous return slightly. This will facilitate extraction of the blood sample (Figure 33–15 ◆).

Figure 33–15 ◆ Heel stick. With a quick, piercing motion, puncture the lateral heel with a microlance. Be careful not to puncture too deeply.

(Continued on next page)

PROCEDURE 33–1   Performing a Heel Stick on a Newborn   continued

NURSING ACTION	RATIONALE
2. Clean the site by rubbing vigorously with 70% isopropyl alcohol swab.	*Friction produces local heat, which aids vasodilation.*
3. Blot the site dry completely with dry gauze square before lancing.	*Alcohol is irritating to injured tissue and it may also produce hemolysis.*
4. With a quick, piercing motion, puncture the lateral heel with a microlancet. Be careful not to puncture too deeply. Optimal penetration is 4 mm.	
5. Wipe the first drop of blood away with the gauze.	*The first drop may be contaminated by skin contact and the blood cells may have been traumatized during the stick. Blood glucose may be lowered by residual alcohol.*

Collecting the Blood Sample

1. Use transfer pipette to place drop of blood on glucose reflectance meter.
2. Use capillary tube for hematocrit testing.

Preventing Excessive Bleeding

1. Apply a folded gauze square to the puncture site and secure it firmly with a bandage.
2. Check the puncture site frequently for the first hour after sampling.

Documentation   Record the findings on the infant's chart

COMPLEMENTARY AND ALTERNATIVE THERAPIES

PAIN RELIEF IN THE NICU

Oral administration of *sucrose* for pain management from procedural pain (heel sticks, venipuncture, IM injections, oral suctioning, etc.) has been introduced in the NICU. The sweetness of the sucrose, a disaccharide, elevates the pain threshold through endogenous opioid release in the CNS (Gibbins & Stevens, 2003). On the anterior part of the tongue, 0.5 to 2 mL of 24% sucrose is administered via a syringe or pacifier approximately 2 minutes before the procedure (Walden & Jorgensen, 2004). Allowing nonnutritive sucking (NNS) with a pacifier aids in the reduction of procedural pain (Gibbins & Stevens, 2003). It is important to be careful with repeated doses of sucrose, as hyperglycemia may arise in the infant. Also, repeated use of sucrose analgesia in preterm infants may affect their neurologic development and behavioral outcomes. Until further research is done, repeated doses of sucrose are not recommended (Mitchell & Waltman, 2003).

maintain a normal blood sugar level. Titrate by decreasing the concentration of parenteral glucose gradually to 5% (D5W), then reducing the rate of infusion to 6 mg/kg/min, then to 4 mg/kg/min, and slowly discontinuing it over 4 to 6 hours. Enteral feeds are increased to maintain an adequate glucose and caloric intake.

Evaluation

Expected outcomes of nursing care include the following:

- The newborn at risk of hypoglycemia is promptly identified, and intervention is started early.
- The newborn's glucose level is stabilized; recovery proceeds without sequelae.

CARE OF THE NEWBORN WITH JAUNDICE

The most common abnormal physical finding in newborns is jaundice (*icterus neonatorum*). Some degree of jaundice, resulting from elevated unconjugated bilirubinemia, occurs in approximately 50% of term infants and 80% of preterm infants (Madan, MacMahon, & Stevenson, 2005). **Jaundice** is a yellowish coloration of the skin and sclera of the eyes that develops from the deposit of yellow pigment bilirubin in lipid/fat-containing tissues, as described in Chapter 28. ∞ Fetal unconjugated bilirubin is normally cleared by the placenta in utero, so total bilirubin at birth is usually less than 3 mg/L unless an abnormal hemolytic process has been present. Postnatally, the infant must conjugate bilirubin (convert a lipid-soluble pigment into a water-soluble pigment) in the liver.

The rate and amount of conjugation of bilirubin depend on the rate of hemolysis, the bilirubin load, the maturity of the liver, and the presence of albumin-binding sites. See

Chapter 28 ∞ for discussion of conjugation of bilirubin. A normal, healthy, full-term infant's liver is usually mature enough and produces enough glucuronyl transferase that the total serum bilirubin concentration does not reach a pathologic level. The diagnosis of pathologic jaundice is given to newborns who exhibit jaundice within the first 24 hours of life; have a total serum bilirubin concentration increase of greater than 0.2 mg/dL/ hour; surpass the 95th percentile on the nomogram for age in hours; or have persistent visible jaundice after 1 week of age in term infants or after 2 weeks in preterm infants.

Physiologic Jaundice

Physiologic or neonatal jaundice is a normal process that occurs during transition from intrauterine to extrauterine life and appears after 24 hours of life. It is typically due to the newborn's increased red cell mass, shorter red cell lifespan (90 days as compared with 120 days in the adult), slower uptake of bilirubin by the liver, lack of intestinal bacteria, and/or poorly established hydration from initial breastfeeding.

Lab tests reveal a predominance of unconjugated bilirubin. The average level of unconjugated bilirubin in cord blood is approximately 2 mg/dL at birth. This level rises to an average of 5 to 6 mg/dL between the third and fifth days of life. The jaundice is usually not visible after 14 days. The pattern of physiologic jaundice differs between breastfed and formula-fed newborns (for further discussion of physiologic jaundice, see "Physiologic Jaundice" in Chapter 28 ∞). Physiologic jaundice remains a common problem for the term newborn and may require treatment with phototherapy.

Pathophysiology of Hyperbilirubinemia

Serum albumin-binding sites are usually able to conjugate enough bilirubin to meet the demands of the normal newborn. However, certain conditions tend to decrease the number or quality of available binding sites. Fetal or neonatal asphyxia and neonatal drugs such as indomethacin decrease the binding affinity of bilirubin to albumin, because acidosis impairs the capacity of albumin to hold bilirubin. Hypothermia and hypoglycemia release FFAs that dislocate bilirubin from albumin. Maternal use of sulfa drugs and salicylates interferes with conjugation or with serum albumin-binding sites by competing with bilirubin for these sites. Finally, premature infants have less albumin available for binding with bilirubin. Neurotoxicity is possible because unconjugated bilirubin has a high affinity for extravascular tissue, such as fatty tissue (subcutaneous tissue) and cerebral tissue.

Bilirubin not bound to albumin is free to cross the blood-brain barrier, damage cells of the CNS, and produce **kernicterus** or **bilirubin encephalopathy** (Juretschke, 2005). *Kernicterus* (meaning "yellow nucleus") usually refers to the deposition of unconjugated bilirubin in the basal ganglia of the brain and to permanent neurologic sequelae of untreated **hyperbilirubinemia** (elevation of bilirubin level).

The classic bilirubin encephalopathy of kernicterus most commonly found with Rh and ABO blood group incompatibility is less common today because of aggressive treatment with phototherapy and exchange transfusions. But cases of kernicterus are reappearing as a result of early discharge and the increased incidence of dehydration (a result of discharge before mother's milk is established when breastfeeding). Current therapy can reduce the incidence of kernicterus encephalopathy but cannot distinguish all infants who are at risk.

Causes of Hyperbilirubinemia

A primary cause of pathologic hyperbilirubinemia is **hemolytic disease of the newborn.** All pregnant women who are Rh negative or who have blood type O (possible ABO incompatibility) should be asked about outcomes of any previous pregnancies, including abortions, and history of blood transfusion. Prenatal amniocentesis with spectrophotographic examination may be indicated in some cases. Cord blood from newborns is evaluated for bilirubin level, which normally does not exceed 5 mg/dL. Newborns of Rh-negative and O blood type mothers are carefully assessed for blood type status, appearance of jaundice, and levels of serum bilirubin.

Alloimmune hemolytic disease, also known as **erythroblastosis fetalis,** occurs when an Rh-negative mother is pregnant with an Rh-positive fetus and maternal antibodies cross the placenta. Maternal antibodies enter the fetal circulation, then attach to and destroy the fetal RBCs. The fetal system responds by increasing RBC production. Jaundice, anemia, and compensatory erythropoiesis result. A marked increase in immature RBCs (erythroblasts) also occurs, hence the designation erythroblastosis fetalis. Because of the widespread use of Rh immune globulin (RhoGAM), the incidence of erythroblastosis fetalis has dropped dramatically.

Hydrops fetalis, the most severe form of erythroblastosis fetalis, occurs when maternal antibodies attach to the Rh site on the fetal RBCs, making them susceptible to destruction; severe anemia and multiple organ system failure result. Cardiomegaly with severe cardiac decompensation and hepatosplenomegaly occur. Severe generalized massive edema (anasarca) and generalized fluid effusion into the pleural cavity (hydrothorax), pericardial sac, and peritoneal cavity (ascites) develop. Jaundice is not present until the newborn period because the bilirubin pigments for the fetus are being excreted through the placenta into the maternal circulation. The hydropic hemolytic disease process is also characterized by hyperplasia of the adrenal cortex and pancreatic islets, which predisposes the infant to neonatal hypoglycemia similar to that of IDMs. These infants also have increased bleeding tendencies due to associated thrombocytopenia and hypoxic damage to the capillaries. Hydrops is a frequent cause of intrauterine death among infants with Rh disease.

ABO incompatibility (the mother is blood type O and the baby is blood type A or B) may result in jaundice, although it rarely results in hemolytic disease severe enough to be clinically diagnosed and treated. Hepatosplenomegaly may be found occasionally in newborns with ABO incompatibility, but hydrops fetalis and stillbirth are rare.

Certain prenatal and perinatal factors predispose the newborn to hyperbilirubinemia. During pregnancy, predisposing

Table 33–3   RISK FACTORS FOR DEVELOPMENT OF SEVERE HYPERBILIRUBINEMIA IN INFANTS OF 35 OR MORE WEEKS' GESTATION (IN APPROXIMATE ORDER OF IMPORTANCE)

Major risk factors

- Predischarge TSB or TcB level in the high-risk zone
- Jaundice observed in the first 24 h
- Blood group incompatibility with positive direct antiglobulin test, other known hemolytic disease (e.g., G6PD deficiency), elevated ETCO$_c$
- Gestational age 35–36 wk
- Previous sibling received phototherapy
- Cephalohematoma or significant bruising
- Exclusive breastfeeding, particularly if nursing is not going well and weight loss is excessive
- East Asian race*

Minor risk factors

- Predischarge TSB or TcB level in the high intermediate-risk zone
- Gestational age 37–38 wk
- Jaundice observed before discharge
- Previous sibling with jaundice
- Macrosomic infant of a diabetic mother
- Maternal age greater than or equal to 25 yr
- Male gender

Decreased risk (these factors are associated with decreased risk of significant jaundice, listed in order of decreasing importance)

- TSB or TcB level in the low-risk zone
- Gestational age greater than or equal to 41 wk
- Exclusive bottle-feeding
- Black race*
- Discharge from hospital after 72 h

* Race as defined by mother's description.

SOURCE: From American Academy of Pediatrics Subcommittee on Hyperbilirubinemia. (2004). Management of hyperbilirubinemia in the newborn infant 35 or more weeks of gestation. *Pediatrics, 114*(1), 297–316 (Table 2, p. 301).

maternal conditions include hereditary spherocytosis, diabetes, intrauterine infections, gram-negative bacilli infections that stimulate production of maternal alloimmune antibodies, drug ingestion (such as sulfas, salicylates, novobiocin, and diazepam), and oxytocin administration. Early prenatal identification of the fetus at risk for Rh or ABO incompatibility allows prompt treatment. (See Chapter 20 ∞ for discussion of in utero management of this condition). Table 33–3 presents risk factors for development of severe hyperbilirubinemia in their approximate order of importance.

In addition to Rh or ABO incompatibility, other newborn conditions predispose to hyperbilirubinemia: polycythemia (central hematocrit 65% or more), pyloric stenosis, obstruction or atresia of the biliary duct or of the lower bowel, low-grade urinary tract infection, sepsis, hypothyroidism, enclosed hemorrhage (cephalhematoma, extensive bruising), asphyxia neonatorum, hypothermia, acidemia, and hypoglycemia. Neonatal hepatitis, atresia of the bile ducts, and GI atresia all can alter bilirubin metabolism and excretion.

DEVELOPING CULTURAL COMPETENCE

ETHNIC VARIATIONS AND JAUNDICE

East Asian infants (Japanese, Chinese, and Filipino ethnic groups) have a higher occurrence of hyperbilirubinemia than Causasian infants. Infants with Asian fathers and Causasian mothers have a higher incidence of jaundice than if both parents are Caucasian. Other ethnic groups at risk for increased bilirubinemia are Navajo, Eskimo, and Sioux Native American newborns; Greek newborns; Separdic-Jewish (oriental ancestry) newborns; and some Hispanic newborns.

The prognosis for a newborn with hyperbilirubinemia depends on the extent of the hemolytic process and the underlying cause. Severe hemolytic disease may result in fetal or early neonatal death from the effects of anemia—cardiac decompensation, edema, ascites, and hydrothorax. Hyperbilirubinemia may lead to kernicterus if not aggressively treated. The resulting neurologic damage may cause death, cerebral palsy, possible mental retardation, or hearing loss, or, to a lesser degree, perceptual impairment, delayed speech development, hyperactivity, muscle incoordination, or learning difficulties.

Clinical Therapy

The best treatment for hemolytic disease is prevention. Prenatal identification of the fetus at risk for Rh or ABO incompatibility will allow prompt treatment. See Chapter 20 ∞ for discussion of in utero management of this condition.

When one or more of the predisposing factors are present, the maternal and neonatal blood types should be tested in the laboratory for Rh or ABO incompatibility. Other necessary laboratory evaluations include Coombs' test, serum bilirubin levels (direct and total), hemoglobin, reticulocyte percentage, white blood cell count, and positive smear for cellular morphology (Table 33–4).

Neonatal hyperbilirubinemia must be considered pathologic if any of the following criteria are met (Bhutani, Johnson, & Keren, 2004):

1. Clinically evident jaundice within the first 24 hours of life
2. Serum bilirubin concentration rising by more than 0.2 mg/dL per hour
3. Total serum bilirubin concentrations exceeding the 95th percentile on the nomogram
4. Conjugated bilirubin concentrations greater than 2 mg/dL or more than 20% of the total serum bilirubin concentration
5. Clinical jaundice persisting for more than 2 weeks in a term newborn

Initial diagnostic procedures are aimed at differentiating jaundice resulting from increased bilirubin production, impaired conjugation or excretion, increased intestinal reabsorption, or a combination of these factors.

Table 33–4   LABORATORY EVALUATION OF THE JAUNDICED INFANT OF 35 OR MORE WEEKS' GESTATION

Indications	Assessments
Jaundice in first 24 h	Measure TcB and/or TSB.
Jaundice appears excessive for infant's age	Measure TcB and/or TSB.
Infant receiving phototherapy or TSB rising rapidly (i.e., crossing percentiles on the nomogram and unexplained by history and physical examination)	Blood type and Coombs' test, if not obtained with cord blood. Complete blood count and smear. Measure direct or conjugated bilirubin. It is an option to perform reticulocyte count, G6PD, and ETCO$_c$, if available. Repeat TSB in 4–24 h depending on infant's age and TSB level.
TSB concentration approaching exchange levels or not responding to phototherapy	Perform reticulocyte count, G6PD, albumin, ETCO$_c$, if available.
Elevated direct (or conjugated) bilirubin level	Do urinalysis and urine culture. Evaluate for sepsis if indicated by history and physical examination.
Jaundice present at or beyond age 3 wk, or sick infant	Total and direct (or conjugated) bilirubin level. If direct bilirubin elevated, evaluate for causes of cholestasis. Check results of newborn thyroid and galactosemia screen, and evaluate infant for signs or symptoms of hypothyroidism.

SOURCE: From American Academy of Pediatrics Subcommittee on Hyperbilirubinemia. (2004). Management of hyperbilirubinemia in the newborn infant 35 or more weeks of gestation. *Pediatrics, 114*(1), 297–316 (Table 1, p. 300).

Because of the shorter lifespan of RBCs in the newborn, a significant bilirubin load is produced. When bilirubin breaks down, carbon monoxide (CO) is released. This production of carbon monoxide is being investigated as a marker in the study of bilirubin production. Measuring end-tidal CO (ETCO) has been shown to provide results similar to laboratory measures of bilirubin (Madan et al., 2005). Other needed laboratory evaluations are Coombs' test, serum bilirubin levels (direct and total), hemoglobin, reticulocyte percentage, white cell count, and positive smear for cellular morphology. The Coombs' test determines whether jaundice is due to Rh or ABO incompatibility. The indirect Coombs' test measures the amount of Rh-positive antibodies in the mother's blood. Rh-positive RBCs are added to the maternal blood sample. If the mother's serum contains antibodies, the Rh-positive RBCs will agglutinate (clump) when rabbit immune antiglobulin is added, which is a positive test result.

The direct Coombs' test reveals the presence of antibody-coated (sensitized) Rh-positive RBCs in the newborn. Rabbit immune antiglobulin is added to the specimen of neonatal blood cells. If the neonatal RBCs agglutinate, they have been coated with maternal antibodies, a positive result.

If the hemolytic process is due to Rh sensitization, laboratory findings reveal the following: (1) an Rh-positive newborn with a positive Coombs' test; (2) increased erythropoiesis with many immature circulating RBCs (nucleated blastocysts); (3) anemia, in most cases; (4) elevated levels (5 mg/dL or more) of bilirubin in cord blood; and (5) a reduction in albumin-binding capacity. Maternal data may include an elevated anti-Rh titer and spectrophotometric evidence of fetal hemolytic process.

If the hemolytic process is due to ABO incompatibility, laboratory findings reveal an increase in reticulocytes. The resulting anemia is usually not significant during the newborn period and is rare later on. The direct Coombs' test may be negative or mildly positive, whereas the indirect Coombs' test may be strongly positive. Infants with a positive direct Coombs' test have increased incidence of jaundice with bilirubin levels in excess of 10 mg/dL. Increased numbers of spherocytes (spherical, plump, mature erythrocytes) are seen on a peripheral blood smear. Increased numbers of spherocytes are not seen on blood smears from Rh disease infants.

Clinical Therapy

Whatever the cause of hyperbilirubinemia, management of these infants is directed toward alleviating anemia, removing maternal antibodies and sensitized erythrocytes, increasing serum albumin levels, reducing serum bilirubin levels, and minimizing the consequences of hyperbilirubinemia. Early discharge of newborns from birthing centers has significantly influenced the diagnosis and management of neonatal jaundice, increasing the emphasis on outpatient and home care management.

Hemolytic disease may be treated with phototherapy, exchange transfusion, and drug therapy. When determining the appropriate management of hyperbilirubinemia due to hemolytic disease, the three variables that must be taken into account are the newborn's (1) serum bilirubin level, (2) birth weight, and (3) age in hours. If a newborn has hemolysis with an unconjugated bilirubin level of 14 mg/dL, weighs less than 2500 g (birth weight), and is 24 hours old or less, an exchange transfusion may be the best management. However, if that same newborn is over 24 hours old, which is past the time where an increase in bilirubin would result from pathologic causes, phototherapy may be the treatment of choice to prevent the possible complications of kernicterus.

PHOTOTHERAPY

Phototherapy is the exposure of the newborn to high-intensity light. It may be used alone or in conjunction with exchange transfusion to reduce serum bilirubin levels. Exposure of the newborn to high-intensity light (fluorescent light bulbs or bulbs in the blue-light spectrum) decreases serum bilirubin levels in the skin by facilitating biliary excretion of unconjugated bilirubin. Phototherapy decreases serum bilirubin levels by changing bilirubin from the nonwater soluble (lipophilic) form to water-soluble byproducts that can then be excreted. When bilirubin absorbs light, three forms of photochemical reaction occur: photo-oxidation, photoisomerization, and structural isomerization. Photo-oxidation is a minor contributor to bilirubin elimination. Structural isomerization is the most important pathway for decreasing serum bilirubin levels. Bilirubin is converted to lumirubin, which is bound to albumin and transported to the

- Use total bilirubin. Do not subtract direct reacting or conjugated bilirubin.
- Risk factors = isoimmune hemolytic disease, G6PD deficiency, asphyxia, significant lethargy, temperature instability, sepsis, acidosis, or albumin < 3.0g/dL (if measured)
- For well infants 35-37 6/7 wk can adjust TSB levels for intervention around the medium risk line. It is an option to intervene at lower TSB levels for infants closer to 35 wks and at higher TSB levels for those closer to 37 6/7 wk.
- It is an option to provide conventional phototherapy in hospital or at home at TSB levels 2-3 mg/dL (35-50mmol/L) below those shown but home phototherapy should not be used in any infant with risk factors.

Figure 33–16 ◆ Guidelines for phototherapy in hospitalized infants of 35 or more weeks' gestation.

Note: These guidelines are based on limited evidence and the levels shown are approximations. The guidelines refer to the use of intensive phototherapy, which should be used when the TSB (total serum bilirubin) exceeds the line indicated for each category. Infants are designated as "higher risk" because of the potential negative effects of the conditions listed on albumin binding of bilirubin, the blood-brain barrier, and the susceptibility of the brain cells to damage by bilirubin.

SOURCE: American Academy of Pediatrics Subcommittee on Hyperbilirubinemia. (2004). Management of hyperbilirubinemia in the newborn infant 35 or more weeks of gestation. *Pediatrics, 114*(1), 297–316 (Fig. 3, p. 304).

liver. It is a stable water-soluble molecule, so it is transferred into the urine and bile for excretion. Photoisomerization occurs when the natural form of bilirubin is exposed to light at a certain wavelength and the bilirubin is converted to a less toxic form. The new isomer, photobilirubin, is created rapidly but is quite unstable. Photobilirubin is bound to albumin, transported to the liver, and incorporated into bile. If it is not quickly eliminated from the bowel, then it can convert back to its original form and return to the bloodstream.

Phototherapy is an intervention that is used more for the prevention of hyperbilirubinemia to halt bilirubin levels from climbing dangerously high. The decision to start phototherapy is based on two factors: gestational age and age in hours. Phototherapy is the most effective in the first 24 to 48 hours of usage; frequently the light can be discontinued during or immediately after this time frame.

Phototherapy plays an important role in preventing a rise in bilirubin levels but does not alter the underlying cause of jaundice, and hemolysis may continue to produce anemia. Many authors have recommended initiating phototherapy "prophylactically" in the first 24 hours of life in high-risk, VLBW, or severely bruised infants. Figure 33–16 ◆ shows guidelines for the use of phototherapy.

Phototherapy can be provided through halogen spotlights (although these are not widely used because of the risk of thermal burns), conventional banks of phototherapy lights, a fiberoptic blanket attached to a halogen light source around the trunk of the newborn, or a combination of these delivery methods. The bank bilirubin lights utilize light in the blue spectrum. This is the most effective source available but can mask cyanosis and causes dizziness and nausea in the staff. With the fiberoptic blanket, the light stays on at all times, and the newborn is accessible for care, feeding, and diaper changes; greater surface area is exposed and there are no thermoregulation issues. The eyes are not covered. Fluid and weight loss are not

complications of this system. Furthermore, it makes the infant accessible to the parents and is less alarming to parents than standard phototherapy. A combination of a fiberoptic light source in the mattress under the baby and a standard light source above may also be used. This is termed *intensive phototherapy*. Intensive phototherapy should reduce the total serum bilirubin (TSB) by 1 to 2 mg/dL within 4 to 6 hours and levels should continue to decline. If this goal is not reached then an exchange transfusion should be considered. Many institutions and pediatricians use fiberoptic blankets for home care.

EXCHANGE TRANSFUSION

Exchange transfusion is the withdrawal and replacement of the newborn's blood with donor blood. It is used to treat anemia with RBCs that are not susceptible to maternal antibodies, remove sensitized RBCs that would be lysed soon, remove serum bilirubin, and provide bilirubin-free albumin and increase the binding sites for bilirubin. Concerns over doing an exchange transfusion are related to the use of blood products and associated potential for HIV infection and hepatitis. If the TSB is at or approaching the exchange level (Figure 33–17 ◆), send blood for immediate type and cross-match. Blood for exchange transfusion is modified whole blood (red cells and plasma) cross-matched against the mother and compatible with the infant.

NURSING CARE MANAGEMENT
Nursing Assessment and Diagnosis

Assessment is aimed at identifying prenatal and perinatal factors that predispose to development of jaundice and identifying jaundice as soon as it is apparent. Clinically, ABO incompatibility presents as jaundice and occasionally as hepatosplenomegaly. Fetal hydrops or erythroblastosis fetalis is rare (see

- The dashed lines for the first 24 hours indicate uncertainty due to a wide range of clinical circumstances and a range of responses to phototherapy.
- Immediate exchange transfusion is recommended if infant shows signs of acute bilirubin encephalopathy (hypertonia, arching, retrocollis, opisthotonos, fever, high pitched cry) or if TSB is ≥5 mg/dL (85 μmol/L) above these lines.
- Risk factors - isoimmune hemolytic disease, G6PD deficiency, asphyxia, significant lethargy, temperature instablity, sepsis, acidosis.
- Measure serum albumin and calculate B/A ratio (See legend)
- Use total bilirubin. Do not subtract direct reacting or conjugated bilirubin
- If infant is well and 35-37 6/7 wk (median risk) can individualize TSB levels for exchange based on actual gestational age.

Figure 33–17 ◆ Transfusion level nomogram.
SOURCE: From American Academy of Pediatrics Subcommittee on Hyperbilirubinemia. (2004). Management of hyperbilirubinemia in the newborn infant 35 or more weeks of gestation. *Pediatrics, 114*(1), 297–316 (Fig. 4, p. 305).

Chapter 20 ∞). Hemolytic disease of the newborn is suspected if the placenta is enlarged, if the newborn is edematous with pleural and pericardial effusion plus ascites, if pallor or jaundice is noted during the first 24 to 36 hours, if hemolytic anemia is diagnosed, or if the spleen and liver are enlarged. The nurse carefully notes changes in behavior and observes for evidence of bleeding. If laboratory tests indicate elevated bilirubin levels, the nurse checks the newborn for jaundice about every 2 hours and records observations.

To check for jaundice in lighter skinned babies, the nurse should blanch the skin over a bony prominence (forehead, nose, or sternum) by pressing firmly with the thumb. After pressure is released, if jaundice is present, the area appears yellow before normal color returns. The nurse should check oral mucosa and the posterior portion of the hard palate and conjunctival sacs for yellow pigmentation in darker skinned babies. Assessment in daylight gives best results, because pink walls and surroundings may mask yellowish tints and yellow light makes differentiation of jaundice difficult. The time of onset of jaundice is recorded and reported. If jaundice appears, careful observation of the increase in depth of color and the infant's behavior is mandatory. The newborn's behavior is assessed for neurologic signs associated with hyperbilirubinemia, which are rare but may include hypotonia, diminished reflexes, lethargy, or seizures.

In addition to visual inspection, reflectance photometers that measure transcutaneous bilirubin (TcB) should be used to screen and monitor neonatal jaundice. Some hospitals have developed a mandatory screening policy for all newborns before discharge using the TcB monitor. If the level comes back as high then a follow-up TSB will be performed. Another portable screening tool is the analysis for ETCO. This analysis allows for rapid identification of newborns with significant hemolytic disease who may be at risk for the sequelae of unconjugated hyperbilirubinemia (American Academy of Pediatrics Subcommittee on Hyperbilirubinemia, 2004).

Nursing diagnoses that may apply to a newborn with jaundice include the following:

- ***Risk for Fluid Volume Deficit*** related to increased insensible water loss and frequent loose stools
- ***Potential for Injury*** related to use of phototherapy
- ***Sensory/Perceptual Alterations*** related to neurologic damage secondary to kernicterus
- ***Risk for Altered Parenting*** related to deficient knowledge of infant care and prolonged separation of infant and parents secondary to illness

Nursing Plan and Implementation

HOSPITAL-BASED NURSING CARE

Hospital-based care is described in Nursing Care Plan: For the Newborn with Hyperbilirubinemia on page 1014. If phototherapy lights are used, expose the newborn's entire skin surface to the light. Minimal covering may be applied over the genitals and buttocks to expose maximum skin surface while still protecting the bedding from soiling. Phototherapy success is measured every 12 hours or daily by serum bilirubin levels (more frequently if there is hemolysis or a higher level before initiation of phototherapy). The lights must be turned off while drawing blood for serum bilirubin levels. Because it is not known whether phototherapy injures the delicate eye structures, particularly the retina, the nurse applies eye patches over the newborn's closed eyes during exposure to banks of phototherapy lights (see Figure 33–18 ◆ in Procedure 33–2: Infant Receiving Phototherapy). Phototherapy is discontinued and the eye patches are removed at least once per shift to assess the eyes for the presence of conjunctivitis. Patches are also removed to allow eye contact during feeding (for social stimulation) or when parents are visiting (to promote parental attachment).

Most phototherapy units will provide this level of irradiance 45 to 50 cm below the lamps. The nurse can use a photometer to measure and maintain desired irradiance levels. Disadvantages of lights are that they create a difficult work environment and can distort an infant's color. A benign transient bronze discoloration of the skin may occur with phototherapy when the infant has elevated direct serum bilirubin levels or liver disease. As a side effect of phototherapy, some newborns develop a maculopapular rash. In addition to assessing the newborn's skin color for jaundice and bronzing, the nurse examines the skin for developing pressure areas. The newborn should be repositioned at least every 2 hours to permit the light to reach all skin surfaces, to prevent pressure areas, and to vary the stimulation to the infant. The nurse keeps track of the number of hours each lamp is used so that each can be replaced before its effectiveness is lost. The nurse must be careful about using ointments under bilirubin lights because they may cause burns.

The newborn's temperature is monitored to prevent hyperthermia or hypothermia. The newborn will require additional fluids to compensate for the increased water loss through the skin and loose stools. Loose stools and increased urine output are the results of increased bilirubin excretion. The infant is observed for signs of dehydration and perianal excoriation.

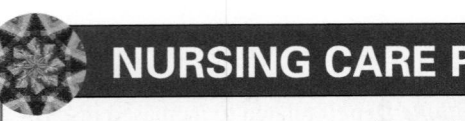

NURSING CARE PLAN

For the Newborn with Hyperbilirubinemia

INTERVENTION	RATIONALE	EXPECTED OUTCOMES
1. Nursing Diagnosis: Impaired Tissue Integrity related to predisposing factors associated with hyperbilirubinemia		
Goal: Babies at risk for jaundice and early signs of jaundice will be identified.		

• Evaluate baby's history for predisposing factors for hyperbilirubinemia.
 	
• Observe color of amniotic fluid at time of rupture of membranes.
• Assess baby for developing jaundice in daylight if possible.
 	
  1. Observe sclera.
 	
  2. Observe skin color and assess by blanching.
 	
  3. Check oral mucosa, posterior portion of hard palate, and conjunctival sacs for yellow pigmentation in dark-skinned newborns.
• Report jaundice occurring within 24 hours of birth.
	• Early identification of risk factors enables the nurse to monitor babies for early signs of hyperbilirubinemia. Acidosis, hypoxia, and hypothermia increase the risk of hyperbilirubinemia at lower bilirubin levels.
	• Amber-colored amniotic fluid indicates hyperbilirubinemia.
	• Early detection is affected by nursery environment. Artificial lights (with pink tint) may mask beginning of jaundice.
	  1. Most visible sign of hyperbilirubinemia is jaundice noted in skin, sclera, or oral mucosa. Onset is first seen on face and then progresses down the trunk.
	  2. Blanching the skin leaves a yellow color to the skin immediately after pressure is released.
	  3. Underlying pigment of dark-skinned infants may normally appear yellow.
		Baby's jaundice is identified early.

2. Nursing Diagnosis: Risk for Fluid Volume Deficit related to phototherapy		
Goal: The infant will not exhibit signs of dehydration and will display appropriate weight gain.		

• Offer feedings every 2 to 3 hr.
  • Breastfeed on demand with no supplementation unless excessive weight loss or increasing TSB with adequate feeding.
• Provide 25% extra fluid intake.
 	
• Assess for dehydration:
  1. Poor skin turgor
  2. Depressed fontanelles
  3. Sunken eyes
  4. Decreased urine output
  5. Weight loss
  6. Changes in electrolytes
	• Adequate hydration increases peristalsis and excretion of bilirubin.
	
	• Replace fluid losses due to watery stools, if under phototherapy.
	• Phototherapy treatment may cause liquid stools and increased insensible water loss, which increases risk of dehydration.
		Baby will have good skin turgor, clear amber urine output of 1–3 mL/kg/hr, six to eight wet diapers/day, and will maintain weight.

NURSING CARE PLAN

For the Newborn with Hyperbilirubinemia continued

INTERVENTION	RATIONALE	EXPECTED OUTCOMES

• Monitor intake and output (I&O).
• Weigh daily.
• Report signs of dehydration.
• Administer IV fluids:
  1. Monitor flow rates.
  2. Assess insertion sites for signs of infection.
	• Prevents fluid overload.
	• IV fluids may be used if baby is dehydrated or in presence of other complications. IV may be started if exchange transfusion is to be done.	

3. Nursing Diagnosis: Potential for Injury related to use of phototherapy

Goal: Baby will not have any corneal irritation/drainage, skin breakdown, or major fluctuations in temperature.

• Cover baby's eyes with eye patches while under phototherapy lights. Cover testes/penis in male infants. • Make certain that eyelids are closed before applying eye patches. • Remove baby from under phototherapy and remove eye patches during feedings. • Inspect eyes each shift for conjunctivitis, drainage, and corneal abrasions due to irritation from eye patches. • Administer thorough perianal cleansing with each stool or change of perianal protective covering. • Provide minimal coverage-only of diaper area. • Avoid the use of oily applications on the skin. • Reposition baby every 2 hours • Observe for bronzing of skin. • Place Plexiglas shield between baby and light. • Monitor baby's skin and core temperature frequently until temperature is stable.	• Protects retina from damage due to high intensity light and testes from damage from heat. • Prevents corneal abrasions. • Provides visual stimulation and facilitates attachment behaviors. • Prevents or facilitates prompt treatment of purulent conjunctivitis. • Frequent stooling increases risk of skin breakdown. Prevents infection. • Provides maximal exposure. Shielded areas become more jaundiced, so maximum exposure is essential. • Prevents superficial burns to skin. • Provides equal exposure of all skin areas and prevents pressure areas. • Bronzing is related to use of phototherapy with increased direct bilirubin levels or liver damage; may last for 2 to 4 months. • Hypothermia and hyperthermia are common complications of phototherapy. • Hypothermia results from exposure to lights, subsequent radiation, and convection losses.	*Baby's eyes are protected, skin is intact, and baby maintains a stable temperature.*

(Continued on next page)

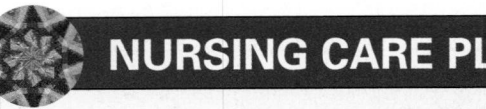

NURSING CARE PLAN

For the Newborn with Hyperbilirubinemia continued

INTERVENTION	RATIONALE	EXPECTED OUTCOMES
• Check axillary temperature with readings on servo-controlled unit on incubator. • Regulate incubator temperature as needed.	• Hyperthermia may result from the increased environmental heat. • Additional heat from phototherapy lights frequently causes a rise in the baby's and incubator's temperatures. Fluctuations in temperature may occur in response to radiation and convection.	

4. Nursing Diagnosis: Risk for Altered Impaired Parenting related to deficient knowledge of infant care and prolonged separation of infant and parents secondary to illness.

Goals: Parents will bond with infant and have realistic expectations about their infant. Parents are comfortable taking their infant home. They are able to demonstrate normal infant care and assessments of possible complications, and they know when to return for follow-up.

INTERVENTION	RATIONALE	EXPECTED OUTCOMES
• Encourage parents to provide tactile stimulation during feeding and diaper changes.	• Newborn has normal needs for tactile stimulation. • Presence of equipment may discourage parents from interacting with newborn.	*The parent will demonstrate ability to perform basic infant care tasks as evidenced by exhibiting appropriate attachment behaviors (i.e., talking and holding infant, feeding infant, and caring for infant under home bili therapy).*

• Encourage cuddling and eye contact during feedings.
• Offer suggestions to comfort restless infant:
  • Nesting when beneath bili lights
  • Talking softly and singing quietly to infant
  • Taped music or tape recording of evening activities from home
  • Rhythmic patting of buttocks
  • Firm, nonstroking touch, assisting with control of extremities
  • Pacifier for nonnutritive sucking
	• Provides opportunity for parents to bond with their newborn.
	• Provides comfort and decreases sensory deprivation.	

• Encourage family/friend support of mother/parents (i.e., meals, rest, child care for siblings, allow expressions of concerns/feelings). • Evaluate additional psychosocial needs. • Discuss rationale for treatment and possible side effects of phototherapy with family (stool changes, increased fluid loss, possible temp instability, slight lethargy, rash, altered sleep-wake patterns).	• Decreases strain on mother/parents by assisting with other responsibilities and allows for additional time with newborn for bonding, care, etc. • Parents may not understand what is happening or why. • Physician preference of treatment modalities may vary. Parents may not understand why their newborn is not receiving a treatment that another with the same condition is receiving.	*Parents verbalize understanding of rationale and possible side effects from phototherapy, parents/family demonstrate safety precautions when caring for infant; parents getting meals, rest, and verbalize support given.*

NURSING CARE PLAN

For the Newborn with Hyperbilirubinemia continued

INTERVENTION	RATIONALE	EXPECTED OUTCOMES

• Instruct family on infant's care while undergoing phototherapy:
  • Safety precautions—bili mask, incubator door closed and latched, covering genitalia per policy.
  • Skin care, cord care, circumcision care as appropriate.
  • Lab draws, rationale I&O.
• Encourage parent/significant other/sibling involvement in infant care as possible.
• Give explanation of equipment being used and changes in bilirubin levels. Allow parents an opportunity to ask questions; reinforce or clarify information as needed.
• Evaluate family's understanding of information.
• As necessary, review role of pumping breasts and offering formula for limited time.
 	
• Assist mother to pump her breasts to maintain milk supply.
	• The etiology of breast milk jaundice remains uncertain. The serum bilirubin levels begin to fall within 48 hr after discontinuation of breastfeeding. Opinion of physicians varies regarding the need for discontinuing breastfeeding.
	• If breastfeeding is temporarily discontinued, assess mother's knowledge of pumping her breasts and provide information and support as needed.	

If the baby is to receive phototherapy at home, parents are taught to record the infant's temperature, weight, fluid I&O, stools, and feedings and to use the phototherapy equipment. In addition, if phototherapy lights are being used, parents must agree that the baby will be exposed to the lights for long periods of time; that they will hold the baby for only short periods for feedings, comforting, and cleansing of the perineal area; and that the room temperature will be regulated to minimize heat loss. The terms *jaundice, hyperbilirubinemia, exchange transfusion,* and *phototherapy* may sound frightening and threatening. Some parents may feel guilty about their baby's condition and think they have caused the problem. Under stress, parents may not be able to understand the physician's or nurse practitioner's first explanations. The nurse must expect that the parents will need explanations repeated and clarified and that they may need help voicing their questions and fears. Eye and tactile

contact with the infant is encouraged. The nurse can coach parents when they visit with the baby. After the mother's discharge, parents are kept informed of their infant's condition and are encouraged to return to the hospital or telephone at any time so that they can be fully involved in the care of their infant. Tell parents that they can expect a rebound of 1 to 2 mg/dL after discontinuation of phototherapy and a follow-up bilirubin test may be done (Watson, 2004).

While the mother is still hospitalized some healthcare facilities may allow phototherapy to be carried out in the mother's room if the only problem is hyperbilirubinemia. The mother must be willing to keep the baby in the room for 24 hours a day; be able to take emergency action, as for choking, if necessary; and complete instruction checklists. Some institutions require that parents sign a consent form. The nurse gives the instructions to the parents but also continues to monitor the

PROCEDURE 33–2 Infant Receiving Phototherapy

NURSING ACTION	RATIONALE

Preparation

- Explain the purpose of phototherapy, the procedure itself (including the need to use eye patches), and possible side effects such as dehydration and skin breakdown from more frequent stooling.
- Note evidence of jaundice in the skin, sclera, and mucous membranes (in infants with darkly pigmented skin). Be sure that recent serum bilirubin levels are available.

The decision to use phototherapy is based on a careful assessment of the newborn's condition over a period of time. The most recent results before starting therapy serve as a baseline to evaluate the effectiveness of therapy.

Equipment and Supplies

Bank of phototherapy lights
Eye patches
Small scale to weigh diapers

Procedure

1. Obtain vital signs including axillary temperature.

   Provides baseline data.

2. Remove all of the infant's clothing except the diaper.

   Exposure of the newborn to high-intensity light (a bank of fluorescent light bulbs or bulbs in the blue-white spectrum) decreases serum bilirubin levels in the skin by aiding biliary excretion of unconjugated bilirubin. Because the tissue absorbs the light, best results are obtained when there is maximum skin surface exposure.

3. Apply eye coverings (eye patches or a bili mask) to the infant according to agency policy. (See Figure 33–18.)

   Eye coverings are used because it is not known if phototherapy injures delicate eye structures, particularly the retina.

4. Place the infant in an open crib or isolette (more commonly used in preterm infants and infants who are sicker) about 45 to 50 cm below the bank of phototherapy lights. Reposition every 2 hours.

   The isolette helps the infant maintain his or her temperature while undressed. Repositioning exposes different areas of skin to the lights, prevents the development of pressure areas on the skin, and varies the stimulation the infant receives.

Figure 33–18 ◆ Infant receiving phototherapy. The phototherapy light is positioned over the incubator. Bilateral eye patches are always used during photo light therapy to protect the baby's eyes.
SOURCE: Courtesy of Lisa Smith-Pedersen, RNC, MSN, NNP.

PROCEDURE 33–2 Infant Receiving Phototherapy   continued

NURSING ACTION	RATIONALE
5. Monitor vital signs every 4 hours with axillary temperatures.	*Temperature assessment is indicated to detect hypothermia or hyperthermia. Deviation in pulse and respirations may indicate developing complications.*
6. Cluster care activities.	
7. Discontinue phototherapy and remove eye patches at least every 2 to 3 hours when feeding the infant and when the parents visit.	*Care activities are clustered to help ensure that the newborn has maximum time under the lights. Eye patches are removed to assess for signs of complications such as excessive pressure, discharge, or conjunctivitis. Patches are also removed to provide some social stimulation and to promote parental attachment.*
8. Maintain adequate fluid intake. Evaluate need for IV fluids.	
9. Monitor intake and output carefully. Weigh diapers before discarding. Record quantity and characteristics of each stool.	*Infants undergoing phototherapy treatment have increased water loss and loose stools as a result of bilirubin excretion. This increases their risk of dehydration.*

CLINICAL TIP

If the area of jaundice about the eyes begins to disappear, it is probable that the eye patches are allowing light to enter and better eye protection is needed.

NURSING ACTION	RATIONALE
10. Assess specific gravity with each voiding. Weigh newborn daily.	*Specific gravity provides one measure of urine concentration. Highly concentrated urine is associated with a dehydrated state. Weight loss is also a sign of developing dehydration in the newborn.*
11. Observe the infant for signs of perianal excoriation and institute therapy if it develops.	*Perianal excoriation may develop because of the irritating effect of diarrhea stools.*
12. Ensure that serum bilirubin levels are drawn regularly according to orders or agency policy. Turn the phototherapy lights off while the blood is drawn.	*Serum bilirubin levels provide the most accurate indication of the effectiveness of phototherapy. They are generally drawn every 12 hours but at least once daily. The phototherapy lights are turned off to ensure accurate serum bilirubin levels.*
13. Examine the newborn's skin regularly for signs of developing pressure areas, bronzing, maculopapular rash, and changes in degree of jaundice.	*Pressure areas may develop if the infant lies in one position for an extended period. A benign, transient bronze discoloration of the skin may occur with phototherapy when the infant has elevated direct serum bilirubin levels or liver disease. A maculopapular rash is another transient side effect of phototherapy that develops occasionally.*
14. Avoid using lotion or ointment on the exposed skin.	*Lotion and ointments on a newborn receiving phototherapy may cause skin burns.*
15. Provide parents with opportunities to hold the newborn and assist in the infant's care. Answer their questions accurately and keep them informed of developments or changes.	*A sick infant is a source of great anxiety for parents. Information helps them deal with their anxiety. Moreover, they have a right to be kept well informed of their baby's status so that they are able to make informed decisions as needed.*

(Continued on next page)

PROCEDURE 33–2 Infant Receiving Phototherapy continued

NURSING ACTION	RATIONALE

16. May also provide phototherapy using lightweight, fiberoptic blankets ("bili blankets"). The baby is wrapped in the blanket, which is plugged into a outlet (Figure 33–19 ◆).

Figure 33–19 ◆ Newborn on fiberoptic "bili" mattress and under phototherapy lights. A combination of fiberoptic light source mattress and standard phototherapy light source may also be used.
NOTE: The color is distorted because of the reflection of the bililight mattress.

With fiberoptic blankets the newborn is readily accessible for care, feedings, and diaper changes. The baby does not get overheated, and fluid and weight loss are not complications of this system. The infant is accessible to the parents and the procedure seems less alarming to parents than standard phototherapy.

Table 33–5   INSTRUCTIONAL CHECKLIST FOR IN-ROOM PHOTOTHERAPY

Explain and demonstrate the placement of eye patches and explain that they must be in place when the infant is under the lights.

Explain the clothing to be worn (diaper under lights, dress and wrap when away from the lights).

Explain the importance of taking the infant's temperature regularly.

Explain the importance of adequate fluid intake.

Explain the charting flow sheet (intake, output, eyes covered).

Explain how to position the lights at a proper distance.

Explain the need to keep the infant under phototherapy except during feeding and diaper changes.

infant's temperature, activity, I&O, and positioning of eye patches (if conventional light banks are used) at regular intervals (Table 33–5).

COMMUNITY-BASED NURSING CARE

Some studies have shown that with early discharge of newborns and their mothers comes an increase in hospital readmission and elevated risk of pathologic hyperbilirubinemia. Home phototherapy use is recommended only if the bilirubin level is plotted on the nomogram and found to be in the "optional phototherapy" range. Any newborn with a level in the higher range should be hospitalized for continual phototherapy and serum bilirubin levels closely monitored on a regular schedule (Bhutani et al., 2004).

Jaundice and its treatment can be very disturbing to parents and may generate feelings of guilt and fear. Reassurance and support are vital especially for the breastfeeding mother, who may question her ability to adequately nourish her newborn. The parents' perception of and/or misconceptions about jaundice can affect parent-infant interactions. The nurse should explain the causes of jaundice and emphasize that it is usually a transient problem and one to which all infants must adapt after birth. It is essential that the impact of cultural beliefs be considered. Some Latina women believe that showing strong maternal emotions during pregnancy and breastfeeding can be detrimental. "Bilis" associated with anger may be blamed by some Latina women for jaundice. Cultural beliefs lead mothers to interpret illness within their cultural framework, especially when left without clear and understood explanations. Maternal reactions can be lessened by careful explanations to the mothers about the diagnosis, prognosis, duration, and management options for jaundice and about the possibility of its recurrence.

If the baby is to receive phototherapy at home, parents are taught to record the infant's temperature, weight, fluid I&O, stools, and feedings and to use the phototherapy equipment. In addition, if phototherapy lights are being used, parents must agree that the baby will be exposed to the lights for long periods of time; that they will hold the baby for only short periods for feedings, comforting, and cleansing of the perineal area; and that the room temperature will be regulated to minimize heat loss. Fiberoptic phototherapy blankets eliminate the need for eye patches, decrease heat loss because the baby is clothed, and provide more opportunities for interaction between the baby and parents. The best method of home phototherapy depends on the cause of the hyperbilirubinemia and the rate of progression of the jaundice. Ongoing monitoring of bilirubin levels is essential with home phototherapy and can be carried out in the home, in the follow-up clinic, or in the clinician's office.

Evaluation

Expected outcomes of nursing care include the following:

- The newborns at risk for development of hyperbilirubinemia are identified, and action is taken to minimize the potential impact of hyperbilirubinemia.

- The baby will not have any corneal irritation or drainage, skin breakdown, or major fluctuations in temperature.

- Parents understand the rationale for, goal of, and expected outcome of therapy.

- Parents verbalize their concerns about their baby's condition and identify how they can facilitate their baby's improvement.

CARE OF THE NEWBORN WITH ANEMIA

Neonatal anemia is often difficult to recognize by clinical evaluation alone. The hemoglobin concentration in a full-term newborn is 15 to 20 g/dL, slightly higher than in premature infants, in whom the mean hemoglobin is 14 to 18 g/dL. Infants with hemoglobin values of less than 14 mg/dL (term) and 13 g/dL (preterm) are usually considered anemic. The most common causes of neonatal anemia are blood loss, hemolysis/erythrocyte destruction, and impaired RBC/erythrocyte production (Bizzarro, Colson, & Ehrenkranz, 2004).

Blood loss (hypovolemia) occurs in utero from placental bleeding (placenta previa or abruptio placenta). Intrapartal blood loss may be fetomaternal, fetofetal, or the result of umbilical cord bleeding. Birth trauma to abdominal organs (adrenal hemorrhage) or the cranium (subgaleal bleed) may produce significant blood loss, and cerebral bleeding may occur because of hypoxia.

Excessive hemolysis of red cells is usually a result of blood group incompatibilities but may be due to infections. The most common cause of impaired red cell production is a genetically transmitted deficiency in glucose-6-phosphate dehydrogenase (G6PD). Anemia and jaundice are the presenting signs.

A condition known as **physiologic anemia of infancy** exists as a result of the normal gradual drop in hemoglobin for the first 6 to 12 weeks of life and corresponds with the decline in fetal hemoglobin. Theoretically, the bone marrow stops production of RBCs in response to higher oxygen levels that result from breathing changes after birth. When the amount of hemoglobin decreases, reaching levels of 10 to 11 g/dL at about 6 to 12 weeks of age (the average is 70 days), the bone marrow begins production of RBCs again, and the anemia disappears.

Anemia in preterm newborns is seen earlier than in term newborns, and increased production of RBCs does not start until hemoglobin is 7 to 9 g/dL. The preterm baby's hemoglobin reaches a low sooner (4 to 8 weeks after birth) than does a term newborn's (6 to 12 weeks) because preterm RBC survival time is shorter than in the term newborn (Diehl-Jones & Askin, 2004). This difference is due to several factors: the preterm infant's rapid growth rate, decreased iron stores, and an inadequate production of erythropoietin (EPO).

Clinical Therapy

Hematologic problems can be anticipated based on the pregnancy history and clinical manifestations. The age at which anemia is first noted is also of diagnostic value. Clinically, light-skinned anemic infants are very pale when they do not have other symptoms of shock and usually have abnormally low RBC counts. In acute blood loss, symptoms of shock may be present, such as pallor, low arterial blood pressure, and a decreasing hematocrit value.

The initial laboratory work-up should include hemoglobin and hematocrit measurements, reticulocyte count, examination of peripheral blood smear, bilirubin determinations, direct Coombs' test of infant's blood, and examination of maternal blood smear for fetal erythrocytes (Kleihauer-Betke test). Clinical management depends on the severity of the anemia and whether blood loss is acute or chronic. The baby should be placed on constant cardiac and respiratory monitoring. Mild or chronic anemia in an infant may be treated adequately with iron supplements alone or with iron-fortified formulas. Frequent determinations of hemoglobin, hematocrit, and bilirubin levels (in hemolytic disease) are essential. In severe cases of anemia, transfusions with O-negative or typed and cross-matched packed red cells are the preferred method of treatment. Management of anemia of prematurity includes treating the causative factor (i.e., antibiotics/antivirals used for infection, steroid therapy for disorders of erythrocyte production), recombinant human erythropoietin (rEPO), and supplemental iron. Blood transfusions (dedicated units of blood) are kept to a minimum.

NURSING CARE MANAGEMENT

The nurse assesses the newborn for symptoms of anemia (pallor). If the blood loss is acute, the baby may exhibit signs of shock (a capillary filling time greater than 3 seconds, decreased pulses, tachycardia, and low BP). Continued observations will be necessary to identify physiologic anemia as the preterm newborn grows. Signs of compromise include poor weight gain, tachycardia, tachypnea, and apneic episodes. The nurse promptly reports any symptoms indicating anemia or shock. The amount of blood drawn for all laboratory tests is recorded in tenths of a milliliter, so that total blood removed can be assessed and replaced by transfusion when necessary. If the newborn exhibits signs of shock, the nurse may need to initiate interventions.

CARE OF THE NEWBORN WITH POLYCYTHEMIA

Polycythemia, a condition in which blood volume and hematocrit values are increased, is observed more commonly in intrauterine growth restricted (IUGR), full-term, or close-to-full-term infants; newborns with placental transfusion caused by delayed cord clamping or cord stripping; infants receiving maternal-fetal or twin-to-twin transfusions; babies who have been exposed to intrauterine hypoxia; and babies of mothers who smoke; suffer from asphyxia, diabetes (IDM), or hypertension; or take propranolol during pregnancy. Other conditions that may present with polycythemia are chromosomal anomalies such as trisomy 21, 18, and 13 and births at altitudes over 5000 feet. The incidence ranges from 1% to 5%, and the condition is uncommon in newborns less than 34 weeks' gestation (Pappas & Delaney-Black, 2004). An infant is considered polycythemic when the central venous hematocrit value is greater than 65% to 70%.

Clinical Therapy

The goal of therapy is to reduce the central venous hematocrit to a range of 55% to 60% in symptomatic infants. To decrease the red cell mass, the symptomatic infant receives a partial exchange transfusion in which blood is removed from the infant and replaced milliliter for milliliter with colloids such as fresh frozen plasma or 5% albumin, or crystalloids such as isotonic saline or Ringer's lactate. The preference is to use crystalloids because of decreased promotion of infection, incidence of necrotizing enterocolitis (NEC), and their hypoallergenic properties. Supportive treatment of presenting symptoms is required until resolution, which usually occurs spontaneously following the partial exchange transfusion.

NURSING CARE MANAGEMENT

The nurse assesses, records, and reports symptoms of polycythemia. The nurse also does an initial screening of the newborn's hematocrit on admission to the nursery. The peak of term newborn's hematocrit will occur at 2 hours of age and begin to drop slowly by 12 to 18 hours. If a capillary hematocrit is done, warming the heel before obtaining the blood helps to decrease falsely high values (see Procedure 33–1: Performing Heel Stick on a Newborn); however, peripheral free-flowing venous hematocrit samples are usually obtained from the antecubital fossa for confirmation.

Many infants are asymptomatic, but as symptoms develop, they are related to the increased blood volume, hyperviscosity (thickness) of the blood, and decreased deformability of RBCs, all of which result in poor perfusion of tissues. The infants have a characteristic plethoric (ruddy) appearance. The most common symptoms observed include the following:

- *Cardiopulmonary:* Tachycardia and congestive heart failure due to the increased blood volume
- *Respiratory:* Respiratory distress with grunting, tachypnea, apnea, pleural effusion, cardiomegaly and cyanosis; increased oxygen need; or hemorrhage in respiratory system due to pulmonary venous congestion, edema, and hypoxemia
- *Gastrointestinal:* Feeding intolerance, NEC, or poor feeding
- *Hematologic:* Hyperbilirubinemia due to increased numbers of RBCs breaking down; thrombocytopenia; or elevated reticulocytes and nucleated RBCs

- *Renal:* Renal vein thrombosis with decreased urine output, hematuria, or proteinuria due to thromboembolism; or renal tubular damage
- *Central nervous system:* Jitteriness, irritability, decreased activity and tone, lethargy, stroke (rare), or seizures due to decreased perfusion of the brain, and increased vascular resistance secondary to sluggish blood flow. (This can result in neurologic or developmental problems.)
- *Endocrine:* Hypoglycemia or hypocalcemia

The nurse observes closely for signs of distress or change in vital signs during the partial exchange. The nurse assesses carefully for potential complications resulting from the exchange such as transfusion overload (which can result in congestive heart failure), irregular cardiac rhythm, bacterial infection, hypovolemia (because of decreased plasma volume), and anemia. Parents need specific explanations about polycythemia and its treatment. The newborn needs to be reunited with the parents as soon after the exchange as the baby's status permits.

CARE OF THE NEWBORN WITH INFECTION

Newborns up to 1 month of age are particularly susceptible to infection, referred to as **sepsis neonatorum,** caused by organisms that do not cause significant disease in older children. Once any infection occurs in the newborn, it can spread rapidly through the bloodstream, regardless of its primary site. The incidence of primary neonatal sepsis is 1 to 8 per 1000 live births (0.1% to 0.8%) (Gerdes, 2004). The risk of mortality is 5% to 15% in this population. Nosocomial infection frequency is less in normal newborn infants and increases for infants in the NICU.

Prematurity and LBW are associated with nosocomial infection rates up to 15 times higher than average. The general debilitation and underlying illness often associated with prematurity necessitates invasive procedures such as umbilical catheterization, intubation, resuscitation, ventilatory support, monitoring, and parenteral alimentation (especially lipid emulsions), and prior broad-spectrum antibiotic therapy.

However, even full-term infants are susceptible because their immunologic systems are immature. They lack the complex factors involved in effective phagocytosis and the ability to localize infection or to respond with a well-defined recognizable inflammatory response. In addition, newborns lack IgM immunoglobulin, which is necessary to protect against bacteria, because it does not cross the placenta (refer to Chapter 28 ∞ for immunologic adaptations in the newborn period).

Most nosocomial infections in the NICU present as bacteremia/sepsis, urinary tract infections, meningitis, or pneumonia. Maternal antepartal infections such as rubella, toxoplasmosis, cytomegalic inclusion disease, and herpes may cause congenital infections and resulting disorders in the newborn. Intrapartal maternal infections, such as amnionitis and those resulting from premature rupture of membranes (PROM) and precipitous birth, are sources of neonatal infection. (See "Care of the Woman with Perinatal Infection Affecting the Fetus" in Chapter 20 ∞ for more detailed information). Passage through the birth canal and contact with microorganisms in the vaginal flora (β-hemolytic streptococci, herpes, *Listeria,* and gonococci) expose the infant to infection (Table 33–6). With infection anywhere in the fetus or newborn, the adjacent tissues or organs are very easily penetrated, and the blood-brain barrier is ineffective. Septicemia is more common in males, except for those infections caused by group B β-hemolytic streptococcus. Gram-negative organisms (especially *E coli, Enterobacter, Proteus,* and *Klebsiella*)

and the gram-positive organism β-hemolytic streptococcus are the most common causative agents. *Pseudomonas* is a common fomite contaminant of ventilatory support and oxygen therapy equipment. Gram-positive bacteria, especially coagulase-negative staphylococci, are common pathogens in nosocomial bacteremias, pneumonias, and urinary tract infections. Other gram-positive bacteria frequently isolated are enterococci and *Staphylococcus aureus* (Gerdes, 2004).

Protection of the newborn from infections starts prenatally and continues throughout pregnancy and birth. Prenatal prevention should include maternal screening for sexually transmitted

Table 33–6   MATERNALLY TRANSMITTED NEWBORN INFECTIONS

Infection	Nursing Assessment	Nursing Plan and Implementation
Group B Streptococcus 1%–2% colonized, with 1 in 10 developing disease Early onset–usually within hours of birth or within first week Late onset–1 week to 3 months	Severe respiratory distress (grunting and cyanosis) May become apneic or demonstrate symptoms of shock Meconium-stained amniotic fluid seen at birth	Early assessment of clinical signs necessary. Assist with x-ray examination—shows aspiration pneumonia or respiratory distress syndrome. Immediately obtain blood, gastric aspirate, external ear canal, and nasopharynx cultures. Administer antibiotics, usually aqueous penicillin or ampicillin combined with gentamicin, as soon as cultures are obtained. Early assessment and intervention are essential to survival.

Syphilis
 	
Spirochetes cross placenta after 16th–18th week of gestation
	Check perinatal history for positive maternal serology
	
	Assess infant for
	
	    Elevated cord serum IgM and FTA-ABS IgM.
	
	    Rhinitis (snuffles)
	
	    Fissures on mouth corners and excoriated upper lip
	
	    Red rash around mouth and anus
	
	    Copper-colored rash over face, palms, and soles
	
	    Irritability
	
	    Generalized edema, particularly over joints; bone lesions; painful extremities
	
	    Hepatosplenomegaly, jaundice
	
	    Congenital cataracts
	
	    SGA and failure to thrive
		Refer to evaluate for blindness, deafness, learning or behavioral problems.
		
		Use isolation techniques, until infants have been on antibiotics for 48 hours.
		
		Administer penicillin.
		
		Provide emotional support for parents because of their feelings about mode of transmission and potential long-term sequelae.

Gonorrhea
 	
Approximately 30%–35% of newborns born vaginally to infected mothers acquire the infection
	Assess for
	
	    Ophthalmia neonatorum (conjunctivitis)
	
	    Purulent discharge and corneal ulcerations
	
	    Neonatal sepsis with temperature instability, poor feeding response, and/or hypotonia, jaundice
		Administer ophthalmic antibiotic ointment (see Drug Guide: Erythromycin [Ilotycln] Ophthalmic
		
		Ointment in Chapter 30 ∞) or, penicillin.
		
		Make a follow-up referral to evaluate any loss of vision.

Herpes Type 2 1–7500 births Usually transmitted during vaginal birth; a few cases of in utero transmission have been reported	Small cluster vesicular skin lesions over all the body Check perinatal history for active herpes genital lesions Disseminated form—DIC, pneumonia, hepatitis with jaundice, hepatosplenomegaly, and neurologic abnormalities. Without skin lesions, assess for fever or subnormal temperature, respiratory congestion, tachypnea, and tachycardia	Carry out careful handwashing and gown and glove isolation with linen precautions. Administer intravenous acyclovir (Zovirax). Make a follow-up referral to evaluate potential sequelae of microcephaly, spasticity, seizures, deafness, or blindness. Encourage parental rooming-in and touching of their newborn. Show parents appropriate handwashing procedures and precautions to be used at home if mother's lesions are active. Obtain throat, conjunctiva, cerebral spinal fluid (CSF), blood, urine, rectal, and lesion cultures to identity herpesvirus type 2 antibiotics in serum IgM fraction. Cultures positive in 24–48 hours.

(Continued on next page)

| Table 33–6 | MATERNALLY TRANSMITTED NEWBORN INFECTIONS | continued |

Infection	Nursing Assessment	Nursing Plan and Implementation
Cytomegalovirus (CMV) Most common cause of congenital infection in the United States—annually infects 10,000–80,000 infants (Enright & Prober, 2004) Transmission occurs in utero, during labor, or may happen postnatally through breast milk	Congenital CMV disease, including intrauterine growth retardation, jaundice, hepatosplenomegaly, petechiae or purpura (blueberry muffin spots), thrombocytopenia, and pneumonia. CNS manifestations are very common and include lethargy and poor feeding, hypertonia or hypotonia, microcephaly, intracranial calcifications, chorioretinitis, and sensorineural deafness	Diagnosis of congenital CMV infection is established by isolating virus from urine, saliva, or tissue obtained during the first 3 weeks of life. All infants in whom the diagnosis is suspected should have a viral culture performed; a CT scan of the brain is particularly important to document the extent of CNS involvement; eye exam and hearing test; close long-term follow-up evaluating for developmental effects.
Oral Candidal Infection (Thrush) Acquired during passage through birth canal	Assess newborn's buccal mucosa, tongue, gums, and inside the cheeks for white plaques (seen 5 to 7 days of age) Check diaper area for bright-red, well-demarcated eruptions Assess for thrush periodically when newborn is on long-term antibiotic therapy	Differentiate white plaque areas from milk curds by using cotton tip applicator (if it is thrush, removal of white areas causes raw, bleeding areas). Maintain cleanliness of hands, linen, clothing, diapers, and feeding apparatus. Instruct breastfeeding mothers on treating their nipples with nystatin. Administer nystatin swabbed on oral lesions 1 hour after feeding or nystatin instilled in baby's oral cavity and on mucosa. Swab skin lesions with topical nystatin.
Chlamydia Trachomatis Acquired during passage through birth canal	Assess for perinatal history of preterm birth Symptomatic newborns present with pneumonia-conjunctivitis after 3–4 days Chronic follicular conjunctivitis (corneal neovascularization and conjunctival scarring)	Instill ophthalmic erythromycin (see Drug Guide: Erythromycin [Ilotycin] Ophthalmic Ointment in Chapter 30 ∞). Make a follow-up referral for eye complications and late development of pneumonia at 4–11 weeks postnatally.

infection and monitoring of rubella titers in women who test negative. Intrapartally, sterile technique is essential. Smears from genital lesions are taken, and placenta and amniotic fluid cultures are obtained if amnionitis is suspected. If genital herpes is present toward term, cesarean birth may be indicated. Local eye treatment with an antibiotic ophthalmic ointment is given to all newborns to prevent damage from gonococcal (occurring 3 days following birth) and possibly chlamydial (occurring 7 to 10 days after birth) infections. Prophylactic antibiotic therapy, for asymptomatic women who test positive for group B streptococcus (GBS) during the intrapartum period, helps prevent early-onset sepsis, decreasing the incidence from 1.5/1000 live births to 0.5/1000 live births (Gerdes, 2004).

Clinical Therapy

Infants with a history of possible exposure to infection in utero (for example, PROM more than 24 hours before birth or questionable maternal history of infection, maternal fever/chorioamnionitis, or high-risk behavior (such as multiple sexual partners or illicit drug use) should have cultures taken as soon after birth as possible (Short, 2004). Cultures are obtained before antibiotic therapy is begun.

1. One blood culture is taken from a peripheral rather than an umbilical vessel because catheters have yielded false-positive results because of contamination. The skin is prepared by cleaning with a unit-specified antiseptic solution and allowed to dry; the specimen is obtained with a sterile needle/syringe. Correct sterile technique will lessen the likelihood of contamination.

2. Spinal fluid culture is done following a spinal tap/lumbar puncture if there are concerns about CNS symptoms/pathology.

3. The specimen for urine culture is best obtained by a suprapubic bladder aspiration or sterile catheterization.

4. Skin cultures are taken of any lesions or drainage from lesions or reddened areas.

5. Nasopharyngeal, rectal, ear canal, conjunctival, and gastric aspirate cultures may be obtained.

Other laboratory investigations include a complete blood count, C-reactive protein (CRP), chest x-ray examination, serology, and Gram stains of cerebrospinal fluid, urine, skin exudate, and umbilicus. White blood cell (WBC) count with differential may indicate the presence or absence of sepsis. A level of 30,000 to 40,000 mm^3 WBC may be normal in the first 24 hours of life, whereas low WBC (less than 5000 to 7500/ mm^3 may be indicative of sepsis. A low neutrophil count and high band (immature white cells) count indicate that an infection is present. Stomach aspirate should be sent for culture and smear if a gonococcal infection or amnionitis is suspected. CRP, an acute-phase reactant protein synthesized in response to inflammation, may or may not be elevated initially. Other inflammatory responses may cause an elevation in the CRP, so it should not be used as the only indicator of infection. Levels will start to increase at 4 to 6 hours following stimulation, peaking at 24 to 48 hours and decreasing as the inflammation resolves (Gerdes, 2004). The CRP may be helpful in watching for improvement once antibiotic therapy is initiated.

Table 33–7   NEONATAL SEPSIS ANTIBIOTIC/ANTIVIRAL THERAPY

Drug	Dose (mg/kg) Total Daily Dose	Schedule for Divided Doses	Route	Comments
Acyclovir (Zovirax)	20 mg/kg	Every 8 hours	IV	Length of treatment is 14 days for skin/eye/mouth (SEM) or 21 days for CNS and disseminated disease: *Herpes*
Ampicillin	50–100 mg/kg	Every 12 hours* Every 8 hours†	IM or IV	Effective against gram-positive microorganisms, *Haemophilus influenzae, Listeria,* and most *Escherichia coli* strains. Higher doses indicated for meningitis. Used with aminoglycoside for synergy.
Cefotaxime	50 mg/kg 100–150 mg/kg/day	Every 12 hours* Every 8 hours	IM or IV	Active against most major pathogens in infants; effective against aminoglycoside-resistant organisms; achieves CSF bactericidal activity; lack of ototoxicity and nephrotoxicity; wide therapeutic index (levels not required); resistant organisms can develop repidly if used extensively; ineffective against *Pseudomonas, Listeria.*
Gentamicin	2.5–3 mg/kg 5–7.5 mg/kg/day	Every 12–24 hours*‡ Every 8–24 hours†	IM or IV	Effective against gram-negative rods and staphylococci; may be used instead of kanamycin against penicillin-resistant staphylococci and *E. coli* strains and *Pseudomonas aeruginosa.* May cause ototoxicity and nephrotoxicity. Need to follow serum levels. Must never be given as IV push. Must be given over at least 30–60 minutes. In presence of oliguria or anuria, dose must be decreased or discontinued. In infants less than 1000 g or 29 weeks, lower dosage 2.5–3 mg/kg/day. Monitor serum levels before administration of second dose.
	4–5 mg/kg/dose (first week of life)	Every 24–48 hours		Peak 5–10 mcg/mL Trough 1–2 mcg/mL
Methicillin	25–50 mg/dose 50–100 mg/kg/day	Every 12 hours* Every 6–8 hours†	IM or IV	Effective against penicillinase-resistant staphylococci. Monitor CBC and UA. Slow IV push.
Nafcillin	25–50 mg/kg 50–100 mg/kg/day	Every 8–12 hours* Every 6–8 hours†	IM or IV	Effective against penicillinase-resistant staphylococci. Caution in presence of jaundice.
Penicillin G (aqueous crystalline)	25,000–50,000 units/kg 50,000–125,000 units/kg/day Up to 400,000 units kg/day for group β strep meningitis	Every 12 hours* Every 8 hours†	IM or IV	Initial sepsis therapy effective against most gram-positive microorganisms except resistant staphylococci; can cause heart block in infants.
Vancomycin	10–20 mg/kg 30 mg/kg/day	Every 12–24 hours*‡ Every 8 hours†	IV	Effective for methicillin-resistant strains (*Staphylococcus epidermidis*); must be administered by slow intravenous infusion to avoid prolonged cutaneous eruption. For smaller infants, less than 1200 g, less than 29 weeks, smaller dosages and longer intervals between doses. Nephrotoxic, especially in combination with aminoglycosides. Slow IV infusion over at least 60 minutes. Peak 25–40 mcg/mL Trough 5–10 mcg/mL

*Up to 7 days of age.

†Greater than 7 days of age.

‡Dependent on gestational age.

Serum IgM levels are elevated (normal level less than 20 mg/dL) in response to transplacental infections. If available, counterimmunoelectrophoresis tests for specific bacterial antigens are performed. In the future repetitive sequence-based polymerase chain reactions (rep-PCR) will be used to identify specific infectious organisms within hours instead of days (Stokowski, 2004). In this test, fragments of DNA are extracted and amplified from infected specimens such as blood or urine. Evidence of congenital infections may be seen on skull x-rays or CT scan for cerebral calcifications (cytomegalovirus or toxoplasmosis), on bone x-rays (syphilis or cytomegalovirus), and in serum-specific IgM levels (rubella). Cytomegalovirus infection is best diagnosed by urine culture.

Because neonatal infection causes high mortality, therapy is instituted before results of the sepsis work-up are obtained. A combination of two broad-spectrum antibiotics, such as ampi-cillin and gentamicin, is given in large doses until a culture with sensitivities results is obtained.

After the pathogen and its sensitivities are determined, appropriate specific antibiotic therapy is begun. Combinations of penicillin or ampicillin and kanamycin have been used in the past, but new kanamycin-resistant enterobacteria and penicillin-resistant staphylococcus necessitate increasing use of gentamicin. Rotating aminoglycosides has been suggested to prevent development of resistance. Use of cephalosporins and, in particular, cefotaxime has emerged as an alternative to aminoglycoside therapy in the treatment of neonatal infections. Duration of therapy varies from 7 to 14 days (Table 33–7). However, if cultures are negative and symptoms subside, antibiotics may be discontinued after 2 days/48 hours of negative blood cultures. Supportive physiologic care may be required to maintain respiratory, hemodynamic, nutritional, and metabolic homeostasis.

NURSING CARE MANAGEMENT
Nursing Assessment and Diagnosis

Symptoms of infection are most often noticed by the nurse during daily care of the newborn (Short, 2004). The infant may deteriorate rapidly in the first 12 to 24 hours after birth if β-hemolytic streptococcal infection is present, with signs and symptoms mimicking RDS. In other cases, the onset of sepsis may be gradual, with more subtle signs and symptoms (Gerdes, 2004). The most common symptoms include the following:

- Subtle behavioral changes—the infant "isn't doing well" and is often lethargic or irritable (especially after first 24 hours), hypotonic, and hypotensive. Color changes may include pallor, duskiness, cyanosis, or a "shocky" appearance. Skin is cool and clammy.

- Temperature instability, manifested most commonly by hypothermia (recognized by a decrease in skin temperature) or, rarely in newborns, hyperthermia (elevation of skin temperature) necessitates a corresponding increase or decrease in incubator temperature to maintain a neutral thermal environment.

- Feeding intolerance is evidenced by a decrease in total intake, abdominal distention, vomiting, poor sucking, lack of interest in feeding, and diarrhea.

- Hyperbilirubinemia.

- Tachycardia initially, followed by spells of apnea/bradycardia.

Signs and symptoms may suggest CNS disease (jitteriness, tremors, seizure activity), respiratory system disease (tachypnea, labored respirations, apnea, cyanosis), hematologic disease (jaundice, petechial hemorrhages, hepatosplenomegaly), or GI disease (diarrhea, vomiting, bile-stained aspirate, hepatomegaly). A differential diagnosis is necessary because of the similarity of symptoms to other more specific conditions.

Nursing diagnoses that may apply to the infant with suspected sepsis neonatorum and the family include the following:

- *Risk for Infection* related to newborn's immature immunologic system

- *Fluid Volume Deficit* related to feeding intolerance

- *Ineffective Family Coping: Compromised* related to present illness resulting in prolonged hospital stay for the newborn

Nursing Plan and Implementation

In the nursery, controlling the environment and preventing acquired infection are the responsibilities of the neonatal nurse. An infected newborn can be isolated effectively in an isolette and receive close observation. The nurse must promote strict handwashing technique for all who enter the nursery, including nursing colleagues; physicians; laboratory, x-ray, and inhalation technicians; and parents. Visits to the nursery area by unnecessary personnel should be discouraged. The nurse assists in the aseptic collection of specimens for laboratory investigations. Scrupulous care of equipment—changing and cleaning incubators at least every 7 days, removing and sterilizing wet equipment every 24 hours, preventing cross-use of linen and other equipment, cleaning sinkside equipment such as soap containers periodically, and taking special care with the open radiant warmers (access without prior handwashing is much more likely than with the closed incubator)—will prevent contamination.

PROVISION OF ANTIBIOTIC THERAPY

The nurse administers antibiotics as ordered by the nurse practitioner or physician. It is the nurse's responsibility to be knowledgeable about the following:

- The proper dose to be administered, based on the weight of the newborn and desired peak and trough levels

- The appropriate route of administration, because some antibiotics cannot be given intravenously

- The appropriate rate of administration

- Admixture incompatibilities because some antibiotics are precipitated by IV solutions or by other antibiotics

- Side effects and toxicity

In the case of term infants who are being treated for infections, neonatal home infusion of antibiotics should be considered as a viable alternative to continued hospitalization. The infusion of antibiotics at home by skilled registered nurses (RNs) facilitates parent-infant bonding while meeting the ongoing healthcare needs of the infant.

PROVISION OF SUPPORTIVE CARE

In addition to antibiotic therapy, physiologic supportive care is essential in caring for a septic infant. The nurse should carry out the following:

- Observe for resolution of symptoms or development of other symptoms of sepsis.

- Maintain a neutral thermal environment with accurate regulation of humidity and oxygen administration.

- Provide respiratory support: Administer oxygen and observe and monitor respiratory effort.

- Provide cardiovascular support: Observe and monitor pulse and blood pressure; observe for hyperbilirubinemia, anemia, and hemorrhagic symptoms.

- Provide adequate calories, because oral feedings may be discontinued because of increased mucus, abdominal distention, vomiting, or aspiration.

- Provide fluids and electrolytes to maintain homeostasis. Monitor weight changes, urine output, and urine specific gravity.

- Observe for the development of hypoglycemia, hyperglycemia, acidosis, hyponatremia, and hypocalcemia.

Restricting parental visits has not been shown to have any effect on the rate of infection and may be harmful to the newborn's psychologic development. With instruction and guidance from the nurse, both parents should be allowed to handle the baby and participate in daily care. Support to the parents is crucial. They need to be informed of the newborn's prognosis as treatment continues and to be involved in care as much as possible. They also need to understand how infection is transmitted.

Evaluation

Expected outcomes of nursing care include the following:

- The risks for development of sepsis are identified early, and immediate action is taken to minimize the development of the illness.
- Appropriate use of aseptic technique protects the newborn from further exposure to illness.
- The baby's symptoms are relieved, and the infection is treated.
- The parents verbalize their concerns about their baby's illness and understand the rationale behind the management of their newborn.

CARE OF THE FAMILY WITH BIRTH OF AN AT-RISK NEWBORN

The birth of a preterm or ill infant or an infant with a congenital anomaly is a serious crisis situation for a family. Throughout the pregnancy, both parents, together and separately, have felt excitement, experienced thoughts of acceptance, and pictured what their baby would look like. Both parents have wished for a perfect baby and feared a damaged, unhealthy one. Each parent and family member must accept and adjust when the fantasized fears become reality.

Parental Responses

Family members have acute grief reactions to the loss of the idealized baby they have envisioned. In a preterm birth, the mother is denied the last few weeks of pregnancy that seem to prepare her psychologically for the stress of birth and the attachment process. Attachment at this time is fragile, and interruption of the process by separation can affect the future mother-child relationship. Parents express grief as shock and disbelief, denial of reality, anger toward self and others, guilt, blame, and concern for the future. Self-esteem and feelings of self-worth are jeopardized.

Feelings of guilt and failure often plague mothers of preterm newborns. They may ask themselves, "Why did labor start? What did I do (or not do)?" A woman may have guilt fantasies and wonder what she may have done to cause the early labor: Was it because I had sex with my husband [a week, 3 days, a day] ago?" "Was it because I carried three loads of wash up from the basement?" "Am I being punished for something I did in the past—even in childhood?"

The period of waiting between suspicion and confirmation of abnormality or dysfunction is a very anxious one for parents

because it is difficult, if not impossible, to begin attachment to the infant if the newborn's future is questionable. During the waiting period, parents need support and acknowledgment that this is an anxious time. They must be kept informed about tests and efforts to gather additional data, as well as efforts to improve their baby's outcome. It is helpful to tell both parents about the problem at the same time with the baby present. An honest discussion of the problem and anticipatory management at the earliest possible time by health professionals help the parents (1) maintain trust in the physician and nurse, (2) appreciate the reality of the situation by dispelling fantasy and misconception, (3) begin the grieving process, and (4) mobilize internal and external support.

Nurses need to be aware that anger is a universal response and that it is best directed outward because holding it in check requires great energy, which is diverted away from grieving and physical recovery from pregnancy and giving birth. Anger may be directed unjustifiably at the physician and/or nurse, at the food, at nursing care, or at hospital regulations and routines. Parents rarely show anger with the baby and such responses can precipitate guilt feelings. Perceived maternal stress may be lessened if information is provided regarding preterm behavioral cues. This empowers the mother and allows her to better care for her child (Thomas, Renaud, & DePaul, 2004). According to Holditch-Davis, Bartlett, Blickman et al. (2003) mothers of preterm babies who have to spend time in a NICU suffer from psychologic distress similar to post-traumatic stress disorder (PTSD). Nurses working with the mothers in the NICU setting have the opportunity to encourage maternal competence and confidence, both during and after hospitalization, by teaching interpretation of their child's behavioral cues, prompting maternal care of the baby while in the NICU, and facilitating expression of their feelings.

PTSD is characterized by three symptoms:

1. Reexperiencing the trauma
2. Avoiding reminders (the mother may not visit her baby)
3. Increased arousal or anxiety

Although reactions and steps of attachment are altered by the birth of these infants, a healthy parent-child relationship can occur. Kaplan and Mason (1974) identified four psychologic tasks as essential for coping with the stress of an at-risk newborn and for providing a basis for the maternal-infant relationship:

1. Anticipatory grief as a psychologic preparation for possible loss of the child while still hoping for his or her survival.
2. Acknowledgment of maternal failure to produce a term or perfect newborn expressed as anticipatory grief and depression and lasting until the chances of survival seem secure.
3. Resumption of the process of relating to the infant, which was interrupted by the threat of nonsurvival. This task may be impaired by a continuous threat of death or abnormality, and the mother may be slow in her response of hope for the infant's survival.

4. Understanding of the special needs and growth patterns of the at-risk newborn, which are temporary and yield to normal patterns.

Solnit and Stark (1961) postulated that grief and mourning of the loss of the loved object—the idealized child—mark parental reactions to an infant with abnormalities. *Grief work,* the emotional reaction to significant loss, must occur before adequate attachment to the actual baby is possible. Parental detachment precedes parental attachment. The parents must first grieve the loss of the wished-for perfect child, and then must adopt the imperfect child as the new love object.

Parental responses to an infant with health problems may also be viewed as a five-stage process (Klaus & Kennell, 1982):

1. *Shock* is felt at the reality of the birth of this baby. This stage may be characterized by forgetfulness, amnesia of the situation, and a feeling of desperation.

2. There is disbelief (*denial*) of the reality of the situation, characterized by a refusal to believe the child has a problem. This stage is exemplified by assertions such as, "It didn't really happen!" "There has been a mistake; it's someone else's baby."

3. *Depression* over the reality of the situation and a corresponding grief reaction follows acceptance of the situation. This stage is characterized by much crying and sadness. Anger may also occur at this stage. A projection of blame on others or on self and feelings of "why me?" are characteristic of this stage.

4. *Equilibrium and acceptance* are characteristic of a decrease in the emotional reactions of the parents. This stage is variable and may be prolonged because of continuing threat to the infant's survival. Some parents experience chronic sorrow in relation to their child.

5. *Reorganization* of the family is necessary to deal with the child's problems. Mutual support of the parents facilitates this process, but the crisis of the situation may precipitate alienation between the mother and father.

Postpartal depression occurs in new mothers from 5% to 25% of the time, and stressful events can exaggerate the problem (Currie & Rademacher, 2004). Fathers also may suffer from depression both before and after the birth of their child, adding to the discord in the family unit and compounding the perceived stress experienced by the mother.

Developmental Consequences

The baby who is born prematurely, is ill, or has a malformation or disorder is at risk for emotional, intellectual, and cognitive development delays. The risk is directly proportional to the seriousness of the problem and the length of treatment.

The necessary physical separation of family and infant and the tremendous emotional and financial burdens adversely affect the parent-child relationship. The recent trend to involve the parents with the newborn early, repeatedly, and over protracted periods of time has done much to facilitate positive parent-child relationships.

Figure 33–20 ◆ Mother of a 26 weeks' gestational age infant with respiratory distress syndrome on a ventilator is getting acquainted with her baby. Physical contact is vital to the bonding process and should be encouraged whenever possible.
SOURCE: Courtesy of Lisa Smith-Pedersen, RNC, MSN, NNP.

The parents must have a clear picture of the reality of the disability and the types of developmental hurdles ahead. Unexpected behaviors and responses from the baby because of his or her problem or disorder can be upsetting and frightening. The demands of care for the child and disputes regarding management or behavior stress family relationships. The entire multidisciplinary team may need to pool their resources and expertise to help parents of children born with problems or disorders so that both parents and children can thrive.

Early and continued involvement may only mean opportunities to look at or stroke the baby (Figure 33–20 ◆). Later, when the mother's and baby's conditions warrant it, the mother should participate in her baby's care (to the extent she is willing) and in planning for the future. This type of involvement facilitates early bonding, attachment, and emotional investment. The parents need a sense of personal success, self-worth, self-esteem, and confidence from the knowledge that they can cope with the situation.

The demands of care of the child and disputes regarding management or behavior stress family relationships. A variety of behavioral patterns may occur. For example, one or more members of the family may make a scapegoat of the child. Another may become the youngster's champion to the exclusion of others. One or the other spouse may feel pushed aside or denied attention and thus may withdraw or leave the family unit. Parents or siblings may feel that their own needs (schooling, material goods, freedom of movement) are being set aside while all assets (financial and other) go to support the one child's needs. Also there may be an increase in child abuse.

NURSING CARE MANAGEMENT
Nursing Assessment and Diagnosis

A positive nurse-family relationship helps information gathering in areas of concern. A concurrent illness of the mother or

Figure 33–21 ◆ Maladaptive and adaptive parental responses during crisis period, showing unhealthy and healthy outcomes.
SOURCE: From P. Grant, *Family & Community Health*, p. 11, fig. 1. Copyright © 1978 Lippincott, Williams & Wilkins.

other family members or other concurrent stress (lack of hospitalization insurance, loss of job, age of parents) may change the family response to the baby. Feelings of apprehension, guilt, failure, and grief that are verbally or nonverbally expressed are important aspects of the nursing history. These observations enable all professionals to be aware of the parental state, coping behaviors, and readiness for attachment, bonding, and caretaking. Appropriate nursing assessments during interviewing and relating to the family include the following:

1. *Level of understanding.* Observations concerning the family's ability to assimilate information given and to ask appropriate questions; the need for constant repetition information

2. *Behavioral responses.* Appropriateness of behavior in relation to information given; lack of response; flat affect

3. *Difficulties with communication.* Deafness (reads lips only); blindness; dysphasia; understanding only a non-English language

4. *Paternal and maternal education level.* Parents who are unable to read or write; parents with eighth–grade-level education; parents with a graduate-level degree or healthcare background

Documentation of such information, gathered through continuing contact and development of a therapeutic family relationship, lets all professionals understand and use the nursing history in providing continuous individual care.

Visiting and caregiving patterns indicate the level or lack of parental attachment. A record of visits, caretaking procedures, affect (in relating to the newborn), and telephone calls from parents is essential. It is important to note serial observations rather than just isolated observations that cause concern. Grant (1978) developed a conceptual framework depicting adaptive and maladaptive responses to parenting of a preterm or less-than-perfect infant (Figure 33–21 ◆).

If a pattern of distancing behaviors evolves, the nurse should institute appropriate intervention. Follow-up studies have found that a statistically significant number of preterm, sick, and congenitally defective infants suffer from failure to thrive, battering, or other disorders of parenting. Early detection and intervention may prevent these aberrations in parenting behaviors from leading to irreparable damage or death.

Nursing diagnoses that may apply to the family of a newborn at risk include the following:

* **Dysfunctional Grieving** related to loss of idealized newborn
* **Fear** related to emotional involvement with an at-risk newborn
* **Altered Parenting** related to impaired bonding secondary to feelings of inadequacy about caretaking activities

Nursing Plan and Implementation

HOSPITAL-BASED NURSING CARE

In their sensitive and vulnerable state, parents are acutely perceptive about others' responses and reactions (particularly non-verbal) to the child. Parents can be expected to identify with the responses of others. Therefore, it is imperative that medical and nursing staff be fully aware of their feelings and come to terms with their own feelings so that they are comfortable and at ease with the baby and the grieving family.

Nurses may feel uncomfortable not knowing what to say to parents or may fear confronting their own feelings as well as those of the parents. Each nurse must work out personal reactions with instructors, peers, clergy, parents, or significant others. It is helpful to have a stockpile of therapeutic questions and statements to initiate meaningful dialog with parents. Opening statements can be as follows: "You must be wondering what could have caused this"; "Are you thinking that you (or someone else) may have done something?"; "How can I help?"; and, "Are you wondering how you are going to manage?" Avoid statements such as, "It could have been worse"; "It's God's will"; "You have other children"; "You are still young and can have more"; and "I understand how you feel." This child is important now.

Support of Parents in Initial Viewing of the Newborn

Before parents see their child, the nurse must prepare them for the visit. It is important to present a positive, realistic attitude regarding the infant. An overly negative, fatalistic attitude further alienates the parents from their infant and retards attachment behaviors. Instead of beginning to bond with their child, the parents will anticipate their loss and the process of grieving. Once started, this process is very difficult to reverse.

Before preparing parents for the first view of their infant, observe the baby. All infants exhibit strengths as well as deficiencies; prepare the parents to see both the deviations and the normal aspects of their infant. The nurse may say, "Your baby is small, about the length of my two hands. She weighs 2 lb 3 oz but is very active and cries when we disturb her. She is having some difficulty breathing but is breathing without assistance and in only 35% oxygen and room air is 21%."

Describe the equipment being used for the at-risk newborn and its purpose before entering the unit. Many NICUs have booklets for parents to read before entering the unit. Through

Figure 33–22 ◆ This 25 weeks' gestational age infant with respiratory distress syndrome may be frightening for her parents to see for the first time because of the technology that is attached to her. SOURCE: Courtesy of Lisa Smith-Pedersen, RNC, MSN, NNP.

explanations and pictures, the parents can be better prepared to deal with the feelings they may experience when they see their infant for the first time (Figure 33–22 ◆).

Upon entering the unit, parents may be overwhelmed by the sounds of monitors, alarms, and respirators, as well as by the unfamiliar language and "foreign" atmosphere. Preparing the parents by having the same healthcare professional(s) accompany them to the unit can be reassuring. The primary nurse and physician caring for the newborn should be with the parents when they first visit the baby. Parental reactions vary, but there is usually an element of initial shock. Providing them with chairs and time to regain composure will assist the parents. Slow, complete, and simple explanations—first about the infant and then about the equipment—allay fear and anxiety.

As parents attempt to deal with the initial stages of shock and grief, they may fail to grasp new information. The parents may need repeated explanations about the procedures, equipment, and the infant's condition on subsequent visits.

Concern about the infant's physical appearance is common, yet may remain unvoiced. Parents may express such concerns as, "He looks so small and red—like a drowned rat." "Why do her genitals look so abnormal?" "Will that awful looking mouth [cleft lip and palate] ever be normal?" Such questions need to be anticipated by the nurse and addressed. Use of pictures, such as of an infant after cleft lip repair, may be reassuring to doubting parents. Knowledge of the development of a "normal" preterm infant will allow the nurse to make reassuring statements such as "The baby's skin may look very red and transparent with lots of visible veins, but it is normal for her maturity. As she grows, subcutaneous fat will be laid down, and these superficial veins will begin to disappear."

The nursing staff set the tone of the NICU. Nurses foster the development of a safe, trusting environment by viewing the parents as essential caregivers, not as visitors or nuisances in the unit. It is important to provide parents privacy when needed and easy access to staff and facilities. An uncrowded and welcoming atmosphere lets parents know, "You are welcome here." However, even in crowded physical surroundings, the nurses can convey an attitude of openness and trust.

A trusting relationship is essential for collaborative efforts in caring for the infant. Use your responses therapeutically to relate to the parents on a one-to-one basis. Each individual has different needs, different ways of adapting to crisis, and different means of support. Professionals must use techniques that are real and spontaneous to them and avoid adopting words or actions that are foreign to them. Nurses must also gauge their interventions to match the parents' pace and needs.

Nurses show concern and support by planning time to spend with the parents, by being psychologically as well as physically present, by encouraging open discussion and grieving, by repetitive explanations (as necessary), by providing privacy as needed, and by encouraging contact with the newborn. Identifying and clarifying feelings and fears decrease distortions in perception, thinking, and feeling. Nurses invest the baby with value in the eyes of the parents when they provide meticulous care to the newborn, talk and coo (especially in the face-to-face position) while holding or providing care to the newborn, refer to the child by gender or name, and relate the newborn's activities ("He took a whole ounce of formula"; "She took hold of the blanket and just wouldn't let go"). Nurses should note the "normal" characteristics and capabilities of each newborn as well as the newborn's needs. The nurse should also learn the baby's name and refer to him or her by name.

Facilitation of Attachment if Neonatal Transport Occurs

Transport to a regional referral center some distance from the parents' community may be necessary. It is essential that the mother see and touch her infant before the infant is transported. Bringing the mother to the nursery or taking the infant in a warmed transport incubator to the mother's bedside will allow her to see the infant before transportation to the center. When the infant reaches the referral center, a staff member should call the parents with information about the infant's condition during transport, safe arrival at the center, and present condition.

Support of parents, with explanations from the professional staff, is crucial. Occasionally, the mother may be unable to see the infant before transport, for example, if she is still under general anesthesia or experiencing postpartum complications such as shock, hemorrhage, or seizures. In these cases, take a photograph of the infant to give to the mother, and provide an explanation of the infant's condition and problems and a detailed description of the infant's characteristics. An additional photograph is also helpful for the father to share with siblings or the extended family. With the increased attention to improved fetal outcome, prenatal maternal transports, rather than neonatal transports, are occurring more frequently. This practice gives the mother of an at-risk infant the opportunity to visit and care for her infant during the early postpartal period.

Promotion of Touching and Parental Caretaking

Parents visiting a small or sick infant may need several visits to become comfortable and confident in their abilities to touch the infant without injuring her or him. Barriers such as incubators, incisions, monitor electrodes, and tubes may delay the mother's development of comfort in touching the newborn. Knowledge of this "normal" delay in touching behavior will enable the nurse to understand parental behavior.

Klaus and Kennell (1982) found a significant difference in the amount of eye contact and touching behaviors of mothers of normal newborns and mothers of preterm infants. Whereas mothers of normal newborns progress within minutes to palm contact of the infant's trunk, the mother of a preterm infant is slower to progress from fingertip to palm contact and from the extremities to the trunk. The progression to palm contact with the infant's trunk may take several visits to the nursery.

Through use of support, reassurance, and encouragement, the nurse can facilitate the mother's positive feelings about her ability and her importance to her infant. Touching facilitates "getting to know" the infant and thus establishes a bond with the infant. Touching as well as seeing the infant helps the mother to realize the "normals" and potentials of her baby (Figure 33–23 ◆).

The nurse can also encourage parents to meet their newborn's need for stimulation. Stroking, rocking, cuddling, singing, and talking should be an integral part of the parents' caretaking responsibilities. Bonding can be facilitated by encouraging parents to visit and become involved in their baby's care (Figure 33–24 ◆). When visiting is impossible, the parents should feel free to phone whenever they wish to receive information about their baby. A warm receptive attitude on the part of the nurse is very supportive. Facilitate parenting by personalizing a baby to the parents, by referring to the infant by name,

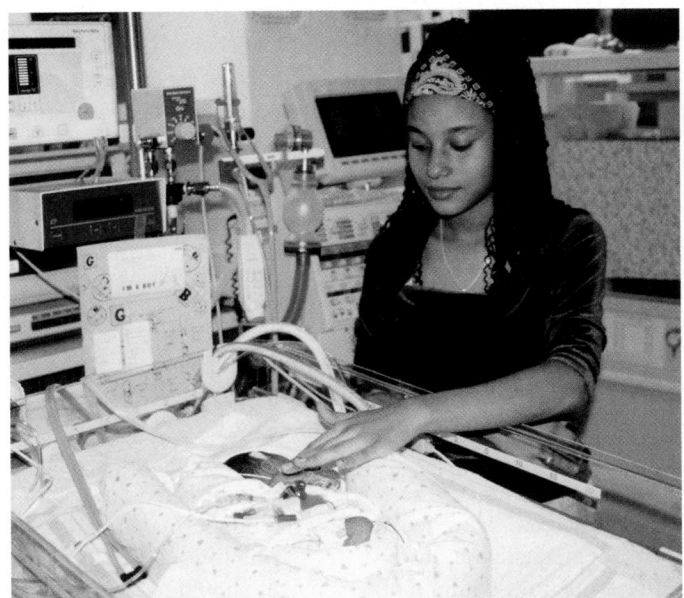

Figure 33–23 ◆ Mother of this 26 weeks' gestational age 600-g baby begins attachment through fingertip touch.
SOURCE: Courtesy of Lisa Smith-Pedersen, RNC, MSN, NNP.

Figure 33–24 ◆ This mother of a 31 weeks' gestational age infant with respiratory distress syndrome is spending time with her newborn and meeting the baby's need for cuddling.
SOURCE: Courtesy of Lisa Smith-Pedersen, RNC, MSN, NNP.

or relating personal behavioral characteristics. Statements such as, "Jenny loves her pacifier," help make the infant seem individual and unique.

The variety of equipment needed for life support is hardly conducive to anxiety-free caretaking by the parents. However, even the sickest infant may be cared for, if only in a small way, by the parents. As a facilitator of parental caretaking, the nurse should promote the parents' success. Demonstration and explanation, followed by support of the parents in initial caretaking behaviors, positively reinforce this behavior. Changing the infant's diaper, giving their infant skin care or oral care, or helping the nurse turn the infant may at first be anxiety provoking for the parents, but they will become more comfortable and confident in caretaking and receive satisfaction from the baby's reactions and their ability "to do something." Complimenting the parents' competence in caretaking also increases their self-esteem, which has received recent "blows" of guilt and failure. *It is vitally important that the parents never be given a task if there is any possibility they will not be able to accomplish it.* Cues that the parents are ready to become involved with the child's care include their reference to the baby by name and their questioning as to amount of feeding taken, sleeping patterns, appearance today, and the like (Loo, Espinosa, Tyler et al., 2003).

The nurse should accept this behavior but continue to remind the parents that it is okay and natural to feel disappointment, a sense of failure, helplessness, or anger. The overprotectiveness and overoptimism are defense mechanisms. To deny the negative feelings only entrenches them further, delays their resolution, and delays realistic planning.

Often mothers of high-risk infants have ambivalent feelings toward the nurse. These feelings may be acted out in criticism of the care being received by the infant, manipulation of staff, or personal guilt. Instead of fostering (by silence) these inferiority feelings within mothers, nurses should recognize such feelings and intervene appropriately to enhance mother-infant attachment. The nurse needs to deal with ambivalent feelings that contribute to a competitive atmosphere. For example, the nurse should avoid making unfavorable comparisons between

the baby's response to parental and nursing caretaking. During a quiet time, it may help for the nurse to encourage the parents to talk about their hopes and fears and to facilitate their involvement in parent groups. Parents are also often anxious when their baby is transferred from the NICU to the "regular nursery." They may feel that their infant is not being cared for as proficiently because the nurses are not at the infant's bedside as often as they were in the NICU. Verbalizations that improve parental self-esteem are essential and easily shared. The nurse can point out that, in addition to physiologic use, breast milk is important because of the emotional investment of the mother. Pumping, storing, labeling, and delivering quantities of breast milk is time-consuming and a "labor of love" for mothers. Positive remarks regarding breast milk reinforce the maternal behavior of caretaking and providing for her infant: "Breast milk is something that only you can give your baby" or "You really have brought a lot of milk today" or "Even small amounts of milk are important, and look how rich it is."

If the infant begins to gain weight while being fed breast milk, it is important to point this correlation out to the mother. Parents should also be advised that initial weight loss with beginning nipple feedings is common because of the increased energy expended when the infant begins active rather than passive nutritional intake.

Encourage parents to provide care for their infant even if the baby is very sick and likely to die. Detachment is easier after attachment because the parents are comforted by the knowledge that they did all they could for their child while he or she was alive.

Facilitation of Family Adjustment

During crisis, maintaining interpersonal relationships is difficult. Yet in a newborn intensive care area, the parents are expected to relate to many different care providers. It is important that parents have as few professionals as possible relaying information to them. A primary nurse should coordinate and provide continuity in the information given to parents. Care providers are individuals and thus will use different terms, inflections, and attitudes. These subtle differences are monumental to parents and only confuse, confound, and produce anxiety. The transfer of the baby from the NICU to a step-down unit or transport back to the home hospital is very anxiety producing for the parents because they must now deal with new healthcare professionals. The nurse not only functions as a liaison between the parents and the wide variety of professionals interacting with the infant and parents, but also offers clarification, explanation, interpretation of information, and support to the parents.

The nurse should encourage the parents to deal with the crisis with help from their support system. The support system attempts to meet the emotional needs and provide support for the family members in crisis and stress situations. Biologic kinship is not the only valid criterion for a support system; an emotional kinship is the most important factor. In our mobile society of isolated nuclear families, the support system may be a next-door neighbor, a best friend, or perhaps a schoolmate. The nurse must search out the significant others in the lives of the parents and help them understand the problems so that they can support the parents.

The impact of the crisis on the family is individual and varied. The nurse obtains information about the family's ability to adapt to the situation through the relationship with the family. To institute appropriate interventions, the nurse should view the birth of the infant (normal newborn, preterm infant, or infant with illness or congenital anomaly) as defined by the family.

Because the family is a unit composed of individuals who must deal with the situation, it is important to encourage open intrafamily communication. The nurse should discourage the family from keeping secrets from one another, especially between spouses, because secrets undermine the trust of their relationship. Well-meaning rationales such as, "I want to protect her," "I don't want him to worry about it," and so on, can be destructive to open communication and to the basic element of a relationship—trust.

Open communication is especially important when the mother is hospitalized apart from the infant. The first person to visit the infant relays information regarding the infant's care and condition to the mother and family. In this situation, the mother has had minimal contact, if any, with her infant. Because of her anxiety and isolation, she may mistrust all those who provide information (the nurse, physician, or extended family) until she can see the infant for herself. This can put tremendous stress on the relationship between spouses. The parents (and family) should be given information together. This practice helps overcome misunderstandings and misinterpretations and promotes mutual "working through" of problems.

The nurse should encourage the entire family—siblings as well as extended relatives—to visit and receive information about the baby. Methods of intervention in assisting the family to cope with the situation include providing support, confronting the crisis, and helping the family understand the reality. Support, explanations, and the helping role must include the extended family, as well as the nuclear family, to aid them in communication and support ties with the nuclear family.

The needs of siblings should not be overlooked. Siblings have been looking forward to the new baby, and they too suffer a degree of loss. Young children may react with hostility and older ones with shame at the birth of an infant with an anomaly. Both reactions make them feel guilty. Parents, preoccupied with working through their own feelings, often cannot give the other children the attention and support they need. Sometimes another child becomes the focus of family tension. Anxiety thus directed can take the form of finding fault or of over concern. This is a form of denial; the parents cannot face the real worry—the infant at risk. After assessing the situation, the observant nurse could see to it that another family member or friend step in and give the needed support to the siblings of the affected baby.

The nurse must respect and facilitate the desires and needs of the individuals involved; differences are tolerable and should be able to exist side by side. The nurse can easily elicit the parents' feelings and the meaning of this experience to them by asking, "How are you doing?" The emphasis is on "you," and the interest must be sincere.

Parents from minority cultures must deal with language barriers and cultural differences that can make feelings of isolation and uncertainty more acute. Healthcare providers have the professional responsibility to be aware of cultural needs of all clients and to ensure that their needs are met. Feelings of isolation and uncertainty influence not only the parent's emotional responses to the ill newborn, but also their use of services and their interaction with health professionals. Hospital cultural interpreters programs can assist families with interactions with staff and provide translation during family meetings, multidisciplinary family conferences, and parent support groups (Shah & Campbell, 2004).

Families with children in the NICU become friends and support one another. To encourage the development of these friendships and to provide support, many units have established parent groups. The core of the groups consists of parents who previously have had an infant in the intensive care unit. Most groups make contact with families within a day or two of the infant's admission to the unit, either through phone calls or visits to the hospital. Early one-on-one parent contacts are more effective than discussion groups in helping families work through their feelings. This personalized method gives the grieving parents an opportunity to share personal feelings about the pregnancy, labor, and birth and their "different from expected" infant with others who have experienced the same feelings and with whom they can identify.

COMMUNITY-BASED NURSING CARE

Predischarge planning begins once the infant's condition becomes stable and indications suggest the newborn will survive. Discharge preparation and care conferences should involve a multidisciplinary team approach (Hummel & Cronin, 2004). NICU nursing staff are the fulcrum for aiding in the transition of high-risk infants from the intensive care unit to the home. Effective open communication with the families during the entire discharge-planning phase of care empowers the families to assume the role of primary caregiver for their children.

Adequate predischarge teaching will help the parents transform their feelings of inadequacy and competition with the nurse into feelings of self-assurance and attachment. From the beginning, the parents should be taught about their infant's special needs and growth patterns. This teaching and involvement are best facilitated by a nurse who has been familiar with the infant and family and who has developed a comfortable and supportive relationship with them. When twins are being discharged, inform parents that cobedding of twins allows for clustering of care and facilitates the parents' ability to spend time with both of their children (Figure 33–25 ◆). Discharge teaching, therefore, is easily facilitated. Cobedding is also a strategy to maximize the synchronization of sleep-wake cycles (Hayward, 2003).

The nurse's responsibility is to provide home care instructions in an optimal environment for parental learning. Learning should take place over time, to avoid the necessity of bombarding the parents with instructions in the day or hour before discharge. Parents often enjoy doing minimal caretaking tasks with gradual expansion of their role.

Many NICUs provide facilities for parents to room in with their infants for a few days before discharge. This allows parents a degree of independence in the care of their infant with the security of nursing help nearby. This practice is particularly

Figure 33–25 ◆ Cobedding of twins facilitates delivery of care and parent interaction with healthcare members. These twins were born at 33 weeks' gestation and required oxygen and gavage feeding while in the NICU.

SOURCE: Courtesy of Lisa Smith-Pedersen, RNC, MSN, NNP.

helpful for anxious parents, parents who have not had the opportunity to spend extended time with their infant, or parents who will be giving complex physical care at home, such as gastrostomy feeding and care (Burd & Burd, 2003).

The families are able to interact with the staff while gradually transitioning to sole caretakers of their medically complex high-risk infant. When discharging a medically fragile infant to home, schedule a predischarge home visit by a public health nurse or home health agency. This predischarge visit evaluates the home for any possible issues that may complicate the parents' ability to care for their at-risk infant, especially if there are multiple monitoring equipment needs.

The basic elements of discharge and home care instruction are as follows:

1. Teach parents routine well-baby care, such as bathing, taking a temperature, preparing formula , and breastfeeding.

2. Help parents learn to do special procedures as needed by the newborn, such as gavage or gastrostomy feedings, tracheostomy or enterostomy care, medication administration, CPR, and operation of an apnea monitor. Before discharge, the parents should be as comfortable as possible with these tasks and should demonstrate independence. Written tools and instructions are useful for parents to refer to once they are home with the infant, but they should not replace actual participation in the infant's care.

3. Make sure that all applicable screening (metabolic, vision, hearing) tests, immunizations, and respiratory syncytial virus (RSV) prophylaxis are done before discharge and that all records are given to the primary care provider and parents.

4. Refer parents to community health and support organizations. The Visiting Nurses Association, public health nurses, or social services can assist the parents in the stressful transition from hospital to home by providing predischarge home visits and then the necessary home teaching and support. Some NICUs have their own parent support groups to help bridge the gap between hospital and home care. Parents can also find support from a variety of community support organizations, such as mothers of twins groups, March of Dimes Birth Defects Foundation, handicapped children services, and teen mother and child programs. Each community has numerous agencies capable of assisting the family in adapting emotionally, physically, and financially to the chronically ill infant. The nurse should be familiar with community resources and help the parents identify which agencies may benefit them.

5. Help parents recognize the growth and development needs of their infant. A developmental care program begun in the hospital can be continued at home, or parents may be referred to an infant development program in the community.

6. Arrange medical follow-up care before discharge. The infant will need to be followed up by a family pediatrician, a well-baby clinic, or a specialty clinic. The first appointment should be made before the infant is discharged from the hospital.

7. Evaluate the need for durable medical equipment for infant care (such as a respirator, oxygen, apnea monitor, feeding pump) in the home. Any extra equipment or supplies should be placed in the home before the infant's discharge.

8. Arrange for neonatal hospice for parents of the medically fragile infant, as needed.

Further evaluation after the infant has gone home is useful in determining whether the crisis has been resolved satisfactorily. The parents are usually given the intensive care nursery's telephone number to call for support and advice. The staff can follow up each family with visits or telephone calls at intervals for several weeks to assess and evaluate the infant's (and parents') progress.

Evaluation

Expected outcomes of nursing care include the following:

- The parents are able to verbalize their feelings of grief and loss.

- The parents verbalize their concerns about their baby's health problems, care needs, and potential outcome.

- The parents are able to participate in their infant's care and show attachment behaviors.

CONSIDERATIONS FOR THE NURSE WHO WORKS WITH AT-RISK NEWBORNS

The birth of a baby with a problem is a traumatic event with the potential for either disruption or growth of the involved family. The NICU staff nurses may never see the long-term results of the specialized, sensitive care they give to parents and their newborns. Their only immediate evidence of effective care may be the beginning of resolution of parental grief; discharge of a recovered, thriving infant to the care of happy parents; and the beginning of reintegration of family life.

Nurses cannot provide support unless they themselves are supported. Working in an emotional environment of "lots of living and lots of dying" takes its toll on staff. NICUs are among the most stressful areas in health care for patients, families, and nurses. Nurses bear most of the stress and largely determine the atmosphere of the NICU. The nurse's ability to cope with stress is the key to creating an emotionally healthy environment and a positive working atmosphere. The emotional needs and feelings of the staff must be recognized and dealt with to enable them to support the parents. An environment of openness to feelings and support in dealing with their own human needs and emotions is essential for personnel.

As caregivers, nurses may be unaware of their need to grieve for their own losses in the NICU. Nurses must also go through the grief work that parents experience. Techniques such

Figure 33–26 ◆ Twins from Figure 33–25 on the happy day of discharge, being held by staff in the NICU. This is what is so rewarding about working in the NICU: healthy babies going home to their family.
SOURCE: Courtesy of Lisa Smith-Pedersen, RNC, MSN, NNP.

as group meetings, individual support, and primary care nursing may assist in maintaining staff mental health. Reunions in some nurseries are beneficial for the families and healthcare professionals so they are able to see the children after discharge.

CHAPTER REVIEW

FOCUS YOUR STUDY

- The sick newborn—whether preterm, term, or postterm—must be managed within narrow physiologic parameters.

- These parameters (respiratory, cardiovascular, and thermal regulation) will maintain physiologic homeostasis and prevent introduction of iatrogenic stress to the already stressed infant.

- The nursing care of the newborn with special problems involves understanding normal physiology, the pathophysiology of the disease process, clinical manifestations, and supportive or corrective therapies. Only with this theoretic background can the nurse make appropriate observations concerning responses to therapy and development of complications.

- Asphyxia results in significant circulatory, respiratory, and biochemical changes in the newborn that make the successful transition to extrauterine life difficult. Asphyxia requires early identification and resuscitative management.

- Newborn conditions that commonly present with respiratory distress and require oxygen and ventilatory assistance are respiratory distress syndrome, transient tachypnea of the newborn, meconium aspiration syndrome, and persistent pulmonary hypertension.

- Management of respiratory problems can result in further respiratory compromising conditions such as pulmonary interstitial emphysema, pneumothorax, and bronchopulmonary dysplasia/chronic lung disease.

- Cold stress sets up the chain of physiologic events of hypoglycemia, pulmonary vasoconstriction, hyperbilirubinemia, respiratory distress, and metabolic acidosis.

- Nurses are responsible for early detection and initiation of treatment for hypoglycemia.

- Differentiation between pathologic and physiologic jaundice is key to early and successful intervention.

- Anemia (decreased amount of red blood cell volume) or polycythemia (excess amount) place the newborn at risk for alterations in blood flow and the oxygen-carrying capacity of the blood.

- Nursing assessment of the septic newborn involves identifying very subtle clinical signs that are also seen in other clinical disease states.

- The nurse is the facilitator for interdisciplinary communication with the parents, identifying their understanding of their infant's care and their needs for emotional support.

- Parents of at-risk newborns need support from nurses and healthcare providers to understand the special needs of their baby and to feel comfortable in an overwhelming and often unfamiliar environment.

EXPLORE MediaLink

http://www.prenhall.com/davidson

NCLEX review questions, case studies, and other interactive resources for this chapter can be found on the Web Site at http://www.prenhall.com/davidson. Click on "Chapter 33" to select the activities for this chapter.

For tutorials including animations and videos, more NCLEX review questions, and an audio glossary, access the accompanying Prentice Hall Nursing MediaLink DVD-ROM in this book.

PRENTICE HALL NURSING MEDIALINK DVD-ROM
Audio Glossary
NCLEX Review
Video: *Infant Receiving Phototherapy*

COMPANION WEBSITE
Additional NCLEX Review
Case Study: *Newborn with Jaundice*
Care Plan Activity: *Infection in a Newborn*
Applications: *Infant with Respiratory Distress Syndrome; Meconium Aspiration Syndrome*
Critical Thinking

CRITICAL THINKING IN ACTION

PHOTOTHERAPY WITH FIBEROPTIC BLANKET

View the Critical Thinking in Action video in Chapter 33 of the DVD-ROM. Then answer the questions that follow.

Rebecca Prince, age 21, G2 now P2, gives birth to a 5-pound baby at 38 weeks' gestation by primary cesarean birth for nonreassuring fetal status. The infant's Apgars are 7 and 9 at 1 and 5 minutes. The infant is suctioned and given free-flow oxygen at birth,

then is admitted to the newborn nursery for transitional care and does well. You are the nurse caring for baby Prince at 36 hours old. You review the newborn's record and note that the baby's blood type is A and his mother's is O. Rebecca wants to breastfeed. You are performing a shift assessment on baby Prince when you observe the infant has a unilateral cephalhematoma and is lethargic. You blanch the skin over the sternum and observe a yellow discoloration of the skin. Lab tests reveal a serum bilirubin level of 12 mg/dL, hematocrit 55%, a mildly positive direct Coombs' test, and a positive indirect Coombs' test. Baby Prince is diagnosed with hyperbilirubinemia secondary to ABO incompatibility and cephalhematoma. You provide phototherapy by fiberoptic blanket around the trunk of the infant and take the baby to his mother's room.

1. How would you explain the purpose of phototherapy with the mother?

2. Describe the care the mother can give to the newborn.

3. Discuss the advantage of the fiberoptic blanket phototherapy for the newborn.

4. Newborns up to 1 month of age are susceptible to organisms that do not cause significant disease in older children. Explore the circumstances that cause susceptibility to infection.

5. Describe how to distinguish between oral thrush and milk curds.

REFERENCES

American Academy of Pediatrics [AAP] & American Heart Association [AHA]. (2006). *Neonatal resuscitation: Instructor manual* (5th ed.). Evanston, IL: Author.

American Academy of Pediatrics (AAP) Committee on Fetus and Newborn & American College of Obstetricians and Gynecologists (ACOG) Committee on Obstetrics. (2002). *Guidelines for perinatal care* (5th ed.). Evanston, IL: Author.

American Academy of Pediatrics Subcommittee on Hyperbilirubinemia. (2004). Management of hyperbilirubinemia in the newborn infant 35 or more weeks of gestation. *Pediatrics, 114*(1), 297–316.

Armentrout, D. (2004). Glucose management. In M. T. Verklan & M. Walden (Eds.), *Core curriculum for neonatal intensive care nursing* (3rd ed., pp. 192–204). St. Louis, MO: Elsevier Saunders.

Askin, D. F., & Diehl-Jones, W. (2004). Assisted ventilation. In M. T. Verklan & M. Walden (Eds.), *Core curriculum for neonatal intensive care nursing* (3rd ed., pp. 536–568). St. Louis, MO: Elsevier Saunders.

Bhutani, V. K., Johnson, L. H., & Keren, R. (2004). Diagnosis and management of hyperbilirubinemia in the term neonate: For a safer first week. *Pediatric Clinics of North America, 51*(4), 843–861.

Bizzarro, M. J., Colson, E., & Ehrenkranz, R. A. (2004). Differential diagnosis and management of anemia in the newborn. *Pediatric Clinics of North America, 51*(4), 1087–1107.

Burd, A., & Burd, R. S. (2003). The who, what, why, and how-to guide for gastrostomy tube placement in infants. *Advances in Neonatal Care, 3*(4), 197–205.

Cloherty, J. P., Eichenwald, E. C., & Stark, A. R. (2004). *Manual of neonatal care* (5th ed.). Philadelphia: Lippincott Williams & Wilkins.

Currie, M. L., & Rademacher, R. (2004). The pediatrician's role in recognizing and intervening in postpartum depression. *Pediatric Clinics of North America, 51*(3), 785–801.

de Ungria, M., & Steinhorn, R. H. (2003). Neonatal resuscitation. In J. J. Sciarra (Eds.), *Gynecology and obstetrics* (Vol. 3, chap. 68, pp. 1–15). Philadelphia: Lippincott Williams & Wilkins.

Diehl-Jones, W., & Askin, D. F. (2004). Hematologic disorders. In M. T. Verklan & M. Walden (Eds.), *Core curriculum for neonatal intensive care nursing* (3rd ed., pp. 728–758). St. Louis, MO: Elsevier Saunders.

Dildy, G. A. (2005). Intrapartum assessment of the fetus: Historical and evidence-based practice. *Obstetrics and Gynecology Clinics of North America, 32*(2), 255–271.

Enright, A. M., & Prober, C. G. (2004). Herpesviridae infections in newborns: Varicella zoster virus, herpes simplex virus, and cytomegalovirus. *Pediatric Clinics of North America, 51*(4), 889–908.

Fanaroff, A. A., Martin, R. J., & Rodriguez, R. J. (2004). Identification and management of problems in the high-risk neonate. In R. K. Creasy & R. Resnik (Eds.), *Maternal-fetal medicine: Principles and practice* (5th ed., pp. 1263–1301). Philadelphia: Saunders.

Farrow, K. N., Fliman, P., & Steinhorn, R. H. (2005). The diseases treated with ECMO: Focus on PPHN. *Seminars in Perinatology, 29*(1), 8–14.

Gelfand, S. L., Fanaroff, J. M., & Walsh, M. C. (2004a). Controversies in the treatment of meconium aspiration syndrome. *Clinics in Perinatology, 31*(3), 445–452.

Gelfand, S. L., Fanaroff, J. M., & Walsh, M. C. (2004b). Meconium stained fluid: Approach to the mother and the baby. *Pediatric Clinics of North America, 51*(3), 655–667.

Gerdes, J. S. (2004). Diagnosis and management of bacterial infections in the neonate. *Pediatric Clinics of North America, 51*(4), 939–959.

Gibbins, S., & Stevens, B. (2003). The influence of gestational age of the efficacy and short-term safety of sucrose for procedural pain relief. *Advances in Neonatal Care, 3*(5), 241–249.

Gomella, T. L., Cunningham, M. D., Eyal, F. G., & Zenk, K. E. (2004). *Neonatology: Management, procedures, on-call problems, diseases, and drugs* (5th ed.). New York: Lange Medical Books/McGraw-Hill.

Grant, P. (1978). Psychological needs of families of high risk infants. *Family and Community Health, 1*(3), 91–102.

Hayward, K. (2003). Cobedding of twins: A natural extension of the socialization process? *American Journal of Maternal/Child Nursing, 28*(4), 260–263.

Hermansen, M. C., & Hermansen, M. G. (2005). Pitfalls in neonatal resuscitation. *Clinics in Perinatology, 32,* 77–95.

Holditch-Davis D., Bartlett, T. R., Blickman, A. L., & Miles, M. S. (2003). Posttraumatic stress symptoms in mothers of premature infants. *Journal of Obstetric, Gynecologic, & Neonatal Nurses, 32,* 161–171.

Hummel, P., & Cronin, J. (2004). Home care of the high-risk infant. *Advances in Neonatal Care, 4* (6), 354–364.

Juretschke, L. J. (2005). Kernicterus: Still a concern. *Neonatal Network, 24*(2), 7–19.

Kaplan, D. M., & Mason, E. A. (1974). Maternal reactions to premature birth viewed as an acute emotional disorder. In H. J. Parad (Ed.), *Crisis intervention.* New York: Family Services Association of America.

Klaus, M. H., & Kennell, J. H. (1982). *Maternal-infant bonding* (2nd ed.). St. Louis, MO: Mosby.

Leuthner, S. R., & Das, U. G. (2004). Low Apgar scores and the definition of birth asphyxia. *Pediatric Clinics of North America, 51*(3), 737–745.

Loo, K. K., Espinosa, M., Tyler, R., & Howard, J. (2003). Using knowledge to cope with stress in the NICU: How parents integrate learning to read the physiologic and behavioral cues of the infant. *Neonatal Networks, 22*(1), 31–37.

Madan, A., MacMahon, J. R., & Stevenson, D. K. (2005). Neonatal hyperbilirubinemia. In H. W. Taeusch, R. A. Ballard, & C. A. Gleason (Eds.), *Avery's diseases of the newborn* (8th ed., pp. 1226–1257). Philadelphia: Elsevier Saunders.

Mitchell, A., & Waltman, P. A. (2003). Oral sucrose and pain relief for preterm infants. *Pain Management Nursing, 4*(2), 62–69. Retrieved from http://www.medscape.com/viewart icle/458592

Pappas, A., & Delaney-Black, V. (2004). Differential diagnosis and management of polycythemia. *Pediatric Clinics of North America, 51*(4), 1063–1086.

Sahni, R., Ammari, A., Suri, M. S., Milisavljevic, V., Ohira-Kist, K., Wung, J. T., et al. (2005). Is the new definition of bronchopulmonary dysplasia more useful? *Journal of Perinatology, 25,* 41–46.

Sasidharan, P. (2004). An approach to diagnosis and management of cyanosis and tachypnea in term infants. *Pediatric Clinics of North America, 51*(4), 999–1021.

Sedin, G. (2004). To avoid heat loss in very preterm infants. *The Journal of Pediatrics, 145,* 720–722.

Shah, M. A., & Campbell, D. (2004). *Transcultural aspects of perinatal health: A resource guide.* Elk Grove Village, IL: American Academy of Pediatrics National Perinatal Association.

Short, M. A. (2004). Guide to a systemic physical assessment in the infant with suspected infection and/or sepsis. *Advances in Neonatal Care, 4*(3), 141–153.

Solnit, A., & Stark, M. (1961). Mourning and the birth of a defective child. *Psychoanalytic Study of the Child, 16,* 505.

Spears, K., Cheney, C., & Zerzan, J. (2004). Low plasma retinol concentrations increase the risk of developing bronchopulmonary dysplasia and long-term respiratory disability in very-low-birth-weight infants. *American Journal of Clinical Nutrition, 80*(6), 1589–1594.

Sperling, M. A., & Menon, R. K. (2004). Differential diagnosis and management of neonatal hypoglycemia. *Pediatric Clinics of North America, 51*(3), 703–723.

Stokowski, L. A. (2004). Rapid identification of infections in the NICU. *Advances in Neonatal Care, 4*(1), 8–9.

Thomas, K. A., Renaud, M. T., & DePaul, D. (2004). Use of the Parenting Stress Index in mothers of preterm infants. *Advances in Neonatal Care, 4*(1), 33–41.

Thureen, P. J., Deacon, J., Hernandez, J. A., & Hall, D. M. (2005). *Assessment and care of the well newborn* (2nd ed.). St. Louis, MO: Elsevier Saunders.

Vohr, B. R., Wright, L. L., Poole, W. K., & McDonald, S. A. (2005). Neurodevelopmental outcomes of extremely low birth weight infants less than 32 weeks' gestation between 1993 and 1998. *Pediatrics, 116,* 635–643.

Walden, M., & Jorgensen, K. M. (2004). Pain management. In C. Kenner & J. M. McGrath (Eds.), *Developmental care of newborns & infants: A guide for health professionals* (pp. 197–222). St. Louis, MO: Mosby.

Watson, R. L. (2004). Gastrointestinal disorders. In M. T. Verklan & M. Walden (Eds.), *Core curriculum for neonatal intensive care nursing* (3rd ed., pp. 643–702). St. Louis, MO: Elsevier Saunders.

Young, T. E., & Mangum, B. (2006). *Neofax* (19th ed.). Raleigh, NC: Acorn.

UNIT 7

Postpartum

CHAPTER
34 Postpartal Family Adaptation and Nursing Assessment

I had heard about the negatives—the fatigue, the loneliness, loss of self. But nobody told me about the wonderful parts: holding my baby close to me, seeing her first smile, watching her grow and become more responsive day by day. How can I describe the way I felt when she stroked my breast while nursing, or looked into my eyes or arched her eyebrows like an opera singer? This was the deepest connection I'd felt to anybody. Sometimes the intensity almost frightened me. For the first time I cared about somebody else more than myself, and I would do anything to nurture and protect her.

~ The Boston Women's Health Collective, The New Our Bodies, Ourselves ~

OBJECTIVES

1. Describe the basic physiologic changes that occur in the postpartum period as a woman's body returns to its prepregnant state.
2. Discuss the psychologic adjustments that normally occur during the postpartum period.
3. Discuss the impact of cultural influence upon the postpartum period.
4. Delineate the physiologic and psychosocial components of a normal postpartum assessment.
5. Summarize the physical and developmental tasks that the mother must accomplish during the postpartum period.
6. Summarize the factors that influence the development of parent-infant attachment.

KEY TERMS

Afterpains 1047
Boggy uterus (uterine atony) 1041
Diastasis recti abdominis 1045
En face 1049
Engrossment 1050
Fundus 1041
Involution 1041
Lochia 1042
Lochia alba 1042
Lochia rubra 1042
Lochia serosa 1042
Maternal role attainment 1048
Newborns' and Mothers' Health Protection Act (NMHPA) 1066
Postpartum blues 1048
Puerperium 1041
Reciprocity 1050
Subinvolution 1042

 MEDIALINK

Additional resources for this content can be found on the Prentice Hall Nursing MediaLink DVD-ROM and on the Companion Website at http://www.prenhall.com/davidson. Click on "Chapter 34" to select the activities for this chapter.

T he **puerperium,** or postpartal period, is the period during which the woman readjusts, physically and psychologically, from pregnancy and birth. It begins immediately after birth and continues for approximately 6 weeks or until the body has returned to a near nonpregnant state.

This chapter describes the physiologic and psychologic changes and adaptations that occur postpartally and the basic aspects of a thorough postpartal assessment.

POSTPARTUM PHYSICAL ADAPTATIONS

Comprehensive nursing assessment is based on a sound understanding of the normal anatomic and physiologic processes of the puerperium. These processes involve the reproductive organs and other major body systems.

Reproductive System
INVOLUTION OF THE UTERUS

The term **involution** is used to describe the rapid reduction in size of the uterus and its return to a condition similar to its nonpregnant state, although it remains slightly larger than it was before the first pregnancy. Specifically, the weight of the uterus decreases from 1000 g in the immediate postpartal period to 500 g at the end of the first week. It reaches 300 g by the end of the second week, finally terminating the involution process with a weight of 100 g or less (Cunningham, Leveno, Bloom et al., 2005).

Following separation of the placenta, the decidua of the uterus is irregular, jagged, and varied in thickness. The spongy layer of the decidua is cast off as lochia, and the basal layer of the decidua remains in the uterus to become differentiated into two layers within the first 48 to 72 hours after birth. The outermost layer becomes necrotic and is sloughed off in the lochia. The layer closest to the myometrium contains the fundi of the uterine endometrial glands, and these glands lay the foundation for the new endometrium. Except at the placental site, this process is completed in approximately 3 weeks. The placental site can take up to 6 to 7 weeks to completely heal (Blackburn, 2003). Bleeding from the larger uterine vessels of the placental site is controlled by compression of the retracted uterine muscle fibers. The clotted blood is gradually absorbed by the body. Some of these vessels are eventually obliterated and replaced by new vessels with smaller lumens.

Rather than forming a fibrous scar in the decidua, the placental site heals by a process of exfoliation. The placental site is undermined by the growth of the endometrial tissue, both from the margins of the site and from the fundi of the endometrial glands left in the basal layer of the site. The infarcted superficial tissue then becomes necrotic and is sloughed off (Blackburn, 2003). *Exfoliation* is one of the most important aspects of involution. If the healing of the placental site left a fibrous scar, the area available for further implantation would be limited, as would the number of possible pregnancies.

With the dramatic decrease in the levels of circulating estrogen and progesterone following placental separation, the uterine cells atrophy, and the hyperplasia of pregnancy begins to reverse. The process is one in which the *size* of the cells decreases markedly; the *number* of cells does not decrease. Proteolytic enzymes are released, and macrophages migrate to the uterus to promote autolysis (self-digestion). Protein material in the uterine wall is broken down and absorbed. The amount of lochia and the speed of involution are not affected by the prophylactic administration of oxytocin (Pitocin) or ergot preparations (Methergine, Ergotrate), which have only short-term effect (Varney, Kriebs, & Gegor, 2004). Factors that enhance involution include an uncomplicated labor and birth, complete expulsion of the amniotic membranes and the placenta, breastfeeding, manual removal of the placenta during a cesarean birth, and early ambulation. Factors that slow uterine involution and the rationale for each factor are listed in Table 34–1.

CHANGES IN FUNDAL POSITION

Immediately following the expulsion of the placenta, the uterus contracts firmly to the size of a large grapefruit. The **fundus** (top portion of the uterus) is situated in the midline of the abdomen, one half to two thirds of the way between the symphysis pubis and the umbilicus (Figure 34–1 ◆). The walls of the contracted uterus are in close proximity and the uterine blood vessels are firmly compressed by the myometrium. Within 6 to 12 hours after birth, the fundus of the uterus rises to the level of the umbilicus because of blood and clots that remain within the uterus and changes in support of the uterus by the ligaments. A fundus that is above the umbilicus and boggy (feels soft and spongy rather than firm and well contracted) is associated with excessive uterine bleeding. As blood collects and forms clots within the uterus, the fundus rises; firm contractions of the uterine muscle are interrupted, causing a **boggy uterus (uterine atony).** When the fundus is higher than expected and is not in midline (usually deviated to the right), distention of the bladder

Table 34–1	FACTORS THAT RETARD UTERINE INVOLUTION
Factor	**Rationale**
Prolonged labor	Muscles relax because of prolonged time of contraction during labor.
Anesthesia	Muscles relax.
Difficult birth	The uterus is manipulated excessively.
Grandmultiparity	Repeated distention of uterus during pregnancy and labor leads to muscle stretching, diminished tone, and muscle relaxation.
Full bladder	As the uterus is pushed up and usually to the right, pressure on it interferes with effective uterine contraction.
Incomplete expulsion of placenta or membranes	The presence of even small amounts of tissue interferes with ability of uterus to remain firmly contracted.
Infection	Inflammation interferes with uterine muscle's ability to contract effectively.
Overdistention of uterus	Overstretching of uterine muscles with conditions such as multiple gestation, hydramnios, or a very large baby may set the stage for slower uterine involution.

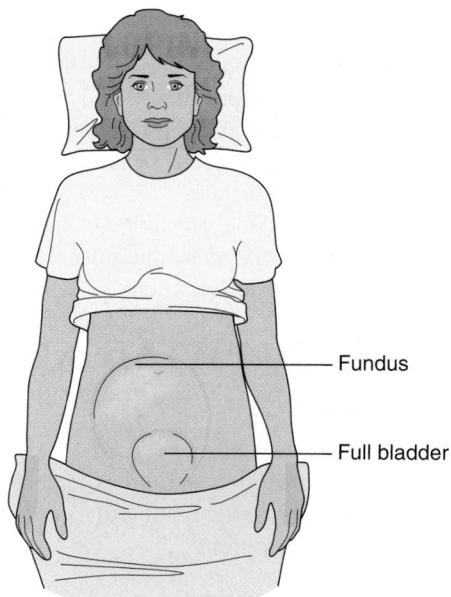

Figure 34–2 ◆ The uterus becomes displaced and deviated to the right when the bladder is full.

Figure 34–1 ◆ Involution of the uterus. (A) Immediately after delivery of the placenta, the top of the fundus is in the midline and approximately two thirds to three-fourths of the way between the symphysis pubis and the umbilicus (B). About 6 to 12 hours after birth, the fundus is at the level of (or one fingerbreadth below) the umbilicus. The height of the fundus then decreases about one fingerbreadth (approximately 1 cm) each day.

should be suspected and the bladder should be emptied immediately and the uterus remeasured (Figure 34–2 ◆). If the woman is unable to void, in-and-out catheterization of the bladder may be required. In the immediate postpartum period many women may not be aware of a full bladder. Because the uterine ligaments are still stretched, a full bladder can move the uterus. By the end of the puerperium these ligaments have regained their nonpregnant length and tension.

After birth, the top of the fundus remains at the level of the umbilicus for about half a day. On the first postpartum day (first day following birth), the top of the fundus is located about 1 cm below the umbilicus. The top of the fundus descends approximately one fingerbreadth (width of index, second, or third finger), or 1 cm, per day until it descends into the pelvis on the 10th day.

If the mother is breastfeeding, the release of endogenous oxytocin from the posterior pituitary in response to suckling may hasten this process. Barring complications, such as infection or retained placental fragments, the uterus approaches its prepregnant size and location by 5 to 6 weeks. In women who had an oversized uterus during the pregnancy (hydramnios, birth of a large-for-gestational-age [LGA] infant, or multiple gestation), the time frame for immediate uterine involution process is lengthened. If intrauterine infection is present, in addition to foul-smelling lochia or vaginal discharge, the uterine fundus descends much more slowly. When infection is sus-

pected, other clinical signs such as fever and tachycardia in addition to delay in involution must be assessed. Any slowing of descent is called **subinvolution** (for further discussion of subinvolution, see Chapter 38 ∞).

LOCHIA

The uterus rids itself of the debris remaining after birth through a discharge called **lochia,** which is classified according to its appearance and contents. **Lochia rubra,** named for the Latin word for *red,* is dark red in color. It is present for the first 2 to 3 days postpartum and contains epithelial cells, erythrocytes, leukocytes, bacteria, shreds of the decidua, and, occasionally, fetal meconium, lanugo, and vernix caseosa. Clotting is often the result of pooling of blood in the upper portion of the vagina. A few small clots (no larger than a nickel) are common, particularly in the first few days after birth. However, lochia should not contain large (plum sized) clots; if it does, the cause should be investigated without delay. **Lochia serosa** is a pinkish color. It follows from about the 3rd to the 10th day. Lochia serosa is composed of serous exudate shreds of degenerating decidua, erythrocytes, leukocytes, cervical mucus, and numerous microorganisms (Blackburn, 2003).

The red blood cell (RBC) component decreases gradually, and a creamy or yellowish discharge persists for an additional week or two. This final discharge, termed **lochia alba** from the Latin word for *white,* is composed primarily of leukocytes, decidual cells, epithelial cells, fat, cervical mucus, cholesterol crystals, and bacteria. Variation in the duration of lochia discharge is not uncommon; however, the trend should be toward a lighter amount of flow and a lighter color of discharge. When the lochia stops, the cervix is considered closed, and chances of infection ascending from the vagina to the uterus decrease.

Like menstrual discharge, lochia has a musty, stale odor that is not offensive. Microorganisms are always present in the vaginal lochia, and by the second day following birth the uterus is contaminated with the vaginal bacteria. Researchers speculate that infection does not develop because the organisms involved are relatively nonvirulent. In addition, by the time the bacteria reach the raw, exposed surface of the uterus, the process of granulation has begun, forming a protective barrier. Any foul smell to the lochia or used perineal pads suggests infection and the need for prompt additional assessment, such as white blood cell (WBC) count and differential and assessment for uterine tenderness and fever.

The total volume of lochia is approximately 225 mL, and the daily volume decreases gradually (Blackburn, 2003). Discharge is greater in the morning because of pooling in the vagina and uterus while the mother lies sleeping. The amount of lochia may also be increased by exertion or breastfeeding. Multiparous women usually have more lochia than first-time mothers. Women who undergo a cesarean birth typically have less lochia than women who give birth vaginally (Blackburn, 2003).

Evaluation of lochia is necessary not only to determine the presence of hemorrhage but also to assess uterine involution. The type, amount, and consistency of lochia determine the state of healing of the placental site, and a progressive color change from bright red at birth to dark red to pink to white or clear should be observed. Persistent discharge of lochia rubra or a return to lochia rubra indicates subinvolution or late postpartum hemorrhage (see Chapter 38 ∞).

The nurse should exercise caution in evaluating bleeding immediately after birth. The continuous seepage of blood is more consistent with cervical or vaginal lacerations and may be effectively diagnosed when the bleeding is evaluated in conjunction with the consistency of the uterus. Lacerations should be suspected if the uterus is firm and of expected size and if no clots can be expressed.

CERVICAL CHANGES

Following birth, the cervix is spongy, flabby, and formless and may appear bruised. The lateral aspects of the external os are frequently lacerated during the birth process (Cunningham et al., 2005). The external os is markedly irregular and closes slowly. It admits two fingers for a few days following birth, but by the end of the first week it will admit only a fingertip.

The shape of the external os is permanently changed by the first childbearing. The characteristic dimplelike os of the nullipara changes to the lateral slit (fish-mouth) os of the multipara. After significant cervical laceration or several lacerations, the cervix may appear lopsided. Because of the slight change in the size of the cervix, a diaphragm or cervical cap will need to be refitted if the woman is using one of these methods of contraception.

VAGINAL CHANGES

Following birth, the vagina appears edematous and gaping and may be bruised. Small superficial lacerations may be evident, and the rugae have been obliterated. The apparent bruising of the vagina is due to pelvic congestion and trauma and will quickly disappear. The hymen, torn and jagged, heals irregularly, leaving small tags called the *carunculae myrtiformes*.

The size of the vagina decreases and rugae return within 3 to 4 weeks (Blackburn, 2003). This facilitates the gradual return

to smaller, although not to nulliparous, dimensions. By 6 weeks, the nonlactating woman's vagina usually appears normal. The lactating woman is in a hypoestrogenic state because of ovarian suppression, and her vaginal mucosa may be pale and without rugae. This may lead to dyspareunia (painful intercourse), which may be reduced by the addition of a water-soluble personal lubricant. Tone and contractibility of the vaginal opening may be improved by perineal tightening exercises (Kegel exercises, discussed in Chapter 16 ∞), which may begin soon after birth. The labia majora and labia minora are looser in the woman who has borne a child than in the nullipara.

PERINEAL CHANGES

During the early postpartal period, the soft tissue in and around the perineum may appear edematous with some bruising. If an episiotomy or laceration is present, the edges should be approximated. Occasionally, ecchymosis occurs, and this may delay healing. Initial healing of the episiotomy or laceration occurs in 2 to 3 weeks after the birth, although complete healing may take up to 4 to 6 months (Blackburn, 2003). Perineal discomfort may be present during this time.

RECURRENCE OF OVULATION AND MENSTRUATION

The return of menstruation and ovulation varies for each postpartum woman. Menstruation generally returns in nonbreastfeeding mothers between 6 and 10 weeks after birth; 50% of the first cycles are anovulatory (Cunningham et al., 2005). The return of ovulation is directly associated with a rise in the serum progesterone level. In nonlactating women the average time to first ovulation is 45 days (range 25 to 72). Overall, 90% of nonlactating mothers resume menstruation within 6 months after birth (Blackburn, 2003).

The return of menstruation and ovulation in breastfeeding mothers is usually prolonged and is associated with the length of time the woman breastfeeds and whether formula supplements are used. If a mother breastfeeds for less than 1 month, the return of menstruation and ovulation is similar to the nonbreastfeeding mother. In women who exclusively breastfeed, menstruation is usually delayed for at least 3 months. Sucking by the infant typically results in alterations in the gonadotropin-releasing hormone (GnRH) production, which is thought to be the cause of amenorrhea (Blackburn, 2003). Although exclusive breastfeeding helps to reduce the risk of pregnancy for the first 6 months after delivery, it should be relied upon only temporarily and if it meets the observed criteria for lactational amenorrhea method (LAM). Furthermore, because ovulation precedes menstruation and women often supplement breastfeeding with bottles and pacifiers, breastfeeding is not considered a reliable means of contraception.

Abdomen

The uterine ligaments (notably the round and broad ligaments) are stretched and require the length of the puerperium to recover. The stretched abdominal wall appears loose and flabby, but it will respond to exercise within 2 to 3 months. In the grandmultipara, in the woman whose abdomen is overdistended, or in the woman whose muscle tone was poor before pregnancy, the

THROUGH THE EYES OF A NURSE

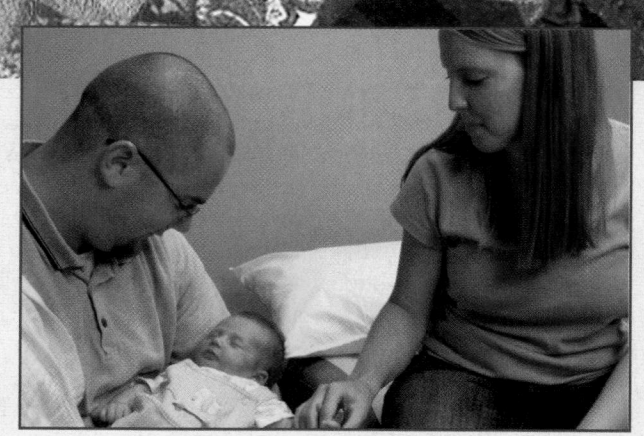

Postpartal Bleeding and Perineal Changes

FAMILY'S EXPERIENCE: Phone call to the birthing unit from a new mother: "I am still feeling some cramping and having vaginal bleeding at this point although it is easing up some. I am concerned because it had gotten lighter but now it seems to have picked up again. My vaginal area seems to feel better but sometimes it is still sensitive when I wipe after urination. Is this normal?"

NURSE'S RESPONSE: "It is normal that the bleeding can increase when your activity level increases. At this point (after 3 to 4 days), the bleeding should be pink in color. You should not be having large clots, although a few small clots may occur. If your bleeding becomes heavy, more than 1 to 2 pads per hour, if there is a foul-smelling odor, or if you have fever or chills, you would need to contact your healthcare provider immediately because those can be warning signs that need further assessing.

"Your uterus will continue to contract in the early postpartum period as a result of *involution*. This helps your uterus return to a prepregnant state and descend behind your pubic bone. You can take an anti-inflammatory medication as directed by your healthcare provider. You may notice that the cramping or afterbirth pains occur commonly with breastfeeding. This is also normal.

"The perineal area will continue to heal in the upcoming weeks. It is not unusual for the area to feel tender and to be sensitive. If the area becomes more painful, red, is warm to the touch, or appears to 'come open,' that could be a sign of an infection or a problem with the incision site. You would want to contact your healthcare provider if any of those things occur. The sutures that were placed after the birth will continue to heal and will dissolve over time. I would continue to use the topical agents you received in the birth setting and to use the sitz bath."

NURSE'S ACTIONS AND RATIONALE:

The nurse reviews the normal physiologic changes associated with the postpartum period. The signs and symptoms of bleeding and infection should be reviewed. The nurse explains the normal physical changes that occur, including involution of the uterus, cessation of lochia, healing of the laceration or episiotomy site, and breast changes related to lactation. Many women find it helpful if the nurse reviews the various changes that occur as the body returns to a prepregnant state.

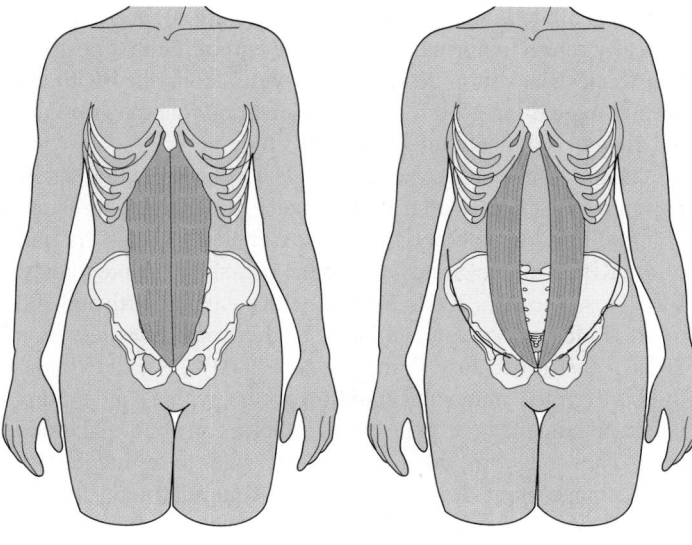

Normal location of rectus   Diastasis recti: separation
muscles of the abdomen   of the rectus muscles

Figure 34–3 ◆ Diastasis recti abdominis, a separation of the musculature, commonly occurs after pregnancy.

abdomen may fail to regain good tone and will remain flabby. **Diastasis recti abdominis,** a separation of the rectus abdominis muscles, may occur with pregnancy, especially in women with poor abdominal muscle tone (Figure 34–3 ◆). If diastasis occurs, part of the abdominal wall has no muscular support but is formed only by skin, subcutaneous fat, fascia, and peritoneum. This may be especially pronounced in women who have undergone a cesarean section, as the rectus abdominis muscles are manually separated to access the uterine muscle. Improvement depends on the physical condition of the mother, the total number of pregnancies, pregnancy spacing, and the type and amount of physical exercise. If rectus muscle tone is not regained, support may be inadequate during future pregnancies. This may result in a pendulous abdomen and increased maternal backache. Fortunately, diastasis usually responds well to exercise, and abdominal muscle tone can improve significantly.

The striae (stretch marks), which occurred as a result of stretching and rupture of the elastic fibers of the skin, take on different colors based on the mother's skin color. The striae of Caucasian mothers are red to purple at the time of birth and gradually fade to silver or white. The striae of mothers with darker skin are darker than the surrounding skin and remain darker. These marks gradually fade after a time but remain visible.

Lactation

During pregnancy, the breasts develop in preparation for lactation as a result of the influence of both estrogen and progesterone. After birth, the interplay of maternal hormones leads to the establishment of milk production (see Chapter 31 ∞).

Gastrointestinal System

Hunger following birth is common, and the mother may enjoy a light meal. Frequently, she is quite thirsty and will drink large amounts of fluid. Drinking fluids helps replace fluid lost during labor, in the urine, and through perspiration.

The bowels tend to be sluggish after birth because of the lingering effects of progesterone, decreased abdominal muscle tone, and bowel evacuation associated with the labor and birth process. Women who have had an episiotomy, lacerations, or hemorrhoids may tend to delay elimination for fear of increasing their pain or in the belief that their stitches will be torn if they bear down. In resisting or delaying the bowel movement, the woman may cause increased constipation and more pain when elimination finally occurs.

The woman with a cesarean birth may receive clear liquids shortly after surgery. Once bowel sounds are present, the diet is quickly advanced to solid food. The woman may experience some initial discomfort from flatulence. This is relieved by early ambulation and use of antiflatulent medications. Chamomile tea and peppermint tea may also be helpful in reducing discomfort from flatulence. It may take a few days for the bowel to regain its tone. The woman who has had a cesarean or a difficult birth may benefit from stool softeners.

Urinary Tract

The postpartum woman has an increased bladder capacity, swelling and bruising of the tissues around the urethra, decreased sensitivity to fluid pressure, and decreased sensation of bladder filling. Consequently, she is at risk for overdistention, incomplete emptying, and buildup of residual urine. Women who have had an anesthetic block have inhibited neural functioning of the bladder and are more susceptible to bladder distention, difficulty voiding, and bladder retention. In addition, immediate postpartal use of oxytocin to facilitate uterine contractions following expulsion of the placenta has an antidiuretic effect. Following cessation of the oxytocin the woman will experience rapid bladder filling (Cunningham et al., 2005).

Urinary output increases during the early postpartal period (first 12 to 24 hours) because of *puerperal diuresis.* The kidneys must eliminate an estimated 2000 to 3000 mL of extracellular fluid with a normal pregnancy, which causes rapid filling of the bladder. Thus adequate bladder elimination is an immediate concern. Women with preeclampsia, chronic hypertension, and diabetes experience even greater fluid retention, and postpartal diuresis is increased accordingly.

If stasis exists, chances increase for urinary tract infection because of bacteriuria and the presence of dilated ureters and renal pelves, which persist for about 6 weeks after birth. A full bladder may also increase the tendency of the uterus to relax by displacing the uterus and interfering with its contractility, leading to hemorrhage. In the absence of infection, the dilated ureters and renal pelves return to prepregnant size by the end of the sixth week.

Hematuria, resulting from bladder or urethral trauma, may occasionally occur after birth, but the presence of lochia may mask this sign. If hematuria occurs in the second or third postpartal week, there may be a bladder infection. Acetone may be present in the urine of women with diabetes or of women with prolonged labor and dehydration. Slight (1+) proteinuria may occur during the first week following birth.

However, proteinuria may be associated with an infectious process (cystitis, pyelitis), so it should be evaluated further. A urine specimen contaminated with lochia may falsely indicate proteinuria, so any specimen should be obtained as a midstream or a catheterized specimen.

Vital Signs

During the postpartal period, with the exception of the first 24 hours, the woman should be afebrile. Epidural anesthesia for labor, which can interfere with heat dissipation, has a direct effect on maternal temperature but rarely results in overt fever (Alexander, 2005). A maternal temperature of up to 38C (100.4F) may occur up to 24 hours after birth as a result of the exertion and dehydration of labor. An increase in temperature to between 37.8C and 39C may also occur during the first 24 hours after the mother's milk comes in (Cunningham et al., 2005). However, in women not meeting these criteria, infection must be considered in the presence of an increased temperature (see Chapter 38 ∞).

Immediately following delivery, many women experience a transient rise in both systolic and diastolic blood pressure, which spontaneously returns to the prepregnancy baseline over the next few days (Varney et al., 2004). A decrease may indicate physiologic readjustment to decreased intrapelvic pressure, or it may be related to uterine hemorrhage. Orthostatic hypotension, as indicated by feelings of faintness or dizziness immediately after standing up, can develop in the first 48 hours as a result of abdominal engorgement that may occur after birth. A low or decreasing blood pressure may reflect hypovolemia secondary to hemorrhage, but it is a late sign. Blood pressure elevations may result from excessive use of oxytocin or vasopressor medications. Because preeclampsia can persist into or occur first in the postpartum period, routine evaluation of blood pressure is needed. If a woman complains of headache, hypertension must be ruled out before analgesics are administered.

Puerperal bradycardia with rates of 50 to 70 beats per minute (bpm) commonly occurs during the first 6 to 10 days of the postpartum period. It may be related to decreased cardiac strain, the decreased blood volume following placental separation, contraction of the uterus, and increased stroke volume. A pulse rate greater than 100 bpm may be indicative of hypovolemia, infection, fear, or pain and requires further assessment.

Blood Values

Blood values should return to the prepregnant state by the end of the postpartal period. Pregnancy-associated activation of coagulation factors may continue for variable amounts of time after birth. This condition, in conjunction with trauma, immobility, or sepsis, predisposes the woman to development of thromboembolism. The incidence of thromboembolism is reduced by early mobilization. Plasma fibrinogen is maintained at pregnancy levels for a week following childbirth, accounting for the higher sedimentation rate observed in the early postpartum period.

Nonpathologic leukocytosis often occurs during labor and in the immediate postpartum period, with WBC counts up to 25,000 to 30,000/mm^3 (Cunningham et al., 2005). WBC values typically return to normal levels by the end of the first postpartum week (Blackburn, 2003). Leukocytosis combined with the normal increase in erythrocyte sedimentation rate may obscure the diagnosis of acute infection at this time.

Hemoglobin and hematocrit levels may be difficult to interpret in the first 2 days after birth because of the changing blood volume. This loss in blood in the first 24 hours accounts for half of the RBC volume gained during the course of the pregnancy. Blood loss averages 200 to 500 mL with a vaginal birth and 700 to 1000 mL with a cesarean birth. Lochia constitutes less than 25% of this blood loss (Varney et al., 2004). As extracellular fluid is excreted, hemoconcentration occurs, with a concomitant rise in hematocrit. A drop in values indicates an abnormal blood loss. The following is a convenient rule to remember: a 2-percentage-point drop in hematocrit equals a blood loss of 500 mL (Varney et al., 2004). After 3 to 4 days, mobilization of interstitial fluid leads to a slight increase in plasma volume. This hemodilution leads to a decrease in hemoglobin, hematocrit, and plasma protein by the end of the first postpartum week. Decreases in plasma volume reach nonpregnant levels by 4 to 6 weeks postpartum (Blackburn, 2003).

Platelet levels typically fall as a result of placental separation. They then begin to increase by the third to fourth postpartum day, gradually returning to normal by the sixth postpartum week. Fibrinolytic activity typically returns to normal during the hours following the birth. The hemostatic system as a whole reaches its normal pregnant status by 3 to 4 weeks postpartum; however, the diameter of deep veins can take up to 6 weeks to return to prepregnant levels (Blackburn, 2003). This is why there is a prolonged risk of thromboembolism in the first 6 weeks following birth.

Cardiovascular Changes

The cardiovascular system undergoes dramatic changes during birth that can result in cardiovascular instability due to an increase in cardiac output. The cardiac output typically stabilizes and returns to pregnancy levels within a hour following birth (Blackburn, 2003). Maternal hypervolemia typically occurs immediately following birth because the maternal circulation has an increase in blood volume that no longer travels through the placenta. Maternal hypervolemia acts to protect the mother from excessive blood loss. Cardiac output declines by 30% in the first 2 weeks and reaches normal levels by 6 to 12 weeks (Blackburn, 2003). Diuresis in the first 2 to 5 days helps to decrease the extracellular fluid and results in a weight loss of 3 kg. Failure to diurese in the immediate postpartum period can lead to pulmonary edema and subsequent cardiac problems. This is seen more commonly in women with a history of preeclampsia or preexisting cardiac problems (Blackburn, 2003).

Neurologic Changes and Conditions

Neurologic problems and disorders can predispose women to higher rates of morbidity and mortality during pregnancy and in the postpartum period. Headaches are the most common neurologic symptoms encountered by postpartum women. It is estimated that up to 40% of postpartum women develop headaches within the first week following birth (Browne & Birnbach, 2003). There may be an increased incidence in headache if the woman had spinal or epidural anesthesia. Migraine headaches, although less frequent during pregnancy, tend to resume in the postpartum period (Shehata & Okosun, 2004). Women with epilepsy are at a 1% to 2% risk of having a seizure in the immediate postpartum period (Tatum, Liporace, Benbadis et al., 2004). It is nine times more likely that a woman will have a seizure during labor or in the first 24 hours after birth than it is during pregnancy (Shehata & Okosun, 2004). Women with multiple sclerosis (MS) and Guillain-Barré syndrome are more likely to have symptoms in the postpartum period than during pregnancy (Wiertlewski, Magot, Drapier et al., 2004). Myasthenia gravis (autoimmune disease) affects the neuromuscular junctions. The increase in symptoms during pregnancy is variable; however, the first month of pregnancy and the first month of the postpartum period are the most critical (Shehata & Okosun, 2004).

Weight Loss

An initial weight loss of 10 to 12 lb occurs as a result of the birth of infant, placenta, and amniotic fluid. Puerperal diuresis accounts for the loss of an additional 5 lb during the early puerperium. By the sixth to eighth week after birth, many women have returned to approximately prepregnant weight if they gained the average 25 to 30 lb. Women often express concern about the slow pace of their postpartum weight loss. Multiparas tend to be more positive than primiparas, probably because the multipara's previous experience has prepared her for the fact that the body does not immediately return to a prepregnant state.

Postpartum Chill

Frequently the mother experiences intense tremors that resemble shivering from a chill immediately after birth. Several theories have been offered to explain this shivering: the result of sudden release of pressure on the pelvic nerves after birth, a response to a fetus-to-mother transfusion that occurred during placental separation, a reaction to maternal adrenaline production during labor and birth, or a reaction to epidural anesthesia. If not followed by fever, this chill is of no clinical concern, but it is uncomfortable for the woman. The nurse can increase the woman's comfort by covering her with a warmed blanket and reassuring her that the shivering is a common, self-limiting situation. If she allows herself to go with the shaking, the shivering will last only a short time. Some women may also find a warm drink helpful. Chills and fever later in the puerperium indicate infection and require further evaluation.

Postpartal Diaphoresis

The elimination of excess fluid and waste products via the skin during the puerperium greatly increases perspiration. Diaphoretic (sweating) episodes frequently occur at night, and the woman may awaken drenched with perspiration. This perspiration is not significant clinically, but the mother should be protected from chilling.

Afterpains

Afterpains occur more commonly in multiparas than in primiparas and are caused by intermittent uterine contractions. Al-

though the uterus of the primipara usually remains consistently contracted, the lost tone of the uterus of the multipara results in alternate contraction and relaxation. This phenomenon also occurs if the uterus has been markedly distended, as with multiple-gestation pregnancies or hydramnios, or if clots or placental fragments were retained. These afterpains may cause the mother severe discomfort for 2 to 3 days following birth. The administration of oxytocic agents (intravenous infusion with Pitocin or oral administration of Methergine) stimulates uterine contraction and increases the discomfort of the afterpains. Because endogenous oxytocin is released when the infant suckles, breastfeeding also increases the severity of the afterpains. A warm water bottle placed against the low abdomen may reduce the discomfort of afterpains. In addition, the breastfeeding mother may find it helpful to take a mild analgesic agent approximately 1 hour before feeding her infant. The nurse can assure the mother that the prescribed analgesic agents are not harmful to the newborn and help improve the quality of the breastfeeding experience. An analgesic agent such as ibuprofen is also helpful at bedtime if the afterpains interfere with the mother's rest.

POSTPARTUM PSYCHOLOGIC ADAPTATIONS

The postpartum period is a time of readjustment and adaptation for the entire childbearing family but especially for the mother. The woman experiences a variety of responses as she adjusts to a new family member, postpartum discomforts, changes in her body image, and the reality that she is no longer pregnant. One young mother described her responses well:

> *I feel like it's the day after Christmas. I'm relieved that everything went well and I have a fine baby, but I feel so let down. I had an image of what childbirth would be like, but everything was a little different. I figured that as soon as I gave birth, I would feel fine. Why didn't someone tell me I would still be sore? The pain didn't magically disappear! When I was pregnant, everyone treated me as though I was a little fragile. Now when people call or visit, all they talk about is the baby. I don't think I'm really jealous, but I do miss the attention. During this past day I've started to realize that my life will never, ever be the same again. I've always wanted to be a mother, but I'm not really sure how to do it. Isn't that strange?*

Taking In and Taking Hold

During the first day or two following birth, the woman tends to be passive and somewhat dependent. The new mother follows suggestions, is hesitant about making decisions, and is still rather preoccupied with her needs. She may have a great need to talk about her perceptions of her labor and birth. This helps her work through the process, sort out the reality from her fantasized experience, and clarify anything that she did not understand. Food and sleep are major needs. In her early work, Rubin (1961) labeled this the *taking-in period.*

By the second or third day after birth, the new mother was observed to be ready to resume control of her body, her mothering, and her life in general. Rubin (1961) labeled this phase as *taking hold.* If she is breastfeeding, the mother may worry about her technique or the quality of her milk. If her baby spits up following feeding, she may view it as a personal failure. She may also feel demoralized by the fact that the nurse or an older family member handles her baby proficiently while she feels unsure and tentative. She requires assurance that she is doing well as a mother. Today's mothers seem to be more independent and adjust more rapidly, exhibiting behaviors of "taking in" and "taking hold" in shorter time periods than those previously identified.

Maternal Role Attainment

Maternal role attainment is the process by which a woman learns mothering behaviors and becomes comfortable with her identity as a mother. The formation of a maternal identity indicates that the woman has attained the maternal role. This process occurs with each child a woman bears. As the mother grows to know this child and forms a relationship with her or him, the mother's maternal identity gradually and systematically evolves, and she "binds in" to the infant (Rubin, 1984).

Maternal role attainment occurs in four stages (Mercer, 1995):

1. The *anticipatory stage* occurs during pregnancy. The woman looks to role models, especially her own mother, for examples of how to mother.

2. The *formal stage* begins when the child is born. The woman is still influenced by the guidance of others and tries to act as she believes others expect her to act.

3. The *informal stage* begins when the mother begins to make her own choices about mothering. The woman begins to develop her own style of mothering and finds ways of functioning that work well for her.

4. The *personal stage* is the final stage of maternal role attainment. When the woman reaches this stage, she is comfortable with the notion of herself as "mother."

In most cases, maternal role attainment occurs within 3 to 10 months following birth. Social support, the woman's age and personality traits, the marital relationship, the presence of underlying anxiety or depression, the woman's previous childcare skills, the temperament of her infant, and the family's socioeconomic status all influence the woman's success in attaining the maternal role (Porter & Hsu, 2003). The postpartal woman faces a number of challenges as she adjusts to her new role (Mercer, 1995):

- For many women, finding time for themselves is one of the greatest challenges. It is often difficult for the new mother to find time to read a book, talk to her partner, or even eat a meal without interruption.

- Women also report feelings of incompetence because they have not mastered all aspects of the mothering role. Often they are unsure of what to do in a given situation.

- The next greatest challenge involves fatigue resulting from sleep deprivation. The demands of nighttime care are tremendously draining, especially if the woman has other children.

- Another challenge the new mother faces involves the feeling of responsibility that having a child brings. Women experience a sense of lost freedom, an awareness that they will never again be quite as carefree as they were before becoming mothers.

- For women with older children, finding time for them is a challenge. Many women feel guilty because the new baby takes up so much of their time. Sibling rivalry or ill feelings about the baby from other children can put additional stress on the mother.

- Mothers sometimes cite the infant's behavior as a problem, especially when the child is about 8 months old. Stranger anxiety develops, the infant begins crawling and getting into things, teething may cause fussiness, and the baby's tendency to put everything in his or her mouth requires constant vigilance by the parent.

Postpartum nurses need to be aware of the long-term adjustments and stresses that the childbearing family faces as its members adjust to new and different roles. Nurses can help by providing anticipatory guidance about the realities of being a parent and by giving the postpartum family parenting literature for reference at home. Ongoing parenting groups give parents an opportunity to discuss problems and become comfortable in their new roles.

Postpartum Blues

The **postpartum blues** consist of a transient period of depression that occurs during the first few days of puerperium in 70% of all postpartum women (Varney et al., 2004). It may be manifested by mood swings, anger, weepiness, anorexia, difficulty sleeping, and a feeling of letdown. This mood change frequently occurs while the woman is still hospitalized, but it may occur at home as well. Changing hormone levels are certainly a factor; an unsupportive environment and insecurity also have been identified as potential causes. In addition, fatigue, discomfort, and overstimulation may play a part. The postpartum blues usually resolve naturally within 10 to 14 days, but if they persist or if symptoms worsen, the woman may need evaluation for postpartum depression (see Chapter 38 ∞).

Importance of Social Support

The psychologic outcomes of the postpartum period are far more positive when the parents have access to a support network. Women and their partners may find that family relationships become increasingly important, but the increased family interaction can be a source of stress. The new parents may also have increasing contact with other parents of small children while contact with coworkers declines. Of great concern are women and their partners who have no family or friends with whom to form a social network. Isolation at a time when the woman feels an increased need for support can result in tremendous stress and is often a contributing factor in situations of postpartum depression, child neglect, or abuse. New-mother support groups are helpful for women who lack a social

DEVELOPING CULTURAL COMPETENCE

MIDDLE EAST INITIAL POSTPARTUM EXPERIENCE

In many patriarchal countries in the Middle East, the new mother and her infant stay with the husband's family following the birth of the infant. Frequent visits from the woman's family are discouraged and may even be viewed as burdensome by the husband's family. Typically, only women visit the new mother during the postpartum period. For the birth of the first baby, the wife's parents are expected to purchase all of the supplies and clothing for the baby.

support system. Attention that their infant receives from family members is a source of satisfaction to the new parents. In many cases, the ties to the woman's family become especially good. Fathers may report that their relationships with their in-laws become far more positive and supportive. But the increased family interaction can be a source of stress, especially for the new mother, who tends to have more contact with the families. Postpartum doulas are professionals trained to help the new mother after the birth of the baby. As a "mother's helper," postpartum doula services are tailored to help the new mother feel as rested as possible and well-nourished, and to place her household in good order so that she can focus her energy on her new baby.

DEVELOPMENT OF FAMILY ATTACHMENT

A mother's first interaction with her infant is influenced by many factors, including her family of origin, her relationships, the stability of her home environment, the communication patterns she has developed, and the degree of nurturing she received as a child. Certain characteristics of the mother are also important:

- *Level of trust.* What level of trust has this mother developed in response to her life experiences? What is her philosophy of childrearing? Will she be able to treat her infant as a unique individual with changing needs that should be met as much as possible?

- *Level of self-esteem.* How much does she value herself as a woman and as a mother? Does she feel generally able to cope with the adjustments of life?

- *Capacity for enjoying herself.* Is the mother able to find pleasure in everyday activities and human relationships?

- *Adequacy of knowledge about childbearing and childrearing.* What beliefs about the course of pregnancy, the capacities of newborns, previous experiences with infants/children, and the nature of her emotions may influence her behavior at first contact with her infant and later?

- *Prevailing mood or usual feeling tone.* Is the woman predominantly content, angry, depressed, or anxious? Is she sensitive to her own feelings and those of others? Will she be able to accept her own needs and to obtain support in meeting them?

- *Reactions to the present pregnancy.* Was the pregnancy planned? Did it go smoothly? Were there ongoing life events that enhanced her pregnancy or depleted her reserves of energy? How were other life roles changed because of her pregnancy and motherhood?

By the time of birth, each mother has developed an emotional orientation of some kind to the baby based on these factors.

Initial Attachment Behavior

New mothers demonstrate a fairly regular pattern of maternal behaviors at first contact with a normal newborn. In a progression of touching activities, the mother proceeds from fingertip exploration of the newborn's extremities toward palmar contact with larger body areas and finally to enfolding the infant with the whole hand and arms. The time taken to accomplish these steps varies from minutes to days. The mother also increases the proportion of time spent in the **en face** position (Figure 34–4 ◆). She arranges herself or the newborn so that she has direct face-to-face and eye-to-eye contact. There is an intense interest in having the infant's eyes open. When the eyes are open, the mother characteristically greets the newborn and talks in high-pitched tones to him or her.

In most instances the mother relies heavily on her senses of sight, touch, and hearing in getting to know what her baby is really like. She tends also to respond verbally to any sounds emitted by the newborn, such as cries, coughs, sneezes, and grunts. The sense of smell may also be involved as well.

While interacting with her newborn, the mother may be experiencing shock, disbelief, and denial. She may state, "I can't believe she's finally here," or, "I felt he was a stranger." However, the mother may express feelings of connectedness between

Figure 34–4 ◆ The mother has direct face-to-face and eye-to-eye contact in the *en face* position.
SOURCE: © Stella Johnson (www.stellajohnson.com).

MEDIALINK

Case Study: Mother-Infant Bonding

the newborn and the rest of the family, either in positive or in negative terms: "She's got your cute nose, Daddy," or "Oh, no! He looks just like the first one, and he was an impossible baby." A mother's facial expression or the frequency and content of her questions may demonstrate concerns about the infant's general condition or normality, especially if her pregnancy was complicated or if a previously born baby was not healthy.

During the first few days after her child's birth, the new mother applies herself to the task of getting to know her baby. This is termed the *acquaintance phase.* If the infant gives clear behavioral cues about needs, the infant's responses to mothering will be predictable, which will make the mother feel effective and competent. Other behaviors that make an infant more attractive to caretakers are smiling, grasping a finger, breastfeeding eagerly, cuddling, and being easy to console.

During this time the newborn is also becoming acquainted. Within a few days after birth, infants show signs of recognizing recurrent situations and responding to changes in routine. To the extent that their mother is their world, they are actively acquainting themselves with her.

CLINICAL TIP

Newborns who require immediate care in a special care or intensive care nursery are sometimes taken from their parents immediately after birth. The separation can interfere with the normal attachment process. The parents should be brought to the nursery as soon as possible to interact with their infant and should be allowed to hold and care for their infant as much as possible. If the infant is in an incubator and cannot be held, encourage the parents to stroke the infant's hand, foot, or cheek. Provide reassurances that this will not hurt their infant and is in fact beneficial.

During the *phase of mutual regulation,* mother and infant seek to deal with the degree of control to be exerted by each in their relationship. In this phase of adjustment, a balance is sought between the needs of the mother and the needs of the infant. The most important consideration is that each should obtain a good measure of enjoyment from the interaction. During the mutual adjustment phase, negative maternal feelings are likely to surface or intensify. Because "everyone knows that mothers love their babies," these negative feelings often go unexpressed and are allowed to build up. If they are expressed, the response of friends, relatives, or healthcare personnel is often to deny the feelings to the mother: "You don't mean that." Some negative feelings are normal in the first few days after birth, and the nurse should be supportive when the mother vocalizes these feelings.

When mutual regulation arrives at the point where both mother and infant primarily enjoy each other's company, reciprocity has been achieved. **Reciprocity** is an interactional cycle that occurs simultaneously between mother and infant. It involves mutual cuing behaviors, expectancy, rhythmicity, and synchrony. The mother develops a new relationship with an individual who has a unique character and evokes a response entirely different from the fantasy response of pregnancy. When reciprocity is synchronous, the interaction between mother and infant is mutually gratifying and is sought and initiated by both partners.

FATHER-INFANT INTERACTIONS

In Western cultures, commitment to family-centered maternity care has fostered interest in understanding the feelings and ex-

DEVELOPING CULTURAL COMPETENCE

MUSLIM PATERNAL ATTACHMENT

In some cultures there may be little involvement of the father in newborn care. In Muslim culture, for example, emphasis on childrearing and infant care activities is on the mother and female relatives. Nurses need to be aware of cultural differences when evaluating a father's interaction with his newborn.

periences of the new father. Evidence suggests that the father has a strong attraction to his newborn and that the feelings he experiences are similar to the mother's feelings of attachment (Figure 34–5 ◆). The characteristic sense of absorption, preoccupation, and interest in the infant demonstrated by fathers during early contact has been termed **engrossment.** Differences in involvement still exist among fathers in Western culture and may be influenced by factors other than culture (e.g., previous experience with paternal role or exposure to male/father role models).

SIBLINGS AND OTHERS

Infants are capable of maintaining a number of strong attachments without loss of quality. These attachments may include siblings, grandparents, aunts, and uncles. The social setting and personality of the individual seem to be significant factors in the development of multiple attachments. Birth centers are especially geared toward the inclusion of the family in the birth process. In the hospital setting, the advent of open visiting hours

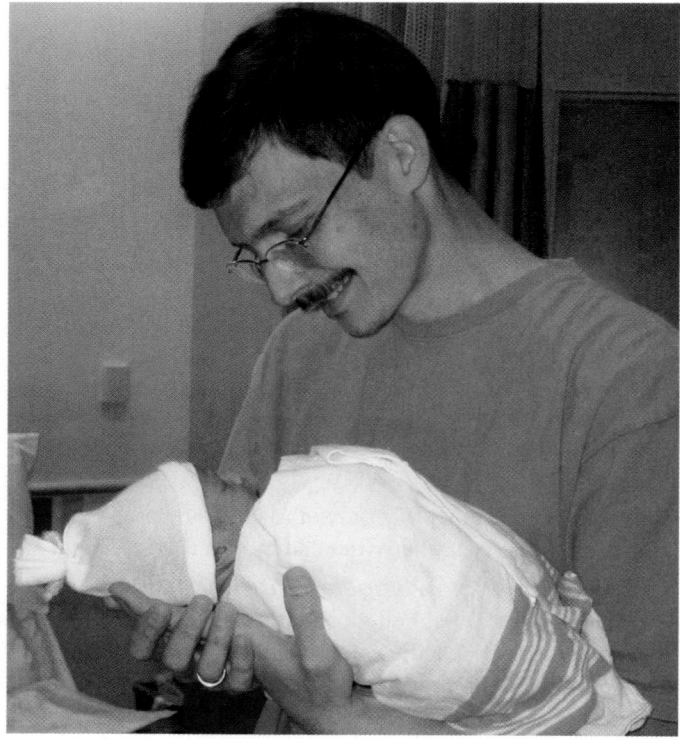

Figure 34–5 ◆ The father experiences strong feelings of attraction during engrossment.

and rooming-in permits siblings and grandparents to participate in the attachment process.

Cultural Influences in the Postpartal Period

Whereas Western culture places primary emphasis on the events of birth, many other cultures place greater emphasis on the post-partum period. For women not of the dominant American culture, the new mother's primary culture, personal values, and level of acculturation can influence her beliefs about her post-partal care. Her expectations regarding food, fluids, rest, hygiene, medications, relief measures, support, and counsel—as well as other aspects of her life—will be influenced by the beliefs and values of her family and cultural group. Sometimes a new mother's wishes will differ from the expectations of the certified nurse-midwife (CNM) or physician or nurse. (See Chapter 2 ∞ for in-depth discussion.)

Nurses belong to a particular ethnoculture and also share in the culture of health care. As a part of the healthcare cultural group, nurses implement practices that support their general beliefs, such as offering food in the recovery period following birth, providing iced fluids, expecting the woman to ambulate as soon as possible, and assuming the woman will want to shower and perhaps wash her hair soon after birth. It is important for nurses to recognize that they are approaching their client's care from their own perspective and that, to individualize care for each mother, they need to assess the woman's preferences, her level of acculturation and assimilation to Western culture, her linguistic abilities, and her educational level (Kim-Goodwin, 2005). In addition, the nurse should have the mother exercise her choices when possible, and support those choices, with the help of cultural awareness and a sound knowledge base.

Although describing the practices of different cultural groups always involves some generalization, it is helpful for nurses to understand some of the possible differences in beliefs and practices. The woman of European heritage may expect to eat a full meal and have a large amount of iced fluids following the birth, in the belief that the food restores energy and the fluids help replace fluid lost during the labor. She may want to ambulate shortly after the birth, shower, wash her hair, and put on a fresh gown. She may expect a relatively short stay in the hospital and may or may not be interested in educational classes. Women of the Islamic faith may have specific modesty requirements; the woman must be completely covered, with only her feet and hands exposed, and no man, other than the husband or a family member, may be alone with her (Al-Oballi Kridli, 2002).

Some cultures emphasize postpartum rituals for mother and baby that are designed to restore the hot-cold balance of the body. Some women of Hispanic, African, and Asian cultures may avoid cold after birth. This prohibition includes cold air, wind, and all water (even if heated). On the other hand, some traditional Mexican women may avoid eating "hot" foods, such as pork, just after the birth of a baby (considered a "hot" experience). It is important to note that each individual or cultural group may define hot and cold conditions as well as hot and cold foods differently. The nurse should ask each woman what she can eat and what foods she thinks would be helpful for healing.

The nurse may encourage family members to bring preferred food and drink for the mother. For more detailed discussion of the hot-cold balance concept, see "Cultural Influences Affecting the Family" in Chapter 2. ∞

In many cultures, the extended family plays an essential role during the puerperium. The grandmother is often the primary helper to the mother and newborn. She brings wisdom and experience, allowing the new mother time to rest as well as giving her ready access to someone who can help with problems and concerns as they arise. It is important to ensure access of all family members during the postpartum period. Visiting rules may be waived to allow family members or authority figures access to the mother and newborn. These practices show respect and foster a blending of old and new behaviors to meet the goals of all concerned (Purnell & Paulanka, 2005). African American mothers model their mothering skills after their older female relatives. In addition, these same older female relatives usually provide child care as needed (Purnell & Paulanka, 2005). People of Jewish faith observe a Sabbath from sundown Friday to sundown Saturday. During this time, Orthodox Jews do not perform any manual labor; for the postpartal woman, this includes turning on or off the lights, pressing the call bell, or raising/lowering the head of the bed (De Sovo, 1997). Jewish clients may also request a kosher diet. Some traditional Jewish couples avoid physical contact while the woman is experiencing any vaginal discharge; thus, the man may be viewed as unsupportive by the staff during the postpartal period (D'Avanzo & Geissler, 2003).

POSTPARTUM NURSING ASSESSMENT

Comprehensive care is based on a thorough assessment, with identification of individual needs or potential problems. (See the accompanying Assessment Guide: Postpartal—First 24 Hours After Birth.)

Risk Factors

Ongoing assessment and client education during the puerperium are designed to meet the needs of the childbearing family and to detect and treat possible complications. Table 34–2 identifies factors that may place the new mother at risk during the postpartum period. The nurse uses this knowledge during the assessment and is particularly alert for possible complications that may occur in an individual because of identified risk factors.

Physical Assessment

There are several principles to remember in preparing for and completing an assessment of the postpartum woman:

- Select the time that will provide the most accurate data. Palpating the fundus when the woman has a full bladder, for example, may give false information about the progress of involution. Ask the woman to void before assessment.

- Provide an explanation of the purposes of regular assessment to the woman.

MEDIALINK   Application: Exploring Cultural Differences Regarding Postpartum Care

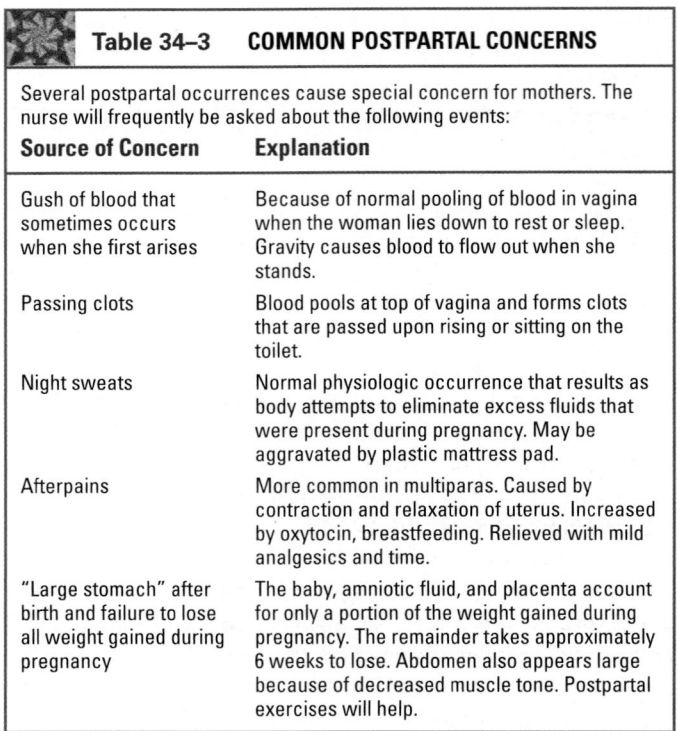

Table 34–2	POSTPARTAL HIGH-RISK FACTORS
Factor	**Maternal Implication**
Preeclampsia	↑ Blood pressure ↑ CNS irritability→ ↑ risk for seizure ↑ Need for bed rest → ↑ risk thrombophlebitis
Diabetes	Need for insulin regulation Episodes of hypoglycemia or hyperglycemia ↓ Healing
Cardiac disease	↑ Maternal exhaustion
Cesarean birth	↑ Healing needs ↑ Pain from incision ↑ Risk of infection ↑ Length of hospitalization
Overdistention of uterus (multiple gestation, hydramnios)	↑ Risk thrombophlebitis (C/S risk) ↑ Risk problems breastfeeding (C/S risk) ↑ Risk of hemorrhage ↑ Risk of anemia ↑ Stretching of abdominal muscles ↑ Incidence and severity of afterpains
Abruptio placentae, placenta previa	Hemorrhage → anemia ↓ Uterine contractility after birth → ↑ infection risk
Precipitous labor (less than 3 hours)	↑ Risk of lacerations to birth canal → hemorrhage
Prolonged labor (greater than 24 hours)	Exhaustion ↑ Risk of hemorrhage Nutritional and fluid depletion ↑ Bladder atony and/or trauma
Difficult birth	Exhaustion ↑ Risk of perineal lacerations ↑ Risk of hematomas ↑ Risk of hemorrhage → anemia
Extended period of time in stirrups at birth	↑ Risk of thrombophlebitis
Retained placenta	↑ Risk of hemorrhage ↑ Risk of infection

Table 34–3	COMMON POSTPARTAL CONCERNS

Several postpartal occurrences cause special concern for mothers. The nurse will frequently be asked about the following events:

Source of Concern	**Explanation**
Gush of blood that sometimes occurs when she first arises	Because of normal pooling of blood in vagina when the woman lies down to rest or sleep. Gravity causes blood to flow out when she stands.
Passing clots	Blood pools at top of vagina and forms clots that are passed upon rising or sitting on the toilet.
Night sweats	Normal physiologic occurrence that results as body attempts to eliminate excess fluids that were present during pregnancy. May be aggravated by plastic mattress pad.
Afterpains	More common in multiparas. Caused by contraction and relaxation of uterus. Increased by oxytocin, breastfeeding. Relieved with mild analgesics and time.
"Large stomach" after birth and failure to lose all weight gained during pregnancy	The baby, amniotic fluid, and placenta account for only a portion of the weight gained during pregnancy. The remainder takes approximately 6 weeks to lose. Abdomen also appears large because of decreased muscle tone. Postpartal exercises will help.

- Ensure that the woman is relaxed before starting; perform the procedures as gently as possible to avoid unnecessary discomfort.
- Record and report the results as clearly as possible.
- Take appropriate precautions to prevent exposure to body fluids.

The physical assessment is an excellent opportunity for client teaching. For example, when assessing the breasts of a lactating woman, the nurse can discuss breast care, breast milk production, the let-down reflex, and breast self-examination. A new mother may be very receptive to instruction on postpartum abdominal tightening exercises when the nurse assesses the woman's fundal height and diastasis. The assessment also provides an excellent time to provide information about the body's postpartum physical and anatomic changes as well as common postpartum concerns (Table 34–3).

Because the time the woman spends in the postpartum unit is limited, nurses should use every available opportunity for client teaching regarding self-care. To assist nurses in recognizing these opportunities, examples of client teaching during the assessment have been provided throughout the following discussion.

VITAL SIGNS

The nurse may organize the physical assessment in a variety of ways. Many nurses choose to begin by assessing vital signs because the findings are more accurate when they are obtained with the woman at rest. In addition, establishing whether the vital signs are within the expected normal range will assist the nurse in determining other assessments that might be needed. For instance, if the temperature is elevated, the nurse considers the time since birth and begins to gather information to determine whether the woman is dehydrated or whether an infection is developing.

Temperature elevations (less than 38C [100.4F]) due to normal processes should last for only 24 hours. The nurse should evaluate any temperature elevation in light of other signs and symptoms and should carefully review the woman's history to identify other factors, such as premature rupture of membranes (PROM) or prolonged labor that might increase the incidence of infection in the genital tract.

Alterations in vital signs may indicate complications, so they are assessed at regular intervals. After an immediate, transient rise after birth, the blood pressure should remain stable. The pulse often shows a characteristic slowness that is no cause for alarm. Pulse rates return to prepregnant norms very quickly unless complications arise.

The nurse informs the woman of the results of the vital signs assessment, providing information regarding the normal changes in blood pressure and pulse. This may also be an opportunity to assess whether the mother knows how to take her own and her infant's temperatures, how to read a thermometer, and how to select a thermometer from the wide variety now available.

ASSESSMENT GUIDE   Postpartal—First 24 Hours after Birth

PHYSICAL ASSESSMENT/ NORMAL FINDINGS	ALTERATIONS AND POSSIBLE CAUSES*	NURSING RESPONSES TO DATA†
VITAL SIGNS		
Blood pressure (BP): Should remain consistent with baseline BP during pregnancy.	High BP (preeclampsia, essential hypertension, renal disease, anxiety).	Evaluate history of preexisting disorders and check for other signs of preeclampsia (edema, proteinuria).
	Drop in BP (may be normal; uterine hemorrhage).	Assess for other signs of hemorrhage (↑ pulse, cool clammy skin).
Pulse: 50–90 bpm. May be bradycardia if 50–70 bpm.	Tachycardia (difficult labor and birth, hemorrhage).	Evaluate for other signs of hemorrhage (↓ BP, cool clammy skin).
Respirations: 16–24/minute.	Marked tachypnea (respiratory disease).	Assess for other signs of respiratory disease.
	Diminished respirations (long-acting epidural narcotics).	
Temperature: 36.2–38C (98–100.4F)	After first 24 hours, temperature of 38C (100.4 F) or above suggests infection.	Assess for other signs of infection: notify physician or certified nurse-midwife.
BREASTS		
General appearance: Smooth, even pigmentation, changes of pregnancy still apparent: one may appear larger.	Reddened area (mastitis).	Assess further for signs of infection.
Palpation: Depending on postpartal day, may be soft, filling, full, or engorged.	Palpable mass (caked breast, mastitis).	Assess for other signs of infection: If blocked duct, consider heat, massage, position change for breastfeeding.
	Engorgement (venous stasis).	Assess for further signs.
	Tenderness, heat, edema (engorgement, caked breast, mastitis).	Report mastitis to physician or certified nurse-midwife.
Nipples: Supple, pigmented, intact; become erect when stimulated.	Fissures, cracks, soreness (problems with breastfeeding), not erectile with stimulation (inverted nipples).	Reassess technique: recommend appropriate interventions.
LUNGS		
Sounds: clear to bases bilaterally.	Diminished (fluid overload, asthma, pulmonary embolus, pulmonary edema)	Assess for other signs of respiratory distress.
ABDOMEN		
Musculature: Abdomen may be soft, have a "doughy" texture; rectus muscle intact.	Separation in musculature (diastasis recti abdominis).	Evaluate size of diastasis: teach appropriate exercises for decreasing the separation.
Fundus: Firm, midline; following expected process of involution.	Boggy (full bladder, uterine bleeding, deviation from midline).	Massage until firm; assess bladder and have woman void if needed; attempt to express clots when firm.
		If bogginess remains or recurs, report to physician or certified nurse-midwife.
May be tender when palpated.	Constant tenderness (infection).	Assess for evidence of endometritis.
Cesarean section incision dressing; dry and intact	Moderate to large amount of blood or serosanguinous drainage on dressing.	Assess for hemorrhage. Reinforce dressing and notify healthcare provider.
LOCHIA		
Scant to moderate amount, earthy odor; no clots.	Large amount, clots (hemorrhage).	Assess for firmness, express additional clots; begin peripad count.
	Foul-smelling lochia (infection).	Assess for other signs of infection; report to physician or certified nurse-midwife.
Normal progression: First 1–3 days: rubra.	Failure to progress normally or return to rubra from serosa (subinvolution).	Report to physician or certified nurse-midwife.
Following rubra: Days 3–10: serosa (alba seldom seen in hospital).		
	*Possible causes of alterations are identified in parentheses.	†This column provides guidelines for further assessment and initial nursing action.

(Continued on next page)

ASSESSMENT GUIDE Postpartal—First 24 Hours after Birth continued

PHYSICAL ASSESSMENT/ NORMAL FINDINGS	ALTERATIONS AND POSSIBLE CAUSES*	NURSING RESPONSES TO DATA†
PERINEUM Slight edema and bruising in intact perineum. *Episiotomy:* No redness, edema, ecchymosis, or discharge, edges well approximated. *Hemorrhoids:* None present; if present, should be small and nontender.	Marked fullness, bruising, pain (vulvar hematoma). Redness, edema, ecchymosis, discharge, or gaping stitches (infection). Full, tender, inflamed hemorrhoids.	Assess size; apply ice glove or ice pack, analgesic and anesthetic sprays; report to physician or certified nurse-midwife. Encourage sitz baths; review perineal care, appropriate wiping techniques. Encourage sitz baths, side-lying position; Tucks pads, anesthetic ointments, manual replacement of hemorrhoids, stool softeners, increased fluid intake.
COSTOVERTEBRAL ANGLE (CVA) TENDERNESS None.	Present (kidney infection).	Assess for other symptoms of urinary tract infection (UTI): obtain clean-catch urine sample; report to physician or certified nurse-midwife.
LOWER EXTREMITIES No pain with palpation; negative Homans' sign.	Positive findings (thrombophlebitis).	Report to physician or certified nurse-midwife.
ELIMINATION *Urinary output:* Voiding in sufficient quantities at least every 4–6 hours; bladder not palpable. *Bowel elimination:* Should have normal bowel movement by second or third day after birth.	Inability to void (urinary retention). Urgency, frequency, dysuria (UTI). Inability to pass feces or hard, small amount of stool (constipation due to fear of pain from episiotomy, hemorrhoids, perineal trauma).	Employ nursing interventions to promote voiding; if not successful, obtain order for catheterization. Report symptoms of UTI to physician or certified nurse-midwife. Encourage fluids, ambulation, roughage in diet; sitz baths to promote healing of perineum; obtain order for stool softener.

CULTURAL ASSESSMENT†	VARIATIONS TO CONSIDER	NURSING RESPONSES TO DATA†
Determine customs and practices regarding postpartum care. Ask the mother whether she would like fluids and ask what temperature she prefers. Ask the mother what foods or fluids she would like. Ask the mother whether she would prefer to be alone during breastfeeding.	Individual preference may include: • Room-temperature or warmed fluids rather than iced drinks. • Special foods or fluids to hasten healing after childbirth. • Some women may be hesitant to have someone with them when their breast is exposed.	Provide for specific request if possible. If woman is unable to provide specific information, the nurse may draw from general information regarding cultural variation. Mexican women may want food and fluids that restore hot-cold balance to the body. Women of European background may ask for iced fluids. Provide privacy as desired by mother.

PSYCHOSOCIAL ASSESSMENT/ NORMAL FINDINGS	VARIATIONS TO CONSIDER*	NURSING RESPONSES TO DATA†
PSYCHOLOGIC ADAPTATION *During first 24 hours:* Passive; preoccupied with own needs; may talk about her labor and birth experience; may be talkative, elated, or very quiet.	Very quiet and passive; sleeps frequently (fatigue from long labor; feelings of disappointment about some aspect of the experience; may be following cultural expectation).	Provide opportunities for adequate rest; provide physical comfort measures; provide nutritious meals and snacks that are consistent with what the woman desires to eat and drink; provide opportunities to discuss birth experience in nonjudgmental atmosphere if the woman desires to do so.
†These are only a few suggestions. It is not our intent to imply this is a comprehensive cultural assessment.	*Possible causes of alterations are identified in parentheses.	†This column provides guidelines for further assessment and initial nursing action.

ASSESSMENT GUIDE   Postpartal—First 24 Hours after Birth continued

Psychosocial Assessment/ Normal Findings	Variations to Consider*	Nursing Responses to Data†
PSYCHOLOGIC ADAPTATION (continued) Usually by 12 hours; beginning to assume responsibility; some women eager to learn; easily feel overwhelmed.	Excessive weepiness, mood swings, pronounced irritability (postpartum blues; feelings of inadequacy; culturally prescribed behavior).	Explain postpartum blues; provide supportive atmosphere; determine support available for mother; consider referral for evidence of profound depression.
ATTACHMENT *En face* position; holds baby close; cuddles and soothes; calls by name; identifies characteristics of family members in infant; may be awkward in providing care. Initially may express disappointment over sex or appearance of infant but within 1–2 days demonstrates attachment behaviors.	Continued expressions of disappointment in sex, appearance of infant; refusal to care for infant; derogatory comments; lack of bonding behaviors (difficulty in attachment, following expectations of cultural/ethnic group).	Provide reinforcement and support for infant caretaking behaviors; maintain nonjudgmental approach and gather more information if caretaking behaviors are not evident.
CLIENT EDUCATION Demonstrates basic understanding of self-care activities and infant care needs; can identify signs of complications that should be reported.	Unable to demonstrate basic self-care and infant care activities (knowledge deficit; postpartum blues; following prescribed cultural behavior and will be cared for by grandmother or other family member).	Identify predominant learning style. Determine whether woman understands English and provide interpreter if needed; provide reinforcement of information through conversation and through written material (remember that some women and their families may not be able to understand written materials because of language difficulties or inability to read); provide information regarding infant care skills that are culturally consistent; give woman opportunity to express her feelings and demonstrate skills taught; consider social service home referral for women who have no family or other support, are unable to take in information about self-care and infant care, and demonstrate no caretaking activities.
	*Possible causes of alterations are identified in parentheses.	†This column provides guidelines for further assessment and initial nursing action.

CLINICAL TIP

During the first few hours after birth, the woman may have some orthostatic hypotension. This will cause her to have a lower blood pressure reading in a sitting position. For the most accurate reading, measure her blood pressure with her in the same position each time, preferably lying on her back with her arm at her side. Because of the propensity for hypotension, the nurse should assist the mother the first few times she attempts to ambulate after delivery.

AUSCULTATION OF LUNGS

The breath sounds should be clear. Women who have been treated for preterm labor or preeclampsia are especially at risk for pulmonary edema (see "Care of Woman with a Hypertensive Disorder" in Chapter 20 ∞).

CLINICAL TIP

An easy way to remember the components specific to the postpartal examination is to remember the term BUBBLEHE: B-breast, U-uterus, B-bladder, B-bowel, L-lochia, E-episiotomy/laceration, H-Homans'/hemorrhoids, and E-emotional.

BREASTS

Before examining the breasts, the nurse dons gloves and then assesses the fit and support of the woman's bra. The nurse provides information about how to select a bra. A properly fitting bra provides support to the breasts and helps maintain breast shape by limiting stretching of supporting ligaments and connective tissue. If the mother is breastfeeding, the straps of the bra should be cloth, not elastic (because cloth has less stretch and provides more support) and easily adjustable. The back should be wide and have at least three rows of hooks to adjust for fit. Traditional nursing bras have a fixed inner cup and a separate half-cup that can be unhooked for breastfeeding while continuing to support the breast. Purchasing a nursing bra one size too large during pregnancy will usually result in a good fit because the breasts increase in size with milk production.

The nurse asks the woman to remove her bra so the breasts can be examined. It is important to note the size and shape of the breasts and any abnormalities, reddened areas, or engorgement. The nurse also palpates the breasts lightly for softness, slight firmness associated with filling, or firmness associated with engorgement, warmth, or tenderness. The nipples are assessed for fissures, cracks, soreness, or inversion. The nurse teaches the woman the characteristics of the breast and explains how to recognize problems such as fissures or cracks in the nipples.

The nurse assesses the nonbreastfeeding mother for evidence of breast discomfort and provides relief measures if necessary. (See discussion of lactation suppression in the nonbreastfeeding mother in Chapter 35 ∞). Breast assessment findings for a nonbreastfeeding woman may be recorded as follows: "Breasts soft, filling, no evidence of nipple tenderness or cracking, nipples everted."

ABDOMEN AND FUNDUS

The woman should void before her abdomen is examined. This practice ensures that a full bladder is not causing displacement of the uterus or any uterine atony; if atony is present, other causes (such as uterine relaxation associated with a regional block, overstretched uterus, or distended bladder) must be investigated.

The nurse determines the relationship of the fundus to the umbilicus and also assesses the firmness of the fundus. The top of the fundus is measured in fingerbreadths above, below, or at the umbilicus. The nurse notes whether the fundus is in the midline or displaced to either side of the abdomen. If not midline, the uterus position should be located. The most common cause of displacement is a full bladder; thus this finding requires further assessment. If the fundus is in the midline but higher than expected, it is usually associated with clots within the uterus. The results of the assessment should then be recorded. (See Procedure 34-1).

While completing the assessment, the nurse teaches the woman about fundal position and how to determine firmness. The mother can be taught to massage her fundus gently if it is not firm.

> **CLINICAL TIP**
>
> Assessing the status of the uterine fundus may be uncomfortable. In addition to explaining the importance of the assessment to the mother, you can show her how to perform frequent light massage of the fundus herself to promote uterine involution. Involving her in her own care encourages her participation. In addition, having her massage her own uterus may lessen bleeding and reduce the need for more thorough massage.

A well-contracted uterus feels as firm as the uterus does during a strong labor contraction. If handled gently, the uterus should not be overly tender. Excessive pain in the uterus during

postpartal examination should alert the nurse to possible uterine infection. If the uterus is not firm, the nurse should gently massage the fundus with the fingertips of the examining hand, and then assess the results. If the uterus becomes firm, the chart should read: "Uterus: boggy → firm with light massage." A good habit for the nurse to develop during the postpartal examination is to have the woman lie flat on her back with her head on a pillow and legs flexed. Then the nurse can release the perineal pad to observe the results of uterine massage based on the amount of expelled blood. Occasionally, oxytocic agents, such as an intravenous Pitocin infusion or methylergonovine maleate (Methergine), need to be administered postpartally to maintain uterine contraction and prevent or treat hemorrhage (see Drug Guide: Methylergonovine Maleate [Methergine] in Chapter 35 ∞).

> **CLINICAL TIP**
>
> During postpartum assessment, a firm uterus typically feels like a grapefruit because the muscles are well contracted. If the uterus loses its ability to contract and begins to relax, it is called boggy. A boggy uterus feels softer, like a sponge, or may become so relaxed that you cannot feel it at all. If the uterus is boggy but you can still feel it, massage it until it becomes firm. If you cannot feel it at all, place the side of one hand just above the woman's symphysis pubis to provide stability. Then place the other hand at the level of the umbilicus. (The fundus may have risen to this level because it is relaxed and filling with blood.) Press deeply into the abdomen and massage in a circular motion. You will usually feel the uterus begin to firm up under your hand. If you do not, move your hand slightly lower on the abdomen, and repeat the process.

A boggy uterus that does not contract with light, gentle massage may need more vigorous massage. The nurse assesses the amount and character of any expelled blood obtained while massaging the fundus. When a woman has postpartal uterine atony (the uterus does not remain firm), the nurse should do the following:

1. Reevaluate for full bladder; if the bladder is full, have the woman void.

2. Question the woman on her bleeding history since the birth or last examination. How heavy does her flow seem? Has she passed any clots? How frequently has she changed pads? Were the pads saturated? Look at the discarded pads.

3. For the breastfeeding mother, put the newborn to the mother's breast for feeding to stimulate oxytocin production.

4. Assess maternal blood pressure and pulse to identify hypotension.

5. Reassess the fundus; if the fundus is still boggy, alert the certified nurse-midwife or physician immediately, because further intervention, such as intravenous fluids and an oxytocic medication, are needed.

In the woman who has had a cesarean birth, the abdominal incision is exquisitely tender. The nurse should palpate the fundus with extreme care and inspect the abdominal incision for signs of healing, such as approximation (absence of separation

PROCEDURE 34–1   Assessing the Status of the Uterine Fundus after Birth

NURSING ACTION	RATIONALE

Preparation

- Explain the procedure, the information it provides, and what it might feel like.
- Ask the woman to void.

A full bladder can cause uterine atony.

- Have the woman lie flat in bed with her head on a pillow. If the procedure is uncomfortable, she may find that it helps to flex her legs.

The supine position prevents falsely high assessment of fundal height. Flexing the legs relaxes the abdominal muscles.

Equipment and Supplies

> **CLINICAL TIP**
> Gloves may be put on before assessing the abdomen and fundus or when you are ready to assess the perineum and lochia.

- A clean perineal pad (see Procedure 34–2)

Procedure

1. Gently place one hand on the lower segment of the uterus. Using the side of the other hand, palpate the abdomen until you locate the top of the fundus.

One hand stabilizes the uterus while the other hand locates the top of the fundus. (Support of the uterus prevents stretching of the ligaments that support the uterus.)

2. Determine whether the fundus is firm. If it is, it will feel like a hard round object (similar to a grapefruit) in the abdomen. If it is not firm, massage the abdomen lightly until the fundus is firm.

A firm fundus indicates that the uterine muscles are contracted and bleeding will not occur.

3. Measure the top of the fundus in fingerbreadths above, below, or at the fundus. See Figure 34–6 ◆.

Fundal height gives information about the progress of involution.

Figure 34–6 ◆ Measuring the descent of the fundus for the woman having a vaginal birth. The fundus is located two fingerbreadths below the umbilicus. Always support the bottom of the uterus during any assessment of fundus.

4. Determine the position of the fundus in relation to the midline of the body. If it is not in the midline, locate it and then evaluate the bladder for distention.

The fundus may deviate from the midline when the bladder is full because the enlarged bladder pushes the uterus aside.

5. If the bladder is distended, use nursing measures to help the woman void. If she is not able to void after a specified period of time, catheterization may be necessary.
6. Measure urine output for the next few hours until normal elimination is established.

During the postpartum as diuresis occurs, the bladder may fill far more rapidly than normal, putting the woman at risk for uterine atony and hemorrhage. (Diminished tone of the uterus may cause loss of the urge to void.)

(Continued on next page)

PROCEDURE 34–1 Assessing the Status of the Uterine Fundus after Birth continued

NURSING ACTION	RATIONALE
7. Assess the lochia (see Procedure 34–2). 8. During the first few hours postpartum, if the fundus becomes boggy frequently or is located high above the umbilicus and the woman's bladder is empty, the uterine cavity may be filled with clots of blood. In this case, do the following: • Release the front of the perineal pad and lay it back so that you can see the perineum and the pad laying between the woman's legs. • Massage the uterine fundus until it is firm. • Keep one hand in position, stabilizing the lower portion of the uterus. With the hand you used to massage the fundus, put steady pressure on the top of the now-firm fundus and see if you are able to express any clots. (Watch the pad between her legs for clots to pass from the vagina.) 9. If measurement of the blood loss is needed, the perineal pads and Chux can be weighed. See Procedure 34–2. 10. Provide the woman with a clean perineal pad. 11. Record findings. Fundal height is recorded in fingerbreadths (e.g., "2 FB ↓ U" or "1 FB U"). If fundal massage was necessary, note that fact: "Uterus boggy → firm with light massage." 12. Communicate bogginess or heavy flow to primary provider.	*If the woman's uterus is filled with blood, it acts as an irritant and the uterus will not remain contracted. When the muscle fibers relax, bleeding results, further aggravating the problem. Pushing on a uterus that is not firm is dangerous because it is possible to cause the uterus to invert, a true emergency.*

between edges of incision), bleeding, and for any signs of infection, including drainage, edema, foul odor, or redness. It is important to document whether internal sutures, steri-strips, or staples are intact. During the assessment, the nurse teaches the woman about her incision. The nurse can also review characteristics of normal healing, incision care, and discuss signs of infection.

LOCHIA

Lochia is then assessed for character, amount, odor, and the presence of clots. The nurse must wear disposable gloves when assessing the perineum and lochia. Nurses may put on the gloves before beginning the assessment, just before assessing the abdomen and fundus, or when they are ready to assess the perineum and lochia. During the first 1 to 3 days, the lochia should be rubra. A few small clots are normal and occur as a result of blood pooling in the vagina. However, the passage of numerous or large clots is abnormal, and the cause should be investigated immediately. After 2 to 3 days, the lochia becomes serosa.

Lochia should never exceed a moderate amount, such as that needed to partially saturate four to eight peri-pads daily, with an average of six. However, because this number is influenced by an individual woman's pad changing practices, as well as the ab-

sorbency of the pad, the nurse must ask about the length of time the current pad has been in use, whether the amount is normal compared with her typical menstrual period, and whether any clots were passed before the examination, such as during voiding. If heavy bleeding is reported but not seen, the nurse asks the woman to put on a clean perineal pad and reassesses the discharge in 1 hour (see Procedure 34-2 and Figure 34–7 ◆).

When a more accurate assessment of blood loss is needed, the perineal pads can be weighed, with 1 g considered equivalent to 1 mL blood.

Clots and heavy bleeding may be caused by uterine relaxation (atony), retained placental fragments, or, rarely, an unknown cervical laceration (seen as heavy bleeding but with firm fundus) that may require further assessment (Table 34–4). Because of the evacuation of the uterine cavity during cesarean birth, women with such surgery usually have less lochia after the first 24 hours than mothers who give birth vaginally. If the woman is at increased risk for bleeding or is actually experiencing heavy flow of lochia rubra, her blood pressure, pulse, and uterus need to be assessed frequently, and the physician may prescribe oxytocin (Pitocin) or methylergonovine maleate (Methergine). See Drug Guide: Methylergonovine Maleate (Methergine) in Chapter 35. ∞

Table 34–4	CHANGES IN LOCHIA THAT CAUSE CONCERN	
Change	**Possible Problem**	**Nursing Action**
Presence of clots	Inadequate uterine contractions that allow bleeding from vessels at the placental site.	Assess location and firmness of fundus. Assess voiding pattern. Record and report findings.
Persistent lochia rubra	Inadequate uterine contractions; retained placental fragments; infection; undetected cervical laceration.	Assess location and firmness of fundus. Assess activity pattern. Assess for signs of infection. Record and report findings.

PROCEDURE 34–2 Evaluating Lochia

NURSING ACTION	RATIONALE

Preparation

- Explain why lochia occurs, why it is assessed, how it is assessed, and how it changes during the postpartum.
- Ask the woman to void.

- Complete the assessment of uterine fundal height and firmness.

- If she has not already done so for the fundal assessment, ask the woman to flex her legs. Then ask her to spread her legs apart. Use the bed sheet as a drape to preserve her modesty.

A full bladder can cause uterine atony and increase the amount of lochia.

In almost all cases, fundal height and firmness are evaluated with an assessment of lochia. This practice provides a more thorough assessment.

This position allows you to see the perineum and the perineal pad more effectively.

Equipment and Supplies

Note: Gloves are put on before assessing the perineum and lochia.

Gloves
Clean perineal pad
Procedure: Clean Gloves

1. Don gloves.
2. Lower the perineal pad and observe the amount of lochia on the pad. Because women's pad-changing practices vary, ask her about the length of time the current pad has been in use, whether the amount is normal, and whether any clots were passed before this examination, such as during voiding.

> **CLINICAL TIP**
> If blood loss exceeds the guidelines given in this chapter, weigh the perineal pads and the chux pads to estimate the blood loss more accurately. Typically, 1 g = 1 mL blood. Because blood can pool below the woman on the chux pad, the pads are included in your assessment.

3. If the woman reports heavy bleeding or clots, ask her to put on a clean perineal pad and then reassess the pad in 1 hour. Also ask her to call you before flushing any clots she passes into the toilet during voiding.
4. When the uterine fundus is firm and stabilized with the nondominant hand, press down on it with the dominant hand while watching to see if any clots are expelled. (See Procedure 34–1, step 8.)
5. Determine the amount of lochia, using the following guide (see Figure 34–7):
   - Heavy amount—Perineal pad has a stain larger than 6 inches in length within 1 hour; 30 to 80 mL lochia.

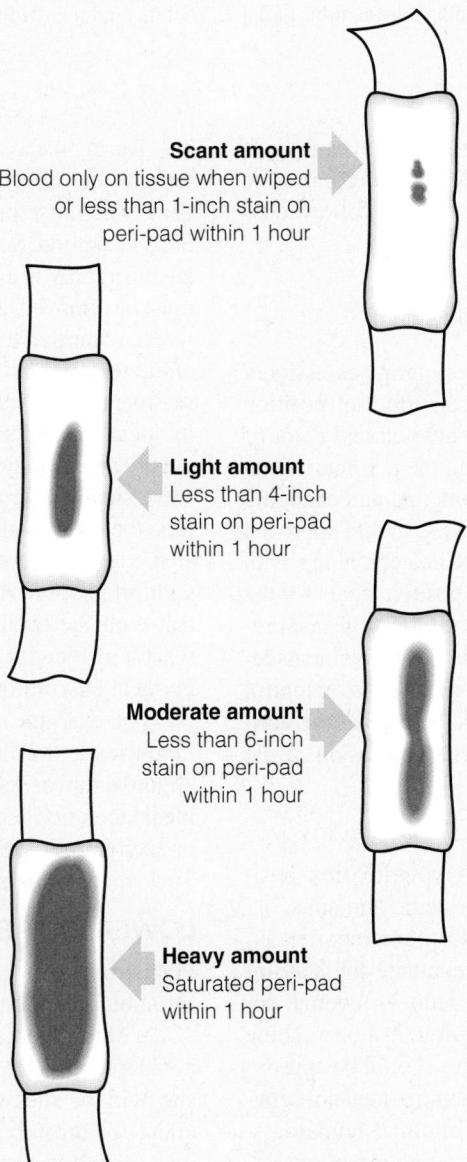

Scant amount
Blood only on tissue when wiped or less than 1-inch stain on peri-pad within 1 hour

Light amount
Less than 4-inch stain on peri-pad within 1 hour

Moderate amount
Less than 6-inch stain on peri-pad within 1 hour

Heavy amount
Saturated peri-pad within 1 hour

During the first 1 to 3 days the woman's lochia should be rubra, which is dark red in color. A few small clots are normal and occur as a result of pooling of blood in the vagina when the woman is lying down. The passage of large clots is abnormal and the cause should be investigated immediately.

Figure 34–7 ◆ Suggested guidelines for assessing lochia volume.
SOURCE: Jacobson, H. "A standard for assessing lochia volume." *American Journal of Maternal/Child Nursing, 10,* 174–175, May-June 1985. Copyright © Lippincott, Williams & Wilkins. Reprinted with permission.

(Continued on next page)

PROCEDURE 34–2 Evaluating Lochia   continued

NURSING ACTION	RATIONALE
• Moderate amount—Perineal pad has a stain less than 6 inches in length within 1 hour; 25 to 50 mL lochia. • Small (light) amount—Perineal pad has a stain less than 4 inches in length after 1 hour; 10 to 25 mL lochia. • Scant amount—Perineal pad has a stain less than 1 inch in length after 1 hour or lochia is only on tissue when the woman wipes.	*Lochia should never exceed a moderate amount such as four to eight partially saturated perineal pads daily. Using a consistent standard for measuring lochia improves the accuracy of the information charted and conveyed to others.*
6. In most cases, a woman is discharged while her lochia is still rubra. Provide her with information about lochia serosa and lochia alba. 7. Record the findings specifically. For example, "Uterus firm, 1 FB ↓ U, Lochia: moderate rubra, no clots passed."	*Accurate discharge information enables the woman to assess herself more accurately and enables her to judge better when to contact her caregiver.*

The odor of the lochia is nonoffensive and never foul. If foul odor is present, so is an infection. When using narrative nursing notes, document the amount of lochia first, followed by character. For example:

• Lochia: moderate rubra

• Lochia: small rubra/serosa

Client teaching that the nurse may address during assessment of the lochia may center on normal changes, effect of position changes on or what can be expected in the amount and color of the flow. Hygienic measures, such as wiping the perineum from front to back and washing her hands after toileting and changing pads, may be reviewed if appropriate. The nurse should approach the timing of teaching hygienic practices delicately, along with the content to be included. By establishing positive goals for the teaching—promoting comfort, enhancing tissue healing, and preventing infection—the nurse can avoid value-laden statements regarding personal beliefs about the need for cleanliness or control of body odor. The nurse should review with the mother the need to notify a healthcare professional if there is regression in the lochia flow pattern (i.e., color or amount).

PERINEUM

The perineum is inspected with the woman lying in Sims' position. The buttock is lifted to expose the perineum and anus.

If an episiotomy was performed or a laceration required suturing, the nurse assesses the wound. To evaluate the state of healing, the nurse inspects the wound for redness, edema, ecchymosis, discharge, and approximation. After 24 hours, some edema may still be present, but the skin edges should be approximated ("glued" together) so that gentle pressure does not separate them. Gentle palpation should elicit minimal tenderness, and there should be no hardened areas suggesting infection. Ecchymosis interferes with normal healing, as does infection. Foul odors associated with drainage indicate infection. Hematomas sometimes occur, although these are considered abnormal. The nurse next assesses whether hemorrhoids are present around the anus. If present, they are assessed for size, number, and pain or tenderness (see Procedure 34-3 and Figure 34–8 ◆).

During the assessment, the nurse talks with the woman to determine the effectiveness of comfort measures that have been used. The nurse provides teaching about the episiotomy or perineal laceration. Some women do not thoroughly understand what an episiotomy is and where it is and may believe that the stitches must be removed, as with other types of surgery. Frequently, when women fear that the stitches must be removed manually, they are afraid to ask about them. While explaining the findings of the assessment, the nurse can provide information about the episiotomy, its location, and signs that are being assessed. In addition, the nurse can casually add that the sutures are special and will dissolve slowly over the next few weeks as the tissues heal. By the time the sutures are dissolved, the tissues are strong, and the incision edges will not separate. This is also an opportunity to teach comfort measures that may be used and reinforce the need to consult with the healthcare provider before using over-the-counter (OTC) medications/supplements if breastfeeding (see "Relief of Perineal Discomfort" in Chapter 35 ∞).

An example of documentation of a perineal assessment might read: "Midline episiotomy; no edema, tenderness, or ecchymosis present. Skin edges are approximated"; or, if a perineal laceration repair, "Skin edges intact, no edema, tenderness or ecchymosis, pain meds helpful. Woman reports sitz bath and Tucks pads or pain relief measures are controlling discomfort."

LOWER EXTREMITIES

Postpartum women are at increased risk for thrombophlebitis, thrombus formation, and inflammation involving a vein (see "Care of the Woman with Postpartal Thromboembolic Disease" in Chapter 38 ∞). If thrombophlebitis occurs, the most likely site will be the woman's legs. Conditions that predispose a client for thrombophlebitis are hypercoaguability, severe anemia, obesity, and traumatic delivery. To assess for thrombophlebitis, the nurse should have the woman stretch her legs out, with the knees slightly flexed and the legs relaxed. The nurse then grasps the foot and dorsiflexes it sharply. The second leg is assessed in the same way. No discomfort or pain should be present. If pain is elicited, the nurse notifies the certified nurse-midwife or physician that the woman has a positive

PROCEDURE 34–3 Postpartum Perineal Assessment

NURSING ACTION	RATIONALE

Preparation

- Explain the purpose and the procedure for assessing the perineum during the postpartum period.
- Complete the assessment of fundal height and lochia as described in Procedures 34-1 and 34-2.
- At this point in a postpartal assessment, the woman is lying on her back with her knees flexed. Her perineal pad has already been lifted away from her perineum to permit inspection of the lochia. If an episiotomy was performed or if the birth was difficult, the woman may be using an ice pack on her perineum to reduce swelling. The ice pack would also have been removed for inspection of the lochia.
- Ask her to turn onto her side with her upper knee drawn forward and resting on the bed (Sims' position).

Typically, perineal assessment follows the fundal and lochial assessment.

When the woman is supine, even with her knees flexed, it is very difficult to expose the posterior portion of the perineum. Thus, Sims' position makes it easiest to inspect the perineum and anal area.

Equipment and Supplies

Clean perineal pad, clean ice pack if desired/needed.
Small light source such as a penlight may be necessary

Procedure: Clean Gloves

1. Use a systematic approach to assessment.

   A systematic approach helps ensure that you do not overlook a significant finding.

2. In evaluating the perineum, begin by asking the woman's perceptions. How does she describe her discomfort? Does it seem excessive to her? Has it become worse since the birth? Does it seem more severe than you would expect?

   Information from the client herself often helps identify developing problems.

(Note: Pain that seems disproportionately severe may indicate that the woman is developing a vulvar hematoma.)

> **CLINICAL TIP**
>
> In evaluating the perineum, use the REEDA scale as a quick reminder of what to assess. Specifically:
>
> R = redness
>
> E = edema or swelling
>
> E = ecchymosis or bruising
>
> D = drainage
>
> A = approximation (how well the edges of an incision—the episiotomy—or a repaired laceration seem to be holding together)

3. After talking with the woman, assess the condition of the tissue. To allow for full visualization, it may be helpful to ask the woman to lift the knee of her upper leg to expose her perineum more fully. In some cases it may help to use the nondominant gloved hand to lift the buttocks and tissue. Note any swelling (edema) and bruising (ecchymosis).
4. Evaluate the episiotomy, if there is one, or any repaired laceration for its state of healing. Is it reddened? Note the edges of the incision. Are they well approximated? Tell the woman that you are going to palpate the incision gently, then do so. Note any areas of hardness. Note whether the incision is warmer to the touch than the surrounding tissue.

The tissue is often traumatized by the birth and mild bruising is not unusual. However, excessive bruising may indicate that a hematoma is developing.

Gentle palpation should elicit minimal tenderness and there should be no redness, warmth, or areas of hardness, which suggest infection. Both bruising and infection interfere with normal healing. Typically, within 24 hours the edges of the incision should be "glued" together (well approximated).

(Continued on next page)

PROCEDURE 34–3 Postpartum Perineal Assessment   continued

NURSING ACTION	RATIONALE
5. During the assessment be alert for odors. Typically the lochia has an earthy, but not unpleasant, smell that is easily identifiable.	*A foul odor associated with drainage often indicates infection.*
6. Finally, assess for hemorrhoids. To visualize the anal area, lift the upper buttocks to fully expose the anal area. (See Figure 34–8.) If hemorrhoids are present, note the size, number, and pain or tenderness.	*Hemorrhoids often develop during pregnancy or labor and can cause considerable discomfort. If hemorrhoids are present, the woman may benefit from available comfort measures.*

Figure 34–8 ◆ Intact perineum with hemorrhoids.

7. During the assessment, talk to the woman about the effectiveness of comfort measures being used. Provide teaching about care of the episiotomy, hemorrhoids, and the like.	*Health teaching is an important part of nursing care. Many women have concerns about the episiotomy and may not know, for example, that the suture used is dissolvable. This is an excellent time to provide information about good healthcare practices in both the short and long term.*
8. Provide the woman with a clean perineal pad. Replenish the ice pack if necessary.	
9. Record findings. For example: "Midline episiotomy; no edema, ecchymosis, or tenderness. Skin edges well approximated. Woman reports pain relief measures are controlling discomfort"; or "Perineal repair, is approximated, minimal edema, no ecchymosis or tenderness; ice pack to perineum relieves pain."	

Homans' sign (see Figure 34–9 ◆). The pain is caused by inflammation of a vessel. The nurse also evaluates the legs for edema by comparing both legs, because usually only one leg is involved. Any areas of redness, tenderness, and increased skin temperature are also noted.

Some facilities have discontinued performing a Homans' sign in the nursing assessment, stating that it is not diagnostic and could lead to an embolus if the clot is dislodged during assessment. Although assessment of Homans' sign is not diagnostic, supporters advocate its use as a screening tool. There are no published reports of an embolus occurring as a result of performing a Homans' sign. In the event of a positive Homans'

sign, diagnosis is made by compression or duplex ultrasonography. Low-dose heparin therapy is used in postpartum women who develop a deep vein thrombosis (Drife, 2003).

Early ambulation is an important aspect of preventing thrombophlebitis. Most women are able to get up shortly after birth or once they have fully recovered from the effects of the regional anesthetic agent, if one has been used. The mother's legs should be assessed for return of sensation following regional anesthesia. The cesarean birth client requires passive range-of-motion exercises until she is ambulating more freely.

Client teaching associated with assessment of the lower extremities focuses on the signs and symptoms of thrombo-

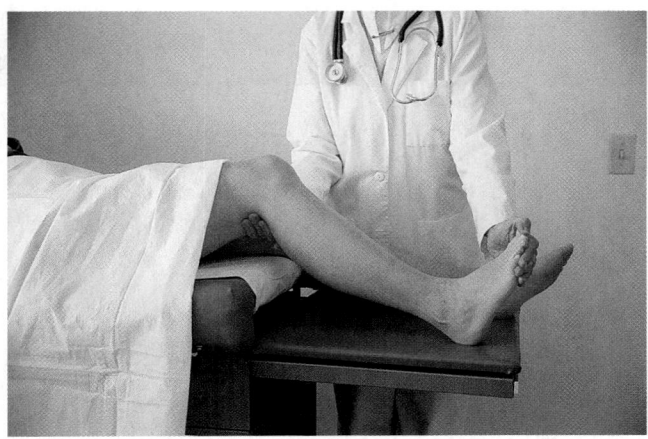

Figure 34–9 ◆ Homans' sign: With the woman's knees flexed, the nurse dorsiflexes the foot. Pain in the foot or leg is a positive Homans' sign.
SOURCE: Photographer, Elena Dorfman.

phlebitis. In addition, the nurse may review self-care measures to promote circulation and prevent thrombophlebitis, such as leg exercises that may be performed in bed, dorsiflexion on an hourly basis while on bed rest, ambulation, avoiding pressure behind the knees, and avoiding crossing the legs.

Usually, the nurse records the results of the assessment on a flowsheet or a summary nursing note. If tenderness and warmth have been noted, they might be recorded as follows: "Tenderness, warmth, slight edema, and slight redness noted on posterior aspect of left calf—positive Homans'. Woman advised to avoid pressure to this area; lower leg elevated and moist heat applied per agency protocol. Call placed to Dr. Garcia to report findings."

ELIMINATION

During the hours after birth, the nurse carefully monitors a new mother's bladder status. A boggy uterus, displaced uterus, or a palpable bladder are a sign of bladder distention and requires nursing intervention.

Following birth, the postpartal woman should be encouraged to void every 4 to 6 hours. The nurse should assess the bladder for distention until the woman is able to completely empty her bladder with each voiding. The nurse may employ techniques to facilitate voiding, such as helping the woman out

COMPLEMENTARY AND ALTERNATIVE CARE

LYSINE

Lysine, an essential amino acid, has been identified as a supplement that decreases the incidence of pain following an episiotomy. Lysine is available as a supplement. The recommended adult dosage is 12 mg/kg of body weight per day. It is present in dietary sources, including meat, cheese, fish, eggs, soybeans, and nuts.

of bed to void, pouring warm water on the vulva, running water in the sink, and encouraging the woman to relax and take deep breaths. The physician will order catheterization when the bladder is distended and the woman cannot void, when she is voiding small amounts (less than 100 mL) frequently, or when no voiding has occurred in 8 hours. Although many physicians or CNMs write orders stating that the woman can be catheterized in 8 hours if she has not voided, the nurse needs to assess the bladder and any voiding pattern frequently before the end of the 8-hour period. Some women may require catheterization sooner. The cesarean birth mother may have an indwelling catheter inserted prophylactically. The nurse should perform the same assessments in evaluating bladder emptying once the catheter is removed.

During the physical assessment, the nurse elicits information from the woman regarding the adequacy of her fluid intake, whether she feels she is emptying her bladder completely when she voids, and any signs of UTI she may be experiencing.

In the same way, the nurse obtains information about the new mother's intestinal elimination and any concerns she may have about it. Many mothers fear that the first bowel movement will be painful and possibly even damaging if an episiotomy has been performed. Often, women have defecated during labor or delivery; therefore, bowel movements normally return within 2 to 3 days after a vaginal delivery. Stool softeners may be ordered to increase bulk and moisture in the fecal material and to allow more comfortable and complete evacuation. Constipation may cause pressure on sutures and increase discomfort and therefore should be prevented. Encouraging ambulation, forcing fluids (up to 2000 mL/day or more), and providing fresh fruits and roughage in the diet enhance bowel elimination and help the woman reestablish her normal bowel pattern.

During the assessment, the nurse may provide information regarding postpartum diuresis, explaining why the woman may be emptying her bladder so frequently. Information about the need for additional fluid intake, with suggestions of specific amounts, may be helpful. The woman should drink at least eight 8-oz glasses of water or juice in addition to other fluids. Breastfeeding mothers will have a higher requirement. The nurse discusses signs of retention and overflow voiding and reviews symptoms of UTI with the mother at this time if it seems an appropriate moment for teaching. The nurse can also review methods of assisting bowel elimination and provide opportunities for the woman to ask questions.

REST AND SLEEP STATUS

Physical fatigue often affects other adjustments and functions of the new mother. The mother requires energy to make the psychologic adjustments to a new infant and to assume new roles. Fatigue is often a highly significant factor in a new mother's apparent disinterest in her newborn. Frequently the woman is so tired from a long labor and birth that everything seems to be an effort.

To avoid inadvertently classifying a very tired mother as one with a potential attachment problem, the nurse should do a psychologic assessment on more than one occasion. After a nap the new mother is often far more receptive to her baby and her

RESEARCH IN PRACTICE

RELATIONSHIPS AMONG INFANT SLEEP PATTERNS, MATERNAL FATIGUE, AND DEVELOPMENT OF DEPRESSIVE SYMPTOMATOLOGY

What is this study about? Postpartum depression is a serious condition with significant prevalence. More than 13% of women will develop a major depressive episode in the first 12 weeks after birth. The etiology of postpartum depression is not clear, but it is widely thought to be a multifactorial process involving biological and psychosocial risk factors. One potential risk factor that has been associated with clinical depression in general—fatigue—has received little attention in the study of postpartum depression. This would be a logical focus for study, as changes to both sleep quality and quantity are dramatic in the postpartum period. This study examined the relationships among infant sleep patterns, maternal fatigue, and the development of postpartum depression.

How was this study done? This longitudinal study (a study over time) was completed on a population of postpartum mothers in Canada. Of 1021 mothers recruited, about 20% were recruited antenatally and the rest during the postpartum period. A reliable, valid assessment tool was used to evaluate if the mother had signs of depression at 1 week postpartum; if so, these mothers were eliminated. A total of 585 mothers remained in the study and completed assessment again at 4 and 8 weeks. Eight sleep outcomes were measured by subject response on a questionnaire that described infant sleep and crying behaviors; how often the infant woke the mother; the quantity and quality of maternal sleep; and the mother's perception of fatigue. The eight outcomes were tested for statistical associations with the degree of depressive symptomatology.

What were the results of the study? At 4 weeks postpartum, a large percentage (82.8%) stated that their infant's sleep pattern allowed them to get a reasonable amount of sleep. Nearly half reported sleeping 7 or more hours in a 24-hour period, and 91% reported that the baby's daytime sleep patterns allowed them to get a break. These numbers improved by 8 weeks postpartum, when more than 60% were sleeping 7 or more hours and only 37% reported they "often" felt tired. Although a minority of the mothers reported serious sleep disturbances, these were, indeed, associated with postpartum depression. The eight outcomes—as a group—were a statistically significant predictive model of risks of postpartum depression. The strongest predictor was maternal perception of fatigue. When analyzed separately, depressed mothers reported that their babies cried more and woke them three or more times a night. Mothers with higher depression scores were more likely to get fewer than 6 hours of sleep in a 24-hour period, and were six times more likely than nondepressed mothers to report that their baby's sleep pattern did not allow them to get enough sleep or get a break.

What additional questions might I have? Mothers were eliminated from study if they were at high risk for depression at 1 week. If these mothers were included as subjects, would these relationships be even stronger? The infant's crying behavior was measured simultaneously with sleeping behavior; could the feelings of inadequacy that accompany infant crying be predictive of postpartum depression separately from fatigue?

How can I use this study? Mothers who report fatigue and sleep disturbances are more likely to report symptoms of depression. Counseling for new mothers should include methods to deal with sleep deprivation, such as using the infant's nap time for a sleep break. Inform mothers that the infant's sleep patterns will continue to improve and that most mothers are sleeping 7 or more hours by the time the baby is 8 weeks old. Be alert for early signs of depressive symptomatology during the postpartum period, particularly if the mother is reporting strong feelings of fatigue, frequent waking on the part of the baby, or the inability to get a break from childcare.

Dennis, C., & Ross, L. (2005). Relationships among infant sleep patterns, maternal fatigue, and development of depressive symptomatology. *Birth, 32*(3),187–193.

surroundings. As part of the postpartal assessment, the nurse evaluates the amount of rest the new mother is getting. If the woman reports difficulty sleeping at night, the nurse should try to determine the cause. If it is simply the strange environment, a warm drink, backrub, or mild sedative may prove helpful. Appropriate nursing measures are indicated if the woman is bothered by normal postpartal discomforts such as afterpains, diaphoresis, or episiotomy or hemorrhoidal pain. The impact of rooming-in on the mother's ability to rest should be assessed. See Chapter 35 ∞ for more detailed discussion of comfort/pain relief measures.

A daily rest period should be encouraged, and hospital activities should be scheduled to allow time for napping. The nurse can also provide information about the fatigue a new mother experiences and strategies to promote rest/sleep at home, and the impact it can have on a woman's emotions and sense of control.

NUTRITIONAL STATUS

Postpartal nutritional status is primarily determined based on information provided by the mother and on direct assessment. During pregnancy the daily recommended dietary allowances call for increases in calories, proteins, and most vitamins and minerals. After birth the nonbreastfeeding mother's dietary requirements return to prepregnancy levels, whereas the lactating mother's requirements increase.

Visiting mothers during mealtime provides an opportunity for unobtrusive nutritional assessment and counseling. The nonbreastfeeding mother should be advised about the need to reduce her caloric intake by about 300 kcal and to return to prepregnancy levels for other nutrients. The breastfeeding mother should increase her caloric intake by about 200 kcal over the pregnancy requirements, or a total of 500 kcal over the nonpregnant requirement. Basic discussion will usually prove helpful, followed by referral as needed. In all cases, the nurse

Table 34–5   DAILY EATING TO ENCOURAGE HEALTHFUL NUTRITION DURING THE POSTPARTAL PERIOD
2–3 servings of milk, yogurt, and cheese group
2–3 servings of meat or protein group
3–5 servings of vegetable group
4 servings of whole grain
2–4 servings of fruit group
6–11 servings of bread, cereal, rice, and pasta group
Fats, oils, and sweets sparingly

should provide literature on nutrition so that the woman will have a source of information following discharge.

The nurse should inform the dietitian of any mother who is a vegetarian, has food allergies or lactose intolerance, or whose cultural or religious beliefs require specific foods. Appropriate meals can then be prepared for her. Many women, especially those who gained more than the recommended number of pounds, are interested in losing weight after birth. The dietitian can design weight reduction diets to meet nutritional needs and food preferences. The nurse may also refer women with unusual eating habits or numerous questions about good nutrition to the dietitian.

New mothers are also advised that it is common practice to prescribe iron supplements for 3 months after birth. Hemoglobin and hematocrit values are then checked at the postpartal visit to detect any anemia.

As a part of the nutritional assessment, the nurse can provide teaching about the nutritional needs of the woman during the postpartal period. See Table 34–5 as well as the discussion in Chapter 18. ∞

Psychologic Assessment

During the first several postpartum weeks, the new mother must accomplish certain physical and developmental tasks:

- Restoring physical condition
- Developing competence in caring for and meeting the needs of her infant
- Establishing a relationship with her new child
- Adapting to altered lifestyles and family structure resulting from the addition of a new member

Adequate assessment of the mother's psychologic adjustment is an integral part of postpartal evaluation. This assessment focuses on the mother's general attitude, feelings of competence, available support systems, and caregiving skills. It also evaluates her fatigue level, sense of satisfaction, and ability to accomplish her developmental tasks.

Some new mothers have little or no experience with newborns and may feel totally overwhelmed. They may show these feelings by asking questions and reading all available material or by becoming passive and quiet because they simply cannot deal with their feelings of inadequacy. Unless a nurse questions the woman about her plans and previous experience in a supportive, nonjudgmental way, the nurse might conclude that the woman is uninterested, withdrawn, or depressed. Clues that may indicate a problem include excessive, continued fatigue; marked depression; excessive preoccupation with physical status or discomfort; evidence of low self-esteem; lack of support systems; marital problems; inability to care for or nurture the newborn; and current family crises (such as illness or unemployment). These characteristics frequently indicate a potential for maladaptive parenting, which may lead to child abuse or neglect (physical, emotional, intellectual) and cannot be ignored. Referrals to public health nurses or other available community resources may provide greatly needed assistance and alleviate potentially dangerous situations.

Assessment of Early Attachment

The nurse in any of the various postpartum settings should periodically observe and note the mother's progress toward attachment. The assessment should include both parents when possible; however, in this section, the behaviors focus primarily on the mother's attachment process. As discussed previously, research shows that fathers experience attachment feelings similar to those experienced by mothers. The following questions can be addressed in the course of nurse-client interaction:

- Is the mother attracted to her newborn? To what extent does she seek face-to-face contact and eye contact? Has she progressed from fingertip touch to palmar contact to enfolding the infant close to her own body? Is attraction increasing or decreasing? If the mother does not exhibit increasing attraction, why not? Do the reasons lie primarily within her, in the baby, or in the environment?

- Is the mother inclined to nurture her infant? Is she progressing in her interactions with her infant?

- Does the mother act consistently? If not, is the source of unpredictability within her or her infant?

- Is her mothering consistently carried out? Does she seek information and evaluate it objectively? Does she develop solutions based on adequate knowledge of valid data? Does she evaluate the effectiveness of her maternal care and make appropriate adjustments?

- Is she sensitive to the newborn's needs as they arise? How quickly does she interpret her infant's behavior and react to cues? Does she seem happy and satisfied with the infant's responses to her efforts? Is she pleased with feeding behaviors? How much of this ability and willingness to respond is related to the baby's nature, and how much to her own?

- Does she seem pleased with her baby's appearance and sex? Is she experiencing pleasure in interaction with her infant? What interferes with the enjoyment? Does she speak to the baby frequently and affectionately? Does she call him or her by name? Does she point out family traits or characteristics she sees in the newborn?

- Are there any cultural factors that might modify the mother's response? For instance, is it customary for the grandmother to assume most of the childcare responsibilities while the mother recovers from childbirth?

Once these questions are addressed and the facts are assembled, the nurse can combine the information with personal intuition and knowledge to answer three more unspoken questions: Is there a problem in attachment? What is the problem? What is its source? The nurse can then devise a creative approach to the problem as it presents itself in the context of a unique, developing mother-infant relationship.

Discharge Assessment and Follow-Up

The **Newborns' and Mothers' Health Protection Act (NMHPA)** of 1996 went into effect January 1, 1998. This law states that a woman who has given birth vaginally in a healthcare setting cannot be forcibly discharged within 48 hours of the time of birth for insurance reasons. A woman who had a cesarean birth is covered by her insurance until 96 hours following the time of giving birth. If a mother with an uncomplicated birth and her physician/caregiver mutually decide that discharge before this time frame is required this can be accomplished. When this occurs it is recommended that the newborn be seen in a follow-up setting within 48 hours.

The final discharge assessment should include a physical examination and appropriate discharge teaching that includes both maternal and newborn care guidelines. The mother's laboratory values are examined. If the mother was nonimmune to rubella, a rubella vaccine is administered before discharge. Rh-negative mothers whose infants are Rh positive need RhoGAM before they go home. If either is given, the nurse documents this in the mother's chart. If referrals, such as to social service programs, support groups, a lactation consultant, or a pediatrician, are needed, they should be provided before the family leaves the facility.

Some obstetricians, CNMs, and nurse practitioners see all postpartal women 1 to 2 weeks after birth in addition to the routine 6-week checkup. These visits provide opportunities for physical assessment as well as assessment of the mother's psychologic and informational needs and needs of the family. The routine physical assessment, which can be made rapidly, focuses on the woman's general appearance, breasts, reproductive tract, bladder and bowel elimination, and any specific problems or complaints. In addition, the nurse should talk with the mother about her diet, fatigue level, family adjustment, and psychologic status. The nurse explores any problems with child care and refers the mother to a pediatric nurse practitioner or pediatrician if needed. Available community resources, including public health department follow-up visits, are mentioned when appropriate. If not already discussed, teaching about family planning is appropriate at this time, and the nurse provides information regarding birth control methods. Women who gave birth vaginally tend to abstain from resuming sexual intercourse for a longer period of time than women who had a cesarean birth. Women who breastfed resumed sexual relations later than those who did not breastfeed.

Postdischarge care for the postpartal woman may be accomplished by home visits or follow-up phone calls, or both. The optimal time for a home visit or follow-up phone call is between 3 and 4 days after birth; this provides opportunities for further assessment of mother and their infants and teaching. (See Assessment Guide: Postpartal—First Home Visit and Anticipated Progress at 6 Weeks in Chapter 36 ∞). During this time period, infections, poor infant feeding, excessive weight loss, jaundice, and other problems become apparent (Simpson & James, 2005). The follow-up phone call is often initiated by a nurse from the postpartal unit of the agency where the mother gave birth. It is made soon after discharge and is designed to provide assessment and, if necessary, care; to reinforce knowledge and provide additional teaching; and to make referrals if indicated. Alternatively, a follow-up phone call from a nurse from the physician or nurse-midwife's office can provide new mothers with a source of support and an opportunity to ask questions. Women who appear to be having adjustment problems should be scheduled for an appointment for further evaluation.

In ideal situations, a family approach involving the father, newborn, and other siblings permits a total evaluation and provides an opportunity for all family members to ask questions and express concerns. In addition, a family approach can sometimes enable the nurse to identify disturbed family patterns more readily and suggest, or even institute, therapeutic measures to prevent future problems of neglect or abuse.

CHAPTER REVIEW

FOCUS YOUR STUDY

- The uterus involutes rapidly, primarily through a reduction in cell size.

- Involution is assessed by measuring fundal height. The fundus is at the level of the umbilicus within a few hours after birth and should decrease by approximately one fingerbreadth per day.

- The placental site heals by a process of exfoliation, so no scar formation occurs.

- Lochia progresses from rubra to serosa to alba and is assessed in terms of type, quantity, and characteristics.

- The abdomen may have decreased muscle tone (flabby consistency) initially. The nurse should assess for diastasis recti abdominis, separation of the rectus abdominis muscles.

- Constipation may develop postpartally because of decreased tone in the abdominal muscles, limited diet, and denial of the urge to defecate because of fear of pain.

- Decreased bladder sensitivity, increased capacity, and postpartal diuresis may lead to problems with bladder elimination. Frequent assessment and prompt intervention are indicated. A fundus that is boggy but does not respond

to massage, is higher than expected, or deviates to the side usually indicates a full bladder.

- Postpartally, a healthy woman should be normotensive and afebrile. Bradycardia is common.

- Postpartally the WBC count is often elevated. Activation of clotting factors predisposes the woman to thrombus formation.

- Psychologic adaptations of the postpartal woman are traditionally described as "taking-in" and "taking-hold."

- In consideration of the client's background, the nurse should recognize and respect cultural variations and individual preferences.

- Postpartal assessment should be completed in a systematic way, usually head to toe, and should include assessment of rest and sleep, nutrition, and attachment. The assessment provides opportunities for informal client teaching.

- In the weeks following birth, the woman's physical condition returns to a nonpregnant state, and she gains competence in caregiving and confidence in herself as a parent.

EXPLORE MEDIALINK

http://www.prenhall.com/davidson

NCLEX review questions, case studies, and other interactive resources for this chapter can be found on the Web Site at http://www.prenhall.com/davidson. Click on "Chapter 34" to select the activities for this chapter.

For tutorials including animations and videos, more NCLEX review questions, and an audio glossary, access the accompanying Prentice Hall Nursing MediaLink DVD-ROM in this book.

PRENTICE HALL NURSING MEDIALINK DVD-ROM

Audio Glossary

NCLEX Review

Videos: *Postpartum Assessment; Through the Eyes of a Nurse—Welcoming the New Arrival at the Postpartal Visit*

COMPANION WEBSITE

Additional NCLEX Review

Case Study: *Mother-Infant Bonding*

Care Plan Activity: *Postpartum Client Requesting Relief*

Applications: *Identifying Strategies to Enhance Father-Infant Interactions; Exploring Cultural Differences Regarding Postpartum Care*

Critical Thinking

CRITICAL THINKING IN ACTION

POSTPARTAL CARE PROCEDURES FOR THE NEW MOTHER

View the Critical Thinking in Action video in Chapter 34 of the DVD-ROM. Then answer the questions that follow.

Janet Burns, a 25-year-old G3 P3, is 2 hours past a low forceps vaginal birth with a right medial lateral episiotomy of a live 8-pound baby boy. You obtain vital signs of BP 118/70, T 98.8F, P 76, R 14. You observe that the fundus is 1 finger above the umbilicus and slightly to the right. Her episiotomy is slightly ecchymotic and well approximated without edema or discharge. Ice has been applied to the episiotomy for the last 20 minutes. Lochia rubra is present and a pad was saturated in 90 minutes. Janet has an intravenous of Ringer's lactate with 10 units of Pitocin infusing at 100 mL/hr in her lower left arm and is complaining of moderate abdominal cramping. Janet's baby is sleeping peacefully in the bassinet next to her bed. She tells you that she is very tired and requests some pain medication so she can sleep for a while.

1. What nursing assessment is of immediate concern?

2. Discuss care of her episiotomy and perineum.

3. What other self-care measures could you advise?

4. Discuss postpartal occurrences that may cause special concern for the mother.

5. Janet expressed concern about her episiotomy healing. What information can you offer?

REFERENCES

Alexander, J. M. (2005). Epidural anesthesia for labor pain and its relationship to fever. *Clinics in Perinatology, 32*(3), 777–787.

Al-Oballi Kridli, S. (2002). Health beliefs and practices among Arab women. *American Journal of Maternal/Child Nursing, 27*(3), 178–182.

Blackburn, S. T. (2003). *Maternal, fetal, & neonatal physiology: A clinical perspective* (2nd ed.). St. Louis, MO: Saunders.

Browne, I. M., & Birnbach, D. J. (2003). Neurocysticercosis: A new differential in the diagnosis of postdural puncture headache. *Anesthesia & Analgesia, 97*(2), 580–582.

Cunningham, F. G., Leveno, K. J., Bloom, S. L., Hauth, J. C., Gilstrap, L. C., & Wenstrom, K. D. (2005). *Williams obstetrics* (22nd ed.). New York: McGraw-Hill.

D'Avanzo, C. E., & Geissler, E. M. (2003). *Cultural health assessment* (3rd ed.). St. Louis, MO: Mosby.

De Sovo, M. R. (1997, August). Keeping the faith: Jewish traditions in pregnancy and childbirth. *Lifelines, 1*(4), 46–49.

Drife, J. (2003). Thromboembolism: Pregnancy: Reducing maternal death and disability. *British Medical Bulletin, 67,* 177–190.

Kim-Goodwin, Y. S. (2005). Postpartum beliefs & practices among non-Western cultures. *American Journal of Maternal/Child Nursing, 28*(2), 75–80.

Mercer, R. T. (1995). *Becoming a mother.* New York: Springer.

Porter, C., & Hsu, H. C. (2003). First time mothers' perceptions of efficacy during the transition to motherhood: Links to infant temperament. *Journal of Family Psychology, 17*(1), 54–64.

Purnell, L. D., & Paulanka, B. J. (2005). *Guide to culturally competent care.* Philadelphia: F. A. Davis.

Rubin, R. (1961). Puerperal change. *Nursing Outlook, 9,* 753.

Rubin, R. (1984). *Maternal identity and the maternal experience.* New York: Springer.

Shehata, H. A., & Okosun, H. (2004). Neurological disorders in pregnancy. *Current Opinion in Obstetrics and Gynecology, 16*(2), 117–122.

Simpson, K. R., & James, D. C. (2005). *Postpartum care: Continuing education for registered nurses and certified nurse-midwives.* White Plains, NY: March of Dimes.

Tatum, W., Liporace, J., Benbadis, S., & Kaplan, P. (2004). Updates on the treatment of epilepsy in women. *Archives of Internal Medicine, 164*(2), 137–145.

Varney, H., Kriebs, J., & Gegor, C. (2004). *Varney's midwifery* (4th ed.). Sudbury, MA: Jones & Bartlett.

Wiertlewski, S., Magot, A., Drapier, S., Malinovsky, J. M., & Pereon, Y. (2004). Worsening of neurologic symptoms after epidural anesthesia for labor in a Guillain-Barré patient. *Anesthesia & Analgesia, 98*(3), 825–827.

35 The Postpartal Family: Needs and Care

Providing family-centered postpartum care is a challenge that requires creativity, patience, and a sincere desire to help families grow and thrive. Individual families come to the unit with a unique set of values, beliefs, life experiences, challenges, gifts, and expectations. The nurse needs to personalize care to meet their special needs in a manner that helps them to nurture one another and their newborn within the context of their family, their community, and the world. The postpartum nurse may provide care to numerous families with a variety of needs and expectations within the space of a few hours, which can require a tremendous expenditure of physical, mental, emotional, and spiritual energy. It has been helpful to remember that while it is simply another day of work for me, it is probably one of the most important days of my clients' lives. The care that I provide shapes their memories of this special time and may affect their health and family processes for many years to come. It is my privilege to be a part of their childbearing experience.

OBJECTIVES

1. Delineate nursing responsibilities for client teaching during the early postpartal period.
2. Discuss appropriate nursing interventions to promote maternal comfort and well-being.
3. Describe the nurse's role in promoting maternal rest and helping the mother to resume gradually an appropriate level of activity.
4. Identify client teaching topics for promoting postpartal family wellness.
5. Compare the nursing needs of a woman who experienced a cesarean birth with the needs of a woman who gave birth vaginally.
6. Summarize the nursing needs of the childbearing adolescent during the postpartal period.
7. Describe possible approaches to sensitive, holistic nursing care for the woman who relinquishes her newborn.
8. Determine the nurse's responsibilities related to early postpartum discharge.

KEY TERMS

Afterpains   1080
Bogginess   1077
Couplet care   1085
Family-centered care   1085
Mother-baby care   1085

Patient-controlled analgesia (PCA)   1092
Relinquishing mother   1096
Skin-to-skin contact   1085

 MEDIALINK

Additional resources for this content can be found on the Prentice Hall Nursing MediaLink DVD-ROM and on the Companion Website at http://www.prenhall.com/davidson. Click on "Chapter 35" to select the activities for this chapter.

Certain premises form the basis of effective nursing care during the postpartal period.

- The best postpartal care is family centered and disrupts the family unit as little as possible. This approach uses the family's resources to support an early and smooth adjustment to the newborn by all family members.
- Knowledge of the range of normal physiologic and psychologic adaptations occurring during the postpartal period allows the nurse to recognize alterations and initiate interventions early. Communicating information about postpartal adaptations to the family facilitates their adjustment to their situation.
- Nursing care is aimed at accomplishing specific goals that ultimately meet individual needs. These goals are formulated after careful assessment and consideration of factors that could influence the outcome of care.

Chapter 34 ∞ provides a thorough discussion of postpartal assessment. This chapter describes nursing care during the immediate postpartal period. Specific nursing responses to the mother's physical needs and the family's psychosociocultural needs are described at length and are summarized in the Clinical Pathway for the Postpartal Period on pages 1071 to 1073.

NURSING CARE DURING THE EARLY POSTPARTAL PERIOD

For most postpartal women, physical recovery proceeds smoothly and is considered a healthy process. Because of this perception, it is all too common for caregivers to think that the woman and her family have no "real" needs and thus no care plan is needed. Nothing can be further from the truth. Every member of the family has needs, although they may not be obvious, especially if educational or emotional.

Nursing Diagnosis

The postpartal family's needs, which should be identified during assessment, are the basis for developing nursing diagnoses. Once a nursing diagnosis is made and recorded, systematic action, as delineated in a nursing care plan or clinical pathway, can be used to meet the identified need.

Often agencies prefer to use only the North American Nursing Diagnosis Association (NANDA) list. Consequently, physiologic alterations form the basis of many postpartal diagnoses. Examples of such diagnoses include the following, which are written in problem, etiology, symptoms (PES) format:

- *Impaired Urinary Elimination* related to tissue trauma as evidenced by (AEB) dysuria or urinary retention
- *Impaired Skin/Tissue Integrity* related to tearing/shearing forces or surgical intervention AEB laceration, episiotomy, and/or surgical incision
- *Pain, Acute,* related to tearing/shearing forces (lacerations), trauma (hematomas), surgical interventions (episiotomy,

incision), and/or muscle fatigue AEB complaints of discomfort

- *Disturbed Sleep Pattern* related to frequent interruption of rest for newborn care
- *Risk for Infection* related to decreased barriers and/or bacterial colonization (lacerations, incision, cervical dilation, prolonged rupture of membranes, positive group Beta Streptococcus [GBS] culture)
- *Risk for Constipation* related to perineal discomfort and decreased peristalsis

Wellness diagnoses related to family coping or instructional needs are also used frequently. Examples of these diagnoses include the following:

- *Health-Seeking Behaviors: Information About Infant* care related to no prior (or recent) experience AEB an expressed desire to understand an infant's needs
- *Readiness for Enhanced Family Coping* related to addition of new family member AEB positive bonding behaviors and successful early adjustment to the new baby

After completing the assessment and diagnosis steps of the nursing process, the nurse identifies desired outcomes and selects nursing interventions that will promote these outcomes.

Nursing Plan and Implementation

Nursing care management is individualized to meet the needs of each postpartal woman, her newborn, and her family. The plan of care needs to consider the newborn's schedule of activities during the day, such as feeding times, because they frequently determine the mother's schedule. Flexibility is crucial because most breastfeeding infants feed on demand at frequent intervals.

An important component of nursing care is client teaching, which is designed to help the woman and her family learn how to perform self-care and provide effective newborn care. Sophisticated, detailed forms and guidelines are often available to assist in health teaching. Such tools are a useful adjunct but cannot take the place of the nurse's client-specific plan. As part of client teaching, the nurse should discuss cultural beliefs, desired outcomes, and goals with the mother as soon as possible on her arrival in the postpartum unit. Examples of these desired client outcomes include the following:

- Mother and baby remain healthy, safe, and free of injury or complications.
- Mother verbalizes comfort.
- Mother tells birth story and verbalizes feelings and concerns regarding the event.
- Mother reviews educational resources for self- and infant care.
- Mother performs appropriate self- and infant care.
- Parent(s) and newborn demonstrate positive bonding behaviors.
- Parents practice principles of infant safety.

CLINICAL PATHWAY For the Postpartal Period

CATEGORY	FIRST 4 HOURS	4–8 HOURS PAST BIRTH	8–24 HOURS PAST BIRTH
Referral	Report from labor nurse if not continuing in an LDR room	Lactation consultation as needed	Home nursing, social work, Women Infant Children (WIC) referral if indicated; coordinate universal hearing and state-required newborn metabolic screening ◆ *Expected Outcomes* Referrals made
Assessments	Postpartum assessments every 30 min × 2, every 1 h × 2, then every 4 h. Includes: • Fundus firm, midline, at or below umbilicus • Lochia rubra less than 2 pad/h; no free flow or passage of clots with massage • Bladder: voids large amounts of urine spontaneously; bladder not palpable following voiding • Perineum: sutures intact; no bulging or marked swelling; no c/o severe pain. Minimal bruising may be present. If hemorrhoids present, no tenseness or marked engorgement; less than 2 cm diameter • Breasts: soft, colostrum present Vital Signs: • BP WNL; no hypotension; not greater than 30 mm systolic or 15 mm diastolic over baseline • Temperature: less than 38C (100.4F) • Pulse: bradycardia normal, consistent with baseline • Respirations: 12–24/min; quiet, easy; lungs CTA Comfort level: less than 3 on scale of 1–10	Continue postpartum assessment every 4 h Breast: evaluate nipple status; should be no evidence of cracks or bruising Observe feeding technique with newborn Vital signs assessment every 8 h; all WNL; report temperature greater than 38C (100.4F) Assess Homans' sign every 8 h Continue assessment of comfort level	Continue postpartum assessment every 4 h Breasts: nipples should remain free of cracks, fissures, bruising Newborn latches and breastfeeds successfully Vital signs assessment every 4 h; all WNL; report temperature greater than 38C (100.4F) Continue assessment of comfort level ◆ *Expected Outcomes* Vital signs WNL, voids QS, postpartum assessment WNL; comfort level: less than 3 on 1–10 scale, involution of uterus in process—fundus may migrate to 1 cm above umbilicus by 12 h; fundal height decreases 1 cm/day thereafter; demonstrates and verbalizes appropriate newborn feeding techniques
Teaching/ psychosocial	Explain postpartum assessments Assist with breastfeeding; discuss benefits and AAP recommendations if undecided Teach self-massage of fundus and expected findings; explain rationale for fundal massage Instruct to call for assistance first time OOB and PRN Demonstrate peri-care, Surgigator, sitz bath PRN Explain comfort measures Begin newborn teaching; bulb suctioning, positioning, feeding, diaper change, cord care, infant security measures Orient to room if transferred from LDR room Provide information on early postpartal period Assess mother/infant attachment Allow skin-to-skin contact Encourage mother to verbalize her birth story Encourage father to bond and provide newborn care	Discuss psychologic changes of postpartum period; facilitate transition through tasks of taking on maternal role Discuss peri-care/hygiene; encourage use of supportive brassiere for breastfeeding or formula-feeding Stress need for frequent rest periods Continue newborn teaching: newborn behavioral states, soothing/comforting techniques, swaddling; return demonstrations indicate woman's understanding Provide opportunities for questions and review; reinforce previous teaching Breastfeeding: nipple care: air-drying, lanolin; proper latch-on technique; Formula-feeding: supportive bra, ice compresses Assess mother/infant attachment	Reinforce previous teaching, complete teaching evaluation Discuss involution; anticipated physical changes in first 2 weeks postpartum; postpartal exercises; need to limit visitors; baby blues; postpartum fatigue; postpartum depression Discuss postpartal nutrition; balanced diet Breastfeeding: • Increase calories by up to 500 kcal over nonpregnant state (200 kcal over pregnant intake) • Explain milk production, let-down reflex, use of supplements, sore nipples, breast pumping, and milk storage Formula-feeding: • Return to nonpregnant caloric intake • Explain formula preparation and storage Discuss birth control options, sexuality Discuss sibling rivalry and plan for supporting siblings at home Discuss pets; suggestions for improving acceptance of infant by pets Discuss fathering experience Emphasize car seat/vehicle safety, SIDS prevention, "never shake a baby" ◆ *Expected Outcomes* Mother verbalizes teaching comprehension Positive bonding and emotional behaviors observed (both parents if present) Provides appropriate self- and infant care.

(Continued on next page)

CLINICAL PATHWAY For the Postpartal Period continued

Category	First 4 Hours	4–8 Hours Past Birth	8–24 Hours Past Birth
Nursing care management and reports	Ice pack to perineum to decrease swelling and increase comfort Straight catheter PRN × 1 if distended or voiding small amounts If continues unable to void or voiding small amounts, insert Foley catheter and notify CNM or physician	Sitz baths PRN If woman Rh– and infant Rh+, RhoGAM work-up; obtain consent; complete teaching Determine rubella status Obtain consent for rubella vaccine if indicated; explain purpose, procedure, implications of vaccine Obtain hematocrit	Continue sitz baths PRN May shower if ambulating without difficulty DC saline lock if present Administer rubella vaccine as indicated ◆ *Expected Outcomes* Using sitz bath; voids QS; lab work WNL; performs ADL without sequelae
Activity	Assistance when OOB first time, then PRN Ambulate ad lib Rests comfortably between assessments	Encourage rest periods Ambulate ad lib; may leave birthing unit after notifying staff of plan to ambulate off unit	Up ad lib ◆ *Expected Outcomes* Ambulates ad lib
Comfort	Institute comfort measures: • Perineal discomfort: peri-care; sitz baths, topical analgesics • Hemorrhoids: sitz baths, topical analgesics, Tucks, side-lying or prone position • Afterpains: prone with small pillow under abdomen; warm shower or sitz baths; ambulation • Administer pain medication PRN	Continue with pain management techniques Offer alternative pain management options: distraction with music, television, visitors; massage; warmed blankets or towels to affected area; using breathing techniques when infant latches on to breast and/or during cramping until medication's action is felt	Continue with pain management techniques ◆ *Expected Outcomes* Comfort level less than 3 on 1–10 scale Verbalizes alternative pain management options
Nutrition	Regular diet Fluid 2000 mL/day	Continue diet and fluids	Continue diet and fluids ◆ *Expected Outcomes* Regular diet/fluids tolerated
Elimination	Voiding large amounts straw-colored urine	Voiding large quantities May have bowel movement	Same ◆ *Expected Outcomes* Voiding QS; passing flatus or bowel movement
Medications	Pain medications as ordered Methergine 0.2 mg every 4–6 h PO if ordered Stool softener Tucks pad PRN, perineal analgesic spray	Continue meds Lanolin to nipples PRN; assist with positioning and latch PRN; saline flush to saline lock (if present) every 8 h or as ordered May take own prenatal vitamins and iron—keep secure from siblings	Continue medications RhoGAM and rubella vaccine administered if indicated ◆ *Expected Outcomes* Vaccines administered; pain controlled Saline lock discontinued (site healthy)
Discharge planning/ home care	Evaluate knowledge of normal postpartum and newborn care Evaluate support systems	Discuss typical newborn schedule; plan for periods of rest Birth certificate paperwork completed Evaluate plans for transporting newborn; car seat available	Review discharge instruction sheet/checklist Describe postpartum warning signs and when to call CNM/physician Provide prescriptions Arrangements for baby pictures as per agency protocol Postpartum and newborn visits scheduled ◆ *Expected Outcomes* Discharged home; mother verbalizes postpartum warning S/S, follow-up appointment times/dates Hearing and metabolic screens completed with follow-up scheduled if needed

CLINICAL PATHWAY For the Postpartal Period continued

CATEGORY	FIRST 4 HOURS	4–8 HOURS PAST BIRTH	8–24 HOURS PAST BIRTH
Family involvement	Identify available support persons Assess family perceptions of birth experience Parenting: demonstrates culturally expected early parenting behaviors	Involve support persons in care, teaching; answer questions Evidence of parental bonding behaviors present	Continue to involve support persons in teaching, involve siblings as appropriate Plans made for providing support to mother following discharge ◆ *Expected Outcomes* Evidence of parental bonding behavior; support persons verbalize understanding of woman's need for rest, good nutrition, fluids, and emotional support

Information is included for both vaginal birth (VB) and cesarean birth (CB). However, because many of the nursing care interventions are the same for either, specific interventions or suggestions related to vaginal birth are designated VB, and those specific to cesarean are designated CB.

ADL, activities of daily living; BP, blood pressure; CB, cesarean birth; CNM, certified nurse-midwife; CTA, clear to auscultation; DC, discontinue; LDR, labor, delivery, and recovery; OOB, out of bed; OR, operating room; PCA, patient-controlled analgesia; PRN, as needed; VB, vaginal birth; WNL, within normal limits; PP, postpartum; QS, quantity sufficient; VS, vital signs; c/o, complaints of; LOS, level of sensation; LOC, level of consciousness; TC&DB, turn-cough and deep breathe; D/C, discharge; S/S, signs and symptoms.

- Mother demonstrates successful breastfeeding and breast care or describes formula preparation for formula-feeding, feeding techniques, and breast care.

- Mother verbalizes sources of support to assist in newborn care and family responsibilities.

- Mother states plan for follow-up health care for self and infant.

- Parent identifies signs/symptoms of maternal or newborn complications and reasons to seek care before routine follow-up visits.

Additional outcomes for the cesarean birth mother include the following:

- Mother states in own words the reason for the cesarean birth and verbalizes feelings related to the event.

- Mother maintains desired comfort level (less than 3 on 1 to 10 scale).

- Mother maintains mobility (up in chair within 12 hours; ambulates within 24).

In summary, all components of nursing care management are designed to achieve the desired outcomes identified for the woman and her family.

COMMUNITY-BASED NURSING CARE

Various services are available to meet the needs of the childbearing family during the immediate postpartal period and beyond. These services range from educational opportunities, such as classes on nutrition, breastfeeding, exercise, infant care and development, and parenting, to specific healthcare programs, such as well-baby checkups, immunization clinics, and family planning services. Some are offered by the birthing unit or private caregivers, some are provided by volunteer and charitable organizations, and some are the domain of city, state, or federal agencies. In all cases, the goal is consistent: to help ensure that the mother, the father (if he is involved), siblings, and the newborn have the opportunity to meet specific healthcare needs regardless of their personal resources.

Home health care is one of the most important forms of community-based nursing care offered to postpartal families. Home care visits and phone contacts (telephone follow-up) help ensure that families have the necessary skills and resources to care for an infant and to meet their own health needs. Because of its importance today in caring for childbearing families, home care is discussed in depth in Chapter 36. ∞

PROMOTION OF EFFECTIVE PARENT LEARNING

Meeting the educational needs of the new mother and her family is one of the primary challenges facing the postpartum nurse. Each woman's educational needs vary according to age, background, culture, experience, and expectations. However, because the mother spends only a brief period of time in the postpartal area, identifying and addressing individual instructional needs can be difficult. Effective education provides the childbearing family with sufficient knowledge to meet many of their own health needs and to seek assistance if necessary.

The nurse assesses the learning needs of the new mother through observation, sensitivity to nonverbal clues, and tactfully phrased questions. For example, "What plans have you made for handling things when you get home?" will elicit a more detailed response than, "Will someone be available to help you at home?" To assess learning needs, some agencies provide a client handout listing the most frequently identified areas of concern for new mothers. The mother checks those that apply to her or writes in concerns not included. The nurse should plan and implement learning experiences in a logical, nonthreatening way based on knowledge of and respect for the family's cultural values and beliefs. For example, Mexican and Vietnamese women frequently wait to breastfeed until after their milk comes in, as they do not believe colostrum is good for the baby (Galanti, 2004). The postpartum nurse needs to be aware of the cultural customs of her clients. Providing education, such as telling the patient about the benefits of colostrum, may be helpful in changing behavior. Unless there is a culturally related activity the nurse believes would be harmful, most cultural customs can be supported and encouraged.

Methods and Timing of Teaching

The educational method the nurse chooses varies. Agencies with many clients and limited staff may rely heavily on structured classes. Smaller units may provide individualized instruction through the use of one-on-one teaching or prepared videotapes. Some agencies use a television channel to show instructional videotapes at scheduled times during the day. Women should have a pencil and paper to jot down questions that arise as they view the material. Afterward, nurses need to be available to clarify material or answer any questions about the content. Because more effective learning occurs when there is sensory involvement and active participation, videotapes (sight and hearing) are more helpful than lecture (hearing only). Demonstration-return demonstration (sight, touch, hearing, and, possibly, smell and taste) is even more effective.

Timing is important in implementing educational activities. The new mother is more receptive to teaching after the first 24 to 48 hours, when she is ready to assume responsibility for her own care and that of her newborn . However, many women are discharged in the early, dependent phase. Because of this, the nurse needs to provide whatever teaching the woman is ready for, with written handouts for future reference.

Timing is also important for new fathers, who are more likely to attend sessions planned for them if they are scheduled in the evening after visiting hours. If material is planned for siblings, late afternoon teaching after school or naps might be more effective.

Content of Teaching

A review of the postpartum learning needs literature by Bowman (2005) found that information regarding stitches, episiotomy, and postpartum complications is a priority for women during the first 3 postpartum days. Information regarding infant feeding and infant illness is a priority during the first postpartum week and continues to be important throughout the postpartum period. Once mothers go home, they also need information regarding mothering, meeting the needs of the family, exercise, and return to nonpregnant status. Most notably, maternal learning needs scatter across a variety of topics and vary depending on the mother's age and whether she is a primipara or multipara. Therefore, it is essential that the teaching content be tailored to the individual mother and family.

Continuing learning needs may be addressed through home visits, in postpartum educational programs, and by nurses in ob-

stetric and pediatric offices. Postpartum nurses should provide written information on a variety of maternal and infant care topics, so parents can refer to them on an as-needed basis following discharge.

Teaching should not be limited to "how-to" activities. Anticipatory guidance is essential in assisting the family to cope with role changes, the realities of a new baby, and potential complications such as infant colic, postpartum fatigue, and postpartum depression. Small-group discussions provide a chance for the new parents to talk about fears and expectations. Questions may arise about sexuality, contraception, child care, and even the grief associated with giving up the fantasized infant in order to accept the actual one.

Although many first-time mothers feel they are well prepared for pregnancy and childbirth, many feel unprepared for the postpartum period (George, 2005). Many women describe the responsibility for a newborn as overwhelming. Additionally, they are surprised at the degree of discomfort and fatigue they feel. These women may need more information about infant care and feeding, especially breastfeeding, as well as more information regarding their own self-care. First-time mothers also express frustration about being overwhelmed with too much information during the short hospital stay followed by abandonment by the healthcare system once they go home. Therefore, it is essential that postpartum nurses make families aware of advice lines, support groups, postpartum educational programs, and other helpful healthcare resources before discharge.

Although second-time mothers are more comfortable with newborn care and know what to expect, their concerns focus on establishing routines that allow them to manage care of older children, maintaining their marital relationship, taking breaks to make time for themselves, and seeking out support with child care. Additionally, they focus on nurturing relationships between each parent and child and between the children (O'Reilly, 2004). Care and teaching for these mothers and families will need to focus on review of self- and newborn care as needed, sibling issues, the marital relationship, sleep patterns and issues, encouraging paternal competence and involvement in newborn care, and identifying sources of support.

Adolescent mothers, clients with cesarean delivery, and parents of newborns with congenital anomalies will have special concerns, as will clients with special needs related to their own physical, mental, or emotional health and abilities. Postpartum nurses need to ensure that special needs families have additional support in place from home care nurses, social workers, chaplains, and other professionals before discharge.

Table 35–1 identifies important topic areas to be included in postpartal client teaching.

Evaluating Learning

Methods for evaluating learning vary according to the objectives and teaching methods. Return demonstrations, question-and-answer sessions, and even programmed instruction are opportunities for evaluating learning, as are formal evaluation tools.

Evaluation of attitudinal or less concrete learning is more difficult. For example, a mother's ability to express her frustrations over an unanticipated cesarean birth or difficulties with

Table 35–1   AREAS TO INCLUDE IN POSTPARTAL TEACHING

Knowledge and Skills to Be Taught	Teaching Method			
	Video	Verbal Only	Verbally Reinforced	Demonstration
Care of the Mother				
Breast care				
Breastfeeding or lactation suppression				
Possible problems and care				
Involutional changes				
Position of fundus				
Afterpains				
Changes in lochia				
Signs of possible problems				
Bladder function				
Fluid needs				
Signs of possible problems				
Bowel function				
Normal patterns				
Dietary assistance				
Perineal care				
Expected healing changes in episiotomy/laceration				
Comfort measures (rinsing with warm water, use of icepacks, use of analgesic/anesthetic spray, sitz bath), home care				
Signs of possible problems				
Rest and activity				
Scheduling rest periods, postpartum fatigue				
Ambulation				
Watching for circulatory problems in legs				
Emotional changes				
Changes in mood, crying, anxiety; "baby blues," postpartum depression				
Care of the Father/Partner				
Emotional changes				
Emotional changes and challenges that may occur				
Encouragement to seek support as needed				
Physiologic and psychologic changes that may occur in the mother and newborn				
Infant care concerns				
Possible supportive measures for the new family				
Care of the Baby				
Infant safety and security measures				
Observing the baby				
General appearance				
Five Senses				
Visual				
Hearing				
Touch				
Smell				
Taste				
Vital signs				
Normal parameters				
How to take a temperature				
Skin				
Coloring				
Normal rashes				
Diaper care				
Elimination cycles of stool/urine				
Normal characteristics				
Signs of diarrhea and treatment				
Signs of constipation and treatment				
Emotional and comforting needs				

(Continued on next page)

Table 35–1   AREAS TO INCLUDE IN POSTPARTAL TEACHING continued

Knowledge and Skills to Be Taught	Teaching Method			
	Video	Verbal Only	Verbally Reinforced	Demonstration
Protective reflexes				
Blinking				
Sneezing				
Swallowing				
Normal reflexes				
Moro				
Fencing				
Head lag				
Stepping				
Feeding the baby				
Schedule				
Breastfeeding				
Positioning, latch, initiating and ending feeding				
Infant cues for feeding				
Identifying problem areas and possible solutions				
Signs of dehydration				
Signs of adequate breastfeeding (output, satiation, weight)				
Formula-feeding				
Positioning				
Preparation of bottles and formula				
Burping or bubbling the baby				
Holding, wrapping, and diapering the baby				
Various holds (cradle, football)				
Securing baby in blanket to provide warmth				
Diapering				
Comparison of reusable (cloth) and single use (paper)				
Methods of diapering and care of soiled diapers				
Perineal skin care				
"Back to sleep!"				
Bathing the baby				
Supplies				
Method				
Safety				
Use of bulb syringe and care if choking				
Sudden Infant Death Syndrome (SIDS) prevention (home *and* child care)				
Prevention of battering/shaken baby injuries				
Prevention of falls				
Childproofing the home				
Positioning				
Car seat/vehicle safety				
Health promotion				
When to call healthcare provider				
Temp				
Diarrhea				
Poor feeding/feeding intolerance				
Malaise/lethargy/"not acting right"				
Protecting baby from infections				
Immunization schedule				
Hearing and metabolic screening				
Aspects of Parenting				
Interaction with newborn				
Newborn behavioral states				
Newborn cues and capacity for interaction				
Parenting needs				
Infant colic				
Acquaintance with individual characteristics of their newborn and possible techniques to use				
Resources available				

breastfeeding as opposed to her desired and expected experience may be the nurse's only clues that learning has occurred. Follow-up phone calls and home visits after discharge may provide additional evaluative information and continue the helping process as the nurse assesses the family's current educational needs and begins planning accordingly.

PROMOTION OF MATERNAL COMFORT AND WELL-BEING

The nurse promotes and restores maternal physical well-being by monitoring the woman's vital signs, cardiovascular status, and elimination. These assessments are discussed in Chapter 34. ∞ The nurse also monitors the status of the woman's uterus and performs nursing activities aimed at relieving specific discomforts, such as an edematous perineum or a distended bladder. In addition, medications may be needed to promote comfort, treat anemia, provide immunity to rubella, and prevent development of antibodies in the nonsensitized Rh-negative woman. Finally, the woman may be experiencing alterations in her emotional well-being. Interventions for these conditions are discussed in this section.

Monitoring Uterine Status

The nurse completes an assessment of the uterus as discussed in Chapter 34. ∞ The assessment interval is every 15 minutes for the first hour after childbirth, every 30 minutes for the next hour, and then hourly for approximately 2 hours. Thereafter, the nurse monitors uterine status every 4 hours, or more frequently if problems arise, such as **bogginess** (softening of the uterus due to inadequate contraction of the muscle tissue), positioning out of midline, heavy lochia flow, or the presence of clots (Table 35–2). The uterus can be assessed every 8 hours from 24 hours postpartum until discharge (Scoggin, 2004).

The amount, consistency, color, and odor of the lochia are monitored on an ongoing basis. Increased bleeding is most often related to uterine atony and responds to emptying the bladder, fundal massage, and expression of any clots. Nipple stimulation can also be utilized to promote contraction of the uterus. Breastfeeding is an ideal and natural way to stimulate oxytocin release and contract a boggy uterus. Bleeding that does not respond readily requires additional evaluation to rule out complications such as retained placenta, lacerations, hemato-

---

Table 35–2   KEY FACTS TO REMEMBER ABOUT MONITORING POSTPARTAL UTERINE STATUS

Position of the Uterine Fundus Following Birth

Immediately after birth: The top of the fundus is in the midline about midway between the symphysis pubis and umbilicus.

Six to 12 hours after birth: The top of the fundus is in the midline and at the level of the umbilicus (may migrate to 1 cm above the umbilicus by the 12-hour point and then descend 1 cm/day).

One day after birth: The top of the fundus is in the midline and one fingerbreadth below the umbilicus.

Second day after birth and thereafter: The top of the fundus remains in the midline and descends about one fingerbreadth per day.

Normal Characteristics of Lochia

Lochia rubra is red and is present for the first 2–3 days.

Lochia serosa is pinkish red or brown and is present from day 3 to day 10.

Lochia alba is creamy white and is present from day 11 to day 14 (may last 3 to 6 weeks).

---

mas, coagulation defects, or uterine inversion. Changes in lochia that need to be assessed further, documented, and reported to the physician or certified nurse-midwife are presented in Table 35–3.

Occasionally a medication such as methylergonovine maleate (Methergine) is prescribed to promote uterine contractions. In some cases an intravenous (IV) infusion of oxytocin (Pitocin) may be necessary if the uterus does not remain firm and uterine bleeding is excessive. The nurse will need to ensure patent IV access in this case. See Drug Guide: Methylergonovine Maleate (Methergine) in this chapter and Drug Guide: Oxytocin (Pitocin) in Chapter 27. ∞ Uterine atony resistant to these drugs can require use of 15-mL carboprost tromethamine (Hemabate). See Table 38–1 regarding the use of uterine stimulants. Postpartum hemorrhage is a life-threatening emergency. The postpartum nurse needs to be particularly vigilant to a uterus that becomes boggy as well as to increases in bleeding throughout the recovery period (MacMullen, Dulski, & Meagher, 2005).

TEACHING FOR SELF-CARE

The nurse teaches the woman to assess her fundus for firmness and position and to massage the fundus gently to promote uterine contraction. In addition, the nurse instructs her to monitor the amount and color of the lochia. Being aware of normal

---

Table 35–3   CHANGES IN LOCHIA THAT CAUSE CONCERN DURING THE EARLY POSTPARTAL PERIOD

Change	Possible Problem	Nursing Action
Presence of clots or excessive bleeding (greater than 2 pads/hour)	Inadequate uterine contractions that allow bleeding from vessels at the placental site. Lacerations, hematomas, coagulation disorders, etc.	Assess location and firmness of fundus—massage prn. Assess voiding pattern—empty bladder. Record and report findings.
Persistent lochia rubra	Inadequate uterine contractions; retained placental fragments; infection.	Assess location and firmness of fundus. Assess activity pattern. Assess for signs of infection. Record and report findings.

DRUG GUIDE   Methylergonovine Maleate (Methergine)

Overview of Action

Methylergonovine maleate (Methergine) is an ergot alkaloid that stimulates uterine and vascular smooth muscle tissue. Because the smooth muscle of the uterus is especially sensitive to this drug, it is used postpartally to stimulate the uterus to contract in order to decrease blood loss by clamping off uterine blood vessels and to promote the involution process. In addition, the drug has a vasoconstrictive effect on all blood vessels, especially the larger arteries. This may result in hypertension, particularly in a woman whose blood pressure is already elevated.

Route, Dosage, and Frequency

Methergine has a rapid onset of action and may be given orally or intramuscularly.

Usual IM dose: 0.2 mg (200 mcg) following expulsion of the placenta. The dose may be repeated every 2–4 hours if necessary (up to 6 doses).

Usual oral dose: 0.2 mg (200 mcg) every 4 to 6 hours (duration varies).

Not for IV use except in extreme emergency—severe hypertension and vasoconstriction may result.

Maternal Contraindications

Pregnancy, hypersensitivity. Use caution in hepatic or renal disease, cardiac disease, hypertension, preeclampsia, sepsis, and lactation (may decrease prolactin levels). Use extreme caution if administered in third stage of labor.

Maternal Side Effects

Hypertension, nausea, vomiting, headache, bradycardia, dizziness, tinnitus, uterine cramps, palpitations, arrhythmias, diaphoresis, dyspnea, chest pain, and allergic reactions may be noted.

Effects on Fetus or Newborn

Because Methergine has a long duration of action and can thus produce tetanic contractions, it **should never be used during pregnancy or before delivery of the fetus,** when it may result in a sustained uterine contraction that may cause injury or death to the mother and/or fetus.

Nursing Considerations

- Monitor fundal height and consistency and the amount and character of the lochia.
- Notify provider if uterus remains boggy despite Methergine administration.
- Assess the blood pressure before and routinely throughout drug administration.
- Inform client that Methergine may cause severe menstrual-like cramps.
- Observe for adverse effects or symptoms of ergot toxicity (ergotism) such as nausea and vomiting, headache, muscle pain, cold or numb fingers and toes, chest pain, and general weakness.
- Provide client/family teaching regarding importance of not smoking during Methergine administration (nicotine from cigarettes leads to constricted vessels and may lead to hypertension), signs of toxicity.

SOURCES: Cunningham et al., 2005; Deglin & Vallerand, 2005.

---

involutional changes will help the woman identify problems. Discharge instructions should specify that women need to call their healthcare provider if their bleeding is equal to or more than two sanitary pads per hour.

Relief of Perineal Discomfort

Many nursing interventions are available for relieving perineal discomfort. Before selecting a method, the nurse needs to have assessed the perineum to determine the degree of edema and other problems. It is also important to ask the woman whether there are special measures that she feels will be particularly effective and to offer her choices when possible. Some cultures believe that the use of "cold" versus "hot" may alter the recovery or spirit of the new mother. These beliefs will affect the choices made by the new mother. The nurse uses disposable gloves while applying all relief measures and washes hands before and after using the gloves.

It is important to use good hygienic practices, such as moving from the front (area of the symphysis pubis) to the back (area around the anus) of the perineum. The nurse should follow this principle when placing ice packs and perineal pads and applying topical anesthetic agents or pain relief products. Avoiding contamination between the anal area and the urethral-vaginal area is essential to prevent infection.

CLINICAL TIP

You may be surprised by how quickly the postpartal woman shows signs of bladder distention, possibly as soon as 1 to 2 hours after childbirth. This is because of normal postpartal diuresis. You can help prevent overdistention by palpating the woman's bladder frequently and encouraging her to void. When urinating the first time after vaginal birth, some mothers may feel the urge to urinate but are unable to begin the flow of urine. Possible interventions include letting her hear running water by turning water on in the sink; running warm water in the sink and having her place one hand in the water; having her place one foot in a basin of warm water; squirting warm water over her perineum using a peri-bottle; and placing a few drops of peppermint oil in the urine collection device ("hat"). Be sure to measure the first few voidings. The amount should be at least 150 mL. If she is still unable to void and catheterization becomes necessary, be prepared for difficulty in visualizing the urethra because of localized swelling and discomfort and tenderness in the area.

PERINEAL CARE

Perineal care after each elimination (urination or defecation) cleanses the perineum and helps promote comfort. Many agencies provide "peri-bottles" that the woman can use to squirt warm tap water over her perineum following elimination. To cleanse her perineum, the woman may use a Surgigator, moist antiseptic towelettes, or toilet paper in a blotting (patting) mo-

CLIENT TEACHING   Care of Episiotomy or Laceration

CLIENT GOALS   At the completion of the teaching, the woman will be able to:

1. Identify the factors that both promote and interfere with wound healing.

2. Summarize self-care activities to promote healing and increase personal comfort.

3. Demonstrate the correct procedure for peri-care and taking a sitz bath.

4. Discuss the judicious use of prescribed analgesics or topical anesthetics as needed.

TEACHING PLAN

CONTENT	TEACHING METHOD
• Describe the process of wound healing. Discuss the risk of contamination of the episiotomy/laceration by bacteria from the anal area.	Discussion helps women understand the importance of good wound care.
• Explain techniques that are used to keep the episiotomy/laceration clean and promote healing such as: 　• Sitz bath 　• Use of peri-bottle following each voiding or defecation 　• Pad change following each elimination and at regular intervals	Focus on open discussion. Demonstrate correct use of the peri-bottle or sitz bath if necessary.
• Describe comfort measures: 　• Ice pack or glove immediately following birth 　• Sitz bath 　• Judicious use of analgesics or topical anesthetics 　• Tightening buttocks before sitting	Focus on discussion and provide an opportunity for questions.
• Identify signs of episiotomy/laceration infection. Advise the woman to contact her caregiver if infection develops.	Encourage discussion and provide printed handouts. Some of this content may also be covered during a small postpartum class.

EVALUATION	DOCUMENTATION
At the end of the teaching session the woman will be able to verbalize the principles of wound healing and episiotomy/laceration care. She will also be able to demonstrate self-care measures such as peri-care, ice packs, taking a sitz bath, and administration of topical anesthetics or analgesics.	Documentation of client teaching should include the teaching information discussed, the client's verbalization of understanding, specific interventions or warning signs that were given, along with the client's understanding of follow-up if needed in the future.

tion. She should be taught to start at the front (area just under the symphysis pubis) and proceed toward the back (area around the anus) to prevent contamination from the anal area. In addition, to prevent contamination, the perineal pad should be applied from front to back, placing the front portion against the perineum first. Perineal pads should be changed regularly to prevent infection.

Teaching for Self-Care

The nurse demonstrates how to cleanse the perineum and assists the woman as necessary, for example, by offering additional information regarding the use of perineal pads. Many women have never used a perineal pad or belt and will need instruction in using them during the postpartal period. (See Client Teach-

ing: Care of Episiotomy or Laceration.) Some women may prefer to use the pads designed for urinary incontinence. The pads are also highly absorbent and are usually self-adherent.

ICE PACK

If an episiotomy is performed at the time of birth or if a laceration occurs, an ice pack is generally applied to reduce edema and numb the tissues, which promotes comfort. In some agencies, chemical ice bags are used. These are usually activated by folding both ends toward the middle. Before applying the ice pack the nurse should ask the woman for permission and consider cultural norms when appropriate. Inexpensive ice bags can be made by filling a disposable glove with ice chips or crushed ice and then tying the top of the glove closed, like a balloon. The gloves should always be wrapped in either a cotton or disposable washcloth to prevent damage to the tissue from excessively cold temperatures. To protect the perineum from burns caused by contact with the ice pack, the disposable glove is first rinsed under running water to remove any powder that may be present and then wrapped in an absorbent towel or washcloth before it is placed against the perineum. To attain the maximum effect of this cold treatment, the ice pack should remain in place approximately 20 minutes and then be removed for about 10 minutes before it is replaced. Ice packs may be continued for as long as necessary. Usually, they are needed for the first 24 hours.

Teaching for Self-Care

The nurse provides information about the purpose of the ice pack, anticipated effects, benefits, possible problems, and ways of preparing an ice pack for home use if edema is present and early discharge is planned.

SITZ BATH

The warmth of the water in the sitz bath provides comfort, decreases pain, and increases circulation to the tissues, which promotes healing and reduces the incidence of infection. Sitz baths may be ordered three times daily (TID) or as needed (PRN). The nurse teaches the mother to fill the disposable sitz bath with water at 102F to 105F or a temperature that is comfortable for her. The nurse instructs the woman to remain in the sitz bath for 20 minutes. It is important for the woman to have a clean towel to pat dry her perineum after the sitz bath and to have a clean perineal pad ready to apply. The woman should be advised to pat her perineal area dry rather than use a more rigorous rubbing technique. The woman should rinse the sitz bath with clean warm water after each use.

Recently, cool sitz baths have gained popularity because they are effective in reducing perineal edema. Until definite research supports one temperature (warm or cold) as more effective, it may be best to offer the woman a choice.

Teaching for Self-Care

The nurse provides information about the purpose and use of the sitz bath, anticipated effects, benefits, possible problems, and safety measures to prevent injury from possible slipping or excessive water temperature. Home use of sitz baths may be recommended for the woman with an extensive episiotomy or laceration; the woman may use either the disposable sitz bath from the birthing unit or her clean bathtub. It is important for the nurse to emphasize that in using a bathtub, the woman should draw only 4 to 6 inches of water, assess the temperature of the water, and use the water only for the sitz, not for bathing. If the woman takes a tub bath, she should release the water, clean the tub, and draw new water before the sitz to prevent infection. The use of a handheld showerhead to irrigate the perineum is another way to cleanse and soothe the traumatized tissue.

TOPICAL AGENTS

Topical anesthetic agents may be used to relieve perineal discomfort. The woman is advised to apply the anesthetic agent after a sitz bath or perineal care. Anesthetic sprays, foams, ointments, or Tucks pads may be ordered for relief of both perineal and hemorrhoidal pain. It is important for the nurse to emphasize that the woman should wash her hands before and after using the topical treatments.

A Cochrane review of eight trials involving 976 women did not find evidence that topical anesthetics provided significantly more short-term relief than placebos (Hedayati, Parsons, & Crowther, 2005). Side effects were not formally measured, but no adverse effects were mentioned that required discontinuation of treatment. Although the scientific evidence supporting their use is not compelling and more research should be accomplished, many institutions do provide local anesthetics to women, and the mothers often anecdotally report increased comfort.

Teaching for Self-Care

The nurse provides information about the anesthetic spray or topical agent. The woman needs to understand the purpose, use, anticipated effects, benefits, and possible problems associated with the product. The nurse can combine an explanation with a demonstration of correct application. A return demonstration is a useful method of evaluating the woman's understanding.

Relief of Hemorrhoidal Discomfort

Some mothers experience hemorrhoidal pain after giving birth. Relief measures include the use of sitz baths, anesthetic ointments, rectal suppositories, or witch hazel pads applied directly to the anal area. Rectal suppositories should not be used by women who have had a fourth-degree laceration during birth.

TEACHING FOR SELF-CARE

The woman may find it helpful to maintain a side-lying position when possible or to tighten her buttocks when sitting down to reduce contact of the perineum with the seat and to avoid prolonged sitting. The mother is encouraged to maintain an adequate fluid intake and is given stool softeners to ensure greater comfort with bowel movements. The hemorrhoids usually disappear a few weeks after birth if the woman did not have them before her pregnancy.

Relief of Afterpains

Afterpains are the pain associated with intermittent uterine contractions that occur as the uterus contracts as it returns to its prepregnant state. A primipara may not notice afterpains, because her uterus is able to maintain a contracted state. Multiparous women and those who have had an overdistended uterus (due to multiple gestation or hydramnios) frequently experience discomfort from afterpains as the uterus intermittently contracts more vigorously. Breastfeeding women are also more likely to experience afterpains than formula-feeding women because of the release of oxytocin when the infant suckles. The nurse can suggest the woman lie prone with a small pillow under the lower abdomen, explaining that the discomfort may be intensified for about 5 minutes but then will diminish greatly, if not completely. The prone position applies pressure to the uterus and therefore stimulates contractions. When the uterus maintains a constant contraction, the afterpains cease. Additional nursing interventions include positioning, ambulation, or administration of an analgesic agent, such as Motrin (ibuprofen), Tylenol (acetaminophen), Tylenol No. 3 (codeine and acetaminophen) or Percocet (oxycodone and acetaminophen). The mother's description of the type and severity of her pain is usually the most reliable method of determining which analgesic agent will best promote the comfort she desires. Many women who are breastfeeding have concerns about the effects of medications on the infant. It is helpful to point out to concerned mothers that mild analgesics such as acetaminophen and ibuprofen pose little risk to their newborns when used judiciously in the short term to allow them the ability to bond and breastfeed in comfort.

TEACHING FOR SELF-CARE

The nurse provides information about the cause of afterpains and methods to decrease discomfort. The nurse also explains any medications that are ordered, expected effect, benefits, possible side effects, and any special considerations such as the possibility of dizziness or sleepiness with particular medications.

Relief of Discomfort from Immobility and Muscle Strain

Discomfort may also be caused by immobility and muscle strain. The woman who pushed for a long time during labor may experience muscular aches. It is not unusual for women to experience joint pains and discomfort in both arms and legs, depending on the effort they exerted during the second stage of labor. Early ambulation is encouraged to help reduce the incidence of complications such as constipation and thrombophlebitis. It also helps promote a general feeling of well-being.

The nurse assists the woman the first few times she gets up during the postpartal period. Fatigue, effects of medications, loss of blood, and possibly even lack of food may cause feelings of dizziness or faintness when the woman stands up. Because this may be a problem during the woman's first shower, the nurse should remain in the room, check the woman frequently, and have a chair close by in case she becomes faint. Dizziness may be aggravated by standing still and by the warmth of the water, so it is best to wait until the woman has shown stability when ambulating and has eaten. The first shower should be somewhat brief. On many postpartal units, ammonia inhalants (referred to as "smelling salts") are taped to the bathroom door for use in case of fainting. During this first shower the nurse instructs the woman in the use of the emergency call button in the bathroom; if she becomes faint during a future shower, she can call for assistance.

TEACHING FOR SELF-CARE

The nurse provides information about ambulation and the importance of monitoring any signs of dizziness or weakness. If she becomes dizzy, the woman should sit down and call for assistance.

Postpartal Diaphoresis

Postpartal diaphoresis (excessive perspiration) may cause discomfort for new mothers. The nurse can offer a fresh dry gown and bed linens to enhance comfort.

Some women may feel refreshed by a shower. It is important to consider cultural practices and realize that some women may prefer not to shower in the first few days following birth. For example, some Hispanic and Asian women prefer to delay showering. Nurses can offer these women a warm washcloth to increase maternal comfort. Because diaphoresis also may lead to increased thirst, the nurse can offer fluids as the woman desires. Again, cultural practices are important to consider. Women of western European background may prefer iced water; Asian women may prefer water at room temperature. The nurse should ascertain the woman's wishes rather than operate solely from the nurse's own values or cultural belief system.

TEACHING FOR SELF-CARE

The nurse provides information about the normal physiologic changes that cause diaphoresis and methods to increase comfort.

Suppression of Lactation in the Nonbreastfeeding Mother

For the woman who chooses not to breastfeed, lactation may be suppressed by mechanical inhibition. Previously, medications were administered to mothers who were not planning on breastfeeding. However, use of these medications was discontinued by the early 1990s because of the potential for adverse side effects. Signs of engorgement usually peak by day 4 and spontaneously resolve by the 10 day postpartum, regardless of treatment. Symptoms of engorgement can be minimized by beginning mechanical methods of lactation suppression as soon as possible after birth. Ideally, this involves having the woman begin wearing a supportive, well-fitting bra within 6 hours after birth. The bra is worn continuously until lactation is suppressed (usually about 7 to 14 days) and is removed only for showers. The bra provides support and eases the discomfort that can occur with tension on the breasts because of fullness.

A comparison of mothers using breast binders and mothers using support bras found that although both groups experienced some engorgement and discomfort that peaked on day 4, the mothers using breast binding reported more complaints of tenderness and milk leakage and required more pharmacologic pain relief measures. The authors recommended that the use of 24-hour support bras be encouraged and the use of breast binders be discouraged (Swift & Janke, 2003).

Although many women report increased comfort with the application of clean cold cabbage leaves and the application of cold compresses (such as bags of frozen vegetables wrapped in cloth), a Cochrane review of eight studies found anti-inflammatory drugs to be the only treatment that significantly improved symptoms (Snowden, Renfrew, & Woolridge, 2005). As noted by Swift & Janke (2003), most research in the past 15 years has focused on the breastfeeding mother, and additional research on the use of nonpharmacologic pain relief measures and methods of lactation suppression in nonbreastfeeding mothers is needed in order to give evidence-based advice to these women.

TEACHING FOR SELF-CARE

The mother is advised to avoid any stimulation of her breasts and nipples by her baby, herself, breast pumps, or her sexual partner until the sensation of fullness has passed (usually about 10 days). Such stimulation will increase milk production and delay the suppression process. Heat is avoided for the same reason, and the mother is encouraged to let shower water flow over her back rather than her breasts. The wearing of a 24-hour support bra, the use of analgesics as prescribed, and the use of cabbage leaves and/or cold compresses should be helpful during this period of time (American Academy of Pediatrics [AAP] & Ameri-

can College of Obstetricians and Gynecologists [ACOG], 2002). Suppression takes only a few days in most cases, but small amounts of milk may be produced up to a month after birth.

Pharmacologic Interventions

Pharmacologic preparations, including pain medications, vaccinations, and Rh immune globulin, are frequently administered in the postpartal period. (See Table 35–4.)

Table 35–4   ESSENTIAL INFORMATION FOR COMMON POSTPARTUM DRUGS

TYLENOL No. 3 (300 mg acetaminophen and 30 mg codeine)

Drug Class: Nonopioid analgesic/opioid analgesic combination.

Dose/Route: Usual adult dose: 1–2 tablets PO every 4 hours PRN.

Indication: For relief of mild to moderate pain.

Adverse Effects: Respiratory depression, apnea, light-headedness, confusion, sedation, dizziness, nausea, vomiting, sweating, dry mouth, constipation, hypotension, facial flushing, suppression of cough reflex, ureteral spasm, urinary retention, pruritus, hepatotoxicity (overdose).

Nursing Implications: Determine whether woman is sensitive to acetaminophen or codeine; has history of impaired hepatic or renal function. Assess pain before and 1 hour after administration. Monitor bowel sounds, respirations, urine output.

Administer with food or milk to minimize gastrointestinal (GI) upset; Warn client that it may cause drowsiness—assistance with newborn care and ambulation may be necessary.

Client Teaching: Inform client about name of drug, expected action, and possible side effects, ask if she has any questions.

Nursing Diagnoses Related to Drug Therapy: *Health-Seeking Behaviors:* Information regarding drug therapy.

Risk for injury related to side effects of drugs.

Constipation related to slowed gastrointestinal activity secondary to effects of medications.

PERCOCET 5/325 (325 mg acetaminophen and 5 mg oxycodone)

Drug Class: Nonopioid analgesic/opioid analgesic combination.

Dose/Route: 1–2 tablets PO every 4 hours PRN.

Indication: For moderate to severe pain. Can be used in aspirin-sensitive women.

Adverse Effects: Acetaminophen: Hepatotoxicity, headache, rash, and hypoglycemia.

Oxycodone: Respiratory depression, confusion, sedation, dizziness, blurred vision, apnea, circulatory depression, orthostatic hypotension, euphoria, facial flushing, sweating, constipation, dry mouth, nausea, vomiting, suppression of cough reflex, ureteral spasm, urinary retention.

Nursing Implications: Determine whether woman is sensitive to acetaminophen or codeine; has bronchial asthma; respiratory depression; convulsive disorder; adrenal insufficiency; renal, hepatic, or pulmonary disease.

Assess pain before and 1 hour after administration. Assess blood pressure, pulse, and respirations before and periodically during administration. Increase fluids and fiber, use stool softener to prevent constipation. Warn client that it may cause sedation—assistance with newborn care and ambulation may be necessary.

Observe woman carefully for respiratory depression if given with barbiturates or sedative/hypnotics or after epidural morphine. Consider that postcesarean-birth woman may have depressed cough reflex, so teaching and encouragement to deep breathe and cough are needed.

Monitor bowel sounds, urine and bowel elimination.

Client Teaching: Teaching should include name of drug, expected effect, possible adverse effects, whether the drug is secreted in the breast milk, encouragement to report any signs of adverse effects immediately.

Nursing Diagnoses Related to Drug Therapy: *Ineffective Breathing Pattern* related to respiratory depression.

Constipation related to slowed gastrointestinal activity secondary to the effects of medications.

RUBELLA VIRUS VACCINE, LIVE (Meruvax 2)

Dose/Route: Single-dose vial, inject subcutaneously in outer aspect of the upper arm.

Indication: Stimulate active immunity against rubella virus.

Adverse Effects: Burning, pain, or stinging at the injection site; fever; about 2–4 weeks later may have rash, malaise, sore throat, or headache.

Nursing Implications: Determine whether woman has sensitivity to neomycin (vaccine contains neomycin), eggs, or gelatin; is immunosuppressed or has received blood transfusions (not to be administered within 3 months of blood transfusion, plasma transfusion, or serum immune globulin). To be given at discharge. Recommend avoiding pregnancy for at least 4 weeks.

Client Teaching: Name of drug, expected effect, possible adverse effects, possible comfort measures to use if adverse effects occur; rubella titer will be assessed in about 3 months. Instruct woman to AVOID PREGNANCY FOR AT LEAST 4 WEEKS following vaccination. Provide information regarding contraceptives and their use.

Nursing Diagnoses Related to Drug Therapy: *Knowledge Deficit* regarding drug therapy. *Health-Seeking Behaviors: Information about Postpartum Contraception* related to an expressed desire to avoid pregnancy following rubella vaccination.

Pain related to rash and malaise.

RhoGAM (Rh immune globulin specific for D antigen)

Dose/Route: Postpartum: One vial (300 mcg) IM within 72 hours of birth. Additional vials may be necessary after fetal-maternal hemorrhage greater than 30 mL as indicated by lab results. Antepartal: One vial (300 mcg) RhoGAM IM at 28 weeks in Rh-negative women; after trauma, amniocentesis, spontaneous or therapeutic abortion, or ectopic pregnancy (50 mcg microdose vial if less than 13 weeks).

Indication: Prevention of sensitization to the Rh factor in Rh-negative women and to prevent hemolytic disease in the newborn in subsequent pregnancies. Mother must be Rh negative, not previously sensitized to Rh factor. Infant must be Rh positive, direct antiglobulin negative.

Adverse Effects: Soreness at injection site, anemia, fever. May decrease response to live virus vaccines such as rubella.

Nursing Implications: Confirm criteria for administration are present. Ensure correct vial is used for the client (each vial is cross-matched to the specific woman and must be carefully checked as with administration of blood products). Ensure client has not already been sensitized. Use cautiously in clients with hypersensitivity to immune globulins or thimerosal. If there is any doubt regarding the infant's blood type or lab studies, the medication should be given.

Inject entire contents of vial.

Client Teaching: Name of drug, expected action, possible side effects; report soreness at injection site to nurse; woman should carry information regarding Rh status and dates of RhoGAM injections with her at all times; explain use of RhoGAM with subsequent pregnancies.

Nursing Diagnoses Related to Drug Therapy: *Health-Seeking Behaviors:* Information about future need for Rh immune globulin related to an expressed desire to understand the long-term implications of her Rh-negative status.

Pain related to soreness at injection site.

Table 35–4   ESSENTIAL INFORMATION FOR COMMON POSTPARTUM DRUGS continued

Motrin, Advil (Ibuprofen)

Drug Class: nonopioid analgesic; nonsteroidal anti-inflammatory drug.

Dose/Route: 400 to 800 mg orally 3–4 times/day (use as an analgesic not to exceed 1200 mg/day; maximum total daily dose for short-term postpartum use may be 2400 mg/day).

Indication: Mild to moderate pain.

Adverse Effects: Headache, dizziness, drowsiness, blurred vision, tinnitus, GI bleeding, hepatitis, constipation, dyspepsia, nausea, vomiting, hematuria, renal failure, arrythmias, edema, hypertension, rashes, prolonged bleeding time, blood dyscrasias, allergic reactions including anaphylaxis.

Nursing Implications: Clients with asthma, aspirin-induced allergy, and nasal polyps are at increased risk for hypersensitivity. Assess pain before and 1 to 2 hours after administration. May cause prolonged bleeding time, which may persist for less than 1 day after discontinuation. Coadministration with opioid

analgesics may have additive effects and permit smaller doses. Administer with food, milk, or antacid to decrease GI upset. May cause drowsiness/dizziness—may require assistance with newborn care and ambulation.

Client Teaching: Name of drug, expected action, possible side effects. Encourage client to drink a full glass of water with medication and to remain upright for 15 to 30 minutes. Instruct not to take it on an empty stomach. Inform client that dosages prescribed for short-term postpartal use are higher than what is recommended for general over-the-counter use of ibuprofen. Ensure that client knows the trade names (Motrin, Advil, etc.) to avoid doubling up on doses. Client should consult with provider before taking other medications or herbal supplements concurrently.

Nursing Diagnosis Related to Drug Therapy: *Health-Seeking Behaviors:* Information regarding drug therapy.

Nausea related to side effects of medication.

SOURCES: Cunningham et al. (2005); Deglin & Vallerand (2005).

RUBELLA VACCINE

Women who are not rubella immune as determined by lab studies should receive the rubella vaccine early in the postpartum period. It is administered before discharge, even if she is breastfeeding (AAP & ACOG, 2002; Centers for Disease Control and Prevention, 2002). Administering the injection just after childbirth is advantageous because the woman is definitely not pregnant and typically does not want another pregnancy within the near future.

Teaching for Self-Care

The nurse needs to ensure that the woman understands the purpose of the vaccine and that she must avoid becoming pregnant for at least 4 weeks (Cunningham et al., 2005; Centers for Disease Control and Prevention, 2002). To ensure that the woman understands, an informed consent is usually signed before administration. Because avoiding pregnancy is so important, counseling regarding contraception is suggested.

RH IMMUNE GLOBULIN (RHOGAM)

All Rh-negative women with Rh-positive babies should receive Rh immune globulin (RhoGAM) within 72 hours after childbirth to prevent sensitization from a fetomaternal transfusion of Rh-positive fetal red blood cells (Cunningham, Leveno, Bloom et al., 2005). See discussion of criteria in Procedure 20–2. ∞

Teaching for Self-Care

The Rh-negative woman needs to understand the implications of her Rh-negative status in future pregnancies. (See Chapter 20 ∞ for a detailed discussion.) The nurse provides opportunities for questions during teaching.

Relief of Emotional Stress

The birth of a child, with the role changes and increased responsibilities it produces, is a time of emotional stress for the new mother. This stress is increased by the tremendous physiologic changes that occur as her body adjusts to a nonpregnant state. Nurses working in maternal-child care should read the works of Reva Rubin (1984) and Ramona Mercer (1986), two of the pioneers of maternal role attainment theory, to better un-

derstand this life transition. Their work is briefly discussed in Chapter 34. ∞

Callister (2004) notes that although nurses are adept at meeting the physiologic and teaching/learning needs of new mothers and their infants, they often overlook the importance of allowing and encouraging new mothers to tell their birth stories. Her study of women's birth stories from around the globe found that sharing the birth story helped a woman to integrate the event into the framework of her life; gave her the opportunity to share a significant experience with the nurse; allowed her the opportunity to discuss fears, concerns, and disappointment related to the event; helped her to understand her strengths; and helped her to feel connected with women across generations. Open-ended questions, active listening, clarification of events, acceptance of the woman's feelings, affirmation of her strengths, and emphasizing that there are no right or wrong answers will encourage the client to share her feelings and to process the event.

During the postpartal period, the mother must adjust to the loss of her fantasized child and accept the child she has borne. This may be more difficult if the child is not of the desired sex or has birth defects. Parents of newborns requiring special care due to congenital anomalies or prematurity will require extra attention and opportunities to share their concerns, fears, and disappointment.

Immediately following the birth (the taking-in period), the mother is dependent and focused inward on bodily concerns. During this time, teaching other than for self-care may not be totally effective. Because early discharge has become so common, however, the nurse should offer classes and information and provide printed handouts for reference as questions arise at home.

Once the woman's self-care needs have been met, her focus will shift to the care of her newborn and her ability as a parent (the taking-hold period). Skillful intervention by the nurse, with continual reassurance that the woman is a successful mother, is vital. During this time the mother is most receptive to teaching, and tactful instruction and demonstration assist her in developing mothering skills. The nurse must carefully avoid "taking over" the infant. By functioning as an adviser and allowing the mother to perform the actual care, the nurse demonstrates confidence in the mother's skill and ability, which in turn increases the mother's self-confidence about her effectiveness as a parent. Recognition and praise of her success help the mother develop feelings of competence in caring for her baby.

Usually the mother is discharged before the onset of mood disturbances and disorders associated with the postpartal period. These include postpartum "baby blues," true postpartum depression, and postpartum psychosis and are described in detail in Chapter 38. ∞

TEACHING FOR SELF-CARE

The nurse should advise the mother that physical, psychologic, and hormonal factors all influence an individual's response to childbirth. It is often helpful to discuss normal adaptations in the postpartum period with both the mother and her partner. This ensures that her partner will be aware of the normal patterns of psychologic responses in the early postpartum period. Normal responses include a brief period of irritability, mood swings, crying spells, and other mood-related symptoms often referred to as "baby blues." Symptoms are relatively mild, and women can be reassured that the emotional lability will be transient, usually resolving within 10 days (Cunningham et al., 2005). Women who experience a longer duration of symptoms should be advised to contact their physician or certified nurse-midwife. The nurse should advise families about symptoms of postpartum depression and emphasize the importance of seeking help should they occur. Anxiety, emotional lability, and irritability may be the presenting symptoms of postpartum depression. Additionally, feelings of loss of self, guilt and shame, eating/sleeping disturbances, and mental confusion may occur (Beck & Indman, 2005). Although there are currently no formal guidelines or evidence-based standards of care regarding how to best educate women about postpartum depression, there is a growing awareness of this entity. Providing anticipatory guidance and questioning women about symptoms at every healthcare contact is recommended (Garg, Morton, & Heneghan, 2005).

PROMOTION OF MATERNAL REST AND ACTIVITY

Following birth, some women feel exhausted and in need of rest. Other women are euphoric and full of psychic energy, ready to retell their experience of birth repeatedly. The nurse evaluates individual needs, always with the goal of providing opportunities for rest. The nurse can provide time for the excited, euphoric woman to air her feelings and then can encourage a period of rest. The nurse may also help the family limit visitors and provide a comfortable sleep chair or bed for the partner.

Relief of Fatigue

Physical fatigue often affects other adjustments and functions of the new mother. For example, there are relationships among fatigue, stress, postpartum depression, immune function, breast milk production, and breast milk biology (Groer, Davis, Casey et al., 2005). The mother requires energy to make the psychologic adjustments to a new infant and to assume new roles. She makes these adjustments more smoothly when she gets ade-

DEVELOPING CULTURAL COMPETENCE

TRADITIONS OF "LYING IN"

Women throughout Asia and Latin America observe a lying-in period after delivery where they rest, stay very warm, and avoid bathing and exercise. Pakistani and East Indian women often have a female family member provide all maternal and infant care except for breastfeeding, and they resist efforts to encourage them to learn or take part in self- and infant care. If they do not have a friend or family member available, they may expect intensive help from their nurse.

quate rest. The nurse can encourage rest by organizing activities to avoid frequent interruptions for the woman. If the new mother chooses, rest times may be arranged by having the newborn remain in the holding nursery for a period of time, or the mother can rest or sleep when the baby is sleeping in her room.

Although fatigue is a common experience for postpartum women, it is important to note that it declines in intensity over the first 2 weeks for most mothers. Persistent fatigue has been implicated as a risk factor for postpartum depression in more than one study. Maternal self-reports of fatigue and perceived stress at 14 days were found to be significantly associated with each other and with postpartum depression at the 28-day point (Corwin, Brownstead, Barton et al., 2005). Therefore, mothers should be counseled to utilize family and friends for support to ensure adequate rest for themselves after discharge and to seek help for fatigue that persists beyond the initial postpartum period.

Although most mothers feel fatigued, they tend to view themselves as healthy and well if they perceive pregnancy and birth as natural processes. Some mothers, however, view the postpartal period as a time of rest. Many cultures have distinct customs that are followed in the postpartum period. Nurses unfamiliar with certain cultural customs may find it stressful if they are expected to perform all maternal-infant care. Most cultural customs can be accommodated if they are not harmful.

TEACHING FOR SELF-CARE

Nearly all new mothers experience some degree of fatigue or sleep deprivation during the postpartum period. Women who have had a cesarean birth are coping with both the constant demands of the baby and their own recovery needs. The nurse should advise the mother to take frequent rest periods, to nap when the baby is napping, and to avoid performing unnecessary chores and activities. It is not uncommon for new mothers to attempt to "do it all" and end up feeling exhausted and irritable. Many women feel self-induced pressure to take care of household chores while the infant is napping. Once a woman becomes sleep deprived, it is difficult to "catch up." The nurse should advise the new mother to take naps and allow others to assist with household tasks. Well-wishing friends who call and ask if anything is needed can be encouraged to prepare a meal or pick up items at the grocery store. The woman will discover that friends and family are usually anxious to provide assistance. It is essential that the nurse help the mother to identify sources of support and to realize the necessity of requesting assistance as needed. Her energy can then be concentrated on caring for herself and the baby.

Resumption of Activity

Ambulation and activity may gradually increase after discharge. The new mother should avoid heavy lifting, excessive stair climbing, and strenuous activity. One or two daily naps are essential and are most easily achieved if the mother sleeps when her baby does.

By the second week at home, the new mother may begin some light housekeeping activities. Although it is customary to delay returning to work for 6 weeks, most women are physically able to resume practically all activities by 4 to 5 weeks when the lochia flow has stopped. Delaying returning to work until after the final postpartal examination will minimize the possibility of problems.

TEACHING FOR SELF-CARE

The nurse can provide the new mother with suggestions for resuming her normal level of activity. Women should be encouraged to limit the number of activities to prevent excessive fatigue, increase in lochia, and negative psychologic reactions, such as feeling overwhelmed. The nurse can encourage the new mother to avoid the temptation to catch up on housework during infant naps, but instead use the time to rest herself. If excessive fatigue or an increase in lochia occurs, the woman should increase rest periods and decrease extra activities.

Postpartal Exercises

The nurse should encourage the woman to begin simple exercises while in the birthing unit and continue them at home, advising her that increased lochia or pain means she should reevaluate her activity and make necessary reductions. Most agencies provide a booklet describing suggested postpartal activities. (Exercise routines vary for women undergoing tubal ligation following birth and for cesarean birth clients.) See Figure 35–1 ◆ for a description of some commonly used exercises. The postpartal woman is more likely to have positive views of her own well-being and less fatigue if she continues to do stretching and/or her own programmed pattern of exercise.

TEACHING FOR SELF-CARE

The nurse should advise the woman to begin Kegel exercises immediately after birth. The nurse can explain that these exercises will assist in returning vaginal tone and preventing urinary leakage. If no complications exist, normal exercise can be initiated at 2 weeks after birth. Women should be advised to take short walks outside if the weather is appropriate. Abdominal exercises can be suggested to retone the abdominal muscles. A regular exercise program including vigorous activities such as running, weight lifting, or competitive sports can usually be initiated after her 6-week postpartum examination or when approved by her physician or certified nurse-midwife.

PROMOTION OF FAMILY WELLNESS AND SHARED PARENTING

A satisfactory maternity experience may have a positive impact on the entire family. The new or expanding family who receives appropriate information and has adequate time to interact with its newest member in a supportive environment will feel more comfortable and secure at home.

In the past, newborns were typically separated from their parents immediately after birth. Today most facilities support **family-centered care,** which is focused on keeping the mother and baby together as much as the mother desires. **Mother-baby care,** or **couplet care** (care of both the mother and her baby), is an important part of the family-centered care approach, in which the infant remains at the mother's bedside and both are cared for by the same nurse. Couplet care allows the nurse to teach and role model and to integrate the entire family into the care of the woman and her infant. It also enables the mother to have time to bond with her baby and learn to care for him or her in a supportive environment. A Cochrane review of 17 studies found that **skin-to-skin contact** between the mother and baby where the naked baby is placed prone on the mother's chest during the first 24 hours has statistically significant positive effects on breastfeeding at 1 and 3 months postpartum (Anderson, Moore, Hepworth et al., 2005). This early contact also promotes bonding and should be encouraged. Many fathers welcome the opportunity to enjoy skin-to-skin contact with their newborns as well, particularly during the immediate recovery from cesarean section or if complications prevent the mother from doing so.

In a mother-baby unit, the newborn's crib is placed near the mother's bed, where she can see her baby easily. The crib should be a self-contained unit stocked with items the parents might require in providing care. A bulb syringe for suctioning the mouth or nares should always be accessible, and the mother and father/partner should be familiar with its use. The mother-baby unit is conducive to a self-demand feeding schedule for both breastfeeding and formula-feeding infants. It is essential that parents be oriented to the facility's infant security procedures and protocols to prevent infant abduction. This can be discussed in prenatal courses and upon admission to the birthing unit, and it will need to be reinforced when the infant begins rooming in.

Mothers are frequently very tired after birth, so the responsibility for providing total infant care could be overwhelming. The mother-baby policy must be flexible enough to permit the mother to return the baby to the nursery if she finds it necessary because of fatigue or physical discomfort. Some mother-baby units also offer return of the newborns to a central nursery at night so the mothers can get more rest. Many agencies have unlimited visiting hours for the father or significant others of the mother's choice. These opportunities to hold and care for the child promote paternal self-confidence and foster paternal attachment. Encouraging fathers to spend the night allows parents to share initial newborn care responsibilities while they still have the support of nursing staff if questions arise.

Figure 35–1 ◆ Postpartal exercises. Begin with 5 repetitions two or three times daily, and gradually increase to 10 repetitions. First day: *A,* Abdominal breathing. Lying supine, inhale deeply, using the abdominal muscles. The abdomen should expand. Then exhale slowly through pursed lips, tightening the abdominal muscles. *B,* Pelvic rocking. Lying supine with arms at sides, knees bent, and feet flat, tighten abdomen and buttocks, and attempt to flatten back on floor. Hold for a count of 10; then arch the back, causing the pelvis to "rock." On the second day, add *C,* Chin to chest. Lying supine with legs straight, raise head and attempt to touch chin to chest. Slowly lower head. *D,* Arm raises. Lying supine, arms extended at a 90-degree angle from body, raise arms so that they are perpendicular and hands touch. Lower slowly. On fourth day, add *E,* Knee rolls. Lying supine with knees bent, feet flat, arms extended to the side, roll knees slowly to one side, keeping shoulders flat. Return to original position, and roll to opposite side. *F,* Buttocks lift. Lying supine, arms at sides, knees bent, feet flat, slowly raise the buttocks, and arch the back. Return slowly to starting position. On sixth day, add *G,* Abdominal tighteners. Lying supine, knees bent, feet flat, slowly raise head toward knees. Arms should extend along either side of legs. Return slowly to original position. *H,* Knee to abdomen. Lying supine, arms at sides, bend one knee and thigh until foot touches buttocks. Straighten leg and lower it slowly. Repeat with other leg. After 2 to 3 weeks, more strenuous exercises, such as sit-ups and side leg raises, may be added as tolerated. Kegel exercises, begun antepartally, should be done many times daily during postpartum to restore vaginal and perineal tone.

A metasynthesis of qualitative research focusing on fatherhood during the early months found that fathers entered the experience with certain expectations and intentions, confronted a reality much different than expected, worked to create their own role as a father, and finally reaped benefits. Although fathers initially held positive views of parenting and wanted to be engaged with their infants, they soon realized that life changed greatly after the birth and that many of their expectations were unrealistic. They did not always immediately bond with their baby, they realized that parenting entailed a huge responsibility, and they often felt helpless and inadequate, particularly if their baby was breastfed. These fathers reported postponing parts of the paternal-infant relationship until weaning occurred. Fathers often felt isolated, without role models or support persons to whom they could turn. Many of them changed their expectations and worked hard to become adept and involved in the care and lives of their infants. Mothers who encouraged paternal involvement strengthened the relationship, and fathers reported emotional rewards related to increased involvement with their infants once the infants responded to them (Goodman, 2005). Although our culture idealistically and theoretically supports involved fathers, new fathers often lack role models, support, and resources. It is imperative that all teaching in the family-centered care unit be directed to both parents at times that are convenient for both and that fathers be encouraged to share their feelings and be actively involved in the childbearing experience. It is also helpful to provide anticipatory guidance for fathers regarding the feelings and situations they may experience, particularly if their baby is breastfed. Encouraging fathers to be involved in infant bathing, the bedtime routine, holding, cuddling, and playing will allow them to develop a relationship and reap the rewards they desire.

Reactions of Siblings

Sibling visitation helps meet the needs of both the siblings and their mother. A visit to the hospital reassures children that their mother is well and still loves them. It also provides an opportunity for the children to become familiar with the new baby. For the mother, the pangs of separation are lessened as she interacts with her children and introduces them to the newest family member.

Most agencies now recognize the importance of providing siblings with opportunities to see their mother and meet the infant during the early postpartal period (Figure 35–2 ◆). Approaches to this issue vary from specified visiting hours for siblings to unlimited visiting privileges.

TEACHING FOR SELF-CARE

Although the parents have prepared the child for the presence of a new brother or sister, the actual arrival of the infant requires some adjustments. Some children may be present for the birth and have an opportunity to spend time with their new sibling and their parents immediately following the birth. They may even remain throughout the woman's hospitalization, especially if it is brief, and all go home as a family.

For the mother who is returning home to small children, it is often helpful to have the father carry the new baby inside. This practice keeps the mother's arms free to hug and hold her older children. She thereby reaffirms her love for them before

Figure 35–2 ◆ The sister of this newborn becomes acquainted with the new family member.
SOURCE: © Stella Johnson (www.stellajohnson.com).

introducing them to their new sibling. Many mothers have found that bringing a doll home with them for the older child is helpful. The child cares for the doll alongside his or her parents, thereby identifying with the parent. This identification helps decrease anger and the need to regress to get attention.

Often older children enjoy working with the parents to care for the newborn. Involvement in care helps the older child develop a sense of closeness to the baby. It also helps the child learn acceptable behavior toward the newborn, feel a sense of accomplishment, and develop tenderness and caring. With constant supervision and assistance as necessary, even very young children can hold the baby or a bottle during feeding.

Regression is a common occurrence even when siblings have been well prepared. The nurse can provide anticipatory guidance so that parents do not become overly upset if their previously toilet-trained child begins to have accidents or requests a bottle.

Regardless of age, an older sibling needs reassurance that he or she is still special to the parents, a truly loved and valued family member. Words of love and praise coupled with hugs and kisses are very important. So, too, is special parent-child time. Both parents should spend quality time in a one-to-one experience with each of their older children. This may require some careful planning, but its worth cannot be overestimated. It confirms the parents' love for the child and often helps the child accept the new baby.

The child, especially one of the opposite sex from the newborn, may raise queries about the appearance of the genitals as compared to his or her own. A simple explanation, such as, "That's what little girls (boys) look like," is often sufficient.

Resumption of Sexual Activity

Nursing interventions in the postpartal period acknowledge that each parent is also a sexual being. Couples were formerly discouraged from engaging in sexual intercourse until 6 weeks postpartum. Currently, the couple is advised to abstain from intercourse until the episiotomy is healed and the lochial flow has stopped (usually by the third to sixth week postpartum). During this period, couples can be encouraged to express their affection

RESEARCH IN PRACTICE

CESAREAN SECTION AND POSTNATAL SEXUAL HEALTH

What is this study about? It is commonly thought that cesarean birth protects sexual function after childbirth, given that perineal trauma is avoided. The protection of sexual function is one rationale given for elective cesarean birth, and these assumptions may contribute to a high cesarean birth rate. Yet little evidence exists regarding the long-term outcomes of cesarean birth, and research about sexual health is particularly lacking. These researchers sought to compare the postnatal sexual health of women who underwent cesarean birth with that of women who experienced vaginal birth.

How was this study done? Data were collected from 796 women giving birth to a live infant at a British teaching hospital over a 6-month period. Only primipara mothers were included in the study to avoid the effects of a previous birth on sexual function. Women were sent a paper questionnaire through the mail 3 and 6 months after the birth. The survey asked the women if they had resumed sexual intercourse, and were asked to describe any sexual problems compared to their prepregnancy sexual health. The mothers were asked specifically about nine sexual problems relative to pain, sexual desire, vaginal complications, or bleeding. Four hundred and eighty four women returned the survey, representing a 61% response rate. One quarter of those returning the survey had a cesarean birth. Tests of relative risk were used to compare characteristics between the two groups.

What were the results of the study? The primary problems reported at 3 months by these women were related to intercourse-related pain, sexual responsiveness, and postcoital problems. Comparing the proportion of women reporting these three groups of problems, mothers with cesarean birth were less affected than those who experienced a vaginal birth. However, only the differences related to pain were statistically significant. The size of these differences increased when specific subgroups were compared. Mothers with instrument-assisted vaginal birth fared the worst, whereas women with cesarean birth reported the fewest problems. There were no differences in sexual function problems between elective and emergent cesarean birth. At 6 months, the proportion reporting each group of problems was statistically equal in the cesarean and vaginal birth groups.

What additional questions might I have? How would these results be different if multiparous mothers had been included? Is there a concern about the accuracy of self-reporting of sexual functioning?

How can I use this study? Contrary to popular assumption, women who experience cesarean birth do not avoid problems associated with postnatal sexual function. Nurses can use this information in preparing teaching plans relative to sexual health in the postpartum period. Women who consider elective cesarean birth based on a rationale of improved postnatal sexual functioning need accurate information about realistic expectations.

Barrett, G., Peacock, J., Victor, C., & Manyonda, I. (2005). Cesarean section and postnatal sexual health. *Birth, 32*(4), 306–311.

---

and love through kissing, holding, and talking. Since postpartum women often experience vaginal dryness due to hormonal changes, some form of lubrication, such as K-Y jelly, may initially be necessary during intercourse. This may continue throughout the period of lactation in breastfeeding mothers because of lower estrogen levels. The female-superior or side-by-side positions for coitus may be preferable because they enable the woman to control the depth of penile penetration.

Breastfeeding couples should be forewarned that during orgasm, milk may spout from the nipples because of the release of oxytocin. Some couples find this pleasurable or amusing; other couples choose to have the woman wear a bra during sexual activity. Breastfeeding the baby before lovemaking may reduce the chance of milk release.

Other factors may inhibit satisfactory sexual experience. The baby's crying may "spoil the mood," the woman's changed body may be unattractive to her or to her partner, and maternal sleep deprivation may interfere with a mutually satisfying experience. Couples may also be frustrated if there are decreased libido or other changes in the woman's physiologic response to sexual stimulation. These changes are due to hormonal changes and may persist for several months.

Maternal fatigue is often a significant factor limiting the resumption of sexual intercourse. Consequently, couples should be encouraged to find a time for lovemaking when both are interested and awake. While interest and desire vary, most couples resume sexual activity within 3 months.

Anticipatory guidance during the prenatal and postnatal periods can forewarn the couple of these eventualities and of their temporary nature. See Client Teaching: Resuming Sexual Activity after Childbirth.

TEACHING FOR SELF-CARE

The nurse should discuss normal sexual changes that frequently occur in the postpartum period. A discussion that includes both partners can facilitate an open dialog between them and can provide an opportunity for questions and answers.

Contraception

Because many couples resume sexual activity before the postpartal examination, family-planning information should be made available before discharge. A couple's decision to use a contraceptive is often motivated by a desire to gain control over the number of children they will conceive or to determine the spacing of future children. In choosing a specific method, consistency of use outweighs the absolute reliability of a given method. The nurse must identify risk factors and contraindications of the various methods to help the couple select a contraceptive method that has practical application and is compatible with the couple's health and physical needs.

CLIENT TEACHING Resuming Sexual Activity after Childbirth

CLIENT GOALS At the completion of the teaching, the couple will be able to:

1. Discuss the changes in the woman's body that affect sexual activity.

2. Formulate alternative approaches to sexual activity based on an understanding of these changes.

3. Identify the length of time it is advisable to wait before resuming sexual activity.

4. Discuss information needed to make contraceptive choices.

TEACHING PLAN

CONTENT

- Present information about changes that may affect sexual activity, including the following:
  - Tenderness of the vagina and perineum
  - Presence of lochia and the healing process
  - Dryness of the vagina
  - Breast tenderness/escape of milk during sex
  - Fatigue

- Discuss healing at the placental site and stress that the presence of lochia indicates that healing is not yet complete. Explain that vaginal dryness may pose a problem because of postpartal hormonal changes. Dryness may be prolonged if woman is breastfeeding, because of low estrogen levels. This can be managed by using a water-soluble lubricant. In most cases, coitus can resume at some point after 2 weeks, depending on the woman's comfort and desire (Cunningham et al., 2005). Explain that escape of milk during sexual activity can be minimized by breastfeeding the baby immediately beforehand.

- Discuss the importance of contraception during the early postpartal period. Provide information on the advantages and disadvantages of different methods, including special considerations for breastfeeding mothers. The woman's body needs adequate time to heal and recover from the stress of pregnancy and childbirth. Couples who are opposed to contraception may choose abstinence at this time.

- Discuss the impact of fatigue and the new baby's schedule on the woman's feelings of desire. Refer the couple to a physician or certified nurse-midwife for additional information if needed.

TEACHING METHOD

Discussion is a logical approach. It may be useful to make a universal statement and link it with a question to determine a couple's initial level of knowledge. For example, "Many women experience vaginal dryness when they resume intercourse for the first several weeks after childbirth. Are you familiar with this change and the cause for it?" Use the information gained during this discussion to determine the depth to which to cover the material.

Provide printed information to clarify content and serve as a resource for the couple following discharge.

Provide samples of different types of contraceptives.

Provide literature on specific contraceptive methods.

Many couples are unprepared for the impact of fatigue and the baby's schedule on lovemaking.

Information enables the couple to anticipate this impact.

EVALUATION

Determine the couple's learning by providing time for discussion and questions. If the couple indicates that they plan to use a particular contraceptive method, you may ask them about aspects of the method to ascertain that they have correct and complete information.

DOCUMENTATION

Documentation of client teaching should include the teaching information discussed, the client's verbalization of understanding, specific interventions or warning signs that were given, along with the client's understanding of follow-up if needed in the future.

Often different methods of contraception are appropriate at different times in the couple's life. Thus they should have a clear understanding of all of the methods available to them so that they can make an appropriate choice. The currently available contraceptive methods are discussed in detail in Chapter 5. ∞

TEACHING FOR SELF-CARE

The nurse should discuss available contraceptive methods with both partners before discharge. Written information should also be provided for the couple to refer to at a later time. The nurse should stress the fact that pregnancy can occur before the first menstrual period returns and that contraception before that time is imperative. The nurse should be frank and open with the couple, answering questions as needed.

Parent-Infant Attachment

Nursing interventions to enhance the quality of parent-infant attachment should be designed to promote feelings of well-being, comfort, and satisfaction. Table 35–5 describes parental attachment behaviors and those that require further assessment. Following are some suggestions for ways of achieving this.

- Determine the childbearing and childrearing goals of the infant's mother and father, and adapt them wherever possible in planning nursing care for the family. This includes considering cultural preferences, and giving the parents choices about their labor and birth experience and their initial time with their new infant.
- Postpone eye prophylaxis for 1 hour after birth to facilitate eye contact between parents and their newborn (eye ointment further clouds the newborn's vision and makes eye contact difficult for the baby).
- Provide private time in the first hour after birth for the new family to become acquainted. Encourage skin-to-skin contact between mother (or father) and baby to promote breastfeeding and bonding.
- Arrange the healthcare setting so that the individual nurse-client relationship can be developed and maintained. A primary nurse can develop rapport and assess the mother's strengths and needs.
- Encourage the mother to tell her birth story. Clarify information for the mother as necessary.
- Encourage the parents to involve the siblings in integrating the infant into the family by bringing them to the birthing center for sibling visits.

- Use anticipatory guidance from conception through the postpartal period to prepare the parents for expected problems of adjustment.
- Include parents in any nursing intervention, planning, and evaluation. Give choices whenever possible.
- Initiate and support measures to alleviate fatigue in the parents.
- Help parents identify, understand, and accept both positive and negative feelings related to the birth, newborn, and overall parenting experience.
- Support and assist parents in determining the personality and unique needs of their infant.

Whenever possible and culturally acceptable, the mother and father should be allowed to care for their baby. This practice gives them a chance to learn their newborn's normal patterns and develop confidence in caring for him or her. It also allows them to spend more uninterrupted time with their infant in the first days of life. Early discharge may be advantageous if mother and baby are doing well, help is available for the mother at home, and the family and certified nurse-midwife or physician agree.

The nurse may observe beginnings of parent-newborn attachment in the first few hours after birth, and when continuing assessments during home visits after discharge. As the nurse assesses attachment, it is important to remember that cultural values, beliefs, and practices will direct child care activities and self-care practices. For example, Vietnamese parents may provide basic care for their infants but refuse to cuddle and show intense interest in them. This reflects their belief that drawing attention to their newborn may attract spirits that will "steal" the newborn by death, and it demonstrates their love and concern for the baby, not their disinterest. Although involving fathers is important in Westernized family centered care, fathers from some Middle Eastern countries do not involve themselves in the

Table 35–5	PARENT ATTACHMENT BEHAVIORS	
Assessment Area	**Attachment**	**Behavior Requiring Assessment and Information**
Care taking	Talks with baby. Demonstrates and seeks eye-to-eye contact. Touches and holds baby "en face." Changes diapers when needed. Baby is clean. Clothing is appropriate for room temperature. Feeds baby as needed, and baby is gaining weight. Positions baby comfortably and checks on baby.	Does not refer to baby. Completes activities without addressing the baby or looking at the baby. Lack of interaction. Does not recognize need for or demonstrate concern for baby's comfort or needs. Feeding occurs intermittently. Baby does not gain weight. Waits for baby to cry and then hesitates to respond.
Perception of the baby	Has knowledge of expected child development. Understands that the baby is dependent and cannot meet parent's needs. Accepts sex of child and characteristics.	Has unrealistic expectations of the baby's abilities and behaviors. Expects love and interaction from the baby. Believes that the baby will fulfill parent's needs. Is strongly distressed over sex of baby or feels that some aspect of the baby is unacceptable.
Support	Has friends who are available for support. Seems to be comfortable with being a parent. Has realistic beliefs of parenting role.	Is alone or isolated. Is on edge, tense, anxious, and hesitant with the baby. Demonstrates difficulty incorporating parenting with own wants and needs.

Please note: These are a few of the behaviors that may be associated with attachment. It is vitally important for the nurse to observe the parents on more than one occasion and to take into consideration individual characteristics, values, beliefs, and customs.

care of infants and young children (Galanti, 2004). Nurses should respect cultural norms and incorporate them into the care of the newborn whenever possible.

TEACHING FOR SELF-CARE

Some parents, especially first-time parents, may feel awkward in their new role. George (2005) found themes of a sense of overwhelming responsibility, confusion regarding role expectations, and the need to reorganize and reprioritize everything in their lives among first-time mothers. It is helpful for the nurse to advise parents that they may experience these feelings as they grow into the parental role and alter their family processes to accommodate the new family member. The nurse should also provide reassurance and advise new parents of normal infant behavior and activity. The nurse assesses attachment before discharge. If the nurse identifies a possible alteration in attachment, the parents can be referred to a new parent support group, parenting classes, or counseling to assist them with their transition into their new roles. The nurse can explain that new attachments are being formed, and like all new relationships, both the infant and the parents are discovering each other. The nurse should discuss possible risk factors of altered attachment such as inability or lack of desire to care for the infant.

NURSING CARE FOLLOWING CESAREAN BIRTH

Preliminary data for 2003 showed a cesarean delivery rate of 27.6% (Martin, Kochanek, Strobino et al., 2005). Nurses need to be adept at addressing the special needs of this growing population of clients. After a cesarean birth, the new mother has postpartal needs similar to those of women who gave birth vaginally. Because she has undergone major abdominal surgery, however, the woman also has nursing care needs similar to those of other surgical clients.

Promotion of Maternal Physical Well-Being after Cesarean Birth

Immobility after the use of narcotic and sedative agents and alterations in the immune response of postoperative clients increase the chances of pulmonary infection. For this reason, the woman is encouraged to cough and deep breathe and to use incentive spirometry every 2 to 4 hours while awake for the first few days following cesarean birth.

Immobility increases the risk of abdominal distention and discomfort, blood clots, deep vein thrombosis, and pulmonary

---

EVIDENCE-BASED PRACTICE

PARENTHOOD EXPERIENCES DURING THE CHILD'S FIRST YEAR

Clinical Question

How can the nurse support mothers and fathers in the experience of parenthood in the first year?

The Evidence

Two researchers conducted an integrative review of qualitative, quantitative, and mixed-method studies. Included were studies that described fathers', mothers', or parents' experiences from the first year of the child's life. Parents could be either experienced or first-time parents. Adolescent parents, ill children, and ill parents were excluded. Application of a systematic search strategy resulted in evaluation of 33 articles. Sixteen studies were qualitative, 14 were quantitative, and 3 were mixed methods. Themes and patterns were identified through statistical and thematic analysis.

What Is Effective?

New parents found the experience of having a baby a profound, life-transforming event. The primary theme identified across these studies was a sense of being overwhelmed. Mothers and fathers both identified the benefits of parenthood, and a sense of being satisfied with the experience. They also reported feeling an overwhelming sense of responsibility for the child, which can cause strain. Mothers described feeling fatigued, drained, and having difficulty finding any time for self-care. Fathers expressed concern about living up to new family demands, but identified with the role of family protector

and provider. Parents reported that assistance in learning how to cope with the added strain was needed.

What Is Unclear?

There were no well-done interventional studies in this analysis. The results are descriptive, as the nursing interventions suggested in the review have not been tested objectively with randomized trials. This evidence should be classified as expert opinion rather than a systematic review.

Best Practice

The nurse should plan interventions that will help the family minimize the experience of strain. Because the primary theme of this experience is a sense of being overwhelmed, the nurse can help the family find resources to support their needs during this demanding time. The authors suggest development of Internet-based resources for the parents during the first year. Access to Internet resources should involve both critical information and support groups, such as chat rooms and discussion boards. Nurses have to provide supportive strategies for both parents, including those that foster fathering and that help women deal with fatigue.

Critical Thinking

What kinds of strategies can help a mother deal with the effects of fatigue? What interventions can support fathering skills?

REFERENCE: Nystrom, K., & Ohrling, K. (2004). Parenthood experiences during the child's first year: Literature review. *Journal of Advanced Nursing, 46*(3), 319–330.

embolisms. Within the first 12 hours postoperatively, unless medically contraindicated, the woman should be assisted to dangle her legs on the side of the bed. The woman should be assisted out of bed within 24 hours. Ambulation should be encouraged at least two to three times a day.

The nurse continues to assess the woman's pain level and provide relief measures as needed. Sources of pain include incisional pain, gas pain, referred shoulder pain, periodic uterine contractions (afterpains), and pain from voiding, defecation, or constipation.

Nursing interventions are oriented toward preventing or alleviating pain or helping the woman cope with pain. The nurse should undertake the following measures:

- Administer analgesic medications as needed, especially during the first 24 to 72 hours. Their use will relieve the woman's pain and enable her to be more mobile and active.
- Promote comfort through proper positioning, backrubs, oral care, and the reduction of noxious stimuli, such as noise and unpleasant odors.
- Encourage the presence of significant others, including other children, and the newborn. This provides distraction from the painful sensations and helps reduce the woman's fear and anxiety. The presence of a significant other provides a watchful presence over the newborn, allowing the baby to stay in the room with the mother while she may not be alert enough to be responsible for this if left alone.
- Encourage the use of breathing, relaxation, and distraction techniques (for example, stimulation of cutaneous tissue) taught in childbirth preparation class.
- Encourage adequate rest periods. This may include limiting excessive visitors and phone calls.
- Encourage early ambulation to prevent abdominal distention that can occur with excess accumulation of gas in the intestines.

Epidural analgesia administered just after the cesarean birth is an effective method of pain relief for most women in the first 24 hours following birth (see Drug Guide: Postpartum Epidural Morphine).

The physician may prescribe **patient-controlled analgesia (PCA).** With this approach, the woman is given a bolus of analgesia, often morphine, at the beginning of therapy. Using a special IV pump system, the woman presses a button to self-administer small doses of the medication as needed. For safety, the pump is preset with a time lockout so that the pump cannot deliver another dose until a specified time has elapsed. Women using PCA feel less anxious and have a greater sense of control with less dependence on the nursing staff. The frequent smaller doses help the woman experience rapid pain relief without grogginess and also eliminate the discomfort of injections. As with any drug therapy, the nurse will monitor the client for side effects and intervene as necessary.

If general anesthesia was used, abdominal distention from the accumulation of gas in the intestines may produce discomfort for the woman during the first postpartal days. Additional measures to prevent or minimize gas pains include leg exercises, abdominal tightening, avoiding carbonated or very hot or cold beverages, and avoiding the use of straws. The woman may find it helpful to lie prone or on her left side. Lying on the left side allows gas to rise from the descending colon to the sigmoid colon so that it can be expelled more readily. Other women report that a rocking chair helps them obtain relief. Medical interventions for gas pain include the use of antiflatulents (such as Mylicon), suppositories, and enemas.

The nurse can minimize discomfort and promote satisfaction as the mother assumes the activities of her new role. Instruction and assistance in assuming comfortable positions when holding or breastfeeding the infant will do much to increase the mother's sense of competence and comfort. Sitting in a chair or tailor fashion in bed, leaning slightly forward with the infant propped on a pillow in her lap, will prevent irritation to the incision. Use of the football hold and side-lying positions may be most comfortable for breastfeeding during the initial postoperative course.

By the first or second day after the cesarean birth, the mother is usually receptive to learning how to care for herself and her infant. Demonstration of proper body mechanics in getting out of bed without the use of a side rail and ways of caring for the infant that prevent strain and torsion on the incision are also indicated. The nurse needs to place special emphasis on home management, encouraging the woman to let others assume responsibility for housekeeping and cooking. Fatigue not only prolongs recovery but also interferes with breastfeeding and mother-infant interaction.

The woman usually does extremely well postoperatively. If spinal or epidural anesthesia was used, the side effects of general anesthesia are absent. Even after general anesthesia, however, most women are ambulating by the day after the surgery. Usually by the second postpartal day, the incision can be covered with plastic wrap so the woman can shower, which seems to provide a mental as well as physical lift. If staples have been used, the incision is sometimes left open to the air, and showering is permitted without covering it. Most women are discharged on the third postoperative day.

Research suggests that women with cesarean births have several special needs following discharge: increased need for rest and sleep; incisional care; assistance with household chores, infant care, and self-care; and relief of pain and discomfort. Nurses need to address these areas during hospitalization and discharge planning. Perhaps one of the most important considerations for cesarean birth mothers is the need to plan for additional assistance at home to enable the new mother to rest and heal.

TEACHING FOR SELF-CARE

The nurse can assist the woman in identifying interventions to relieve discomfort or pain. The woman should be encouraged to take pain medication regularly, engage in frequent rest periods, avoid prolonged activity, and observe for signs of "overdoing it" (such as discomfort and fatigue). The nurse should advise the woman that recovery after a surgical procedure involves healing time and that fatigue and soreness are common symptoms of too much activity too quickly. The nurse can assist the family in

DRUG GUIDE   Postpartum Epidural Morphine

Overview of Obstetric Action

Epidural morphine is used to provide relief of pain associated with cesarean births, extensive episiotomies, or third- and fourth-degree lacerations. Epidural morphine pain relief results directly from its effect on the cerebral and spinal opiate receptors (it depresses pain impulse transmission). Morphine binds opiate receptors, thereby altering both the perception of and emotional response to pain. Women experience little or no discomfort or pain during recovery and for up to 24 hours afterward. There is no motor or sympathetic block. Onset of analgesia is slower than with fentanyl, but duration is longer.

Route, Dosage, and Frequency

Five milligrams of morphine is injected through a catheter into the epidural space by the anesthesia provider, providing pain relief for about 24 hours. If a second dose is required (up to a total of 10 mg/24 hr), the dose would be given by the anesthesia provider (not postpartum nurses).

Maternal Contraindications

Allergy/hypersensitivity to morphine.

Maternal Side Effects

Most common: pruritus, urinary retention, nausea, and vomiting.

Late-onset respiratory depression (rare but may occur 8–12 hours after administration).

Confusion, sedation, headache, hypotension, bradycardia, and flushing are possible. Side effects can be managed with naloxone.

Neonatal Effects

More research is needed.

Nursing Considerations

* Obtain history: sensitivity (allergy) to morphine.
* Assess vital signs, orientation, level of consciousness, motor function, sensation, reflexes, skin color, breath sounds, depth and rate of respirations, catheter insertion site, and ability to void (unless Foley in place).
* Monitor and evaluate analgesic effect. Ask client about comfort level and notify anesthesiologist of inadequate pain relief.
* Check catheter (if still present) to ensure it is intact and not leaking.
* Assess for pruritus (scratching and rubbing, especially around face and neck).
* Administer comfort measures for narcotic-induced pruritus, such as lotion, backrubs, cool/warm packs, or diversional activities. Give prn medications as prescribed if needed.
* If allergic reaction (urticaria, edema, or respiratory difficulties) occurs, administer naloxone or diphenhydramine per physician standing order.
* Provide comfort measures for nausea/vomiting, such as frequent oral hygiene or gradual increase of activity; administer prescribed prn medications as needed.
* Assess postural blood pressure and heart rate before ambulation.
* Assist client with her first ambulation and then as needed.
* Provide assistance/supervision with newborn care.
* Assess respiratory function every 1 to 2 hours for 24 hours, then every 2 to 8 hours as needed. Also assess level of consciousness and mucous membrane color. May need to monitor client via apnea monitor for 24 hours.
* Assess bladder for distention if unable to void. Assist client to void. Catheterization may be necessary if unresolved.
* Inform client that headaches related to epidurals are uncommon, but occasionally occur 2 to 5 days after administration. Bed rest in a quiet dark room, caffeine, and hydration may help. Call anesthesia provider as needed. Blood patch can be administered by anesthesia if unresolved.

SOURCES: Cunningham et al., 2005; Deglin & Vallerand, 2005; Nystedt, Edvardsson, & Willman, 2004; Roman & Cabaj, 2005.

---

identifying resources for assisting the new mother at home, such as assistance from friends and family, cleaning services, or food delivery services.

Promotion of Parent-Infant Interaction after Cesarean Birth

Many factors associated with cesarean birth may hinder successful and frequent maternal-infant interaction. These include the physical condition of the mother and newborn and maternal reactions to stress, anesthesia, and medications. The mother and her infant may be separated after birth because of hospital routines, prematurity, or neonatal complications. A healthy infant born by an uncomplicated cesarean birth is no more fragile than an infant born vaginally. Many agencies are beginning to provide time for the family together in the operating room if the mother's and infant's conditions permit, but some agencies still automatically place cesarean birth newborns in a high-risk nursery for a time.

Signs of depression, anger, or withdrawal in the cesarean birth mother may indicate a grief response to the loss of the fantasized vaginal birth experience. Fathers as well as mothers may experience feelings of "missing out," guilt that the surgery was the result of something they did "wrong," and even jealousy toward another couple who had a vaginal birth. The cesarean birth couple may also feel guilty that they are considering their personal needs and not simply the welfare of the infant.

Newborn Safety Following Cesarean Birth

One of the primary concerns regarding the nursing care of the couplet is the promotion of safety. Mothers who have experienced cesareans, particularly unanticipated ones that follow lengthy labors, may be fatigued, sleep deprived, and under the influence of medications that alter their level of consciousness. Vigilant attention must be paid to the mother's level of awareness and ability to stay awake when holding her infant, providing care, and

RESEARCH IN PRACTICE

EARLY COMPARED WITH DELAYED ORAL FLUIDS AND FOOD AFTER CESAREAN SECTION

What is this study about? Food and fluids are frequently withheld after abdominal surgery for a set period of time or until the return of propulsive bowel sounds or the passing of flatus or stool. There are wide variations in practice regarding this issue following cesareans, ranging from early introduction to delays of 24 hours or more. Therefore, a review was completed to assess the effect of early versus delayed introduction of food and fluids following cesarean sections.

How was this study done? The authors reviewed six clinical trials comparing the effect of early versus delayed introduction of fluids and/or food on clinical outcome measures such as nausea, vomiting, crampy abdominal pain, bloating, abdominal distention, bowel action on day 3, return of bowel sounds and action, ketosis, blood sugars, duration of intravenous fluids, breastfeeding success, client satisfaction, fatigue, need for analgesia, ambulation, and time spent in hospital. Early introduction was defined by the individual researchers in each trial—usually within 6 to 8 hours or less.

What were the results of the study? The trials found no evidence to justify standing policies that restrict oral fluids or food following uncomplicated cesarean sections. Early introduction was associated with reduced time to first food intake, reduced time to return of bowel sounds, reduced postoperative hospital stay (after regional anesthetics), and a trend toward reduced abdominal distention. No significant differences were found with respect to nausea, vomiting, time to bowel action, time to passing flatus, paralytic ileus, and number of postoperative analgesic doses. No data were available on outcome measures such as duration of intravenous hydration, biochemical changes, client satisfaction, fatigue, and breastfeeding. The authors point out that although the review does not include large enough numbers to exclude the possibility of a rare adverse event related to early introduction, all outcomes showing significant differences are in favor of the early introduction of fluids and food.

What additional questions might I have? How does the withholding of fluids and food affect nutrition and postoperative tissue healing? How does the withholding of fluids and food affect the mother's perception of the event and her energy level, particularly in cases where cesarean section followed a long labor?

How can I use this study? Because early introduction of fluids and food has not been shown to cause problems and may even speed recovery, nurses should initiate discussions and change regarding policies and standing orders that restrict fluids and food after uncomplicated cesarean sections. Because standing orders often allow introduction of fluids and food as tolerated, the nurse should offer them as the client desires, not according to preconceived ideas or dated practices. The nurse can reassure postoperative clients that fluids and foods can be consumed as desired and tolerated without fear of adverse consequences.

Mangesi, L., & Hofmeyr, G. J. (2005). Early compared with delayed oral fluids and food after cesarean section. *The Cochrane Database of Systematic Reviews. The Cochrane Library, Copyright 2005, The Cochrane Collaboration.* Volume (3), 2005, (no page #). Date of Most Recent Update: 29 May 2002. Date of Most Recent Substantive Update: 20 May 2002.

breastfeeding. Some mothers will require constant support and observation to complete these activities safely, particularly if the father is sleep deprived as well. Nursing units should have risk management guidelines in place to assist nurses in their assessment and support of these clients (Mahlmeister, 2005).

The nurse can support the parents in a variety of ways. Initially, nurses must work through their own feelings about cesarean birth. The nurse who considers a vaginal birth "normal" and refers to it as such indicates that a cesarean birth is "abnormal," rather than simply an alternative method. Thus language and terminology, though seemingly insignificant, can convey to the couple negative messages about their cesarean birth experience.

The nurse should offer positive support to the couple. The cesarean birth couple may need the opportunity to tell their story repeatedly to work through their feelings. The nurse can provide factual information about their situation and support the couple's effective coping behaviors. The nurse should provide the parents with choices by allowing them to participate in decision making about the options available to them.

The presence of the father or significant other during the birth process positively influences the woman's perception of the birth event. His or her presence not only reduces the woman's fears but also enhances her sense of control and en-

ables the couple to share feelings and respond to one another with touch and eye contact. Later they have the opportunity to relive the experience and fill in any gaps or missing pieces. This is especially valuable if the mother has had general anesthesia. The father or significant other can take pictures, hold the baby, and foster the discovery process by directing the mother's attention to details about her newborn.

The perception of and reactions to a cesarean birth experience depend on how the woman defines that experience. Her reality is what she perceives it to be. If the woman's attitude is more positive than negative, successful resolution of subsequent stressful events is more likely. Because the definition of events is transitory in nature, the possibility of change and growth is present. Often the mothering role is perceived as an extension of the childbearing role, and inability to fulfill expected childbearing behavior (vaginal birth) may lead to parental feelings of role failure and frustration. The nurse can help families alter their negative definitions of cesarean birth and bolster and encourage positive perceptions.

TEACHING FOR SELF-CARE

The nurse should advise the mother that she is able to hold, cuddle, lift, and feed her infant despite her surgical incision. The nurse can assist the woman in finding positions that are comfortable for holding and feeding the baby. Upon discharge, the woman should be encouraged to care for the infant and allow family members or friends to assist with household duties rather than infant care practices.

NURSING CARE OF THE POSTPARTAL ADOLESCENT

The birth rate for teenage mothers has fallen by one third since 1991, with 41.7 births per 1000 females age 15 to 19 in 2003 (Martin et al., 2005). However, the postpartum nurse will provide care for a number of adolescent mothers, some of whom are very young. The transition to motherhood can be stressful for adult women, and the teen mother has fewer life experiences and resources from which to draw and cope with the transition.

Adolescent mothers have the same basic physical care needs as older mothers. They usually recover without difficulty, as they are young and healthy. However, some adolescents may not have a working knowledge of their own anatomy and physiology or the related terminology, and they may require special assistance with postpartum hygiene and care. The nurse should provide clear and explicit instructions, use diagrams if possible, check for understanding, and reinforce teaching as needed (Montgomery, 2003). Contraceptive counseling is necessary, and the nurse should ensure that the teen has a plan or prescription in place and that she understands how to use the contraceptive before discharge.

The nurse has many opportunities for teaching the adolescent parents about their newborn in the postpartal unit. Because the nurse serves as a role model, the manner in which she handles the baby greatly influences the young mother. The father, if involved, should be included in as much of the teaching as possible. Although the grandmother or another family member may plan to assist with or provide much of the newborn care in some cases, the nurse should always ensure that the adolescent mother has the knowledge and demonstrates the skills to provide care for her newborn before discharge. Working with the adolescent mother and her family requires sensitivity on the nurse's part. The adolescent will need family support, and the nurse should work with the entire family to promote healthy and positive interactions during this time (Montgomery, 2003).

A newborn physical examination performed at the bedside gives the adolescent immediate feedback about the newborn's health and shows her methods of handling an infant. The nurse can teach as the examination progresses, giving the new mother information about the fontanelles, cradle cap, shampooing the newborn's hair, and so on. The nurse might also use this time to teach the young mother about infant stimulation techniques. Because adolescent mothers tend to concentrate their interactions in the physical domain, they need to comprehend the importance of verbal, visual, and auditory stimulation for newborns as well.

Performing an examination at the bedside also gives the adolescent permission to explore her baby, which she may have been hesitant to do. A Brazelton neonatal assessment (see Chapter 29 ∞) will help the mother understand the newborn's response to stimuli, a key factor in the adolescent's response to

the individuality of her newborn once she goes home. Parents who have some idea of what to expect from their infants will be less frustrated with the newborn's behavior.

The adolescent mother appreciates positive feedback about her fine newborn and her developing maternal responses. This praise and encouragement will increase her confidence and self-esteem.

Group classes for adolescent mothers should include infant care skills, information about growth and development, infant feeding, well-baby care, and danger signals in the ill newborn. If classes are offered in the hospital during the postpartum stay, the adolescent mother should be strongly encouraged to attend. If the child's father is involved, he should also be encouraged to attend and participate. The nurse can correct misconceptions and unrealistic expectations about growth and development.

During the postpartal period, the adolescent may have special needs, depending on her level of maturity, support systems, and cultural background. Stiles (2005) found that adolescent mothers perceive some of their primary needs to include assistance with child care so they can work and/or attend school; assistance with transportation to school, work, and healthcare appointments; financial support; emotional support from someone who will listen without judging; knowledge regarding newborn care and illness; and knowledge regarding self-care in the areas of formal education, relationships, stress management, self-discipline, birth control, time management, and financial planning. The adolescent mothers in her study described their goals as happiness, independence, and career. They indicated that they needed support from peers, professionals, and the child's father to meet their goals. The strategies they used to meet their goals included support groups, life skills education, formal education, and jobs. It will be helpful for the postpartum nurse to explore these issues with the adolescent mother and her family to determine what types of support and resources are in place for her and what additional referrals may be helpful.

Ideally, teenage mothers should visit adolescent clinics where mother and baby are assessed for several years after birth. In this way, classes on parenting, vocational guidance, and school attendance can be followed closely. School systems' classes for young mothers are an excellent way of helping adolescents finish school and learn how to parent at the same time. Support groups and programs should address the issues discussed above and meet at a time and place that is welcoming and allows the mother (and father) to attend. Although the teen mother may already attend or have a plan to attend a local program accessed during the prenatal period, the postpartum nurse should be aware of local programs and support groups offered through schools and healthcare organizations and make referrals as needed.

In the event that a woman decides to keep an unwanted child, the nurse should be aware of the potential for parenting problems. Families with unwanted children are more prone to crisis than others, although in many cases parents grow to love their child after attachment occurs. The nurse should be ready to initiate crisis management strategies or make appropriate referrals as the need arises. Assessment and follow-up by social workers should be coordinated before discharge.

NURSING CARE OF THE WOMAN WHO RELINQUISHES HER INFANT

Relinquishing mothers are those who choose to give their infants up for adoption. Typically these mothers are young or unmarried, or both. Some relinquishing mothers are living in poverty or simply unable to care for another child, whereas others do not have the desire or emotional maturity to be mothers. Relinquishment may also involve complex psychosocial issues such as rape, incest, conception outside the current relationship, domestic violence, or the threat of abandonment by her partner if the mother keeps the child.

Although there is much research on the experience of adoptees and adoptive families, there is little written on the experience of relinquishing mothers. Clearly, more studies are needed to provide optimal care for this population of clients. Qualitative research by Kobokovich (2002) found that relinquishing mothers described their experience as one that was difficult and caused grief. The mothers also felt relief, however. They expressed concern about their baby's well-being and expressed a desire to keep their baby but added that some factor impeded their ability to do so. Nurses caring for relinquishing mothers and their babies offered the mothers as much control as possible, worked to be supportive and nonjudgmental, provided mementos if asked, and created a protective and caring environment for the mother. Nurses voiced uncertainty regarding the pros and cons of interaction between the relinquishing mother and the baby. Uncertainty in the mother raised tension and a sense of caution in the nurses.

Uncertainty regarding how to care for relinquishing mothers may be a source of anxiety for labor and delivery nurses, particularly those who are inexperienced. In some cases, the relinquishing mother may receive only physical care while providers fail to acknowledge or address her emotional needs. It is essential to use active listening, provide nonjudgmental support, show concern and compassion, and personalize care as needed for the relinquishing mother. When she is admitted to the birthing unit, the staff should be informed about the mother's decision to relinquish the infant. Any special requests regarding the birth should be respected, and the woman should be encouraged to express her emotions. If the woman is accompanied by family members or a significant other, the nurse provides support to them throughout the experience as well. If no support person is present, the nurse acts as the primary support person and ensures that the woman has a clear understanding of all that occurs. Following the birth, the nurse should honor the mother's decision as to whether she desires to see and hold her newborn. The nurse should support the mother with her presence or allow privacy as requested.

In cases in which the birth mother has already established a relationship with the intended adoptive parents, both sets of parents may be present for the delivery. The nurse will need to take cues from the birth mother as to how to best provide support for all involved, remembering that meeting the needs of the birth mother is his or her primary responsibility at this time.

Although some relinquishing mothers may feel mostly relief, others will experience feelings of grief and loss. Most often, a complex combination of feelings will be present. Although there is abundant research and support available to individuals and couples experiencing loss due to miscarriage, stillbirth, or death, there is much less in regard to the experience of relinquishment. It is essential that nurses allow and encourage these clients to explore and voice their feelings and that nurses provide support as needed. See Chapter 37 ∞ regarding nursing care of parents experiencing grief and loss.

> *The decision to give up my baby was by far the most difficult and heart-wrenching thing I ever did! I was a college freshman and Shane was a senior football player. When I found out I was pregnant he dropped me without another thought. I was away at college and was so ashamed. I wanted to tell my Mom but I just couldn't disappoint my parents. I skipped going home at Spring Break and went into labor 3 weeks later. After I had the baby (a little boy), I went back to my dorm 9 hours later. I never told anyone. To this day, no one knows the secret I hold and the sadness it carries.*

After the birth, the nurse can ask the mother if she wishes to remain on the postpartum unit or if she would prefer to be cared for on another unit. The mother's choice should be supported. Many mothers who relinquish their infants may opt for a shortened hospital stay. Nurses should facilitate discharge instructions in the immediate postpartum period. Charitable and religious organizations that assist birth mothers with the experience of adoption often provide support to these mothers throughout the prenatal and postpartum experience. If she is not already connected in this way, the mother may benefit from a referral to a therapist or clergy person if she desires additional support beyond what she expects to receive from family and friends.

DISCHARGE INFORMATION

The postpartum stay allowed by most third-party payers has decreased dramatically in recent years. Hospital stays that were measured in weeks in the 1940s are now measured in hours. Postpartum nursing care that has traditionally included a strong focus on the adjustments of the mother, newborn, and family is very difficult to accomplish because of the brief length of stay. Mothers and newborns are being discharged before many of their important postbirth healthcare needs can be addressed. These include establishing breastfeeding, ruling out infections, supporting infant-family bonding, and client teaching. Home health services are increasingly being recognized as a cost-effective means of meeting the postbirth needs of mothers and newborns. Home care of the postpartal family is the subject of Chapter 36. ∞

Ideally, preparation for discharge begins the moment a woman enters the unit to give birth. Nursing efforts should be directed toward assessing the couple's knowledge, expectations, and beliefs and then providing anticipatory guidance and teaching accordingly (see Table 35–1). Because teaching is one of the primary responsibilities of the postpartum nurse, many agencies have elaborate teaching programs and classes. Before the actual

Figure 35–3 ◆ The nurse provides discharge instructions to the mother and father before discharge.

discharge, however, the nurse should spend time with the couple to determine whether they have any last-minute questions (Figure 35–3 ◆). In general, discharge teaching should include at least the following:

1. The woman should contact her caregiver if she develops any of the signs of possible complications:

   a. Sudden persistent or spiking fever (greater than 100.4F) or chills

   b. Change in the character of the lochia—foul smell, return to bright red bleeding, excessive amount (more than two pads per hour)

   c. Evidence of mastitis, such as breast tenderness, reddened areas, malaise, fever, chills

   d. Evidence of thrombophlebitis, such as calf pain, tenderness, redness

   e. Evidence of urinary tract infection, such as urgency, frequency, burning on urination

   f. Evidence of infection in an incision (either episiotomy or cesarean), such as redness, edema, pain or discomfort, discharge, or lack of approximation

   g. Continued severe or incapacitating postpartal depression, inability to care for self or baby, feelings of self-harm, or anxiety

   h. Severe pelvic pain

2. The woman should review the literature she has received that explains recommended postpartum exercises, the need for adequate rest, the need to avoid overexertion initially, and the recommendation to abstain from sexual intercourse until lochia has ceased. The woman may take a shower and may continue sitz baths at home if she desires.

3. The woman should be given the phone numbers of the postpartum unit, lactation consultant, and nursery and be encouraged to call if she has any questions, no matter how simple.

4. The woman should receive information on local agencies or support groups, such as La Leche League and Mothers of Twins, that might be of particular assistance to her.

5. Both breastfeeding and formula-feeding mothers should receive information geared to their specific nutritional needs. They should also be told to continue their vitamin and iron supplements until their postpartal examination.

6. The woman should have a scheduled appointment for her postpartal examination and for her infant's first well-baby examination before they are discharged.

7. The mother should clearly understand the correct procedure for obtaining copies of her infant's birth certificate.

8. The new parents should be able to provide home care for their infant and should know when to anticipate that the cord will fall off, when the infant will need his or her first immunizations, and so on. They should also be comfortable feeding and handling the baby and should be aware of basic safety considerations, including the need to use a car seat whenever the infant is in a car, sudden infant death syndrome (SIDS) prevention, and prevention of shaken baby injuries. These topics are covered in Chapter 36. ∞

9. The parents should be aware of signs and symptoms in the infant that indicate possible problems and whom they should contact about them.

The nurse can also use this final period to reassure the couple of their ability to be successful parents, stressing the infant's need to feel loved and secure. The nurse can also urge parents to talk to each other and work together to solve any problems that may arise.

The nurse addresses follow-up visits when appropriate. If not already discussed, teaching about family planning is appropriate at this time, and the nurse can provide information regarding birth control methods.

In ideal situations, a family approach involving the father, infant, and possibly other siblings would permit a total evaluation and provide an opportunity for all family members to ask questions and express concerns. In addition, a family approach can enable the nurse to identify disturbed family patterns more readily and initiate interventions to prevent future problems of neglect or abuse.

EVALUATION

Anticipated outcomes of comprehensive nursing care of the postpartal family include the following:

- The mother and infant remain healthy, safe, and free of injury or complications.

- The mother verbalizes comfort and uses self-comfort measures as appropriate.

- The mother verbalizes feelings and concerns related to the birth event and her newborn.

- The mother performs appropriate self-care measures.
- The new parents demonstrate safe and effective care of their baby.
- The parents and newborn display positive bonding behaviors.
- The couple demonstrates successful breastfeeding (or parents describe safe formula preparation and feeding).
- The mother is rested and verbalizes understanding of the importance of gradual return to activities.
- The mother identifies sources of support to assist with newborn care and family responsibilities.
- The mother states plan for follow-up health care for herself and her infant.
- The mother identifies signs/symptoms of maternal/newborn complications and reasons to seek care before routine follow-up visits.

- The cesarean birth mother states in her own words the reason for the cesarean birth and verbalizes feelings.
- The cesarean birth mother verbalizes comfort and maintains mobility.
- The adolescent mother has been supported physically and emotionally.
- The woman relinquishing her newborn verbalizes the rationale for her decision and demonstrates acceptance of her decision.
- In summary, all components of nursing care are designed to achieve the desired outcomes identified for the woman and her family.

CHAPTER REVIEW

FOCUS YOUR STUDY

- Effective parent learning requires precise timing of teaching, as well as choice of a teaching method that is effective for the family, such as videotapes, return-demonstration, and so on. Content on self-care, infant care, and anticipatory guidance is important.
- Postpartum discomfort may be due to a variety of factors, including an edematous perineum, an episiotomy or extension, engorged hemorrhoids, hematoma formation, afterpains, immobility, diaphoresis, sore nipples, or engorged breasts. Various self-care approaches are helpful in promoting comfort. Cultural values are incorporated in providing care to the new family.
- Lactation may be suppressed by mechanical techniques.
- The first day or two following birth are marked by maternal behaviors that are more dependent and oriented to the woman's comfort. Thereafter the woman becomes more independent and ready to assume responsibility.
- The new mother requires opportunities to discuss her childbirth experience with an empathetic listener.
- Maternal rest is promoted by advising the woman to take frequent rest periods, nap when the baby is napping, avoid unnecessary activities, and use her social support system. Ambulation and activity should be resumed gradually.

- Rooming-in provides the childbearing family with opportunities to interact with their new member during the first hours and days of life. This enables the family to develop some confidence and skill in a "safe" environment.
- Sexual intercourse may resume once the episiotomy has healed and lochia has stopped. Couples should be forewarned of possible changes; for example, the vagina may be "dry," fatigue may inhibit the level of desire, or the woman's breasts may leak milk during orgasm.
- Following cesarean birth, a woman has the nursing care needs of a surgical client in addition to her needs as a postpartum client. She may also require assistance in working through her feelings if the cesarean birth was unexpected.
- Postpartally, the nurse evaluates the adolescent mother in terms of her level of maturity, available support systems, cultural background, and existing knowledge and then plans care accordingly.
- The mother who decides to relinquish her baby needs emotional support. She should be able to decide whether to see and hold her baby and should have any special requests regarding the birth honored.

- Before discharge, the nurse should give the couple any information necessary for the woman to provide appropriate self-care. They should have a beginning skill in caring for their newborn and should be familiar with warning signs of possible complications for mother or baby. Printed

information is valuable in helping couples deal with questions that may arise at home.

- Because of the trend toward early discharge, follow-up care is more important than ever. Many approaches are used, especially home visits.

EXPLORE MediaLink

http://www.prenhall.com/davidson

NCLEX review questions, case studies, and other interactive resources for this chapter can be found on the Web Site at http://www.prenhall.com/davidson. Click on "Chapter 35" to select the activities for this chapter.

For tutorials including animations and videos, more NCLEX review questions, and an audio glossary, access the accompanying Prentice Hall Nursing MediaLink DVD-ROM in this book.

PRENTICE HALL NURSING MEDIALINK DVD-ROM

Audio Glossary

NCLEX Review

Video: *Through the Eyes of a Nurse—Welcoming the New Arrival at the Postpartal Visit*

COMPANION WEBSITE

Additional NCLEX Review

Case Studies: *Perineal Discomfort; Postpartum Client*

Care Plan Activity: *Postpartal Care Following Cesarean Birth*

Applications: *Perineal Discomfort; Clinical Pathway to Promote Family Wellness; Caring for the Postpartum Adolescent; Discharge Planning*

Critical Thinking

CRITICAL THINKING IN ACTION

POSTPARTUM CONCERNS

View the Critical Thinking in Action video in Chapter 35 of the DVD-ROM. Then answer the questions that follow.

Wendy Calahan, a 31-year-old G3, P2, gave birth to an 8.5-pound baby boy by primary cesarean birth for failure to progress. The baby's Apgar score was 9 and 9 at 1 and 5 minutes. The baby was admitted to the newborn nursery for transitional observation. Wendy was transferred to the postpartum unit where you assume her care. You introduce yourself and orient her to the

room. You perform an initial assessment, with all findings within normal limits. Wendy tells you she is very tired and would like to rest while her baby is in the nursery. Her husband and family have left the hospital after spending time with her in the recovery room but will return later. She admits she is disappointed that she could not give birth vaginally even though she pushed for 2 hours. She says, "This baby was just too big."

1. How would you discuss with Wendy the need for frequent assessments after birth?

2. Explain "maternity or baby blues."

3. Explore activities to minimize maternity blues.

4. Discuss concerns of a woman experiencing her second pregnancy.

5. Discuss behaviors that inhibit paternal attachment.

REFERENCES

American Academy of Pediatrics (AAP) & American College of Obstetricians and Gynecologists (ACOG). (2002). *Guidelines for perinatal care* (5th ed.). Elk Grove Village, IL: Author.

Anderson, G. C., Moore, E., Hepworth, J., & Bergman, N. (2005). Early skin-to-skin contact for mothers and their healthy newborn infants. *The Cochrane Database of Systematic Reviews (CDSR), 3.*

Beck, C. T., & Indman, P. (2005). The many faces of postpartum depression. *Journal of Obstetric, Gynecologic, & Neonatal Nursing, 34*(4), 569–576.

Bowman, K. G. (2005). Postpartum learning needs. *Journal of Obstetric, Gynecologic, & Neonatal Nursing, 34*(4), 438–443.

Callister, L. C. (2004). Making meaning: Women's birth narratives. *Journal of Obstetric, Gynecologic, & Neonatal Nursing, 33*(4), 508–518.

Centers for Disease Control and Prevention. (2002). Recommended adult immunization schedule—United States, 2002–2003. *Morbidity and Mortality Weekly Report, 5*(1), 904–906.

Corwin, E. J., Brownstead, J., Barton, N., Heckard, S., & Morin, K. (2005). The impact of fatigue on the development of postpartum depression. *Journal of Obstetric, Gynecologic, & Neonatal Nursing, 34*(5), 577–585.

Cunningham, F. G., Leveno, K. J., Bloom, S. L., Hauth, J. C., Gilstrap, L. C., & Wenstrom, K. D. (2005). *Williams obstetrics* (22nd ed.). New York: McGraw-Hill.

Deglin, J. H., & Vallerand, A. H. (2005). *Davis's drug guide for nurses* (9th ed.). Philadelphia: F. A. Davis.

Galanti, G. (2004). *Caring for patients from different cultures* (3rd ed.). Philadelphia: University of Pennsylvania Press.

Garg, A., Morton, S., & Heneghan, A. (2005). A hospital survey of postpartum depression education

at the time of delivery. *Journal of Obstetric, Gynecologic, & Neonatal Nursing, 34*(5), 587–594.

George, L. (2005). Lack of preparedness: Experiences of first-time mothers. *American Journal of Maternal/Child Nursing, 30*(4), 251–255.

Goodman, J. H. (2005). Becoming an involved father of an infant. *Journal of Obstetric, Gynecologic, & Neonatal Nursing, 34*(2), 190–200.

Groer, M., Davis, M., Casey, K., Short, B., Smith, K., & Groer, S. (2005). Neuroendocrine & immune relationships in postpartum fatigue. *American Journal of Maternal/Child Nursing, 30*(2), 133–138.

Hedayati, H., Parsons, J., & Crowther, C. A. (2005). Topically applied anaesthetics for treating perineal pain after childbirth. *The Cochrane Database of Systematic Reviews* (3).

Kobokovich, L. J. (2002). *The nature of infant relinquishment as described by two voices: The relinquishing mother and the obstetrical nurse.* Unpublished doctoral dissertation, University of Rhode Island.

MacMullen, N. J., Dulski, L. A., & Meagher, B. (2005). Red alert: Perinatal hemorrhage. *American Journal of Maternal/Child Nursing, 30*(1), 46–51.

Mahlmeister, L. R. (2005). Couplet care after cesarean delivery: Creating a safe environment for mother and baby. *Journal of Perinatal and Neonatal Nursing, 19*(3), 212–214.

Mangesi, L., & Hofmeyr, G. J. (2005). Early compared with delayed oral fluids and food after caesarean section. *The Cochrane Database of Systematic Reviews, 3.*

Martin, J. A., Kochanek, K. D., Strobino, D. M., Guyer, B., & MacDorman, M. F. (2005). Annual summary of vital statistics—2003. *Pediatrics, 115*(3), 619–634.

Mercer, R. (1986). *First-time motherhood—experiences from teens to forties.* New York: Springer.

Montgomery, K. S. (2003). Nursing care for pregnant adolescents. *Journal of Obstetric, Gynecologic, & Neonatal Nursing, 32*(2), 249–257.

Nystedt, A., Edvardsson, D., & Willman, A. (2004). Epidural analgesia for pain relief in labour and childbirth—a review with a systematic approach. *Journal of Clinical Nursing, 13*(4), 455–466.

O'Reilly, M. M. (2004). Achieving a new balance: Women's transition to second-time parenthood. *Journal of Obstetric, Gynecologic, & Neonatal Nursing, 33*(4), 455–462.

Roman, M., & Cabaj, T. (2005). Epidural analgesia. *Medsurg Nursing, 14*(4), 257–259.

Rubin, R. (1984). *Maternal identity and the maternal experience.* New York: Springer.

Scoggin, J. (2004). Physical and psychological changes. In S. Mattson & J. Smith (Eds.), *AWHONN core curriculum for maternal-newborn nursing* (3rd ed., pp. 371–386). St. Louis, MO: Elsevier Saunders.

Snowden, H. M., Renfrew, M. J., & Woolridge, M. W. (2005). Treatments for breast engorgement during lactation [Review]. *The Cochrane Database of Systematic Reviews (CDSR), 3.*

Stiles, A. S. (2005). Parenting needs, goals, & strategies of adolescent mothers. *American Journal of Maternal/Child Nursing, 30*(5), 327–333.

Swift, K., & Janke, J. (2003). Breast binding . . . is it all that it's wrapped up to be? *Journal of Obstetric, Gynecologic, & Neonatal Nursing, 32*(3), 332–339.

CHAPTER

36 Home Care of the Postpartal Family

Working as a home care nurse with an early discharge program is the most fulfilling job I have ever had. It is an honor and a privilege to be allowed into the home to share this special time with childbearing families. When I offer breastfeeding support, help new parents to access the resources they need, or recognize a problem and ensure timely follow-up, I know that I am making a difference in their lives. The appreciation expressed by the families and the healthcare providers I serve is a gift that I receive.

OBJECTIVES

1. Explain the history of the controversy surrounding length of stay.
2. Discuss the components of postpartal home care.
3. Identify the main purposes of home visits during the postpartum period.
4. Summarize actions the nurse should take to ensure personal safety during a home visit.
5. Delineate aspects of fostering a caring relationship in the home.
6. Describe assessment, care of the newborn, and reinforcement of parent teaching in the home.
7. Discuss maternal and family assessment and anticipated progress after birth.
8. Identify appropriate nursing interventions for women who are experiencing breastfeeding difficulties.
9. Identify postpartum resources that are available to new families.

KEY TERMS

Active alert state 1114
Bed sharing 1113
Cosleeping 1113
Crying state 1114
Deep sleep 1114
Drowsy state 1114
Late preterm infant 1102

Light sleep 1114
Postpartal home care 1103
Quiet alert state 1114
Shaken baby injuries 1116
Sudden infant death syndrome (SIDS) 1112
Weaning 1128

MEDIALINK

Additional resources for this content can be found on the Prentice Hall Nursing MediaLink DVD-ROM and on the Companion Website at http://www.prenhall.com/davidson. Click on "Chapter 36" to select the activities for this chapter.

Home care is an essential component of perinatal nursing care, particularly as caregivers struggle to find an appropriate balance between providing quality client care and managing escalating healthcare costs. The hospital length of stay (LOS) following childbirth proved controversial during the last years of the 20th century. Consumers often requested early discharge as an alternative to home delivery in the 1980s. The average LOS decreased further during the early 1990s in an effort to contain healthcare costs, with third-party payers reimbursing only a 24-hour stay following an uncomplicated vaginal delivery. Professional organizations questioned the safety of this trend during the mid-1990s, and Congress responded with the Newborns' and Mothers' Health Protection Act (NMHPA) of 1996 (American Academy of Pediatrics [AAP] Committee on Fetus and Newborn, 2004; Meara, Kotagal, Atherton et al., 2004).

ROLE OF LENGTH OF STAY AND PROFESSIONAL GUIDELINES AND RECOMMENDATIONS IN POSTPARTAL HOME CARE

The NMHPA was signed into law in 1997 and took effect in January 1998. Although the bill does not prohibit earlier discharge, it provides for a guaranteed minimum stay of up to 48 hours following an uncomplicated vaginal birth and 96 hours following an uncomplicated cesarean birth at the discretion of the new mother and her healthcare provider (AAP Committee on Fetus and Newborn, 2004). Despite numerous studies, findings are inconclusive as to whether a shortened LOS is harmful or beneficial to childbearing families. For example, a study of mother-baby couplets during an 8-year period in Massachusetts suggested that increases in diagnosis of jaundice and feeding problems following changes in LOS were not caused by the shortened stay but were instead a result of heightened vigilance and identification of these problems on postpartal day 3 or 4 (Madden, Soumerai, Lieu et al., 2004). Also, according to a Cochrane review of eight trials involving 3600 women, the benefits and risks of early discharge after childbirth for mothers of healthy babies are uncertain because of poor-quality studies (Brown, Small, Faber, et al., 2002).

The AAP and the American College of Obstetricians and Gynecologists (ACOG) have developed guidelines for LOS and follow-up care for mothers and newborns. A home visit or follow-up telephone call by a healthcare provider such as a lactation nurse within 48 hours of discharge is recommended for mothers with a shortened hospital stay. An examination by a healthcare provider is recommended within 48 hours of discharge for newborns who go home before 48 hours of age. The exam may be completed in the home by personnel competent in newborn assessment, provided that the results are reported to the physician that day (AAP & ACOG, 2002; AAP Committee on Fetus and Newborn, 2004). Optimal timing of discharge needs to be determined by considering the medical, social, and financial factors in each case. Suggested discharge criteria and recommendations for follow-up after early discharge are found in Table 36–1.

Despite AAP guidelines and legislation regarding discharge and recommended follow-up, a California study found that many newborns continue to be discharged early and that most of them do not receive the recommended follow-up after early discharge. This was particularly true with vulnerable newborns from families with low incomes, Latina background, Medicaid coverage, and English language barriers. The study did find that home visits were more likely to be timely than were office visits, perhaps because they eliminated obstacles such as lack of transportation, lack of sibling care, and difficulty accessing appointments (Galbraith, Egerter, Marchi et al., 2003).

The American Nurses Association (ANA) advocates for an initial home visit model of postpartum care, and this model has been supported by the AAP. The home visit overcomes transportation and child care issues for healing mothers and allows them to breastfeed without interruption. A study by Paul, Phillips, Widome et al. (2004) found home nursing visits within 48 hours after discharge to be highly cost-effective by reducing subsequent hospital-based services for jaundice and dehydration. This was true regardless of LOS, and the authors recommended routine home nursing visits for **every** newborn to improve compliance with AAP follow-up guidelines and the overall quality of care for all newborns and their parents.

A nursing home visit for nursing mothers also meets the recommendations set forth by the AAP Subcommittee on Hyperbilirubinemia in 2004. The recommendations include follow-up within the first few days following discharge to assess the infant's well-being and for the presence or absence of jaundice during the time of highest risk at 72 to 96 hours of life. These assessments may require two visits for infants discharged early (one between 24 and 72 hours of life and one at 72 to 120 hours of life), and one follow-up visit for infants who stay in the hospital for at least 48 hours. The visit(s) should include assessment of the weight and percent change since birth, adequacy of intake, voiding and stooling patterns, and the presence or absence of jaundice. Clinical judgment should be used to determine the need for a bilirubin test (AAP Subcommittee on Hyperbilirubinemia, 2004).

The Association of Women's Health, Obstetric, and Neonatal Nurses (AWHONN) convened an expert panel and launched a multiyear initiative in 2005 to improve the health care of late preterm infants through education of healthcare providers and parents (AWHONN, 2005). These **late preterm infants,** born between 34 and 37 weeks of gestation, are at increased risk for respiratory distress syndrome, temperature instability, hypoglycemia, hyperbilirubinemia, apnea, bradycardia, neurodevelopmental delays, and feeding problems (Jenkins, 2005; Wang, Dorer, Fleming et al., 2004). Although research will need to be accomplished, it is likely that home care nursing could cost-effectively enhance the care of this population of vulnerable infants through parent education and follow-up.

Table 36–1   MINIMAL CRITERIA FOR DISCHARGE OF NEWBORNS

1. Antepartum, intrapartum, and postpartum course for both the mother and the newborn is uncomplicated.

2. Vaginal delivery.

3. Singleton birth at 38 to 42 weeks' gestation, with birth weight appropriate for gestational age according to appropriate intrauterine growth curves.

4. Newborn's vital signs are normal and stable for 12 hours before discharge.
   - Respiratory rate less than 60/min
   - Heart rate 100 to 160 /min
   - Axillary temperature of 36.1 to 37C (97 to 98.6F) in an open crib with appropriate clothing

5. Newborn has urinated and passed at least one stool.

6. Newborn has completed at least two successful feedings.
   - Documentation has been made regarding the newborn's ability to coordinate sucking, swallowing, and breathing while feeding.
   - If breastfeeding, a knowledgeable caregiver has observed and documented latch, feeding, and maternal/infant response.

7. Physical exam reveals no abnormalities requiring continued hospital stay.

8. No evidence of excessive bleeding from the circumcision site for the previous 2 hours.

9. No evidence of significant jaundice in the first 24 hours.

10. Mother's knowledge, ability, and confidence to care for the newborn are documented to include teaching of the following:
    - Condition of the newborn
    - Assessment of breastfeeding to include maternal knowledge of adequate newborn output
    - Care of the cord, skin, and genitals as well as temperature assessment and measurement
    - Maternal knowledge of signs of illness and common problems, particularly jaundice
    - Instruction in newborn safety to include car seat use and positioning for sleep

11. Family or other support persons and healthcare providers are available to the couplet during the first few days following discharge.

12. Instructions given to follow in the event of a complication or emergency.

13. Lab data have been reviewed to include maternal syphilis, hepatitis B virus surface antigen, and HIV; umbilical cord or newborn blood type and direct Coombs' if indicated.

14. Required screening tests have been accomplished; if a test was performed before 24 hours of milk feeding, a plan for repeat must be in place in accordance with local or state policy.

15. Initial hepatitis B vaccine has been administered or an appointment made for its administration.

16. A physician-directed source of continuing medical care for both mother and baby has been identified; appropriate follow-up is scheduled.

17. Family, environmental, and social risk factors have been assessed. If risk factors are present, the discharge should be delayed until resolved or a plan is in place to safeguard the infant. Factors may include but not be limited to untreated parental substance use, positive maternal or infant toxicology results, history of child abuse or neglect, mental illness in a parent who is in the home, lack of social support, no fixed home, untreated domestic violence, adolescent mother—especially with other risk factors.

Recommended follow-up for infants with a shortened hospital stay of less than 48 hours should include the following within 48 hours of discharge:

Weigh the infant.

Assess the newborn's general health, hydration, and degree of jaundice; identify any new problems.

Review feeding pattern and technique; observe breastfeeding for position, latch-on, and swallowing.

Assess historical evidence of stool and urine patterns for adequacy.

Assess quality of mother-newborn interaction and details of newborn behavior.

Reinforce maternal or family education in neonatal care, particularly feeding and sleep position.

Review results of laboratory tests performed at discharge.

Perform screening tests as required by the state and others as clinically indicated.

Identify a plan for healthcare maintenance, including a method for obtaining emergency services, preventive care and immunizations, periodic evaluations and physical examinations, and necessary screening.

SOURCES: Adapted from American Academy of Pediatrics (AAP) & American College of Obstetricians and Gynecologists (ACOG). (2002). *Guidelines for Perinatal Care* (5th ed.). Elk Grove Village, IL; American Academy of Pediatrics, American College of Obstetricians and Gynecologists. Guidelines for perinantal care. 5th ed. Elk Grove Village (IL): AAP; Washington, DC: ACOG; 2002.

CONSIDERATIONS FOR THE HOME VISIT

In planning a home visit, the nurse should clearly understand the purpose of the visit and identify the maximum amount of content to be addressed. Other important considerations include ways of creating and fostering relationships with families, techniques for preplanning and executing the visit while maintaining safety, documenting the visit, and ensuring telephone follow-up.

The postpartal home visit differs from community health visits in that only one or two visits are typically planned, and long-term follow-up by the nurse is not anticipated. Although the postpartal home visit is comprehensive, it is specifically focused on a postpartal family's needs and care.

Because of the established guidelines for discharge of the mother and baby (refer to Table 36–1), the nurse can logically expect to find certain levels of health and wellness. However, because the status of the mother and newborn can change, the nurse should stay alert for deviations from the norm.

Purpose and Timing of the Home Visit

Home care for the postpartal family focuses on assessment, teaching, and counseling. The visit frequently occurs on the third to sixth day of life, depending on when the couplet was discharged. This time frame encompasses the potential peak times for newborn jaundice and maximal weight loss, and it meets the 2004 recommendations set forth by the AAP Subcommittee on Hyperbilirubinemia (2004) discussed earlier. Additionally, by this time the milk should be coming in, and breastfeeding is either going well or problems are becoming apparent. Parents frequently have new and different questions, having spent a couple of days and nights caring independently for their newborn since discharge.

Postpartal home care provides opportunities for expanding information and reinforcing self- and infant care techniques initially presented in the birth setting. The home setting provides an opportunity for the nurse and family to interact in a more relaxed environment, one in which the family has control of the setting. It also provides an invaluable opportunity for the nurse to assess home safety in the setting where the family will grow together. In some instances, a home provides unique challenges in assessing and enhancing the woman's self-care and infant care, and the nurse has many opportunities to exercise critical thinking and develop creative options with the family.

Fostering a Caring Relationship with the Family

Although the nurse in the birthing center strives to enhance family autonomy and control, the inherent atmosphere of the institutional environment may cause the new mother and family to feel unempowered. It is important for the professional nurse to recognize that the parameters of the home visit are different in many ways from those of the hospital or birthing center environment. In the home, the family has control of their environment and the nurse is an invited visitor. The nurse can rely on the same characteristics of a caring relationship that have been integral to hospital-based practice—regard for clients, genuineness, empathy, and establishment of trust and rapport—but the relationship may take on new elements as the nurse moves into the home setting for the first time (Table 36–2).

CLINICAL TIP

When visiting a culturally diverse family the nurse may be invited to take part in specific rituals or customs. Whenever possible, the nurse should accept the invitation and join the mother and other family members. Willingness to accept the family's customs will assist the care provider in establishing a positive relationship with the family and signifies acceptance of cultural diversity.

Table 36–2	FOSTERING A CARING RELATIONSHIP
Demonstrated Goal	**Approaches to Achieve Goal**
Regard	Introduce yourself to the family. Call the family members by their surnames until you have been invited to use the given or a less formal name. Ask to be introduced to other members of the family who are present. Allow the mother or spokesperson to assume this role. Use active listening. Maintain objectiveness. Ask permission before sitting.
Genuineness	Mean what you say. Make sure that your verbal and nonverbal messages are congruent. Be nonjudgmental. Don't make assumptions about individuals or settings. Always strive to demonstrate caring behaviors. Be prepared for the visit, honestly answer questions and provide information, and be truthful. If you don't know the answer to a question, tell the client you will find the information and report back.
Empathy	Listen to the mother and family without judgment, trying to view events and circumstances from their point of view. Be attentive to what the birthing experience means to them so that you will understand their concerns from their perspective. Remember, empathy denotes understanding, not sympathy.
Trust and rapport	Do what you say you will do. Be prepared for the visit and be on time. Notify the family if running late because of client care. Follow up on any areas that are needed.

Planning the Home Visit

Before the home visit, the nurse prepares by identifying the purpose of the visit and gathering anticipated materials and equipment. Communication with the primary healthcare provider(s) and a thorough review of inpatient records gives the nurse an understanding of current needs and any special concerns for each individual mother-baby couplet. A personal contact while the woman is still in the birth setting or a previsit telephone call is used to arrange the appointment with the woman and her family. During the previsit contact it is important for the nurse to identify clearly the purpose and goals of the visit, to let the client know approximately how long the visit will take, and to begin establishing a rapport.

Maintaining Safety

In the past, nurses were viewed as a mainstay of communities and could move in most settings without fear or concern for safety. However, in current times some communities are not safe for visiting nurses. Risks noted by home care nurses include isolated locations, illegal drugs, threatening animals, gangs, vandalism, inadequate lighting, guns, verbal abuse, robberies, inappropriate sexual comments, adverse weather and road conditions, unsanitary conditions, violent lifestyles, and clients without phones (Brillhart, Kruse, & Heard, 2004; Sylvester & Reisener, 2002). Thus it is important for the nurse to follow some basic safety rules when conducting a home visit. Specifically, the nurse should:

- Confirm the address, and ask for directions during the previsit contact
- Trace out the route to the client's home on a map or the Internet before leaving for the visit, and take the map along
- Provide a daily schedule of visits, including client addresses and phone numbers, to supervisors
- Notify an instructor or supervisor when leaving for a visit and check in as soon as the visit is completed
- Carry a cellular phone with the battery charged at all times
- Carry a phone card or enough change to make a call from a pay phone in case of poor cellular transmission in some locations
- Ensure that the vehicle used for visits is well maintained and has sufficient fuel
- Wear a name tag and carry identification
- Carry a flashlight, particularly for night visits
- Carry food and water for the nurse's personal use
- Avoid wearing expensive jewelry
- Before starting out (or before arriving at the home) lock personal belongings in the trunk of the car, out of sight
- Call clients when the nurse is on the way to confirm that they are home and that they are expecting the nurse
- Pay attention to the body language of anyone present during the visit, not just the client
- Request that threatening or sexually inappropriate behavior stop immediately

- Be aware of personal body language and how it might be interpreted (for example, avoid crossing arms or shoving hands in pockets; remain calm and convey a sense of respect at all times)

- Leave the home immediately if a weapon is visible and the client or family member refuses requests to put it away

- Ask clients to keep threatening pets secured in a different area of the home during the visit

- Request that clients and family members avoid the use of illegal substances during the visit

- If a situation arises that feels unsafe or if the previous requests are not honored, terminate the visit

- Always have car keys in the nurse's hand before returning to the vehicle

- Lock the doors and drive away upon return to the vehicle at the completion of visits—do not sit in the vehicle to chart

A more extensive list of safety precautions for home care nurses, including specific recommendations for extreme weather conditions and inadequate housing conditions, is provided by Brillhart et al. (2004).

It may be helpful to drive around neighborhoods known to be unsafe before making an initial visit to identify potential cues to violence and to determine whether extra security is necessary. If the visit is in an area that seems very unsafe, it may be wise for two nurses to go together or for the nurse to be accompanied by a security officer. Nurses should avoid entering areas where violence is in progress. In such cases, they should return to the car and contact the appropriate authorities by calling 911.

Many agencies that provide home care services have established violence prevention programs to help ensure safety. A protective services escort program developed at The Cincinnati Children's Hospital Medical Center Home Health Care & Starshine is described by Morris, Krueger, & Yaross (2004). Some agencies have all clients sign a contract at the onset of services that specifies expectations and client responsibilities to ensure a safe environment for the visit. They inform clients that failure to honor the contract will result in loss of home care services (Sylvester & Reisener, 2002). Other agencies respond with specific contracts only as necessary on a case-by-case basis. Because postpartum home care frequently involves only one visit, it may be helpful to discuss safety expectations during the previsit telephone contact. Home care nurses should be familiar with their agency policies and notify supervisors if safety issues requiring agency support are present.

Most people are more comfortable in familiar settings and have some hesitation in entering other residential areas. It is always important for nurses to be aware of their surroundings and the people who are nearby. First home visits may feel uncomfortable because they are unfamiliar, but with experience comfort increases (Figure 36–1 ◆).

Carrying Out the Home Visit

When the door is answered, the nurse should introduce herself or himself and confirm that the location is correct. The nurse may tactfully request to be introduced to others present if this infor-

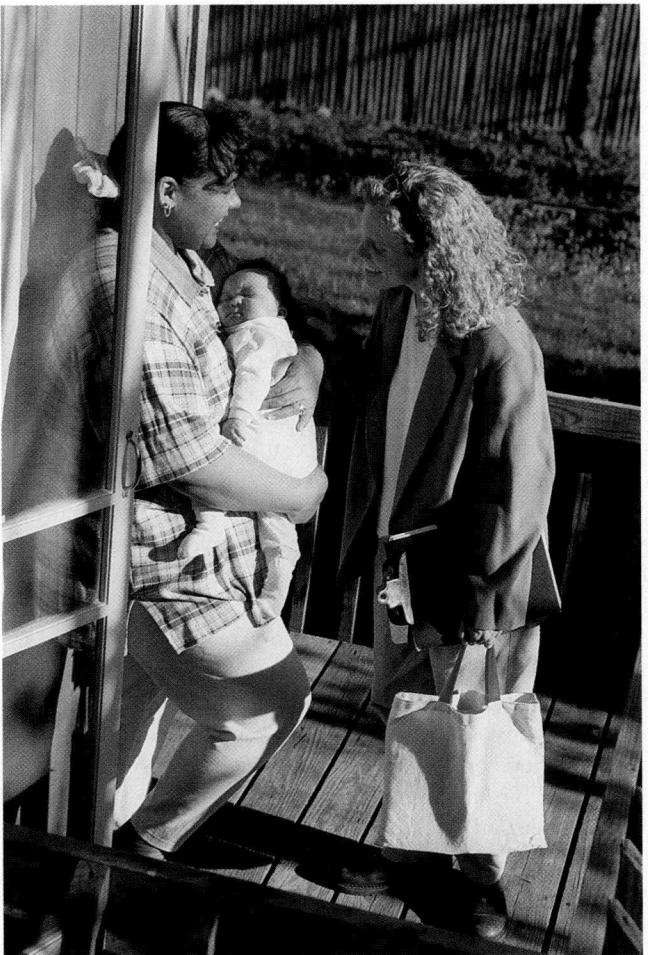

Figure 36–1 ◆ Nurse arriving for a home visit.

mation is not offered. If a place to sit is not indicated, the nurse may inquire, "Where is the best place to sit so that we can talk for a while?" In some homes, the mother or family may offer refreshments, and this may be an important aspect of welcoming a visitor. In this case, it is beneficial to the relationship to accept the refreshment graciously. Other culturally appropriate customs should be respected in the home setting whenever possible.

Many agencies have developed a uniform assessment tool to be used during postpartum home visits. This ensures that the nurse completes a physical assessment of both the mother and the newborn; assesses infant feeding and weight; evaluates maternal psychosocial adjustment, parental bonding, parenting behaviors, family adaptation, and coping skills; and determines environmental strengths and risk factors. Based on these assessments the nurse may do any of the following:

- Provide direct physical care.
- Carry out client and family teaching.
- Consult with the physician, midwife, or a specialist, such as a lactation consultant.
- Refer the woman or family to appropriate community agencies.
- Schedule additional home visits or telephone follow-up.

Because home care nursing is practiced geographically independently from the healthcare facility, the nurse needs to have excellent assessment skills and be adept at noticing variations from the norm. Critical thinking and problem-solving skills are necessary. Communication with the families and the appropriate healthcare providers is essential in the coordination of required treatment and follow-up.

The remainder of the chapter focuses on specific aspects of newborn and maternal care that are assessed, addressed, and evaluated during the home visit.

HOME CARE: THE NEWBORN

When the family provides care for their newborn, the nurse can instill confidence by giving them positive feedback. If the family encounters problems, the nurse can suggest alternatives and serve as a role model. Each newborn has variations in normal physiologic responses and in growth and development patterns. Parents need to learn to interpret these changes in their child. To help parents care for their newborn at home, some physicians encourage prenatal pediatric visits to establish contact before the birth. Public health nurses have long been involved as guides in newborn care and parent education. Some birthing units are now expanding their primary care functions to the new family to include one home visit by the nurse who cared for the family in the birthing unit. The birthing unit nursery staff may also make themselves available as a 24-hour telephone resource for the new family who needs additional support and consultation during the first few days at home with their newborn. Routine well-baby visits should be scheduled with the clinic, pediatric nurse practitioner, or physician.

The family should have been taught all necessary caregiving methods before discharge. However, during the home visit the nurse may use a checklist to determine that the family clearly understands the material. If not, the nurse should complete pertinent teaching. Parents are frequently overwhelmed, sensory overloaded, and exhausted during their short hospital stay and will require a review of initial teaching. A comprehensive literature review by Bowman (2005) found that infant feeding and recognition of illness were the most important learning needs during the first 7 days postpartum. Therefore, the home care nurse will want to address those issues. The nurse also needs to review with the couple all areas for understanding and to answer any questions they may have, making sure that the mother has the phone number and address of, and any specific instructions from, the certified nurse-midwife or nurse practitioner or physician and lactation consultant. Having the nursery phone number is also reassuring to a new family. The nurse encourages them to call with questions.

Physical Assessment of the Newborn at Home

In the home, a newborn physical exam is performed to assess vital signs as well as the skin and the respiratory, cardiovascular, gastrointestinal, genitourinary, musculoskeletal, and neurologic body systems. The infant's behavioral state and the parent-infant interaction should be assessed as well. An exam of the in-

fant's fontanelles, eyes, ears, mouth, nose, neck, color, evidence of jaundice, umbilical cord, circumcision if done, reflexes, hydration, nutritional status and feeding history, elimination of urine and stool, activity, sleep-wake cycles, weight, and percentage of change from birth weight should be documented under the appropriate body systems (AAP Committee on Fetus and Newborn, 2004; Tappero & Honeyfield, 2003). See Chapter 29 ∞ for a complete newborn assessment. Another excellent resource for newborn assessment is *Physical Assessment of the Newborn: A Comprehensive Approach to the Art of Physical Examination* (Tappero & Honeyfield, 2003).

The home visit is the time to ensure that the appropriate screening exams as required by the state have been accomplished and to obtain the blood for screening if still needed. If the newborn did not pass a universal hearing screen before discharge, the nurse should ensure that the parents have a plan to accomplish the required screening or audiology follow-up. The nurse will also assess and reinforce knowledge related to infant care as detailed in the following paragraphs.

Positioning and Handling

The nurse demonstrates methods of positioning and handling the newborn as needed. When the newborn is out of the crib, one of the following holds can be used (Figure 36–2 ◆). The cradle hold is frequently used during feeding. It provides a sense of warmth and closeness, permits eye contact, frees one of the adult's hands, and provides security because the cradling protects the newborn's body. Extra security is provided by gripping the thigh with the hand while the arm supports the newborn's body. The upright position provides security and a sense of closeness and is ideal for burping. One hand should support the neck and shoulders while the other hand holds the buttocks or is placed between the newborn's legs. The newborn may also be held upright in a cloth sling carrier that gently holds the baby against the mother's or father's chest and frees the hands for other tasks. The football hold frees one of the caregiver's hands and permits eye contact. This hold is ideal for shampooing, carrying, or breastfeeding. It frees the caregiver to talk on the telephone, answer the door, or do the myriad tasks that await attention at this busy time.

Skin Care and Bathing

The skin maintains temperature and serves as a barrier between the newborn and the environment. It is also a potential portal of entry for environmental toxins and infectious agents. Keeping the skin healthy and intact is essential to the newborn's health. The requirements of infant skin care include effective cleansing, effective moisturizing, and maintenance of an effective barrier against external irritants (Hopkins, 2004). The following section uses information from the AWHONN Neonatal Skin Care Guidelines (AWHONN, 2001). Hopkins (2004) endorses the AWHONN guidelines, whereas Walker, Downe, & Gomez (2005) note that the guidelines regarding emollients were evaluated primarily in preterm infants, and that the use of emollients, soaps, and lotions in term newborns requires further study.

Although it is difficult to be familiar with every product on the market, the home care nurse should encourage parents to

A   B   C

Figure 36–2 ◆ Various positions for holding an infant. *A,* Cradle hold. *B,* Upright position. *C,* Football hold.

read the labels on over-the-counter skin care products. Alcohol, hexachlorophene, iodine-containing compounds, eutectic mixtures of local anesthetics, and lindane are among the topical agents that have been associated with toxicity (Mancini, 2004). Therefore, parents will want to avoid use of products containing these agents.

An actual bath demonstration is the best way for the nurse to provide information to parents. Because excess bathing and use of soap removes natural skin oils and dries out the newborn's sensitive skin, bathing should be done only two to three times per week. A mild, nonmedicated soap may be used as needed. Cleansing agents with a neutral pH that are preservative-free are recommended. Because soap can be drying to the skin, it need not be used at every bath or in excess. Sponge baths have traditionally been recommended for the first 2 weeks or until the umbilical cord completely falls off and the umbilicus has healed; this is the method that many new parents are comfortable using.

The type of bathing recommended before separation of the cord is controversial. Simon and Simon (2004) reported three cases of omphalitis after nonantiseptic whole-body baths for newborns were instituted at one facility. A different study of 51 tub-bathed babies and 51 sponge-bathed babies found that the tub-bathed babies experienced significantly less temperature loss and significantly increased contentment throughout the bath. Their mothers rated their own pleasure with the bath significantly higher as well. No differences in cord healing scores or maternal confidence were found between the two groups. No cord infections occurred in either group. The authors recommended tub bathing as safe and pleasureable for healthy term newborns (Bryanton, Walsh, Barrett et al., 2004).

Some agencies use a tub bath for the bath demonstration. Additionally, many birthing units and agencies provide videos for parents to watch before bathing their baby for the first time,

Table 36–3	BATH SUPPLIES
Washcloths (2)	Petrolatum product if indicated
Towels (2)	Cotton balls
Blankets (2)	Diapers
Unperfumed mild soap	Clean clothes
Shampoo	

as a home visit does not usually allow time for a nurse demonstration and a parent return demonstration of a bath. See Client Teaching: Newborn Bathing.

Supplies can be kept in a plastic bag or some type of container to eliminate the necessity of hunting for them each time (Table 36–3). At home, the family may want to use a small plastic dishpan, a clean kitchen or bathroom sink, or a large bowl as the baby's tub. Commercial plastic baby tubs are not necessary, but some parents prefer to purchase them.

Before starting, if no one else is at home, the parent may want to take the phone off the hook and place a sign on the door to avoid being disturbed. Having someone home during the first few baths is helpful, because that person can retrieve forgotten items, attend to interruptions, and provide moral support. The room should be warm and free of drafts. It is important to have supplies gathered before beginning, as the caregiver will not be able to turn away or break hand contact with the newborn once he or she is positioned for the bath.

SPONGE BATH

After the supplies are gathered, the tub (or any of the containers mentioned) is filled with water that is warm to the touch. Even though the newborn will not be placed in the tub, the bath giver carefully tests the water temperature with an elbow or forearm.

CLIENT TEACHING Newborn Bathing

CLIENT GOALS   At the completion of the teaching, the family will be able to:

1. Identify safety concerns related to sponge and tub baths for newborns.
2. List appropriate supplies for bathing.

3. Demonstrate proper bathing procedures for both sponge and tub baths.
4. Discuss the use of appropriate skin care agents for newborn use.

TEACHING PLAN

TEACHING METHOD

Clarify information related to sponge bathing and tub bathing for safe newborn bathing. Explain that the proper environment is needed for newborn safety and comfort.

Encourage the mother to assemble supplies before beginning the newborn bath to avoid cold exposure, and ensure that proper supplies are being used.

Demonstrate proper technique and encourage the family to ask questions as they arise. Help instill confidence in new parents.

Clarify the need for appropriate cleansing agents for newborns.

CONTENT

Describe the proper environment (including safety factors) for sponge and tub bathing for newborns.

Identify proper bathing supplies that are needed for both sponge and tub baths.

Demonstrate sponge bathing.

Discuss and demonstrate tub bathing using an infant model.

Explain the need for neutral pH, fragrance-free, and dye-free cleansing products for newborn use.

EVALUATION

At the end of the teaching session the woman and family will be able to verbalize the principles of proper bathing for the newborn. They will be able to demonstrate the proper techniques to ensure safety during both sponge and tub baths.

DOCUMENTATION

Document the information that was given, the type of teaching method used, indicate if the client performed a bath, if it was demonstrated, or if verbal or written directions were given. Verbalization of understanding and clarification of any information should be documented. Safety issues and instructions should also be documented.

Families may also choose to purchase a thermometer to help them determine when the bath water is approximately 37.8C (100F) and safe to use. Soap should not be added to the water. The newborn should be wrapped in a blanket, with a T-shirt and diaper on, to keep him or her warm and secure. The newborn can be placed on a flat protected surface, such as a counter or in a bassinet adjacent to the container of water. Parents should be reminded never to leave an infant unattended on an elevated surface or near any amount of water. Parents should be encouraged to keep one hand on their infant at all times and to keep their eyes on their infant at all times while positioned for a bath.

To start the bath, the adult wraps a washcloth around the index finger once. Each eye is gently wiped from inner to outer canthus. This direction prevents the potential for clogging the tear duct at the inner canthus, where the eye naturally drains. A different portion of the washcloth is used for each eye to prevent cross-contamination. Cotton balls can also be used for this purpose, using a new one for each eye. Some eye swelling and drainage may be present the first few days after birth as a result of the eye prophylaxis.

The bath giver washes the ears next by wrapping the washcloth once around an index finger and gently cleaning the exter-

nal ear and behind the ear. Cotton swabs are never used in the ear canal because it is possible to put the swab too far into the ear and damage the eardrum. In addition, the swab may push any discharge farther down into the ear canal.

The caregiver then wipes the remainder of the baby's face with the soap-free washcloth. Many babies start to cry at this point. The face should be washed every day and the mouth and chin wiped off after each feeding.

The neck is washed carefully but thoroughly with the washcloth. A mild soap may now be used. Formula or breast milk and lint collect in the skinfolds of the neck, so it may be helpful to sit the newborn up, supporting the neck and shoulders with one hand while washing the neck with the other hand.

The bath giver now unwraps the blanket, removes the T-shirt, and wets the chest, back, and arms with the washcloth. The bath giver may then lather the hands with a mild infant skin cleanser and wash the baby's chest, back, and arms. Soap is rinsed off with the wet washcloth, and the upper part of the body is dried with a towel or blanket. The newborn's upper body is then wrapped with a clean, dry blanket to prevent heat loss.

Next the bath giver unwraps the newborn's legs, wets them with the washcloth, and lathers, rinses, and dries them well. If the newborn has dry skin, a small amount of an emollient such as petrolatum or Aquaphor may be used. Products without perfumes or dyes are recommended. Ointments are thought to be better than lotions for dry, cracked feet and hands. Baby oil is not recommended because it clogs skin pores. Families should be warned that baby powder can cause serious respiratory problems for the baby if it is inhaled and therefore should not be used.

The genital area is cleansed after each wet or dirty diaper. Females are washed from the front of the genital area toward the rectum to avoid fecal contamination of the urethra and thus the bladder. Newborn females often have a thick, white mucous discharge or a slight bloody discharge from the vaginal area. This discharge is normal for the first 1 to 2 weeks after birth. The mucus may come off if wiped gently after diaper changes but should not be intentionally scrubbed off.

Parents of uncircumcised males should cleanse the penis daily. Even minimal retraction of the foreskin is not advised (see in-depth discussion of care of uncircumcised male babies in Chapter 30 ∞). Males who have been circumcised also need their penis cleansed daily. A very wet washcloth is squeezed above the baby's penis, allowing clear water to run over the circumcision site. The area is gently patted or fanned dry. A mild soap may be used and then rinsed off beginning several days after the circumcision. A small amount of an emollient such as petrolatum, petrolatum-impregnated gauze, or Aquaphor may be applied during each diaper change for the first 24 to 48 hours. Emollients promote comfort and healing and prevent adherence of the diaper to the site. It is important to avoid using ointments if a Plastibell is in place because ointments may cause the Plastibell ring to slip off the penis too early. The Plastibell usually falls off within 5 to 8 days. If it does not, the family needs to call the healthcare provider.

The newborn should be wrapped in a terry cloth bath towel or bath blanket and gently patted dry at the end of the bath to promote skin integrity and prevent heat loss. It is particularly important that the cord be thoroughly dried if it has become wet during the bath.

The last step in bathing is washing the hair (although some prefer to do this step first). The newborn is swaddled in a dry blanket, leaving only the head exposed, and held in the football hold with the head tilted slightly downward. A cup or cupped hand may be used to pour warm water over the newborn's head, taking care to avoid the eyes and ear canals. Parents should avoid placing the infant's head directly under running water, as changes in water temperature could cause burns or discomfort. The hair is moistened and lathered with a small amount of shampoo. A very soft brush may be used to massage the shampoo over the entire head, including the fontanelles, which families often call the "soft spots." The hair is then rinsed and toweled dry. Oils or lotions are not used on the newborn's head unless prescribed by a healthcare provider.

TUB BATHS

The newborn's face, eyes, ears, and neck can be washed and dried before undressing him or her for the tub bath. A large, clean kitchen or bathroom sink, plastic container, or commer-

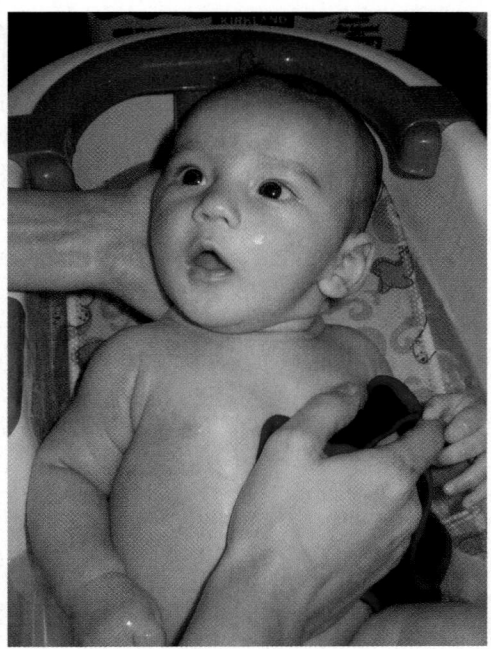

Figure 36–3 ◆ When bathing the newborn, the caregiver must support the head. Wet babies are very slippery.

cial infant tub that allows the baby to be immersed to the neck may be used as the infant's tub. A washcloth can be placed in the bottom of the container to prevent slippage. It is particularly important to keep the room warm and draft-free, because the infant's clothes will be removed for the duration of the bath. The infant should be held securely at all times (Figure 36–3 ◆). Commercial infant tubs often support the infant's head and neck. Parents can support the infant's neck on their nondominant forearm while using that hand to grasp the infant's distal shoulder and arm. Alternatively, the nondominant elbow can be used to support the neck, and the nondominant hand can be used to grasp the infant's distal thigh, using the cradle position. Cleansing can be accomplished quickly with a mild infant skin cleanser without having to turn the infant from front to back (Bryanton et al., 2004).

Because wet newborns are slippery, some parents pull a cotton sock (with holes cut out for the fingers) over the supporting arm to provide a "nonskid" surface. The newborn's body is washed with a soapy washcloth or hand. To wash the back, the bath giver places the noncradling hand on the newborn's chest with the thumb under the newborn's arm closest to the adult. Gently tipping the newborn forward onto the supporting hand frees the cradling arm to wash the back. After the bath, the newborn is lifted out of the tub in the cradle position, dried well, and wrapped in a dry blanket. If the cord has not fallen off, it should be thoroughly dried before recovering with clothing. The hair is then washed in the same way as for a sponge bath.

The nurse must educate parents that infants and young children can drown even in small amounts of water. It is paramount that adults not allow the infant to be immersed above the neck and that they keep the infant safe by maintaining hand, arm, and eye contact with the infant at all times during the tub bath.

Cord Care

The cord stump generally falls off in 5 to 15 days. Until then it is considered to be a healing wound and a potential route of entry for pathogens. Colonization of the cord by pathogenic bacteria allows for the potential to develop omphalitis, necrotizing fasciitis, septicemia, or focal infections, which can be fatal if untreated (Zupan, Garner, & Omari, 2004).

A variety of methods of cord care are used in different facilities throughout the United States. Antimicrobial agents such as bacitracin or triple dye are applied at some hospitals. Concerns related to the appearance and potential risks of using triple dye have resulted in many units using dry cord care—simply spot cleaning the periumbilical area with mild soap and water as needed and keeping it dry (Janssen, Selwood, Dobson et al., 2003). Alcohol used alone has not been shown to prevent bacterial colonization and infection of the cord (AAP & ACOG, 2002).

Regardless of the cord care practices employed in the local setting, the home care nurse should emphasize the importance of keeping the umbilical cord stump clean and dry. The diaper should be folded down to allow air to circulate around the cord and the periumbilical area should be exposed to air or covered loosely with clean clothes. Handwashing is imperative before and following infant care. The parents should consult their healthcare provider immediately if redness, swelling, inflammation, or exudate with a foul odor appears around the umbilicus or if the area remains unhealed 2 to 3 days after the cord stump has sloughed off.

Nail Care

The nails of the newborn are seldom cut in the birthing center. During the first days of life, the nails may adhere to the skin of the fingers, and cutting is contraindicated. Within a week the nails separate from the skin and frequently break off. If the nails are long or if the newborn is scratching his or her face, the nails may be gently filed using a newborn file. This is most easily done while the infant is asleep. Newborn socks or mittens may be used to cover the newborn's hands and prevent facial scratching.

Dressing the Newborn

Newborns need to wear a T-shirt, diaper (diaper cover if using cloth diapers), and a sleeper. At home, the amount of clothing the newborn wears is determined by the temperature. Families who maintain their home at 60F to 65F should dress the infant more warmly than those who maintain a temperature of 70F to 75F.

Newborns should wear a head covering outdoors to protect their sensitive ears from drafts and to prevent heat loss. A blanket can also be wrapped around the baby, leaving one corner free to place over the head for added protection while outdoors or in crowds. The nurse must advise families about the ease with which a newborn's skin can burn when exposed to the sun. To prevent sunburn, the newborn should remain shaded, wear a light layer of clothing, or be protected with sunscreen specifically formulated for infants. Many healthcare professionals, however, recommend avoiding sunscreen until the infant is at least 6 months old.

Diaper shapes vary and are subject to personal preference. Prefolded and disposable diapers are usually rectangular. Cloth diapers may also be triangular or kite-folded. Extra material is placed in front for males and toward the back for females to increase absorbency.

Baby clothing should be laundered separately with a mild soap or detergent. Diapers are generally presoaked before washing. All clothing should be rinsed twice to remove soap and residue and to decrease the possibility of rash. Some newborns may not tolerate clothing treated with fabric softeners added to the washer or dryer.

Temperature Assessment, Fever, and Illness

As the nurse prepares to teach parents about taking their baby's temperature, it is important to provide opportunities for discussion and demonstration. Families often need a review of how to take their infant's temperature and when to call their primary healthcare provider.

> **CLINICAL TIP**
>
> Dressing a newborn baby with a T-shirt may be quite a challenge. The T-shirt is first pulled over the baby's head. The next challenge is getting the arms in the sleeves, because the newborn grasps at the fabric of the T-shirt as you try to pull it over the hands and arms. It helps to put your hand through the right sleeve of the T-shirt and hold the baby's right hand. Then pull the sleeve over your hand. Repeat the same movements for the left sleeve.

The parents may want to discuss their choice of temperature measurement and type of thermometer with their primary healthcare provider. It is also helpful for nurses to periodically check thermometer availability at local retailers and review current literature and manufacturers' literature.

A review of various temperature measurement studies by Kayman (2003) noted that all methods had limitations. The tympanic membrane thermometer was noted to have significant problems with fit and orientation of the instrument in very young infants. Although mercury-containing glass thermometers are a very reliable method of measuring core temperature in infants, the risks outweigh the benefits. Breakage of mercury thermometers has caused symptomatic mercury poisoning in children and adults, and improper disposal contributes to environmental contamination. *Mercury thermometers should not be used or kept in homes* and should be disposed of at a hazardous waste collection site. A variety of programs in which citizens turn in mercury thermometers in exchange for digital thermometers have been used throughout the country (Shoemaker & Ghaemghami, 2003). The nurse should ask parents if they are aware of the hazards of mercury thermometers during the safety assessment and inform parents of local programs or hazardous waste facilities where the thermometers may be turned in.

Parents need to take the newborn's temperature only when signs of illness are present. Although axillary temperatures are used to determine temperature stability and readiness for discharge in healthy newborns (AAP & ACOG, 2002), a review of pediatric literature finds that rectal temperatures are recommended when evaluating fever in infants (Kayman, 2003; Kourtis, Sullivan & Sathian, 2004). Some parents are comfortable taking rectal temperatures, whereas others prefer using the axillary method. Many healthcare providers will verify an axillary temperature with a rectal measurement when evaluating an infant for fever.

Traditionally, a rectal temperature of 38C (100.4F) has been considered a fever. Because newborns under 90 days of age, and particularly those under 30 days of age, are at high risk for systemic infections such as sepsis and meningitis, the nurse should tell parents to see their healthcare provider if their newborn has a rectal temperature of 100.4F or greater or an axillary temperature of 99.4F or greater (Brook, 2003; Kayman, 2003; Kourtis et al. (2004). It will be important for the parents to document the measured temperature, time of measurement, and the method used.

Parents need to be informed that newborns with systemic infection may not be febrile but may exhibit more subtle manifestations such as temperature instability, poor feeding, abdominal distention, inability to tolerate feedings, apnea, or alterations in behavior such as irritability or lethargy (Witt, 2004). A baby who is feeding poorly or just not acting right may be exhibiting signs of potentially serious infection. Therefore, parents of young infants should call their primary care provider immediately for any signs of illness and/or fever, rather than treating the infant at home.

Parents of older babies will want to discuss the management of colds, flu, teething, constipation, diarrhea, and other common ailments with their clinician before they occur. Although fevers in otherwise healthy older babies do not necessarily require treatment with antipyretics, their healthcare provider can make recommendations regarding over-the-counter analgesics and antipyretic medications, such as acetaminophen or ibuprofen, to increase comfort as necessary.

Aspirin is infrequently used since it was noted to be associated with Reye's syndrome in children with varicella or influenza. Although some healthcare providers recommend alternating ibuprofen and acetaminophen, this practice has not been demonstrated to be useful or safe through research. Because a combination of the two cannot be safely recommended at this time, nurses should educate parents that treatment with a single antipyretic is recommended. Additionally, parents should be encouraged to discuss therapeutic safe doses with their healthcare provider (Carson, 2003; Kayman, 2003).

Stools and Urine

The appearance and frequency of a newborn's stools can cause concern for parents. The nurse prepares them by discussing and showing pictures of meconium stools and transitional stools and by describing the difference between breast milk and formula stools. Although each baby develops his or her own stooling patterns, parents can get an idea of what to expect (see Figure 28–12 ∞).

- Babies can be expected to have at least one meconium stool on the first day of life and at least two during the second 24 hours. Three to four stools can be expected each day by

3 to 5 days of age, and three to six stools per day on days 5 through 7 and thereafter (AAP Section on Breastfeeding, 2005). Stools progress from meconium on the first 2 days to transitional (greenish-brown) stools, to mushy yellow and seedy. Once breastfeeding is well established, usually by 1 month of age, individual babies vary in their stooling patterns. Constipation is unlikely to occur in newborns receiving only breast milk. Infrequent stooling in the first few weeks may indicate inadequate milk intake.

- Formula-fed babies may have only 1 or 2 stools a day; they are more formed and yellow or yellow-brown.

The parents may also be shown pictures of a constipated stool (small, pelletlike) and diarrhea (watery, loose, green, or perhaps blood-tinged). Families should understand that a green color is common in transitional stools so that they do not mistake transitional stools for diarrhea during the first week of a newborn's life.

Babies normally void (urinate) at least once in the first 24 hours and at least twice in the second 24 hours. At least three to five voids can be expected on days 3 through 5 and four to six voids on days 5 through 7 (AAP Section on Breastfeeding, 2005). By the fifth day of life and thereafter, the newborn can be expected to have five or more wet diapers per day. Fewer may indicate the newborn needs more fluids. Frequency of voiding is easy to assess with cloth diapers. Parents who use superabsorbent single-use disposable diapers may have difficulty determining voiding patterns because the surface of the diaper feels dry. The liquid pools inside the filling of the diaper. Parents can pull the top layer off to check whether the filling is saturated. Although pink or orange uric acid crystals may be found in the diaper during the first few days of life, the presence of crystals beyond the third or fourth day may indicate inadequate hydration.

DIAPER CARE

The diaper area should be cleansed and well dried with each diaper change to prevent diaper rash. Frequent diaper changes that allow the infant to spend short periods of time air-drying with the diaper off help to prevent maceration and irritation. Even with proper care many babies experience some type of diaper rash. This can take the form of contact dermatitis, a nonimmunologic reaction to the friction, occlusion, moisture, urine, feces, and chemicals in the diaper environment. Less commonly, it may be a form of allergic contact dermatitis related to fragrances or dyes in the diapers. It is often difficult clinically to distinguish between the two (Alberta, Sweeney, & Wiss, 2005).

Moisturizers such as petrolatum provide protection from wetness and promote healing of mildly irritated skin. Generous application of a protective skin barrier containing zinc oxide is recommended to prevent further injury if diaper rash occurs. Fecal material should be removed with each diaper change, but the skin barrier should be maintained if possible and reapplied.

If the ointment does not help the rash, families using single-use (disposable) diapers should try another brand. Alberta et al. (2005) described five cases where use of dye-free diapers markedly improved the skin in young children suspected to have allergen contact dermatitis related to diaper dyes. If the family uses cloth diapers, a different mild detergent, more thorough rinsing, and hanging them in the sun to dry may alleviate the problem. If the rash persists, parents should discuss the problem with their nurse practitioner or physician, because it may be due to a yeast or fungal infection. In this case, the provider may prescribe an appropriate topical agent.

Sleeping

When, where, and for how long their baby sleeps are common concerns of parents. The following sections address SIDS prevention, crib safety, cosleeping, and the proper positioning of a baby for sleep. The newborn's sleep/wake states are then described.

SIDS PREVENTION

Sudden infant death syndrome (SIDS) is defined as "the sudden unexpected death of an infant less than 1 year of age, with onset of the fatal episode apparently occurring during sleep, that remains unexplained after a thorough investigation, including performance of a complete autopsy and review of the circumstances of death and the clinical history" (Krous, Beckwith, Byord et al., 2004, p. 237). As discussed later in this chapter, *babies should sleep on their backs* as recommended by the AAP. In 2005, a number of recommendations were published by the AAP to prevent SIDS deaths.

The AAP recommends a "standard" sleep surface such as a firm crib mattress that is covered with a sheet specifically designed for infants. Soft crib materials and makeshift bedding composed of pillows, comforters, sheepskin, quilts, or similar items should not be used and should be removed from the crib. Infant toys, stuffed animals, and loose blankets and sheets should all be removed. If a blanket is used, it should be secured by tucking it under the mattress. Blankets should be inspected to ensure they are not covering the infant's face. Blankets should not come higher than chest level on a sleeping infant. Parents may be advised to instead use sleep clothing or sleep sacks to reduce the danger from unsecured blankets. Nurses should educate parents about the need to maintain proper temperature for the infant, because overheating is also a risk factor for SIDS. Recent recommendations have included keeping the infant in close proximity to the parents (within the same room but not in the same bed) to reduce the incidence of SIDS (Barclay & Lie, 2005).

Recent studies show that women who smoke while pregnant have a much greater incidence of having a baby die of SIDS than do nonsmokers (Barclay & Lie, 2005). Smoking should be avoided in the home and around children to minimize SIDS risk as well as the numerous additional risks of secondhand smoke. Adequate ventilation in and around the crib should be provided.

The AAP also recommends giving infants a pacifier when napping or sleeping, because the use of pacifiers has decreased the incidence of SIDS (Barclay & Lie, 2005). Parents should be advised that the pacifier does not need to be reinserted once it falls out after the infant has fallen asleep. The pacifier should not be coated with sweet substances or sugar, and it should be cleaned and replaced frequently. Infants who do not wish to use a pacifier should not be forced to do so (Barclay & Lie, 2005).

These recommendations are for healthy infants, and parents should follow them unless otherwise directed by their healthcare provider in response to a particular medical condition. Nurses have the opportunity to assess for risk factors in the home environment and to educate families, particularly clients in groups at high risk for SIDS. Parents can be encouraged to attend infant cardiopulmonary resuscitation (CPR) classes, especially if there is a family history of SIDS, prematurity, or another health problem.

The SIDS rate in African Americans continues to remain higher than that in other races. Shields, Hunsaker, Muldoon, colleagues (2005) found that black parents were significantly more likely than whites to bed share at both 1 and 6 months of age and significantly less likely to place infants in the supine position at 6 months of age. Practices recommended to reduce the racial disparity in SIDS deaths include back sleeping, use of firm mattresses, avoidance of loose bedding, avoidance of parental smoking, and avoidance of overheating infants (Unger, Kemp, Wilkins et al., 2003). The home care nurse should emphasize these recommendations to this vulnerable population.

Bed sharing often occurs in low-income families when there is no access to a safe crib (Unger et al., 2003). Bed sharing on soft surfaces or with individuals other than the mother, particularly with siblings, is associated with higher risk. Home health nurses should work with local agencies and charitable organizations to make approved cribs accessible to low-income families.

CRIB SAFETY

During the home visit, the nurse discusses with the family their newborn's sleeping arrangements, and observes the crib, bassinet, cradle, mat, or other devices. If possible, the nurse should observe the infant while sleeping to ensure all safety precautions are being followed.

Parents will want to make certain that their infant's crib meets all federal safety standards as set by the Consumer Product Safety Commission and ASTM (formerly the American Society for Testing and Materials) (Barclay & Lie, 2005). The crib headboard and footboard should be solid, with no large designs cut out of the wood, as the infant's head could become entrapped in them. Crib slats should be no more than 2 3/8 inches apart. If the crib is older and painted, ensure that the paint is nonlead based. If there is any doubt, the crib should not be used unless it is stripped and painted with new enamel. It is important for parents to be aware that safety regulations today are different from those in years past and that there are safety issues with the use of an old crib.

Mattresses should fit snugly to prevent entrapment and suffocation and should always be lowered to a level at which the infant cannot fall out. Parents should always leave the side rails up when the baby is in the crib, even if they are in the room. Parents should inspect the crib regularly to determine whether it is in safe working order, with no splinters, sharp edges, or loose parts.

COSLEEPING

Cosleeping or **bed sharing** refers to an infant sleeping in close social and/or physical contact with a committed caregiver (usually the mother). Cosleeping may include sharing any surface, such as a mat, futon, or floor. Bed sharing is just one form of cosleeping (Academy of Breastfeeding Medicine [ABM], 2003). The practice of maternal-infant cosleeping has for centuries been the norm in many cultures, and it has become a topic of heated debate in the United States.

In 2005, the AAP created recommendations that included a statement that cosleeping with infants may put them at risk for SIDS. A number of studies over the past few years have found problems with entrapment, suffocation, and overlaying by larger individuals when infants cosleep on surfaces not intended for infant sleep (Mesich, 2005). The AAP has, since 1997, strongly discouraged bed sharing on soft surfaces or in situations with caregivers who smoked or had used alcohol or drugs (Shields et al., 2005).

As the debate continues, home healthcare nurses should review the most recent studies and recommendations. It is important for nurses to make parents aware of AAP recommendations so they can make informed decisions regarding their newborn's safety within the context of their culture, personal beliefs, and living situation. Following extensive reviews of literature on both sides of the issue, Mesich (2005), Quillin and Glenn (2004), and the ABM (2003) all developed advice for parents regarding safety measures for newborn sleep environments. The following list incorporates their separate recommendations for those families who practice cosleeping with their infants:

- Place infant on the "Back to Sleep"!
- If the infant breastfeeds in a side-lying position, move the infant to his or her back after nursing.
- Place the infant on a firm mattress, never on comforters, pillows, sofas, daybeds, or waterbeds.
- Adult beds are not designed to meet federal safety standards for infants and do have potential risks.
- If the infant is to sleep on an adult bed, the mattress should be moved to the floor to prevent falls.
- Headboards, footboards, and side rails should be removed to prevent wedging or entrapment.
- Remove all cords, ties, or other strangulation risks from the environment.
- Use a tightly fitting fitted sheet on the surface where an infant sleeps.
- Do not smoke in the home during or after pregnancy.
- Mothers who smoke should not cosleep with their infants.
- Remove all decorative pillows, stuffed animals or toys, or blankets that could impair the baby's breathing.
- Avoid down or fluffy comforters, pillows, sheepskins, bean bags, or quilts on top of or under the baby.
- Ensure plenty of ventilation to the infant and avoid overbundling.
- Never cosleep with an infant after the use of alcohol, depressants, sedatives, or illegal substances.
- Cosleeping is best limited to the mother and the infant.
- Mothers greater than 175 pounds have a higher risk of overlaying while cosleeping.

PROPER POSITIONING FOR SLEEP

Newborns and infants should always be placed in the supine position to sleep, as recommended by the AAP since 1992 (Figure 36–4 ◆). If the infant breastfeeds in a side-lying position, move the infant back to his or her back after nursing. National SIDS rates have decreased more than 40% since the AAP's "Back to Sleep" campaign began. Although there were initial concerns that supine sleeping may result in increases in aspiration, a review of vital statistics data found no evidence of increased risk of death from aspiration as a result of the "Back to Sleep" campaign. In fact, the mortality rate for aspiration-related deaths has dropped since 1991 as well. These findings are similar to those in other countries that have initiated supine sleeping campaigns (Malloy, 2002).

However, an increase in the number of children with cranial asymmetry, particularly unilateral flattening of the occiput, has been noted since the "Back to Sleep" campaign began. Parents should therefore be counseled within the newborn's first 2 to 4 weeks of life to place their infant in the prone position to allow "tummy time" *while the infant is awake and under their direct observation*. This position will promote upper shoulder girdle strength and will help to prevent the development of flat areas on the occiput.

Parents can also be taught to alternate their infant's head position from right to left each night when placing the newborn

Figure 36–4 ◆ Infants should be placed on their backs when sleeping.

supine for sleep. Periodically changing the infant's orientation to outside activity such as the bedroom door will encourage the infant to use more than one head position to sleep and rest. This can be accomplished by placing the infant at alternate ends of the crib or bassinet (Persing, James, Swanson et al., 2003).

The home care nurse can demonstrate these positions for the parents, reinforce the importance of supine sleep in relation to SIDS prevention, and give parents other ideas for carrying and positioning, such as the use of front packs, backpacks, and slings. Parents should be encouraged to read and follow all product information provided by the manufacturer. Many parents express concern about the newborn's choking or spitting up if placed supine after feedings. The nurse can encourage parents to hold their infants upright or place them on their side after feedings, provided the newborn remains under their direct observation. Although the side position is safer than the prone position, the supine position (lying wholly on the back) carries the lowest risk of SIDS and is preferred when the infant is unobserved (AAP & ACOG, 2002).

Bullock, Mickey, Green et al. (2004) found that, despite the AAP guidelines, many practicing maternal-child nurses continue to use lateral or a combination of lateral and supine positioning for newborns in the hospital. These findings are consistent with previous studies. Because nurses are important role models for postpartum families, the home care nurse bears the responsibility of ensuring that parents are properly educated on "Back to Sleep."

Finally, infants who routinely sleep supine face an even greater risk for SIDS when placed prone for sleep. Some licensed child care providers do not observe or even have an awareness of the recommendations for supine sleep (Moon & Oden, 2003; Moon, Weese-Mayer, & Silvestri, 2003). Because many mothers return to the workforce during the first year of their newborn's life, it is essential that parents educate caregivers and family members who will care for the newborn in their absence about the importance of "Back to Sleep" and insist that it is practiced with their child.

Sleep-Wake States

The newborn demonstrates several different sleep-wake states after the initial periods of reactivity. It is not uncommon for a newborn to sleep almost continuously for the first 2 to 3 days following birth, awakening only for feedings every 3 to 4 hours. Some newborns bypass this stage of deep sleep and require only 12 to 16 hours of sleep. The parents need to know that this is normal.

Sleep states include **deep sleep** and **light sleep.** During *deep sleep* the infant will be nearly still except for occasional startles, twitches, and sucking. The infant will arouse to intense stimuli, and care and feeding at this time will be frustrating. *Light sleep* makes up the highest proportion of newborn sleep and usually precedes awakening. It is characterized by some body movements, rapid eye movements (REM), and brief fussing or crying. The infant may arouse, remain in light sleep, or return to deep sleep in response to stimuli. Infants are not usually ready to feed in this state.

Awake states include **drowsy, quiet alert, active alert,** and **crying states.** *Drowsy* infants open and close their eyes,

but the eyes appear glazed and the face is often still. They may return to sleep or awaken further in response to stimuli. The *quiet alert state* is characterized by a brightening of the eyes and face. Infants are most attentive to their environment in this state and provide positive feedback to caregivers. It is usually easiest to initiate feeds during this state (Karl, 2004). The *active alert state* brings about an increase in facial and body movement, with periods of fussiness occurring. The infant in this state has increased sensitivity to disturbing stimuli, and intervention to console the infant at this point is beneficial.

Crying is evidenced by increased motor activity, grimaces, eyes tightly closed or open, and extreme responsiveness to stimuli. Infants may be able to console themselves, or they may require consoling from a caregiver.

For newborns, crying is a spontaneous response to unpleasant stimuli, and their only means of expressing their needs vocally. After 2 or 3 days, newborns settle into individual patterns and families learn to distinguish different tones and qualities of this newborn's cry. The amount of crying is also highly individual. Some newborns cry as little as 15 to 30 minutes in 24 hours, or as long as 2 or more hours. When crying continues after such causes as discomfort or hunger are eliminated, the newborn may be comforted by swaddling, rocking, or other reassuring activities. There is some indication that newborns who are held more tend to be calmer and cry less when not being held. Some parents may be afraid that holding will "spoil" the newborn, and need reassurance that is not the case. On the contrary, picking babies up when they cry teaches them that adults are responsive to them. This helps build a sense of trust in humankind. Of course, the nurse documents and assesses any crying, and provides teaching and referrals as necessary. See Table 36–4 for the characteristics and caregiving implication of each state.

It was so exciting to go home with our new baby. That first day went quite well and Joe and I felt that we were on our way as new parents. Our son had been fed and diapered a number of times and it was now time for bed. When we snuggled him in his bassinet, he lay quietly and didn't cry. Then we looked at each other, and at the same time said, 'What if we don't hear him in the middle of the night?' We went on to bed but with much trepidation. Our baby's first cry in the night woke us immediately. We both sat up and simultaneously said, 'There he is!'

After a few weeks, we could laugh at the anxiety we had during those first few days. I'm sure all new parents must have had similar experiences.

Injury Prevention

Unintentional injuries are the leading cause of death in children, accounting for 44.5% of all deaths between the ages of 1 and 19 in 2002 (Martin, Kochanek, Strobino et al., 2005). An analysis of pediatric injuries found falls, poisoning, transportation, foreign body, and fires/burns (in that order) to be the leading causes of injury resulting in hospitalization or death in children from birth to 3 years. Leading causes of injury by age group were falls from height between 0 and 2 months, battering from 3 to 5 months, falls from furniture at 6 to 8 months, nonairway foreign body at 9 to 11 months, and hot liquid and vapor injuries at 12

Table 36–4   INFANT SLEEP AND AWAKE STATES*

Infant States	Physical Characteristics	Body Activity	Eye Movements	Facial Movements	Breathing Pattern	Responses	Caregiver Implications
Sleep States Quiet sleep (also known as deep sleep)	Anabolic, restorative sleep, increased cell mitosis and replication, lowered oxygen consumption, release of growth hormone.	Typically still, may occasionally startle or twitch.	None	None or may have occasional sucking movements.	Slow and regular.	Only intense or disturbing stimuli will arouse infant, threshold to stimuli is high.	Difficult to arouse for feedings. Teach parents to time feedings when infant is in a more responsive state. Infant may arouse slightly if an attempt is made to awaken but typically returns to the quiet sleep state.
Active sleep (also known as light sleep or rapid eye movement [REM] state)	Processing and recording information. Often linked to learning. Is the highest proportion of sleep and precedes awakening.	Some body movements.	REM, eyelids flutter beneath closed eyelids.	May smile or make fussing or crying noises.	Irregular.	More responsive to internal stimuli (hunger) and external stimuli (such as being picked up by caregiver). When stimulated may arouse, return to quiet sleep, or remain in active sleep.	Inexperienced care providers may attempt to feed when infant makes normal crying sounds.
Awake States Drowsy	May return to sleep or awaken further.	Smooth movements with variable activity level. May experience mild startles intermittently.	Eyes may open and close. May appear heavy-lidded, or eyes may appear like slits.	May have no facial movements and appear still, or may have some facial movements.	Irregular.	Usually reacts to stimuli but may be slowed. May change to other states such as quiet alert, active alert, or crying.	To stimulate infant, provide verbal, sight, or oral stimulation. If left alone, infant may return to a sleep state.
Quiet alert	Attentive to environment, focus attention on stimuli.	Minimal	Eyes bright and wide.	Attentive appearance.	Regular.	Most attentive, focus attention on stimuli.	In the first hours after birth, may experience intense alertness before going into a long sleeping period. This state increases in intensity as the infant becomes older. Providing stimuli will help maintain an active alert state or a drowsy or active-alert state. Infant provides pleasure and positive feedback to care providers. Good time to feed infant.
Active alert	Infant's eyes are open, not as bright as in quiet alert. More body activity than in a quiet alert state.	Smooth movements may be interspersed with mild startles from time to time.	Eyes open with a gazed, dull appearance.	May be still with or without facial movements.	Irregular.	Reacts to stimuli with delayed responses to stimuli, or may change to quiet alert or crying state.	Infant may be fussy and become more sensitive to stimuli, may become more and more active and start crying. If fatigue or caregiver interventions disturb this state, infant may return to a drowsy or sleep state.
Crying	Communication tool, response to unpleasant stimuli from environment or internal stimuli. Characterized by intense crying for more than 15 seconds.	Increased motor activity, skin color changes to darkened appearance, red, or ruddy.	Eyes may be tightly closed or open.	Grimaces	More irregular than in other states.	Very responsive to internal or external unpleasant stimuli.	Indicates that the infant's limits have been reached. May be able to console himself or herself and return to an alert or sleep state, or may need intervention from caregiver.

* A *state* is a group of characteristic behaviors and physiologic changes that occur together in a regular pattern.

SOURCE: March of Dimes. (2003). *Understanding the behavior of term infants.* White Plains, NY: Author.

to 17 months. Poisoning by medication led the causes of injury from 18 to 35 months. Both battering and neglect rates were highest among infants 0 to 2 months and 3 to 5 months of age. Bathtub submersions peaked at age 6 to 11 months. Young children had the highest injury rate between 15 and 17 months, coinciding with their independent mobility, exploratory behavior, and hand-to-mouth activity (Agran, Anderson, Winn et al., 2003). It is helpful to keep these causes of injury in mind when counseling new parents regarding safety in the home.

During the home visit, the nurse observes the environment and identifies changes that need to be made to childproof the home. For example, accessible electrical outlets can cause severe injury or death. Childproof covers should be installed to decrease the risk of electrocution. Unattended pots and pans on stoves can easily be pulled over, scalding or seriously burning young children. The nurse can advise the family to install a stove guard (a plastic partition that prevents small children from touching hot stoves or pulling down pots or pans). Handles should also be turned inward and should not protrude over the edge of the stove. Poisonous substances and medications should be secured. It is essential that the parents understand never to leave a baby unattended on any elevated surface and that they understand never to shake a baby. It is important for nurses to be aware of the impact they can have on the safety of families through the use of home visits.

SHAKEN BABY INJURIES

Shaken baby injuries, which are any injuries acquired by an infant as a result of being shaken or hit, are a major focus of prevention for home healthcare nurses. The AAP has made a number of recommendations to address and prevent shaken baby injuries, including home visitation programs and any other child abuse prevention efforts that prove efficacious. A hospital-based program educating parents on the dangers of violent infant shaking and recommending alternative responses to infant crying significantly decreased the incidence of abusive head injuries among infants of parents who received the information (Dias, Smith, deGuehey et al., 2005). In another study, five postnatal home visits by nurse-midwives to teenage mothers resulted in a reduction in adverse neonatal outcomes such as infant death, severe nonaccidental injury, and nonvoluntary foster care (Quinlivan, Box, & Evans, 2003). Home visits provide an ideal opportunity to educate parents regarding safety and injury prevention, shaken baby injuries, and the hazards of abuse and neglect. Home visits are also the ideal time to provide appropriate resources and referrals.

INFANT COLIC AS A PARENTAL STRESSOR

Infant colic is manifested by persistent, unexplained, inconsolable crying, and is a source of great distress to new parents. A literature review by Ellett, Schuff, and Davis (2005) found that infant colic occurs in 15% to 25% of infants. It often emerges at 2 to 3 weeks of age, peaks in intensity by age 6 weeks, and may continue until the infant is 3 to 6 months of age. It occurs equally in both genders and across races, ethnicities, and socioeconomic classes. Their qualitative research

found that parents described the experience as unforgettable, exhausting, and frustrating. Support from spouses, friends, family members, and healthcare providers was essential, and parents without support felt very isolated. Although most parents reported that the infants grew to develop normally and were often very intelligent, a number of parents noted that the experience strained the marital relationship and that the family processes were disrupted for some time afterward.

It is important for nurses to provide new parents with anticipatory guidance regarding the symptoms of infant colic and the strain that it can cause in family relationships. Parents should be encouraged to seek help from their infant's healthcare provider as well as support from family and friends if colic occurs. It is also important to reassure parents that the condition does resolve in time and that newborns go on to develop normally. Home care nurses should be aware of local support groups and/or hotlines for colic and share these resources with all new parents.

Newborn Screening and Immunization Program

Before the newborn and mother are discharged from the hospital, the nurse informs parents about the normal screening tests for newborns and tells them when to return for further tests if needed. The home care nurse ensures that the blood specimens have been obtained and may obtain a specimen as necessary.

Newborn screening tests detect disorders that cause mental retardation, physical handicaps, or death if left undiscovered. Disorders that can usually be detected from a drop of blood obtained by a heel stick on the second or third day include galactosemia, congenital adrenal hyperplasia, congenital hypothyroidism, phenylketonuria (PKU), and sickle cell anemia. Parents should be instructed that a second blood specimen will often be required from the newborn after 7 to 14 days. It must be clarified that an abnormal test result is not diagnostic. More definitive tests must be performed to verify the results. It is important to follow protocols that incorporate state laws about newborn testing.

If additional tests are positive, treatment is initiated. These conditions may be treated by dietary means or by administering missing hormones. The inborn conditions cannot be cured, but they can be treated. They are not contagious, but they may be inherited (see Chapter 32 ∞).

The nurse should ensure that the family has information regarding the current childhood immunization schedule and has plans to begin or continue immunizations. The nurse should be familiar with current recommendations and should share information about immunizations with the family as necessary.

HOME CARE: THE MOTHER AND FAMILY

Home care of the mother and family involves performing an assessment of the mother and family as well as discussing breastfeeding concerns.

RESEARCH IN PRACTICE

AN INTERVENTION PROGRAM FOR FAMILIES WITH IRRITABLE INFANTS

What is this study about? Colic, referred to as irritable infant syndrome, can disturb the parent-child relationship and cause parents to doubt their parenting skills. It is thought to be due to dysfunction in the infant's ability to self-regulate sleep-wake cycles due to central nervous system immaturity. Irritable infants are easily overstimulated; as they become overwhelmed, they cannot self-soothe or reduce their arousal level sufficiently. As a result, they give inconsistent clues to parents as to what they require. Parents may unwittingly reinforce the irritable behavior by unproductive strategies to soothe the baby. This study was conducted to describe and evaluate a home-based nursing intervention program called REST. The intervention includes parent education and support in recognizing infant behaviors and responding in an effective manner.

How was this study done? This study was a randomized controlled trial conducted in two geographic sites. A sample of 164 full-term, healthy infants were recruited if they had symptoms of excessive unexplained irritability or colic between the ages of 2 and 6 weeks. The infants were randomly assigned to either a treatment group that received the homebound intervention, or a control group that received routine home care. There were four interventions relative to the infant and four for the parents. The four primary nursing interventions in the REST program for parents are: *reassurance* about the infant's health and the parent's competence; *empathy* through listening and acknowledging the challenges of parenting these high-need infants; *support* as an advocate and resource for parents in obtaining assistance and creating a support network; and *time-out* that legitimizes the parent's critical need for self-care. The infant-based REST strategies included: *regulation* to help these infants regulate their behavior and prevent overstimulation; *entrainment* in which the infant's sleep-wake cycles are synchronized with environmental conditions; *structure* and repetition that creates a predictable, soothing pattern of events; and *touch* that includes various infant holds and positions and encourages skin-to-

skin contact. These skills were taught over four home visits. All parents were asked to complete a weekly assessment of their infant's amount of crying and level of fussiness using a reliable, valid scale.

What were the results of the study? Initial unexplained infant crying in both treatment and control groups was reported to almost 6 hours per day when the study began. The hours of crying declined as the child approached 8 weeks of age in both groups. However, the infants who received the home-based intervention had a steeper decline in both the amount of crying and the degree of fussiness. On average, infants in the intervention program cried 1.3 hours per day, compared with 3 hours per day in the control group. Parents reported that irritability was resolved in less than 1 hour for 62% of the intervention group, while only 29% of the control group was able to resolve irritability within an hour. Qualitative comments solicited from the parents provided anecdotal information that the parents reported benefits from the attention, instruction, and support received during the interventional home visits.

What additional questions might I have? Do these outcomes apply to babies who are not full term and are not healthy? Were there any negative outcomes reported from either the intervention or the parent's responses to the interventions? Did the increased attention alone—from the number of home visits to the intervention alone—create a difference in the outcome?

How can I use this study? Infant irritability syndrome, or colic, is a frustrating condition that makes new parents doubt their abilities as parents. Interventions that can reduce both the amount of unexplainable crying and irritability in an infant can enhance the parenting experience. Early discharge for new mothers from the acute care setting makes it difficult to teach more than basic infant care skills. Home visits dedicated to helping parents deal with an irritable infant can improve the quality of the experience of having a newborn baby.

Keefer, M., Barboxa, G., Froese-Fretz, A., Kotzer, A., & Lobo, M. (2005). An intervention program for families with irritable infants. *American Journal of Maternal/Child Nursing, 30*(4), 120–126.

Assessment of the Mother and Family at Home

During the home visit, the nurse can complete ongoing postpartum assessment following discharge. The initial goal is to assess the woman's perceptions of her current circumstances, her recovery from childbirth, her adjustment and that of her partner to parenthood, the newborn's condition, family-newborn bonding, and any problems or concerns the woman may have. The nurse asks specifically about the following areas: (1) progression of lochia (color, amount of flow, presence of foul odor or clots); (2) fever or malaise; (3) dysuria or difficulty voiding; (4) pain in the pelvis or perineum; (5) painful, reddened hot spots or shooting pains in the breasts during or between feedings; and (6) areas of redness, edema, tenderness, or warmth in the legs. The nurse also talks

with the mother about her diet, fatigue level, ability to rest and sleep, pain management, signs of postpartal complications, activity level, sexuality issues, self-care ability, social support system, and any pertinent cultural or religious practices related to postpartum or newborn care. Before performing the physical assessment, the nurse ensures privacy. The physical assessment focuses on maternal physical adaptation, which is assessed by evaluating vital signs, breasts, abdominal musculature, bowel and bladder elimination patterns, fundal height and location, the perineum, lochia, edema, and laboratory values.

The psychologic assessment focuses on attachment, adjustment to the parental role, maternal emotions, sibling adjustment, and educational needs. When appropriate, the nurse mentions available community resources, including the public health department, which can be used for follow-up visits. In ideal situations, a family approach involving the presence of the father and any siblings provides an opportunity to observe family interactions and opportunities for all family members to ask questions and express concerns. In addition, this approach may bring to the surface any questionable family interaction pattern, such as one suggestive of abuse or neglect; the nurse can consider further referral if needed. See Assessment Guide: Postpartal—First Home Visit and Anticipated Progress at Six Weeks.

If information about family-planning options has not been addressed previously, the nurse provides it at this time and answers any questions the woman or her partner may have about methods of birth control and their sexual relationship.

POSTPARTUM FATIGUE

Postpartum fatigue is a major concern that may trouble new mothers for as long as 19 months postpartum. It is characterized by feelings of exhaustion and decreased capacity for physical and mental work. Based on her research and a review of the literature, Troy (2003) summarizes physical, psychologic, and situational factors that can contribute to maternal postpartum fatigue. Physical factors include length of labor, type of delivery, blood loss associated with delivery, anemia, hormonal shifts, wound or episiotomy healing, pain, and breastfeeding. Psychologic factors include sleep difficulties, nonsupportive partner, and depression. Situational factors include infant care responsibilities, multiple roles, length of postpartum hospital stay, lack of assistance with child care and/or housework, more than one child at home, returning to work outside the home, and child care difficulties.

Although more research needs to be done, there are relationships among fatigue, stress, postpartum depression, immune function, breast milk production, and breast milk biology in new mothers (Groer, Davis, Casey et al., 2005). Although mothers often expect to feel some fatigue during pregnancy, they are frequently caught off guard by the depth and duration of postpartum fatigue. George (2005) found that new mothers expressed surprise and distress at the amount of pain and fatigue they experienced postpartum. Postpartum fatigue affects not only the health of the couplet but the family processes as well.

The home care nurse can inform mothers that fatigue may be a significant problem and stress the need for good nutrition and periods of uninterrupted sleep if possible. Using family and friends for assistance with responsibilities, limiting visitors, and using an answering machine or voicemail will allow for more rest. The nurse can also reinforce continued use of prescribed prenatal vitamins and iron, particularly if the client is breastfeeding.

During the home visit, the nurse continues to provide teaching to the mother and her family and describes self-care measures as needed. The nurse also reviews the signs of developing illness with the woman and her partner. If signs of potential complications are present, the nurse completes a more in-depth evaluation and determines whether it is necessary for the woman to see her primary care provider.

Breastfeeding Concerns Following Discharge

The U.S. Department of Health and Human Services (HHS) Office on Women's Health (OWH), along with other federal agencies and professional organizations, developed the HHS Blueprint for Action on Breastfeeding. The blueprint recommendations have been translated into the National Breastfeeding Awareness Campaign to promote breastfeeding among first-time parents. The goal of this campaign is aligned with that of *Healthy People 2010*—to increase initial breastfeeding rates to 75% and 6-month rates to 50% by 2010 (Lewis, 2003).

Breastfeeding benefits maternal as well as newborn health and results in cost savings for parents, insurers, and employers. Therefore, it has a high economic as well as medical value for society (Lewis, 2003). However, most mothers are discharged before breastfeeding is well established and many require anticipatory guidance and support in order to continue once they go home. Chezem, Friesen, and Boettcher (2003) found a correlation between breastfeeding knowledge and the duration of breastfeeding and achievement of breastfeeding goals. Therefore, time is well spent when educating clients on the benefits and techniques related to breastfeeding.

George (2005) found that all first-time mothers experienced feelings of unpreparedness to care for themselves and their infants following discharge. Many had questions about newborn care, particularly breastfeeding, but they felt that there was too much information to absorb during their hospital stay. Because many mothers discontinue breastfeeding as a result of problems and concerns early on, the home visit is the ideal time to promote continuation of breastfeeding. The home care nurse has the opportunity to not only reinforce initial breastfeeding teaching and answer questions, but also to observe an episode of breastfeeding in the home environment where it will continue until weaning. Guidance and support can be individualized according to the mother's specific needs and living situation. There are numerous books and references available to assist nurses in the care of breastfeeding couplets. See Table 36–5 for more detailed information.

The AAP recommends that all breastfeeding newborns be seen by a pediatrician or other knowledgeable healthcare professional at 3 to 5 days of age to assess weight and to have a physical exam to include assessment of jaundice and hydration, maternal breastfeeding status, infant elimination, and formal observation of a breastfeeding session (AAP Section on Breastfeeding, 2005). A home visit a few days after discharge meets these requirements and can identify at-risk infants before they lose excessive weight and at a time when intervention can correct most breastfeeding problems before they become complicated by insufficient milk. The home health nurse can assess the infant and the breastfeeding process, provide appropriate education to promote breastfeeding, and initiate referrals to a lactation consultant or primary healthcare provider as needed. Additionally, the nurse can provide individualized support and encouragement as desired by the client.

ASSESSMENT GUIDE   Postpartal—First Home Visit and Anticipated Progress at Six Weeks

PHYSICAL ASSESSMENT/ NORMAL FINDINGS	ALTERATIONS AND POSSIBLE CAUSES*	NURSING RESPONSES TO DATA†
VITAL SIGNS		
Blood pressure: Return to normal prepregnant level.	Elevated blood pressure (anxiety, essential hypertension, renal disease), preeclampsia (can occur postpartum).	Review history, evaluate normal baseline; refer to physician/certified nurse midwife (CNM) if necessary.
Pulse: 60–90 bpm (or prepregnant normal rate).	Increased pulse rate, tachycardia, chest pain (excitement, anxiety, blood loss, cardiac disorders).	Count pulse for full minute, note irregularities; marked tachycardia or beat irregularities require additional assessment and possible physician/CNM referral.
Respirations: 12–24/min.	Marked tachypnea or abnormal patterns (respiratory or cardiac disorders).	Evaluate for respiratory disease or cardiac complications; refer to physician/CNM if necessary.
Temperature: 36.6C–37.6C (98F–99.6F).	Increased temperature (infection or engorgement).	Assess for signs and symptoms of infection or disease state.
WEIGHT		
2 days: Possible weight loss of 12–20+ lb.	Minimal weight loss (fluid retention, preeclampsia).	Evaluate for fluid retention, edema, deep tendon reflexes, and blood pressure elevation.
6 weeks: Returning to normal prepregnant weight.	Retained weight (excessive caloric intake).	Determine amount of daily exercise. Provide dietary teaching. Refer to dietitian if necessary for additional dietary counseling.
	Extreme weight loss (excessive dieting, inadequate caloric intake).	Discuss appropriate diets, refer to dietitian for additional counseling if necessary; reinforce need for up to 500 additional kcal/day when breastfeeding.
BREASTS		
Nonbreastfeeding: 2 days: May have mild tenderness; small amount of milk may be expressed. 6 weeks: Soft, with no tenderness; return to prepregnant size.	Some engorgement (incomplete suppression of lactation). Redness; hardened area, marked tenderness (mastitis). Palpable mass (tumor).	Engorgement may be seen in nonbreastfeeding mothers. Advise client to wear a supportive, well-fitted bra, avoid very warm showers, avoid pumping or any stimulation of breasts, use ice packs for comfort, evaluate for signs and symptoms of mastitis.
Breastfeeding: Full, with prominent nipples; lactation established.	Cracked, fissured nipples (improper latch). Redness, marked tenderness, hardened area (mastitis or abscess). Palpable mass (plugged milk duct, tumor).	Counsel about nipple care. Observe infant feeding. Evaluate client condition, evidence of fever; refer to physician/CNM for initiation of antibiotic therapy, if indicated. A breastfeeding mother should examine her breasts monthly, after feeding, when breasts are empty; if palpable mass is felt, refer to physician for further evaluation. For breast engorgement accompanied by erythema, instruct the mother to 1. Keep breast empty by frequent feeding. 2. Rest when possible with breasts elevated. 3. Take prescribed pain relief med. 4. Drink adequate fluids. If symptoms persist for more than 24 hours, or if accompanied by fever greater than 100.4, or flu-like symptoms, redness, instruct her to call her physician/CNM.
	*Possible causes of alterations are identified in parentheses.	†This column provides guidelines for further assessment and initial intervention.

(Continued on next page)

ASSESSMENT GUIDE   Postpartal—First Home Visit and Anticipated
Progress at Six Weeks continued

PHYSICAL ASSESSMENT/ NORMAL FINDINGS	ALTERATIONS AND POSSIBLE CAUSES*	NURSING RESPONSES TO DATA†
ABDOMINAL MUSCULATURE		
2 days: Improved firmness, although "bread dough" consistency is not unusual, especially in multipara. Striae pink and obvious.	Marked relaxation of muscles.	Evaluate exercise level; provide information on appropriate exercise program.
Cesarean incision healing.	Drainage, redness, tenderness, pain, edema (infection).	Evaluate for infection; refer to physician/CNM if necessary.
6 weeks: Muscle tone continues to improve; striae may be beginning to fade, may not achieve a silvery appearance for several more weeks; linea nigra fading.		
ELIMINATION PATTERN		
Urinary Tract: Return to prepregnant urinary elimination routine.	Urinary incontinence, especially when lifting, coughing, laughing, and so on (urethral/perineal trauma, hormonal influences, cystocele).	Assess for cystocele; instruct in appropriate muscle tightening exercises; refer to physician/CNM.
	Pain or burning when voiding, urgency and/or frequency, pus or white blood cells (WBC) in urine, pathogenic organisms in culture (stinging may be due to lacerations/episiotomy; urinary tract infection).	Evaluate for urinary tract infection; obtain clean-catch urine; refer to physician/CNM for treatment if indicated.
Routine urinalysis within normal limits (proteinuria disappeared).	Sugar or ketone in urine—may be some lactose present in urine of breastfeeding mothers (diabetes).	Evaluate diet; assess for signs and symptoms of diabetes; refer to physician/CNM.
Bowel Habits: 2 days: May be some discomfort with defecation, especially if client had severe hemorrhoids or third- or fourth-degree extension.	Severe constipation or pain when defecating (trauma or hemorrhoids).	Discuss dietary patterns; encourage fluid, adequate roughage. Continue use of stool softener if necessary to prevent pain associated with straining; continue sitz baths, periods of rest for severe hemorrhoids; assess healing of episiotomy and/or lacerations; severe constipation may require administration of laxatives, stool softeners, and an enema if not contraindicated (check with physician/CNM).
6 weeks: Return to normal prepregnancy bowel elimination.	Marked constipation (inadequate fluid/fiber intake).	See previously discussed interventions.
	Fecal incontinence or constipation (rectocele).	Assess for evidence of rectocele; instruct in muscle tightening exercises; refer to physician/CNM.
REPRODUCTIVE TRACT		
Lochia: 2 days: Lochia rubra or lochia serosa, scant amounts, fleshy odor.	Excessive amounts and/or large clots (nonfirm uterus), foul odor (infection), passing tissue (possible retained placenta).	Assess for evidence of infection and/or failure of the uterus to descend and decrease in size; refer to physician/CNM.
6 weeks: No lochia, or return to normal menstruation pattern.	See above.	See above.
Fundus and Perineum 2 days: Fundus is at least two fingerbreadths below the umbilicus; uterine muscles still somewhat lax; introitus of vagina lacks tone—gapes when intra-abdominal pressure is increased by coughing or straining.	Uterus not decreasing in size appropriately or extremely tender (infection).	Assess fundus for firmness and/or signs of infection; refer to physician/CNM if indicated.
Episiotomy and/or lacerations healing; no signs of infection; may have some bruising and tenderness.	Evidence of redness, severe pain, poor tissue approximation in episiotomy and/or laceration (wound infection).	Continue perineal hygiene care; refer to physician or CNM as necessary.
6 weeks: Uterus almost returned to prepregnant size with almost completely restored muscle tone.	Continued flow of lochia, failure to decrease appropriately in size (subinvolution).	Assess for evidence of subinvolution and/or infection; refer to physician for further evaluation and treatment if necessary.
	*Possible causes of alterations are identified in parentheses.	†This column provides guidelines for further assessment and initial intervention.

ASSESSMENT GUIDE   Postpartal—First Home Visit and Anticipated Progress at Six Weeks continued

PHYSICAL ASSESSMENT/ NORMAL FINDINGS	ALTERATIONS AND POSSIBLE CAUSES*	NURSING RESPONSES TO DATA†
HEMOGLOBIN AND HEMATOCRIT LEVELS 6 weeks: Hemoglobin (Hb) 12 g/dL; Hematocrit (Hct) 37% ±5%	Hb less than 12 g/dL; Hct 32% (anemia).	Assess nutritional status, assess for signs or symptoms of anemia, begin (or continue) supplemental iron; for marked anemia (Hb less than or equal to 9 g/dL) additional assessment and/or physician/CNM referral may be necessary.
ATTACHMENT Bonding process demonstrated by soothing, cuddling, and talking to infant; appropriate feeding techniques; eye-to-eye contact; touching; calling infant by name.	Failure to bond demonstrated by lack of behaviors associated with bonding process, calling infant by nickname that promotes ridicule, inadequate infant weight gain, infant is dirty, hygienic measures are not being maintained, severe diaper rash, failure to obtain adequate supplies to provide infant care (malattachment).	Provide counseling; talk with the woman about her feelings regarding the infant; provide support for the caretaking activities that are being performed; refer to public health nurse or social worker for continued home visits; refer if abuse or neglect is suspected.
Parent interacts with infant and provides soothing, caretaking activities.	Parent is unable to respond to infant needs (inability to recognize needs, inadequate education and support, fear, family stress).	Provide support for caretaking activities observed; provide information regarding caretaking activities, such as responding to infant cry; methods of wrapping infant; methods of soothing the infant such as swaddling, rocking, increasing stimuli by singing to the infant or decreasing stimuli by putting infant to rest in quiet room; methods of holding the infant; differences in the cry. Identify support system such as friends, neighbors; provide information regarding community resources and support groups; reinforce "Never shake a baby."
Parents express feelings of comfort and success with the parent role.	Evidence of stress and anxiety (difficulty moving into or dealing with the parent role).	Provide support and encouragement; provide information regarding progression into parent role and assist parents in talking through their feelings; refer to community resources and support groups.
Woman is in the informal or personal stage of maternal role attainment.	Woman is still greatly influenced by others, has not developed an image or style of her own (woman remains in the anticipatory stage).	Provide role modeling for the woman in working through problem solving with the infant, provide encouragement as she thinks through decisions and develops her sense of problem solving; encourage her to make decisions regarding infant care; provide positive reinforcement.
ADJUSTMENT TO PARENTAL ROLE Parents are coping with new roles in terms of division of labor, financial status, communication, readjustment of sexual relations, and adjusting to new daily tasks.	Inability to adjust to new roles (immaturity, extremes of maternal age, inadequate education and preparation, ineffective communication patterns, inadequate support, current family crisis).	Provide counseling, provide anticipatory guidance, refer to parent groups.
EDUCATION Mother understands self-care measures.	Inadequate knowledge of self-care (inadequate education).	Provide education and counseling.
Parents are knowledgeable regarding infant care.	Inadequate knowledge of infant care (inadequate education).	
Siblings are adjusting to new baby.	Excessive sibling rivalry.	
Parents have a method of contraception.	Birth control method not chosen.	
	*Possible causes of alterations are placed in parentheses.	†This column provides guidelines for further assessment and initial nursing intervention.

EVIDENCE-BASED PRACTICE

SCREENING FOR POSTPARTUM DEPRESSION

Postpartum depression (PPD) can result in significant personal suffering and can have devastating effects on maternal-infant health. It frequently goes undiagnosed, despite multiple contacts with various healthcare providers during the first postpartum year, because women are not questioned about symptoms. It is essential for nurses to encourage new mothers to tell their stories and to talk openly about their feelings, emotions, and coping mechanisms (Clemmens, Driscoll, & Beck, 2004). Although an in-depth discussion of postpartum depression and the use of a formal screening tool is beyond the scope of this chapter, it is essential that home care nurses be competent to recognize symptoms of this entity and to provide anticipatory guidance to new mothers.

Clinical Question

How can home care nurses screen for PPD?

The Evidence

A number of qualitative studies published during the 1990s identified themes of "loss of self," "sense of loneliness," "obsessive thoughts," "feelings of insecurity," and "sleeplessness," as unique components of PPD that differ from those of generic depression. Subsequently, the Postpartum Depression Screening Scale (PDSS) was developed to screen for this entity. Multiple analyses and use of the PDSS since 2000 have found it to be a reliable and valid screening tool for PPD, particularly in the areas of sleep disturbances, anxiety, and cognitive impairment, which may not always be detected by the use of standard screening tools for generic depression. Consequently, these symptoms may be mistaken as part of normal maternal postpartum adaptation rather than indicators of evolving PPD (Clemmens et al., 2004).

Best Practice

New mothers should be questioned about mood and anxiety problems at every healthcare contact and should receive anticipatory

guidance regarding symptoms of PPD, so that they feel comfortable discussing feelings of PPD if they evolve later in the postpartum course. Nurses should be particularly attentive to the symptoms mentioned earlier, in addition to symptoms of generic depression such as feelings of sadness, fatigue, thoughts of self-harm, and loss of appetite.

The home visit provides a private, comfortable setting in which to encourage the mother to discuss feelings openly. The authors suggest opening with a comment similar to the following, *"Many women have shared with me that they have a difficult time with emotions during the postpartum period. Are you having any difficulties, problems, or feelings that you would like to talk about?"* (Clemmens et al., 2004, p. 185).

It is essential the the nurse listen attentively and nonjudgmentally. Reports of sleeplessness, anxiety, and cognitive impairment must be taken seriously, and appropriate referrals should be made through the mother's primary care provider. Home care nurses should be familiar with the PDSS and discuss use of the tool with local physicians and advanced practice nurses. Resources regarding the PDSS are noted below:

- Beck, C., & Gable, R. (2000). Postpartum depression screening scale: Development and psychometric testing. *Nursing Research, 49*(5), 272–282.
- Beck, C., & Gable, R. (2001). Comparative analysis of the performance of the postpartum depression screening scale with two other depression instruments. *Nursing Research, 50*(4), 242–250.
- Beck, C., & Gable, R. (2001). Further validation of the postpartum depression screening scale. *Nursing Research, 50*(3), 155–164.
- Beck, C., & Gable, R. (2002). *The Postpartum Depression Screening Scale Manual.* Los Angeles: Webster Psychological Association.
- Clemmens, D., Driscoll, J. W., & Beck, C. T. (2004). Postpartum depression as profiled through the postpartum depression screening scale. *American Journal of Maternal/Child Nursing, 29*(5), 180–185.

BREASTFEEDING ASSESSMENT

The nurse should observe a feeding episode, if possible, to assess for correct position, maternal and infant feeding cues, latch-on, position, let-down, sucking pattern, nipple condition, infant response, and maternal response. The nurse can assess the parents' ability to identify infant feeding cues such as rooting, hand-to-mouth movements, sucking, opening of mouth in response to stimulation, and infant transition from sleep to drowsy to quiet alert states. Various tools are available to assess the breastfeeding session, including the LATCH Scoring Table provided in Chapter 31. ∞ Assessment of the mother's ability to perceive infant satiety cues such as a gradual decrease in sucking, pulling away and releasing the nipple, relaxation, sleep, contentment, and a small amount of milk visible in the mouth can be accomplished at this time as well.

CONCERNS RELATED TO THE BREASTFEEDING INFANT

According to AAP criteria, the infant's weight should remain within 10% of his or her birth weight and the infant should feed at least 8 to 10 times per day by the fourth day of life. The infant should have at least three voids and at least three stools per 24 hours by the third day of life. Infants with a weight loss of more than 7% or inadequate output require more extensive evaluation of breastfeeding to correct potential problems (AAP Section on Breastfeeding, 2005).

The nurse can assist the couplet experiencing a 7% to 9% infant weight loss with techniques to increase milk production and promote better milk transfer. The nurse will provide assistance with breastfeeding techniques as needed, encourage breastfeeding every 2 hours for the next 24 hours, and may

Table 36–5   BREASTFEEDING PROBLEMS AND REMEDIES

Nipples Not Graspable

Flat or inverted nipples
- Use nipple tug and roll to increase protractility.
- Form the nipple before breastfeeding by hand shaping and ice before feeding.
- As a last resort, use nipple shield for first few minutes of feeding to draw out nipple; then place baby on breast.

Engorged breasts
- Treat engorgement by relieving fullness with hand expression of milk before breastfeeding and instituting frequent feedings so nipple is more prominent.

Large breasts
- Support breast with opposite hand, or use rolled towel under breast to bring nipple to the level of baby's mouth.
- Use C-hold to make nipple accessible to baby.

Engorgement

Missed or infrequent feedings
- Breastfeed frequently (every 1½–2 hours). Minimum of eight feedings and 160 minutes of suckling/24 hr.
- Massage and hand express or pump to empty breasts completely when feedings are missed or when a full feeling develops in breasts and baby is not available or willing to feed.

Breasts not emptied at feedings
- Breastfeed long enough to empty breasts. Do not interrupt the first side—allow the newborn to actively nurse 20 to 25 minutes on the first side then offer the second.
- If baby will not feed long enough to empty breasts, hand express or pump after feeding.

Inadequate let-down
- Use relaxation techniques, massage, and warm or cool compresses before breastfeeding.
- Relax in warm shower with water running from back over shoulders and breasts, hand expressing to relieve fullness.
- If due to anxiety, try to eliminate the source of tension.

Baby sleepy or not eager to feed
- Use rousing techniques (e.g., unwrap blanket, change diaper, vestibular stimulation, skin-to-skin).
- Pre-express milk onto nipple or baby's lips to entice baby.
- Avoid use of bottles of water or formula; these will decrease baby's willingness to suckle.

Inadequate Let-Down

Let-down not well established
- Give the baby ample time at the breast (at least 15 to 20 minutes per side) to allow for let-down and complete emptying.
- Breastfeed in a quiet spot away from distractions.
- Massage breasts before breastfeeding.
- Drink juice, water, tea (minimize caffeine) before and during breastfeeding.
- Condition let-down by setting up a routine for beginning feedings.
- Use relaxation and breathing techniques.
- Stimulate the nipple manually before breastfeeding.
- Concentrate thought on the baby and milk flow; turn on a faucet so that the sound of running water helps stimulate let-down.
- Use synthetic oxytocin nasal spray several times during a feeding. (This should condition let-down within 24 hours. Then it is no longer needed. Spray must be prescribed by a doctor.)

Mother overtired or overextended
- Nap or rest when the baby rests.
- Use side-lying position.
- Breastfeed the baby in bed at night.
- Simplify daily chores; set priorities.

Mother tense, pressured
- Identify the causes of tensions and eliminate or minimize them.
- Decrease fatigue.

Mother caught in cycle of little milk, worry, less milk
- Try all the previous actions.
- Develop confidence in mothering skills. (A home visit by a counselor may help.)

Plugged Ducts

Poor positioning; unknown
- Try a variety of positions for complete emptying.

Incomplete emptying of breast
- Breastfeed at least 10 minutes per side after let-down. Do not interrupt first side, allow baby to decide.
- Alternate breastfeeding positions.
- If baby does not empty breasts, pump or express milk after feedings.

External pressure on breast
- Use larger size bras, insert bra extender, or go braless. Loosen clothing.
- Use nursing bra instead of pulling up conventional bra to breastfeed to avoid pressure on ducts.
- Avoid bunching up sweater or nightgown under arm during breastfeeding.

Sore/Cracked Nipples

Poor positioning; improper latch or sucking
- Alternate breastfeeding positions throughout the day.
- Bring the baby close to feed so the baby does not pull on the breast.
- Place the nipple and some of the areola in the baby's mouth.
- Check to ensure the baby is latched on and taken off the breast properly.
- Check to ensure the nipple is back far enough in the baby's mouth.
- Hold the baby closely during feeding so the nipple is not constantly being pulled.
- Check alignment; examine mother and baby for anatomic variations

Baby chewing or nuzzling onto nipple
- Form the nipple for the baby.
- Set up a pattern of getting the baby onto the breast using the rooting reflex.

Baby sucking on end of nipple
- Ensure the nipple is way back in the baby's mouth by getting the baby properly onto the breast.
- Check for an inverted nipple.
- Check for engorgement.

Baby chewing his or her way off the nipple (nipple being pulled out of baby's mouth at end of feeding)
- Remove the baby from the breast by placing a finger between the baby's gums to ensure suction is broken.
- End feeding when the baby's suckling slows, before he or she has a chance to chew on the nipple.

(Continued on next page)

Table 36–5 BREASTFEEDING PROBLEMS AND REMEDIES continued	
Sore/Cracked Nipples (continued) **Baby overly eager to nurse** • Breastfeed more often. • Pre-express milk to hasten let-down, avoiding vigorous suckling. **Dry colostrum or milk causing nipple to stick to bra or breast pads** • Moisten bra or pads before taking off so as not to remove keratin. **Nipples not allowed to dry** • Remove plastic liners from milk pads. • Air dry breast completely after nursing. • Change milk pads frequently. • Use breast shells.	**Improper use of breast shield** • Use shield only to draw out nipple; then have the baby breastfeed. • Longer term use of shields should be supervised by experienced registered nurses (RNs) or lactation consultants (LCs) noting infant's nutrition/hydration/output. **Nipple skin not resistant to stress** • Improve diet, especially adding fresh fruits and vegetables and vitamin supplements. • Eliminate or decrease use of sugary foods, alcohol, caffeine, cigarettes. • Check use of cleansing or drying agents. **Natural oils removed or keratin layers broken down by drying agents (soap, alcohol, shampoo, deodorant)** • Eliminate irritants. • Wash breasts with water only.

SOURCE: Adapted from Lauwers, J., & Woessner, C. *Counseling the Nursing Mother: A Reference Handbook for Health Care Providers and Lay Counselors,* 2nd ed. Garden City Park, NY: Avery, © 1990, pp. 385–397.

recheck the newborn's weight the next day. Alternatively, if breastfeeding technique is correct and the milk is just starting to come in, a reliable mother may be taught what to look for in the next 24 to 48 hours and to call if feedings or output fall behind. The newborn's primary healthcare provider should be notified regarding a weight loss of more than 9%. Lactation problems beyond the expertise of the nurse require a lactation consultant and/or provider referral.

Newborns frequently require assistance in awakening to feed at least 8 times a day during the first week of life. Although the quiet alert state is ideal for latch-on, many newborns do not have the ability to transition to this state independently at this point. The nurse can utilize knowledge of newborn behavioral states as recommended by Karl (2004) to assist the mother with techniques to awaken a sleepy baby, calm a crying infant, or calm an overstimulated infant who has closed down to additional stimuli.

Techniques that are helpful in arousing a sleepy baby to the quiet alert state include undressing, changing the diaper, lightly touching, speaking, turning on lights, and placing the baby skin-to-skin on the mother's chest. Vestibular stimulation may be used where the mother supports the baby's buttocks in one hand and the baby's neck in the other and gently rocks the newborn up and down from lying to sitting and facing the mother.

Overaroused newborns who are crying or who exhibit closed down behaviors such as furrowed eyebrows, tightly closed eyes, and tensed muscles require calming techniques to bring them to a quiet alert state. Calming techniques include lowering the lights and noise level, talking or singing softly, massaging, and wrapping the baby snugly in a flexed position with the hands near the mouth. Vestibular stimulation and skin-to-skin contact are frequently helpful in this situation as well. Once the baby is calm and awake, the mother can position the baby at the breast and encourage nursing (Karl, 2004).

Many mothers have concerns related to their breast milk supply. The nurse can educate and reassure the mother regarding the signs of adequate transfer. The baby should feed at least 8 to 12 times in 24 hours for a total of at least 160 to 180 min-

utes of active suckling per day during the first 2 weeks. Audible swallowing should be heard. The mother's nipple should be moist, and mother and baby should be satisfied at the end of feedings. The baby's lips and mucous membranes should look moist. The baby should pass at least three to five loose yellow stools per day by day 4 or 5, and the baby should have at least six very wet diapers with clear urine each day by 1 week of age. Additionally, the baby should return to birth weight by the 2-week well-baby visit (Smith & Riordan, 2005).

The satiated baby will be content at the end of feedings with arms extended and very relaxed. A small amount of milk may be visible at the side of the mouth. If all of the previous criteria are met, the nurse can feel confident in telling the mom that the baby is "getting enough" and that exclusive breastfeeding is the ideal diet for the baby until 6 months of age.

Recommendations at this point would be to continue nursing on demand, at least every 3 hours, and to expect the baby to demand more frequent feedings during growth spurts. The mother can allow the baby who is actively sucking and swallowing to nurse for as long as desired on the first side and then for as long as the baby desires on the second side to encourage consumption of the high-fat hind milk. The mother will need to take the newborn in for periodic weight checks, well-baby exams, and immunizations as directed by the infant's provider. As recommended by the AAP (AAP Section on Breastfeeding, 2005), the parents will want to discuss with their provider vitamin D supplementation within the first 2 months and adding additional foods at 6 months.

The home care nurse will occasionally discover a breastfed baby with a weight loss of up to 7% in a normal newborn. Infants experiencing breastfeeding difficulties whose weight loss is greater than 7% may need supplementation. A call to the pediatrician from the client's home is warranted to discuss the issue. Because it is important to begin rehydrating the newborn as soon as possible, the home care nurse may need to help a client who has planned only to feed from the breast to formulate an interim contingency plan. The nurse can assist her with pumping or hand expressing. The expressed breast milk can be fed to the newborn from a cup, bottle, or syringe, depending on the mother's preference. Expressed breast milk is the ideal intervention. However, if the mother does not have enough breast milk, the nurse will find it necessary to assist the mother with preparation of formula until her supply is adequate and the baby is rehydrated. Therefore, it is important that the home care nurse be familiar with infant formulas and be ready to help the mother follow package instructions correctly. The use of infant formula is discussed later in this chapter.

CONCERNS RELATED TO MATERNAL BREASTFEEDING DIFFICULTIES AND FORMULA-FEEDING

In addition to problems with milk transfer and concerns about milk supply, many new mothers have breastfeeding difficulties, including leaking, nipple soreness, cracked nipples, breast engorgement, and plugged ducts. The nurse can assess for these complications at the home visit and provide interventions to decrease maternal discomfort.

Nipple Soreness

Mothers should be counseled to expect sensations of massaging and stretching as the infant elongates the nipple during nursing. This may be uncomfortable when the infant initially latches for feedings, but the discomfort should decrease after the first few seconds of nursing. Nipple soreness is a common complaint and frequent reason for early discontinuation of breastfeeding. The nipples may exhibit erythema, edema, abrasions, fissures, cracks, bruises, blisters, and bleeding. This early transient discomfort is usually due to mechanical trauma, and it peaks between the third and sixth days. Poor latch and/or suck are the primary causes of mechanical trauma. Therefore, observation of feeding and assistance with proper positioning and latching technique are essential to the prevention and treatment of soreness (Morland-Schultz & Hill, 2005; Smith & Riordan, 2005).

The baby's position at the breast is a critical factor in nipple soreness. The mother's hand should be off the areola, and the baby should be tummy to tummy and facing the mother's chest, with ear, shoulder, and hip aligned. The nose is near or just touching the breast, and the lips should be flanged out. The gums are on the areola, and the tongue is over the bottom gum and cupping the nipple. (See Figures 31–8 through 31–11 in Chapter 31 ∞).

Because the area of greatest stress to the nipple is in line with the newborn's chin and nose, nipple soreness may be decreased by encouraging the mother to rotate positions when feeding the infant. Changing positions alters the focus of greatest stress and promotes more complete breast emptying. Although some mothers are initially hesitant to try the side-lying position, this is frequently a helpful position to use when difficulty in latching is encountered. Additionally, as noted by Troy (2003), the use of the side-lying position has been empirically tested and has been shown to be associated with significantly less postpartum fatigue than use of the sitting positions.

Nipple soreness due to mechanical trauma is frequently related to the infant's sucking pattern or to anatomical variations of the newborn's oral cavity or the mother's nipples. Nipple characteristics such as their size and ability to elongate may affect comfort during sucking. Retracted or inverted nipples may rub on the baby's palate even when properly positioned, resulting in pain. The size and shape of the infant's oral cavity may affect the sucking pattern and comfort. A short or tight newborn lingual frenulum (ankyloglossia or tongue-tie) can cause discomfort as well. Because the use of artificial nipples on bottles or pacifiers can affect the newborn's suck, their use should be discouraged if possible (Smith & Riordan, 2005).

An observation of the feed should assess the baby's oral cavity for anatomical concerns as well as the ability to open the mouth wide enough to attain a deep latch. When latched, the lips should be flanged out, and the newborn should cover as much of the areola as possible. Turning the lips under can cause pain and inadequate transfer of milk. The mother can be taught to observe this and to apply gentle upward pressure on the newborn's upper lip and gentle downward pressure on the infant's chin to correct the position as needed. To prevent trauma, the mother should also be taught to gently insert her finger between the infant's gums to break the latch before removing the baby from the breast.

While nursing, the baby can be expected to suck rapidly at the beginning and more slowly toward the end of a feeding. Sucking should be quiet, with swallowing heard every two to three sucks. The baby's cheeks should be full and rounded. Movement should be seen at the jawline. Dimpling at the cheek may be indicative of a poor or shallow latch or an unusual movement of the tongue. The presence of clicking, smacking, or slurping may indicate an improper seal or suck, and the infant should be re-latched (Smith & Riordan, 2005). Persistent clicking may be heard if the infant has ankyloglossia (tongue-tie).

Finally, the mother's nipple will be elongated at the end of a feeding, but it should be the same shape as at the beginning. Nipples that are angled, creased, or distorted at the end of feedings indicate anatomical variations or latch problems. Intervention is required if distorted nipples are painful (Smith & Riordan, 2005).

The nurse can instruct the mother in a number of measures to promote comfort and healing and to prevent skin breakdown. Washing the breasts with warm water and avoiding drying soaps is recommended. Simply keeping the nipples clean and dry is adequate for many mothers. Alternatively, warm water compresses can be applied followed by air-drying (Figure 36–5 ◆). Another natural and inexpensive method involves applying expressed breast milk to the nipples and areola followed by air-drying at the end of each feeding. Gently massaging or pumping the breast before feedings stimulates let-down and flow and may be helpful in decreasing initial latch-on pain related to vigorous nursing. The mother can also apply an ice compress to the nipples just before feeding to decrease sensation (Smith & Riordan, 2005). The use of hairdryers and heat lamps is no longer recommended (Mohrbacher & Stock, 2003).

Products such as purified anhydrous lanolin and hydrogel dressings have been used with success in treating sore nipples. Although high infection rates occurred in one study of glycerin-based hydrogel, no infections were noted in a subsequent study of water-based hydrogel (Smith & Riordan, 2005). Application of a lanolin product such as Lansinoh provides a moisture barrier,

Figure 36–5 ◆ Air-drying the nipples can help prevent cracking and fissures.

which prevents scab formation. Lansinoh does not require removal before feedings (Mohrbacher & Stock, 2003).

If a woman finds that her bra or clothing rubs against her nipples and adds to her discomfort, she may find it helpful to use breast shells between feedings. It is not helpful to limit nursing time at the breast. This may actually increase discomfort related to engorgement and have a negative effect on milk production and infant nutrition. In severe cases where the mother is unable to tolerate breastfeeding until the nipple improves, the mother will need to pump or hand-express the breast milk (Smith & Riordan, 2005).

The most important factor in decreasing pain is educating the mother on proper latch-on techniques. Anticipatory guidance and informing clients that many mothers experience nipple discomfort on days 3 through 6 and that the discomfort usually improves markedly by the end of the first week should be helpful in encouraging new mothers to continue breastfeeding, knowing that an end to the discomfort is in sight (Morland-Schultz & Hill, 2005).

The home care nurse can make recommendations for interventions for clients with sore nipples. It is essential that the nurse read the product literature and current research on products recommended by the providers and lactation consultants in the local area. Additionally, the nurse should remind the mother that small amounts of any product applied to her nipples will be ingested by her newborn. Therefore, she will want to consult her primary care provider or a lactation consultant before applying commercial products.

The nurse should talk with a lactation consultant or provider if the client's comfort is severe enough to require

temporary use of a nipple shield and/or pumping rather than nursing. Nipple shields should be used only under close monitoring, as they can potentially affect milk transfer and have a negative impact on the infant. Nipple pain that does not resolve after a week may indicate infection or other problems and should be referred to a provider so the appropriate therapy can be prescribed.

Flat or Inverted Nipples

Many women with flat or inverted nipples have the fear that they will be unable to breastfeed. This is not usually the case. Pregnancy and previous breastfeeding often lessen the inversion to the point that it is not an issue with subsequent babies. Breastfeeding mothers with flat or inverted nipples may experience difficulties after discharge if breastfeeding was not successfully established before leaving the hospital. Frequently, positioning the infant well back on the areola will be enough to promote the suckling that stretches and elongates the nipple during feedings. Exercising the nipple before latching loosens the tissue and helps to separate adhesions that cause retraction or inversion. The nurse can teach the mother to stimulate and shape the nipple just before feeding. A cold cloth will evert a flat nipple. Inverted nipples can be shaped by the mother by placing her thumb 1 1/2 to 2 inches behind the nipple and pulling back into her chest. As noted previously, use of the side-lying position is helpful. The wearing of breast shells and Hoffman's exercises are not effective and are no longer recommended (Riordan, 2005a). The nurse can also recommend use of a pump to evert the nipple just before latch-on. A thin silicone nipple shield can be utilized during the initial latch and removed once the baby has suckled enough to elongate the nipple. Rubber or latex nipple shields are not recommended.

Breast Engorgement

A distinction exists between breast fullness and engorgement. All lactating women experience a transitional fullness at first, initially because of venous congestion and later because of accumulating milk. However, this fullness generally lasts only 24 hours, the breasts remain soft enough for the newborn to suckle, and there is no pain. Severely engorged breasts are hard, painful, and warm, and may appear taut and shiny. Engorgement may occur as a result of infrequent feedings, delayed initiation of feedings, use of supplements, time-limited feedings, and removing the baby from the first side to ensure feeding from both breasts at each feeding (Riordan & Hoover, 2005; Snowden, Renfrew, & Woolridge, 2005).

Treatments employed for engorgement may include warm compresses or showers for a short time just before nursing, cold compresses or frozen bags of vegetables applied to breasts after feedings, cabbage compresses, breast massage and milk expression, ultrasound, anti-inflammatory medications, and pumping. Many women anecdotally express increased comfort with the use of cold compresses, frozen vegetable bags, and the judicious use of cabbage leaves. However, a Cochrane review of eight studies found anti-inflammatory drugs to be the only treatment that significantly improved engorgement symptoms (Riordan & Hoover, 2005; Snowden et al., 2005).

Engorgement can be accompanied by a fever up to 101F. Although unrelieved engorgement and stasis are not necessarily associated with mastitis, they do lead to involution and decreased milk synthesis (Smith & Riordan, 2005). Frequent feedings for a minimum of 160 minutes of nursing every 24 hours are essential to the prevention and treatment of engorgement (Riordan & Hoover, 2005). Although pumping is sometimes discouraged in this situation for fear that it will increase milk production, it is necessary to pump if the infant is unable to nurse to empty the breasts. A technique described as areolar compression by Miller and Riordan (2004) and reverse pressure softening by Cotterman (2004) is recommended before pumping or attempting to latch if severe breast and alveolar edema is present. It will be helpful for home care nurses working with breastfeeding mothers to review these references and to work with a lactation consultant to learn this technique as well as to learn more about the use of commercial breast pumps and manual expression of breast milk.

Plugged Ducts

Some mothers experience plugging of one or more ducts. Manifested as an area of tenderness or lumpiness in an otherwise well woman, plugging may be relieved by the use of heat and massage. The nurse can encourage the mother to massage her breasts from her chest wall forward to the nipple while standing in a warm shower or following the application of moist heat to the breast. The mother should then breastfeed her infant, starting on the affected breast to promote drainage. Frequent breastfeeding and the use of a variety of positions to ensure complete emptying help prevent the problem (Riordan, 2005a). If these interventions do not relieve the tenderness or if lumpiness remains, a breast pump may be effective in unplugging the duct. The client should also be encouraged to wear a comfortable bra and loose, nonrestrictive clothing. Interventions for commonly occurring breastfeeding problems can be found in Table 36–5.

Mastitis

Plugged ducts increase the risk for mastitis, an inflammatory condition of the breast. Stress and fatigue, cracked nipples, and an abundant milk supply are associated with mastitis as well. Symptoms of mastitis include fever (greater than 100.4F); a hot, red, tender area on the breast; and flulike symptoms. Treatment of mastitis includes continued breastfeeding, application of moist heat, increased fluids, rest, analgesics, and antibiotics as prescribed if necessary (Riordan, 2005a).

Effect of Medications and Alcohol

Analgesics are appropriate as directed by a primary healthcare provider. Avoidance of breastfeeding while the drug levels are peaking in maternal plasma minimizes the amount received by the infant. The peak concentration varies from drug to drug, and it may be difficult to time this during the first week of breastfeeding. Nursing ideally occurs frequently, and the mother may require analgesics to nurse comfortably. Hale (2005) points out that the nonsteroidal anti-inflammatory drug (NSAID) ibuprofen is cleared for infant use and that its levels in milk are generally subclinical. Because most drugs do pass into the breast

Table 36–6   REFERENCES FOR NURSES WHO WORK WITH BREASTFEEDING CLIENTS

Briggs, G. G., Freeman, R. K., & Yaffe, S. J. (2005). *Drugs in pregnancy and lactation* (7th ed.). Baltimore: Lippincott, Williams & Wilkins.

Hale, T. D. (2002). *Medications and mothers' milk* (10th ed.). Amarillo, TX: Pharmasoft Medical.

Lawrence, R. A., & Lawrence, R. M. (2005). *Breastfeeding—a guide for the medical profession.* Philadelphia: Elsevier Mosby.

Mohrbacher, N., & Stock, J. (2003). *The breastfeeding answer book* (3rd rev. ed). Schaumburg, IL: La Leche League International.

Newman, J., & Pitman, T. (2000). *The ultimate breastfeeding book of answers.* Roseville, CA: Prima. (Member of Crown Publishing, a division of Random House, Inc.)

Riordan, J. (2005). *Breastfeeding and human lactation.* Boston: Jones & Bartlett.

milk, the mother will want to check with her provider before taking medications. The nurse will want to check the use of specific drugs in references such as those listed in Table 36–6.

Although alcohol use was considered acceptable in the past, it is no longer recommended for breastfeeding women. Alcohol levels in breast milk parallel those found in maternal plasma, peaking 30 to 60 minutes after consumption. Mothers who do occasionally drink while lactating should be advised to consume the alcohol after breastfeeding rather than shortly before a feeding in order to minimize the amount the infant receives (Menella, 2002).

Breastfeeding and the Working Mother

Many new mothers return to the workplace by the time their babies are 3 months old, and most mothers in the United States return to work, at least part time, by the time their babies are 6 months old. The idea of managing breastfeeding in addition to all their other responsibilities is frightening, and some mothers choose not to breastfeed at all because of these concerns. The home care nurse can help the woman to explore options and solve problems related to breastfeeding in the workplace to promote continuation (Tully, 2005).

The earlier the breastfeeding mother returns to work, the more often she will need to pump her breasts to express the breast milk. Recommendations for mothers who are using a breast pump can be found in Table 31–3. ∞ Because milk production follows the principle of supply and demand, if breasts are not pumped, the milk supply will decrease. The nurse can review pumping and storage of breast milk with the mother. An electric pump and double collection system is optimal for the working mother. Working mothers can also obtain printed materials on pumping, storage, working while breastfeeding, and related issues from lactation consultants and breastfeeding support groups, such as La Leche League. The mother will want to begin pumping at some point after breastfeeding is established, and she will want to introduce expressed milk from the bottle at least a week before the baby will need to take it from a care provider (Tully, 2005).

The nurse can also discuss methods of maintaining breast milk supply such as relaxation, stress reduction, proper nutrition, adequate fluid intake, and frequent nursing during the

MEDIALINK

Application: Maintaining Lactation after Returning to Work

evenings, in the mornings, and on days off. The nurse and client can explore options such as pumping at work, visiting the infant or having the infant brought to work during the mother's lunch, and having the child care provider give expressed breast milk (Tully, 2005).

Night breastfeeding presents a dilemma. It may help a working mother maintain her milk supply, but it may also contribute to fatigue. Quillin and Glenn (2004) found that total hours of sleep did not differ between breastfeeding and bottle-feeding mothers at 4 weeks postpartum, but the breastfeeding mothers were up and down more in the night and probably took naps to catch up. Depending on the rigidity and demands of the mother's work schedule, the nurse can explore options with the mother to promote the continuation of breastfeeding as much as possible during the first year of life. As noted earlier, use of the side-lying position is less fatiguing.

Weaning

Weaning is a process that begins with the introduction of sources of nutrition other than breastmilk and ends with the last breastfeeding. Weaning may be gradual, deliberate, or abrupt (Riordan, 2005b). The decision to *wean* the baby from the breast may be made for a variety of reasons, including family or cultural pressures, changes in the home situation, work schedules, pressure from the woman's partner, or a personal opinion about when weaning should occur. For the woman who is comfortable with breastfeeding and well informed about the process, the appropriate time to wean her infant will become evident if she is sensitive to the child's cues. Often weaning falls between periods of great developmental activity for the child, when interest in exploring the environment grows and interest in the breast decreases (Lawrence & Lawrence, 2005). A child may spontaneously wean during a subsequent pregnancy. The infant who is weaned before 12 months should be given iron-fortified newborn formula, not cow's milk (AAP & ACOG, 2002).

If weaning is timed to respond to the child's cues, and if the mother is comfortable with the timing, it can be accomplished with less difficulty than if the process begins before mother and child are ready emotionally. Nevertheless, weaning is a time of emotional separation for mother and baby; it may be difficult for them to give up the closeness of their breastfeeding sessions. The nurse who is understanding about this possibility can help the mother see that her infant or toddler is growing up and plan other comforting, consoling, and play activities to replace breastfeeding.

For both mother and baby, a gradual approach is the easiest and most comforting way to wean the child from breastfeedings (Riordan, 2005b). During weaning, the mother can substitute one cup feeding or bottle-feeding for one breastfeeding session for a period of time so that her breasts gradually produce less milk. Eliminating the breastfeedings associated with meals first facilitates the mother's ability to wean the infant, because satiation with food lessens the desire for milk. Over a period of several weeks she can substitute more cup feedings or bottle-feedings for breastfeedings until only the morning and night feedings remain. These feedings often continue for several months and gradually come to a stop (Lawrence & Lawrence, 2005). The slow method of weaning

prevents breast engorgement, allows infants to alter their eating methods at their own rates, and provides time for psychologic adjustments in both mother and baby. If a baby initiates weaning during the first year of life and the mother wishes to continue breastfeeding, she can often work through this with the help of a lactation consultant.

Cultural Considerations Related to Breastfeeding

Cultures vary tremendously in their initiation of breastfeeding, support persons important to the continuation of breastfeeding, and weaning practices. Despite increases in breastfeeding in the United States, minority women still breastfeed at lower rates than white women. Many immigrants breastfeed less than family members from their native countries after moving to the United States. Black women, in particular, breastfeed at low rates (Lewis, 2003). Lack of family support decreases the likelihood that the woman will continue breastfeeding once she goes home, so it is important to find out the important support persons for breastfeeding in each cultural context.

Although cultural considerations related to each group are beyond the scope of this chapter, it is important for the home care nurse to individualize care for minority women by incorporating their cultural beliefs and practices related to breastfeeding. For further discussion regarding cultural influences on infant feeding practices, see Chapter 2. ∞ Another excellent reference is Chapter 24 ∞, "The Cultural Context of Breastfeeding," in *Breastfeeding and Human Lactation* (Riordan, 2005b).

Breastfeeding Referrals and Social Support

Support from the woman's family and social contacts is very important with regard to the initiation and continuation of breastfeeding. Weissinger (2002) highly recommends referral to local support groups where women can learn over time and observe role models to enhance their breastfeeding experience. The home care nurse should be familiar with local lay support groups and encourage breastfeeding mothers to contact them.

Formula-Feeding

The Food and Drug Administration (FDA) recommends using commercially prepared formulas as an alternative to breastmilk if the mother is unable to breastfeed (Lewis, 2003). Some mothers need or choose to feed their infants formula because of their own health status or personal choice. It is important for the home care nurse to assist and offer them support. If the mother does not have a health history that precludes her from breastfeeding, it may be helpful to explore the reasons for her decision. Some mothers have chosen bottle-feeding because of lack of education about the benefits of breastfeeding, misconceptions about breastfeeding, or lack of support. If that is the case and the mother desires help with breastfeeding, lactation can still be established at this time with proper support. If the mother needs or chooses to formula-feed, it is important for the nurse to support her choice and to answer any questions she may have regarding formula-feeding.

A systematic review and examination of the literature on reconstitution of breast milk substitutes for term newborns by Renfrew, Ansell, and Macleod (2003) found only five studies eligible for inclusion. All were published between 1985 and 1991. No studies had been published since 1991, which is of concern because of the large number of formula-fed infants worldwide. All the studies found errors in reconstitution. Although over-concentration was most common, underconcentration occurred as well.

Most substitutes in this country are available in ready-to-feed, liquid concentrate, and powder forms. Many parents reconstitute the powder, as it is the most economical formulation. Chronic overconcentration can result in hypernatremic dehydration, whereas underconcentration can result in water intoxication and undernourishment. Therefore, it is important to emphasize the importance of mixing the formula exactly as the package directs. Although cold tap water is acceptable for reconstitution in this country, parents should run the water for at least 1 minute before use to clear any lead from water in the pipes (Morin, 2005). Parents with well water will want to use distilled water until they have the water checked by the health department for safety (Hand, 2005).

It will be helpful for the home care nurse to check the area where the formula is prepared and the bottles are stored. Bottles and nipples can be washed in the top rack of the dishwasher or in hot soapy water, then rinsed and air-dried upside down in a clean area. Hand towels should not be used. Sterilizing is not necessary for healthy newborns. Handwashing is imperative before preparing formula and handling the nipples and bottles. Product storage recommendations should be followed, expiration dates should be honored, and parents should date and time the bottles when prepared. Prepared formula should be refrigerated and used within 48 hours. Formula that remains in a bottle at the end of a feeding should always be discarded (Hand, 2005). Although many parents use clean bottles from previous babies or from friends because of economic constraints, they will probably want to purchase new nipples that are supple and intact. It is preferable that the same type of nipple be used consistently for the baby at each feeding.

OTHER TYPES OF FOLLOW-UP CARE

Other types of follow-up care may include return home visits, telephone follow-up, and postpartal classes or support groups.

Return Visits

If the mother and family and physician or certified nurse-midwife have chosen discharge earlier than 48 hours after vaginal birth, the mother may, in some states, request a total of three visits. In such cases, the nurse would schedule the first visit about 24 hours after discharge and then space out the other two visits over the next week. In other instances, the nurse may schedule additional home visits based on the findings of the first home visit and the follow-up phone call.

Telephone Follow-Up

The postpartum home care nurse usually makes a follow-up phone call a few days after the home visit. During the call, the nurse may provide additional information, address questions or areas of confusion, and make referrals.

Some families may be offered or may request a telephone follow-up at the time of discharge. A mutually agreeable time is set for the call, typically within 3 days of discharge, or earlier if desired. Calls typically last about 20 minutes and are pre-planned and goal directed.

To perform an effective telephone assessment, the nurse must be able to listen skillfully, use open-ended questions, and wait for answers. The nurse projects a warm, caring attitude so that the mother feels comfortable talking to a faceless caller. When assessment reveals signs of an initial or recurring postpartum complication, the nurse refers the woman to her primary care provider for further evaluation.

The plan of care developed and implemented during a telephone conversation is limited to supportive counseling, teaching, and referral. The new mother may have many questions, especially about newborn care, and is generally at a high level of learning readiness. The nurse can answer the woman's questions and use the questions as a "stepping stone" for further teaching. Many communities have established 24-hour advice lines for new parents to call when they have questions or need support. In areas where help lines are not available, parents may be directed to call the birthing center. If birthing center nurses field parent phone calls, they should follow established protocols regarding the advice to be given and the documentation required. In either case, the home care nurse provides the number so that it is readily accessible for the family.

Postpartal Classes and Support Groups

Postpartal classes are becoming more common as caregivers recognize the continuing needs of the childbearing family. In many instances, classes are prepared to meet the specific needs of a variety of families so that, for example, single mothers and adolescent mothers can attend class with peers. A series of structured classes may focus on topics such as parenting, postpartal exercise, or nutrition, or there may be loosely structured group sessions that address mothers' concerns as they arise. Such classes offer chances for the new mother to socialize, share her concerns, and receive encouragement. Because baby-sitting arrangements may be difficult or expensive, it is desirable to provide child care for siblings.

Some cities offer breastfeeding or new-parent support groups through birthing centers or hospitals or as a community effort. Once again, the support group provides an opportunity for parents to interact with one another and to share information and experiences.

Many parents look to Internet resources for additional information on parenting and newborn care. Internet sites can be devised by anyone, so the quality, usefulness, and accuracy of the information may vary. Nurses have an opportunity to assist parents in evaluating the reliability of the information they find. Criteria that suggest Internet information is reliable and high in quality include affiliation with a university medical or nursing school; inclusion of the authors' credentials, education, board certification, and affiliations; referencing of information; currency of information; similarity of information when compared with other sources; and easy accessibility (Beyea, 2002).

CHAPTER REVIEW

FOCUS YOUR STUDY

- The Newborns' and Mothers' Health Protection Act took effect in January 1998, and provides for a guaranteed minimum stay of up to 48 hours following an uncomplicated vaginal birth and 96 hours following an uncomplicated cesarean birth. The AAP recommends that all infants discharged before 48 hours be examined within 48 hours after discharge, and, ideally, that all newborns be seen at the 3- to 5-day point for weight, hydration, intake and output, and jaundice screening. Home care nursing meets this requirement.

- The overall goal of postpartal home visits is to enhance opportunities for smooth transition of the new family. The home visit provides opportunities for assessment, teaching, breastfeeding support, and fostering a caring relationship with new families.

- In planning the home visit, the nurse needs to take precautions to maintain safety, such as carrying a cellular phone, notifying supervisors of location of visit, keeping personal belongings out of sight, assessing the neighborhood and home for signs of danger, and, if present, terminating the visit.

- Physical assessment of the newborn during a home visit includes assessments of vital signs, weight, overall color including jaundice, assessment of body systems, intake/output, hydration, umbilical cord and circumcision, newborn nutrition, newborn safety, parent education, and attachment.

- Teaching goals during home visits include reinforcing daily newborn care, including demonstrations of positioning and handling, sponge and tub bathing, nail care, and dressing; discussing temperature assessment and signs of illness; assisting with newborn feeding; discussing expected newborn output; discussing newborn behavioral states; promoting safe and appropriate newborn sleeping, including SIDS prevention; promoting crib safety; encouraging childproofing of the home environment; discussing prevention of unintentional injuries and abuse; and encouraging newborn screening and immunization.

- The physician or pediatric nurse practitioner should be notified if there is evidence of redness around the newborn's umbilicus, if there is bright red bleeding or puslike drainage near the cord stump, or if the umbilical site remains unhealed.

- A primary risk factor for sudden infant death syndrome (SIDS) is sleeping in the prone position. New guidelines in 2005 discouraged cosleeping, smoking in pregnancy, and smoking after birth. Further recommendations include placement of the infant crib in close proximity to the parents' bed and the use of pacifiers as measures to further prevent SIDs.

- State-mandated screening is performed on all newborns in the first 1 to 3 days, with a second blood specimen drawn after 7 to 14 days.

- Universal hearing screening is performed on all newborns. Newborns who do not pass the screening should receive diagnostic testing by age 3 months and interventions by age 6 months as necessary.

- Signs of illness in mothers include pain or burning with urination, passage of clots or placental tissue, excessive pelvic or perineal pain, chest pain, difficulty breathing, excessive or foul-smelling lochia, failure of fundus to descend at the anticipated rate, temperature of 100.4F or above, elevation of blood pressure, tenderness, redness, or pain in the legs or breasts, and feelings consistent with postpartum depression.

- Difficulties with breastfeeding include sore, cracked, flat, or inverted nipples; breast engorgement; plugged ducts; and mastitis.

- Breastfeeding mothers require information on effects of alcohol and various medications on breast milk; pumping; weaning; and breastfeeding referrals and social support.

- Return visits, telephone follow-up, classes, and support groups can provide valuable information and support to new mothers and their families.

EXPLORE MediaLink

 http://www.prenhall.com/davidson

NCLEX review questions, case studies, and other interactive resources for this chapter can be found on the Web Site at http://www.prenhall.com/davidson. Click on "Chapter 36" to select the activities for this chapter.

For tutorials including animations and videos, more NCLEX review questions, and an audio glossary, access the accompanying Prentice Hall Nursing MediaLink DVD-ROM in this book.

 PRENTICE HALL NURSING MEDIALINK DVD-ROM
Audio Glossary
NCLEX Review
Video: *Through the Eyes of a Nurse—Welcoming the New Arrival at the Postpartal Visit*

 COMPANION WEBSITE
Additional NCLEX Review
Case Study: *Follow-Up with the Client at Home*
Care Plan Activity: *Breastfeeding Pain*
Applications: *Positioning and Handling the Newborn; Maintaining Lactation after Returning to Work*
Critical Thinking

CRITICAL THINKING IN ACTION

HOME POSTPARTUM VISIT

View the Critical Thinking in Action video in Chapter 36 of the DVD-ROM. Then answer the questions that follow.

 Jane Benne, age 23, G1 gave birth by cesarean for cephalopelvic disproportion to a healthy 7 pound 1 ounce baby boy 5 days ago. You are making a home visit 2 days after Jane was discharged from the hospital to her two-story home. When you arrive the baby is sleeping in a bassinet in Jane's bedroom on the second level. Jane has been trying to breastfeed and complains to you of sore nipples and swollen breasts. She is also having problems getting the baby to latch on and says that she has

been supplementing her baby's feedings with a bottle because she is afraid her baby is not getting enough milk from her breasts alone. She also mentions that the baby seems more satisfied after she gives the bottle and seems to sleep longer. You ask her how she has been feeling, and she tells you that she is very tired and upset about her body not making enough milk to feed her child. You assess Jane's breasts and find them to be full and firm, but the nipples are cracked and blistered.

1. What is your focus in the home postpartum visit?
2. What counseling can you give Jane regarding her sore nipples?
3. What suggestion do you give Jane regarding supplemental bottle-feedings?
4. Explain your assessment of Jane's abdominal incision and provide suggestions for healing.
5. How would you discuss the baby's voiding patterns to ensure adequate hydration?

REFERENCES

Academy of Breastfeeding Medicine (ABM). (2003). *Clinical protocol number 6—guideline on cosleeping and breastfeeding.* Retrieved September 11, 2005, from http://www.bfmed.org/protocol/proto6.html.

Agran, P. F., Anderson, C., Winn, D., Trent, R., Walton-Haynes, L., & Thayer, S. (2003). Rates of pediatric injuries by 3-month intervals for children 0 to 3 years of age [Electronic version]. *Pediatrics, 111*(6), e683–e692.

Alberta, L., Sweeney, S. N., & Wiss, K. (2005). Diaper dye dermatitis [Electronic version]. *Pediatrics, 116*(3), e450–e452.

American Academy of Pediatrics (AAP) Committee on Fetus and Newborn. (2004). Hospital stay for healthy term newborns. *Pediatrics, 113*(5), 1434–1436.

American Academy of Pediatrics (AAP) Section on Breastfeeding. (2005). Breastfeeding and the use of human milk. *Pediatrics, 115*(2), 496–506.

American Academy of Pediatrics (AAP) Subcommittee on Hyperbilirubinemia. (2004). Management of hyperbilirubinemia in the newborn infant 35 or more weeks of gestation. *Pediatrics, 114*(1), 297–316.

American Academy of Pediatrics (AAP) & American College of Obstetricians and Gynecologists (ACOG). (2002). *Guidelines for perinatal care* (5th ed.). Elk Grove Village, IL: Author.

Association of Women's Health, Obstetric, and Neonatal Nurses (AWHONN). (2001). *Evidence-based clinical practice guideline–neonatal skin care.* Washington, DC: Author.

Association of Women's Health, Obstetric, and Neonatal Nurses (AWHONN). (2005). AWHONN news and views: Caring for the near-term infant. *AWHONN Lifelines, 9*(4), 336–337.

Barclay, L., & Lie, D. (2005). American Academy of Pediatrics updates guidelines to reduce incidence of SIDS. *Medscape Medical News.* Retrieved December 13, 2005, from http://www.medscape.com/viewarticle/514267

Beyea, S. C. (2002). Finding patient safety Internet resources. *Association of Perioperative Registered Nurses Journal, 75*(6), 1171–1173.

Bowman, K. G. (2005). Postpartum learning needs. *Journal of Obstetric, Gynecologic, & Neonatal Nursing, 34*(4), 438–443.

Brillhart, B., Kruse, B., & Heard, L. (2004). Safety concerns for rehabilitation nurses in home care. *Rehabilitation Nursing, 29*(6), 227–229.

Brook, I. (2003). Unexplained fever in young children: How to manage severe bacterial infection. *British Medical Journal, 327*(7234), 1094–1097.

Brown, S., Small, R., Faber, B., Krastev, A., & Davis, P. (2002). Early postnatal discharge from hospital for healthy mothers and term infants. *The Cochrane Database of Systematic Reviews, 3.*

Bryanton, J., Walsh, D., Barrett, M., & Gaudet, D. (2004). Tub bathing versus traditional sponge bathing for the newborn. *Journal of Obstetric, Gynecologic, & Neonatal Nursing, 33*(6), 704–712.

Bullock, L. F. C., Mickey, K., Green, J., & Heine, A. (2004). Are nurses acting as role models for the prevention of SIDS? *American Journal of Maternal/Child Nursing, 29*(3), 172–177.

Carson, S. M. (2003). Alternating acetaminophen and ibuprofen in the febrile child: Examination of the evidence regarding efficacy and safety. *Pediatric Nursing, 29*(5), 379–382.

Chezem, J., Friesen, C., & Boettcher, J. (2003). Breastfeeding knowledge, breastfeeding confidence, and infant feeding plans: Effects on actual feeding practices. *Journal of Obstetric, Gynecologic, & Neonatal Nursing, 32*(1), 40–57.

Clemmens, D., Driscoll, J. W., & Beck, C. T. (2004). Postpartum depression as profiled through the postpartum depression screening scale. *American Journal of Maternal/Child Nursing, 29*(3), 180–185.

Cotterman, K. J. (2004). Reverse pressure softening: A simple tool for easier latching during engorgement. *Journal of Human Lactation, 20*(2), 227–237.

Dias, M. S., Smith, K., deGuehery, K., Mazur, P., Li, V., & Shaffer, M. L. (2005). Preventing abusive head trauma among infants and young children: A hospital-based, parent education program [Electronic version]. *Pediatrics, 115*(4), e470–e477.

Ellett, M., Schuff, E., & Davis, J. B. (2005). Parental perceptions of the lasting effects of infant colic. *American Journal of Maternal/Child Nursing, 30*(2), 127–132.

Galbraith, A. A., Egerter, S. A., Marchi, K. S., Chavez, G., & Braveman, P. A. (2003). Newborn early discharge revisited: Are California newborns receiving recommended postnatal services? *Pediatrics, 111*(2), 364–371.

George, L. (2005). Lack of preparedness— Experiences of first-time mothers. *American Journal of Maternal/Child Nursing, 30*(4), 251–255.

Groer, M., Davis, M., Casey, K., Short, B., Smith, K., & Groer, S. (2005). Neuroendocrine & immune relationships in postpartum fatigue. *American Journal of Maternal/Child Nursing, 30*(2), 133–138.

Hale, T. W. (2005). Drug therapy and breastfeeding. In J. Riordan (Ed.), *Breastfeeding and human lactation* (3rd ed., pp. 137–166). Boston: Jones & Bartlett.

Hand, B. (2005). Bottle feeding your baby— Part 3. Retrieved September 14, 2005, from http://www.babyfit.com/myspark/articles.asp?id=

Hopkins, J. (2004). Essentials of newborn skin care. *British Journal of Midwifery, 12*(5), 314–317.

Janssen, P. A., Selwood, B. L., Dobson, S. R., Peacock, D., & Thiessen, P. N. (2003). To dye or not to dye: A randomized, clinical trial of a triple dye/alcohol regime versus dry cord care. *Pediatrics, 111*(1), 15–20.

Jenkins, A. W. (2005). Near-term, but still a preemie–Speaking up for infants born a little too early. *AWHONN Lifelines, 9*(4), 295–297.

Karl, D. J. (2004). Using principles of newborn behavioral state organization to facilitate breastfeeding. *American Journal of Maternal/Child Nursing, 29*(5), 292–298.

Kayman, H. (2003). Management of fever: Making evidence-based decisions. *Clinical Pediatrics, 42*(5), 383–392.

Kourtis, A. P., Sullivan, D. T., & Sathian, U. (2004). Practice guidelines for the management of febrile infants less than 90 days of age at the ambulatory network of a large pediatric health care system in the United States: Summary of new evidence. *Clinical Pediatrics, 43*(1), 11–16.

Krous, H. F., Beckwith, J. B., Byard, R. W., Rognum, T. O., Bajanowski, T., Corey, T., et al. (2004). Sudden infant death syndrome and unclassified sudden infant deaths: A definitional and diagnostic approach. *Pediatrics, 114*(1), 234–238.

Lawrence, R. A., & Lawrence, R. M. (2005). *Breastfeeding—A guide for the medical profession.* Philadelphia: Elsevier Mosby.

Lewis, C. (2003). HHS blueprint to boost breast-feeding. *FDA Consumer, 37*(3), 12–17.

Madden, J. M., Soumerai, S. B., Lieu, T. A., Mandl, K. D., Zhang, F., & Ross-Degnan, D. (2004). Length-of-stay policies and ascertainment of postdischarge problems in newborns. *Pediatrics, 113*(1), 42–49.

Malloy, M. H. (2002). Trends in postneonatal aspiration deaths and reclassification of sudden infant death syndrome: Impact of the "back to sleep" program. *Pediatrics, 109*(4), 661–665.

Mancini, A. J. (2004). Skin. *Pediatrics, 113*(4), 1114–1119.

Martin, J. A., Kochanek, K. D., Strobino, D. M., Guyer, B., & MacDorman, M. F. (2005). Annual summary of vital statistics—2003. *Pediatrics, 115*(3), 619–634.

Meara, E., Kotagal, U. R., Atherton, H. D., & Lieu, T. A. (2004). Impact of early newborn discharge legislation and early follow-up visits on infant outcomes in a state Medicaid population. *Pediatrics, 113*(6), 1619–1627.

Menella, J. A. (2002). Alcohol use during lactation: The folklore versus the science. In K. Auerbach (Ed.), *Current issues in clinical lactation: 2002* (pp. 3–9). Boston: Jones & Bartlett.

Mesich, H. M. (2005). Mother-infant co-sleeping—Understanding the debate and maximizing infant safety. *American Journal of Maternal/Child Nursing, 30*(1), 30–37.

Miller, V., & Riordan, J. (2004). Treating postpartum breast edema with areolar compression. *Journal of Human Lactation, 20*(2), 223–226.

Mohrbacher, N., & Stock, J. (2003). *The breastfeeding answer book* (3rd rev. ed.). Schaumburg, IL: La Leche League International.

Moon, R. Y., & Oden, R. P. (2003). Back to sleep: Can we influence child care providers? *Pediatrics, 112*(4), 878–882.

Moon, R. Y., Weese-Mayer, D. E., & Silvestri, J. M. (2003). Nighttime child care: Inadequate sudden infant death syndrome risk factor knowledge, practice, and policies. *Pediatrics, 111*(4), 795–799.

Morin, K. (2005). Information parents need about preparing formula. *American Journal of Maternal/Child Nursing, 30*(5), 334.

Morland-Schultz, K., & Hill, P. D. (2005). Prevention of and therapies for nipple pain: A systematic review. *Journal of Obstetric, Gynecologic, & Neonatal Nursing, 34*(4), 428–437.

Morris, R., Krueger, C., & Yaross, D. (2004). Better safe than sorry—One agency's successful safety and security strategies. *Home Healthcare Nurse, 22*(6), 417–422.

Paul, I. M., Phillips, T. A., Widome, M. D., & Hollenbeak, C. S. (2004). Cost-effectiveness of postnatal home nursing visits for prevention of hospital care for jaundice and dehydration. *Pediatrics, 114*(4), 1015–1022.

Persing, J., James, H., Swanson, J., Kattwinkel, J., Committee on Practice and Ambulatory Medicine, Section on Plastic Surgery, and Section on Neurological Surgery. (2003). Prevention and management of positional skull deformities in infants. *Pediatrics, 112*(1), 199–202.

Quillin, S. I. M., & Glenn, L. L. (2004). Interaction between feeding method and co-sleeping on maternal-newborn sleep. *Journal of Obstetric, Gynecologic, & Neonatal Nursing, 33*(5), 580–588.

Quinlivan, J. A., Box, H., & Evans, S. F. (2003). Postnatal home visits in teenage mothers: A randomised controlled trial. *The Lancet, 361*(9361), 893–900.

Renfrew, M. J., Ansell, P., & Macleod, K. L. (2003). Formula feed preparation: Helping reduce the risks; a systematic review. *Archives of Disease in Childhood, 88*(10), 855–858.

Riordan, J. (2005a). Breast-related problems. In J. Riordan (Ed.), *Breastfeeding and human lactation* (3rd ed., pp. 247–275). Boston: Jones & Bartlett.

Riordan, J. (2005b). The cultural context of breastfeeding. In J. Riordan (Ed.), *Breastfeeding and human lactation* (3rd ed., pp. 713–728). Boston: Jones & Bartlett.

Riordan, J., & Hoover, K. (2005). Perinatal and intrapartum care. In J. Riordan (Ed.), *Breastfeeding and human lactation* (3rd ed., pp. 185–216). Boston: Jones & Bartlett.

Shields, L. B. E., Hunsaker, D. M., Muldoon, S., Corey, T. S., & Spivack, B. S. (2005). Risk factors associated with sudden unexplained infant death: A prospective study of infant care practices in Kentucky [Electronic version]. *Pediatrics, 116*(1), e13–e20.

Shoemaker, P. A., & Ghaemghami, J. (2003). Protecting the public from mercury exposure: Success through microexchange events. *American Journal of Public Health, 93*(12), 1997–1999.

Simon, N. P., & Simon, M. W. (2004). Changes in newborn bathing practices may increase the risk for omphalitis. *Clinical Pediatrics, 43*(8), 763–767.

Smith, L. J., & Riordan, J. (2005). Postpartum care. In J. Riordan (Ed.), *Breastfeeding and human lactation* (3rd ed., pp. 217–245). Boston: Jones & Bartlett.

Snowden, H. M., Renfrew, M. J., & Woolridge, M. W. (2005). Treatments for breast engorgement during lactation [Review]. *The Cochrane Database of Systematic Reviews, 3.*

Sylvester, B. J., & Reisener, L. (2002). Scared to go to work: A home care performance improvement initiative. *Journal of Nursing Care Quality, 17*(1), 71–82.

Tappero, E. P., & Honeyfield, M. E. (2003). *Physical assessment of the newborn—A comprehensive approach to the art of physical examination* (3rd ed.). Santa Rosa, CA: NICU INK.

Troy, N. W. (2003). Is the significance of postpartum fatigue being overlooked in the lives of women? *American Journal of Maternal/Child Nursing, 28*(4), 252–257.

Tully, M. R. (2005). Working and breastfeeding—Helping moms and employers figure it out. *AWHONN Lifelines, 9*(3), 198–203.

Unger, B., Kemp, J. S., Wilkins, D., Psara, R., Ledbetter, T., Graham, M., et al. (2003). Racial disparity and modifiable risk factors among infants dying suddenly and unexpectedly [Electronic version]. *Pediatrics, 111*(2), e127–e131.

Walker, L., Downe, S., & Gomez, L. (2005). Skin care in the well term newborn: Two systematic reviews. *Birth, 32*(3), 224–228.

Wang, M. L., Dorer, D. J., Fleming, M. P., & Catlin, E. A. (2004). Clinical outcomes of near-term infants. *Pediatrics, 114*(2), 372–376.

Weissinger, D. (2002). Last step first. In K. Auerbach (Ed.), *Current issues in clinical lactation* (pp. 69–73). Boston: Jones & Bartlett.

Witt, C. (2004). Management of neonatal infection, sepsis, and complications. In D. F. Askin (Ed.), *Infection in the neonate: A comprehensive guide to assessment, management, and nursing care* (pp. 143–162). Santa Rosa, CA: NICU INK.

Zupan, J., Garner, P., & Omari, A. A. A. (2004). Topical umbilical cord care at birth [Review]. *The Cochrane Database of Systematic Reviews (CDSR), 3.*

CHAPTER
37

Grief and Loss in the Childbearing Family

Again, they searched for a heartbeat. The high-tech monitor was silent—there was no heartbeat. No one would say the words, so I did. "So, you mean, my daughter is dead?" "Yes," the nurse answered. She stared at me a moment and then looked away. "I'm going to leave you alone for a little while. I'll be back shortly." She handed my husband a form on a clipboard and asked him to fill it out. . . . It was still morning, only two hours since we had arrived at the doctor's office. **Could the whole world change that quickly?**

~ *Lorraine Ash,* Life Touches Life: A Mother's Story of Stillbirth and Healing ~

OBJECTIVES

1. Discuss perinatal loss including etiology, diagnosis, and the nurse's role in facilitating the family's mourning process.
2. Describe the physical, cognitive, emotional, behavioral, and spiritual responses experienced during grieving associated with perinatal loss.
3. Explore the personal and societal issues that may complicate responses to perinatal loss.
4. Identify nursing diagnoses and interventions to meet the special needs of parents and their families related to perinatal loss and grief.
5. Differentiate between helpful and nonhelpful responses in caring for families experiencing perinatal loss and grief.

KEY TERMS

 MEDIALINK

Additional resources for this content can be found on the Prentice Hall Nursing MediaLink DVD-ROM and on the Companion Website at http://www.prenhall.com/davidson. Click on "Chapter 37" to select the activities for this chapter.

Perinatal loss is death of a fetus or infant from the time of conception through the end of the newborn period 28 days after birth. This chapter discusses the family's experience of perinatal loss and the nurse's role in facilitating the family's mourning process. Although not independently addressed, care of the family experiencing the death of their infant in the newborn period is inclusive. Causes and clinical aspects of spontaneous abortion (miscarriage) in the antepartal period are discussed in Chapter 15 ∞; this section discusses causes and clinical aspects of intrauterine fetal death (IUFD) after 20 weeks' gestation, often referred to as *stillbirth* or *fetal demise.*

Perinatal loss is a tragic event for the couple experiencing it and the family who loves them. Compounding the tragedy are the many misconceptions surrounding perinatal loss, a lack of grief education afforded healthcare personnel, and clinical interventions that are out of step with current research. One of the biggest misconceptions about perinatal loss is that it is not as relevant as other losses because of the lack of interaction with the infant. In reality, this could not be further from the truth. Studies have shown that about 90% of couples believe that the loss of their infant was the worst thing that ever happened to them, and more than 80% believe that the death caused a significant decrease in their ability to function (Uren & Wastell, 2002). With regard to education, studies assessing the comfort level of nurses assisting families experiencing perinatal loss clearly demonstrated that many nurses are still uncomfortable with death and dying and that more education is needed and, indeed, greatly desired (Chan, Wu, Day, & Chan, 2005; Rock, 2004). Finally, in recent years there has been a paradigm shift in the field of grief and bereavement concerning the components of a "normal" mourning process and when and where intervention is warranted. Much of what has become the traditional standard of care for bereaved individuals has come into question as new research sheds light on the inefficacy of predetermined early and intense intervention. This chapter focuses on providing frameworks for understanding grief and loss, guidelines for effectively responding to a grieving family, and specific nursing interventions for the family experiencing perinatal loss in the clinical setting.

COMMON CAUSES OF PERINATAL LOSS

The incidence of fetal death after 20 weeks in the United States is 6.8 per 1000 total births, accounting for 50% of all perinatal deaths (fetal and neonatal) (Magann, Chauhan, Bofill et al., 2002). More than 80% of stillbirths occur before term, with more than 50% occurring before 28 weeks' gestation (Cunningham, Leveno, Bloom et al., 2005). The cause may be unknown, or it may result from any of a number of physiologic maladaptations, including preeclampsia or eclampsia, abruptio placentae, placenta previa, diabetes, congenital anomalies, renal disease, cord accidents, fetal growth restriction, and alloimmunization. Perinatal loss associated with birth defects can occur if the fetus is exposed to teratogens late in the pregnancy (Blackburn, 2003) (Table 37–1).

Table 37–1	FACTORS ASSOCIATED WITH PERINATAL LOSS
Fetal Factors	Preeclampsia/eclampsia
Chromosomal disorders	Advanced maternal age
Birth defects not chromosomal in nature	Hereditary thrombophilias
	Antiphospholipid syndrome
Anencephaly, open neural tube defects, isolated hydrocephalus, congenital heart defects	Uterine rupture
	RH disease
Nonimmune hydrops	Ascending bacteria from the vagina
Infections	
Complications of multiple gestations	**Placental and Other Factors**
	Placenta previa
Maternal Factors	Abruptio placentae
	Cord accident
Prolonged pregnancy	Premature rupture of membranes
Diabetes	Unknown factors
Chronic hypertension	

Perinatal loss in industrialized countries has declined in recent years as early diagnosis of congenital anomalies and advances in genetic testing techniques have increased the use of elective termination (Liu, Joseph, & Wen, 2002). Surprisingly, other reproductive advances have increased the incidence of fetal death. It appears that fetal death occurs more frequently in monochorionic twins and twins conceived by assisted reproductive technologies (Skeie, Froen, Vege et al., 2003). In addition, certain genetic testing procedures such as amniocentesis and chorionic villus sampling (CVS) can actually cause fetal loss (Papp & Papp, 2003).

In developing countries, infection plays a significant role in fetal deaths, accounting for 10% to 25% of all fetal demises (Goldenberg & Thompson, 2003). Ascending bacterial organisms include *Escherichia coli,* group B streptococci, and *Ureaplasma urealyticum.* These infections can occur either before or after the membranes have ruptured, resulting in fetal demise. Viral causes of fetal demise include parvovirus and coxsackievirus. *Toxoplasma gondii, Listeria monocytogenes,* and the organisms that cause leptospirosis, Q fever, and Lyme disease have also been identified as causative factors for stillbirth. Untreated syphilis is associated with a high stillbirth rate, as is malaria infection when contracted for the first time by the mother during the pregnancy (Goldenberg & Thompson, 2003). These infections carry a much higher morbidity and mortality rate in developing countries.

Paternal causes of fetal death are also being examined. One recent study determined that paternal exposure to pesticides resulted in a high rate of fetal anomalies and fetal deaths (Regidor, Ronda, Garcia et al., 2004).

Certain maternal conditions can also be associated with higher rates of fetal death. Past maternal exposure to certain bacterial and viral antigens can produce an autoimmune response that can result in fetal death (Blackwell, Romero, Chaiworapongsa et al., 2003). Women with acquired and immune thrombophilia have higher rates of miscarriage and fetal demise than those without hematologic alterations (Alonso,

Soto, Urgelles et al., 2002). Women who lack the endothelial cell protein C receptor are more prone to thrombosis within the placenta, resulting in an increased incidence of fetal loss (Gu, Crawley, Ferrell et al., 2002).

MATERNAL PHYSIOLOGIC IMPLICATIONS

Prolonged retention of the dead fetus may lead to the development of disseminated intravascular coagulation (DIC), also called consumption coagulopathy, in the mother. After the release of thromboplastin from the degenerating fetal tissues into the maternal bloodstream, the extrinsic clotting system is activated, triggering the formation of multiple tiny blood clots. Fibrinogen and factors V and VII are subsequently depleted, and the woman begins to display symptoms of DIC. Fibrinogen levels begin a linear descent 3 to 4 weeks after the death of the fetus and continue to decrease in the absence of appropriate medical intervention.

Besides DIC, other adverse outcomes can also occur if the onset of labor and subsequent birth are delayed. Women with prolonged retention of a dead fetus are more prone to infection. A resulting infection can cause endometritis or sepsis. The longer the pregnancy continues, the higher the incidence of maternal infection.

Although immediate induction is routinely performed, there may be situations in which induction is delayed, such as maternal refusal or the presence of a multiple gestation. In these cases, fibrinogen levels are monitored weekly or biweekly to recognize and prevent progressive coagulopathy from occurring (Lindsey, 2002).

Clinical Therapy

When fetal death has occurred, abdominal x-ray examination may reveal Spalding's sign, an overriding of the fetal cranial bones. In addition, maternal estriol levels fall. Diagnosis of IUFD is confirmed by absence of heart action on ultrasound. Without medical intervention, most women have spontaneous labor within 2 weeks of fetal death. The once common practice of waiting for the onset of labor has largely been abandoned in recent years, because the risks of complications increase with delaying the birth. In 25% of all fetal deaths, the cause remains unknown even after an autopsy. The specific cause is more difficult to identify if the time since the death is prolonged. Prompt birth increases the ability to identify the cause of death.

In modern practice, most women with a diagnosed fetal demise are given the option of waiting a few days or scheduling an induction procedure immediately. Most women will elect for an induction within a day or 2 of the final diagnosis. The mode of induction depends on the gestational age of the fetus, the readiness of the cervix, and previous mode of birth. In women who have had a previous cesarean birth, a repeat cesarean may be performed, because the use of Pitocin or prostaglandin agents can increase the risk of a uterine rupture. Women with an unfavorable cervix may be given vaginal prostaglandin agents, misoprostol, or laminara tents. Women less than 28 weeks' gestation are typically given prostaglandin E_2 (PGE$_2$) 20 mg vaginal suppositories every 4 to 6 hours or oral or vaginal misoprostol 200 mcg every 4 to 6 hours until spontaneous labor occurs (Lindsey, 2002). Because PGE$_2$ suppositories can cause severe vomiting and diarrhea, women are commonly pretreated with antiemetic and antidiarrheal preparations to prevent or lessen these unpleasant side effects (Lindsey, 2002). Laminaria tents are made from the stems of brown seaweed, which are cut, shaped, dried, sterilized, and packaged in specific sizes. Laminaria tents work by drawing water out of the cervical tissue, allowing the cervix to soften and dilate. They are commonly used to dilate the cervix in preterm gestations when induction is warranted.

POSTBIRTH EVALUATION

Identifying the causative factor of fetal loss assists many families in progressing through the mourning process. Information obtained from a postmortem examination or postmortem studies can provide vital information related to the cause of the fetal death, the possibility for reoccurrence, and closure for the couple. The types of studies and tests performed depend on the parents' past history, medical history, and the couple's preferences for the depth of testing desired. Chromosome studies should be considered if the couple has a history of other second- or third-trimester losses or if either parent has a suspected balanced translocation or mosaic chromosomal pattern (Lindsey, 2002).

If an intra-amniotic infection is the suspected cause, cultures of both the placenta and the fetus should be obtained. If specific infections are being considered, both IgM and IgG antibodies should be drawn to determine if an acute infectious process has occurred.

All stillborn infants should have a careful visual inspection at the time of birth for obvious defects or abnormalities. The placenta and membranes should also be closely examined and the placenta should be sent to pathology for further testing. The umbilical cord should be inspected for true knots, a velamentous insertion, lack of Wharton's jelly, or a short cord to determine if a cord accident was the cause. If a specific cause is suspected, blood tests and x-rays can be performed (Lindsey, 2002). An autopsy is the best mechanism to determine the cause of death; however, in the event that the parents decline an autopsy, magnetic resonance imaging (MRI) can also provide detailed information (Lindsey, 2002).

Most practitioners perform a complete blood count (CBC) and antibody screen upon admission. Because diabetes is a causative factor, a random or postpartum glucose level can be obtained to rule out this cause. Additional maternal factors can also be evaluated. Additional tests that may be performed are listed in Table 37–2.

THE EXPERIENCE OF LOSS

The term **bereavement** comes from a root term meaning to be "deprived of something" or to be left "desolate or alone." To be bereaved simply means to have suffered the *event of loss* (Corr, Nabe, & Corr, 2003). **Grief** is an individual's *reaction to the loss,* including physical symptoms, thoughts, feelings, functional limitations, and spiritual responses. Grief reactions may be immediate or delayed, exaggerated or stunted, and highly

Table 37–2	TESTS TO DETERMINE CAUSE OF FETAL LOSS		

Fetal Testing	Maternal Testing
Fetal blood tests and x-rays	Diabetes testing
Autopsy or magnetic resonance imaging (MRI)	Complete blood count (CBC) with platelet count
Placental studies	Kleihauer-Betke test
Chromosomal studies (if indicated)	Abnormal antibody testing (lupus anticoagulant, anticardiolipin antibodies)
	Thyroid stimulating hormone (TSH) levels
	Infectious disease testing (rubella, syphilis, malaria, toxoplasmosis, cytomegalovirus)
	Hereditary thrombophilia testing
	Toxicology testing

variable. Though often used interchangeably, **mourning** is the *process* by which individuals incorporate the experience into their lives and is influenced by many factors, including personality, gender, family dynamics, and social, religious, and cultural norms (DeSpelder & Strickland, 2005). Mourning may be manifested by certain behaviors and rituals, such as weeping or visiting a gravesite, which help the person experience, accept, and adjust to the loss. The unanticipated loss of an expected child can be devastating and traumatic for parents. Though most people eventually regain a sense of purpose and adjust well, some suffer long-lasting and destructive consequences. "Studies suggest that 15% to 25% of women who experience perinatal loss have enduring adjustment problems and many seek professional help to guide them through this difficult time" (Bennett, Litz, Lee et al., 2005, p. 180). Bennett et al. suggest that there is nothing in a person's background to prepare him or her for the abrupt transition from a joyous event to the sorrow of perinatal loss. Perinatal loss is also unique in that the parents have not had experiences with the child that was to be, and attachment is based mostly upon hopes and dreams for the future relationship. There is an old saying that puts it into perspective, "When you lose your parents, you lose your past; when you lose your spouse, you lose your present; and when you lose your child, you lose your future."

Society typically does not offer the kind of support for perinatal loss that is offered for other, more recognized losses. This places perinatal loss in the category of disenfranchised grief. **Disenfranchised grief,** as defined by Kenneth Doka (2002), is grief that is not supported by the usual societal customs. Perinatal loss is sometimes referred to as a "silent loss" because of this phenomenon of disenfranchising grief. People are uncomfortable discussing the loss with the parents and often pull away when their support is most needed. "The loss of a child and all the child has to offer, compounded with the societal attitude discounting the loss and the potential withdrawal of social support, may leave the bereaved parents feeling distraught and alone at a time that was supposed to be full of happiness" (Bennett et al., 2005, p. 181). Parents struggle to come to terms with the devas-

tation of the loss and are often confused and bewildered as to how to make that happen. The nurse caring for a family experiencing perinatal loss can take positive steps to help facilitate the family's mourning process and help them begin their journey to recovery.

FRAMEWORKS FOR UNDERSTANDING PERINATAL LOSS

There have been a plethora of models and theories postulated over the years attempting to explain grief and loss, and at present there is no real consensus as to which models should serve as the cornerstones of theory and teaching. Worth noting is the **dual process model** (Stroebe & Schut, 1999) that is a view of grief encompassing two competing facets: loss and restoration. The loss orientation is concerned with the individual's need to confront the reality of the loss, and the restoration orientation seeks to regain balance and temper the pain of grief. With respect to perinatal loss specifically, however, there are two theories that may provide the best framework for the nurse seeking to understand and assess the grieving family in his or her care. **Attachment theory,** first developed by John Bowlby in 1969 and revisited by Weiss (2001) and Shaver and Tancredy (2001), begins with the basic premise that human beings are biologically predisposed to bond with emotionally significant persons in their lives. The grief response as seen through the lens of attachment theory is a state of separation anxiety brought on by the disruption in the attachment bond. The intensity of the grief response displayed by parents experiencing perinatal loss can be assessed to some extent by determining the level of attachment to the anticipated infant. For mothers, there are nine events that are important to the formation of attachment to her baby:

1. Planning the pregnancy
2. Confirming the pregnancy
3. Accepting the pregnancy
4. Feeling fetal movement
5. Accepting the fetus as an individual
6. Giving birth
7. Seeing the baby
8. Touching the baby
9. Giving care to the baby (Bennett et al., 2005; Klaus & Kennell, 1976).

Helpful questions to assess the first five levels of attachment could include topics such as naming of the baby, future plans, nursery preparations, and personal stories of the pregnancy. Additionally, there are psychologic processes related to becoming a parent that can help to identify those parents who have a strong level of attachment. These are noted in Table 37–3.

Recent studies have demonstrated the need for continuing bonds as a means to remain connected to the deceased infant (Boerner & Heckhausen, 2003; Klass, Silverman, & Nickman, 1996; Talbot, 2002). Therefore, the goal of recovery, as related

Table 37–3   PSYCHOLOGIC PROCESS OF BECOMING A PARENT
Feelings of procreativity or generativity
A sense of continuity through the generations
Responses to quickening and bodily changes
Fears and expectations about the coming baby
The impact of this exciting process on expectant parents' relationship at home
Changes that the baby will bring to their careers and to their lives in general
Attachment to real and idealized aspects of the infant
Self-esteem building

SOURCE: Reprinted from *Loss During Pregnancy or in the Newborn Period: Principles of Care with Clinical Cases and Analyses*, 1997, p. 7. Reprinted with permission of the publisher, Jannetti: Publications, Inc., East Holly Avenue, Box 56, Pitman, NJ 08071-0056. Phone (856) 256-2300; FAX (856) 589-7463. (For more information, visit the Web site at www.ajj.com).

to attachment theory, is for the grieving parent to find a way to maintain the bond with the deceased infant while at the same time acknowledging that the infant is not physically present for future interactions.

The second theory centers on a search for meaning. Robert Neimeyer (2000, 2005) argues that meaning reconstruction is one of the most important aspects of the process for bereaved individuals. Simply put, **meaning reconstruction** focuses on redefining ourselves and how we interact with the world after a significant loss. There is no question that the unexpected loss of a baby can precipitate a crisis of meaning for the parents. Are they still parents? How do they readapt to the world without their child in it? "As meaning is organized by core purposes, which are intimately linked with our attachments, the loss of a primary attachment is likely to be the most disruptive form of loss" (Uren & Wastell, 2002). In recent studies (Attig, 1996; Uren & Wastell, 2002) a large percentage of parents (61%) were troubled by the question, "Why me?" and a whopping 70% to 85% found themselves searching for meaning early in the loss. Evidence supporting the conceptualization of parental bereavement as a crisis of meaning is plentiful (Attig, 1996, 2004; Gamino & Sewell, 2004; Wheeler, 2001). However, it has also been suggested that some individuals do not seek meaning; that of those who do, less than half are able to find it; and that even when they do, the tendency is to continue searching (Davis, Wortman, Lehman et al., 2000). Other studies showed that a significant factor of influence is the particular meaning construct the person places on the loss. People who tend to find positive constructs within the loss fare better than those who tend toward negative constructs (Gamino & Sewell, 2004). Neimeyer concluded, partly in response to the Davis study, that when [parents] are struggling with meaning making, it is important to facilitate the process; but if they are not, the caregiver should not initiate the process. The goal of recovery, as related to meaning reconstruction, is a positive change in self-identity by assigning the loss a meaning, thereby allowing the individual to assimilate the loss into her or his world.

Once there is an understanding of the frameworks for the mourning process, or the rationale behind the grief, the phases

or tasks of mourning can be addressed. It is important to note here that for purposes of this discussion, only the early responses, or first phases and tasks of mourning, are identified, as these are the ones the nurse is most likely to encounter in the clinical care setting. The first two phases or tasks of mourning have been described by various theorists as shock and numbness, denial, acute phase, protest, disorientation, searching and yearning, accepting the reality of the death, and confronting or working through the pain of grief (Bowlby, 1969; Kay, Roman, & Schulte, 1997; Worden, 2002). In the first phase, alternately termed shock and numbness, denial, acute, or protest phase, there is a protective brain mechanism at work that activates to prevent us from taking in too much damaging information at one time and going into "meltdown." For a couple experiencing perinatal loss, this might manifest itself in *denial of* the death of the fetus or infant. Even when the initial healthcare provider suspects fetal demise, the couple is hoping that a second opinion may be different. Some couples may not be convinced of the death until they see and hold the dead infant after birth. As the first task associated with mourning is to accept the reality of the loss, holding the infant may help the couple to begin to accept the fact that the death has indeed occurred. The second phase, alternately described as disorientation or searching and yearning, is often characterized by intense emotions. *Anger*, resulting from feelings of loss, loneliness, and, perhaps, guilt, is common in this phase. The anger may be projected at significant others and healthcare team members. The mother may attempt to identify a specific event that caused the death and may blame herself. The second task of mourning, as described by J. William Worden (2002), is to work through or confront the pain of grief. This is easier said than done as many parents express doubts of their ability to withstand the pain of the devastating loss. Attempts to avoid this task are common but usually time limited. As the couple and their family begin to accept the reality of the death and confront the pain of their loss, many normal manifestations of grief may be present. The nurse should be familiar with these normal reactions, so that abnormal or complicated reactions can be identified when present. See Table 37–4.

SPECIAL ISSUES FOR CONSIDERATION

There are many factors that will influence a couple's response to perinatal loss, including individual factors such as age, gender, and personality type. A teenage couple is going to respond very differently than a couple in their 30s, men and women tend to respond differently, and emotional personalities will display differently than stoic personalities. Family dynamics will greatly factor into the grief response. Is this family chaotic in nature, is there a leader, do they have open communication or closed and guarded interactions, do they deny the reality of the event and pretend it isn't happening? Culture and religion will influence the couple's reaction in either a negative or positive manner. Socioeconomic status will play a role in that for some people, grief is a luxury. If they are more concerned with other children at home, or putting food on the table, their grief will most likely be delayed to a time when they have the resources

Table 37–4   NORMAL PHYSICAL, COGNITIVE, EMOTIONAL, BEHAVIORAL, AND SPIRITUAL EARLY RESPONSES TO LOSS

Physical	Cognitive	Emotional	Behavioral	Spiritual
Physical signs and symptoms of shock	Denial, disbelief	Sadness	Withdrawal	Blaming God
Palpitations	Confusion	Anger/rage	Dependence	Hostility toward God
Shortness of breath	Sense of unreality	Guilt/self-reproach	Fear of being alone	Lack of meaning or direction
Difficulty sleeping	Disorientation	Anxiety	Memorializing the loss	Wishing to join the deceased
Nausea/vomiting	Time confusion	Numbness	Disorientation	Isolation
Loss of appetite	Vigilance or obliviousness	Flat affect	Sleep and appetite disturbances	Feelings of betrayal
Dry mouth	Focused or detached	Indifference	Absent-minded behavior	Hopelessness
Feeling of emptiness in the pit of the stomach	Poor concentration	Withdrawn or explosive	Dreams of the deceased	Destruction or strengthening of beliefs
Weakness/lethargy	Preoccupation	Repetitive storytelling	Crying/sighing	Feelings of being punished
Tightness in throat	Sense of presence	Loneliness	Restlessness	Acceptance as "Divine Will"
Sighing	Hallucinations of the deceased infant	Yearning/nostalgia	Avoidant behaviors	Assigning of deceased infant as "angel" in heaven
Fatigue			Treasuring of mementos	
Oversensitivity to light and sound				
"Aching" arms				

Data from DeSpelder, L. A., & Strickland, A. L. (2005). *The last dance: Encountering death and dying* (7th Ed.). New York: McGraw Hill; Eutsey, D. E., et al., Eds. (2001). *Palliative care: Patient and family counseling manual.* Gaithersburg: Aspen Publishers, Inc.; Schneider, J. M. (1994). *Finding my way: Healing and transformation through loss and grief.* Colfax: Seasons Press; Worden, J. W. (2002). *Grief counseling and grief therapy: A handbook for the mental health practitioner* (3rd ed.). New York: Springer Publishing Company, Inc.

to deal with it. Finally, there are special circumstances that will influence the grief response. Early pregnancy loss has a special form of grief attached, fetal reduction and multifetal pregnancy loss entail separate and distinct issues, and grief from infertility is a largely ignored segment of the grieving population. Each of these components bears further discussion.

Individual and Family Issues

AGE

Age plays a major role in grief reactions. Couples in their 30s may feel that they are running out of time for childbearing; however, they are most likely to have living children at the time of the loss, which may somewhat soften the blow in the long run. Couples in their 20s may be experiencing their first significant death, yet often have the sense that they still have time to have another child. With regard to age, adolescent parents probably pose the greatest challenge to nursing interventions.

According to the National Center for Health Statistics (2005), the birth rate for 2004 for females aged 15 to 19 was 41.2 births per 1000. When adolescents become pregnant, 70% have mixed feelings or do not want to be pregnant and only 41% view themselves as pregnant with a "baby" (Wheeler, 1997). The adolescent who attaches meaning to her pregnancy has the highest rate of grief reaction and life impact. Wheeler's study (1997) showed that grief responses of adolescents were also affected by age of the adolescent, the gestational age at the time of the loss, and the length of time since the loss. Those who were 16 years and younger reported more physical and emotional responses to the loss than did the older adolescents, and those whose losses occurred after 14 weeks' gestation reported more sensitivity to the lack of social support afforded them following the loss.

Though adolescents have a mature concept of death, it is often clouded by their sense of invulnerability, an "It can't happen to me" mentality (Corr et al., 2003). Adolescents rely heavily on peer support and have a natural mistrust of authority figures, which can make assisting them more difficult. It is important to remember that adolescents are already experiencing major life changes, and the death of an infant can have a profound impact on their development. For many adolescents, a pregnancy loss may be the first time they are experiencing the psychologic impact of grief, and normal adolescent growth and development must be taken into consideration when assessing the impact of grief responses (Wheeler & Austin, 2000). Nursing care of the adolescent parent experiencing perinatal loss requires patience and understanding on the part of the nurse. Adolescent parents should be treated with respect and offered the same consideration as adult grievers. They should not be forced into any particular mode of response, but allowed to dictate their own needs within the experience. Gentle and honest guidance are often all that are needed to ensure a healthy nurse-client interaction.

FAMILY DYNAMIC

Family dynamics and the presence or lack of cohesion will greatly factor into a couple's grief response. Families who are chaotic and have poor interfamily communication skills are often fractured and of little support to the couple experiencing the loss. Families who demonstrate strong familial ties and open group interaction tend to fare better in the long run. The most difficult family dynamic to assess and assist is the "lie and deny" family. This is the family who deals with bad news and loss events as though they have not occurred. If they do not talk about it, it did not happen. As a necessary component for the beginning of a healthy mourning process is to accept the reality of the death, the nurse is placed in the tenuous position of mediator between medical personnel and the family who does not want to hear anything negative. It is important to discern the possible causes for denial before proceeding. Denial is a normal and necessary process in the beginning of the mourning process, and the family may just need more time to assimilate the difficult information. Persistent denial, however, can be addressed by a gentle review of the facts of the situation with an emphasis on past tense verbiage when discussing the infant.

GENDER ISSUES

Historically, most of the research regarding grief and bereavement has been done on women. As a result, many stereotypes developed regarding how men and women cope with loss. The latest research by Martin and Doka (2000), however, has identified a new model for the two major coping styles and reveals a more effective means of supporting the griever. The current model identifies the two dominant styles of coping as "intuitive" and "instrumental." People with **intuitive styles of coping** generally feel their way through loss and prefer care with an emphasis on emotional and psychosocial support. People with **instrumental styles of coping** generally use more cognitive skills to navigate loss and value care that includes an emphasis on problem solving (Corr et al., 2003; Martin & Doka, 2000). It is important for the nurse to be aware that although gender *influences* mourning, it does not *determine* the experience for the bereaved.

For intuitive grievers, the nurse may initiate discussion of thoughts and feelings concerning the loss. Mobilization of support from nonjudgmental family and friends is generally appreciated, and providing resource materials that include support groups and the opportunity for networking is usually welcome. The nurse should share with the intuitive griever that enlisting the support of others with whom they can talk rather than relying solely on their spouse is favorable for both partners. The nurse should also share that spouses are commonly unable to be emotionally available to each other following loss. The nurse should normalize the lack of emotional accessibility and provide reassurance that the relationship is not doomed to fail because of the death of an infant.

For the instrumental griever, the nurse should specifically address that a parent who seems detached and unaffected by the loss is not uncaring. It is common for men to fall into this category, as they frequently experience pregnancy through the mother and, when traditionally trained, believe they are not supposed to emote but be strong for their partner (Worden, 2002). The parent who is an instrumental griever may not mention the infant, talk about the loss, or view pictures. He or she may resist when the partner shows emotion or attempts to engage him or her in conversation regarding the loss. Instrumental grievers tend to be more active as well as more vocal in assigning blame and commonly use explosive emotion to obtain desired results. Contrary to traditional thought, instrumental grievers are not unhealthy in their response to loss, yet they are often criticized for their behavior. Because of their perceived strength, they rarely receive validation and support from others. In supporting instrumental mourners, the nurse should keep in mind that they

value acceptance, acknowledgment of their pain, information regarding the loss, what to expect in the aftermath, and tasks that are connected to the loss.

The nurse should inform bereaved couples that both styles of grieving are acceptable and should be honored. Intuitive grievers (most often women) should understand that instrumental grievers may not show emotion or wish to talk about the loss, but are mourning in their own way. Instrumental grievers (most often men) should understand that intuitive grievers will need to talk about the event and help to provide avenues for that outlet. The nurse can instill a measure of hope by reassuring parents that although they may feel as if they cannot bear the pain of the loss, it will not always remain so intense.

OTHER FEATURES OF BEREAVED INDIVIDUALS

In addition to age, family traits, and gender issues, Parkes and Weiss (1983) identified overall features of bereaved individuals that place them at increased risk for pathologic or complicated grief reactions. These features include insecurity, anxiety, or low self-esteem; previous psychiatric history; excessive anger and guilt; a physical disability/illness; previous unresolved losses; inability to express emotion; and concurrent problems of living. Parkes and Weiss also identified features of the bereaved's circumstances that will put them at risk; these include an unsupportive or unavailable family, lack of social/religious or other supports, and low socioeconomic status.

Societal Issues
SPIRITUALITY

In times of crisis, spirituality brings comfort and strength to some people, and for many it is the single most important factor in quality of life (Swensen, Fuller, & Clements, 1993). For others, a life crisis may precipitate a spiritual crisis and catalyze a complete redefining of the belief system, though the new belief system is often stronger than the one previously ascribed to (Frantz, Farrell, & Trolley, 2005).

Religion and spirituality are not one and the same. **Spirituality** is defined as the human search for meaning and connectedness to life, others, God, the universe, and transcendence. **Religion** is defined as structured efforts conducted in a systematic approach to attain holiness (Balk, 2004). Religious practices are based upon the level of a person's assimilation into the particular religion and are too varied and numerous to define for standards of care. With regard to specific religious practices, it is prudent for the nurse simply to ask the family how they can best be assisted in meeting their religious needs.

A recent study identified six themes affecting the spiritual needs of bereaved parents: honest exchange of information, empathy and presence, continuing bonds, spiritual rites, attachment with others, and grief support (Meert, Thurston, & Briller, 2005). The nurse can facilitate the spiritual needs of the couple by providing an atmosphere of acceptance regarding spiritual rites and encouraging the couple's use of spiritual writings, prayers, and observances. Questions that solicit the spiritual viewpoint of the couple regarding the loss can allow release of parental distress concerning spiritual matters. It is important for

DEVELOPING CULTURAL COMPETENCE

GRIEF RESPONSES AND INTERACTIONS

- Cultural background often plays a large part in determining the emotional response of the grieving couple. Cultures that are stoic in nature can be the most difficult to assist. The underlying cause of stoicism usually stems from three possible sources: shock, denial, or family/cultural background. It is important to ascertain the underlying cause so that appropriate interventions, where warranted, can take place.

- In male-dominant cultures, mothers experiencing perinatal loss may tend to dwell more on their "failure" as a woman to successfully reproduce. The nurse should reassure these women (while respecting cultural beliefs) that nothing they did or did not do affected the outcome. A reiteration of known medical causes is often helpful as well.

- In cultures in which the extended family is the couple's main form of support, it is important to allow as much interaction as possible within the confines of the clinical environment. Family support is often the greatest source of comfort to the grieving couple and, therefore, should be respected and encouraged.

- A basic rule of thumb for cultural issues is to remember that curiosity is okay; avoidance is not. If you are not sure what the family needs, simply ask them how you can help to accommodate their wishes. Families appreciate an honest and caring attitude.

the nurse not to answer rhetorical questions, but allow the parents to process their own thoughts and feelings concerning meaning, purpose, and significance of the life and death of their infant. It is also important for the nurse to distinguish between his or her own personal beliefs and those of the parents. Some healthcare professionals get defensive and critical when the spiritual needs of the parents conflict with their own spiritual viewpoint. Recognition of personal limitations is healthy and providing care is not exclusive to direct delivery. The nurse acts as a family advocate by offering to contact the couple's clergyperson, spiritual advisor, or the hospital chaplain. Research confirms that providing effective spiritual care to a parent during loss and bereavement is valuable in facilitating healthy parental mourning (Meert et al., 2005).

Specific Circumstance

INFERTILITY

Nearly seven million people in the United States suffer from infertility, yet fewer than 50% of people who could be successfully treated will access treatment, mostly because of the lack of insurance coverage and lack of knowledge regarding their options (Isaacs, 2005). Infertility is diagnosed when partners have

been unable to conceive while having unprotected sexual intercourse for approximately 12 months (Swanson, Karmali, Powell et al., 2003). A common misconception regarding infertility centers on its being a wholly female problem, when in actuality one third can be attributed to male factors. Another common misconception is that it is most often caused by waiting too late in life, when in reality the impact in the 20 to 34 age range is almost equal to that in the 35 to 44 age range. Infertility is far more likely to be the result of a physical or genetic abnormality (Isaacs, 2005).

Infertility is not an episode, but an ongoing struggle for those who are caught in its grasp. The focus of treatment for infertility is a correct diagnosis, appropriate treatment, and successful live birth, yet infertility brings with it grief and loss issues that affect all realms of the couple's life. Not only are the medical and physical components extremely challenging, but the loss of infertility goes largely unrecognized by the usual support systems, placing it within the disenfranchised grief category. In the early phase, the clients are trying to assimilate the diagnosis of infertility and what the diagnosis actually means for them. Then they are faced with a gamut of decisions and difficulties: treatment available; method that is best for them; when to begin; repercussion of choices; risk involved; waiting; menstrual cycles; pregnancy; failed pregnancy; surgery; hormone treatments; in vitro fertilization (IVF); hospitalization(s); psychologic roller coaster; spiritual impact; the strain on finances and primary, secondary, familial, and workplace relationships; and, finally, when to discontinue treatment.

In supporting the client dealing with infertility, the nurse should assess where the client is in the process and respond accordingly. The nurse should be compassionate, give accurate and honest information, validate the many losses incurred, and support whatever decisions the couple makes regarding the continuation of treatment or decision to stop treatment. The nurse should not avoid the couple, offer pat answers or reasons for the infertility or the outcome, or relay unsolicited stories of others' successes or failures (Flowers, 2003). For couples finally experiencing a pregnancy following infertility treatment, there may be heightened anxiety for which additional reassurances will need to be offered.

EARLY PREGNANCY LOSS

Early pregnancy loss, whether by ectopic or molar pregnancy, blighted ovum, or spontaneous abortion, is devastating for many couples. It is important to note that approximately 75% of women view early pregnancy loss as the death of an infant, whereas only 25% view it as merely a life event (Swanson-Kaufman, 1986). As attachment is based on the level of emotional bonding, it is necessary for the nurse to assess the situation in order to respond to actual client needs and validate the loss for those who view the event as the death of their baby. Compounding early pregnancy loss is the extraordinary guilt the couple typically harbors, especially the mother. Mothers will often blame themselves, whether by commission or omission, particularly in cultures where a woman's status is dominated by themes of motherhood and childrearing. The nurse should reassure the couple that they did not do anything to precipitate the

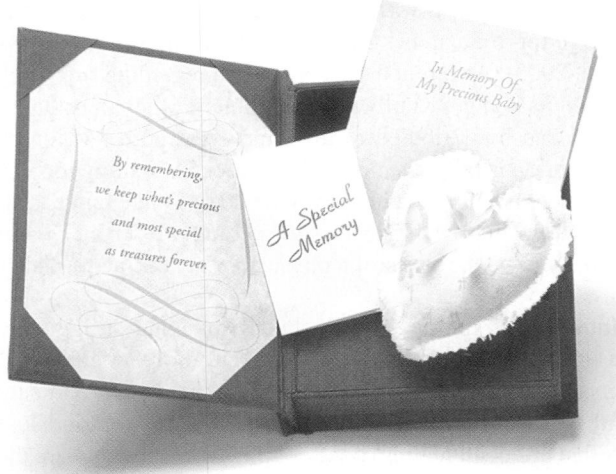

Figure 37–1 ◆ Early pregnancy remembrance box.
SOURCE: © 2006 Gundersen Luthern Medical Foundation, Inc.
www.bereavementservices.org.

loss, and provide support materials specific to the type of loss incurred and what to expect in the immediate aftermath.

Assessment of future pregnancies will need to be dealt with gently, as some couples have no desire to try again. Healthcare professionals sometimes find it easier and more comfortable to refocus on something other than the loss; however, that tends to minimize the loss event and isolate the griever. Even if the parents are expressing an interest in trying again, it is important not to focus exclusively on the future pregnancy, but to provide opportunities to address the current loss (Hess, 2004). The nurse should prepare the couple for the fact that family members and friends will often underestimate the impact of the loss and may offer well-meaning, though often harmful, remarks or platitudes in an attempt to ease emotional pain. An early pregnancy remembrance box (a remembrance journal, sachet pillow, and a baby ring) provides a sensitive and caring way to give parents something to take with them that contains memories of their baby (Figure 37–1 ◆). This is a common reaction in early pregnancy loss, as they may have not known about the pregnancy or feel as if the couple "didn't know the baby." The nurse should reassure the parents that they have a right to their feelings, thoughts, emotions, and reactions to the loss.

MULTIFETAL PREGNANCY LOSS

In 2002, the U.S. live twin birth rate was 31 per 1000, and the high-order multiple-birth rate was 184 per 100,000 births (Martin, Hamilton, Sutton et al., 2003). Twins are 5 times, and multiples 12 times, more likely to die in their first year than singletons (Martin et al., 2003). Multifetal pregnancy loss (MPL) may occur by spontaneous abortion, elective termination for unwanted pregnancy, selective reduction for fetal malformation, or selective reduction in high-risk multiple pregnancy to provide a greater chance of survival for remaining embryos. The loss of an infant in a multiple pregnancy may also occur by intrauterine demise, twin-to-twin transfusion syndrome, complications of monoamniotic twinning, placental problems, adverse intrapartum events, delayed interval delivery, postoperative complications, and the effects of prematurity (Pector, 2004). Parents whose multiples die have an increased risk of prolonged or delayed grief (Pector & Smith-Levitin, 2002).

There are many aspects of multifetal pregnancy loss that have historically been overlooked by healthcare professionals. Some of the predominant issues affecting parents are traumatic impact of diagnoses of malformation or birth defects, options and impact of difficult decisions, sudden death of an infant, fear and anxiety for surviving infants, prospect of infertility because of previous abortions, last attempt at IVF or such fertility intervention, guilt, cohabitation of mourning and joy, and resurgence of the body's remembering on special days and holidays (Keefe-Cooperman, 2004–2005; Kersting, Dorsch, Krevlich et al., 2005; Pector, 2004).

In supporting bereaved parents caring for surviving infant(s) in the loss of a multiple, the nurse should resist the urge to suggest the parents refocus on the positive aspect of having surviving siblings. Statements inferring that the death was meant to be, the death allowed the other infant(s) to live, or the child who died would have had a compromised quality of life should never be made. The nurse should understand that the couple will have difficulty mourning their loss as they attempt to balance emotions of joy and sadness while caring for the surviving infant(s). Parents will often imagine what the deceased infant would have looked liked, what kind of personality the infant would have developed, and what the relationship with siblings would have been. They may harbor feelings of guilt if they feel relief for not having to care for numerous infants. The nurse should support parents by addressing these distinctive concerns and prepare them for the unique issues related to multifetal loss before they leave the hospital (Pector, 2004).

When creating visual memories for bereaved parents, an effort should be made to take pictures of the multiples together. The nurse should ask parents how they prefer to address surviving infants, for example, twins, triplets, quadruplets, and so forth. Additionally, the nurse should ask the couple whether or not they wish to delay funeral services until the mother is able to attend the ceremony. If the couple desires a delay, the nurse should contact appropriate disciplines to arrange for the delay in disposition of fetal remains (Pector, 2004). The nurse should prepare the mother for the likelihood of her body missing and remembering the baby immediately after delivery, while caring for surviving infant(s), and surrounding special days, milestones, and holidays. Finally, the nurse should be aware of the risk for complicated bereavement and refer the couple for appropriate support via resource materials (Keefe-Cooperman, 2004–2005).

NURSING CARE MANAGEMENT
Nursing Assessment and Diagnosis
THE CLINICAL SETTING

Cessation of fetal movement reported by the mother to the nurse is frequently the first indication of fetal death. It is followed by a gradual decrease in the signs and symptoms of pregnancy.

Fetal heart tones are absent, and fetal movement is no longer palpable. Once fetal demise is established, the nurse assesses the family members' ability to adapt to their loss. Open communication between the mother, her partner, and the healthcare team members contributes to a realistic understanding of the medical condition and its associated treatments. The nurse may discuss prior experiences the family has had with loss and what they feel were their perceived coping abilities at that time. Identifying the family's social supports and resources is also important.

Perinatal loss may also occur in the intrapartum period as a result of an intrapartum complication, such as an unresolved shoulder dystocia, prolapsed umbilical cord, abruptio placentae, or other complication. In such emergency situations, healthcare team members often focus on the physical needs of the mother and an attempt to save the fetus' life. Commonly, it is not until the infant is delivered that the family is advised a perinatal death has occurred. Thus, the parents are faced with the sudden and completely unanticipated death of their infant. The most common response is protest or disbelief.

Although the physician or certified nurse-midwife (CNM) informs the family of the death, the nurse continues one-on-one care with the family, providing both physical and emotional support throughout this crucial period. The nurse assists the family in the mourning process and explores their immediate wishes for viewing and holding their deceased (Figure 37–2 ◆).

MEMORIES TO HOLD CHECKLIST   SARASOTA MEMORIAL HOSPITAL

Mother's Name: _____ Father's Name: _____

Address: _____

Please verify address and phone number listed on face sheet with family

Phone Number: _____ Best time to call: _____

Gravida: _____ Para: _____ Estimated Due Date: _____ Previous Loss: _____

Date/time Delivered: _____ ❑ Vaginal ❑ C-Section Gest. Age: _____

Infant's Name: _____ Sex: ❑ Male ❑ Female Weight: _____

Sibling Name(s)/Age: _____

Support People: _____

Do you wish to be notified of MTH Meetings and Annual Memorial Service?. . . . . ❑Yes ❑ No

Do you speak English? . . . . ❑Yes ❑ No

Notification of:

    Social Worker. . . . . ❑Yes ❑ No Initials: _____

    Clergy . . . . ❑Yes ❑ No Initials: _____

    Memories to Hold, x-2468 . . . . ❑Yes (Required) Initials: _____

Services Provided:

    Baptism . . . . ❑Yes ❑ No Initials: _____

    Saw baby at delivery. . . . . ❑Yes ❑ No Initials: _____

    Touched/Held baby . . . . ❑Yes ❑ No Initials: _____

      Mother . . . . ❑Yes ❑ No Initials: _____

      Father . . . . ❑Yes ❑ No Initials: _____

      Siblings . . . . ❑Yes ❑ No Initials: _____

      Grandparents . . . . ❑Yes ❑ No Initials: _____

Mementos Offered: (See Below)   **Mementos Declined by Patient:** ❑ Yes

    Footprints/Handprints/Weight/Length record,

    Lock of hair/crib card/I.D. bracelet/tape measure . . . . . . ❑ Given to Parents ❑To MTH Initials: _____

    Remembrance of Blessing/Baptism . . . . ❑ Given to Parents ❑To MTH Initials: _____

    Photos taken: (clothed, unclothed)

      Polaroid. . . . . ❑ Given to Parents ❑To MTH Initials: _____

      First Foto Co. . . . . ❑ Placed in Mailer ❑To MTH Initials: _____

    Name of Funeral Home selected: _____

MTH Brochure given to: ❑ Mother ❑ Father ❑ Other: _____

Discussed grief process: ❑ Mother ❑ Father ❑ Other: _____

Face Sheet and Yellow Copy tubed to MTH at Station# 46: ❑Yes

Patient Signature: _____ Date: _____

Staff Signature: _____ Date: _____

MTH Counselor Assigned: _____
                                                    OFFICE USE

705820 2/03   White – Chart   Yellow –Tube 46   Pink – Physician or SCPHD

Figure 37–2 ◆ Memories to Hold Checklist.
SOURCE: Sarasota Memorial Hospital, Sarasota, FL.

Nursing diagnoses that may apply include the following (Wilkinson, 2005):

- **Anticipatory Grieving** related to the imminent loss of a child
- **Powerlessness** related to lack of control in current situational crisis
- **Compromised Family Coping** related to death of a child/unresolved feelings regarding perinatal loss
- **Interrupted Family Processes** related to fetal demise
- **Hopelessness** related to sudden, unexpected fetal loss
- **Risk for Spiritual Distress** related to intense suffering secondary to unexpected fetal loss

Nursing Plan and Implementation

It happened early in my pregnancy. The heart that was beating so strongly only a week before was now gone and my dream was over. While waiting for a D & C in the emergency department of a local hospital, Brahms lullaby began playing over the hospital sound system. I understand that birth is a joyous event for most people, but I couldn't believe that they had overlooked the obvious; there were women like me for whom a lullaby, in that moment, brought intense pain into an already difficult situation. I just wish they would have thought of that.

~A BEREAVED PARENT~

Most facilities have an established protocol to follow in the event of perinatal death. It typically provides a holistic focus for family-centered nursing care. It is important that the entire healthcare team is notified so multidisciplinary care can be initiated. When fetal death has been confirmed before admission, the entire staff on the unit is informed so they can avoid making inappropriate remarks. Many facilities have a symbol, such as a card with a leaf or a cluster of flowers, that is placed on the mother's door so all staff is aware of the loss (Figure 37–3 ◆). This is something that should be discussed with the family before placement, as some may view the symbol as an identification of them as "damaged." As is stated throughout

Figure 37–3 ◆ Door card.
SOURCE: © 2006 Gundersen Luthern Medical Foundation, Inc.
www.bereavementserivces.org.

RESEARCH IN PRACTICE

THE ROLE OF CAREGIVERS AFTER A STILLBIRTH: VIEWS AND EXPERIENCES OF PARENTS

What is this study about? A stillbirth is a traumatic event for both parents and caregivers. Caregivers need to give parents information about the situation, advise the parents about next steps, and support the parents by creating a trusting relationship that can help parents through bereavement. The objective of this study was to determine the ways that caregivers can support parents in the event of a stillbirth so that they are able to grieve for the loss of their child.

How was this study done? This qualitative study involved semistructured interviews of 24 couples and 7 single mothers who had experienced a stillbirth at greater than 28 weeks' gestation. An initial interview was conducted using an interview guide that explored attachment to the stillborn child, clinic management of the situation, the parents' own sense of control, and the grieving process. A second interview focused on questions that arose from the first interview that needed further clarification. The interviews were transcribed in their entirety and analyzed using qualitative content analysis. Intercoder reliability was established through independent verification of the coding guidelines.

What were the results of the study? The parents described six caregiver behaviors that were crucial during the period following a stillbirth. The six behaviors were support in chaos; support in meeting with and separating from the baby; support in bereavement; explanation of the stillbirth; organization of the care; and understanding the nature of grief. The quality of "support in chaos" included structured information about how to cope with the baby's death and with meeting the baby. The parents noted that it was helpful to have some moments to recover after finding out the fetus had died but before receiving information about the birth. Support for meeting with and separating from the baby required that the caregiver provide concrete support for the process of spending time with the child. It was important to these parents not to be rushed or judged in terms of the time they wanted with the baby; some parents spent up to 7 hours with the child before separating from him or her. To be supported in

both events—meeting and separating from the baby—was identified as critical by these parents. Support in bereavement included support by both professional caregivers and laypersons, such as clergy. The explanation of the stillbirth included ways of dealing with parental guilt, as well as the importance of finding a medical explanation for the death. Organization of care focused on care options, including having adequate sick leave and obtaining special antenatal care for subsequent pregnancies, that is, that caregivers for subsequent births are aware the parents have experienced a stillbirth. Finally, the quality of understanding the nature of grief includes facing the grief and understanding that the essence of the sorrow will never end, but rather become part of the parents' shared history. Parents clearly emphasized that a stillbirth changed the parents' experiences of life.

What additional questions might I have? These data were collected between 4 and 6 years after the stillbirth. Although this gave the parents some perspective on the event, would these responses be different if the stillbirth were more recent? Are these experiences different for couples and for single mothers?

How can I use this study? The emotional attitudes demonstrated by caregivers are significant in helping bereaved parents cope with the death of a baby. It is important for the nurse to establish a relationship of trust between themselves and the parents. The parents need to be given time to react to information given to them during the process of learning about a fetal death and the subsequent birth. A basic knowledge of care management for parents of stillborn children is essential for caregivers, because they are in a unique position to facilitate the process of grieving for the baby. Nurses can help the parents establish an attachment to the baby, to give them time with the child, and to support them in their grief process. The parents of a stillborn child are influenced by the caregivers' emotional attitudes in critical moments during this difficult time.

Saflund, K., Sjogran, B., & Wredling, R. (2004). The role of caregivers after a stillbirth: Views and experiences of parents. *Birth, 31*(2), 132–137.

the chapter, it is important to allow the family to dictate their own experience.

AVOIDING THE USE OF CLICHÉS

Inappropriate remarks are a hallmark of uniformed interactions, even though the intent behind them is honorable. The nurse should become familiar with statements that are helpful in facilitating the family's mourning process. Although grieving people often say that it is easier to forgive less-than-helpful remarks than it is to forgive those who do not reach out to them at all, the use of clichés can be harmful. The nurse can facilitate a healthy mourning process for the family by using active listening techniques and avoiding the use of clichés. Sitting in silence with a family is often the most helpful form of intervention available. For a list of helpful versus nonhelpful statements with rationales, see Table 37–5.

CLINICAL TIP

No matter who you are or how much nursing experience you have, when an expectant family is in pain because of their loss, and you feel you do not know the right thing to say, "I'm so sorry, I don't know what to say" is a start.

FACILITATING THE FAMILY'S MOURNING PROCESS

As mentioned at the opening of this chapter, there has been a recent paradigm shift in the field of grief and bereavement with regard to what constitutes a "normal" mourning process and when and where early intervention is warranted. The standard of care has been centered on the notion that early and intense grief responses should be encouraged and even elicited for healing to begin. Current research, however, has determined that

Table 37–5   NONHELPFUL VERSUS HELPFUL INTERACTIONS WITH GRIEVING FAMILIES

Nonhelpful	Helpful	Rationale
You're young; you can try again. At least you have your other children.	I know you'll miss [Sara] and no one will ever take her place in your heart.	Saying that they can try again diminishes the current pain they are in. Saying that no one can ever take the deceased infant's place validates the loss as real and the infant as unique.
At least you didn't know him/her yet.	I'm sure you had many hopes and dreams for the future.	Never start a sentence with the words "at least." It diminishes whatever follows. Speaking of future plans validates the loss of the hoped-for child and the dreams that will never be.
It's a blessing in disguise.	I don't know why this terrible thing has happened to you. I just want you to know that I care and want to help you through it.	Statements like, "It's a blessing in disguise" are often said when there are deformities involved. There is no adequate explanation for the family as to why this tragedy has befallen them and none should be offered. Instead, reassurance that they will not be alone should be given.
God needed another angel in heaven.	I'm so sorry this is happening to you. You are a good person and this is a terrible thing to have to go through. I'm here to listen if you would like to talk about it.	The family may make this statement as an indication of their belief system, and that is perfectly acceptable. It is not acceptable, however, for the nurse to impose her or his own belief system upon the family. It is much more effective to address the issue at hand (they are in pain) and reassure them of your caring presence.

many people are naturally resilient and will recover in their own time, without the benefit of assistance (Balk, 2004; Bonanno, 2004; Lang, Goulet, Aita et al., 2001; Lang, Goulet, & Amsel, 2003; Miller, 2003; Moskowitz, Folkman, & Acree, 2003). For instance, stoic responses, when exhibited as a result of familial or cultural traits, are not always counterproductive and may not need intervention in order for the person to begin the path to recovery. Furthermore, not only is early intervention not always necessary, it can even be harmful in some instances (Bonnano, Weriman, Lehman et al., 2002; Hughes, Turton, Hopper et al., 2002; Hughes & Riches, 2003; Murray, Terry, Vance et al., 2000). Although the research confirms that traumatic grief is usually best assisted by early intervention, perinatal loss does not *always* fall into this category, which leads to the current quandary: When is early intervention warranted and effective? The debate continues, but for the nurse caring for a family experiencing perinatal loss, avoiding the trap of "cookie cutter" responses is not difficult if *simple, caring guidelines* are followed rather than *rigid* rules. This will ensure the family is treated as a unique entity and allow them to dictate their own experience.

THE CARING THEORY

The classic caring model, developed by Swanson (1991), has sustained the test of time and is as relevant today as when it was originally developed. Perhaps because of its lack of rigidity and concentration wholly on the overall *attitude* of the caregiver, it can best serve as a solid foundation for good nursing practice related to bereavement care. The **caring theory** consists of five attributes of the caregiver: (1) knowing, (2) being with, (3) doing for, (4) enabling, and (5) maintaining belief.

Knowing is defined as attempting to understand the event as it has meaning in the life of the parents. A thorough nursing assessment will facilitate the nurses' understanding of the significance of the loss to the parents. Nurses who operate from a level of knowing are perceived as sensitive, knowledgeable, and ap-

propriate. Nurses who do not are often perceived as distant, cold, and uncaring. *Being with,* or being emotionally present, is the nurse's ability to reach beyond professionalism and give of herself or himself as a human being, *Doing for* is a restating of the golden rule. It means that the nurse does for the parents as she or he would have things done for her or him in the same situation. This does not mean detail by detail, as every family is unique in their needs; rather, this is an overall, treat-them-as-you-would-your-own-family type of behavior. *Enabling* means facilitation of the parents' passage through life transitions and unfamiliar events. Enabling encompasses all of the interventions listed throughout the text regarding perinatal loss and places the caregiver in the role of facilitator. Finally, *maintaining belief* is defined as believing in the parents' capacity to get through the event and face a future with meaning. The nurse who ascribes to this model of care well serves the needs of bereaved parents by compassionately helping them in the midst of their pain and imprinting positive memories to sustain them.

THE ART OF RESPONDING

Employing the caring theory of behavior, the nurse can then look to the responding model as a set of guidelines for successful interactions with grieving families. Keeping in mind the uniqueness of each situation, the **responding model** is offered to give the nurse an overall set of guidelines for effectively interacting with families experiencing perinatal loss (see Table 37–6). The specific elements of the model are addressed throughout the rest of the chapter and within the nursing care plan.

PREPARING THE FAMILY FOR THE BIRTH AND DEATH

Upon arrival to the facility, the couple with a known or suspected fetal demise should immediately be placed in a private room. When possible, the woman should be in a room that is farthest away from other laboring women. Care should be taken not to

Table 37–6   THE ESSENTIAL ELEMENTS OF
***RESPONDING* EFFECTIVELY TO THE NEEDS OF GRIEVING**
FAMILIES

Recognition and Validation of the Loss
Emotional Availability
Spiritual and Cultural Accommodation
Physical Presence
Open Communication
Normalization of Grief Reactions
Decision-Making Assistance
Interdisciplinary Involvement
Nonjudgmental Attitude
Genuine Caring

SOURCE: Shields, K. (2005). *Preparing the Family for the Birth and Death.* Healing Through Hope. Used with permission.

leave the couple in the waiting room with other expectant parents or visitors waiting for news from other women in labor. The nurse should sit down for a moment, offer an introduction, and acknowledge the loss in the event of a known demise or impending death. A simple statement such as "My name is Brenda and I'll be your nurse today; I'm so sorry; this must be so hard for you. I'd like to help you through it," will go a long way toward establishing a relationship of trust between the nurse and the parents.

The couple should be allowed to remain together as much as they wish. The nurse provides privacy as needed and maintains a supportive environment. The couple should be given complete information about what to expect and what will happen. Questions should be encouraged and answered. The nurse stays with the couple so they do not feel alone and isolated; however, cues that the couple wants to be alone should be assessed continuously. Some couples may want outside support, such as family members or friends, to be present during the labor. The nurse facilitates the couple's wishes.

When possible, the same nurse should provide care for the couple so that a therapeutic relationship can be established. As the relationship develops, the nurse provides solace by listening to the couple without offering explanations. The nurse also provides ongoing opportunities for the couple to ask questions. It is not uncommon for the family to ask the same questions repeatedly. This is part of the initial process. Clear explanations and straightforward answers should be provided and the parents treated equally in giving of information. The nurse also arranges for other members of the multidisciplinary team to interact with the family. The team should take great care to avoid inflicting further trauma on the couple by displaying conflicting words and behavior, such as using a falsely cheerful tone of voice while their body language clearly indicates sorrow (Trulsson & Rädestad, 2004). The nurse offers to contact the hospital chaplain or another cleric for them, and a social worker should also be involved. The nurse typically coordinates members of the multidisciplinary team so that a comprehensive plan of care can be initiated.

The nurse explains details of the plan of care and allows the family to ask questions and make decisions for their labor and birth preferences. The availability of anesthesia and analgesia should be reviewed. The woman typically can have pain medication whenever she desires. The nurse facilitates the participation of the woman and her partner in the labor and birth process.

It is important to remember that, in contrast to a typical birth experience, the birth of a stillborn infant marks both the beginning and the end. For this reason, it is imperative that the couple and family have all wishes and preferences respected. The family may be overwhelmed and may have difficulty making decisions in this period. The nurse can strengthen the couples' ability to cope by providing a warm atmosphere of acceptance. The nurse must assist the couple in exploring their feelings and help them to make decisions about who will be present and what rituals will occur during and following the birth. Examples of birth preferences include:

- Use of music, dimmed lighting, or other environmental preferences
- Laboring or birthing in a specific position
- Having the infant placed on the mother's chest immediately after birth
- Allowing the father to cut the umbilical cord
- Having other family members or friends present at the birth

Sometimes couples worry that others may view their preferences as "strange" or "wrong." Reassure the family that it is their experience and that there are no right or wrong feelings or wishes.

The couple may have waves of overwhelming grief, disbelief, or sadness. Encourage them to experience the grief that they feel, but do not force the issue. It is not uncommon for one partner to attempt to put on a "brave front," feeling that, by showing grief, he or she will make the other partner feel worse. It is also not uncommon for partners to have intense feelings that they feel unable to share. Encourage partners to express their emotions freely to the extent they are able. Help them understand that they may each experience different feelings.

SUPPORTING THE FAMILY IN DECISION MAKING

It is important to remember that the family will need guidance *throughout* the process. The couple should be offered simple choices all along the way to help them retain as much control over their situation as possible. Advocates of seeing the stillborn infant believe that viewing assists in dispelling denial and enables the couple to progress to the next step in the mourning process; however, at least one recent study may indicate otherwise. Researchers concluded that adverse outcomes such as higher anxiety levels were reported in higher numbers in mothers who held the infant than in mothers who only saw the infant or did not see or hold the infant (Hughes et al., 2002). One potential explanation for this finding is the possibility that if nurses who are uncomfortable with death and dying are rigidly following standard bereavement checklists rather than recognizing the uniqueness of each situation, the mother and father may be forced into uncomfortable situations they are not properly prepared for. Another proposed explanation is that when the parents view and hold the infant, further bonding occurs, which leads to a more intense grief reaction. Until more conclusive

Figure 37–4 ◆ Parents holding their deceased infant.
SOURCE: Ash, L. (2004). *Life touches life: A mother's story of stillbirth and healing.* Troutdale, OR: New Sage Press, Inc.

studies are reported, the nurse should offer the couple the opportunity to see and hold the infant, assess possible motivations behind negative responses (such as a fear of the unknown), and reassure the couple that *any decision they make for themselves is the right one.* Additionally, the nurse should not allow pressure from others to be put upon the couple to either see and hold or not see and hold their stillborn infant. If they choose to see their stillborn infant, prepare the couple for what they will see by saying "she is going to feel cold," "he is going to be blue," or other appropriate statements. If the parents have shared with you the name they had chosen for their baby, use that name in discussing the baby; for example, "Jessie's face is bruised." If the couple is hesitant to view the infant out of a fear of what the infant will look like, offering a Polaroid picture will sometimes help to allay their fears. The picture should always be taken after the postmortem care is complete and the infant is readied for holding (Figure 37–4 ◆).

> *I looked at the picture of Victoria that the counselor had given Bill so I knew what she looked like. Bill and I decided we would meet with Victoria separately, and then together. After that we would have the baptism with the two of us and my parents present. My mother-in-law, whose second baby had been stillborn, did not want to participate. Already it was clear that grieving had many ways to express itself, and I began to understand that everybody's way was right.*
>
> ~LIFE TOUCHES LIFE~

CLINICAL TIP

Allow the family to dictate their own experience. A compassionate, caring presence and gentle guidance are often all that is needed to facilitate the family's mourning process.

POSTMORTEM CARE

Properly preparing the infant for viewing is an essential step in the process. Stillborn infants are often misshapen, and the skin can be discolored or in a state of maceration. **Maceration** is the process of tissue breakdown, which begins from the moment an undelivered infant dies. It is characterized by sloughing of the

skin, which can help determine the interval between death and delivery of the infant; that is, the more sloughing, the greater length of time between the demise and delivery (Pauli, 2005). When bathing the infant for viewing, care should be taken to cause as little additional disruption to the skin as possible. A gloved hand is preferable to a washcloth for these infants. After bathing, the infant should be placed in a suitable-sized gown and then wrapped in a blanket. A hat can be applied to cover birth defects. This allows the parents an opportunity to view the infant before seeing the birth defect. Many parents will eventually remove the covering to inspect the infant; however, applying a covering allows them time to adjust to the appearance at their own pace. In cases of extreme maceration, the parents should be fully informed of the condition of the skin, so that they can decide for themselves if they want to see, hold, and/or fully uncover the infant. Couples will often look to assisting medical and nursing personnel for the "correct" attitude toward their stillborn infant. The nurse should carefully monitor personal reactions and display acceptance of the choices the parents make. For step-by-step postmortem care instructions, see Table 37–7.

> *I watched as my mother handed my baby back to the bereavement counselor, as the counselor nestled Victoria gently amid the blankets in the wheeled hospital cart, as the cart moved out of the room. I knew I would never see her again. There was nothing the staff could do to stop the rapid decomposition of her body after that. The process, they said, already had begun, which is why I did not unwrap my baby from her clothes. I did not want to see that. I wanted to remember her as whole.*
>
> ~LIFE TOUCHES LIFE~

Some families will hold their infant for a short time before returning him or her to the nurse, whereas others will wish to spend a great deal of time with their infant. The nurse allows the infant to remain with the family for as long as the family desires.

SUPPORTING SIBLINGS AND EXTENDED FAMILY MEMBERS

Some couples may want other family members, friends, or their other children to be with them in their experience and possibly view and hold the infant. The nurse acts as an advocate to ensure that the family's wishes are respected. Siblings will respond according to their age and maturity level. Children younger than 7 may not recognize that the death is permanent, whereas older children may respond with concern for the parents' well-being. It is normal for them to slightly regress in social and cognitive behaviors when under stress. Children should be included as much as desired by the parents and should be told the truth in a simple, honest, and age-appropriate manner, avoiding the use of euphemisms when describing death and the aftermath. A **euphemism** is a substituted word or expression with a more pleasant association than the one which, although more direct, is considered to be harsher (Corr et al., 2003). Children will, quite normally, need reassurance of two things: that they are still going to be taken care of and that nothing they did caused the event to happen. In facilities in which child life

Table 37–7   POSTMORTEM CARE

Document time of death per physician.

Gather supplies per hospital protocol.

Appropriate forms.

Bathing—2 basins, absorbent pads, diapers, clothing, washcloths, hat.

Memory kit—memory card with foot or handprint area, memory box.

Morgue kit—identification tags, pads for wrapping, paperwork.

Remove tubes and wires when applicable.

Cap and leave all indwelling tubes and catheters if autopsy is to be performed.

Plug endotracheal tube (E.T.) with cotton ball and tape over opening to hold in place and prevent seepage.

Bathe and dress fetus/infant.

Offer parents opportunity to assist with bathing and dressing infant as appropriate (if infant is stillborn, skin maceration may be traumatic for parents).

With gloved hands, place infant in lukewarm basin of water.

Rinse if skin breakdown is present; if skin integrity is intact, rub gently with washcloth. Soap is optional; based also on integrity of skin.

Place fetus/infant in second basin of lukewarm water to rinse.

Gently pat dry. Do not use scented (especially baby products) lotions or powders.

If seepage present from nasal cavity, place petroleum jelly in nostrils.

Diaper and dress fetus/infant in outfit provided either by parents, hospital, or volunteer organization. Consider the use of a hat, particularly where deformity is present.

Take pictures.

Cover imperfections and deformities where applicable.

Use mementos in pictures when available.

Use soft, yet vibrant, colors in background or consider black and white photos.

Place fetus/infant in a flattering and comforting position (different for every infant).

Offer parents opportunity to participate in picture taking, but do not force the issue.

If desired by parents, wrap in warm blanket and present infant for holding.

Prepare parents before holding fetus/infant by telling them what they will see, feel, and smell.

Offer a picture before holding.

Model normal nurturing behavior for parents.

Offer time alone with infant and check back frequently within previously specified time frame.

After holding, remove clothing for weight and measurements, footprints, handprints, memory card, and lock of hair (when applicable).

Prepare fetus/infant for pathology/morgue/family transport according to hospital protocol.

For morgue care:

Complete all hospital paperwork.

Place infant in supine position on top of folded diapers and pad to maintain body position and prevent disfigurement.

Use neck and body rolls to help with alignment.

Wrap infant according to hospital protocol.

Take memory box and bereavement information to parents.

Memory box should include pictures, ID bracelet, memory card, other personal items, and bereavement clothes.

Bereavement information should include pamphlets on grief and loss as well as local and national resources for support and information.

Document the events leading up to and following the death including:

Time and pronouncement of death with physician's name.

Placement of tubes and catheters.

Postmortem care.

Comfort measures and bereavement care provided to family.

Preparation and transport to morgue.

---

specialists are present, their help can be elicited to assist the family in preparing the children for the death and provide an outlet for the children during the event.

Extended family members, especially grandparents, are "doubly" grieving as they suffer through the pain their children are experiencing and the loss of their grandchild. They will have varied reactions, from the extreme of attempting to completely control the process for their child to a display of total passivity. Most reactions fall somewhere in the middle of the continuum. The nurse can help to validate the grandparents' grief by acknowledging the difficulty of their position and extending her support to them as well as to the parents. Even grandparents who are blaming, questioning, or demanding can be made a part of the team when approached in a nondefensive, nonjudgmental, and aid-enlisting manner.

Family support has been shown to be a major comfort to couples in families in which there is open communication and honest interaction. Less intense grief over time has been reported in families who are able to express their emotions with one another as compared with more stoic families (Traylor, Hayslip, Kaminski, et al., 2003). The nurse should provide every opportunity for family cohesion throughout the process, encouraging as much participation and interaction as desired by the couple.

ACTUALIZING THE LOSS: PROVIDING MEMORIES

In a fetal demise, the nurse should remember that mementos are some of the few memories the parents have to provide them comfort after the death of their baby. Every effort should be made to offer as many quality mementos as possible, such as pictures and hand or footprint molds and cards (Figure 37–5 ◆). Most facilities prepare a remembrance box or package for the family to take home. This typically consists of a photograph taken of the infant or the family, a card with the baby's footprints, a crib card, identification band, a lock of hair, and, possibly, a blanket or clothing worn by the infant. In the event that the couple declines the package, it is common for the hospital to retain these items for a specific period of time in case they change their minds.

PROVIDING DISCHARGE CARE

The family usually has three options open to them for disposition of the fetus or infant's body. The first is a traditional burial. Many funeral homes offer reduced fees for infant burial services. The family should contact the funeral home directly to make arrangements. Some families may wish to bury their infant on private land. This is state, county, and locally dictated

Figure 37–5 ◆ Memory Box.
SOURCE: © 2006 Gundersen Luthern Medical Foundation, Inc.
www.bereavementservices.org.

and it is up to the family to ascertain any restrictive ordinances as to transportation and burial. Hospitals with comprehensive bereavement programs in place usually have access to this information. The second option is cremation at a funeral home. Families will need to decide what to do with the cremains. The third option, and not one generally recommended, is hospital disposition. **Hospital disposition** at most facilities is incineration at regular intervals, usually with other body parts, and the family does not have the option to obtain the ashes. Some institutions, especially private and/or religiously affiliated facilities, offer mass burial options for hospital disposition, but not many. In the last decade or so, a few programs have been initiated that offer more individualized burial options for infants designated for hospital disposition (Figure 37–6 ◆). These programs are usually a coordinated effort between facilities within a specific area and one of the local funeral homes and cemeteries that serve their community. The program is usually offered at little or no charge to the family. Whatever option the family decides upon, the nurse should support their decision and assist them in any way possible to achieve their goal for disposition and/or funeral services.

After the birth, the couple can be given the option of an early discharge (as early as 6 to 8 hours after the birth). Facility protocol will dictate where mothers are transferred after a perinatal loss. Some hospitals have the woman remain on the labor and delivery unit, whereas others will give the mother the option of choosing a postpartum room or one on a medical unit. If the mother is transferred to a postpartum unit, care is given to put her in a room far away from other rooms and the newborn nursery. Again, it is imperative that all staff members, as well as student nurses, be notified of the mother's status (see Figure 37–3).

Discharge focuses on the physical considerations and adaptation of the mother and emotional considerations of the couple. Postpartum directions for follow-up care should be provided. Written materials should be provided and a phone number for questions can be given. The woman should also be given information on her milk coming in and interventions to follow to decrease the discomfort associated with engorgement.

Additional information should be given on the mourning process (Figure 37–7 ◆). The nurse can prepare the couple to return home by stressing that others may not know what to say, and that even loved ones may make inappropriate comments because they do not know how to respond to grief and loss. This can

Figure 37–6 ◆ Baby Rest.
SOURCE: Healing Through Hope.

Figure 37–7 ◆ Bereavement literature.
SOURCE: Healing Through Hope.

EVIDENCE-BASED PRACTICE

SUPPORTING PARENTS THROUGH THE AFTERMATH OF STILLBIRTH

Clinical Question

Women who experience a stillbirth face one of the most devastating events that can affect a family. How can the nurse provide appropriate support to parents in the aftermath of a stillbirth in both the short and long term?

The Evidence

It is commonly qualitative researchers who investigate the meaning of this devastating experience for parents. A qualitative synthesis of the literature about the aftermath of stillbirth reveals examination of both the immediate issues and the longer-term considerations, including the unique experiences of subsequent pregnancies. Four qualitative studies were appraised and their findings synthesized to determine the common experiences of families after stillbirth, and the ways in which healthcare practitioners can support the family in both the short and long term after this devastating event.

What Is Effective?

For all women, the aftermath of a stillbirth is an emotionally laden, high-anxiety period of their life. The experience affects virtually all aspects of a woman's life, including her relationship with her existing children, her marital adjustment, and her community. There is little that any individual can do to lessen the impact of this grief, but supporting the parents in bringing to bear their personal coping mechanisms can help. Allowing parents their grief rituals is an important supportive action the nurse can take. Parents will grieve in very personal ways, and the nurse must value the individuality of the experience. Giving the parents a safe place and time to express their grief is critical. Nurses should make an effort to listen to the perspectives of parents in order to assist them in coming to terms with their loss. Women who experience pregnancy subsequent to stillbirth have a powerful personal history that changes their life and

their experience of future childbearing as well. These women need reassurance, control, and choices during the subsequent pregnancy. These particular mothers report a need for the caregivers to know of the history of stillbirth, and to be sensitive that the subsequent pregnancy will involve substantial emotional and psychologic energy.

What Is Unclear?

It does not appear that psychologic or psychosocial interventions on the part of caregivers are effective in the short term. While these are not randomized trials, none of these researchers reported actions that relieved the grief and pain of these parents, but rather focused on interventions that nurses can apply to help parents cope with the ongoing work of grieving.

Best Practice

The nurse should recognize the devastating nature of a stillbirth event for the entire family. Parents should be supported in their unique and individual methods of dealing with this event. Long-term considerations require sensitivity on the part of caregivers that any subsequent pregnancies will be fraught with emotional and psychologic challenges, and should assume that a previous stillbirth will affect the ways that parents deal with subsequent pregnancies.

Critical Thinking

How should the nurse alter the plan of care for a mother who has experienced a previous stillbirth and is experiencing a subsequent birth?

REFERENCES: Brin, D. (2004). The use of rituals in grieving for a miscarriage or stillbirth. *Women and Therapy, 27*(3), 123–132.

Burkhammer, M., Anderson, G., & Chiu, S. (2004). Grief, anxiety, stillbirth, and perinatal problems. *Journal of Obstetric, Gynecological, & Neonatal Nursing, 33*(6), 774–782.

Cosgrove, L. (2004). The aftermath of pregnancy loss: A feminist critique of the literature and implications for treatment. *Women and Therapy, 27*(3), 107–122.

Keith, P. (2005). *Women's experience of livebirth after stillbirth.* Unpublished doctoral dissertation, University of British Columbia.

prepare the couple for the reactions of others. If there are siblings, each will usually progress through age-appropriate grieving. Provide the parents with information about normal grief reactions, both psychologic and physiologic. The couple should be given information regarding depression as a normal part of grieving. Couples may feel empty and lost and may experience physical symptoms such as sleep disturbances, weight loss or gain, listlessness, fatigue, hyperactivity, inability to concentrate, and a lack of motivation. The onset of the symptoms of depression often coincides with the time when other people have moved on and withdrawn support for the couple, making it harder for them to cope. The couple should be informed that depression following perinatal loss is normal and unless debilitating or prolonged need not be medicated or treated and will subside in time. If depression is prolonged, outside help should be sought. Additionally, as the

mourning process ensues, families should be encouraged to implement cultural, religious, or social customs that will assist them in their grief. The nurse should advise the family that certain upcoming milestones, such as holidays, future birthdays, baby showers, Mother's Day, Father's Day, and other social events may trigger their grief. The family can better cope with these events if they are adequately prepared. Finally, the couple should be advised not to make any major life change decisions in the first year following the death, whenever possible. Making major life changes compounds grief reactions by adding other losses (such as moving away from the familiar) on top of the loss of infant, resulting in often complicated mourning.

When caring for a family suffering from a perinatal loss, it is important to remember that the nurse experiences many of the same grief reactions as the parents of a stillborn infant. It is important to have colleagues and family members available for counseling and support.

Following discharge, some families may need closure of the intrapartum event to continue their mourning process. A consultation can be scheduled with the practitioner who cared for them during the pregnancy and birth. Families may also wish to read the results of tests performed during the intrapartum period and the autopsy report. The couple should be provided with a copy of the medical record and encouraged to ask questions, express their feelings, and ask for clarification.

Families are routinely referred for counseling services after a perinatal loss has occurred. A counselor who specializes in perinatal issues can provide expertise and assist the couple in their grieving. Partners should be allowed to verbalize fears and concerns about future pregnancies. When appropriate, referrals to genetic counselors, religious support persons, and social service agencies also should be provided.

Besides referral information, the woman should receive scheduled follow-up phone calls to assess the family's functioning and their progress with grief work. During these follow-up phone calls, pertinent information can be given and additional resources can be identified.

REFERRING THE FAMILY TO COMMUNITY SERVICES

Although most facilities have an established protocol for families experiencing perinatal loss, more comprehensive programs are being established in communities to provide a step-by-step intervention program to assist these families. Community support groups that focus on perinatal loss can provide an important support network and resources. Specialized groups, such as those focused on early pregnancy loss, stillbirth, and perinatal loss associated with specific congenital anomalies, allow families the opportunity to interact with peers who have lost infants under similar circumstances. The nurse provides the group name, contact person (if possible), and phone number. Bereavement materials such as *When Hello Means Goodbye* by Schwiebert and Kirk (1985), *The Bereaved Parents' Survival Guide* by Rothman (1999), *Unsupported Losses* by Ilse (1994), *Empty Arms* by Ilse (1996), and *Another Baby? Maybe ...* by Ilse and Doerr (1996) can also be provided.

Internet technology has allowed large numbers of individuals to share resources and information and participate in online support groups. Internet resources can be effective for all families and may be the only resources available for families in rural underserved areas. A study by Capitulo (2004) found that online perinatal loss support groups were "cultures," in that they had distinct beliefs, behaviors, norms, and attitudes that set a pattern of behavior for members of the online community. They were very helpful in allowing mothers to interact with other mothers in similar circumstances.

Specialized community outreach programs are another community resource that can provide assistance to grieving families. One example is an early community intervention program that provides counseling to parents whose fetus has a known lethal congenital anomaly. In perinatal hospice programs, parents are given the opportunity to explore options, such as elective termination or waiting for the onset of spontaneous labor or a medically indicated induced labor. For families wishing to continue their pregnancies, the program typically assigns a multidisciplinary team who provides compassionate care, ongoing counseling, referral to support groups, and spiritual guidance (Calhoun, Napolitano, Terry et al., 2003).

CARE OF THE COUPLE WHO HAS EXPERIENCED LOSS IN A PREVIOUS PREGNANCY

Couples who have had a previous perinatal loss typically enter a subsequent pregnancy with conflicting feelings and may experience ambivalence, fear, and anxiety. Many times, their past experience is relived when another pregnancy occurs. Some couples conceive soon after a loss, whereas others wait years. Some couples enter a subsequent pregnancy with grief work largely completed, whereas others are still experiencing unresolved grief.

The nurse caring for a couple who has had a previous loss needs to be kind, compassionate, and patient. Couples need specific information and clear explanations of all prenatal information. Referrals to a genetic counselor should be made when appropriate. Some couples may wish to have a consultation with a perinatologist. If unresolved grief issues are present or the family experiences extreme anxiety, counseling may be beneficial.

Interventions to decrease anxiety can help the couple tremendously. At the first visit, an early ultrasound can be performed to verify the presence of the fetal heart. In early pregnancy, women may be fearful when first-trimester pregnancy symptoms begin to resolve. It may be helpful for these women to come in for weekly visits for a period of time simply to hear the fetal heartbeat. This intervention may continue to be helpful until the woman begins to feel fetal movement. Throughout the pregnancy, the office or clinic nurse can play a key role by providing reassurance and answering questions that the woman may have.

Women with a previous loss typically receive additional antepartum testing throughout the pregnancy. Ultrasounds can be used to provide reassurance and assess fetal growth and development, placental functioning, and cord variations. Non-stress testing and biophysical profiles can be performed weekly after 32 weeks to ensure fetal well-being. Fetal kick counts should be initiated at 28 weeks and continue until the birth occurs. Women with a previous loss should be delivered at their expected date of birth or when the pregnancy is at term and should not go over their due date, because placental functioning can decline in postdate pregnancies.

Evaluation

Caring for a family experiencing perinatal loss is a challenging, yet rewarding, opportunity for the nurse who offers his or her humanity, concern, and acceptance. There is nothing quite like helping a family through one of the most difficult events of their lives. The reward is often greater for the giver than for those who are receiving, because the important life lessons learned and the sense of accomplishment achieved when reaching out to others in need is rarely rivaled. Nurses should remember to

MediaLink Application: Pregnancy after a Miscarriage

MediaLink Perinatal Loss Resources

MediaLink Case Study: Family with Perinatal Loss

process their own grief reactions so that they remain healthy responders for the next family in need.

Expected outcomes of nursing care for the family experiencing perinatal loss include the following:

- Family members feel free to express their feelings about the death of their baby if they desire to do so.
- Family members participate in decision making regarding preferences for the labor, birth, and the immediate postpartum period.

- Family members participate in the decision of whether to see their baby and other decisions about the baby.
- The family has resources available for continued support.
- Family members know the community resources available and have names and phone numbers to use if they choose.

Nursing care of a family experiencing perinatal loss is further described in the accompanying Nursing Care Plan.

NURSING CARE PLAN

For a Family Experiencing Perinatal Loss

INTERVENTION	RATIONALE	EXPECTED OUTCOMES
1. Nursing Diagnosis: Emotional Distress related to perinatal loss as evidenced by crying/sadness, irritability/anger, guilt responses and/or fear		
Goal: The client will verbalize thoughts and feelings associated with the loss, and understand the factual events surrounding the loss. The client begins to form a trust relationship with the nurse and freely asks for and accepts support provided by nursing staff.		
• Normalize the experience by assuring parents that there is no right or wrong way to express grief.	• Grief reactions encompass a broad spectrum of thoughts and emotions. Providing a nonjudgmental, supportive environment validates the grief response, thereby establishing a trust relationship, which helps to facilitate a healthy mourning process.	*The client and family acknowledge the loss as evidenced by verbalizing an understanding of the factual events surrounding the loss and openly expressing thoughts and feelings regarding the loss in a safe and constructive manner.*
• Crying. Offer tissues while allowing free expression of emotion.	• Crying is a normal reaction to the loss event and offering tissues is a tangible form of acceptance.	*The client and family begin to form a trust relationship as evidenced by freely asking for, and accepting support provided by nursing staff, and relating to the nurse in an environment of acceptance.*
• Anger. Avoiding defensiveness, state the obvious and enlist the parent's assistance in exploring possible sources of, and solutions to, their anger.	• Anger, as a part of the grief response, usually stems from the frustration at the circumstances and should not be taken personally. Allowing for the free expression of anger, as well as remaining neutral in responses will help to defuse the situation. Utilizing a team approach will assist the client in viewing hospital personnel as partners in care, rather than adversaries.	
• Guilt responses. Reframe the event in a reality-based forum, reassuring the parents that they did nothing to precipitate the loss.	• Guilt is a predominant feature of grief following loss, especially in parents experiencing the death of an infant. Reality testing, a companion of the factual information versus the parents' perceptions of culpability, assists them in coming to the conclusion that they did the best they could in the circumstance.	

NURSING CARE PLAN

For a Family Experiencing Perinatal Loss continued

INTERVENTION	RATIONALE	EXPECTED OUTCOMES
• Fear. Provide honest, simple explanations of what to expect before, during, and after the loss event.	• Families can cope with even the most extreme situations when they are properly in an honest and forthright manner. Maintaining a close presence while providing factual information will help alleviate feelings of fear and isolation. Offering simple choices allows clients to maintain a semblance of control over their circumstances.	

2. Nursing Diagnosis: Disruption of Family Systems related to sudden, unexpected crisis of perinatal loss

Goal: The client and family are able to maintain familial cohesion necessary for returning to homeostasis.

INTERVENTION	RATIONALE	EXPECTED OUTCOMES
• Gather information regarding the family *familial* and the surrounding loss event before initial interaction. • Determine the extent of the family's knowledge regarding the situation before initial interaction. • Assess the family's internal resources necessary for maintaining family cohesion by active listening and asking open-ended questions regarding normal coping styles. • Mobilize family and hospital support systems.	• Effective intervention requires an extensive knowledge of the situation at hand. Failure to gather essential facts can precipitate a negative interaction with the family, leading to a breakdown in communication. • Effective crisis intervention always begins with the point of the family's knowledge and bridges from which they know to what you need them to know. Presenting the facts in an orderly fashion with increasing detail will help the family process difficult information. • Asking open-ended questions will help to identify the family's resources for coping. Identifying the family's internal resources allows the nurse to utilize the family's unique strengths and normal coping mechanisms in dealing with crisis and loss. This will help them regain equilibrium as a family unit. • The family support system is preferable because of the comfort factor associated with familiarity and the consistency of long-term support. The hospital support system is supplementary to the family support system and can provide additional resources and support for individual family members, thereby strengthening the family unit.	*The client and family maintain the cohesion necessary for returning to homeostasis as evidenced by openly interacting, supporting, and communicating needs within the family and using family and hospital/community support systems as needed.*

CHAPTER REVIEW

FOCUS YOUR STUDY

- Perinatal loss poses a major nursing challenge to provide support and care for the parents.

- Perinatal loss is a tragic and often traumatic event in the life of most families experiencing it.

- Fetal death after 20 weeks accounts for 50% of all fetal deaths per year, with 50% of those deaths occurring before 28 weeks' gestation.

- Bereavement is the *event* of the loss, grief is the *reaction* to that loss, and mourning is the *process* by which we incorporate the loss into our lives through the use of individual, cultural, religious, and social norms.

- Up to 25% of women will need professional help to facilitate their mourning process following the death of their infant.

- Attachment theory with regard to perinatal loss is based upon the premise that human beings are biologically predisposed to bond with emotionally significant persons in their lives and the grief response is a state of separation anxiety brought on by the disruption in the attachment bond.

- For mothers, there are nine events that are important to the formation of attachment to her infant. They are (1) planning the pregnancy, (2) confirming the pregnancy, (3) accepting the pregnancy, (4) feeling fetal movement, (5) accepting the fetus as an individual, (6) giving birth, (7) seeing the baby, (8) touching the baby, and (9) giving care to the baby.

- Meaning reconstruction focuses on redefining ourselves and how we interact with the world after a significant loss. The goal of recovery, as related to meaning reconstruction, is a positive change in self-identity by assigning the loss a meaning, thereby allowing the individual to assimilate the loss into her or his world.

- There are many normal physical, cognitive, emotional, behavioral, and spiritual early responses to loss. The recognition of normal responses helps to identify the presence of abnormal or exaggerated responses.

- There are many factors that will influence a couple's response to perinatal loss, including individual and family personality traits, and social, cultural, and religious customs.

- Cessation of fetal movement reported by the mother to the nurse is frequently the first indication of fetal death. The nurse continues one-on-one care with the family, providing both physical and emotional support throughout this crucial period.

- The nurse can facilitate a healthy mourning process for the family by using active listening techniques and avoiding the use of clichés. Sitting in silence with a family is often the most helpful form of intervention available.

- Traditionally, it was believed that early and intense grieving was necessary for healing, but recent studies show that many people are naturally resilient and will not necessarily grieve initially or intensely.

- The caring theory places the emphasis of care on the attitude adopted by the nurse toward the grieving family as paramount to successful intervention and includes knowing, doing for, enabling, and maintaining belief.

- The responding model describes 10 behaviors and actions necessary for effective interaction with the grieving family and includes recognition of the loss, emotional availability, spiritual and cultural accommodation, physical presence, open communication, normalization of grief reactions, decision-making assistance, interdisciplinary involvement, nonjudgmental attitude, and genuine caring.

- Upon arrival to the facility, the nurse should make introduction, acknowledge the loss, and establish the beginnings of a trust relationship with the family.

- The nurse functions as advocate for the family in organizing interdisciplinary involvement, maintaining continuity of care, offering the opportunity for open communication, and ensuring that the family's wishes regarding their loss experience are honored.

- Couples experiencing perinatal loss should be offered the opportunity to participate in postmortem care and to view, hold, and name their baby. In the event a couple declines the opportunity, the nurse should assess for fear of the unknown as a motivating factor and take steps to alleviate that fear. The couple should never be coerced into viewing and holding their infant if they do not choose to do so, and the nurse should display a nonjudgmental, accepting attitude regardless of the decision made by the couple.

- Siblings and extended family members should be included in the plan of care to whatever extent the couple wishes. Children should be given information in an honest and age-appropriate manner, and grandparents should be recognized for the "double" grief they are experiencing through the pain of their child and death of their grandchild.

- Mementos are important links for the family to their deceased infant. A memory box should be offered with as many personal items of the infant as possible. Hand and/or footprint cards are especially desired items.

- Follow-up care should include bereavement materials and community support information as well as a telephone call to assess the family's well-being and provide any further desired information.

- Couples experiencing pregnancy following a loss can be expected to have higher levels of fear and anxiety and will need to be treated with care and concern. Information may need to be repeated and details of time lines provided to raise the comfort level of the couple.

EXPLORE MEDIALINK

http://www.prenhall.com/davidson

NCLEX review questions, case studies, and other interactive resources for this chapter can be found on the Web Site at http://www.prenhall.com/davidson. Click on "Chapter 37" to select the activities for this chapter.

For tutorials including animations and videos, more NCLEX review questions, and an audio glossary, access the accompanying Prentice Hall Nursing MediaLink DVD-ROM in this book.

PRENTICE HALL NURSING MEDIALINK DVD-ROM
Audio Glossary
NCLEX Review

COMPANION WEBSITE
Additional NCLEX Review
Care Plan Activity: *Family with Perinatal Loss*
Case Study: *Family with Perinatal Loss*
Applications: *Grief; Pregnancy after a Miscarriage*
Critical Thinking

CRITICAL THINKING IN ACTION

PERINATAL GRIEF

View the Critical Thinking in Action video in Chapter 37 of the DVD-ROM. Then answer the questions that follow.

Marguerite, a 25-year-old married woman, is admitted for delivery of a stillborn baby girl. Through tears, Marguerite shares that she has named the baby, Alicia, after her grandmother. She has already decorated the nursery with the many gifts she received at her baby shower. Marguerite apolo-

gizes for "crying so much" and frequently expresses a fear that her husband, John, may blame her for Alicia's death because she worked until the time of the final ultrasound. She wonders aloud if he would be right. She communicates a desire to see and hold Alicia, but is very fearful of how the baby will look and whether people will think that she is morbid for wanting to hold a dead baby. Marguerite apologizes again for crying and shares that she does not know who else to talk to because no one seems to understand what she is going through.

1. What should the nurse helping families through the crisis of perinatal loss know about grief in general?

2. What should the nurse know about the unique nature of perinatal loss?

3. What types of nursing behaviors will facilitate the family's mourning process?

REFERENCES

Alonso, A., Soto, I., Urgelles, M. E., Corte, J. R., Rodriquez, M. J., & Pinto, C. R. (2002). Acquired and inherited thrombophilia in women with unexplained fetal losses. *American Journal of Obstetrics & Gynecology, 187*(5), 1337–1342.

Ash, L. (2004). *Life touches life: A mother's story of stillbirth and healing.* Troutdale, OR: New Sage Press.

Attig, T. (1996). *How we grieve: Relearning the world.* New York: Oxford University Press.

Attig, T. (2004). Meanings of death seen through the lens of grieving. *Death Studies, 28,* 341–360.

Balk, D. E. (2004). Recovery following bereavement: An examination of the concept. *Death Studies, 28,* 361–374.

Bennett, S. M., Litz, B. T., Lee, B. S., & Maguen, S. (2005). The scope and impact of perinatal loss: Current status and future directions. *Professional Psychology: Research and Practice, 36*(2), 180–187.

Blackburn, S. T. (2003). *Maternal, fetal, and neonatal physiology: A clinical perspective* (2nd ed.). Philadelphia: Saunders.

Blackwell, S., Romero, R., Chaiworapongsa, T., Refuerzo, J., Gervasi, M. T., Yoshimatsu, J., et al. (2003). Unexplained fetal death is associated with changes in the adaptive limb of the maternal immune response consistent with prior antigenic exposure. *Journal of Maternal-Fetal and Neonatal Medicine, 14*(4), 241–246.

Boerner, K., & Heckhausen, J. (2003). To have and have not: Adaptive bereavement by transforming mental ties to the deceased. *Death Studies, 27,* 199–226.

Bonnano, G. A. (2004). Loss, trauma, and human resilience: Have we underestimated the human capacity to thrive after extremely aversive events? *American Psychologist, 59*(1), 20–28.

Bonnano, G. A., Wortman, C. B., Lehman, D. R., Tweed, R. G., Haring, M., Sonnega, J., et al. (2002). Resilience to loss and chronic grief: A prospective study from pre-loss to 18 months post-loss. *Journal of Personality and Social Psychology, 83,* 1150–1164.

Bowlby, J. (1969). *Attachment and loss: Attachment* (Vol. 1). New York: Basic Books.

Calhoun, B. C., Napolitano, P., Terry, M., Bussey, C., & Hoeldtke, N. J. (2003). Perinatal hospice: Comprehensive care for the family of the fetus with a lethal condition. *Journal of Reproductive Medicine, 48*(5), 343–348.

Capitulo, K. L. (2004). Perinatal grief online. *American Journal of Maternal/Child Nursing, 29*(5), 305–311.

Chan, M. F., Wu, L. H., Day, M. C., & Chan, S. H. (2005). Attitudes of nurses toward perinatal bereavement: Findings from a study in Hong Kong. *Journal of Perinatal and Neonatal Nursing, 19*(3), 240–252.

Corr, C. A., Nabe, C. M., & Corr, D. M. (2003). *Death and dying: Life and living* (4th ed.). Belmont, CA: Thomson/Wadsworth.

Cunningham, F. G., Leveno, K. J., Bloom, S. L., Hauth, J. C., Gilstrap, L. C., & Wenstrom, K. D. (2005). *Williams obstetrics* (22nd ed.). New York: McGraw-Hill.

Davis, C. G., Wortman, C. B., Lehman, D. R., & Silver, R. C. (2000). Searching for meaning in loss: Are clinical assumptions correct? *Death Studies, 24,* 497–540.

DeSpelder, L. A., & Strickland, A. L. (2005). *The last dance: Encountering death and dying* (7th ed.). New York: McGraw Hill.

Doka, K. J. (Ed.). (2002). *Disenfranchised grief: New directions, challenges, and strategies for practice.* Champaign, IL: Research Press.

Eutsey, D. E., & DiLima, S. N. (Eds.). (2001). *Palliative care: Patient and family counseling manual.* Gaithersburg, MD: Aspen.

Flowers, L. (2003). *Infertility: Finding God's peace in the journey.* Eugene, OR: Harvest House.

Frantz, T. T., Farrell, M. M., & Trolley, B. C. (2005). Positive outcomes of losing a loved one. In R. A. Neimeyer (Ed.), *Meaning reconstruction & the experience of loss* (pp. 193, 194). Washington, DC: American Psychological Association.

Gamino, L. A., & Sewell, K. W. (2004). Meaning constructs as predictors of bereavement adjustment: A report from the Scott & White Grief Study. *Death Studies, 28,* 397–421.

Goldenberg, R. L., & Thompson, C. (2003). The infectious origins of stillbirth. *American Journal of Obstetrics & Gynecology, 189*(3), 861–873.

Gu, J. M., Crawley, J. T., Ferrell, G., Zhang, F., Li, W., Esmon, N. L., et al. (2002). Disruption of the endothelial cell protein C receptor gene in mice causes placental thrombosis and early embryonic lethality. *Journal of Biological Chemistry, 277*(45), 4335–4343.

Hess, R. F. (2004). Dimensions of women's long-term postabortion experience. *American Journal of Maternal/Child Nursing, 29*(3), 193–198.

Hughes, P., Turton, P., Hopper, E., & Evans, C. (2002). Assessment of guidelines for good practice in psychosocial care of mothers after stillbirth: A cohort study. *Lancet, 360* (9327), 114–118.

Hughes, P., & Riches, S. (2003). Psychological aspects of perinatal loss. *Current Opinion in Obstetrics and Gynecology, 15,* 107–111.

Ilse, S. (1994). *Unsupported losses: Ectopic pregnancy, molar pregnancy, and blighted ovum.* Saint Paul, MN: deRuyter-Nelson.

Ilse, S. (1996). *Empty arms.* Maple Plain, MN: Wintergreen Press.

Ilse, S., & Doerr, M. W. (1996). *Another baby? Maybe . . . Thirty questions on pregnancy after loss.* Maple Plain, MN: Wintergreen Press.

Isaacs, J. C. (2005). The patient voice in infertility. *AWHONN Lifelines, 9*(5), 363–364.

Kay, J., Roman, B., & Schulte, H. M. (1997). Pregnancy loss and the grief process. In J. R. Woods & J. L. Esposito (Eds.), *Loss during pregnancy or in the newborn period: Principles of care with clinical cases and analyses* (pp. 5–36). Pittman, NJ: Jannetti.

Keefe-Cooperman, K. (2004–2005). A comparison of grief as related to miscarriage and termination for fetal abnormality. *OMEGA, 50*(4), 281–300.

Kersting, A., Dorsch, M., Kreulich, C., Reutemann, M., Ohrmann P., Baez, E., et al. (2005). Trauma and grief 2–7 years after termination of pregnancy because of fetal anomalies—A pilot study. *Journal of Psychosomatic Obstetrics & Gynecology, 26*(1), 9–14.

Klass, D., Silverman, P. R., & Nickman, S. L. (1996). *Continuing bonds: New understandings of grief.* Philadephia: Taylor & Francis.

Klaus, M. H., & Kennell, J. H. (1976). *Maternal-infant bonding.* St. Louis, MO: Mosby.

Lang, A., Goulet, C., Aita, M., Giguere, V., Lamarre, H., & Perrreault, E. (2001). Weathering the storm of perinatal bereavement via hardiness. *Death Studies, 25,* 297–512.

Lang, A., Goulet, C., & Amsel, R. (2003). Lang and Goulet Hardiness Scale: Development and testing on bereaved parents following the death of their fetus/infant. *Death Studies, 27,* 851–880.

Lindsey, J. L. (2002). *Evaluation of fetal death.* Retrieved May 13, 2004, from http://www.emedicine.com/med/topic3235.htm#section-bibliography

Liu, S., Joseph, K. S., & Wen, S. W. (2002). Trends in fetal and infant deaths caused by congenital anomalies. *Seminars in Perinatology, 26*(4), 268–276.

Magann, E. F., Chauhan, S. P., Bofill, J. A., Waddell, D., Rust, O. A., & Morrison, J. C. (2002). *Maternal morbidity and mortality associated with intrauterine fetal demise: Five year experience at a tertiary referral hospital.* Paper presented at the 70th annual meeting of the Central Association of Obstetricians and Gynecologists, Maui, HI.

Martin, J. A., Hamilton, B. E., Sutton, P. D., Ventura, S. J., Menacker, F., & Kirmeyer, S. (2003). Births: Final data for 2002. National Vital Statistics Report. *National Center for Health Statistics, 52*(10), 1–14.

Martin, T. L., & Doka, K. J. (2000). *Men don't cry . . . Women do.* Philadelphia: Brunner/Mazel.

Meert, K. L., Thurston, C. S., & Briller, S. H. (2005). The spiritual needs of parents at the time of their child's death in the pediatric intensive care unit and during bereavement: A qualitative study. *Pediatric Critical Care Medicine, 6*(4), 420–427.

Miller, E. D. (2003). Reconceptualizing the role of resiliency in coping and therapy. *Journal of Loss and Trauma. 8,* 239–246.

Moskowitz, J. T., Folkman, S., & Acree, M. (2003). Do positive psychological states shed light on recovery from bereavement? Findings from a 3-year longitudinal study. *Death Studies, 27,* 471–500.

Murray, J. A., Terry, D. J., Vance, J. C., Battistutta, D., & Connolly, Y. (2000). Effects of a program of intervention on parental distress following infant death. *Death Studies, 24*(4), 275–305.

National Center for Health Statistics. (2005). *Preliminary birth data for 2004. Health E-Stats.* Retrieved December 23, 2005, from http://www.cdc.gov/nchs/pressroom/05facts/prelimbirths04.htm

Neimeyer, R. A. (2000). Searching for the meaning of meaning: Grief therapy and the process of reconstruction. *Death Studies, 24,* 541–558.

Neimeyer, R. A. (2005). *Meaning reconstruction & the experience of loss.* Washington, DC: American Psychological Association.

Papp, C., & Papp, Z. (2003). Chorionic villus sampling and amniocentesis: What are the risks in current practice? *Current Opinion in Obstetrics and Gynecology, 15*(2), 159–165.

Parkes, C. M., & Weiss, R. S. (1983). *Recovery from bereavement.* New York: Basic Books.

Pauli, R. M. (2005). *Maceration and the timing of intrauterine death.* Retrieved November 25, 2005, from http://www.wisc.edu/wissp/wisspers/jan95001.htm

Pector, E. A. (2004). Views of bereaved multiple-birth parents on life support decisions, the dying process, and discussions surrounding death. *Journal of Perinatology, 24,* 4–10.

Pector, E. A., & Smith-Levitin, M. (2002). Mourning and psychological issues in multiple birth loss. *Seminars in Neonatology, 7*(3), 247–256.

Regidor, E., Ronda, E., Garcia, A. M., & Dominguez, V. (2004). Paternal exposure to agricultural pesticides and cause specific fetal death. *Occupational & Environmental Medicine, 61*(4), 334–339.

Rock, J. V. (2004). *Comfort levels of obstetric nurses caring for parents who have experienced a perinatal loss/stillborn infant* (dissertation). Ann Arbor, MI: ProQuest Information and Learning.

Rothman, J. C. (1999). *The bereaved parents' survival guide.* New York: Continuum.

Schneider, J. M. (1994). *Finding my way: Healing and transformation through loss and grief.* Colfax, WI: Seasons Press.

Schwiebert, P., & Kirk, P. (1985). *When hello means goodbye.* Eugene, OR: Health Sciences University.

Shaver, P., & Tancredy, C. (2001). Emotion, attachment, and bereavement: A conceptual commentary. In M. S. Stroebe, R. O. Hansson, W. Stroebe, & H. Schut (Eds.), *Handbook of bereavement research: Consequences, coping and care* (pp. 63–88). Washington DC: American Psychological Association.

Shields, K. (2005). *Preparing the family for the birth and death.* Lakewood Ranch, FL: Healing Through Hope.

Skeie, A., Froen, J. F., Vege, A., & Stray-Pedersen, B. (2003). Cause and risk of stillbirth in twin pregnancies: A retrospective audit. *Acta Obstetricia et Gynecologica Scandinavica, 82*(11), 1010–1016.

Stroebe, M., & Schut, H. (1999). The dual process model of coping with bereavement: Rationale and description. *Death Studies, 23,* 197–224.

Swanson, K. M. (1991). Empirical development of a middle range theory of caring. *Nursing Research, 40*(3), 161–166.

Swanson, K. M., Karmali, Z. A., Powell, S. H., & Pulvermakher, F. (2003). Miscarriage effects on couples' interpersonal and sexual relationships during the first year after loss: Women's perceptions. *Psychosomatic Medicine, 65,* 902–910.

Swanson-Kaufman, K. (1986). Caring in the instance of unexpected early pregnancy loss. *Topics in Clinical Nursing, 8*(2), 37–46.

Swensen, C. H., Fuller, S., & Clements, R. (1993). Stages of religious faith and reactions to terminal cancer. *Journal of Psychology and Theology, 23*(4), 261–265.

Talbot, K. (2002). *What forever means after the death of a child.* London: Brunner-Routledge.

Traylor, E. S., Hayslip, B., Kaminski, P. L., & York, C. (2003). Relationships between grief and family system characteristics: A cross lagged longitudinal analysis. *Death Studies, 27,* 575–601.

Trulsson, O., & Rädestad, I. (2004). The silent child—Mothers' experiences before, during, and after stillbirth. *Birth, 31*(3), 189–195.

Uren, T. H., & Wastell, C. A. (2002). Attachment and meaning-making in perinatal bereavement. *Death Studies, 26,* 279–308.

Weiss, R. (2001). Grief, bonds, and relationships. In M. S. Stroebe, R. O. Hansson, W. Stroebe, & H. Schut (Eds.), *Handbook of bereavement research: Consequences, coping and care* (pp. 47–62). Washington DC: American Psychological Association.

Wheeler, I. (2001). Parental bereavement: The crisis of meaning. *Death Studies, 25,* 51–66.

Wheeler, S. R. (1997). Adolescent pregnancy loss. In J. R. Woods & J. L. Esposito (Eds.), *Loss during pregnancy or in the newborn period: Principles of care with clinical cases and analyses* (pp. 387–410). Pittman, NJ: Jannetti.

Wheeler, S. R., & Austin, J. (2000). The loss response list: A tool for measuring adolescent grief responses. *Death Studies, 24,* 21–34.

Wilkinson, J. M. (2005). *Nursing diagnosis handbook* (8th ed.). Upper Saddle River, NJ: Prentice Hall.

Worden, J. W. (2002). *Grief counseling and grief therapy: A handbook for the mental health practitioner* (3rd ed.). New York: Springer.

CHAPTER
38
The Postpartal Family at Risk

We are surviving. Just. Why don't they give the Croix de Guerre to people who can go without more than 2 hours total daily sleep for 5 weeks? I thought babies ate at 6–10–2–6–10–2—mine does. He also eats at 5–7–9–11 and 4–8–12. I am getting rather used to going around with my breasts hanging out. They are either drying from the last feed or getting ready for the next one. But the love—I never knew, never imagined that I would love him like this. This incredible feeling of boundless, endless love—a wish to protect his innocence from ever being hurt or wounded or scratched. And that awful, horrible, mad feeling in the first week that you'll never be able to keep anything so precious and so vulnerable alive.

~ *The Boston Women's Health Collective,*
The New Our Bodies, Ourselves ~

KEY TERMS

Early (primary) postpartal hemorrhage 1159
Endometritis (metritis) 1166
Late (secondary) postpartal hemorrhage 1159
Mastitis 1173
Pelvic cellulitis (parametritis) 1166
Peritonitis 1166
Postpartum blues (adjustment reaction with depressed mood) 1184
Postpartum depression (postpartum major mood disorder) 1184
Postpartum psychosis 1184
Puerperal infection 1165
Puerperal morbidity 1166
Subinvolution 1163
Thrombophlebitis 1176
Uterine atony 1159

OBJECTIVES

1. Describe assessment of the woman for predisposing factors, onset, signs, and symptoms of various postpartum complications to facilitate early and effective management of complications.

2. Incorporate preventive measures for various complications of the postpartal period into nursing care of the postpartum woman.

3. List the causes of and appropriate nursing interventions for hemorrhage during the postpartal period.

4. Develop a nursing care plan that reflects knowledge of etiology, pathophysiology, and current clinical management for the woman experiencing postpartal hemorrhage, reproductive tract infection, urinary tract infection, mastitis, thromboembolic disease, or a postpartal psychiatric disorder.

5. Evaluate the mother's knowledge of self-care measures, signs of complications to be reported to the primary care provider, and measures to prevent recurrence of complications.

6. Identify ways to provide continuity of nursing care for women with postpartum complications in the community setting.

MEDIALINK

Additional resources for this content can be found on the Prentice Hall Nursing MediaLink DVD-ROM and on the Companion Website at http://www.prenhall.com/davidson. Click on "Chapter 38" to select the activities for this chapter.

The postpartal period is typically envisioned as a smooth, uneventful time, somewhat anticlimactic, that follows the anticipation of pregnancy and the excitement and work of labor and birth—and often it is, despite the challenges of new parenthood and integration of a new person into the family. Short maternity hospitalization—1.5 days after vaginal childbirth and 2.5 days following cesarean childbirth—may wrongly reinforce the notion that the postpartum recovery is speedy and uncomplicated. Early postpartum discharge challenges the nurse to impart anticipatory information about normal postpartum recovery.

However, it is equally important for the nurse to be aware of physical or emotional complications that may develop postpartally, and to teach the family the signs of such complications; findings to report to the physician or certified nurse-midwife (CNM); and preventive measures, if available. Written instructions to supplement any discussion will be of great value in the early weeks at home with a newborn, when life can be chaotic and verbal instructions may be forgotten. The family should have telephone numbers for postpartum follow-up services and other resources for getting answers to questions. By communicating an attitude of willingness to answer questions and listen to concerns, the nurse enhances the family's comfort in making calls later for what they might otherwise perceive as "too trivial to bother someone about."

When a telephone follow-up or an examination at the home visit provides evidence of a developing complication, the nurse shares these findings or impressions with the woman, and they mutually plan an appropriate next step. In the case of telephone follow-up, the nurse usually counsels the woman to notify her physician or CNM, being prepared to schedule an appointment immediately if risk assessment indicates. The nurse who identifies a complication at the home visit will need to communicate the clinical findings to the physician or CNM and document them and any interventions for the permanent record. Complications, by their very nature, suggest the need for immediate collaborative management and are by their nature inherently stressful. Postpartum complications sometime necessitate readmission of the postpartum client to the hospital, thereby disrupting the family and adding concerns not only about her health but the way in which infant care will be managed. The most common complications of the postpartal period are hemorrhage, infection, thromboembolic disease, and postpartum psychiatric disorders. These are the focus of this chapter.

CARE OF THE WOMAN WITH POSTPARTAL HEMORRHAGE

Hemorrhage in the postpartum period is described as either early (immediate or primary) or late (delayed or secondary) postpartal hemorrhage. **Early (primary) postpartal hemorrhage** occurs in the first 24 hours after childbirth. **Late (secondary) postpartal hemorrhage** occurs from 24 hours to 6 weeks after birth. Postpartal hemorrhage continues to be a cause of significant maternal mortality and morbidity and accounts for 10.5% of maternal deaths attributable to pregnancy-related hemorrhage in the United States (Rebarker & Roman, 2003).

The traditional definition of postpartal hemorrhage has been a blood loss of greater than 500 mL following childbirth. This definition is being questioned, because careful quantification indicates that the average blood loss in a vaginal birth is actually greater than 500 mL, and the average blood loss after cesarean childbirth exceeds 1000 mL (Poole & White, 2005). Clinical estimates of blood loss tend to underestimate actual loss by up to 50%. Some clinicians believe that postpartal hemorrhage can be objectively and reliably defined as a decrease in the hematocrit of 10% between the time of admission and the time postbirth. Clinical estimation of blood loss at childbirth may be difficult because blood mixes with amniotic fluid and is obscured as it oozes onto sterile drapes or is sponged away; without vigilance, it may be difficult over the next hours to appreciate the significance of slow, steady blood loss. As the amount of blood loss increases, as in the case of hemorrhage, estimates are likely to be even less accurate. Moreover, postpartal hemorrhage may occur intra-abdominally, into the broad ligament, or into hematomas arising from genital tract trauma, wherein the blood loss is concealed. Given the increased blood volume of pregnancy, the clinical signs of hemorrhage—such as decreased blood pressure (BP), increasing pulse, widening pulse pressure (BP), thirst, restlessness, and decreasing urinary output—do not appear until as much as 1800 to 2100 mL has been lost, shortly before the woman becomes hemodynamically unstable (Gilbert & Harmon, 2003).

CLINICAL TIP

Women who are natural redheads tend to experience heavier bleeding after childbirth. Consequently, they should be assessed frequently for signs of postpartum hemorrhage and hypovolemia.

Early (Primary) Postpartal Hemorrhage

At term, blood volume and cardiac output have increased so that 20% of cardiac output, or 600 mL per minute, perfuses the pregnant uterus, supporting the developing fetus. When the placenta separates from the uterine wall, the many uterine vessels that have carried blood to and from the placenta are severed abruptly. The normal mechanism for hemostasis after expulsion of the placenta is contraction of the interlacing uterine muscles to occlude the open sinuses that previously brought blood into the placenta. Absence of prompt and sustained uterine contraction (uterine atony) can cause significant blood loss. Other causes of postpartal hemorrhage include laceration of the genital tract; episiotomy; retained placental fragments; vulvar, vaginal, or subperitoneal hematomas; uterine inversion; uterine rupture; problems of placental implantation; and coagulation disorders.

UTERINE ATONY

Uterine atony (relaxation of the uterus) is a common cause of early postpartum hemorrhage (Cunningham, Gant, Leveno et al., 2005). As many as 1 in every 20 new mothers will experience some degree of uterine atony. Although uterine atony can occur after any childbirth, its contributing factors include the following:

- Overdistention of the uterus due to multiple gestation, polyhydramnios, or a large infant (macrosomia)

- Dysfunctional or prolonged labor, which indicates that the uterus is contracting abnormally
- Oxytocin augmentation or induction of labor
- Grandmultiparity, because stretched uterine musculature contracts less vigorously
- Use of anesthesia (especially halothane) or other drugs such as magnesium sulfate, calcium channel blockers such as nifedipine, or tocolytics like terbutaline (Brethine), any of which cause the uterus to relax
- Prolonged third stage of labor—more than 30 minutes
- Preeclampsia
- Asian or Hispanic heritage
- Operative birth (includes vacuum extraction or forceps-assisted births)
- Retained placental fragments
- Placenta previa

Hemorrhage from uterine atony may be slow and steady or sudden and massive. The blood may escape vaginally or collect in the uterus, evident as large clots. The uterine cavity may distend with up to 1000 mL or more of blood, while the perineal pad and linen protectors remain suspiciously dry. A treacherous feature of postpartal hemorrhage is that maternal vital signs may not change until significant blood loss has occurred because of the increased blood volume associated with pregnancy. The woman with preeclampsia is an exception to this finding because she does not have the normal hypervolemia of pregnancy and cannot tolerate even normal postchildbirth blood loss (Cunningham et al., 2005).

Ideally, postpartal hemorrhage is prevented, beginning with adequate prenatal care, good nutrition, avoidance of traumatic procedures, risk assessment, early recognition, and management of complications as they arise. Any woman at risk should be typed and cross-matched for blood and have intravenous (IV) lines in place with needles suitable for blood transfusion (18-gauge minimum). Excellent labor management and childbirth techniques are imperative.

After expulsion of the placenta, the fundus is palpated to ensure that it is firmly contracted. If it is not firm, fundal massage is performed until the uterus contracts. Fundal massage is painful for the woman who has not received regional anesthesia; she will need explanations for why this uncomfortable procedure is necessary and support as massage is initiated. If bleeding is excessive, the clinician will likely order IV oxytocin at a rapid infusion rate and may elect to do a bimanual massage (Figure 38–1 ◆). Table 38–1 summarizes critical nursing information about the use of uterine stimulants. The need for IV fluid replacement and transfusion is determined on the basis of hemoglobin and hematocrit results and coagulation studies.

Conservative management includes uterine stimulants to contract the atonic musculature. Oxytocin, ergotamine, and prostaglandin are most often used. Misoprostol, best known to the obstetric community for its use in labor induction and medical abortion, is being used to prevent and treat uterine atony after failed attempts to control bleeding with oxytocics. Misoprostol used rectally is absorbed quickly and causes uterine con-

A

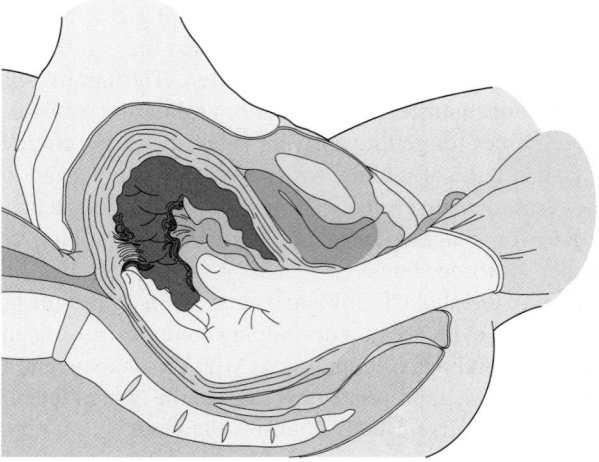

B

Figure 38–1 ◆ *A,* Manual compression of the uterus and massage with the abdominal hand usually will effectively control hemorrhage from uterine atony. *B,* Manual removal of placenta. The fingers are alternately abducted, adducted, and advanced until the placenta is completely detached. Both procedures are performed only by the medical clinician.
SOURCE: Adapted from Cunningham, F. G., MacDonald, P. C., & Gant, N. F. (eds.). (1989). *Williams obstetrics* (18th ed., pp. 417–418). Norwalk, CT: Appleton & Lange.

traction within minutes (Rebarker & Roman, 2003). When conservative measures do not successfully control bleeding, surgical intervention is required. In order of increasing invasiveness, surgical procedures include uterine balloon tamponade, selective radiographic-guided pelvic arterial embolization, uterine suturing techniques, ligation of the uterine or hypogastric arteries, and, as last resort, hysterectomy, which clearly ends childbearing (Ornan, White, Pollak et al., 2003).

Uterine packing, common in the past in cases of postpartum hemorrhage, has been used less often out of concerns of concealed hemorrhage and uterine overdistention that might actually increase bleeding. Instead, physicians in many clinical settings are resorting to uterine balloon tamponade, using large Foley catheters or Sengstaken-Blakemore tubes to control bleeding. Both these tubes have open tops, which permit any continuous drainage from the uterus to be visualized even as pressure tamponade is effectively controlling bleeding.

Table 38–1   UTERINE STIMULANTS USED TO PREVENT AND MANAGE UTERINE ATONY

Drug	Dosing Information	Contraindications	Expected Effects	Side Effects
Oxytocin (Pitocin, Syntocinon)	IV use: 10–40 units in 500–1000 mL crystalloid fluid at 50 milliunits/min administration rate. Onset: immediate. Duration: 1 h. **IV bolus administration not recommended.** IM use: 10–20 units. Onset: 3–5 min. Duration: 2–3 h.	None for use in postpartum hemorrhage.	Rhythmic uterine contractions that help to prevent or reverse postpartal hemorrhage caused by uterine atony.	Uterine hyperstimulation, mild transient hypertension, water intoxication rare in postpartum use.
Methylergonovine maleate (Methergine)	IM use: 0.2 mg every 2–4 h. Onset: 2–5 min. Duration: 3 h (for 5 dose maximum). PO use: 0.2 mg every 6–12 h. Onset: 7–15 min. Duration: 3 h (for 1 week). **IV administration not recommended.**	Women with labile or high blood pressure or known sensitivity to drug, cardiac disease.	Sustained uterine contractions that help to prevent or reverse postpartal hemorrhage caused by uterine atony; management of postpartal subinvolution.	Hypertension, dizziness, headache, flushing/hot flashes, tinnitus, nausea and vomiting, palpitations, chest pain. Overdose or hypersensitivity is recognized by seizures; tingling and numbness of fingers and toes from vasoconstrictive effect, leading rarely to gangrene; hypertension; weak pulse; chest pain.
Ergonovine maleate (Ergotrate Maleate)	IM use: 0.2 mg every 2–4 h. Onset 7 min. Duration: 3 h (5 dose maximum). PO use: 0.2 mg every 6–12 h. Onset: 15 min. Duration: 3 h (for 2–7 days). **IV administration not recommended.**	Women with labile or high blood pressure or known sensitivity to drug.	Sustained uterine contractions that help to prevent or reverse postpartal hemorrhage caused by uterine atony; management of postpartal subinvolution.	Hypertension, dizziness, headache, nausea and vomiting, chest pain. Hypersensitivity is noted by systemic vasoconstrictive effects: seizure, chest pain, and tingling and numbness of fingers and toes that leads rarely to gangrene.
Prostaglandin (PGF$_{2a}$, Hemabate, Prostin/15M)	IM use: 0.25 mg repeated up to maximum 5 doses; may be repeated every 15–90 min, up to 8 doses. Physician may elect to administer by direct intramyometrial injection.	Women with active cardiovascular, renal, liver disease, or asthma or with known hypersensitivity to drug.	Control of refractory cases of postpartal hemorrhage caused by uterine atony; generally used after failed attempts at control of hemorrhage with oxytocic agents.	Nausea, vomiting, diarrhea, headache, flushing, bradycardia, bronchospasm, wheezing, cough, chills, fever.

Implications for Nursing Management of the Postpartal Woman Receiving Uterine Stimulants

- Assess fundus for evidence of contraction and amount of uterine bleeding at least every 10–15 min for 1–2 h after administration, then every 30–60 min until stable. **More frequent assessments are determined by the woman's condition or by orders of the physician or certified nurse-midwife.**
- Weigh pads for objective estimate of blood loss.
- Monitor blood pressure and pulse every 15 min for at least 1 h after administration, then every 30–60 min until stable.
- Note expected duration of action of drug being administered, and take care to recheck fundus at that time for adequate tone.
- When the drug is ineffective, the fundus remains atonic (boggy or uncontracted), and bleeding continues, massage the fundus. If massage fails to cause sustained contraction, notify the physician or certified nurse-midwife immediately.
- Monitor woman for signs of known side effects of the drug; report to physician or certified nurse-midwife if side effects occur.

- Remind the woman and her support person that uterine cramping is an expected result of these drugs and that medication is available for discomfort. Administer analgesic medications as needed for pain relief. Provide nonpharmacologic comfort measures. If analgesic medication ordered is insufficient for pain relief, notify the physician or certified nurse-midwife.

When Prostaglandin Is Used
- Check temperature every 1–2 h and/or after chill. Administer antipyretic medication as ordered for prostaglandin-induced fever.
- Auscultate breath sounds frequently for signs of adverse respiratory effects.
- Assess for nausea, vomiting, and diarrhea. Administer antiemetic and antidiarrheal medications as ordered. (In some settings, women are premedicated with these drugs.)

LACERATIONS OF THE GENITAL TRACT

Early postpartum hemorrhage also may be associated with lacerations of the perineum, vagina, or cervix. Several factors predispose women to higher risk of reproductive tract lacerations:

- Nulliparity
- Epidural anesthesia
- Precipitous childbirth (less than 3 hours)

- Macrosomia
- Forceps- or vacuum-assisted birth
- Use of oxytocin

Thorough inspection of the genital tract by the birth attendant allows recognition and timely repair of most lacerations. Genital tract lacerations should be suspected when vaginal bleeding persists in the presence of a firmly contracted uterus.

The nurse who suspects a laceration should notify the clinician so that the laceration can be immediately sutured to control hemorrhage and repair the integrity of the reproductive tract.

Episiotomies can be a source of postpartal blood loss. Episiotomy is an underappreciated source because of slow, steady bleeding. The risk for bleeding is increased with mediolateral episiotomies.

Nurses who care for postpartum clients are wise to appreciate that most morbidity and mortality from postpartum hemorrhage are not only due to catastrophic bleeding episodes but may also occur from delayed recognition and ineffective management of slow, steady blood loss.

RETAINED PLACENTAL FRAGMENTS

Retained placental fragments may be a cause of early postpartal hemorrhage and are also the most common cause of late hemorrhage. Retention of fragments is usually attributable to partial separation of the placenta during massage of the fundus before spontaneous placental separation, so this practice should be avoided.

Following birth, the placenta should always be inspected for intactness and evidence of missing fragments or cotyledons on the maternal side and for vessels that traverse to the edge of the placenta outward along the membranes of the fetal side. The latter finding may indicate succenturiate placenta and a retained lobe. Uterine exploration by the physician may be required at that time to remove missing fragments (see Figure 38–1B ◆). This cause should be immediately suspected if bleeding persists and no lacerations are noted. Sonography may be used to diagnose retained placental fragments. Curettage, formerly a standard treatment, is now thought by some to traumatize the implantation site, thereby increasing bleeding and the potential for uterine adhesions. It may be necessitated by the degree of hemorrhage, however (Cunningham et al., 2005).

VULVAR, VAGINAL, AND PELVIC HEMATOMAS

Hematomas occur as a result of injury to a blood vessel from birth trauma, often without noticeable trauma to the superficial tissue, or from inadequate hemostasis at the site of repair of an incision or laceration. The soft tissue in the area offers little resistance, and hematomas containing 250 to 500 mL of blood may develop rapidly. Hematomas may be vulvar (involving branches of the pudendal artery), vaginal (especially in the area of the ischial spines), vulvovaginal, or subperitoneal. The latter are rare but most dangerous because of the large amount of blood loss that can occur without clinical symptoms until the woman becomes hemodynamically unstable. Subperitoneal hematomas involve the uterine artery branches or vessels in the broad ligaments.

Risk factors for hematomas include the following: preeclampsia, use of pudendal anesthesia, first full-term birth, precipitous labor, prolonged second stage of labor, macrosomia, forceps- or vacuum-assisted births, and history of vulvar varicosities. Frequent assessment of the perineum of the woman under the effects of regional anesthesia is important. Once the effects of anesthesia have subsided, vaginal and vulvar hematomas are generally associated with perineal pain, often intense and sometimes disproportionate to the objective findings observed.

If the hematoma is localized in the posterior vaginal area, rectal pressure may also be a presenting complaint. Hematomas that develop in the upper vagina may cause difficulty voiding because of pressure against the urinary meatus or urethra. Rather than automatically attributing complaints of perineal pain to the presence of an episiotomy, the nurse should examine the perineal area for signs of hematomas: ecchymosis, edema, tenseness of tissue overlying the hematoma, a fluctuant mass bulging at the introitus, and extreme tenderness to palpation. Estimating the size on first assessment of the perineum enables the nurse to better identify increases in size and the potential blood loss. The nurse notifies the physician or CNM if a hematoma is suspected.

Hematomas less than 5 cm in size and nonexpanding are managed expectantly with ice packs and analgesia. They usually resolve over several days. For larger hematomas and those that expand, surgical management is usually required: the hematoma is evacuated, the bleeding vessel ligated, and the wound closed, with or without vaginal packing. An indwelling urinary catheter may be necessary because voiding may be impossible if packing is placed.

The initial sign of subperitoneal hematoma may be hypovolemic shock; however, the woman may also complain of severe pelvic pain, flank pain, or abdominal distention. A parametrial mass may be identified on bimanual examination. Expectant management with serial ultrasonography and hematocrit may be possible. In rare cases, angiographic embolization or ligation of the hypogastric vessels may be required to manage the hemorrhage associated with postpartal hematomas.

The hematoma site is an ideal medium for proliferation of flora normally present in the genital tract. Consequently, broad-spectrum antibiotics are usually ordered to prevent infection or abscess.

The nurse can decrease the risk of vulvar or vaginal hematoma by applying an ice pack to the woman's perineum during the first hour after birth and intermittently thereafter for the next 8 to 12 hours. If a small hematoma develops despite preventive measures, a sitz bath after the first 12 hours will aid fluid absorption once bleeding has stopped and will promote comfort, as will the judicious use of analgesic agents.

UTERINE INVERSION

Uterine inversion, a prolapse of the uterine fundus to or through the cervix so that the uterus is, in effect, turned inside out after birth, is a rare (the incidence is 1 in 2000 or more) but life-threatening cause of postpartal hemorrhage (Shevell & Malone, 2003). Although not always preventable, uterine inversion is often associated with these factors: fundal implantation or abnormal adherence of the placenta, weakness of the uterine musculature or other uterine abnormalities, protracted labor, uterine relaxation secondary to anesthesia or drugs such as magnesium sulfate, and excess traction on the umbilical cord or vigorous manual removal of the placenta. Most cases of uterine inversion are managed by immediate repositioning of the uterus within the pelvis by the physician.

UTERINE RUPTURE

Spontaneous rupture of the uterus is rare in the United States but continues to be seen in developing countries where emergency surgery for obstructed labors may be less immediately accessible. The woman with a ruptured uterus will have acute, severe abdominal pain, with minimal to diffuse external bleeding. Concealed hemorrhage may occur in the abdominal cavity or broad ligaments, undetected until the woman becomes symptomatic from hypovolemic shock. Risk factors for uterine rupture include prior uterine surgery, including cesarean birth; fetal malpresentation; grandmultiparity; operative vaginal birth; and oxytocic induction of labor. With uterine rupture, immediate surgery is required with fluid and blood replacement as needed.

ABNORMAL PLACENTAL IMPLANTATION

Normally, a layer of decidual tissue separates the proliferating placental villi from the myometrium at the site of placental implantation. A defect in the formation of this decidual layer, possibly related to a poor blood supply, can contribute to a placenta that directly adheres to the myometrium (placenta accreta) or penetrates deeply into the myometrium (placenta increta). See Chapter 27. ∞ Abnormally adherent placentas are rare in normal pregnancies but occur in 5% of women with placenta previa, especially those with cesarean births. Placenta accreta accounts for the majority of retained placental fragments. Even if successfully removed, uncontrollable hemorrhage is possible and requires immediate intervention.

COAGULATION DISORDERS (COAGULOPATHIES)

Coagulopathies should be suspected when postpartal bleeding persists with no identifiable cause. Preexisting coagulation defects, such as von Willebrand disease and idiopathic thrombocytopenic purpura, should have been identified prenatally and managed in consultation with a hematologist. A consumptive coagulopathy such as disseminated intravascular coagulation (DIC) may occur during pregnancy as a result of preeclampsia, amniotic fluid embolism, sepsis, abruptio placentae, or prolonged intrauterine fetal demise syndrome. Coagulopathy can also result from excessive blood loss (Poole & White, 2005). Oozing from a puncture site or development of petechiae may be initial clues of coagulopathy. Coagulation studies (prothrombin time, partial thromboplastin time, platelet count, fibrinogen level, and fibrin split products) should be assessed immediately (Poole & White, 2005).

Late (Secondary) Postpartal Hemorrhage

Although early postpartal hemorrhage most often occurs within hours of birth, delayed hemorrhage occurs most often within 1 to 2 weeks after childbirth, most frequently as a result of subinvolution of the placental site or retention of placental tissue. Blood loss at this time may be excessive but rarely poses the same risk as that from immediate postpartal hemorrhage. Late postpartum hemorrhage is much less common but can be extremely stressful for the woman and her family who are at home by this time.

The site of placental implantation is always the last area of the uterus to regenerate after childbirth. In the case of subinvolution, adjacent endometrium and the decidua basalis fail to regenerate to cover the placental site. Deficiency of immunologic factors has been implicated as a cause. Faulty implantation in the less vascular lower uterine segment, retention of placental tissue, or infection may contribute to subinvolution. With **subinvolution,** the postpartum fundal height is greater than expected. In addition, lochia often fails to progress from rubra to serosa to alba normally. Lochia rubra that persists longer than 2 weeks postpartum is highly suggestive of subinvolution (Cunningham et al., 2005). Some women report scant brown lochia or irregular heavy bleeding. Leukorrhea, backache, and foul-smelling lochia may occur, if infection is a cause. There may be a history of heavy early postpartal bleeding or difficulty in expulsion of the placenta.

When portions of the placenta have been retained in the uterus, bleeding continues because normal uterine contraction that constricts the bleeding site is prohibited. Presence of placental tissue within the uterus can be confirmed by pelvic ultrasonography. Occasionally the placental fragment becomes necrotic over time and, when it separates from the uterus, hemorrhage occurs suddenly.

Subinvolution is most commonly diagnosed during the routine postpartal examination at 4 to 6 weeks. The woman may relate a history of irregular or excessive bleeding or describe the symptoms listed previously. An enlarged, softer-than-normal uterus, palpated bimanually, is an objective indication of subinvolution. Treatment includes oral administration of methylergonovine maleate (Methergine) 0.2 mg orally every 3 to 4 hours for 24 to 48 hours (see Drug Guide: Methylergonovine Maleate Methergine in Chapter 35 ∞). When uterine infection is present, antibiotics are also administered. The woman is reevaluated in 2 weeks. If retained placenta is suspected or other treatment is ineffective, curettage may be indicated (Cunningham et al., 2005).

NURSING CARE MANAGEMENT
Nursing Assessment and Diagnosis

Careful and ongoing assessment of the woman during labor and birth and evaluation of her prenatal history will help identify factors that put her at risk for postpartal hemorrhage. Following birth, periodic assessment for evidence of bleeding is a major nursing responsibility. Regular and frequent assessment of fundal height and evidence of uterine tone or contractility will alert the nurse to the possible development or recurrence of hemorrhage. Careful observation and documentation of vaginal bleeding are important to determine whether further medical intervention is needed. This assessment can be done visually, by pad counts, or by weighing the perineal pads. In cases of excess bleeding, nurses should be alert for signs of impending hypovolemic shock and the development of coagulation problems, such as DIC.

MediaLink   Case Plan Activity: Postpartal Perineal Pain

Nursing diagnoses that may apply when a woman experiences postpartal hemorrhage include the following:

- *Health-Seeking Behaviors* related to lack of information about signs of delayed postpartal hemorrhage
- *Fluid Volume Deficit* related to blood loss secondary to uterine atony, lacerations, hematomas, coagulation disorders, or retained placental fragments

Nursing Plan and Implementation

Clearly, postpartum hemorrhage can be life threatening and requires immediate management. Nonfatal hemorrhage can result in significant morbidity when blood loss is considerable: hypovolemic shock, DIC, renal failure, hepatic failure, and adult respiratory distress syndrome (Ornan et al., 2003). Nurses should be vigilant for these problems and intervene immediately, seeking physician consultation, as needed.

If the nurse detects a soft, boggy uterus, it is massaged until firm. If the uterus is not contracting well and appears larger than anticipated, the nurse may express clots during fundal massage. Once clots are removed, the uterus tends to contract more effectively.

If the woman seems to have a slow, steady, free flow of blood, the nurse begins weighing the perineal pads (1 mL = 1 g) and monitors the woman's vital signs at least every 15 minutes—more frequently if indicated. If the fundus is displaced upward or to one side because of a full bladder, the nurse encourages the woman to empty her bladder—or catheterizes her if she is unable to void—to allow for efficient uterine contractions.

When there are risk factors for postpartal hemorrhage or frequent fundal massage has been necessary to sustain uterine contractions, the nurse should maintain the vascular access (IV) initiated during labor in case additional fluid or blood becomes necessary. Sometimes physicians and CNMs write orders that specify "discontinue IV after present bottle." The astute postpartum nurse will assess the consistency of the fundus and the presence of normal versus excessive lochia before discontinuing the infusion. If the assessments are not reassuring, the nurse continues the IV and notifies the physician or CNM.

CLINICAL TIP

As you know, bogginess indicates that the uterus is not contracting well, which results in increased uterine bleeding. This blood may remain in the uterus and form clots or may result in increased flow. In assessing the amount of blood loss, you must first massage the uterus until it is firm and then express clots. Do not be misled by the fact that a woman has a firm uterus. Significant bleeding can occur from causes other than uterine atony. To accurately determine the amount of blood loss, it is not sufficient to assess only the peri-pad. You should also ask the woman to turn on her side so you can assess underneath her for pooling of blood.

In most settings, postpartum collection of blood for hemoglobin and hematocrit determination is routine. The nurse reviews these findings when available, compares them to the admission baseline, and notifies the physician or CNM if the hematocrit has decreased by 10 percentage points or more. In cases where there is risk of postpartal hemorrhage and blood has

been cross-matched earlier, the nurse checks that blood is available in the blood bank.

The nurse evaluates the woman for signs of anemia, such as fatigue, pallor, headache, thirst, and orthostatic changes in pulse or BP, and reviews the results of all hematocrit determinations. All medical interventions, IV infusions, blood transfusions, oxygen therapy, and medications such as uterine stimulants are monitored as necessary and evaluated for effectiveness. Urinary output should be monitored to determine adequacy of fluid replacement and renal perfusion, with amounts less than 30 mL per hour reported to the physician. The nurse also helps the woman plan activities so that adequate rest is possible.

The woman who is experiencing anemia and fatigue related to hemorrhage may need assistance with self-care and progressive ambulation for several days. When she is able to be out of bed to shower, use of a shower chair permits independence while providing a measure of safety should the woman experience weakness or dizziness. The emergency call light should be easily accessible.

The mother may find it difficult to care for her baby because of the fatigue associated with blood loss. The nurse can often find ways to promote attachment while still recognizing the health needs of the mother. The mother may require additional assistance in caring for her infant. If she has IV lines in place, even carrying the newborn may be awkward. For the mother who feels compelled to do as much as possible, the nurse may also need to "give permission" to the mother to return her infant to the nursery so she can have adequate periods of uninterrupted rest.

If the father of the child is involved in the birth experience, including him in the plan of care is a productive strategy. He supports the mother's recovery by helping to meet her physical needs while encouraging her to rest. The mother is likely to feel less concern over her limited opportunities for newborn care if she can witness the father's interactions with and care for the newborn. The couple may wish for arrangements to be made for the father to stay in the hospital room, sleeping on a cot and eating with the mother so that limited rooming-in with the newborn is still an option. In that way, even if the mother is too fatigued to care for the infant, she can enjoy the infant's presence and initiate bonding. The extent to which the father becomes involved with the care of the mother and baby must be carefully balanced with his need to be rested for the extra responsibilities he will assume when his partner and newborn child are discharged from the hospital.

TEACHING FOR SELF-CARE

The woman and her family or other support persons should receive clear, preferably written, explanations of the normal postpartal course, including changes in the lochia and fundus and signs of abnormal bleeding. Instructions for the prevention of bleeding should include fundal massage, ways to assess the fundal height and consistency, and inspection of the episiotomy and lacerations, if present. The woman should receive instruction in perineal care. The woman and her family are advised to contact their caregiver if any of the following occur: excessive or bright red bleeding (saturation of more than one pad per hour), a boggy

Table 38–2	SIGNS OF POSTPARTAL HEMORRHAGE

Excessive or bright red bleeding

A boggy fundus that does not respond to massage

Abnormal clots

Any unusual pelvic discomfort or backache

Persistent bleeding in the presence of a firmly contracted uterus

Rise in the level of the fundus of the uterus

Increased pulse or decreased BP

Hematoma formation or bulging/shiny skin in the perineal area

fundus that does not respond to massage, abnormal clots, leukorrhea, high temperature, or any unusual pelvic or rectal discomfort or backache. See Table 38–2. If iron supplementation is ordered, instructions for proper dosage should be provided to enhance absorption and avoid constipation and nausea.

COMMUNITY-BASED NURSING CARE

For most postpartal women, routine discharge instructions include advice such as: "You take care of the baby, and let someone else care for you, the family, and the household." Because of her fatigue and weakened condition, the woman who experienced postpartal hemorrhage may be unable even to care for her newborn unassisted. The caregivers at home need clear, concise explanations of her condition and needs for recovery. For example, all should understand the woman's need to rest and to be given extra time to rest after any necessary activity.

To ensure her safety, the woman should be advised to rise slowly to minimize the likelihood of orthostatic hypotension. Until she regains strength, the mother should be seated when holding the newborn.

The person who assumes responsibility for grocery shopping and meal preparation will need advice about the importance of including foods high in iron in the daily menus. Having the woman indicate her preferences from a list of such foods will promote cooperation with the diet. The nurse also explains the rationale for continuing medications containing iron.

The woman should continue to count perineal pads for several days so she can recognize any recurring problem with excessive blood loss. The debilitated condition and anemia associated with hemorrhage increase the woman's risk of puerperal infection. She and her caregivers should use good handwashing technique and minimize exposure to infection in the home. They should be given a list of signs of infection and should understand the importance of alerting the physician immediately should signs occur.

A sense of emergency often exists in the event of late postpartal hemorrhage. Because it commonly occurs 1 to 2 weeks after birth, the couple is generally at home, involved in the day-to-day activities demanded by their new roles, when the unexpected, excessive bleeding begins. Quick decisions about child care arrangements must often be made so that the mother can return to the hospital. Both mother and father are likely to be alarmed by the excessive bleeding and concerned about her prognosis. There will be additional worries about separation from the newborn, especially when the mother is breastfeeding.

The father may find himself torn between the needs of the mother and those of the newborn. Ideally, arrangements can be made to minimize separation of the family members.

In addition to meeting the woman's physical needs, the nurse will assess the couple for impending crisis by addressing these factors: (1) What is their perception of the current situation? Is the perception realistic? (2) What coping strategies have been helpful in previous difficult circumstances? Are they in use at this time, and are they effective? (3) What degree of support do they have from significant others? Do they have necessary resources? Providing realistic information, offering to call those in their support network, and exploring effective coping strategies can be of immeasurable value as they try to maintain a sense of balance in this difficult situation.

Evaluation

Expected outcomes of nursing care include:

- Signs of postpartal hemorrhage are detected quickly and managed effectively.
- Maternal-infant attachment is maintained successfully.
- The woman is able to identify abnormal changes that might occur following discharge and understands the importance of notifying her caregiver if they develop.

CARE OF THE WOMAN WITH A REPRODUCTIVE TRACT INFECTION OR WOUND INFECTION

Because shortened inpatient stays are the norm in maternity care, women will likely be discharged following childbirth before clinical signs of puerperal infection are evident. Consequently, hospital-based nurses are challenged to analyze the woman's history and clinical course for risk assessment and to recognize the sometimes early subtle signs of infection so that discharge may be delayed as needed. Before discharge, the nurse advises the woman about preventive measures and signs of infection. Community and home care nurses review the prenatal and birth record for continuity of risk assessment, conduct physical assessment for objective findings of infection, collect specimens as ordered for diagnosing infection, and collaborate with the primary caregiver in managing infection.

Puerperal infection is an infection of the reproductive tract associated with childbirth that occurs at any time up to 6 weeks postpartum. The most common postpartal infection is metritis (endometritis), which is limited to the uterus. Indeed, the cause of postpartal fever is presumed to be metritis until proven otherwise. However, infection can spread by way of the lymphatic system and circulatory system to become a progressive disease resulting in parametrial cellulitis and peritonitis. The woman's prognosis is directly related to the stage of the disease at the time of diagnosis, the causative organism, and the state of her health and immune system.

The standard definition of **puerperal morbidity** established in 1919 by the Joint Committee on Maternal Welfare is a temperature of 38C (100.4F) or higher, with the temperature occurring on any 2 of the first 10 days postpartum, exclusive of the first 24 hours, and when taken by mouth by a standard technique at least four times a day. However, serious infections can occur in the first 24 hours or may cause only persistent low-grade temperatures. Therefore, careful assessment of all postpartal women with elevated temperatures is essential.

Routine antibiotic prophylaxis for cesarean childbirth has significantly reduced infection rates. Antibiotic therapy alone has not caused the decrease in overall postpartal morbidity and mortality that is seen today. Aseptic technique, fewer traumatic operative births, a better understanding of labor dystocia, improved surgical intervention, and a population that is generally at less risk from malnutrition and chronic debilitative disease have also contributed to this reduction.

The vagina and cervix of approximately 70% of all healthy pregnant women contain pathogenic bacteria that, alone or in combination, are sufficiently virulent to cause extensive infections. Although the uterus is considered a sterile cavity before rupture of the fetal membranes, bacterial contamination of amniotic fluid with the membranes still intact at term is more common than previously believed and may contribute to premature labor. Following rupture of the membranes and during labor, contamination of the uterine cavity by vaginal or cervical bacteria can easily occur. Other factors must also be present for infection to occur, such as the change to an alkaline pH postpartally that favors growth of aerobes. Uterine infections are relatively uncommon following uncomplicated vaginal births, but they continue to be a major source of morbidity for women who give birth by cesarean.

Postpartal Uterine Infection

Postpartal uterine infection is known variously as metritis, endometritis, endomyometritis, and endoparametritis. Because the infection involves the decidual lining of the uterus, the myometrium, and parametrial tissue, some authorities are proposing the terminology *metritis with parametrial cellulitis* (Cunningham et al., 2005). Risk factors for postpartal uterine infection include the following:

- Cesarean birth is the single most significant risk (20 times greater than in vaginal births) (Gibbs, Sweet, & Duff, 2004)
- Prolonged premature rupture of the amniotic membranes (PPROM)
- Prolonged labor preceding cesarean birth
- Multiple vaginal examinations during labor
- Compromised health status (low socioeconomic status, anemia, obesity, smoking, use of illicit drugs or alcohol, poor nutritional state)
- Use of fetal scalp electrode or intrauterine pressure catheter for internal monitoring during labor
- Obstetric trauma—episiotomy, laceration of perineum, vagina, or cervix

- Chorioamnionitis
- Preexisting bacterial vaginosis or *Chlamydia trachomatis* infection
- Instrument-assisted childbirth—vacuum or forceps
- Manual removal of the placenta
- Lapses in aseptic technique by surgical staff
- Diabetes mellitus (infection is four times more common than in nondiabetic women (Minkoff & Gibbs, 2003)

ENDOMETRITIS (METRITIS)

Endometritis or **metritis,** an inflammation of the endometrium, occurs postpartally in 1% to 3% of women who give birth vaginally and up to 27% of women who give birth by cesarean (Minkoff & Gibbs, 2003). After expulsion of the placenta, the placental site provides an excellent culture medium for bacterial growth. The site in the contracted uterus is a round, dark red, elevated area of 4 cm, with a nodular surface composed of numerous veins, many of which may become occluded because of clot formation. The remaining portion of the decidua is also susceptible to infection because of its thinness (approximately 2 mm) and its large blood supply. The cervix presents a bacterial breeding ground because of multiple small lacerations attending normal labor and spontaneous birth.

Both aerobic and anaerobic organisms cause metritis, which is often polymicrobial (Minkoff & Gibbs, 2003). See Table 38–3 for a list of common causative organisms.

Clinical findings of metritis in the initial 24 to 36 hours postpartum tend to be related to group B streptococcus (GBS). Late-onset postpartal endometritis/metritis is most commonly associated with genital mycoplasmas and *Chlamydia trachomatis*. These microbes have a longer replication time and latency period than other bacteria and are not consistently eradicated by antibiotics used for early postpartal infections.

In mild cases of metritis, the woman generally has vaginal discharge that is bloody, foul smelling, and either scant or profuse. In more severe cases, she also has uterine tenderness; sawtooth temperature spikes, usually between 38.3C (101F) and 40C (104F); tachycardia; and chills. Foul-smelling lochia is cited as a classic sign of endometritis, but in the case of infection with β-hemolytic streptococcus, the lochia may be scant, serosanguineous, and odorless (Gibbs et al., 2004).

PELVIC CELLULITIS (PARAMETRITIS)

Pelvic cellulitis (parametritis) is infection involving the connective tissue of the broad ligament or, in more severe forms, the connective tissue of all the pelvic structures. The infection generally ascends upward in the pelvis by way of the lymphatic vessels in the uterine wall but may also occur if pathogenic organisms invade a cervical laceration that extends upward into the connective tissue of the broad ligament—a direct pathway into the pelvis.

A pelvic abscess may form in postpartal **peritonitis** (infection involving the peritoneal cavity) and is most commonly found in the uterine ligaments, the cul-de-sac of Douglas, and the subdiaphragmatic space. Parametritis may be a secondary result of pelvic thrombophlebitis. This condition occurs when

Table 38–3	COMMON CAUSATIVE ORGANISMS IN METRITIS	
Aerobes	**Anaerobes**	
• Group A, B, D streptococcus	• *Peptostreptococcus*	
• Enterococcus	• *Clostridium* species	
• *Staphylococcus* species	• *Bacteroides* species	
• *Escherichia coli*	• *Chlamydia trachomatis*	
• *Klebsiella pneumoniae*	• Genital *mycoplasma*	
• *Proteus mirabilis*		

the clot, usually in the right ovarian vein, becomes infected, and the wall of the vein breaks down from necrosis, spilling the infection into the connective tissues of the pelvis.

A woman suffering from parametritis may demonstrate a variety of symptoms, including marked high temperature (38.9C to 40C or 102F to 104F), chills, malaise, lethargy, abdominal pain, subinvolution of the uterus, tachycardia, and local and referred rebound tenderness. If peritonitis develops, the woman will be acutely ill with severe pain; marked anxiety; high fever; rapid, shallow respirations; pronounced tachycardia; excessive thirst; abdominal distention; nausea; and vomiting.

Perineal Wound Infections

Given the degree of bacterial contamination that occurs with normal vaginal birth, it is surprising that more women do not have infections of the episiotomy or repaired lacerations of perineum, vagina, or vulva. Good aseptic technique is the likely rationale. When perineal wound infection does occur, it is recognized by the classic signs: redness, warmth, edema, purulent drainage, and, later, gaping of the previously approximated wound. Local pain may be severe. Infected perineal wounds, like other infected wounds, are treated by the draining purulent material. Sutures are removed, and the wound is left open. A regimen of broad-spectrum antibiotics is used. When the surface of the wound is free of infectious exudate and tissue granulation is evident, the mother returns for secondary closure of the wound under regional anesthesia.

Cesarean Wound Infections

The infection rate following cesarean births is 3% to 5%, with the highest rate occurring after emergency cesarean births because there is more traumatization of the tissue (Gibbs et al., 2004). Predisposing factors include obesity, diabetes mellitus, prolonged postpartal hospitalization, PROM, metritis, prolonged labor, anemia, steroid therapy, and immunosuppression (Gibbs et al., 2004). Signs of an abdominal wound infection, which may not be evident until after discharge, include erythema; warmth; skin discoloration; edema; tenderness; purulent drainage, sometimes mixed with serosanguineous fluid; or gaping of the wound edges. Fever, pain, malodorous lochia, and other systemic signs of infection are also common. Abdominal distention and decreased bowel sounds may be noted. Culture of wound drainage commonly reveals mixed pathogens.

Clinical Therapy

The infection site and causative organism are diagnosed by careful history and complete physical examination, blood tests, aerobic and anaerobic endometrial cultures (although this may be of limited value, because multiple organisms are usually present), and urinalysis to rule out urinary tract infection (UTI). When a localized infection develops, it is treated with antibiotics, sitz baths, and analgesics as necessary for pain relief. If an abscess has developed or a stitch site is infected, the suture is removed, and the area is allowed to drain. Packing the wound with saline gauze twice to three times daily, using aseptic technique, allows removal of necrotic debris when packing is removed. Broad-spectrum antibiotic coverage is used to treat postpartal wound infections. Cephalosporins, penicillinase-resistant penicillin, and vancomycin are commonly used with anaerobic coverage by clindamycin or ampicillin/sulbactam (Cunningham et al., 2005; Newton, 2003).

The incidence of metritis has been reduced by prophylactic administration of antibiotics to women undergoing cesarean childbirth. Metritis, once diagnosed, is treated by the administration of antibiotics (Minkoff & Gibbs, 2003). With appropriate antibiotic coverage, improvement should occur within a few days. Antibiotics are generally continued until the woman is afebrile for 24 to 48 hours. The route and dosage are determined by the severity of the infection. Careful monitoring is also necessary to prevent the development of a more serious infection.

Parametritis and peritonitis are treated with IV antibiotics. Broad-spectrum antibiotics effective against the most common causative organisms are chosen initially until the results of culture and sensitivity reports are available. If multiple organisms are present, the approach to antibiotic therapy is continued unless no improvement is observed; then the antibiotic is changed. Antibiotics are generally continued until the woman has been afebrile for 48 hours. Oral antibiotics are rarely needed on discharge.

An abscess is frequently manifested by the development of a palpable mass and may be confirmed with ultrasound. An abscess usually requires incision and drainage to avoid rupture into the peritoneal cavity and the possible development of peritonitis. After drainage of the abscess, the cavity may be packed with iodoform gauze to promote drainage and facilitate healing.

The woman with a severe systemic infection is acutely ill and may require care in an intensive care unit. Supportive therapy includes maintenance of adequate hydration with IV fluids, analgesic medications, ongoing assessment of the infection, and possibly continuous nasogastric suctioning if paralytic ileus develops.

NURSING CARE MANAGEMENT
Nursing Assessment and Diagnosis

The nurse should inspect the woman's perineum every 8 to 12 hours for signs of early infection. The REEDA scale helps the nurse remember to consider *r*edness, *e*dema, *ec*chymosis, discharge, and approximation. Any degree of induration (hardening) should be immediately reported to the clinician.

Fever, malaise, abdominal pain, foul-smelling lochia, larger than expected uterus, tachycardia, and other signs of infection should be noted and reported immediately so that treatment can begin. The white blood cell (WBC) count, a usual objective measure of infection, cannot be used reliably because of the normal increase in WBCs during the postpartum period; a WBC count of 14,000 to 16,000 mm^3 is not an unusual finding. An increase in WBC level of more than 30% in a 6-hour period, however, is indicative of infection.

Nursing diagnoses that may apply to the woman with a puerperal infection include the following:

- *Risk for Injury* related to the spread of infection
- *Pain* related to the presence of infection
- *Deficient Knowledge* related to lack of information about condition and its treatment
- *Risk for Altered Parenting* related to delayed parent-infant attachment secondary to woman's pain and other symptoms of infection

Nursing Plan and Implementation

HOSPITAL-BASED NURSING CARE

Careful attention to aseptic technique during labor, birth, and postpartum is essential.

The nurse caring for a woman during the postpartal period is responsible for teaching the woman self-care measures that are helpful in preventing infection. The woman should understand the importance of good perineal care, hygiene practices to prevent contamination of the perineum (such as wiping from front to back, changing perineal pads after voiding), and thorough handwashing. Once edema and perineal pain are under control, the nurse can also encourage sitz baths, which are cleansing and promote healing. Adequate fluid intake, coupled with a diet high in protein and vitamin C, which are necessary to promote wound healing, also helps prevent infection.

If the woman has a draining wound or purulent lochia, it is especially important that those in contact with soiled items and linens practice good handwashing. Clear, concise instructions about wound care and how to discard soiled dressings appropriately must be provided to safeguard the woman and her caregivers.

If the woman is seriously ill, ongoing assessment of urine specific gravity and intake and output is necessary. The nurse also carefully administers antibiotics as ordered and regulates the IV fluids rate. Ongoing assessment of the woman's condition is vital to detect subtle changes in her health status. The nurse also recognizes the woman's comfort needs related to hygiene, positioning, oral care, and pain relief.

Promoting maternal-infant attachment can be difficult with the acutely ill woman. The nurse may provide pictures of the infant and keep the mother informed of the infant's well-being. Mementos, such as a footprint, a note written by the father "from the baby," or a videotape of the baby can be comforting to the mother during their separation. If she feels up to it, the new mother will also benefit from brief visits with her newborn.

The woman who wishes to breastfeed when her condition allows can maintain lactation by pumping her breasts regularly. Understanding that the opportunity to breastfeed is simply delayed, not eliminated, by the infectious process may improve the woman's morale.

The partner of a seriously ill woman will be concerned about her condition and torn about spending time with her and with their newborn. Because maternal-infant bonding may be compromised, father-newborn bonding can be especially important. See Nursing Care Plan: The Woman with a Puerperal Infection.

COMMUNITY-BASED NURSING CARE

The woman with a puerperal infection needs assistance when she is discharged from the hospital. If the family cannot provide this home assistance, a referral to home care services is needed. Home care services should be contacted as soon as puerperal infection is diagnosed so that the nurse can meet with the woman for a family and home assessment and development of a home care plan.

The family needs instruction in the care of a newborn, including feeding, bathing, cord care, immunizations, and significant observations that should be reported. A well-baby appointment should be scheduled. The woman who wishes to breastfeed when her condition allows can maintain lactation by pumping her breasts regularly. The mother needs to understand that the opportunity to breastfeed is simply delayed, not eliminated, by the infectious process; this may improve the woman's morale. Breastfeeding mothers receiving antibiotics should be instructed to inspect the infant's mouth for signs of thrush and to report the finding to their physician.

The mother should be instructed regarding activity, rest, medications, diet, and signs and symptoms of complications, and she should be scheduled for a return medical visit. She needs to know the importance of taking the entire course of prescribed antibiotics even though she may begin to feel better before the bottle is empty. She also needs to be informed about the importance of pelvic rest; that is, she should not use tampons or douches nor have intercourse until she has been examined by the physician and told it is safe to resume those activities.

Evaluation

Expected outcomes of nursing care include:

- The infection is quickly assessed, and treatment is instituted successfully without further complications.
- The woman understands the nature of the infection and the purpose of therapy; she carries out any ongoing antibiotic therapy necessary after discharge.
- Maternal-infant attachment is maintained.

CARE OF THE WOMAN WITH A URINARY TRACT INFECTION

Urinary tract infection (UTI) is common in the postpartum period. The woman is at increased risk of developing urinary tract problems because of the normal postpartal diuresis, increased

NURSING CARE PLAN

For the Woman with a Puerperal Infection

INTERVENTION	RATIONALE	EXPECTED OUTCOMES
1. Nursing Diagnosis: Risk for Spread of Infection related to traumatized tissues		
Goal: *The woman will be free of complications associated with infection.*		
• Encourage the woman, staff, and family members to adhere to a strict handwashing policy.	• Handwashing kills bacteria and prevents cross-contamination.	• *The woman will be free of complications associated with infection as evidenced by practicing behaviors that prevent the spread of infection and promote timely wound healing.*
• Review the woman's prenatal, intrapartal, and postpartal records for underlying problems that could contribute to poor wound healing or increased risk for spread of infection. Monitor blood pressure, pulse, respiration, and temperature.	• Identifying underlying problems gives the caregiver an opportunity to initiate preventive measures that will promote healthy wound healing and stop the spread of infection. Obtain baseline data; signs and symptoms of septic shock produce a decrease in blood pressure and an increase in respirations. Temperature increase of 38C/100.4F or greater on any 2 days after the first 24 hours indicates infection.	
• Instruct the woman on proper perineal care including: wiping perineum from front to back after voiding, washing the perineum after voiding and defecating, and changing peri-pads frequently, always followed by handwashing.	• Proper perineal care techniques enhance good hygiene and assist in removing urine and fecal contaminants from perineum. Changing peri-pads frequently decreases skin contact with a moist medium that favors bacteria growth.	
• Encourage a well-balanced diet with adequate protein, calories, and vitamin C.	• Protein and vitamin C are essential nutrients for tissue healing and repair.	
• Encourage the woman to consume 2000 mL of fluid a day.	• Maintains hydration and increases circulating volume.	
• Encourage use of the sitz bath, Surgigator, or the perineal light two to four times a day for at least 10–15 minutes.	• Moist or dry heat to the perineum increases localized blood flow, promotes healing, and provides comfort.	
• Encourage early ambulation.	• Enhances circulation and drainage of lochia.	
• Assess and report signs and symptoms of infection in perineum including: erythema, edema, discharge, pain, and approximation of wound edges (REEDA).	• Identifying signs and symptoms of infection early allows for prompt treatment and healing.	
Collaborative: Obtain lab work as ordered by the physician including: culture and sensitivity, complete blood count (CBC) with differential, and WBC count.	• Identifies abnormal lab values for early intervention. In addition, identifies infection and its causative organism for appropriate antibiotic treatment.	

(Continued on next page)

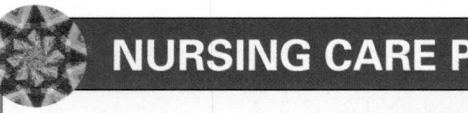

NURSING CARE PLAN

For the Woman with a Puerperal Infection continued

INTERVENTION	RATIONALE	EXPECTED OUTCOMES
• Administer antibiotic therapy as ordered by the physician. • Promote wound drainage by assisting physician in opening the wound if necessary. Also, if the wound is greater than 2–3 cm, pack with iodoform gauze. • Report signs and symptoms of severe infections: foul-smelling lochia, uterine subinvolution, uterine tenderness, severe lower abdominal pain, elevated temperature, elevated WBC count, general malaise, chills, lethargy, tachycardia, nausea and vomiting, and abdominal rigidity.	• Fights infection and helps prevent the spread of further infection. • Iodoform gauze is used to maintain patency of wound opening. This promotes drainage and prevents abscesses from developing. • Reporting signs and symptoms of severe infections early allows for initiation of appropriate therapy by the physician and prevents further spread of the invading pathogen.	

2. Nursing Diagnosis: Pain related to the infection process

Goal: *The woman will be free of pain or have a level of relief that is acceptable.*

• Assess pain location and intensity; have the woman describe on a scale from 1 (mild) to 10 (severe). Assess nonverbal signs of pain, including facial grimacing and agitation. • Teach the woman to request or take analgesic before pain is severe. • Encourage the woman to discuss anxiety and fears. • Encourage frequent rest periods and decrease disturbing environmental stimuli. • Promote relaxation by encouraging diversional activities and the use of exercises including: radio/television, reading, guided imagery, deep breathing techniques, massage, visualization, and meditation. **Collaborative:** Administer analgesics as ordered by the physician, evaluating the response to the analgesic and any adverse effects in a timely manner.	• Assesses the need for pain management and evaluates interventions already implemented. • Allows timing of medication for effective relief. The effects of IV analgesia are almost immediate; the effects of intramuscular (IM) analgesics occur in 20–30 min, while those of oral medications are 30–45 min. • Reduces anxiety/fear and may decrease the woman's perception of pain. • Frequent rest periods will conserve client's energy. Increasing environmental stimuli may increase client's pain perception. • Promotes relaxation and refocuses woman's attention away from the intensity of pain. • Relieves pain and interrupts the pain, fear, tension cycle to facilitate relaxation.	• *Woman is free of pain or has an acceptable level of pain as evidenced by verbalization of pain relief and the exhibition of a relaxed demeanor.*

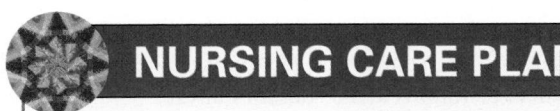

NURSING CARE PLAN

For the Woman with a Puerperal Infection continued

INTERVENTION	RATIONALE	EXPECTED OUTCOMES
3. Nursing Diagnosis: Risk for Altered Parent/Infant Attachment related to pain secondary to maternal infection and/or separation from infant to minimize exposure		
Goal: *Mother will have no problems bonding with infant and assuming responsibility for the care of the infant.*		
• Provide quality time for mother and infant contact.	• Aids in the bonding process.	• *Mother will bond with the infant as evidenced by exhibiting appropriate attachment behaviors when interacting with infant, providing care to self and infant, and verbalization of understanding of the parenting role.*
• Encourage the partner or family members to give the woman videos and pictures of the infant if the mother's condition requires separation from the infant.	• Promotes bonding and gives the mother reassurance that the infant is being cared for.	
• Encourage the partner and family members to become involved with the care of the infant and verbalize interaction to the mother.	• Allows the mother to feel as though she is involved in the care of the infant.	
• Encourage the mother to feed (breast or bottle) infant if her condition is stable. If the mother is unable to breastfeed, encourage and assist her in pumping her breasts to maintain milk production.	• Hands-on participation in the infant's care gives mother a positive outlook.	
• Assess maternal support systems.	• As the mother is recovering, she will need assistance in household organization and personal care.	
Collaborative: Offer referrals to home health services, doula services, and/or support groups.	• Ensures the woman's well-being, and identifies problems that may require intervention	

bladder capacity, decreased bladder sensitivity from stretching or trauma, and possible inhibited neural control of the bladder following the use of general or regional anesthesia and contamination from catheterization. It is important that the mother empty her bladder completely with each voiding.

Overdistention of the Bladder

Overdistention occurs postpartally when the woman is unable to empty her bladder, usually because of trauma or the effects of anesthesia. Women who have not sufficiently recovered from the effects of anesthesia cannot void spontaneously, and catheterization is necessary. After the effects of anesthesia have worn off, if the woman cannot void, postpartal urinary retention is highly indicative of UTI. Other risk factors for urinary retention after childbirth include nulliparity, instrumental delivery, and prolonged labor (Yip, Shota, Pang et al., 2005).

CLINICAL TIP

Postpartum urinary retention is often defined as "the absence of spontaneous urination within 6 hours of a vaginal delivery or within 6 hours after removal of an indwelling catheter post-Cesarean delivery." The astute nurse will watch the woman's bladder for signs of retention—not the clock! As urinary retention promotes uterine atony and a subsequent increase in bleeding and also contributes to the possibility of UTI, timely intervention is crucial.

CLINICAL THERAPY

Overdistention in the early postpartal period is often managed by draining the bladder with a straight catheter as a one-time measure. If the overdistention recurs or is diagnosed later in the postpartal period, an indwelling catheter may be ordered for 24 hours. An alternate urinary retention protocol involves bladder ultrasound scans with intervention based on the amount of urine volume. For example, if the volume is greater than 400 mL, the bladder is drained and the catheter removed, whereas if the volume is 400 mL or less, a spontaneous void is awaited for 1 hour, after which another scan is performed (Yip et al., 2005).

NURSING CARE MANAGEMENT
Nursing Assessment and Diagnosis

The overdistended bladder appears as a large mass, reaching sometimes to the umbilicus and displacing the uterine fundus upward. There is increased vaginal bleeding, the fundus is boggy, and the woman may complain of cramping as the uterus attempts to contract. Some women also experience backache and restlessness. Nursing diagnoses that may apply when a woman has difficulties due to overdistention include the following:

- *Risk for Infection* related to urinary stasis secondary to overdistention
- *Urinary Retention* related to decreased bladder sensitivity and normal postpartal diuresis

Nursing Plan and Implementation

Diligent monitoring of the bladder during the recovery period and preventive health measures greatly reduce the chance for overdistention of the bladder. Encouraging the mother to void spontaneously and helping her use the toilet, if possible, or the bedpan if she has received conductive anesthesia, prevents overdistention in most cases. The nurse assists the woman to a normal position for voiding (i.e., sitting with the legs and feet lower than the trunk) and provides privacy to encourage voiding. The woman should be medicated for whatever pain she may be having before attempting to void because pain may cause a reflex spasm of the urethra. Perineal ice packs applied after birth will minimize any edema, which may interfere with voiding. Pouring warm water over the perineum or having the woman void in a sitz bath may also be effective.

If catheterization becomes necessary, careful, meticulous, aseptic technique should be employed during catheter insertion. The vagina and vulva are traumatized to some degree by vaginal birth, and edema is common. This edema may obscure the urinary meatus; therefore, the nurse needs to be extremely careful in cleansing the vulva and inserting the catheter. It is imperative to discard a catheter that has inadvertently been introduced into the vagina and thus contaminated. Because catheterization is an uncomfortable procedure as a result of the postpartal trauma and edema of the tissue, the nurse should be careful and gentle not only in inserting the catheter but also in handling and cleaning the perineal area.

If the amount of urine drained from the bladder reaches 900 to 1000 mL, the catheter should be clamped and taped firmly to the woman's leg. The nurse should carefully document the procedure, including taking the woman's vital signs before and after the procedure and noting her responses. After an hour, the catheter may be unclamped and placed on gravity drainage. This technique protects the bladder and avoids rapid intra-abdominal

decompression. When the indwelling catheter is removed, a urine specimen is often sent to the laboratory. The tip of the catheter may also be removed and sent for culture.

Evaluation

Expected outcomes of nursing care include:

- The woman voids adequately to meet the demands of the increased fluid shifts during the postpartal period.
- The woman does not develop infection due to stasis of urine.
- The woman actively incorporates self-care measures to decrease bladder overdistention.

Cystitis (Lower Urinary Tract Infection)

Retention of residual urine, bacteria introduced at the time of catheterization, and a bladder traumatized by childbirth combine to provide an excellent environment for the development of cystitis. *Escherichia coli* has been demonstrated to be the causative agent in most cases of postpartal cystitis and pyelonephritis (in both lower and upper UTI). In most cases, the infection ascends the urinary tract from the urethra to the bladder. If cystitis is not treated, the infection can spread to the kidneys (pyelonephritis) because vesiculoureteral reflux forces contaminated urine into the renal pelvis.

CLINICAL THERAPY

When cystitis is suspected, a clean-catch midstream urine sample is obtained for microscopic examination, culture, and sensitivity tests. The specimen may require collection by the nurse with the woman on a bedpan because few postpartal women can collect a true midstream, clean-catch specimen without contaminating the specimen with lochia. A catheterized specimen is avoided when possible because of the increased risk of infection. When the bacterial concentration is greater than 100,000 colonies of the same organism per milliliter of fresh urine, infection is generally present. Counts between 10,000 and 100,000 may also suggest infection, particularly if clinical symptoms are noted.

In the clinical setting, antibiotic therapy is often begun before culture and sensitivity reports are available. Frequently used antibiotics include a preparation of trimethoprim-sulfamethoxazole–double strength (Bactrim DS, Septra DS), one of the short-acting sulfonamides, nitrofurantoin (Macrodantin), or, in the case of sulfa allergy, ampicillin or amoxicillin-clavulanic acid. The antibiotic is changed later if indicated by the results of the sensitivity report (Poggi & Kapernick, 2003). Antispasmodic or urinary analgesic agents, such as phenazopyridine hydrochloride (Pyridium), may be given to relieve discomfort.

Pyelonephritis (Upper Urinary Tract Infection)

Pyelonephritis is an infection of the upper urinary tract. In most cases, the infection has ascended from the lower urinary tract. It occurs more commonly on the right, although both kidneys may be affected. If untreated, the renal cortex may be damaged and kidney function impaired.

CLINICAL THERAPY

When pyelonephritis is diagnosed, IV antibiotic therapy is begun immediately. If sensitivity reports so indicate, the antibiotic can be changed later. Bed rest and careful monitoring of intake and output are necessary to detect the development of bacterial shock. Fluids are encouraged. Antispasmodic, analgesic, and antipyretic medications are given to relieve discomfort. The woman usually continues to take antibiotics for 2 to 4 weeks after clinical and bacteriologic response. A clean-catch urine culture should be obtained 2 weeks after completion of therapy and then periodically for the next 2 years. An IV pyelogram may be ordered in 2 to 4 months to identify any residual renal damage.

Continuation of breastfeeding during therapy is limited only by the degree of the mother's malaise and clinical discomfort. For the breastfeeding mother, the antibiotic should be selected carefully to avoid problems for the infant via the milk.

NURSING CARE MANAGEMENT
Nursing Assessment and Diagnosis

Symptoms of cystitis often appear 2 to 3 days after birth. The initial symptoms of cystitis may include frequency, urgency, dysuria, and nocturia. Hematuria and suprapubic pain may also be present. A slightly elevated temperature may occur, but systemic symptoms are often absent.

When a UTI progresses to pyelonephritis, systemic symptoms usually occur, and the woman becomes acutely ill. Symptoms include chills, high fever, flank pain (unilateral or bilateral), nausea, and vomiting, in addition to all the signs of lower UTI. Costovertebral angle tenderness on palpation and pain also may or may not be present. The nurse obtains a urine culture so that sensitivity tests can identify the causative organism.

Nursing diagnoses that may apply if a woman develops a UTI postpartally include the following:

- *Pain* with voiding related to dysuria secondary to infection
- *Health-Seeking Behaviors* related to need for information about self-care measures to prevent UTI

Nursing Plan and Implementation

Screening for asymptomatic bacteriuria in pregnancy should be routine. Frequent emptying of the bladder during labor and postpartum should be encouraged to prevent overdistention and trauma to the bladder. Catheterization technique and nursing actions to prevent overdistention (previously discussed) also apply. The woman with pyelonephritis must understand the importance of follow-up care after discharge to prevent recurrence or further complications.

TEACHING FOR SELF-CARE

The nurse should advise the postpartal woman to continue good perineal hygiene following discharge, to maintain a good fluid intake (at least 8 to 10 8-oz glasses daily) especially of water,

and to empty her bladder whenever she feels the urge to void, but at least every 2 to 4 hours while awake. Once sexual intercourse is resumed, the new mother should void before (to prevent bladder trauma) and following intercourse (to wash contaminants from the vicinity of the urinary meatus). Wearing cotton-crotch underwear to facilitate air circulation also reduces the risk of UTI.

Acidification of the urine is thought to aid in preventing and managing UTI. The nurse thus advises the woman to avoid carbonated beverages, which increase alkalinity of urine, and to drink cranberry, plum, apricot, and prune juices and take vitamin C, which increase the acidity of urine (Gilbert & Harmon, 2003).

Evaluation

Expected outcomes of nursing care include:

- The woman identifies the signs of UTI and her condition is treated successfully.
- The woman uses self-care measures to prevent the recurrence of UTI as part of her personal hygiene routine.
- The woman continues with any long-term therapy or follow-up.
- Maternal-infant attachment is maintained; the woman is able to care for her newborn effectively.

CARE OF THE WOMAN WITH MASTITIS

Mastitis is a unilateral infection of the breast connective tissue that occurs primarily in lactating women. The incidence of febrile mastitis is 3% to 5% of breastfeeding women (Hager, 2004). The usual causative organisms are *Staphylococcus aureus, Haemophilus parainfluenzae, H. influenzae, E. coli,* and *Streptococcus* species. Infectious mastitis is a more serious infection with fever, chills; headache; flulike muscle aches and malaise; and a warm, reddened, painful area of the breast, often wedge-shaped because of septal distribution of connective tissue (Figure 38–2 ◆). Because symptoms rarely occur before the second to fourth week postpartum, birthing unit nurses often are not fully aware of how uncomfortable and acutely ill the woman may be; they must ensure that all breastfeeding women are taught preventive techniques, ways of recognizing it, and the appropriate response of immediate notification of their physician or CNM.

The infection usually begins when bacteria invade the breast tissue after it has been traumatized in some way (see the factors commonly associated with mastitis in Table 38–4). Milk serves as a favorable medium for the invasive bacteria to multiply; thus, milk stasis is another risk factor (Mass, 2004). The most common source of the causative organism is the infant's nose and throat, although other sources include the hands of the mother or birthing unit personnel and the woman's circulating blood. Infants of women with mastitis generally remain well.

In some cases, *Candida albicans* is the causative organism of mastitis, entering the breast through a small fissure or abrasion on the nipple; the baby will often have thrush, a candidal

Figure 38–2 ◆ Mastitis. Erythema and swelling are present in the upper outer quadrant of the breast. Axillary lymph nodes are often enlarged and tender. The segmental anatomy of the breast accounts for the demarcated, often V-shaped wedge of inflammation.

Table 38–4   FACTORS ASSOCIATED WITH DEVELOPMENT OF MASTITIS

Milk stasis

Failure to change infant position to allow emptying of all lobes
Failure to alternate breasts at feedings
Poor suck
Poor let-down

Actions that promote access/multiplication of bacteria

Poor handwashing technique
Improper breast hygiene
Failure to air-dry breasts after breastfeeding
Use of plastic-lined breast pads that trap moisture against nipple

Breast/nipple trauma

Incorrect positioning for breastfeeding
Poor latch-on
Failure to rotate position on nipple
Incorrect or aggressive pumping technique

Obstruction of ducts

Restrictive clothing
Constricting bra
Underwire bra

Change in number of feedings/failure to empty breasts

Attempted weaning
Missed feeding
Prolonged sleeping, including sleeping through the night
Favoring side of nipple soreness

Lowered maternal defenses

Fatigue
Stress

infection of the mouth. There may be a history of a recent course of antibiotics in the woman. Signs include late-onset nipple pain, followed by shooting pain between feedings, often radiating to the chest wall (Mass, 2004). Eventually, the skin of the affected breast may become pink, flaking, and pruritic. Women may notice a yeasty odor to their milk. Unless the mother and her newborn are treated for *Candida*, recolonization will occur when breastfeeding is resumed. Pacifiers and pump equipment in contact with *Candida* should be boiled for 20 minutes, and clothing in contact with the breast should be laundered in dilute bleach solution (Mass, 2004).

Clinical Therapy

Diagnosis is usually based on history and physical examination, although culture and sensitivity testing of breast milk may be done. Some clinicians question the worth of milk culture because it is not ductal tissue that is infected and recommend antibiotic coverage empirically based on the most common etiologic organisms. If a culture of the breast milk is ordered either for initial diagnosis or with recurrence or failed treatment of mastitis, it is more reliable with a midstream-type collection process. The nipple is washed first; then the first 3 mL of breast milk are manually expressed and discarded, after which the actual specimen is collected. A leukocyte count of 1 million/mL and a bacterial count greater than 10,000/mL are diagnostic (Hager, 2004).

Treatment of mastitis involves bed rest for at least 24 hours; increased fluid intake (at least 2 to 3 L/day); a supportive bra; frequent breastfeeding; local application of warm, moist heat; and analgesics that are compatible with breastfeeding. Nonsteroidal anti-inflammatory agents are recommended to treat both fever and inflammation. Also a course of 7 to 10 days of antibiotics, usually a penicillinase-resistant penicillin or cephalosporin, is appropriate (Betzold, 2005).

Candidal infections can be especially stubborn. Initial treatment generally involves antifungal creams or ointments once or twice daily. Oral Diflucan is excreted in breast milk but is not considered toxic to the infant and can be used if other agents fail. Women should be instructed to cleanse their nipples with warm water and allow air-drying before application of the antifungal medication. For the woman who prefers to avoid medication, an alternative treatment is cleansing of the nipples with a solution of 1 tablespoon of vinegar in 1 cup of water or 1 teaspoon of baking soda in 1 cup of water, followed by air-drying.

Improved outcome, a decreased duration of symptoms, and decreased incidence of a breast abscess result if the breasts continue to be emptied by either breastfeeding or pumping. Thus, continued breastfeeding is recommended in the process of mastitis. The plan of care should include contacting the woman within 24 hours of initiation of treatment to ensure that symptoms are subsiding.

Ten percent of cases will progress to abscess formation if mastitis remains untreated, treatment fails, or the infant is abruptly weaned. Abscess is more common when there is a lag

COMPLEMENTARY AND ALTERNATIVE THERAPIES

PROBIOTICS

Probiotics are a category of dietary supplements consisting of beneficial microorganisms (*pro* means "for" and *biotic* means "life" versus *antibiotic,* which literally means "against life"). Probiotics compete with disease-causing microorganisms in the gastrointestinal tract. When antibiotics are taken, they kill many of the beneficial bacteria that exist naturally in the digestive tract. Supplementing with probiotics after a course of antibiotics is frequently prescribed by nutritionists and complementary practitioners. Commonly used probiotics include *Lactobacillus acidophilus* and *Bifidobacterium bifidum;* there are other species of *Lactobacillus* and *Bifidobacterium* that have been shown to be effective in such conditions as diarrhea and vaginal infections (Reid & Bocking, 2003). *Bifidobacterium* also competes against *Candida albicans.* Probiotics can be taken in the form of powder, capsules, and suppositories, or in fermented milk products such as yogurt or *kefir.*

of 24 hours or more between onset of symptoms and when the woman seeks care (Mass, 2004). Breast abscess may require incision and drainage and IV antistaphylococcic antibiotics (Gibbs et al., 2004).

NURSING CARE MANAGEMENT
Nursing Assessment and Diagnosis

Daily assessment of breast consistency, skin color, surface temperature, nipple condition, and presence of pain is essential to detect early signs of problems that may predispose to mastitis. The mother should be observed breastfeeding her baby to ensure use of proper technique.

If an infection has developed, the nurse should assess for contributing factors such as cracked nipples, poor hygiene, engorgement, supplemental feedings, change in routine or infant feeding pattern, abrupt weaning, or lack of proper breast support so that these factors may be corrected as part of the treatment plan.

Nursing diagnoses that may apply to the woman with mastitis include the following:

- *Health-Seeking Behaviors* related to lack of information about appropriate breastfeeding practices
- *Ineffective Breastfeeding* related to pain secondary to development of mastitis

Nursing Plan and Implementation

Preventing mastitis is far simpler than treating it. Ideally, mothers should be instructed in proper breastfeeding technique prenatally. The nurse should help the mother breastfeed soon after birth and should review correct technique. Comanagement of breastfeeding between the nurse and a certified lactation spe-

cialist is often possible. All women, even those not breastfeeding, are encouraged to wear a good supportive bra at all times to avoid milk stasis, especially in the lower lobes.

Meticulous handwashing by the breastfeeding mother and all personnel is the primary measure for preventing epidemic nursery infections and subsequent maternal mastitis. Prompt attention to mothers who have blocked milk ducts eliminates stagnant milk as a growth medium for bacteria. If the mother finds that one area of her breast feels distended, she can rotate the position of her infant for breastfeeding, manually express milk remaining in the breast after feeding (usually only necessary if the infant is not sucking well), or massage the caked area toward the nipple as the infant suckles. Mothers who have developed mastitis can apply warm, moist compresses to the affected area before breastfeeding. The nurse encourages the mother to breastfeed frequently, starting with the unaffected breast until let-down occurs in the affected breast, then encourages feeding from the affected breast until it is emptied completely. After breastfeeding, the mother can leave a small amount of milk on each nipple to prevent cracking and allow nipples to air dry. Early identification of and intervention for sore nipples are also essential, as is prompt assessment of the breastfeeding mother's breasts when thrush is discovered in her newborn's mouth.

DISCHARGE PLANNING AND HOME CARE TEACHING

The nurse stresses to the breastfeeding woman the importance of adequate breast and nipple care to prevent the development of cracks and fissures, a common portal for bacterial entry. For a detailed discussion of breastfeeding, see "Breastfeeding Concerns Following Discharge" in Chapter 36. ∞

The woman should be aware of the importance of regular, complete emptying of the breasts to prevent engorgement and stasis. She should also understand the role of let-down in successful breastfeeding, correct positioning of the infant on the nipple, proper latch-on, and the principles of supply and demand. If the mother is taking antibiotics, she needs to understand the importance of completing the full course of antibiotics, even if the infection seems to clear quickly. Infants tolerate the small amount of antibiotics in breast milk without difficulty. The infant should also be checked for possible colonization with the same bacteria present in the mother's breast (Poggi & Kapernick, 2003). Breastfeeding mothers who will be returning to work outside the home need information on how to do so successfully. Because mastitis tends to develop following discharge, it is important to include information about signs and symptoms in the discharge teaching and printed materials (Table 38–5). All flulike symptoms should be considered a sign of mastitis until proved otherwise. If symptoms develop, the woman should contact her caregiver immediately, because prompt treatment helps to avoid abscess formation.

COMMUNITY-BASED NURSING CARE

The home care nurse who suspects mastitis on the basis of assessment findings refers the woman to the physician. The nurse may be asked to obtain a sample of breast milk to be cultured for the causative organism.

Table 38–5   COMPARISON OF FINDINGS OF ENGORGEMENT, PLUGGED DUCT, AND MASTITIS

Characteristics	Engorgement	Plugged Duct	Mastitis
Onset	Gradual, immediately postpartum	Gradual, after feedings	Sudden, after 10 days
Site	Bilateral	Unilateral	Usually unilateral
Swelling and heat	Generalized	May shift, little or no heat	Localized, red, hot, and swollen
Pain	Generalized	Mild but localized	Intense but localized
Body temperature	Less than 38.4C (101.1F)	Less than 38.4C (101.1F)	Greater than 38.4C (101.1F)
Systemic symptoms	Feels well	Feels well	Flulike symptoms

SOURCE: Reprinted from *Breastfeeding: A guide for the medical profession,* 5th ed., by R. A. Lawrence & R. M. Lawrence, p. 276, Copyright 1999, with permission from Elsevier.

If the mother feels too ill to breastfeed or develops an abscess that prevents breastfeeding, the home care nurse can help the mother obtain an appropriate breast pump to help her maintain lactation and can provide opportunities for demonstration and return demonstration of pumping. The nurse can assist the mother to deal with her feelings about temporarily being unable to breastfeed. Referral to a lactation consultant or to La Leche League can be invaluable to the woman's physical and emotional adjustment to mastitis.

Evaluation

Expected outcomes of nursing care include:

* The woman is aware of the signs and symptoms of mastitis.
* The woman reports her signs and symptoms of mastitis early, and it is treated successfully.
* The woman can continue breastfeeding if she chooses.
* The woman understands self-care measures she can use to prevent recurrence of mastitis.

CARE OF THE WOMAN WITH POSTPARTAL THROMBOEMBOLIC DISEASE

Thromboembolic disease may occur antepartally, but it is generally considered a postpartal complication. *Venous thrombosis* refers to formation of a blood clot (thrombus formation) at an area of impeded blood flow in a superficial or deep vein. When the thrombus is formed in response to inflammation in the vein wall, it is termed **thrombophlebitis.** Pulmonary embolism, a rare, life-threatening condition, occurs when thrombi formed in the deep leg veins are carried to the pulmonary artery, obstructing pulmonary blood flow to one or both lungs. These vascular occlusive processes—venous thrombosis, thrombophlebitis, septic pelvic thrombophlebitis, and pulmonary embolism—are known as thromboembolic diseases (Laros, 2004).

Three major causes of thromboembolic disease are hypercoagulability of blood, venous stasis, and injury to the epithelium of the blood vessel. Changes in the woman's coagulation system in pregnancy contribute to hypercoagulability, and compression of the common iliac vein by the gravid uterus leads to venous stasis. These factors increase the risk of this phenome-

Table 38–6   FACTORS ASSOCIATED WITH INCREASED RISK OF THROMBOEMBOLIC DISEASE

* Cesarean birth
* Immobility
* Obesity
* Cigarette smoking
* Previous thromboembolic disease
* Trauma to extremity (can include injury from incorrect positioning or prolonged interval in stirrups during labor)
* Varicose veins
* Diabetes mellitus
* Advanced maternal age
* Inherited coagulation disorders
* Multiparity
* Anemia
* Exogenous hormone use (oral contraceptives, hormone replacement therapy)
* Malignancy
* Inherited coagulation pathway deficiency
* Factor V Leiden mutation
* Antithrombin III deficiency
* Protein C deficiency
* Protein S deficiency
* Prothrombin mutation (G20210A)
* Hyperhomocysteinemia

non in pregnant and postpartum women approximately fivefold (Laros, 2004). Superficial vein thrombophlebitis complicates the general childbearing period for 1 in 500 to 750 women. Deep vein thrombosis (DVT), which is more serious, occurs most commonly in postpartum women between postpartum days 10 to 20. These types are discussed shortly. Factors associated with increased risk of thromboembolic disease are identified in Table 38–6. Factors contributing directly to the development of thromboembolic disease postpartally include (1) increased amounts of certain blood clotting factors; (2) postpartal thrombocytosis (increased quantity of circulating platelets and their increased adhesiveness); (3) release of thromboplastin substances from the tissue of the decidua, placenta, and fetal membranes; and (4) increased amounts of fibrinolysis inhibitors. Because women are at risk for thromboembolic disease during the childbearing period, attention should be given to measures that might prevent this complication (Table 38–7).

Table 38–7   MEASURES TO DECREASE RISK OF THROMBOEMBOLIC DISEASE IN CHILDBEARING WOMEN

Antepartum Measures	Intrapartum Measures	Postpartum Measures
Advise woman to avoid sedentary lifestyle and to exercise as possible (walking is ideal).	Encourage ambulation unless contraindicated in early labor.	Encourage early ambulation.
Recommend plenty of fluids to avoid dehydration.	Later, encourage leg exercises.	For clients on bed rest, advise or assist with turning and leg exercises every 2 hours (woman may be encouraged to rotate ankles and to "write baby's name in air with toes").
Advise to quit smoking.	Do not gatch bed or use pillows under knees.	
Teach to avoid prolonged standing or sitting in one position or sitting with legs crossed.	Pad stirrups.	Encourage fluids to avoid dehydration.
Encourage elevation of legs when sitting.	Ensure correct positioning in stirrups that minimizes pressure on the popliteal area.	Advise no smoking.
Teach to avoid tight knee-high hose or other constrictive garments.	Limit time in stirrups as possible. After cesarean birth, initiate leg/foot exercises as soon as possible (in recovery).	Use antiembolism stockings with those at risk. Pneumatic compression stockings may be ordered after cesarean birth until ambulation occurs.
Encourage to take frequent breaks during long car trips to walk around, thereby preventing prolonged venous stasis.	Use antiembolism stockings for women at risk of DVT.	Advise against prolonged sitting and crossing legs.
		Encourage elevation of legs while sitting.

Women with inherited thrombophilias are at significantly greater risk of thromboembolism than women without these conditions. The inherited thrombophilias are a heterogenous group of conditions. Recognized inherited thrombophilias include factor V Leiden and prothrombin G20210A gene mutations, antithrombin III, protein S, and protein C deficiencies. In these conditions, several regulatory proteins that act as inhibitors in the coagulation cascade are deficient, exacerbating hypercoagulability and contributing to recurrent venous thromboembolism. Inherited coagulopathies may present as venous thrombosis at any age. Most are transmitted by autosomal-dominant inheritance and affect predominantly Caucasian European populations, rarely those with Asian or African ethnic background. A personal or family history of thrombosis is not uncommon, nor is a history of adverse pregnancy outcomes, such as severe pregnancy-induced hypertension, placental abruption, intrauterine growth retardation, or fetal loss after 20 weeks (Doyle & Monga, 2004; Paidas, De-Hui, & Arkel, 2004). These women may require therapeutic levels of low-molecular-weight or unfractionated heparin throughout pregnancy and continued heparin therapy, followed by warfarin sodium (Coumadin) for at least 6 weeks postpartum (Lockwood, 2002).

Superficial Leg Vein Disease

Superficial thrombophlebitis is far more common postpartally than during pregnancy. Often the clot involves the saphenous veins. This disorder is more common in women with preexisting varices (enlarged veins), although it is not limited to these women. They may also occur as a sequelae to IV catheterization. Symptoms—tenderness in a portion of the vein, some local heat and redness, normal temperature or low-grade fever, and, occasionally, slight elevation of the pulse—usually become apparent about the third or fourth postpartal day. A tender palpable cord may be noted along a portion of the vein. Treatment involves application of local heat, elevation of the affected limb, bed rest and analgesic agents, and the use of elastic support hose. Anticoagulants are usually not necessary unless complications develop. Pulmonary embolism is extremely rare. There is generally little risk beyond discomfort. If improvement

is not evident or deep vein involvement is suspected, appropriate diagnostic measures are taken and serve as a basis for treatment decisions (Doyle & Monga, 2004).

Deep Vein Thrombosis

DVT or thrombophlebitis is more frequently seen in women with a history of thrombosis. Certain obstetric complications such as polyhydramnios, preeclampsia, and operative birth are associated with an increased incidence. After a clinical diagnosis of DVT, a woman's risk in a subsequent pregnancy increases.

Clinical manifestations may include edema of the ankle and leg and an initial low-grade fever often followed by high temperature and chills. Other findings include tenderness or pain, a palpable cord, changes in limb color, and difference in limb circumference of more than 2 cm. Depending on the vein involved, the woman may complain of pain in the popliteal and lateral tibial areas (popliteal vein), entire lower leg and foot (anterior and posterior tibial veins), inguinal tenderness (femoral vein), or pain in the lower abdomen (iliofemoral vein). Homans' sign (Figure 38–3 ◆) may or may not be positive. A positive Homans' sign is a specific finding but has a low sensitivity for helping diagnose DVT (Aronson, Chelmow, & Lee, 2003). Most DVTs occur in the left leg. Because of reflex arterial spasm, sometimes the limb is pale and cool to the touch—the so-called *milk leg* or *phlegmasia alba dolens*—and peripheral pulses may be decreased.

Septic Pelvic Thrombophlebitis

Septic pelvic thrombophlebitis is a complication that develops in conjunction with infections of the reproductive tract and is more common in women who have had a cesarean birth. Infection ascends upward along the venous system, and thrombophlebitis develops in the uterine, ovarian, or hypogastric veins (Cunningham et al., 2005). This diagnosis is suspected with clinical findings resembling metritis that fail to respond to antibiotics. Abdominal or flank pain, or both, sometimes accompanied by guarding, occurs on the second or third day postpartum with fever and tachycardia. Bimanual exam may or may not reveal a parametrial mass; the uterus is generally exquisitely

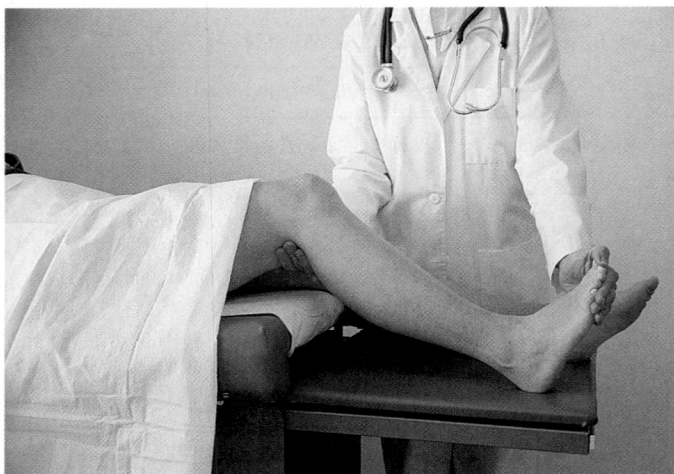

Figure 38–3 ◆ Homans' sign. With the client's knee flexed to decrease the risk of embolization, the nurse dorsiflexes the client's foot. Pain in the foot or leg is a positive Homans' sign.
SOURCE: Photographer, Elena Dorfman.

tender. On occasion, paralytic ileus develops. Treatment consists of anticoagulation and antibiotic therapy. Fever generally resolves within 48 to 72 hours of heparin therapy. Resolution of fever with heparin anticoagulation allows a presumptive diagnosis to be made (Laros, 2004).

Pulmonary Embolism

Pulmonary embolism (PE) is a particularly catastrophic event with a high mortality rate; most fatalities occur within 30 minutes; however, early recognition and prompt action can decrease the mortality rate significantly. Although the incidence of DVT in pregnancy is now believed to be almost comparable with that of postpartum DVT, PE develops most commonly in postpartal women. The most common risk factors are proximal DVT and recurrent thromboembolic disease. Diagnosis may be difficult because the most common clinical findings include nonspecific signs and symptoms such as dyspnea, chest pain, cough with hemoptysis, cyanosis, tachypnea and tachycardia, syncope, or sudden hypotension. The nurse who recognizes these findings, especially in a woman at risk, should alert the woman's physician immediately, as time can be critical. Elevating the head of the woman's bed may facilitate ease of breathing; oxygen by facemask at 8 to 10 L per minute is often used. Narcotics may be ordered for pain and to decrease anxiety, thereby decreasing the respiratory effort. Chest x-ray, arterial blood gases, and electrocardiogram (ECG) may be ordered to rule out other diagnoses; if the initial tests do not diagnose some other cause for symptomatology, ventilation-perfusion (V/Q) lung scanning may be ordered. If the results are not diagnostic and the woman is clinically stable, an ultrasound or magnetic resonance imaging (MRI) may be done of the lower extremities to assess for DVT. In some cases, a computed tomography (CT) scan or pulmonary angiography, an invasive procedure, may be used to diagnose PE. The primary treatment is anticoagulation with standard or low molecular weight heparins (LMWH). In some cases, thrombolytics (streptokinase or urokinase) or an embolectomy may be used.

Clinical Therapy

Because cases of thromboembolic disease are seldom clear-cut, diagnosis involves a variety of approaches, such as client history and physical examination, occlusive cuff impedance plethysmography (IPG), Doppler ultrasonography, and contrast venography (increased circumference of affected extremity). In questionable cases, contrast venography provides the most accurate diagnosis of DVT; unfortunately, it is not practical for multiple examinations or prospective screening and may itself induce phlebitis. Positive D-dimer has a high sensitivity in nonpregnant women but is not a reliable marker because of the wide variation in normal lab values in the pregnant population (Doyle & Monga, 2004).

Treatment involves the administration of IV heparin, using an infusion pump to permit continuous, accurate infusion of medication. Strict bed rest and elevation of the affected leg are required, and analgesics are given as necessary to relieve discomfort. If fever is present, deep thrombophlebitis is suspected, and the woman is also given antibiotic therapy. In most cases thrombectomy (surgical removal of the clot) is not necessary.

Once the symptoms have subsided (usually in several days), the woman may begin walking while wearing elastic support stockings. IV heparin is continued until prothrombin time reaches 1.5 to 2, and treatment with sodium warfarin (Coumadin) is begun. The woman will continue on Coumadin for 2 to 6 months at home. While taking warfarin, prothrombin times are assessed periodically to maintain correct dosage levels.

NURSING CARE MANAGEMENT
Nursing Assessment and Diagnosis

The nurse carefully assesses the woman's history for factors predisposing to development of thrombosis or thrombophlebitis. In addition, as part of regular postpartal assessment, the nurse is alert to any client complaints of pain in the leg, inguinal area, or lower abdomen because such pain may indicate DVT. The nurse also assesses the woman's legs for evidence of edema, temperature change, or pain with palpation.

Nursing diagnoses that may apply to a postpartal woman with thromboembolic disease include the following:

- *Altered Tissue Perfusion in Periphery* related to obstructed venous return
- *Pain* related to tissue hypoxia and edema secondary to vascular obstruction
- *Risk for Altered Parenting* related to decreased maternal-infant interaction secondary to bed rest and intravenous lines
- *Altered Family Processes* related to illness of family member
- *Deficient Knowledge* related to self-care after discharge on anticoagulant therapy

Nursing Plan and Implementation

Women with varicosities should be evaluated for the need for support hose during labor and postpartum. Adequate fluid intake is necessary during labor to avoid dehydration. Because trauma is often a factor in the development of thrombophlebitis, the nurse avoids keeping the woman's legs elevated in stirrups for prolonged periods. If stirrups are used, they should be comfortably padded and adjusted to provide correct support and prevent pressure on popliteal vessels. Early ambulation is encouraged following birth, and the use of the knee gatch on the bed should be avoided. Women confined to bed following a cesarean birth are encouraged to perform regular leg exercises to promote venous return.

Once the diagnosis of DVT is made, the nurse maintains the heparin therapy, provides for appropriate comfort measures, and monitors the woman closely for signs of PE. The nurse also assesses for evidence of bleeding related to heparin and keeps the antagonist for heparin, protamine sulfate, readily available.

The nurse instructs the woman to avoid prolonged standing or sitting, because these positions contribute to venous stasis. She is also instructed to avoid crossing her legs because of the pressure it causes. The nurse also advises her to take frequent breaks, such as when taking car trips and while working if she sits most of the day. Walking is acceptable because it promotes venous return. The woman is reminded to identify her history of thrombosis or thrombophlebitis to her physician during subsequent pregnancies so that preventive measures may be instituted early (Crowther & McCourt, 2005).

Women discharged on warfarin sodium should be taught about the drug and safety factors associated with its use. Clients need to be educated about foods high in vitamin K (Table 38–8) and the need to strive for consistent daily intake. In moderation, these foods can remain a part of the daily diet. When the dietary intake of such foods decreases significantly, there is a risk of bleeding. Many multivitamins contain vitamin K; clients on warfarin may take them but should do so consistently. Vitamin C doses up to 500 mg per day and vitamin E doses up to 400 international units per day are considered safe; higher doses can affect coagulation. While taking anticoagulants, the woman will be asked to undergo frequent coagulant tests to guide dosing. Point-of-care testing is now available to decrease the inconvenience of going into a laboratory environment for testing. Home self-testing involves a single capillary finger stick (Coaguchek, ProTime, Avocet) to test thromboplastin-mediated clotting expressed as prothrombin time (PT) or international normalized ratio (INR). The risk of bleeding increases significantly when

the INR is greater than 4 (Zajac, 2004). Bleeding should be reported if it fails to stop within 10 minutes. The nurse encourages the woman to carry a MedicAlert card in case of emergency to inform all healthcare providers (including dentists) that she is taking anticoagulants, and to have vitamin K available in case of bleeding.

Women who are discharged on warfarin must understand the purpose of the medication and be alert to signs of hemorrhage, such as bleeding gums, epistaxis, petechiae or ecchymosis, or evidence of blood in the urine or stool. Because careful monitoring is important, the woman should clearly understand the need to keep scheduled appointments for PT assessment. Certain medications, such as aspirin and other nonsteroidal anti-inflammatory drugs, increase anticoagulant activity, so they should be avoided. In fact, while she is taking warfarin the woman should check for possible medication interaction before taking *any* other medication. Binge alcohol use inhibits warfarin metabolism; an occasional alcoholic beverage does not affect coagulation adversely. Many herbals affect the efficacy of warfarin; for example, garlic, ginger, and ginkgo prolong PT and should be avoided. The nurse should encourage the woman to carry a MedicAlert card in case of emergency and to inform all medical care providers, including dentists, that she is taking anticoagulants. She should also have vitamin K available in case bleeding occurs. See the Nursing Care Plan: The Woman with Thromboembolic Disease for specific nursing care measures.

COMMUNITY-BASED NURSING CARE

Because the mother with postpartal thromboembolic disease will depend on others for much of her initial home care, it is helpful for the father to be involved in preparations for discharge. The nurse should provide ample opportunities to answer questions and clarify instructions, verbally and in writing. The nurse will evaluate the extent to which both mother and father have understood instructions regarding the plan of care. It is especially important before discharge to assess the couple's plans to ensure complete bed rest for the mother. They might explore ways for her to maintain bed rest and still spend quality time with her newborn and any other children. For example, young children can sit on the bed for storytelling or play quiet games, and the newborn's crib can be placed adjacent to the mother's bed.

The father may be assuming multiple roles in the circumstances—household manager, parent, worker, and caregiver. Fatigue is inevitable. There may be financial concerns as a result of prolonged health care or his extended time away from work to care for the family. Many concerns will not surface until the couple returns home and fully comprehends the reality of their situation. For that reason it is valuable to provide them with an accessible resource and to plan telephone or home visit follow-up care. Signs of postpartum thrombophlebitis may not occur until after discharge from the birthing unit. Consequently, all couples must be taught about the signs and symptoms and to appreciate the importance of reporting them immediately and of not massaging the affected leg. If signs and symptoms occur after discharge, a short readmission might be required. Every effort is made in that case to allow mother, father, and newborn to remain together.

Table 38–8	FOODS HIGH IN VITAMIN K
• Basil	• Lettuce
• Broccoli	• Mint
• Brussels sprouts	• Mustard greens
• Cabbage	• Parsley
• Canola oil, soybean oil, mayonnaise	• Peppers
• Cauliflower	• Spinach
• Chives	• Tea (both green and black)
• Collard greens	• Turnips
• Coriander	• Watercress
• Kale	

MEDIALINK   Case Study: Postpartal Thromboembolic Disease

NURSING CARE PLAN

The Woman with Thromboembolic Disease

INTERVENTION	RATIONALE	EXPECTED OUTCOMES
1. Nursing Diagnosis: Ineffective Tissue Perfusion: Peripheral related to interruption of venous blood flow secondary to complications of labor and birth		
Goal: *The woman's presenting signs and symptoms are relieved.*		
• Assess, record, and report signs of thrombophlebitis. • Assess leg for edema, peripheral pulse, temperature, color, and tenderness every 8 hours. Initially note presence of palpable cord.	• Early detection of developing thrombophlebitis permits prompt treatment. As the thrombus increases in size, signs of obstruction also increase. Assessment provides baseline data that may be used to monitor success of treatment. • Edema/swelling, diminished or absent peripheral pulse, pallor, cool skin temperature, and tenderness are symptoms of DVT and indicate dysfunction of peripheral circulation in the lower extremities. Measure circumference of lower leg to monitor for swelling. Peripheral pulses in both legs should be palpated for pulse rate, pulse strength to allow for comparison. A lower extremity cool to the touch may be due to reflex arterial spasm.	• *Woman will have increased venous return from lower leg as evidenced by decreased edema in lower leg, negative Homans' sign, and no pain or tenderness in lower leg.*
• Assess Homans' sign every 8 hours.	• Normally there is no pain or discomfort associated with this procedure. Pain is caused by inflammation of the vessel. If pain is elicited the nurse documents the response as a positive Homans' sign and reports findings to the physician.	
• Maintain bed rest during the acute phase.	• Bed rest is ordered to decrease the possibility that a portion of the clot will dislodge and result in pulmonary embolism.	
• Provide warm, moist soaks as ordered.	• Warmth promotes blood flow to affected area.	
• Maintain limb in elevated position.	• Elevation of affected limb promotes venous return and helps decrease edema.	
• Initiate progressive ambulation following the acute phase and provide properly fitting elastic stockings before ambulation.	• Elastic stockings or "TEDs" help prevent pooling of venous blood in lower extremities. • Woman may begin to ambulate within a few days when symptoms subside.	
Collaborative: Administer intravenous heparin as ordered, by continuous intravenous drip, heparin lock, or subcutaneously, including: 1. Monitor IV or heparin lock site for patency, signs of infiltration, or signs of infection.	• Heparin does not dissolve blood clot but is administered to prevent further clotting and improve tissue perfusion. It is safe for breastfeeding mothers because heparin is not excreted in breast milk.	

NURSING CARE PLAN

The Woman with Thromboembolic Disease continued

INTERVENTION	RATIONALE	EXPECTED OUTCOMES

2. Obtain international normalized ratio (INR) and partial thromboplastin time (PTT) per physician order and review before administering heparin.
3. Observe for signs of anticoagulant overdose with resultant bleeding including:
  a. Hematuria
  b. Epistaxis
  c. Ecchymosis or petechiae
  d. Bleeding gums
  e. Nose bleeds
  f. Bruising disproportionate to injury
  g. Cuts, scratches, injection, or venipuncture sites that bleed excessively
4. Provide protamine sulfate, per physician order, to combat bleeding problems related to heparin overdose.
 	
5. Monitor and report any signs of pulmonary embolism.
6. Initiate or support any emergency treatment.
 	
7. Obtain prothrombin time (PT) and review before beginning warfarin. Repeat periodically per physician order.
	• Protamine sulfate is a heparin antagonist, given intravenously, which is almost immediately effective in counteracting bleeding complications caused by heparin overdose.
	• Pulmonary embolism is a major complication of DVT/thrombophlebitis.
	• Signs and symptoms may occur suddenly and require immediate emergency treatment; prognosis is related to size and location of embolism.
	• PT is the test most commonly used to monitor the blood of clients receiving warfarin.	

2. Nursing Diagnosis: Pain related to tissue hypoxia and edema secondary to vascular obstruction

Goal: *Woman will obtain relief of pain or experience level of pain which is acceptable.*

• Administer analgesics per physician order. Notify physician if pain is not relieved. • Observe or report disruptive effects of pain on emotions and behavior. • Provide supportive nursing comfort measures such as backrubs, provision of quiet time for sleep, diversional activities, or imagery.	• Analgesics act to relieve pain and enable the woman to rest. Aspirin or ibuprofen products are contraindicated because they inhibit platelet adhesiveness. Acetaminophen may be ordered by the physician. • Once pain decreases, client is more likely to ambulate, which will help increase venous return and decrease edema.	• *Woman will have reduction in pain as evidenced by a pain level less than 5 at all times.*

(Continued on next page)

NURSING CARE PLAN

The Woman with Thromboembolic Disease continued

INTERVENTION	RATIONALE	EXPECTED OUTCOMES
3. Nursing Diagnosis: Risk for Impaired Parenting related to decreased maternal-infant interaction secondary to bed rest and IVs		
Goal: *Woman will demonstrate evidence of positive physical and social interaction with newborn.*		

• Maintain mother-infant attachment when mother is on bed rest:
  1. Provide frequent contacts for mother and infant; modified rooming-in if possible by having the crib placed close to the mother's bed and nurse checks often to help mother lift or move infant.
  2. Encourage mother to continue feeding infant.
	• Maternal-infant attachment is enhanced by frequent contact and opportunities to interact.	• Woman will develop attachment bonds as evidenced by physical interactions: good eye contact, touching the baby, holding baby close, attempting to comfort baby, and kissing baby and social interactions: calling baby by name, making positive comments about baby, asking questions about baby, asking questions about baby care, and talking to baby.

4. Nursing Diagnosis: Interrupted Family Processes related to illness of family member		
Goal: *Woman and her family will cope effectively with her illness.*		

• Encourage woman to express her concerns to her partner. Assist couple in planning ways to manage while woman is hospitalized and after her discharge.
 	
• Encourage partner or support person to bring other children to the hospital to visit mother and meet new sibling.
• Encourage partner or support person to bring in family pictures and notes from other children. Encourage phone calls.
• Contact social services if indicated to obtain additional assistance for family if needed.
	• Illness of any family member impacts the entire family. This is especially true when the family situation is such that the mother is the primary nurturer and she is absent. Family members attempt to continue their own roles while also assuming the tasks of the missing mother. This can result in crisis.	• Woman expresses assurance that her family misses her but is coping effectively as evidenced by:
		  • Family visits woman frequently.
		  • Woman and family verbalize plan for division of family tasks while the woman is hospitalized, and understanding of potential needs of woman once released from hospital.

5. Nursing Diagnosis: Health-Seeking Behaviors related to lack of information about DVT/thrombophlebitis, its treatment, preventive measures, and the medication, warfarin.		
Goal: *Woman will understand her condition, its treatment, safety during treatment, and long-term implications.*		

• Provide information (both verbal and written supplements) about the woman's condition, its treatment regimen, the importance of compliance, and safety factors. Provide contact information that the woman can access 24/7.	• Such discussion is essential to help the woman understand the condition, her medication, and its implications. She must have a clear understanding to be able to provide effective self-care.	• Woman has health promotion knowledge as evidenced by:
		  • Woman verbalizes understanding of ways to avoid circulatory stasis, need to wear supportive stockings, medications dosage and side effects, and the importance of a balanced diet.
		  • Woman verbalizes understanding of signs and symptoms of bleeding that need to be reported to healthcare provider.

NURSING CARE PLAN

The Woman with Thromboembolic Disease continued

INTERVENTION	RATIONALE	EXPECTED OUTCOMES
• Discuss ways of avoiding circulatory stasis such as avoiding prolonged standing, sitting, crossing legs, and wearing restrictive clothing. • Discuss safety precautions necessary while taking LMWH and warfarin (extra care with knives, razors, and other sharp objects; care around animals in the home that may scratch or bite; wear MedicAlert bracelet identifying that she is on anticoagulant therapy). • Advise use of soft toothbruth. • Advise to routinely inspect her body for evidence of bleeding. • Advise to monitor menstrual flow, as it may be increased. • Teach importance of compliance with warfarin therapy and interactions of vitamin K with warfarin, and check for interactions when starting new medications. • Teach woman and partner to advise all healthcare providers, including dentists, that she is taking anticoagulants. • If LMWH is being used at home, teach proper sterile technique for self-injection and safe disposal of syringes. • Teach importance of consistent level of vitamin K intake while on warfarin and foods high in vitamin K to facilitate planning.	• Prolonged sitting, standing, and crossing legs should be avoided, as these activities decrease venous return. • Anticoagulation places woman at risk of excessive bleeding and requires increased attention to safety issues that typically do not pose a significant risk. During warfarin therapy, INR levels are monitored regularly to minimize risks. • Warfarin interacts with numerous medications that either increase or decrease its effectiveness. • INR levels are monitored initially to facilitate dosage decisions. Once consistent effects are obtained, LMWH may be used without laboratory monitoring. With warfarin therapy, INR results will be monitored and dosage managed on the basis of lab results. • Vitamin K interacts with warfarin. A consistent (balanced) intake of foods with vitamin K minimizes the problem of interaction.	

Evaluation

Expected outcomes of nursing care include:

- The woman seeks treatment for her thrombophlebitis early and is managed successfully without further complications.

- At discharge, the woman is able to explain the purpose, dosage regimen, and necessary precautions associated with any prescribed medications, such as anticoagulants.

- The woman can discuss self-care measures and ongoing therapies (such as the use of elastic stockings) that are indicated.

- The woman has bonded successfully with her newborn and is able to care for the baby effectively.

CARE OF THE WOMAN WITH A POSTPARTUM PSYCHIATRIC DISORDER

The relationship of affective disorders to childbirth is reflected in the fact that the rate of admission to a psychiatric hospital is greater during the year after childbirth than at any other time in a woman's life.

Types of Postpartum Psychiatric Disorders

Many types of psychiatric problems may occur in the postpartum. Their classification is a subject of some controversy. The

Diagnostic and Statistical Manual of Mental Disorders (American Psychiatric Association, 2000) has added a postpartum-onset specifier to the mood disorder diagnostic category of psychiatric disorders. It is proposed that postpartum psychiatric disorders be considered one diagnosable syndrome with three subclasses: (1) adjustment reaction with depressed mood, (2) postpartum psychosis, and (3) postpartum major mood disorder. The incidence, etiology, symptoms, treatment, and prognosis vary with each subclass.

ADJUSTMENT REACTION WITH DEPRESSED MOOD

Adjustment reaction with depressed mood is commonly known as **postpartum blues,** or as *maternal* or *"baby" blues.* It occurs in as many as 50% to 75% of mothers and is characterized by mild depression interspersed with happier feelings (Beck, 2006). Postpartum blues typically occur within a few days after the baby's birth and are self-limiting, lasting from a few hours to 10 days or longer. The depression is more severe in primiparas than in multiparas and seems related to the rapid alteration of estrogen, progesterone, and prolactin levels after birth. New mothers experiencing postpartum blues commonly report feeling overwhelmed, unable to cope, fatigued, anxious, irritable, and oversensitive. A key feature is episodic tearfulness, often without an identifiable reason. Not uncommonly, when asked why she is crying, this woman responds that she does not know. Cunningham et al. (2005, p. 705) speculate that several factors contribute to the blues:

- Emotional letdown that follows labor and childbirth
- Physical discomfort typical in the early postpartum
- Fatigue
- Anxiety about caring for the newborn after discharge
- Fears about her physical attractiveness

Validating the existence of this phenomenon, labeling it as a real but normal adjustment reaction, and providing reassurance can offer a measure of relief. Measures that promote comfort and rest, opportunities to share her childbirth story, assistance with self and infant care, information, and family support are helpful. The partner should be encouraged to watch for and report signs that the new mother is not returning to a more normal mood but is instead slipping into a deeper depression.

POSTPARTUM PSYCHOSIS

Postpartum psychosis, which has an incidence of 1 to 2/1000, usually becomes evident within the first 1 to 3 months postpartum (Beck, 2006). Although relatively rare, these disorders gain considerable national attention in the media when there is an incident of infanticide associated with them. Symptoms include agitation, hyperactivity, insomnia, mood lability, confusion, irrational thoughts and behaviors, difficulty remembering or concentrating, and poor judgment, as well as delusions and hallucinations, which tend to be related to the infant. With appropriate treatment, improvement is seen in 95% of women in 2 to 3 months. There is an increased recurrence rate in subsequent pregnancies (Parry, 2004).

Risk factors include (1) previous puerperal psychosis; (2) history of bipolar (manic-depressive) disorder; (3) prenatal stressors, such as lack of social support, lack of a partner, and low socioeconomic status; (4) obsessive personality; and (5) a family history of a mood disorder. Treatment may include hospitalization, antipsychotic medications, sedatives, electroconvulsive therapy, removal of the infant, social support, and psychotherapy.

Postpartum psychosis is considered an emergency because of the risk of suicide and/or infanticide (Beck, 2006). The psychotic woman may experience delusions or hallucinations that support her perceptions that the infant should not be allowed to live. For example, she may believe that her newborn is evil and will harm her other children, or she may believe that her newborn would be "better off dead" than living in such an evil world. She may contemplate suicide because she believes that her child would be better off without a mother than with her as such a "terrible, crazy mother." Illogical thinking or evidence of bonding difficulties may serve as cues to infanticide and suicide risk; however, this assessment is often challenging because of the lucidity seen in some psychotic clients.

Treatment usually involves admission to an inpatient psychiatric unit. Mood stabilizers and neuroleptic agents are generally used for symptom management.

POSTPARTUM MAJOR MOOD DISORDER

Postpartum major mood disorder, also known as **postpartum depression,** develops in about 7% to 30% of all postpartal women (Parry, 2004). Although it may occur at any time during the first year postpartum, the greatest risks occur around the fourth week, just before the initiation of menses, and upon weaning. Surprisingly, it is not always associated with depression during pregnancy.

Many of the symptoms of this major depression are indistinguishable from serious depression at other times: sadness, frequent crying, insomnia or excessive sleeping, appetite change, difficulty concentrating and making decisions, feelings of worthlessness, obsessive thoughts of inadequacy as a person and parent, lack of interest in usual activities (including sexual relations), and lack of concern about personal appearance. Persistent anxiety further contributes to the woman's feeling of being out of control. Irritability and hostility toward others, including the newborn, may be evident. Beck (1993) described these debilitating symptoms as "teetering on the edge" between sanity and insanity. Women participating in Beck's qualitative research on postpartum depression described a sense of living their daily life in a sort of fog, from which they believed they would never emerge. Once they improved, they often grieved over the time lost with their newborns while in this "fog." The duration of symptoms varies but as many as half continue to be symptomatic at 6 months. Some women continue to suffer for the entire postpartum year (Goodman, 2004b).

Risk factors for postpartum depression include the following:

- Primiparity
- Ambivalence about maintaining the pregnancy
- History of postpartum depression or bipolar illness

- Lack of social support
- Lack of a stable and supportive relationship with parents (especially her father, as a child) or partner
- The woman's dissatisfaction with herself, including body image problems and eating disorders
- Poverty
- Depression during pregnancy
- Complications of delivery
- Loss of newborn
- Age (adolescence increases risk)

Alcohol has depressive effects as can "coming down from" illicit drugs such as amphetamines and cocaine. Some prescription medications widely used by postpartum women can also cause depression. These include certain contraceptives, drugs used to treat gastroesophageal reflux and peptic ulcer disease, and several others. Women with postpartum depression are at risk of suicide, most prominently as they enter or exit the deeply depressed state. In a deep depression, the woman is unlikely to be able to plan and carry out suicide. For that reason, signs of improvement in depression should be celebrated with some caution.

Whereas the woman with postpartal psychosis may attempt suicide because of illogical thought processes, the woman with major depression attempts suicide because her suffering is so great that dying seems a more favorable option than continuing to live in such pain. She may also attempt suicide to save her newborn from some perceived or real threat—including the threat that she herself might harm the baby. The risk of suicide is greater in those who have attempted suicide previously, have a specific plan, and can access the means or weapon identified within the plan. The more specific the plan, the greater is the probability of an attempt.

Clinical Therapy

Women with a history of postpartum psychosis or depression or other risk factors should be referred to a mental health professional for counseling and biweekly visits between the second and sixth week postpartum for evaluation. Medication, individual or group psychotherapy, and practical assistance with child care and other demands of daily life are common treatment measures for both disorders; however, specific therapies used may vary.

Treatment of postpartum depression is not unlike treatment of any significant depression: psychotherapy and antidepression medications, usually the selective serotonin reuptake inhibitors. The woman and her partner should be reminded that antidepressants may take several weeks to have an effect. It is important to realize that many of the drugs used in treating postpartum psychiatric conditions may be contraindicated in breastfeeding women.

Support groups have proved to be successful adjuncts to such treatment. Within a support group of postpartal women and their partners, a couple may feel consolation that they are not alone in their experience. Moreover, the support group provides a forum for gaining information about postpartum depression, learning stress reduction measures, and experiencing renewed self-esteem and support. The most effective support groups provide for safe child care to facilitate attendance. If a support group is not available locally, the woman and her family may be encouraged to contact Depression After Delivery (DAD), now a national Web-based support network that provides education and volunteers, or Postpartum Support International. The Mills Depression and Anxiety Symptom-Feeling Checklist also is available online. This checklist focuses on symptoms and feelings the postpartum woman has experienced over the previous 2-week interval, using a Likert-type scale (0 = not at all to 3) most of the time. The woman is advised to contact her healthcare provider immediately if she marks symptoms and feelings highlighted in red—those that relate to harm to herself or the infant.

Treatment of postpartum psychosis is directed at the specific type of psychotic symptoms displayed and may include lithium, antipsychotics, or electroconvulsive therapy in combination with psychotherapy, removal of the infant, and social support.

NURSING CARE MANAGEMENT
Nursing Assessment and Diagnosis

Assessment for factors predisposing a client to postpartum depression or psychosis should begin prenatally (Beck, 2002). Questions designed to detect problems can be included as part of the routine prenatal history interview or questionnaire. Women with a personal or family history of psychiatric disease, particularly postpartum depression or psychosis, need prenatal instructions on the signs and symptoms of depression and may need additional emotional support. Ideally the assessment should be completed each trimester to update a pregnant woman's risk status (Beck, 2002). If the assessment has not been done previously, the nurse assesses the woman for predisposing factors during her labor and postpartum stay.

Becoming a mother is idealized by most societies as a joyful event. Consequently, the woman who experiences depression, instead of joy, often suffers silently because she feels guilty and hesitant to disclose her honest feelings with family and caregivers. Some women believe that admission of emotional difficulty and mothering inadequacy will be used against them and that their children will be taken away. Before assessment for evidence of depression, the nurse can give voice to this societal myth of joyful motherhood, giving the woman permission to share negative feelings and thoughts she might be having.

The first-time mother who has anticipated a period of adjustment with a newborn may not realize that her feelings are not part of the normal transition to motherhood. The woman may develop symptoms in advance of her follow-up visit to the obstetrician or pediatrician, complicating choice of healthcare provider for some.

Several depression scales are available for assessing postpartum depression. The routine use of a screening tool in a matter-of-fact approach significantly increases the diagnosis.

The Edinburgh Postnatal Depression Scale (Table 38–9) is likely the most widely used screening tool for postpartum depression in large populations of women. The tool has been validated, computerized, and used in telephone screening. Mothers who score above 12 on the Edinburgh Postnatal Depression Scale are likely to be suffering from postpartum depression. Another tool is Beck's (2002) revised Postpartum Depression Predictors Inventory (PDPI-Revised). This tool is also a practical and simple screening checklist for use during routine care with all postpartal women to identify those who might be experiencing postpartum depression so that early management might be initiated (Table 38–10). No matter what approach the nurse uses to assess for postpartum depression, enabling the woman's voice to be heard about her feelings of maternal role transition and how she is adjusting in this vulnerable time is of inestimable value (Hanna, Jarman, & Savage, 2004). Listening to her story provides a critical emic (insider's) view of her circumstances as opposed to an etic (outsider's) view.

In providing daily care, the nurse observes the woman for objective signs of depression—anxiety, irritability, poor concentration, forgetfulness, sleeping difficulties, appetite change, fatigue, and tearfulness—and listens for statements indicating feelings of failure and self-accusation. Severity and duration of symptoms should be noted. Behavior and verbalization that are bizarre or seem to indicate a potential for violence against herself or others, including the infant, are reported as soon as possible for further evaluation.

The nurse needs to be aware that many normal physiologic changes of the puerperium are similar to symptoms of depression (lack of sexual interest, indecisiveness, appetite change, sleep disturbance, and fatigue). It is essential that observations be as specific and as objective as possible and that they be carefully documented.

Beck and Indman (2005) found that anxiety was a prominent feature of illness for some women and suggested that women be assessed for their level of anxiety, particularly regarding infant care. Because of the strong association of interrupted sleep and postpartum depression and the finding that severe fatigue was an excellent predictor of postpartum depression (Corwin, Brownstead, Barton et al, 2005; Huang, Carter, & Guo, 2004), assessing fatigue level at 2 weeks postpartum by telephone may be helpful in predicting depression risk early. Restorative sleep improves one's ability to cope and make decisions, thereby producing a sense of better self-control. A central challenge for nursing is identifying women at risk of suicide. Like others with psychologic disorders, the postpartum woman is likely ambivalent about suicide, and may be "rescuable" if suicide ideation is assessed and timely action follows. Assessment of suicide risk reflects the standard of care; contrary to myth, asking a depressed woman about suicidal thoughts does not increase her risk, but it may save her life. Introducing the issue of suicide can be as simple as saying something like, "I'm concerned about the amount of emotional pain you're feeling, and I'm wondering whether you've ever thought of hurting yourself." Ambivalence about suicide is likely to make the woman answer candidly. A suicide prevention contract may be established with the woman to exact an agreement

Table 38–9   EDINBURGH POSTNATAL DEPRESSION SCALE

In the past 7 days:

1. I have been able to laugh and see the funny side of things
   - As much as I always could
   - Not quite so much now
   - Definitely not so much now
   - Not at all

2. I have looked forward with enjoyment of things
   - As much as I ever did
   - Rather less than I used to
   - Definitely less than I used to
   - Hardly at all

*3. I have blamed myself unnecessarily when things went wrong
   - Yes, most of the time
   - Yes, some of the time
   - Not very often
   - No, never

4. I have been anxious or worried for no good reason
   - No, not at all
   - Hardly ever
   - Yes, sometimes
   - Yes, very often

*5. I have felt scared or panicky for no very good reason
   - Yes, quite a lot
   - Yes, sometimes
   - No, not much
   - No, not at all

*6. Things have been getting on top of me
   - Yes, most of the time I haven't been able to cope at all
   - Yes, sometimes I haven't been coping as well as usual
   - No, I have been coping quite well
   - No, I have been coping as well as ever

*7. I have been so unhappy that I have had difficulty sleeping
   - Yes, most of the time
   - Yes, sometimes
   - Not very often
   - No, not at all

*8. I have felt sad or miserable
   - Yes, most of the time
   - Yes, quite often
   - Not very often
   - No, not at all

*9. I have been so unhappy that I have been crying
   - Yes, most of the time
   - Yes, quite often
   - Only occasionally
   - No, never

*10. The thought of harming myself has occurred to me
   - Yes, quite often
   - Sometimes
   - Hardly ever
   - Never

NOTE: Response categories are scored 0, 1, 2, and 3 according to increased severity of the symptoms. Items marked with an asterisk are reverse scored (3, 2, 1, 0). The total score is calculated by adding together the scores for each of the 10 items. A score above the threshold of 12–13 out of 30 indicates with 86% sensitivity that the woman is suffering from postpartum depression.

SOURCE: Cox, J. L., Holden, J. M., & Sagovsky, R. (1987). Detection of postnatal depression: Development of the 10-item Edinburgh Postnatal Depression Scale. *British Journal of Psychiatry, 150,* 782–786. Users may reproduce the scale without further permission provided they respect copyright by quoting the names of the authors, the title, and the source of the paper in all reproduced copies.

Table 38–10 POSTPARTUM DEPRESSION PREDICTORS INVENTORY (PDPI)—REVISED AND GUIDE QUESTIONS FOR ITS USE

During Pregnancy

Marital status — Check One
1. Single — O
2. Married/cohabitating — O
3. Separated — O
4. Divorced — O
5. Widowed — O
6. Partnered — O

Socioeconomic status
- Low — O
- Middle — O
- High — O

Self-esteem	Yes	No
Do you feel good about yourself as a person?	O	O
Do you feel worthwhile?	O	O
Do you feel you have a number of good qualities as a person?	O	O

Prenatal depression
1. Have you felt depressed during your pregnancy? — O / O
   If yes, when and how long have you been feeling this way?
   If yes, how mild or severe would you consider your depression?

Prenatal anxiety
- Have you been feeling anxious during your pregnancy? — O / O
  If yes, how long have you been feeling this way?

Unplanned/unwanted pregnancy
- Was the pregnancy planned? — O / O
- Is the pregnancy unwanted? — O / O

History of previous depression
1. Before this pregnancy, have you ever been depressed? — O / O
   If yes, when did you experience this depression?
   If yes, have you been under a physician's care for this past depression? — O / O
   If yes, did the physician prescribe any medication for your depression? — O / O

Social support
1. Do you feel you receive adequate emotional support from your partner? — O / O
2. Do you feel you receive adequate instrumental support from your partner (e.g., help with household chores or baby-sitting)? — O / O
3. Do you feel you can rely on your partner when you need help? — O / O
4. Do you feel you can confide in your partner? (repeat same questions for family and again for friends) — O / O

Marital satisfaction
1. Are you satisfied with your marriage (or living arrangement)? — O / O
2. Are you currently experiencing any marital problems? — O / O
3. Are things going well between you and your partner? — O / O

Life stress
1. Are you currently experiencing any stressful events in your life such as:
   - Financial problems — O / O
   - Marital problems — O / O
   - Death in the family — O / O
   - Serious illness in the family — O / O
   - Moving — O / O
   - Unemployment — O / O
   - Job change — O / O

(Continued on next page)

Table 38–10   POSTPARTUM DEPRESSION PREDICTORS INVENTORY (PDPI)—REVISED AND GUIDE QUESTIONS FOR ITS USE   continued

After delivery, add the following items

	Yes	No
Child care stress		
1. Is your infant experiencing any health problems?	O	O
2. Are you having problems with your baby feeding?	O	O
3. Are you having problems with your baby sleeping?	O	O
Infant temperament		
1. Would you consider your baby irritable or fussy?	O	O
2. Does your baby cry a lot?	O	O
3. Is your baby difficult to console or soothe?	O	O
Maternity blues		
1. Did you experience a brief period of tearfulness and mood swings during the 1st week after delivery?	O	O

COMMENTS:

_____

_____

_____

_____

that she will seek help immediately if she begins to consider self-harm. For example, the nurse might say, "Promise me that should you begin to feel as if you are going to hurt yourself, you will telephone me or the hot line immediately—that you will not act without talking to someone." Because of the hope this offers, the woman is likely to respond by seeking help; she does not want to renege on a promise she made to a nurse who has shown such caring for her.

If a woman admits that she has thought of hurting herself, assessment of the risk that she will follow through is imperative. The mnemonic **SAL** is useful for risk assessment: Is there a **S**pecific plan with a designated time? Is there an **A**ccessible weapon or other means? How **L**ethal is the method identified in the plan? A specific plan that identifies a highly lethal method that is immediately accessible is evidence of very high risk of suicide. Immediate intervention is critical; emergency psychiatric hospitalization is likely necessary. Those considered a threat to themselves or others may be admitted to involuntary hospitalization for a minimum of 48 hours until further evaluation is complete.

Family members of the depressed woman should also be alert to signals that she may be intent on self-harm; they must be advised that threats should always be taken seriously. Cues to suicide that might be noted by family are comments such as "I don't deserve to live," "Life is no longer worth living," or "You won't have to worry about me for long." Someone who is considering suicide may also telephone or write family or friends to say good-bye or give away prized possessions. Family members should be told to be especially vigilant for suicide when the woman seems to be feeling better.

Possible nursing diagnoses that may apply to a woman with a postpartum psychiatric disorder include the following:

- *Ineffective Individual Coping* related to postpartum depression
- *Risk for Altered Parenting* related to postpartal mental illness
- *Risk for Violence* against self (suicide), newborn, and other children related to depression.

Nursing Plan and Implementation

Nurses working in antepartal settings or teaching childbirth classes play indispensable roles in helping prospective parents appreciate the lifestyle changes and role demands associated with parenthood. Offering realistic information and anticipatory guidance and debunking myths about the perfect mother or perfect newborn may help prevent postpartum depression. Social support teaching guides are available for nurses to help postpartum women explore their needs for postpartum support.

The nurse should alert the mother, partner, and other family members to the possibility of postpartum blues in the early days after birth and reassure them of the short-term nature of the condition. Symptoms of postpartum depression should be described and the mother encouraged to call her healthcare provider if symptoms become severe, if they fail to subside quickly, or if at any time she feels she is unable to function. Encouraging the mother to plan how she will manage at home and providing concrete suggestions on how to cope will aid in her adjustment to motherhood. Table 38–11 indicates suggestions that serve as primary prevention for postpartum depression.

EVIDENCE-BASED PRACTICE

PREVENTION OF POSTPARTUM DEPRESSION

Clinical Question

What psychologic, psychosocial, and/or pharmacologic interventions are effective in preventing postpartum depression?

The Evidence

Three systematic reviews were conducted that appraised the evidence regarding interventions to prevent postpartum depression. One review focused only on psychologic and psychosocial interventions. These reviewers evaluated 15 trials involving more than 7600 women. A second review assessed the effects of pharmacologic agents given in the early postpartum period as a prophylactic measure. These reviewers independently assessed two randomized trials, both of which had small samples (40 women total). The third review was an integrative review of nursing interventions. These authors summarized the findings from 11 randomized trials and qualitative studies.

What Is Effective?

In general, the effectiveness of psychologic or psychosocial interventions was not demonstrated as effective in preventing postpartum depression. Overall, the women who received a psychosocial intervention were equally likely to develop postpartum depression as those receiving standard care. Antenatal classes focusing on postpartum depression were repeatedly shown to have no preventive effect. Trials evaluating in-hospital psychologic support before discharge provide evidence that these services are ineffective. Interventions focused only on the postpartum component were more effective than those that incorporated an antenatal component. The reviewers speculate that antenatal preventive activities are not effective because it is difficult to predict which women will later develop postpartum depression. Routine administration of antidepressants in the postpartum period—specifically Nortriptyline and Sertraline—did not reduce the incidence of depression. The reviewers do not recommend the routine use of prophylactic antidepressant medications, particularly for mothers who are breastfeeding. However, there were some indications that certain types of interventions may be effective. Individually based interventions were the most promising, particularly those delivered at home by a professional nurse or nurse-midwife.

What Is Unclear?

Although the reviewers suggest that identifying mothers "at risk" assisted in the prevention of postpartum depression, there is no current consistency in the identification of women "at risk." A review of antenatal screening tools suggests that there are no measurement tools with documented predictive validity, a requirement for determining the chance of a future event. The reviewers could not document the effectiveness of individual intensive psychotherapy or lay support groups, as none of the trials addressed these interventions.

Best Practice

Currently, there is no evidence to recommend antenatal classes about depression, early postpartum follow-up, or in-hospital psychologic debriefing. The nurse should help identify mothers who may be at risk for postpartum depression, but in-hospital preventive activities are not effective. Individually based interventions delivered by professional nurses in the new mother's home are the most effective. Routine administration of prophylactic antidepressants should be avoided.

Critical Thinking

What kind of behaviors would indicate to the nurse that a mother was at risk for postpartum depression? How can the nurse give the new mother information about recognition of signs of postpartum depression and resources for help if it is needed?

REFERENCES: Dennis, C., & Creedy, D. (2004). Psychosocial and psychological interventions for preventing postpartum depression. *The Cochrane Database of Systematic Reviews* (4). Article No.: CD001134.pub2.

Driscoll, J. (2006). Postpartum depression: The state of the science. *Journal of Perinatal and Neonatal Nursing, 20*(1), 40–3.

Howard, L., Hoffbrand, S., Henshaw, C., Boath, L., & Bradley. E. (2005). Antidepressant prevention of postnatal depression. *The Cochrane Database of Systematic Reviews* (2). Article No.: CD001168.pub2.

COMMUNITY-BASED NURSING CARE

Home visits, especially for early discharge families, are invaluable to fostering positive adjustments for the new family constellation. Telephone follow-up at 2 to 3 weeks postpartum to ask whether the mother is experiencing difficulties is also helpful. Monitoring for signs of depression or performing brief screening at well-child follow-ups also can be valuable for early identification and timely intervention (Chaudron, Szilagyi, Kitzman et al., 2004).

In all women, the presence of three symptoms on one day or one symptom for 3 days may signal serious postpartum depression and requires immediate referral to a mental health professional. Immediate referral should also be made if rejection of the infant or threatened or actual aggression against the infant has occurred. In such cases, the newborn is never left unattended with the mother. Depression does appear to interfere with optimal mothering; there is less interaction between mother and child, more mood and cognitive development problems, and more visits to the doctor in these children (Beck, 2002). A diagnosis of postpartum depression or other psychiatric disorder will pose major problems for the family, especially the father. The symptoms of these disorders are difficult to witness and may be harder to understand than physical problems such as hemorrhage or infection. The father may feel hurt by his partner's hostility and may worry that she is becoming insane, or be baffled by her mood swings and lack of concern

MEDIALINK

Postpartum Support

Table 38–11   PRIMARY PREVENTION STRATEGIES FOR POSTPARTUM DEPRESSION

1. Celebrate childbirth but appreciate that it is a life-changing transition that can be stressful—at times it can seem overwhelming. Share your feelings with each other and/or others.

2. Consider keeping a journal where you write down feelings. Not only is it emotionally cathartic, it provides a great memory book.

3. Appreciate that you do not have to know everything to be a good parent—it is okay to seek advice during this transition.

4. Connect to others who are parents—use them as a support and information network.

5. Set a daily schedule and follow it even if you do not feel like it. Structuring activity helps counteract inertia that comes with feeling sad or unsettled.

6. Prioritize daily tasks. Decide what must be done and what can wait. Try to get one major thing done every day. Remember, you do not always have to look like a magazine fashion model.

7. Remember that you do not have to entertain or care for everyone who drops by. Doing something for someone else, however, often tends to make you feel better.

8. If someone volunteers to help you with tasks or baby care, take them up on it. While your volunteer is in action, do something pleasurable or get some rest.

9. Maintain outside interests. Plan some time every day—even if it's just 15 minutes—to do something exclusively for "you" that is pleasurable.

10. Eat a healthful diet. Limit alcohol. Quit smoking. Get some exercise. (All of these can positively affect the immune system.)

11. Get as much sleep as possible. Rest whenever you can, such as when the baby is napping. If you have other young children, bring them onto your bed to read or play quietly while you lie down.

12. Limit major changes (moves, job changes, etc.) the first year insofar as possible.

13. Spend time with others.

14. If things get overwhelming, and you feel yourself slipping into depression, reach out to someone for help.

15. Attend a postpartum support group if one is available. Consider also an international program:

SOURCE: From Postpartum Support International (PSI) Copyright © PSI. Reprinted with permission.

about herself, the newborn, or household responsibilities. He may be troubled by their lack of intimacy or deteriorating communication. Certainly, he has cause for concern about how the newborn and any other children are being affected. There may be very real practical matters to handle—running the household; managing the children, including the totally dependent newborn; and caring for the mother—added to his usual routines and work responsibilities. It is not surprising that even in the most supportive families, relationships may suffer in response to these circumstances. It is often a family member who in desperation makes contact with the healthcare agency. This is especially difficult when the mother is reluctant to admit she is suffering emotional difficulty or is too ill to recognize her own needs. The integration of the newborn into the family and care of the newborn and other children can be further compromised by co-occurrent postpartum depression in fathers. An examination of research studies citing incidences of paternal postpartum depression indicates 24% to 50% incidence of depression among men whose partners were experiencing postpartum depression (Goodman, 2004b).

Information, emotional support, and assistance in providing or obtaining care for the infant may be needed. The nurse can assist family members by identifying community resources and making referrals to public health nursing services and social services. Postpartum follow-up is especially important, as well as visits from a psychiatric home health nurse.

Evaluation

Expected outcomes of nursing care include:

- The woman's signs of depression are identified and she receives therapy quickly.

- The newborn is cared for effectively by the father or another support person until the mother is able to provide care.

- The mother and newborn will remain safe.

- The newborn is integrated into the family.

CHAPTER REVIEW

FOCUS YOUR STUDY

- Nursing assessment and intervention play a large role in preventing postpartum complications.

- The main causes of early postpartal hemorrhage are uterine atony, lacerations of the vagina and cervix, and retained placental fragments. Late postpartum hemorrhage most

often originates from retained placental fragments and, though not usually as catastrophic as early hemorrhage, may require readmission.

- The most common postpartal infection is metritis, which is limited to the uterine cavity.

- A postpartal woman is at increased risk for developing urinary tract problems because of normal postpartal diuresis, increased bladder capacity, decreased bladder sensitivity from stretching or trauma, and, possibly inhibited neural control of the bladder following the use of anesthetic agents.

- Mastitis is an inflammation of the breast often caused by *Staphylococcus aureus, Escherichia coli,* and *Streptococcus* species. Mastitis is seen primarily in breastfeeding women. Symptoms seldom occur before the second to fourth postpartal week. Continuation of breastfeeding is recommended as part of the treatment plan.

- Thromboembolic disease originating in the veins of the leg, thigh, or pelvis may occur antepartally or postpartally and carries with it the potential for creating a life-threatening pulmonary embolus.

- Although many different types of psychiatric problems may be encountered in the postpartal period, postpartum blues is the most common. Postpartum blues episodes occur frequently in the week after birth, are associated with hormonal fluctuations, and are typically transient.

- Risk factors for postpartum depression should be screened for during each trimester of pregnancy and during the immediate postpartum period. Nurses should be alert to the risk of suicide and infanticide in cases of severe postpartum depression or psychosis.

- Telephone calls and home visits are effective measures for extending comprehensive care into the home setting of the postpartal family at risk. Support groups in which child care is available also can be an invaluable community service by professional nurses.

EXPLORE MediaLink

http://www.prenhall.com/davidson

NCLEX review questions, case studies, and other interactive resources for this chapter can be found on the Web Site at http://www.prenhall.com/davidson. Click on "Chapter 38" to select the activities for this chapter.

For tutorials including animations and videos, more NCLEX review questions, and an audio glossary, access the accompanying Prentice Hall Nursing MediaLink DVD-ROM in this book.

PRENTICE HALL NURSING MEDIALINK DVD-ROM

Audio Glossary

NCLEX Review

COMPANION WEBSITE

Additional NCLEX Review

Case Study: *Postpartal Thromboembolic Disease*

Care Plan Activity: *Postpartal Perineal Pain*

Applications: *Postpartum Hemorrhage; Caring for the Client with Mastitis*

Critical Thinking

CRITICAL THINKING IN ACTION

HIV-POSITIVE MOTHER AND INFANT: SUPPORTIVE CARE

View the Critical Thinking in Action video in Chapter 38 of the DVD-ROM. Then answer the questions that follow.

Betty Jones, a 32-year-old G4 P2012, is admitted to the postpartum unit after a precipitous birth of a preterm (35 weeks' gestation) 1814-g baby girl followed by a postpartum tubal ligation. Betty's vital signs and postpartum assessment are within

normal limits. She has an abdominal dressing, which is dry and intact, and she is able to void. Her IV with 10 units of Pitocin is infusing well in her lower left arm. She admits to 3 on a pain scale of 10. Betty admits to active use of crack cocaine throughout her pregnancy, and smoked it most recently 5 hours before she gave birth. She is HIV positive with a CD4 count of 726 cells/mm^3 and was treated with zidovudine during the pregnancy, labor, and birth. She also has a history of genital herpes and had been treated for chlamydia during the pregnancy. Her infant has been admitted to the special care nursery because of her preterm status. Betty anticipates her baby will be taken into foster care when discharged from the nursery. Wishing to establish as much of a relationship with her infant as possible before that happens, she asks if she can breastfeed the baby while she is in the hospital.

1. What is your response to Betty's request to breastfeed her infant?

2. Over the course of the first postpartum day, Betty appears lethargic and spends most of her time sleeping. After her evening visitors leave, you observe that she is highly energetic and excitable. Would urine testing be useful to help determine if Betty has used cocaine this evening?

3. Discuss supportive nursing care for infants born of HIV-positive mothers.

4. Betty wishes for an early discharge from the hospital. What physical criteria must be met before leaving the hospital?

5. Discuss when she should contact her physician or CNM after her discharge.

REFERENCES

American Psychiatric Association (APA). (2000). *Diagnostic and statistical manual of mental disorders: DSM-IV-TR* (4th ed.). Washington, DC: Author.

Aronson, M. P., Chelmow, D., & Lee, S. B. (2003). Intraoperative and postoperative complications of gynecologic surgery. In A. H. DeCherney & L. Nathan (Eds.), *Current obstetrics & gynecologic: Diagnosis & treatment* (9th ed., pp. 838–855). New York: Lange Medical Books/McGraw-Hill.

Beck, C. T. (1993). Teetering on the edge: A substantive theory of postpartum depression. *Nursing Research, 42*(1), 42–48.

Beck, C. T. (2002). Revision of the postpartum depression predictors inventory. *Journal of Obstetric, Gynecologic, & Neonatal Nursing, 31*(4), 394–402.

Beck, C. T. (2006). Postpartum depression: It isn't just the blues. *American Journal of Nursing, 106*(5), 40–51.

Beck, C. T., & Indman, P. (2005). The many faces of postpartum depression. *Journal of Obstetric, Gynecologic, Neonatal Nursing, 34*(5), 569–576.

Betzold, C. M. (2005). Infections of the mammary ducts in the breastfeeding mother. *Journal for Nurse Practitioners, 1*(1), 15–22.

Chaudron, L. H., Szilagyi, P. G., Kitzman, H. J., Wadkins, H. I. M., & Conwell, Y. (2004). Detection of postpartum depressive symptoms by screening at well-child visits. *Pediatrics, 113*(3, Pt. 1), 551–558.

Corwin, E. J., Brownstead, J., Barton, N., Heckard, S., & Merin, K. (2005). The impact of fatigue on the development of postpartum depression. *Journal of Obstetric, Gynecologic, & Neonatal Nursing, 34*(5), 577–586.

Crowther, M., & McCourt, K. (2005). Venous thrombolism: A guide to prevention and treatment. *The Nurse Practitioner, 30*(8), 26–29, 32–34, 45.

Cunningham, F. G., Gant, N. F., Leveno, K. J., Gilstrap, L. C., III, Hauth, J. C., & Wenstrom, K. D. (2005). *Williams obstetrics* (22nd ed.). New York: McGraw-Hill.

Doyle, N. M., & Monga, M. (2004). Thromboembolic disease in pregnancy. *Obstetrics and Gynecology Clinics of North America, 31*, 319–344.

Gibbs, R. S., Sweet, R. L., & Duff, W. P. (2004). Maternal and fetal infectious disorders. In R. K. Creasy & R. Resnik (Eds.), *Maternal-fetal medicine: Principles and practice* (5th ed., pp. 741–800). Philadelphia: Saunders.

Gilbert, E. S., & Harmon, J. S. (2003). *Manual of high risk pregnancy and delivery* (3rd ed.). St. Louis, MO: Mosby.

Goodman, J. H. (2004a). Paternal postpartum depression, its relationship to maternal postpartum depression, and implications for family health. *Journal of Advanced Nursing, 45*(1), 26–35.

Goodman, J. H. (2004b). Postpartum depression beyond the early postpartum period. *Journal of Obstetric, Gynecologic, & Neonatal Nursing, 33*(4), 410–420.

Hager, W. D. (2004). Managing mastitis. *Contemporary OB/GYN, 49*, 33–47.

Hanna, B., Jarman, H., & Savage, S. (2004). The clinical application of three screening tools for recognizing post-partum depression. *International Journal of Nursing Practice, 10*(2), 72–79.

Huang, C., Carter, P. A., & Guo, J. (2004). A comparison of sleep and daytime sleepiness in depressed and non-depressed mothers during the early postpartum period. *Journal of Nursing Research, 12*(4), 287–295.

Laros, R. K. (2004). Thromboembolic disease. In R. K. Creasy & R. Resnik (Eds.), *Maternal-fetal medicine: Principles and practice* (5th ed., pp. 845–857). Philadelphia: Saunders.

Lockwood, C. J. (2002). Inherited thrombophilias in pregnant patients: Detection and treatment paradigm. *American College of Obstetrics and Gynecology, 99*(2), 333–341.

Mass, S. (2004). Breast pain: Engorgement, nipple pain and mastitis. *Clinical Obstetrics and Gynecology, 47*(3), 676–682.

Minkoff, H. L., & Gibbs, R. S. (2003). Obstetric and perinatal infections. In J. R. Scott, R. S. Gibbs, B. Y. Karlan, & A. F. Haney (Eds.), *Danforth's obstetrics and gynecology* (9th ed., pp. 339–364). Philadelphia: Lippincott Williams & Wilkins.

Newton, E. R. (2003). Antibiotics in maternal-fetal medicine. In J. J. Sciarri (Ed.), *Gynecology and obstetrics* (Vol. 3, pp. 1–34). Philadelphia: Lippincott Williams & Wilkins.

Ornan, D., White, E., Pollak, J., & Tal, M. (2003). Pelvic embolization for intractable postpartum hemorrhage: Long-term follow-up and implications for fertility. *American College of Obstetrics and Gynecology, 102*(5), 904–910.

Paidas, M. J., De-Hui, W. K., & Arkel, Y. S. (2004). Screening and management of inherited thrombophilias in the setting of adverse pregnancy outcomes. *Clinics in Perinatology, 31*, 783–805.

Parry, B. L. (2004). Management of depression and psychoses during pregnancy and the puerperium. In R. K. Creasy & R. Resnik (Eds.), *Maternal-fetal medicine: Principles and practice* (5th ed., pp. 1193–1200). Philadelphia: Saunders.

Poggi, S. B. H., & Kapernick, P. S. (2003). Postpartum hemorrhage & the abnormal puerperium. In A. H. DeCherney & L. Nathan (Eds.), *Current obstetrics & gynecologic: Diagnosis & treatment* (9th ed., pp. 531–552). New York: Lange Medical Books/McGraw-Hill.

Poole, J. H., & White, D. (2005). *Obstetrical emergencies for the perinatal nurse* (2nd ed.). White Plains, NY: March of Dimes.

Rebarker, A., & Roman, A. S. (2003, March). Seven ways to control postpartum hemorrhage. *Contemporary OB/GYN, 34*–41.

Reid, G., & Bocking, A. (2003). The potential for probiotics to prevent bacterial vaginosis and preterm labor. *American Journal of Obstetrics & Gynecology, 189*(4), 1202–1208.

Shevell, T., & Malone, F. D. (2003). Management of obstetrical hemorrhage. *Seminars in Perinatology, 27*(1), 86–104.

Yip, S. K., Shota, D., Pang, M. W., & Day, L. (2005). Postpartum urinary retention. *Obstetrics and Gynecology, 106*(3), 602–606.

Zajac, P. M. (2004). Going with the flow: Warfarin. *Nursing Made Incredibly Easy, 2*(4), 52–57.

APPENDICES

APPENDIX A

Common Abbreviations in Maternal-Newborn and Women's Health Nursing

AC	Abdominal circumference		CPD	Cephalopelvic disproportion *or* Citrate-phosphate-dextrose
accel	Acceleration of fetal heart rate		CRL	Crown-rump length
AFAFP	Amniotic fluid alpha-fetoprotein		CRNP	Certified registered nurse practitioner
AFI	Amniotic fluid index		C/S	Cesarean section (or C-section)
AFP	Alpha-fetoprotein		CST	Contraction stress test
AFV	Amniotic fluid volume		CT	Chlamydia
AGA	Average for gestational age		CVA	Costovertebral angle
AI	Amnioinfusion		CVS	Chorionic villus sampling
AMOL	Active management of labor		D&C	Dilatation and curettage
AOP	Apnea of prematurity *or* Anemia of prematurity		D&E	Dilatation and evacuation
ARBOW	Artificial rupture of bag of waters		decels	Deceleration of fetal heart rate
AROM	Artificial rupture of membranes		DFMR	Daily fetal movement response
ART	Artificial reproductive technology		dil	Dilatation
BAT	Brown adipose tissue (brown fat)		DTR	Deep tendon reflexes
BBOW	Bulging bag of water		DV	Domestic violence
BBT	Basal body temperature		EAB	Elective abortion
BL	Baseline (fetal heart rate baseline)		ECMO	Extracorporal membrane oxygenator
BOW	Bag of waters		EDB	Estimated date of birth
β-hCG	Beta-human chorionic gonadotropin		EDC	Estimated date of confinement
BPD	Biparietal diameter *or* Bronchopulmonary dysplasia		EDD	Estimated date of delivery
BPP	Biophysical profile		EFM	Electronic fetal monitoring
BRB	Bright red bleeding *or* Breakthrough bleeding		EFW	Estimated fetal weight
BR CA	Breast cancer		EIA	Enzyme immunoassay
BSE	Breast self-examination		ELF	Elective low forceps
BSST	Breast self-stimulation test		ELISA	Enzyme-linked immunosorbent assay
CC	Chest circumference *or* Cord compression		EP	Ectopic pregnancy
CEI	Continuous epidural infusion		epis	Episiotomy
C–H	Crown-to-heel length		FAD	Fetal activity diary
CID	Cytomegalic inclusion disease		FAE	Fetal alcohol effects
CLD	Chronic lung disease		FAS	Fetal alcohol syndrome
CM	Certified midwife		FBD	Fibrocystic breast disease
CMV	Cytomegalovirus		FBM	Fetal breathing movements
CNM	Certified nurse-midwife		FBS	Fetal blood sample *or* Fasting blood sugar test
CNP	Certified nurse practitioner		FCC	Family-centered care
CNS	Clinical nurse specialist		FECG	Fetal electrocardiogram
CP	Chest pain		FeSO$_4$	Ferrous sulfate (iron supplement)
CPAP	Continuous positive airway pressure		FHR	Fetal heart rate

FHT	Fetal heart tones	**LBW**	Low birth weight
Fhx	Family history	**LDR**	Labor, delivery, and recovery room
FL	Femur length	**LGA**	Large for gestational age
FMC	Fetal movement count	**LH**	Luteinizing hormone
FMR	Fetal movement record	**LHRH**	Luteinizing hormone-releasing hormone
FPG	Fasting plasma glucose test	**LMA**	Left-mentum-anterior
FSE	Fetal scalp electrode	**LML**	Left mediolateral (episiotomy)
FSH	Follicle-stimulating hormone	**LMP**	Last menstrual period *or* Left-mentum-posterior
FSHRH	Follicle-stimulating hormone-releasing hormone	**LMT**	Left-mentum-transverse
FSPO$_2$	Fetal arterial oxygen saturation	**LOA**	Left-occiput-anterior
G or grav	Gravida	**LOF**	Low outlet forceps
GC	Gonorrhea	**LOP**	Left-occiput-posterior
GDM	Gestational diabetes mellitus	**LOS**	Length of stay
GIFT	Gamete intrafallopian transfer	**LOT**	Left-occiput-transverse
GnRF	Gonadotropin-releasing factor	**L/S**	Lecithin/sphingomyelin ratio
GnRH	Gonadotropin-releasing hormone	**LSA**	Left-sacrum-anterior
GTD	Gestational trophoblastic disease	**LSP**	Left-sacrum-posterior
GTPAL	Gravida, term, preterm, abortion, living children; a system of recording maternity history	**LST**	Left-sacrum-transverse
		MAS	Meconium aspiration syndrome
HA	Head-abdominal ratio or headache	**mec**	Meconium
HAI	Hemagglutination-inhibition test	**mec st**	Meconium stain
HC	Head compression	**MLE**	Midline episiotomy
hCG	Human chorionic gonadotropin	**MSAFP**	Maternal serum alpha-fetoprotein
hCS	Human chorionic somatomammotropin (same as hPL)	**MUGB**	4-methylumbelliferyl quanidinobenzoate
		multip	Multipara
HIV	Human immunodeficiency virus	**NEC**	Necrotizing enterocolitis
HMD	Hyaline membrane disease	**NGU**	Nongonococcal urethritis
hMG	Human menopausal gonadotropin	**NP**	Nurse practitioner
hPL	Human placental lactogen	**NSCST**	Nipple stimulation contraction stress test
HPV	Human papilloma virus	**NST**	Nonstress test *or* Nonshivering thermogenesis
HRT	Hormone replacement therapy		
HSV	Herpes simplex virus	**NSVD**	Normal sterile vaginal delivery
ICSI	Intracytoplasmic sperm injection	**NTD**	Neural tube defect
IDM	Infant of a diabetic mother	**NTE**	Neutral thermal environment
IPG	Impedance phlebography	**OA**	Occiput anterior
ISAM	Infant of a substance-abusing mother	**OC**	Oral contraceptive
IU	International units	**OCPs**	Oral contraceptive pills
IUD	Intrauterine device	**OCT**	Oxytocin challenge test
IUFD	Intrauterine fetal death	**OF**	Occipitofrontal diameter of fetal head
IUGR	Intrauterine growth restriction	**OFC**	Occipitofrontal circumference
IUPC	Intrauterine pressure catheter	**OGTT**	Oral glucose tolerance test
IUS	Intrauterine system	**OM**	Occipitomental (diameter)
IVF	In vitro fertilization	**OP**	Occiput posterior
LADA	Left-acromion-dorsal-anterior	**p**	Para
LADP	Left-acromion-dorsal-posterior	**Pap smear**	Papanicolaou smear
LBC	Lamellar body count	**PCA**	Patient-controlled analgesia

PDA	Patent ductus arteriosus	**SMB**	Submentobregmatic diameter
PEEP	Positive end-expiratory pressure	**SOB**	Suboccipitobregmatic diameter *or* Shortness of breath
PG	Phosphatidylglycerol *or* Prostaglandin	**SPA**	Sperm penetration assay
PID	Pelvic inflammatory disease	**SRBOW**	Spontaneous rupture of bag of waters
Pit	Pitocin	**SROM**	Spontaneous rupture of membranes
PKU	Phenylketonuria	**STD**	Sexually transmitted disease
PMS	Premenstrual syndrome	**STI**	Sexually transmitted infection
PNV	Prenatal vitamins	**STS**	Serologic test for syphilis
PPHN	Persistent pulmonary hypertension	**SVE**	Sterile vaginal examination
Premie	Premature infant	**TAB**	Therapeutic abortion
primip	Primipara	**TC**	Thoracic circumference
PROM	Premature rupture of membranes	**TCM**	Transcutaneous monitoring
PSI	Prostaglandin synthesis inhibitor	**TDI or THI**	Therapeutic donor insemination (*H* designates mate is donor)
PUBS	Percutaneous umbilical blood sampling	**TET**	Tubal embryo transfer
RADA	Right-acromion-dorsal-anterior	**TOL**	Trial of labor
RADP	Right-acromion-dorsal-posterior	**TORCH**	Toxoplasmosis, rubella, cytomegalovirus, herpesvirus hominis type 2
RDS	Respiratory distress syndrome		
REM	Rapid eye movements	**TSS**	Toxic shock syndrome
RIA	Radioimmunoassay	**u**	Umbilicus
RLF	Retrolental fibroplasia	**UA**	Uterine activity
RMA	Right-mentum-anterior	**UAC**	Umbilical artery catheter
RMP	Right-mentum-posterior	**UAU**	Uterine activity units
RMT	Right-mentum-transverse	**UC**	Uterine contraction
ROA	Right-occiput-anterior	**UPI**	Uteroplacental insufficiency
ROM	Rupture of membranes	**US**	Ultrasound
ROP	Right-occiput-posterior *or* Retinopathy of prematurity	**VBAC**	Vaginal birth after cesarean
		VDRL	Venereal Disease Research Laboratories
ROT	Right-occiput-transverse	**VIP**	Voluntary interruption of pregnancy
RRA	Radioreceptor assay	**VLBW**	Very low birth weight
RSA	Right-sacrum-anterior	**VVC**	Vulvovaginal candidiasis
RSP	Right-sacrum-posterior	**WIC**	Special Supplemental Nutrition Program for Women, Infants, and Children
RST	Right-sacrum-transverse		
SAB	Spontaneous abortion	**ZIFT**	Zygote intrafallopian transfer
SET	Surrogate embryo transfer		
SGA	Small for gestational age		
SIDS	Sudden infant death syndrome		

APPENDIX B

Conversions and Equivalents

TEMPERATURE CONVERSION

(Fahrenheit temperature − 32) × 5/9 = Centigrade temperature
(Centigrade temperature × 9/5) + 32 = Fahrenheit temperature

SELECTED CONVERSION TO METRIC MEASURES

Known Value	Multiply by	To find
inches	2.54	centimeters
ounces	28	grams
pounds	454	grams
pounds	0.45	kilogram

SELECTED CONVERSION FROM METRIC MEASURES

Known Value	Multiply by	To find
centimeters	0.4	inches
grams	0.035	ounces
grams	0.0022	pounds
kilograms	2.2	pounds

CONVERSION OF POUNDS AND OUNCES TO GRAMS

Pounds \ Ounces	0	1	2	3	4	5	6	7	8	9	10	11	12	13	14	15
0	—	28	57	85	113	142	170	198	227	255	283	312	340	369	397	425
1	454	482	510	539	567	595	624	652	680	709	737	765	794	822	850	879
2	907	936	964	992	1021	1049	1077	1106	1134	1162	1191	1219	1247	1276	1304	1332
3	1361	1389	1417	1446	1474	1503	1531	1559	1588	1616	1644	1673	1701	1729	1758	1786
4	1814	1843	1871	1899	1928	1956	1984	2013	2041	2070	2098	2126	2155	2183	2211	2240
5	2268	2296	2325	2353	2381	2410	2438	2466	2495	2523	2551	2580	2608	2637	2665	2693
6	2722	2750	2778	2807	2835	2863	2892	2920	2948	2977	3005	3033	3062	3090	3118	3147
7	3175	3203	3232	3260	3289	3317	3345	3374	3402	3430	3459	3487	3515	3544	3572	3600
8	3629	3657	3685	3714	3742	3770	3799	3827	3856	3884	3912	3941	3969	3997	4026	4054
9	4082	4111	4139	4167	4196	4224	4252	4281	4309	4337	4366	4394	4423	4451	4479	4508
10	4536	4564	4593	4621	4649	4678	4706	4734	4763	4791	4819	4848	4876	4904	4933	4961
11	4990	5018	5046	5075	5103	5131	5160	5188	5216	5245	5273	5301	5330	5358	5386	5415
12	5443	5471	5500	5528	5557	5585	5613	5642	5670	5698	5727	5755	5783	5812	5840	5868
13	5897	5925	5953	5982	6010	6038	6067	6095	6123	6152	6180	6209	6237	6265	6294	6322
14	6350	6379	6407	6435	6464	6492	6520	6549	6577	6605	6634	6662	6690	6719	6747	6776
15	6804	6832	6860	6889	6917	6945	6973	7002	7030	7059	7087	7115	7144	7172	7201	7228
16	7257	7286	7313	7342	7371	7399	7427	7456	7484	7512	7541	7569	7597	7626	7654	7682
17	7711	7739	7768	7796	7824	7853	7881	7909	7938	7966	7994	8023	8051	8079	8108	8136
18	8165	8192	8221	8249	8278	8306	8335	8363	8391	8420	8448	8476	8504	8533	8561	8590
19	8618	8646	8675	8703	8731	8760	8788	8816	8845	8873	8902	8930	8958	8987	9015	9043
20	9072	9100	9128	9157	9185	9213	9242	9270	9298	9327	9355	9383	9412	9440	9469	9497
21	9525	9554	9582	9610	9639	9667	9695	9724	9752	9780	9809	9837	9865	9894	9922	9950
22	9979	10007	10036	10064	10092	10120	10149	10177	10206	10234	10262	10291	10319	10347	10376	10404

APPENDIX C

Spanish Translations of English Phrases*

This appendix includes phrases you might find helpful in working with families during pregnancy, labor, and birth, and after the birth. There are many ways to phrase questions. We have chosen some statements we consider essential and have tried to phrase them in a straightforward way. The phrases are designed to help you in situations in which translation is not possible at the moment.

This list begins with introductory statements, which are presented in a logical conversational flow. The remaining phrases are arranged according to the phases of pregnancy and birth during which they are most applicable.

Essential Introductory Phrases

Hello
I am a nurse.
I am a student nurse.
My name is _____.
What is your name?

What name should I call you?

Thank you
Please
Is someone here with you?
Does he (she) speak English?
Goodbye

Frases Introductoras Esenciales

Hola
Soy enfermera (enfermero).[†]
Soy estudiante de enfermería.
Mi nombre es _____.
Me llamo _____.
¿Cuál es su nombre?
¿Cómo se llama?
¿Cómo quiere que la llamemos?
¿Cómo quiere ser llamada?
Gracias
Por favor
¿Hay alquien aquí con usted?
¿Habla él (ella) inglés?
Adiós

Phrases for the Antepartal Period

Are you taking any medications now?
Show me the medicine bottles please.
Have you ever had trouble with your blood pressure?
When was the first day of your last period?

Have you had any spotting or bleeding since your last period?
Have you been on birth control pills?
When did you stop taking them?
Do you have an intrauterine device (IUD)?
How many times have you been pregnant?
Are you having any problems with your pregnancy?
Is there anything that is worrying you?
I would like to take your blood pressure.
I would like to take your pulse.
I would like to take your temperature.
I would like to listen to your heart and lungs.
I would like to check your uterus.
Please urinate in this cup and leave it in the bathroom.
Please stand up.
Please sit down.
Please lie down.

Frases para el Periodo Prenatal

¿Está tomando algunas medicinas ahora?
Por favor, muéstreme los frascos.
¿Ha tenido problemas alguna vez con la presión arterial?
¿Cuál fue el primer día de su última regla?
¿Cuál fue el primer día de su última menstruación?
¿Ha sangrado o ha tenido manchas de sangre desde su última regla?
¿Ha estado tomando píldoras anticonceptivas?
¿Cuándo dejó de tomarlas?
¿Usa un aparato intrauterino?
¿Cuántas veces ha estado usted embarazada?
¿Tiene problemas con su embarazo?
¿Hay algo o alguna cosa que la preocupe?
Quisiera tomarle la presió arterial.
Quisiera tomarle el pulso.
Quisiera tomarle la temperatura.
Quisiera escucharle el corazon y los pulmones.
Quisiera examinarle el útero.
Puede orinar en este vaso y dejarlo en el baño.
Por favor, levántese.
Por favor, siéntese.
Por favor, acuéstese.

*Prepared by Elizabeth Medina, Ph.D., Associate Professor of Spanish, Regis University, Denver, Colorado.

†In Spanish, nouns that end in *a* indicate female gender; nouns that end in *o* indicate male gender.

Phrases Related to Client Safety

I would like to talk to you alone.
Are you safe at home?
Are you afraid of your partner?
During your pregnancy, has your partner hit, slapped, kicked, or punched you?

How many times?
Do you have someone for support?

Questions the Mother or Father May Ask

How big is my baby?
How much does the baby weigh now?
When will I feel my baby move?

Phrases for the Intrapartal Period

Note: Review the essential introductory phrases for beginning a conversation.
Are you having labor pains?
Are you having contractions?
Are you having pain?
Do you need medicine for pain?
Do you need to urinate?
This is a bedpan to urinate in.
Can I help you to the bathroom?
Do you need to have a bowel movement?

Has your bag of water broken?
Have you had any bright-red bleeding during your pregnancy?
How many births have you had?
I need to do a vaginal examination.
I will help you.
I will stay with you.
Please pant. I will show you how.
Do not push now.
Push now.
Stop pushing.

The doctor needs to do a cesarean birth.
This is medicine for your pain. You will feel better soon.
When is your baby supposed to be born?
January
February
March
April
May
June
July
August
September
October
November
December
What is your doctor's name?

Frases Relacionadas con la Seguridad del Cliente

Quisiera hablar a solas con usted.
¿Sufre de peligros en casa?
¿Le tiene miedo a su compañero?
Durante su embarazo,
¿la ha golpeado?
¿la ha abofeteado?
¿la ha pateado? o
¿le ha dado puñetazos?
¿Cuántas veces?
¿Cuénta con alguien que la pueda ayudar?

Posibles Preguntas que Madres o Padres Hacen

¿De qué tamaño es el (la) bebé?
¿Cuánto pesa el bebé ahora?
¿Cuándo lo (la) voy a sentir moverse?

Frases Durante el Parto

Nota: Repase las frases introductoras para comenzar una conversación.
¿Tiene dolores de parto?
¿Tiene contracciones?
¿Tiene dolores?
¿Necesita medicina para el dolor?
¿Necesita orinar?
Aquí tiene el bacín (la chata) (el pato) para orinar.
¿La ayudo a ir al baño?
¿Necesita mover el vientre (obrar)? Necesita "Hacer caca"— coloquial
¿Se le ha roto la bolsa de agua(s)?
¿Ha tenido algún sangramiento de color rojo durante su embarazo?
¿Cuántos niños le han nacido?
Necesito hacerle un examen vaginal.
La voy a ayudar.
Me quedaré con usted.
Por favor, jadee. Le voy a mostrar cómo.
No puje ahora.
Puje ahora.
Pare de pujar.
No puje más.
El doctor le va a hacer una operación cesárea.
Esta medicina es para el dolor. Va a sentirse mejor pronto.
¿Cuando está supuesto a nacer el bebé?
enero
febrero
marzo
abril
mayo
junio
julio
agosto
septiembre
octubre
noviembre
diciembre
¿Cuál es el nombre de su doctor?

What is your midwife's name?	¿Cuál es el nombre de su comadrona (partera)?
Your baby is having some trouble now.	El bebé está pasando por algunos problemas.
	El bebé está sufriendo algunas dificultades.
I need to put this oxygen mask on you. It will help your baby. It may smell funny, but it is OK.	Le voy a poner esta máscara de oxígeno.
	Va a ayudar al bebé.
	Huele extraño, pero no hay problemas.
Please turn on your left side.	Por favor voltéese al lado izquierdo.
Please turn on your right side.	Por favor voltéese al lado derecho.
Your baby is OK.	El bebé está bien.

Phrases for the Postpartal Period and the Newborn Area

Note: Review the essential introductory phrases for beginning a conversation.

Frases para el Periodo Despues del Parto y el Area del Recien Nacido

Nota: Repase las frases introductoras para comenzar una conversación.

Are you hungry?	¿Tiene hambre?
Are you thirsty?	¿Tiene sed?
Are you cold?	¿Tiene frío?
Are you tired?	¿Está cansada?
I am going to put antibiotic ointment in the baby's eyes.	Le voy a poner al bebé un ungüento antibiótico alrededor de los ojos.
It will help protect your baby from some infections.	Lo (la) va a proteger contra algunos infecciones.
I am going to take some blood from your baby's foot to check the blood sugar and hemocrit.	Le voy a sacar sangre del pie al bebé para determinar el azúcar de la sangre y el hematocrítico.
If your baby begins to spit up, please turn him (her) on his (her) side.	Si el bebé comienza a vomitar, colóquelo (colóquela) de costado.
It may help to position your baby like this.	Lo (la) ayudará— si lo coloca así.
	Lo (la) ayudaría—si lo colocara así.
I would like to suggest that you clean your nipples this way before you breastfeed your baby.	Es bueno que se lave los pezones de esta manera antes de darle el pecho al bebé.
It is better that you clean your baby's cord this way.	Es mejor para el bebé que le lave el ombligo de esta manera.
It is better that you bathe your baby this way.	Es mejor que lo (la) bañe de esta manera.
It is better that you clean your baby's penis this way.	Es mejor que le limpie el pene así.
I would like to suggest that you fold the diaper this way.	Le sugiero que doble el pañal así.
I would like to suggest that you fasten the diaper this way.	Le sugiero que asegure el pañal así.
Take the baby's temperature this way.	Tómele la temperatura así.
I need to check (your breasts, your uterus, your flow, your stitches, your legs and feet).	Necesito examinarle (los pechos, el útero, el flujo, los puntos, las piernas y los pies).
I need to feel your uterus.	Necesito examinarle el útero.
I need to massage your uterus.	Necesito darle un masaje en la región del útero.
Place your baby on its side.	Coloque al bebé de costado.
Place the baby's used diapers here.	Coloque aquí los pañales usados.
Please rub your uterus every half hour to keep it firm.	Necesita darse un masaje en la región del útero cada media hora para mantenerlo firme. Le voy a mostrar
I will show you how.	cómo.
Would you like to see your baby now?	¿Quiere ver a su bebé ahora?
Would you like me to help you feed your baby?	¿Quiere que le ayude a alimentarlo (la)?
Your baby needs a car seat to go home in.	El (la) bebé necesita un asiento para bebé en el automóvil.

Special Neonatal Needs

Necesidades del Recien Nacido

We are giving your baby oxygen.	Le vamos a dar oxígeno al (a la) bebé.
Your baby is having problems breathing.	El (la) bebé tiene problemas al respirar.
Your baby needs extra help.	El (la) bebé necesita ayuda especial.
Your baby needs to go to a special care nursery.	El (la) bebé necesita ir a la sala de cuidados especiales para bebés.

APPENDIX D

Guidelines for Working with Deaf Clients and Interpreters

1. First, remember that it requires trust on the part of the client to allow nonsigning caregivers and an interpreter into her life.

2. It is important to use a registered interpreter. Medical interpreters are registered with the Registry of Interpreters for the Deaf. Although family members and friends may offer to interpret, it is best to use registered medical interpreters because they are required to translate the clients' and nurses' words accurately without adding in any other opinion.

3. Greet the client and family with a handshake and body posture that indicates welcome. You may point to your name tag and use the American Sign Language (ASL) alphabet cards to spell out your name. The client may wish to select cards to indicate her name. It is especially important as you work together to make the effort to provide a greeting as you would with speaking clients; greetings help develop rapport.

4. Once the interpreter is present, continue to look at the client and speak directly to her. There will be a temptation to look at the interpreter, and it will help to remember that you are speaking to the client.

5. Avoid phrasing your words as if you are talking to the interpreter (e.g., "Can you tell her. . . ?"). Instead, phrase your questions as you do with speaking clients (e.g., "I'm going to ask you some questions now.").

6. Depend on the deaf client to ask questions.

7. Look at the client's face for signs of difficulty in understanding. Deaf clients have a behavior of "gesturing" that involves shaking their heads as if to indicate "yes" even when they do not understand. If the client is nodding "yes," ask her to repeat the directions you have just given.

8. Be as direct as possible. Keep to what you want to know or what you want to convey. Speak in short sentences, using nontechnical words. Avoid colloquial or slang words. Be sure to explain what you want to do before you do it. For instance, tell her you want to start an IV and explain the equipment. Then, with her permission, start the IV.

9. Be aware that deaf clients may have difficulty understanding when to take medications. It will be helpful to associate taking medications or completing some treatment or activity with meals. (For instance, while showing her the two capsules she is to take when she goes home, tell her to take the two capsules at breakfast and another two capsules at bedtime.) Avoid saying "take two capsules at 8:00 A.M., 2:00 P.M., and 12:00 A.M."

10. The difference in interpreting time may also affect obtaining a history. It is best to begin with a specific event in the past and work forward.

What to Do Until the Interpreter Arrives

1. Role-play as much as possible.

2. Demonstrate what you want the client to do or what you want to do.

3. Be resourceful.

4. Remember that some deaf clients can read lips. Some may read written language, but use care in assuming the client understands.

What to Do to Prepare for Working with a Deaf Client

1. Contact local agencies that work with deaf clients to see what resources are available. Ask about classes in ASL. Being able to use some basic signs will be very helpful while waiting for an interpreter to arrive.

2. Read to learn more about the deaf culture. Contact your local agency or the National Information Center on Deafness, Silver Springs, Maryland, to get suggestions on books you might read.

3. Investigate your health facility. What is available to assist you? Look for videos used for teaching in the maternal-child unit and note if they have captions. Remember that many deaf clients do not read written language, so it will be important to review the content of the video with an interpreter present.

Prepared with the kind assistance of Mr. Gerald Dement, Interpreter Coordinator, Pikes Peak Center on Deafness, Colorado Springs, Colorado.

Sign Language for Healthcare Professionals

Ache (or pain) Allergic* Bathroom

Better Congratulate (or praise) Constipate*

Dizzy Drink Faint

*Indicates signs that are in manually signed English. Those without an asterisk are in American Sign Language.

Feel

Headache

Lie down

Medicine

Name

Nauseous

No

Nurse

Pain

Please

Put on

Sick

Stay

Stomachache*

Thank you (or good)

Thirsty

Vomit

Want

Yes

APPENDIX F

Actions and Effects of Selected Drugs During Breastfeeding*

Anticoagulants

Coumarin derivatives (warfarin, dicumarol): Relatively safe to use; only small amount in breast milk; check PTT.

Heparin and derivatives (Lovenox): Does not cross into breast milk; check PTT.

Anticonvulsants

Phenytoin (Dilantin), phenobarbital: Generally considered safe; if high doses of phenobarbital are ingested, may cause drowsiness; short-acting phenobarbiturates (secobarbital) preferred, because they appear in lower concentration in milk.

Magnesium sulfate: Lactogenesis may be delayed.

Antidepressants

SSRI class:

Fluoxetine (Prozac), fluvoxamine: Effect on newborn unknown but may be of concern.

Tricyclic antidepressants (doxepin): Sedation, potential respiratory arrest in infant.

Antihistamines

Diphenhydramine (Benadryl), Claritin, Allegra: May cause decreased milk supply; infant may become drowsy or irritable.

Clemastine (Tavist): Contraindicated.

Antihypertensives

β adrenergic blockers:

Atenolol, acebutolol: Cyanosis.

Tenormin: Hypotension, bradycardia.

Antimetabolites

Unknown, probably long-term anti-DNA effect on the infant; potentially very toxic.

Antimicrobials

Aminoglycosides: May cause ototoxicity or nephrotoxicity if given for more than 2 weeks.

Ampicillin: Skin rash, candidiasis; diarrhea.

Azithromycin: No risk to newborn.

Chloramphenicol (rarely used): Possible bone marrow suppression; too low a dose for Gray syndrome; refusal of breast.

Erythromycin: Accumulates in breast milk, idiopathic hypertrophic pyloric stenosis.

Methacycline: Possible inhibition of bone growth; may cause discoloration of the teeth; use should be avoided.

Metronidazole (Flagyl): Possible neurologic disorders or blood dyscrasias; delay breastfeeding for 12 hours after dose.

Penicillin: Possible allergic response; candidiasis.

Quinolones (synthetic antibiotics): Can cause arthropathies.

Sulfonamides: May cause hyperbilirubinemia; use contraindicated until infant is over 1 week old.

Tetracycline: Long-term use and large doses should be avoided; may cause tooth staining or inhibition of bone growth.

Antithyroids

Thiouracil: Contraindicated during lactation; may cause goiter or agranulocytosis.

Propylthiouracil: Safe; monitor infant thyroid function.

Barbiturates

Phenothiazines: May produce sedation.

Bronchodilators

Aminophylline: May cause insomnia or irritability in the infant.

Leukotriene inhibitors (Zyflo, Accolate): Potential tumorigenicity.

Caffeine

Excessive consumption may cause jitteriness or wakefulness.

Cardiovascular

Clonidine (Catapres): Reduces milk volume.

Methyldopa: Increases milk volume.

Propranolol (Inderal): May cause hypoglycemia; possibility of other blocking effects, especially if infant has renal or liver dysfunction.

Quinidine: May cause arrhythmias in infant.

Reserpine (Serpasil): Nasal stuffiness, lethargy, or diarrhea in infant.

Corticosteroids

Adrenal suppression may occur with long-term administration of doses greater than 20 mg/day.

Diuretics

Furosemide (Lasix): Not excreted in breast milk.

Thiazide diuretics (Esidrix, HydroDIURIL, Oretic): Safe but can cause dehydration, reduce milk production.

*Based on data from Riordan, J., & Auerbach, K. J. (2005). *Breastfeeding and human lactation* (3rd ed., pp. 146–166). Boston: Jones & Bartlett; Briggs, G. G., Freeman, R. K., & Yaffe, S. J. (2005). *Drugs in pregnancy and lactation* (7th ed.). Baltimore: Williams & Wilkins; Hale, T. (2004). *Medications and mothers' milk* (11th ed.). Amarillo, TX: Pharmasoft Publishing; Committee on Drugs, American Academy of Pediatrics. (2001). The transfer of drugs and other chemicals into human milk. *Pediatrics, 108* (3), 776.

Heavy Metals

Gold: Potentially toxic; gold salts—compatible with breastfeeding.

Lead: Excreted in breast milk; high maternal levels can affect neuropsychologic development.

Mercury: Excreted in the milk and hazardous to infant.

Hormones

Androgens: Suppress lactation.

Thyroid hormones: May mask hypothyroidism.

Laxatives

Peri-Colace, Dulcolax: Relatively safe.

Milk of magnesia, Metamucil: Relatively safe.

Narcotic analgesics

Codeine: Accumulation may lead to neonatal depression.

Meperidine: Avoid use. May lead to neonatal depression.

Morphine: Long-term use may cause newborn addiction.

Nonnarcotic Analgesics, NSAID

Acetaminophen (Tylenol): Relatively safe for short-term analgesia.

Ibuprofen (Motrin): Safe.

Propoxyphene (Darvon): May cause sleepiness and poor breastfeeding in infant.

Salicylates (aspirin): Safe after first week of life; monitor PTT.

Oral Contraceptives

Combined estrogen/progestin pills: Significantly decrease milk supply; may alter milk composition; may cause gynecomastia in male infants.

Progestin only (DMPA, Norplant): Safe if started after lactation is established.

Radioactive Materials for Testing

Gallium citrate (67G): Insignificant amount excreted in breast milk; no breastfeeding for 2 weeks.

Iodine: Contraindicated; may affect infant's thyroid gland.

$^{125}I:$ Discontinue breastfeeding for 24 hours.

$^{131}I:$ Breastfeeding should be discontinued until excretion is no longer significant; may be resumed after 10 days.

Technetium-99m: Discontinue breastfeeding for 24 hours (half-life = 6 hours).

Sedatives/Tranquilizers

Diazepam (Valium): May accumulate to high levels; may increase neonatal jaundice; may cause lethargy, weight loss, and poor suck.

Lithium: Contraindicated; may cause neonatal flaccidity and hypotonia.

Smoking Cessation

Nicotine patch (Nicoderm, Nicotrol): Irritability, abnormal sleep patterns, poor feeding.

Bupropion (Zyban, Wellbutrin): No effect on breastfeeding.

Substance Abuse

Alcohol: Potential motor developmental delay; mild sedative effect.

Amphetamines: Controversial; may cause irritability, poor sleeping pattern.

Cocaine, crack: Extreme irritability, tachycardia, vomiting, apnea.

Marijuana: Drowsiness.

Heroin: Tremors, restlessness, vomiting, poor feeding.

Nicotine (smoking): Shock, vomiting, diarrhea, decreased milk production.

APPENDIX G

Selected Maternal-Newborn Laboratory Values

NORMAL MATERNAL LABORATORY VALUES

Test	Nonpregnant Values	Pregnant Values
Hematocrit	37%–47%	32%–42%
Hemoglobin	12–16 g/dL**	10–14 g/dL**
Platelets	150,000–350,000/mm³	Significant increase 3–5 days after birth (predisposes to thrombosis)
Partial thromboplastin time (PTT)	12–14 seconds	Slight decrease in pregnancy and again in labor (placental site clotting)
Fibrinogen	250 mg/dL	400 mg/dL
Serum glucose		
Fasting	70–80 mg/dL	65 mg/dL
2-hour postprandial	60–110 mg/dL	Less than 140 mg/dL
Total protein	6.7–8.3 g/dL	5.5–7.5 g/dL
White blood cell total	4500–10,000/mm³	5000–15,000/mm³
Polymorphonuclear cells	54%–62%	60%–85%
Lymphocytes	38%–46%	15%–40%

**At sea level

NORMAL TERM NEONATAL CORD BLOOD LABORATORY VALUES

Test	Normal Values
Hematocrit	43%–63%*
Hemoglobin	14–20 g/dL
Platelets	150,000–350,000/mm³
Reticulocyte	3%–7%
White blood cell total	10,000–30,000/mm³
White blood cell differential	
Polymorphonuclear (segs)	40%–80%
Lymphocytes	20%–40%
Monocytes	3%–10%
Serum glucose	45–96 mg/dL*
Serum electrolytes	
Sodium	126–166 mEq/L*
Potassium	5.6–12.0 mEq/L*
Chloride	98–110 mEq/L*
Carbon dioxide	13–29 mmol/L
Bicarbonate	18–23 mEq/L
Calcium	8.2–11.1 mg/dL
Total protein	4.8–7.3 g/dL

Note: Adapted from Fanaroff, A. A., & Martin, R. J. (Eds.). (2002). *Neonatal-perinatal medicine* (7th ed.). St. Louis, MO: Mosby.

*All laboratory values are approximate. Consult your local laboratory for guidelines as to normal values.

GLOSSARY

Abdominal effleurage Gentle stroking used in massage.

Abortion Loss of pregnancy before the fetus is viable outside the uterus; miscarriage.

Abruptio placentae (ab-rŭp´shē-ō pla-sen´tē) Partial or total premature separation of a normally implanted placenta.

Abstinence Refraining voluntarily, especially from indulgence in food, alcoholic beverages, or sexual intercourse.

Acceleration Periodic increase in the baseline fetal heart rate.

Acculturation The process by which people adapt to a new cultural norm.

Acini cells Secretory cells in the human breast that create milk from nutrients in the bloodstream.

Acme Peak or highest point; time of greatest intensity (of a uterine contraction).

Acquaintance and date rape Rape in which the assailant is someone with whom the victim has had previous nonviolent interaction (acquaintance rape) or which occurs between a dating couple. Date rape is a form of acquaintance rape.

Acquired immunodeficiency syndrome (AIDS) An immunologic disorder caused by infection with the human immunodeficiency virus (HIV) and characterized by increasing susceptibility to opportunistic infections and rare cancers.

Acrocyanosis Cyanosis of the extremities.

Acrosomal reaction Breakdown of the hyaluronic acid in the corona radiata by enzymes from the heads of sperm; allows one spermatozoon to penetrate the ovum zona pellucida.

Active acquired immunity Formation of antibodies by the pregnant woman in response to illness or immunization.

Active alert state Alert state marked by an increase in facial and body movement, with periods of fussiness occurring. The infant in this state has increased sensitivity to disturbing stimuli.

Active management of labor (AMOL) Medical protocol for augmentation of labor that includes (1) a strict criterion for labor admission, (2) early amniotomy, (3) high-dose oxytocin infusion for inefficient labor contractions, and (4) a commitment to provision of continuous nursing care.

Acupressure (sometimes called *Chinese massage*) Therapy using pressure from the fingers and thumbs to stimulate pressure points.

Acupuncture Therapy using very fine (hairlike) stainless steel needles to stimulate specific acupuncture points depending on the client's medical assessment and condition.

Adequate intake (AI) A value cited for a nutrient when there are not sufficient data to calculate an estimated average requirement.

Adnexa Adjoining or accessory parts of a structure, such as the uterine adnexa: the ovaries and fallopian tubes.

Adolescence Period of human development initiated by puberty and ending with the attainment of young adulthood.

Afterbirth Placenta and membranes expelled after the birth of the infant, during the third stage of labor. Also called *secundines*.

Afterpains Cramplike pains due to contractions of the uterus that occur after childbirth. They are more common in multiparas, tend to be most severe during breastfeeding, and last 2 to 3 days.

Alcohol-related birth defect (ARBD) Birth defects and cognitive difficulties occurring in infants born to mothers who drink.

Alpha-fetoprotein (AFP) A fetal protein produced in the yolk sac for the first 6 weeks of gestation and then by the fetal liver.

Alternative therapy Any procedure or approach that is used in place of conventional medicine.

Alveoli Small units of the breast tissue in which milk is synthesized by the alveolar secretory epithelium.

Amenorrhea Suppression or absence of menstruation.

Amniocentesis Removal of amniotic fluid by insertion of a needle into the amniotic sac; amniotic fluid is used to assess fetal health or maturity.

Amnioinfusion Procedure used to infuse a sterile fluid (such as normal saline) through an intrauterine catheter into the uterus in an attempt to increase the fluid around the umbilical cord to decrease or prevent cord compression during labor contractions; also used to dilute thick meconium-stained amniotic fluid.

Amnion The inner of the two membranes that form the sac containing the fetus and the amniotic fluid.

Amnionitis Infection of the amniotic fluid.

Amniotic fluid The liquid surrounding the fetus in utero. It absorbs shocks, permits fetal movement, and prevents heat loss.

Amniotic fluid embolism Amniotic fluid that has leaked into the chorionic plate and entered the maternal circulation.

Amniotic fluid index (AFI) A method of reporting fluid volume. The AFI is calculated by dividing the maternal abdomen into four quadrants with the umbilicus as the reference point. Then the deepest vertical pocket is measured. These measurements are summed to calculate the AFI.

Amniotomy (am-nē-ot´ō -mē) The artificial rupturing of the amniotic membrane.

Ampulla The outer two-thirds of the fallopian tube; fertilization of the ovum by a spermatozoon usually occurs here.

Androgen Substance producing male characteristics, such as the male hormone testosterone.

Android pelvis Male-type pelvis.

Antepartum Time between conception and the onset of labor; usually used to describe the period during which a woman is pregnant.

Anterior fontanelle Diamond-shaped area between the two frontal and two parietal bones just above the newborn's forehead.

Anthropoid pelvis Pelvis in which the anteroposterior diameter is equal to or greater than the transverse diameter.

Apgar score A scoring system used to evaluate newborns at 1 minute and 5 minutes after birth. The total score is achieved by assessing five signs: heart rate, respiratory effort, muscle tone, reflex irritability, and color. Each of the signs is assigned a score of 0, 1, or 2. The highest possible score is 10.

Apnea A condition that occurs when respirations cease for more than 20 seconds, with generalized cyanosis.

Areola Pigmented ring surrounding the nipple of the breast.

Aromatherapy The use of certain essential oils, derived from plants, whose odor or aroma is believed to have a therapeutic effect.

Artificial rupture of membranes (AROM) Use of a device such as an amnihook or allis forceps to rupture the amniotic membranes.

Assimilation Phenomenon in which a minority group completely changes its cultural identity to become part of the majority culture.

Assisted reproductive technology (ART) Term used to describe the highly technologic approaches used to produce pregnancy.

Attachment Enduring bonds or relationship of affection between persons.

Attachment theory A framework for understanding perinatal loss that begins with the basic premise that human beings are biologically predisposed to bond with emotionally significant persons in their lives.

Attitude In perinatal care, the relationship of the fetal parts to each other.

Autosome A chromosome that is not a sex chromosome.

Ayurveda The classical system of Hindu medicine. The term *ayurveda* means the knowledge of how to live a vital, healthful life.

Babinski reflex Reflex found normally in infants under 6 months of age in which the great toe dorsiflexes when the sole of the foot is stimulated.

Bacterial vaginosis A bacterial infection of the vagina, formerly called *Gardnerella vaginalis* or *Hemophilus vaginalis,* characterized by a foul-smelling, grayish vaginal discharge that exhibits a characteristic fishy odor when 10% potassium hydroxide (KOH) is added. Microscopic examination of a vaginal wet prep reveals the presence of "clue cells" (vaginal epithelial cells coated with gram-negative organisms).

Bag of waters (BOW) The membrane containing the amniotic fluid and the fetus.

Ballottement (bal-ot-maw´) A technique of palpation to detect or examine a floating object in the body. In obstetrics, the fetus, when pushed, floats away and then returns to touch the examiner's fingers.

Barlow maneuver A test designed to detect subluxation or dislocation of the hip. A dysplastic joint will be felt to be dislocated as the femur leaves the actabulum.

Barr body Deeply staining chromatin mass located against the inner surface of the cell nucleus. It is found only in normal females. Also called *sex chromatin.*

Basal body temperature (BBT) The lowest waking temperature.

Baseline rate The average fetal heart rate observed during a 10-minute period of monitoring.

Baseline variability Changes in the fetal heart rate that result from the interplay between the sympathetic and the parasympathetic nervous systems.

Battledore placenta Placenta in which the umbilical cord is inserted on the periphery rather than centrally.

Bed sharing An infant sleeping in close social and/or physical contact with a committed caregiver (usually the mother). Also called *cosleeping.*

Bereavement To have suffered the *event* of loss.

Beta human chorionic gonadotropin (Beta hCG) A product of the trophoblast or placenta that is detected through serum testing and is a very accurate marker of the presence of pregnancy and placental health.

Bilirubin encephalopathy See *Kernicterus.*

Bimanual palpation Examination of the pelvic organs by placing one hand on the abdomen and one or two fingers of the other hand into the vagina.

Biofeedback The use of monitoring devices to help individuals learn to control their autonomic responses.

Biophysical profile (BPP) Assessment of five variables in the fetus that help to evaluate fetal risk: breathing movement, body movement, tone, amniotic fluid volume, and fetal heart rate reactivity.

Birth center A setting for labor and birth that emphasizes a family-centered approach rather than obstetric technology and treatment.

Birth defects Structural abnormalities present at birth.

Birth plan A written document prepared by the expectant parents that is used to identify available options in the birth setting.

Birthing room A room for labor and birth with a relaxed atmosphere.

Birth preference plan Decisions made by the expectant couple about aspects of the childbearing experience that are most important to them.

Birth rate Number of live births per 1000 population.

Bishop score A prelabor scoring system to assist in predicting whether an induction of labor may be successful. The total score is achieved by assessing five components: cervical dilatation, cervical effacement, cervical consistency, cervical position, and fetal station. Each of the components is assigned a score of 0 to 3, and the highest possible score is 13.

Blastocyst The inner solid mass of cells within the morula.

Bloody show Pink-tinged mucus secretions resulting from rupture of small capillaries as the cervix effaces and dilates.

Body stalk Future umbilical cord; structure that attaches the embryo to the yolk sac and contains blood vessels that extend into the chorionic villi.

Bogginess The softening of the uterus due to inadequate contraction of the muscle tissue.

Boggy uterus A term used to describe the uterine fundus when it is not firmly contracted after the birth of the baby and in the early postpartum period; excessive bleeding occurs from the placental site, and maternal hemorrhage may occur.

Bonding Process of parent-infant attachment occurring at or soon after birth.

Brachial palsy Partial or complete paralysis of portions of the arm resulting from trauma to the brachial plexus during a difficult birth.

Braxton Hicks contractions Intermittent painless contractions of the uterus that may occur every 10 to 20 minutes. They occur more frequently toward the end of pregnancy and are sometimes mistaken for true labor signs.

Brazleton's neonatal behavioral assessment A brief examination used to identify the infant's behavioral states and responses.

Breasts Mammary glands.

Breast self-examination (BSE) A manual examination conducted monthly by a woman to evaluate her own breasts for signs of masses, changes, nipple discharge, or evidence of abnormalities.

Breech presentation A birth in which the buttocks and/or feet are presented instead of the head.

Broad ligament The ligament extending from the lateral margins of the uterus to the pelvic wall; keeps the uterus centrally placed and provides stability within the pelvic cavity.

Bronchopulmonary dysplasia (BPD)/chronic lung disease of prematurity (CLD) Chronic pulmonary disease of multifactorial etiology characterized initially by alveolar and bronchial necrosis, which results in bronchial metaplasia and interstitial fibrosis. Appears in x-ray films as generalized small, radiolucent cysts within the lungs.

Brown adipose tissue (BAT) Fat deposits in newborns that provide greater heat-generating activity than ordinary fat. Found around the kidneys, adrenals, and neck; between the scapulas; and behind the sternum. Also called *brown fat.*

Calorie Amount of heat required to raise the temperature of 1 kg of water 1 degree centigrade.

Capacitation Removal of the plasma membrane overlying the spermatozoa's acrosomal area with the loss of seminal plasma proteins and the glycoprotein coat. If the glycoprotein coat is not removed, the sperm will not be able to penetrate the ovum.

Caput succedaneum (kap´ut suk_s"ĕ -dáne-um) Swelling or edema occurring in or under the fetal scalp during labor.

Cardinal ligaments The chief uterine supports, suspending the uterus from the side walls of the true pelvis.

Cardinal movements of labor The positional changes of the fetus as it moves through the birth canal during labor and birth. The positional changes are descent, flexion, internal rotation, extension, restitution, and external rotation.

Cardiopulmonary adaptation Adaptation of the newborn's cardiovascular and respiratory systems to life outside the womb.

Caring theory Consists of five attributes of the caregiver: (1) knowing, (2) being with, (3) doing for, (4) enabling, and (5) maintaining belief.

Cephalhematoma (sef´ăl-hé-mă-tōmă) Subcutaneous swelling containing blood found on the head of an infant several days after birth; it usually disappears within a few weeks to 2 months.

Cephalic presentation Birth in which the fetal head is presenting against the cervix.

Cephalopelvic disproportion (CPD) A condition in which the fetal head is of such a shape or size, or in such a position, that it cannot pass through the maternal pelvis.

Certified nurse-midwife (CNM) An RN who has received special training and education in the care of the family during childbearing and the prenatal, labor and birth, and postpartal periods. After a period of formal education, the nurse-midwife takes a certification test to become a CNM.

Certified registered nurse (RNC) A registered nurse who has shown expertise in a specific field by passing a national certification examination.

Cervical cap A cup-shaped device placed over the cervix to prevent pregnancy.

Cervical dilatation Process in which the cervical os and the cervical canal widen from less than 1 cm to approximately 10 cm, allowing birth of the fetus.

Cervical funneling A cone-shaped indentation in the cervical os which is common in cases of cervical incompetence.

Cervical ripening Softening of the cervix; occurs normally as a physiologic process before labor or is stimulated to occur through the process of induction of labor.

Cervix The "neck" between the external os and the body of the uterus. The lower end of the cervix extends into the vagina.

Cesarean birth Birth of fetus accomplished by performing a surgical incision through the maternal abdomen and uterus.

Chadwick's sign Violet bluish color of the vaginal mucous membrane caused by increased vascularity; visible from about the fourth week of pregnancy.

Chemical conjunctivitis Irritation of the mucous membrane lining of the eyelid; may be due to instillation of silver nitrate ophthalmic drops.

Child abuse Nonaccidental physical or threatened harm, including mental or emotional injury, sexual abuse, and sexual exploitation.

Child neglect Failure by parents or other custodians to meet the medical, emotional, physical, or supervisory needs of a child.

Chiropractic Third largest independent health profession found in the United States. Uses spinal manipulation to address abnormal nerve transmission (subluxation) caused by misalignment of the spine.

Chlamydial infection Caused by *Chlamydia trachomatis,* this infection is the most common bacterial sexually transmitted infection in the United States.

Chloasma (klō-az´mă) **(melasma gravidarum)** Brownish pigmentation over the bridge of the nose and the cheeks during pregnancy and in some women who are taking oral contraceptives. Also called *mask of pregnancy.*

Chorioamnionitis (kō'rē -ō-am´nē -ō-ī´tis) An inflammation of the amniotic membranes stimulated by organisms in the amniotic fluid, which then becomes infiltrated with polymorphonuclear leukocytes.

Chorion The fetal membrane closest to the intrauterine wall that gives rise to the placenta and continues as the outer membrane surrounding the amnion.

Chorionic villus sampling (CVS) Procedure in which a specimen of the chorionic villi is obtained from the edge of the developing placenta at about 8 weeks' gestation. The sample can be used for chromosomal, enzyme, and DNA tests.

Chromosomes The threadlike structures within the nucleus of a cell that carry the genes.

Circumcision Surgical removal of the prepuce (foreskin) of the penis.

Circumoral cyanosis Bluish appearance around the mouth.

Circumvallate (ser-kŭm-val´ăt) **placenta** A placenta with a thick, white fibrous ring around the edge.

Civil unions Legally recognized partnerships that involve rights and responsibilities comparable with those enjoyed by married couples. Often used by same-sex couples.

Cleavage Rapid mitotic division of the zygote; cells produced are called *blastomeres.*

Client Person seeking assistance from professionals who have the special skills and knowledge the individual lacks.

Client advocacy An approach to client care in which the nurse educates and supports the client and protects the client's rights.

Climacteric The period of time that marks the cessation of a woman's reproductive function; the "change of life," or menopause.

Clinical nurse specialist (CNS) A nurse possessing a master's degree and specialized knowledge and competence in a specific clinical area.

Clitoris Female organ homologous to the male penis; a small oval body of erectile tissue situated at the anterior junction of the vulva.

Coitus interruptus Method of contraception in which the male withdraws his penis from the vagina before ejaculation.

Cold stress Excessive heat loss resulting in compensatory mechanisms (increased respirations and nonshivering thermogenesis) to maintain core body temperature.

Colostrum (kō -los´trŭm) Secretion from the breast before the onset of true lactation; contains mainly serum and white blood corpuscles. It has a high protein content, provides some immune properties, and cleanses the newborn's intestinal tract of mucus and meconium.

Colposcopy The use of an instrument inserted into the vagina to examine the cervical and vaginal tissues by means of a magnifying lens.

Combined oral contraceptives (COCs) Commonly called birth control pills or "the pill," COCs are a form of contraception that uses a combination of a synthetic estrogen and a progestin.

Comparable worth The standard that the same wages should be paid for different types of work that require comparable skills, responsibility, education, and experience.

Complementary therapy Any procedure or product that is used together with conventional medical treatment.

Conception Union of male sperm and female ovum; fertilization.

Conceptional age The number of complete weeks since the moment of conception. Because the moment of conception is almost impossible to determine, conceptional age is estimated at 2 weeks less than gestational age.

Condom A rubber sheath that covers the penis to prevent conception or disease.

Conduction Loss of heat to a cooler surface by direct skin contact.

Condyloma (kon-di-lō'mă) Wartlike growth of skin, usually seen on the external genitals or anus. There are two types, a pointed variety and a broad, flat form usually found with syphilis.

Condylomata acuminata Known also as genital or venereal warts, they are a common sexually transmitted infection caused by the human papilloma virus (HPV).

Conjugate Important diameter of the pelvis, measured from the center of the promontory of the sacrum to the back of the symphysis pubis. The diagonal conjugate is measured and the true conjugate is estimated.

Conjugate vera The true conjugate, which extends from the middle of the sacral promontory to the middle of the pubic crest.

Contraception The prevention of conception or impregnation.

Contraction Tightening and shortening of the uterine muscles during labor, causing effacement and dilatation of the cervix; contributes to the downward and outward descent of the fetus.

Contraction stress test (CST) A method of assessing the reaction of the fetus to the stress of uterine contractions. This test may be utilized when contractions are occurring spontaneously or when contractions are artificially induced by oxytocin challenge test (OCT) or breast self-stimulation test (BSST).

Convection Loss of heat from the warm body surface to cooler air currents.

Coombs' (kōōmz) **test** A test for antiglobulins in the red cells. The indirect test determines the presence of Rh-positive antibodies in maternal blood; the direct test determines the presence of maternal Rh-positive antibodies in fetal cord blood.

Cordocentesis Also called percutaneous umbilical blood sampling (PUBS), a technique used to obtain pure fetal blood from the umbilical cord while the fetus is in utero, which is used for diagnosis of hemophilias, hemoglobinopathies, fetal infections, chromosome abnormalities, nonimmune hydrops, and isoimmune hemolytic disorders, as well as assessment of fetal hemoglobin and hematocrit for calculation of transfusion requirements in the second and third trimesters.

Cornua The elongated portions of the uterus where the fallopian tubes open.

Corpus The upper two thirds of the uterus.

Corpus luteum A small yellow body that develops within a ruptured ovarian follicle; it secretes progesterone in the second half of the menstrual cycle and atrophies about 3 days before the beginning of menstrual flow. If pregnancy occurs, the corpus luteum continues to produce progesterone until the placenta takes over this function.

Cosleeping An infant sleeping in close social and/or physical contact with a committed caregiver (usually the mother).

Cotyledon (kot-i-lē´don) One of the rounded portions into which the placenta's uterine surface is divided, consisting of a mass of villi, fetal vessels, and an intervillous space.

Couplet care A family-centered approach for maternal-child nursing where both the mother and her baby are cared for by the same nurse, with the baby remaining at the mother's bedside. Also called mother-baby care.

Couvade (kū-vahd´) In some cultures, the male's observance of certain rituals and taboos to signify the transition to fatherhood.

Crack A form of freebase cocaine that is smoked.

Crisis intervention Actions taken by the nurse to help the client deal with an impending, potentially overwhelming crisis; regain his or her equilibrium; grow from the experience; and improve coping skills.

Critical thinking Intellectual processes that include separating fact from opinion, identifying prejudices and stereotypes that may influence interpretation of information, exploring differing ideas and views, and arriving at conclusions or insights.

Crowning Appearance of the presenting fetal part at the vaginal orifice during labor.

Crying state A state in the infant sleep/awake cycle in which the infant exhibits increased motor activity, grimaces, eyes that are tightly closed or open, and extreme responsiveness to stimuli.

Cultural beliefs Those beliefs that reflect the predominating values, attitudes, and practices accepted by a population, community, or ethnic group.

Cultural competency Referring to the skills and knowledge necessary to appreciate, understand, and work with individuals from different cultures.

Culture The beliefs, values, attitudes, and practices that are accepted by a population, community, or an individual.

Cycle of violence A theory that postulates that battering takes place in a cyclic fashion through three phases: the tension-building phase, the acute battering incident, and the tranquil phase (honeymoon period).

Cystocele The downward displacement of the bladder, which appears as a bulge in the anterior vaginal wall.

Deceleration Periodic decrease in the baseline fetal heart rate.

Decidua (dē-sid´ yū ă) Endometrium or mucous membrane lining of the uterus in pregnancy that is shed after childbirth.

Decidua basalis The part of the decidua that unites with the chorion to form the placenta. It is shed in lochial discharge after childbirth.

Decidua capsularis The part of the decidua surrounding the chorionic sac.

Decidua vera (parietalis) Nonplacental decidua lining the uterus.

Decrement Decrease or stage of decline, as of a contraction.

Deep sleep State of sleep in which the infant will be nearly still except for occasional startles, twitches, and sucking.

Depo-Provera A long-acting, injectable progestin contraceptive.

Descriptive statistics Statistics that describe or summarize a set of data.

Desquamation (des-kwă-mā´ shǔn) Shedding of the epithelial cells of the epidermis.

Diagonal conjugate Distance from the lower posterior border of the symphysis pubis to the sacral promontory; may be obtained by manual measurement.

Diaphragm A flexible disk that covers the cervix to prevent pregnancy.

Diastasis (dī-as´tă-sis) **recti** (rek´ti) **abdominis** Separation of the recti abdominis muscles along the median line. In women, it is seen with repeated childbirths or multiple gestations. In the newborn, it is usually caused by incomplete development.

Dietary reference intakes (DRIs) Specific allowances for pregnant and lactating women, DRIs are subdivided into the recommended dietary allowance (RDA) and adequate intake (AI).

Dilatation and curettage (D&C) Stretching of the cervical canal to permit passage of a curette, which is used to scrape the endometrium to empty the uterine contents or to obtain tissue for examination.

Dilatation of the cervix Expansion of the external os from an opening a few millimeters in size to an opening large enough to allow the passage of the infant.

Diploid number of chromosomes Containing a set of maternal and a set of paternal chromosomes; in humans, the diploid number of chromosomes is 46.

Disability Impairment in one or more of five function categories: cognition, communication, motor abilities, social abilities, or patterns of interactions.

Disassociation relaxation A pattern of active relaxation in which the woman learns to tighten one area of the body and then relax other areas simultaneously. This relaxation pattern is very effective for some women during labor.

Disenfranchised grief Grief that is not supported by the usual societal customs.

Domestic partnership A mechanism by which public and private employers can provide insurance coverage and pension-rights benefits to the partners of gay and lesbian employees.

Domestic violence Defined as the collective methods used to exert power and control by one individual over another in an adult intimate relationship. Forms of abuse typically fall into three categories: psychologic abuse, physical abuse, and sexual abuse.

Doula A supportive companion who accompanies a laboring woman to provide emotional, physical, and informational support and acts as an advocate for the woman and her family.

Down syndrome An abnormality resulting from the presence of an extra chromosome number 21 (trisomy 21); characteristics include mental retardation and altered physical appearance. Formerly called *mongolism.*

Drowsy awake state Awake state in which infants open and close their eyes although the eyes appear glazed and the face is often still. They may return to sleep or awaken further in response to stimuli.

Drowsy state A state in the infant sleep/awake cycle that occurs between light sleep and the quiet alert state. It is marked by infants opening and closing their eyes, but the eyes appear glazed and face is often still. They may return to sleep or awaken further in response to stimuli.

Drug-exposed infant The newborn of an alcoholic or drug-addicted woman.

Drug-facilitated sexual assault A sexual assault in which the perpetrator uses alcohol or other drugs to sedate his intended victim.

Dual process model A view of grief encompassing two competing facets: loss and restoration. The loss orientation is concerned with the individual's need to confront the reality of the loss, and the restoration orientation seeks to regain balance and temper the pain of grief.

Dubowitz tool A clinical gestational age assessment tool.

Ductus arteriosus A communication channel between the main pulmonary artery and the aorta of the fetus. It is obliterated after birth by rising PO_2 and changes in intravascular pressure in the presence of normal pulmonary functioning. It normally becomes a ligament after birth but sometimes remains patent (patent ductus arteriosus, a treatable condition).

Ductus venosus A fetal blood vessel that carries oxygenated blood between the umbilical vein and the inferior vena cava, bypassing the liver; it becomes a ligament after birth.

Duncan's mechanism Occurs when the maternal surface of the placenta rather than the shiny fetal surface presents upon birth.

Duration The time length of each contraction, measured from the beginning of the increment to the completion of the decrement.

Dysfunctional uterine bleeding (DUB) A condition characterized by anovulatory cycles with abnormal uterine bleeding that does not have a demonstrable organic cause.

Dysmenorrhea Painful menstruation.

Dyspareunia Painful intercourse.

Dystocia (dis-tō´sē-ă) Difficult labor due to mechanical factors produced by the fetus or the maternal pelvis or due to inadequate uterine or other muscular activity.

Early adolescence A term referring to adolescents who are age 14 and under.

Early decelerations Periodic change in fetal heart rate pattern caused by head compression; deceleration has a uniform appearance and early onset in relation to maternal contraction.

Early (primary) postpartal hemorrhage See *Postpartal hemorrhage.*

Eclampsia (ek-lamp´sē-ă) A major complication of pregnancy. Its cause is unknown; it occurs more often in the primigravida and is accompanied by elevated blood pressure, albuminuria, oliguria, tonic and clonic convulsions, and coma. It may occur during pregnancy (usually after the 20th week of gestation) or within 48 hours after childbirth.

Ectoderm Outer layer of cells in the developing embryo that gives rise to the skin, nails, and hair.

Ectopic pregnancy Implantation of the fertilized ovum outside the uterine cavity; common sites are the abdomen, fallopian tubes, and ovaries. Also called *oocyesis.*

Effacement Thinning and shortening of the cervix that occurs late in pregnancy or during labor.

Effleurage (e-fler-ahz´) A light stroking movement of the fingertips over the abdominal area during labor; used to provide distraction during labor contractions.

Ejaculation Expulsion of the seminal fluids from the penis.

Elder abuse Any deliberate action or lack of action that causes harm to an elderly person.

Electronic fetal monitoring (EFM) A method of placing a fetal monitor on the fetus in order to obtain a continuous tracing of the FHR, which allows many characteristics of the fetal heart rate to be observed and evaluated.

Emancipated minors Minors who are legally considered to have assumed the rights of an adult. An adolescent may be considered emancipated if he or she is self-supporting and living away from home, married, pregnant, a parent, or in the military.

Embryo The early stage of development of the young of any organism. In humans the embryonic period is from about 2 to 8 weeks' gestation and is characterized by cellular differentiation and predominantly hyperplastic growth.

Embryonic membranes The amnion and chorion.

Endoderm The inner layer of cells in the developing embryo that give rise to internal organs such as the intestines.

Endometrial biopsy Procedure providing information about the effects of progesterone produced by the corpus luteum after ovulation and endometrial receptivity.

Endometriosis Ectopic endometrium located outside the uterus in the pelvic cavity. Symptoms may include pelvic pain or pressure, dysmenorrhea, dispareunia, abnormal bleeding from the uterus or rectum, and sterility.

Endometritis (metritis) Infection of the endometrium.

Endometrium (en´dō-me´ tre-ŭm) The mucous membrane that lines the inner surface of the uterus.

En face An assumed position in which one person looks at another and maintains his or her face in the same vertical plane as that of the other.

Engagement The entrance of the fetal presenting part into the superior pelvic strait and the beginning of the descent through the pelvic canal.

Engorgement Vascular congestion or distention. In obstetrics, the swelling of breast tissue brought about by an increase in blood and lymph supply to the breast, preceding true lactation.

Engrossment Characteristic sense of absorption, preoccupation, and interest in the infant demonstrated by fathers during early contact with their infants.

Entrainment Phenomenon in which a newborn moves in rhythm to adult speech.

Environmental toxins Chemical compounds found in air, food, and water, whose bioaccumulation can lead to adverse health effects.

Epidural block Regional anesthesia effective through the first and second stages of labor.

Episiotomy (ĕ-piz-ē-ot´o-mē) Incision of the perineum to facilitate birth and to avoid laceration of the perineum.

Epstein's (ep´stīnz) **pearls** Small, white blebs found along the gum margins and at the junction of the hard and soft palates; commonly seen in the newborn as a normal manifestation.

Erb-Duchenne paralysis (Erb's palsy) Paralysis of the arm and chest wall as a result of a birth injury to the brachial plexus or a subsequent injury to the fifth and sixth cervical nerves.

Erythema toxicum Innocuous pink papular rash of unknown cause with superimposed vesicles; it appears within 24 to 48 hours after birth and resolves spontaneously within a few days.

Erythroblastosis fetalis Hemolytic disease of the newborn characterized by anemia, jaundice, enlargement of the liver and spleen, and generalized edema. Caused by isoimmunization due to Rh incompatibility or ABO incompatibility.

Essure Method of permanent sterilization that requires no surgical incision. Under hysteroscopy, a stainless steel micro-insert is placed into each proximal section of the fallopian tube.

Estimated date of birth (EDB) During a pregnancy, the approximate date when childbirth will occur; the "due date."

Estrogens The hormones estradiol and estrone, produced by the ovary.

Ethnicity A social identity that is associated with shared beliefs, behaviors, and patterns.

Ethnocentrism An individual's belief that the values and practices of his or her own culture are the best ones.

Euphemism A substituted word or expression with a more pleasant association than the one which, although more direct, is considered to be harsher.

Evaporation Loss of heat incurred when water on the skin surface is converted to a vapor.

Evidence-based practice An approach to problem solving and decision making based on the consideration of data from research, statistical analysis, quality measures, risk management measurements, and other sources of reliable information.

Exchange transfusion The replacement of 70% to 80% of circulating blood by withdrawing the recipient's blood and injecting a donor's blood in equal amounts, for the purpose of preventing the accumulation of bilirubin or other by-products of hemolysis in the blood.

External cephalic version (ECV) Procedure involving external manipulation of the maternal abdomen to change the presentation of the fetus from breech to cephalic.

External os The opening between the cervix and the vagina.

Fallopian tubes Tubes that extend from the lateral angle of the uterus and terminate near the ovary; they serve as a passageway for the ovum from the ovary to the uterus and for the spermatozoa from the uterus toward the ovary. Also called *oviducts* and *uterine tubes.*

False labor Contractions of the uterus, regular or irregular, that may be strong enough to be interpreted as true labor but that do not dilate the cervix.

False pelvis The portion of the pelvis above the linea terminalis; its primary function is to support the weight of the enlarged pregnant uterus.

Family Two or more persons who are joined together by bonds of sharing and emotional closeness and who identify themselves as being part of a family.

Family assessment The process by which a nurse collects data regarding a family's current level of functioning, support systems, sociocultural influences, home and work environment, type of family, family structure, and needs.

Family-centered care An approach to health care based on the concept that a hospital can provide professional services to mothers, fathers, and infants in a homelike environment that would enhance the integrity of the family unit.

Family development The changes that families experience over time, including changes in relationships, communication patterns, roles, and interactions.

Family planning Actions an individual or a couple takes to avoid a pregnancy, to space future pregnancies for a specific reason, or to gain control over the number of children conceived.

Family power The individual who has either the potential or actual ability to change the behavior of other family members.

Family roles The specific roles of individuals within a family unit. Examples of roles include breadwinner, homemaker, mother, father, social planner, and family peacemaker.

Family values A system of ideas, attitudes, and beliefs about the worth of an entity or a concept that consciously or unconsciously bind together the members of the family in a common culture.

Fecundability The ability to become pregnant.

Female condom A thin, disposable polyurethane sheath with a flexible ring at each end that is placed inside the vagina and serves to prevent sperm from entering the cervix, thus preventing conception.

Female genital mutilation (FGM) Also known as *female genital cutting, female circumcision,* and *genital circumcision,* the practice of removing all or parts of a girl's or women's genitalia for cultural reasons.

Female reproductive cycle (FRC) The monthly rhythmic changes in sexually mature women.

Feminization of later life Worldwide trend for women to comprise a majority of the elderly population.

Feminization of poverty Term used to describe the fact that, in the United States, women comprise a majority of the adult poor.

Ferning capacity Formation of a palm-leaf pattern by the crystallization of cervical mucus as it dries at mid-menstrual cycle. The formation can be helpful in determining time of ovulation. Observed via microscopic examination of a thin layer of cervical mucus on a glass slide. This pattern is also observed when amniotic fluid is allowed to air dry on a slide and is a useful and quick test to determine whether amniotic membranes have ruptured.

Fertility awareness-based (FAB) methods Also known as natural family planning, fertility awareness-based methods are founded on an understanding of the changes that occur throughout a woman's ovulatory cycle. All these methods require periods of abstinence and recording of certain events throughout the cycle; cooperation of the partner is important.

Fertility rate Number of births per 1000 women aged 15 to 44 in a given population per year.

Fertilization Impregnation of an ovum by a spermatozoon; conception.

Fetal acoustic stimulation test (FAST) A fetal assessment test that uses sound from a speaker, bell, or artificial larynx to stimulate acceleration of the fetal heart; may be used in conjunction with the nonstress test.

Fetal activity diary (FAD) A method for tracking fetal activity taught to pregnant women.

Fetal alcohol effects (FAE) The less severe fetal manifestations of maternal alcohol ingestion, including mild to moderate cognitive problems and physical growth retardation.

Fetal alcohol syndrome (FAS) Syndrome caused by maternal alcohol ingestion and characterized by microcephaly, intrauterine growth restriction, short palpebral fissures, and maxillary hypoplasia.

Fetal attitude Relationship of the fetal parts to one another. Normal fetal attitude is one of moderate flexion of the arms onto the chest and flexion of the legs onto the abdomen.

Fetal blood sampling Blood sample drawn from the fetal scalp (or from the fetus in breech position) to evaluate the acid-base status of the fetus.

Fetal bradycardia A fetal heart rate less than 120 beats per minute during a 10-minute period of continuous monitoring.

Fetal death Death of the developing fetus after 20 weeks' gestation. Also called *fetal demise.*

Fetal distress Evidence that the fetus is in jeopardy, such as a change in fetal activity or heart rate.

Fetal fibronectin (fFN) A glycoprotein that is produced by the trophoblast and fetal tissues whose presence between 20 and 34 weeks' gestation is a strong predictor of preterm birth associated with preterm spontaneous rupture of membranes.

Fetal heart rate (FHR) The number of times the fetal heart beats per minute; normal range is 120 to 160.

Fetal lie Relationship of the cephalocaudal axis (spinal column) of the fetus to the cephalocaudal axis (spinal column) of the woman. The fetus may be in a longitudinal or transverse lie.

Fetal movement record (FMR) See *Fetal activity diary (FAD).*

Fetal position Relationship of the landmark on the presenting fetal part to the front, sides, or back of the maternal pelvis.

Fetal presentation The fetal body part that enters the maternal pelvis first. The three possible presentations are cephalic, shoulder, and breech.

Fetal scalp blood sample A collection of fetal blood collected via the vagina from the fetal head by making a small nick with a scalpel and collecting a blood sample that is used to identify the fetal acid-base status and determine if hypoxia is occurring during labor.

Fetal tachycardia A fetal heart rate of 160 beats per minute or more during a 10-minute period of continuous monitoring.

Fetoscope An adaptation of a stethoscope that facilitates auscultation of the fetal heart rate.

Fetoscopy A technique for directly observing the fetus and obtaining a sample of fetal blood or skin.

Fetus The child in utero from about the seventh to ninth week of gestation until birth.

Fibrocystic breast changes Benign breast changes characterized by bilateral, cyclic breast pain and breast nodularities that may be unilateral or bilateral, and often in the upper outer quadrants of the breasts.

Fibrocystic breast disease Benign breast disorder characterized by a thickening of normal breast tissue and the formation of cysts.

Fimbria Any structure resembling a fringe; the fringelike extremity of the fallopian tubes.

Folic acid An important vitamin directly related to the outcome of pregnancy and to maternal and fetal health.

Follicle-stimulating hormone (FSH) Hormone produced by the anterior pituitary during the first half of the menstrual cycle, stimulating development of the graafian follicle.

Fontanelle (fon´tănel´) In the fetus, an unossified space, or soft spot, consisting of a strong band of connective tissue lying between the cranial bones of the skull.

Foramen ovale Special opening between the atria of the fetal heart. Normally, the opening closes shortly after birth; if it remains open, it can be repaired surgically.

Forceps Obstetric instrument occasionally used to aid in childbirth.

Forceps-assisted birth A birth in which a set of instruments, known as forceps, are applied to the presenting part of the fetus to provide traction or to enable the fetal head to be rotated to an occiputanterior position. Forceps-assisted birth is also known as *instrumental delivery, operative delivery,* or *operative vaginal delivery.*

Forceps marks Reddened areas over the cheeks and jaws caused by the application of forceps. The red areas usually disappear within 1 to 2 days.

Foremilk Breast milk obtained at the beginning of the breastfeeding episode.

Fourth trimester First several postpartal weeks during which the woman returns to an essentially prepregnant state and becomes competent in caring for her newborn.

Frequency The time between the beginning of one contraction and the beginning of the next contraction.

Fundus The upper portion of the uterus between the fallopian tubes.

Galactorrhea Nipple discharge.

Gamete (gam´ēt) Female or male germ cell; contains a haploid number of chromosomes.

Gamete intrafallopian transfer (GIFT) Retrieval of oocytes by laparoscopy; immediately combining oocytes with washed, motile sperm in a catheter; and placement of the gametes into the fimbriated end of the fallopian tube.

Gametogenesis The process by which germ cells are produced.

General anesthesia A state of induced unconsciousness that may be achieved through intravenous injection, inhalation of anesthetic agents, or a combination of both methods.

Genotype The genetic composition of an individual.

Gestation (jes-tā´shŭn) Period of intrauterine development from conception through birth; pregnancy.

Gestational age The number of complete weeks of fetal development, calculated from the first day of the last normal menstrual cycle.

Gestational age assessment tools Systems used to evaluate the newborn's external physical characteristics and neurologic and/or neuromuscular development to accurately determine gestational age. These replace or supplement the traditional calculation from the woman's last menstrual period.

Gestational diabetes mellitus (GMD) A form of diabetes of variable severity with onset or first recognition during pregnancy.

Gestational trophoblastic disease (GTD) Disorder classified into two types: benign (hydatidiform mole) and malignant.

Gonadotropin-releasing hormone (GnRH) A hormone secreted by the hypothalamus that stimulates the anterior pituitary to secrete FSH and LH.

Gonadotropins Hormones that stimulate the gonads (ovaries in women or testes in men).

Gonorrhea A sexually transmitted infection caused by the bacterium *Neisseria gonorrhoeae.*

Goodell's sign Softening of the cervix that occurs during the second month of pregnancy.

Graafian follicle The ovarian cyst containing the ripe ovum; it secretes estrogens.

Grasping reflex Normal newborn reflex elicited by stimulating the palm with a finger or object, resulting in newborn firmly holding on to the finger or object.

Gravida (grav´i-dă) A pregnant woman.

Grief An individual's *reaction* to loss, including physical symptoms, thoughts, feelings, functional limitations, and spiritual responses.

Grief work The inner process of working through or managing the bereavement.

Guided imagery A state of intense, focused concentration used to create compelling mental images. It is sometimes considered a form of hypnosis.

Gynecoid pelvis Typical female pelvis in which the inlet is round instead of oval.

Habituation (ha-bit-chū-ā´shŭn) Infant's ability to diminish innate responses to specific repeated stimuli.

Haploid number of chromosomes Half the diploid number of chromosomes. In humans there are 23 chromosomes, the haploid number, in each germ cell.

Harlequin sign A rare color change that occurs between the longitudinal halves of the newborn's body, such that the dependent half is noticeably pinker than the superior half when the newborn is placed on one side; it is of no pathologic significance.

Hatha yoga The physical branch of yoga; in the United States, it is commonly practiced for wellness, illness prevention, and healing.

Hegar's sign A softening of the lower uterine segment found upon palpation in the second or third month of pregnancy.

HELLP syndrome A cluster of changes including *h*emolysis, *e*levated *l*iver enzymes, and *l*ow *p*latelet count; sometimes associated with severe preeclampsia.

Hemolytic disease of the newborn *Hyperbilirubinemia* secondary to Rh incompatibility.

Herpes genitalis A lifelong, recurrent sexually transmitted infection caused by the herpes simplex virus (HSV).

Heterozygous A genotypic situation in which two different alleles occur at a given locus on a pair of homologous chromosomes.

Hindmilk Breast milk released after initial let-down reflex; high in fat content.

Homeopathy Term derived from the Greek word *homos,* meaning "the same," and describing a healing system that uses as remedies minute dilutions of substances that, if ingested in larger amounts, would produce effects *similar* to the symptoms of the disorder being treated.

Homozygous A genotypic situation in which two similar genes occur at a given locus on homologous chromosomes.

Hormone replacement therapy (HRT) Administration of hormones, usually estrogen and a progestin, to alleviate the symptoms of menopause.

Hospital disposition The incineration at regular intervals of a dead fetus or infant's body, usually with other body parts.

Human chorionic gonadotropin (hCG) A hormone produced by the chorionic villi and found in the urine of pregnant women. Also called *prolan.*

Human immunodeficiency virus (HIV) A virus that causes a progressive disease that ultimately results in the development of acquired immunodeficiency syndrome (AIDS).

Human placental lactogen (hPL) A hormone synthesized by the syncytiotrophoblast that functions as an insulin antagonist and promotes lipolysis to increase the amounts of circulating free fatty acids available for maternal metabolic use.

Hydatidiform (hī-da-tid´i-form) **mole** Degenerative process in chorionic villi, giving rise to multiple cysts and rapid growth of the uterus, with hemorrhage.

Hydramnios (hī-dram´nē-os) An excess of amniotic fluid, leading to overdistention of the uterus. Frequently seen in diabetic pregnant women, even if there is no coexisting fetal anomaly. Also called *polyhydramnios.*

Hydrops fetalis See *Erythroblastosis fetalis.*

Hydrotherapy Type of therapy that makes use of hot or cold moisture in any form. Hydrotherapy is used to relax muscles, promote rest, decrease pain, reduce swelling, promote healing, cleanse wounds and burns, reduce fever, lessen cramps, and improve well-being.

Hyperbilirubinemia (hī-per-bil´i-rū-bi-nē´mē-ă) Excessive amount of bilirubin in the blood; indicative of hemolytic processes due to blood incompatibility, intrauterine infection, septicemia, neonatal renal infection, and other disorders.

Hyperemesis gravidarum Excessive vomiting during pregnancy, leading to dehydration and starvation.

Hyperventilation Rapid breathing that occurs over a prolonged period of time resulting in an imbalance of oxygen and carbon dioxide that can result in tingling or numbness in the tip of nose, lips, fingers, or toes; dizziness; spots before the eyes; or spasms of the hands or feet (carpal-pedal spasms).

Hypnosis Whether guided by a trained hypnotherapist or self-induced, a state of great mental and physical relaxation during which a person is very open to suggestions.

Hypoglycemia Abnormally low level of sugar in the blood.

Hysterectomy Surgical removal of the uterus.

Hysterosalpingogram Result of testing by instillation of radiopaque substance into the uterine cavity to visualize the uterus and fallopian tubes.

Hysterosalpingography (HSG) Testing by instillation of radiopaque substance into the uterine cavity to visualize the uterus and fallopian tubes.

Hysteroscopy Use of a special endoscope to examine the uterus.

Inborn error of metabolism A hereditary deficiency of a specific enzyme needed for normal metabolism of specific chemicals.

Incompetent cervix The premature dilatation of the cervix, usually in the second trimester of pregnancy.

Increment Increase or addition; to build up, as of a contraction.

Induction of labor The process of causing or initiating labor by use of medication or surgical rupture of membranes.

Infant A child under 1 year of age.

Infant mortality rate Number of deaths of infants under 1 year of age per 1000 live births in a given population per year.

Infant of diabetic mother (IDM) At-risk infant born to a woman previously diagnosed as diabetic or who develops symptoms of diabetes during pregnancy.

Infant of substance-abusing mother (ISAM) Formerly called infant of an addicted mother, an infant born to a mother who abuses or is addicted to drugs or alcohol.

Inferential statistics Statistics that allow an investigator to draw conclusions about what is happening between two or more variables in a population and to suggest or refute causal relationships between them.

Infertility Diminished ability to conceive.

Informed consent A legal concept that protects a person's rights to autonomy and self-determination by specifying that no action may be taken without that person's prior understanding and freely given consent.

Infundibulopelvic ligament Ligament that suspends and supports the ovaries.

Instrumental style of coping A style of coping by which persons generally use more cognitive skills to navigate loss and value care that includes an emphasis on problem solving.

Integrative medicine An approach that combines mainstream medical therapies with complementary therapies for which there is some high-quality scientific evidence of safety and effectiveness.

Intensity The strength of a uterine contraction during acme.

Internal os An inside mouth or opening; the opening between the cervix and the uterus.

Internal version Procedure used for the vaginal birth of a second twin. The obstetrician inserts a hand into the uterus, grasps the feet of the fetus, and changes the fetus from a transverse to a breech presentation.

Intrapartum The time from the onset of true labor until the birth of the infant and expulsion of the placenta.

Intrauterine device (IUD) Small metal or plastic form that is placed in the uterus to prevent implantation of a fertilized ovum.

Intrauterine drug-exposed infants Infants exposed while in the uterus to drugs of abuse taken by their mother.

Intrauterine fetal surgery Surgery performed on a fetus to correct anatomic lesions that are not compatible with life if left untreated.

Intrauterine growth restriction (IUGR) Fetal undergrowth due to any etiology, such as intrauterine infection, deficient nutrient supply, or congenital malformation. A term used to describe fetuses falling below the 10th percentile in ultrasonic estimation of weight at a given gestational age.

Intrauterine pressure catheter (IUPC) A catheter that can be placed through the cervix into the uterus to measure uterine pressure during labor. Some types of catheters may be inserted for the purpose of infusing warmed saline to add additional intrauterine fluid when oligohydramnios is present.

Intrauterine resuscitation Interventions initiated when nonreassuring fetal heart rate patterns are noted; they are directed at improving intrauterine blood flow.

Introitus Opening or entrance into a cavity or canal such as the vagina.

Intuitive style of coping A style of coping by which persons generally feel their way through loss and prefer care with an emphasis on emotional and psychosocial support.

In vitro fertilization (IVF) Procedure during which oocytes are removed from the ovary, mixed with spermatozoa, fertilized, and incubated in a glass petri dish; then up to four viable embryos are placed in the woman's uterus.

Involution Rolling or turning inward; the reduction in size of the uterus following childbirth.

Ischial spines Prominences that arise near the junction of the ilium and ischium and jut into the pelvic cavity; used as a reference point during labor to evaluate the descent of the fetal head into the birth canal.

Isthmus The straight, narrow part of the fallopian tube with a thick muscular wall and an opening (lumen) 2 to 3 mm in diameter; the site of tubal ligation. Also, a constriction in the uterus that is located above the cervix and below the corpus.

Jaundice Yellow pigmentation of body tissues caused by the presence of bile pigments. See also *Physiologic jaundice*.

Karyotype The set of chromosomes arranged in a standard order.

Kegel exercises Perineal muscle tightening that strengthens the pubococcygeus muscle and increases its tone.

Kernicterus (ker-nik´ter-ŭs) An encephalopathy caused by deposition of unconjugated bilirubin in brain cells; may result in impaired brain function or death.

Kilocalorie (kcal) Equivalent to 1000 calories, it is the unit used to express the energy value of food.

Klinefelter syndrome A chromosomal abnormality caused by the presence of an extra X chromosome in the male. Characteristics include tall stature; sparse pubic and facial hair; gynecomastia; small, firm testes; and absence of spermatogenesis.

Labor The process by which the fetus is expelled from the maternal uterus. Also called *childbirth, confinement,* or *parturition.*

Labor augmentation The stimulation of uterine contractions when spontaneous contractions have failed to result in progressive cervical dilation or descent of the fetus.

Labor induction The stimulation of uterine contractions before the spontaneous onset of labor, with or without ruptured fetal membranes, for the purpose of accomplishing birth.

Lactase deficiency (lactose intolerance) A condition characterized by difficulty digesting milk and dairy products. Results from an inadequate amount of the enzyme lactase, which breaks down the milk sugar lactose into smaller digestible substances.

Lactation The process of producing and supplying breast milk.

Lacto-ovovegetarians Vegetarians who include milk, dairy products, and eggs in their diets and occasionally fish, poultry, and liver.

Lactose intolerance A condition in which an individual has difficulty digesting milk and milk products.

Lactovegetarians Vegetarians who include dairy products but no eggs in their diets.

La Leche League Organization that provides information on and assistance with breastfeeding.

Lamaze method A method of childbirth preparation.

Lanugo (lă-nū´ gō) Fine, downy hair found on all body parts of the fetus, with the exception of the palms of the hands and the soles of the feet, after 20 weeks' gestation.

Laparoscopy Procedure that enables direct visualization of pelvic organs.

Large for gestational age (LGA) Excessive growth of a fetus in relation to the gestational time period.

Last menstrual period (LMP) The last normal menstrual period experienced by the woman before pregnancy; sometimes used to calculate the infant's gestational age.

Late adolescence A term referring to adolescents who are ages 18 to 19 years.

Late decelerations Symmetrical decrease in fetal heart rate beginning at or after the peak of the contraction and returning to baseline only after the contraction has ended, indicating possible uteroplacental insufficiency and potential that the fetus is not receiving adequate oxygenation.

Late preterm infant An infant born between 34 and 37 weeks of gestation.

Late (secondary) postpartal hemorrhage See *Postpartal hemorrhage.*

Lecithin/sphingomyelin (les´i-thin sfing´gō-mī´ĕ -lin) **(L/S) ratio** Lecithin and sphingomyelin are phospholipid components of surfactant; their ratio changes during gestation. When the L/S ratio reaches 2:1, the fetal lungs are thought to be mature and the fetus will have a low risk of respiratory distress syndrome (RDS) if born at that time.

Leiomyoma A benign tumor of the uterus, composed primarily of smooth muscle and connective tissue. Also referred to as a myoma or a fibroid.

Leopold's maneuvers A series of four maneuvers designed to provide a systematic approach whereby the examiner may determine fetal presentation and position.

Let-down reflex Pattern of stimulation, hormone release, and resulting muscle contraction that forces milk into the lactiferous ducts, making it available to the infant. Also called *milk ejection reflex.*

Leukorrhea Mucous discharge from the vagina or cervical canal that may be normal or pathologic, as in the presence of infection.

Lie Relationship of the long axis of the fetus and the long axis of the pregnant woman. The fetal lie may be longitudinal, transverse, or oblique.

Lightening Moving of the fetus and uterus downward into the pelvic cavity.

Light sleep State that makes up the highest proportion of newborn sleep and precedes awakening; characterized by some body movements, rapid eye movements (REM), and brief fussing or crying.

Linea nigra (lin´ē -ă ni´gră) The line of darker pigmentation extending from the umbilicus to the pubis noted in some women during the later months of pregnancy.

Local anesthesia Injection of an anesthetic agent into the subcutaneous tissue in a fanlike pattern.

Lochia (lō´kē-ă) Maternal discharge of blood, mucus, and tissue from the uterus; may last for several weeks after birth.

Lochia alba White vaginal discharge that follows lochia serosa and that lasts from about the 10th to the 21st day after birth.

Lochia rubra Red, blood-tinged vaginal discharge that occurs following birth and lasts 2 to 4 days.

Lochia serosa Pink, serous, and blood-tinged vaginal discharge that follows lochia rubra and lasts until the 7th to 10th day after birth.

Luteinizing hormone (LH) Anterior pituitary hormone responsible for stimulating ovulation and for development of the corpus luteum.

Maceration The process of tissue breakdown that begins from the moment of death.

Macrosomia (mak-rō-sō´mē-ă) A condition seen in newborns of large body size and high birth weight (more than 4000 to 4500 g [8 lb, 13 oz to 9 lb, 14 oz]), such as those born of prediabetic and diabetic mothers.

Malposition An abnormal position of the fetus in the birth canal.

Malpresentation A presentation of the fetus into the birth canal that is not "normal"—that is, brow, face, shoulder, or breech presentation.

Mammogram A soft-tissue radiograph of the breast without the injection of a contrast medium.

Massage therapy Manipulation of the soft tissues of the body to reduce stress and tension, increase circulation, diminish pain, and promote a sense of well-being.

Mastitis Inflammation of the breast.

Maternal mortality rate The number of maternal deaths from any cause during the pregnancy cycle per 100,000 live births.

Maternal role attainment Process by which a woman learns mothering behaviors and becomes comfortable with her identity as a mother.

Maternal serum alpha-fetoprotein (MSAFP) Screening test performed between 16 and 22 gestational weeks that utilizes the multiple markers (the "triple screen") of alpha-fetoprotein (AFP), human chorionic growth hormone (hCG), and urine estriol (uE3) to screen pregnancies for neural tube defect, Down syndrome, and trisomy 18.

Mature milk Breast milk that contains 10% solids for energy and growth.

McDonald's sign A probable sign of pregnancy characterized by an ease in flexing the body of the uterus against the cervix.

Meaning reconstruction A framework for understanding perinatal loss that focuses on redefining ourselves and how we interact with the world after a significant loss. The goal of recovery, as related to meaning reconstruction, is a positive change in self-identity by assigning the loss a meaning, thereby allowing the individual to assimilate the loss into her or his world.

Meconium Dark green or black material present in the large intestine of a full-term infant; the first stools passed by the newborn.

Meconium aspiration syndrome (MAS) Respiratory disease of term, postterm, and SGA newborns caused by inhalation of meconium or meconium-stained amniotic fluid into the lungs; characterized by mild to severe respiratory distress, hyperexpansion of the chest, hyperinflated alveoli, and secondary atelectasis.

Meiosis The process of cell division that occurs in the maturation of sperm and ova that decreases their number of chromosomes by one half.

Melasma gravidarum See *Chloasma.*

Menarche (me-nar´kē) Beginning of menstrual and reproductive function in the female.

Mendelian inheritance A major category of inheritance whereby a trait is determined by a pair of genes on homologous chromosomes. Also called *single gene inheritance.*

Menopause The permanent cessation of menses.

Menorrhagia Excessive or profuse menstrual flow.

Menstrual cycle Cyclic buildup of the uterine lining, ovulation, and sloughing of the lining occurring approximately every 28 days in nonpregnant females.

Mentum The chin.

Mesoderm The intermediate layer of germ cells in the embryo that gives rise to connective tissue, bone marrow, muscles, blood, lymphoid tissue, and epithelial tissue.

Metrorrhagia Abnormal uterine bleeding occurring at irregular intervals.

Middle adolescence A term referring to adolescents who are ages 15 to 17 years.

Milia (mil´ē-ă) Tiny white papules appearing on the face of a newborn as a result of unopened sebaceous glands; they disappear spontaneously within a few weeks.

Milk/plasma ratio The comparison of the concentration of substances in the breast milk and the maternal blood serum.

Miscarriage See *Spontaneous abortion.*

Mitosis Process of cell division whereby both daughter cells have the same number and pattern of chromosomes as the original cell.

Molding Shaping of the fetal head by overlapping of the cranial bones to facilitate movement through the birth canal during labor.

Mongolian spot Dark, flat pigmentation of the lower back and buttocks noted at birth in some infants; usually disappears by the time the child reaches school age.

Moniliasis Yeastlike fungal infection caused by *Candida albicans.*

Monosomies A genetic condition that occurs when a normal gamete unites with a gamete that is missing a chromosome.

Mons pubis (monz pu´bis) Mound of subcutaneous fatty tissue covering the anterior portion of the symphysis pubis.

Morning sickness A term that refers to the nausea and vomiting that a woman may experience in early pregnancy. This lay term is sometimes used because these symptoms frequently occur in the early part of the day and disappear within a few hours.

Moro reflex Flexion of the newborn's thighs and knees accompanied by fingers that fan, then clench, as the arms are simultaneously thrown out and then brought together, as though embracing something. This reflex can be elicited by startling the newborn with a sudden noise or movement. Also called the *startle reflex.*

Morula Developmental stage of the fertilized ovum in which there is a solid mass of cells.

Mosaicism Condition of an individual who has at least two cell lines with differing karyotypes.

Mother-baby care Also called couplet care, a family-centered care approach in which the infant remains at the mother's bedside and both are cared for by the same nurse.

Mottling (mot´ling) Discoloration of the skin in irregular areas; may be seen with chilling, poor perfusion, or hypoxia.

Mourning The *process* by which individuals incorporate the loss experience into their lives, it is influenced by many factors including personality, gender, family dynamics, and social, religious, and cultural norms.

Mucous plug A collection of thick mucus that blocks the cervical canal during pregnancy. Also called *operculum.*

Multigravida (mŭl-tē-grav´i-dă) Woman who has been pregnant more than once.

Multipara (mŭl-tip´ă-ră) Woman who has had more than one pregnancy in which the fetus was viable.

Multiple pregnancy More than one fetus in the uterus at the same time.

Music therapy Form of sound therapy using one or more musical instruments and improvisations or musical compositions. *Sound therapy* is based on the premise that when the body is exposed to the correct sound frequency (including some very low and very high frequencies that humans cannot normally hear) the body restores itself.

Myometrium Uterine muscular structure.

Nägele's rule A method of determining the estimated date of birth (EDB): after obtaining the first day of the last menstrual period, subtract 3 months and add 7 days.

Naturopathy A healing system that employs various natural means of preventing and treating human disease, such as foods, herbs, rest, etc. (Also called *natural medicine.*)

Neonatal morbidity The risk of death during the newborn period—the first 28 days of life.

Neonatal mortality rate Number of deaths of infants in the first 28 days of life per 1000 live births.

Neonatal mortality risk The chance of death within the newborn period.

Neonatal transition The first few hours of life, in which the newborn stabilizes his or her respiratory and circulatory functions.

Neonatology The specialty that focuses on the management of at-risk conditions of the newborn.

Neutral thermal environment (NTE) An environment that provides for minimal heat loss or expenditure.

Nevus (nē´vŭs) **flammeus** (flaem´iŭs) Large port-wine stain.

Nevus vasculosus "Strawberry mark": raised, clearly delineated, dark-red, rough-surfaced birthmark commonly found in the head region.

New Ballard score (NBS) A postnatal gestational age assessment tool, it is a refinement of a previous Ballard score tool with added criteria for more accurate assessment of the gestational age of newborns between 20 and 28 weeks' gestation and less than 1500 g.

Newborn Infant from birth through the first 28 days of life.

Newborn screening tests Tests that detect inborn errors of metabolism that, if left untreated, cause mental retardation and physical handicaps.

Newborns' and Mothers' Health Protection Act (NMHPA) Legislation which states that women who have given birth vaginally cannot be forcibly discharged from the hospital within 48 hours of the time of birth for insurance reasons. Cesarean birth mothers are covered by their insurance for 96 hours following the time of birth.

Nidation Implantation of a fertilized ovum in the endometrium.

Nipple A protrusion about 0.5 to 1.3 cm in diameter in the center of each mature breast.

Nipple preparation Prenatal activities designed to toughen the nipple in preparation for breastfeeding.

Nonmendelian (multifactorial) inheritance The occurrence of congenital disorders that result from an interaction of multiple genetic and environmental factors.

Nonstress test (NST) An assessment method by which the reaction (or response) of the fetal heart rate to fetal movement is evaluated.

Nuchal cord Term used to describe the umbilical cord when it is wrapped around the neck of the fetus.

Nuchal folds The accumulation of fluid between the posterior cervical spine and the overlying skin in the fetal neck identified during an ultrasound examination.

Nuchal translucency testing A combination of an ultrasound and maternal serum test that is used to screen fetuses between 11 weeks and 1 day and 13 weeks and 6 days to determine if a fetus is at risk for a chromosomal disorder, such as Down syndrome (trisomy 21) and trisomy 18.

Nulligravida (nŭl-i-grav´i-dă) A woman who has never been pregnant.

Nullipara A woman who has not given birth to a viable fetus.

Nurse practitioner A professional nurse who has received specialized education in either a master's degree program or a continuing education program and thus can function in an expanded role.

Obstetric conjugate Distance from the middle of the sacral promontory to an area approximately 1 cm below the pubic crest.

Oligohydramnios (ol´i-gō-hī-dram´nē-os) Decreased amount of amniotic fluid, which may indicate a fetal urinary tract defect.

Oocyte Early primitive ovum before it has completely developed.

Oogenesis Process during fetal life whereby the ovary produces oogonia, cells that become primitive ovarian eggs.

Oophoritis Infection of the ovaries.

Ophthalmia (of-thal´mē-ă) **neonatorum** Purulent infection of the eyes or conjunctiva of the newborn, usually caused by gonococci.

Oral contraceptives Birth control pills that work by inhibiting the release of an ovum and by maintaining a type of mucus that is hostile to sperm.

Orientation Infant's ability to respond to auditory and visual stimuli in the environment.

Ortolani maneuver A manual procedure performed to rule out the possibility of developmental dysplastic hip.

Osteoporosis A condition most common in postmenopausal women that is characterized by decreased bone strength related to diminished bone density and bone quality. It is thought to be associated with lowered estrogen and androgen levels. Osteoporosis puts an individual at increased risk for fractures of the hip, forearm, and vertebrae.

Ovarian ligaments Ligaments that anchor the lower pole of the ovary to the cornua of the uterus.

Ovary Female sex gland in which the ova are formed and in which estrogen and progesterone are produced. Normally there are two ovaries, located in the lower abdomen on each side of the uterus.

Ovulation Normal process of discharging a mature ovum from an ovary approximately 14 days before the onset of menses.

Ovum Female reproductive cell; egg.

Oxygen toxicity Excessive levels of oxygen therapy that result in pathologic changes in tissue.

Oxytocin Hormone normally produced by the posterior pituitary, responsible for stimulation of uterine contractions and the release of milk into the lactiferous ducts.

Oxytocin challenge test (OCT) See *Contraction stress test.*

Palpation The technique of assessing a uterine contraction by touch.

Pap smear Procedure to detect the presence of cancer of the uterus by microscopic examination of cells gently scraped from the cervix.

Para (par´ă) A woman who has borne offspring who reached the age of viability.

Parametritis Inflammation of the parametrial layer of the uterus.

Parent-newborn attachment Close affectional ties that develop between parent and child. See also *Attachment.*

Passive acquired immunity Transfer of antibodies (IgG) from the mother to the fetus in utero.

Patient-controlled analgesia (PCA) A method of pain control where anesthesia, usually morphine or meperidine, is initially administered by the anesthesiologist and subsequent doses are self-administered by pushing a button controlled by a special IV pump system.

Pedigree Graphic representation of a family tree.

Pelvic cavity Bony portion of the birth passages; a curved canal with a longer posterior than anterior wall.

Pelvic cellulitis (parametritis) Infection involving the connective tissue of the broad ligament or, in severe cases, the connective tissue of all the pelvic structures.

Pelvic diaphragm Part of the pelvic floor composed of deep fascia and the levator ani and the coccygeal muscles.

Pelvic floor Muscles and tissue that act as a buttress to the pelvic outlet.

Pelvic inflammatory disease (PID) An infection of the fallopian tubes that may or may not be accompanied by a pelvic abscess; may cause infertility secondary to tubal damage.

Pelvic inlet Upper border of the true pelvis.

Pelvic outlet Lower border of the true pelvis.

Pelvic tilt Also called *pelvic rocking;* exercise designed to reduce back strain and strengthen abdominal muscle tone.

Penis The male organ of copulation and reproduction.

Percutaneous umbilical blood sampling (PUBS) See *Cordocentesis.*

Perimenopause A term referring to the period of time before menopause during which the woman moves from normal ovulatory cycles to cessation of menses.

Perimetrium The outermost layer of the corpus of the uterus. Also known as the serosal layer.

Perinatal loss Death of a fetus or infant from the time of conception through the end of the newborn period 28 days after birth.

Perinatal mortality rate The number of neonatal and fetal deaths per 1000 live births.

Perinatology The medical specialty concerned with the diagnosis and treatment of high-risk conditions of the pregnant woman and her fetus.

Perineal (per´i-nē-ăl) **body** Wedge-shaped mass of fibromuscular tissue found between the lower part of the vagina and the anal canal.

Perineum (per´i-nē´ŭm) The area of tissue between the anus and scrotum in a man or between the anus and vagina in a woman.

Periodic breathing Sporadic episodes of apnea, not associated with cyanosis, that last for about 10 seconds and commonly occur in preterm infants.

Periods of reactivity Predictable patterns of newborn behavior during the first several hours after birth.

Peritonitis Infection involving the peritoneal cavity.

Persistent occiput-posterior (OP) position Malposition of the fetus in which the fetal occiput is posterior in the maternal pelvis.

Persistent pulmonary hypertension of the newborn (PPHN) Respiratory disease resulting from right-to-left shunting of blood away from the lungs and through the ductus arteriosus and patent foramen ovale.

Phenotype The whole physical, biochemical, and physiologic makeup of an individual as determined both genetically and environmentally.

Phenylketonuria (fen´il-kē´tō-nū´rē-ă) A common metabolic disease caused by an inborn error in the metabolism of the amino acid phenylalanine.

Phosphatidylglycerol (PG) (fos-fă-tī´dĭl-glis´er-ol) A phospholipid present in fetal surfactant after about 35 weeks' gestation.

Phototherapy The treatment of jaundice by exposure to light.

Physiologic anemia of infancy A harmless condition in which the hemoglobin level drops in the first 6 to 12 weeks after birth, then reverts to normal levels.

Physiologic anemia of pregnancy Apparent anemia that results because during pregnancy the plasma volume increases more than the erythrocytes increase.

Physiologic jaundice A harmless condition caused by the normal reduction of red blood cells, occurring 48 or more hours after birth, peaking at the 5th to 7th days, and disappearing between the 7th and 10th days.

Pica The eating of substances not ordinarily considered edible or to have nutritive value.

Placenta (plă-sen´tă) Specialized disk-shaped organ that connects the fetus to the uterine wall for gas and nutrient exchange. Also called *afterbirth*.

Placenta accreta Partial or complete absence of the decidua basalis and abnormal adherence of the placenta to the uterine wall.

Placenta increta A high-risk condition that occurs when the placenta attaches to the uterine wall and invades or attaches itself within the myometrium.

Placenta percreta A high-risk condition that occurs when the placenta penetrates the myometrium, sometimes attaching to peritoneal structures within the abdominal cavity, where the removal of the uterus (hysterectomy) is sometimes necessary.

Placenta previa Abnormal implantation of the placenta in the lower uterine segment. Classification of type is based on proximity to the cervical os: *total*—completely covers the os; *partial*—covers a portion of the os; *marginal*—is in close proximity to the os.

Platypelloid pelvis An unusually wide pelvis, having a flattened oval transverse shape and a shortened anteroposterior diameter.

Podalic version Type of version used to turn a second twin during a vaginal birth.

Polar body A small cell resulting from the meiotic division of the mature oocyte.

Polycystic ovarian syndrome (PCOS) The most common endocrine disorder affecting women of reproductive age, marked by menstrual dysfunction, androgen excess, obesity, hyperinsulinemia, and infertility.

Polycythemia An abnormal increase in the number of total red blood cells in the body's circulation.

Polydactyly (pol-ē-dak´ti-lē) A developmental anomaly characterized by more than five digits on the hands or feet.

Polypharmacy The act of taking multiple drugs to treat symptoms, when the etiology of the symptoms is actually a side effect from one or more prescribed medications.

Positive signs of pregnancy Indications that confirm the presence of pregnancy.

Postcoital emergency contraception (EC) A form of combined hormonal contraception that is used when a woman is worried about pregnancy because of unprotected intercourse, rape, or possible contraceptive failure (e.g., broken condom, slipped diaphragm,

missed oral contraceptives, or too long a time between Depo-Provera injections).

Postcoital test (PCT) An examination that evaluates the cervical mucus, sperm motility, sperm-mucus interaction, and the sperm's ability to negotiate the cervical mucus barrier. Also called *Sims-Huhner test*.

Postconception age periods Period of time in embryonic/fetal development calculated from the time of fertilization of the ovum.

Postmature newborn See *Postterm newborn*.

Postmaturity See *Postterm newborn*.

Postpartal hemorrhage A loss of blood of greater than 500 mL following birth. The hemorrhage is classified as *early* if it occurs within the first 24 hours and *late* if it occurs after the first 24 hours.

Postpartal home care Home visits for postpartal families occurring in the home setting. This provides opportunities for expanding information and reinforcing self- and infant care techniques initially presented in the birth setting.

Postpartum After childbirth.

Postpartum blues A maternal adjustment reaction occurring in the first few postpartal days, characterized by mild depression, tearfulness, anxiety, headache, and irritability.

Postpartum depression (postpartum major mood disorder) Severe depression that occurs within the first year after giving birth with increased incidence at about the fourth week postpartum, just before resumption of menses, and upon weaning.

Postpartum psychosis Psychosis occurring within the first 3 months after birth.

Postterm labor Labor that occurs after 42 weeks' gestation.

Postterm newborn Any infant born after 42 weeks' gestation.

Postterm pregnancy Pregnancy that lasts beyond 42 weeks' gestation.

Post-traumatic stress disorder (PTSD) Intense psychologic distress resulting from a traumatic event and evidenced by recurrent, intrusive thoughts; flashbacks, persistent avoidance of stimuli associated with the trauma; a generalized feeling of "numbness"; and persistent signs of arousal.

Precipitous birth (1) Unduly rapid progression of labor. (2) A birth in which no physician is in attendance.

Precipitous labor Labor lasting less than 3 hours.

Preeclampsia (prē-ē-klamp´sē-ă) Toxemia of pregnancy, characterized by hypertension, albuminuria, and edema. See also *Eclampsia*.

Premature infant See *Preterm infant*.

Premature rupture of the membranes (PROM) See *Rupture of membranes (ROM)*.

Premenstrual dysphoric disorder (PMDD) A disorder associated with the luteal phase of the menstrual cycle (2 weeks before onset of menses) in which a woman experiences five or more affective (emotional) or somatic (physical) symptoms, which are relieved with menstruation and have occurred during most cycles during the previous year.

Premenstrual syndrome (PMS) Cluster of symptoms experienced by some women, typically occurring from a few days up to 2 weeks before the onset of menses.

Prenatal education Programs offered to expectant families, adolescents, women, or partners to provide education regarding the pregnancy, labor, and birth experience.

Prep Shaving of the pubic area.

Presentation The fetal body part that enters the maternal pelvis first. The three possible presentations are cephalic, shoulder, and breech.

Presenting part The fetal part present in or on the cervical os.

Presumptive signs of pregnancy Symptoms that suggest but do not confirm pregnancy, such as cessation of menses, quickening, Chadwick's sign, and morning sickness.

Preterm infant Any infant born before 38 weeks' gestation.

Preterm labor Labor occurring between 20 and 38 weeks of pregnancy. Also called *premature labor*.

Primigravida (pr ī-mi-grav´i-dă) A woman who is pregnant for the first time.

Primipara (pr ī-mip´ă-ră) A woman who has given birth to her first child (past the point of viability), whether or not that child is living or was alive at birth.

Probable signs of pregnancy Manifestations that strongly suggest the likelihood of pregnancy, such as a positive pregnancy test, enlarging abdomen, and positive Goodell's, Hegar's, and Braxton Hicks signs.

Professional nurse A person who has graduated from an accredited basic program in nursing, has successfully completed the nursing licensure examination (NCLEX), and is currently licensed as a registered nurse (RN).

Progesterone A hormone produced by the corpus luteum, adrenal cortex, and placenta whose function is to stimulate proliferation of the endometrium to facilitate growth of the embryo.

Progressive relaxation A relaxation technique that involves relaxing first one portion of the body and then another portion, until total body relaxation is achieved; may be used during labor.

Prolactin A hormone secreted by the anterior pituitary that stimulates and sustains lactation in mammals.

Prolapsed umbilical cord Umbilical cord that becomes trapped in the vagina before the fetus is born.

Prolonged decelerations Decelerations in which the FHR decreases from the baseline for 2 to 10 minutes.

Prolonged labor Labor lasting more than 24 hours.

Prostaglandins Complex lipid compounds synthesized by many cells in the body.

Pseudomenstruation Blood-tinged mucus from the vagina in the newborn female infant; caused by withdrawal of maternal hormones that were present during pregnancy.

Psychologic disorders Abnormal mental or emotional conditions characterized by alterations in thinking, mood, or behavior.

Ptyalism Excessive salivation.

Puberty The developmental period between childhood and the attainment of adult sexual characteristics and functioning.

Pubic Pertaining to the pubes or pubis.

Pubis Pertaining to the pubes or pubic area.

Pudendal (pyū-den´dăl) **block** Injection of an anesthetizing agent at the pudendal nerve to produce numbness of the external genitals

and the lower one third of the vagina to facilitate childbirth and permit episiotomy if necessary.

Puerperal infection Infection of the reproductive tract associated with childbirth and occurring any time up to 6 weeks postpartum.

Puerperal morbidity A maternal temperature of 38C (100.4F) or higher on any 2 of the first 10 postpartal days, excluding the first 24 hours. The temperature is to be taken by mouth at least four times per day.

Puerperium (pyū-er-pēr´ē-ŭm) The period after completion of the third stage of labor until involution of the uterus is complete, usually 6 weeks.

Quickening The first fetal movements felt by the pregnant woman, usually between 16 and 18 weeks' gestation.

Quiet alert state Alert state characterized by a brightening of the eyes and face. Infants are most attentive to their environment in this state and provide positive feedback to caregivers.

Radiation Heat loss incurred when heat transfers to cooler surfaces and objects not in direct contact with the body.

Rape Sexual activity, often intercourse, against the will of the victim.

Rape trauma syndrome A term that refers to a variety of symptoms, clustered in phases, that a rape survivor experiences following an assault.

Reciprocal inhibition The principle that it is impossible to feel relaxed and tense at the same time; the basis for relaxation techniques.

Reciprocity An interactional cycle that occurs simultaneously between mother and infant. It involves mutual cuing behaviors, expectancy, rhythmicity, and synchrony.

Recommended dietary allowances (RDA) Government recommended allowances of various vitamins, minerals, and other nutrients.

Reflexology Form of massage involving the application of pressure to designated points or reflexes on the client's feet, hands, or ears using the thumb and fingers.

Regional analgesia The temporary and reversible loss of sensation produced by injecting an anesthetic agent (called a local anesthetic) into an area that will bring the agent into direct contact with nervous tissue.

Regional anesthesia Injection of local anesthetic agents so that they come into direct contact with nervous tissue.

Reiki Tibetan-Japanese hand-mediated therapy designed to promote healing, reduce stress, and encourage relaxation. During Reiki sessions, practitioners place their hands on or above specific problem areas and transfer energy from themselves to their clients in order to restore the balance of the client's energy fields.

Relaxin A water-soluble protein secreted by the corpus luteum that causes relaxation of the symphysis and cervical dilatation.

Religion An institutionalized system that shares a common set of beliefs and practices.

Relinquishing mothers Those mothers who choose to give their infants up for adoption.

Respiratory distress syndrome (RDS) Respiratory disease of the newborn characterized by interference with ventilation at the alveolar level, thought to be caused by the presence of fibrinoid deposits lining the alveolar ducts. Formerly called *hyaline membrane disease*.

Responding model A set of guidelines for successful interactions with grieving families.

Retained placenta Retention of the placenta beyond 30 minutes after birth.

Retinopathy (ret-i-nop´ă-thē) **of prematurity (ROP)** Formation of fibrotic tissue behind the lens; associated with retinal detachment and arrested eye growth, seen with hypoxemia in preterm infants.

Rh factor Antigens present on the surface of blood cells that make the blood cell incompatible with blood cells that do not have the antigen.

Rh immune globulin (RhoGAM) An anti-Rh *(D)* gamma globulin given after birth to an Rh-negative mother of an Rh-positive fetus or child. Prevents the development of permanent active immunity to the Rh antigen.

Rhythm method The timing of sexual intercourse to avoid the fertile time associated with ovulation.

Risk factors Any findings that suggest the pregnancy may have a negative outcome, for either the woman or her unborn child.

Roles Patterns of behavior normatively defined and expected of an occupant of a given social position.

Rooting reflex An infant's tendency to turn the head and open the lips to suck when one side of the mouth or cheek is touched.

Round ligaments Ligaments that arise from the side of the uterus near the fallopian tube insertion to help the broad ligament keep the uterus in place.

Rugae (rū´gē) Transverse ridges of mucous membranes lining the vagina that allow the vagina to stretch during the descent of the fetal head.

Rupture of membranes (ROM) Rupture may be PROM (premature), SROM (spontaneous), or AROM (artificial). Some clinicians may use the abbreviation RBOW (rupture of bag of waters).

Sacral promontory A projection into the pelvic cavity on the anterior upper portion of the sacrum; serves as an obstetric guide in determining pelvic measurements.

Salpingitis Infection of the fallopian tubes.

Saltatory pattern A fetal heart rate pattern of marked or excessive variability.

Scalp stimulation A test used during labor to assess fetal well-being by pressing a fingertip on the fetal scalp. A fetus not under excessive stress will respond to the digital stimulation with heart rate accelerations.

Scarf sign The position of the elbow when the hand of a supine infant is drawn across to the other shoulder until it meets resistance.

Schultze's mechanism Expulsion of the placenta with the shiny, or fetal, surface presenting first.

Secondary infertility Condition in which couples are unable to conceive after one or more successful pregnancies.

Self-quieting ability Infant's ability to use personal resources to quiet and console himself or herself.

Semen Thick whitish fluid ejaculated by the male during orgasm and containing the spermatozoa and their nutrients.

Sepsis neonatorum Infections experienced by a newborn during the first month of life.

Sex chromosomes The X and Y chromosomes, which are responsible for sex determination.

Sexual assault A broad term that refers to a variety of types of unwanted sexual touching or penetration without consent, from unwanted sexual contact or touching of an intimate part of another person to forced anal, oral, or genital penetration.

Sexually transmitted infection (STI) Refers to infections ordinarily transmitted by direct sexual contact with an infected individual. Also called *sexually transmitted disease.*

Shaken baby injuries Injuries acquired by an infant as a result of being shaken or hit.

Show A pinkish mucus discharge from the vagina that may occur a few hours to a few days before the onset of labor.

Simian line A single palmar crease frequently found in children with Down syndrome.

Sims-Huhner test See *Postcoital test (PCT).*

Sinusoidal baseline A fetal heart rate pattern consisting of a series of cycles that are extremely smooth and regular in amplitude and duration.

Situational contraceptives Contraceptive methods that involve no prior preparation (e.g., abstinence or coitus interruptus).

Skin turgor Elasticity of skin; provides information on hydration status.

Skin-to-skin contact Physical contact between the mother and baby whereby the naked baby is placed prone on the mother's chest during the first 24 hours.

Small for gestational age (SGA) Inadequate weight or growth for gestational age; birth weight below the 10th percentile.

Sonohysterography Transvaginal ultrasound during or after the introduction of sterile saline that defines the uterine cavity contour and readily demonstrates even small intrauterine lesions.

Spermatogenesis The process by which mature spermatozoa are formed, during which the number of chromosomes is halved.

Spermatozoa Mature sperm cells of the male animal, produced by the testes.

Spermicides A variety of creams, foams, jellies, and suppositories that, when inserted into the vagina before intercourse, destroy sperm or neutralize any vaginal secretions and thereby immobilize sperm.

Spinal block Injection of a local anesthetic agent directly into the spinal fluid in the spinal canal to provide anesthesia for vaginal and cesarean births.

Spinnbarkheit The elasticity of the cervical mucus that is present at ovulation.

Spirituality A belief in a transcendent power pertaining to the spirit or soul

Spontaneous abortion Abortion that occurs naturally. Also called *miscarriage.*

Spontaneous rupture of membranes (SROM) The breaking of the "water" or membranes marked by the expulsion of amniotic fluid from the vagina.

Station Relationship of the presenting fetal part to an imaginary line drawn between the pelvic ischial spines.

Sterilization An inclusive term that refers to surgical procedures that permanently prevent pregnancy. In the male, sterilization is achieved through a procedure called a vasectomy. In the female, sterilization is done by tubal ligation.

Stillbirth The birth of a dead infant.

Striae (strī´ă) Stretch marks; shiny purplish lines that appear on the abdomen, breasts, thighs, and buttocks of pregnant women as a result of stretching the skin.

Subconjunctival hemorrhage (sŭb´kon-jŭnk-tī´văl hem´ŏ-rij) Hemorrhage on the sclera of a newborn's eye, usually caused by changes in vascular tension during birth.

Subdermal implants Capsules implanted in the woman's upper underarm that prevent ovulation in most women.

Subfertility A couple who has difficulty conceiving because both partners have reduced fertility.

Subinvolution (sŭb-in-vō-lū´shŭn) Failure of a part to return to its normal size after functional enlargement, such as failure of the uterus to return to normal size after pregnancy.

Sucking reflex Normal newborn reflex elicited by inserting a finger or nipple in the newborn's mouth, resulting in forceful, rhythmic sucking.

Sudden infant death syndrome (SIDS) The sudden death of an infant; the primary cause of infant death beyond the neonatal period in the United States.

Supine hypotensive syndrome (vena caval syndrome, aortocaval compression) A condition that can develop during pregnancy when the enlarging uterus puts pressure on the vena cava when the woman is supine. This pressure interferes with returning blood flow and produces a marked decrease in blood pressure with accompanying dizziness, pallor, and clamminess, which can be corrected by having the woman lie on her left side.

Surfactant (ser-fak´tănt) A substance composed of phospholipid, which stabilizes and lowers the surface tension of the alveoli during extrauterine respiratory exhalation, allowing a certain amount of air to remain in the alveoli during expiration.

Suture Fibrous connection of opposed joint surfaces, as in the skull.

Symphysis pubis Fibrocartilaginous joint between the pelvic bones in the midline.

Syndactyly (sin-dak´ti-lē) Malformation of the fingers or toes in which there may be webbing or complete fusion of two or more digits.

Syphilis A chronic, sexually transmitted infection caused by the spirochete *Treponema pallidum.*

Taboos Behaviors or objects that are avoided by individuals or groups.

Telangiectatic nevi (tel-an´jē-ek-tat´ik nē´v ī) **(stork bites)** Small clusters of pink-red spots appearing on the nape of the neck and around the eyes of infants; localized areas of capillary dilatation.

Teratogens Nongenetic factors that can produce malformations of the fetus.

Term The normal duration of pregnancy.

Testes The male gonads, in which sperm and testosterone are produced.

Testosterone The male hormone; responsible for the development of secondary male characteristics.

Therapeutic abortion Medically induced termination of pregnancy when a malformed fetus is suspected or when the woman's health is in jeopardy.

Therapeutic insemination Procedure to produce a pregnancy in which sperm obtained from a woman's husband or from a donor is deposited in the woman's vagina.

Therapeutic touch Complementary therapy grounded in the belief that people are a system of energy with a self-healing potential. The therapeutic touch practitioner, often a nurse, unites his or her energy field with that of the client, directing it in a specific way to promote well-being and healing.

Thrombophlebitis Inflammation of a vein wall, resulting in thrombus.

Thrush A fungal infection of the oral mucous membranes caused by *Candida albicans.* Most often seen in infants; characterized by white plaques in the mouth.

Tocolysis Use of medications to arrest preterm labor.

Tonic neck reflex Postural reflex seen in the newborn. When the supine infant's head is turned to one side, the arm and leg on that side extend while the extremities on the opposite side flex. Also called the *fencing position.*

TORCH An acronym used to describe a group of infections that represent potentially severe problems during pregnancy. *TO,* toxoplasmosis; *R,* rubella; *C,* cytomegalovirus; *H,* herpesvirus.

Total serum bilirubin Sum of conjugated (direct) and unconjugated (indirect) bilirubin.

Touch relaxation A relaxation technique that involves relaxing an area of one's body as another person provides a "touch" cue to that specific area. Touch relaxation is very effective during labor contractions.

Toxic shock syndrome (TSS) Infection caused by *Staphylococcus aureus,* found primarily in women of reproductive age.

Traditional Chinese medicine System of medicine developed more than 3000 years ago in China that seeks to ensure the balance of energy, which is called *chi* or *qi* (pronounced "chee"). Chi is thought to maintain health and vitality and enable the body to carry out its physiologic functions.

Transitional milk Breast milk produced from the end of colostrum production until about 2 weeks postpartum.

Transvaginal ultrasound A follicular monitoring test that is used in women undergoing induction cycles, for timing ovulation for insemination and intercourse, for retrieving oocytes for in vitro fertilization, and for monitoring early pregnancy.

Transverse diameter The largest diameter of the pelvic inlet; helps determine the shape of the inlet.

Transverse lie A lie in which the fetus is positioned crosswise in the uterus.

Trichomonas vaginalis A parasitic protozoan that may cause inflammation of the vagina, characterized by itching and burning of vulvar tissue and by white, frothy discharge.

Trichomoniasis A sexually transmitted infection caused by *Trichomonas vaginalis,* a microscopic motile protozoan that thrives in an alkaline environment.

Trimester Three months, or one third of the gestational time for pregnancy.

Trisomy The presence of three homologous chromosomes rather than the normal two.

Trophoblast The outer layer of the blastoderm that will eventually establish the nutrient relationship with the uterine endometrium.

True pelvis The portion that lies below the linea terminalis, made up of the inlet, cavity, and outlet.

Trunk incurvation (Galant reflex) Reflex resulting from the stroking of the spine that causes the pelvis to turn to the stimulated side.

Tubal embryo transfer (TET) Procedure in which eggs are retrieved and incubated with the man's sperm then transferred back into the women's body at the embryo stage.

Tubal ligation Sterilization of a woman accomplished by transecting or occluding the fallopian tubes.

Turner syndrome A number of anomalies that occur when a woman has only one X chromosome. Characteristics include short stature; little sexual differentiation; webbing of the neck, with a low posterior hairline; and congenital cardiac anomalies.

Ultrasound High-frequency sound waves that may be directed, through the use of a transducer, into the maternal abdomen. The ultrasonic sound waves reflected by the underlying structures of varying densities allow identification of various maternal and fetal tissues, bones, and fluids.

Umbilical cord (ŭm-bil´i-kăl kōrd) The structure connecting the placenta to the umbilicus of the fetus and through which nutrients from the woman are exchanged for wastes from the fetus.

Urinary tract infection (UTI) Significant *bacteriuria* in the presence of symptoms.

Uterine atony Relaxation of uterine muscle tone following birth.

Uterine inversion Prolapse of the uterine fundus through the cervix into the vagina; may occur just before or during expulsion of the placenta; associated with massive hemorrhage, requiring emergency treatment.

Uterosacral ligaments Ligaments that provide support for the uterus and cervix at the level of the ischial spines.

Uterus The hollow muscular organ in which the fertilized ovum is implanted and in which the developing fetus is nourished until birth.

Vacuum extraction An obstetric procedure used to assist in the birth of a fetus by applying suction to the fetal head with a soft suction cup attached to a suction bottle (pump) by tubing and placing the device against the occiput of the fetal head.

Vagina The musculomembranous tube or passageway located between the external genitals and the uterus of a woman.

Vaginal birth after cesarean (VBAC) Practice of permitting a trial of labor and possible vaginal birth for women following a previous cesarean birth for nonrecurring causes such as fetal distress or placenta previa.

Variability Baseline fluctuations of two cycles per minute or greater in the FHR and classified by the visually quantified amplitude of peak-to-trough in beats per minute.

Variable deceleration Periodic change in fetal heart rate caused by umbilical cord compression; decelerations vary in onset, occurrence, and waveform.

Vasa previa Condition occurring when the fetal vessels course through membranes and are present at the cervical os. Although this is a rare cause of antepartum bleeding, it has a high rate of fetal death.

Vasectomy Surgical removal of a portion of the vas deferens (ductus deferens) to produce infertility.

Vegan A "pure" vegetarian; one who consumes no food from animal sources.

Vena caval syndrome Symptoms of dizziness, pallor, and clamminess that result from lowered blood pressure when a pregnant woman lies supine and the enlarged uterus presses on the vena cava. Also known as supine hypotensive syndrome.

Vernix caseosa (ver´niks kā´sē-ō-să) A protective, cheeselike, whitish substance made up of sebum and desquamated epithelial cells that is present on the fetal skin.

Version Turning of the fetus in utero.

Vertex The top or crown of the head.

Viability The potential for the pregnancy to result in a live birth.

Vibroacoustic stimulation (VAS) Application of device delivering 90 dB of sound and vibration for 1 to 3 seconds to the mother's abdomen to stimulate movement in the fetus, thereby accelerating the fetal heart rate. (Also called FAST for fetal acoustic stimulation test or VST for vibroacoustic stimulation test.)

Vicarious trauma (also called secondary trauma effect) A condition that can occur as a result of working with people who are trauma victims.

Visualization Complementary therapy in which a person goes into a relaxed state and focuses on or "visualizes" soothing or positive scenes such as a beach or a mountain glade. Visualization helps reduce stress and encourage relaxation.

Vulva The external structure of the female genitals, lying below the mons veneris.

Vulvovaginal candidiasis (VVC) Also called moniliasis or yeast infection, VVC is a genital infection most often caused by *Candida albicans*.

Weaning The process of discontinuing breastfeeding and accustoming an infant to another feeding method.

Wharton's (hwar´tunz) **jelly** Yellow-white gelatinous material surrounding the vessels of the umbilical cord.

Zona pellucida Transparent inner layer surrounding an ovum.

Zygote A fertilized egg.

Zygote intrafallopian transfer (ZIFT) Retrieval of oocytes under ultrasound guidance, followed by in vitro fertilization and laparoscopic replacement of fertilized eggs into the fimbriated end of the fallopian tube.

INDEX

Page numbers followed by *f* indicate figures and those followed by *t* indicate tables or special features. The titles of special features (e.g., Chapter Review, Critical Thinking in Action, Evidence-Based Practice, Research in Practice) are also capitalized.

NURSING EXCELLENCE

Success in Skills, Review, & Test Preparation

Excellence in Nursing Skills

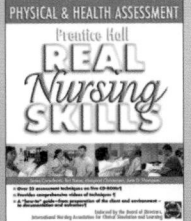

Prentice Hall's Real Nursing Skills on CD-ROMs

Prentice Hall Real Nursing Skills series offers you the complete foundation for competency in performing clinical skills. The CD-ROMs provide comprehensive procedures demonstrated in hundreds of videos, animations, illustrations, and photographs. These skills CD-ROMs are designed to help you visualize how to perform each skill and understand the concepts and rationales for each skill.

Basic Nursing Skills:
94 skills on 5 CD-ROMs. 2005, ISBN: 0-13-191526-6
Intermediate & Advanced Nursing Skills:
84 skills on 5 CD-ROMs. 2005, ISBN: 0-13-119344-9
Physical & Health Assessment Nursing Skills:
25 skills on 5 CD-ROMs. 2006, ISBN: 0-13-191525-8
Maternal-Newborn & Women's Health Nursing Skills:
24 skills on 2 CD-ROMs. 2005, ISBN: 0-13-191527-4
Pediatric Nursing Skills:
65 skills on 3 CD-ROMs. 2006, ISBN: 0-13-191524-X
Critical Care Nursing Skills:
35 skills on 2 CD-ROMs. 2005, ISBN: 0-13-119264-7

Excellence in NCLEX-RN® Review

2008, ISBN 0-13-119599-9

Prentice Hall's Comprehensive Review for NCLEX-RN® is designed specifically to help you achieve nursing excellence by simplifying your review and making the most of your valuable study time. This review book is uniquely organized according to the April 2007 NCLEX-RN® Test Plan, providing you with both a comprehensive content review and practice questions in sections covering * Safe, Effective Care Environment * Health Promotion * Physiological Integrity, and * Psychosocial Integrity. Throughout this book, you will find:

• **Memory Aids** that help you remember key concepts.
• **NCLEX® Alerts** that identify critical concepts you are likely to see on the NCLEX-RN®.
• **Check Your NCLEX® IQ** boxes that help you to assess your readiness for the NCLEX-RN® on the topics covered in the chapter.
• **Practice Tests** at the end of the chapter that review the concepts from that chapter and provide comprehensive rationales and test-taking strategies to help you find the right answers.

The **NCLEX-RN® Test Prep CD-ROM** that comes with your book simulates the test-taking environment by allowing you to practice questions on the computer. It contains all the questions in the book PLUS thousands of additional questions. You can choose to practice in Study, Quiz, or Exam modes, and you will receive detailed reports that will help you focus your preparation for NCLEX-RN®.

For additional information and resources

FOR THE NEXT GENERATION

Success in Skills, Review, & Test Preparation

Excellence in Testing

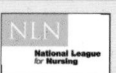

Prentice Hall and the National League for Nursing are pleased to offer you unique practice tests that correlate directly to your Prentice Hall Nursing textbooks. Each test is a comprehensive examination intended for students who have completed their course work and provides feedback regarding comprehension of the course content. The access code gives you access to two unique practice tests—use them to prepare for your course final exams or for NCLEX-RN®. Go to the website below and search for the **National League for Nursing** to find practice tests in any of your core nursing courses or to accompany the **Prentice Hall Reviews & Rationales Series.**

Excellence in Course Review

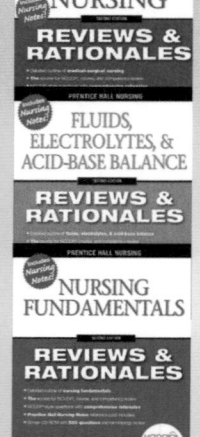

The **Prentice Hall Nursing Reviews & Rationales Series** will help you achieve nursing excellence by simplifying your review and making the most of your valuable study time for both your nursing courses and for the NCLEX-RN®. Each book in the series provides a comprehensive review of course content across the curriculum, as well as hundreds of practice questions with rationales and test-taking strategies in Pre- and Post-Tests and on the CD-ROM that comes with each book. This is the only review series that offers you a tear-out review card, **Prentice Hall NursingNotes,** and an audio review, **VangoNotes,** for additional purchase to play on your MP3 player.

Fundamentals & Nursing Skills, 2nd Ed.	2008	0-13-224078-5
Medical-Surgical Nursing, 2nd Ed.	2008	0-13-178970-8
Nutrition & Diet Therapy, 2nd Ed.	2007	0-13-243712-0
Fluids, Electrolytes, & Acid-Base Balance, 2nd Ed.	2007	0-13-224079-3
Pathophysiology, 2nd Ed.	2008	0-13-178972-4
Pharmacology, 2nd Ed.	2008	0-13-243710-4
Maternal-Newborn Nursing, 2nd Ed.	2007	0-13-178973-2
Child Health Nursing, 2nd Ed.	2007	0-13-243711-2
Mental Health Nursing, 2nd Ed.	2008	0-13-224077-7

Hear it. Get it.
www.vangonotes.com

please visit www.MyPearsonStore.com